Therapeutic Communication Techniques *Review these techniques in Chapter 18.*

Acknowledging:	Gives nonjudgmental recognition to a client for a certain behavior or contributio the client
Clarifying:	Asks for additional information to ensure understanding of the message sent; a about what you have just said?" indicates that understanding the client's message is important to the nurse
Focusing:	Focuses the client on information that is pertinent and helps the client expand on that information; this technique directs the client towards information that is important
Giving information:	Provides specific information to a client either with or without the client's request
Offering self:	Offers the nurse's presence without attaching any expectations or conditions about the client's behavior during that time
Restating or paraphrasing:	Ensures the nurse understands the message sent; utilizing this technique the nurse repeats the main thought of the message sent
Reflecting:	Redirects the content of a client's message back to the client for further thought or consideration
Summarizing:	May be used at the end of an interaction to identify material discussed; it helps to sort out relevant information from irrelevant
Using silence:	Allows for quiet time without conversation for several seconds or minutes to allow for reflection about the discussion that just occurred, to reduce tension, or to gather thoughts about how to proceed

PHYSIOLOGICAL INTEGRITY: Basic Care and Comfort

Basic Care and Comfort makes up 9–15% of the questions on the NCLEX-PN® exam.

Key Testing Strategies

- Use principles of administering basic physiological care to clients when answering questions in this part of the test plan.
- When questions address a client's mobility, select answers that will preserve muscle tone and joint function and prevent contractures or skin breakdown.
- Keep principles of safety in mind when answering questions about the use of assistive devices, such as canes, walkers, and crutches.
- Promote good nutrition by selecting meal choices that are balanced and that address any diet restrictions, such as low sodium or reduced fat.
- Use principles of gravity when considering how to position the clients or when working with clients who have drainage or wound tubes.

Sample Topics for Basic Care and Comfort Questions

Assistive devices	Nutrition and oral hydration
Elimination	Personal hygiene
Mobility/immobility	Rest and sleep
Nonpharmacological comfort interventions	

Safety Precautions During Oxygen Therapy

Review these precautions in Chapter 26

- Place cautionary signs reading, "No Smoking: Oxygen in Use" on client's door, at head or foot of bed, and on oxygen equipment.
- Instruct the client and visitors about the danger of smoking when oxygen is in use. If necessary, remove matches, lighters, and ashtrays.
- If oxygen therapy is used at home, instruct family members or caregivers to smoke only outside. If smoking is permitted, teach visitors to use smoking room.
- Avoid materials that generate static electricity such as woolen blankets and synthetic fabrics; instead use cotton fabrics.
- Avoid use of volatile, flammable substances such as acetone in nail polish removers, alcohol, ether, and oils near clients using oxygen.
- Remove any friction type or battery operated gadgets, devices, or toys.
- Make sure electric devices such as radios, razors, and televisions are in good working order to prevent short-circuit sparks.
- Ensure that electric monitoring equipment and suction machines are properly grounded. Disconnect any ungrounded equipment.
- Know location of fire extinguishers and be able to use them properly; know location of oxygen meter turn-off value.

Therapeutic Diets *Review information about these diets in Chapter 25*

Regular diet	High-residue/high-fiber diet
Clear liquids	Low-residue/low-fiber
Full liquids	Carbohydrate controlled
Pureed diet	Fat controlled
Dysphagia diet	Protein controlled
Soft diet	Gastric bypass diet
Mechanical soft diet	Restricted diets (gluten, tyramine, others)
Bland diet	

Types of Dressings *Review these dressings in Chapter 26*

Dressing Type	Description
Gauze	Plain or impregnated with an antimicrobial • Packs and fills wound • Absorbs drainage • Used for full- and partial-thickness wounds with drainage • May be apply dry, wet-to-moist, and wet-to-wet
Transparent	Adhesive membrane that is occlusive to liquids and bacteria • Protects wound and promotes autolytic debridement (the removal of dead tissue from a wound) • Impermeable to bacteria • Op-Site and Tegaderm are examples
Composite dressing	Contains an absorbent pad and an adhesive covering • Purpose is to absorb drainage Advantage is that it only has to be changed three times a week
Hydrocolloids	Adhesive made of gelatin • Is occlusive to microorganisms and liquids and promotes absorption of wound exudates Enhances autolysis of necrotic tissue within wound bed • Duo-Derm and Tegasorb are examples
Hydrogel	Water or glycerin is primary component of this nonadherent dressing• Maintains moist wound surface and provides some absorption Permeable to oxygen and can fill dead spaces in a wound • Secondary nonadhesive dressing may be required
Calcium alginates	Pad made of seaweed fibers • Purpose is to absorb larger amounts of drainage
Exudate absorbers	Semipermeable polyurethane foam dressings that absorb large amounts of exudates while keeping the wound moist • Nonadherent
Absorptive or filler dressings	Absorb moderate amounts of drainage • Duo-Derm paste is an example

PHYSIOLOGICAL INTEGRITY: Pharmacological Therapies

Pharmacological Therapies makes up 11–17% of the questions on the NCLEX-PN® exam.

Key Testing Strategies

- Use knowledge of drug action, intended effects and key side and adverse effects to answer a question about a specific medication.
- For questions addressing medication history, do not forget to ask about over-the-counter and herbal supplements as well as prescription medications.
- Double-check drug dosages and make sure the answer passes the common sense test (e.g., answer for a subcutaneous dose should not be more than 1 milliliter for an adult).
- Look for certain prefixes and suffixes in drug names to help identify the drug if the name is unfamiliar.

Sample Topics for Pharmacological and Parenteral Therapies Questions

Adverse effects/contraindications/ side effects/interactions	Medication administration
Blood and blood products	Parenteral/intravenous therapies
Central venous access devices	Pharmacological agents/actions
Dosage calculation	Pharmacological pain management
Expected actions/outcomes	Total parenteral nutrition

Calculating Medication Dosages

Formula 1

$$\frac{\text{dose ordered (desired)}}{\text{dose on hand (have)}} \times \text{amount available (quantity)} = \text{amount to give}$$

Formula 2 (ratio and proportion)

$$\frac{\text{dose ordered}}{\text{dose on hand}} = \frac{x}{\text{quantity available}}$$

Formula 3 (dimensional analysis)

Rule 1: Multiplying one side of an equation by a conversion factor will not change the value of the equation.

Rule 2: Set up the problem so that all labels cancel from the numerator and denominator except the label desired in the answer.

Calculating IV Drip Rates

$$\frac{\text{volume (of fluid)}}{\text{time (in minutes)}} \times \text{drop factor} = \text{flow rate}$$

Steps for Calculating Pediatric Medication Dosages

1. Convert the child's weight from pounds (lb) to kilograms (kg); 1 kg = 2.2 lb.
2. Calculate the safe total daily dose in mg/kg or in mcg/kg for a child of this weight as recommended in a standard drug reference book (mg/kg recommended × weight in kg). Then calculate the amount of one dose (total daily dose divided by the number of doses/day).
3. Compare the ordered dose to the recommended dose and determine if the dose is safe.
4. If the dose is safe, calculate the amount of one dose using one of the medication dosage formulas shown. If unsafe, consult prescriber before administering.

Reducing the Risk of Medication Errors

- Question any medication order that is not written clearly, has an unusual dose, or is not in keeping with treatment for client's known health problems.
- Prepare medications in a quiet area away from noise and distractions.
- Check client drug allergies before giving medications; if there is no notation in the allergy section(s) of the medical record, STOP and be sure to obtain allergy history prior to administration. Verify order for a medication that is questionable based on allergy history before administration.
- Be knowledgeable about medications: various names, correct dosage ranges, method of administration, and side/adverse effects.
- Have another nurse check dosage of parenteral medications (such as heparin, digoxin, and insulin) that could pose immediate harm to client if given incorrectly.
- Be aware of drug–food and drug–drug interactions to reduce risk of either ineffective treatment or toxic effects. Sometimes interactions reduce drug's effectiveness and sometimes they heighten its effect.
- Identify client correctly by asking client to state his or her name; checking identification bracelet is the next best method if client is nonverbal. Be especially careful when there are two clients or more in room. Use two unique identifiers per agency policy.
- If client questions a medication or states it is different than one taken at home, STOP and recheck medication order and client history. Verify order as necessary before proceeding to administer.
- Carefully and promptly document medication administration.
- Check results of ordered therapeutic drug levels as soon as they are expected to be available and report results promptly.
- Teach clients and significant others/family members about medications well in advance of discharge so they are prepared for safe self-administration following discharge.

Memory Aid for Drugs by Generic Name Prefix, Root, or Suffix*

Syllable in Generic Name	Interpretation	Examples by Generic Name
-ase, -plase	Thrombolytic agent (-ase usually indicates enzyme)	alteplase, anistreplase, reteplase, streptokinase, tenecteplase
-azole	Antifungal antimicrobial	itraconazole, fluconazole, clotrimazole, miconazole
cef-, ceph-	Cephalosporin, antibiotic; check allergy to this class and penicillins	cefazolin, cephalexin, cefotetan, ceftazidime, ceftriazone
-cillin	Penicillin, antibiotic; check allergy	amoxicillin, penicillin, piperacillin, ticarcillin, nafcillin, oxacillin
-cycline	Tetracycline, antibiotic	doxycycline, minocycline, tetracycline
-dipine	Calcium channel blocker, antianginal, antihypertensive	amlodipine, nicardipine, nifedipine, felodipine
-dronate	Bisphosphonate, bone resorption inhibitor	alendronate, etidronate, pamidronate, risedronate
-floxacin	Fluoroquinolone, antibiotic	ciprofloxacin, levofloxacin, norfloxacin, sparfloxacin
-micin, -mycin	Aminoglycoside, antibiotic**	gentamicin, kanamycin, netilmicin, tobramycin
nitr-, -nitr-	Nitrate, vasodilator, antianginal	nitroglycerin, isosorbide dinitrate
-olol, -lol	Beta adrenergic blocker, antihypertensive and/or antianginal	propranolol, atenolol, metoprolol, nadolol, labetalol, timolol
-parin	Anticoagulant, heparin or heparinoid	heparin, dalteparin, enoxaparin
-phylline	Xanthine type of bronchodilator	aminophylline, theophylline
-prazole	GI proton pump inhibitor, antiulcer	omeprazole, lansoprazole

Age-Related Changes *Review these changes in Chapter 17*

Skin: Subcutaneous tissue loss and dermal thinning, leading to wrinkling; increase in lentigines (brown age spots); hair thins and loses pigment; nail growth slows and nails may become thicker; skin tissue is more fragile

Sensory/perceptual: Visual acuity changes; ocular changes lead to increased astigmatism (presbyopia), increased sensitivity to glare, decreased ability to adjust to darkness; cataracts may develop; eyelids lose elasticity; ear canal narrows with calcification of ossicles and increased cerumen, resulting in progressive hearing loss (presbycusis); reduced ability to smell and discriminate odors; sense of taste decreases (especially to sense sweet taste); touch sensation changes with reduced ability to sense heat and cold

Neurological: Conduction speeds of neuron firing and transmission decrease; memory retrieval is slower; sleep stages 2–4 shorten, leading to a decrease in deep sleep; proprioception decreases

Musculoskeletal: Muscles atrophy; joint cartilage deteriorates; intervertebral disks atrophy, resulting in a loss of height of 1–3 inches

Pulmonary: Chest wall becomes rigid; thoracic muscles weaken; ciliary activity decreases; delivery and diffusion of O_2 to tissues decreases

Cardiovascular: Cardiac output and stroke volume decrease; valves stiffen; conductivity is altered; blood vessels are less elastic, leading to increasing blood pressure

Renal: Decreased glomerular filtration rate and creatinine clearance; possible residual urine or nocturia

Gastrointestinal: Thirst decreases; swallowing time is delayed; possible loss of teeth; decreased saliva; decreased gastric enzymes; weaker intestinal walls

Endocrine: Slowed basal metabolism; insulin levels increase but insulin sensitivity decreases

Genital: Males: prostate enlarges (often benign); decreased sperm protection
Females: vaginal dryness and atrophy

Immune: First sign of infection in an older adult may be a fall; temperature pattern may be lower than younger adult with the same infection

Psychosocial Integrity

Psychosocial Integrity makes up 7–13% of the questions on the NCLEX-PN® exam.

Key Testing Strategies

- For communication questions, select answers that use therapeutic communication techniques and eliminate options that represent communication blocks.
- If a question suggests that a client is at risk for abuse, assess the client without caregivers present and be aware of mandatory reporting laws.
- When responding to a client's communication, look for options that address the client's concern or issue.
- When answering questions of a psychosocial nature when all options seem of equal importance, follow the SEAs: **s**afety, **e**xpressing feelings, and **a**ssisting with problem solving.

Sample Topics for Psychosocial Integrity Questions

Abuse/neglect	Mental health concepts
Behavioral interventions	Religious and spiritual influences on health
Chemical and other dependencies	Sensory/perceptual alterations
Coping mechanisms	Stress management
Crisis intervention	Support systems
Cultural diversity	Therapeutic communication
End-of-life care	Therapeutic environment
Family dynamics	
Grief and loss	

Components of a Mental Status Exam

General Appearance	Appears stated age? Hygiene? Body odors? Dressed to season? Layered? Cleanliness?
Orientation	Person, place, time, and situation?
Thought Process	Clear, coherent, appropriate to topic? Concentration? Hallucinations or delusions?
Memory	Short-term (What did you have for breakfast?), long-term (Who is the president, and the president before that?)
Judgment	Appropriate? Safe? Impaired? Poor?

Communication Techniques to Avoid

Review these techniques in Chapter 18

Self-disclosure	Giving personal opinions or advice
Inattentive listening	Prying to satisfy personal curiosity
Overuse of medical jargon	Changing the subject

Suicide Precautions

When a client is acutely or actively suicidal, the following precautions should be taken:

- If not already hospitalized, someone should stay with the client until he or she can be admitted to prevent self-harm and maintain the safety of the client.
- Remove all sharp or dangerous objects from the client and the immediate vicinity, including knives or forks, scissors, mirrors, glass, and other objects that could be used for self-harm.
- Remove clothing that could be used as a tourniquet to cause self-harm, including belts of all kinds, neckties, stockings, handbags with long straps, etc.
- Remove all substances that could be ingested to toxic levels, including alcohol, recreational drugs, and medications. Keep client's medications locked.
- Ensure that the client swallows all pills, tablets, or other oral forms of medication, so that they are not kept in the cheek and then stored for later overdose.
- Keep the client in seclusion under one-to-one supervision while actively suicidal; explain in a gentle manner that this is for the client's safety until he or she is able to resist suicidal urges.
- Monitor a client who is not under one-to-one supervision with a nursing unit staff member every 10 to 15 minutes on an irregular schedule of observation.

Ensuring Your Safety on the Psychiatric Unit

1. Never be with a client by yourself. Alert staff to your whereabouts at all times.
2. Always have the ability to exit; do not put yourself in a position where your back is toward a closed-in area without an escape route.
3. Dress in casual clothes. Avoid sexually provocative clothing. Avoid having too much skin exposed.
4. Psychotic clients generally experience three delusional themes: 1) sexual, 2) political, and 3) religious. Avoid these topics unless you are experienced in managing them.
5. Remember that staff members are trained in managing client behavioral problems. Obtain the assistance of more experienced staff members when encountering unsafe situations early in practice.
6. Avoid wearing necklaces or other items that can be used as a weapon strangle. Wear closed-toe shoes. Do not wear loop earrings (or rings).
7. Remember safety first. Always listen to your primary or gut instinct. Enlist the aid of other staff to help in maintaining control.

Syllable in Generic Name	Interpretation	Examples by Generic Name
-pril	Angiotensin converting enzyme (ACE) inhibitor, antihypertensive	captopril, enalapril, fosinopril, lisinopril, quinapril
sal-, -sal-	Contains salicylate; check allergy to salicylates or aspirin	salsalate (nonopioid analgesic), sulfasalazine (GI anti-inflammatory)
-sartan	Angiotensin II receptor antagonist, antihypertensive	candesartan, eprosartan, losartan, valsartan
-sone, -lone, pred-	Corticosteroid	prednisone, betamethasone, dexamethasone, cortisone, triamcinolone, prednisolone
-statin	HMG-Coenzyme A reductase inhibitor, lipid lowering agent	atorvastatin, fluvastatin, lovastatin, pravastatin, simvastatin
sulfa-	Sulfonamide, antibiotic; check allergy to sulfa	sulfacetamide, sulfamethoxazole
-terol	Adrenergic type of bronchodilator	albuterol, formoterol, levabuterol, pirbuterol, salmeterol
-tidine	Histamine H2 antagonist (GI), antiulcer	cimetidine, ranitidine, famotidine, nizatidine
-triptan	Vascular headache suppressant, serotonin (5-HT1) agonist	almotriptan, naratriptan, sumatriptan, zolmitriptan
-vir	Antiviral antiinfective	acyclovir, cidofovir, famciclovir, gangciclovir, valacyclovir
-zepam, -zolam	Benzodiazepine, antianxiety, sedative/hypnotic	diazepam, lorazepam, oxazepam, alprazolam, midazolam
-zosin	Peripherally acting anti-adrenergic, antihypertensive	doxazocin, prazosin, terazosin

*This is not an exhaustive list and may not be inclusive of every drug in each category.
**This category does not include erythromycin, azithromycin, or clarithromycin, all of which are a macrolide type of antibiotic.

PHYSIOLOGICAL INTEGRITY: Reduction of Risk Potential

Reduction of Risk Potential makes up 9–15% of the questions on the NCLEX-PN® exam.

Key Testing Strategies

- Memorize common laboratory values and use them to answer questions about specific laboratory test results.
- Always ask if a female client of childbearing age is pregnant before she has x-rays taken.
- Remove all metal objects before a client has an x-ray.
- Ask about allergies to contrast dyes, iodine, and shellfish before a client undergoes a diagnostic test using injectable contrast material.
- Recall that clients cannot wear or have imbedded metal (prostheses, for example) to be eligible for magnetic resonance imaging (MRI).

Key Assessments in the Immediate Post-surgical Period

Review these assessments in Chapter 44

- Adequacy of airway
- Adequacy of ventilation
- Cardiovascular status
- Level of consciousness
- Presence of protective reflexes (e.g., gag, cough)
- Activity, ability to move extremities
- Skin color (pink, pale, dusky, blotchy, cyanotic, jaundiced)
- Fluid status: intake and output, status of IV infusions (type of fluid, rate, amount in container, patency of tubing), signs of dehydration or fluid overload
- Condition of operative site, dressing and presence of drainage
- Patency of and character and amount of drainage from catheters, tubes, and drains
- Discomfort (i.e., pain) (type, location, and severity), nausea, vomiting
- Safety (e.g., necessity for side rails, call bell within reach)

Sample Topics for Reduction of Risk Potential Questions

Diagnostic tests	Potential for complications from surgical procedures and health alterations
Laboratory values	System-specific assessments
Potential for alterations in body systems	Therapeutic procedures
Potential for complications of diagnostic tests/treatments/procedures	Changes/abnormalities in vital signs

Vital Signs by Age

Age	Heart Rate Range & (Avg) in bpm*	Respiratory Rate Range in rpm**	Median Blood Pressure (mm Hg)***
Newborn (NB)–1 mo	NB 110–170 (120) 1 mo 90–130 (110)	30–60	NB 73/55 1 mo 86/52
6 months–1 year	80–130 (110)	6 mo 24–36 1 yr 20–40	6 mo 90/53 1 yr 90/56
2 years	70–120 (100)	20–40	90/56
3–5 years	70–120 (100)	20–30	92/55
6–9 years	70–110 (90)	16–22	6 yrs 96/57 9 yrs 100/61
10–15 years	60–100 (85)	16–20	10 yrs 100/61 12 yrs 107/64 15 yrs 114/65
18 years	60–100 (85)	12–20	121/70

*Beats per minute
**Respirations per minute; higher when awake; slower during sleep
***Blood pressure varies by gender as well as age

Normal Arterial Blood Gas Values

Review Chapter 50 for additional information on acid base imbalances.

Arterial Blood Gas Parameter	Normal Value
pH	7.35–7.45
PCO_2	35–45 mm Hg
HCO_3^-	22–26 mEq/ L
PO_2	80–100 mm Hg

Centers for Disease Control and Prevention (CDC) Precautions *Review these precautions to prevent the spread of microorganisms in Chapter 7*

Tier 1: Standard Precautions

Handwashing
Gloves
Face protection (mask, goggles, face shield)
Gowns and other protective apparel
Others

Tier 2: Transmission Based Precautions

Airborne Precautions: Use when small (<5 μm) pathogen-infected droplet nuclei may remain suspended in air over time and travel distances greater than 3 feet. *Examples: varicella, measles, tuberculosis*

Droplet Precautions: Use with large (>5 μm) pathogen-infected droplets that travel 3 feet or less via coughing, sneezing, etc. or during procedures (suctioning). *Examples: Haemophilus influenzae, Neisseria meningitides, others*

Contact Precautions: Use with known or suspected microorganisms transmitted by direct hand-to-skin client contact or indirect contact with surfaces or care items in the environment. *Examples: Clostridium difficile, diphtheria (cutaneous), herpes simplex (mucocutaneous or neonatal), impetigo, pediculosis, scabies, zoster (disseminated, immunocompromised host), viral/hemorrhagic infections (Ebola, Lassa, Marburg), others*

Health Promotion and Maintenance

Health Promotion and Maintenance makes up 7–13% of the questions on the NCLEX-PN® exam.

Key Testing Strategies

- Make note of whether the client's age is identified in the question. If so, the question may be determining ability to apply concepts of normal growth and development.
- Because health promotion often involves client education, be prepared to apply principles of teaching and learning to questions in this area.
- When determining interventions to enhance a client's wellness, consider options that promote healthy nutrition, regular exercise, proper weight maintenance, proper rest, and avoidance of harmful chemicals, such as nicotine, and risk-taking behaviors, such as not wearing a seat belt.

Sample Topics for Health Promotion and Maintenance Questions

Aging process
Ante/intra/postpartum and newborn care
Data collection techniques
Developmental stages and transitions
Health and wellness
Health promotion/disease prevention
Health screening
High-risk behaviors
Lifestyle choices
Self-care

Health Screening for Cancer

Remember to use CAUTION to recognize possible signs of cancer:

Change in bowel or bladder habits
A sore that does not heal
Unusual bleeding or discharge
Thickening or lump in breast or elsewhere
Indigestion or difficulty in swallowing
Obvious change in a wart or mole
Nagging cough or hoarseness

Source: From the American Cancer Society.

Techniques of Data Collection

Review these techniques in Chapter 15

- Inspection: utilizes observation to obtain important information about a client's state of health; have adequate lighting to visually inspect the body without distortions or shadows; lighting can be sunlight or artificial
- Palpation: uses the sensation of touch and pressure of the hands and fingers to determine masses, elevations, temperature, organ position, and any abnormal findings; can be light or deep depending on the area of the body being examined
  - Light palpation is 1 cm in depth
  - Deep palpation is about 4 cm in depth
  - Deep palpation should occur after light palpation
- Percussion: a skill in which the finger of one hand touches or taps a finger of the other hand to generate vibration, which in turn produces a specific, diagnostic sound; the sound changes as the practitioner moves from one area to the next
- Auscultation: uses the sense of hearing to identify sounds produced by the body; some sounds can be heard and identified without a stethoscope; others can only be identified in a quiet environment with a stethoscope

ABCD Rule for Evaluating a Suspicious Skin Lesion

A = Asymmetry (one half of lesion does not match the other half)
B = Border irregularity (edges are blurred, jagged, or have a notched appearance)
C = Color variation is present or has a dark black color change
D = Diameter is greater than 6 millimeters in size

Adult Reference Range for Common Laboratory Tests

Coagulation Studies	*Prothrombin time (PT):* 10–13 seconds; 1.5–2.0 times the control in seconds for anticoagulant therapy *Activated partial thromboplastin time (APTT):* 20–35 seconds (1.5–2.5 times the control in anticoagulant therapy) *Partial thromboplastin time (PTT):* 60–70 seconds; 1.5–2.5 times the control in anticoagulant therapy *International normalized ratio (INR):* 2.0–3.0 for most anticoagulation needs
Electrolytes	*Sodium (Na^+):* 135–145 mEq/L; *Potassium (K^+):* 3.5–5.1 mEq/L *Chloride (Cl^-):* 95–105 mEq/L *CO_2 combining power:* 22–30 mEq/L; 22–30 mmol/L *Calcium, total (Ca^{++}):* 4.5–5.5 mEq/L, 9–11 mg/dL, 2.3–2.8 mmol/L *Calcium (ionized):* 4.25–5.25 mg/dL, 2.2–2.5 mEq/L, 1.1–1.24 mmol/L *Magnesium (Mg^{++}):* 1.5–2.5 mEq/L, 1.8–3.0 mg/dL
Glucose	*Fasting (FBS):* 70–110 mg/dL (serum, plasma); 60–100 mg/dL (whole blood); 70–120 mg/dL (elderly); panic values: < 40 or > 700 mg/dL *Fingerstick glucose (self-monitoring device):* 60–100 mg/dL
Hematology	*White blood cells (WBC):* 5000–10,000 microliter or 4500–11,500/mm^3 *Neutrophils:* 1935–7942 (absolute count) or 45–75% *Red blood cells (RBC):* 4.5–5.3 million or (10^6)/mm^3 (men), 4.1–5.1 million or (10^6)/mm^3 (women) *Hemoglobin (Hgb):* 13.0–18.0 grams/100 mL (men), 12–16 grams/100 mL (women) *Hematocrit (Hct):* 37–49% (men), 36–46% (women) *Platelet count:* 150,000–400,000/mm^3 (or microliter)
Renal Function Studies	*Blood urea nitrogen (BUN):* 5–25 mg/dL *Serum creatinine:* 0.5–1.5 mg/dL
Therapeutic Drug Levels	*Digoxin (Lanoxin):* 0.5–2.0 ng/mL; *Phenytoin (Dilantin):* 10–20 mcg/mL *Theophylline derivatives:* 10–20 mcg/mL or 10–20 mg/mL

PHYSIOLOGICAL INTEGRITY: Physiological Adaptation

Physiological Adaptation makes up 9–15% of the questions on the NCLEX-PN® exam.

Key Testing Strategies

- Think about the underlying pathophysiology when selecting interventions to assist a client with a health problem affecting a particular body system.
- Remember when a client's status is deteriorating rapidly, follow the ABCs—airway, breathing, and circulation.
- When evaluating the condition of a client with a particular health problem, use knowledge of normal findings or the client's usual baselines as a gauge as to the effectiveness of care.

Sample Topics for Physiological Adaptation Questions

Alterations in body systems	Medical emergencies
Fluid and electrolyte imbalances	Pathophysiology
Hemodynamics	Unexpected response to therapies
Illness management	

Glasgow Coma Scale *See Chapter 53 for review of neurological disorders.*

Assessment	Response	Score*
Eyes open (record C if eyes are closed by swelling)	Spontaneously	4
	To speech	3
	To pain	2
	No response	1
Best motor response (record best upper arm response)	Obeys commands	6
	Localized pain	5
	Flexion-withdrawal	4
	Abnormal flexion	3
	Abnormal extension	2
	No response	1
Best verbal response (record T if an endotracheal tube is in place)	Oriented	5
	Confused	4
	Inappropriate words	3
	Incomprehensible sounds	2
	No response	1
Total Score:		___

*A higher score indicates a higher level of functioning.
Source: LeMone, P., Burke, K., & Bauldoff, G. (2012). *Medical surgical nursing: Critical thinking in patient care* (5th ed.). Upper Saddle River, NJ: Pearson Education, Inc., p. 1421.

Symptom Analysis

A Are there any associated symptoms with the chief complaint?
P What was the provoking incident (aggravating factor[s]) that caused the symptom, if any?
Q What is the quality of the symptom? Is it burning, throbbing, aching, stabbing, other?
R Where is the region of symptom? Does it radiate? Does anything relieve the symptom?
S How severe is the symptom? (intensity, quantity)
T What is the timing of the symptom? When does it occur; how long does it last? (pattern, duration)

Neurovascular Status: checking the "6 Ps"

Pain: is there pain or discomfort in the extremity?
Pallor: is the skin color paler than normal or baseline?
Polar: is the skin cooler to the touch than normal or baseline in the area?
Paresthesia: are there any unusual sensations, such as numbness or tingling?
Paralysis: is the extremity without movement or weaker than normal or baseline?
Pulse: is the affected pulse (or pulses) diminished or absent?

Nursing Care of the Client in a Cast

See Chapter 57 for review of musculoskeletal disorders.

- Casts made from plaster of Paris should not get wet and cast padding should not be removed; if cast becomes soiled, clean with a damp cloth. Casts made of synthetic material dry more quickly and allow mobility in less than an hour.
- Smooth rough edges to prevent skin injury; explain that no foreign objects should be inserted into the cast (sticks, food crumbs, etc.) to prevent skin breakdown.
- Avoid covering a new plaster cast with blanket or plastic for extended periods (air cannot circulate, and heat builds up in cast).
- Turn client from side to side (using palms, not fingertips) every 2 hours to facilitate drying for the first 24 to 72 hours.
- Apply ice for the first 24 hours over fracture site to control edema, ensuring that ice is securely contained to avoid wetting cast.
- Elevate extremity above the level of the heart to promote venous return for the first 24 hours after application.
- Encourage active range of motion (AROM) to joints above and below immobilized extremity.
- Report to health care provider: increasing pain in immobilized extremity, excessive swelling and discoloration of exposed limb, burning or tingling under cast, sores, or foul odor under cast.

Informed Consent *Review these guidelines in Chapter 4*

- Requirements of client: has mental capacity to consent; it is voluntarily done; and client understands treatment and information presented
- Requirements of health care provider (performing treatment, procedure, or surgery): shares information about planned treatment, procedure or surgery, its associated risks and benefits, and alternatives to treatment; gives client opportunity to ask questions and have them answered
- If a client waives right to informed consent, document this in the medical record
- If client is deemed incompetent to make informed decisions about health care in court of law, a court-apporinted guardian makes these decisions
- Informed consent for minors is obtained from parent or legal guardian, except in emergency situations, when minor is married or emancipated from parents, or with special needs for care, such as with sexually transmitted disease or pregnancy

Upholding HIPAA (Health Information Portability and Accountability Act) *Review these guidelines in Chapter 4*

- Protect personal identifying information (such as name, social security number, date of birth) and information about diagnosis or treatment
- Share information only with individuals involved directly in client's care, payment for care, and/or management of client's care
- Verify identify of persons asking for client information
- Dispose of confidential documents in accord with agency policy (such as shredder, locked recycle bin)
- Keep contents of medical record out of public view by placing in a secure area and turning computer screens displaying client data away from general view
- Discuss client's care only in areas where cannot be overheard

SAFE AND EFFECTIVE CARE ENVIRONMENT: Safety and Infection Control

Safety and Infection Control makes up 11–17% of the questions on the NCLEX-PN® exam.

Key Testing Strategies

- Questions that focus on assessing the home environment of a client may be seeking to determine knowledge of risks to safety in the home, such as risk of falls (e.g., throw rugs, no night lights, handrails, or bathroom safety bars) or risk of fire (e.g., oxygen in the home, frayed electrical cords, lack of smoke detectors).
- When answering a question that addresses an infectious disease, consider that the question may be determining knowledge of precautions to prevent disease transmission, and discriminate the need to use contact, airborne, or droplet precautions.
- When answering a question that addresses a client with a compromised immune system or who is receiving chemotherapy, consider that the question may be determining whether the client has a need for neutropenic precautions (for low white blood cell count) or thrombocytopenic precautions (for low platelet count).

Sample Topics for Safety and Infection Control Questions

Accident/injury prevention	Reporting of incident/event/ irregular occurrence/variance
Emergency response plan	Safe use of equipment
Ergonomic principles	Security plan
Error prevention	Standard/precautions/transmission-based precautions/surgical asepsis
Handling hazardous and infectious materials	Use of restraints/safety devices
Home safety	

4 Steps to Maintain Client Safety During a Fire
Review these steps in Chapter 6

Remove clients from danger
Activate the fire alarm
Contain the fire
Evacuate the area
(do horizontal evacuation if possible before vertical evacuation)

Fall Risk Factors in Older Adults *Review these guidelines in Chapter 17*

Intrinsic Age-Related Changes	Intrinsic Disease Related Changes	Extrinsic Risk Factors
Gait (step length and height)	Orthostatic hypotension	Floor surface; waxed, scatter rugs, tears in carpeting
Gait (symmetry and path)	Dehydration	Steps uneven, without hand rails
Balance when sitting	Cardiac arrhythmias and anemias	Edges and curbing without contrasting colors
Balance when standing	Urinary tract and other infections	Dim lighting, bright lights that cause glare
Balance when turning	Osteoporosis and fractures	Bathrooms without grab bars and tub or shower seats
Stability	Hypoglycemia	High-heeled shoes
Cognition	Seizures, TIA, CVA, adverse effects of medication, delirium	Clutter

Principles of Surgical Asepsis *Review these principles in Chapter 7*

- All objects used in a sterile field must be sterile.
- Sterile objects that touch unsterile objects become unsterile.
- Sterile items that are out of vision or below waist level are considered unsterile.
- Sterile objects can become unsterile by prolonged exposure to airborne microorganisms.
- Fluids flow in the direction of gravity.
- Moisture that passes through a sterile object exerts capillary action to draw microorganisms from unsterile surfaces above or below to the sterile surface.
- The edges of a sterile field are considered unsterile.
- The skin is unsterile and cannot be sterilized.
- Conscientiousness, alertness, and honesty are essential qualities in maintaining surgical asepsis.

Rule of Nines for Calculating Burn Injury

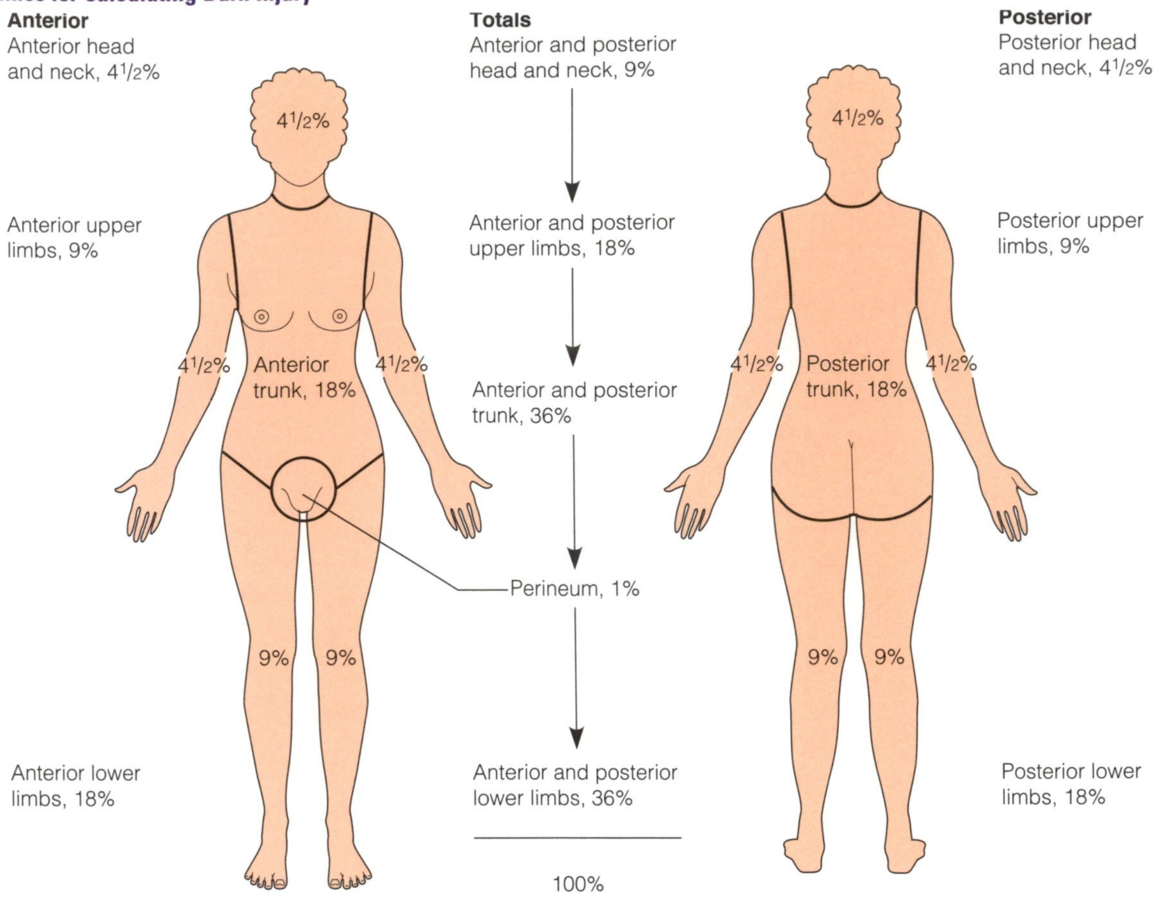

Clinical Manifestations of Renal Failure *See Chapter 54 for review of renal disorders.*

Body System	Clinical Manifestations	Cause of Manifestations
Cardiovascular	Hypervolemia, hypertension, tachycardia, arrhythmias, congestive heart failure, pericarditis	Increased fluid volume, build-up of metabolic wastes, chronic hypertension, change in renin-angiotension mechanism
Hematologic	Anemia, leukocytosis, decreased platelet function, thrombocytopenia	Decreased production of erythropoietin and RBCs, decreased survival of RBCs, decreased platelet activity; blood loss through dialysis and bleeding
Gastrointestinal	Anorexia, nausea, vomiting, abdominal distention, diarrhea, constipation, bleeding	Build-up of uremic toxins, electrolyte imbalances, changes in platelet activity, conversion of urea to ammonia by saliva
Neurologic	Lethargy, confusion, convulsions, stupor, coma, sleep disturbances, behavioral changes, muscle irritability	Uremic toxins, electrolyte imbalances, cerebral swelling caused by fluid shifts
Dermatologic	Pallor, pigmentation, pruritus, ecchymosis, excoriation, uremic frost	Anemia, decreased activity of sweat glands, dry skin, phosphate deposits on skin
Urinary	Decreased urine output, decreased specific gravity, proteinuria, casts and cells in the urine	Damage to the nephron
Skeletal	Osteoporosis, renal rickets, joint pain	Decreased calcium absorption, decreased phosphate excretion

PEARSON *Nursing Notes*

Preparing for the NCLEX-PN® Exam*

SAFE AND EFFECTIVE CARE ENVIRONMENT: *Coordinated Care*

Coordinated Care makes up 13–19% of the questions on the NCLEX-PN® exam.

Key Testing Strategies:

- Recognize questions that require priority setting through words in the question such as first, initial, best, most important, essential, and most therapeutic.
- When answering questions related to delegation to caregivers, such as unlicensed assistive personnel (UAPs), recall that the task being delegated needs to be part of that caregiver's skill set and that the other rights of delegation must be upheld.
- Immediately eliminate distracters that violate client rights or ethical principles.

Sample Topics for Coordinated Care Questions

Advance directives	Continuity of care
Advocacy	Establishing priorities
Client care assignments	Ethical practice
Client rights	Informed consent
Concepts of management and supervision	Legal responsibilities
Confidentiality	Performance improvement (quality improvement)
Consultation with members of the health care team	Referral process
	Resource management

Essential Rights of Delegation *Review these 'rights' in Chapter 5*

1. **Right Task:** Nurses determine those activities team members may perform. For each situation, the nurse must consider the client's condition, the complexity of the activity, the UAP's capabilities, and the amount of supervision the nurse will be able to provide.
2. **Right Circumstances:** The nurse evaluates the individual clients and the individual UAPs and matches the two. The nurse assesses the client's needs, looks at the care plan, and considers the setting, ensuring that UAPs have the proper resources, equipment, and supervision to work safely.
3. **Right Person:** The nurse follows organizational policies, which are congruent with state law, in determining the appropriate staff to which to delegate a nursing activity.
4. **Right Direction and Communication:** The nurse needs to communicate the acceptable tasks and activities. The nurse needs to clearly understand the organization's policies and procedures to carry out effective delegation. In turn, staff nurses need to direct UAPs' actions and communicate clearly about each delegated task. Nurses must be specific about how and when UAPs should report back to them. Nurses should feel comfortable asking, *Do you know how to do this? Where did you learn? How many times have you done it in the past? Where is your experience documented?*
5. **Right Supervision and Evaluation:** Nurse managers must ensure that each unit has adequate staffing and time, identify the task inherent to each staff role, and evaluate the impact of the organization's nursing service on the community. The delegating nurse then must supervise, guide, and evaluate the UAPs' task implementation. The nurse must ensure that UAPs meet expectations and must intervene if they aren't performing well.

Strategies for Setting Priorities in Clinical Practice *Review these strategies in Chapter 5*

Guiding Principles	First Priority	Second Priority
Physiology Maslow's Hierarchy of Needs theory	**Airway, breathing, and circulation** Physiological (primary) needs: air, breathing, circulation, water, food (oxygen therapy, circulatory support, IV hydration, nutrition, critical lab values, treatment of pain)	Safety and security (primary) needs: prevention of falls, reorientation to surroundings, abnormally high or low values that are not critical, may include some client teaching (e.g. insulin administration)
Policies and Procedures	Activities governed by agency policy or procedure that involves strict timelines (e.g., restraints, falls, stat medications)	Activities governed by policy or procedure that directly affect client care (e.g., non-stat, regularly scheduled medications, dressings)
Care activities related to clinical condition of client	Life-threatening or potentially life-threatening occurrences (adverse changes in VS, change in LOC, potential for respiratory or circulatory collapse); often unanticipated	Activities essential to safety: life-saving medications and equipment that protect clients from infections or falls
Medication or IV therapy priorities	Medications that prevent or treat physiological distress (e.g., analgesics, updrafts or inhalers); medications ordered more frequently (e.g., every 4 hours) because late medication delivery could affect next dose; IV therapy for hydration in clients who are NPO because of nonfunctional GI tract	Medications that prevent reoccurrences of symptoms of disease processes (such as digoxin or antibiotics); medications ordered once per shift, routine maintenance of IV therapy or heparin/saline lock care

Ethical Principles and Decision-making *Review these principles in Chapter 4*

Autonomy	Beneficence
Accountability	Justice
Fidelity	Veracity
Confidentiality	Nonmaleficence

*Based on the April 2011 Test Plan

Priority Cardiac Dysrhythmias *Review Chapter 52 for additional information about cardiac dysrhythmias.*

Rhythm/ECG Appearance	ECG Characteristics	Management
Supraventricular Rhythms		
Sinus tachycardia 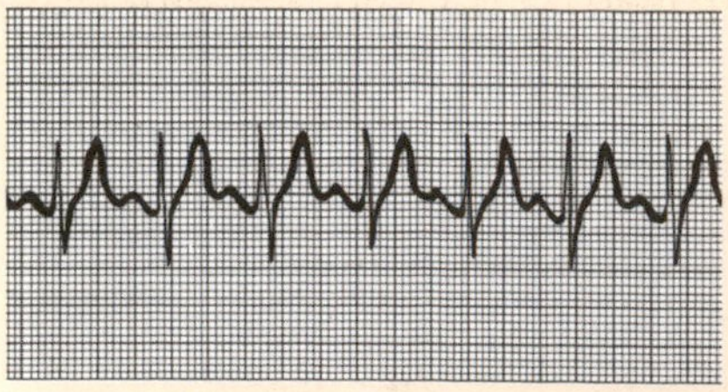	Rate: 101 to 150 bpm Rhythm: regular P:QRS ratio is 1:1 (with very fast rates, P wave may be hidden in preceding T wave) PR interval: 0.12–0.20 sec QRS complex: 0.06–0.10 sec	Treat only if client is experiencing symptoms or is at risk for myocardial damage; treat underlying cause (e.g., hypovolemia, fever, pain); beta blockers or verapamil may be used
Sinus bradycardia 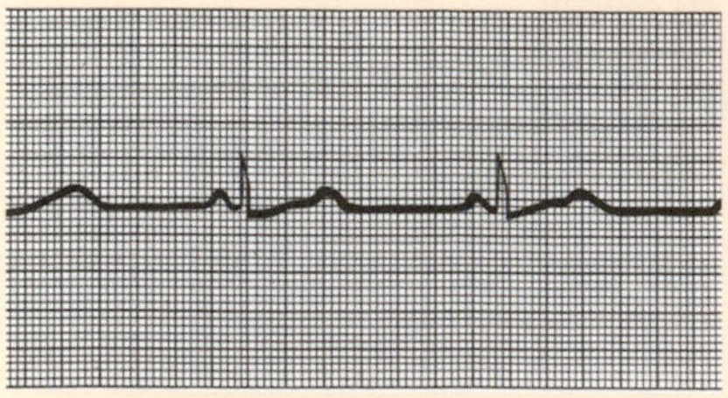	Rate: less than 60 bpm Rhythm: regular P:QRS ratio is 1:1 PR interval: 0.12–0.20 sec QRS complex: 0.06–0.10 sec	Treat only if client is experiencing symptoms; intravenous atropine and/or pacemaker therapy may be used
Atrial fibrillation 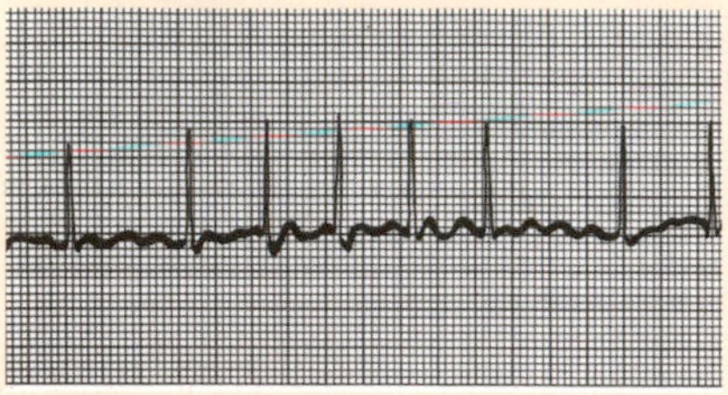	Rate: atrial 300–600 bpm (too rapid to count); ventricular 100–180 bpm in untreated clients Rhythm: irregularly irregular P:QRS ratio is variable PR interval: not measured QRS complex: 0.06–0.10 sec	Synchronized cardioversion; medications to reduce ventricular response rate: verapamil, propranolol, digoxin, anticoagulant therapy to reduce risk of clot formation and stroke
Ventricular Rhythms		
Premature ventricular contractions (PVC) 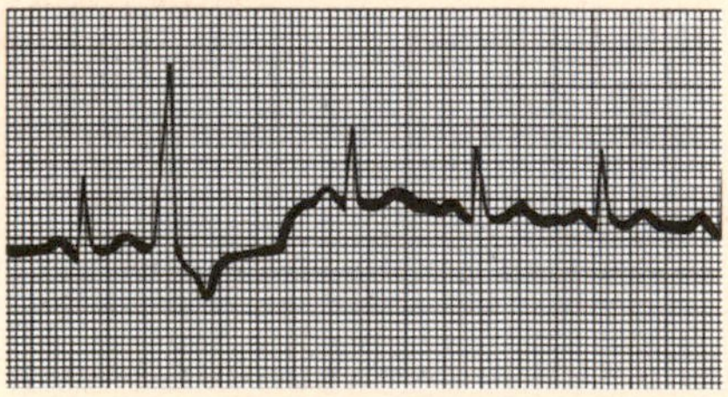	Rate: variable Rhythm: irregular, with PVC interrupting underlying rhythm and followed by a compensatory pause P:QRS ratio: no P wave noted before PVC PR interval: absent with PVC QRS complex: wide (greater 0.12 sec), bizarre in appearance; differs from normal QRS complex	Treat if client is experiencing symptoms; advise against stimulant use (caffeine, nicotine); drug therapy includes intravenous lidocaine, procainamide, quinidine, propranolol, phenytoin, bretylium
Ventricular tachycardia (VT or V tach) 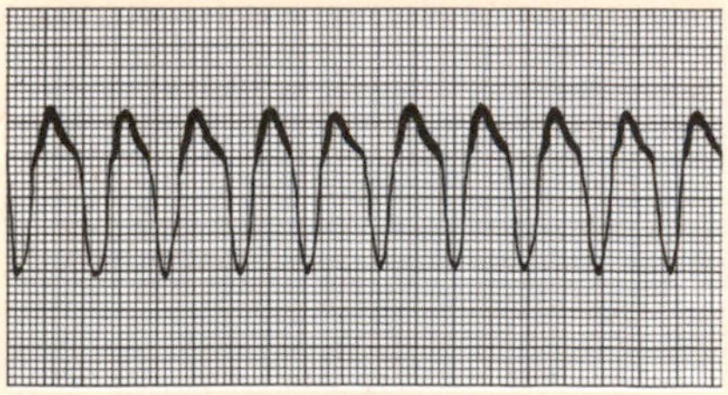	Rate: 100–250 bpm Rhythm: regular P:QRS ratio: P waves usually not identifiable PR interval: not measured QRS complex: 0.12 sec or greater; bizarre shape	Treat if VT is sustained or if client is experiencing symptoms; treatment includes intravenous procainamide or lidocaine and/or immediate defibrillation if the client is unconscious or unstable
Ventricular fibrillation (VF or V fib) 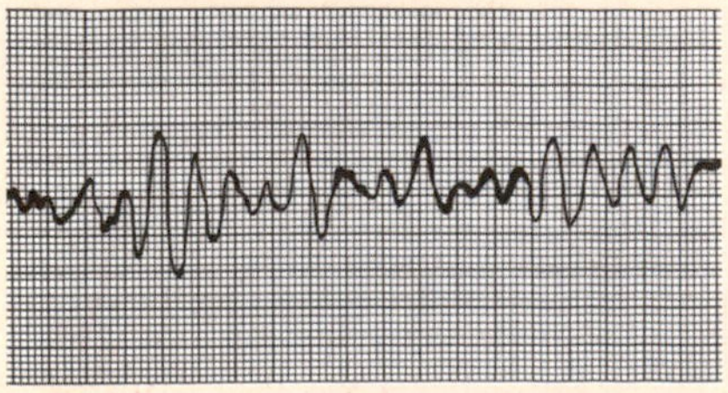	Rate: too rapid to count Rhythm: grossly irregular P:QRS ratio: no identifiable P waves PR interval: none QRS: bizarre, varying in shape and direction	Immediate defibrillation

PEARSON

COMPREHENSIVE REVIEW FOR NCLEX-PN®

SECOND EDITION

REVIEWS & RATIONALES

Mary Ann Hogan, MSN, RN
Clinical Assistant Professor
University of Massachusetts–Amherst
Amherst, Massachusetts

with Julie Skrabal, MSN, RN
Assistant Professor
BryanLGH College of Health Sciences
Lincoln, Nebraska

PEARSON

Boston Columbus Indianapolis New York San Francisco Upper Saddle River
Amsterdam Cape Town Dubai London Madrid Milan Munich Paris Montréal Toronto
Delhi Mexico City São Paulo Sydney Hong Kong Seoul Singapore Taipei Tokyo

Director, Nursing Program Solutions: Maura Connor
Executive Editor: Jennifer Farthing
Editorial Assistant: Deirdre MacKnight
Developmental Editor: Victoria Gaudette
Director of Digital Product Development: Alex Marciante
Media Product Manager: Travis Moses-Wesphal
Director of Media Production: Ally Graesser
Media Production: Rachel Collett
Managing Editor: Patrick Walsh
Director of Marketing: David Gesell
Senior Marketing Manager: Phoenix Harvey
Retail Marketing: Laura Huisking
Marketing Coordinator: Michael Sirinides
Composition: GEX Publishing Services
Printer/Binder: Courier Printing, Westford, MA
Cover Printer: Lehigh-Phoenix Color, Hagerstown, MD

Library of Congress Cataloging-in-Publication Data
Hogan, Mary Ann, MSN.
Comprehensive review for NCLEX-PN / Mary Ann Hogan ; with Julie Skrabal. — 2nd ed.
p. ; cm. — (Pearson reviews & rationales)
Includes bibliographical references and index.
ISBN-13: 978-0-13-262141-0 (pbk.)
ISBN-10: 0-13-262141-X (pbk.)
I. Skrabal, Julie. II. Title. III. Series: Pearson nursing reviews & rationales series.
[DNLM: 1. Nursing Care—Examination Questions. WY 18.2]
610.73076—dc23

2011042093

10 9 8 7 6 5 4 3 2 1

PEARSON

ISBN-13: 978-0-13-262141-0
ISBN-10: 0-13-262141-X

Contents

Preface

INTRODUCING: *PEARSON COMPREHENSIVE REVIEW FOR NCLEX-PN®*, Second Edition

This volume of the popular *Pearson Nursing Reviews & Rationales* series is designed to serve as the ultimate study guide to prepare you for the NCLEX-PN® exam. It provides a comprehensive outline review of the essential content areas tested on the NCLEX-PN® exam, including commonly occurring health problems that have predictable outcomes, contributing to the interdisciplinary team in a variety of settings, and providing competent care guided by use of ethical and legal principles. This book incorporates these topics throughout, and provides practice questions simulating the level of difficulty on the actual NCLEX-PN® exam.

The NCLEX-PN® exam is organized according to the categories and subcategories of client needs, integrating the concepts you learned in nursing school. While most other books provide a review of nursing concepts by course area, we integrate these concepts into the categories of client needs as they would be found on the actual NCLEX-PN® exam.

For example, in ***Pearson Comprehensive Review for NCLEX-PN®***, all of the concepts related to health problems commonly encountered in both medical-surgical and pediatric nursing are brought together in the body systems chapters in section 9 on Physiological Adaptation. Similarly, the important concepts while working with healthy individuals (such as growth and development, lifestyle management, health screening, age-related changes, nutrition, and healthy mothers and newborns) are brought together in the chapters in section 4 on Health Promotion and Maintenance. This unique organization allows you to study for specific sections of the test based on the results of any predictor tests for the NCLEX-PN® exam that you have taken.

WHAT YOU NEED TO KNOW ABOUT THE NCLEX-PN® EXAMINATION

Upon graduation from a nursing program, successful completion of the NCLEX-PN® licensing examination is required to begin a professional nursing practice. The NCLEX-PN® exam is a Computer Adaptive Test (CAT) that ranges in length from 85 to 205 individual (stand-alone) test items, depending on your performance during the examination. The blueprint for the exam is reviewed and revised every three years by the National Council of State Boards of Nursing using results of a job analysis study of new graduate nurses practicing within the first six months after graduation. Each question on the exam is coded to a *Client Need Category* and an *Integrated Process.*

Client Need Categories

There are four categories of client needs, and each exam will contain a minimum and maximum percent of questions from each category. The *Client Needs* categories according to the NCLEX-PN® Test Plan effective April 2011 are as follows:

- **Safe and Effective Care Environment**
  - Coordinated Care (13–19%)
  - Safety and Infection Control (11–17%)
- **Health Promotion and Maintenance (7–13%)**
- **Psychosocial Integrity (7–13%)**
- **Physiological Integrity**
  - Basic Care and Comfort (9–15%)
  - Pharmacological Therapies (11–17%)
  - Reduction of Risk Potential (9–15%)
  - Physiological Adaptation (9–15%)

Integrated Processes

The integrated processes identified on the NCLEX-PN® Test Plan with condensed definitions, are as follows:

- **Nursing Process (Clinical Problem-Solving Process):** a scientific approach to client care that includes data collection, planning, implementation, and evaluation
- **Caring:** interaction of the practical/vocational nurse and clients, families, and significant others in an atmosphere of mutual respect and trust. In this collaborative environment, the practical/vocational nurse provides support and compassion to help achieve desired therapeutic outcomes
- **Communication and Documentation:** verbal and/or nonverbal interactions between the practical/vocational nurse and clients, families, significant others, and members of the health care team. Events and activities associated with client care are validated in written and/or electronic records that reflect standards of practice and accountability in the provision of care
- **Teaching and Learning:** facilitation of the acquisition of knowledge, skills, and attitudes to assist in promoting positive changes in behavior

More detailed information about this examination may be obtained by visiting the National Council of State Boards of Nursing website at **http://www.ncsbn.org** and viewing the 2011 *NCLEX-PN® Examination Test Plan for the National Council Licensure Examination for Practical Nurses.*[1]

PREPARING FOR THE NCLEX-PN® EXAMINATION

Study Tips

Using this book should help simplify your review. To make the most of your valuable study time, follow these simple but important suggestions:

1. **Use a weekly calendar to schedule study sessions.**
   - Outline the timeframes for all of your activities (home, school, appointments, etc.) on a weekly calendar.
   - Find the "holes" in your calendar—the times when you can plan to study. Add study sessions to the calendar at times when you can expect to be mentally alert, and then follow your plan!
2. **Create the optimal study environment.**
   - Eliminate external sources of distraction, such as television, telephone, etc.
   - Eliminate internal sources of distraction, such as hunger, thirst, or dwelling on items or problems that cannot be worked on at the moment.
   - Take a break for 10 minutes or so after each hour of concentrated study both as a reward and an incentive to keep studying.
3. **Use pre-reading strategies to increase comprehension of chapter material.**
   - Skim read the headings in the chapter; they identify chapter content.
   - Read the definitions of key terms, which will help you learn new words to comprehend chapter information.
   - Review all graphic aids (figures, tables, boxes, memory aids); they are often used to explain important points in the chapter.
4. **Read the chapter thoroughly but at a reasonable speed.**
   - Comprehension and retention are actually enhanced by not reading too slowly.
   - Do take the time to reread any section that is unclear to you.

[1]National Council of State Boards of Nursing, Inc. NCLEX Examination Test Plan for National Council Licensure Examination for Practical Nurses. Effective April, 2011. Retrieved from https://www.ncsbn.org/2011_PN_TestPlan.pdf

5. **Summarize what you have learned.**
   - Use the accompanying online resource, NursingReviewsandRationales.com, to test yourself with thousands of *NCLEX-PN*®-style practice questions.
   - Review again any sections that correspond to questions you answered incorrectly or incompletely.

Test-Taking Strategies

Every question in the book and on the accompanying Nursing Reviews & Rationales website provides test-taking strategies that enable you to select the correct answer by breaking down the question, even if you don't know the correct response. Use the following strategies to increase your success in testing situations:

- Get sufficient sleep and have something to eat before taking a test. Take deep breaths during the test as needed. Remember, the brain requires oxygen and glucose as fuel. Avoid concentrated sweets before a test, however, to avoid rapid upward and then downward surges in blood glucose levels.
- Read each question carefully, identifying the stem, all options, and any critical words or phrases in either the stem or options.
  - Critical words in the stem such as "most important" indicate the need to set priorities, since more than one option is likely to contain a statement that is technically correct.
  - Remember that the presence of absolute words such as "never" or "only" in an answer option is more likely to make that option incorrect.
- Determine who is the client in the question; often this is the person with the health problem, but it may also be a significant other, relative, friend, or another nurse.
- Decide whether the stem is a true response stem or a false response stem. With a true response stem, the correct answer will be a true statement, and vice-versa.
- Determine what the question is really asking, sometimes referred to as the core issue of the question. Evaluate all answer options in relation to this issue, and not strictly to the "correctness" of the statement in each individual option.
- Eliminate options that are obviously incorrect, then go back and reread the stem. Evaluate the remaining options against the stem once more to make a final selection.
- If two answers seem similar and correct, try to decide whether one of them is more global or comprehensive. If one option includes the alternative option within it, it is likely that the more global option is the correct answer.

HOW YOUR BOOK PREPARES YOU FOR SUCCESS ON THE NCLEX-PN® EXAMINATION

***Pearson Comprehensive Review for NCLEX-PN*®, Second Edition** helps you prepare for the NCLEX-PN® exam in three ways:

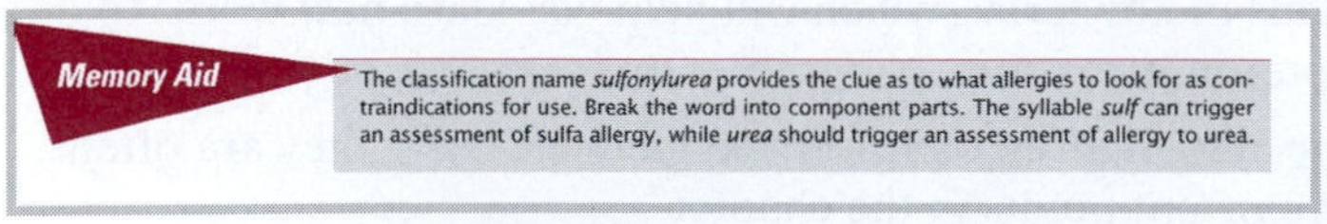

Memory Aid

The classification name *sulfonylurea* provides the clue as to what allergies to look for as contraindications for use. Break the word into component parts. The syllable *sulf* can trigger an assessment of sulfa allergy, while *urea* should trigger an assessment of allergy to urea.

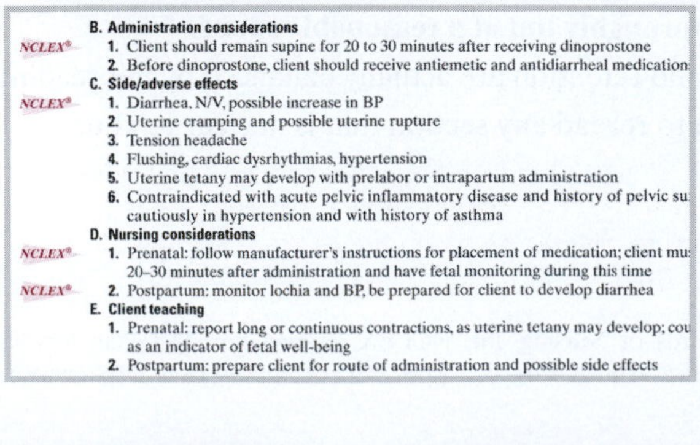

B. **Administration considerations**
NCLEX® 1. Client should remain supine for 20 to 30 minutes after receiving dinoprostone
2. Before dinoprostone, client should receive antiemetic and antidiarrheal medication
C. **Side/adverse effects**
NCLEX® 1. Diarrhea, N/V, possible increase in BP
2. Uterine cramping and possible uterine rupture
3. Tension headache
4. Flushing, cardiac dysrhythmias, hypertension
5. Uterine tetany may develop with prelabor or intrapartum administration
6. Contraindicated with acute pelvic inflammatory disease and history of pelvic su cautiously in hypertension and with history of asthma
D. **Nursing considerations**
NCLEX® 1. Prenatal: follow manufacturer's instructions for placement of medication; client mu 20–30 minutes after administration and have fetal monitoring during this time
NCLEX® 2. Postpartum: monitor lochia and BP, be prepared for client to develop diarrhea
E. **Client teaching**
1. Prenatal: report long or continuous contractions, as uterine tetany may develop; cou as an indicator of fetal well-being
2. Postpartum: prepare client for route of administration and possible side effects

1. Highlights critical concepts on the NCLEX-PN® Exam

One key to your success on the NCLEX-PN® exam will be focusing your review on nursing concepts and interventions typically incorporated into test questions. Your book has a few devices to help you familiarize with these topics so you can better manage your review time.

- **Memory Aid boxes** tie specific content from the review outline to the Test Plan. These boxes provide you with hints or suggestions about how to remember these concepts for easy recall during testing.

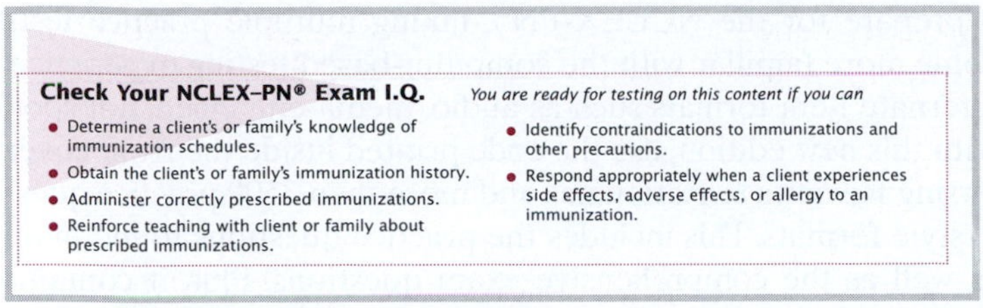

- **NCLEX® Alert** identifies concepts that are likely to be tested on the NCLEX-PN® exam. Be sure to learn the information highlighted wherever you see this icon.
- **Check Your NCLEX-PN® Exam I.Q.,** found at the end of each chapter, provides an opportunity for you to assess your readiness for the NCLEX-PN® exam on the topics covered in the chapter.

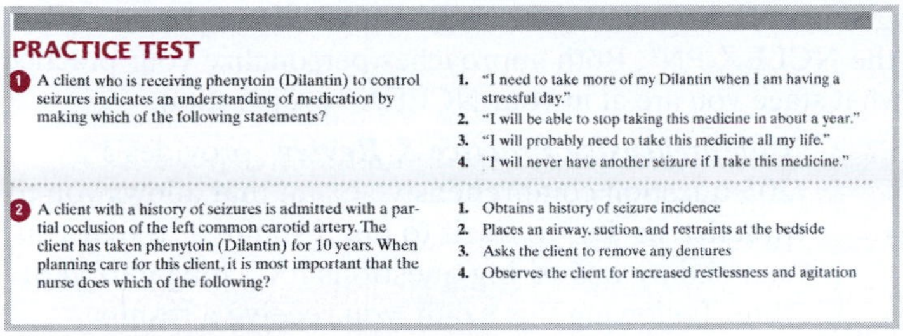

2. Provides practice opportunities

Most faculty tell students they must practice thousands of questions before taking the NCLEX-PN® exam. This book and online Nursing Reviews & Rationales provides you with thousands of questions using alternate item types found on the NCLEX® exam so you can approach your practice review in a variety of ways.

- **Practice Test** sections provide a quiz at the end of each chapter to test your mastery of the concepts in that chapter.

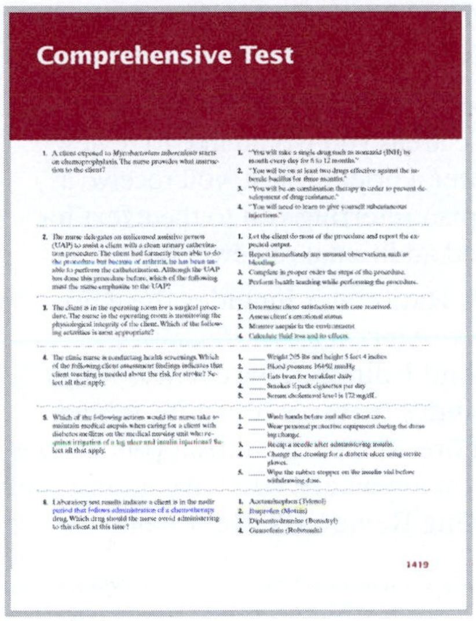

- **Comprehensive Exam** at the end of the book contains 205 questions. This exam helps you build your endurance in case you have to answer questions for an extended time during the real exam.
- New **Nursing Reviews & Rationales** online includes an additional 3500 questions, which give you ample opportunities to practice NCLEX®-style questions and assess your readiness for the actual exam. Please see below for more information about this powerful review website.

3. Hones your test-taking skills

An important part of preparing for the NCLEX-PN® exam is understanding the questions asked and knowing how best to answer them. This book provides you with feedback to build these important skills.

- **Answers & Rationales** are provided following the Practice Test at the end of each chapter and on the Nursing Reviews & Rationales website. For every question, you will see a comprehensive rationale for the correct and incorrect choices, because it is important for you to understand why an answer option is correct or incorrect.
- **Test-Taking Strategies** are highlighted in the Answers & Rationales section of the book and on the Nursing Reviews & Rationales website. Since you cannot skip questions on the NCLEX-PN® exam, you need to learn how to select the correct answer even if you don't recognize it immediately. These strategies break down each question and show you how to select the correct choice.
- ***Pearson Nursing Notes*** cards offer a quick review of testing strategies and frequently used information organized by the categories of client needs. These tear-out cards are designed to be useful also in the clinical setting, when quick and easy access to information is so important.

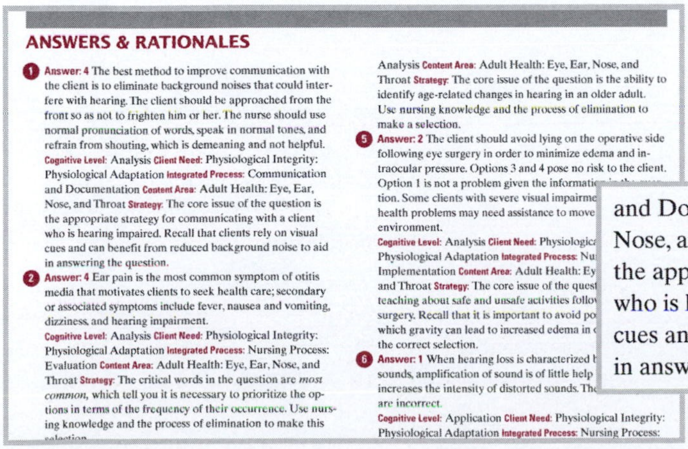

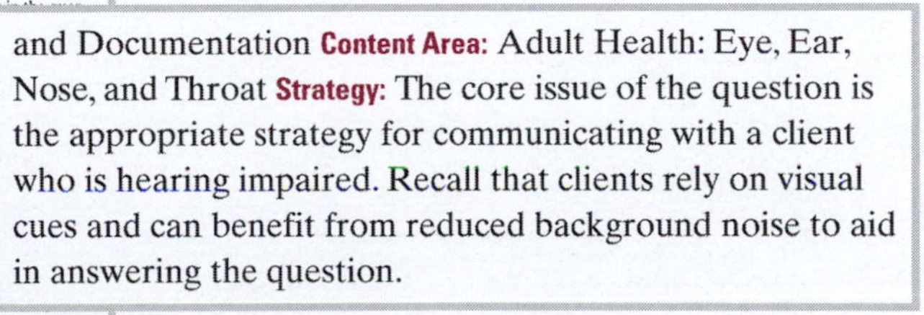

Nursing Reviews & Rationales and eText Online

For those who want to prepare for the NCLEX-PN®, taking multiple practice tests online will help you become more familiar with the computer-based testing experience, especially for the new alternate item formats such as audio, media-enhanced, hot spot, and exhibit questions. With this new edition, use the code printed inside the front cover of the book to access Nursing Reviews & Rationales and more than 3500 practice questions using all NCLEX®-style formats. This includes the practice questions found in all chapters of the book as well as the comprehensive exam questions. Plus, it contains thousands of NEW questions to help you further evaluate your readiness for the exam and hone your test-taking skills. Nursing Reviews & Rationales allows you to choose two ways to prepare for the NCLEX-PN®. Both approaches personalize your practice experience according to what stage you are at in your NCLEX® preparation:

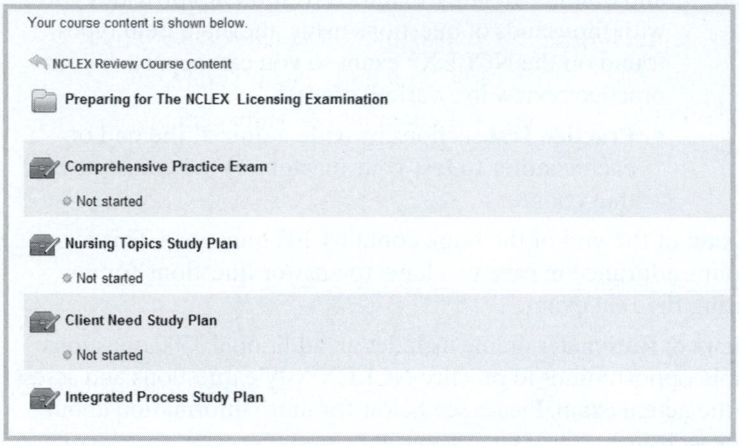

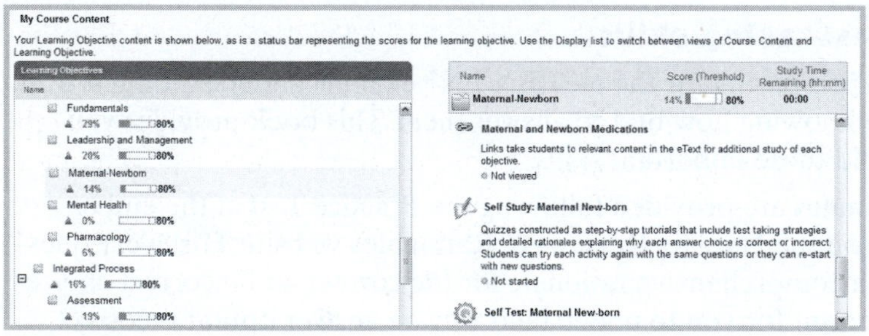

Comprehensive Practice & Review provides a 205-question comprehensive exam that allows you to practice pacing yourself to build stamina so that you can endure answering questions for a long period of time. Following this exam, you receive a results report, a personalized study plan, and links to the eText to help you focus your review with additional opportunities to test yourself.

Nursing Topics Review allows you to select which specific nursing topic areas you would like to review and test yourself. After a brief pretest, you receive a personalized study plan referring you to the eText for areas where you need additional review.

Nursing Reviews & Rationales includes the eText version of *Pearson Comprehensive Review of NCLEX-PN®*, Second Edition. This eText is fully searchable and includes features like note-taking, highlighting, and more. The eText allows you to take your review with you anywhere you have an internet connection to Nursing Reviews & Rationales.

ABOUT PEARSON REVIEWS & RATIONALES SERIES

This popular series is the complete foundation for success within the classroom, in clinical settings, and on the NCLEX-PN® exam. Each topical volume offers a concentrated review of core content from across the nursing curriculum, while providing hundreds of practice questions and comprehensive rationales. The *only* review series offering a tear-out reference card and additional audio reviews, the complete series includes the following volumes:

- Anatomy & Physiology
- Nursing Fundamentals
- Nutrition and Diet Therapy
- Fluids, Electrolytes, & Acid–Base Balance
- Medical-Surgical Nursing
- Pathophysiology
- Pharmacology
- Maternal-Newborn Nursing
- Child Health Nursing
- Mental Health Nursing
- Health & Physical Assessment
- Community Health Nursing
- Leadership & Management
- Comprehensive Review for NCLEX-PN®
- Comprehensive Review for NCLEX-RN®

Audio Reviews for Students On the Go

Study on the go with **VangoNotes**. Just download chapter reviews from your text and listen to them on any mp3 player. Now wherever you are—whatever you're doing—you can study by listening to the following for each chapter of the Prentice Hall Nursing Reviews & Rationales Series:

- **Big Ideas:** Your "need to know" for each chapter
- **Practice Test:** A gut check for the Big Ideas—tells you if you need to keep studying
- **Key Terms:** Audio "flashcards" to help you review key concepts and terms

VangoNotes are **flexible**; download all the material directly to your player, or only the chapters you need. And they're **efficient**. Use them in your car, at the gym, walking to class, wherever. So get yours today. And get studying.

VangoNotes are available for purchase and download at www.vangonotes.com.

Acknowledgments

This book is a monumental effort of collaboration. Without the contributions of many individuals, this book and online Nursing Reviews & Rationales would not have been possible. Thank you to all the contributors and reviewers who devoted their time and talents to this book, including the newly licensed practical nurses who contributed to Chapter 3. Their work will surely help students prepare for success on the NCLEX-PN® exam.

We owe a special debt of gratitude to the wonderful team members at Pearson for their enthusiasm for this project, as well as their good humor, expertise, and encouragement as the series developed. Maura Connor, Director of Nursing Program Solutions, was unending in her creativity, support, encouragement, and belief in the need for this series. Victoria Gaudette, Developmental Editor, and Jennifer Farthing, Executive Editor, devoted many long hours to coordinating different facets of this project, and tirelessly and cheerfully encouraged our efforts as well. Their high standards and attention to detail contributed greatly to the final "look" of this book. Product Manager Travis Moses-Wesphal and Media Production Manager Rachel Collett were extremely helpful in developing Nursing Reviews & Rationales and the accompanying eText online. Editorial Assistant Deirdre MacKnight helped to keep the project moving forward on a day-to-day basis, and we are grateful for their efforts as well. A very special thank you goes to the designers of the book and the production team, led by Patrick Walsh, Managing Production Editor, who brought the ideas and manuscript into final form.

Thank you to the team at GEX Publishing Services, led by Project Managers Micah Petillo and Ashley Lewis, for the detail-oriented work of revising this book. We greatly appreciate the hard work, attention to detail, and spirit of collaboration.

Mary Ann also wishes to thank her nursing students, past and present, who continually search for knowledge to provide the best care possible to patients. Their work, today and in the future, is of the most important kind! Finally, Mary Ann acknowledges and gratefully thanks her children, who sacrificed hours of their time together, to bring the second edition of this book to publication. Their love and support kept her energized and focused.

Mary Ann Hogan
Julie Skrabal

About the *Authors*

Mary Ann Hogan, MSN, RN has been a nurse educator for over 25 years, currently as a Clinical Associate Professor at the University of Massachusetts, Amherst. She has taught in diploma, associate degree, and baccalaureate nursing programs. A former item writer for the CAT NCLEX-RN® exam, Ms. Hogan has been teaching review courses throughout New England for the last 20 years. She also has contributed to a number of publications in the areas of adult health, pharmacology, and fundamentals of nursing. She is a member of the American Nurses Association, Massachusetts Association of Registered Nurses, and the Beta Zeta at-large chapter of Sigma Theta Tau, the International Honor Society for Nursing.

Julie Skrabal, MSN, RN has been an assistant professor at BryanLGH College of Health Sciences in Lincoln, Nebraska since 2002, where she actively serves on curriculum and assessment committees and is the faculty advisor for the local student nurses' association. Ms. Skrabal is a member of the Nu Rho-at-Large chapter of Sigma Theta Tau, the National League for Nursing, and the Nebraska League for Nursing where she serves on the Board of Directors. She is also a member of the American Nurses Association. In addition, Ms. Skrabal is pursuing her doctorate at College of Saint Mary in Omaha, Nebraska.

CONTRIBUTORS TO FIRST EDITION

Kim Attwood, MSN
Moravian University
Bethlehem, PA
Chapter 19 Cultural Awareness

Sharon Beasley, MSN, RN
Technical College of the Lowcountry
Beaufort, SC

Donna Bowles, MSN, EdD, RN
Indiana University Southeast
New Albany, IN

Barbara Carranti, MS, RN, CNS
Le Moyne College
Syracuse, NY

Jo Anne Carrick, MSN, RN, CEN
The Pennsylvania State University
Sharon, PA
Chapter *64 Basic Life Support*

Maureen Clusky, DNSc, RN
Bradley University
Peoria, IL
Chapter 6 *Injury Prevention, Disaster Planning, and Protecting Client Safety*

Julie Eggert, MSN, PhD
Clemson University
Clemson, SC
Chapter *24 End-of-Life Care*

Latrell Fowler, RN, PhD
Florence Darlington Technical College
Florence, SC
Chapter *16 Promoting Healthy Lifestyle Choices*

Rebecca Gesler, MSN, RN
Spalding University
Louisville, KY

Margaret Gingrich, RN, MSN
Harrisburg Area Community College
Harrisburg, PA
Chapter 42 Common Laboratory Tests

Marilyn Greer, MS, RN
Rockford College
Rockford, IL

Kathleen Haubrich, PhD, RN
Miami University
Hamilton, OH

Judith Herrman, PhD, RN
University of Delaware
Newark, DE

Kathy Keister, PhD, RN
Miami University
Middletown, OH
Chapter 7 *Preventing and Controlling Infection*

Virginia Lester, RN, MSN
Angelo State University
San Angelo, TX
Chapter *13 Lifespan Growth and Development, Chapter 27 Maintaining Function of Tubes and Drains, Chapter 43 Common Diagnostic Tests and Procedures, Chapter 44 Perioperative Care*

Debra S. McKinney, MSN, MBA/HCM, RN
TESST College
Alexandria, VA

Donna M. Nickitas, RN, PhD, CNAA, BC
Hunter College
New York, NY
Chapter *5 Leadership and Management*

Lilli Raffeldt, RN, MA
Three Rivers Community College
Norwich, CT
Chapter *17 Age-Related Care of Older Adults*

Samir Samour, MSN, RN
Midlands Technical College
Columbia, SC
Chapter *30 Intravenous Therapy*

Kim Serroka, MSN, RN
Youngstown State University
Youngstown, OH
Chapter *14 Providing Immunizations*

Priscilla Simmons, EdD APRN, BC
Eastern Mennonite University
Lancaster, PA
Chapter *42 Common Laboratory Tests*

Nancy Wagner, MSN, RN
Youngstown State University
Youngstown, OH
Chapter *14 Providing Immunizations*

REVIEWERS FOR FIRST EDITION

Faculty

Mike Aldridge, MSN, RN, CCRN, CNS
The University of Texas at Austin
Austin, TX

Louise A. Aurilio, RNC, Ph.D., CNA
Youngstown State University
Youngstown, OH

Tatayana Bogopolskiy, ANRP
Florida International University
Miami, FL

Mary T. Boylston, RN, EdD
Eastern University
St. Davids, PA

Vera C. Brancato, EdD, MSN, RN, BC
Kutztown University
Kutztown, PA

Tracey Carlson, MSN, RNC
Kent State University
Kent, OH

Fang-yu Chou, RN,PhD
San Francisco State University
San Francisco, CA

Harvey "Skip" Davis, RN, PhD, CARN, PHN
San Francisco State University
San Francisco, CA

Peggy Davis, MSN, RN, CNS
The University of Tennessee at Martin
Martin, TN

Letty Chan Domingo, MSN, RN, CRNP, CEN
Temple University
Philadelphia, PA

Mary L. Dowell, PhD, RNC
University of Mary Hardin-Baylor
Belton, TX

Marilyn S. Fetter, PhD, RN, CS
Villanova University
Villanova, PA

Julie Pearson Floyd, APRN, BC
The University of Tennessee at Martin
Martin, TN

Dina Faucher, RN, PhD, APRNBC, OCN, CHt
Apollo College/US Education Corporation
Phoenix, AZ

Joni C. Goldwasser, RN, MSN, CEN
Radford University
Radford, VA

Rebecca Crews Gruener, RN, MS
Louisiana State University at Alexandria
Alexandria, LA

Sandra Gustafson, MA, RN
Hibbing Community College
Hibbing, MN

Patricia K. Hawley, MEd
Ferris State University
Mecosta Osceola Career Center
Big Rapids, MI

Susan P. Holmes, RN, MSN, CRNP
Auburn University
Auburn, AL

Katherine M. Howard MS, RN, BC
Raritan Bay Medical Center
Perth Amboy, NJ

Barbara Konopka, MSN, RN, CCRN, CEN
Penn State University
Dunmore, PA

Darcus Margarette Kottwitz, MSN, RN
Fort Scott Community College
Fort Scott, KS

Sandra S. Meeker, RN, MSN
Central Texas College
Killeen, TX

Zahra Nowbahari, MAS, BSN, PHN, RN, DSD
San Diego City College
San Diego, CA

Mary Pihlak, PhD, RN
University of Mary Hardin-Baylor
Belton, TX

Beth Hogan Quigley, RN, MSN, CRNP
University of Pennsylvania
Philadelphia, PA

Linda L. Rather, RN, MSN, MS
Neosho County Community College
Chanute, KS

Anita K. Reed, MSN, RN
Saint Joseph's College
Lafayette, IN

Linda Snell, DNS, WHNP-C
SUNY College at Brockport
Brockport, NY

Marianne F. Swihart, RN, MEd, MSN
Pasco-Hernando Community College
New Port Richey, FL

Patricia R. Teasley, APRN, BC
Central Texas College
Killeen, TX

Sheila Upshaw, RN/ADN
University of Arkansas at Monticello
Crossett, AR

Loretta Wack, RN, BSN, MSN
Blue Ridge Community College
Weyers Cave, VA

Gerry Walker, MSN, RN
Park University
Parkville, MO

Leanne M. Waterman, MS, APRN, BC, FNP
Onondaga Community College
Syracuse, NY

Dorothy Williams, MSN, RN
Baptist Health System
San Antonio, TX

Linda S. Williams, MSN, RNBC
Jackson Community College
Jackson, MI

Kim C. Wright, MSN, RN
Amarillo College
Amarillo, TX

The NCLEX-PN® Licensing Examination 1

In this chapter

Passing the National Council Licensing Examination for Practical/Vocational Nurses (NCLEX-PN®) is the last threshold you will cross after completing nursing school to enter the world of professional nursing. Congratulations, you are well on your way! Although you may be nervous or even frightened about taking this test, it is not intended to be a barrier to keep you from your goal. Rather, its purpose is to safeguard the public trust—to ensure that nurses caring for clients are minimally competent and safe for practice. When framed in such a way, it doesn't sound so bad, does it? Then why is the exam so often viewed as a hurdle to be jumped?

The answer partially lies in the construction of the test—it is not like many tests you often took in nursing school. This chapter helps you gain a greater understanding of the NCLEX-PN® exam, developed by the National Council of State Boards of Nursing (NCSBN). By reducing the fear of the unknown, it may help lessen the anxiety about this exam. Chapter 2 provides more information about how to deal with test anxiety and how to use effective test-taking strategies.

COMPUTERIZED ADAPTIVE TESTING: WHAT IS IT?

Computerized adaptive testing (CAT) is a method of test administration in which the computer randomly generates a test question from the test item pool and, after the first question, selects the next question based on your ability to answer the previous one. If the question is answered correctly, the next question is at a similar or higher level of difficulty. If the question is answered incorrectly, the next question is at a similar or lower level of difficulty. This process continues with each subsequent question. Because the questions are tailored to the individual, no two test takers will receive the same test. CAT also assures that anyone who takes the exam more than once never receives the same question twice within a prescribed period of time.

CAT explains why some people are able to answer the minimum number of questions (85) while others must take up to the maximum (205). In essence, successful test takers who can answer difficult questions will have a shorter but harder test, while those who can answer easier questions can expect a longer test.

A key difference between a tradional paper-and-pencil test and a CAT is that with CAT, each question must be answered in the order presented before the test taker can proceed to the next question. Thus, questions cannot be "skipped" to be returned to later. Although being "forced" to answer a question may be unnerving to the test taker who typically skips questions, it is actually beneficial. Why? Because in skipping and returning to questions, more answers are changed from correct to incorrect than are changed from incorrect to correct, according to student reports.

The overall goal of CAT is to evaluate your ability to remain consistently above or below a predetermined passing standard. The computer will continue to select test items from the test bank until

- The requirements of the test plan have been met (see next section) and
- The computer has determined with 95% confidence statistically that your ability is either clearly above or clearly below the passing standard, or
- The maximum 205 questions have been answered, or
- The maximum time limit (5 hours) has been reached.

At this point, the computer will shut down and the examination is ended. Many test takers have mixed feelings at this time. Some are glad it is over, while others wish the computer would keep generating questions.

AN OVERVIEW OF THE NCLEX-PN® TEST PLAN

The test plan is designed to measure the knowledge, abilities, and skills needed by an entry-level nurse in order to practice safely and effectively (NCSBN, 2009). Each question in the test bank is written according to a two-part framework, including *Client Needs* and *Integrated Processes*. Each question is also written at a specific level of cognitive ability.

Cognitive Ability Level

Bloom's taxonomy for the cognitive domain of learning (Bloom et al., 1956, Anderson & Krathwohl, 2001) is used as the measure for coding the difficulty level of an individual test item in terms of its design. Four of the cognitive levels are remembering, understanding, applying, and analyzing. Because nursing is an applied human discipline that requires critical thinking and clinical decision making, most questions on the licensing exam for practical/vocational nurses are written at either the applying or analyzing levels (see Box 1–1 and Box 1–2 for samples). Thus, these questions are often more difficult than test questions on teacher-generated tests, which are likely to contain a greater number of questions at the remembering and understanding levels.

Box 1–1

Sample Question Illustrating Applying Cognitive Level

The nurse has an order to administer a daily dose of sodium warfarin (Coumadin) 5 mg by mouth. Prior to preparing this medication, the nurse would make note of which laboratory test result drawn at 0600 today?

___ **1.** Hematocrit (Hct) 42%
___ **2.** Hemoglobin (Hgb) 12.8 mg/dL
___ **3.** Partial thromboplastin time (PTT) 49 seconds
___ **4.** International normalized ratio (INR) 2.6

Answer: 4

A question written at the applying level of difficulty requires you to consider nursing knowledge that is relevant to the question and use it to make a nursing judgment. In this question, the relevant nursing knowledge is that effectiveness of warfarin is evaluated by noting the results of the INR or prothrombin time (PT, which is not an answer choice in this question).

Box 1–2

Sample Question Illustrating Analyzing Cognitive Level

The nurse on a medical nursing unit has been notified of an external disaster with an estimated 30 clients being brought to the emergency department. The nurse is asked to develop a list of clients on the unit that could be discharged. Which client would the nurse place at the top of the triage list for discharge?

___ **1.** A 39-year-old client who underwent laparoscopic cholecystectomy 24 hours ago and reports right shoulder pain rated as a 4 on a scale of 1 to 10
___ **2.** A 54-year-old client with draining venous leg ulcer and a temperature of 100.8°F
___ **3.** A 76-year-old client with chronic obstructive pulmonary disease with an oxygen saturation of 89% while wearing oxygen at 2 liters/minute
___ **4.** An 82-year-old client who underwent pacemaker insertion 4 hours ago and whose cardiac monitor shows ventricular paced rhythm with no failure to capture

Answer: 1

A question written at the analyzing level of difficulty generally requires you to

- Consider multiple sets of information to make a nursing decision, and/or
- Make nursing judgments using ordinary nursing knowledge in unusual circumstances.

In this question, the nurse needs to use knowledge about which client is the most stable in order to make a decision. The situation is also unusual because nurses are not frequently involved in disasters in everyday nursing practice. Considering stability, you would not discharge first the client in option 3 (airway) or the client in option 2 (risk of infection). The client in option 4 still has potential for developing complications postprocedure, so you would discharge first the client in option 1 who had surgery 24 hours ago. Because it is a laparoscopic procedure, referred shoulder pain is expected, and the client could be taught effective pain management strategies.

Client Needs

The framework for the test plan must identify nursing competencies that apply to all clients across all care settings. With this in mind, the NCSBN developed the test framework of Client Needs. There are four categories of Client Needs: *Safe and Effective Care Environment*, *Health Promotion and Maintenance*, *Psychosocial Integrity*, and *Physiological Integrity*. Two categories—*Safe and Effective Care Environment* and *Physiological Integrity*—are further divided into subcategories on the test plan. All test takers receive the same percentage of questions from each category or subcategory in the test plan, regardless of the length of an individual test (see Table 1–1). These percentages took effect April 1, 2011.

Table 1–1 Overview of the 2011 NCLEX-PN® Test Plan

Client Need Category/Subcategory	Percentage of Questions
Safe and Effective Care Environment	
Coordinated Care	13–19%
Safety and Infection Control	11–17%
Health Promotion and Maintenance	7–13%
Psychosocial Integrity	7–13%
Physiological Integrity	
Basic Care and Comfort	9–15%
Pharmacological and Parenteral Therapies	11–17%
Reduction of Risk Potential	9–15%
Physiological Adaptation	9–15%

Safe and Effective Care Environment

This category contains two subcategories: *Coordinated Care* and *Safety and Infection Control*. The *Coordinated Care* subcategory contains questions that evaluate your knowledge, skills, and ability to collaborate with health care team members to facilitate effective client care (NCSBN, 2011). The *Safety and Infection Control* subcategory contains questions that evaluate your ability to contribute to the protection of clients and health care personnel from health and environmental hazards (NCSBN, 2011). The topics included in each of these subcategories are outlined in Box 1–3.

Box 1–3

Sample Topics for Safe and Effective Care Environment

Coordinated Care

Advance directives

Advocacy

Client care assignment

Client rights

Collaboration with interdisciplinary team

Concepts of management and supervision

Confidentiality/Information security

Continuity of care

Establishing priorities

Ethical practice

Informed consent

Information technology

Legal rights and responsibilities

Performance improvement (quality improvement)

Referral process

Resource management

Safety and Infection Control

Accident/error/injury prevention

Emergency response plan

Ergonomic principles

Handling hazardous and infectious materials

Home safety

Reporting of incident/event/irregular occurrence/variance

Restraints and safety devices

Safe use of equipment

Security plan

Standard precautions/Transmission-based precautions/Surgical asepsis

Health Promotion and Maintenance

This category has no subcategories in the test plan. It contains questions that evaluate your ability to provide nursing care for clients that incorporates knowledge of expected stages of growth and development and prevention and/or early detection of health problems (NCSBN, 2011). The topics included in this category are outlined in Box 1–4.

Box 1–4

Sample Topics for Health Promotion and Maintenance

- Aging process
- Ante/intra/postpartum and newborn care
- Data collection techniques
- Developmental stages and transitions
- Health promotion/disease prevention
- High-risk behaviors
- Lifestyle choices
- Self-care

Box 1–5

Sample Topics for Psychosocial Integrity

- Abuse/neglect
- Behavioral management
- Chemical and other dependencies
- Coping mechanisms
- Crisis intervention
- Cultural awareness
- End-of-life concepts
- Grief and loss
- Mental health concepts
- Religious and spiritual influences on health
- Sensory/perceptual alterations
- Stress management
- Support systems
- Therapeutic communication
- Therapeutic environment

Psychosocial Integrity

This category also has no subcategories. It contains questions that evaluate your ability to provide care that assists with promotion and support of the emotional, mental, and social well-being of clients (NCSBN, 2011). The topics included in this category are outlined in Box 1–5.

Physiological Integrity

This category has four subcategories: *Basic Care and Comfort*, *Pharmacological and Parenteral Therapies*, *Reduction of Risk Potential*, and *Physiological Adaptation* (NCSBN, 2011). The *Basic Care and Comfort* subcategory contains questions that evaluate your knowledge and ability to provide comfort to clients and assistance in performing their activities of daily living. The *Pharmacological and Parenteral Therapies* subcategory addresses your knowledge and ability to provide care related to medication administration and monitor clients who are receiving parenteral therapies. The *Reduction of Risk Potential* subcategory addresses your ability to take action to reduce the potential for clients to develop complications or health problems related to treatments, procedures, or existing conditions. The *Physiological Adaptation* subcategory addresses your ability to participate in providing care for clients with acute, chronic, or life-threatening physical health conditions (NCSBN, 2011). Topics included in each of these subcategories are outlined in Box 1–6.

Integrated Processes

The Integrated Processes category forms the second part of the framework of the test plan for the NCLEX-PN® examination. The four processes are the clinical problem-solving process (nursing process), caring, communication and documentation, and teaching/learning. Because these processes are considered foundational to nursing practice, they are integrated throughout the Client Need categories; however, there are no specific percentages attached to each Integrated Process in the test plan.

TEST INNOVATIONS: ALTERNATE ITEM FORMATS

Alternate item formats were designed to provide ways, other than standard multiple-choice questions, to measure competence for entry-level nursing practice (NCSBN, 2011). As part of its own ongoing quality improvement program, NCSBN continually looks to the future to design, field test, and implement innovative methods for assessing entry-level nurse

Box 1-6

Sample Topics for Physiological Integrity

Basic Care and Comfort	Reduction of Risk Potential
Assistive devices	Changes/abnormalities in vital signs
Elimination	Diagnostic tests
Mobility/immobility	Laboratory values
Nonpharmacological comfort interventions	Potential for alterations in body systems
Nutrition and oral hydration	Potential for complications of diagnostic tests/treatments/procedures
Personal hygiene	Potential for complications from surgical procedures and health alterations
Rest and sleep	Therapeutic procedures
Pharmacological and Parenteral Therapies	**Physiological Adaptation**
Adverse effects/contraindications/side effects/interactions	Alterations in body systems
Dosage calculation	Basic pathophysiology
Expected actions/outcomes	Fluid and electrolyte imbalances
Medication administration	Medical emergencies
Pharmacological pain management	Radiation therapy
	Unexpected response to therapies

competence. In so doing, NCSBN holds itself to the same high professional standards as other health-oriented organizations that hold the public trust. Types of alternate item questions being developed by NCSBN include the following:

- Hot spot (the candidate clicks on a specific area of an image or graphic to answer the question)
- Fill-in-the-blank (the candidate types in a number after performing a calculation)
- Multiple response (the candidate clicks on as many responses as apply to the question)
- Chart/exhibit (the candidate clicks on the "exhibit" button and then views information contained in three tabs to use in answering the question)
- Drag-and-drop/ordered response (the candidate uses the mouse to place in order a sequence of actions based on a client situation)
- Audio (the candidate listens to a recording using a headset prior to answering the question)
- Graphic option (the candidate answers a multiple choice question by clicking on a graphic as the answer)

Alternate item format questions are scored as either correct or incorrect in the same way standard multiple-choice questions are scored. More information about alternate item format questions can be found on the website for the National Council of State Boards of Nursing at http://www.ncsbn.org. At least 400 alternate item format questions can be found in this book and on the accompanying website to provide you with ample opportunity to practice these types of questions.

Remember that any question on the exam may contain a picture, chart, table, or graphic to use when answering the question. Multiple-choice questions that contain such enhancements are not necessarily alternate item format.

BEHIND THE SCENES: THE TEST DEVELOPMENT PROCESS

The test plan for the NCLEX-PN® examination is developed considering the content of Nurse Practice Acts in the various U.S. states and territories and the rules and regulations of the various boards of nursing. A practice (job) analysis study is also done every 3 years to assess what activities entry-level nurses perform in the clinical setting within the first 6 months after graduation. The test plan is then modified after reviewing the results of the latest study and considering other data already mentioned.

In a separate process, the passing standard for the examination is also reviewed on a 3-year cycle in the same year that the revised test plan is approved. In April 2011, the passing standard was raised to –0.27 logits from –0.37 logits, a mathematical "line" above which the test candidate must remain to pass the exam. As an example, test takers who can answer difficult questions correctly remain easily above the line (and will thereby also take a shorter test). Those who can answer easier questions correctly can also pass as long as they remain above the line, but they must answer more questions to do so. The most important point is that as long as the computer is generating questions, it has *not* determined failure, so answer each question thoughtfully and carefully.

To ensure that the exam reflects current clinical practice, new test questions are continually added to the test bank, and outdated questions are discarded or modified. After a question is written and reviewed, it is pilot tested during actual examinations. For this reason, 25 of the first 85 questions on any licensing examination do not calculate into the passing score. Because you will not know which questions they are, it is critical to answer all questions carefully.

New test items are written by a pool of volunteer item writers. Item writers are extensively screened by the NCSBN and are registered nurses who hold a master's degree or higher; often they are nurse educators. A review panel (consisting of content experts who work in clinical settings) also looks at all questions developed by the item writers to ensure they reflect current nursing practice before being included in the test item pool.

REGISTERING FOR THE EXAM

The Registration Process

To be eligible to take the NCLEX-PN® examination following graduation, you must complete two processes simultaneously. The first is to apply for licensure to the Board of Nursing in the state or territory in which you wish to be licensed. The second is to register to take the licensing examination with the test service vendor, currently Pearson VUE.

Fill out the state licensure application completely and carefully, and be sure to submit the correct application fee (varies from state to state) in an approved form of payment. If the form is completed incorrectly, or if the proper fee is not enclosed using the correct form of payment, the application will be returned to you, which in turn will delay your ability to take the examination. After receiving your application, the Board of Nursing will determine your eligibility for licensure (based on state law) and notify the test service once you are authorized for admission to the licensing examination.

At the same time that you apply to a state Board of Nursing for licensure, you will register for the NCLEX-PN® examination with the test service. There is a separate registration fee for the test service. You can register on the Internet at the NCLEX® Candidate website (http://www.pearsonvue.com/nclex). You can also register by mail or by telephone using the directions in the *NCLEX-PN® Examination Candidate Bulletin* obtained through your school of nursing or on the Web at http://www.ncsbn.org.

Once you are authorized by a state Board of Nursing to take the examination, an Authorization to Test (ATT) form will be mailed to you, or it will be e-mailed to you if you included an e-mail address on your registration form. The ATT is valid for a time period specified by the Board of Nursing in which you seek licensure (average is 90 days, with a range of 60 to 365 days). Once you receive the ATT, you can schedule an examination appointment. If you do not receive an ATT within 4 weeks of registration, or if you lose the ATT card once it is sent, report this to the NCLEX® Candidate Test Service according to the directions in the *NCLEX® Examination Candidate Bulletin.*

Scheduling an Examination Appointment

After receiving the ATT, schedule the appointment for the exam promptly, even if you do not plan to take it immediately. This will provide you with the best selection of test dates and times from which to choose. Remember that postgraduation, there are many people seeking to fill the appointment slots, so popular time slots fill up quickly. Also, if you wait until your ATT is almost ready to expire, the test center may not be as able to seat you easily. First-time applicants must be offered an appointment within 30 days of telephoning or e-mailing the test service; repeat candidates can be offered an appointment in 45 days.

Make sure you have an ATT form before you attempt to schedule an appointment. It contains information needed to make the appointment, including your test authorization number, candidate identification number, and expiration date. When you choose your test date, be sure you have 5 hours available (the maximum length of the test).

If you need to change your appointment, you must call the test center at least 24 hours (1 full business day) in advance. For example, if your appointment is for Tuesday at 1:00 p.m., you must call on or before 1:00 p.m. on Monday. For appointments scheduled on Saturday, Sunday, or Monday, you must call by the appropriate time on Friday.

THE TEST CENTER: WHAT TO EXPECT

Getting to the Test Center

Before the day of your appointment, take a test drive to the test center to become familiar with the route and parking availability. Do this at the same time of day you will be driving to your exam, which will give you an idea of traffic conditions and road construction or other delays that may occur at that time of day. Tell family or friends who might accompany you on the actual test day that they will not be allowed to remain in the test center waiting area or to talk to you at any time during the examination.

Be sure to arrive at the test center 30 minutes prior to your appointment. If not, you may have to forfeit your appointment and reschedule it at a later date for an additional fee. The test service will report to the appropriate Board of Nursing any candidate who does not test on the date and time scheduled (due to late arrival or absence). Do not bring textbooks or other study materials into the test center; these are prohibited and could lead to dismissal from the test center or cancellation of your results.

Test Center Procedures

On arrival, you must present your ATT, a valid picture identification that has your signature, and a secondary form of identification that has your signature. It is critical that your name on the ATT and the picture identification match. You then must provide your signature. You will be photographed and a digital fingerprint and palm vein pattern scan will be recorded as additional identity protection measures.

A small storage locker will be provided for your use for personal belongings. Again, you are not allowed to bring books or study materials with you. If you bring a cell phone to the test center, do *not* use it when you take a break because cell phones can be used to access study materials through the Internet. It may be helpful to bring a small snack and/or drink if you take a break during the test, but you may not bring them into the actual testing area.

The test administrator will provide you with a short orientation before escorting you to a computer terminal. After you are admitted to the testing area, the test administrator (proctor) will give you erasable note boards for your use during the test. They must remain in the room and will be collected after the test.

The Actual NCLEX-PN® Examination

The examination may take up to 5 hours to complete. This includes time needed for a short tutorial, and any breaks. If you take a break, you must leave the testing area and have your identity verified by fingerprint and palm vein scan for readmission. All breaks count against your testing time. There is no minimum or maximum time that you must spend on each question, but maintaining a steady pace (averaging about one question every 80 seconds) during the test will help ensure that you do not run out of time. This is just an average, however; you may be able to answer some questions more quickly, and some may take longer. It is most important to do the best you can with each question that appears on the screen.

The first 85 questions of the examination will contain 25 questions that are being pretested (pilot tested). The computer may shut down at any time after 85 questions and up to 205 questions. Again, remember that as long as the computer is generating questions, you have not failed! Maintain concentration and give each question your full and thoughtful attention.

Some people are afraid they will select an incorrect answer accidentally while taking the exam. You do not need to worry about this. Once you select an answer, the computer will not generate another question until you confirm your selection. Until you confirm, you are able to change your answer as many times as you wish. It is only when you confirm your answer that it is finalized and a new question appears. A word of caution here: it is far more common to change the correct answer to an incorrect one because of self-doubt than the reverse. Change answers only for a good reason!

Once the computer shuts down, you will be given a brief computerized questionnaire about the testing experience. When you finish, the test administrator will collect the note boards and dismiss you from the test center.

GETTING THE RESULTS: WHAT NEXT?

You did it! You've taken the test, and you are probably both relieved and nervous at the same time. Your examination is scored twice (for quality control), once by the computer at the test site and again after the examination record has been transmitted to Pearson VUE (usually within 4 to 6 hours). The results are usually made available electronically to the appropriate Board of Nursing in approximately 6 to 8 hours, and results are mailed from the Board of Nursing to the candidates in a variable amount of time, but within approximately 4 weeks.

In a majority of states and jurisdictions, an unofficial report of your result may be obtained for a fee after the test at http://www.pearsonvue.com/nclex or by calling the NCLEX® Quick Results line at 1-900-776-2539 (1-900-77-NCLEX). Check the NCSBN website (http://www.ncsbn.org) to see whether the state in which you have applied for licensure utilizes this service. Do remember that results obtained in this way are unofficial and do not authorize you to begin practicing as a registered nurse. Only the official results from the Board of Nursing allow you to begin practice.

What if you did not pass? Don't give up hope! The Board of Nursing will send you a copy of your results, which will indicate whether you scored above, near, or below the passing standard on each area of the test plan. Talk to a trusted mentor (who is familiar with the NCLEX-PN® exam) and develop a study plan before retesting. Some excellent practicing nurses did not pass on the first try, so stay focused on your goal.

How long will you have to wait to retest? The NCSBN has reduced the waiting period from 90 days to 45 days. Currently, 46 of 59 jurisdictions allow the 45-day wait period. See the NCSBN website (https://www.ncsbn.org/1225.htm) for more information. Check with your Board of Nursing as needed to verify the retake period.

References

Anderson, L., & Krathwohl, D. (Eds.). (2001). *A taxonomy for learning, teaching, and assessing. A revision of Bloom's taxonomy of educational objectives.* New York: Addison-Wesley Longman.

Bloom, B., Engelhart, M., Furst, E., Hill, W., & Krathwohl, D. (1956). *Taxonomy of educational objectives: The classification of educational goals. Handbook I. Cognitive domain.* New York: David McKay.

National Council of State Boards of Nursing, Inc. (2010, March) *2009 LPN/VN practice analysis: Linking the NCLEX-PN® examination to practice.* Chicago: Author.

National Council of State Boards of Nursing (2011). *2011 NCLEX-PN® Detailed Test Plan: Item Writer/Item Reviewer/Nurse Educator Version.* Chicago: Author.

National Council of State Boards of Nursing, Inc. Website: http://www.ncsbn.org

Test Yourself

Are you ready for the NCLEX-PN® or course exams? Use the practice tests on the companion website to check.

Test Preparation and Test-Taking Strategies 2

In this chapter

By successfully passing the courses in your nursing program, you have already shown that you have acquired a set of test-taking skills. Some of you may say, "Yes, that's true for me," while others may say, "Well, I did pass, but I always struggle with tests. I'm not looking forward to the licensing exam!" This chapter helps you use the test-taking skills you currently have and build on them to increase your success on the NCLEX-PN® licensing examination.

PHYSICAL AND PSYCHOLOGICAL PREPARATION FOR TEST TAKING

Many nurses say that life during nursing school was a constant juggling act, trying to balance school schedules, study times, and work responsibilities, as well as family and personal needs. However, life after graduation but prior to licensure does not automatically get much simpler. The school schedule is gone, but work schedules, study time, and family and personal needs are still part of your life.

One critical difference, though, is that you have graduated! This alone shows that you have what it takes, and you must now focus on your final preparation for the licensing exam. A critical step in preparing for the exam is to regain the lost balance in your life, physically and mentally. Physical balance means focusing on diet, rest and sleep, and exercise. Mental balance is achieved by creating a schedule in which you spend the right amount of energy at the right times doing the right things.

Diet

It is easy to give lip service to good nutrition, but it is another thing to follow through. Take time now to pay attention to what you eat and how you plan meals. Get back to the basics of eating regular, balanced meals and nutritious snacks. Three small, light, and nutrient-packed meals are so much better than one large meal at the end of the day (when you are famished and more likely to eat almost anything). Choose low-fat and low-calorie snacks. Make sure you have enough whole grains and fiber, and drink six to eight glasses of water per day. Cut back on caffeine and drinks with sugar, and keep alcohol intake low. Even after a few days, you should feel a difference in both your energy level and your ability to focus.

Rest and Sleep

This is another area that probably got short-changed during nursing school. Most people know how many hours of sleep they need to feel rested, usually between 6 and 8 hours per night. Find out what is right for you, and get the sleep you need. Again, you will quickly reap the rewards of increased stamina, energy, and ability to concentrate.

Exercise and Diversional Activity

Most people have some form of physical activity or exercise that they enjoy. Exercise is not only good for the body, it is a stress reliever as well. Pick an activity that you enjoy (aerobic is great!) and do it regularly. Aerobic exercise will increase your energy, provide a break from studying, and generally benefit your overall health. If you do not really like vigorous exercise, try walking. It is healthy and can be adjusted to any time and distance, depending on the schedule of your day.

Sometimes we all need mental relaxation, which is where diversional activities come into play. As you prepare for the licensing exam, take time to see a movie, go out to eat, visit with friends, or do something else that is fun and makes you happy. This gives you a mental as well as a physical break from studying. Again, when you do not feel short-changed in another area of your life, you are more likely to focus better during your study time.

GENERAL STUDY AND PREPARATION TIPS

The Importance of Self-Assessment

There are two areas of self-assessment that will help you succeed on the NCLEX-PN® licensing examination. The first is to understand your preferred learning style(s), and the second is to understand your relative strengths and areas that need further development before you take the examination.

How Do You Learn Best?

The literature abounds with research about various learning styles, but this discussion focuses on how you use your senses for learning. If you are a visual learner (i.e., you learn best by seeing things), then form a mental picture of what you are studying or the scenario presented in the test question. Look carefully at pictures and diagrams. You may also enjoy reviewing materials on videotape. If you are an auditory learner, then use audiotapes, an MP3 player, or read material out loud as you do your review. Keep in mind, though, that you will not be able to read questions aloud during the exam. If you are a kinesthetic learner, then you learn best by doing. You might find it helpful to write down things as you study. For example, you might make flash cards with hard-to-remember facts. The act of writing may help you to retain the information better. The flash cards will also be handy to review when you have unexpected spare minutes in your schedule.

What Are Your Relative Strengths and Weaknesses?

Before you make a formal plan for NCLEX-PN® examination preparation, take a few minutes to honestly appraise your areas of relative strength. Write down in order from lowest to highest your nursing content areas of strength. Examples are maternity, child health, psychiatric–mental health, medical surgical, and leadership. If you took any standardized tests that provided results according to the Client Needs subcategory of the NCLEX-PN® Test Plan, write down the areas from lowest to highest in terms of how you scored. An example might be Pharmacological and Parenteral Therapies, Reduction of Risk Potential, Health Promotion and Maintenance, Psychosocial Integrity, Physiological Adaptation, Basic Care and Comfort, Coordinated Care, and Safety and Infection Control. This information will form the basis for a formal study plan.

Develop a Study Plan

To make an effective study plan, first determine a target date for testing. Then calculate the number of weeks you have for preparation. Many people take anywhere from 4 to 8 weeks to prepare, but this varies depending on the person's ability, perceived need for study, and availability of appointments near the target test date.

Create a calendar for those weeks that you plan to study. Block off one day per week that you will *not* devote at all to exam preparation. This will help ensure you keep that mental balance we discussed. Next, block off work schedules, appointments, and other commitments you may have. The holes remaining in your calendar are the times that you have available for review and study. Plan to review approximately 2 hours per day, or longer if you have the stamina and feel that you need the extra time. Actual preparation time may vary widely among graduates.

Map out what areas you will review each week according to the lists you developed. Write into the calendar the areas to review, beginning with the areas in which you scored lowest and spacing the material out over the weeks you have available. Allow more time to review weaker areas, and less time for areas of identified strength. This will allow you to concentrate your efforts most on areas that need development; If you run short on time, your areas of strength are the ones that have the least review.

Use this book to guide your review. This book was specifically designed to help you understand how the content blocks that you learned in school fit into the structure of Client Needs in the NCLEX-PN® Test Plan. On average, you should spend approximately one-third of your time initially reviewing content in the various chapters, with the other two-thirds of the time devoted to answering questions. For areas that are more difficult, it may be closer to half and half for review and questions. As a rule, do not use class notes or reread your textbooks. Refer back to them only to clarify any areas of confusion or difficulty. Carefully read the answer rationales as well as the test-taking strategies to increase your retention and fine-tune your test-taking abilities. As you progess, you will spend less time on review and more on questions. Try to plan your review sessions for hours that you are normally alert.

Practice tests will also be an important part of your preparation. These are best scheduled on your days off when you have additional study time. In nursing school, your average tests were probably 50 to 100 questions in length. For the NCLEX-PN® exam, you may need to answer 205 questions. Because you can pass taking the maximum number of questions, it is important to have the stamina to answer each question well. To build your test-taking concentration and endurance, integrate a comprehensive review test once per week into your plan, increasing the number of questions each time. Try to work your way from 100 to 125, then to 150, and so on. Try to answer 205 consecutive questions at least once or twice before your test date. Tests you took in nursing school prepared you to "sprint to the bus stop," but the licensing exam might be more like "running a marathon." You need to be able to stay strong and concentrate through the whole test. Be ready to go the distance! A sample calendar for exam preparation over a 6-week period of time might look like the plan outlined in Table 2–1.

Table 2–1 Sample 6-Week Exam Preparation Calendar

Sunday	Monday	Tuesday	Wednesday	Thursday	Friday	Saturday
6/5 Relax	6/6 (Work) Pharm	6/7 Pharm	6/8 (Work) Pharm	6/9 (Work) Pharm	6/10 (Work) Pharm	6/11 Pharm
6/12 Relax	6/13 (Work) Coordinated Care	6/14 (Work) Coordinated Care	6/15 Coordinated Care	6/16 (Work) Coordinated Care	6/17 (Work) Coordinated Care	6/18 Wedding
6/19 Relax	6/20 (Work) Health Promotion and Maintenance	6/21 (Work) Health Promotion and Maintenance	6/22 (Work) Health Promotion and Maintenance	6/23 (Work) Birthday party in evening!	6/24 Basic Care and Comfort	6/25 Basic Care and Comfort
6/26 Relax	6/27 (Work) Safety and Infection Control	6/28 (Work) Safety and Infection Control	6/29 Reduction of Risk Potential	6/30 (Work) Reduction of Risk Potential	7/1 (Work) Reduction of Risk Potential	7/2 (Work) Psych
7/3 Relax	7/4 (Work) Psych	7/5 Physiological Adaptation	7/6 (Work) Physiological Adaptation	7/7 (Work) Physiological Adaptation	7/8 (Work) Physiological Adaptation	7/9 Physiological Adaptation
7/10 Relax	7/11 (Work) 125-question comprehensive test and review wrong answers	7/12 (Work) 175-question comprehensive test and review wrong answers	7/13 (Work) 205-question comprehensive test and review wrong answers	7/14 Relax; no review!	7/15 NCLEX-PN exam date	7/16 Relax and celebrate

Comprehensive = all test plan areas; Pharm = Pharmacological and Parenteral Therapies; Psych = Psychosocial Integrity

Create a Study Environment

Find a household area that is relatively free of foot traffic and distractions such as television, radio, and the like. Set this area up as your temporary study center. Turn off the telephone and cell phone if you need to. Also turn off other programs on your computer to avoid the "blinging" noises of instant messages and other pop-ups.

Before you begin a review session, make sure you have created an optimal "internal" study environment as well. Make sure you are not hungry or thirsty. Take a few minutes to relax and take a deep breath to clear your mind; this will help you gather your attention for the task at hand and erase any issues that you cannot deal with right now. Get focused and go to work! Plan to take a 10-minute break after each 50 to 60 minutes of concentrated review. This will serve both as a reward and as an incentive to go back to studying.

Stick to the Plan and Know What to Do When You Do Not

Try hard to stick to your plan. If you get behind, it is not the end of the world, but review your calendar to see what the problem is. Was the calendar unrealistic, or did you not follow it? Rearrange your calendar if need be and figure out what you must do psychologically if procrastination is the problem. Remember, this period of time is an investment in yourself; do not use it poorly or throw it away! If you get very far behind, consider whether rescheduling the test is in your best interest.

TEST-TAKING STRATEGIES

Read the Entire Question but Only the Question

Every test question contains all the information you need to know to answer the question. Each question contains three parts:

- The first part presents case-related information about the client in a few sentences or less.
- The second part asks you a specific question about the case provided; these first two parts are sometimes collectively called the question stem, although technically the second part is the stem.

- The third part consists of the answer options. In a standard multiple-choice question there are four options labeled 1 through 4; you must select one of these as the answer. In an alternative item format question; the third part may require typing in numbers, clicking on a diagram, arranging priorities, or selecting more than one option.

It is important to read every word in the question, one at a time. Do not speed read the question, and do not read into the question anything that is not there. It is easy to read into questions based on your personal experience or the experience of others. Resist the urge to choose your answer based on specific real-world experiences. This exam represents the ideal world, and the case situation in the question may or may not closely resemble the one with which you have experience. For each question you answer, remember the client in the question is your only client, and you have all the supplies and materials you need to deliver care.

Reinterpret the Question to Identify the Core Issue

After you read the question stem but before you read the options, take a moment to reword the question in your head to help you identify the core issue of the question. The core issue is the specific skill, ability, or point of knowledge that is needed to make the correct answer selection. Identifying the core issue may prevent you from getting distracted by the options and making an incorrect choice. See Box 2–1 for an example of a reworded stem.

Focus on the Client in the Question

In most questions, the actual client presented is the subject of the question, but sometimes the question is really asking about a significant other, family member or friend, or even another health team member. As you read each question, deliberately determine who is the real client in the question, and choose the option that helps you to answer accordingly.

Find Critical Words in the Question

Critical words in the question help you to discriminate what you need to focus on while answering the question because they put the question into a specific context. The critical words may relate to time, probability, and sequencing of actions or priority setting, as shown in Box 2–2. Be sure to notice these words as you read, because they will help you to discard options that are incorrect answer choices.

Be Alert for Words That Are Red Flags

We do not live in an all-or-nothing world, and nursing practice is not an all-or-nothing endeavor. Watch for words that oversimplify the decision-making process in nursing practice. Examples of these words are *all*, *every*, *none*, *never*, *always*, *cannot*, *must not*, and *only*. You may recognize these words more quickly and easily as you practice answering questions.

On the other hand, words that are not so extreme could indicate the option is correct. Options that contain words such as *often*, *usually*, *likely to*, and *probably* warrant closer examination because they could be part of a correct choice.

Identify Positive and Negative Words in Question Stems

Positive or negative words in the question stem help you decide whether to choose an option that is a true statement or one that is a false statement as it relates to the case situation. Many questions on the exam will be worded in the affirmative; fewer will use negative words. Consider the following examples, which ask about an identical core issue (discharge teaching information following tonsillectomy) but use positive and negative words that lead to entirely different answers:

- Positive: A 10-year-old child is being discharged to home following tonsillectomy. The nurse determines that the child's caregiver **understands** discharge teaching points after the caregiver makes which statement?

Box 2–1

The Core Issue of the Question

Sample question stem:
A 39-year-old female client is scheduled for discharge following right mastectomy with breast reconstruction. The nurse places highest priority on reinforcing which teaching point before discharge?

Sample reworded question stem:
What is the most important client teaching point for a client going home after mastectomy and breast reconstruction?

Box 2–2

Examples of Critical Words in a Question

Time: early, late, the day before, the day of, the day after, just prior to, immediately following, 1 hour after (or *x* hours after)

Probability: most likely, least likely, at highest risk, at lowest risk

Sequencing of actions (priority setting): initial, first, immediately, highest priority, most appropriate

- Negative: A 10-year-old child is being discharged to home following tonsillectomy. The nurse determines that the child's caregiver **needs further reinforcement** related to discharge teaching after the caregiver makes which statement?

In the first example, the correct answer would be an option that is a true statement about a point of discharge teaching, while in the second, the correct answer would be the option that contains a false statement. Note how easy it could be to make an incorrect choice by missing the negative words "needs further reinforcement." Note also that the real client in this question is the child's caregiver, not the child who had surgery.

Eliminate Incorrect Options

Whenever you decide that an option is incorrect, immediately eliminate it as an answer choice. Each time you eliminate such an option, you increase the probability of ultimately choosing the correct answer. For example, if you do not know an answer and randomly choose from among four options, you have a 25% chance of getting the right answer. If you can eliminate one, leaving three to choose from, your odds of success are increased to 33%. If you can narrow down the choices to two options, you now have a 50% chance of making the correct choice. On the NCLEX-PN® exam, however, it is likely that more than one option or all of them may seem to be correct, so read on to the next section for more test-taking strategies.

Carefully Examine Options with Similarities

If you read a question to which you do not know the answer, look for similarities either between the stem and one option or between two of the options. Some possibilities are outlined below, with suggestions to guide your thought process.

Similarities between the Stem and an Option

If the stem of the question and one of the options contain a similar idea, action, word, or emotion, then that option could be the correct answer. Consider this option carefully as you read all the options and prepare to make a selection.

Similarities between Two or More Options

This could be a little trickier. If two or more options seem to have a similar idea, action, or response, examine them carefully. If they are essentially saying the same thing but using different words, then neither of them can be correct and you must eliminate them both (or all). If, however, they seem to be saying similar things but one option is more encompassing or global than the other option, it is possible that the more encompassing option is the correct answer choice. You can recognize the encompassing option because it contains the main thought of the other option plus some others within it. Reread the question and all viable choices to help you decide if this should be your selection. Examples of questions to which this strategy could apply are questions about communication processes, interdisciplinary care, or taking action in an emergency.

Recognize the Need to Prioritize

This is a very important test-taking strategy. Because many questions are written at the analysis level of difficulty, expect to get a reasonable number of questions in which all of the options are technically correct actions or responses. You must decide what is the best action or response for that client and situation. Questions such as these require you to engage in priority setting. Universal strategies for prioritizing in nursing are outlined in the following sections.

Maslow's Hierarchy of Needs

Examine the question and analyze if Maslow's Hierarchy of Needs theory applies. When a question or option seems relevant, recall that physiological needs (air/oxygen, water, food, sleep) come first, followed by safety needs. Secondary or psychosocial needs are addressed only after physiological and safety needs are met.

The ABCs: Airway, Breathing, and Circulation

This strategy is very straightforward. Airway takes priority, followed by breathing, and then circulation. Remember that oxygen saturation could refer to either airway or breathing and that hypovolemia and hemorrhage relate to circulation.

Least Stable or Most at Risk for Complications

When choosing between which client to visit, assess, or care for first, remember that the correct answer is most likely to be the client that is the least stable of all clients presented or, if all are stable, then the one who is most at risk for developing a serious complication. These questions can be difficult to answer. To make the correct choice for such a question, you must understand a variety of client health problems and their significance, and you must understand principles of clinical decision making. For this reason, it is very important to review pathophysiology, nursing management, and client education for a wide variety of health problems.

Time/Scheduling

For some questions, priority setting may be guided by events that are time-bound. In questions that involve clients who have specific discharge times or have immediate preoperative or preprocedure status, consider whether the core issue of the question is caring for this client before other stable clients, using time as the priority.

Use the Clinical Problem Solving Process (Nursing Process) Effectively

Data Collection

Since data collection is the first step of the nursing process, consider when you read a question whether the correct answer is likely to focus on data collection. In general, when questions ask for your first nursing action, look to see how much data is presented in the case situation. If there is no data or just a single piece of datum, the correct option is more likely to be one that gathers more subjective or objective data. If, on the other hand, you have a complete set of data presented to you, an option that reflects further data collection or data collection of a low-priority item is not as likely to be correct.

Analysis level questions require critical thinking and clinical decision-making skills. These questions present physiological or psychosocial data in the case situation and ask you to interpret the information so you can take action based on the data or respond in a therapeutic way to the data. In any event, you need to draw the correct conclusions from the data in order to select the correct answer. Analysis level questions are often difficult because they require interpretation of multiple pieces of data.

Planning

The planning step of the nursing process involves assisting in developing a plan of care, setting goals and/or establishing outcomes, and determining priorities of care. Because the plan must be communicated to others in the health care team, these questions may also involve interdisciplinary communication and collaboration.

Implementation

Questions that address the implementation step of the nursing process are action-oriented. They require you to carry out interventions; reinforce client teaching; communicate with clients, families, and interdisciplinary team members; and document care. These types of questions are also often combined with priority setting, so again you need to use clinical decision-making skills in selecting an option.

Evaluation

Questions that address this step of the nursing process require you to assist in determing whether a client has met the expected outcomes of care. They may require you to assist in determining the following:

- Whether the plan of care has been effective
- Whether a client has achieved the goals of care (returned to normal status or client's baseline)
- Whether a client or family member understands how to care for a client following discharge (diet, activity, medications, and follow-up care)
- Whether the client has adequate knowledge of the underlying health problem
- Whether unlicensed assistive personnel are performing care correctly
- Whether revisions to the plan of care are necessary

Because they involve clinical judgment and decision making, these questions are also more likely to be written at an analysis rather than application level of difficulty.

Strategies for Subsections of the Test Plan

Although there are many ways to write questions that address each part of the test plan, certain types of questions seem to naturally align with specific parts of the test plan. These types of questions include those utilizing communication and scientific principles and those addressing pharmacology.

Communication

Questions addressing communication have a natural affinity for the Psychosocial Integrity category of Client Needs. These questions require you to apply therapeutic communication skills. The correct answer will contain the most therapeutic statement, focus on the client's feelings, and/or assist the client to work toward therapeutic goals. Although communication strategies and communication blocks were part of your foundational nursing curriculum, they warrant review and practice. Questions related to communication may have several options that seem similar in some ways, but different in others. You must be able to choose which one is *most* therapeutic.

Use of Scientific Principles

The use of everyday scientific principles is an all but unheard-of strategy for answering test questions. Yet, scientific principles play a key role in assisting you to answer some questions that are typically part of the Physiological Integrity category of Client Needs. Consider, for example, how gravity may affect your answers to questions about positioning clients, troubleshooting IV flow rate problems, and monitoring various tubes and drains. Consider how concepts of pressure affect your answers to questions about flail chest, mechanical ventilation, intracranial pressure, the Valsalva maneuver, stopping bleeding, and so on. If you visualize these options in terms of how they are affected by pressure, you may be able to eliminate one or more incorrect options.

Pharmacology

When answering questions related to pharmacology, look at both the generic name and the trade name provided. If you recognize the drug, use your knowledge about it to answer the question. If not, try next to determine what classification the medication belongs to by looking at the syllables in the name. For example, a medication that ends in *-mycin* is either an antibacterial agent or antitumor antibiotic. If you cannot determine the classification, try to look for hints in the case situation, such as the client's diagnosis. If none of these strategies work, look for other words in the question that provide clues.

Read the Memory Aid boxes contained in the pharmacology chapters in this book to learn common prefixes and suffixes that will help you recognize drugs more easily on sight. Also use general principles of medication administration, such as the following:

- Administer medications in the doses ordered without changing the dose or discontinuing the medication; you may need to withhold a single dose for a specific reason, such as withholding digoxin (Lanoxin) for a pulse rate of 48, or withholding metoprolol (Lopressor) for a blood pressure less than 90 systolic.
- Question an order if any part of the order is missing or unclear.
- Look for endings such as XL, SR, and others that indicate a medication is sustained release; if present, do not crush or break the medication and do not allow the client to chew it.
- Do not allow a client to take over-the-counter medications with a prescribed medication without checking with the physician first.
- Teach clients to avoid drinking alcohol while taking medications; this is especially true for medications that are central nervous system (CNS) depressants because alcohol also depresses the nervous system.

References

Katz, J., Carter, C., Kravits, S., Bishop, J., & Block, J. (2010). *Keys to nursing success,* Revised edition. (3rd ed.). Upper Saddle River, NJ: Prentice Hall.

National Council of State Boards of Nursing (2011). *2011 NCLEX-PN® Detailed Test Plan: Item Writer/Item Reviewer/Nurse Educator Version.* Chicago: Author.

National Council of State Boards of Nursing, Inc. Website: http://www.ncsbn.org

Test Yourself

Are you ready for the NCLEX-PN® or course exams? Use the practice tests on the companion website to check.

3 The NCLEX-PN® Examination through the Candidates' Eyes

This chapter gives you an opportunity to hear directly from a few graduates who took the NCLEX-PN® licensing exam. Some basic questions were posed to them; the questions and their responses are outlined below. Each person has a unique perspective, and each one is valid, just as your own will be. Take and use what you can from them. They all wish you well! Thanks to the following graduates listed in alphabetical order, who shared their words of wisdom.

Sandra De Los Rios, LPN
Sarah Elwood, LPN
Dina Faucher, LPN

What did you do to prepare in the months and weeks prior to the NCLEX-PN® exam and how useful do you believe your strategies were?

LPN 1, First-time pass at 91 questions: I found preparing for the NCLEX-PN® exam to be most challenging, especially figuring out what to study and how to study it. Ninety percent of the time I used computerized tests like the ones we used throughout my program. I appreciated the tests that provided questions and answers best. After graduating I continued to take these computer tests for review and that was about 90% of my strategy. I literally answered hundreds of questions before taking the exam. I started slowly, answering 20 questions from each category, and would check my answers and take notes on the questions I missed. I slowly increased the number of questions I answered each day. Some days I might have only concentrated on one subject, and then I would study the areas where I performed poorly. I would change categories every few days and increase the number of questions I answered. I had to get used to taking computerized exams and the possibility of having to answer more than 200 questions. Another thing that was helpful was studying with a friend. We both used different review books and read questions back and forth to one another. I felt like she might think of things to review that I would not think of on my own.

I had a few key strategies I used when preparing for and taking the exam that helped me choose the correct answers. First, I remembered to keep the ABCs (airway, breathing, and circulation) in mind when choosing an answer. Next, I placed safety as another key concept when reviewing answers. Finally, someone once told me to "remove the boulder first" and it helped to point me to the correct answer. By "remove the boulder" I mean that if a boulder rolled down the hill and landed on my foot, before considering any other first aid responses my first concern would be to remove the boulder. This would take priority over bandaging my foot or planning care for my injured foot. Therefore, in questions that asked what my first priority would be I would think about fixing the problem before doing anything else. A nursing instructor told me to remember that the NCLEX-PN® exam tests your nursing skills, so answers that involve calling the physician or getting the respiratory therapist are probably the wrong answers. Instead, look for an answer that involves your nursing skills first and settle only on an answer that involves other team members if there are no other choices that seem right. Finally, think textbook. The NCLEX-PN® exam tests how things should be done, not the real world method. Do not answer as if you are in the real world, but instead answer the way the textbooks taught you to do things.

LPN 2, First-time pass at 85 questions: I studied using a published review book.

LPN 3, First-time pass at 105 questions: I was fortunate to have acquired the NCLEX-PN® review book early in my nursing program and I used it to study for actual exams during school. Each module I would use the book and study. This enabled me to feel very confident and prepared by the time I graduated because I studied and learned throughout the program and only had to review to prepare for the NCLEX-PN® exam.

What was the actual testing center like? Did anything surprise you?

LPN 1: The testing center was very nice. I wasn't sure what to expect, thinking it might be a huge open room, but it was just a small room in a small office building. The room had about 7–10 cubicles with computers in each one. The atmosphere was very comfortable.

LPN 2: The testing center was very secure and all personal belongings had to be placed in a locker. Every time someone entered or left the testing area, they had to use the fingerprint on their index finger to open the door.

LPN 3: The testing center was very professional and the people who were there expected professionalism from those coming to take the test. I was surprised that the facility was so strict about what you could take into the exam area. They had me store my personal items in a locker and the only thing I could enter the actual testing room with was the writing instrument and paper the center provided.

How did you handle the stress of taking the exam and the waiting period until you received your results?

LPN 1: Taking the exam was nerve-wracking. I kept watching the question counter at the bottom of the screen, waiting to answer 85 questions. I know everyone says you shouldn't determine pass or fail by the number of questions you are given, but others have told me it is a good indicator—the closer to 85 you get, the better chance you have of passing. The waiting period was awful! They tell you your results will be posted within 48 hours of taking the exam and they mean almost 48 hours to the minute. The entire second day I kept calling the 900 number to see if my results were posted, and when they weren't posted yet, my anxiety level would climb. I would advise you to save yourself the stress and wait until around the time you finished the exam before calling the 900 number. When I left the testing center, I believed I had failed the exam. I was not confident in myself and it was the most awful feeling in the world. The uncertainty was unbelievably scary. I honestly cried when I got my results and discovered I had passed!

LPN 2: I handled the stress by talking to friends and family.

LPN 3: I was nervous and excited at the same time. I remember stopping soon after beginning the exam and thinking, "Well, here I am! The day is finally here! I have been waiting and working for this for the last two years." I took a deep breath, smiled, and reminded myself to savor the moment and really feel what I was going through. This helped me relax and, better yet, have fun with what I was experiencing. I felt good after taking the test and this made waiting for results a lot easier.

What words of advice do you have for future graduates preparing for the NCLEX-PN® licensing exam?

LPN 1: Remember to study while you are in school. Once you graduate, it is not as much about learning as it is about applying what you learned. You need to review and prepare for the exam but don't stress yourself studying for hours every day. Instead, take two to three hours a few days per week to focus on your weak areas. Create mnemonics to help aid in reviewing and memorizing facts.

LPN 2: Don't spend too much time on any one question. Go with your first instinct when choosing the correct answer. Don't change your morning routine the day of the exam because that could increase your stress level.

LPN 3: Acquire an NCLEX® exam review book as early in your nursing program as possible. Use this as a tool during school while preparing for exams or finals. This is a great way to familiarize yourself with critical-thinking formatted questions. I believe this is how I acquired such good grades during school and it made the actual licensing exam easier for me.

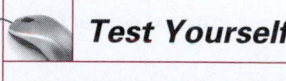

Test Yourself

Are you ready for the NCLEX-PN® or course exams? Use the practice tests on the companion website to check.

4 Legal and Ethical Nursing Practice

In this chapter

Cross Reference

Other chapters relevant to this content area are

Leadership and Management — Chapter 5

I. ETHICS, MORALS, AND VALUES

A. ***Ethics***

1. A branch of philosophy that seeks to utilize a body of knowledge to determine what is right or wrong

NCLEX®

2. **ANA Code of Ethics for Nurses**
   - **a.** Developed by American Nurses Association (ANA) to provide guidance to nurses and protection for clients and families
   - **b.** Guidelines delineate values and standards for professional practice
   - **c.** Key elements include compassion and respect, commitment, advocacy, and **accountability** when working with clients, families, and communities, as well as responsibility to the profession

B. Morals

1. Personal philosophy based on what is right or wrong, good or bad
2. Applying ethics is a practical way of putting morals into practice; it aids decision making and problem solving
3. Ethical considerations define morals essential to practice

C. Values

1. Are personally and professionally developed and based on philosophy and principles
2. Define actions and reactions to issues and problems
3. Provide guidance in determining actions; socialization and experiences help mold personal value system

II. ETHICAL PRINCIPLES AND DECISION MAKING

NCLEX®

A. Ethical principles (see Table 4–1)

B. Ethical decision making

1. Nursing is based on ethics of care, including medical indications, client preferences, quality of life, and contextual factors

Memory Aid

All interactions, even ordinary ones, between client and nurse utilize principles of ethical behavior. Learn these principles to be able to engage in effective decision making as a nursing professional.

Table 4–1 Ethical Principles Important in Nursing

Autonomy	Freedom to make decisions that affect self and to take action for self; is self-governing; includes four basic elements: respect for others, ability to determine personal goals, complete understanding of choice, and freedom to implement plan or choice
Nonmaleficence	To do no harm, either intentional or unintentional
Beneficence	To act in the best interest of others; to contribute to the well-being of others; includes client advocacy; has three major components: to promote good, prevent harm or evil, and remove harm or evil
Justice	Fair, equitable, and appropriate treatment; resources are distributed equally to all
Fidelity	Remaining faithful to ethical principles and ANA Code of Ethics for Nurses; keeping commitments and promises
Veracity	To tell the truth, which has an added benefit of promoting trust between client and nurse
Accountability	Being answerable to self and others for one's actions; includes the concept of responsibility, a specific type of accountability for duties performed within a specific role

2. Nurses are required to make numerous ethical decisions every day; differences in clients' values, culture, and lifestyles may present nurses and other health care providers with ethical dilemmas
3. The perspective of principalism in ethics ignores the socioeconomic and cultural contexts and is too abstract to have practical application in clinical practice

III. LEGAL PARAMETERS OF NURSING PRACTICE

A. Overview

1. Practice of nursing must be done within confines of law; nurses must know law and parameters of nursing license
2. *NCLEX®* Legal limits of nursing are dictated by state and federal laws and guidelines and are regulated by each state's Board of Nursing (see Table 4–2)
3. Good Samaritan laws: designed to protect those who aid victims in emergencies; statutes vary among states; care rendered must be free of charge and done in good faith; will not protect nurse when there is gross negligence; once aid is offered, must stay with victim until stable or another provider with equal or greater training takes over
4. Health Information Portability and Accountability Act (HIPAA): mandates confidentiality (to maintain privacy of client and family and avoid disclosure of client data or personal information); confidentiality is also part of ANA Code of Ethics for Nurses

B. Licensure

1. Credential determined by state boards of nursing; qualifies individual to perform designated skills and services; requires completion of a nursing curriculum that leads to successful passage of a licensing examination in order to be issued
2. *NCLEX®* **Nurse Practice Act** determines the scope of practice for a professional nurse in a specific state
   - **a.** Establishes guidelines by which nurses can perform skills or services
   - **b.** Is a set of state statutes (rules and regulations) that provide guidance to professional nurses
   - **c.** Establishes educational, examination, and behavioral standards for nurses that protect public
   - **d.** To enforce requirements, each state has a Board of Registration in Nursing to oversee implementation of Nurse Practice Act by nurses across care delivery settings

C. Sanctions against nursing license

1. Boards of nursing in state of licensure can deny, suspend, or revoke license to practice as registered nurse on basis of authority granted in state statute
2. *NCLEX®* Possible reasons for disciplinary action or sanction
   - **a.** Unprofessional conduct
   - **b.** Conduct that could negatively affect public health and welfare
   - **c.** Accepting and carrying out assignments incorrectly or with insufficient preparation
   - **d.** Physical or verbal abuse of client
   - **e.** Breach of confidentiality
   - **f.** Improper delegation of care that places client at risk for harm
   - **g.** Failure to maintain accurate client record or falsifying client record
   - **h.** Abandonment; leaving an assignment without proper notification and approval
   - **i.** Failure to engage in continuing education activities as required by state statute

Table 4–2 Types of Laws Affecting Nurses

Type of Law	Description	Examples
Constitution	Law of the land; defines structure, power, and limits of government; guarantees fundamental rights and liberty; other laws may not infringe on constitutional rights	Due process, equal protection
Statutory laws	Laws enacted by legislative branch of government; regulatory agencies are established through statutes	Nurse Practice Acts, guardianship codes, informed consent, living wills, abuse reporting, sexual harassment, Good Samaritan Acts
Common laws	Judge-made law, derived from court decisions that establish a precedent by which other cases are judged	Resolution of a dispute between two parties
Administrative laws	Authority of administrative agencies to create rules and regulations to enforce statutory laws	Rules and regulations of a State Board of Nursing
Criminal law	Laws affecting safety and welfare of public	Homicide, theft, arson, sexual assault, euthanasia
Private or civil law	Law that applies to relationships between private individuals; includes contract law and tort law	*Contract law:* Between nurse and client/employer/insurance or client and agency *Tort law:* Negligence/malpractice, slander/libel, invasion of privacy, abandonment, false imprisonment

IV. LIABILITY IN NURSING PRACTICE

A. Liability: nurses are responsible and accountable for incorrect or inappropriate actions or inactions

NCLEX® **B. *Negligence*: unintentional failure to act as a reasonable person in similar circumstance would act that results in injury to another; elements include the following**

1. Duty: nurse has responsibility to care for and watch over client as a component of employment; duty indicates legal relationship between client and nurse
2. Breech of duty: nurse fails to complete this duty; this can include acts of commission (activities nurse did) or omission (activities nurse failed to do)
3. Injury occurred: client has suffered physical, emotional, or financial injuries
4. Proximate cause: there is a reasonably close causal connection between nurse's conduct and resulting injury
5. Actual loss or damage resulting from conduct

C. *Malpractice*: negligence by a professional; professional failure to carry out or perform duties that result in injury to another; acting outside one's scope of practice

1. Boundaries of malpractice are defined by statute, rules, and educational requirement
2. Malpractice is usually filed as a civil tort; a court finding of guilty usually results in restitution
3. Nurses may carry personal malpractice insurance to provide for restitution if malpractice occurs
4. Rarely are malpractice charges filed as criminal charges (in which a guilty verdict results in punishment, either jail or capital punishment)

D. Miscellaneous legal charges

1. Assault: threat of harm or unwanted contact with client that causes the client fear
2. Battery: a purposeful touching of client without that client's consent
3. Invasion of privacy: can result from violations of confidentiality
4. Fraud: deliberately deceiving client for purpose of unlawful gains
5. Defamation of character: sharing client information with a third party that results in damage to client's reputation; can occur in the form of slander (oral) or libel (in writing)
6. False imprisonment
   a. Prohibiting a client from leaving a health care facility with no legal justification
   b. Using chemical or physical restraints without satisfactory clinical evidence of need

NCLEX® **E. Nursing activities to reduce risk of liability**

1. Practice within provisions of state Nurse Practice Act
2. Follow ANA Code of Ethics for Nurses and standards of professional practice
3. Treat every client with kindness and respect

4. Maintain confidentiality by not sharing client information with a third party without client's consent; do not share chart or medical record information without written client consent and then do so only in accordance with agency policies and procedures; see also next item
5. Avoid violations of HIPAA
   a. Protect client's personal identifying information (such as name, Social Security number, date of birth) and information about diagnosis or treatment
   b. Share information only with individuals involved directly in client's care, payment for care, and/or management of client's care
   c. Verify identity of persons asking for client information
   d. Dispose of confidential documents in accordance with agency policy (such as shredder, locked recycle bin)
   e. Keep contents of medical record out of public view
   f. Discuss client's care only in areas where conversation cannot be overheard
6. Document client assessments, interventions, and events factually and timely in medical record
7. Document on appropriate "against medical advice" forms when a competent client refuses care despite explanations about the benefits of that care
8. Maintain skills and knowledge base by completing continuing education programs
9. Recognize personal strengths and weaknesses; seek help when facing new experiences and job requirements

V. SAFEGUARDING CLIENT RIGHTS

A. Client rights

1. Patient's Bill of Rights communicates to clients and health care workers that clients are entitled to specific rights during care
2. Key rights include confidentiality (see previous discussion), informed consent, and others listed in following text that affect client self-determination

NCLEX® **B. Informed consent**

1. A legal protection of client's right to choose type of care desired and make own decisions about health care
2. Required before care is provided except in an emergency situation or when client is unresponsive (assumption is that client would consent if able)
3. Must meet three requirements: client has mental capacity to consent; it is voluntarily done; and client understands treatment and information presented by provider of treatment
4. Information shared in process of obtaining consent consists of condition requiring treatment, purpose of proposed treatment, procedure, surgery, or other care; associated risks and benefits; and alternatives to treatment including their advantages and disadvantages; client has opportunity to ask questions and hear answers
5. Obtaining informed consent is responsibility of health care provider performing treatment, procedure, or surgery
6. Nurses may witness signature of client on appropriate consent form validating that client is signing the form and has no further questions; does not indicate provision of information by nurse or understanding by client
7. Occasionally clients do not want to hear details of planned procedures but do wish to consent to them; clients may waive right to informed consent, but waiver must be documented in medical record
8. Special considerations in informed consent
   a. If client is deemed by court of law incompetent to make informed decisions about health care, a court-appointed guardian makes these decisions
   b. Informed consent for minors is obtained from parent or legal guardian except in emergency situations, when minor is married or emancipated from parents, or with special needs for care, such as with sexually transmitted infection or pregnancy

Memory Aid

The chart of a typical hospitalized client could have up to three types of consents: the general consent for treatment signed at admission, a consent for a surgical procedure or other invasive procedure, and a consent for anesthesia.

C. Privileged communication versus duty to disclose

1. Communications between clients and health care workers cannot be shared with others outside health care team (such as in court of law) unless client consents
2. Duty to disclose is health care professional's obligation to warn identified individuals if a client has made a credible threat to harm such individuals

NCLEX® **D. Advance directives**

1. Two common forms of advance directives are a living will or health care proxy
   a. Living will outlines medical treatment client wishes to refuse (e.g., intubation) if client unable to communicate wishes at that time
   b. Health care proxy (also called durable power of attorney for health care) appoints someone (usually family or trusted friend) to make health care decisions if client unable to do so
   c. Some forms combine living will and durable power of attorney into one document, which is witnessed by two people or notarized
2. Advance directives provide guidance to the health care team and are followed if client's decision-making powers become impaired
3. Copy of advance directive must be placed in medical record
4. Health care provider is notified of advance directive so that written orders are consistent with client wishes

NCLEX® **E. Organ/tissue donation**

1. Clients 18 years of age or older may choose to donate organs
2. Consent can be given through will, advance directive, or donor card
3. Decision can be made in advance when client is alive and competent or by family at time of death
4. All 50 states utilize Uniform Anatomical Gift Act to procure cadaver organs for transplant
5. Transplant considerations
   a. Bereaved family must be approached with compassion by defined personnel in requesting a discussion on organ donation
   b. Goal is to assist those in need of transplant with organ necessary to prolong life
   c. Clinical death is defined as having no brain waves, no spontaneous breathing, and no superficial or deep reflexes
   d. Transplant team recovers organs after consent is obtained

VI. SAFEGUARDING LEGAL PROFESSIONAL PRACTICE

A. Health care provider orders

1. Determine prescriptive course of treatment for health care team; guide course of action for client and family
2. Typically include orders for medications, diet, activity, diagnostic and laboratory testing, and procedures or treatments
3. Nurses must legally carry out these orders unless believed to be inaccurate
4. Nurse is obligated to question or clarify an order that is illegible, unclear, or possibly inappropriate or inaccurate

NCLEX® **B. Incident reports**

1. Each agency develops a policy or protocol for reporting accidents, unusual occurrences, or other incidents involving clients, which are not in keeping with usual agency operation
2. Incident reports are communication tools that provide information to risk managers and administration about potential areas of exposure to liability; they may be used in legal cases
3. Incident reports are used to identify problems and develop solutions to prevent same incident from happening again
4. When completing an incident report, fill out form in accurate, complete, and factual manner; include client name and other identifying information, date/time/place of incident, facts (no opinions or conclusions), client's account of incident using quotation marks, witnesses, and if applicable, equipment number or medication name and dosage
5. Do not place copy in client record or make reference to incident report in client record
6. Do record facts of incident in medical record

C. Risk management

1. A program designed to protect client and nurse from harm and protect organization from liability related to harm
2. A comprehensive risk management program includes organizational commitment to employee health and safety, a comprehensive worksite risk analysis, employee participation, and hazard prevention and control, including waste management

D. Reporting to external authorities or governing bodies

NCLEX®
1. Nurses and physicians are required to report specific communicable diseases to public health department

NCLEX®
2. Nurses and physicians are also required to report evidence of crimes (such as homicide, suicide, inflicted injury such as stab or gunshot wounds, and abuse) to police

NCLEX®
3. Nurses need to confidentially report suspected chemical abuse by a co-worker to supervisor; administration will notify state board of nursing for investigation; priority issue in this type of case is treatment
4. Under state and federal law, nurses as well as any other employee can report sexual harassment to supervisor or higher administration; consists of any unwelcome statements or behavior of a sexual nature
5. Unsafe working conditions need to be reported under Occupational Safety and Health Act (OSHA) regulations

VII. SPECIAL ETHICAL AND LEGAL CONSIDERATIONS IN PSYCHIATRIC MENTAL HEALTH SETTINGS

A. Client autonomy and liberty

1. Must be ensured by treatment in least restrictive setting by active client participation in treatment
2. Voluntary admission occurs when a client consents to confinement in hospital and signs a document indicating as much
3. Commitment, or involuntary admission, may be done if client is a danger to self or others; some states also have criterion of preventing significant physical or mental deterioration for involuntary admission

B. Competency

1. A legal determination that a client can make reasonable judgments and decisions about treatment and other significant areas of personal life
2. An adult is considered competent unless a *court* rules client incompetent; in such cases, a guardian is appointed to make decisions on client's behalf
3. Clients who are committed are still capable of participating in health care decisions

NCLEX®
C. Informed consent: clients in mental health settings do not relinquish right to informed consent upon admission; may still accept or refuse specific aspects of treatment or care

D. Confidentiality: extremely important also in psychiatric mental health nursing

1. Federal rules apply to confidentiality regarding chemical dependence; staff cannot disclose admission or discharge information
2. Some states require written consent before human immunodeficiency virus (HIV) tests may be performed; states have laws regarding when HIV test results or diagnosis of acquired immunodeficiency syndrome (AIDS) may be disclosed; this occurs regardless of psychiatric or nonpsychiatric health care setting

Check Your NCLEX-PN® Exam I.Q.

You are ready for testing on this content if you can

- Articulate ethical and legal issues in nursing practice that affect clients or families.
- Identify appropriate actions to promote ethical and legal nursing care.
- Evaluate the outcomes of interventions used to promote ethical and legal nursing care.
- Apply principles of confidentiality to client care situations.
- Identify actions to uphold client rights.
- Provide information to clients and families about advance directives.

PRACTICE TEST

1 An adult female ambulatory care client receiving an oral anticoagulant is given aspirin for a headache while visiting a neighbor, who is a nurse. The client subsequently has a bleeding episode because of a drug interaction. The legal nurse consultant interprets that which necessary elements of malpractice are missing from this case? Select all that apply.

1. Breech of duty
2. Duty owed
3. Injury experienced
4. Causation between nurse's action and injury
5. Intent to cause harm or injury

2 The health care provider orders a medication in a dose that is considered toxic. The nurse administers the medication to the client, who later suffers a cardiac arrest and dies. What consequence can the nurse expect from this situation? Select all that apply.

1. The health care provider can be charged with negligence, being the person who ordered the dose.
2. As the employing agency, only the hospital can be charged with negligence.
3. The nurse and physician may be terminated from employment to prevent a charge of negligence to the hospital.
4. Negligence will not be charged, as this event could happen to any reasonable person.
5. The nurse can be charged with negligence for administering the toxic dose.

3 A nurse and teacher are discussing legal issues related to the practice of their professions. The teacher asks what the functions are of the Nurse Practice Act (NPA) in that state. The nurse would include which thoughts in a response? Select all that apply.

1. Accredit schools of nursing
2. Enforce ethical standards of behavior
3. Protect the public
4. Define the scope of nursing practice
5. Determine liability insurance rates

4 The nurse working in an acute care environment would utilize which strategies to reduce the risk of malpractice litigation? Select all that apply.

1. Discuss any errors with the client and family in detail.
2. Keep incident reports on file.
3. Maintain expertise in practice.
4. Offer opinions to clients when the situation warrants.
5. Report unsafe staffing levels to supervisor.

5 A client is referred to a surgeon by the general practitioner. After meeting the surgeon, the client decides to find a different surgeon to continue treatment. The nurse supports the client's action, utilizing which ethical principle?

1. Beneficence
2. Veracity
3. Autonomy
4. Privacy

6 A nurse forgets to administer a client's diuretic and the client experiences an episode of pulmonary edema. The charge nurse would consider the medication error to constitute negligence because the situation contains which element?

1. Purposeful failure to perform a health care procedure
2. Unintentional failure to perform a health care procedure
3. Act of substituting a different medication for the one ordered
4. Failure to follow a direct order by a physician

7 A client asks why a diagnostic test has been ordered and the nurse replies, "I'm unsure but will find out for you." When the nurse later returns and provides an explanation, the nurse is acting under which principle?

1. Nonmaleficence
2. Veracity
3. Beneficence
4. Fidelity

8 An individual has a seizure while walking down the street. During the seizure, a nurse from a physician's office is noticed driving past without stopping to assist. The individual sues the nurse for negligence but fails to win a judgment for which reason?

1. The nurse had no duty to the individual.
2. The nurse did what most nurses would do in the same circumstance.
3. The nurse did not cause the client's injuries.
4. The nurse was off-duty at that time.

9 A client with cancer has decided to discontinue further treatment. Although the nurse would like the client to continue treatment, the nurse recognizes the client is competent and supports the client's decision using which ethical principle?

1. Justice
2. Fidelity
3. Autonomy
4. Confidentiality

10 A staff nurse who is concerned about maintaining client confidentiality would take which action while carrying out assigned duties?

1. Read the records of clients not assigned to the nurse to become more familiar with disease processes.
2. Share information about a client with nurses from the unit to which the client may eventually be transferred.
3. Allow the client's family members to review the medical record to obtain answers to their questions.
4. Share information about the client with those involved in planning nursing care.

PRACTICE TEST

ANSWERS & RATIONALES

1 **Answer: 1, 2 Rationale:** There was no breach of duty because there was no official nurse–client relationship, which accompanies an employment situation. There was no nurse–client relationship because the nurse was acting as a neighbor and not in an employment capacity. Thus, there can be no duty owed. There was injury experienced because of this event. The bleeding was caused by the interaction of the aspirin with the anticoagulant. Intent is not a necessary element of malpractice, because malpractice can occur because of unintended actions as well. **Cognitive Level:** Analyzing **Client Need:** Coordinated Care **Integrated Process:** Nursing Process: Evaluation **Content Area:** Fundamentals **Strategy:** Use the process of elimination. The wording of the question indicates more than one option is correct, and the focus is on *necessary elements* that must be present. First eliminate *intent to cause harm or injury*, since this is not necessary to a charge of malpractice. Next note that there is no duty owed, and because of this, there can be no breach of duty, to choose these two options as the necessary missing elements.

2 **Answer: 1, 5 Rationale:** Health care providers who prescribe incorrect dosages of medications are liable for their errors. The nurse is open to a charge of negligence for failing to verify and question the incorrect dose. The hospital can be sued as the responsible employing agency, but the health care provider and the nurse can also be charged with negligence. Terminating the health care provider and nurse from employment would not stop a lawsuit charging negligence for employee actions that have already taken place. Prescribing and administering incorrect doses are not considered events that routinely happen to "reasonable person." **Cognitive Level:** Applying **Client Need:** Coordinated Care **Integrated Process:** Nursing Process: Implementation **Content Area:** Fundamentals **Strategy:** The wording of the question indicates that more than one option is correct. Choose the response that holds both individuals accountable, since the nurse failed to question an incorrect dose and the health care provider ordered the incorrect dose.

3 **Answer: 3, 4 Rationale:** A state's NPA serves to protect the public by setting minimum qualifications for nursing in relation to skills and competencies. One way it fulfills responsibility to protect the public is by defining the scope of nursing practice in that state. The state board of nursing approves schools to operate but does not accredit them. The state board of nursing does not enforce ethical standards. A state NPA has no role in setting liability insurance rates for nurses. **Cognitive Level:** Applying **Client Need:** Coordinated Care **Integrated Process:** Nursing Process: Implementation **Content Area:** Fundamentals **Strategy:** Use the process of elimination and basic nursing knowledge to answer the question. The wording of the question indicates that more than one option is correct and that the correct responses are worded as true statements.

4 **Answer: 3, 5 Rationale:** Maintaining expertise in practice by keeping up to date in knowledge and skills aids in reducing the risk of malpractice claims by fostering continued competence in practice. Unsafe staffing levels can result in a higher incidence rate of errors, which could later lead to charges of malpractice. Thus, reporting such situations so they can be prevented should be beneficial. Discussing errors in detail with the client and family does not reduce the risk of a malpractice claim. Incident reports should be kept on file but do not decrease the risk of malpractice litigation. The nurse should not offer opinions at any time as this is not part of therapeutic communication. **Cognitive Level:** Applying **Client Need:** Coordinated Care **Integrated Process:** Nursing Process: Implementation **Content Area:** Fundamentals **Strategy:** Focus on malpractice as the concept being tested. Recall that maintaining expertise is the best way to reduce personal risk and that reporting unsafe staffing situations may help reduce general agency risk by preventing omissions or errors due to insufficient numbers of caregivers to do the work required during the shift.

5 **Answer: 3 Rationale:** Autonomy is the right of individuals to take action for themselves. Beneficence is an ethical principle to do good and applies when the nurse has a duty to help others by doing what is best for them. Veracity refers to truthfulness. Privacy is the nondisclosure of information by the health care team. **Cognitive Level:** Applying **Client Need:** Coordinated Care **Integrated Process:** Nursing Process: Implementation **Content Area:** Fundamentals **Strategy:** The core issue of the question is the ability to interpret which ethical principle is operating in a specific situation. Eliminate privacy because it does not apply to the situation as described. Eliminate beneficence and veracity next because they focus on the obligation of the nurse rather than on a right of the client.

6 **Answer: 2 Rationale:** Negligence is the unintentional failure of an individual to perform or not perform an act that a reasonable person would or would not do in the same or similar

ANSWERS & RATIONALES

circumstances. A purposeful failure to perform a procedure would be the opposite of negligence, which is unintentional. Substituting a different medication does not fit the description of the situation in the question. Failure to follow a direct order does not fit the description in the situation in the question. **Cognitive Level:** Applying **Client Need:** Coordinated Care **Integrated Process:** Nursing Process: Evaluation **Content Area:** Fundamentals **Strategy:** Two options are opposites, which is a clue that one of them may be correct. Choose unintentional failure to carry out a procedure over purposeful failure because it matches the definition of negligence.

7 **Answer: 4** **Rationale:** Fidelity means being faithful to agreements and promises. This nurse is acting on the client's behalf to obtain needed information and report it back to the client. Nonmaleficence is the duty to do no harm. Veracity refers to telling the truth for example, not lying to a client about a serious prognosis. Beneficence means doing good, such as by implementing actions (e.g., keeping a salt shaker out of sight) that benefit a client (heart condition requiring sodium-restricted diet). **Cognitive Level:** Understanding **Client Need:** Coordinated Care **Integrated Process:** Caring **Content Area:** Fundamentals **Strategy:** Use the process of elimination. The correct answer is the one that matches the description in the stem; that is, the nurse made a promise to a client and kept it, which constitutes fidelity.

8 **Answer: 1** **Rationale:** To be guilty of negligence, the nurse must have a relationship with the client that involves a duty to provide care. The relationship is usually a component of employment. The nurse did not necessarily do what others would do in this situation. Although the nurse did not cause the client's injuries, it does not prevent the nurse from assisting in this situation. Although the nurse was off-duty, the nurse could have assisted if motivated to do so. **Cognitive Level:** Understanding **Client Need:** Coordinated Care **Integrated Process:** Nursing Process: Implementation **Content Area:** Fundamentals **Strategy:** Use the process of elimination and nursing knowledge. The correct answer recognizes that the nurse was not in the role of employee at the time of the incident, removing the requirement of acting on the client's behalf.

9 **Answer: 3** **Rationale:** Autonomy refers to the right to make one's own decisions, which is the principle supported in this situation. Justice refers to fairness. Fidelity refers to trust and loyalty. Confidentiality refers to the right to privacy of personal health information. **Cognitive Level:** Understanding **Client Need:** Coordinated Care **Integrated Process:** Caring **Content Area:** Fundamentals **Strategy:** Use the process of elimination. The wording of the question indicates that only one option is correct and that you need to select the principle that is consistent with the circumstances in the question.

10 **Answer: 4** **Rationale:** Client confidentiality is maintained when the nurse shares client information only with those currently involved in the plan of care. Staff should only access information about clients currently assigned to their care and should not access information about other clients on the unit not assigned to them. Client information should not be shared with nurses who are not currently working with the client. Family members would need approval from the client and the health care provider prior to reviewing a medical record. **Cognitive Level:** Applying **Client Need:** Coordinated Care **Integrated Process:** Communication and Documentation **Content Area:** Fundamentals **Strategy:** Select the response that protects the client's information, but allows communication necessary for the delivery of quality care.

Key Terms to Review

accountability p. 18
ANA Code of Ethics for Nurses p. 18
ethics p. 18
malpractice p. 20
negligence p. 20
Nurse Practice Act p. 19

References

American Nurses Association (2004). *Code for nurses with interpretative statements.* Kansas City, MO.

Berman, A., & Snyder, S. (2012). *Kozier & Erb's fundamentals of nursing: Concepts, process, and practice* (9th ed.). Upper Saddle River, NJ: Pearson Education, Inc.

Davis, A., Fowler, M., & Aroskar, M. (2010). *Ethical dilemmas & nursing practice* (5th ed.). Upper Saddle River, NJ: Pearson Education, Inc.

Guido, G. (2010). *Legal and ethical issues in nursing* (5th ed.). Upper Saddle River, NJ: Pearson Education, Inc.

Test Yourself

Are you ready for the NCLEX-PN® or course exams? Use the practice tests on the companion website to check.

Leadership and Management

5

In this chapter

Cross Reference

Other chapters relevant to this content area are

Injury Prevention, Disaster Planning, and Protecting Client Safety Chapter 6
Coping with Stressors Chapter 20

I. HEALTH CARE SETTINGS

A. Types of health care settings

1. Hospitals
2. Long-term care
3. Ambulatory
4. Home health care
5. Temporary service
6. Managed health care organizations

B. Types of managed care organizations

1. Health maintenance organization (HMO)
2. Preferred provider organization (PPO)
3. Point of service (POS)

C. Types of HMOs

1. Staff model
2. Independent practice associations
3. Group model
4. Network model

II. HEALTH CARE MANAGEMENT

A. *Health maintenance organizations (HMOs)*

1. A configuration of health care agencies that provide basic and supplemental health maintenance and treatment services to voluntary enrollees who prepay a fixed periodic fee without regard to either in-patient or out-patient services used
2. Formally established through federal legislation to reorganize health care services to slow increases in health care costs and control utilization of services
3. NCLEX® Geographically organized system that provides enrollees with an agreed-on package of health maintenance and treatment services
4. Types of HMOs
   a. Staff model: physicians are HMO employees and are paid a salary
   b. Independent practice associations: physicians maintain individual or group practices but contract with an HMO to serve enrollees for a negotiated fee
   c. Group model: HMO contracts with a multispecialty group to provide enrollee services for a negotiated fee
   d. Network model: HMO contracts with two or more IPAs, independent or group practices, to provide enrollee services at a fixed monthly fee per enrollee, called **capitation**

NCLEX® B. *Managed care*

1. A health care plan that brings delivery and financing functions into one entity in contrast to a fee for service
2. Objective is to restructure health care services to
   a. Enhance cost containment by decreasing unnecessary services
   b. Maintain quality
   c. Facilitate management of client care needs
   d. Promote timely and appropriate care
3. Providers must submit written justification and request prior approval for diagnostic tests and interventions or to extend a client's length of stay
4. See Box 5–1, Key Objectives of Managed Care

NCLEX® C. Case management

1. Organizes client care by major diagnoses and focuses on attaining predetermined client outcomes within specific time frames
2. Advantages
   a. All professionals are equal members of team
   b. Emphasis is on managing interdisciplinary outcomes
   c. Promotes continuity of care
3. Disadvantage: requires essential baseline data be available to team members; role is still in process with job descriptions varying among institutions

D. Nursing care delivery systems

1. Functional nursing
   a. Began in the mid-1940s
   b. NCLEX® Client needs are defined by tasks to be allocated to RNs, LPNs, and unlicensed assistive personnel (UAPs) and coordinated by a charge nurse
   c. Advantages: efficient and effective at regularly performed tasks and financially advantageous for organization
   d. Disadvantages: fragmentation of care, absence of a holistic view of client, time-consuming communications, problems with follow-up
2. Primary nursing
   a. NCLEX® Primary nurse designs, implements, and is accountable for nursing care of clients with delegation of care to an associate nurse
   b. Care is given by primary nurse and associates

Box 5–1

Key Objectives of Managed Care

Cost containment	Administrative efficiency
Some forms of rationing	Contracting efficiency
Efficiency of care	Managing care
Less duplication	Appropriateness of care

c. Advantages: having a knowledge-based practice model; decentralization of nursing care decisions, authority, and responsibility to staff nurse; decrease in number of unlicensed personnel; enhanced family satisfaction with care; and high level of accountability
d. Disadvantages: it requires excellent communication between nurses, and continuity of care and accountability may be challenged; it is costly for institutions to hire highly skilled nurses

3. Team nursing
a. Most common nursing care delivery system in United States
NCLEX®
b. A team of nursing personnel provides total care to a group of clients
c. Advantages: allows use of non-RN staff and coordination of activities requiring more than one person; team leader is a skilled practitioner; it is cost-effective for agency; and client satisfaction with care is increased
d. Disadvantages: communication is time consuming; continuity of care may be decreased, role confusion and resentment can occur, and reporting mechanism is to only one person

E. *Shared governance* model of practice

1. Principles of shared governance include partnerships, equity, accountability, and ownership; the structure demands participation in ownership
2. Characterized by decentralized power sharing and decision making; interdisciplinary team building; activities and conferences; organizational priorities are accomplished through a series of committees
3. Four committees generally set policies and address organizational issues (one representative for each committee from each nursing unit)
a. Nursing practice
b. Quality improvement
c. Education (ensures continuing education requirements and staff competency)
d. Management of the organization's service-specific areas such as general medical-surgical, maternal–child, critical care, intermediate care, and ancillary services such as employee and family health, radiology, and cardiac catherization
4. An overall coordinating council composed of a chairperson elected by nursing staff, a clinical nurse specialist, and four chairs of housewide councils

III. ORGANIZATIONAL SKILLS

A. *Time management* allows nurse to determine how best to prioritize client care, decide outcomes, and perform most important nursing interventions first

1. Time management is a set of skills that encourages and supports most effective and productive uses of time
2. Effective time management means becoming outcome oriented, not task oriented
a. Identify long-term goals and divide them into achievable outcomes
b. Write down all long-term goals and outcomes
c. Goals and outcomes should remain fluid, flexible, and changeable to situation at hand

B. Common symptoms of poor time management

1. Irritability and stress
2. Fatigue
3. Difficulty concentrating and forgetfulness
4. Disorganization and inability to complete tasks

C. How to organize nursing care shift responsibilities and activities

1. Arrange nursing care environment with efficient access to supplies, equipment, and client-designated areas
2. Use previous shift's report to determine tasks and priorities
3. Develop a shift action plan that includes expected outcomes that are optimal and reasonable with a statement that includes by what time interventions will be completed
4. Make assignments indicating who will perform the interventions
5. Implement shift action plan beginning with initial client care rounds
a. Making client care rounds: a rapid information-gathering process
b. Schedule treatments and monitoring: firm time commitment for treatments and monitoring
c. Plan for appropriate equipment and supplies to be available for care
6. Evaluate outcomes and re-examine shift action plan
a. Ask whether optimal outcomes were achieved; if not, why not?
b. Determine if there were staffing problems or client care crises
c. Ask whether realistic outcomes were set, and if not, why not?
d. Identify lessons learned from this shift action plan and determine what can be applied in future
e. Make appropriate change when similar problems occur

IV. ESTABLISHING PRIORITIES OF CARE

NCLEX®

A. Frameworks for determining priorities of client care (see Table 5–1)

1. ABCs: airway, breathing, and circulation
2. Maslow's hierarchy of needs
3. Agency policies and procedures
4. Time
5. Client and family preferences
6. Care related to client acuity
7. Priorities in medication therapy

B. More stable versus less stable client

1. Attend to least stable client first (whose condition is changing or deteriorating)
2. Clients who become unstable may have dramatic signs (such as bleeding, shock, or cardiopulmonary arrest) but could exhibit more subtle signs; watch for gradual trends in data, such as deteriorating vital signs, declining urine output, decreasing level of consciousness
3. When all clients are stable, attend first to client most likely to become unstable or who is at risk for greatest complications because of disease process

Table 5–1 Strategies for Priority Setting in Clinical Practice

Guiding Principles	First Priority	Second Priority	Third Priority
ABCs	Airway, breathing, and circulation	—	—
Maslow's Hierarchy of Needs theory	Physiological (primary) needs: air, breathing, circulation, water, food (oxygen therapy, circulatory support, IV hydration, nutrition, critical lab values, treatment of pain)	Safety and security (primary) needs: prevention of falls, reorientation to surroundings, abnormally high or low values that are not critical; may include some client teaching (e.g., insulin administration)	Secondary needs: activities and care that support "love and belonging," self-esteem (includes ability for self-care and self-management of health problem), and self-actualization; includes routine client teaching and psychosocial support
Policies and procedures	Activities governed by agency policy or procedure that involve strict timelines (e.g., restraints, falls, stat medications)	Activities governed by policy or procedure that directly affect client care (e.g., non-stat, regularly scheduled medications, dressings)	Activities not affecting client care or that might be delegated to another (e.g., checking falls, temperature of unit refrigerator, code cart check, emptying laundry bags)
Time	Clients with highly time-bound therapies (e.g., OR, stat x-ray); tasks that can be fully completed in less than 2 minutes if no competing priority present; necessary time-bound care for admission or discharge clients	Clients with scheduled therapies that need to be completed within a 2- to 4-hour window; routine client teaching	Clients with scheduled therapies that need to be completed once during the shift
Client and family preferences	Clients or families in physical or psychological distress	Clients or families with concerns about status or nursing care	Routine client and family psychological preferences or requests
Care activities related to clinical condition of client	Life-threatening or potentially life-threatening occurrences (adverse changes in VS, change in LOC, potential for respiratory or circulatory collapse); often unanticipated	Activities essential to safety: life-saving medications and equipment that protect clients from infections or falls	Activities essential to the plan of care leading to outcomes of symptom relief or healing (that if omitted would slow client recovery; e.g., nutrition, positioning, ambulation)
Medication or IV therapy priorities	Medications that prevent or treat physiological distress (e.g., analgesics, updrafts, or inhalers); medications ordered more frequently (e.g., every 4 hours) because late medication delivery could affect next dose; IV therapy for hydration in clients who are NPO because of nonfunctional GI tract	Medications that prevent reoccurrences of symptoms of disease processes (e.g., digoxin, antibiotics); medications ordered once per shift; routine maintenance of IV therapy or heparin/saline lock care	Medications that maintain normal organ system functioning (e.g., stool softener); medications ordered daily or twice daily; site and dressing changes for IV therapy

NCLEX®

C. General client problems that usually indicate priority

1. Fresh postoperative clients (newly arrived on nursing unit from postanesthesia care)
2. Clients whose status has deteriorated from baseline (vital signs, level of consciousness, neurovascular status)
3. Clients exhibiting signs of shock (hypovolemic, hemorrhagic, cardiogenic, distributive)
4. Clients who have allergic reactions
5. Clients who have chest pain
6. Clients who have returned from diagnostic procedures and require temporary, more intensive monitoring, including assessing for complications
7. Clients who verbalize unexpected or unusual symptoms (such as new or suddenly increased acute pain, blurred vision, sudden weakness or paralysis)
8. Clients who have equipment or tubing malfunction or accident (such as disconnection of IV line, central line, chest tube; or alarms ringing on mechanical ventilator or cardiac monitor)
9. Lower priority clients are often those whose main needs include teaching, which is not as time bound unless individual circumstances indicate otherwise

V. SUPERVISION AND DELEGATION

NCLEX®

A.

1. A **supervisor** is any individual having authority from employer to hire, transfer, suspend, lay off, recall, promote, discharge, assign, reward, or discipline other employees
2. **Supervising** is the provision of guidance or direction, evaluation, and follow-up of nursing personnel for accomplishment of a delegated nursing task
3. Supervisors are responsible for
   - a. A competent and disciplined staff
   - b. Clear directions and communication
   - c. Timely follow-up to ensure prompt execution of delegated activities and orders
   - d. Active listening skills
   - e. A thorough scope of technical knowledge of supervised work
   - f. Demonstrating fairness and respect toward all
   - g. Feedback for work well done and resolution of problems and conflicts

NCLEX®

B. *Delegation*

1. Delegation is use of nursing personnel to accomplish a desired objective through allocation of authority and responsibility; involves, as part of assigning work, asking another to do some aspect of client care
2. Delegation is
   - a. A complex process and crucial management skill
   - b. Retaining accountability for number and diversity of caregivers
   - c. Knowing capacity and qualification level of each practitioner for doing work
   - d. Accomplishing nursing tasks efficiently using appropriate resources
   - e. Knowing intricacy of relationship among nursing team, client, and environment
3. See Box 5–2 for guidelines on delegation
4. NCLEX® National Council of State Boards in Nursing (NCSBN) defines delegation as transferring to a competent individual authority to perform a selected nursing task in a selected situation

Box 5–2

How to Delegate

1. Identify a suitable person (LPN/LVN or UAP) for the task who has the appropriate skill set.
2. Prepare the person. Explain the task clearly. Make sure that you are understood.
3. Keep in touch with the person for support and to monitor progress while allowing sufficient time and opportunity to complete the task.
4. Retain responsibility for knowing the outcome of the delegation; be specific about data or results to report back.
5. Praise and acknowledge a job well done.

NCLEX® **C. Delegation of nursing activities**

1. LPN/LVNs can delegate nursing care activities to unlicensed assistive personnel (UAPs) based on competency of UAP, including educational knowledge and skill levels
2. Clearly identify outcomes or expectations of each assigned nursing task or activity, including
   a. Standard of care
   b. Time frame for assignment completion
   c. Limitations regarding performance of task (see Box 5–3 for concepts to consider in determining when to delegate); LPN/LVN can delegate authority but cannot delegate responsibility and therefore must ensure UAPs are practicing in a competent manner
3. Do not delegate the following to UAPs:
   a. Initial or subsequent data collection during work shift
   b. Interventions that require knowledge and skill beyond UAP training, including reinforcement of client teaching

NCLEX® **D. Principles of delegation**

1. Only authority, but not ultimate responsibility, can be delegated
2. All delegated tasks must be clearly assigned and continuously clarified
3. Know the job responsibilities of staff and what can and cannot be delegated
4. Set clear parameters around how much authority is needed to accomplish a task; delegate just enough authority to accomplish assigned task successfully
5. Be sure delegated task is completed as assigned
6. Delegation requires ongoing follow-up and evaluation; obtain feedback on assigned tasks upon completion
7. For delegation to occur, three elements must be present
   a. Delegator
   b. Delegatee
   c. Task or activity to be accomplished

NCLEX® **E. The delegation process to other LPN/LVNs and UAPs**

1. Determine and identify task and level of responsibility of each task
2. Evaluate delegatee's fit with assigned task
3. Decide what level of supervision is needed and describe expectations
4. Reach agreement on performance and outcome
5. Provide continuous feedback—monitor performance and adjust accordingly

F. Inappropriate delegation

NCLEX®
1. **Underdelegation**: delegator does not think that UAP can perform or complete an assignment or does not transfer full authority
2. **Reverse delegation:** team members request that LPN/LVN complete task because of inability or unwillingness to perform designated task or procedure

NCLEX®
3. **Overdelegation**: delegator becomes overwhelmed by situation and loses control by delegating inappropriate tasks; tasks that are beyond their scope of practice should not be delegated to UAPs

NCLEX® **G. Five rights of delegation**

1. NCSBN (1995) outlines five rights of delegation (see Box 5–4, The Essential Rights of Delegation)
2. Registered nurses (RNs) retain responsibility for caring for clients who require skilled assessment, whose status is changing or at risk for changing, and who require teaching
3. LPN/LVNs may be delegated care of clients who are medically stable, but have higher levels of acuity or require performance of skills beyond UAP training
4. LPNs/LVNs may collect data to report to RN but are not responsible for same level of client assessment that RN conducts
5. Routine nursing care and basic nursing procedures may be delegated to UAPs; nursing care activities that require ongoing assessment, interpretation, or clinical decision making that cannot be separated from the activity itself should not be delegated to a UAP

Box 5–3

Concepts to Consider before Delegating

1. Understand need to keep the client safe and protected from potential harm.
2. Ensure the delegated activity is routine and has a predictable outcome.
3. Ensure the client is medically stable or has a stable chronic condition.
4. Ensure that agency policies and procedures allow such delegation and that delegated activities are consistent with the delegatee's job description.

Box 5–4

The Essential Rights of Delegation

1. **Right Task:** Nurses determine those activities team members may perform. For each situation, nurse must consider client's condition, complexity of activity, UAP's capabilities, and amount of supervision nurse can provide.
2. **Right Circumstances:** Nurse evaluates individual clients and UAPs and matches the two. Nurse assesses client's needs, looks at care plan, considers the setting, and ensures that UAPs have proper resources, equipment, and supervision to work safely.
3. **Right Person:** Nurse follows organizational policies, which are congruent with state law, in determining appropriate staff to which to delegate a nursing activity.
4. **Right Direction and Communication:** Nurse needs to clearly understand organization's policies and procedures to carry out effective delegation. (Nurse needs to direct UAPs' actions and communicate clearly about each delegated task being specific about how and when UAPs should report back). Nurse should feel comfortable asking, *Do you know how to do this? Where did you learn? How many times have you done it in the past? Where is your experience documented?*
5. **Right Supervision and Evaluation:** Nurse managers ensure that each unit has adequate staffing and time, identify tasks inherent to each staff role, and evaluate impact of organization's nursing service on the community. Delegating nurse must supervise, guide, and evaluate UAPs' task implementation, ensure that UAPs meet expectations, and intervene if not performing well.

VI. INTERDISCIPLINARY CONSULTATION AND REFERRALS

A. *Interdisciplinary* describes situations in which various disciplines are involved in reaching a common goal, and each representative of a discipline brings own expertise to situation

NCLEX® **B. Interdisciplinary consultation requires**

1. Cooperation, integration, and modification of efforts by contributing disciplines
2. Acknowledgment by participants to take into account contributions of other teams members in making their own contribution
3. Understanding of intersecting lines of communication and collaboration that may emerge from these contributions

C. Interdisciplinary care team: works together with client/family in planning client care from each team member's discipline-specific perspective

1. Discipline-specific perspectives are shared through staff conferencing and consultation
2. Collaboration helps team members gain new insights for addressing problems
3. Collaboration promotes development of a holistic plan for client

D. Key components of interdisciplinary care team

1. Team members understand, appreciate, and collaborate with other disciplines and providers
2. Team members make decisions about services in collaboration with client and other discipline(s) rather than dividing care decisions by discipline or setting
3. Team members have a thorough understanding of their own profession

E. *Consultation* involves communication with another nurse or other health care professional (i.e., dietitian, pharmacist) about an aspect of client care

1. This type of communication is facilitated in agencies where employees enjoy collaborative work relationships with other health team members
2. Nursing units that use interdisciplinary rounds on clients have created an environment that fosters this type of communication

F. Referrals: often nurses are integral in assisting and coordinating client care that requires referrals

1. The term referral may include any of these definitions
   a. A formal process that authorizes an HMO member to get care from a specialist or hospital; most HMOs require clients to get a referral from their primary care provider (PCP) before seeing a specialist
   b. May be either an informal suggestion from one provider for client to see another provider
   c. The recommendation by a PCP and/or health plan for a member to receive care from a different provider or facility

d. A process in which a health care provider recommends that a client see a medical professional with advanced knowledge of a certain medical specialty or technique (such as heart disease or dermatology)
e. The process of sending a client from one practitioner to another for consultation, diagnostic intervention, and/or treatment; health plans may require a designated PCP to authorize a referral for specialty services to be reimbursed

2. In managed care, a health plan member must first contact PCP to obtain medical services unless it is an emergency; together, the member and PCP decide if member needs to see a specialist or obtain special services; this is also called *preauthorization*

VII. LEADERSHIP

A. Overview of leadership

1. Contemporary nursing **leadership** is about engaging people, building relationships, and influencing change; it is not only about formal titles, job duties, and functions
2. The terms leader, administrator, supervisor, and **manager** are sometimes used interchangeably; they are different but complementary
3. NCLEX® A **leader** is a person who possesses personal traits that enable her or him to personally move others constructively and ethically to positively impact client/family care or to achieve a goal or vision
4. Leadership is a(n)
   a. Exercise of power, influence, and responsibility
   b. Attempt to change the behavior of another
   c. Art of getting others to want to do what one deems important
   d. Ability to cope with change and be flexible in varied situations
   e. Ability to mentor others toward higher levels

B. To be a leader, one must earn respect and trust of another

1. Without respect and trust of others, leader will have no followers
2. Effective leaders understand various types of followers
   a. Effective follower
   b. Alienated follower
   c. Yes follower
   d. Shy follower
   e. Passive-aggressive follower
   f. Independent follower
3. For followers to grow and flourish, nurse leader must provide
   a. Personal attention: support and guidance in foreseeing problems and challenges
   b. Role modeling: encouragement of self-management, assessment, openness, and forthrightness
   c. Precepting: to assist, approach, and coach in a timely and appropriate manner
   d. Mentoring: to invest by sharing expertise and experience with others

C. Formal versus informal leadership

1. NCLEX® **Formal leadership** is bestowed by employing organization and described in a job description; it provides for influence through
   a. Legitimate authority
   b. Power of position
   c. Ability to reward and punish
2. NCLEX® **Informal leadership** does not provide an official organizational title but informal leader can substantially influence others through thoughtful and convincing ideas, knowledge, status, and personal skills

D. Attributes of effective leaders

1. Consider their position a responsibility rather than a rank or privilege (see Box 5–5, Effective Leadership)
2. Desire strong associates and encourage them, push them, and glory in their success
3. Articulate organization's vision in a manner that stresses values of followers
4. Involve followers in deciding how to achieve organization's vision
5. Support followers' efforts to realize vision by providing coaching, feedback, and role modeling and by recognizing and rewarding success

E. A nurse leader's first objective is to assist and support professional clinical practice environment for nurses by

1. Putting clients first
2. Focusing on client safety
3. Enhancing care quality
4. Improving client care outcomes

Box 5-5

Effective Leadership

Is a responsibility rather than rank and privilege.

Is knowing that when things go wrong, and often they do, leaders do not blame others.

Is acknowledging that leaders are ultimately responsible for their words and actions.

Is having strong and competent associates whom the leader encourages, coaches, and provides with ongoing evaluation and feedback.

F. Theories of leadership and management

1. Behavioral theories (introduced in early 1930s)
   - **a.** Focused on the abilities and behaviors of leaders, including what leaders do
   - **b.** Personal traits provide only a portion of leader capacity
   - **c.** Leadership evolves through education, training, and life experiences
   - **d.** **Autocratic leadership**: based on belief that individuals are motivated by power, authority, and need for approval; an autocratic leader makes all decisions, uses coercion and punishment, and is uncollegial
   - **e.** **Democratic leadership**: based on belief that individuals are motivated by internal drives and impulses, desire active participation in decisions, and desire to get tasks done; democratic leadership promotes participation and majority rule for goal setting
   - **f.** **Laissez-faire leadership**: based on belief that individuals are motivated by internal drives and impulses; need to be left alone to make decisions about how to complete work; leader provides no direction or facilitation
   - **g.** **Bureaucratic leadership**: based on belief that individuals are motivated by external forces; leader trusts either followers or self to make decisions; relies on organizational policies and rules to identify goals and direct work flow
   - **h.** Behavioral theory involves initiating structured behaviors that managers use to organize and define work goals, work patterns and methods, channels of communication, and roles
   - **i.** Behavioral theory includes consideration of behaviors that show mutual trust, respect, friendship, warmth, and rapport between leader and followers
2. Situational leadership theory considers follower's readiness and willingness to perform a designated task; leadership styles can be categorized according to readiness and ability of follower to perform task
   - **a.** Telling style (S1—high task, low relationship) is used for followers who are unable and unwilling to perform, or insecure about performing assigned task
   - **b.** Selling style (S2—high task, high relationship) is used for followers who are unable but willing to perform, or confident in performing task
   - **c.** Participating style (S3—low task, high relationship) is used for followers who are both able and willing to perform, and have confidence in performing task
3. Quantum leadership theory: a contemporary theory in which leader is viewed as an influential facilitator and followers assume an active role in decision making
   - **a.** Leadership is a shared activity
   - **b.** Information is freely disseminated to followers and clients
   - **c.** Leaders are expected to be expert communicators and possess strong interpersonal skills
   - **d.** Followers are equitable and accountable partners in client care outcomes
   - **e.** Quantum leadership evolves from concepts of chaos theory; reality is constantly shifting; levels of complexity are constantly changing; movement reverberates throughout system; roles are fluid and outcome oriented
4. Charismatic leadership
   - **a.** Leaders possess powerful personal qualities, such as charm, persuasiveness, personal power, self-confidence, extraordinary ideas, and strong convictions
   - **b.** Leader's personality arouses affection and emotional commitment, and drives and advances vision, mission, and goals
5. **Transactional leadership**
   - **a.** Built on principles of social exchange, in which individuals expect to give and receive rewards
   - **b.** Exchange process between leaders and followers is economic, where workers perform according to policy and procedures to maximize self-interests and rewards
   - **c.** Leaders are most successful when they understand and meet followers' needs

d. Exchange between leader and follower continues until exchange of performance and reward is no longer valuable
e. Uses incentives to enhance follower loyalty and performance
f. Is aimed at maintaining equilibrium or status quo
g. Fosters interpersonal dependence

6. **Transformational leadership**
a. Emphasizes interpersonal relationships and inspires followers
b. Not concerned with the status quo
c. Focuses on merging motives and values
d. Generates followers' commitment to leader's vision
e. Fosters followers' inborn desires to pursue higher values and ideals
f. Encourages followers to exercise leadership
g. Uses power to instill a belief that followers can accomplish exceptional things

7. Shared leadership
a. Founded on principles of empowerment, participation, and transformational leadership
b. No one person or leader possesses all knowledge and ability
c. Elements of shared leadership include relationships, dialogs, partnerships, and understanding boundaries
d. Different issues call for different responses
e. Shared leadership allows for appropriate leadership to emerge in relation to current problems and issues as they arise

8. **Servant leadership**
a. Focuses on desire to serve others and is based upon principles of caring
b. In the desire to serve, one can be called upon to lead—hence the name *servant leadership*
c. A servant leader seeks to address others' needs as priority
d. Nurse leaders provide care and compassionate service to others

VIII. MANAGEMENT CONCEPTS AND SKILLS

NCLEX® **A. Management process**

1. A manager is an individual employed by organization who is responsible and accountable for efficiently accomplishing organizational goals
2. Responsibilities include
a. Effectively accomplishing goals of organization
b. Coordinating tasks and integrating resources
c. Using functions of planning, organizing, supervising, staffing, evaluating, and negotiating
d. Clarifying organizational structure
e. Evaluating client care outcomes and providing feedback
f. Coping with complexity

B. Functions of management process: planning, organizing, leading, and controlling

1. Planning and setting a direction
a. Sets goals and decides course of action through an inductive process
b. Gathers data and looks for patterns
c. Builds relationships and links to help explain issues, goals, expectations, and so on
d. Creates visions and strategies for organization's future
2. Organizing and aligning people
a. Identifies work to be accomplished and goals to be achieved
b. Hires right person for right work
c. Creates interdependence by getting people to move in same direction
d. Delegates authority by talking to those who can help implement the vision and those who can block implementation
e. Coordinates work of others
3. Leading and getting others to believe the message
a. Influences others to get job done
b. Keeps message clear
c. Communicates with integrity and trustworthiness
d. Molds the culture and maintains morale
e. Insists on consistency between words and deeds

4. Controlling
    a. Sets standards for accomplishing organization's goals and activities
    b. Determines means to measure performance and makes sure that quality lapses are spotted immediately
    c. Evaluates performance and provides feedback

IX. PERFORMANCE IMPROVEMENT AND QUALITY ASSURANCE

A. History of quality assurance (QA)

1. Emerged in health care in the 1950s as an inspection approach to ensure minimum standards in health care institutions
2. Emphasized "doing the right thing" and was not proactive in preventing problems before they occurred
3. Focused on clinical aspects of a provider's care, often in response to an identified problem

B. Total quality management (TQM)

1. Began in the 1950s also and incorporates principles of QA, but focuses on customer satisfaction rather than on "doing it right"
2. Integrated into health care delivery in the 1980s

NCLEX® **C. Definition of quality**

1. Meeting or exceeding expectations of customers
2. Meeting and exceeding standards
3. Achieving planned outcomes

NCLEX® **D. Quality management principles**

1. TQM
    a. Customer/client focus: recognizing customers and their needs
    b. Total organizational involvement: all employees are involved in the process
    c. Use of quality tools and statistics for measurement: decisions are supported by data
    d. Identification of key processes that support continuous quality improvement (CQI)
2. See Box 5–6, Ways to Enhance Quality Nursing Care

NCLEX® **E. Components of quality management**

1. Comprehensive quality management plan
2. Structure, process, and outcome benchmarks
3. Performance appraisals

Box 5–6

Ways to Enhance Quality Nursing Care

1. **Seek to provide nursing care with the outcome of a continuous healing relationship.** Nursing care is responsive at all times (24 hours a day, every day), and access to nursing care should be provided over the Internet, by telephone, and by other means in addition to face-to-face visits.
2. **Provide nursing care based on client needs and values.** Nursing care should be designed to meet the most common types of needs as well as to respond to individual client choices and preferences.
3. **Remember that the client is the source of information.** Clients are given the necessary information and the opportunity to exercise the degree of control they choose over health care decisions that affect them.
4. **Nursing care requires shared knowledge and the free flow of information.** Clients have access to their own nursing and medical information and to clinical knowledge. The health team communicates effectively and shares information with clients and their families.
5. **Nurses use evidence-based decision making.** Clients receive care based on the best available scientific knowledge.
6. **Safety is a key feature in all aspects of nursing care.** Clients are kept safe and are protected from injury caused by the care system. Reducing risk and ensuring safety requires all team members to pay greater attention to systems that help prevent errors.
7. **Nurses anticipate client needs.** Nursing staff anticipate client needs rather than simply react to events.
8. **Nurses understand the essential need to cooperate with other clinicians.** Nurses and other clinicians actively collaborate and communicate to ensure an appropriate exchange of information and coordination of care.

4. Intradisciplinary assessment and improvement
5. Interdisciplinary assessment and improvement

F. Methods of quality management in health care

1. Nursing audits
2. Peer review
3. Utilization review
4. Outcomes management

NCLEX®

G. Measuring outcomes

1. **Indicators** are a measurement or flag used as a guide to monitor, assess, and improve the quality of client care, support services, and organizational functions affecting client outcomes
2. Nurse-sensitive indicators are measurements of client care that are sensitive to nursing interventions, such as
   - a. Maintenance of skin integrity
   - b. Pressure ulcer prevalence rate
   - c. Fall injury rate
   - d. Medication incident rate
   - e. Restraint utilization rate
   - f. Client satisfaction for pain management
   - g. Client satisfaction with overall nursing care
   - h. Nurse satisfaction
   - i. Failure to rescue

H. Types of indicators

NCLEX®

1. Structure indicator: describes characteristics of a setting that support and have an impact on care (e.g., availability of approved least restraint devices on a unit, RN-to-client ratio)

NCLEX®

2. Process indicator
   - a. Measures an activity that is carried out in caring for clients
   - b. Focuses on nature and amount of nursing care provided during hospital stay (e.g., rate of clients placed on fall prevention program)

NCLEX®

3. Outcome indicator
   - a. Describes client's status at a defined time following care interventions
   - b. Measures result of nursing care and process (examples: pressure ulcer prevalence rate, fall injury rate)
   - c. Nursing outcomes are key indicators to show impact of nursing care on positive client outcomes; indicators that most reflect the effect of nursing care are staff mix, total nursing care hours provided per client day, pressure ulcers, client falls, client satisfaction, nosocomial infections, and nurse satisfaction

I. Six Sigma

1. A quality management program that uses mostly quantitative data to monitor progress
2. Has specific themes of customer (client) focus: data driven, process emphasis, proactive management, boundary-less collaboration, aim for perfection while tolerating failure
3. Unique features: greater management involvement in process, more connection between departments, and tolerance for failure as a necessary condition for creativity

Check Your NCLEX–PN® Exam I.Q.

You are ready for testing on this content if you can

- Describe the various health care settings.
- Monitor time management priorities.
- Request interdisciplinary consultation and referrals.
- Provide effective leadership and management to nursing care personnel.
- Demonstrate effective leadership strategies.
- Describe the management process.
- Effectively delegate nursing activities.
- Incorporate performance improvement into clinical nursing practice.

PRACTICE TEST

1 A nurse who has been in practice for 6 months is due for the first performance evaluation. In preparation, the nurse should evaluate personal performance during the first 6 months of employment against which standard?

1. ANA standards of care
2. State nurse practice act
3. Written job description
4. Organization's standard of clinical care

2 The charge nurse on the night shift reports that the narcotic count is incorrect. The nurse has spoken to the responsible staff nurse and believes that substance abuse by the nurse is the cause. If substance abuse proves to be the cause of the incorrect count, what is the most appropriate next step?

1. Recount the narcotics with the staff nurse and take disciplinary action.
2. Ask the staff nurse to leave the unit and report the incident to the American Nurses Association.
3. Complete an incident report and report findings to the pharmacy and nursing administration.
4. Submit the findings to the Council on Nursing Practice.

3 The nurse on the skilled nursing facility quality improvement team has been asked to evaluate nursing care on the nurse's assigned unit. After deciding to ask other nursing staff for assistance in this effort, what would be most appropriate for the nurse to initially ask staff to do?

1. Track the number of supplies used by clients on the unit.
2. Document the time spent on direct client care.
3. Administer a client and family satisfaction survey.
4. Monitor clients and report acuity daily.

4 A nurse is about to make first rounds after receiving an intershift report at 3 p.m. In what order should the nurse see the following clients? Place the options in order. All options must be used.

1. A 54-year-old client 4 hours post–cardiac catheterization who has mild discomfort at the access site
2. A client newly diagnosed with diabetes mellitus who needs reinforcement of sick day management guidelines
3. A client who arrived 30 minutes ago from the postanesthesia care unit
4. A client who is ready for discharge but will not have transportation home available until 5 p.m.
5. A client with pneumonia who has received two doses of IV antibiotics and has an oxygen saturation of 93%

5 An LPN/LVN in a skilled nursing facility is delegating care of clients to the certified nursing assistant (CNA) and another licensed practical nurse (LPN). Which tasks should the delegating LPN/LVN give the CNA and LPN?

1. CNA: Measure vital signs; LPN/LVN: Give oral medications on assigned clients
2. CNA: Change a dressing on an infected wound; LPN/LVN: Administer subcutaneous medications
3. CNA: Ambulate a client who had a stroke; LPN/LVN: Administer a newly ordered IV piggyback medication
4. CNA: Measure vital signs; LPN/LVN: Complete a head-to-toe assessment on a newly admitted client

6 An LPN/LVN is working with three clients. One client is receiving IV push morphine for left shoulder pain rated as 7 on a scale of 0–10; a second has an oral order of digoxin (Lanoxin) and furosemide (Lasix) for heart failure (HF); the third is stable and has vitamins ordered to improve wound healing. What task should the LPN/LVN request be completed by the registered nurse (RN)?

1. The administration of IVP morphine for the client with pain
2. The administration of oral meds for the client with HF
3. The administration of vitamins for the stable client with wounds
4. The LPN/LVN should administer medications for all clients.

7 A nurse is caring for a group of clients. One client is scheduled to go to the operating room (OR) in one hour. The second client needs information on nursing homes, and the third client needs to provide a urine specimen. The nurse has not documented on any clients. What should the nurse do first?

1. Obtain the urine specimen.
2. Provide the client with nursing home information.
3. Document care provided for all clients.
4. Prepare the client for the operating room.

PRACTICE TEST

8 A nurse is caring for a group of clients. Which client takes priority?

1. A 67-year-old client with a history of congestive heart failure (CHF)
2. A 20-year-old client with sickle-cell anemia and a low hemoglobin level
3. A 50-year-old client with pneumonia and oxygen saturation 95% with oxygen at 2 L/min
4. An 80-year-old client with dehydration and a BP of 92/60 mm Hg

9 A staff nurse is receiving report on assigned clients. The client in bed 1 has congestive heart failure (CHF); the client in bed 2 has multiple pressure ulcers; the client in bed 3 has a chest tube to treat a pleural effusion; and the client in bed 4 has pneumonia. The nurse decides to collect data on the client in bed 3 with a pleural effusion and chest tube. What framework for determining priorities of care is this nurse using?

1. ABCs: airway, breathing, circulation
2. Priorities in medication therapy
3. Client and family preferences
4. Time management and organization

10 After receiving intershift report, in what order would the nurse see assigned clients?

1. Client with chronic pain requesting pain meds
2. Client with diarrhea who needs to be cleaned
3. Client who is due for a dressing change
4. Client who requires suctioning

ANSWERS & RATIONALES

1 **Answer: 3 Rationale:** The best way that the nurse can effectively self-evaluate job performance is to compare individual performance against the written job description. Job descriptions identify responsibilities of the position and activities that the staff member may perform. The ANA standards of care can be used as universal guidelines for practice in any setting, but they are not specific to one agency or job description. The state nurse practice act is a set of general standards that assist nurses in knowing what tasks are within the scope practice within that jurisdiction; they are not specific to one setting. Standards of clinical care would form the foundation for part of the nurse's evaluation, but not the entire professional role. **Cognitive Level:** Analyzing **Client Need:** Coordinated Care **Integrated Process:** Nursing Process: Evaluation **Content Area:** Leadership and Management **Strategy:** The core issue of the question is knowledge of appropriate reference points when preparing for employee evaluations. Use knowledge that the job description provides specific direction for practice in an institution to make a selection.

2 **Answer: 3 Rationale:** An incident report must be completed because of the inaccurate narcotic count. Narcotics are controlled substances and fall under federal law and regulation. Both the pharmacy and nursing administration must be notified. It is unnecessary to recount the narcotics, although agency policy for discipline needs to be undertaken. The American Nurses Association, through the Code of Ethics for Nurses, provides guidance to nurses and protection for clients and their families but does not have the authority to discipline nurses. This finding must be reported to the state board of nursing by nursing administration. Individual state boards of nursing identify the legal boundaries of nursing practice, including disciplinary action, through nurse practice acts (which differ among the states). **Cognitive Level:** Applying **Client Need:** Coordinated Care **Integrated Process:** Nursing Process: Planning **Content Area:** Leadership and Management **Strategy:** Agency policies and procedures and state nurse practice acts dictate the course of action for drug diversion by nurses. Recall that nursing administration would communicate with outside agencies to aid in eliminating incorrect options.

3 **Answer: 3 Rationale:** Client satisfaction surveys are an important tool to monitor and evaluate client and family needs. This information helps health care organizations meet those needs. Tracking supplies provides information that can be used in preparing a budget. Documenting time spent on direct client care provide information useful in planning a budget or unit staffing requirements. Information on client acuity is useful in planning for unit staffing requirements. **Cognitive Level:** Applying **Client Need:** Coordinated Care **Integrated Process:** Nursing Process: Planning **Content Area:** Leadership and Management **Strategy:** The core issue of the question is quality management. The purpose of quality management is to improve performance and meet client needs. Consider that the best way to assess client satisfaction with care is to ask the client directly.

4 **Answer: 3, 5, 1, 4, 2 Rationale:** Priority setting can be implemented using a variety of models. The client who is post operative should be seen first because the client is newly arrived on the unit and is at greatest risk of becoming unstable or experiencing a change in clinical condition. The client with pneumonia should be seen second because the infection involves the airway, although oxygen saturation levels are higher than the critical value of 90% or less.

The client who is 4 hours post–cardiac catheterization should be seen third to evaluate the site and conduct general assessment of the affected extremity, once the clients who are potentially unstable or having airway/breathing problems are attended to. The client who will be discharged should be seen fourth because this client is stable but there is a need to determine that there are no last-minute needs or issues. The client who needs teaching should be seen fifth because this is not a physiological need and this activity may be more time-intensive. **Cognitive Level:** Analyzing **Client Need:** Coordinated Care **Integrated Process:** Nursing Process: Planning **Content Area:** Leadership and Management **Strategy:** Determine which client is at greatest risk of becoming unstable to choose the postanesthesia client, followed by assessing the client whose airway is potentially at risk. The client who had cardiac catheterization could become unstable but has been on the unit for 4 hours, so this client can be seen third. The client scheduled for discharge should be checked fourth, because it will not take long to complete the discharge procedure and address any remaining issues or concerns. The client needing reinforcement of teaching will need the most time and can be planned for last.

5 **Answer: 1** **Rationale:** The scope of practice and most job descriptions for CNAs include vital signs. It is within the scope of practice for the LPN/LVN to administer oral medications. In some facilities, CNAs are allowed to change simple dressings, but they should not change dressings on infected wounds. The scope of practice for LPN/LVNs allows them to administer subcutaneous medications. CNAs are allowed to ambulate clients; however, LPN/LVNs may not be allowed to administer IV medications.. CNAs are able to measure vital signs but LPNs do not complete admissions assessments; an RN would be called to the unit for this activity. **Cognitive Level:** Applying **Client Need:** Coordinated Care **Integrated Process:** Nursing Process: Planning **Content Area:** Leadership and Management **Strategy:** Use knowledge of delegation and scope of practice to select the correct answer.

6 **Answer: 1** **Rationale:** The administration of IVP morphine for the client with pain is within the scope of practice for the registered nurse, but not in the scope of practice for the LPN/LVN. Administration of oral medications for the client with HF is within the scope of an LPN/LVN, although this client will also need assessment by the RN due to the pathophysiology of HF. The administration of vitamins is within the scope of practice for the LPN/LVN. The LPN/LVN will not be able to administer IV medications. **Cognitive Level:** Applying **Client Need:** Coordinated Care **Integrated Process:** Nursing Process: Planning **Content Area:** Leadership and Management **Strategy:** Use knowledge of delegation and the process of elimination to select the correct answer.

7 **Answer: 4** **Rationale:** The nurse should consider urgent or time-bound issues such as surgeries first. The client who is scheduled for surgery needs special preparation prior to the surgery. This is a priority that takes precedence over the urine specimen, documentation, and client education. Routine activities such as obtaining a urine specimen have lower priority than urgent or emergent problems. Routine activities such as client education have lower priority than urgent or emergent problems. Routine activities such as documentation have lower priority than urgent or emergent problems. **Cognitive Level:** Applying **Client Need:** Coordinated Care **Integrated Process:** Nursing Process: Implementation **Content Area:** Leadership and Management **Strategy:** Use nursing knowledge and strategies for prioritization to make the correct selection.

8 **Answer: 4** **Rationale:** The older adult client with dehydration and a low BP is in physiological distress and could go into multiple-organ failure due to fluid loss. The major organs might not receive adequate perfusion. This client is a priority over the other clients. The client who has a history of CHF is not represented as being actively in CHF. Most clients with sickle cell anemia have low hemoglobin levels and the question does not specify lab values. Based on the information provided, the middle-aged client with pneumonia is not in distress. **Cognitive Level:** Analyzing **Client Need:** Coordinated Care **Integrated Process:** Nursing Process: Implementation **Content Area:** Leadership and Management **Strategy:** Use the ABCs (airway, breathing, and circulation) of priority of care and the process of elimination to make the correct selection.

9 **Answer: 1** **Rationale:** The nurse is using the ABCs of priority to plan care for the day. The client with a pleural effusion is not able to fully expand the affected lung and has a compromised respiratory system, making this client a priority. Priorities in medication therapy are not being set in this scenario. Priorities in client and family preferences are not being set in this scenario. Time management is not being used, as the nurse is organizing the priorities by using the ABCs of care. **Cognitive Level:** Applying **Client Need:** Coordinated Care **Integrated Process:** Nursing Process: Implementation **Content Area:** Leadership and Management **Strategy:** Use the ABCs (airway, breathing, and circulation) of prioritization and nursing knowledge to make the correct choice.

10 **Answer: 2, 3, 4, 1** **Rationale:** The client who requires suctioning has an issue with the airway, which is a priority in care. The client in pain would require attention second after the client who has a problem with airway because pain is considered the fifth vital sign and pain has physiological consequences for the client. The client with diarrhea and need for skin care third because there is a potential risk for skin breakdown (however, this also could be delegated to another caregiver for faster attention if this was an option). The client who is due for the dressing change would be last because this is a routine care activity and does not indicate an acute need by the client. **Cognitive Level:** Analyzing **Client Need:** Coordinated Care **Integrated Process:** Nursing Process: Data Collection **Content Area:** Leadership and Management **Strategy:** Think ABCs and the basis for life. Which one of the options could be potentially life-threatening if not addressed first?

Key Terms to Review

autocratic leadership p. 35
bureaucratic leadership p. 35
capitation p. 28
consultation p. 33
delegation p. 31
democratic leadership p. 35
formal leadership p. 34
health maintenance organization (HMO) p. 28
indicators p. 38
informal leadership p. 34
interdisciplinary p. 33
laissez-faire leadership p. 35
leader p. 34
leadership p. 34
managed care p. 28
manager p. 34
overdelegation p. 32
reverse delegation p. 32
servant leadership p. 36
shared governance p. 29
supervising p. 31
supervisor p. 31
time management p. 29
transactional leadership p. 35
transformational leadership p. 36
underdelegation p. 32

References

American Nurses Association. (2001). *Code of ethics.* Washington, DC: Author.

Berman, A., Snyder, S., & McKinney, D. (2011). *Nursing basics for clinical practice.* Upper Saddle River, NJ: Pearson Education, Inc.

Blais, K. K., & Hayes, J. S. (2011). *Professional nursing practice: Concepts and Perspectives* (6th ed.). Upper Saddle River: NJ: Pearson Education, Inc.

Delegation of UAP Issues: Delegation Documents. Council of State Boards on Nursing. Retrieved December 29, 2005, from http://www.ncsbn.org/public/regulation/delegation_documents.htm

Grohar-Murray, M. E., DiCroce, H. R., & Langan, J. (2011). *Leadership and management in nursing* (4th ed.). Upper Saddle River, NJ: Pearson Education, Inc.

Hansten, R. I., & Jackson, M. (2009). *Clinical delegation skills: A handbook for professional practice* (4th ed.). Sudbury, MA: Jones & Bartlett.

Institute of Medicine. 2001. *Crossing the quality chasm: A new health system for the 21st century*. Washington, DC: National Academy Press.

Motacki, K., & Burke, K. (2010). *Nursing delegation and management of patient care*. St. Louis, MO: Elsevier.

National Council of State Boards of Nursing. *Delegation: Concepts and decision making process* (1995). Position Paper. Retrieved October 18, 2011, from https://www.ncsbn.org/323.htm

Sullivan, E. J. (2009). *Effective leadership and management in nursing* (7th ed). Upper Saddle River, NJ: Pearson Education, Inc.

Test Yourself

Are you ready for the NCLEX-PN® or course exams? Use the practice tests on the companion website to check.

Injury Prevention, Disaster Planning, and Protecting Client Safety

6

In this chapter

Cross Reference

Other chapters relevant to this content area are

Preventing and Controlling Infection — Chapter 7

I. ACCIDENT PREVENTION ACROSS THE LIFE SPAN

NCLEX®

A. Infant safety depends on actions of parents and infant caretakers; anticipatory guidance at well-baby check-ups is an opportunity for nurse to educate parents

1. Place infants on back after eating and while sleeping; this will not increase risk of aspiration and will reduce risk of sudden infant death syndrome (SIDS)
2. Rapid changes in development and acquisition of new motor skills put infants at increased risk for injury from falls from tables, beds, high chairs, infant seats, and so on
3. Place infants riding in a car in a rear-facing car restraint system in back seat; use a rear-facing restraint system until child is 1 year old and at least 20 pounds (current law)
4. Because of their inability to communicate, infants are at risk for burns from applications of heat to skin, such as from a hot water bottle or other heated device
5. Carefully select infant furniture paying special attention to current safety standards
   a. Infants may be trapped by crib slats spaced too far apart
   b. Infants or young children may be poisoned by lead paint on antique furniture (normal serum lead level is < 10 mg/dL; lead level 10–19 mg requires environmental history; higher levels require treatment to reduce or prevent neurological deficits)

NCLEX®

B. Toddlers are most frequently prone to accidents and injury due to increased physical mobility and intellectual curiosity

1. Store medications, cleaning supplies, and poisons in locked cabinets to prevent poisonings in a curious toddler; have poison control phone number readily available to caregiver and posted on telephone
2. Current law is to place car safety seats for toddlers in back seat and may be forward-facing after toddler has reached 1 year of age and 20 pounds; safety seats are used until child's shoulders are above the harness or ears have reached top of seat; when a child outgrows system, a booster seat with a lap/shoulder belt is required; latest American Academy of Pediatrics (AAP) recommendation is to keep toddler rear-facing until age 2 or reaching highest weight or height allowed by car seat manufacturer; thereafter, toddlers should use rear-facing car seat with a harness for as long as possible, up to highest weight/height allowed by manufacturer, followed by a booster seat

3. Toddlers explore all objects with their mouths; assess toys for small parts; avoid giving foods such as hard candy, peanuts, and chewing gum to prevent choking and aspiration
4. Burns in toddlers occur because of chewing on electrical wires, pulling hot liquids from tables or stove tops, and touching space heaters; keep electrical outlets covered and keep handles of pans on stove tops facing inward
5. Drowning is a leading cause of death in toddlers; accompany children at all times when in and around water in bathtub, wading pool, or swimming pool

NCLEX®

C. School-age children are at risk for injury at home and in community, as a school-age child spends increased time away from parent or caregiver

1. Teach and model pedestrian and bicycle safety to children at this age; bicycle helmets can prevent head injury to children biking, rollerblading, or skateboarding
2. Place children under 12 years or under 4 feet 9 inches in rear seat of a car with a belt-positioning booster seat until vehicle seat belt fits properly; then use lap and shoulder seat belts thereafter; keep all children younger than age 13 years in rear seat of vehicle; never allow children to ride in the bed of a pickup truck or open, unsecured area of an automobile, such as a station wagon or van
3. Teach school-age children principles of fire safety; injury can occur from experimentation with matches, lighters, and fireworks; school-age children can participate in implementing a school or home fire escape plan; teach to "stop, drop, and roll" if clothing catches fire
4. Teach school-age children principles of water safety; swimming lessons and life jackets are necessary for boating and swimming; children should never swim without adult supervision
5. Include in safety education for children to play in safe areas, avoid strangers, recognize unwelcome touch, and obey traffic signals

NCLEX®

D. Adolescent injury and death may be very violent in nature; newly found independence, feelings of invincibility and immortality, and access to motor vehicles can lead to accidents with injury

1. Encourage courses in driver's education; seat belt regulations should be role modeled and enforced by parents
2. Teach adolescents dangers of alcohol and substance use
3. Adolescents may be injured in sports-related accidents; encourage protective sporting gear for organized and impromptu sporting events
4. Review water safety principles because adolescents can overestimate endurance when swimming
5. Adolescents benefit from information about sexual health, including information about sexually transmitted infections and pregnancy prevention (birth control)

E. Adult safety concerns can be related to home, workplace, and leisure activities

1. Encourage working adults to participate in occupational health programs offered in workplace; musculoskeletal injury is most frequent workplace injury
2. Hazardous conditions and toxic substances may occur in workplace; educate employees in **OSHA** (Occupational Safety and Health Administration) regulations and guidelines for use of safety devices and handling hazardous substances
3. Alcohol consumption is involved in 40% of deaths from motor vehicle accidents, making it important to have community education programs about hazards of drinking and driving; other drugs that cause impairment pose similar risks
4. NCLEX® Firearms in the home may lead to accidental injury or death; encourage owners to attend firearm safety class and store all firearms and ammunition in a locked cabinet
5. Residents in some neighborhoods may be at risk for crime and injury; assess for access to police and fire services
6. NCLEX® Residential fires account for the majority of fire-related injuries; teach that homes should have smoke detectors, a fire extinguisher in the kitchen, and a fire evacuation plan

F. Older adults may experience a decrease in strength, vision, hearing, and cognitive ability that could lead to accidents or injury; evaluate homes for safety hazards

1. NCLEX® Falls are the leading cause of accidents in older adults
    a. Stairwells should be well lit
    b. Small scatter rugs, runners, and mats should not be used
    c. Bathrooms and showers/tubs should have grab bars
    d. Furniture, floors, and passageways should be free of clutter
2. Home modifications may be necessary to accommodate safe use of wheelchairs or walkers
3. Clients taking some medications may have decreased cognitive abilities or impaired judgment; encourage them to ask for assistance with activities of daily living
4. NCLEX® Neighbors, police, and fire officials should be made aware of older adults with disabilities living alone

5. Decrease in temperature regulation may increase risk of hyperthermia or hypothermia; be careful with use of space heaters; be sure older adults have fans or air conditioners in summer heat
6. Older adults may be prey to strangers and criminals who can inflict physical and financial injury; caution them against letting strangers into their homes or responding to telephone calls, e-mails, or letters asking for money or personal information
7. Motor vehicle accidents are of concern for older adults; frequent assessment of driving ability is required; loss of driving privileges can mean a loss of independence

II. ERROR PREVENTION IN HEALTH CARE SETTINGS

A. Medication errors are most frequent type of medical error in hospital setting; Institute of Medicine (IOM) has widely publicized the problem of hospital deaths caused by medication error

1. Types of untoward medication events
   a. Medication error involves wrong client, medication, dose, time, or route
   b. **Adverse reaction** is an undesired effect of a prescribed medication, whether a severe side effect or a toxicity
   c. **Toxic reaction** occurs when prescribed medication dosage is excessive or poisonous to an individual; this may be due to client's size, health condition, or other medications being taken
   d. Side effects are actions or effects of drugs other than that desired
   e. **Idiosyncratic reaction** is an unusual response to a drug that may be unrelated to dose; reaction may or may not reoccur if medication is given again
   f. Hypersensitivity or allergic reactions may range from mild rashes to life-threatening anaphylaxis; this reaction will reoccur and could get worse with each subsequent exposure

NCLEX®

2. Nursing interventions to prevent medication errors
   a. Know agency medication administration system; follow protocols
   b. Be familiar with medication resources at agency
   c. Ensure client information (e.g., height, weight, allergies) is accessible to health care providers, clinicians, and pharmacists
   d. Verify medication orders; do not transcribe orders that contain unapproved or nonstandard abbreviations until clarified
   e. Use standard hours and times for medication administration
   f. Be familiar with side effects or possible adverse reactions; observe for these on an ongoing basis
   g. Ask a nurse colleague to double-check complex dosage calculations
   h. Do not interrupt nurses giving medications, which can lead to errors during administration
   i. Check client identification bracelet before administering medication; ask client to verbalize name and date of birth (or other method of checking two unique identifiers) according to agency policy; additional measures are needed with blood administration
   j. Stop and double-check medication if client questions appearance or dose
   k. Report and document any error or variation in medication administration process

B. Allergies or an allergic response to an allergen can be life-threatening for a client

1. Include allergies in all health histories; ask about allergies to medications, food, tape, latex, or soap; document type and severity of reaction to allergen

NCLEX®

2. Allergies to seafood may alert nurse to a potential allergy to iodine-based dyes used in radiologic procedures
3. Document all allergies on medical records, lab records, pharmacy records, client identification bracelet, and bedside nameplate

III. INJURY PREVENTION IN HEALTH CARE SETTINGS

NCLEX®

A. Client safety can be at risk when admitted to a health care agency; assess risk factors for each client upon admission and identify methods to reduce possibility of injury

B. Risk for falls is most common in infants and elderly clients; implement a fall prevention program for those at risk

1. Assess ability to ambulate and transfer
2. Orient client to nurse call system and encourage use
3. Be sure nurse call system is within reach
4. Keep bedside table and chair near bed

NCLEX®

5. Keep hospital bed in low position
6. Do not use full-length bed side-rails for confused clients; do not leave confused client alone—evaluate need for constant companion
7. Keep crib side-rails up when child is unattended

8. Encourage use of nonskid footwear
9. Keep room tidy and free of clutter
10. NCLEX® Use a bed or chair monitoring device if necessary for clients at risk for falls

C. *Restraints* are devices used to limit client mobility

1. Restraints can be physical or chemical
2. Purposes of restraints
   a. Reduce risk of client injury from falls
   b. Prevent interruption of therapy such as traction or IV infusions
   c. Prevent a confused or agitated client from removing life support
   d. Reduce risk of injury to others by an agitated client
3. NCLEX® There are legal implications related to use of restraints because they limit client freedom
   a. A written order is needed to restrain a client
   b. Order must include reason for restraint and time period; PRN restraint orders are prohibited
   c. A nurse may apply physical restraints; however, health care provider must evaluate client within an agency-prescribed time period, which may be as soon as 1 hour; verify hospital policy and follow it
4. NCLEX® Assess and document condition of a restrained client hourly; remove restraints, assess skin, and allow or assist client to reposition per agency policy
5. Bed side-rails
   a. Are considered restraints
   b. NCLEX® Half or three-quarter rails may be better than full length rails for confused or agitated clients who may be injured climbing over rail; keep bed in lowest position
6. NCLEX® Jacket, belt, or extremity restraints
   a. Apply only as specified by manufacturer; never tie them to a movable part of a bed or chair
   b. Use a half-bow knot for easy release when attaching restraint to bed or chair
   c. Check for adequate circulation when using restraints; maintain two finger widths between client and restraint
7. Try creative nursing measures to prevent use of physical or chemical restraints
   a. Orient client to surroundings
   b. Encourage family, friends, or a sitter to stay with client
   c. Keep confused clients near nursing station
   d. Provide confused clients with diversionary activities
   e. Maintain frequent toileting routine
   f. Reposition or ambulate frequently if appropriate
   g. Evaluate client medications for undesirable effects
   h. Use relaxation techniques such as music, aroma therapy, and books on tape

D. Seizure precautions protect client in case of seizure activity; clients are at risk for injury if they experience seizures

1. Explain purpose of seizure precautions
2. Pad head and side-rails of bed with blankets and linens to prevent injury
3. NCLEX® Keep suction and oxygen equipment near bed; use oxygen mask after seizure activity has ceased
4. Do not attempt to insert anything into mouth of client during seizure (bitestick, airway)
5. Do not attempt to restrain or limit movement during a seizure; instead remove objects that could lead to client harm

E. Fire safety

1. Preventive measures for hospital or agency
   a. Staff needs to be aware of safety precautions and fire prevention practices
   b. Know categories of fire and correct type of extinguisher to use for each
   c. Participate in practice fire drills and evacuation procedures
2. NCLEX® Use the acronym RACE to recall what to do in an actual fire

Memory Aid

Use the mnemonic RACE to remember in order the four steps to maintain client safety during a fire.
Remove clients from danger.
Activate the fire alarm.
Contain the fire.
Evacuate the area (horizontal evacuation should be done before vertical evacuation if possible).

3. Preventive measures for home
   a. Focus on teaching emergency phone numbers, maintaining smoke alarms and fire extinguishers, importance of family fire drills, careful disposal of burning cigarettes and use of matches, grease fire prevention
   b. Teach precautions during an actual fire: close windows and doors to contain fire, cover nose and mouth with damp cloth when leaving a smoke-filled area, and stay as close as possible to ground

F. **Employee safety**
1. Is a responsibility of each employee
2. Occupational Safety and Health Administration (OSHA), a federal agency, regulates workplaces to protect health of employees
3. **Bloodborne pathogen** exposure is a health hazard for many employees in a health care setting; OSHA has issued written standards that include recommendations from the Centers for Disease Control and Prevention (**CDC**) regarding standard precautions (see also Chapter 7 on preventing and controlling infections)
   a. Standard precautions are techniques used with all clients to decrease risk of exposure to pathogens
   b. Gloves and face and eye protection will help protect health care workers from bloodborne pathogens
   c. Nurses may be required to have a vaccine for hepatitis B or influenza, or sign a declination refusing vaccines
4. Needlestick precautions, when properly used, protect health care workers
   NCLEX® a. Do not recap needles and do not bend or break needles before disposal
   NCLEX® b. Ensure that sharps containers are in each client room and medication area
   c. Needle-free technology should be provided by employers
   d. Each health agency must have a needle/sharps injury protocol in case of injury; report all injuries and follow protocol for self-protection
   e. Many institutions now use needleless devices or syringes with needles that retract after use to prevent exposure
5. Environmental infection control can protect employees and clients from exposure to pathogens; CDC sets infection control standards for health care agencies
   a. Employees may be annually tested for tuberculosis
   b. Laundry and medical waste are regulated by environmental infection control guidelines: laundry and items soiled with blood or body fluids must be identified by biohazard markers such as red bags

NCLEX® 6. Latex allergy is an actual or potential hazard for health care workers and clients
   a. Latex rubber is used in many medical products but most frequently in gloves used in health care settings
   b. Always ask clients about latex allergies; be sure latex-free gloves are available
   c. Provide a latex-free cart that includes latex-free tourniquets, IV tubing and IV supplies, and other items for clients with a latex allergy

NCLEX® 7. Hazardous chemicals pose a safety threat in many areas of a health care setting
   a. Material Safety Data Sheets (**MSDS**) are OSHA-required informational handouts that describe any and all chemical agents in an employment setting
   b. Employees are required to be trained in use of MSDS
   c. All chemicals must be properly labeled and have a corresponding MSDS
   d. Read and be aware of all information related to chemicals before handling or cleaning spills; a few examples of chemicals in health care settings are antineoplastic (chemotherapy) drugs, cleaning supplies, and pesticides
   NCLEX® e. In case of a chemotherapy drug spill, restrict access to area of spill and contact environmental services or other department per protocol; if nurse must clean spill, refer to MSDS protocol on unit (see Box 6–1)

IV. INCIDENT REPORTS

A. Overview
1. Is an agency record of an accident or other event in the health care agency that is not consistent with hospital policy; may also be called unusual occurrence report or variance report
2. Agencies have specific forms to report these events, such as accidents, falls, needle sticks, client infections, medication errors, or missing personal property
3. For the protection of client and nurse, it is vital to report all incidents

Box 6–1

Procedure for Chemotherapy Drug Spill

1. Restrict access to area of the spill.
2. Obtain a chemotherapy spill kit (gloves, gown, goggles, detergent, sponges, labeled container for disposal).
3. Use absorbent sponges to absorb spill.
4. Clean surface with designated cleanser.
5. Dispose of all supplies in approved container.
6. Wash hands.
7. Cleanse all skin exposed to chemotherapy agent—both client and staff.
8. Document the occurrence.

NCLEX®

B. Procedure for incident reporting

1. Prevent further injury and provide care for client, visitor, or employee
2. Notify health care provider immediately and take orders for interventions that may limit further harm
3. File report as soon as possible; person filing report may or may not be the person responsible for or involved in incident
4. Identify client, visitor, employee, and all witnesses to event
5. State objective facts of incident; do not draw conclusions or lay blame
6. Be specific—list name of medication or equipment involved
7. Document facts of incident in client's record also; do not document in client record that an incident report was filed
8. The policy for incident reporting is unique to each health care agency; review and follow specific agency policy for incident reporting

V. DISASTER PLANNING AND EMERGENCY RESPONSE

A. Disasters and emergencies are traumatic events that can affect an individual, family, community, or nation; nurses and health care providers are instrumental in disaster preparedness, disaster response, and client care in community and hospital settings

1. Disasters may be natural or man-made; disasters vary by predictability, frequency, preventability, imminence, and destructive potential
2. Natural disasters such as hurricanes and floods generally allow time for planning and evacuation; disasters such as earthquakes and tornadoes do not but are predictable in certain areas of the country; residents and health care providers should be encouraged to prepare
3. Man-made disasters are usually less predictable; explosions, fires, airline accidents, radiation emergencies, bioterrorism, and toxic chemical releases occur randomly; however, plans can be made by health care providers and emergency response personnel to have trained resources to take action
4. The Federal Emergency Management Agency (FEMA) is a government agency that has a National Response Plan; it provides states and local communities guidelines for reporting threats and incidents and for assessment, response, and recovery during disasters; nurses are part of disaster planning and response at federal, state, and local levels
5. Purpose of disaster planning is to decrease community vulnerability and to assure available resources if a disaster occurs

B. Planning for any type of disaster must start with individuals and families; one community health nurse role is to educate and guide citizens in preparedness

1. Families must have a communication plan; emergency phone numbers should be carried by all family members; establish a place to meet in an emergency
2. Be prepared to shut off all utilities in home; water may be precious after a disaster; electricity and natural gas may pose a safety threat
3. A package of vital records should be readily available when evacuating a home; identification, health and immunization records, insurance policies, deeds, and cash or traveler checks would be needed during and after an evacuation

NCLEX®

4. Identify special family needs; make an emergency kit; have extra medications and food items for dietary requirements; have extra batteries for medical devices
5. Make plans for homebound pets; pets are not usually allowed in shelters; leave food and water; attach proper pet identification
6. Encourage family members to learn CPR and first aid

C. *The Joint Commission* (formerly known as JCAHO) requires hospitals to have a disaster plan and to periodically practice response to plan

1. Plan should include policy and procedures for administration, nursing and patient service, medical staff, security, medical records, engineering, laboratory, and radiology, as well as the following:
   - **a.** Notification and communication of disaster
   - **b.** Assessment of hospital resources
   - **c.** Personnel recall system/transportation plan
   - **d.** Establishment of a facility command center
   - **e.** Maintenance of accurate records
   - **f.** Communication and public relations
   - **g.** Equipment and resupply
2. Nurses are responsible for knowing their role in disaster response and are part of committees that design and evaluate hospital plan; nursing tasks during a disaster may include the following:
   - **a.** Assess nursing unit for resources—staff, beds, and equipment
   - *NCLEX®* **b.** Assess current clients for discharge in case of increased need of hospital/nursing services by high acuity/injured clients
   - **c.** Activate staff recall plan
   - **d.** Communicate with hospital disaster control center
   - *NCLEX®* **e.** Assess disaster victims for extent of injury; this is called **triage**
   - **f.** Render first aid
   - **g.** Provide treatment based on protocols

D. Triage

1. Triage is a French word meaning "to sort"; in case of emergency, nurses may be asked to triage injured or ill clients to identify those in need of emergent, urgent, or nonurgent care; LPN/LVNs may be asked to assist the RN with triage
2. Primary survey focuses on airway, breathing, circulation, and neurological disability/deficits (ABCD)
   - **a.** Clear and open the airway
   - **b.** Assess for respiratory distress
   - **c.** Assess quality of ventilation (rate, color, auscultate lungs)
   - **d.** Check pulses for quality and rate
   - **e.** Assess for external bleeding
   - **f.** Take blood pressure
   - **g.** Assess level of consciousness and pupillary response, weakness or paralysis of extremities

Memory Aid

Remember ABCD to recall the components of the primary survey for a victim of trauma: Airway, Breathing, Circulation, Disability (deficits)

3. The secondary survey is initiated after initiating lifesaving interventions
   - **a.** Measure and record a full set of vital signs
   - **b.** Remove all of client's clothing
   - **c.** Do a complete health history and physical examination
   - **d.** Identify family members
   - **e.** Administer comfort measures or pain medication if appropriate

Check Your NCLEX-PN® Exam I.Q.

You are ready for testing on this content if you can

- Identify client developmental and environmental factors that may lead to accidents or injury.
- Provide care and teaching to the client at risk for accident or injury.
- Protect the client who is at risk for injury.
- Utilize restraints safely, effectively, and only when necessary, such as when less restrictive measures are unsuccessful.
- Accurately identify situations requiring completion of an incident or unusual occurrence report.
- Explain personal and professional actions to take for disaster preparedness.
- Effectively utilize triage concepts in an emergency or disaster situation.

PRACTICE TEST

1 The nurse determines that a new mother is in greatest need of having teaching about infant care and safety reinforced when the mother makes which statement?

1. "I am pretty sure that I am going to breastfeed my baby."
2. "After feeding, I should put my baby on her tummy to prevent choking."
3. "Solid foods are unnecessary during the baby's first 4–6 months."
4. "I should wake my baby up every 3–4 hours for feeding."

2 A newborn is scheduled for discharge from the birthing center tomorrow. When reinforcing teaching to the new parents about car seats, which characteristics of infant restraint systems would the nurse include as essential for the newborn? Select all that apply.

1. Forward-facing
2. Rear-facing
3. In the back seat
4. In the front seat
5. Of a solid and neutral color

3 Which snack would the nurse appropriately offer the hospitalized toddler?

1. Crackers
2. Peanuts
3. Grapes
4. Cereal bar

4 What is the best method for the nurse to use to encourage the use of bicycle helmets by school-age children?

1. Advocate for legislation on helmet laws.
2. Teach parents to role-model helmet use while riding bicycles.
3. Verbally reprimand children who report not wearing helmets while riding.
4. Recommend the parents purchase stylish helmets to increase compliance.

5 A nurse is explaining information related to accidents and injuries to high school students. Which topic is most important to include?

1. Occupational-related injuries at work
2. Motor vehicle-related injuries
3. Fall-related injuries
4. Injury due to residential fires

6 The nurse is visiting an older adult client with diabetes mellitus. The nurse becomes concerned and reinforces safety education when which of the following occurs?

1. Neighbors bring a warm lunch to client
2. Children install air conditioners in kitchen and bedroom
3. Grandchildren place baskets of folded laundry by bedroom door
4. Client stores diabetic testing supplies on kitchen table

7 The nurse preceptor observes the new LPN/LVN administering medications. The preceptor concludes there is a risk for medication error when the new LPN/LVN takes which action?

1. Answers a physician's page while passing medications
2. Uses military time for documentation
3. Asks for help with a dosage calculation
4. Does not give a medication that the client questions

8 The nurse would ask a client scheduled for a venogram about allergy to which substance before the procedure?

1. Peanuts
2. Shellfish
3. Eggs
4. Meat tenderizer

9 The nurse calculates a dose of a medication for subcutaneous injection to be 4.5 mL. Rechecking the calculation yields the same result. What is the next best action that the nurse should take?

1. Verify the written order.
2. Call the prescriber.
3. Call the pharmacist.
4. Ask another nurse to check the dosage calculation.

10 Which of the following medication orders should the nurse question?

1. Morphine sulfate (Morphine) 4 mg IV every 3–4 hours as needed for pain
2. Ceftriaxone (Rocephin) IVPB every 8 hours
3. Furosemide (Lasix) 40 mg po daily
4. Metoprolol (Lopressor) 50 mg po twice a day

11 The nurse has applied elbow splints on a confused client to prevent the client from removing the intravenous (IV) line. Which of the following interventions is required?

1. Document appearance of client's IV site every hour.
2. Remove elbow splints every 8 hours.
3. Ask for renewal of physician's restraint order every 72 hours.
4. Observe and document client's condition at least every hour.

12 A Code Red (fire) has been announced on the hospital unit. What is the nurse's first response?

1. Remove clients in danger from the fire.
2. Contain the fire.
3. Report fire to other staff.
4. Extinguish the fire.

13 A client on the hospital unit has fallen. Place the nursing interventions in order of priority. All options must be used.

1. Identify all witnesses.
2. Call the physician.
3. Collect data and provide urgent care.
4. Notify the charge nurse.
5. Fill out the incident report.

14 Which information would the nurse omit from written documentation when a reportable incident has occurred?

1. Names of witnesses on incident report
2. Nursing interventions in medical record
3. Time physician was called on incident report
4. That an incident report was submitted in medical record

15 A major portion of a construction project has collapsed. The emergency department (ED) has been notified that numerous victims are being transported to the ED. In the ED, with what activity should the LPN/LVN assist the RNs?

1. Determining department resources—staff, beds, equipment
2. Implement personnel recall system.
3. Discharge stable clients
4. Set up a temporary morgue

16 The nurse should explain to the mother of a 12-month-old infant that by current law, a forward-facing infant seat is safest once the infant weighs at least ____ pounds. Record your answer, rounding to the nearest whole number.

Fill in your answer below:
____ pounds

17 The nurse is communicating with a client who continues to return to a violent relationship saying, "There is nothing I can do." What is the nurse's best response?

1. "You do have some choices; let's sit together and explore them."
2. "If you return you are at risk for further abuse."
3. "Here is the number of the crisis hotline."
4. "Do you have family or friends who can help?"

18 The LPN/LVN is volunteering at the local grammar school. Which finding by the nurse regarding the behavior of one of the children may indicate physical neglect?

1. Not following instructions well
2. Boisterous activity
3. Stealing or hoarding food
4. Sudden onset of enuresis

19 Which type of physical restraint is most appropriate for the nurse to apply with an order to a client who is confused and pulling at an incisional dressing?

1. Mitt restraint
2. Limb restraint
3. Belt restraint
4. Wrist restraint

20 When determining the effectiveness of a restraint, it is most important for the nurse to document which item?

1. Behavior and response of the client's family to the restraint
2. Exact time the restraint is removed
3. Nurse's interactions with the client while the client is in the restraint
4. Client's behavior while in the restraint

21 The nurse is reinforcing safety measures for a parent of a child who has been treated for accidental ingestion of acetaminophen (Tylenol). The nurse recognizes that the parent has understood the information when the parent makes which statements? Select all that apply.

1. "I will use warning stickers like Mr. Yuk on all medicine containers."
2. "I will buy products with childproof caps."
3. "I will keep magnesium citrate available."
4. "I will put the Poison Control Center phone number by every phone."
5. "I will keep activated charcoal in the house and use it readily if needed."

ANSWERS & RATIONALES

1 **Answer: 2** **Rationale:** Infants should always be put to sleep on the back, indicating the need for further teaching about newborn care and safety. Breastfeeding is a nutrition choice. Solid foods are not needed in the first 4 to 6 months of infancy. Newborns do sleep frequently and should be awakened every 3–4 hours for feeding. **Cognitive Level:** Analyzing **Client Need:** Safety and Infection Control **Integrated Process:** Nursing Process: Evaluation **Content Area:** Maternal-Newborn **Strategy:** The wording of the question guides you to look for a false statement as the correct response. Use the process of elimination and nursing knowledge.

2 **Answer: 2, 3** **Rationale:** An infant child restraint system should always be in the back seat and rear-facing. After a child is 1 year of age and weighs 20 pounds, the seat may be in the rear and front-facing by law, although new guidelines recommend keeping a child rear-facing until age 2. Although bright colors are stimulating to an infant, the color of the system does not matter. **Cognitive Level:** Applying **Client Need:** Safety and Infection Control **Integrated Process:** Teaching and Learning **Content Area:** Child Health **Strategy:** Choose between opposites, since usually one of each is correct. Use the process of elimination and nursing knowledge of infant safety measures to make appropriate selections.

3 **Answer: 1** **Rationale:** Crackers are of a soft consistency when chewed and swallowed. Toddlers can easily choke on small foods such as peanuts, popcorn, and grapes. Toddlers can choke on firm-consistency foods such as cereal bars. **Cognitive Level:** Applying **Client Need:** Safety and Infection Control **Integrated Process:** Nursing Process: Implementation **Content Area:** Child Health **Strategy:** Note that the question is determining risk for choking and select the option that has a food that will dissolve easily in the mouth.

4 **Answer: 2** **Rationale:** Parent role models of behavior are most effective in fostering good habits in children. Legislative action provides legal support for helmet use, but this is not a direct motivator for children. Stylish helmets and reprimands for lack of use may be effective on a case by case basis, but make less of an impression than positive role modeling. **Cognitive Level:** Applying **Client Need:** Safety and Infection Control **Integrated Process:** Nursing Process: Planning **Content Area:** Child Health **Strategy:** Note the critical word *best*, indicating that all answers could be correct, but one is better than the others. Consider that legislation is a positive step but may not change behaviors. Reprimanding is a negative behavior. The style of helmet may be effective but may not be realistic for all families depending on financial circumstances.

5 **Answer: 2** **Rationale:** Driving a car and having the independence to ride with friends are important milestones for high school-age adolescents. In addition to being inexperienced, some adolescents experiment with alcohol and drugs, putting them at increased risk for motor vehicle accidents. Occupational injury is a risk for the working adult. Falls are risk factors for the older adult. Residential fires can affect any age. **Cognitive Level:** Analyzing **Client Need:** Safety and Infection Control **Integrated Process:** Nursing Process: Implementation **Content Area:** Child Health **Strategy:** Use knowledge of the principles of growth and development to aid in answering this question.

6 **Answer: 3** **Rationale:** Laundry baskets that are set on the floor will pose a risk for falling for the older client. All hallways, floors, stairways, and furniture should be free of clutter. Neighbors bringing lunch for the elderly client is a good safety intervention. Family controlling the climate for the elderly client is a good safety intervention. Keeping diabetic supplies on a kitchen table with easy access will facilitate diabetic testing. **Cognitive Level:** Applying **Client Need:** Safety and Infection Control **Integrated Process:** Nursing Process: Data Collection **Content Area:** Fundamentals **Strategy:** Focus on the critical word *safety* and choose the option that poses a risk to the client. Recall that older adults are at increased risk for falls, so this should guide your thought process as you make a selection.

7 **Answer: 1 Rationale:** The nurse should never interrupt the medication administration process, because this increases the risk for errors. Military time is frequently used by institutions for documentation. The nurse should always ask for assistance with dosage calculations when in doubt. The nurse should never give a medication that a client questions; instead, recheck the order, dosage, and medication, and give the client an explanation. **Cognitive Level:** Analyzing **Client Need:** Safety and Infection Control **Integrated Process:** Nursing Process: Implementation **Content Area:** Fundamentals **Strategy:** Focus on the risk for error and select the option that poses a threat to the safe administration of medications.

8 **Answer: 2 Rationale:** Iodine is used in many radiological procedures. Shellfish allergies may be an indicator of iodine allergy. Peanuts, eggs, and meat tenderizer do not pose a risk of cross-sensitivity to iodine. **Cognitive Level:** Applying **Client Need:** Safety and Infection Control **Integrated Process:** Nursing Process: Data Collection **Content Area:** Fundamentals **Strategy:** Knowledge of radiological procedures must be applied. In addition, recall that allergy to iodine or shellfish commonly applies to radiological procedures.

9 **Answer: 1 Rationale:** If a calculated dose seems unrealistic, refer to and verify the original written order. Be careful to read abbreviations and dosage correctly. Asking another nurse to check the dose, or calling the prescriber or pharmacist are correct interventions, but not the first intervention, because the first step in the medication process is the writing of the order. **Cognitive Level:** Analyzing **Client Need:** Safety and Infection Control **Integrated Process:** Nursing Process: Implementation **Content Area:** Fundamentals **Strategy:** Read all options carefully. Apply the six rights of medication administration.

10 **Answer: 2 Rationale:** The ceftriaxone order does not have a medication dosage listed. All other options have required information for dispensing medications. **Cognitive Level:** Applying **Client Need:** Safety and Infection Control **Integrated Process:** Nursing Process: Planning **Content Area:** Fundamentals **Strategy:** The critical words in the stem of the question are *should the nurse question.* This indicates that the correct answer is an incorrect item. Consider the elements of a valid medication order, and choose the option that has an element missing.

11 **Answer: 4 Rationale:** The client should be checked at least hourly, and the nurse must document client status. The IV site should be checked every hour, but documentation may be done only once per shift unless a problem occurs. Because restraints may impede circulation, they should be removed according to agency policy, which is generally every 1–2 hours rather than every 8 hours. Physical restraints impede a client's freedom; their use needs to be ordered every 24 hours. **Cognitive Level:** Applying **Client Need:** Safety and Infection Control **Integrated Process:** Nursing Process: Implementation **Content Area:** Fundamentals **Strategy:** Utilize knowledge of common policy and procedures for use of physical restraints. Always consider an answer that contains data collection as an option.

12 **Answer: 1 Rationale:** The primary responsibility of the nurse is client safety. Removing a client from danger should be the priority. Next the alarm should be sounded. The nurse and others can then contain and possibly extinguish the fire. **Cognitive Level:** Analyzing **Client Need:** Safety and Infection Control **Integrated Process:** Nursing Process: Implementation **Content Area:** Fundamentals **Strategy:** The priority option is client focused. The other options are fire focused. Remember the mnemonic RACE (remove, alarm, contain, extinguish).

13 **Answer: 4, 3, 1, 2, 5 Rationale:** The primary actions of the nurse are emergency data collection and first aid. If the nurse notifies the charge nurse, there will be nursing help to contact the physician and speak with witnesses. After caring for the client and monitoring the situation, the nurse is prepared to fill out the incident report. **Cognitive Level:** Analyzing **Client Need:** Safety and Infection Control **Integrated Process:** Nursing Process: Implementation **Content Area:** Fundamentals **Strategy:** Focus on the client first. Then obtain additional help, collect data, and do the paperwork last.

14 **Answer: 4 Rationale:** The medical record belongs to the client and should contain all facts related to the client and the incident. The incident report belongs to the hospital and should contain all facts and supportive data related to the client and the incident. The medical record should not refer to the incident report. **Cognitive Level:** Applying **Client Need:** Safety and Infection Control **Integrated Process:** Nursing Process: Implementation **Content Area:** Fundamentals **Strategy:** Use knowledge of policy and procedure regarding incident reports to analyze this situation.

15 **Answer: 1 Rationale:** The nurses must first assist the RN to determine current ED resources. No decisions can be made without a comprehensive environmental assessment of staff, beds, and equipment. The other options are not as encompassing, and a comprehensive environmental assessment is needed with a possible impending disaster. **Cognitive Level:** Analyzing **Client Need:** Safety and Infection Control **Integrated Process:** Nursing Process: Data Collection **Content Area:** Fundamentals **Strategy:** Choose the option that is the most comprehensive or global of the option choices.

16 **Answer: 20 Rationale:** By current law, the infant must weigh at least 20 pounds in order to be safe in a forward-facing infant seat and must be 1 year or older. **Cognitive Level:** Applying **Client Need:** Safety and Infection Control **Integrated Process:** Teaching and Learning **Content Area:** Child Health **Strategy:** Because this item is a standard, it is necessary to commit this information to memory. A quick way to remember this requirement is that the number 20 is also the number of fingers and toes on an infant.

17 **Answer: 1 Rationale:** Helping the client to explore alternatives helps empower this client who is feeling powerless. Powerlessness is common in victims of ongoing violence, as the emotional component of the violence instills terror and helplessness. The client is ashamed and demoralized, criticized and controlled by the perpetrator, who often makes numerous serious threats and convinces the victim that there is no hope of escape. Teaching about further risk of violence, providing and/or mobilizing resources are appropriate interventions, but they will not be effective if the client feels powerless to act. **Cognitive Level:** Analyzing **Client Need:** Psychosocial Integrity **Integrated Process:** Communication and Documentation **Content Area:** Mental Health **Strategy:** Recognize the powerlessness of the client and choose an option that will allow the client to take action to combat this feeling and achieve a feeling of competence and control.

18 **Answer: 3 Rationale:** Children who are physically neglected will often steal and hoard food because of inadequate nutrition. The child's level of physical activity and response to discipline may be indicators of emotional or physical abuse. A sudden onset of enuresis is one possible indication of sexual abuse. **Cognitive Level:** Applying **Client Need:** Safety and

Infection Control **Integrated Process:** Nursing Process: Data Collection **Content Area:** Child Health **Strategy:** Look carefully at the options. Identify the one that has to do with meeting basic needs. This child has been neglected and is trying to cope with that and provide for own basic needs.

19 **Answer: 1 Rationale:** A mitt restraint is appropriate for a client who is confused and picking at dressings and tubes. It allows the client to continue to move around freely. A limb restraint would not necessarily prevent picking at the dressing; instead, it would prevent movement of the client and may agitate a confused client. A belt restraint would not necessarily prevent picking at the dressing; instead, it would prevent movement of the client and may agitate a confused client. A wrist restraint would not necessarily prevent picking at the dressing; instead, it would prevent movement of the client and may agitate a confused client. **Cognitive Level:** Applying **Client Need:** Safety and Infection Control **Integrated Process:** Nursing Process: Implementation **Content Area:** Fundamentals **Strategy:** Recall that it is important to assess the need for the restraint and to not restrain more than necessary.

20 **Answer: 4 Rationale:** It is imperative for the nurse to assess and document the client's behavior while the client is in restraints. This will help to determine whether the client has a continued need for restraints. Family response to the client's restraints can be documented, but is not as critical as documenting the client's behavior. The exact time the restraints are removed should be documented, but this does not help evaluate the effectiveness of the restraint. Nurses' interactions with the restrained client can be documented, but is not as critical as documenting the client's behavior. **Cognitive Level:** Analyzing **Client Need:** Safety and Infection Control **Integrated Process:** Communication and Documentation **Content Area:** Fundamentals **Strategy:** Choose the response that is totally client focused. Client safety is always the nurse's primary focus.

21 **Answer: 1, 2, 4 Rationale:** Using warning stickers like Mr. Yuk to teach the child to avoid these items will help to keep substances from being ingested. Using childproof caps will inhibit the child from opening medicine containers. An important aspect of teaching is to inform parents to contact the Poison Control Center or 911 for instructions on the appropriateness of care following ingestion of substances. Magnesium citrate is not used in the home setting for treatment of poisonings. Activated charcoal is not used in the home setting for treatment of poisonings. **Cognitive Level:** Applying **Client Need:** Safety and Infection Control **Integrated Process:** Nursing Process: Evaluation **Content Area:** Child Health **Strategy:** Knowledge of the ways to avoid childhood poisoning will help to choose the correct answers.

Key Terms to Review

adverse reaction p. 45
bloodborne pathogen p. 47
CDC p. 47
idiosyncratic reaction p. 45
The Joint Commission p. 49
MSDS p. 47
OSHA p. 44
restraint p. 46
toxic reaction p. 45
triage p. 49

References

American Academy of Pediatrics (March, 2011). *Car safety seats: Information for families 2011*. Retrieved July 1, 2011, from http://www.healthychildren.org/English/safety-prevention/on-the-go/Pages/Car-Safety-Seats-Information-for-Families.aspx

Berman, A., & Snyder, S. (2012). *Kozier & Erb's fundamentals of nursing: Concepts, process, and practice*. (9th ed.). Upper Saddle River, NJ: Pearson Education, Inc.

Clark, M. J. (2008). *Community health nursing: Advocacy for population health* (5th ed.). Upper Saddle River, NJ: Pearson Education, Inc.

Consumer Product Safety Commission (n.d.). *Older consumers safety checklist*. Retrieved June 8, 2010, from http://www.cpsc.gov/CPSCPUB/PUBS/705.pdf

Deglin, J. H., & Vallerand, A. H. (2010). *Drug guide for nurses*. Philadelphia: FA Davis.

Federal Emergency Management Agency (n.d.). *Are you ready? Emergency planning and checklists*. Retrieved June 8, 2010, from http://www.fema.gov/areyouready/emergency_planning.shtm

Healthy People 2010 (n.d.). Retrieved June 8, 2010, from http://www.healthypeople.gov

Institute of Medicine of the National Academies (n.d.). Retrieved June 8, 2010, from http://www.iom.edu

Langhorn, M., Fulton, J. & Otto, S. (2007). *Oncology nursing* (5th ed.). St. Louis, MO: Elsevier.

Lewis, S. M., Dirksen, S. R., Heitkemper, M. M., & Bucher, L. (2011). *Medical surgical nursing: Assessment and management of clinical problems* (8th ed.). St. Louis, MO: Elsevier.

Mothershead, J. L. (n.d.). *Disaster planning*. Retrieved June 8, 2010, from http://www.emedicine.com/emerg/topic718.htm

U.S. Department of Labor Occupational Safety and Health Administration (n.d.). *Bloodborne pathogens and needlestick prevention*. Retrieved June 8, 2010, from http://www.osha.gov/SLTC/bloodbornepathogens/index.html

Test Yourself

Are you ready for the NCLEX-PN® or course exams? Use the practice tests on the companion website to check.

ANSWERS & RATIONALES

Preventing and Controlling Infection

7

In this chapter

Cross Reference

Other chapters relevant to this content area are

Intravenous Therapy Chapter 30
Perioperative Care Chapter 44
Respiratory Disorders Chapter 51
Oncological Disorders Chapter 61
Communicable or Infectious Diseases Chapter 63

I. STANDARD PRECAUTIONS

NCLEX® **A.** ***Chain of infection* comprises six elements that must occur for infection to develop**

1. Etiologic agent: any pathogen capable of causing infection; causative agents include bacteria, virus, fungi, protozoa, rickettsiae, and helminths
2. Reservoir: favorable environment in which infectious organism grows and reproduces; reservoir may be animate (humans, animals, insects) or inanimate (food, water, soil, equipment); blood and respiratory, gastrointestinal (GI), reproductive, and urinary tracts serve as reservoirs in humans
3. Portal of exit from reservoir: route by which microorganism leaves reservoir; portal of exit can be breaks in skin, the blood, and respiratory, GI, reproductive, and urinary tracts in humans
4. Method of transmission: mode by which microorganism is transferred from reservoir to host; transfer occurs by three mechanisms: direct, indirect, and airborne transmission
   a. Direct contact involves physical transfer of causative agent from person to person; routes of direct transmission include touching, kissing, biting, and sexual intercourse; transmission can also occur through droplets when person talks, coughs, sneezes, or spits, but only when source is within 3 feet of susceptible host
   b. Indirect contact involves transfer from reservoir to susceptible host via either a vehicle or a vector; vehicle-borne transmission requires inanimate object to serve as mode of transmission; intermediary agent, such as an animal or insect, is required in vector-borne transmission
   c. Airborne transmission involves transport of droplet nuclei or dust bearing infectious agent by air currents
5. Portal of entry to susceptible host: route by which infectious agent enters susceptible host; examples include breaks in skin and respiratory, GI, reproductive, and urinary tracts
6. Susceptible host: individual at increased risk for infection; infection occurs when infectious agent overwhelms host's defenses against infection (Figure 7–1)

NCLEX® **B.** ***Standard precautions***

1. Represent first tier of Centers for Disease Control and Prevention (CDC) guidelines for isolation precautions
2. NCLEX® Reduce risk of transmission of infection, protecting both health care providers and clients from recognized and unrecognized sources

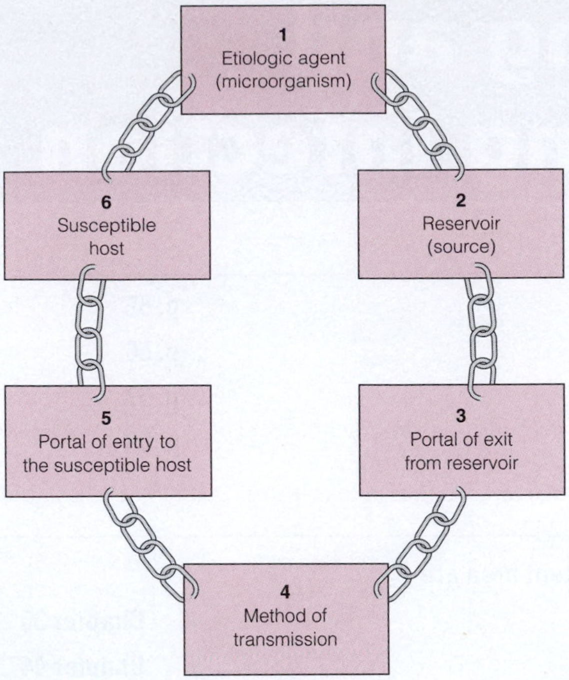

Figure 7–1

Links in the chain of infection.

NCLEX®

3. Are used in providing care to all clients regardless of medical diagnosis or setting
4. Applies to blood, all body fluids, excretions, and secretions except sweat regardless of whether blood is visible or whether skin and mucous membranes are not intact

C. Standard precautions include hand hygiene and use of *personal protective equipment (PPE)*

1. Hand hygiene: most effective way to prevent spread of microorganisms; perform before and after each client contact, immediately following exposure to blood and/or other body fluids and contaminated items, and before and after donning gloves; wash hands with plain (nonantimicrobial) soap and water or use waterless alcohol-based hand rub
2. PPE is equipment worn by health care providers to prevent transmission of microorganisms
   a. Gloves (clean, nonsterile): worn to protect hands when exposure to blood, body fluids, secretions, excretions, and contaminated items is likely; used for touching mucous membranes and nonintact skin; change gloves if they become torn or heavily soiled, even between procedures on same client; avoid adjusting PPE or touching noncontaminated items with contaminated gloves; remove promptly after use and wash hands
   b. Gown: worn to protect health care provider's skin and clothing; used during procedures and care activities when splashing or spraying of blood, body fluids, secretions, and excretions is possible
   c. Mask: worn to protect mucous membranes of nose and mouth; should fully cover nose and mouth; used during care activities when splashes or sprays of blood, body fluids, secretions, and excretions can be expected
   d. Eye protection: goggles are worn to protect eyes; do not use personal glasses as a substitute for goggles; face shield is worn to protect face, including eyes, nose, and mouth, and should cover forehead, extending below chin and wrapping around each side of face; eye protection is used during care activities when splashes or sprays of blood, body fluids, secretions, and excretions are likely

D. Procedures for using PPE

NCLEX®

1. Donning PPE: perform hand hygiene immediately before donning PPE; don PPE before coming in contact with client, usually outside client's room; don gown first, followed by mask, then eye protection, then gloves

NCLEX®

2. Removing PPE: remove carefully at doorway of client's room; remove gloves first, followed by mask, then gown, then eye protection; discard contaminated PPE in appropriate container; perform hand hygiene immediately after removing PPE

II. MEDICAL ASEPSIS

NCLEX®

A. General principles

1. **Medical asepsis** involves practices, such as hand hygiene and use of PPE, to reduce the number and limit the spread of microorganisms

2. Is also known as clean technique; objects are designated as "clean" (nearly free of microorganisms) or "dirty" (contaminated)
3. Used in implementing nonsterile procedures, such as taking vital signs, nasogastric tube insertion, and tube feeding administration

B. Disposal of contaminated equipment and supplies is conducted in accordance with institution policies and procedures

1. Linens: handle soiled linen as little as possible in a manner that prevents exposure to own skin, mucous membranes, and clothing; contain soiled linens in a bag before removal from client's room
2. Dishes: no special considerations are needed; some facilities may use disposable dishes for convenience
3. Syringes, needles, and sharps: avoid recapping needles or detaching needles from syringes; dispose of items in a rigid, puncture-resistant container immediately after use
4. Equipment (thermometers, blood pressure equipment): dedicated equipment is used for clients with transmission-based precautions; discard single-use (disposable) items immediately after use in an appropriate manner; reusable (nondisposable) equipment must be cleaned and decontaminated before use with other clients

NCLEX®
5. Lab specimens: place specimen in a leak-proof container with a biohazard label; then place container in a sealed plastic bag

NCLEX®
6. Transportation of clients with infections: avoid transporting clients with infections to other areas of hospital; if transportation is necessary, take precautions to prevent spread of infection to others; a client with respiratory infection should wear a mask; a client with an infected wound should have wound covered; notify personnel in receiving department of client's infection

III. SURGICAL ASEPSIS

A. General principles

1. **Surgical asepsis** involves practices to maintain objects and areas free of microorganisms
2. Is also known as sterile technique; objects are designated as "sterile" (completely free of microorganisms) or "nonsterile" (contaminated)
3. Used in implementing sterile procedures, such as intravenous therapy and urinary catheterization

NCLEX® **B. Principles and practices of surgical asepsis are listed in Table 7–1**

Table 7–1 Principles and Practices of Surgical Asepsis

Principles	Practices
All objects used in a sterile field must be sterile.	All articles are sterilized appropriately by dry or moist heat, chemicals, or radiation before use.
	Always check a package containing a sterile object for intactness, dryness, and expiration date. Sterile articles can be stored for only a prescribed time, after which they are considered unsterile. Consider as unsterile any package that appears already open, torn, punctured, or wet.
	Storage areas should be clean, dry, off the floor, and away from sinks.
	Before using a package, always check chemical indicator of sterilization, which is often a tape used to fasten the package or contained inside the package (indicator changes color during sterilization as an indicator of the sterilization process). If the color change is not evident, consider the package unsterile. If commercially prepared sterile packages do not have indicators, they are marked with the word *sterile*.
Sterile objects become unsterile when touched by unsterile objects.	Handle sterile objects that will touch open wounds or enter body cavities only with sterile forceps or sterile gloved hands.
	Discard or resterilize objects that come into contact with unsterile objects.
	Whenever the sterility of an object is questionable, assume the article is unsterile.
Sterile items that are out of vision or below the waist level of the nurse are considered unsterile.	Once left unattended, a sterile field is considered unsterile.
	Always keep sterile objects in view. Nurses do not turn their backs on a sterile field.
	Only the front part of a sterile gown (from the waist to the shoulder) and 2 inches above the elbows to the cuff of the sleeves are considered sterile.
	Always keep sterile gloved hands in sight and above waist level; touch only objects that are sterile.
	Sterile draped tables in the operating room or elsewhere are considered sterile only at surface level.
	Once a sterile field becomes unsterile, it must be set up again before proceeding.

(continued)

Table 7–1 Principles and Practices of Surgical Asepsis *(continued)*

Principles	Practices
Sterile objects can become unsterile by prolonged exposure to airborne microorganisms.	Keep doors closed and traffic to a minimum in areas where a sterile procedure is being performed because moving air can carry dust and microorganisms. Keep areas in which sterile procedures are carried out as clean as possible by frequent damp cleaning with detergent germicides to minimize contaminants in the area. Keep hair clean and short or enclose it in a net to prevent hair from falling on sterile objects. Microorganisms on the hair can make a sterile field unsterile. Wear surgical caps in operating rooms, delivery rooms, and burn units. Refrain from sneezing or coughing over a sterile field. This can make it unsterile because droplets containing microorganisms from the respiratory tract can travel 1 m (3 ft). Some agencies recommend that masks covering the mouth and the nose should be worn by anyone working over a sterile field or an open wound. Nurses with mild upper respiratory tract infections refrain from carrying out sterile procedures or wear masks. When working over a sterile field, keep talking to a minimum. Avert the head from the field if talking is necessary. To prevent microorganisms from falling over a sterile field, refrain from reaching over a sterile field unless sterile gloves are worn and refrain from moving unsterile objects over a sterile field.
Fluids flow in the direction of gravity.	Unless gloves are worn, always hold wet forceps with the tips below the handles. If tips are held higher than the handles, fluid can flow onto the handle and become contaminated by the hands. When the forceps are again pointed downward, the fluid flows back down and contaminates the tips. During a surgical hand wash, hold the hands higher than the elbows to prevent contaminants from the forearms from reaching the hands.
Moisture that passes through a sterile object draws microorganisms from unsterile surfaces above or below to the sterile surface by capillary action.	Sterile, moisture-proof barriers are used beneath sterile objects. Liquids (sterile saline or antiseptics) are frequently poured into containers on a sterile field. If they are spilled onto the sterile field, the barrier keeps the liquid from seeping beneath it. Keep the sterile covers on sterile equipment dry. Damp surfaces can attract microorganisms in the air. Replace sterile drapes that do not have a sterile barrier underneath when they become moist.
The edges of a sterile field are considered unsterile.	A 2.5 cm (1 in.) margin at each edge of an opened drape is considered unsterile because the edges are in contact with unsterile surfaces. Place all sterile objects more than 2.5 cm (1 in.) inside the edges of a sterile field. Any article that falls outside the edges of a sterile field is considered unsterile.
The skin cannot be sterilized and is unsterile.	Use sterile gloves or sterile forceps to handle sterile items. Prior to a surgical aseptic procedure, wash hands to reduce the number of microorganisms on them.
Conscientiousness, alertness, and honesty are essential qualities in maintaining surgical asepsis.	When a sterile object becomes unsterile, it does not necessarily change in appearance. The person who sees a sterile object become contaminated must correct or report the situation. Do not set up a sterile field ahead of time for future use.

Source: Berman, A., & Snyder, S. *Kozier & Erb's fundamentals of nursing: Concepts, process, and practice* (9th ed.), © 2012, p. 701. Reprinted by permission of Pearson Education, Inc., Upper Saddle River, NJ 07458.

IV. TRANSMISSION-BASED PRECAUTIONS

A. *Transmission-based precautions* are measures to limit spread of pathogenic microorganisms

NCLEX®

B. *Airborne precautions*

1. Involves spread of infection through airborne droplet nuclei smaller than 5 microns, evaporated droplets that remain suspended in air for long periods of time, or dust particles containing infectious agent
2. Because microorganisms can be widely spread by air currents, special air handling and ventilation are needed

3. Examples of diseases include rubeola (measles), varicella (chicken pox), and tuberculosis
4. Use standard precautions and mask; use other PPE as appropriate for expected risk of exposure
   a. For tuberculosis, wear particulate respirator mask that is fit-tested to individual nurse
   b. For other airborne diseases such as rubeola or varicella, susceptible persons should not enter client's room; if entry is unavoidable, respiratory protection must be worn
   c. Individuals immune to rubeola or varicella do not need to wear respiratory protection
5. Place client in private, negative–air pressure room with 6 (older construction) to 12 (renovations or new construction) air exchanges per hour; air is exhausted directly to outdoors or recirculated through HEPA filtration before return
6. If private room is not possible, client may be placed in room with another client (cohorted) who has an infection with same microorganism but no other infection
7. Client should remain in room with door closed
8. If transportation of client to other hospital departments is unavoidable, client should wear surgical mask
9. Visitors should wear mask appropriate to type of infection at all times

NCLEX®

C. Droplet precautions

1. Involves spread of infection by particle droplets larger than 5 microns that can be generated when client coughs, sneezes, talks, laughs, and so on
2. Examples of diseases include diphtheria (pharyngeal), mycoplasma pneumonia, rubella, pertussis, mumps, streptococcal pharyngitis, pneumonia, and scarlet fever
3. Use standard precautions; mask is required when providing care or if within 3 feet of client; use other PPE as appropriate
4. Place client in private room; if private room is not possible, client may cohorted with another client who has same infection but no additional infections
5. Client should remain in room; if transportation of client to other hospital departments is unavoidable, client should wear surgical mask; notify personnel in receiving department of client's infection
6. Door to room may remain open
7. Visitors should wear mask if within 3 feet of client and should try to maintain distance of 3 feet whenever possible

NCLEX®

D. Contact precautions

1. Involves spread of infection by contact with client or contact with items in client's environment
2. Examples of diseases include skin infections (scabies, pediculosis, herpes simplex or zoster), hepatitis A, and wound, GI or urinary infections, including those with multi–drug resistant organisms, such as **methicillin-resistant *Staphylococcus aureus* (MRSA)** and **vancomycin-resistant enterococcus (VRE)**
3. Use standard precautions; gloves are required; wear gown when contact with infected secretions is expected; use other PPE as appropriate for expected risk of exposure
4. Place client in private room; if private room is not possible, client may be cohorted with another client who has same infection
5. Door to room may remain open
6. Limit transportation of client to other hospital departments; infected wound should be securely covered; notify personnel in receiving department of client's infection
7. Dedicate equipment for client care (such as stethoscope or sphygmomanometer) to a single client or cohort of clients; if such items must be used to care for other clients, adequately clean and disinfect them first

E. Multiple precautions

1. A client is not limited to one set of transmission-based precautions; rather, precautions are implemented based on specific need
2. For example, a client with measles who has a wound infected with MRSA would require both airborne and contact precautions
3. Clients with severe acute respiratory syndrome (SARS) require the use of both airborne and contact precautions; SARS is a highly infectious viral infection that is transmitted by airborne respiratory droplets and by touching surfaces and objects contaminated with infectious droplets

Check Your NCLEX–PN® Exam I.Q. *You are ready for testing on this content if you can*

- Describe the chain of infection.
- Explain the principles of standard precautions.
- Correctly don and remove personal protective equipment.
- Distinguish between medical and surgical asepsis.
- Explain principles of medical and surgical asepsis.
- Compare and contrast transmission-based airborne, droplet, and contact precautions.
- Identify infectious diseases that require transmission-based precautions.

PRACTICE TEST

1 The nurse would perform which actions when washing hands as part of medical asepsis before caring for a client in an outpatient clinic? Select all that apply.

1. Wash hands with the hands held higher than the elbows
2. Adjust temperature of water to the hottest possible
3. Scrub hands and nails with a scrub brush for 5 minutes
4. Use a clean paper towel to turn water off
5. Rub vigorously using firm, circular motions

2 The nurse's forearm becomes splattered with blood while inserting an intravenous catheter. What action should the nurse take?

1. Wash blood away with isopropyl alcohol
2. Wipe blood away with a tissue
3. Flush forearm with hot water, letting water flow from elbow toward fingers.
4. Wash forearm with soap and water

3 The nurse would take which action to protect the client from infection at the portal of entry?

1. Place sputum specimen in a biohazard bag for transport to the lab
2. Empty Jackson-Pratt drain using sterile technique
3. Dispose of soiled gloves in waste container
4. Wash hands after providing client care

4 Which actions by the nurse comply with core principles of surgical asepsis? Select all that apply.

1. Wash hands before and after client care
2. Keep sterile field in view at all times
3. Wear personal protective equipment
4. Add contents to sterile field holding package 6 inches above field
5. Consider outer 1.5 inches of sterile field as contaminated

5 Which precaution would the nurse implement when admitting a client with herpes zoster to the nursing unit?

1. Airborne precautions
2. Contact precautions
3. Droplet precautions
4. Neutropenic precautions

6 A client with tuberculosis asks the nurse if visitors will need to wear masks. What response by the nurse is most accurate?

1. "Everyone who enters your room must wear a mask to protect themselves from tuberculosis."
2. "Masks would not be necessary for visitors who have had tuberculosis before."
3. "It is less important for your family to wear masks, since they live in close contact with you."
4. "Only visitors who are at risk for tuberculosis need to wear a mask."

7 The nurse is leaving the room of a client who has methicillin-resistant Staphylococcus aureus (MRSA) microorganisms in a wound and the urine. Place the following personal protective equipment in order of removal. All options must be used.

1. Eye protection
2. Gloves
3. Mask
4. Gown

8 A client with suspected severe acute respiratory syndrome (SARS) arrives at the emergency department. Which physician order should the nurse implement first?

1. Airborne and contact precautions
2. IV D_5NS at 100 mL/hr
3. Nasopharyngeal culture for reverse-transcription polymerase chain reaction
4. Sputum for enzyme immunoassay testing

9 A client with vancomycin-intermediate-resistant *Staphylococcus aureus* (VISA) is admitted to the nursing unit. What type of precautions should the nurse institute?

1. Standard precautions
2. Neutropenic precautions
3. Droplet precautions
4. Contact precautions

10 The nurse would implement which of the following as a requirement of care specific to the client who has tuberculosis?

1. Disposal of needles and syringes in a rigid, puncture-proof container
2. Handwashing after removing contaminated gloves
3. Wearing a gown if splashing is possible
4. A private room with negative air flow

11 The nurse would expect to institute transmission-based precautions for a client with which infection?

1. Pneumonia caused by *Pseudomonas aeruginosa*
2. *Pneumocystis carinii* pneumonia
3. A sacral wound contaminated by *Escherichia coli*
4. A draining leg wound with methicillin-resistant *Staphylococcus aureus*

12 A client asks, "How did I get scarlet fever?" What would be the nurse's best response?

1. "Scarlet fever is transmitted through sexual intercourse."
2. "You can get scarlet fever if you share contaminated needles or get a blood transfusion."
3. "Most people get it by eating contaminated food."
4. "You inhaled infected droplets in the air."

13 The nurse is assisting a client who has methicillin-resistant *Staphylococcus aureus* in collecting a clean-catch urine specimen. Which protective equipment is unnecessary?

1. N95 particulate respirator
2. Gown
3. Eye protection
4. Gloves

14 The nurse is preparing to irrigate a wound infected with vancomycin-resistant enterococci (VRE). What personal protective equipment (PPE) would the nurse wear?

1. Gloves, gown, and particulate respirator
2. Gloves and surgical mask
3. Gloves, eye protection, and shoe covers
4. Gloves, gown, eye protection, and surgical mask

15 The nurse assigned to the respiratory care unit is working with four clients who have pneumonia. The nurse expects that the client infected with which organism would be assigned to a private room on the nursing unit?

1. Penicillin-resistant *Streptococcus pneumoniae* pneumonia
2. *Pseudomonas aeruginosa* pneumonia
3. *Pneumocystis carinii* pneumonia
4. *Legionella pneumophila* pneumonia

16 The nurse is caring for a client with hepatitis A. Which client statements indicate that teaching reinforced by the nurse about disease transmission was effective? Select all that apply.

1. "We must avoid kissing."
2. "We can use the same bath towels."
3. "We must avoid eating with the same utensils."
4. "We must wear masks."
5. "No special precautions are needed."

17 The nurse would take which actions to comply with principles of medical asepsis? Select all that apply.

1. Wash hands before and after assisting client with personal hygiene
2. Wear gown and gloves when working with client on contact precautions
3. Re-cap needle after administering insulin
4. Insert needle into rubber port of a previously used multidose vial without swabbing it with alcohol
5. Use surgical facemask while working with client who has tuberculosis

18 The nurse is preparing to enter the room of a client with pneumonia caused by penicillin-resistant *Streptococcus pneumoniae* (PRSP). The client has a tracheostomy and requires suctioning. Put the following personal protective equipment in order of donning. All options must be used.

1. Eye protection
2. Gloves
3. Mask
4. Gown

19 The nurse is preparing to leave the room of a client on transmission-based precautions. Place in the correct order the steps the nurse would follow to remove personal protective equipment and perform hand hygiene. All options must be used.

1. Remove gown.
2. Remove gloves.
3. Remove mask.
4. Remove eye protection.
5. Wash hands.

20 Several clients are being admitted to the hospital unit at one time. There is only one private room available. Which client has the highest priority for being admitted to this private room?

1. Client admitted for elective surgery who requested a private room prior to admission
2. Client with a large infected abdominal wound
3. Client who has a communicable respiratory infection
4. Client under the age of 12

ANSWERS & RATIONALES

1 **Answer: 4, 5** **Rationale:** A paper towel is used to shut off the faucet because the faucet is considered contaminated. Rubbing vigorously using firm, circular motions creates friction on the skin to assist in cleansing. The hands are considered to be more contaminated than the elbows, and the hands should be held down so water flows from least contaminated to most contaminated. Hot water can result in burns to the nurse. Warm water protects from burns and removes less protective skin oil than hot water. A surgical scrub is performed for over 5 minutes, while in medical asepsis hands are washed for at least 10-15 seconds. **Cognitive Level:** Applying **Client Need:** Safety and Infection Control **Integrated Process:** Nursing Process: Implementation **Content Area:** Fundamentals **Strategy:** The core issue of the question is utilization of medical asepsis. Recall basic principles of care and use the process of elimination to make a selection.

2 **Answer: 4** **Rationale:** Washing the skin with the combination of soap and water will remove the blood through mechanical friction. While alcohol can kill bacteria, it cannot kill viruses and fungi. Tissues would not adequately remove the blood. Hot water can burn the nurse, and water alone is inadequate in removing the blood. **Cognitive Level:** Applying **Client Need:** Safety and Infection Control **Integrated Process:** Nursing Process: Implementation **Content Area:** Fundamentals **Strategy:** The core issue of the question is the most effective means of reducing the risk of bloodborne disease transmission after contact with the skin. Recall principles of medical asepsis and use the process of elimination to make a selection.

3 **Answer: 2** **Rationale:** Using sterile technique to empty wound drains is aimed at interrupting the portal-of-entry link in the chain of infection. By using sterile technique, the nurse reduces the risk of introducing pathogens into the client's wound via the drain. Proper handling of specimens interrupts the chain of infection at the reservoir link. Disposing of gloves properly and washing hands after providing care breaks the chain of infection at the mode of transmission link. **Cognitive Level:** Applying **Client Need:** Safety and Infection Control **Integrated Process:** Nursing Process: Implementation **Content Area:** Fundamentals **Strategy:** Knowledge of the chain of infection is required. The portal of entry has to be a route whereby microorganisms can enter the client, so select the option that is directly in contact with the client.

4 **Answer: 2, 4** **Rationale:** Keeping the sterile field in view and holding items 6 inches above the sterile field are core principles of surgical asepsis. Washing hands before and after providing care and wearing personal protective equipment are core principles of medical asepsis. The outer 1 inch of a sterile field is considered contaminated, not 1.5 inches. **Cognitive Level:** Analyzing **Client Need:** Safety and Infection Control **Integrated Process:** Nursing Process: Implementation **Content Area:** Fundamentals **Strategy:** The core issue of the question is the ability to discriminate between medical and surgical asepsis and to choose correct interventions that support surgical asepsis. Use these principles and the process of elimination to make a selection.

5 **Answer: 2** **Rationale:** Herpes zoster is caused by the herpes virus varicella zoster. It can be transmitted by direct contact with the client. It is not transmitted via droplets or air currents. Neutropenic precautions are not indicated, because the client is not at risk for contracting an infection from the nurse or other individuals. **Cognitive Level:** Applying **Client Need:** Safety and Infection Control **Integrated Process:** Nursing Process: Implementation **Content Area:** Fundamentals **Strategy:** Herpes zoster is a viral skin infection. Specific knowledge of the types of transmission-based precautions is needed to select the correct answer. Eliminate airborne and droplet precautions because herpes zoster is not transmitted on air currents. Next, eliminate neutropenic precautions, which are used with immunocompromised clients.

6 **Answer: 1** **Rationale:** Tuberculosis is highly contagious and spread by inhalation of airborne droplets. Airborne precautions would be initiated, requiring everyone to wear a special particulate respirator fit-tested mask. Individuals who have had tuberculosis in the past can be re-exposed and develop the active form of the disease again. **Cognitive Level:** Applying **Client Need:** Safety and Infection Control **Integrated Process:** Communication and Documentation **Content Area:** Fundamentals **Strategy:** Look for similarities among the options in order to eliminate choices. In this case, the incorrect options are similar in that they suggest certain individuals would not be required to wear masks.

7 **Answer: 4, 1, 2, 3** **Rationale:** Gloves are removed first because they would be most contaminated. The mask would be removed next, followed by the gown. Eye protection is removed last, followed by washing the hands. **Cognitive Level:** Analyzing **Client Need:** Safety and Infection Control **Integrated Process:** Nursing Process: Implementation **Content Area:** Fundamentals **Strategy:** Remember that removal of PPE should occur in order of most contaminated to least contaminated items.

8 **Answer: 1** **Rationale:** SARS is a highly contagious viral respiratory illness that is spread by close person-to-person contact. SARS is transmitted by airborne respiratory route and by touching surfaces and objects contaminated with the virus. Instituting infection-control measures would be the first priority of the nurse. This action would protect both health care workers and other clients in the emergency department. Then all other interventions can be safely implemented. **Cognitive Level:** Analyzing **Client Need:** Safety and Infection Control **Integrated Process:** Nursing Process: Implementation **Content Area:** Fundamentals **Strategy:** The critical word *first* indicates all of the answers are correct and the nurse needs to set priorities. The first priority is to implement measures that protect the client and/or nurse—instituting airborne and contact precautions.

9 **Answer: 4** **Rationale:** Clients with antibiotic-resistant microorganisms must be isolated with transmission-based precautions. The organism is transmitted via close person-to-person direct contact and by touching contaminated surfaces and objects. Standard precautions are used with all clients, regardless of medical diagnosis. Reverse isolation (neutropenic precautions) is instituted for immunocompromised clients. This organism is not transmitted via droplet nuclei. **Cognitive Level:** Applying **Client Need:** Safety and Infection Control **Integrated Process:** Nursing Process: Implementation **Content Area:** Fundamentals **Strategy:** The critical words *vancomycin-intermediate* and *vancomycin-resistant* suggest the microorganism is difficult to eradicate, indicating that it is highly contagious. Eliminate standard and neutropenic, as they are not disease-specific precautions. Select contact over droplet, recalling that *Staphylococcus aureus* is a microorganism that is commonly found on skin.

10 **Answer: 4** **Rationale:** The client with tuberculosis can spread the infection by breathing, and requires a private room and airborne precautions. Proper equipment disposal, handwashing, and wearing protective equipment as indicated are precautions that would be implemented with any client, regardless of medical diagnosis. **Cognitive Level:** Applying **Client Need:** Safety and Infection Control **Integrated Process:** Nursing Process: Implementation **Content Area:** Fundamentals **Strategy:** The critical word *specific* suggests that the correct option must apply to a client with tuberculosis and is not a general measure used for all clients. Next, consider that this is transmitted by the airborne route to make the correct selection.

11 **Answer: 4** **Rationale:** Transmission-based precautions are required for all antibiotic-resistant microorganisms regardless of their mode of transmission. The other options indicate the need for medical and surgical asepsis in the care of the client but not the use of transmission-based precautions. **Cognitive Level:** Applying **Client Need:** Safety and Infection Control **Integrated Process:** Nursing Process: Planning **Content Area:** Fundamentals **Strategy:** The critical words *methicillin-resistant* indicate a microorganism that is difficult to eradicate. Eliminate each of the incorrect options after visualizing each situation because they can be managed by use of standard precautions.

12 **Answer: 4** **Rationale:** Scarlet fever is transmitted by particle droplets larger than 5 microns. Scarlet fever is not transmitted through sexual intercourse or the blood, or by consuming contaminated food. **Cognitive Level:** Applying **Client Need:** Safety and Infection Control **Integrated Process:** Communication and Documentation **Content Area:** Fundamentals **Strategy:** Begin by recalling that scarlet fever is transmitted by droplets. With this in mind, use the process of elimination to select the client situation that is compatible with the mode of transmission.

13 **Answer: 1** **Rationale:** Methicillin-resistant *Staphylococcus aureus* requires transmission-based contact precautions. Eye protection would be worn to protect the mucous membranes of the eyes when splatters of body fluids or excretions are possible. A gown would be worn when the nurse is in direct contact with the client. Contact precautions require gloves. N95 respirators are needed when caring for the client with tuberculosis, so it is inappropriate for this scenario. **Cognitive Level:** Applying **Client Need:** Safety and Infection Control **Integrated Process:** Nursing Process: Planning **Content Area:** Fundamentals **Strategy:** The critical word *unnecessary* suggests that all but one of the answers are correct. Using the process of elimination, look for the choice that identifies personal protective equipment that is not needed for contact precautions.

14 **Answer: 4** **Rationale:** An infection with vancomycin-resistant enterococci (VRE) requires transmission-based contact precautions. Since the nurse will be irrigating the wound and splatters of body fluids or exudates are possible, eye protection and surgical mask should be worn to protect the mucous membranes of the eyes, nose, and mouth. A gown would be worn when the nurse is in direct contact with the client. Contact precautions require gloves. Shoe covers are unnecessary. **Cognitive Level:** Applying **Client Need:** Safety and Infection Control **Integrated Process:** Nursing Process: Implementation **Content Area:** Fundamentals **Strategy:** Wound infections require contact precautions. Look for the option that identifies the correct PPE to be used with contact precautions. Eliminate options with particulate respirators and shoe covers, since these are unnecessary. Choose the option containing eye protection because the risk for splatters exists.

15 **Answer: 1** **Rationale:** While each option contains "pneumonia," the causative agent is different for each. An organism that is "resistant" is a pathogenic microorganism that is difficult to treat and requires droplet precautions. **Cognitive Level:** Applying **Client Need:** Safety and Infection Control **Integrated Process:** Nursing Process: Implementation **Content Area:** Fundamentals **Strategy:** Note the critical word *resistant* in the correct option. This provides a clue that the infection is difficult to treat and requires specific additional infection control practices, in this instance droplet precautions. The pneumonias in the other options do not require transmission based precautions.

16 **Answer: 1, 3** **Rationale:** Hepatitis A is an infectious disease transmitted by the fecal–oral route. Standard precautions are mandatory. Contact precautions are instituted if the client is incontinent of stool. Family members should avoid close contact with the client. They should not kiss the client or use the same eating utensils and bath towels. Masks are not necessary because the disease is not transmitted by the respiratory tract. **Cognitive Level:** Analyzing **Client Need:** Safety and Infection Control **Integrated Process:** Teaching and Learning **Content Area:** Fundamentals **Strategy:** The critical word *effective* indicates that options that are correct are the ones that should be selected. Knowledge of how hepatitis A is transmitted is necessary. The fecal–oral route of transmission eliminates the choices with bath towels and masks, and no need for special precautions. The correct options are similar in that they limit close contact with the client.

17 **Answer: 1, 2** **Rationale:** Washing hands before and after assisting a client with personal hygiene, and wearing a gown and gloves when working with a client on contact precautions are core principles of medical asepsis. Re-capping the needle after administering insulin violates principles of medical asepsis. Inserting a needle into the rubber port of a previously used multidose vial without swabbing it with alcohol violates principles of surgical asepsis. Using a surgical facemask while working with a client who has tuberculosis violates principles of transmission-based precautions for a client with tuberculosis. The nurse should wear an N95 (fit-tested) mask instead of a simple surgical mask. **Cognitive Level:** Applying **Client Need:** Safety and Infection Control **Integrated Process:** Nursing Process: Implementation **Content Area:** Fundamentals **Strategy:** Knowledge of medical versus surgical asepsis is essential to answer this question. Note that handwashing, gowns and gloves use medical aseptic technique, while recapping and not wiping do not. Also discard surgical face mask because it addresses transmission-based precautions and is an incorrect statement.

18 **Answer: 3, 4, 2, 1** **Rationale:** The gown is applied first, as it takes the most time to don. The mask is donned next, followed by eye protection. These items can be more securely applied with ungloved hands. Gloves are donned last, so the gloves can be pulled up to cover the cuffs of the gown. **Cognitive Level:** Applying **Client Need:** Safety and Infection Control **Integrated Process:** Nursing Process: Implementation **Content Area:** Fundamentals **Strategy:** Rationalize the ordering based on nursing knowledge of standard precautions and surgical asepsis. Visualize the procedure to aid in choosing correctly.

19 **Answer: 3, 1, 2, 4, 5** **Rationale:** Gloves are removed first, as they would be the most contaminated. The mask would be removed next, followed by the gown. Eye protection is removed last, followed by handwashing. **Cognitive Level:** Applying **Client Need:** Safety and Infection Control **Integrated Process:** Nursing Process: Implementation **Content Area:** Fundamentals **Strategy:** Washing the hands is last. Removal of gloves is first, as the gloves would be the most contaminated.

20 **Answer: 3** **Rationale:** The client with the airborne infection can spread this infection simply by breathing and requires isolation in a private room. This client with a request has no medical need for a private room. The client with the abdominal wound would not be as likely to spread this organism when the wound is dressed. The client who is 12 years old has no demonstrated medical need for a private room. **Cognitive Level:** Applying **Client Need:** Safety and Infection Control **Integrated Process:** Nursing Process: Implementation **Content Area:** Fundamentals **Strategy:** The critical term is highest priority. Recall CDC precaution guidelines to enable you to make safe room assignments.

Key Terms to Review

airborne precautions p. 58
chain of infection p. 55
medical asepsis p. 56
methicillin-resistant *Staphylococcus aureus* (MRSA) p. 59
personal protective equipment (PPE) p. 56
standard precautions p. 55
surgical asepsis p. 57
transmission-based precautions p. 58
vancomycin-resistant enterococci (VRE) p. 59

ANSWERS & RATIONALES

References

Berman, A., & Snyder, S. (2012). *Kozier & Erb's fundamentals of nursing: Concepts, process, and practice* (9th ed.). Upper Saddle River, NJ: Pearson Education.

Elkin, M. K., Perry, A. G., & Potter, P. A. (2008). *Nursing interventions and clinical skills* (4th ed.). St. Louis: Elsevier.

Francis J. Curry National Tuberculosis Center (n.d.). Airborne infection isolation rooms (AIIRs). Retrieved June 9, 2010, from http://www.nationaltbcenter.edu/TB_IC/docs/07AIIR.pdf

LeMone, P., & Burke, K., & Bauldoff, G. (2011). *Medical-surgical nursing: Critical thinking in client care* (5th ed.). Upper Saddle River, NJ: Pearson Education, Inc.

Perry, A., & Potter, P. (2010). *Clinical nursing skills and techniques* (7th ed.). St. Louis, MO: Elsevier.

Siegel, J.D., Rhinehart, E., Jackson, M., Chiarello, L., and the Healthcare Infection Control Practices Advisory Committee. *2007 Guideline for isolation precautions: Preventing transmission of infectious agents in healthcare settings*. Retrieved June 8, 2010, from http://www.cdc.gov/ncidod/dhqp/pdf/isolation2007.pdf

Smith, S. F., Duell, D. J., & Martin, B. C. (2012). *Clinical nursing skills: Basic to advanced skills* (8th ed.). Upper Saddle River, NJ: Pearson Education, Inc.

World Health Organization (2009). *WHO Guidelines on hand hygiene in health care*. Retrieved June 9, 2010, from http://whqlibdoc.who.int/publications/2009/9789241597906_eng.pdf

Test Yourself

Are you ready for the NCLEX-PN® or course exams? Use the practice tests on the companion website to check.

8 Reproduction, Family Planning, and Infertility

In this chapter

Cross Reference

Other chapters relevant to this content area are

I. THE MALE AND FEMALE REPRODUCTIVE SYSTEMS

A. Female internal structures

1. Vagina: muscular, membranous tube that connects external genitalia with cervix; also called birth canal; provides passageway for sperm, menstrual flow, and delivery of fetus
2. Uterus: hollow muscular organ that sheds endometrium with menstrual cycles and holds fetus during pregnancy; consists of fundus (superior portion), body (middle), and cervix (inferior)
3. Fallopian tubes: connect each ovary to uterus; ciliated to transport ovum or zygote; parts are isthmus (attached to uterus), ampulla (middle), and infundibulum (has fingerlike fimbriae reaching toward ovary)
4. Ovaries: almond-sized glands that secrete estrogen and progesterone; release one mature follicle and ovum per menstrual cycle from menarche to menopause, except during pregnancy

B. Functions of female structures

NCLEX®

1. Oogenesis: all oocytes are present at birth; ovum matures via meiosis under influence of follicle-stimulating hormone (FSH); luteinizing hormone (LH) transforms follicle into corpus luteum, which maintains pregnancy by producing progesterone; ovaries produce estrogen and progesterone in both pregnant and nonpregnant states
2. Menstruation occurs when ovum is not fertilized and corpus luteum disintegrates; endometrium becomes ischemic as progesterone and estrogen levels drop in last week of menstrual cycle, leading to sloughing of myometrium
3. Conception occurs in fallopian tube when a 23-chromosome–containing spermatozoon enters a 23-chromosome–containing ovum and produces a 23-chromosome-pair–containing diploid zygote
4. Pregnancy: cleavage (rapid mitotic division of zygote) creates a blastocyst, which in turn becomes a multicellular solid ball of 16 cells (morula); further division leads to trophoblast stage, when it implants within endometrium
5. Secretion production: cervical secretions become elastic and stretchy during ovulation to facilitate sperm transport toward ovum; endometrial secretions are rich in glycogen to nourish developing embryo until placental circulation is in place

C. Age-related changes of female reproductive system

1. Menses begin during puberty, stimulated by estrogen and progesterone

NCLEX®

2. Menopause is characterized by 1 year of amennorhea and occurs on average at age 50; postmenopausal changes of reproductive tract include thinning and atrophy of external and internal structures

D. Male internal structures

1. Testes: two lobular, oval glands located within scrotum where spermatogenesis takes place via meiosis
2. Epididymis: tubelike duct arising from top of each testis and ending in vas deferens
3. Vas deferens: connects epididymis to prostate gland
4. Prostate gland: encircles urethra just below bladder, producing alkaline fluid that is released during ejaculation
5. Seminal vesicles: lobular glands located just superior to prostate; produce seminal fluid (secreted during ejaculation to support sperm metabolism, motility)
6. Urethra: tube that passes through prostate and connects bladder and urethral meatus; also is passage for ejaculate
7. Semen: male ejaculate comprised of spermatozoa and glandular secretions; milky white in color; average volume from 2 to 5 mL

E. Functions of male structures

NCLEX®

1. Spermatogenesis takes place in testes; spermatozoa then proceed through epididymal tubules where motility and fertility develop, and are stored in reservoir of epididymis
2. Ejaculation is a series of muscular contractions that release spermatozoa and seminal fluid through penis
3. Urination also takes place through urethra in penis
4. Secretion production: prostate and seminal glands create a milky-white fluid that nourishes spermatozoa during and after ejaculation

F. Age-related changes of male reproductive system

1. Puberty: serum testosterone levels greatly increase, which stimulates elongation and thickening of penile shaft, spermatozoa production, and enlargement of testes and scrotum
2. Spermatozoa count, motility, and morphology begin to decrease in middle age
3. External organs atrophy in older adults

II. FERTILITY

A. Female components

NCLEX®

1. Primary infertility occurs before ever conceiving; secondary infertility occurs after a pregnancy
2. Menstrual cycle: follicular phase is days 1 to 14 of cycle, incorporating menstrual phase (menses) and proliferative phase (beginning of endometrial thickening); variations in menstrual cycle length are caused by variations in length of follicular phase; luteal phase is days 15 to 28 of cycle and includes secretory phase (endometrium secretes glycogen to prepare for implantation of fertilized ovum) and ischemic phase (beginning of endometrial breakdown after no fertilization); luteal phase is always 12 to 14 days long

NCLEX®

3. Ovulation: an ovum begins to mature during follicular phase as a result of FSH; at onset of luteal phase, a blisterlike graafian follicle appears and enlarges on surface of ovary under influence of FSH and LH; ovum oozes out of follicle; ruptured follicle becomes corpus luteum, which disintegrates if fertilization does not occur or creates progesterone if fertilization does occur; a body fat percentage of

14% or more is needed to support ovulation (estrogen is stored in body fat); less than 14% body fat will result in irregular menses or amenorrhea

4. Cervical mucus: becomes more plentiful, with a thinner and more stretchy consistency, and forms columns during ovulation to facilitate transport of sperm into uterus; cervical mucus production can be impeded by surgery for abnormal Pap smears
5. Uterine structure: abnormalities result in unhealthy myometrium and fewer healthy places for successful embryo implantaton; abnormalities include a septum (a fibrous, vertical, wall-like structure in center of uterine body), a unicornate uterus (one-sided, banana-shaped uterus), or a bicornate uterus (two banana-shaped uteri side by side, curving away from each other; may end at one cervix or have two cervices and vaginas)
6. Hormones
   - NCLEX® a. Estrogen: produced by ovaries, especially ovarian follicle during ovulation; responsible for development of secondary sex characteristics at puberty; peaks in follicular phase of menstrual cycle; inhibits FSH and LH production
   - b. Progesterone: secreted by corpus luteum; peaks during luteal phase; stimulates FSH and LH secretion; responsible for endometrial thickening
   - c. FSH: anterior pituitary hormone that matures one ovarian follicle each cycle
   - d. LH: anterior pituitary hormone that completes maturation of ovarian follicle; ovulation occurs 10 to 12 hours after LH peaks
7. Fallopian tube must be patent for sperm to reach ovum and for fertilized ovum to reach uterus; scarring can occur from an infection, such as a ruptured appendix during adolescence or **pelvic inflammatory disease (PID)**, an infection of uterus and fallopian tubes; cilia in fallopian tubes (which propel ovum toward oncoming sperm) have decreased motility in cigarette smokers, thus decreasing fertility

B. Male components

1. Sperm production: at least 50% of sperm must have normal form for optimal fertility; normal levels are greater than 20 million sperm per milliliter of ejaculate; at least 50% of sperm should have normal motion patterns; decreased sperm count and motility can be caused by increased scrotal temperature (from frequent hot tub or sauna use, tight clothing, or varicocele); heavy alcohol, marijuana, or cocaine use; scrotal trauma; mumps during adulthood; developmental factors; and cigarette smoking
2. Testosterone is primary hormone responsible for libido, sperm production, ability to achieve and maintain erection, and ejaculation
3. Erections must be maintained long enough for ejaculation to occur in vagina and near cervix for optimal fertility
4. Ejaculation must occur and contain sufficient numbers of healthy sperm to achieve fertility

III. INFERTILITY

A. Common diagnostic studies for infertility

1. NCLEX® **Basal body temperature (BBT)** or resting body temperature: obtained by taking oral temperature daily prior to arising from bed and graphing results on a month-long graph; a sudden dip occurs on day before ovulation and is followed by a rise of 0.5 to 1.0°F, which indicates ovulation; this rise remains until menstruation begins; **fertility awareness** includes monitoring BBT and cervical mucus changes to detect ovulation
2. Serum hormone testing: venous blood levels of FSH and LH in infertile women indicate ovarian function
3. Postcoital exam: couple has intercourse 8 to 12 hours prior to exam, 1 or 2 days before expected ovulation; a 10-mL syringe with catheter attached is used to collect a specimen of vaginal secretions, which are examined for signs of infection, number of active and nonmotile spermatozoa, sperm–mucus interaction, and consistency of cervical mucus
4. **Endometrial biopsy**: obtaining an endometrial tissue sample; client is positioned on exam table in lithotomy position; provider inserts vaginal speculum to visualize cervix; a paracervical block is first administered to decrease cramping and pain; a sample of endometrium is obtained to check for a luteal phase defect (lack of progesterone)
   - a. Preprocedure care includes assisting client (after undressing below waist and applying gown) onto exam table and advising client that she will feel crampy discomfort both during paracervical block administration and during aspiration
   - b. Postprocedure care should include providing sanitary napkins for client (vaginal bleeding will occur) and assessing client for a vasovagal response (sudden fainting caused by hypotension induced by vagus nerve stimulation) prior to arising from exam table

5. Hysterosalpingogram (HSG): detects uterine anomalies (septate, unicornate, or bicornate structures) and tubal anomalies or blockage; after client is sedated or anesthetized, iodine-based radiopaque dye is instilled via catheter into uterus and tubes to outline these structures, and x-rays are taken
6. Laparoscopy: carried out under general or epidural anesthesia; three-puncture approach (umbilicus and suprapubic areas) often used to introduce instruments into abdomen, which is insufflated with carbon dioxide; laparoscope is then used to view pelvic structures or perform surgical procedures
7. Male semen analysis: client ejaculates into specimen container, and ejaculate is examined microscopically for number, morphology, and motility of sperm
8. Male and female partner: antisperm antibody evaluation of cervical mucus and ejaculate are tested for agglutination (indicates secretory immunological reactions are occurring between cervical mucus and spermatozoa)

B. Psychological factors associated with infertility

NCLEX® 1. Many couples experience shame, guilt, blame, or grief stages during diagnosis and treatment of infertility

NCLEX® 2. Nurse should facilitate communication between couple and provide information on resources for coping with infertility, such as support groups; professional counseling may help some couples

C. Collaborative management of infertility

1. Educational needs of infertile couple often include
   a. Performing various procedures (e.g., semen collection or postcoital exam)
   b. Understanding results of tests and assessments
   c. Self-monitoring during medication administration
   d. Understanding how assisted reproductive technologies (ART) are performed
2. Hormonal therapy is used to induce ovulation in preparation for in vitro fertilization; client and/or partner must learn subcutaneous and/or intramuscular injection techniques
3. Medications such as clomiphene citrate (Clomid, Serophene) and single-dose hCG are used to induce ovulation in cases of anovulatory menstrual cycles (menstrual cycles without ovulation) or to achieve multiple ova prior to in vitro fertilization (see also Chapter 56); risks of ovulation induction include multiple births and ovarian hyperstimulation, which can result in enlarged ovaries, abdominal distention, pain, and occasionally ovarian cysts
4. Sperm washing for intrauterine insemination (IUI): client's ejaculate is centrifuged to concentrate spermatozoa, rinsed in saline to remove seminal fluid, and are again centrifuged and used for either in vitro or intrauterine artificial insemination

NCLEX® 5. Intrauterine insemination is a form of **artificial insemination** whereby
   a. Sperm collected within 3 hours of masturbation are inserted via catheter into uterus
   b. Donor sperm may be used if male partner's sperm count or motility is low or for single women who desire to become pregnant; sperm donor identity is kept confidential

6. **In vitro fertilization (IVF)**: multiple ova are harvested via large-bore needle and syringe transvaginally under ultrasound guidance; ova are then mixed with spermatozoa, and up to four resultant embryos are returned to uterus 2 to 3 days later; extra embryos can be frozen for later implantation; side effects include ovarian cysts, multiple births, and ovarian hyperstimulation
   a. Preprocedure care: instruct client to give synthetic FSH injections subcutaneously in abdomen, thigh, or upper arm to stimulate ova production for 5 to 6 days preprocedure; give sedation for ova retrieval procedure; observe client for 2 hours after egg retrieval, and instruct to limit activity for next 24 hours
   b. Postprocedure care following embryo placement in uterus includes instructing client to have minimal activity for 24 hours; progesterone supplementation is commonly prescribed
7. Other specialized fertilization procedures
   a. Gamete intrafallopian transfer (GIFT): harvested ova and sperm are mixed and placed via large-bore needle and syringe under ultrasound guidance into ovarian end of fallopian tube
   b. Tubal embryo transfer (TET): in vitro fertilized embryos are placed into fallopian tube via large-bore needle and syringe under ultrasound guidance; performed 42 to 72 hours after egg retrieval
   c. Zygote intrafallopian transfer (ZIFT): ova fertilized in vitro are placed into fallopian tube via large-bore needle and syringe under ultrasound guidance; performed 18 to 24 hours after egg retrieval
   d. Micro-epididymal sperm aspiration (MESA) is a microsurgical technique to obtain a specimen of sperm from epididymis; done as an outpatient procedure under sedation and/or local anesthesia
   e. Percutaneous epididymal sperm aspiration (PESA) utilizes a small needle under local anesthesia to aspirate sperm from epididymis

IV. GENERAL CONSIDERATIONS IN FAMILY PLANNING AND CONTRACEPTION

A. Overview

1. Goal of family planning is to assist clients with reproductive decision making; enable client control to prevent pregnancy, limit number of children, space time between children, and/or voluntarily interrupt pregnancy as desired
2. Legal issues related to family planning and contraception
   a. Laws pertaining to provision of contraceptives to minors without parental consent vary among states
   b. Some states may require consent from client's spouse for sterilization and voluntary interruption of pregnancy
   c. Because of potentially serious complications associated with many contraceptive methods, informed consent is obtained; document information provided and client's understanding of information

NCLEX®

3. The mnemonic BRAIDED (see Memory Aid) may be useful when counseling a client about family planning and contraceptive methods

Memory Aid

Use the mnemonic BRAIDED to recall important considerations regarding consent for contraceptive use:

- **B** Benefits: information about advantages
- **R** Risks: information about disadvantages
- **A** Alternatives: information about other available methods
- **I** Inquiries: opportunity for the client to ask questions
- **D** Decisions: opportunity for client to make or change a decision
- **E** Explanations: information about selected method and its use
- **D** Documentation: information given and client understanding

V. NATURAL METHODS OF FAMILY PLANNING

A. Natural methods are safe, situational methods requiring self-awareness and self-control to be effective

B. Types of natural family planning methods

1. Abstinence: avoiding sexual intercourse

NCLEX®

   a. Advantages: safe, free, and available to all; 100% effective in preventing pregnancy and sexually transmitted infections (STIs) when consistently practiced; can be initiated at any time; encourages communication between partners
   b. Disadvantage: both partners must practice self-control
   c. Client education: teach alternative methods of obtaining sexual pleasure; provide positive feedback to clients who desire and maintain abstinence
2. Coitus interruptus (withdrawal)
   a. Requires male to withdraw penis from female's vagina when urge to ejaculate occurs and ejaculate away from external female genitalia
   b. Clients must utilize self-control because most pleasurable moment during intercourse may coincide with time to withdraw penis
   c. Advantages: can be practiced at any time during menstrual cycle; is free
   d. Disadvantages: least reliable contraceptive method; some pre-ejaculatory fluid (which may contain sperm) may escape from penis during excitement phase prior to ejaculation; at peak sexual excitement, exercising self-control may be difficult
   e. Client education: before intercourse male should urinate and wipe off tip of penis to decrease risk of sperm entering vagina; conception may occur if pre-ejaculatory fluid containing sperm enters introitus; spermicide or postcoital contraceptive may be needed if female partner is exposed to sperm

VI. FERTILITY AWARENESS METHODS OF FAMILY PLANNING

A. Overview

1. These methods are based on an understanding of woman's ovulation cycle and timing of sexual intercourse
2. All methods attempt to identify period of female fertility and avoid unprotected intercourse during that time

3. Advantages: free, safe, and acceptable to couples whose religious beliefs prohibit other methods; increases awareness of woman's body; encourages couple communication; can prevent or plan a pregnancy
4. Disadvantages: requires extensive initial counseling and education; may interfere with sexual spontaneity; may be difficult or impossible for women with irregular menstrual cycles; offers no protection against STIs if used alone; theoretically reliable but less effective in actual use

B. *Calendar method*

1. Also known as rhythm method; based on assumptions that ovulation occurs 14 days (plus or minus 2 days) prior to next menses, sperm are viable for up to 7 days, and ovum is viable for up to 3 days
2. Client education: teach woman to first keep a menstrual calendar for 6 to 8 months to identify shortest and longest cycles; using first day of menses as first day of cycle, calculate fertile period by subtracting 18 days from length of shortest cycle through length of longest cycle minus 11 days; counsel to avoid intercourse during fertile period

C. Basal body temperature (BBT) method

1. Based on thermal shift in menstrual cycle; temperature drops just prior to ovulation, rises and fluctuates at a higher level until 2 to 4 days prior to next menses, then falls if no conception
2. Client education
   a. Teach client to measure temperature with a BBT thermometer, which shows tenths of a degree, and record findings on a temperature chart
   NCLEX® b. Teach client to take temperature each morning prior to arising or beginning activity
   c. Counsel to avoid intercourse on day temperature drops and for 3 days after temperature rises
   d. Inform client that reliability can be affected by a decrease in BBT too small to detect, factors that raise or lower BBT (such as illness, stress, fatigue, consuming alcohol the prior evening, or sleeping in a heated waterbed) and that intercourse just prior to drop in BBT may result in pregnancy

D. Cervical mucus method

1. Also known as ovulation or Billings method; based on cervical mucus changes that occur during menstrual cycle; effectiveness same as BBT method
2. Client education
   a. Teach client to assess cervical mucus daily for amount, color, consistency, and viscosity
   NCLEX® b. Counsel to avoid intercourse when client first notices cervical mucus becoming more clear, elastic, and slippery and for about 4 days after
   c. Convey sensitivity as women who are uncomfortable touching their genitals may find this method unacceptable
   d. Instruct client that cervical mucus can be affected by douches and vaginal deodorants, semen, blood and discharge from vaginal infections, antihistamine drugs, and contraceptive gels, foams, film, or suppositories

E. *Symptothermal method*

1. The symptothermal method involves assessing multiple indicators of ovulation, recording findings and coital history on a menstrual calendar, then abstaining from intercourse during fertile period; provides no protection against STIs
2. Client education
   a. Instruct client to assess and record BBT and condition of cervical mucus as primary indicators of ovulation
   b. Teach client to recognize and record secondary indicators of ovulation: increased libido, abdominal bloating, midcycle abdominal pain (Mittelschmerz), breast or pelvic tenderness, pelvic or vulvar fullness, slight dilatation of cervical os, and softer cervix located higher in vagina

VII. MECHANICAL METHODS OF CONTRACEPTION

A. Overview

1. Provide a physical or chemical barrier to block sperm from entering cervix
2. Some barrier devices are made from latex and should be avoided by those with latex allergies

B. *Male condom*

1. A sheath made of latex, plastic, or natural membranes, which is placed over erect penis to collect semen
2. Client education
   a. Check package expiration date, and if past date, use another condom
   NCLEX® b. Avoid using oil-based lubricants, but contraceptive foam or water-based lubricants may be used

c. Put on condom by placing it on tip of erect penis, leaving enough room at tip to collect sperm, then unrolling condom from tip to base of erect penis

NCLEX®

d. After intercourse, client should hold rim of condom while withdrawing erect penis from vagina to prevent leakage

e. Inspect used condom for tears or holes because these will decrease effectiveness

f. Discard used condom in a disposable waste container; do not flush in toilet

3. Advantages
   - a. Males can participate in contraception
   - b. Sexual intercourse may be prolonged
   - c. Condoms are available in a variety of sizes and styles at low cost
   - d. Partners can participate in placing condom to enhance enjoyment
   - e. All condoms except those made of natural skins offer protection against pregnancy and STI; natural skin condoms have pores, which can allow passage of viruses and do not protect against STIs

4. Disadvantages
   - a. Penis must be erect before placing condom
   - b. To prevent spillage of semen, male must withdraw after ejaculating, while penis is still erect
   - c. Condoms can rupture or leak, increasing potential for semen to escape into vagina
   - d. Oil-based lubricants can decrease condom's effectiveness
   - e. Condoms are for single use only
   - f. Misplacement, perineal/vaginal irritation, or dulled penile sensation may occur

C. *Female condom*

1. A thin, polyurethane sheath with flexible rings at each end, which covers cervix, lines vagina, and partially shields perineum

2. Client education
   - a. Insert closed end of condom into vagina so ring fits loosely against cervix
   - b. Have partner insert penis into open end leaving approximately 1 inch of sheath from flexible ring outside of introitus
   - NCLEX® c. After intercourse, before woman stands up, remove condom by squeezing and twisting outer ring to close sheath while gently pulling it from vagina

3. Advantages
   - a. May be inserted up to 8 hours before intercourse
   - b. Clients who are sensitive to latex can use female condom
   - c. Both partners are protected against STIs during intercourse
   - d. Female condoms are available without a prescription
   - e. Use of lubricants will not decrease effectiveness
   - f. Breastfeeding women can safely use condoms

4. Disadvantages
   - a. May twist or slip during intercourse
   - b. If penis is placed outside of condom, effectiveness is jeopardized
   - c. Improper removal results in risk of ejaculate leaking out of condom
   - d. Outer ring may irritate external genitalia
   - e. High cost, noise produced with intercourse, or altered sensation are unacceptable for some couples
   - f. Initially, insertion may be difficult or awkward

D. *Spermicide*

1. The approved spermicidal agent in U.S. is nonoxynol-9(N9); allergic response is possible

2. Forms a chemical barrier preventing pregnancy by killing sperm or neutralizing vaginal secretions; is available as a cream, jelly, foam, vaginal film, and suppository

3. When N9 is used with a diaphragm or condom, contraceptive and antimicrobial benefits increase

4. Client education
   - a. Apply N9 inside vagina and close to cervix before placing penis near introitus
   - NCLEX® b. N9 must be applied with each act of sexual intercourse
   - NCLEX® c. Contraceptive foam, cream, and gel are effective immediately, while contraceptive film and suppository are effective 15 minutes after insertion into vagina
   - d. When used alone, effectiveness is no longer than 1 hour

5. Advantages
   - a. No prescription is required
   - b. May be used alone, with a diaphragm, or with a condom

c. Foam, gel, and suppository may add additional lubrication and moisture
d. The penis can remain in vagina following ejaculation
e. Method is safe for breastfeeding women
f. A variety of forms offers clients additional choices

6. Disadvantages
a. May be irritating to one or both clients or be perceived as messy
b. May interfere with spontaneity, as it is inserted before each act of intercourse and may require an interval of time before onset of action
c. Does not protect against STIs if used alone without additional barrier method

E. ***Diaphragm***

1. A dome-shaped appliance made of latex (or silicone if latex allergy) with a flexible rim that fits over cervix; used with spermicidal cream or jelly; prevents sperm from entering cervix
2. Client education
a. Utilize models and visual aids to demonstrate insertion and removal
b. Teach proper insertion: apply about a teaspoon of spermicidal cream or jelly around rim and inside cup; squeeze sides of diaphragm together, insert through vagina, place side of device containing spermicide over cervix, and push upper edge under symphysis pubis
c. Teach proper removal by grasping rim to dislodge from cervix and pulling down to remove through vagina
d. Encourage client to practice insertion and removal when health care provider is present to check for proper placement in vagina
NCLEX® e. Diaphragm should be left in place at least 6 hours after coitus
NCLEX® f. If diaphragm is placed more than 4 hours prior to intercourse or if coitus is desired again within 6 hours, a condom should be used or additional spermicide should be used without disturbing diaphragm
NCLEX® g. Remove at least once during a 24-hour period to decrease risk of toxic shock syndrome
h. Clean diaphragm with mild soap and water and inspect for tears, punctures, and thinning; avoid using oil-based lubricants, which weaken the latex; replace diaphragm if any damage is observed
i. Air dry device thoroughly and store in carrying case away from light and heat
j. Avoid use during menses or when abnormal vaginal discharge is present to decrease risk of toxic shock syndrome
k. Contact health care provider for any warning signs listed in Table 8–1

3. Advantages
a. Gives woman control
b. Provides some protection against STIs
c. A partner may insert diaphragm if client has trouble with placement or as part of foreplay
d. Contains no hormones and is safe for breastfeeding client
e. Penis can remain inside vagina after ejaculation

4. Disadvantages
a. Must be fitted by a qualified health care provider and replaced annually
NCLEX® b. Refitting may be needed following pregnancy or 10- to 15-pound weight gain or loss
c. Some clients may have difficulty learning to correctly place diaphragm

NCLEX® 5. Contraindications
a. A history of urinary tract infections; pressure of diaphragm on urethra may interfere with complete bladder emptying and increase risk of infection from urine stasis
b. A history of toxic shock syndrome; if left in place for a long period of time, diaphragm may increase risk of infection

F. ***Cervical cap***

1. A small, cup-shaped device that fits over cervix, is held in place by suction, and acts as a barrier between sperm and cervix; has many similarities to diaphragm
2. Client education
a. Teach client to apply spermicide inside cap
NCLEX® b. Insert cap at least 20 minutes but not longer than 4 hours prior to intercourse
c. May be left in place up to 48 hours
NCLEX® d. Reapplication of spermicide with repeated intercourse is not needed
e. Do not use cap during menses or if abnormal vaginal discharge is present
NCLEX® f. Contact health care provider for warning signs described in Table 8–1

3. Advantages of cervical cap are similar to those of diaphragm
4. Disadvantages
   a. May be more difficult to fit because of limited sizes; some clients may have difficulty inserting and removing cervical cap

NCLEX®

   b. Must be fitted by a qualified health care provider and should be replaced annually; clients must be rechecked for fit following pregnancy or 10- to 15-pound weight gain or loss; effectiveness is reduced for parous women

G. ***Vaginal contraceptive sponge***
1. A small, round synthetic sponge with nonoxynol-9 spermicide; has a concave or cupped area on cervical side and a loop for easy removal on other
2. Client education
   a. Moisten sponge with water prior to insertion to activate spermicide
   b. Place concave side of sponge next to cervix
   c. Leave sponge in place for at least 6 hours after intercourse
   d. Remove by pulling polyester loop on convex side of sponge downward and out of vagina

Table 8–1 Warning Signs and Symptoms Associated with Various Methods of Contraception

Method	Warning Signs and Symptoms
Cervical cap, diaphragm, and contraceptive sponge	Toxic shock syndrome: elevation of temperature >101.4°F, diarrhea and vomiting, weakness and faintness, muscle aches, sore throat, sunburn-type rash Difficult or painful urination Abdominal or pelvic fullness Foul-smelling vaginal discharge
IUD	Acronym **PAINS** **P**—Period late (pregnancy), abnormal spotting or bleeding **A**—Abdominal pain, pain with intercourse **I**—Infection exposure (STI), abnormal vaginal discharge **N**—Not feeling well, fever >100.4°F, chills **S**—String missing, shorter or longer than usually felt
Oral contraceptives	Acronym **ACHES** **A**—Abdominal pain **C**—Chest pain, cough, and/or shortness of breath **H**—Headaches, dizziness, weakness, or numbness **E**—Eye problems (blurring or change in vision) and speech problems **S**—Severe leg, calf, and/or thigh pain
Vasectomy	Fever >100.4°F Excessive pain Difficulty urinating Redness, swelling, bruising, drainage, or skin edges of the incision that are not closed Bleeding at the site
Tubal ligation	Fever >100.4°F Excessive pain Difficulty with defecation or urination Nausea or vomiting Redness, swelling, bruising, drainage, or skin edges of the incision that are not closed

e. The sponge provides protection up to 24 hours and for repeated acts of intercourse; remove by 24-hour time limit to reduce risk of toxic shock syndrome
f. Contact health care provider for warning signs listed in Table 8–1
3. Advantages: same as for diaphragm; plus low cost and no prescription
4. Disadvantages: some clients perceive sponge as bulky or awkward when in place, or uncomfortable during intercourse; effectiveness is reduced for parous women

H. ***Intrauterine device (IUD)***
1. Triggers spermicidal-type reaction that prevents fertilization and has local inflammatory effects on endometrium
2. Types of IUDs available in United States
NCLEX® a. Copper T380A (ParaGard) can be left in place for 10 years
b. Levonorgestrel-releasing intrauterine system (LNG-IUS or Mirena) can be left in place 5 years
c. Preferred candidates for use include women in a stable monogamous relationship (low risk for STI) with no history of pelvic inflammatory disease (PID) and with healthy uterine anatomy
3. Client education
a. Cramping or intermittent bleeding may occur for 2 to 6 weeks after insertion
b. The first few menses after placement may be irregular
c. Follow-up examination is suggested in 4 to 8 weeks
NCLEX® d. Check for presence of string protruding through cervix by inserting a finger into vagina once a week for first month and then after each menses
NCLEX® e. Counsel client to contact health care provider if exposed to STI or warning signs known as PAINS develop, as listed in Table 8–1

Memory Aid

Use the mnemonics embedded in Table 8–1 to remember the warning signs for complications of selected contraceptive methods.

4. Advantages
a. Are highly effective and provide continuous contraceptive protection
b. Do not interact with medications
c. Are a good contraceptive option for women who cannot use hormone contraceptives, are breast-feeding, or are smokers over age 35
5. Disadvantages
a. Must be inserted by a qualified health care professional
b. May cause discomfort, bleeding, and cramping during and between menses
NCLEX® c. Uterus may perforate during insertion
d. May be expelled spontaneously
e. Does not protect clients from acquiring STIs

VIII. HORMONAL METHODS OF CONTRACEPTION

A. ***Combined oral contraceptives*** **(COCs or birth control pills) act by inhibiting release of an ovum, blocking cyclical release of gonadotropin-releasing hormone, and changing cervical mucus**
1. Typical combined oral contraceptives contain both estrogen and progestin and are available in 21-day and 28-day packages
2. Extended oral contraceptives (Seasonique, Seasonale) are 91-day regimens in which client takes active pill daily for 84 days, followed by inactive pill for 7 days, during which client has menses
3. Progestin-only pill, also known as a mini-pill, does not contain estrogen, contains less progestin than combination pills, and may be used by lactating women, women with mild hypertension, and those experiencing side effects from oral contraceptives containing estrogen
4. Client education
a. When starting oral contraceptives, begin pills on first Sunday after onset of menses and take one pill at same time each day
b. If a 28-day pack is prescribed or client is taking progestin-only pills, do not skip days between packages
c. Clients using a 21-day pack should wait 7 days before starting next cycle of pills
NCLEX® d. If one progestin-only contraceptive pill is missed at any time during cycle, take it immediately and take next pill at regular time; any time a pill is missed, use an additional method of contraception through end of that cycle

NCLEX® e. If one combination oral contraceptive pill is missed at any time during cycle, take missed pill immediately and take next pill at the regular time, and no back-up method is needed; if two pills are missed during first 2 weeks, take two pills for next 2 days and resume taking pills on regular schedule; if two pills are missed during the third week, take one pill daily until Sunday, then begin a new pack on Sunday without missing any days; if three or more pills are missed at any time, take one pill daily until Sunday, then begin a new pack on Sunday without missing any days; if two or more pills are missed at any time, use a back-up method for 1 week or consider emergency postcoital contraception if unprotected intercourse occurs

NCLEX® f. Observe for side effects of oral contraceptives, which can be estrogen related (such as thromboembolic disease, headache, fluid retention, and nausea) or progestin related (including acne, increased HDL cholesterol level, depression, and hirsutism)

NCLEX® g. Contact health care provider immediately if warning signs develop, which are remembered using the mnemonic ACHES; see Table 8–1

5. Advantages
   a. Use of method is not directly related to act of sexual intercourse
   b. Menstrual periods are usually more regular and predictable; amount of menstrual flow and premenstrual symptoms are decreased
   c. Incidence or degree of iron-deficiency anemia may be reduced
   d. Are safe throughout reproductive years for women who do not smoke
   e. Noncontraceptive benefits include a decreased risk of ectopic pregnancy, fibrocystic breast disease, and ovarian and endometrial cancers; improvement of acne; and some protection against development of functional ovarian cysts
6. Disadvantages
   a. Progestin-only pill: risk of ectopic pregnancy is increased; are more likely to cause irregular bleeding or amenorrhea
   b. COCs offer no protection against STIs
   c. Clients need to remember to take a pill at same time each day
   d. NCLEX® Clients with preexisting medical problems may not be candidates for this method
   e. COCs may decrease effectiveness of insulin and oral anticoagulants such as warfarin (Coumadin)
   f. NCLEX® Effectiveness may be decreased when taken with other drugs, such as phenytoin (Dilantin), carbamazepine (Tegretol), primidone (Mysoline), topirimate (Topamax), griseofulvin (Grisactin), rifampin (Rifadin), ampicillin (Omnipen), and tetracycline (Achromycin)
7. Contraindications
   a. COCs should not be taken by women with a history of thromboembolic or cardiovascular disorders, breast cancer, or estrogen-dependent neoplasms
   b. COCs should not be used if woman is currently pregnant, lactating for less than 6 weeks, smokes more than 20 cigarettes per day and is over 35 years old, has headaches with focal neurological symptoms, has prolonged immobility or surgery on legs, has hypertension higher than 160/100 or diabetes mellitus for 20 years or more with vascular disease

B. Other combined hormonal methods

1. Contraceptive skin patch (Ortho Evra): applied weekly to one of four sites (abdomen, buttocks, upper outer arm or trunk but not breasts); during week 4 no patch is worn and menses occurs
2. Vaginal contraceptive ring (Nuvaring) is a soft flexible ring inserted into vagina for 3 weeks and delivers low-dose, sustained release contraceptive hormone; removed for week 4 and menses occurs

C. *Subdermal implants*

1. Consist of silastic capsules containing levonorgestrel, a progestin, implanted subdermally into upper inner arm during first 7 days of menstrual cycle; prevent ovulation and stimulate production of thick cervical mucus, preventing penetration by sperm
2. Client education
   a. Inform of possible side effects such as spotting, irregular bleeding, amenorrhea, weight gain, headache, fluid retention, mood changes, and depression
   b. Teach signs and symptoms of infection indicating need for postprocedure followup
3. Advantages: not user-dependent for effectiveness; provides continuous contraception not related to sexual intercourse; does not contain estrogen; effective within 24 hours and for up to 5 years
4. Disadvantages: requires minor surgery to insert and remove implants; may be visible under skin; irregular or prolonged menses may be unacceptable to client; cost may be prohibitive; offers no protection against STIs; slightly higher failure rates have been reported in women weighing more than 154 pounds in fifth year of use

D. Long-acting progestin injections

1. Medroxyprogesterone acetate (Depo-Provera) is a long-acting progestin that blocks luteinizing hormone surge, suppresses ovulation and thickens cervical mucus to prevent penetration of sperm
2. Client education
   - **a.** Inform of potential side effects such as menstrual irregularities, headache, weight gain, breast tenderness, and depression
   - **b.** Follow 3-month injection regimen to maintain contraceptive effects; subsequent dose must be given 80 to 90 days after previous dose for continuous contraceptive protection
   - **c.** Counsel client to contact health care provider for warning signs of ACHES identified in Table 8–1
   - **d.** Note black box warning to reevaluate use after 2 years for other contraceptive options because of interference with calcium
   - **e.** Teach client to use dietary calcium supplements
3. Advantages: contraception is not related to sexual intercourse; safe for lactating women; does not contain estrogen; requires administration only every 3 months
4. Disadvantages: injection must be repeated within 80 to 90 days to maintain effectiveness; clients with cardiovascular disorders or breast cancer are not candidates for use; return of fertility may be delayed up to 1 year after stopping method

E. *Emergency postcoital contraception*

1. Indicated when there is concern about pregnancy because of unprotected intercourse or when a contraceptive method fails
2. Because it is an emergency method, it should not be used on a frequent or regular basis
3. Levonorgestrel, the only one currently available in U.S., should be initiated as soon as possible after unprotected intercourse or contraceptive failure
4. Is sometimes called "morning-after pill," which is deceiving because dose should be taken as soon as possible after intercourse and a second dose 12 hours later

IX. SURGICAL METHODS OF CONTRACEPTION

A. Overview

1. Surgical contraceptive methods: result in voluntary sterilization of male or female
2. Surgical consent: obtained after risks and benefits of specific method are explained

B. *Vasectomy*

1. A form of sterilization in which vas deferens is resected through small incisions made in each side of scrotum to block passage of sperm
2. Client education
   - **a.** Procedure takes about 15 to 20 minutes and can be performed in a clinic setting under local anesthesia
   - **b.** Client should not drive immediately after procedure; should have someone drive him home after discharge and remain with him for 24 hours postprocedure
   - **c.** Rest with minimal activity for 48 hours; avoid strenuous activity for 1 week
   - **d.** Avoid tub baths for 48 hours
   - **e.** Wear a scrotal support to increase comfort
   - *NCLEX®* **f.** Use ice packs intermittently to minimize discomfort and swelling
   - **g.** Sitz baths can be used after 48 hours
   - *NCLEX®* **h.** Contact health care provider if warning signs develop, as listed in Table 8–1
   - **i.** Sterility is not achieved until semen is free of sperm, about 4 to 6 weeks or 6 to 36 ejaculations; until then, use another contraceptive method
   - **j.** Two or three semen samples should be analyzed to verify sterility prior to resuming unprotected intercourse
   - **k.** Semen should be rechecked at 6 and 12 months to verify stertility has been maintained
   - **l.** Advantages: effectiveness rate is 99.85%; recovery time is short; simpler, safer, and more effective than female sterilization; complications are rare; sexual function is not affected; is cost-effective and convenient
   - **m.** Disadvantages: although reversal may be possible, this method is considered permanent; potential complications are adverse reaction to anesthesia, infection, bleeding, sperm granuloma, or spontaneous reanastomosis of vas deferens with restored fertility

C. *Tubal ligation*

1. Fallopian tubes are accessed via two small incisions into abdomen and visualized using a laparoscope, then cut, tied, cauterized, or banded to block passage of sperm and prevent ovum from becoming fertilized

NCLEX®

2. Client education
   a. Out-patient procedure takes about 30 minutes; is performed under regional or general anesthesia
   b. May need to restrict food and fluid intake for several hours prior to procedure, especially if general anesthesia is planned
   c. May experience pain for several days after procedure
   d. Avoid tub baths for 48 hours and driving, lifting, and strenuous activity for 1 week
   e. Contact health care provider if warning signs develop, as listed in Table 8–1
3. Advantages: permanent and effective in preventing pregnancy; may be performed at any time (immediately after childbirth is optimal because uterus is enlarged and fallopian tubes are easy to identify); sexual function and spontaneity are not affected
4. Disadvantages: requires outpatient surgery; potential complications are adverse reaction to anesthesia, infection, and bleeding; if pregnancy occurs after tubal ligation, risk of ectopic pregnancy increases; reversal of procedure may not be possible; occasional changes in menstrual pattern: posttubal ligation syndrome

Check Your NCLEX–PN® Exam I.Q.

You are ready for testing on this content if you can

- Provide support to a client and partner during infertility assessment and treatment.
- Use knowledge from biologic and social sciences in discussions with clients contemplating contraception and family planning.
- Gauge the client's readiness to use contraception.
- Determine the client's preferences for contraceptive methods.
- Describe risks and contraindications to selected contraceptive methods.

PRACTICE TEST

1 The client has been diagnosed with Trichomonas vaginitis. The nurse reinforces that this infection can affect fertility by which of the following?

1. Using glycogen in vaginal secretions, leaving no nutrition for spermatozoa
2. Blocking fallopian tubes, which prohibits spermatozoa from reaching an ovum
3. Decreasing pH of vaginal secretions, thus destroying most spermatozoa
4. Increasing temperature inside the vagina, which decreases sperm motility

2 The nurse is concerned that which viral infection, if experienced by an adult male, may cause infertility?

1. Varicella zoster
2. Rubella
3. Influenza
4. Mumps

3 What information would the nurse gather before scheduling a client's endometrial biopsy?

1. Usual length of menstrual cycle
2. Blood type and Rh factor
3. Presence of any metal implants
4. Last type of birth control used

4. The client has an obstruction between the uterus and fallopian tubes. In obtaining a health history, the nurse collects information about which possible etiology?

1. Rubella infection prior to adolescence
2. Pelvic inflammatory disease caused by gonorrhea
3. Smoking two packs of cigarettes per day
4. Ingestion of 2 ounces of alcohol daily

5. Which statement by a client could indicate a potential problem for a couple planning to use coitus interruptus as a means of birth control?

1. "I really don't want to get pregnant right now, so we need a very effective method."
2. "I think I can always pull out before I ejaculate."
3. "We don't have any other sex partners."
4. "We want a contraceptive method that is inexpensive and completely natural."

6. Which client statement indicates that reinforcement of teaching about cervical mucus changes as an indicator of ovulation has been understood?

1. "If my cervical mucus is yellowish and thick, I am probably fertile."
2. "The thin, clear mucus will block sperm from getting to my cervix."
3. "If my cervical mucus is thick and white, I will need to avoid intercourse or use a backup method of contraception."
4. "If my cervical mucus is thin and stretchable, I am probably fertile."

7. The client, who is married and has three children, has come to the family planning clinic asking about a birth control method that is most effective and sanctioned by the Roman Catholic Church. What would be the nurse's best suggestion?

1. Billings or cervical assessment method
2. Ovulation testing kit
3. Symptothermal method
4. Basal body temperature (BBT) method

8. The client is interested in using female condoms and wants to know if there are any disadvantages. What is the nurse's best response?

1. "The female condom provides good protection against pregnancy but not against sexually transmitted infections (STIs)."
2. "The female condom may be difficult to insert and may be uncomfortable to both partners."
3. "The female condom is very effective; let me arrange to get you a prescription."
4. "The female condom is made of latex and should not be used by those with latex allergies."

9. Which client being seen in the outpatient clinic would be the best candidate for insertion of an intrauterine device (IUD)?

1. A client who is married, has one child, and wants to get pregnant in about 6 months
2. A client who is unmarried, has no children, and has numerous sexual partners
3. A client who is married, has two children, and does not want more children for at least 3 years
4. A client who is unmarried, has one child, and has a history of pelvic inflammatory disease (PID)

10. The client, a 16-year-old female, has come to the clinic for contraception after recently becoming sexually active. The client states that several friends use spermicides and asks about their advantages and disadvantages. What is the nurse's best response?

1. "If you want an effective method, you should choose something else."
2. "It is a very convenient method to use overall and you will be able to insert the spermicide up to 4 hours before intercourse."
3. "Spermicides cause very few problems for the majority of people, and they are almost 100% effective."
4. "Spermicides may or may not be a good choice; they have a failure rate of about 21% and offer some protection against sexually transmitted infections."

PRACTICE TEST

11 In teaching a client about the risk of toxic shock syndrome associated with diaphragm use, the nurse should tell the client to take which action to decrease her risk?

1. Leave the diaphragm in place for 36–48 hours after intercourse.
2. Avoid using soap when cleaning the device.
3. Wear latex or rubber gloves when handling the device.
4. Seek treatment of any vaginal infection before reusing the device.

12 The client has come to the clinic to discuss contraception. If discovered during the nurse's assessment, what data would be a contraindication to use of the cervical cap?

1. History of blood clots
2. Age greater than 35 years
3. Abnormal Pap smear 6 months ago
4. Elevated liver enzymes

13 In reinforcing client teaching about factors that can decrease the effectiveness of oral contraceptives, which item should be included by the nurse?

1. Antibiotic use
2. Weight gain
3. Amenorrhea
4. Iron-deficiency anemia

14 A 2-day postpartum client is interested in a contraceptive method that is not associated with intercourse and will not interfere with lactation. The nurse concludes that which method may be best for this client?

1. Progestin-only oral contraceptives (mini-pills)
2. Female condoms
3. Diaphragm
4. Triphasic pills

15 A client has been admitted as an outpatient for a tubal ligation. Following the procedure, the client should be told to expect which of the following?

1. Hot flashes and other hormonally associated symptoms
2. Heavier bleeding with menstruation
3. Possible mild pain for a few to several days
4. Change in sexual function

16 A man has decided to take total responsibility for birth control and elects to have a vasectomy. What information about this procedure would the nurse reinforce with the client?

1. Epididymis will be removed so spermatozoa can become mobile.
2. Urethra will be severed to prevent ejaculation.
3. Prostate gland will be removed to create a more acidic environment hostile to sperm.
4. Vas deferens will be cut or cauterized to prevent sperm from being transported.

17 The client is a long-distance runner, with 9.0% body fat. Which of the following data would the nurse expect to collect when speaking with this client?

1. Regular menses, and a BBT that indicates ovulation
2. Irregular menses, and a BBT that shows ovulation
3. Regular menses, and a BBT that indicates lack of ovulation
4. Irregular menses, and a BBT that indicates lack of ovulation

18 The nurse concludes that a client needs additional information when the client makes which statement about what the couple needs to do to become pregnant?

1. "We need to have intercourse on the 14th day of my menstrual cycle."
2. "Have intercourse when my basal body temperature rises."
3. "Have intercourse every other day during the week before and after ovulation."
4. "Abstain from intercourse for the month prior to the month we want to conceive."

19 The nurse reinforces the physician's explanation that a client with fallopian tube blockage would be a candidate for which method of achieving pregnancy?

1. Natural family planning
2. In vitro fertilization
3. Tubal ligation
4. Sperm washing

20 The nurse assisting in the women's health clinic determines that which clients would be appropriate candidates for use of emergency postcoital contraception? Select all that apply.

1. Had unprotected intercourse 4 days ago
2. Took her oral contraceptive 7 hours late
3. Removed her cervical cap 40 hours after intercourse
4. Had her last Depo-Provera injection 4 months ago
5. Had been sexually assaulted the previous day

21 Which statements indicate to the nurse that a male client understands how to correctly apply a condom? Select all that apply.

1. "I need to put it on before the penis is erect."
2. "I should unroll the condom, then place it on the penis."
3. "When putting on the condom, I need to leave some space at the tip to collect the sperm."
4. "I can use oil-based lubricants if needed."
5. "I can use a water-based lubricant if needed."

ANSWERS & RATIONALES

1 **Answer: 3** **Rationale:** Vaginal fluid pH is slightly alkaline, as is semen. Spermatozoa cannot survive in an acidic environment. Trichomonas vaginitis increases the acidity of the vaginal and cervical secretions, thus reducing the number of viable sperm. The microorganisms do not use glycogen. The microorganisms do not block the fallopian tubes, as by definition this infection is in the vagina. The microorganisms are not able to increase the temperature inside the vagina. **Cognitive Level:** Applying **Client Need:** Health Promotion and Maintenance **Integrated Process:** Teaching and Learning **Content Area:** Adult Health **Strategy:** Look for the option that is a true statement and use knowledge of pathophysiology to eliminate incorrect distractors.

2 **Answer: 4** **Rationale:** Mumps in adult males can cause permanent blockage of the vas deferens, contributing to or resulting in infertility. Varicella, rubella and influenza do not have this effect. **Cognitive Level:** Applying **Client Need:** Health Promotion and Maintenance **Integrated Process:** Nursing Process: Planning **Content Area:** Adult Health **Strategy:** Look for the option that exerts this effect and use knowledge of pathophysiology to eliminate incorrect distracters.

3 **Answer: 1** **Rationale:** The nurse assesses the first day of the last normal menstrual period and the menstrual cycle length. Endometrial biopsy is performed on days 21–27 of the menstrual cycle to assess endometrial response to progesterone and development of luteal phase endometrium. It is unnecessary to assess for blood type and Rh factor, metal implants, or most recent type of birth control used. **Cognitive Level:** Applying **Client Need:** Health Promotion and Maintenance **Integrated Process:** Nursing Process: Data Collection **Content Area:** Adult Health **Strategy:** Eliminate implants first as irrelevant and then blood type because excessive bleeding requiring transfusion is not expected. Recall the relationship between the menstrual cycle and biopsy procedure to choose length of cycle over birth control method.

4 **Answer: 2** **Rationale:** Infectious processes of the reproductive tract such as PID may result in tubal scarring and therefore tubal blockage. Rubella infection in childhood usually results in the development of active immunity to the disease. Smoking and alcohol present health risks to the woman but not related to tubal patency. **Cognitive Level:** Analyzing **Client Need:** Health Promotion and Maintenance **Integrated Process:** Nursing Process: Data Collection **Content Area:** Adult Health **Strategy:** Look for an association between blockage in the reproductive system and a condition that is causally related to this. Recall that inflammation and infection can lead to scarring and obstruction in the body. Choose PID over rubella of because of its association with inflammation.

5 **Answer: 1** **Rationale:** Because some semen is released before ejaculation, coitus interruptus has an 18% failure rate and would not be considered a very effective method for a couple wanting to avoid pregnancy. An ability to withdraw before ejaculation is necessary for coitus interruptus to be effective, so the client's statement would be consistent with successful use of this method. Not having other sex partners has no effect on choice of coitus interruptus as a contraceptive method. Coitus interruptus has no cost and is completely natural. **Cognitive Level:** Analyzing **Client Need:** Health Promotion and Maintenance **Integrated Process:** Nursing Process: Data Collection **Content Area:** Adult Health **Strategy:** The critical words in the question are *potential problem*, guiding you to look for a statement that corresponds to a negative aspect of coitus interruptus. With this in mind, each incorrect option can be systematically eliminated.

6 **Answer: 4** **Rationale:** Thin and clear cervical mucus indicates a rising level of estrogen and impending ovulation. Stretchability of the cervical mucus, or spinnbarkeit, is indicative of the fertile period and promotes motility of the sperm. Thick cervical mucus occurs during the infertile period when sexual intercourse is unlikely to result in pregnancy. **Cognitive Level:** Analyzing **Client Need:** Health Promotion and Maintenance **Integrated Process:** Nursing Process: Evaluation **Content Area:** Adult Health **Strategy:** The critical word *understood* indicates the correct option is also a correct statement. Use knowledge of physical changes during ovulation to make a selection, or use logic to reason that sperm are more motile through thinner liquids than thicker liquids.

7 **Answer: 3** **Rationale:** The symptothermal method combines cervical mucus and BBT measurements and results in a lower failure rate than either BBT or cervical mucus as a single assessment of the fertile period. This method is completely natural and congruent with beliefs of this religious group. Ovulation testing kits do not give enough warning of ovulation to prevent pregnancy. **Cognitive Level:** Analyzing **Client Need:** Health Promotion and Maintenance **Integrated Process:** Nursing Process: Planning **Content Area:** Adult Health **Strategy:** Note the word *best*, which indicates more than one

option, could be true. In this question, eliminate ovulation testing first as least timely, and choose symptothermal method over Billings and BBT methods because the symptothermal method is comprehensive and includes these other options.

8 **Answer: 2 Rationale:** Made of polyurethane, the female condom does not require a prescription but can be difficult to insert, and can cause discomfort. It is effective against both STIs and pregnancy. **Cognitive Level:** Applying **Client Need:** Health Promotion and Maintenance **Integrated Process:** Communication and Documentation **Content Area:** Adult Health **Strategy:** Note the critical word *disadvantages* to focus your selection. Eliminate first the option referring to a prescription because a prescription is not necessary. Eliminate the option that says it is only good at protecting against pregnancy next because it is an effective barrier against STIs, and eliminate the option containing latex as a false statement.

9 **Answer: 3 Rationale:** An IUD is a long-tem method of contraception usually recommended for women who have been pregnant and are in a monogamous relationship so that they are at a low risk for sexually transmitted infection. The clients in the incorrect options have one or more factors that should guide them to select a different contraceptive method. **Cognitive Level:** Analyzing **Client Need:** Health Promotion and Maintenance **Integrated Process:** Nursing Process: Planning **Content Area:** Adult Health **Strategy:** Use knowledge of advantages and disadvantages of this birth control method to evaluate the options. Eliminate the options with PID and three sexual partners because of the risk for infection, and choose the client desiring pregnancy in 3 years instead of 6 months because the method is for long-term, not short-term use.

10 **Answer: 4 Rationale:** Spermicides have a failure rate of 21%, and do offer some protection against sexually transmitted infections. Other key information needed is the sexual history of the client and her partner(s) to more accurately assess risk for STIs. The nurse should not provide advice to the client. Spermicides must be used within 30 minutes of intercourse. Spermicides have a failure rate of 21%. **Cognitive Level:** Applying **Client Need:** Health Promotion and Maintenance **Integrated Process:** Communication and Documentation **Content Area:** Adult Health **Strategy:** Note the focus of the question is on advantages and disadvantages of spermicide use. Eliminate options containing false statements first and then eliminate the option that provides advice to the client.

11 **Answer: 4 Rationale:** The client should seek treatment for any new vaginal infections before reusing the device. The woman should remove the device within 24 hours of intercourse. The diaphragm should be cleaned with soap and water. When removing a diaphragm used for contraception, the woman should wash her hands with soap and water, but it is not necessary to wear gloves. **Cognitive Level:** Applying **Client Need:** Health Promotion and Maintenance **Integrated Process:** Nursing Process: Implementation **Content Area:** Adult Health **Strategy:** The positive wording of the question indicates that the correct answer contains a true statement. Use nursing knowledge and the process of elimination to reject the incorrect options, which are false statements.

12 **Answer: 3 Rationale:** Long-term exposure to secretions, spermicides, and bacteria trapped inside the cervical cap can lead to abnormal Pap smear results. Because this client already has a history of an abnormal Pap smear, a different contraceptive method should be explored. A history of blood clots, maternal age, and elevated liver enzymes are not contraindications to using a cervical cap. **Cognitive Level:** Analyzing **Client Need:** Health Promotion and Maintenance **Integrated Process:** Nursing Process: Planning **Content Area:** Adult Health **Strategy:** Note the critical word *contraindication*, which indicates a negative question stem. Next, select the option that would pose a risk to this client with regard to use of a cervical cap.

13 **Answer: 1 Rationale:** Antibiotic use can decrease the effectiveness of oral contraceptives. Oral contraceptives can help prevent iron-deficient anemia by decreasing menstrual blood flow. Weight gain and anemia are not related to the effectiveness of birth control pills. **Cognitive Level:** Applying **Client Need:** Health Promotion and Maintenance **Integrated Process:** Nursing Process: Implementation **Content Area:** Adult Health **Strategy:** Note the critical phrase *decrease the effectiveness*, and use the process of elimination and nursing knowledge to make a selection. Recall as a general principle that medications can adversely interact, which is the basis for this question.

14 **Answer: 1 Rationale:** Progestin-only pills are safe for lactating women. The use of female condoms is associated with sexual intercourse. The use of a diaphragm is associated with sexual intercourse. Oral contraceptives with a combination of estrogen and progestin are not recommended in the first 6 weeks of lactation. In addition, the long-term effects on the infant are not known. **Cognitive Level:** Applying **Client Need:** Health Promotion and Maintenance **Integrated Process:** Nursing Process: Planning **Content Area:** Adult Health **Strategy:** Note the critical phrase *not associated with intercourse*, which eliminates female condoms and diaphragm. Choose progestin-only contraceptives because they estrogen-free and thus contain fewer hormones to which a breastfeeding infant would be exposed.

15 **Answer: 3 Rationale:** Some clients report mild pain after the procedure, which is usually relieved with analgesics. Hormonal symptoms such as hot flashes are not typical after tubal ligation. Changes in menstruation, such as heavy bleeding, are not typical after tubal ligation. Changes in sexual function are not typical after tubal ligation. **Cognitive Level:** Applying **Client Need:** Health Promotion and Maintenance **Integrated Process:** Nursing Process: Implementation **Content Area:** Adult Health **Strategy:** The wording of the question indicates that the correct answer is an option that is a true statement. Use knowledge that this is a minor surgical procedure and the process of elimination to make your selection.

16 **Answer: 4 Rationale:** The scrotal portion of the vas deferens is surgically incised or cauterized. Sperm are still produced, but they can no longer be squeezed from the storage site (epididymis) into the urethra for ejaculation. The epididymis is not excised during this procedure. Severing the urethra would prevent passage of urine from the bladder as well as semen and would not be considered. The prostate gland is not excised during this procedure. **Cognitive Level:** Applying **Client Need:** Reduction of Risk Potential **Integrated Process:** Teaching and Learning **Content Area:** Adult Health **Strategy:** The critical words are *vasectomy* and *teach the client.* Use knowledge of the male reproductive system and vasectomy to choose the correct answer.

17 **Answer: 4 Rationale:** Fourteen percent body fat is considered adequate to have regular menses and regular ovulation. A client with less than 10% body fat will ovulate and

ANSWERS & RATIONALES

menstruate very irregularly if at all. **Cognitive Level:** Applying **Client Need:** Health Promotion and Maintenance **Integrated Process:** Nursing Process: Data Collection **Content Area:** Maternal-Newborn **Strategy:** Critical words are *long-distance runner* and *9.0% body fat*. Use knowledge of physiology of menstrual cycle and ovulation to answer the question.

18 **Answer: 4** **Rationale:** Abstinence decreases the likelihood of becoming pregnant and indicates a need for further teaching. This increases the likelihood of conception by timing intercourse around the expected time of ovulation. **Cognitive Level:** Analyzing **Client Need:** Health Promotion and Maintenance **Integrated Process:** Teaching and Learning **Content Area:** Maternal-Newborn **Strategy:** Critical words are *needs further teaching*, indicating an incorrect response from the client. Use knowledge of the normal menstrual cycle to eliminate incorrect options.

19 **Answer: 2** **Rationale:** Tubal blockage will prohibit sperm from traveling through the fallopian tubes to reach an ovum and fertilize it. In vitro fertilization involves harvesting ova and placing them with sperm in a petri dish. The resultant embryos are then returned to the uterus. Natural family planning when the client has a fallopian tube blockage would not result in pregnancy. Tubal ligation would not result in pregnancy; it would prevent it. Sperm washing when the client has a fallopian tube blockage would not result in pregnancy. **Cognitive Level:** Applying **Client Need:** Health Promotion and Maintenance **Integrated Process:** Nursing Process: Planning **Content Area:** Maternal-Newborn **Strategy:** Critical words in the stem of the question are *fallopian tube blockage* and *achieve pregnancy*. Use knowledge of anatomy and physiology and methods of artificial insemination to choose correctly.

20 **Answer: 4, 5** **Rationale:** Emergency postcoital contraception must be initiated within 72 hours of unprotected intercourse, sexual assault, or method failure. Oral contraceptives may be taken up to 12 hours late and cervical caps may be left in up to 48 hours without compromising safety. Depo-Provera is given every 80–90 days, after which a repeat dose is needed or emergency postcoital contraceptive protection is indicated. **Cognitive Level:** Analyzing **Client Need:** Health Promotion wand Maintenance **Integrated Process:** Nursing Process: Data Collection **Content Area:** Maternal-Newborn **Strategy:** Critical words are *candidate* and *emergency postcoital contraception*. Knowledge of emergency postcoital indications is necessary to answer the question correctly.

21 **Answer: 3, 5** **Rationale:** The male condom is placed when the penis is erect, then rolled down. Leaving space at the end of the condom to collect semen can prevent breakage or spillage after ejaculation. Water-based lubricants can be used to provide additional comfort, if needed. Oil-based lubricants are contraindicated. **Cognitive Level:** Analyzing **Client Need:** Health Promotion and Maintenance **Integrated Process:** Teaching and Learning **Content Area:** Maternal-Newborn **Strategy:** The wording of the question is positive, indicating that the correct options are true statements about points of client education. Use nursing knowledge to select these options.

Key Terms to Review

References

Davidson, M., London, M., & Ladewig, P. (2012). *Olds' maternal newborn nursing and women's health across the lifespan* (9th ed.). Upper Saddle River, NJ: Pearson Education, Inc.

Ladewig, P., London, M., Moberly, S., & Davidson, M. (2010). *Contemporary maternal-newborn nursing care* (7th ed.). Upper Saddle River, NJ: Pearson Education, Inc.

London, M., Ladewig, P., Ball, J., Bindler, R., & Cowen, K. (2011). *Maternal & child nursing care* (3rd ed.). Upper Saddle River, NJ: Pearson Education, Inc.

Perry, S., Hockenberry, M., Lowdermilk, D., & Wilson, D. (2010). *Maternal child nursing care* (4th ed.). St. Louis, MO: Elsevier.

Planned Parenthood Federation of America. Birth Control. Retrieved June 13, 2010, from http://www.plannedparenthood.org/birth-control-4211.htm

Test Yourself

Are you ready for the NCLEX-PN® or course exams? Use the practice tests on the companion website to check.

9 Uncomplicated Antenatal Care

In this chapter

Cross Reference

Other chapters relevant to this content area are

Reproduction, Family Planning, and Infertility	**Chapter 8**
Uncomplicated Labor and Delivery Care	**Chapter 10**
Uncomplicated Postpartum Care	**Chapter 11**
Uncomplicated Newborn Care	**Chapter 12**
Complicated Antenatal Care	**Chapter 45**
Complicated Labor and Delivery Care	**Chapter 46**
Complicated Postpartum Care	**Chapter 47**
Complicated Newborn Care	**Chapter 48**

I. ESSENTIAL CONCEPTS OF PREGNANCY

A. *Estimated date of birth (EDB),* or due date: can be determined by several methods

NCLEX®

1. **Naegele's Rule**: take first day of last menstrual period, subtract 3 months, and add 7 days; this date is most accurate when woman remembers last menstrual period, has menses every 28 days, and was not taking oral contraceptives
2. **McDonald's method** uses uterine size to indicate gestational age by measuring, in centimeters (cm), distance from symphysis pubis to top of uterine fundus
    - **a.** This distance, **fundal height**, correlates well with number of weeks' gestation between 22 and 34 weeks
    - **b.** Formula for calculating gestational age based on fundal height:

$$\frac{\text{distance in centimeters} \times 8}{7} = \text{total weeks of gestation}$$

    - **c.** Prediction of EDB using this method can be affected by maternal height, irregular fetal growth, multiple gestation, and abnormal amounts of amniotic fluid

NCLEX®

3. **Quickening**, feeling of fetal movement by mother, usually occurs between 16 and 18 weeks; because of wide range of times quickening is experienced, this method gives a less accurate EDB

4. Auscultation of fetal heart rate (FHR) can occur as early as 8 weeks' gestation using an ultrasonic Doppler device but is more commonly heard between 10 and 12 weeks; this variation can result in a less accurate date
5. Ultrasound examination estimates EDB when date of last menstrual period is unknown or uterine size is inconsistent with EDB calculated with Naegele's rule or McDonald's method

NCLEX®

B. ***Gravida* and *para***

1. Gravida and para are terms to describe a woman's childbearing history
2. Gravida is number of times woman has been pregnant
3. Para is number of infants delivered after 20 weeks' gestation, born dead or alive; multiple births count as one delivery regardless of number of infants delivered
4. TPAL (see Memory Aid) is a more detailed description of para

Memory Aid

Use the mnemonic TPAL to remember the detailed description of parity (para)
T number of **T**erm infants born after 37 completed weeks
P number of **P**reterm infants born between 20 and 37 weeks
A number of pregnancies that end in spontaneous or therapeutic **A**bortion prior to 20 weeks
L number of **L**iving children

II. SIGNS AND SYMPTOMS OF PREGNANCY

NCLEX®

A. ***Presumptive signs of pregnancy***

1. Subjective signs and symptoms that the woman reports (see Table 9–1)
2. May or may not be associated with pregnancy

NCLEX®

B. ***Probable signs of pregnancy***

1. Objective signs and symptoms noted by examiner (see Table 9–1)
2. May or may not be associated with pregnancy

C. ***Positive signs of pregnancy***

1. Diagnostic signs and symptoms noted by examiner (see Table 9–1)
2. Can only be associated with pregnancy

III. NURSING CARE DURING FIRST PRENATAL VISIT

A. **First prenatal visit**

1. Determine why woman is seeking care; perform complete health history and physical examination
2. History taking should include
   a. Weight, nutrition, and exercise pattern
   b. Over-the-counter (OTC), prescription, and illicit drug use
   c. Allergies and potential teratogens
   d. History of surgery or present disease states, especially those with known implications for pregnancy, such as viral infections, diabetes, hypertension, cardiovascular disease, renal problems, and thyroid or bleeding disorders
   e. Gynecologic history including date of last Papanicolaou (Pap) smear, previous infections, age at menarche, and menstrual, contraceptive, and obstetric histories

Table 9–1 Signs and Symptoms of Pregnancy

Category	Signs and Symptoms
Presumptive signs	Amenorrhea, nausea and vomiting, fatigue, urinary frequency, breast changes, quickening
Probable signs	Hegar's sign, McDonald's sign, enlargement of abdomen, pigmentation changes, abdominal striae, ballottement, positive pregnancy test, palpation of fetal outline
Positive signs	Fetal heartbeat, fetal movement palpable by examiner, visualization of the fetus by ultrasound

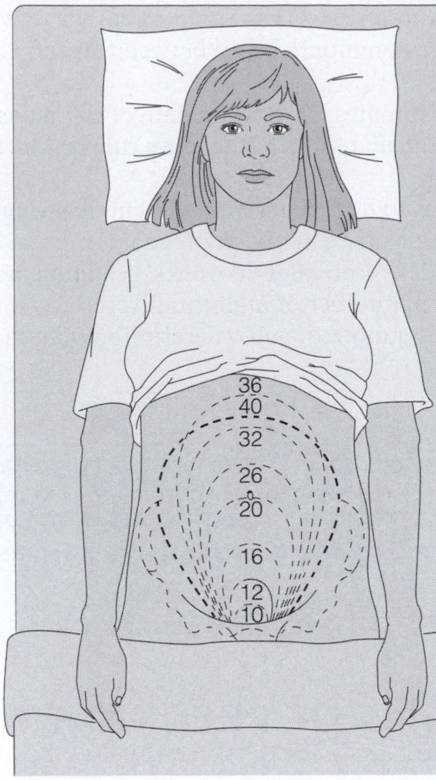

Figure 9–1

Fundal height changes during pregnancy.

3. Physical data collection
    a. **Fetal heart rate** (FHR): fetal heart beats per minute, heard by fetoscope (beginning at about 16 weeks) or by ultrasonic Doppler device (beginning at about 8 weeks); is useful in determining gestational age and fetal well-being; normally ranges from 120 to 160 beats per minute (NCLEX®)
    b. Fundal height, a measurement from symphysis pubis to top of uterine fundus (in cm), helps assess gestational age and fetal growth (see Figure 9–1) (NCLEX®)
    c. Complete maternal physical examination includes vital signs; height and weight; thyroid; heart and breath sounds; and reproductive organs including pelvic musculature, size of uterus, and adequacy of pelvis for delivery (NCLEX®)
    d. Laboratory assessment includes hematocrit and hemoglobin, blood type, Rh and irregular antibody, rubella titer, tuberculin skin test, renal function tests, urinalysis and culture, screening for sexually transmitted infections (STIs), and Pap test; offer of HIV test (see section that follows)
4. Psychosocial data collection (NCLEX®)
    a. Emotions such as excitement, anxiety, and/or ambivalence about pregnancy
    b. Available support systems
    c. Stability and functional level of client's immediate and extended family
    d. Economic support adequate for housing, daily needs, and medical expenses
    e. Cultural preferences including practices to be used or avoided during pregnancy, preference of caregiver gender, and preferred support person(s)
5. Collaborative management
    a. Prepare client for physical exam by stating what to expect
    b. Provide information about prenatal care program, setting, and personnel
    c. Provide information about physiologic changes to be expected in pregnancy as well as danger signs to report

B. Laboratory and diagnostic testing during first prenatal visit

1. Testing done at initial visit can be analyzed for abnormal results; intervention can be implemented immediately or at follow-up visits, as indicated
2. Complete blood count (CBC): provides information on hematologic and other body systems; advantages include being inexpensive, easy to perform, and quickly available results; for individual tests, normal results, and changes in pregnancy, see Table 9–2

Table 9–2 Complete Blood Count

Test	Normal Results	Changes in Pregnancy
Red blood cell count	4.2–5.4 million/mm^3	5–6.25 million/mm^3
Hemoglobin	12–16 grams/dL	>11grams/dL
Hematocrit	37–47%	>33%
Mean corpuscular volume	80–95/cubic micrometer	none
Mean corpuscular hemoglobin	27–31/picogram	none
Mean corpuscular hemoglobin concentration	32–36 grams/dL packed RBCs	none
White blood cell (WBC) count	5000–10,000/mm^3	5000–15,000/mm^3
Polymorphonuclear cells	55–70% of WBCs	60–85% of WBCs
Lymphocytes	20–40% of WBCs	15–40% of WBCs
Platelet count	150,000–400,000/mm^3	none until 3–5 days after delivery

3. Blood group and Rh typing
   a. Purpose: to determine client's blood group and Rh status so that fetus at risk for developing erythroblastosis fetalis or hyperbilirubinemia in neonatal period may be identified
   NCLEX® b. Significant results: type O or Rh negative mothers may require further fetal or infant testing
4. Urinalysis: collect fresh urine specimen in urine container; if culture is to be done, collect midstream clean-catch specimen
   a. pH may be decreased with poor glucose metabolism and ketone acids in urine
   NCLEX® b. Specific gravity may be increased with dehydration caused by excessive vomiting as seen in hyperemesis gravidarum
   c. Color should be pale yellow to amber depending on foods ingested and concentration
   NCLEX® d. Glucose reabsorption is impaired in pregnancy resulting in spilling of glucose in urine at a blood glucose level of 160 mg/dL
   NCLEX® e. Protein may normally be found in urine during pregnancy at a level of trace to +1 using dipstick method; increased protein may indicate preeclampsia
   NCLEX® f. White blood cells (WBCs) or nitrites can indicate possible urinary tract infection, which can place client at risk for preterm labor
   g. Casts, which are formed from clumps of materials or cells in renal distal and collecting tubules, form when urine is acidic and concentrated; can be associated with proteinuria and stasis in renal tubules
   NCLEX® h. Ketones may indicate diabetes mellitus and hyperglycemia
   i. Urine culture can identify women with asyptomatic bacteriuria; greater than 10,000 bacteria/mL urine indicates urinary tract infection
   j. Urine toxicology can screen for illicit drug use
5. **TORCH infections**: a group of infections caused by viruses and protozoa that cause serious fetal problems when contracted by mother during pregnancy; each letter represents a different infection: **T**oxoplasmosis, **O**ther infections (usually hepatitis), **R**ubella, **C**ytomegalovirus, and **H**erpes simplex virus; see sections that follow
6. Toxoplasmosis
   a. Cause: infection with toxoplasmosis protozoan
   b. Transmission: infection in mother is associated with consuming infested undercooked meat and poor hand hygiene after handling cat litter; fetal infection occurs if mother acquires toxoplasmosis after conception and passes it to fetus via placenta
   c. Diagnosis: is made by serologic testing; indirect fluorescent antibody test is most commonly used; IgG titers greater than 1:256 suggest a recent infection, whereas IgM titers greater than 1:256 indicate an acute infection
   d. Maternal effects: flu-like symptoms in acute phase
   e. Fetal/neonatal effects: miscarriage is likely in early pregnancy; in neonates central nervous system (CNS) lesions can result in hydrocephaly, microcephaly, chronic retinitis, and seizures
7. Other infections, usually hepatitis virus
   a. Cause: infection with hepatitis A virus (HAV) or hepatitis B virus (HBV); HBV is most common in fetus

b. Transmission: HAV is spread by droplets or hands and is associated with poor handwashing after defecation; transmission to fetus is rare but can occur; HBV transmission to fetus can occur via placenta, but usually occurs when infant is exposed to blood and genital secretions during labor and delivery
c. Diagnosis: radioimmunoassay and enzyme-linked immunosorbent assay methods are used to detect HAV antibodies; elevated IgM antibody in the absence of IgG antibody indicates probable acute hepatitis; elevated IgG in the absence of IgM indicates a convalescent or chronic stage of HAV; HBV is detected through hepatitis B surface antigen (HbsAg)
d. Maternal effects: fever, malaise, nausea, and abdominal discomfort; may be associated with liver failure
NCLEX® e. Fetal/neonatal effects: preterm birth, hepatitis infection, and intrauterine fetal death

8. Rubella, sometimes called German measles or 3-day measles
a. Cause: infection with rubella virus
NCLEX® b. Transmission: infection is spread by droplet
c. Diagnosis: IgG antibodies to rubella are measured to determine client's rubella immunity status; a titer of 1:10 or greater indicates that woman is immune to rubella; a titer of 1:8 or less indicates minimal or no immunity
d. Maternal effects: fever, rash, and mild lymphedema
NCLEX® e. Fetal/neonatal effects: miscarriage, congenital anomalies, and death

9. Cytomegalovirus (CMV)
a. Cause: exposure to CMV
NCLEX® b. Transmission: respiratory droplet, semen, cervical and vaginal secretions, breast milk, placental tissue, urine, feces, and banked blood; most common mode is respiratory droplet; workers in daycare centers, institutions for mentally retarded, and health settings are especially at risk
c. Diagnosis: a viral culture is most definitive diagnostic tool; CMV antibodies indicate a recent infection; a fourfold increase in CMV titer in paired sera drawn 10 to 14 days apart usually indicates an acute infection
d. Maternal effects: asymptomatic illness, cervical discharge, and mononucleosis-like syndrome
NCLEX® e. Fetal/neonatal effects: fetal death or severe generalized disease with hemolytic anemia and jaundice, hydrocephaly or microcephaly, pneumonitis, hepatosplenomegaly, and deafness

10. Herpes simplex virus (HSV)
a. Cause: exposure to HSV
NCLEX® b. Transmission: HSV type II is a an STI transmitted by exposure to vesicular lesions on penis, scrotum, vulva, perineum, perianal region, vagina, or cervix; infant is usually infected during exposure to lesion in birth canal; infant is most at risk during primary infection in mother
c. Diagnosis: viral culture is used for definitive diagnosis; serologic tests have a lower accuracy
d. Maternal effects: blisters, rash, fever, malaise, nausea, and headache
NCLEX® e. Fetal/neonatal effects: miscarriage, preterm labor, or stillbirth; transplacental infection is rare but can cause skin lesions, intrauterine growth restriction (IUGR), mental retardation, and microcephaly
f. Significant results: vaginal delivery is recommended if client has no visible lesions or prodromal symptoms; if visible lesions or prodromal symptoms are present, cesarean delivery is indicated

11. **Sexually transmitted infections (STIs)** are caused by bacteria, viruses, protozoa, or ectoparasites and include human papillomavirus (HPV), human immunodeficiency virus (HIV), group B streptococcus (GBS), syphilis, gonorrhea, and chlamydia; all sexual partners of clients with STIs should be contacted and treated, as indicated; see sections that follow

12. HPV
NCLEX® a. Cause/transmission: sometimes called genital or venereal warts; spread through sexual contact; neonates can acquire infection during birth; can be prevented now by Gardasil vaccine
b. Diagnosis: direct visualization of warts and confirmation by biopsy
c. Maternal effects: symptoms depend on viral strain but can include genital lesions, chronic vaginal discharge, pruritis, and cervical dysplasia; some strains are asymptomatic
d. Fetal/neonatal effects: juvenile laryngeal papillomata

13. HIV
NCLEX® a. Cause/transmission: primarily through exchange of body fluids, including semen, blood, or vaginal secretions; neonatal transmission can occur transplacentally and is less likely if mother receives treatment during pregnancy; transmission can also occur via contact at time of delivery or through breast milk
b. Diagnosis: made with a reactive enzyme immunoassay (EIA) and a positive Western blot or immunofluorescence assay; the p24 antigen capture assay can diagnose neonatal HIV infection as early as 2 to 6 weeks after infection, detect HIV before seroconversion, and determine progression of AIDS; viral cultures provide best diagnostic tool for neonates; but are expensive and require 4 to 6 weeks for results

c. Maternal effects: opportunistic diseases including *Pneumocystis carinii* pneumonia, candida esophagitis, and wasting syndrome; HSV and CMV infections are also common; fever, headache, night sweats, malaise, generalized lymphadenopathy, myalgias, nausea, diarrhea, weight loss, sore throat, and rash are associated with seroconversion

NCLEX® d. Fetal/neonatal effects: asymptomatic at birth followed by opportunistic infections, immunodeficiency, failure to thrive, parotitis, lymphadenopathy, hepatosplenomegaly, fever, chronic diarrhea, dermatitis, thrush, and death

e. Test procedure: after explaining test to client, obtain an informed consent; clients may remain anonymous through use of number identification

14. Group B streptococcus (GBS)
   a. Cause/transmission: considered normal vaginal flora, found in 10–30% of healthy pregnant women; transmitted vertically from birth canal of infected mother to fetus
   NCLEX® b. Diagnosis: current recommendations are to screen all women at 36 to 37 weeks' gestation with a GBS culture
   c. Maternal effects: preterm labor, chorioamnionitis, premature rupture of membranes, urinary tract infections, and postpartum infections
   d. Fetal/neonatal effects: neonatal meningitis, sepsis, and septic shock; early onset GBS has a significant infant mortality rate
15. Syphilis
   NCLEX® a. Cause/transmission: caused by *Treponema pallidum*, a motile spirochete transmitted through microscopic abrasions in subcutaneous tissue; primarily transmitted via sexual intercourse, but also by kissing, biting, or oral–genital sex; transmission to fetus can occur via placenta at any time during pregnancy
   b. Diagnosis: microscopic examination of primary and secondary lesion tissue; serology is used for diagnosis during latency and late infection; women should be screened at first prenatal visit and possibly again late in third trimester with VDRL (Venereal Disease Research Laboratories) or the RPR (rapid plasma reagin) test; if either is positive, diagnosis is confirmed with a fluorescent treponemal antibody absorption (FTA-ABS) test
   c. Maternal effects: during acute stage, a chancre develops on skin near infection; second stage is marked by lymphadenopathy and rash on palms of hands and soles of feet; the latent stage, which can last up to 5 years, is asymptomatic; disease can progress to a tertiary stage that involves central nervous system (CNS), cardiovascular, and ocular signs and symptoms; infection can cause miscarriage or premature labor
   NCLEX® d. Fetal/neonatal effects: CNS damage, hearing loss, or death
16. Gonorrhea
   a. Cause/transmission: caused by *Neisseria gonorrhoeae*, an aerobic, gram-negative diplococci bacteria, transmitted by all types of sexual activity; neonates can acquire infection by exposure to bacteria in birth canal
   NCLEX® b. Diagnosis: screen all pregnant women at initial prenatal visit and at-risk women again at 36 weeks' gestation using a Thayer-Martin culture of endocervix, rectum, or pharynx
   c. Maternal effects: sometimes asymptomatic but can cause purulent endocervical discharge, menstrual irregularities, pelvic or lower abdominal pain, and premature rupture of membranes
   NCLEX® d. Fetal/neonatal effects: preterm birth, neonatal sepsis, IUGR, and ophthalmia neonatorum, which can cause blindness
17. Chlamydia
   a. Cause/transmission: the *Chlamydia trachomatis* bacteria is spread through sexual contact; Centers for Disease Control and Prevention (CDC) recommends screening of asymptomatic, high-risk women
   b. Diagnosis: by cultures; are expensive, require special transport and storage, and take up to 10 days
   c. Maternal effects: although usually asymptomatic, infection can cause bleeding, mucoid or purulent cervical discharge, PID, or dysuria
   NCLEX® d. Fetal/neonatal effects: conjunctivitis, pneumonia, and ophthalmia neonatorum

IV. NURSING CARE DURING SUBSEQUENT PRENATAL VISITS

NCLEX® **A. Frequency of follow-up prenatal visits**
1. Every 4 weeks during first 28 weeks' gestation
2. Every 2 weeks until 36 weeks
3. Every week until delivery

B. Collaborative management
1. Visits should include observation of maternal and fetal well-being and reinforcing teaching

Table 9–3 Danger Signs in Pregnancy

Danger Sign	Possible Cause
Gush of fluid from vagina	Rupture of membranes
Vaginal bleeding	Abruptio placentae, placenta previa, bloody show
Abdominal pain	Premature labor, abruptio placentae
Temperature > 101°F	Infection
Persistent vomiting	Hyperemesis gravidarum
Visual disturbances	Hypertension, preeclampsia
Edema of hands and face	Hypertension, preeclampsia
Severe headache	Hypertension, preeclampsia
Epigastric pain	Preeclampsia
Dysuria	Urinary tract infection
Decreased fetal movement	Compromised fetal well-being

2. Instruct mother concerning physical changes associated with pregnancy, such as quickening (first fetal movements felt) and colostrum production, as well as danger signs of pregnancy, presented in Table 9–3
3. NCLEX® Collect data to determine changes from baseline measurement of vital signs, weight gain, nutritional status, and presence of glucose and/or protein in urine
4. Collect clean-catch urine specimen at each visit to detect glucose (diabetes mellitus), protein (preeclampsia), and nitrites and leukocytes (urinary infection)
5. Measure maternal hemoglobin monthly for iron-deficiency anemia
6. NCLEX® Monitor fetus at each visit for growth as measured by fundal height, movement, and heart rate
7. NCLEX® Measure blood level of alpha-fetoprotein at 16 to 18 weeks to screen for fetal neural tube defects; measure maternal blood glucose level at 24 to 28 weeks to screen for gestational diabetes (see sections to follow)

C. Diagnostic tests during subsequent prenatal visits

1. **Quadruple screening test** includes measurement of **alpha-fetoprotein (AFP)**, human chorionic gonadotropin (hCG), unconjugated estriol (uE3), and inhibin A
   a. During pregnancy, AFP leaks from fetus's body into amniotic fluid and is absorbed into maternal circulation; hCG, uE3, and inhibin A are placental hormones
   b. This blood test is usually performed between 15 and 22 weeks' gestation but is most accurate at 16 to 18 weeks
   c. NCLEX® Findings: increased maternal serum AFP levels may indicate neural tube defects or other body wall defects, threatened abortion, fetal distress, or death; decreased maternal AFP levels may indicate trisomy 21 (Down syndrome) or fetal wastage; changes in hormonal levels can support AFP
   d. Interfering factors: multiple pregnancy, incorrect estimate of gestational age
   e. Follow-up: abnormal levels may indicate a need for a repeat test, ultrasound, or assessment of amniotic fluid using amniocentesis
2. NCLEX® **Triple-screen test** includes AFP, hCG, and uE3, but does not include inhibin A
3. **Glucose tolerance test (GTT)** to screen pregnant clients for gestational diabetes; generally completed between 24 and 28 weeks' gestation
   a. Test procedure: after test is explained to client, a 50-gram oral glucose load is provided; time of day or time since last meal is not a factor; venous plasma glucose is measured 1 hour after glucose load
   b. NCLEX® Findings: a level greater than 130–140 mg/dL after 1 hour (depending on lab) is considered abnormal
   c. Follow-up: clients with an abnormal GTT results should have a 3-hour, 100-gram oral GTT to diagnose gestational diabetes
4. **Oral glucose tolerance test (OGTT)**
   a. Test procedure: client eats high-carbohydrate diet for 3 days before test; on day of test, she fasts for 8 hours (overnight), and a fasting serum glucose is obtained; following the fast, 100 grams of oral glucose is administered and glucose levels are measured at 1, 2, and 3 hours
   b. NCLEX® Findings: gestational diabetes is diagnosed if two or more results are abnormal (see Table 9–4); results are borderline if one value is abnormal and OGTT is then repeated in 1 month
5. **Ultrasound**: sound waves with a frequency higher than 20,000 Hz produce a three-dimensional view and pictorial image to identify maternal and fetal tissues, bones, and fluids; screen for anomalies, assess

Table 9–4 Abnormal Oral Glucose Tolerance Test Results

Time	Abnormal Result
Fasting	greater than 95 mg/dL
1 hour	greater than 180 mg/dL
2 hour	greater than 155 mg/dL
3 hour	greater than 140 mg/dL

Table 9–5 Childbirth Education Topics by Trimester

Trimester	Educational Topic
First	Physical and psychosocial changes of pregnancy Self-care in pregnancy Protecting and nurturing the fetus Choosing a care provider and birth setting Prenatal exercise Relief of common early pregnancy discomforts
Second	Planning for breastfeeding Sexuality in pregnancy Relief of common later-pregnancy discomforts
Third	Preparation for childbirth Development of a birth plan

fetal well-being, and establish gestational age; results can be used to decide whether to continue pregnancy or terminate because of fetal abnormalities

NCLEX®
a. Transvaginal ultrasound used primarily during first trimester; eliminates need for full bladder and gives clearer images in obese clients; some clients are embarrassed or uncomfortable with vaginal insertion of probe; contraindicated in clients with latex allergies as probe is covered with a latex condomlike sac

NCLEX®
b. Abdominal ultrasound provides a safe, noninvasive fetal assessment, but is best done when client's bladder is full; this can result in discomfort

c. Viability is determined by measurement of fetal heart activity; this is possible at 6 to 7 weeks' gestation with real-time echo scan; fetal death can be determined by absence of heart activity as well as scalp edema and maceration

d. Gestational age can best be established during first 20 weeks' gestation because fetal growth rate is fairly consistent during this time; body part assessed is based on development; measurement of gestational sac is done at about 8 weeks, and crown-rump measurement is done at 7 to 14 weeks; with greater than 12 weeks' gestation, biparietal diameter (BPD) and femur length are measured

e. Fetal growth is assessed by serial measurements of BPD and femur length; assists health care provider to distinguish between IUGR and inaccurate dating of pregnancy

D. Childbirth education

1. Childbirth classes provide information on pregnancy and childbirth to facilitate families in optimal decision making; topics are timed during pregnancy; see Table 9–5
2. Classes can be planned for special groups such as grandparents, siblings, adolescents, and clients who will deliver by cesarean section
3. Exercise is an important topic for childbirth education; encourage women to participate in regular (three times per week) exercise during pregnancy
    a. Benefits of exercise include maintaining muscle tone and bowel function and having fewer complications during labor and delivery

NCLEX®
    b. Exercises especially helpful for childbirth include pelvic tilt, partial sit-ups, Kegel exercises, and exercises to stretch inner thigh muscles
4. Classes on preparation for birth process provide information on selection of birthing method and relaxation techniques
    a. Commonly taught birthing methods: Lamaze, Kitzinger, and Bradley methods of prepared childbirth; see Table 9–6

NCLEX®
    b. Relaxation techniques commonly taught for use in labor include touch, breathing, disassociation, and progressive relaxation

Table 9–6 Comparison of Common Birthing Methods

Method	Characteristics	Breathing Techniques
Lamaze	Uses education about fetal growth and changes associated with pregnancy along with training in exercises that strengthen muscles used during labor and delivery to decrease fear and help mother cope with pain of labor	Patterned, paced
Bradley	Relies on partner or husband to coach laboring woman; promotes relaxation through abdominal breathing and exercises	Primarily abdominal
Kitzinger	Prepares woman for birth through use of sensory memory and Stanislavsky acting method to teach relaxation	Chest breathing with abdominal relaxation

Table 9–7 Management of Discomforts in Early Pregnancy

Discomfort	Management
Nausea and vomiting	Avoid strong odors; drink carbonated beverages; avoid drinking while eating; eat crackers or toast before getting out of bed; eat small frequent meals; avoid spicy or greasy foods
Breast tenderness	Wear a well-fitting, supportive bra
Urinary frequency	Increase daytime fluid intake; decrease evening fluid intake; empty bladder as soon as urge is felt
Fatigue	Plan rest period or nap during day; go to bed as early as possible
Ptyalism	Use gum, mints, hard candy, or mouthwash
Nasal stuffiness/bleeding	Use cool air vaporizer

Table 9–8 Management of Discomforts in Late Pregnancy

Discomfort	Management
Heartburn	Eat small, frequent meals; avoid spicy or greasy foods; refrain from lying down immediately after eating; use low-sodium antacids
Constipation	Increase fluid and fiber intake; exercise regularly; develop regular bowel habits; use stool softeners as needed
Hemorrhoids	Avoid constipation; apply topical anesthetics, ointments, or ice packs; use sitz baths or warm soaks; reinsert into rectum, if necessary
Backache	Practice good body mechanics; practice pelvic tilt exercise; avoid high heels, heavy lifting, overfatigue, and excessive bending or reaching
Leg cramps	Dorsiflex feet; apply heat to affected muscle; evaluate calcium-to-phosphorus ratio in diet
Varicose veins	Elevate legs; wear support hose; avoid crossing legs at the knee, restrictive clothing, and standing for long periods of time
Ankle edema	Practice frequent dorsiflexion of feet; avoid standing for long periods of time; elevate legs when sitting or resting
Faintness	Arise slowly; avoid prolonged standing; maintain hematocrit and hemoglobin
Flatulence	Avoid gas-forming foods; chew food thoroughly; establish regular bowel habits

5. Classes focused on knowledge needed post delivery include postpartum self-care, newborn care, infant stimulation, and infant safety needs

E. **Management of common discomforts of pregnancy**

1. Discomforts occur because of physiologic or anatomic changes of pregnancy; they differ from trimester to trimester

NCLEX® 2. While not dangerous, they constitute a significant problem for client and present an opportunity for nursing intervention (see Tables 9–7 and 9–8)

V. PHYSIOLOGICAL CHANGES OF PREGNANCY

A. **Reproductive**

1. Uterus: during pregnancy takes on an ovoid shape and increases in capacity from 10 mL to 5 L; primarily caused by an increase in size of cells (hypertrophy) in response to estrogen, and distention

caused by growing fetus; by end of pregnancy, uterus and its contents require up to one-sixth of total maternal blood flow

NCLEX®

2. Cervix: under influence of estrogen, secretes mucus that forms a plug at opening of endocervical canal to limit bacteria entering uterus; increased blood flow to cervix results in **Goodell's sign** (softening of cervix) and **Chadwick's sign** (bluish color of cervix during pregnancy)
3. Vagina: under influence of estrogen, vaginal mucosa thickens and connective tissue relaxes; vaginal secretions thicken and increase in amount during pregnancy; the pH is acidic, 3.6 to 6.0
4. Breasts: estrogen and progesterone cause breasts to increase in size and number of glands; **colostrum** (a thin bluish-white secretion high in protein and immune properties) is produced and may be expressed during last trimester

B. Cardiovascular

1. Cardiac output increases 30–40% over nonpregnant output with an increase in pulse of 10 to 15 beats/minute
2. Peak time for cardiac problems occurs around 28 weeks
3. Pulmonary and peripheral vascular resistance decreases 40–50%, resulting in decreased BP throughout first and second trimesters; in third trimester, begins to increase to prepregnant levels; postural hypotension may result as pregnant uterus presses on pelvic and femoral vessels, limiting blood return to heart

NCLEX®

4. Vena cava syndrome results as gravid uterus compresses vena cava, causing decreased blood flow to right atrium and decreased BP
   a. Symptoms include pallor, dizziness, and clammy skin
   b. Prevent or treat by positioning woman on left side or with a pillow under right hip
5. Blood volume increases 45% over prepregnant levels
   a. Red blood cells (RBCs) increase 18–30% depending on amount of iron supplementation
   b. Plasma volume increases 50%
   c. The greater increase in plasma over RBCs results in physiologic anemia and is seen as a 7% decrease in hematocrit

C. Respiratory

1. Volume of air breathed increases 30–40% because of decreased airway resistance that occurs in response to progesterone
2. Intrathoracic volume remains unchanged even though enlarged uterus presses up on diaphragm, because rib cage flares and chest circumference increases

D. Neurologic: no known changes

E. Musculoskeletal

1. Relaxation of pelvic joints results in classic "waddling" gait often seen in pregnancy

NCLEX®

2. Physiologic lordosis develops as curvature of lumbar spine increases to compensate for weight of gravid uterus; can result in low back pain
3. Diastasis recti, separation of rectus abdominis muscle, can result as uterus enlarges

F. Gastrointestinal (GI)

1. During first trimester, human chorionic gonadotropin (hCG) increases and can cause nausea and vomiting

NCLEX®

2. Increased progesterone levels relax smooth muscles, resulting in decreased peristalsis as noted by bloating, reflux of gastric secretions, and constipation; GI problems are worsened as gravid uterus presses on intestines
3. Constipation and increased pressure on blood vessels in rectum can lead to hemorrhoids

G. Renal

1. In first trimester, gravid uterus presses on bladder, causing urinary frequency; relieved in second trimester by uterus moving up into abdominal area; frequency returns in third trimester as presenting part presses on bladder
2. Glomerular filtration increases 50% during second trimester and remains elevated until delivery; kidneys may not be able to reabsorb all filtered glucose, resulting in glycosuria

H. Integumentary

1. Increased estrogen levels may lead to areas of increased skin pigmentation, especially in areas already highly pigmented such as areola, nipples, and vulva
   a. **Chloasma**, mask of pregnancy, is an increase in pigmentation on forehead and around eyes; is seen most often in women of color and is aggravated by sun exposure
   b. **Linea nigra** is a darkly pigmented line that extends from umbilicus to pubic area
   c. **Striae gravidarum**, or stretch marks, appear as reddish streaks on trunk and thighs; result from stretching of connective tissue caused by increased adrenal steroid levels; generally change to a shiny gray-white color after delivery but do not disappear

2. Sweat and sebaceous gland activity increases during pregnancy

I. Endocrine

1. Metabolism
   a. Average weight gain is 3 to 5 pounds in first trimester and 12 to 15 pounds in each following trimester
   b. Water retention occurs because of increased sex hormones and decreased serum protein
2. Hormones in pregnancy
   a. hCG is secreted by trophoblast early in pregnancy and stimulates progesterone and estrogen production; it is thought to support pregnancy and cause nausea and vomiting in first trimester
   b. Human placental lactogen (hPL), also known as chorionic somatomammotropin, is an insulin antagonist that promotes lipolysis, resulting in increased circulating free fatty acids available for maternal metabolic use
   c. Estrogen and progesterone are produced by corpus luteum for first 7 weeks of pregnancy and then by placenta; estrogen stimulates uterine development to support fetal growth and stimulates ductal system of breast for lactation; progesterone maintains endometrium, decreases uterine contractility, stimulates development of breast acini and lobules, and causes relaxation of smooth muscle
   d. Relaxin, primarily made by corpus luteum, decreases uterine contractility, contributes to softening of cervix, and has long-term effects on collagen
   e. Prostaglandins, lipids that are found throughout female reproductive system, contribute to decrease seen in placental vascular system, and probably contribute to onset of labor

VI. NUTRITIONAL NEEDS

A. Factors affecting maternal nutrition requirements

1. Prepregnancy nutritional status: women who are underweight or overweight may need more or less calories respectively for adequate fetal weight gain
2. Maternal age: adolescent mothers may need increased caloric intake for both maternal and fetal growth
3. Maternal parity: number of pregnancies and interval between them can affect nutritional needs

B. General principles of maternal nutrition

NCLEX® 1. Healthy pregnant woman requires an additional 300 calories per day

NCLEX® 2. Other nutritional requirements are increased during pregnancy, including protein, vitamins (especially folate), minerals, and trace elements; many health care providers recommend taking a prenatal vitamin supplement to ensure adequate intake and reduce risk of birth defects associated with folic acid (vitamin B_6) deficiency

NCLEX® 3. Appropriate pregnancy weight gain averages 25 to 35 pounds for women with a normal prepregnant weight
   a. 10 to 13 pounds in first 20 weeks
   b. About 1 pound per week after 20th week

4. Maternal weight gain is distributed to a variety of structures, including fetus, placenta, and amniotic fluid (11 pounds); uterus (2 pounds); blood volume (4 pounds); breast tissue (3 pounds); and maternal stores (5 to 10 pounds)

C. Lactose intolerance

1. Results from insufficient levels of lactase, an enzyme that breaks down lactose in dairy products into glucose and galactose (simple sugars)

NCLEX® 2. Leads to nausea and vomiting, epigastric discomfort, abdominal cramping and distention, and loose stools

NCLEX® 3. Lactase may be replaced by adding it as a liquid to milk or by chewing a tablet before ingesting milk products

4. Dairy products that may be better tolerated include cheese and yogurt, or milk products in cooked form
5. Lactose-free products are also available

D. Vegetarianism

1. Intake should include unrefined grains, legumes, nuts, fruits, and vegetables

NCLEX® 2. Strict vegetarians (vegans) need to eat adequate amounts and combinations of proteins to be able to synthesize complete proteins; combinations should include whole-grain foods and legumes, nuts and legumes, and nuts and whole-grain foods

3. Ovovegetarians may add eggs to diet to help meet protein requirement
4. Lacto-ovovegetarians may use milk and eggs

NCLEX® 5. All clients eating a vegetarian diet should take a daily supplement of vitamin B_{12} (cyanocobalamin)

E. **Pica**
1. A condition of eating items that are not foods or have no nutritional value
2. Leads to iron-deficiency anemia
3. Commonly ingested substances are clay, dirt, and ice
4. Can affect all socioeconomic levels, although impoverished clients are more at risk

VII. PSYCHOSOCIAL NEEDS OF PREGNANCY

A. **Role changes:** occur as decisions are made as to whether mother will continue or return to work and who will meet household responsibilities

B. **Anxieties:** related to birthing process, well-being of mother and baby, and finances

C. **Family strengths in coping with psychosocial changes of pregnancy**
1. Communication skills
2. Ability to resolve conflict and reach compromise
3. Willingness to seek and utilize support systems

D. **Collaborative management**
1. Discuss with client psychosocial processes that occur during pregnancy, such as role changes, anxieties related to well-being of mother and infant, and additional financial responsibilities
2. Explore family coping mechanisms, communication skills, and support systems

Check Your NCLEX-PN® Exam I.Q.

You are ready for testing on this content if you can

- Collect data about the physiological status of a pregnant client.
- Calculate an expected delivery date.
- Collect data about the psychosocial needs of a pregnant client.
- Monitor results of maternal and fetal diagnostic tests.
- Provide antenatal care to a client.
- Provide instructions about self-care during the antenatal period.

PRACTICE TEST

1 The client has come to the clinic for her first prenatal visit. During the pelvic examination, the examiner indicates that the vaginal mucosa has a bluish color. The nurse documents which finding as positive?

1. Hegar's sign
2. Goodell's sign
3. McDonald's sign
4. Chadwick's sign

2 With regard to normal changes in the reproductive system during pregnancy, the nurse should reinforce teaching to the pregnant client about which of the following?

1. Vaginal secretions will increase and thicken.
2. Uterus will grow by adding many new cells.
3. Breasts will become red and hard.
4. Cervix will begin to dilate during the second trimester.

3 What would the nurse include when describing to a pregnant client the normal changes in the cardiovascular system during pregnancy?

1. Her pulse rate will decrease.
2. She may experience dizziness if she lies on her back.
3. She will have a decrease in red blood cells.
4. She may experience a feeling of fullness in her chest.

4 During a prenatal visit in the second trimester, which item reported by the client would be a cause for concern?

1. Thirst and urinary frequency
2. +1 deep tendon reflexes
3. Constipation
4. Backache in the lower sacral area

5 The nurse is assisting with a health care provider exam of a client who is at 12 weeks' gestation. The nurse would expect the examiner to find the fundus at which location at this time?

1. 3 cm below the sternum
2. The level of the umbilicus
3. The level of the symphysis pubis
4. 3 cm below the umbilicus

6 What would the prenatal clinic nurse conclude to be a contraindication for maternal serum alpha-fetoprotein testing for a pregnant client?

1. Being at 25 weeks' gestation
2. Client would not consider termination of pregnancy
3. Client has no family history of neural tube defects
4. Client had ultrasound at 8 weeks' gestation

7 At the first prenatal visit, the client reveals that her last menstrual period began March 18 (03.18). The nurse calculates her estimated date of delivery to be ______________. Provide a numerical answer using format month.day (i.e., July 10 = 07.10).

Fill in your answer below:

____

8 The nurse concludes by which client statement that the pregnant client best understands prenatal nutrition education?

1. "I understand that if I don't eat foods with folic acid, my baby will have birth defects."
2. "I understand that eating citrus fruits, especially oranges, will help me meet my need for folic acid."
3. "I understand that if my level of folic acid is low, it could cause my baby to have a neural tube defect."
4. "I understand that I should limit my intake of folic acid because it can build up in the liver and cause birth defects."

9 A pregnant client, who is a vegetarian, is concerned about her folic acid intake and asks the nurse to recommend some foods that she should include in her diet. Which of the following should the nurse recommend?

1. Peanuts
2. Hamburger
3. Bananas
4. Apple juice

10 The pregnant client has been started on an iron supplement. What information should be included by the nurse as a priority when sharing information about the iron supplement?

1. It should be taken 30 minutes after eating a full meal.
2. It is better absorbed if taken with a liquid containing vitamin C.
3. It will eliminate the need for prenatal vitamins.
4. It should be taken at the same time as the prenatal vitamin.

11 The pregnant client tells the nurse that she is lactose-intolerant. When considering the health care provider's recommendation of a calcium supplement, what data should the nurse gather?

1. History of kidney stones
2. Presence of leg cramps
3. Color of mucous membranes and conjunctiva
4. Resting heart rate

12 When assisting with a client's first prenatal assessment, the nurse discovers that the client has not had a second vaccination for measles, mumps, and rubella. What is the best plan for this client?

1. Administer the vaccine during this visit
2. Wait until the third trimester to administer the vaccine
3. Administer the vaccine following delivery
4. Omit the vaccine because these are childhood diseases not acquired by adults

13 The pregnant client, who is at 34 weeks' gestation, calls the prenatal clinic reporting cramping pain in her abdomen. After the diagnosis of Braxton-Hicks contractions is made, the nurse should give the client which recommendation?

1. "Go to bed and wait for your real labor to begin."
2. "Empty your bladder frequently and change positions if these contractions are bothering you."
3. "Avoid using your Lamaze breathing with these contractions because it might precipitate preterm labor."
4. "Just ignore these contractions; we will let you know if there is a problem."

14 The client, who is at 37 weeks' gestation, reports joint pain especially in the lower back and pelvic area. What is the best reply by the nurse?

1. "I'm afraid you are just going to have to put up with that for a few more weeks."
2. "Sleeping flat on your back may help with the pain."
3. "Aspirin taken every 3–4 hours will be the best thing to relieve this pain."
4. "It may help to apply a heating pad to the painful area for 15–20 minutes."

15 In reviewing the chart of a prenatal client, which client finding would be considered by the nurse to be a probable sign of pregnancy?

1. Fetal heartbeat on ultrasound
2. Amenorrhea
3. Positive pregnancy test
4. Chloasma

16 The client is planning to breastfeed and asks the nurse what she should do to prepare. The nurse explains that the client can do which of the following?

1. Wash her nipples with water daily
2. Apply lanolin daily in the last trimester
3. Rub the nipples briskly with a towel twice a day
4. Perform the pinch test daily

17 What information, if revealed to the nurse during a prenatal visit, would indicate an increased risk for exposure to cytomegalovirus?

1. Caring for a cat and litter box
2. Working at a day care center
3. Using IV drugs several years ago
4. Giving blood twice yearly

18 Which of the following, if noted by the nurse, would indicate a need for delivery by cesarean section?

1. Positive herpes culture at the first prenatal visit; client asymptomatic at the time of delivery
2. History of genital herpes lesions; at the time of delivery, prodromal symptoms present but no lesions
3. Oral fever blisters at the time of delivery
4. Genital herpes lesion 1 month prior to delivery; no symptoms at the time of delivery

19 What would the nurse anticipate as follow-up in the plan of care for a pregnant client who is diagnosed with a sexually transmitted infection?

1. Contacting and treating all sexual partners
2. Delivery by cesarean section
3. Amniocentesis for assessment of genetic damage
4. Close monitoring of hematocrit and hemoglobin throughout pregnancy

20 Which of the following, if reported to the nurse by a pregnant client prior to collection of a gonorrhea culture, would result in postponing specimen collection?

1. Recent diagnosis and treatment for herpes
2. Persistent vaginal discharge
3. Douching 3 days ago
4. Is currently menstruating

21 The client has come to the prenatal clinic reporting repeated nausea and vomiting. The nurse would look to which laboratory finding for the best information about the client's hydration status?

1. Hematocrit
2. Platelet count
3. Urine specific gravity
4. IgG level

22 Which of the following statements by the pregnant client indicates to the nurse an understanding of the client's nutritional needs during the second and third trimester? Select all that apply.

1. "I will need to increase my intake of protein."
2. "I will need to increase my daily intake by 500–600 calories per day."
3. "I will need to increase my intake of calcium so that it is double my phosphorus intake."
4. "I will need to decrease my intake of iodine."
5. "I will need to increase my iron and may even need a prenatal iron supplement."

23 The nurse considers which data collected regarding a pregnant client is the best indicator of normal fetal growth?

1. Maternal weight gain 7 pounds at 22 weeks' gestation
2. Fundal height 22 centimeters at 25 weeks' gestation
3. Maternal waist circumference 41 inches at 36 weeks' gestation
4. Maternal intake 1500 calories per day

24 A client comes to the clinic for her first prenatal visit and reports that July 10 was the first day of her last menstrual period. Using Naegele's rule, the nurse calculates the estimated date of birth for the client to be __________. Provide a numerical answer using format month.day (i.e., July 10 = 07.10).

Fill in your answer below:

____

25 The client, who is at 36 weeks' gestation, calls the prenatal clinic because she is concerned about a thin, bluish-white fluid leaking from her breasts. What is an appropriate response by the nurse? Select all that apply.

1. "This probably indicates an infection in your breasts. You will need to come into the office."
2. "This usually happens when you are going into premature labor. You should go to the hospital."
3. "This normally occurs as your breasts prepare for breastfeeding. You should continue to wear a good-fitting bra."
4. "This is an indication that you may have some problems with breastfeeding. I will have the lactation consultant call you."
5. "The fluid is colostrum and normally leaks from the breast during the last trimester of pregnancy."

ANSWERS & RATIONALES

1 **Answer: 4 Rationale:** Beginning around the fourth week of pregnancy, vasocongestion in the pelvic area results in a bluish color to the vulva, vagina, and cervix, known as Chadwick's sign. Hegar's sign is a softening of the lower uterine segment. Goodell's sign is a softening of the cervix. McDonald's sign is an ease in flexing the body of the uterus against the cervix. **Cognitive Level:** Analyzing **Client Need:** Health Promotion and Maintenance **Integrated Process:** Nursing Process: Data Collection **Content Area:** Maternal-Newborn **Strategy:** The critical words in the question are *first prenatal visit* and *bluish color*. Use the process of elimination and knowledge of the changes in cervical mucosa in early pregnancy to make your selection.

2 **Answer: 1 Rationale:** During pregnancy, increased estrogen production results in an increased amount and thickening of vaginal secretions. The uterus grows by cell hypertrophy, not by adding more cells. Red and hard breasts or a cervix dilating during the second trimester are not normal findings. **Cognitive Level:** Applying **Client Need:** Health Promotion and Maintenance **Integrated Process:** Teaching and Learning **Content Area:** Maternal-Newborn **Strategy:** Note the critical words *normal changes during pregnancy*. Eliminate cervical dilation and reddened breasts first because they are abnormal. Use concepts of physiology to choose vaginal secretions over new uterine cells.

3 **Answer: 2 Rationale:** Pressure on the vena cava from the gravid uterus may cause a decrease in blood flow to the right atrium and result in a decrease in blood pressure. Dizziness is a symptom of hypotension. The pulse rate could stay the same or increase as the workload of the heart increases during the course of pregnancy. There is an increase in the number of red blood cells to meet physiological demand. A feeling of fullness in the chest is not a cardiovascular change during pregnancy, although abdominal fullness occurs as the pregnancy progresses. **Cognitive Level:** Applying **Client Need:** Health Promotion and Maintenance **Integrated Process:** Teaching and Learning **Content Area:** Maternal-Newborn **Strategy:** Note the critical words *normal changes*, *cardiovascular*, and *pregnancy*. With these in mind, eliminate both decreased pulse rate and RBCs as incorrect. Choose dizziness over chest fullness by recalling concepts of maternal and fetal circulation.

4 **Answer: 1 Rationale:** Urinary frequency usually disappears in the second trimester. Thirst and urinary frequency may be signs of developing gestational diabetes and warrant further investigation. Deep tendon reflexes are noted during a physical examination by the health care provider and are not reported to a health care provider by the client. Constipation is a typical finding because of the pressure exerted by the growing fetus. Backache in the lower sacral area can occur because of changing posture associated with the growing fetus. **Cognitive Level:** Analyzing **Client Need:** Health Promotion and Maintenance **Integrated Process:** Nursing Process: Data Collection **Content Area:** Maternal-Newborn **Strategy:** Note the critical words *cause for concern*, which indicates the correct answer is an option that is an abnormal finding. Eliminate constipation and backache first, since they are typical symptoms that may be associated with pregnancy. Choose thirst and urinary frequency over deep tendon reflexes because

these symptoms are clearly abnormal and are also subjective data that are reported by the client.

5 **Answer: 3 Rationale:** By the 12th week of gestation, the uterus should have increased in size to be palpable at the symphysis pubis. Factors affecting this finding include abnormal fetal growth or the presence of a multiple gestation. **Cognitive Level:** Analyzing **Client Need:** Health Promotion and Maintenance **Integrated Process:** Nursing Process: Data Collection **Content Area:** Maternal-Newborn **Strategy:** To answer this question correctly, recall the expected physiological changes during pregnancy. Use nursing knowledge and the process of elimination to make your selection.

6 **Answer: 1 Rationale:** This test, which measures the level of maternal serum alpha-fetoprotein, is most sensitive between 16 and 18 weeks' gestation. However, it can be performed at up to 22 weeks' gestation. Knowledge of fetal anomalies can help a client determine need for possible pregnancy termination or need for added services after delivery. **Cognitive Level:** Analyzing **Client Need:** Health Promotion and Maintenance **Integrated Process:** Nursing Process: Planning **Content Area:** Maternal-Newborn **Strategy:** Note the critical word *contraindication*. This means the correct answer is an option that is a false statement. Use knowledge of the purpose of the test to eliminate each of the incorrect options.

7 **Answer: 12.25 Rationale:** According to Naegele's rule, the estimated date of birth can be calculated by subtracting 3 months from the beginning date of the last menstrual period and then adding 7 days to that date. **Cognitive Level:** Applying **Client Need:** Health Promotion and Maintenance **Integrated Process:** Nursing Process: Data Collection **Content Area:** Maternal-Newborn **Strategy:** Specific knowledge of Naegele's rule is needed to answer the question. Use knowledge of this rule and mathematical/calculating ability to determine the appropriate due date.

8 **Answer: 3 Rationale:** Maternal folic acid deficiency has been linked to infant neural tube defects. Maternal folic acid deficiency has been linked to infant neural tube defects. Folic acid may be obtained from prenatal vitamin supplements as well as foods: citrus fruits are high in vitamin C. Folic acid should be supplemented during pregnancy to help prevent neural tube defects. **Cognitive Level:** Analyzing **Client Need:** Health Promotion and Maintenance **Integrated Process:** Nursing Process: Evaluation **Content Area:** Maternal-Newborn **Strategy:** Note the critical words *best understands*, which indicates that the correct answer is also a correct statement. First, eliminate the option that indicates birth defects will occur because that level of certainty is unrealistic. Choose correctly between the remaining options, recalling either that neural tube defects are associated with low folic acid or because oranges are not an especially good source of folic acid.

9 **Answer: 1 Rationale:** Both peanuts and hamburger are good sources of folic acid, but since the client is a vegetarian, peanuts are a better recommendation. Bananas and apple juice do not contain significant amounts of folic acid. **Cognitive Level:** Applying **Client Need:** Health Promotion and Maintenance **Integrated Process:** Nursing Process: Implementation **Content Area:** Maternal-Newborn **Strategy:** Use the process of elimination and knowledge of nutrition to answer this question. Eliminate hamburger first because the client is a vegetarian, and eliminate bananas and apple juice because they are fruit or fruit products. Nuts are better sources of folic acid.

10 **Answer: 2 Rationale:** Iron is absorbed best on an empty stomach (not after a full meal) and in the presence of vitamin C. It may or may not be taken at the same time as other vitamin supplementation. It does not replace the need for other vitamins. **Cognitive Level:** Applying **Client Need:** Health Promotion and Maintenance **Integrated Process:** Nursing Process: Planning **Content Area:** Maternal-Newborn **Strategy:** First, recall that iron intake does not eliminate the need for other vitamins. Next recall that a full meal may decrease iron absorption. Choose between the remaining two options by recalling the beneficial effect of vitamin C on iron absorption.

11 **Answer: 1 Rationale:** Increased calcium intake can lead to formation of kidney stones. A calcium supplement is not expected to affect leg cramps, color of mucous membranes and conjunctiva, or resting heart rate. **Cognitive Level:** Analyzing **Client Need:** Health Promotion and Maintenance **Integrated Process:** Nursing Process: Data Collection **Content Area:** Maternal-Newborn **Strategy:** Recall that calcium is a salt, and use this information to recall that salts can form crystals, which can in turn lead to kidney stones.

12 **Answer: 3 Rationale:** The measles, mumps, and rubella vaccine contains live, attenuated virus and could cause disease and harm to the fetus during pregnancy. It should be given after delivery, and the woman should avoid conceiving for 3 months. **Cognitive Level:** Analyzing **Client Need:** Health Promotion and Maintenance **Integrated Process:** Nursing Process: Planning **Content Area:** Maternal-Newborn **Strategy:** The issue in this question is immunization safety during pregnancy. The vaccine does need to be administered, so choose the option that considers the live attenuated viral nature of the vaccine.

13 **Answer: 2 Rationale:** Braxton-Hicks contractions are probably caused by stretching of the myometrium. They are usually relieved by position changes, frequent emptying of the bladder, resting in a lateral recumbent position, and walking or light exercise. Continuous bedrest until true labor begins is not necessary. Lamaze breathing is helpful for some women in managing discomfort that can be associated with Braxton-Hicks contractions. Clients are not advised to ignore symptoms; instead the nurse would focus on teaching the client how to recognize true labor. **Cognitive Level:** Applying **Client Need:** Health Promotion and Maintenance **Integrated Process:** Communication and Documentation **Content Area:** Maternal-Newborn **Strategy:** The question addresses the issue of client teaching about Braxton-Hicks contractions. The wording of the question indicates the correct answer is a true statement. Recall that emptying the bladder and position changes help to relieve this discomfort.

14 **Answer: 4 Rationale:** Heat may relieve pain caused by increased joint mobility resulting from hormonal changes. Aspirin should be avoided in the last trimester because it increases bleeding time. Telling the client to just put up with it is not a therapeutic communication. Sleeping flat on the back may not be helpful for maternal–fetal circulation because the gravid uterus may cause pressure on the great vessels in the abdomen. The client should lie on one side; often the left is advised. **Cognitive Level:** Applying **Client Need:** Health Promotion and Maintenance **Integrated Process:** Communication and Documentation **Content Area:** Maternal-Newborn **Strategy:** Recall principles of heat and cold therapy and therapeutic communication to choose correctly.

15 **Answer: 3 Rationale:** Probable signs of pregnancy are those that are detected by the examiner and are usually related to the physical signs of pregnancy. Amenorrhea and chloasma are reported by the client (presumptive signs) and can be caused by conditions other than pregnancy. Fetal heartbeat on ultrasound is a positive sign of pregnancy. **Cognitive Level:** Analyzing **Client Need:** Health Promotion and Maintenance **Integrated Process:** Nursing Process: Data Collection **Content Area:** Maternal-Newborn **Strategy:** Specific knowledge of the different classifications of signs of pregnancy is needed to answer this question. If you recall that *probable* is the middle category, it may help you to eliminate positive and possible signs.

16 **Answer: 1 Rationale:** The use of water to wash the nipples can help avoid irritation that could lead to nipple cracking or trauma. Daily use of lanolin on the nipples during the last trimester is unnecessary. Rubbing the nipples briskly could cause trauma. The pinch test is to determine if nipples are inverted and need only be done one time. **Cognitive Level:** Applying **Client Need:** Health Promotion and Maintenance **Integrated Process:** Nursing Process: Implementation **Content Area:** Maternal-Newborn **Strategy:** Use nursing knowledge to answer the question. It may also be helpful to recall general principles of skin care and avoidance of skin trauma, which helps eliminate each of the incorrect options.

17 **Answer: 2 Rationale:** Day care workers are frequently exposed to the virus. Exposure to cat litter can result in toxoplasmosis exposure. IV drug use increases the risk for HIV or hepatitis. Giving blood does not increase the client's risk. **Cognitive Level:** Analyzing **Client Need:** Health Promotion and Maintenance **Integrated Process:** Nursing Process: Data Collection **Content Area:** Maternal-Newborn **Strategy:** Use the process of elimination and knowledge of transmission of viral infections to answer this question. Eliminate giving blood first as unrelated to acquiring infection. Eliminate the option with cat litter next because the organism in toxoplasmosis is not a virus. Choose working in a day care center over past use of IV drugs because there is more risk of exposure.

18 **Answer: 2 Rationale:** Indications for cesarean section are presence of a herpes lesion or prodromal symptoms. If there are no herpes symptoms or lesions, a vaginal delivery is recommended. **Cognitive Level:** Analyzing **Client Need:** Health Promotion and Maintenance **Integrated Process:** Nursing Process: Evaluation **Content Area:** Maternal-Newborn **Strategy:** Specific knowledge related to risk of delivery with herpes infection is needed to answer the question. Use concepts of time and direct contact with lesions to eliminate the incorrect options.

19 **Answer: 1 Rationale:** All partners have been exposed and should be made aware, tested, and treated as indicated. Cesarean section would be appropriate only if there were symptoms of a herpes lesion or prodromal symptoms. Genetic assessment and more-than-routine monitoring of hematocrit and hemoglobin are not indicated. **Cognitive Level:** Applying **Client Need:** Health Promotion and Maintenance **Integrated Process:** Nursing Process: Implementation **Content Area:** Maternal-Newborn **Strategy:** Use knowledge of principles of communicable disease transmission to answer the question. The client in the question is actually the sexual partner(s), not the fetus.

20 **Answer: 4 Rationale:** Menstrual blood can affect the results of a gonorrheal culture. Douching within 24 hours can affect results, but diagnosis/treatment of herpes and persistent vaginal discharge would not affect the results, and therefore do not interfere with specimen collection. **Cognitive Level:** Applying **Client Need:** Health Promotion and Maintenance **Integrated Process:** Nursing Process: Planning **Content Area:** Maternal-Newborn **Strategy:** Use general knowledge of specimen collection procedures to answer the question. Visualize each option and choose the one that could physically alter the test results.

21 **Answer: 3 Rationale:** Urine specific gravity is a measure of the concentration of particles in the urine. Urine specific gravity rises when the client is dehydrated. Hematocrit would also rise when the client is dehydrated, but is an indirect measure. Hemoglobin measurements are not as greatly affected. Platelet count and IgG levels are not affected. **Cognitive Level:** Applying **Client Need:** Health Promotion and Maintenance **Integrated Process:** Nursing Process: Data Collection **Content Area:** Maternal-Newborn **Strategy:** Note the critical word *best* in the question, which means that more than one value could be affected. Use knowledge of laboratory indicators of dehydration to eliminate platelet count and IgG level. Then choose urine specific gravity over hematocrit because it is a more direct measurement of fluid balance.

22 **Answer: 1, 5 Rationale:** Protein and iron intake in pregnancy must increase to meet the needs of the growing fetus. Calcium requirements increase at the same rate as phosphorus. Caloric needs increase, but only about 300 calories per day. Iodine requirements increase during pregnancy. **Cognitive Level:** Applying **Client Need:** Health Promotion and Maintenance **Integrated Process:** Teaching and Learning **Content Area:** Maternal-Newborn **Strategy:** Recall specific concepts of nutrients needed during pregnancy to help answer the question correctly.

23 **Answer: 2 Rationale:** In singleton births with fetal growth within normal limits, fundal height in centimeters multiplied by 8 and divided by 7 should correlate with gestational age in weeks. This weight gain may be insufficient depending on maternal weight before pregnancy. Maternal waist circumference is not measured, and could be influenced by other factors such as maternal weight and number of fetuses being carried. A caloric intake of 1500 calories per day may be insufficient at 22 weeks to meet the needs of the growing fetus. A 1500-calorie diet is often a weight-reduction diet. **Cognitive Level:** Analyzing **Client Need:** Health Promotion and Maintenance **Integrated Process:** Nursing Process: Evaluation **Content Area:** Maternal-Newborn **Strategy:** Remember that from about 22–34 weeks' gestation, fundal height correlates well with weeks of gestation, plus or minus 2 cm. The question also contains the critical word *best*, which means one option is better than the others.

24 **Answer: 04.17 Rationale:** Using Naegele's rule, the estimated date of birth is calculated by subtracting 3 months from the first day of the last menstrual period and then adding 7 days to that date. **Cognitive Level:** Analyzing **Client Need:** Health Promotion and Maintenance **Integrated Process:** Nursing Process: Data Collection **Content Area:** Maternal-Newborn **Strategy:** Recall Naegele's rule to calculate the answer to this question.

25 **Answer: 3, 5 Rationale:** The fluid leaking from her breasts is colostrum. It normally leaks from the breasts during the last trimester. The client should wear a supportive bra. **Cognitive Level:** Analyzing **Client Need:** Health Promotion and Maintenance **Integrated Process:** Teaching and Learning **Content Area:** Maternal-Newborn **Strategy:** Recall normal changes to the breast during pregnancy and associated teaching needs to help to answer this question.

Key Terms to Review

alpha-fetoprotein (AFP) p. 90
Chadwick's sign p. 93
chloasma p. 93
colostrum p. 93
estimated date of birth (EDB) p. 84
fetal heart rate p. 86
fundal height p. 84
glucose tolerance test (GTT) p. 90
Goodell's sign p. 93
gravida p. 85
linea nigra p. 93
McDonald's method p. 84
Naegele's rule p. 84
oral glucose tolerance test (OGTT) p. 90
para p. 85
positive signs of pregnancy p. 85
presumptive signs of pregnancy p. 85
probable signs of pregnancy p. 85
Quadruple screening test p. 90
quickening p. 84
sexually transmitted infections (STIs) p. 88
striae gravidarum p. 93
TORCH infections p. 87
triple-screen test p. 90
ultrasound p. 90

References

Davidson, M., London, M., & Ladewig, P. (2012). *Olds' maternal newborn nursing and women's health across the lifespan* (9th ed.). Upper Saddle River, NJ: Pearson Education, Inc.

Kee, J. (2010). *Laboratory and diagnostic tests* (8th ed.). Upper Saddle River, NJ: Pearson Education, Inc.

Ladewig, P., London, M., & Davidson, M. (2010). *Contemporary maternal-newborn nursing care* (7th ed.). Upper Saddle River, NJ: Pearson Education, Inc.

London, M., Ladewig, P., Ball, J., Bindler, R., & Cowen, K. (2011). *Maternal & child nursing care* (3rd ed.). Upper Saddle River, NJ: Pearson Education, Inc.

Perry, S., Hockenberry, M., Lowdermilk, D., & Wilson, D. (2010). *Maternal child nursing care* (4th ed.). St. Louis, MO: Elsevier.

Test Yourself

Are you ready for the NCLEX-PN® or course exams? Use the practice tests on the companion website to check.

10 Uncomplicated Labor and Delivery Care

In this chapter

Cross Reference

Other chapters relevant to this content area are

Reproduction, Family Planning, and Infertility	Chapter 8
Uncomplicated Antenatal Care	Chapter 9
Uncomplicated Postpartum Care	Chapter 11
Uncomplicated Newborn Care	Chapter 12
Complicated Antenatal Care	Chapter 45
Complicated Labor and Delivery Care	Chapter 46
Complicated Postpartum Care	Chapter 47
Complicated Newborn Care	Chapter 48

I. NURSING CARE OF THE LABOR AND DELIVERY CLIENT

A. Physiologic safety

1. The laboring client is actually two clients—mother and newborn
2. Nursing care focuses on physiologic safety of both

B. Psychological safety

1. Nursing care focuses on mother and includes fear, comfort, partner involvement, parental attachment to newborn, and past experiences
2. Primigravida women experience fear of unknown and often have longer labors
3. Multigravida women can expect a shorter labor with subsequent pregnancies but may have memories of perceived bad experiences from previous births

C. Maternal history: determine a history of abuse, assault, and violence because such experiences often manifest as extreme fear and tension during labor process or vaginal examinations

D. Cultural background

1. Must be understood to provide a safe and acceptable birthing environment for childbearing family
2. Some common nursing actions may be cultural taboos for a particular client and affect parents' view of child throughout life

E. Educational preparation for labor by client and her support person(s)

1. Varies from formal prenatal classes to information passed through generations
2. Address any misconceptions about birthing process or sensations to expect during birth in a nonjudgmental manner that informs and supports birthing family

F. Electronic fetal monitoring

1. Provides computer-assisted auditory and visual monitoring of fetal heart rate (FHR) and uterine contractions (UC)
2. FHR monitoring continuously records FHR on upper portion of monitor strip

NCLEX®
3. External monitoring: an ultrasound transducer is placed over fetal back and detects movements of fetal heart; fetal or maternal movement and maternal obesity may interfere with obtaining a continuous reading
4. Internal monitoring
   a. An **internal fetal scalp electrode** is inserted through cervix (must be at least 2 cm dilated with ruptured membranes) and attached to epidermis of presenting part, providing a direct electrocardiogram (ECG) of fetal heart
   b. Is unaffected by maternal obesity, maternal or fetal movement; thick fetal hair may prevent adequate insertion on a cephalic presentation

NCLEX®
5. **Baseline fetal heart rate** is average heart rate between contractions; measured in beats per minute (bpm); normal range: 110 to 160; bradycardia: < 110; tachycardia: > 160

NCLEX®
6. **Accelerations**: transient increases in FHR
   a. Nonperiodic (spontaneous): symmetric, uniform, not related to contractions, occur in response to fetal movement and indicate fetal well-being
   b. Periodic: occur with contractions and may indicate decreased amniotic fluid or mild umbilical cord compression
7. Decelerations are categorized as early, late, or variable

NCLEX®
8. **Early deceleration**: decrease in FHR beginning at onset of contraction and returning to baseline by end of contraction with lowest rate at peak of contraction
   a. Caused by fetal head compression; usually benign
   b. Nursing interventions: vaginal examination to determine if fetus is descending in pelvis; if fetus is not descending, notify health care provider

NCLEX®
9. **Late decelerations** begin after contraction starts, with lowest rate occurring after peak of contraction and returning to baseline after end of contraction
   a. Caused by uteroplacental insufficiency; always considered ominous
   b. Nursing interventions focus on maintaining oxygenation: reposition client to left lateral, administer oxygen by mask at 7 to 10 L/min, correct hypotension by increasing IV fluid rate or administering medications, discontinue oxytocin if being administered, and report to health care provider
10. Uterine contraction monitoring documents contraction frequency, duration, and intensity on lower half of monitor strip
    a. External monitoring: tocodynamometer is placed on maternal abdomen near fundus; accurate only for documenting contraction frequency and duration; affected by fetal or maternal movement, transverse or oblique lie, and maternal abdominal fat: a thin woman's mild contractions may look strong on monitor strip, while an obese woman's strong contractions may not be detected at all
    b. Internal monitoring is accomplished through an **intrauterine pressure catheter (IUPC)**, a wire with pressure gauge on one end or a saline-filled tube, which is inserted through cervix and past presenting part into amniotic fluid in uterus; increase in intrauterine pressure is measured in mm Hg; cervix must be at least 2 to 3 cm dilated with ruptured membranes before an IUPC can be inserted

II. THE LABOR PROCESS

A. Initiation of labor: comes about from an interplay of factors, including distension of uterus causing irritability and contractility, and hormonal influence of prostaglandins, oxytocin, fetal cortisol, estrogen, and progesterone

NCLEX®
B. True versus false labor: differentiated by cervical change: effacement and dilatation

C. Factors of labor: passageway, passenger, powers, and psyche

1. *Passageway* is maternal bony pelvis comprised of innominate bones (ilium, ischium, and pubis), sacrum and coccyx
   a. False pelvis lies above pelvic brim, supports increasing weight of enlarging pregnant uterus, and directs presenting part into true pelvis below
   b. True pelvis consists of inlet, midpelvis, and outlet and represents bony limits of birth canal; adequacy of each part, measured as transverse and anterior–posterior (AP) diameters, must be sufficient to allow passage of fetus
   c. Four pelvic types are gynecoid, android, anthropoid, and platypelloid (see Table 10–1); type and diameters of pelvis influence fetal descent, progression of labor, and type of delivery
2. *Passenger* refers to fetus

NCLEX® a. **Attitude** is relationship of fetal parts to one another; normal attitude is flexion of neck, arms, and legs

NCLEX® b. **Lie** is relationship of cephalocaudal axis of fetus to cephalocaudal axis of mother; is either longitudinal (or vertical, most common) or transverse (lateral)

NCLEX® c. **Presentation** is fetal part entering pelvis first; most common is cephalic (with subcategories of vertex, military, brow or face presentation), but breech (subtypes of complete, frank, or footling) and shoulder (also called transverse lie) can also occur

NCLEX® d. **Position** is relationship of fetal presenting part to maternal pelvis; a three-letter notation describes fetal position: see memory aid box; most common positions at delivery are ROA (right occiput anterior) and LOA (left occiput anterior)

Table 10–1 Pelvic Types

Pelvic Type	Incidence	Inlet	Midpelvis	Outlet	Implications for Birth
Gynecoid	50%	Round, adequate diameters	Round, adequate diameters	Wide transverse, long anterior–posterior (AP) diameters	Occiput anterior most common, NSVD favorable
Android	20%	Heart-shaped, angulated	Short AP diameter	Short AP diameter	Slow descent, arrest of labor, operative birth more common
Anthropoid	25%	Ovoid, long AP diameter	Rounded, adequate diameters	Narrow transverse diameter	Occiput anterior or posterior, NSVD favorable
Platypelloid	5%	Ovoid, wide transverse diameter	Rounded, wide transverse diameter	Wide transverse, short AP diameter	Occiput posterior more common, NSVD not favorable

Memory Aid

Use the mnemonics in 2 and 3 to help remember fetal position:

1. **R** or **L:** **r**ight or **l**eft; direction that presenting part of fetus faces
2. **AMOS:** **a**cromion process, **m**entum, **o**cciput, **s**acrum; the landmark of the fetal presenting part
3. **PAT:** **p**osterior, **a**nterior, **t**ransverse; the relationship of the landmark of the presenting part to the front, back, or side of pelvis

NCLEX® e. **Engagement** occurs when largest diameter of presenting part reaches pelvic inlet and can be detected by vaginal exam; termed *floating* if it is directed toward pelvis but can easily be moved out of inlet; termed *ballotable* when presenting part dips into inlet but can be displaced with upward pressure by examiner's fingers; termed *engaged* if fixed in pelvic inlet and cannot be displaced

f. **Station** is relationship of presenting part to pelvic ischial spines; measured in centimeters (cm) above (–1 to –5 station), at (0 station), or below (+1 to +4 station) ischial spines (see Figure 10–1)

3. Powers include primary and secondary forces of labor
   a. Primary forces: involuntary contractions of uterine muscle fibers, which are stimulated by a pacemaker located in upper uterine segment
   b. Phases of contractions: increment (building-up), acme (peak), and decrement (letting-up) followed by a resting phase (nadir) to facilitate uteroplacental–fetal reoxygenation

NCLEX® c. Frequency of contractions: time in seconds or minutes from onset of one contraction to onset of next

NCLEX® d. Intensity: strength of contraction at acme, which can be palpated as mild, moderate, or strong; detected with a fetal monitor externally; or measured internally in mm Hg

NCLEX® e. Duration: length of contraction measured in seconds from beginning of increment to end of decrement

f. With each contraction, muscles of upper uterine segment shorten and exert longitudinal traction on cervix, causing **effacement** (thinning and drawing up of internal os and cervical canal into uterine side walls); measured from 0 to 100%; in primigravidas, effacement usually precedes dilatation; in multigravidas, they normally occur simultaneously

g. As uterus elongates with contractions, fetal body straightens and exerts pressure against lower uterine segment and cervix; **dilatation** or opening of cervix results; is measured from 0 to 10 cm, and allows for birth of fetus

h. Secondary powers: voluntary use of abdominal muscles during second stage of labor to facilitate descent and delivery of fetus

Figure 10–1

Stations of fetal descent measured in centimeters.

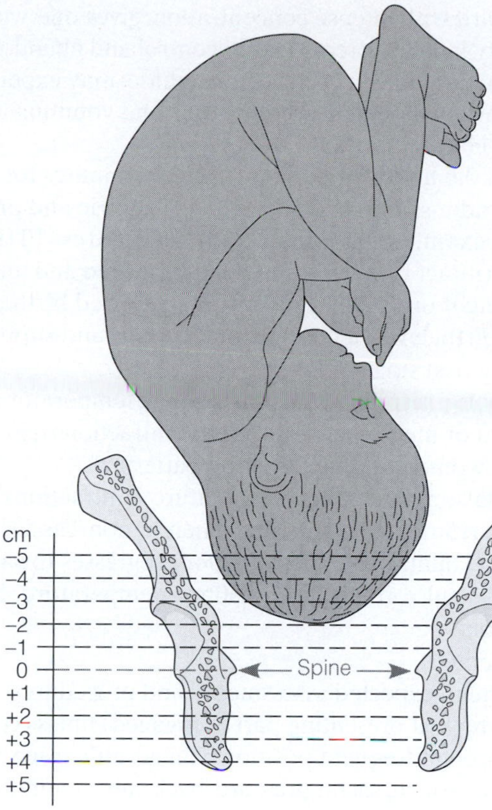

4. Psyche: psychological component of childbearing; excitement, fear, perceived loss of control, anxiety are common emotions during labor and delivery
   a. Extreme emotions such as fear result in muscular tension, which can create more pain from friction between working uterus and tense abdominal muscles or impede descent of fetus when pelvic and perineal muscles are tense rather than relaxed when pushing
   b. Psyche can also manifest physiologically as increased maternal blood pressure (BP), pulse, and respiratory rates occur with fear, excitement, and anxiety
   c. Lack of knowledge and preparation for childbirth can negatively affect psyche

III. THE STAGES OF LABOR

A. First stage

1. Extends from onset of true labor to complete dilatation of cervix (0 to 10 cm) and is divided into three phases: latent, active, and transition

NCLEX®

2. Latent phase
   a. 0 to 3 centimeters dilated, little descent occurs
   b. Contractions usually begin irregularly and become more regular, with increasing frequency and duration and intensity (from mild to moderate)
   c. Client is usually relieved labor has started; can recognize and express anxiety; may be happy, excited, and talkative; and changes position without reminder
   d. Average duration is 8.6 hours for nulliparas and 5.3 hours for multiparas

NCLEX®

3. Active phase
   a. 4 to 7 centimeters dilated, effacement and descent are progressive
   b. Contractions usually every 2 to 3 minutes, 60 seconds in duration, and moderate to strong intensity
   c. Client is usually serious, intense, has a need for increased concentration, answers questions in short phrases between contractions; fatigue increases and woman becomes more dependent; pain increases, relaxation is more difficult, and woman may need reminders to change positions
   d. Average duration is 4.6 hours for nulliparas and 2.4 hours for multiparas

NCLEX®

4. Transition phase
   a. 8 to 10 centimeters dilated, effacement is completed, and descent increases
   b. Contractions every 1½ to 2 minutes, lasting 60 to 90 seconds, strong intensity

c. Client is working hard with intense concentration; gives one-word answers to questions only between contractions; anxiety increases, fears loss of control and abandonment, senses helplessness; relaxation is difficult as contraction time exceeds resting phase; may experience intense low abdominal, pelvic, and rectal discomfort from fetal descent; nausea and vomiting are common; may need reminders to empty bladder and change position

d. Average duration is 3.6 hours for nulliparas and 30 minutes for multiparas

5. Data collection upon admission: review medical, obstetric and prenatal history; labor status (contractions, vaginal examination if indicated), fetal status (FHR, variability, periodic changes), status of membranes (intact or if ruptured, length of time and amount, color, odor), maternal vital signs, laboratory testing if ordered (Hgb and UA), desired birth plan including cultural considerations, preparation for childbirth, level of comfort and coping, and support system

NCLEX®

6. Data collection during first stage of labor

a. Latent phase: BP, pulse, respirations q1h if normal; temperature q4h if normal or membranes intact and q2h if abnormal or membranes ruptured; contractions q30 min; FHR q1hr for low-risk women or q30min if high-risk women or nonreassuring pattern

b. Active phase: BP, pulse, respirations, temperature, contractions same as latent phase; FHR q30min for low-risk women or q15min for high-risk women or nonreassuring pattern; look for bloody mucus or "show" from cervical dilatation as active labor progresses toward transition

c. Transition phase: BP, pulse, respirations q30min; temperature same as latent phase; contractions q15min, FHR q15min

7. Collaborative management

a. Orient to environment, expected assessments, and procedures

b. Encourage ambulation (if presenting part is engaged) unless contraindicated

NCLEX®

c. Provide comfort through frequent position change, effluerage, focal point, hydrotherapy, caregiver presence, therapeutic touch, sacral pressure, back rub, or administration of analgesia as requested by client and ordered by health care provider

d. Encourage voiding q2h

e. Monitor labor progress and fetal well-being

NCLEX®

f. Provide ice chips and clear liquids to prevent dehydration

g. Teach, reinforce, or support use of relaxation, visualization, or breathing patterns

NCLEX®

h. Encourage rest between contractions

i. Document and provide continuing status reports to health care provider

B. Second stage

NCLEX®

1. Extends from complete dilatation of cervix to delivery of fetus; accompanied by involuntary efforts to expel fetus and low-pitched, guttural, grunting sounds

2. Many women initially feel renewed energy because they can voluntarily work with contractions to push out fetus; over time can be exhausting work

3. Normal duration is up to 3 hours for nulliparas and up to 30 minutes for multiparas

4. **Cardinal movements**: adaptations that fetus undertakes to maneuver through pelvis during labor and birth; in most common presentation, occiput, movements occur in the following order:

a. *Engagement* of presenting part occurs

b. *Descent* of fetus into pelvis

c. *Flexion* of fetal head; (descent and flexion often occur simultaneously)

d. ***I****nternal* ***R****otation* of fetal head takes place to accommodate maternal pelvis so that anterior–posterior (AP) diameter of fetal head (largest diameter of fetus) aligns with AP dimension of maternal pelvis

e. *Extension* of fetal head occurs as it comes under maternal symphysis pubis and emerges from vagina

f. ***R****estitution* occurs as fetal head turns 45 degrees to untwist neck after head has delivered

g. ***E****xternal* ***R****otation* is viewed as head turns an additional 45 degrees as second-largest fetal diameter (lateral diameter of fetal shoulders) rotates into alignment with AP dimension of maternal pelvis

h. *Expulsion* occurs as anterior shoulder slips beneath symphysis pubis, which facilitates delivery of body

Memory Aid

Use the following mnemonic phrase to assist in remembering the cardinal movements, using the first letter of each cardinal movement to begin a word: ***E****very* ***d****arn* ***f****ool* ***in*** ***R****otterdam* ***e****ats* ***r****otten* ***e****gg* ***r****olls* ***e****veryday.*

5. **Crowning**: outward perineal bulging and thinning and opening of vagina that occurs as fetal presenting part presses downward onto perineum and becomes visible prior to delivery; process is slower in nulliparous client than multiparous client

NCLEX®

6. Assisting with nursing care
   - a. BP, pulse, and respirations q5–q15min
   - b. Contractions palpated continuously
   - c. FHR q15min if low risk, q5min if high risk, and if nonreassuring pattern, monitor continuously
   - d. Monitor fetal descent, cardinal fetal movements, and crowning

NCLEX®

7. Collaborative management
   - a. Position comfortably for pushing and birth; encourage rest and relaxation between contractions
   - b. Comfort measures: cool cloth to forehead, support legs while pushing, provide encouragement to push
   - c. Ice chips and clear fluids to prevent dehydration
   - d. Empty bladder, straight catheter if bladder distended or unable to void
   - e. Local infiltration of anesthetic agent for birth by health care provider
   - NCLEX® f. **Episiotomy**: surgical incision into perineum to enlarge vaginal opening; usually done during or just prior to crowning; medically indicated in presence of fetal distress, but often performed to prevent tearing of perineal tissues because lacerations have irregular edges and are more difficult to repair
   - g. Types of episiotomy: midline (1- to 3-cm incision straight back from vagina toward rectum), mediolateral (4- to 5-cm incision from vagina obliquely toward one buttock)
   - h. Lacerations to perineum or surrounding tissues may occur during childbirth; see Box 10–1 for degrees of laceration; 3rd- and 4th-degree lacerations most commonly occur after midline episiotomy is performed
   - i. Document in client record: time of birth, gender, position, nuchal cord if present, and medications administered

C. Third stage

1. Extends from birth of newborn to delivery of placenta; average duration is 30 minutes for nulliparas and multiparas
2. Maternal data collection
   - NCLEX® a. BP, pulse, and respirations q5min
   - b. Uterine fundus maintains tone and contraction pattern to deliver placenta by decreasing surface volume of uterus and shearing placenta from uterine wall
   - c. Monitor for signs of placental separation: uterus rises up in abdomen; uterine volume shrinks as a result of contractions creating a gush of blood vaginally as uterine contents are expelled; as placenta is separating and beginning to be expelled, umbilical cord protrudes further from vagina and appears to lengthen
3. Fetal data collection
   - a. **Apgar score**: quick method to determine fetal adaptation to extrauterine life; five criteria are scored at 1 and 5 minutes after birth with 0, 1, or 2 points given for each criteria (see Table 10–2); Apgar scores of 8 or greater indicate need for minimal intervention (nasopharyngeal suction and oxygen near face); scores of 4 to 7 indicate need for oropharyngeal suctioning, tactile stimulation, and oxygen administration; scores of 3 or less indicate need for resuscitation
   - b. Respirations: normally 30 to 60, may be irregular
   - c. Apical pulse: 110 to 160, may be irregular and may be as high as 180 when crying
   - d. Temperature (skin): above 97.8°F (36.5°C)
   - e. Umbilical cord: normally two arteries and one vein
   - f. Gestational age assessment: consistent with expected date of delivery
   - g. Physical assessment: abbreviated exam done to detect visible congenital anomalies
4. Collaborative management
   - a. Encourage mother to rest and relax while awaiting delivery of placenta

Box 10–1

Degrees of Laceration

1st degree: involves only epidermal layers; if no bleeding, may not need repair

2nd degree: epidermal and muscle/fascia involvement, which requires suturing

3rd degree: extends into rectal sphincter

4th degree: extends through rectal mucosa

NCLEX®
b. Immediate care of newborn: place in a modified Trendelenburg position, suction nose and oropharynx (bulb syringe or DeLee mucus trap), provide and maintain warmth (dry immediately with warm blankets, skin-to-skin contact with mother covered with warm blankets, radiant heat source, cap)
c. Assist parents in seeing and holding newborn to begin attachment
d. Document time of placental delivery, appearance and intactness of placenta, mechanism of placental expulsion, and estimated delivery blood loss (averages 250 to 500 mL)
e. Administer oxytocic agent as ordered
f. Consider cultural practices in disposal of placenta

D. Fourth stage (immediate recovery phase)

1. Includes first 1 to 4 hours after delivery; is actually part of postpartal period
2. Data collection: BP, pulse, respirations, fundus, lochia and perineum per agency protocol; usually q15min for 1 hour; q30min for 2 hours; q60min for 1 hour (NCLEX®)
3. Collaborative management
   a. Episiotomy or lacerations are repaired
   b. Provide comfort: clean gown, warm blanket, position of comfort, ice to perineum if sutures or edema present, analgesia as requested and ordered
   c. Help parents to explore newborn and initiate breastfeeding if desired and if mother and baby are stable (NCLEX®)
   d. Provide fluids and regular diet as tolerated; consider cultural preferences
4. Outcome is that maternal and newborn well-being are maintained; family unit is supported and participates in birth process as desired

IV. PAIN MANAGEMENT DURING BIRTH

A. Analgesia and anesthesia: can decrease or eliminate pain during birthing process when nonpharmacologic methods of pain relief are ineffective

B. Type of analgesia or anesthesia

1. Determined by obstetric history of client, stage and phase of labor, rate of progression in labor, and preferences of client and health care provider
2. Regional differences in use of particular methods or medications exist

NCLEX® **C. Nonpharmacologic methods of pain relief**

1. Position changes to decrease weight of fetus on area of most intense pain
2. Hydrotherapy by standing or sitting in a warm shower or reclining in a tub
3. Breathing techniques to prevent breath-holding and facilitate oxygen and carbon dioxide exchange; use of a focal point for concentration
4. Relaxation through verbal instruction, massage, soft music, or therapeutic touch

D. Pharmacologic methods of pain relief

1. Analgesics decrease perception of pain; goal is maximum pain relief with minimal risk; must consider effect on woman, fetus, and contractions (see also Table 10–3 for advantages, disadvantages, and nursing implications of various pain relief methods)
2. All systemic drugs cross placental barrier in varying amounts; analgesia given too early may prolong labor and depress fetus; analgesia given too late may cause neonatal respiratory depression with no benefit to woman (NCLEX®)
3. Intravenous synthetic agonist-antagonist opioids: nalbuphine hydrochloride (Nubain) and butorphanol tartrate (Stadol) most commonly used in active phase of first stage of labor
4. Intrathecal opioids: morphine sulphate (Morphine) or fentanyl citrate (Fentanyl) injected into L4–L5 or L5–S1 subarachnoid space

Table 10–2 Apgar Scoring

	Color (Appearance)	Heart Rate (Pulse)	Reflex Irritability (Grimace)	Muscle Tone (Activity)	Respiratory Effort (Respirations)
0 Points	Blue, pale	Absent	Absent	Absent	Absent
1 Point	Blue extremities, pink body	< 100	Grimace	Some flexion of extremities	Slow, irregular
2 Points	Completely pink	≥ 100	Vigorous cry	Active motion	Good cry

5. Lumbar **epidural block**: provides temporary and reversible loss of sensation by injection into area with direct contact to nerve tissue; needle and catheter introduced at L4–L5 or L5–S1 level; local anesthetics such as bupivacaine hydrochloride (Marcaine) or lidocaine hydrochloride (Xylocaine) injected; provides either regional analgesia or anesthesia depending on dose injected
6. **Paracervical block**: a type of regional anesthesia; local anesthetic agent injected into lateral aspects of cervix during active or transition phases
7. **Pudendal block**: local anesthetic agent injected into lateral vaginal walls near ischial spines to anesthetize pudendal nerve; administered during second stage in preparation for cutting and repairing an episiotomy
8. Local infiltration: local anesthetic agents are injected into tissues of perineum to provide anesthesia for episiotomy incision or repair and suturing of lacerations

Table 10–3 Pharmacological Pain Relief Methods During Labor

Pharmacological Pain Relief Method	Advantages	Disadvantages	Nursing Implications
Intravenous opioids	RN administration, rapid onset of pain relief, easy to administer, relatively short duration	May ↓ contraction frequency and intensity, crosses placenta resulting in neonatal respiratory depression, short duration may not give adequate pain control during first or prolonged labor	Do not give opioid agonist-antagonist if narcotic dependency as immediate withdrawal will occur that can lead to seizures
Intrathecal opioids	Excellent pain control occurring within several minutes, lasts several hours, rarely results in neonatal respiratory depression, easier and faster than epidural for both provider and client	Undesirable for rapidly progressing labor or transition phase; may stop urge to push; must be injected by anesthesia personnel and is uncomfortable; client must hold still during injections; spinal headache may occur if CSF leaks through dura at injection site	Monitor for common side effects, including nausea, pruritus, urinary retention, muscle spasms at site of injection
Lumbar epidural block	Excellent pain relief, re-dosing possible, no neonatal respiratory depression results, may provide a few hours of postpartum pain relief as well as during labor and delivery	Undesirable for rapidly progressing labor or transition phase; must be inserted by anesthesia personnel; usually causes numbness of lower extremities, limiting mobility; ↓ contraction frequency and intensity; ↓ or eliminates urge to push; relaxation of musculature below site of injection often results in failure of fetus to accomplish internal rotation, necessitating an operative birth	Monitor urine output because retention requiring indwelling urinary catheter may result Monitor BP because maternal hypotension commonly results from vasodilation; avoid supine position
Paracervical block	Rapid onset of pain relief, no neonatal respiratory depression, can be given during transition, relatively easy to administer	Systemic absorption of drug through vascular cervix, excessive bleeding from cervix, ↓ or absent urge to push	FHR drop (bradycardia) can result from systemic absorption
Pudendal block	Provides excellent anesthesia of perineum, rarely needs second dose, provides a few hours of postpartum pain relief	Must inject along presenting part, creating ↓ vaginal pressure and discomfort for client; eliminates urge to push	Monitor client safety because ↓ sensation in lower extremities affects mobility
Local tissue infiltration	Easy to administer, provides a few hours of postpartum pain relief	Reinjection may be needed to obtain complete anesthesia with extensive lacerations or large episiotomies	Loss of sensation may ↓ urge or ability to urinate

Check Your NCLEX-PN® Exam I.Q. *You are ready for testing on this content if you can*

- Monitor the physiological status of a client in labor.
- Teach relaxation methods during labor.
- Measure fetal heart rate.
- Describe the delivery of a newborn.
- Provide effective support, information-sharing, and nursing care to a client in labor.

PRACTICE TEST

PRACTICE TEST

1 After walking for 30 minutes, the laboring client now has blood-tinged mucus on her underpad. Which of the following is the most appropriate interpretation by the nurse?

1. The fetus has had a bowel movement.
2. The amniotic sac has ruptured.
3. The client has fallen while walking and sustained internal injury.
4. The cervix is opening more rapidly.

2 After administration of an epidural block for labor analgesia, the client's blood pressure decreases from 130/75 to 90/50. The nurse should assist the woman to do which of the following?

1. Lie in a supine position
2. Assume a semi-Fowler's position
3. Empty her bladder
4. Turn to the side, to a left lateral position

3 The nurse understands that which of the following is the most accurate method for collecting data about the frequency, duration, and strength of contractions of a woman in active labor?

1. Abdominal palpation
2. Tocodynamometer
3. Intrauterine pressure catheter (IUPC)
4. Client's description

4 The nurse concludes that the use of nonpharmacologic pain management techniques have been helpful to the client after observing which of the following?

1. Decreased short-term variability in the fetal heart rate
2. Increased maternal blood pressure and pulse
3. Decreased muscle tension in the arms and face
4. Increased frequency of contractions

5 The nurse who is assisting in implementing a plan of care for a laboring client with pain would incorporate which of the following concepts?

1. Childbirth pain is caused only by physical factors.
2. The expression of pain is universal.
3. Having the presence of a supportive partner eliminates pain.
4. Labor pain has physiologic and psychologic components.

6 The nurse assisting in the care of a client with a prolonged latent phase of labor includes which of the following as a priority measure?

1. Encouraging rest and relaxation through the playing of soft music
2. Monitoring IV hydration with lactated Ringer's solution or 5 percent dextrose
3. Continuous internal fetal monitoring of the fetal response to contractions
4. Measuring maternal blood pressure, temperature, and pulse every 15 minutes

7 The client's fetal heart rate (FHR) is 150 before a contraction begins. During the contraction, the FHR falls to 110 and returns to baseline 30 seconds after the contraction ends. What is the priority nursing action in response to this finding?

1. Place the client into a semi-Fowler's position.
2. Administer oxygen by nasal cannula at 2 liters per minute.
3. Insert a Foley catheter and measure urinary output.
4. Place the client in left lateral position.

8 When assisting in the care of an adolescent in labor, the nurse should address which of the following concerns?

1. Misconceptions of the functions of various body parts
2. The pregnant adolescent's nutritional needs
3. Reliability of her boyfriend as a support person
4. Appropriateness of names for her newborn that she has chosen

9 The laboring client is 8 centimeters dilated, 100% effaced, with vertex presenting at +2 station. The fetal heart rate gradually slows during each contraction, returning to baseline by the end of the contraction. The nurse concludes that which of the following is occurring?

1. The umbilical cord is becoming compressed.
2. There is uteroplacental insufficiency.
3. The fetal head is becoming compressed.
4. The fetus is moving between contractions.

10 A woman is admitted to the birth unit. She is bearing down uncontrollably with contractions and says, "The baby is coming!" What is the priority action of the nurse, who is alone in the room at this time?

1. Telephone the health care provider.
2. Put on gloves and prepare for immediate birth.
3. Obtain a medical and obstetric history.
4. Assess maternal vital signs and fetal heart rate.

11 The laboring client has begun to make guttural, grunting sounds during contractions. The nurse assisting in this client's care should now include which nursing intervention?

1. Inspect the perineum to see if it is bulging outward.
2. Encourage the client's husband to go and eat now.
3. Remind the client about breastfeeding soon after delivery.
4. Measure the client's blood pressure and temperature.

12 A primigravida client is in the second stage of labor. The nurse recognizes that reinforcement of the teaching plan has been effective when the client makes which statement?

1. "I'll push two or three times and the baby will be born."
2. "It's not the baby, I have to have a bowel movement."
3. "I know I'll have to push a while. This is hard work."
4. "My doctor will come and pull the baby out now."

13 The newly delivered infant has been placed on the mother's abdomen. What is the nurse's priority nursing intervention for the newborn?

1. Dry off the infant with blankets or towels.
2. Apply identification bracelets and obtain footprints.
3. Estimate the newborn's gestational age.
4. Use the bulb syringe to clear the mouth and nose of mucus if needed.

14 A laboring client's membranes spontaneously rupture. What should be the nurse's first action?

1. Note the fetal heart rate.
2. Encourage the woman to ambulate.
3. Document the color, odor, and amount of amniotic fluid.
4. Prepare for imminent delivery of the newborn.

15 The multiparous client is 9 centimeters, 100% effaced, at a 2 station, with strong contractions every 2–3 minutes lasting 70 seconds. What action should the nurse take at this time?

1. Call the client's health care provider.
2. Offer the client pain medication.
3. Encourage the client to be up and walking.
4. Assist in preparing for imminent delivery.

16 The nurse should include which elements when collecting psychosocial data regarding the laboring client? Select all that apply.

1. Cultural practices
2. Plans for naming the child
3. Fetal heart rate monitoring
4. Socioeconomic status of the family
5. Expectations of the experience

17 The nurse reinforces with a pair of expectant parents about cardinal movements, or changes in position, that occur as the fetus with a cephalic presentation passes through the birth canal. Order the cardinal movements in proper sequence for the nurse's presentation. All options must be used.

1. Expulsion
2. External rotation
3. Flexion
4. Internal rotation
5. Restitution

18 The nurse assisting in the maternity unit would implement which intervention as part of fourth-stage nursing care for a client who delivered an infant? Select all that apply.

1. Application of ice beginning 4 hours after delivery
2. Ice pack to the perineum for up to 60 minutes per application
3. Inspection of the perineum every 15 minutes for the first hour after birth
4. Instructions to avoid intercourse for at least 12 weeks
5. Ice packs to be applied for 20–30 minutes and removed for at least 20 minutes

19 Which observation by the maternal newborn nurse would indicate a sign of impending placental separation and expulsion?

1. Steady trickle of blood with an unchanged cord length
2. No bleeding with lengthening of the cord
3. Small gush of blood with lengthening of the cord
4. Small gush of blood with an unchanged cord length

20 The nurse assisting in the maternity unit notes that earlier in the shift, the fetal heart rate (FHR) was 140 beats/minute and the baseline has now risen to 170. The nurse would investigate which factors as possible causes for the higher baseline readings? Select all that apply.

1. Maternal fever
2. Narcotic administration
3. Fetal movement
4. Utero-placental insufficiency
5. Fetal distress

ANSWERS & RATIONALES

1 **Answer: 4 Rationale:** Bloody mucus is often called bloody show and becomes more profuse during the late active phase and into the transition phase of the first stage of labor and during the second stage of labor. Fetal bowel movements are not blood-tinged. Rupture of the amniotic sac would produce a clear, watery fluid. There is no correlation of blood-tinged mucus during labor with injury sustained through walking. **Cognitive Level:** Analyzing **Client Need:** Health Promotion and Maintenance **Integrated Process:** Nursing Process: Evaluation **Content Area:** Maternal-Newborn **Strategy:** Note the critical word *blood-tinged* and associate this with progression in labor. Recall that exercise such as walking hastens labor. Both of these concepts should guide you to select cervical dilation as the answer.

2 **Answer: 4 Rationale:** Vasodilation occurs with epidural analgesia and anesthesia, which can result in hypotension. The client who is hypotensive after epidural administration should be turned to a left lateral position and have the IV fluid rate increased to increase the circulation to the fetus and increase circulating volume, respectively. Lying supine allows the gravid uterus to place pressure on the aorta and can reduce further the circulation to the fetus. A semi-Fowler's position could worsen the hypotension. Emptying the bladder will not alleviate the hypotension. **Cognitive Level:** Applying **Client Need:** Health Promotion and Maintenance **Integrated Process:** Nursing Process: Implementation **Content Area:** Maternal-Newborn **Strategy:** The issue of the question is the appropriate action that counteracts a side effect of epidural analgesia. Recall that opioid analgesics often cause vasodilation, which can be counteracted by proper positioning.

3 **Answer: 3 Rationale:** Internal contraction monitoring through the use of an intrauterine pressure catheter will objectively measure the contractions in mm of Hg and is the most accurate method of contraction monitoring. Abdominal palpation will give limited information about uterine contractions, especially if the client is either very thin or obese. The tocodynamometer, or external uterine transducer, will detect the onset and end of contractions in most women but does not assess intensity of the contractions. Additionally, if the client is either very thin or obese, the fetal monitor tracing will either exaggerate the contractions or minimize them. The client's description of the contractions will be influenced by her culturally based expression of pain as well as by her previous pain experiences and pain threshold. **Cognitive Level:** Analyzing **Client Need:** Health Promotion and Maintenance **Integrated Process:** Nursing Process: Data Collection **Content Area:** Maternal-Newborn **Strategy:** Note the critical words *most accurate method*, which tell you that more than one option may be partially or totally correct but that one option is best. Evaluate each option and make your choice based on the method (IUPC) that is closest to the source (fetus and uterus).

4 **Answer: 3 Rationale:** Objective signs of pain relief include decreased muscle tension as evidenced by unclenched fists; relaxed facial muscles and decreased grimacing, frowning, or creasing of the brow; and slightly lowered blood pressure, pulse rate, and respiratory rate. Frequency of uterine contractions would not be affected by relieving pain through nonpharmacological methods. **Cognitive Level:** Analyzing **Client Need:** Health Promotion and Maintenance **Integrated Process:** Nursing Process: Evaluation **Content Area:** Maternal-Newborn **Strategy:** The issue of the question is a satisfactory outcome of nonpharmacological methods of pain relief. With this in mind, use knowledge of general signs of pain relief to make your selection. Eliminate short-term variability and contractions first because they are not evidence of pain relief, then eliminate maternal blood pressure and pulse, because they would decrease rather than increase with pain relief.

5 **Answer: 4 Rationale:** The pain of labor and childbirth has both physiologic and psychologic components. A support person's presence has been shown to decrease the perceived pain of childbearing. However, the expression of pain through nonverbal cues or verbalizations is highly culturally based (not universal), having been learned in early childhood. **Cognitive Level:** Applying **Client Need:** Health Promotion and Maintenance **Integrated Process:** Nursing Process: Planning **Content Area:** Maternal-Newborn **Strategy:** Note that two options are essentially the opposite of each other. When two options are opposites, often one of them is correct. Choose the one that is more comprehensive.

6 **Answer: 1 Rationale:** Prolonged latent phase of labor is defined as greater than 20 hours in primigravida women and greater than 14 hours in multigravida women. Encouraging rest and relaxation during this phase will help the client have enough energy to push effectively during the second stage of labor. Music is often used effectively to induce relaxation. Encouraging a well-rested client to ambulate will also facilitate the latent phase. Intravenous hydration is given to

women who are unable to take oral fluids. Internal monitoring is indicated if labor is being augmented or induced, the amniotic fluid is meconium-stained, or there is evidence of fetal distress by external monitoring. During the first stage of labor, maternal vital signs are obtained every hour. **Cognitive Level:** Applying **Client Need:** Health Promotion and Maintenance **Integrated Process:** Nursing Process: Planning **Content Area:** Maternal-Newborn **Strategy:** Note the critical word *priority* in the question. This tells you some or all options may be partially or totally correct, but one is most important. First eliminate maternal vital signs every 15 minutes as unnecessary. Then eliminate internal fetal monitoring because external monitoring may be equally effective. Choose correctly between the remaining options because there is no indication that the client cannot tolerate fluids and also because of the words *prolonged latent phase* in the question.

7 **Answer: 4** **Rationale:** Late decelerations are caused by uteroplacental insufficiency and are always ominous. To optimize uteroplacental blood flow and therefore fetal oxygenation, the client should be positioned on her left side. Oxygen is appropriate but would be administered via mask at 7–10 liters per minute. A Foley catheter is unrelated to the fetus's needs at this time. **Cognitive Level:** Applying **Client Need:** Health Promotion and Maintenance **Integrated Process:** Nursing Process: Implementation **Content Area:** Maternal-Newborn **Strategy:** Determine what the question is testing, which is uteroplacental insufficiency. With this mind, reposition the client because it is more effective in increasing delivery of oxygen and blood flow to the fetus.

8 **Answer: 1** **Rationale:** Adolescents commonly misunderstand the functions of their body parts and additional teaching may be needed so the adolescent client in labor understands how birthing will take place. Because the client is in labor, it is too late to address nutritional needs of pregnancy. The role of the nurse is to be informative, supportive, but never judgmental. Thus, the reliability of the boyfriend is not an assessment that the labor and delivery nurse should perform. The role of the nurse is to be informative, supportive, but never judgmental. Thus, the appropriateness of names chosen is not an assessment that the labor and delivery nurse should perform. **Cognitive Level:** Applying **Client Need:** Health Promotion and Maintenance **Integrated Process:** Nursing Process: Planning **Content Area:** Maternal-Newborn **Strategy:** The issue of the question is age-appropriate care of the adolescent during labor. Choose the option that addresses lack of knowledge. Eliminate those that are not timely, do not address the client's current needs, or that could create distance between the client and nurse, depending on the conversation.

9 **Answer: 3** **Rationale:** Gradual decelerations that begin and end with contractions are early decelerations and are caused by fetal head compression. Variable decelerations result from umbilical cord compression and are characterized by a sudden drop from baseline during contractions with a sudden return to baseline as the contraction ends. Late decelerations are caused by uteroplacental insufficiency and are characterized by gradual decrease in the fetal heart rate after the contraction begins, and gradual return to baseline after the contraction has ended. Fetal movement usually results in fetal heart rate accelerations. **Cognitive Level:** Applying **Client Need:** Health Promotion and Maintenance **Integrated Process:** Nursing Process: Evaluation **Content Area:** Maternal-Newborn **Strategy:** Specific knowledge of the relationship between fetal monitoring results and the effect on the fetus is needed to answer this question. Note that the data indicate the changes are occurring during contractions, when the head would be compressed against the lower pelvic structures.

10 **Answer: 2** **Rationale:** Delivery appears imminent and priority should be given to the safety of the woman and her newborn through a controlled and attended birth. Another person can be summoned to contact the health care provider and perform assessments. The history provides helpful information but can be obtained at a later time. **Cognitive Level:** Applying **Client Need:** Health Promotion and Maintenance **Integrated Process:** Nursing Process: Implementation **Content Area:** Maternal-Newborn **Strategy:** The situation in the question is urgent and requires immediate action by the nurse. Eliminate options that are assessments, and choose the option that addresses the immediate physiological and safety needs of the mother and fetus.

11 **Answer: 1** **Rationale:** The second stage of labor begins when the cervix is completely dilated and pushing begins. Most women make a low-pitched, guttural, grunting sound when they push spontaneously. The nurse should immediately inspect the perineum for bulging and the appearance of the presenting part. If neither of these is occurring, the nurse should perform a vaginal examination to assess for complete dilatation of the cervix. Because delivery is more imminent once the second stage of labor begins, it would be better for the client if the husband does not leave at this time. The focus of the nurse at this time is the client's progress toward delivery, not teaching. There is no specific need to assess blood pressure or temperature at this time. **Cognitive Level:** Applying **Client Need:** Health Promotion and Maintenance **Integrated Process:** Nursing Process: Planning **Content Area:** Maternal-Newborn **Strategy:** The issue of this question is accurate interpretation of onset of the second stage of labor. Knowing that pushing is characteristic of this stage, recall it is important for the husband to be present at this time. Eliminate the option with teaching next because it is not timely. Choose inspection of the perineum as the appropriate assessment because it addresses the status of the fetus during the pushing stage.

12 **Answer: 3** **Rationale:** The average duration of the second stage of labor for primigravidas is 2 hours. Many women feel rectal pressure, as if they were having a bowel movement, as the baby descends deeper into the pelvis. The use of vacuum extraction or forceps to assist delivery is not routine. **Cognitive Level:** Applying **Client Need:** Health Promotion and Maintenance **Integrated Process:** Teaching and Learning **Content Area:** Maternal-Newborn **Strategy:** The wording of the question indicates that the correct answer is a statement that is true. Use knowledge of the second stage of labor to systematically eliminate each of the incorrect options.

13 **Answer: 4** **Rationale:** Although all of the nursing actions presented are important after delivery, clearing the airway is the highest physiologic need and ensures safe adaptation to the extrauterine environment. **Cognitive Level:** Applying **Client Need:** Health Promotion and Maintenance **Integrated**

Process: Nursing Process: Implementation **Content Area:** Maternal-Newborn **Strategy:** The critical word in the question is *priority*, which indicates that one intervention is more important than the others to be completed first. Recall that physiological needs take priority over psychosocial needs, and make a final selection that addresses the airway.

14 **Answer: 1 Rationale:** The nurse should immediately assess the fetal heart rate to detect changes, which may be associated with prolapse of the umbilical cord. Ambulation is appropriate if the fetal heart is determined to be within normal parameters and the presenting part is engaged. Documentation is important but is not the priority intervention. The membranes may rupture at any time during labor; preparing for delivery may not be indicated at this time. **Cognitive Level:** Analyzing **Client Need:** Health Promotion and Maintenance **Integrated Process:** Nursing Process: Planning **Content Area:** Maternal-Newborn **Strategy:** The critical word in the question is *first*, which indicates that one intervention is more important than the others at this time. Choose the option that protects the fetus after membrane rupture, and recall that this does not mean that delivery is imminent.

15 **Answer: 4 Rationale:** Multiparous women in the transition phase of the first stage of labor with strong regular contractions will progress to the second stage of delivery very quickly. The nurse should prepare for delivery. The health care provider should be notified prior to this time to ensure his or her presence for delivery. Analgesia is inappropriate this late in labor because it may cause fetal sedation and respiratory depression. Most women prefer to lie down during transition. In addition, safety of the fetus cannot be promoted in an upright ambulatory position if there is a precipitous delivery. **Cognitive Level:** Analyzing **Client Need:** Health Promotion and Maintenance **Integrated Process:** Nursing Process: Implementation **Content Area:** Maternal-Newborn **Strategy:** The question gives assessment findings indicating imminent delivery. Eliminate options that are not timely or that do not promote client safety at this time.

16 **Answer: 1, 5 Rationale:** Knowing what culture the client comes from, and how traditional she is with her cultural beliefs and practices, is important to understand, as it may dictate labor and birthing practices that the client will want to follow, as well as the client's response to pain. The expectations of the experience are important in order to try to integrate realistic ones into the labor plan or help to establish realistic ones that can be explored. Plans to name the child are not relevant at this time. FHR monitoring is not part of the psychosocial assessment. Plans to name the child and the socioeconomic status of the family are not relevant at this time. **Cognitive Level:** Analyzing **Client Need:** Health Promotion and Maintenance **Integrated Process:** Nursing Process: Data Collection **Content Area:** Maternal-Newborn **Strategy:** Eliminate naming the child first because this does not directly relate to psychosocial assessment. Eliminate fetal heart rate because it does not focus on psychosocial assessment and socioeconomic status because financial resources do not provide insight into beliefs, practices, or coping strategies at the time of birth.

17 **Answer: 5, 4, 1, 2, 3 Rationale:** In order, the cardinal movements (position changes) of the fetus are engagement, descent, flexion, internal rotation, extension, restitution, external rotation, and expulsion. These movements represent the normal adaptation of the fetus in a cephalic presentation to the maternal pelvis and facilitate vaginal birth. **Cognitive Level:** Analyzing **Client Need:** Health Promotion and Maintenance **Integrated Process:** Nursing Process: Planning **Content Area:** Maternal-Newborn **Strategy:** Recall the memory aid *Every darn fool in Rotterdam eats rotten egg rolls everyday*. The first letters of each word in the memory aid represent the first letter of each of the cardinal movements of the fetus in a cephalic position.

18 **Answer: 3, 5 Rationale:** Frequent inspection for redness, swelling, tenderness, and hematoma is essential to fourth-stage nursing care. Pain relief begins with immediate application of ice. Ice packs should be applied for 20–30 minutes and removed for at least 20 minutes. If ice is applied for more than 30 minutes, vasodilation and edema may occur. Clients are usually advised to wait until bleeding stops and stitches heal (about 3 weeks) before resuming sexual activity, but this teaching would be part of the client's discharge instructions, and is not appropriate during the fourth stage of labor. **Cognitive Level:** Applying **Client Need:** Health Promotion and Maintenance **Integrated Process:** Nursing Process: Implementation **Content Area:** Maternal-Newborn **Strategy:** The critical issue in this question is time-related. The fourth stage of labor is a time of critical physiologic adaptation and requires frequent assessment. The correct answer is the option that includes a true statement about nursing action at this time.

19 **Answer: 3 Rationale:** As the uterus contracts and the placenta begins to shear off the uterine wall and be expelled, a small gush of blood occurs from the uterine contractions emptying the uterus. In addition, the cord will lengthen as the placenta is released from the uterine wall and moves toward the cervix prior to expulsion. **Cognitive Level:** Analyzing **Client Need:** Health Promotion and Maintenance **Integrated Process:** Nursing Process: Data Collection **Content Area:** Maternal-Newborn **Strategy:** The critical words in this question are *separation* and *expulsion*. As the placenta and cord are expelled, more of the umbilical cord becomes visible. Eliminate two options that are false regarding cord change. Then consider that blood flow would temporarily increase to make the final selection.

20 **Answer: 1, 5 Rationale:** An increase in fetal heart rate baseline can be an indication of fetal distress, as well as maternal fever. Narcotics may decrease the short-term variability but do not affect the baseline. Fetal movement will create an acceleration of the fetal heart rate. Utero-placental insufficiency causes late decelerations. **Cognitive Level:** Analyzing **Client Need:** Physiological Adaptation **Integrated Process:** Nursing Process: Data Collection **Content Area:** Maternal-Newborn **Strategy:** Eliminate options that are obviously incorrect; narcotics are CNS depressants, movement temporarily increases heart rate, and utero-placental insufficiency causes periodic late decelerations.

Key Terms to Review

accelerations p. 103
Apgar score p. 107
attitude p. 104
baseline fetal heart rate p. 103
cardinal movements p. 106
crowning p. 107
dilatation p. 104
early deceleration p. 103
effacement p. 104
engagement p. 104
epidural block p. 109
episiotomy p. 107
internal fetal scalp electrode p. 103
intrauterine pressure catheter (IUPC) p. 103
late deceleration p. 103
lie p. 104
paracervical block p. 109
position p. 104
presentation p. 104
pudendal block p. 109
station p. 104

References

Adams, M., & Cook, R. (2010). *Pharmacology: Connections to nursing practice.* Upper Saddle River, NJ: Pearson Education, Inc.

Davidson, M., London, M., & Ladewig, P. (2012). *Olds' maternal newborn nursing and women's health across the lifespan* (9th ed.). Upper Saddle River, NJ: Pearson Education, Inc.

Ladewig, P., London, M., & Davidson, M. (2010). *Contemporary maternal-newborn nursing care* (7th ed.). Upper Saddle River, NJ: Pearson Education, Inc.

London, M., Ladewig, P., Ball, J., Bindler, R., & Cowen, K. (2011). *Maternal & child nursing care* (3rd ed.). Upper Saddle River, NJ: Pearson Education, Inc.

Perry, S., Hockenberry, M., Lowdermilk, D., & Wilson, D. (2010). *Maternal child nursing care* (4th ed.). St. Louis, MO: Elsevier.

Ward, S., & Hisley, S. (2009). *Maternal-child nursing care: Optimizing outcomes for mothers, children, and families.* Philadelphia, PA: F.A. Davis.

Test Yourself

Are you ready for the NCLEX-PN® or course exams? Use the practice tests on the companion website to check.

11 Uncomplicated Postpartum Care

In this chapter

Cross Reference

Other chapters relevant to this content area are

Reproduction, Family Planning, and Infertility **Chapter 8**
Uncomplicated Antenatal Care **Chapter 9**
Uncomplicated Labor and Delivery Care **Chapter 10**
Uncomplicated Newborn Care **Chapter 12**
Complicated Antenatal Care **Chapter 45**
Complicated Labor and Delivery Care **Chapter 46**
Complicated Postpartum Care **Chapter 47**
Complicated Newborn Care **Chapter 48**

I. PHYSICAL CHANGES DURING POSTPARTUM PERIOD

A. *Involution*

1. Reduction in uterine size after delivery to prepregnant size, caused by uterine contractions that constrict and occlude underlying blood vessels at placental site
2. NCLEX® Table 11–1 presents factors that slow or hasten this process during **puerperium**, the 6-week period after delivery

B. *Fundus*

1. Top portion of uterus is a palpable indicator of involution
2. If contractions of uterine muscle are interrupted, a **boggy uterus** (one that is soft, relaxed) results and is likely to cause hemorrhage

C. Lochia

1. NCLEX® Discharge of blood and debris after delivery; types include **lochia rubra**, **lochia serosa**, and **lochia alba**
2. Characteristics of lochia are shown in Table 11–2
3. Should not contain large clots
4. Total volume is 240 to 270 mL, and daily volume gradually decreases
5. NCLEX® Amount may be increased by exertion or breastfeeding
6. Pooling in uterus or vagina may occur while reclining, with increased bleeding upon arising
7. NCLEX® Unexplained increase in amount or reappearance of lochia rubra is abnormal

Table 11-1 Factors That Influence Involution

Factors That Enhance Involution	Factors That Slow Involution
Uncomplicated labor and delivery	Prolonged labor and difficult delivery
Breastfeeding	Anesthesia
Early ambulation	Grand multiparity
Complete expulsion of placenta and membranes	Retained placental fragments or membranes
	Full urinary bladder
	Infection
	Overdistention of the uterus

D. *Afterpains*

NCLEX®
1. Caused by intermittent uterine contractions following delivery
2. Occur in all women but are more painful in multiparous and breastfeeding women

E. Cervix

1. Soft, irregular, and edematous; may appear bruised with multiple small lacerations
2. Closes to 2 to 3 cm after several days, admits a fingertip after 1 week
3. Shape permanently changes after first delivery from round, dimplelike os of nullipara to lateral slitlike os of multiparous woman

F. Vagina

1. Smooth walls, edematous with multiple small lacerations
2. Client should be free from perineal pain within 2 weeks
3. NCLEX® Low estrogen levels postpartum lead to decreased vaginal lubrication and vasocongestion for 6 to 10 weeks, which can result in painful intercourse

G. Abdominal wall

1. Abdominal wall soft and flabby with decreased muscle tone
2. Striae, or stretch marks, that were red during pregnancy will fade to silver or white in Caucasian women; darker-skinned women will have darker striae
3. **Diastasis recti**, separation of rectus muscles of abdomen, may improve postpartum depending on physical condition, number of pregnancies, and type and amount of exercise

H. Cardiovascular

1. Returns to prepregnant state within 2 weeks
2. The 40% increase in blood volume during pregnancy is lost primarily by diuresis
3. NCLEX® First 48 hours postpartum pose greatest risk of complications for clients with heart disease
4. Blood pressure should remain consistent with pregnancy baseline
5. Bradycardia of 50 to 70 beats per minute is common during first 6 to 10 days; tachycardia would occur with increased blood loss, temperature elevation, or difficult, prolonged labor and birth
6. Increased fibrinogen continues for 1 week with increased erythrocyte sedimentation rate (ESR) and risk for thrombophlebitis

Table 11-2 Characteristics of Lochia

Type	Occurrence	Appearance	Composition
Lochia rubra	1–3 days	Dark red, bloody; fleshy, musty, stale odor that is nonoffensive; may have clots smaller than a nickel	Blood with small amounts of mucus, shreds of decidua, epithelial cells, leukocytes; may contain fetal meconium, lanugo, or vernix caseosa
Lochia serosa	4–10 days	Pink or brownish; watery; odorless	Serum, erythrocytes, shreds of degenerating decidua, leukocytes, cervical mucus, numerous bacteria
Lochia alba	11–21 days, up to 6 wks if lactating	Yellow to white; may have slightly stale odor	Leukocytes, decidual cells, epithelial cells, fat, cervical mucus, cholesterol, bacteria

NCLEX®
7. Increased white blood cells (WBCs) up to 30,000/mm^3 does not necessarily mean infection or may mask signs of infection; an increase of more than 30% in 6 hours indicates pathology
8. Decreased hemoglobin is related to amount of blood lost during delivery; should return to prelabor value in 2 to 6 weeks depending on degree of decrease
9. Hematocrit increases by third to fifth day postpartum related to diuresis; a drop indicates abnormal blood loss

I. Urinary

1. Increased bladder capacity and decreased bladder tone lead to decreased sensation and increased risk of urinary retention and infection
2. (NCLEX®) Postpartum diuresis of 2 to 3 L increases output in first 12 to 24 hours after delivery and accounts for a 5-pound weight loss
3. Increased glomerular filtration rate assists in diuresis
4. (NCLEX®) A full bladder displaces uterus, increasing risk of uterine atony and postpartum hemorrhage
5. Fluids are also lost through diaphoresis with increased perspiration most commonly occurring at night

J. Gastrointestinal

1. Hunger and thirst are common following birth
2. (NCLEX®) Risk for constipation increases because of decreased peristalsis, use of opioid analgesics, dehydration and decreased mobility during labor, and fear of pain with defecation
3. Risk for hemorrhoids increases due to pressure from pushing during second stage of labor

K. Endocrine

1. Estrogen and progesterone levels drop rapidly after delivery of placenta
2. Menstruation usually resumes at 7 to 9 weeks for nonlactating women with 90% experiencing a menstrual period by 12 weeks; first cycle is usually anovulatory
3. (NCLEX®) Ovulation and menstruation return time is prolonged in lactating women and affected by length of time the woman breastfeeds and whether formula supplements are used; may vary from 2 to 18 months
4. Lactation
   a. Nipple stimulation leads to oxytocin release from pituitary gland; this stimulates release of prolactin from pituitary gland, which causes production of milk and the **let-down reflex**, release of milk by contractions of alveoli of breast
   b. **Colostrum** is first milk secreted and is rich in protein and immunoglobulins
   c. (NCLEX®) Primary **engorgement** occurs on second or third day as supply of blood and lymph in the breast is increased and transitional milk is produced
   d. (NCLEX®) Mature milk is produced after 2 weeks and appears watery and slightly bluish in color, similar to skim milk

II. PSYCHOSOCIAL CHANGES DURING POSTPARTUM PERIOD

A. Phases of maternal adjustment

1. Taking-in phase: first 3 days postpartum; needs to discuss labor and delivery; preoccupied with own needs; passive and dependent; touches and explores infant
2. Taking-hold phase: third to tenth day postpartum: obsessed with body functions; rapid mood swings; anticipatory guidance most effective now
3. Letting-go phase: 10 days to 6 weeks postpartum; mothering functions established; sees infant as a unique person

NCLEX® **B. *Bonding*** (also known as attachment)

1. Process by which parents form an emotional relationship with their infant over time
2. Mother explores infant first with fingertips, then palms, and finally enfolding newborn with whole hands and arms
3. Holds infant in **en face** position, face-to-face position, about 20 cm apart and on same plane
4. Uses a soft, high-pitched tone of voice
5. **Engrossment** is father's absorption, preoccupation, and interest in infant shortly after birth, which can be stimulated by witnessing birth

NCLEX® **C. *Postpartum blues*:** a maternal adjustment reaction

1. Transient depression usually occurs between second and third postpartum days and/or within first 2 weeks postpartum
2. Probably related to changes in hormone levels, fatigue, and psychological stress related to infant dependency

3. Experienced to some degree by a majority of women
4. Characterized by mood swings, anger, tearfulness, feeling let down, anorexia, and insomnia
5. Usually resolves spontaneously; may need evaluation for postpartum depression if symptoms persist or are severe

III. NURSING CARE OF POSTPARTUM CLIENT

A. General considerations with postpartum data collection

1. Evaluate prenatal and intrapartal history for risk factors
2. Provide privacy and encourage client to void prior to data collection
3. *NCLEX®* Position client in bed with head flat for most accurate findings
4. Proceed in a head-to-toe direction
5. Measure vital signs with woman at rest for better accuracy; will determine need or priority for other measurements
   - a. *NCLEX®* Temperature: above 100.4°F after first 24 hours may indicate an infection; may be elevated initially after delivery related to dehydration
   - b. *NCLEX®* Pulse: normal range postpartum is 50 to 80 beats per minute; report a rate greater than 100 to health care provider
   - c. Respirations: normal range is 16 to 24 breaths/min
   - d. Blood pressure: monitor for orthostatic hypotension; monitor more closely if client has a history of preeclampsia
6. Women who experience operative procedures, cesarean delivery, or tubal ligation have postpartum needs similar to those with vaginal births and of postoperative clients; monitor breath sounds and have client cough and deep breathe

B. Assisting with postpartum data collection: using nine components of assessment (see Memory Aid)

1. Breasts
   - a. Determine if mother is breast- or bottle-feeding
   - b. Palpate for engorgement or tenderness
   - c. Inspect nipples for redness, cracks, and erectility if nursing
2. Uterus (see Figure 11–1)
   - a. Gently place nondominant hand on lower uterine segment just above symphysis pubis; dominant hand palpates top of fundus
   - b. *NCLEX®* Determine uterine firmness, height of fundus, and position of fundus in relation to midline of abdomen
   - c. Correlate fundal location with expected descent of 1 cm each postpartum day
   - d. *NCLEX®* Inspect any abdominal incisions, cesarean delivery, or tubal ligation, for REEDA (see Memory Aid): redness, edema, ecchymosis, discharge, and approximation of skin edges

Memory Aid

Use the mnemonic BUBBLE-HEB to aid in remembering the nine components of postpartum assessment:

B—Breasts
U—Uterus
B—Bladder
B—Bowel
L—Lochia
E—Episiotomy or perineal lacerations
H—Homan's sign
E—Emotional status
B—Bonding

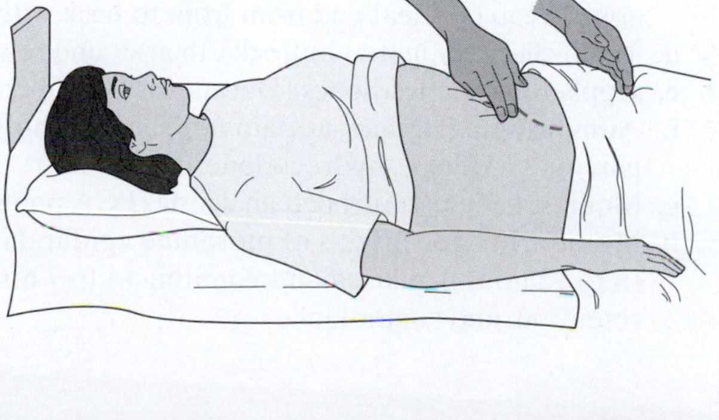

Figure 11–1
Measuring the descent of the fundus.

Memory Aid

Use the mnemonic REEDA to remember components of an episiotomy/wound assessment:
R—Redness
E—Edema
E—Ecchymosis
D—Discharge
A—Approximation of skin edges

3. Bladder
   - NCLEX® **a.** Client should void within 6 to 8 hours after delivery
   - **b.** Monitor for frequency, burning, or urgency (could indicate urinary tract infection)
   - **c.** Evaluate ability to completely empty bladder
   - **d.** Palpate for bladder distention if questionable ability to void or completely empty bladder
4. Bowel
   - **a.** Monitor for passage of flatus
   - **b.** Inspect for distention
   - **c.** Auscultate bowel sounds in all four quadrants for postoperative clients
5. NCLEX® Lochia
   - **a.** Inspect type, quantity, amount, and odor
   - **b.** Correlate findings with expected characteristics of bleeding
   - **c.** Cesarean-delivered women may have less lochia
6. NCLEX® Episiotomy or perineal lacerations
   - **a.** Inspect perineum for REEDA (redness, edema, ecchymosis, discharge, approximation of skin edges)
   - **b.** Inspect for hemorrhoids
7. **Homan's sign**
   - NCLEX® **a.** Pain in calf upon dorsiflexion of foot is recorded as a positive sign and may indicate thrombophlebitis
   - **b.** Inspect for pedal edema, redness, or warmth; if abnormal changes are present, assess pedal pulse
8. Emotional status
   - **a.** Note if emotions are appropriate for situation
   - **b.** Determine phase of postpartum psychological adjustment
   - **c.** Be alert for signs of postpartum blues
9. Bonding: describe how parents interact with infant

C. Collaborative management

1. Prevent hemorrhage
   - **a.** Collect data about risk factors
   - **b.** Keep bladder empty
   - NCLEX® **c.** Gently massage fundus if boggy; teach self-massage of uterus
   - **d.** Administer oxytocic medications if ordered: oxytocin (Pitocin), methylergonovine maleate (Methergine), ergonovine maleate (Ergotrate)
   - **e.** Monitor for side effects of oxytocics if administered; hypotension with rapid IV bolus of Pitocin, hypertension with Methergine and Ergotrate
2. Promote comfort
   - NCLEX® **a.** Apply ice to perineum 20 min on/10 min off for first 24 hours
   - NCLEX® **b.** Encourage sitz bath, warm or cool three times a day and prn (as needed) after first 12 to 24 hours
   - NCLEX® **c.** Teach client to perform perineal care after every elimination: squirt or pour warm water over perineum; blot dry from front to back to prevent tissue trauma and contamination from anal area; apply clean perineal pad from front to back without touching surface in contact with client
   - **d.** Teach client to tighten buttocks, then sit and relax muscles
   - **e.** Apply topical anesthetics (Dermaplast or Americaine spray) or witch hazel compresses (Tucks)
   - **f.** Administer analgesics; acetaminophen (Tylenol), nonsteroidal antiinflammatory agents (ibuprofen), narcotics (codeine, hydrocodone, oxycodone)
   - **g.** Monitor patient-controlled analgesia (PCA pump) as needed
   - NCLEX® **h.** Monitor for side effects of morphine epidural if administered: late-onset respiratory depression (8 to 12 hours), nausea and vomiting (4 to 7 hours), itching (within 3 and up to 10 hours), urinary retention, and somnolence

NCLEX®

3. Promote bowel elimination
   a. Encourage early and frequent ambulation
   b. Encourage increased fluids and fiber
   c. Administer stool softeners as ordered; suppositories are contraindicated if client has a third- or fourth-degree perineal laceration involving rectum
   d. Teach client to avoid straining; normal bowel pattern returns in 2 to 3 weeks
4. Urinary elimination
   a. Encourage voiding every 2 to 3 hours even if no urge is felt
   b. Catheterize as ordered for urinary retention; indwelling urinary catheter for 12 to 24 hours after cesarean delivery
5. Promote successful establishment of lactation and breastfeeding if desired
   a. Utilize well-fitting bra for continuous support of breasts
   b. Teach breast care, including no use of soap and air drying nipples after feedings
   c. (NCLEX®) Encourage nursing on demand every 2 to 4 hours, awakening infant during day and allowing to sleep at night
   d. (NCLEX®) Advise mother to nurse 10 to 15 minutes on first breast and until infant lets go of second; alternate breast used first and rotate positions
   e. Suggest football hold or side-lying position for mothers with cesarean delivery or tubal ligation to avoid discomfort caused by weight of infant on abdominal incision
   f. Provide help with positioning, latching on, and breaking suction when done nursing for women nursing multiple births
6. Promote successful suppression of lactation and successful bottle-feeding
   a. Utilize snug bra or breast binder continuously for 5 to 7 days to prevent engorgement
   b. Avoid heat and stimulation of breasts
   c. Apply ice packs for 20 min four times a day if engorgement occurs
   d. (NCLEX®) Encourage demand feedings every 3 to 4 hours, awakening infant during day and allowing to sleep at night
7. Explore impact of culture on feeding practices and support family choices as illustrated in Table 11–3
   a. Amount of contact and degree of closeness between mother and newborn is often culturally determined
   b. Culture may influence how long breastfeeding continues
   c. Feeding practices vary across cultures
8. Promote rest and gradual return to activity
   a. Organize nursing care to avoid frequent interruptions
   b. Plan maternal rest periods when infant is expected to sleep
   c. Teach client to resume activity gradually over 4 to 5 weeks; avoid lifting, stair-climbing, and strenuous activity
   d. Encourage simple postpartum exercises, per orders, to strengthen muscles affected by childbearing; Kegel exercises tighten perineum by alternately stopping and starting flow of urine; strengthen abdomen by raising chin to chest and doing knee rolls and buttocks lifts
   e. Increased lochia or pain indicates overexertion; modify exercise plan
9. (NCLEX®) Promote adequate nutritional intake
   a. Encourage lactating mothers to add 500 kcal/day to prepregnancy diet; bottle-feeding mothers should return to prepregnancy diet

Table 11–3 Cultural Influences on Infant Feeding

Cultural Group	Infant Feeding Practice
North American and European	Exposing the breast is indecent; weaning is a sign of infant development
Hmong (southeast Asian)	Breast- and bottle-feeding may be combined; expressing or pumping breast milk is unacceptable
Mexican American, Filipino, Navajo, Vietnamese	Colostrum is not offered to the newborn
African American	Plentiful feeding is emphasized; solids are introduced early
Muslim	Breastfeeding is encouraged to 2 years of age

b. Encourage fluid intake of 2000 mL/day
c. Continue administration of prenatal vitamins and iron, as ordered; iron is best absorbed in presence of vitamin C and may increase constipation

10. Promote psychological well-being
    a. Plan nursing care based on phase of psychological adjustment and degree of dependence/independence; provide choices whenever possible
    b. Encourage and support expression of feelings, positive and negative, without guilt
    c. Encourage client to tell story of her labor and birth to integrate expectations and fantasies with reality
    d. *NCLEX®* Provide recognition and praise for self- and infant-care activities
11. Promote family well-being
    a. Provide an environment that supports family unity and promotes attachment to newborn
    b. *NCLEX®* Encourage rooming-in, presence of family members
    c. Assist parents in preparing siblings with realistic expectations of newborn; involve siblings in infant care
    d. Explain to parents that sibling regression is common
    e. *NCLEX®* Advise couple to resume sexual activity after episiotomy has healed and lochia has stopped, about 3 weeks after delivery; level of sexual interest and activity may vary, additional water-soluble lubrication may be needed, and breast milk may be released with orgasm
    f. Provide information regarding contraception before discharge, assist couple to select a method compatible with health needs and individual preferences; a diaphragm or cervical cap must be refitted after delivery; oral contraceptives containing estrogen may interfere with lactation
12. *NCLEX®* Give Rho (D) gamma globulin (Rhogam, RhIG, Gamulin) if needed to prevent Rh sensitization and future hemolytic disease of newborn
    a. Confirm woman is a candidate: Rh-negative mother not sensitized (negative indirect Coombs test), Rh-positive newborn not sensitized (negative direct Coombs test), and no known maternal allergy to globulin preparations
    b. Administer 300 mcg IM within 72 hours of delivery
13. *NCLEX®* Give rubella vaccine to provide active immunity for mother and avoid fetal malformations if disease is contracted during a future pregnancy
    a. Confirm woman is a candidate: titer of less than 1:8 (not immune); no known allergy to neomycin
    b. Administer 0.5 mL subcutaneously prior to discharge
    c. If woman is a candidate for both Rhogam and rubella vaccine, delay rubella vaccine at least 6 weeks, and preferably 3 months, to avoid drug interaction and reduced rubella immunity
    d. Explain that client should avoid pregnancy for at least 3 months following vaccination; vaccine contains live virus and can adversely affect fetus; side effects include burning and stinging at injection site, warmth and redness, mild symptoms of disease
14. *NCLEX®* Reinforce teaching about postpartum warning signs to report
    a. Bright red bleeding saturating more than one pad per hour or passing large clots
    b. Temperature greater than 100.4°F
    c. Chills
    d. Excessive pain
    e. Reddened or warm areas of breast
    f. Reddened or gaping episiotomy, foul-smelling lochia
    g. Inability to urinate; burning, frequency, or urgency with urination
    h. Calf pain, tenderness, redness, or swelling

Check Your NCLEX–PN® Exam I.Q.

You are ready for testing on this content if you can

- Perform a postpartum assessment.
- Collect data regarding postpartum complications.
- Perform postpartum care.
- Reinforce postpartum discharge instructions.
- Incorporate cultural considerations into postpartum care.

PRACTICE TEST

1 A goal on the nursing care plan is "to facilitate parent–infant bonding." The nurse assisting in the care of the client should give priority to which nursing intervention to help the client attain this goal?

1. Provide assistance and encouragement with rooming-in.
2. Encourage the parents to join a new parent support group.
3. Keep the newborn in the nursery at night to allow the parents to rest.
4. Show the parents infant-care skills to increase their confidence.

2 A postpartum client who delivered 3 hours ago states, "I feel all wet underneath." What should be the initial action of the nurse?

1. Determine when she last voided.
2. Ask the client to rate her discomfort on a 1–10 scale.
3. Perform perineal care.
4. Have the client roll over to assess her lochia flow.

3 After delivering a 9-pound, 10-ounce baby, a client who is a gravida 5, para 5 is admitted to the postpartum unit. What would be a priority in delivering nursing care to this client?

1. Palpate the fundus because she is at risk for uterine atony.
2. Offer fluids, since multiparas generally dehydrate faster during labor.
3. Perform passive range of motion on extremities because she is at risk for thromboembolism.
4. Collect data about the client's diet because she is at risk for anemia.

4 Although a client initially wanted to breast-feed, she has now decided to bottle-feed her newborn. The nurse recognizes that reinforcement of teaching regarding breast care has been effective when the client makes which statement?

1. "I'll pump 2–3 times each day until my milk supply decreases."
2. "I'll rub lotion on my breasts if they are sore."
3. "I'll soak my breasts in a warm tub twice daily for the first week."
4. "I'll wear a snug bra continuously until my breasts are soft again."

5 When explaining to a new mother how to breastfeed, the nurse should include which information?

1. Wash the nipples with soap and water twice daily.
2. Begin nursing with the right breast at each feeding.
3. Slide a finger into the baby's mouth to break suction before removing from the breast.
4. Supplement the baby with formula every 12 hours until the milk supply is established.

6 The nurse is assisting in caring for a client who delivered vaginally 2 hours ago. The client's fundus is firm at 1 centimeter below the umbilicus and vital signs are stable. She received morphine IV 4 hours ago for labor pain. The nurse should question which new order from the physician?

1. Sitz bath 20 minutes TID
2. Bathroom privileges
3. Regular diet
4. RhoGAM for an Rh-negative client

7 The nurse assisting in the care of clients in the maternity unit should notify the physician immediately of which finding upon data collection?

1. Three pea-sized clots passed 4 hours after delivery
2. Musty odor to lochia 48 hours postpartum
3. Scant amount of rubra lochia after cesarean delivery
4. Firm uterus with steady trickle of blood 2 hours after delivery

8 Three hours after a vaginal delivery, the client reports increased perineal pain. What should the nurse do first?

1. Inspect the perineum
2. Administer analgesia as ordered
3. Apply ice to the perineum
4. Perform perineal care

PRACTICE TEST

9. The nurse notes that the postpartum client is Rh-negative and her baby is Rh-positive. Which maternal laboratory result should the nurse review next in determining if the client is a candidate for RhoGAM?

1. Hemoglobin
2. Direct Coombs' test
3. Indirect Coombs' test
4. Bilirubin

10. A postpartum client's hemoglobin is 9.2 mg/dL after delivery, and she has been instructed to take an iron supplement at home. The nurse should include which information when reinforcing client teaching about this medication?

1. Call the physician if your stools become black.
2. Take your iron with a glass of orange juice.
3. Don't drive a car while taking this medication.
4. Diarrhea is a common side effect of iron pills.

11. The nurse is reinforcing client teaching to a new mother about how to breast-feed her infant. Which intervention should the nurse carry out when sharing these instructions?

1. Place pillows under the baby's buttocks to elevate the hips while nursing.
2. Reposition the baby with the hips rotated away from the mother's abdomen.
3. Encourage the mother to use the football hold exclusively.
4. Provide positive feedback to the mother for correctly positioning the infant at the breast.

12. A new mother calls the clinic 4 days after delivery. She is breastfeeding and is concerned that her baby is not getting enough milk. What is the most important question for the nurse to ask this mother?

1. "How many wet diapers has your baby had in the last 24 hours?"
2. "Do you have any red or tender areas on the breasts?"
3. "Are your nipples sore or bleeding?"
4. "Do your breasts tingle when you begin nursing?"

13. A nurse is reinforcing instructions to a new mother about how to care for herself after delivery. Which statement should the nurse make during this discussion?

1. "Call your physician if you experience night sweats."
2. "Wait one week before resuming sexual intercourse."
3. "Change your perineal pad twice daily."
4. "Your diaphragm will need to be refitted."

14. A postpartum client's hemoglobin is 10.5 mg/dL. The nurse should encourage the client to include which food item in her diet?

1. Whole wheat bread
2. Red meat
3. Yellow vegetables
4. Skim milk

15. A postpartum client asks the nurse to remind her what to do to strengthen her perineal muscles. The nurse shares with the client to do which of the following?

1. Try to start and stop the flow of urine.
2. Bear down as though having a bowel movement.
3. Gently squeeze the uterus while pushing downward on the fundus.
4. Straighten the leg and point the toes toward the head.

16. In preparing to care for a postpartum client who delivered 2 days ago, the nurse should expect the client to exhibit which behavior?

1. Ask questions about infant care.
2. Hesitate in making decisions.
3. Need help with hygiene and ambulation.
4. Request the baby be fed in the nursery at night.

17. What interventions would the nurse expect to be in the care plan of a client who has a midline episiotomy with a third-degree laceration? Select all that apply.

1. Increase fiber in diet.
2. Administer bisacodyl (Dulcolax) suppository prn.
3. Increase fluid intake.
4. Administer an oral stool softener.
5. Administer an enema.

18 The nurse palpates the uterus of a client immediately after delivery. Where does the nurse expect to feel the fundus? Select the correct area on the image shown. Draw an "X" in the correct area on the image shown.

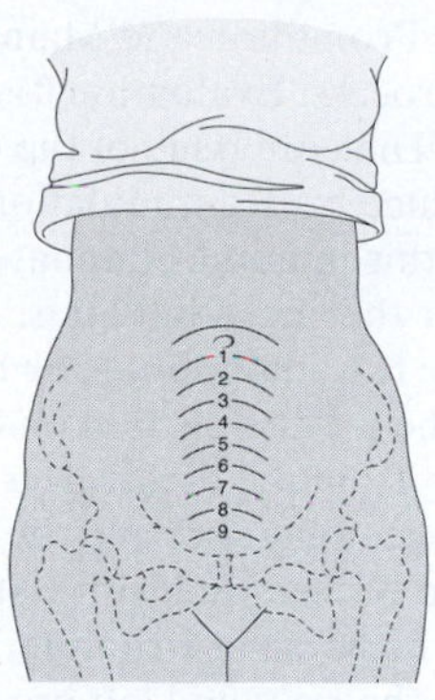

19 The nurse is preparing to reinforce instructions to a new mother about when it is acceptable to resume sexual intercourse postpartum. What items should the nurse include in the discussion? Select all that apply.

1. Use petroleum jelly for vaginal lubrication.
2. An intrauterine device (IUD) is appropriate for birth control in the early postpartum period.
3. Wait until episiotomy has healed and lochia has stopped before resuming intercourse.
4. Refrain from intercourse until first menstrual period after delivery is completed.
5. A water-soluble lubricant may be used if necessary.

20 The nurse is caring for a client who has decided not to breastfeed. What elements should the nurse include when reinforcing client teaching to promote suppression of lactation? Select all that apply.

1. Applying warm compresses
2. Pumping the breasts
3. Applying ice bags
4. Using medication to suppress lactation
5. Binding the breasts, either with a snug bra or binder

ANSWERS & RATIONALES

1 **Answer: 1** **Rationale:** Bonding occurs best when parents have direct and prolonged contact with their newborn in a supportive environment. Although the other answers may be appropriate, they would not be the priority in facilitating bonding. **Cognitive Level:** Applying **Client Need:** Health Promotion and Maintenance **Integrated Process:** Nursing Process: Implementation **Content Area:** Maternal-Newborn **Strategy:** The word *priority* in the question indicates that more than one or all options may be partially or totally correct. Identify the critical issue as parent–infant bonding. Compare each option in terms of its ability to stimulate attachment, and then use the process of elimination to make a final selection.

2 **Answer: 4** **Rationale:** It is possible that a significant amount of lochia could pool beneath the client after delivery. The highest priority at this time is risk for hemorrhage, and this should be the initial point of data collection. Noting time of last voiding and perineal care could then follow. Rating discomfort is irrelevant to the question as stated. **Cognitive Level:** Analyzing **Client Need:** Health Promotion and Maintenance **Integrated Process:** Nursing Process: Data Collection **Content Area:** Maternal-Newborn **Strategy:** The critical word *initial* in the question indicates that more than one or all actions are potentially correct, but one is better than the others. Focus on the ABCs (airway, breathing, and circulation) and on the risk of hemorrhage to make your selection.

3 **Answer: 1** **Rationale:** Uterine atony is the most common cause of early postpartum hemorrhage. This client is at greater risk for hemorrhage because she had an overdistended uterus with a large baby, and she is a grand multipara. Parity does not influence dehydration. The client may be at risk for thromboembolism, but there is no indication passive range of motion should be implemented rather than early ambulation. Nutritional assessment is important, but there is no indication the client is anemic and this action is not the priority for the client. **Cognitive Level:** Applying **Client Need:** Health Promotion and Maintenance **Integrated Process:** Nursing Process: Implementation **Content Area:** Maternal-Newborn **Strategy:** The critical word *priority* in the question indicates that more than one or all actions are potentially correct, but one is better than the others. Consider that the core issue of the question is uterine atony and associated risk of hemorrhage. Then focus on the ABCs (airway, breathing, and circulation) and on the risk of hemorrhage to make your selection.

4 **Answer: 4** **Rationale:** Mothers who are bottle-feeding should be encouraged to suppress milk production by wearing a snug bra or breast binder, applying cold compresses, and avoiding breast stimulation until primary engorgement subsides. Pumping the breasts and applying lotion to them are forms of breast stimulation that should be avoided. Applying heat via a warm bath will also stimulate the breasts and should not be done. **Cognitive Level:** Analyzing

Client Need: Health Promotion and Maintenance **Integrated Process:** Nursing Process: Evaluation **Content Area:** Maternal-Newborn **Strategy:** The core issue of the question is measures that will reduce breast stimulation and milk production. With this in mind, eliminate options that contain mechanical or thermal stimulants.

5 **Answer: 3 Rationale:** It is important for a breastfeeding mother to break the infant's suction on the nipple before removing the baby from the breast. This will help prevent the nipples from becoming sore and the skin from cracking. The nipples should be cleansed with water after each feeding, but soaps can be harsh or irritating. The client should alternate between the right and left breasts for first use at each feeding. Milk production and supply is enhanced when no supplementation is used. **Cognitive Level:** Applying **Client Need:** Health Promotion and Maintenance **Integrated Process:** Nursing Process: Implementation **Content Area:** Maternal-Newborn **Strategy:** The wording of the question indicates that there is one clearly correct answer. Use nursing knowledge to systematically eliminate each incorrect option based on appropriate breastfeeding techniques.

6 **Answer: 1 Rationale:** Application of heat to the perineum 2 hours after delivery will cause vasodilation, and increase the client's risk of edema and hematoma formation. Ice should be applied for the first 24 hours. Other interventions presented are appropriate. **Cognitive Level:** Analyzing **Client Need:** Health Promotion and Maintenance **Integrated Process:** Nursing Process: Implementation **Content Area:** Maternal-Newborn **Strategy:** The core issue of the question is knowledge of the effects of heat and cold on a client who is newly postpartum. Note the critical word *question*, which tells you the correct answer is an incorrect item. Eliminate each item that is an acceptable part of care and choose the option that increases the client's risk through application of heat instead of cold.

7 **Answer: 4 Rationale:** A steady trickle of blood in the presence of a firm uterus could indicate the presence of a vaginal or cervical laceration. The physician should be notified immediately so further evaluation can be initiated. The other findings are normal. **Cognitive Level:** Analyzing **Client Need:** Health Promotion and Maintenance **Integrated Process:** Nursing Process: Evaluation **Content Area:** Maternal-Newborn **Strategy:** The critical words *notify . . . immediately* indicate the correct answer is an abnormal finding. Use nursing knowledge and the process of elimination to make a selection. The words *steady trickle of blood* are also a strong clue that this is the correct answer.

8 **Answer: 1 Rationale:** The first step of the nursing process is data collection. Increased perineal pain in a client with a vaginal delivery could be a normal process as delivery anesthetics administered locally wear off. It could also indicate abnormal processes, such as the development of a hematoma. Further data collection for this client is needed prior to intervention. **Cognitive Level:** Analyzing **Client Need:** Health Promotion and Maintenance **Integrated Process:** Nursing Process: Data Collection **Content Area:** Maternal-Newborn **Strategy:** Analyze the question to determine that there is not enough information to guide nursing intervention. When more information is needed, an option that provides for further assessment is a good choice.

9 **Answer: 3 Rationale:** An indirect Coombs' test assesses for the presence of Rh antibodies in the maternal blood. Direct Coombs' test and bilirubin tests are conducted on the newborn. Hemoglobin is not a determinant for the administration of RhoGAM. **Cognitive Level:** Analyzing **Client Need:** Health Promotion and Maintenance **Integrated Process:** Nursing Process: Data Collection **Content Area:** Maternal-Newborn **Strategy:** The core issue of the question is the effect of an Rh-positive newborn on an Rh-negative mother. Use nursing knowledge to select the laboratory test that will directly evaluate the mother rather than the newborn.

10 **Answer: 2 Rationale:** Iron absorption is enhanced when taken with vitamin C, and orange juice is a good source of vitamin C. Darker-colored stools and constipation (not diarrhea) are common side effects of iron administration. Iron should not cause impaired judgment or dizziness that would impair safety while driving. **Cognitive Level:** Applying **Client Need:** Health Promotion and Maintenance **Integrated Process:** Nursing Process: Implementation **Content Area:** Maternal-Newborn **Strategy:** The core issue of the question is knowledge of administration and effects of iron as a supplement. Use the process of elimination and knowledge of basic mineral supplements to make the selection.

11 **Answer: 4 Rationale:** The baby should be positioned with the head midline and with the abdomen toward the mother's abdomen. Positive reinforcement will facilitate the development of maternal competence and confidence in infant care. **Cognitive Level:** Applying **Client Need:** Health Promotion and Maintenance **Integrated Process:** Nursing Process: Planning **Content Area:** Maternal-Newborn **Strategy:** The core issue of this question is proper breastfeeding techniques. Use factual information to systematically eliminate each incorrect option. The wording of the question tells you that only one option contains a true statement.

12 **Answer: 1 Rationale:** Once the mother's milk comes in, typically after the third postpartum day, breastfed babies should have 6–8 wet diapers each day. This would indicate the baby is getting enough milk. The other options address the mother, not the intake of the newborn. Red, tender areas or sore, bleeding nipples contribute to infection such as mastitis. Tingling is often used to describe the feeling mothers experience with the letdown reflex. **Cognitive Level:** Analyzing **Client Need:** Health Promotion and Maintenance **Integrated Process:** Nursing Process: Data Collection **Content Area:** Maternal-Newborn **Strategy:** Analyze the question and determine that the core issue is how to evaluate whether an infant is getting sufficient milk intake while breastfeeding. Then systematically eliminate any option that focuses on the mother instead of the infant.

13 **Answer: 4 Rationale:** Diaphragms need to be refitted after each delivery and a change in body weight of greater than 10–15 pounds. Night sweats are common and need not be reported. Sexual intercourse can be safely resumed once

the episiotomy is healed and the lochia stops in about 3 weeks. Perineal pads should be changed after each elimination. **Cognitive Level:** Applying **Client Need:** Health Promotion and Maintenance **Integrated Process:** Communication and Documentation **Content Area:** Maternal-Newborn **Strategy:** The core issue of this question is self-care and self-management following delivery. The wording of the question indicates the correct answer is a true statement. Use nursing knowledge to systematically eliminate each incorrect option.

14 **Answer: 2** **Rationale:** A hemoglobin level of 10.5 is low and indicates anemia. Because of this, the client should eat foods high in iron, such as red meat. The other foods are important to a well-balanced diet but are not high in iron. **Cognitive Level:** Analyzing **Client Need:** Health Promotion and Maintenance **Integrated Process:** Nursing Process: Implementation **Content Area:** Maternal-Newborn **Strategy:** The core issues of the question are laboratory indicators of anemia and dietary treatment. Knowledge of both concepts is needed to answer the question. As a strategy, however, recall that hemoglobin contains iron; use this knowledge to make a dietary selection from the options presented.

15 **Answer: 1** **Rationale:** Kegel exercises are designed to strengthen the muscles of the perineum. By alternately tensing and releasing the muscles of the perineum, as if to start and stop the flow of urine, muscle tone and strength are enhanced. Bearing down is the opposite type of exercise for this set of muscles. Squeezing the uterus and dorsiflexing the foot, straightening the leg, and pointing the toes toward the head are incorrect statements of technique. **Cognitive Level:** Applying **Client Need:** Health Promotion and Maintenance **Integrated Process:** Nursing Process: Implementation **Content Area:** Maternal-Newborn **Strategy:** The core issue of the question is specific knowledge of Kegel exercises. As a strategy, however, choose the option that helps to tighten the perineal floor, which is weakened by pregnancy and childbirth.

16 **Answer: 1** **Rationale:** By the second or third postpartum day, mothers are moving into the taking-hold phase of adjustment and are eager to care for the baby and self independently. The other behaviors are characteristic of the taking-in phase, which occurs earlier and reflects greater dependence on the part of the mother. **Cognitive Level:** Analyzing **Client Need:** Health Promotion and Maintenance **Integrated Process:** Nursing Process: Planning **Content Area:** Maternal-Newborn **Strategy:** The core issue of this question is the progression of maternal behaviors in the days following delivery. The wording of the question indicates the correct option is an expected behavior for that time period. Use nursing knowledge to make a selection.

17 **Answer: 1, 3, 4** **Rationale:** A third- or fourth-degree perineal laceration involves the rectal sphincter, therefore suppositories, enemas, and rectal exams are contraindicated until the rectum heals. Increased fiber and fluids or use of stool softeners is appropriate to promote bowel elimination in all postpartum clients. **Cognitive Level:** Applying **Client Need:** Physiological Adaptation **Integrated Process:** Nursing Process: Implementation **Content Area:** Maternal-Newborn **Strategy:** The wording of the question indicates the correct option(s) are also appropriate interventions. Incorrect options would contain inaccurate nursing actions or jeopardize client safety and restoration of health. Use knowledge of management of a third- or fourth-degree laceration to make your selection(s).

18 **Answer:**

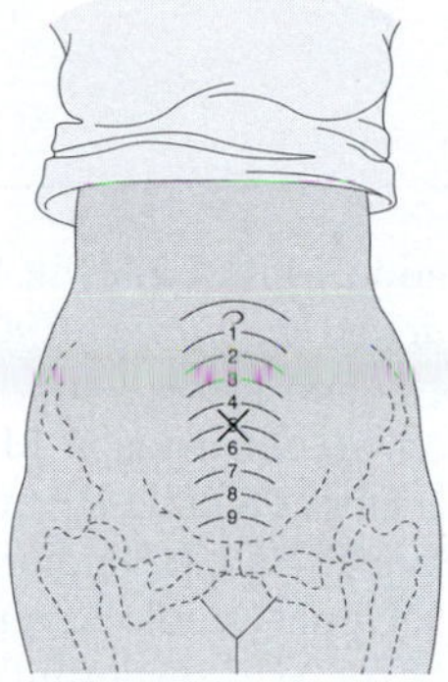

Rationale: Immediately after expulsion of the placenta, the uterus is firmly contracted, about the size of a grapefruit. The fundus is located in the abdominal midline halfway between the symphysis pubis and umbilicus. Within 6–12 hours after delivery, the fundus rises to a level of the umbilicus. The top of the fundus then descends the width of a fingerbreadth each day until it descends into the pelvis by about 2 weeks, when it is no longer palpable. **Cognitive Level:** Applying **Client Need:** Physiological Adaptation **Integrated Process:** Nursing Process: Implementation **Content Area:** Maternal-Newborn **Strategy:** Recall the physiologic process of uterine involution and the changes in fundal position after delivery.

19 **Answer: 3, 5** **Rationale:** Having sexual intercourse before the episiotomy is healed or the lochia has stopped increases the risk of infection. Water-soluble lubricants can be used, if necessary. An IUD is contraindicated during the early postpartum period. **Cognitive Level:** Applying **Client Need:** Health Promotion and Maintenance **Integrated Process:** Teaching and Learning **Content Area:** Maternal-Newborn **Strategy:** Use the process of elimination and look for a statement that is true. Knowledge of client teaching for resumption of sexual activity after delivery will help to answer the question correctly.

20 **Answer: 3, 5** **Rationale:** Binding the breasts, either with a snug bra or binder, and applying cold to the breasts will help suppress lactation. Milk supply is stimulated by expressing milk and applying heat to the breasts. Medications to suppress lactation are not recommended. **Cognitive Level:** Applying **Client Need:** Health Promotion and Maintenance **Integrated Process:** Teaching and Learning **Content Area:** Maternal-Newborn **Strategy:** Knowledge of the ways to suppress lactation in the nonbreastfeeding mother will help to answer the question correctly. Correct answers are options that include a true statement about a point of client education.

Key Terms for Review

afterpains p. 117
boggy uterus p. 116
bonding p. 118
colostrum p. 118
diastisis recti p. 117
en face p. 118
engorgement p. 118
engrossment p. 118
fundus p. 116
Homan's sign p. 120
involution p. 116
let-down reflex p. 118
lochia alba p. 116
lochia rubra p. 116
lochia serosa p. 116
postpartum blues p. 118
puerperium p. 116

References

Davidson, M., London, M., & Ladewig, P. (2012). *Olds' maternal newborn nursing and women's health across the lifespan* (9th ed.). Upper Saddle River, NJ: Pearson Education, Inc.

Ladewig, P., London, M., & Davidson, M. (2010). *Contemporary maternal-newborn nursing care* (7th ed.). Upper Saddle River, NJ: Pearson Education, Inc.

London, M., Ladewig, P., Ball, J., Bindler, R., & Cowen, K. (2011). *Maternal & child nursing care* (3rd ed.). Upper Saddle River, NJ: Pearson Education, Inc.

Perry, S., Hockenberry, M., Lowdermilk, D., & Wilson, D. (2010). *Maternal child nursing care* (4th ed.). St. Louis, MO: Elsevier.

Ward, S., & Hisley, S. (2009). *Maternal-child nursing care: Optimizing outcomes for mothers, children, and families*. Philadelphia, PA: F.A. Davis.

Test Yourself

Are you ready for the NCLEX-PN® or course exams? Use the practice tests on the companion website to check.

Uncomplicated Newborn Care

12

In this chapter

Cross Reference

Other chapters relevant to this content area are

Reproduction, Family Planning, and Infertility **Chapter 8**
Uncomplicated Antenatal Care **Chapter 9**
Uncomplicated Labor and Delivery Care **Chapter 10**
Uncomplicated Postpartum Care **Chapter 11**
Complicated Antenatal Care **Chapter 45**
Complicated Labor and Delivery Care **Chapter 46**
Complicated Postpartum Care **Chapter 47**
Complicated Newborn Care **Chapter 48**

I. IMMEDIATE CARE OF HEALTHY NEWBORN

A. Physical exam and data collection

NCLEX® 1. Vital signs and newborn measurement (see Table 12–1)

2. Pain data collection: intermittent crying not lasting more than 60 seconds, not high-pitched, quiets easily, and no tears noted

3. Collaborative management

NCLEX® a. Maintain newborn on radiant warmer or in isolette with servocontrol to maintain skin temperature 36.4 to 37°C (97.5 to 98.6°F)

b. Allow infant to assume a flexed position to decrease skin surface area exposed to environment (reduces heat loss)

c. Monitor axillary and skin probe temperature per institution's protocol

NCLEX® d. Monitor respirations for tachypnea and skin color changes for mottling; use bulb syringe or suction device as appropriate to remove secretions from nose and/or mouth

4. Outcomes: at 2 hours of age newborn maintains axillary temperature of 97.5–98.6°F, heart rate of 110–160/min, respirations 30–60/min with no distress, has pink skin color, and remains in flexed position

B. General examination (performed in cephalocaudal or head to toe manner within 4 hrs of birth)

1. Head

a. One quarter of body size, molding of fontanels and suture spaces, round, and moves easily from left to right and up to down

b. Symmetric exception may be caused by birth trauma—that is, **caput succedaneum** (swelling of soft tissue under scalp that subsides within a few days) or **cephalhematoma** (collection of blood between cranial bone and periosteum; absorbs spontaneously in about 6 weeks)

c. Anterior and posterior fontanels should be open, with posterior closing sooner (8 to 12 weeks) than anterior (by 18 months)

Table 12–1 Newborn Vital Signs and Measurements

Vital Sign or Measurement	Normal Range	Comments
Heart rate	110–160 beats/min	Irregular, especially when crying, and possible functional murmur; may be as high as 170 when crying or as low as 100 when sleeping; count apical pulse for one full minute
Respirations	30–60 breaths/min	May have short periods of apnea, irregular; cry is vigorous and loud; may elevate slightly when crying, but report respirations over 60/min (tachypnea) 2 hours after delivery or under 30/min (bradypnea); count for 1 full minute
Temperature	36.4–37°C (97.5–98.6°F) axillary	Stabilizes about 8 to 10 hours after birth; poor thermostability results from heat loss via *convection* (loss to cooler air currents), *radiation* (indirect heat transfer from body to cooler surfaces), *evaporation* (from wet skin), and *conduction* (direct heat loss to cooler objects)
Blood pressure	90–60/50–40 mm Hg	Varies with changes in activity and blood volume; more accurate when newborn is resting; increases to 100/50 by day 10
Weight	2500–4500 grams (5 lb, 8 oz–8 lb, 13 oz)	Average 3405 grams (7 lb, 8 ounces [oz]); influenced by race and maternal size and age; expect physiologic weight loss of 5–10% for term newborns and up to 15% if preterm
Length	46–56 cm (18–22 in)	Average 50 cm (20 in); place newborn flat on back with legs extended to measure; normal newborn legs are flexed and tense
Head circumference	32–37 cm (12.5–14.5 in)	Average 33–35 cm (13–14 in); is about 2 cm (0.8 in) larger than chest circumference; place measuring tape over most prominent part of occiput and bring forward just above eyebrows
Chest circumference	30–35 cm (12–14 in)	Average 32 cm (12.5 in); place measuring tape at lower edge of scapulas and bring forward across nipple line

2. Hair: smooth with texture variations according to ethnic background, grows toward face, high above eyebrow
3. Face: symmetric features and movement; eyebrows and eyelashes present
4. Eyes
   a. Clear blue or slate blue-gray in color
   b. Pupils equal and reactive to light, blink reflex present, sclera is bluish white
   c. May have subconjunctival hemorrhage (small broken tiny capillaries on sclera, will disappear in few weeks)
   d. Edematous eyelids
   e. Lacrimal structures (tearing) functions at about 2 months
5. Nose: patent nares bilaterally, no discharge, may have flat bridge, sneezing done to clear nostrils
6. Mouth
   a. Symmetrical when cries, hard palate intact, uvula midline, reflexes present
   NCLEX®
   b. **Rooting reflex** (infant turns to side stimulated and opens mouth to suck); **sucking reflex** (when object placed in mouth or touches lips)
   c. May have **Epstein's pearls** (small white specks, inclusion cysts, on gum ridges), tongue not protruding
7. Ears: well-formed notch of ear on straight line with outer canthus of eye
8. Neck: short, freely movable, has **tonic neck reflex** or fencer position (when head is turned to one side, extremities on same side extend and extremities on opposite side flex)
9. Chest
   a. Clavicles straight and intact, barrel-shaped chest with bilateral expansion on inspiration
   b. Breath sounds clear
   c. Heart rate auscultated at border of left sternum extending left to midclavicle; regular rate and rhythm
   NCLEX®
   d. Point of maximum impulse (PMI) lateral to midclavicular line at third to fourth intercostal space
10. Breasts: nipples symmetrical, may have whitish discharge or supernumerary (extra small) nipples on chest surface
11. Abdomen
    a. Soft, dome-shaped, round, some laxness of muscles, moves with respirations
    b. Bowel sounds when relaxed

c. Umbilical cord is white, gelatinous with two arteries and one vein, clamped with no foul odor
d. Femoral pulses palpable and equal, no bulges or nodes along bilateral inguinal areas

12. Genitalia
    a. Male: pendulous scrotum with rugae, testes descended into scrotum, penis with urinary meatus at tip of glans on ventral surface of penile shaft
    NCLEX® b. Female: labia minora may have **vernix caseosa** (white, cheesy protective covering that decreases as gestational age increases) and smegma in creases, labia majora normally covers labia minora and clitoris, discharge (blood-tinged mucus) may be present because of maternal hormones
13. Extremities and trunk
    a. Trunk: short, flexed, synchronized movement
    b. **Trunk incurvation** (Galant reflex): newborn lies prone, and when side is stroked, pelvis turns to stimulated side
    c. Hips: stable with no clicks or snaps upon movement
    d. To rule out hip dislocation, **Barlow's maneuver** adducts legs over hips and a snap is felt as femur leaves the acetabulum; with **Ortolani's maneuver**, the hip joint is abducted and lifted, and a click is felt as femur enters acetabulum
    e. Arms: equal in length with symmetrical movement; **grasp reflex** present, newborn grasps when object is placed in hand; nonmovement may indicate **Erb-Duchenne paralysis** or **Erb's palsy**; newborn inability to move upper arms or asymmetric Moro response may be caused by damage to fifth and sixth cervical roots of brachial plexus; five digits on each hand with normal palmar creases, nails present
    f. Legs: equal length, bowed, well-flexed, symmetric skin folds, peripheral pulses present
    NCLEX® g. Feet: creases on soles, may have "positional" clubfoot caused by intrauterine position but should be able to turn toward midline; **plantar grasp**—pressure on soles of feet elicits curling of toes; **Babinski reflex**—stroking sole upward and across ball of foot elicits fanning and extension of toes, disappears at 12 months
    NCLEX® h. Back: spine straight and flexible, may have small **pilonidal dimple**, a small dimple at base of spine but without connection to spinal cord
    i. Anus: patent, well-placed, may have meconium stool
14. Skin
    a. Color consistent with ethnic background, pink-tinged
    NCLEX® b. **Acrocyanosis**: bluish discoloration of hands and feet may be present
    c. May have mottling: lacy pattern of dilated blood vessels under skin caused by fluctuation of general circulation
    NCLEX® d. May have **milia**—obstructed secretions of sebaceous glands
    e. May have **Mongolian spots**—bluish pigmented areas on dorsal area of buttocks; most common in Asian, African, or Hispanic descent
    f. May have **lanugo**—downy, fine hair of fetus between 20 weeks and birth, noticeably found on shoulders, forehead, and cheeks
    g. May have Harlequin's sign—a deep red color over one side of body while other side remains pale; results from vasomotor disturbance

C. Gestational age determination using Ballard tool

1. Data collection that evaluates six neuromuscular and six physical characteristics; performed during first few hours after birth
2. A score of 1 to 5 is assigned to each characteristic and total score correlates to gestational age: that is, a term newborn given a score of 3 for each characteristic scores 18 for neuromuscular assessment and 18 for physical characteristics; total of 36 points correlates to 38+ weeks' gestation
3. Rating is marked on a graph with newborn's birth weight, length, and head circumference to classify newborn based on maturity and intrauterine growth
4. An overall rating below 10th percentile indicates infant is *small for gestational age (SGA);* between 10th and 90th percentile is *appropriate for gestational age (AGA);* above 90th percentile is *large for gestational age (LGA)*
5. Determining ratings for each of subscores
    a. Wear gloves when touching newborn after birth prior to first bath
    b. First evaluate observable characteristics without disturbing newborn, then proceed to characteristics that require more handling of infant
    c. Maternal conditions such as gestational hypertension, diabetes, and maternal analgesia and anesthesia in intrapartal period may affect some gestational age components

d. Neuromuscular maturity: during first 24 hours, newborn nervous system is unstable; reflexes and data collection depend on brain centers; results may be unreliable and need to be repeated in 24 hours
e. Physical maturity: not influenced by labor and birth and do not change significantly within first 24 hours after birth
f. Skin: opaque texture, few distinct larger veins, dry, some peeling
g. Lanugo: minimal, decreases as gestational age increases
h. Plantar surface: a reliable indicator of gestational age in first 12 hours of life; beginning at top of foot, creases should cover at least two-thirds of entire foot surface
i. Breast: using forefinger and middle finger, gently measure breast tissue diameter in millimeters (mm); should be 5–10 mm at term; nipple should be raised above skin level
j. Eye/ear: eyes are open and clear; ears—when top and bottom of pinna are folded over each other, pinna will spring back quickly when released; upper two-thirds of pinna incurves
k. Male genitalia: testes descended, scrotum pendulous and covered with rugae
l. Female genitalia: labia majora increases with gestation and nearly covers clitoris at 36 to 40 weeks; at 40 weeks, majora cover labia minora and clitoris

II. PHYSIOLOGIC CHANGES AFTER BIRTH

A. Cardiovascular

1. Expansion of lungs occurs with first breath; increases pulmonary blood flow and decreases pulmonary vascular resistance
2. Increased aortic pressure and decreased venous pressure present: clamping of umbilical cord increases vascular resistance, and aortic blood pressure increases
3. Increased systemic pressure and decreased pulmonary artery pressure occur because of loss of placenta; lung expansion increases pulmonary blood flow and dilates pulmonary vessels; pulmonary vascular beds open and perfuse other body systems
4. The **foramen ovale** (opening that previously connected right and left atria), functionally closes in about 1 to 2 hours and anatomically closes in a few weeks to 1 year, increasing left atrial pressure; some shunting may occur early in transition and with crying
5. The **ductus arteriosus** (in fetal circulation, an anatomic shunt between pulmonary artery and arch of aorta) closes, reversing blood flow, so now blood flows from aorta to pulmonary artery because of increased left arterial pressure
6. The **ductus venosus** closes (in fetal circulation, shunts arterial blood into inferior vena cava); results in redistribution of blood and cardiac output; closure forces perfusion of liver

B. Respiratory

1. Initial respirations are triggered by physical, sensory, and chemical factors
   a. Physical: effort is required to expand lungs and fill collapsed alveoli; changes in pressure gradient
   b. Sensory: temperature, noise, light, sound
   c. Chemical: changes in blood (decreased O_2 level, increased CO_2 level, decreased pH) as a result of transitory asphyxia during delivery
2. *NCLEX®* Newborn is an obligatory nose-breather, and any obstruction will cause respiratory distress; ability to maintain respiratory function is influenced by a large heart that reduces lung space and weak intercostal muscles, horizontal ribs, and high diaphragm, which restrict space available for lung expansion
3. Collaborative care
   a. Monitor respirations for any signs of respiratory distress (increased rate, audible grunting, nasal flaring, retractions) per institutional protocol; normal limits are 30 to 60/min
   b. *NCLEX®* Monitor color of skin, oral area, and extremities for any signs of hypoxia
   c. Keep newborn on warmer for closer observation
   d. *NCLEX®* Keep infant NPO if respirations are above 60/min
   e. Maintain oral area free from mucus or emesis
4. Outcomes: newborn's respirations are within normal limits, color is pink, temperature stable with no signs of respiratory distress

C. Neurologic

1. Newborn's brain is 25% of adult size and nerve fiber myelination is incomplete
2. Newborn exhibits uncoordinated movements, labile temperature regulation, poor control over musculature, easy startling, and tremors of extremities
3. Newborn reflexes are important indicators of normal development; these include **Moro reflex** (elicited by startling newborn; flexion of thighs and knees and fingers that fan, then clench as arms are thrown

out then brought together) and previously discussed Babinski grasp, plantar grasp, sucking, and tonic neck reflexes

4. Periods of reactivity: pattern of behavior during first several hours after birth

NCLEX®
   a. First period of reactivity: 30 to 60 minutes after birth; awake and alert; may display nursing and attachment behaviors with random diffuse movements
   b. Period of inactivity to sleep phase: activity diminishes, heart and respiratory rates decrease, and newborn enters sleep phase lasting from a few minutes to 2 to 4 hours; will be difficult to awaken
   c. Second period of reactivity: awakes from deep sleep, lasts 4 to 6 hours; close observation is required for changes in heart rate, respiration, and color

D. Musculoskeletal

1. Newborn should have full range of motion—when extremities are fully extended, they should return to a flexed position
2. Any variations should be further investigated

E. Gastrointestinal

1. Digestive enzymes are active at birth and can support extrauterine life by 36 to 38 weeks' gestation
2. Necessary muscular and reflex developments for transporting food are present at birth
3. Digestion of protein and carbohydrates is easily accomplished, but fat digestion and absorption are poor due to absence of pancreatic enzymes
4. Little saliva is manufactured until 3 months
5. An immature lower esophageal sphincter often leads to regurgitation or spitting up

NCLEX®

6. **Meconium**, stool that contains bile, epithelial cells, and amniotic cells, is excreted within 24 hours in 90% of healthy newborns
7. Wide variations occur among newborns regarding interest in food

F. Genitourinary

1. Functioning nephrons are complete by 34 to 36 weeks' gestation
2. Glomerular filtration rate (reabsorption and filtration) is low; therefore, newborn may tend to reabsorb sodium and excrete large amounts of water

NCLEX®

3. Decreased ability to excrete drugs and excessive fluid loss can lead to acidosis and fluid imbalance; uric acid crystals may cause a reddish stain in diaper

G. Hepatic

1. If mother's iron intake has been adequate, iron stores are sufficient through fifth month of extrauterine life; iron supplements may be given after this age
2. Liver controls amount of circulating unconjugated bilirubin, a pigment derived from hemoglobin that is released with breakdown of red blood cells

NCLEX®

3. Unconjugated bilirubin can leave vascular system and permeate other extravascular tissues (e.g., skin, sclera, oral mucous membranes), causing a yellow color termed jaundice or icterus
4. Because unconjugated bilirubin binds to albumin (protein) and is eliminated in stools, early and increased feeding may be encouraged to promote increased excretion of stool
5. Collaborative care
   a. Record intake (oral and parental) and output (weigh diapers) every 2 to 4 hours
   b. Monitor for adequate hydration; skin turgor, specific gravity with each voiding, noting quality and characteristics of urine

NCLEX®
   c. Phototherapy; maintain "bili-mask" over eyes, check eyes for pressure from mask
   d. Monitor diaper area for skin breakdown and rash
6. Outcomes: newborn feeds every 2 to 3 hours with balanced intake and output; skin is elastic; oral mucous membranes are moist; urine is clear, straw-colored, and passes bili-stools 6 times in 24 hours; bili-mask positioned over eyes if used; diaper area is clean with no skin breakdown

H. Integumentary

1. Maturity of skin increases with gestational age, and mature skin is better able to protect newborn from heat loss and infection
2. Skin color depends on activity level, temperature, hematocrit levels, and race
3. Plethora is a ruddy (red) appearance and usually indicates a hematocrit greater than 65% and should be evaluated; monitor a polycythemic infant closely for cyanosis, respiratory distress, hypoglycemia, and jaundice

NCLEX®

4. When infant cries, skin becomes bright red because of immature capillary system; acrocyanosis is common

I. Immune system

1. Of three major types of immunoglobulins (IgG, IgA, and IgM), only IgG crosses placenta; therefore, infants receive passive immunity from mother in form of IgG near end of gestation, or passive acquired immunity
2. Infants eventually produce antibodies (active acquired immunity) beginning at about 3 months, but IgA is missing from respiratory, urinary, and GI tract until approximately 4 to 6 months of age unless newborn is breastfed or until infant produces own antibodies
3. Breastfed infants receive antibodies from breast milk for as long as breastfeeding continues, and thereby receive protection from many infectious diseases, including influenza, mumps, and chickenpox
4. Use standard precautions and aseptic technique when caring for newborn; wear gown during care and do not assign caregivers with infections to newborns

III. NEWBORN NUTRITION

A. Nutrition guidelines

1. A healthy newborn needs 90–120 kcal/24 hr of nutrition and 140–160 mL/kg/24 hr of fluid intake
2. Weight gain is 4 to 8 oz/week; weight doubles by 6 months of age and triples by 1 year

B. Guidelines for formula/bottle-feeding

1. Formula meets energy and nutrient requirements of newborn/infants, but does not have immunologic properties and digestibility of human milk
2. Standard formulas are available in three types
   - **a.** Concentrated liquid: diluted with water at a 1:1 ratio
   - **b.** Powder: mixed with water, usually 1 scoop to 60 mL water
   - **c.** Ready-to-feed: can be poured directly into a bottle; must be refrigerated once opened and discarded after 24 hours
   - **d.** The American Academy of Pediatrics (AAP) recommends that infants be given formula or breast milk until 12 months of age
   - NCLEX® **e.** Soy formulas are available if infant cannot tolerate cow's milk protein and lactose, and hypoallergenic (hydrolysate) formulas are available for infants with an allergic response to standard formulas
3. Preparation of formula
   - **a.** Aseptic sterilization: supplies are sterilized separately from formula by boiling in water for 20 minutes
   - **b.** Terminal sterilization: formula is poured into unsterilized bottles and sterilized together for 25 minutes
   - **c.** With sanitary conditions, bottles and formula are not routinely sterilized, but all equipment is cleaned thoroughly, including top of can of formula
   - **d.** Formula may be warmed to room temperature in a container of warm water; never warm bottles in a microwave; hot spots may develop and burn infant's mouth or throat; heating also changes nutritional composition of formula
4. Feeding techniques
   - **a.** Hold infant close with head elevated
   - **b.** Keep bottle tipped so that nipple remains full of formula
   - NCLEX® **c.** Never prop bottle or put infant to bed with a bottle in mouth; propping can cause aspiration and middle ear infections
   - **d.** Discard any formula left in bottle because of risk of bacterial growth

C. Guidelines for breastfeeding

1. Influences on supply and demand (infant need)
   - **a.** Maternal supply is related to frequency of feedings until about 3 to 4 weeks when the milk supply is well established; thereafter, critical factor for supply to meet demand is breast emptying
   - **b.** Infants self-regulate their intake and control breast milk production by the degree to which they "empty" breast; a lactating breast is never "emptied" completely, but infant chooses how much to take
2. The suckling sequence and proper **latch-on**
   - **a.** Nipple and areola are drawn into mouth enough for lips to cover 1–1.5 inches of areola
   - **b.** Jaw should move up and down in a rhythmic motion during milk transfer; ears may wiggle; cheeks should be full and rounded, not sucked in
   - **c.** Upper and lower lips should be flanged
   - **d.** Tongue should be troughed—cup-shaped, beginning at bottom of mouth and extending over lower alveolar ridge; in this way, tongue draws nipple in and presses it against hard palate, forming a teat; tongue then humps up from back to front of areola in a rolling movement for milk transfer

NCLEX®

3. Frequency of feedings: increasing frequency will not increase supply unless transfer of milk is successfully occurring; audible swallowing is best indicator of milk transfer; swallowing is more frequent as more milk is transferred
   - **a.** Schedules should not be imposed on breastfeeding newborns because they have a stomach capacity of about 30 mL, and breast milk is more easily digested than artificial milk (formula)
   - **b.** Breastfeeding infants should be fed when hunger cues (rooting, sucking on fists) are displayed, which may be 90 mins to 3 hrs after last feeding; crying is last sign of hunger
   - **c.** Night feedings are necessary during first 6 to 8 weeks; fat content of breast milk is high in evening, which may help infant to consume more calories and feel more satiated; infants who consume more calories during day may have longer stretches of sleep at night
4. Duration of feedings
   - **a.** Limiting time at breast will not minimize or prevent sore nipples; sore nipples are almost always caused by incorrect positioning at breast or poor latch-on
   - **b.** Mothers should watch infant, not the clock; what infant is doing at breast is a better indicator of milk transfer than time spent there
   - **c.** Newborns/infants with different sucking styles take different amounts of time to complete a feeding, anywhere from 10 to 30 minutes; foremilk is milk that is produced and stored between feedings, looks like skimmed milk—bluish in tint—and usually has less fat content than hindmilk, which is produced during and released at end of a feeding and looks much richer, with a yellowish tint
   - **d.** Signs of satiation are slowing of audible swallowing; pauses between sucking bursts; infant takes self off breast; hunger cues disappear; infant is relaxed, drowsy, sleeping

NCLEX®

5. Good positioning for feeding is critical for proper latch-on and effective suckling
   - **a.** Maternal body position starts with good posture: straight back, pillows under arms (and under infant), feet touching floor or a footstool beneath feet
   - **b.** Hand position: in early weeks, breast should be supported using C-hold or scissor-hold hand position; use caution that fingers do not cover lactiferous sinuses or areola that infant needs to take into mouth; later on, infant will be able to support breast after initial latch-on
   - **c.** Cradle hold: infant is in chest-to-chest position, facing breast close enough to touch with nose and chin, with shoulder resting slightly lower on mother's forearm; mother's hand supports infant's buttocks, opposite hand supports breast
   - **d.** Side-lying position: infant is lying alongside mother with a rolled-up blanket behind infant and a pillow behind mother to maintain position; suggested for nighttime feedings and mothers who had cesarean births
   - **e.** Football or clutch position: infant is positioned in mother's arm with head, back, and shoulders in palm of hand; infant is tucked up under mother's arm, lining up infant's lips with nipple
6. Breastfeeding support is necessary for beginning and continuing breastfeeding
   - **a.** Encourage use of breastfeeding support groups or telephone hotlines at hospitals
   - **b.** Lactation consultants are trained and certified to provide assistance to breastfeeding mothers who experience problems
   - **c.** La Leche League is an international breastfeeding support and information group, with local groups often meeting in neighborhoods

NCLEX®

   - **d.** Hospitals and birthing centers that subscribe to World Health Organization's (WHO) Baby Friendly Hospital promote "Ten Steps to Successful Breastfeeding" and stop distribution of breast milk substitutes (Box 12–1)

D. Outcomes

1. Infant gains 0.5 to 1 oz per day, doubles weight by age 6 months and triples weight by 1 year
2. Infant has 8 to 10 wet or soiled diapers per day and is alert and responsive

IV. NURSING CARE OF HEALTHY NEWBORN

A. Eye prophylaxis after birth

1. May be done immediately after birth or delayed up to 1 hour (to allow eye contact that facilitates parent–newborn bonding); prevents ophthamalia neonatorum, caused by *Neiserria gonorrhoeae* and *Chlamydia trachomatis*
2. Commonly used solutions are erythromycin (0.5%) and tetracycline (1%) ophthalmic ointment
3. Eye prophylaxis can cause chemical conjunctivitis with possible edema, inflammation, and discharge; clears within 24–48 hrs

Box 12-1

Ten Steps to Successful Breastfeeding

Every facility providing maternity services and care for newborn infants should

1. Have a written breastfeeding policy routinely communicated to all health care staff.
2. Train all health care staff in the skills necessary to implement this policy.
3. Inform all pregnant women about the benefits and management of breastfeeding.
4. Help mothers initiate breastfeeding within a half-hour of birth.
5. Show mothers how to breastfeed and how to maintain lactation even if they are separated from their infants.
6. Give newborn infants no food or drink other than breast milk unless it is medically indicated.
7. Practice rooming-in—allow mothers and infants to stay together—24 hours a day.
8. Encourage breastfeeding on demand.
9. Give no artificial teats or pacifiers (also called dummies or soothers) to breast-feeding infants.
10. Foster the establishment of breastfeeding support groups and refer mothers to them on discharge from the hospital or clinic.

B. Preventing hemorrhagic disorders after birth

1. Newborn cannot synthesize own vitamin K_1 phytonadione until intestinal bacteria are present
2. Give prescribed vitamin K_1 phytonadione (Aqua-MEPHYTON) 0.5 to 1.0 mg IM in middle third of vastus lateralis muscle (lateral aspect) as a one-time dose

C. Screening for phenylketonuria (PKU)

1. Instruct that screening is done before hospital discharge and repeated in 7–14 days
2. *NCLEX®* Newborn should be taking breast milk or formula for 24 hours prior to screening so that there is sufficient protein intake

D. Bathing

1. Teach parent to use mild soap and to give sponge bath every other day or twice weekly for first two weeks; this prevents skin dryness and allows time for umbilical cord to fall off and for umbilicus to heal
2. Demonstrate bath and provide ample time for new parents to practice skills
3. Plan bath for a time prior to feeding and ensure a warm room temperature
4. Principle of care is to bathe from cleanest area to dirtiest
   a. Clean eyes from inner to outer canthus to reduce risk of clogging at tear duct, followed by ears, rest of face, neck, chest, back, arms, legs, and finally perineum
   b. Use care when cleaning areas with skin folds, such as neck, axillae, genitals, and peri area
5. Explain that bath time provides excellent opportunity for parent–infant interaction
6. Once tub bathing begins, only 3–4 in of water is needed; teach parents to be cautious because infant skin is slippery when wet

E. Cord care

1. Keep cord clean and dry; cord clamp may be removed after 24 hours
2. Inspect cord for yellowish discharge, odor, or swelling, and report if noted
3. Perform cord care in hospital according to agency protocol; many variations of care exist, including triple dye and antimicrobial agents such as Bacitracin or 70% alcohol
4. Before discharge teach parents to clean base of cord stump with cotton balls 2 to 3 times daily during diaper change; do not apply unclean substances to cord; recent research suggests use of alcohol on cord stump does not promote faster cord stump separation
5. *NCLEX®* Fold diaper down below cord stump to avoid covering it, prevent soiling of area, and enhance drying
6. Instruct to use sponge baths and avoid submerging cord in water until it falls off (in 7 to 14 days)
7. Observe for cultural practices related to umbilical cord care, such as binding of abdomen; if such a practice is necessary, recommend sanitary method such as use of clean gauze

F. Circumcision care

1. Inspect circumcision for signs of hemorrhage every 30 mins for 2 hrs after procedure
2. Observe first voiding to detect urinary obstruction from penile edema or injury
3. Apply petrolatum and gauze following procedure and for first few diaper changes to reduce further bleeding unless Plastibell is used

4. Plastibell remains in place and should fall off within 8 days; no ointments or creams are used while in place, but may be used after it falls off; consult health care provider if it remains in place after 8 days
5. For either type of circumcision, a yellowish film indicates presence of normal granulation tissue
6. Use hygiene measures to reduce risk of infection; report signs of infection such as increased swelling, drainage, or absence of urine flow

G. Care of uncircumcised penis

1. Foreskin and glans are two layers of cells that separate fully between 3 and 5 years of age
2. Explain to parent not to force foreskin back over glans for cleansing
3. Explain that when separation does occur, foreskin may be gently retracted daily for gentle cleansing with soap and water

H. Clothing

1. Instruct how to swaddle (wrap) an infant, which helps maintain body temperature, provide a sense of closeness and security, and perhaps quiet a crying infant
2. Dress infant in layers to avoid overheating or chilling
3. Cover infant's head in cool/cold weather to minimize heat loss when outdoors
4. Wash baby clothing with mild soap or detergent separate from other laundry; rinse clothing twice to remove soap and residue and reduce risk of rash

I. Newborn safety (see Box 12–2)

Box 12–2

Maintaining Newborn Safety in Hospital

- Compare names and numbers on identification bracelets of mother and newborn before giving newborn to parent.
- Allow only people with proper birthing unit picture identification to remove newborn from hospital room.
- Teach parents to
  - Report any suspicious people on birthing unit to staff.
  - Avoid leaving newborn alone in room, such as during showering or walking in hall; have a family member watch newborn or return newborn to nursery.
  - Avoid lifting newborn if weak, faint, or unsteady on feet; call for assistance.
  - Watch and keep hand on newborn whenever out of crib.
- To protect against infection, do not allow visitors who have a cold, contagious illness, draining skin sores, or diarrhea.
- At discharge, place infant in rear-facing, federally approved infant car seat in back seat of car.

Check Your NCLEX–PN® Exam I.Q.

You are ready for testing on this content if you can

- Explain healthy newborn characteristics.
- Provide care to the healthy newborn.
- Assist the client in learning skills needed to perform newborn care.
- Observe client's ability to care for newborn.
- Reinforce discharge teaching about newborn care.
- Appreciate cultural differences related to aspects of newborn care.

PRACTICE TEST

1 A 6-hour-old infant passes an unformed, black, tarlike stool. What conclusion should the nurse draw from this finding?

1. It is meconium stool that is expected at this time.
2. It is meconium stool expected at the time of birth.
3. It is a transitional stool expected at this time.
4. It is a transitional stool that is expected later.

PRACTICE TEST

2 A newborn's father expresses concern that his baby does not have good control of his hands and arms. The nurse would explain which concept in response to the client, using wording that the client can understand?

1. Neurologic function progresses in a head-to-toe, proximal-to-distal fashion.
2. Purposeful, uncoordinated movements of the arms are abnormal.
3. Mild hypotonia is expected in the upper extremities.
4. Asymmetric muscle tone is not unusual.

3 When caring for a newborn, the nurse must be alert for what potential sign of cold stress?

1. Decreased activity level
2. Increased respiratory rate
3. Hyperglycemia
4. Shivering

4 Which physical finding upon data collection would the nurse record as part of a newborn's gestational age assessment?

1. Umbilical cord moist to touch
2. Anterior and posterior fontanels nonbulging
3. Plantar creases present on anterior two-thirds of sole
4. Milia present on bridge of nose

5 When reinforcing client instruction on breastfeeding, the nurse includes that the amount of breast milk the mother produces is directly related to which of the following?

1. Her newborn's sucking stimulus
2. Her breast size
3. Her newborn's weight
4. Her nipple erectility

6 The first-time parents of a healthy term newborn are very anxious. The mother asks why the baby's hands are clenched, and why the knees and elbows are bent. What should the nurse include in an explanation to the parents?

1. The baby's muscle tone will relax when he is stimulated appropriately.
2. Placing the baby in a supine position will decrease his flexed posture.
3. Parental anxiety causes the baby's tension and flexed posture.
4. Flexion is the normal position for the newborn.

7 Which action by a new postpartum client indicates to the nurse the need for further reinforcement of instruction in breastfeeding technique?

1. Holds the breast with four fingers along the bottom and thumb on top
2. Leans forward to bring her breast toward the baby
3. Stimulates the rooting reflex, then inserts the nipple and areola into the newborn's mouth
4. Checks the placement of the newborn's tongue before breastfeeding

8 The nurse observes that when a newborn is supine and the head is turned to one side, the extremities straighten to that side while the opposite extremities flex. How would the nurse document this finding?

1. Tonic neck reflex
2. Moro reflex
3. Cremasteric reflex
4. Babinski reflex

9 The nurse anticipates that a newborn male, estimated to be 39 weeks' gestation, would exhibit which characteristic?

1. Extended posture when at rest
2. Testes descended into the scrotum
3. Abundant lanugo over his entire body
4. The ability to move his elbow past his sternum

10 If a newborn does not pass meconium during the first 36 hours of life, what is the most appropriate next action by the nurse?

1. Observe the anal area for fissures.
2. Notify the physician.
3. Increase the amount of oral feedings.
4. Measure the abdominal girth.

11 A new mother asks the nurse, "Why are my baby's hands and feet blue?" When making a reply, the nurse uses which term to describe this common and temporary condition?

1. Acrocyanosis
2. Erythema neonatorum
3. Harlequin color
4. Vernix caseosa

12 Which suggestion would the nurse make to the mother of a breastfeeding newborn as the best way for the mother to help resolve the infant's physiologic jaundice?

1. Switching permanently to formula
2. Giving supplemental water feedings
3. Increasing the frequency of breastfeeding sessions
4. Feeding the newborn nothing by mouth

13 A new mother who is breastfeeding her infant asks the nurse, "What kind of stools will my baby have, and how many will there be during the next month?" What would be the best response by the nurse?

1. "One or two well-formed yellow-orange stools per day."
2. "As many as 6–10 small, loose, yellow stools per day."
3. "A well-formed brown stool at least every other day."
4. "Frequent loose, green stools."

14 During a physical exam of a newborn with developmental hip dysplasia, which data collection findings would the nurse expect to obtain? Select all that apply.

1. Symmetrical gluteal folds
2. Limited adduction of the affected leg
3. Absent femoral pulse when the hip is flexed and the leg is abducted
4. Limited abduction of the affected leg
5. Asymmetrical gluteal folds

15 A newborn undergoing phototherapy for jaundice experiences increased urine output and loose stools. The nurse should take which action at this time?

1. Decrease the amount of time the baby is in phototherapy.
2. Recognize this as a normal occurrence needing no intervention.
3. Provide extra fluids to prevent dehydration.
4. Institute contact isolation.

16 A term newborn weighs 3,405 grams (7 pounds, 8 ounces). The parents question how rapidly their baby should grow. Which response by the nurse is correct?

1. "Your baby's birth weight should triple by 6 months."
2. "Most babies gain about 4–7 ounces a week during the first six months."
3. "Most babies gain a pound a month for the first six months."
4. "Most babies gain a pound a week for the first six months."

17 The nurse conducts a neurological examination of the newborn. What findings indicate the need for further evaluation? Select all that apply.

1. Asymmetrical fine jumping movements of the leg and arm muscles
2. Fanning and hyperextension of the toes when the sole is stroked upward from the heel
3. Grasping a finger placed in the neonate's palm
4. Muscle flaccidity not relieved by holding the newborn
5. Weak but effective sucking movements

18 A postpartum client is bottle-feeding her newborn. What would the nurse tell the client about regurgitation of small amounts of formula? Select all that apply.

1. Take a rectal temperature to check for fever.
2. Recognize this as a normal occurrence.
3. Discontinue feedings for 6–8 hours.
4. Report this promptly to the pediatrician.
5. Understand that this may result from overfeeding.

19 The nurse recognizes that a postpartum client is using good bottle-feeding technique after observing which behavior? Select all that apply.

1. Keeps the nipple full of formula throughout the feeding
2. Props the bottle on a rolled towel
3. Points the bottle at the infant's tongue
4. Enlarges the nipple hole to allow for a steady stream of formula to flow
5. Keeps the infant close with head elevated

20. The nurse is performing data collection on a newborn. Which infant manifestation is not a response that would result from reflex testing by the nurse?

1.
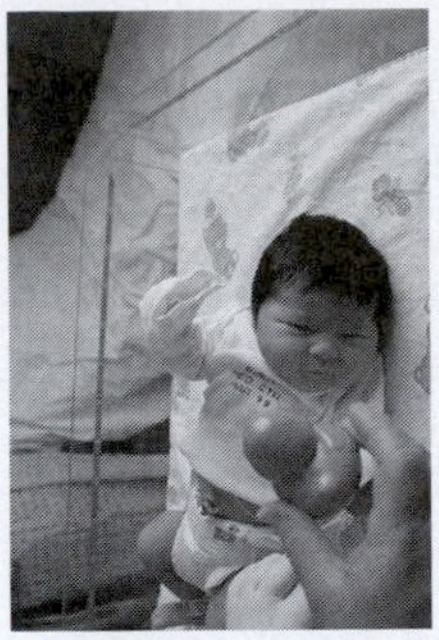

2.
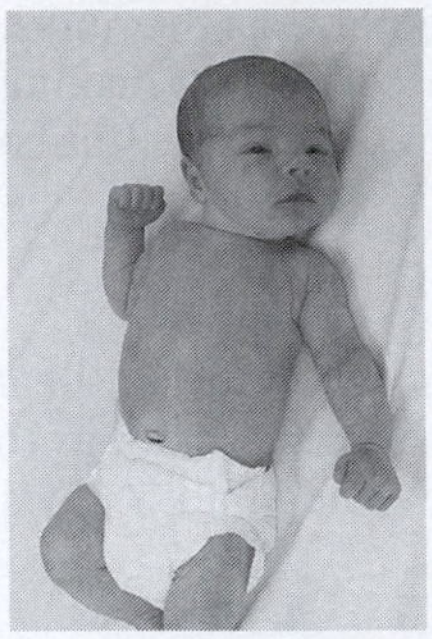

3.
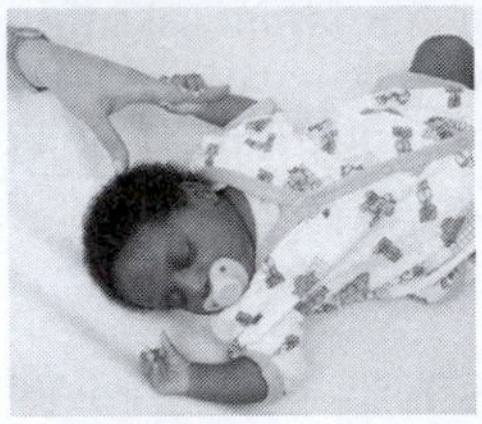

4.
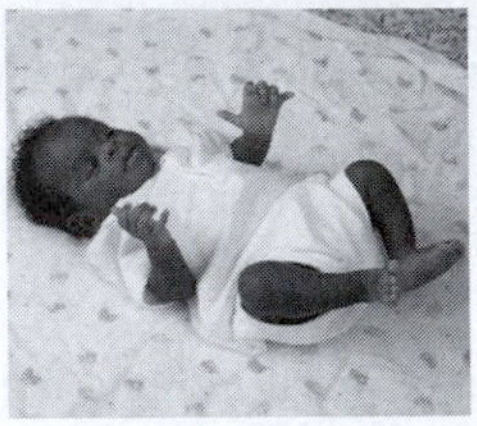

ANSWERS & RATIONALES

1. **Answer: 1 Rationale:** Meconium stools are tarry, black, or dark green, and are usually passed within 8–24 hours of birth. It is unusual to pass meconium at birth, unless there has been hypoxia or trauma. Transitional stools are thinner in consistency, with a brown-to-green appearance, and consist of part meconium and part fecal material. They are expected a few days later, after food has been digested. **Cognitive Level:** Analyzing **Client Need:** Health Promotion and Maintenance **Integrated Process:** Nursing Process: Evaluation **Content Area:** Maternal-Newborn **Strategy:** The core issues of the question are recognition and identification of meconium stool. The wording of the question indicates that only one option is correct. Use nursing knowledge to make a selection.

2. **Answer: 1 Rationale:** The newborn body grows in a head-to-toe fashion; therefore, uncoordinated movements of the hands and arms are expected and are normal. Mild hypertonia might be noted, and muscle tone should be symmetric. Diminished tone or asymmetric movement could indicate neurological dysfunction. **Cognitive Level:** Analyzing **Client Need:** Health Promotion and Maintenance **Integrated Process:** Nursing Process: Implementation **Content Area:** Maternal-Newborn **Strategy:** The core issue of the question is discriminating between normal and abnormal motor movements of a newborn. Use knowledge of growth and development to make your selection.

3. **Answer: 2 Rationale:** When an infant is stressed by cold, oxygen consumption increases, and the increased respiratory rate is a response to the need of oxygen. Additional signs of cold stress are increased activity level and crying, and hypoglycemia as glucose stores are depleted. Newborns are unable to shiver as a means to increase heat production. **Cognitive Level:** Analyzing **Client Need:** Health Promotion and Maintenance **Integrated Process:** Nursing Process: Data Collection **Content Area:** Maternal-Newborn **Strategy:** This question is eliciting knowledge of manifestations of cold stress. Make a connection between increased metabolic need (oxygen) without shivering and increased supply of oxygen (increased respiratory rate) to make a correct choice.

4. **Answer: 3 Rationale:** Plantar creases are part of the physical maturity rating on the gestational age assessment. Umbilical cord, fontanels, and milia may be observed but are not part of the gestational age assessment. **Cognitive Level:** Applying **Client Need:** Health Promotion and Maintenance **Integrated Process:** Nursing Process: Data Collection **Content Area:** Maternal-Newborn **Strategy:** The critical words in the question are *gestational age*. Eliminate umbilical cord and fontanels, which should be typical findings for all infants. From this point, use the process of elimination and nursing knowledge to eliminate milia.

5. **Answer: 1 Rationale:** Prolactin and oxytocin, two hormones necessary for breast milk production and letdown, are released from the stimulus of the newborn suckling. The mammary gland of each breast is composed of 15–20 lobes (where milk is produced and travels to the nipple) arranged around the nipple. Breast size is related to adipose tissue. Neither newborn weight nor nipple erectility is directly related to breast milk production. **Cognitive Level:** Applying **Client Need:** Health Promotion and Maintenance **Integrated Process:** Nursing Process: Evaluation **Content Area:** Maternal-Newborn **Strategy:** The wording of this question is straightforward and direct. Use nursing knowledge and the process of elimination to make a selection.

6. **Answer: 4 Rationale:** The full-term infant exhibits greater-than-90-degree flexion of the extremities, and clenched fists. Stimulation will not relax the muscle tone. Placing the infant in a supine position will not decrease the flexed position. Parental anxiety does not cause the flexed position. **Cognitive Level:** Analyzing **Client Need:** Health Promotion and Maintenance **Integrated Process:** Nursing Process: Planning **Content Area:** Maternal-Newborn **Strategy:** The core issue of the question is a rationale for musculoskeletal status of the newborn. Use knowledge of growth and development, and the process of elimination, to answer the question.

7. **Answer: 2 Rationale:** The newborn should be brought to the breast, not the breast to the newborn; therefore, the mother would need further demonstration and teaching to correct

this ineffective action. Holding the breast with four fingers along the bottom and the thumb on top, checking for rooting reflex, and checking the newborn's tongue position are correct actions for successful breastfeeding. **Cognitive Level:** Applying **Client Need:** Health Promotion and Maintenance **Integrated Process:** Nursing Process: Implementation **Content Area:** Maternal-Newborn **Strategy:** Note the critical words *further instruction*, which indicates the correct answer has incorrect information in it. Evaluate the truth of each option presented, and select the option that contains false information.

8 **Answer: 1 Rationale:** The tonic neck reflex, or fencing position, refers to the position the newborn assumes when supine with the head turned to one side. The extremities on that side will extend, and the extremities on the opposite side will flex. The Moro reflex occurs when the newborn is startled and responds by abducting and extending arms, with fingers fanning out and the arms forming a "C." The cremasteric reflex refers to retraction of the testes when chilled, or when the inner thigh is stroked. The Babinski reflex refers to the flaring of the toes when the sole of the foot is stroked upward. **Cognitive Level:** Applying **Client Need:** Health Promotion and Maintenance **Integrated Process:** Nursing Process: Data Collection **Content Area:** Maternal-Newborn **Strategy:** The core issue of this question is knowledge of the normal reflexes of a newborn. Use knowledge of growth and development, and the process of elimination, to make a selection.

9 **Answer: 2 Rationale:** A full-term male infant will have both testes in his scrotum, with rugae present. Good muscle tone results in a more flexed posture when at rest and inability to move his elbow past midline. Only a moderate amount of lanugo is present, usually on the shoulders and back. **Cognitive Level:** Applying **Client Need:** Health Promotion and Maintenance **Integrated Process:** Nursing Process: Data Collection **Content Area:** Maternal-Newborn **Strategy:** The core issue of this question is knowledge of physical findings of an infant according to gestational age. Use knowledge of physical growth and development of the newborn to eliminate each of the incorrect options.

10 **Answer: 4 Rationale:** The first meconium stool should be passed within the first 24 hours after birth; if not, the abdominal girth should be measured to evaluate distention and the possibility of obstruction. The presence of anal fissures will not prevent the passage of a meconium stool. Notifying the physician will not provide more information. Increasing the amount of feedings will not provide more information, and if there is an obstruction, will complicate that problem. **Cognitive Level:** Analyzing **Client Need:** Health Promotion and Maintenance **Integrated Process:** Nursing Process: Implementation **Content Area:** Maternal-Newborn **Strategy:** Note the critical words *not* and *first 36 hours*. This tells you that there is a problem with the infant's gastrointestinal status. When the nurse has only one piece of assessment data, often it is important to gather more assessment data unless the situation represents an emergency, which is not the case in this question.

11 **Answer: 1 Rationale:** Acrocyanosis is a bluish discoloration of the hands and feet and may be present in the first few hours after birth, but resolves as circulation improves. Erythema appears as a rash on newborns, usually after 24–48 hours of life. Harlequin color results as a vasomotor disturbance, lasting 1–20 seconds, which is transient in nature and not of clinical consequence. Vernix caseosa is a cheeselike substance that protected the newborn's skin while in utero. **Cognitive Level:** Applying **Client Need:** Health Promotion and Maintenance **Integrated Process:** Nursing Process: Planning **Content Area:** Maternal-Newborn **Strategy:** Note the key words *new mother* in the stem of the question to determine that the infant is a newborn. From there, use the process of elimination and knowledge of newborn physical assessment findings to make a selection.

12 **Answer: 3 Rationale:** Physiologic jaundice is best treated by more frequent feedings to increase stooling and the excretion of bilirubin. Switching to formula undermines the mother's feeling of her ability to provide nutrition for the newborn and may result in too-early weaning. Supplemental water may lead the infant to take less breast milk, delay the breast milk supply, and cause the bilirubin level to increase. Withholding food from the newborn will provide inadequate nutrition and cause bilirubin levels to increase. **Cognitive Level:** Applying **Client Need:** Health Promotion and Maintenance **Integrated Process:** Nursing Process: Implementation **Content Area:** Maternal-Newborn **Strategy:** The core issue of the question is what interventions a new mother can use to decrease physiologic jaundice. Eliminate options that contain the extreme words *permanently* and *nothing*. Choose the option that provides nutrition, not just hydration, for the newborn infant.

13 **Answer: 2 Rationale:** Breastfed infants will have 6–10 small, loose yellow stools per day during the first few months. They are not brown, green, or well-formed. Meconium may have a greenish color to it, but it is not a permanent color. **Cognitive Level:** Applying **Client Need:** Health Promotion and Maintenance **Integrated Process:** Communication and Documentation **Content Area:** Maternal-Newborn **Strategy:** The core issue of the question is normal bowel elimination patterns for a newborn infant who is breastfeeding. A simple way to remember this is to remember that they are yellow, liquid, and frequent.

14 **Answer: 3, 4, 5 Rationale:** Abduction is limited in the affected leg. The nurse would also find asymmetrical gluteal folds and an absent femoral pulse when the affected leg is abducted. **Cognitive Level:** Analyzing **Client Need:** Physiological Adaptation **Integrated Process:** Nursing Process: Data Collection **Content Area:** Maternal-Newborn **Strategy:** The core issue of the question is abnormal assessment findings associated with hip dysplasia. Eliminate normal findings and discriminate between abduction and adduction to make your selections.

15 **Answer: 3 Rationale:** Infants undergoing phototherapy will need additional fluids to compensate for the increased fluid loss through the skin and loose stools. Decreasing the time in phototherapy needs a physician's order. Losing excess fluid can cause dehydration leading to a life-threatening event. Instituting contact isolation is not necessary as there is no risk of infection from the stools. **Cognitive Level:** Applying **Client Need:** Physiological Adaptation **Integrated Process:** Nursing Process: Implementation **Content Area:** Maternal-Newborn **Strategy:** Recognize these assessment findings as expected for a newborn undergoing phototherapy but increasing the risk for dehydration. The correct answer would be the option that contains a nursing action to decrease the risk for dehydration.

16 **Answer: 2 Rationale:** Most infants, whether breastfed or formula-fed, average a weight gain of 4–7 ounces per week during the first six months. An infant's weight triples by 1 year. A pound a month for six months is an insufficient weight gain. One pound

per week for the first six months represents an excessive weight gain. **Cognitive Level:** Applying **Client Need:** Health Promotion and Maintenance **Integrated Process:** Teaching and Learning **Content Area:** Maternal-Newborn **Strategy:** Knowledge of the normal weight gain for the infant will aid in choosing the correct answer.

17 **Answer: 1, 4** **Rationale:** The usual position of the infant is partially flexed, and all movements should be symmetrical. Any absent, asymmetrical, or fine jumping movements suggest nervous system disorders and indicate the need for further evaluation. A weak sucking effort in the newborn would be considered adequate as long as it is effective. Common reflexes found in the normal newborn include the Babinski or plantar reflex (fanning and hyperextension of the toes when the sole is stroked upward from the heel toward the ball of the foot) and the grasping reflex (in which a newborn grasps onto an object that is placed in the palm of the hand). **Cognitive Level:** Applying **Client Need:** Health Promotion and Maintenance **Integrated Process:** Nursing Process: Data Collection **Content Area:** Maternal-Newborn **Strategy:** This question is worded as a negative statement. The correct answer would be the options that contain abnormal assessment findings that warrant further investigation.

18 **Answer: 2, 5** **Rationale:** Small amounts of regurgitation of formula are common, often caused by "overfeeding" or an immature cardiac sphincter. Regurgitation of formula is not necessarily a sign of infection, or a reason to take a temperature, or discontinue a feeding. Vomiting or forceful or persistent expulsion of formula should be further investigated. **Cognitive Level:** Applying **Client Need:** Health Promotion and Maintenance **Integrated Process:** Nursing Process: Planning **Content Area:** Maternal-Newborn **Strategy:** Because the wording in the stem of the question is positive, the correct option(s) will all be true statements. Knowledge of normal newborn care related to bottle-feeding will aid in answering this question correctly.

19 **Answer: 1, 5** **Rationale:** Keeping the infant close with head elevated is an optimal position for bottle-feeding. Keeping the nipple full of formula prevents the infant from sucking air. Propping the bottle and enlarging the nipple opening can cause aspiration of formula. Pointing the bottle at the infant's tongue could cause the infant to gag and vomit. **Cognitive Level:** Analyzing **Client Need:** Health Promotion and Maintenance **Integrated Process:** Nursing Process: Evaluation **Content Area:** Maternal-Newborn **Strategy:** The question is worded positively, indicating that the correct options are also correct actions. Use principles related to prevention of aspiration to help make your selections.

20 **Answer: 1** **Rationale:** This option illustrates visual capacity and not a reflex. The activity measures the newborn's orientation through the ability to be alert to, to follow, and to fixate on appealing and attractive complex visual stimuli. This option illustrates the tonic neck reflex. This option illustrates the palmar grasp reflex. This option illustrates the Moro reflex. **Cognitive Level:** Analyzing **Client Need:** Physiological Adaptation **Integrated Process:** Nursing Process: Data Collection **Content Area:** Maternal-Newborn **Strategy:** The core concept of the question is recognition of the reflexes present in newborn assessment. Use nursing knowledge to select the correct answer.

Key Terms to Review

References

Davidson, M., London, M., & Ladewig, P. (2012). *Olds' maternal newborn nursing and women's health across the lifespan* (9th ed.). Upper Saddle River, NJ: Pearson Education, Inc.

Ladewig, P., London, M., & Davidson, M. (2010). *Contemporary maternal-newborn nursing care* (7th ed.). Upper Saddle River, NJ: Pearson Education, Inc.

London, M., Ladewig, P., Ball, J., Bindler, R., & Cowen, K. (2011). *Maternal & child nursing care* (3rd ed.). Upper Saddle River, NJ: Pearson Education, Inc.

Perry, S., Hockenberry, M., Lowdermilk, D., & Wilson, D. (2010). *Maternal child nursing care* (4th ed.). St. Louis, MO: Elsevier.

Ward, S., & Hisley, S. (2009). *Maternal-child nursing care: Optimizing outcomes for mothers, children, and families*. Philadelphia, PA: F.A. Davis.

Test Yourself

Are you ready for the NCLEX-PN® or course exams? Use the practice tests on the companion website to check.

Lifespan Growth and Development 13

In this chapter

Cross Reference

Other chapters relevant to this content area are
Providing Immunizations Chapter 14
Promoting Healthy Lifestyle Choices Chapter 16
Age-Related Care of Older Adults Chapter 17
End-of-Life Care Chapter 24
Pediatric Dosage Calculation and Medication Administration Chapter 29
Maternal and Newborn Medications Chapter 31

I. INTRODUCTION TO GROWTH AND DEVELOPMENT

A. Patterns of growth and development

1. Each person displays definite predictable patterns of growth and development that are universal and basic to all human beings
2. Individual differences: although sequence is predictable, variations exist in rates of growth at which people reach developmental milestones
3. Directional trends: growth and development follow a specific pattern
   a. **Cephalocaudal development**: proceeds from head downward through body toward feet (head to tail)
   b. **Proximodistal development**: proceeds from center of body outward to extremities (near to far)
   c. **Differentiation**: development from simple operations to more complex activities and functions
4. Sequential trends: is orderly; each person normally passes through every stage
   a. Each stage is affected by preceding stage and affects stages that follow
   b. **Critical periods**: time period in which person is especially responsive to certain environmental effects; sometimes called sensitive periods
   c. Positive and negative stimuli enhance or defer achievement of a skill or function

B. Factors influencing development (see Table 13–1)

Table 13–1 Factors Influencing Development

Factor	Influence
Genetics	A family history of diseases may be inherited by unique genes linked to specific disorders; chromosomes carry genes that determine physical characteristics, intellectual potential, and personality
Nutrition	Greatest influence on physical growth and intellectual development; adequate nutrition provides essentials for physiologic needs, which promote health and prevent illness
Prenatal and environmental factors	Nutritional status in utero and exposures in utero such as alcohol, smoking, infections, drugs; also environmental exposures, such as radiation and chemicals
Family and community	A stimulating family environment helps individual reach his or her potential; family structure and community support services influence environment and thereby growth and development
Cultural factors	Customs, traditions, and attitudes of cultural groups influence growth and development regarding physical health, social interaction, and assumed roles

II. GROWTH AND DEVELOPMENT THEORIES

NCLEX® **A. Stages of Piaget's theory of cognitive development (see Table 13–2)**

Table 13–2 Stages of Piaget's Theory of Cognitive Development

Stage	Characteristics
Sensorimotor (birth to 2 years)	1. Infant learns about world through senses and motor activity 2. Progresses from reflex activity through simple repetitive behaviors to imitative behaviors 3. Develops a sense of "cause and effect" 4. Language enables child to better understand the world 5. Curiosity, experimentation, and exploration result in the learning process 6. Object permanence is fully developed
Preoperational (2 to 7 years)	1. Forms symbolic thought 2. Exhibits egocentrism—inability to understand another's position or put himself or herself in the place of another 3. Unable to understand conservation (e.g., clay shapes, glasses of liquid) 4. Increasing ability to use language 5. Play becomes more socialized 6. Can concentrate on only one characteristic of an object at a time (centration)
Concrete operational (7 to 11 years)	1. Thoughts become increasingly logical and coherent 2. Able to shift attention from one perceptual attribute to another (decentration) 3. Concrete thinkers: view things as black or white, right or wrong, no in between or gray areas 4. Able to classify and sort facts, do problem solving 5. Acquires conservation skills
Formal operations (11 years to death)	1. Able to logically manipulate abstract and unobservable concepts 2. Adaptable and flexible 3. Able to deal with contradictions 4. Uses scientific approach to problem solve 5. Able to conceive the distant future

NCLEX®

B. Stages of Erikson's theory of psychosocial development (see Table 13–3)

Table 13–3 Stages of Erikson's Theory of Psychosocial Development

Stage	Characteristics
Trust vs. mistrust (birth to 1 year)	1. Task of first year of life is to establish trust in people providing care 2. Mistrust develops if basic needs are inconsistently or inadequately met
Autonomy vs. shame and doubt (1 to 3 years)	1. Increased ability to control self and environment 2. Practices and attains new physical skills, developing autonomy 3. Symbolizes independence by controlling body secretions, saying "no" when asked to do something, and directing motor activity 4. If successful, develops self-confidence and willpower; if criticized or unsuccessful, develops a sense of shame and doubt about own abilities
Initiative vs. guilt (3 to 6 years)	1. Explores physical world with all senses, initiates new activities, and considers new ideas 2. Initiative is demonstrated when child is able to formulate and carry out a plan of action 3. Develops a conscience 4. If successful, develops direction and purpose; if criticized, leads to feelings of guilt and a lack of purpose
Industry vs. inferiority (6 to 12 years)	1. Middle years of childhood; displays development of new interests and involvement in activities 2. Learns to follow rules 3. Acquires reading, writing, math, and social skills 4. If successful, develops confidence and enjoys learning about new things; if compared to others, may develop feeling of inadequacy; inferiority may develop if too much is expected
Identity vs. role confusion (12 to 18 years)	1. Rapid and marked physical changes 2. Preoccupation with physical appearance 3. Examines and redefines self, family, peer group, and community 4. Experiments with different roles 5. Peer group very important 6. If successful, develops confidence in self-identity and optimism; if unable to establish meaningful definition of self, develops role confusion
Intimacy vs. isolation (early adulthood)	1. Depends on strong sense of self-accomplishment in adolescence 2. Extends beyond sexual relations to broader view of psychosocial intimacy with a partner, parents, children, or friends 3. Searches for continuity, regularity, or unity in meaningful relationships rather than for relationships with little commitment
Generativity vs. stagnation (middle adulthood)	1. Includes a sense of productivity 2. Reaches and attains goals 3. Engages in critical self-review 4. Lack of achievement of developmental goal leads to stagnation and self-absorption
Ego integrity vs. despair (older adulthood)	1. Honest acceptance of life that has passed and current stage of life 2. At peace with self 3. Includes achieving an identity apart from work, acceptance of bodily changes without preoccupation, and acceptance of death

III. PRENATAL DEVELOPMENT

NCLEX® **A. Physical growth and development (see Table 13–4)**

Table 13–4 Overview of Fetal Development by Gestational Age in Weeks

Weeks	Length & Weight	Neurological and Musculoskeletal Systems	Cardiovascular and Respiratory Systems	Gastrointestinal and Genitourinary Systems	Endocrine, Integumentary and Immune Systems, Eye/Ear
2–3	2 mm crown-to-rump (C-R)	Groove forms along middle back; neural tube forms from closure of groove	Blood circulation begins; tubular heart begins to form in 3rd week; nasal pits form	Liver begins to function; kidneys begin to form	***Endo:*** thyroid tissue forms ***Eyes:*** optic cup and lens pit formed; pigment in eyes ***Ears:*** auditory pit closes
4	4–6 mm C-R; 0.4 grams	Anterior neural tube closes to form brain; posterior closure forms spinal cord; limb buds noted	Tubular heart beats (28 days); primitive RBCs circulate	Oral cavity forms; primitive jaws present; esophagus and trachea begin to divide; stomach forms; esophagus and intestine become tubular; pancreatic/liver ducts forming	***Eyes:*** primitive eye is present ***Ears:*** primitive ear is present
6–7	**6 wks:** 12 mm C-R **7 wks:** 18 mm C-R	**6 wks:** Brain becomes differentiated with cranial nerves present at week 5; bone rudiments present; primitive skeleton forming; muscle mass begins to develop; skull and jaw ossification begins	**6 wks:** Heart chambers present (atrial division at 5 weeks); blood cell groups identifiable; trachea, bronchi, lung buds present **7 wks:** Fetal heartbeats detectable; diaphragm separates abdominal/ thoracic cavities	**6 wks:** Oral/nasal cavities and upper lip formed; liver starts to form RBCs; embryonic sex glands appear **7 wks:** Tongue separates; palate folds; stomach in final form; bladder and urethra separate from rectum; sex glands become testes or ovaries	**6 wks:** ***Ear:*** formation of external, middle, and inner ear continues **7 wks:** ***Eyes:*** optic nerve formed, eyelids present, lens thickens
8	2.5–3 cm C-R; 2 grams	Digits formed; skeletal cells differentiate further; ossification begins in cartilaginous bones; muscle development in head, trunk, and limbs allows some movement	Development of heart and fetal circulation complete	Lip fusion complete; rotation in mid-gut; anal membrane has perforated; external male and female genitalia appear similar until end of 9th week	***Ear:*** external, middle, and inner ear assuming final forms
10	5–6 cm crown-to-heel (C-H); 14 grams	Neurons appear at caudal end of spinal cord; brain has basic divisions; nail growth begins in fingers/ toes	By 9th week, RBCs produced in liver	Lips separate from jaw; palate folds fuse; developing intestines are enclosed in abdomen; bladder sac formed; testosterone physical characteristics at 8–12 wks (males)	***Endo:*** Islets of Langerhans differentiated ***Eyes:*** lids fused closed
12	8 cm C-R; 11.5 cm C-H; 45 grams	Clear outline of miniature bones (12–20 wks); process of ossification established; involuntary muscles in viscera appear	Lungs acquire definitive shape	Mouth palate completed; muscles in gut appear; bile secretion begins; liver produces most of RBCs	***Skin:*** delicate, pink ***Endo:*** thyroid secretes hormones; insulin present in pancreas ***Immune:*** lymphoid tissue in thymus gland

Table 13–4 Overview of Fetal Development by Gestational Age in Weeks (*continued*)

Weeks	Length & Weight	Neurological and Musculoskeletal Systems	Cardiovascular and Respiratory Systems	Gastrointestinal and Genitourinary Systems	Endocrine, Integumentary and Immune Systems, Eye/Ear
16	13.5 cm C-R; 15 cm C-H; 200 grams	Teeth begin to form hard tissue for central incisors	Fetal heart tones audible with fetoscope at 16–20 weeks	Hard and soft palate differentiating; gastric and intestinal glands developing; intestines start to collect meconium; kidneys assume shape and organization; able to note sex	***Skin:*** scalp hair appears; body has lanugo; visible blood vessels beneath transparent skin; sweat glands developing ***Eyes, ears, nose:*** formed
20	25 cm C-H; 435 grams (6% fat)	Spinal cord myelination begins; teeth begin to form hard tissue for canine and first molar (lateral incisors at 18 wks); lower limbs have final relative proportions	Fetal heart tones audible; primitive respiratorylike movements begin; iron is stored in blood; bone marrow important	Fetus sucks and swallows amniotic fluid; peristalsis begins	***Skin:*** lanugo covers entire body; brown fat and vernix caseosa begin to form ***Endo:*** iron is stored; bone marrow functioning, fetal antibodies detectable ***Immune:*** fetal IgG levels detectable
24	28 cm C-H; 780 grams	Brain appears mature; teeth begin to form 2nd molars	Resp. movements occur (24–40 wks), nostrils reopen, alveoli appear and begin to produce surfactant, gas exchange possible	Testes descend into inguinal ring (males)	***Skin:*** reddish and wrinkled ***Immune:*** IgG at mature levels ***Eyes:*** structurally complete
28–32	**28 wks:** 35 cm C-H; 1200–1250 grams **32 wks:** 38–43 cm C-H; 2000 grams	**28 wks:** Nervous system begins regulation of some bodily processes **32 wks:** More reflexes present	Viability is reached at 26–27 weeks; if born now, intensive care is needed to support respirations	Testes descend into inguinal canal and upper scrotum (males)	**28 wks: *Eyes:*** eyelids open ***Skin:*** adipose tissue begins to accumulate; eyebrows and eyelashes develop
36–40	**36 wks:** 42–48 cm C-H; 2500–2750 grams **40 wks:** 48–52 cm C-H; 3200+ grams (16% fat)	**36 wks:** Ossification centers present in distal femur	**38 wks:** Lecithin-sphingomyelin (L/S) ratio approaches 2:1 (less risk of respiratory distress from inadequate surfactant if born)	**36 wks:** small scrotum with few rugae (males), final descent of testes into upper scrotum (36–40 wks), labia majora/minora equally prominent (females) **40 wks:** rugous scrotum (males); labia majora well-developed and cover the smaller labia minora and clitoris (females)	**36 wks: *Skin:*** pale, lanugo disappearing, hair fuzzy/wooly, few sole creases, increased vernix caseosa (36–40 wks) ***Ears:*** lobes soft with little cartilage **40 wks: *Skin:*** smooth, pink; vernix in skinfolds, silky hair, lanugo on shoulders and upper back, nails extend to tips of digits, creases cover sole ***Ears:*** lobes firmer, increased cartilage

NCLEX®

B. Highlights of development of concern to parents

1. Fetal heart begins to beat at 4 weeks
2. All body organs formed by 8 weeks
3. Fetal heart sounds heard by Doppler device at 8 to 12 weeks
4. Gender can be seen and has appearance of baby at 16 weeks
5. Heartbeat heard with a fetoscope and mother feels movement (quickening); assumes a favorite position in utero; head hair, eyebrows, and eyelashes present at 20 weeks
6. Weighs approximately 1 lb 10 oz and activity is increasing; fetal respiratory movements begin at 24 weeks
7. Surfactant needed for breathing at birth is formed, and baby is two-thirds final size at 28 weeks
8. Fingernails and toenails formed and subcutaneous fat appears; baby appears less red and wrinkled at 32 weeks
9. Baby fills uterus and gets antibodies from mother at 38 to 40 weeks

IV. INFANT GROWTH AND DEVELOPMENT

A. Neonatal period (birth to 1 month)

1. General appearance: newborn's head is one quarter of body length; is top heavy with short lower extremities
2. NCLEX® Weight: 6 to 8 lb; gains 5 to 7 oz (142 to 198 grams) weekly for first 6 months
3. Height: 20 in. (50 cm); grows 1 in. (2.5 cm) monthly for first 6 months
4. Head circumference: 33 to 35 cm (13 to 14 in.); head circumference is greater than chest circumference

B. Growth during infancy (1 to 12 months)

1. NCLEX® Weight: doubles birth weight in 6 months; triples birth weight in 1 year
2. Height: increases 50% by 1 year
3. Head growth is rapid; brain increases in weight 2.5 times by 1 year
   a. Head circumference exceeds chest circumference
   b. NCLEX® Posterior fontanel closes at 2 to 3 months
   c. Anterior fontanel closes by 12 to 18 months
4. NCLEX® Reflexes present at birth
   a. Moro: startle reflex elicited by loud noise or sudden change in position
   b. Tonic neck: elicted when infant lies supine and head is turned to one side; infant will assume a "fencing position"
   c. Gag, cough, blink, pupillary: protective reflexes
   d. Grasp: infant's hands and feet will grasp when hand or foot is stimulated
   e. Rooting: elicited when side of mouth is touched, causing infant to turn to that side
   f. Babinski: fanning of toes when sole of foot is stroked upward
5. Reflexes that appear during infancy
   a. Parachute: involves extension of arms when suspended in prone position and lowered suddenly
   b. Landau: when infant is suspended horizontally, head is raised
   c. Labyrinth righting: provides orientation of head in space
   d. Body righting: when caregiver turns hips to the side, the body follows
6. NCLEX® Gross motor development: developmental maturation in posture, head balance, sitting, creeping, standing, and walking
   a. Gains head control by 4 months
   b. Rolls from back to side by 4 months
   c. Rolls from abdomen to back by 5 months
   d. Rolls from back to abdomen by 6 months
   e. Sits alone without support by 8 months
   f. Stands holding furniture by 9 months
   g. Crawls (may go backward initially) by 10 months
   h. Creeps with abdomen off floor by 11 months
   i. Cruises (walking upright while holding furniture) by 10 to 12 months
   j. Can sit down from upright position by 10 to 12 months
   k. Walks well with one hand held by 12 months
7. NCLEX® Fine motor development: use of hands and fingers to grasp objects
   a. Hand predominantly closed at 1 month
   b. Desires to grasp at 3 months
   c. Two-handed, voluntary grasp at 5 months

d. Holds bottle, grasps feet at 6 months
e. Transfers from hand to hand by 7 months
f. Pincer grasp established by 10 months
g. Neat pincer grasp (e.g., picks up raisin) with thumb and finger by 12 months

8. Sensory development
a. Hearing and touch well developed at birth
b. Sight not fully developed until 6 years; differentiates light and dark at birth; prefers human face; smiles at 2 months
c. Usually searches and turns head to locate sounds by 2 months
d. Has taste preferences by 6 months
e. Responds to own name by 7 months
f. Able to follow moving objects; visual acuity 20/50 or better; amblyopia ("lazy eye") may develop by 12 months
NCLEX® g. Can vocalize four words by 1 year

9. Nutrition
a. Human breast milk is easily digested and most complete
b. Iron-fortified commercial formulas used for bottle-feeding closely resemble nutritional content of human milk; recommended for first 12 months
NCLEX® c. Solids are introduced no sooner than 6 months to avoid exposure to allergens
d. Iron-fortified rice cereal is introduced first because of its low allergenic potential
e. Deciduous "baby" teeth erupt by 5 to 6 months; lateral incisors erupt first; increase in drooling and saliva; may be accompanied by slight elevated temperature
f. Gradual weaning from breast to bottle to cup during second 6 months of infancy
g. Juices may be introduced, diluted 1:1 at 6 months; preferably given by a cup
h. Introduction of fruits, vegetables, and meats (one food each week is recommended to identify any allergy)
i. Junior foods or chopped table foods introduced by 12 months
NCLEX® j. Limit intake of formula to no more than 32 oz per 24 hours to avoid iron-deficiency anemia

NCLEX® 10. Safety
a. Infants up to 20 lb (9 kg) and age 1 year should be restrained by law in a rear-facing car seat in back seat of car; the American Academy of Pediatrics recommends keeping toddlers in a rear-facing direction until they reach 2 years or the maximum height and weight allowed by car seat manufacturer
b. Keep side-rails of crib up
c. Never leave infant unattended on table, bed, or in bathtub
d. Check temperature of bath water, formula, and foods
e. Avoid giving bottles at naps or bedtime (may cause dental caries)
f. Parents should learn injury prevention, including aspiration of foreign objects (buttons, toys, peanuts, hotdogs), suffocation (plastic bags, strangulation), falls, poisonings, and burns (electric cords, wall outlets, radiators, pots and pans on stoves)

NCLEX® 11. Play (solitary)
a. Provide black/white contrasts for premature and newborn infants
b. Hang mobile 8 to 10 inches from infant's face
c. Provide sensory stimuli (bath water) and tactile stimuli (feel of various shapes of objects), large toys, balls
d. Expose to environmental sounds: rattles, musical toys
e. Use variety of primary-colored objects during infancy
f. Place unbreakable mirror in crib for infants to focus on own face
g. Provide toys that let infants practice skills to grasp and manipulate objects
h. Vocalization provides pleasure in relationships with people (smiling, cooing, laughing)

V. TODDLER GROWTH AND DEVELOPMENT

A. Period from 1 to 3 years of age
B. Weight: growth rate slows considerably; weight is 4 times the birth weight by 2½ years
C. Height: at 2 years, height is 50% of future adult height
D. Head circumference: 19½ to 20 in. (49 to 50 cm) by 2 years; increases only 3 cm in second year; achieves 90% of adult-sized brain by 2 years
NCLEX® **E. Anterior fontanel closes by 18 months**
NCLEX® **F. Gross motor development:** still clumsy at this age

1. Walks without help (usually by 15 months)
2. Jumps in place by 18 months
3. Goes up stairs (with 2 feet on each step) by 24 months
4. Runs fairly well (wide stance) by 24 months

NCLEX® **G. Fine motor development**

1. Uses cup well by 15 months
2. Builds a tower of two cubes by 15 months
3. Holds crayon with fingers by 24 to 30 months
4. Good hand–finger coordination by 30 months
5. Copies a circle by 3 years

H. Sensory development

1. Binocular vision well developed by 15 months
2. Knows own name by 12 months; refers to self
3. Identifies geometric forms by 18 months
4. Uses short sentences by 18 months to 2 years
5. Follows simple directions by 2 years
6. Able to speak 300 words by 2 years
7. Remembers and repeats 3 numbers by 3 years

I. *Object permanence* is knowledge that an object or person continues to exist when not seen, heard, or felt

J. Ritualistic behavior is exhibited during toddler period; *ritualism* is toddler's need to maintain sameness and reliability; provides sense of comfort

NCLEX® **K. Nutrition**

1. Growth slows at age 12 to 18 months; thus appetite and need for intake decrease
2. Toddlers are picky, ritualistic eaters
3. Avoid more than 32 oz formula or milk/day to prevent iron-deficiency anemia
4. Avoid large pieces of food such as hot dogs, grapes, cherries, peanuts
5. Able to feed self completely by 3 years
6. Deciduous teeth (approx. 20) are present by 2½ to 3 years
7. Teach good dental practices (brushing, fluoride)

NCLEX® **L. Safety**

1. Continue to use car seat properly; the American Academy of Pediatrics recommends placing toddlers in a rear-facing car seat in the back seat of car until they reach age two or they exceed car seat manufacturer height and weight limits for rear-facing seat; children over the age of 1 and over 20 lb may be placed in forward-facing car seats with harness straps at or above shoulders per current law
2. Supervise indoor play and outdoor activities
3. Teach that use of ipecac for accidental ingestions is no longer recommended
4. Teach injury prevention
   a. Childproof home environment: stairways, cupboards, medicine cabinet, outlets
   b. Suffocation: plastic bags, pacifier, toys, unused refrigerators
   c. Burns: ovens, heaters, sunburns; check water and food temperature
   d. Falls: stairs, windows, balconies, walkers
   e. Aspiration/poisonings: medications, cleaners, chemicals; store harmful substances out of reach

NCLEX® **M. Play (parallel)**

1. Begins as imaginative and make-believe play; may imitate adult in play
2. Provide blocks, wheel toys, push toys, puzzles, crayons to develop motor and coordination abilities
3. Toddlers enjoy repetitive stories and short songs with rhythm

VI. PRESCHOOL GROWTH AND DEVELOPMENT

A. Period from 3 to 5 years of age; tricycle by 3 years

B. Weight: growth is slow and steady; gains 4 to 5 lb/year

C. Height: increases 2 to 3 in/year

D. Motor

1. Rides tricycle by 3 years
2. Skips and hops on one foot by 4 years
3. Throws and catches ball well by 5 years
4. Balances on alternate feet by 5 years
5. Knows 2100 words by 5 years

NCLEX® 6. Increased strength and refinement of fine and gross motor abilities

E. Nutrition
1. Similar to toddlers' eating patterns
2. Demonstrates food preferences: likes and dislikes
3. Influenced by others' eating habits
4. Caloric requirement: 90 kcal/kg/day
5. Reinforce good dental hygiene: regular exams, brushing, fluoride, less concentrated sugar

NCLEX® **F. Safety**
1. Use belt-positioning booster seat with car's lap and shoulder belt when child exceeds manufacturer's height and weight limits on forward-facing car seat; all children younger than 13 years should sit in back seat of vehicle
2. Able to learn safety habits
3. Teach injury prevention such as traffic safety, risks with strangers, fire prevention/safety, water safety/drowning

NCLEX® **G. Play (associative)**
1. Enjoys imitative and dramatic play (imitates same sex role in play)
2. Provide toys to develop motor and coordination skills (tricycle, clay, paints, swings, sliding board)
3. Parental supervision of television
4. Enjoys sing-along songs with rhythm

VII. SCHOOL AGE GROWTH AND DEVELOPMENT

A. Period from 6 to 12 years of age
B. Weight: steady, slow growth; gains approximately 5 lb/yr
C. Height: increases 1 to 2 in/year; boys and girls differ little at first, but by end of period girls gain more weight and height compared to boys
D. Motor/sensory develop
1. Bones grow faster than muscles and ligaments develop
2. Susceptible to greenstick fractures
3. Movements become more limber, graceful, and coordinated
4. Have greater stamina and energy
5. Vision 20/20 by 6 to 7 years; myopia may appear by 8 years

E. Nutrition
1. Risk of obesity in this age group
2. NCLEX® Identify those above 95th and below 5th percentiles in weight and height on plotted growth charts
3. Requirement of 85 kcal/kg/day
4. Tendency to eat "junk" foods, empty calories
5. Secondary sex characteristics begin at 10 years in girls; 12 years in boys
6. Loses first deciduous teeth at age 6; by age 12 has all permanent teeth, except final molars

NCLEX® **F. Safety**
1. Incidence of accidents/injuries less likely
2. Teach proper use of sports equipment
3. Discourage risk-taking behaviors (smoking, alcohol, drugs, sex)
4. Introduce sex education
5. Teach injury prevention: bicycle safety, firearms, smoking education, hobbies/handicrafts

NCLEX® **G. Play (cooperative)**
1. Comprehends rules and rituals of games
2. Enjoys team play, which helps instill values and develop sense of accomplishment
3. Enjoys athletic activities such as swimming, soccer, hiking, bicycling, basketball, baseball, football
4. Provide construction toys: puzzles, erector sets, small interlocking blocks
5. Good eye–hand coordination: interested in video and computer games (needs monitoring and time limits)
6. Enjoys music, adventure stories, competitive activities

VIII. ADOLESCENT GROWTH AND DEVELOPMENT

A. Period from 13 to 18 years of age
B. Weight: rapid period of growth causes anxiety; girls gain 15 to 55 lb (7 to 25 kg); boys gain 15 to 65 lb (7 to 29 kg)
C. Height: attain final 20% of mature height; girls: height increases 3 in/year, slows at menarche, stops at 16 years; boys: height increases 4 in/year, growth spurt approximately at 13 years, slows in late teens

NCLEX® **D. Puberty**
1. Related to hormonal changes
2. Apocrine glands become active; adolescent may develop body odor

3. Appearance of acne on face, back, trunk
4. Development of secondary sex characteristics: girls experience breast development, menarche (average age 12½ yrs), pubic hair; boys experience enlargement of testes (13 years), increase in scrotum and penis size, nocturnal emission, pubic hair, vocal changes, possibly gynecomastia

E. Nutrition

1. **Growth spurt**: brief period of rapid increase in growth
2. "Hollow leg stage": appetite increases
3. Nutrition requirements: 60 to 80 kcal/kg/day (approximately 1500 to 3000 kcal/day at 11 to 14 yrs and 2100 to 3900 kcal/day at 15 to 18 years)
4. At risk for fad diets; food choices influenced by peers
5. Require increased calcium for skeletal growth
6. Continue emphasis on prevention of caries and good dental hygiene
7. Final molars erupt at end of adolescence; orthodontia common dental need

NCLEX® **F. Safety**

1. Accidents: leading cause of death (motor vehicle accidents, sports, firearms)
2. Provide drug and alcohol education
3. Provide sex education
4. Discourage risk-taking activities
5. Adolescents may display lack of impulse control, reckless behaviors, sense of invulnerability
6. Reinforce health promotion: breast self-exam (BSE), testicular self-exam (TSE)
7. Teach injury prevention
   a. Proper use of sports equipment (protective gear)
   b. Diving, drowning
   c. Provide driver's education
   d. Use of seat belts
   e. Violence prevention
   f. Crisis intervention (stress, depression, eating disorders)
   g. Provide information about the risks of body piercing
8. Reinforce rules when necessary

NCLEX® **G. Play/activities**

1. Enjoy sports, school and peer group activities (movies, dances, eating out, music, videos, computers)
2. Interest in heterosexual relationships common

IX. ADULT GROWTH AND DEVELOPMENT

A. Consists of young adulthood (18–35 years), middle adulthood (36–64 years), and older adulthood (65 years and older)

B. See Chapter 17 for discussion of needs of older adults

NCLEX® **C. Weight:** stabilizes in adulthood, although risks of overweight and obesity may apply based on lifestyle and eating habits

D. Height: stabilized

E. Young adulthood generally considered to be healthiest time of life

F. Physical strength, coordination, endurance, and speed of response are at maximal levels

G. Nutrition

1. Nutrient needs influenced by activity level and body size
2. Nutritional needs increase during pregnancy and lactation
3. Decreased fat intake, and increased intake of fruits, vegetables, and fiber recommended to promote healthy lifestyle (see Chapter 16)

NCLEX® **H. Safety**

1. Accidents, injuries, and acts of violence are frequent causes of death
2. Injury prevention methods similar to adolescence: proper use of safety and sports equipment, seat belts, and reduction of personal risk behaviors

NCLEX® **I. Leisure activities**

1. Should include healthy form of exercise most days of week (see Chapter 16)
2. May take a wide variety of forms depending on personal interests
3. Leisure activities should be encouraged for personal enjoyment and as means to reduce stress

X. CHILD'S REACTION TO ILLNESS AND HOSPITALIZATION

A. Infants and toddlers

1. Parent–child relationship is disturbed
2. Unpredictable routine of hospital promotes feelings of distrust

3. Infants and toddlers experience **separation anxiety**, which is distress behavior observed between ages of 6 and 30 months when separated from familiar caregivers; it peaks around 15 months
4. Stages of separation anxiety include protest (child appears sad, agitated, angry, inconsolable, watches desperately for parents to return), despair (child appears sad, hopeless, withdrawn; acts ambivalent when parents return), and detachment (child appears happy, interested in environment, becomes attached to staff members; may ignore parents)

NCLEX®

5. Goal of nursing interventions is to preserve child's trust
   a. Reassure child that parents will return
   b. Provide "rooming in" to encourage parent–child attachment
   c. Have parents leave a personal article, picture, or favorite toy with child
   d. Maintain usual routine and rituals, whenever possible
   e. Allow choices, whenever possible, to return control to parent and child

NCLEX®

6. Responses to pain
   a. Infants will have increases in blood pressure and heart rate and decrease in arterial oxygen saturation
   b. Harsh, tense, or loud crying
   c. Facial grimacing, flinching, thrashing of extremities
   d. Toddlers will verbally indicate discomfort ("no," "ouch," "hurts")
   e. Generalized restlessness, uncooperative, clings to family member

NCLEX®

7. **Regression**: use of behavior representative of an earlier stage of development, often used to cope with stress or anxiety
   a. Result is lack of control, frustration, possible return to bottle-feeding, temper tantrums, incontinence
   b. Help parents to understand changes in behavior; avoid punishment

B. Preschoolers

1. Major fears
   a. Mutilation: have general lack of understanding of body integrity
   b. Intrusive procedures: will misinterpret words; have active imagination
2. Very egocentric and present-oriented
3. Perceive illness as punishment; associate own actions with disease; may believe hospitalization is punishment for bad behavior

NCLEX®

4. Some degree of separation anxiety still exists; may become uncooperative, develop nightmares, become withdrawn or aggressive

NCLEX®

5. Nursing interventions
   a. Encourage parents to participate in child care
   b. Allow child to express feelings
   c. Give simple explanations; avoid medical terminology
   d. Provide **therapeutic play** (planned play techniques that provide an opportunity for children to deal with fears and concerns about illness or hospitalization)
   e. Allow child to manipulate and play with equipment
   f. Maintain trusting relationship with parents and child; allow time for questions
   g. Praise child, focus on the desired behavior, give rewards (stickers)
6. May show signs of regression to toddlerhood (such as loss of bowel/bladder control)

NCLEX®

7. Response to pain
   a. All children have a major fear of needles; preschoolers will deny pain to avoid an injection
   b. Restless, irritable, cries, kicks with experiences of pain
   c. Able to describe location and intensity of pain

C. School-age children

1. Major fears
   a. Pain and bodily injury
   b. Loss of control
   c. Fears often related to school, peers, and family
2. Ask relevant questions, want to know reasons for procedures, tests
3. Have a more realistic understanding of disease
4. Become distressed over separation from family and peers

NCLEX®

5. Nursing interventions
   a. Communicate openly and honestly; explain rules
   b. Clarify any misconceptions
   c. Encourage participation in care to maintain sense of control and independence
   d. Provide visiting for siblings and peers

e. Use age-appropriate therapeutic play to provide an opportunity for children to deal with fears and concerns about illness or hospitalization
f. Art therapy to assist child to express feelings
g. Provide explanations; use visual aids such as diagrams, models, and body outlines
h. Praise child; focus on desired behavior

NCLEX® 6. Response to pain
a. Able to describe pain; concerned with disability and death
b. Girls express pain more often than boys do
c. Demonstrate overt behaviors: biting, kicking, crying, and bargaining
d. Cues to pain: facial expression, silence, false sense of being "okay"

D. Adolescents
1. Major fears: loss of independence and/or identity, body image disturbance, rejection by others
2. Separation from peers is a source of anxiety
3. Physical appearance has major influence on how adolescents perceive themselves
4. Behaviors seen with loss of control: anger, withdrawal, uncooperative, power struggles
5. Reluctant to ask questions; question competency of others, verify answers with more than one person to determine if others are truthful
6. Often believe they are invincible, nothing can hurt them, resulting in risk-taking and noncompliant behaviors

NCLEX® 7. Nursing interventions
a. Involve adolescent in plan of care
b. Support relationships with family and peers
c. Provide consistent and truthful explanations; can use abstract terms
d. Accept emotional outburts
e. Promote communication between adolescents and parents

NCLEX® 8. Response to pain
a. Associate pain with being different from peers
b. May exhibit projected confidence, conceited attitude; withdraws, rejects others
c. Increased muscle tension and body control
d. Understand cause and effect; able to describe pain

XI. CHILD'S REACTION TO DEATH AND DYING

A. Infants and toddlers
1. Both lack an understanding of concept of death

NCLEX® 2. Infants react to loss of caregiver with behaviors such as crying, sleeping more, and eating less
3. Aware someone is missing; may experience separation anxiety

NCLEX® 4. Toddlers may develop fearfulness, become more attached to remaining parent, cease walking and talking

B. Preschoolers
1. View death as temporary and reversible
2. Magical thinking and **egocentricity** (preoccupied with own interests and needs; self-centered) lead to belief that dead person will come back
3. View death as a punishment; believe bad thoughts and actions cause death
4. First exposure to death is frequently death of a pet

NCLEX® 5. Common behaviors: nightmares, bowel and bladder problems, crying, anger, out-of-control behaviors

NCLEX® 6. Preschoolers will ask a lot of questions, may display fascination with death

C. School-age children
1. View death as irreversible, but not necessarily inevitable
2. By age 10, understand death is universal and will happen to them
3. May believe death serves as a punishment for wrongdoing
4. May deny sadness, attempt to act like an adult

NCLEX® 5. Common behaviors: difficulty with concentration in school, psychosomatic complaints, acting-out behaviors

D. Adolescents
1. View death as irreversible, universal, and inevitable
2. Seen as a personal but distant event
3. Develop a better understanding between illness and death

NCLEX® 4. Sense of invincibility conflicts with fear of death

NCLEX®

5. Common behaviors: feelings of loneliness, sadness, fear, depression; acting out behaviors may include risk-taking, delinquency, suicide attempts, promiscuity

E. Adults (see Chapter 24, "End-of-Life Care")

Check Your NCLEX–PN® Exam I.Q.

You are ready for testing on this content if you can

- Describe expected physical, cognitive, psychosocial, and moral stages of development.
- Compare the developmental stage of a client to norms.
- Plan appropriate nursing care based on client's developmental stage.
- Modify nursing care based on developmental stage of client.
- Identify achievement of developmental milestones.

PRACTICE TEST

1 The nurse wants to reduce the stress of a hospitalized, chronically ill 8-year-old child. Which approach by the nurse is most likely to improve the child's coping ability? Select all that apply.

1. Allow 24-hour open visitation with peers.
2. Provide care specifically designed for a school-age child.
3. Have tutoring postponed until discharge.
4. Caution against making any decisions while hospitalized.
5. Offer the child some choices for activities such as bathing or ambulating.

2 An inexperienced mother is playing with her 8-month-old in the playroom. The nurse has discussed with the mother toys that are developmentally appropriate for the child. The nurse will conclude that the mother has understood the nurse's information when the mother selects which type of toy? Select all that apply.

1. A set of blocks
2. A wagon
3. A puzzle with large pieces
4. A rattle
5. A soft ball

3 The nurse is caring for a 7-year-old child scheduled for surgery in the morning. While reinforcing preoperative teaching, the nurse would choose which aid to enhance the child's learning about the perioperative experience?

1. Videotape
2. Colorful brochure
3. Doll or puppet
4. A visit from the surgeon

4 The parents of a 16-month-old ask when they should begin toilet training. Which of the following should be included in a response by the nurse? Select all that apply.

1. When the child walks well
2. When the child is able to sit alone without support
3. When the child enters preschool
4. When the child has a dry diaper throughout the night
5. When the child can pull pants up and down

5 The grandparents of a 2½-year-old ask what would be an appropriate toy to buy their grandson. Which toy should the nurse recommend? Select all that apply.

1. A play telephone
2. A 54-piece puzzle
3. A paint-by-number set
4. A musical mobile
5. A small tricycle

6 The pediatric nurse would avoid using therapeutic play with a hospitalized 6-year-old at which times? Select all that apply.

1. During preoperative teaching
2. At bedtime
3. Before a diagnostic test
4. During a bedside procedure
5. When the child is stressed

7 The nurse working in a sexually transmitted infection (STI) clinic uses communication skills to collect data from clients and to provide health information. When developing rapport with a new adolescent client, it is important for the nurse to use which approach?

1. Consistently give honest information.
2. Have the parents present if at all possible.
3. Use jargon when communicating with the adolescent.
4. Allow the adolescent to smoke if desired during the conversation.

8 The Denver Developmental Screening Test has shown a 6-month-old infant is delayed in gross motor development. What activities by the nurse would best help the child reach the expected developmental level? Select all that apply.

1. Encouraging the child to stand
2. Talking to the child
3. Propping the child in a sitting position
4. Encouraging the child to hold a rattle
5. Pulling the child to a sitting position

9 The nurse needs to obtain a height on a 3-year-old child as a part of routine health screening. To obtain an accurate measurement, the nurse should instruct the child to do which of the following?

1. Lie down in a supine position.
2. Remove shoes and stand upright with head erect.
3. Stand with his or her feet wide apart.
4. Face the wall while being measured.

10 Four children recently admitted to the hospital unit have parents who will not be able to spend much time with them. The nurse would be most concerned with adjustment to hospitalization and separation from parents in the infant or child of which age?

1. 2 months old
2. 13 months old
3. 8 years old
4. 14 years old

11 A toddler is admitted for severe anemia, which is found to be dietary in nature. What recommendation would the nurse make to the parents to enhance dietary iron intake to promote healthy growth and development?

1. Limit milk to no more than 32 oz/day.
2. Increase fat-soluble vitamins in the diet.
3. Include grains and legumes in the daily intake.
4. Limit foods that are high in protein in the daily caloric requirement.

12 The mother of a neonate states she is concerned about her relationship with the infant. She says the baby goes to anyone and doesn't seem to care if she is present or not. The nurse explains that prior to developing a dependence on the mother the infant must develop which of the following?

1. Ritualistic behavior
2. Egocentrism
3. Conservation
4. Object permanence

13 The nurse discusses swimming pool safety with the parents of 4-year-old twins. Which statement identifies that more instruction is needed? Select all that apply.

1. "We remove all toys from the pool area when not in use."
2. "The twins wear flotation devices when they are in the pool by themselves."
3. "We never go in the house for more than a minute when the twins are in the pool."
4. "We always tell the twins not to run by the pool."
5. "Our children are enrolled in swimming classes."

14 The nurse prepares to transport a sedated 2-year-old from the pediatric unit to the endoscopy department. Taking into consideration the child's developmental stage and safety, what should the nurse use to transport the child to the area?

1. Padded wagon
2. Small wheelchair
3. High-top crib
4. Gurney (stretcher)

15 A 50-year-old female comes to the clinic with complaints of fatigue, breast tenderness, change in sex drive, constipation, and abdominal bloating. What would the nurse include when reinforcing client teaching about management of this condition?

1. A psychiatric consult, increased estrogen/progesterone therapy, and increased amounts of red meat in the diet
2. A meal plan with six small meals including a decrease in caffeine, salt, and sugar and an increase in water and grains, and an exercise plan outlining a mild exercise program
3. Hypnotics, fluid restriction, diversional therapy, and increased dairy products
4. A need to share feelings with the family, avoid exercise, and increase rest periods

16 When planning a menu for the older adult client, the nurse should limit which types of foods?

1. Low-fat dairy products
2. Whole-grain products
3. Alternate proteins
4. Refined carbohydrates

17 When discussing health promotion with young working adults, the nurse should focus prevention measures on which disorder?

1. Heart disease
2. Hypoglycemia
3. Obesity
4. Cancer

18 The nurse considers that which physical change commonly associated with aging is most likely to require a reduction in medication dosage for an older adult client? Select all that apply.

1. Increased rate of drug retention
2. Decreased total body fluid proportionate to body mass
3. Decreased efficiency in drug distribution
4. Decreased rate of drug metabolism by the liver
5. Significant weight gain

19 The nurse discusses the risk of aspiration with the parents of an 18-month-old. The nurse recommends the parents avoid giving their child which food items?

1. Oranges, crackers, and applesauce
2. Apples, fruit juice, and raisins
3. Cherries, peanuts, and hard candy
4. Oat cereal circles, toast, and bananas

20 The parent of a 6-month-old infant is concerned that the infant's anterior fontanel is still open. The nurse would explain to the parent that further evaluation is needed if the anterior fontanel is still open after how many months?

Fill in your answer below:

_____ months

PRACTICE TEST

ANSWERS & RATIONALES

ANSWERS & RATIONALES

1 **Answer: 2, 5** **Rationale:** Age-specific care is care that better meets the developmental needs of the hospitalized child. Providing opportunity for choices is beneficial for the child to achieve some sense of control while being hospitalized. Although visitation of peers is important, open visitation is usually recommended only for family members. Depending on the status of the child's illness and resources available, tutoring may be recommended. Mutual decision making is beneficial for the child and family. **Cognitive Level:** Applying **Client Need:** Health Promotion and Maintenance **Integrated Process:** Nursing Process: Planning **Content Area:** Foundational Sciences **Strategy:** Use the process of elimination. Critical words in the question are *8-year-old*, which lead you to look for an option that matches the needs of a child of this age group.

2 **Answer: 1, 5** **Rationale:** Objects that can be grasped and banged together, such as blocks, develop manipulation skills and are most appropriate for an 8-month-old infant. Pleasure is experienced from the feel and sounds of these activities. Throwing or rolling a ball helps the infant to develop gross motor skills and is appropriate for this age. A wagon may be used by preschoolers and toddlers. A large-piece puzzle may be used by preschoolers and toddlers. Rattles are recommended for infants ages 1 to 6 months. **Cognitive Level:** Applying **Client Need:** Health Promotion and Maintenance **Integrated Process:** Nursing Process: Evaluation **Content Area:** Foundational Sciences **Strategy:** Use the process of elimination and knowledge of growth and development to answer the question. The question indicates that more than one option may be correct. The correct answers match the physical development level of the child with the skills ability needed to use the toy.

3 **Answer: 3** **Rationale:** The use of a doll or puppet may decrease a 7-year-old child's anxiety and fear if the nurse uses such aids to explain what is expected. Videotapes are useful with explanations to adolescents. Brochures are useful with explanations to adolescents. A visit from the surgeon is informative primarily with the parents. **Cognitive Level:** Applying **Client Need:** Health Promotion and Maintenance **Integrated Process:** Nursing Process: Implementation **Content Area:** Foundational Sciences **Strategy:** Use the process of elimination and knowledge of growth and development to answer the question. The core issue of the question is the most effective method of teaching to use with a school-age child.

4 **Answer: 1, 5** **Rationale:** Children must have the physical and developmental capabilities to begin toilet training. They should be able to stand and walk well, pull pants up and down, recognize the urge to urinate or defecate, and be able to wait until they reach the potty chair. **Cognitive Level:** Analyzing **Client Need:** Health Promotion and Maintenance **Integrated Process:** Nursing Process: Planning **Content Area:** Foundational Sciences **Strategy:** Use the process of

elimination and knowledge of growth and development. The core issue of the question is physical and mental readiness for toilet training. The wording of the question indicates more than one option is likely to be correct.

5 **Answer: 1, 5 Rationale:** Toddlers enjoy such toys as a play telephone, which allows them to practice imitative behaviors and fine motor skills. Manipulation of toys such as a tricycle develops gross motor abilities in toddlers. More complex puzzles, such as those with 54 pieces, are recommended for school-age children. Paint-by-number sets are recommended for school-age children. Musical mobiles are appropriate for infants. **Cognitive Level:** Applying **Client Need:** Health Promotion and Maintenance **Integrated Process:** Nursing Process: Implementation **Content Area:** Foundational Sciences **Strategy:** Use the process of elimination and knowledge of growth and development. The core issue of the question is knowledge of appropriate play items for a toddler.

6 **Answer: 2, 4 Rationale:** Play is not recommended at bedtime to maintain a restful environment, or when the child needs to remain quiet, such as during a procedure. A quiet and calm environment will promote sleep. Play is a very effective teaching intervention. It is often used before surgery and diagnostic tests to aid understanding of these events. Play is therapeutic to help the child express feelings during stressful times. **Cognitive Level:** Applying **Client Need:** Health Promotion and Maintenance **Integrated Process:** Teaching and Learning **Content Area:** Foundational Sciences **Strategy:** Use the process of elimination and knowledge of growth and development. The core issue of the question is that therapeutic play must be used at appropriate times and in appropriate ways to be effective.

7 **Answer: 1 Rationale:** Nurses are credible sources of information, support, and encouragement that can help adolescents cope with challenges. To develop trust, honest and accurate information must be given to the client. The adolescent should be given the choice to have parents present because of the nature of the health problem, but treatment for STIs can be given without parental consent. The nurse should use appropriate language rather than jargon when communicating with clients. The client should not smoke during discussions with the nurse for general health reasons. **Cognitive Level:** Applying **Client Need:** Health Promotion and Maintenance **Integrated Process:** Communication and Documentation **Content Area:** Foundational Sciences **Strategy:** Use the process of elimination and knowledge of growth and development. The core issue of the question is knowledge that honest communication builds trust in a therapeutic relationship, regardless of age. A concept that also applies is knowledge related to issues of informed consent for an adolescent.

8 **Answer: 3, 5 Rationale:** Propping the child in a sitting position helps to develop self-righting behaviors. Pulling the child to a sitting position allows neck muscles to support the head and also aids with sitting. It is too early to begin assistance with standing. Talking to the child promotes language development. Handling a rattle involves fine-motor behavior. **Cognitive Level:** Analyzing **Client Need:** Health Promotion and Maintenance **Integrated Process:** Nursing Process: Planning **Content Area:** Foundational Sciences **Strategy:** Use the process of elimination and knowledge of growth and development to answer the question. The core issue of the question is the abilities of a 6-month-old infant.

9 **Answer: 2 Rationale:** It is recommended that the child's height be measured with a stadiometer. The correct procedure is to have the child remove his or her shoes and stand erect facing the examiner, holding the head erect. Shoulders, buttocks, and heels should touch the back of the wall. **Cognitive Level:** Applying **Client Need:** Health Promotion and Maintenance **Integrated Process:** Nursing Process: Implementation **Content Area:** Foundational Sciences **Strategy:** Use the process of elimination and knowledge of growth and development to answer the question. The correct answer is the one that incorporates proper technique based on the child's developmental level.

10 **Answer: 2 Rationale:** The 13-month-old will experience toddler hospitalization reaction, which is primarily related to separation from the parents. The 2-month-old has not recognized object permanence and will not suffer from the hospitalization as long as his or her needs are met in a consistent fashion. The 8-year-old and the 14-year-old are accustomed to separation from parents and working with new adults. **Cognitive Level:** Analyzing **Client Need:** Health Promotion and Maintenance **Integrated Process:** Nursing Process: Data Collection **Content Area:** Foundational Sciences **Strategy:** Use the process of elimination and knowledge of growth and development to answer the question. The core issue of the question is recognition of the client that is most at risk for separation anxiety from parents during hospitalization.

11 **Answer: 1 Rationale:** Excessive milk consumption should be discouraged, especially more than 1 liter/day (32 oz), since it is a poor source of iron. Fat-soluble vitamins will not increase absorption or utilization of iron. Although grains and legumes are good sources of nutrients, they are not especially high in iron. Foods high in protein should be encouraged, and especially food proteins of animal origin and organ meats, such as liver. **Cognitive Level:** Applying **Client Need:** Health Promotion and Maintenance **Integrated Process:** Teaching and Learning **Content Area:** Foundational Sciences **Strategy:** Use the process of elimination and knowledge of nutrition, growth, and development to answer the question. The correct answer is the one that would either decrease the intake of iron-poor foods or increase the intake of iron-rich foods.

12 **Answer: 4 Rationale:** Object permanence is the knowledge that an object or person continues to exist when not seen, heard, or felt. The baby will not attach to a single person, even the mother, until he or she is aware of the mother's existence. Ritualistic behavior, egocentrism, and conservation do not address this phenomenon. **Cognitive Level:** Applying **Client Need:** Health Promotion and Maintenance **Integrated Process:** Teaching and Learning **Content Area:** Foundational Sciences **Strategy:** Use the process of elimination and knowledge of growth and development to answer the question. The core issue of the question is knowledge that a young infant has not developed an awareness of object permanence.

13 **Answer: 2, 3 Rationale:** Flotation devices are not a substitute for supervision by an adult. Young children should never be left unattended in a swimming pool. The other options describe appropriate parental behaviors to support safety in the area of swimming pools. **Cognitive Level:** Analyzing **Client Need:** Health Promotion and Maintenance **Integrated Process:** Nursing Process: Evaluation **Content Area:** Foundational Sciences **Strategy:** Use the process of elimination and knowledge of growth and development. The critical words *need further instruction* guide you to choose options that represent safety hazards to 4-year-olds using a pool.

14 **Answer: 3** **Rationale:** Toddlers should be transported in a high-top crib with side rails up to ensure safety. The sedated toddler is at risk for falls. A wagon, wheelchair, or gurney will not eliminate the risk of fall injury to a sedated toddler. **Cognitive Level:** Applying **Client Need:** Safety and Infection Control **Integrated Process:** Nursing Process: Planning **Content Area:** Foundational Sciences **Strategy:** Use the process of elimination and knowledge of growth and development. The correct option is one that prevents the child from slipping out of the transport device while under sedation.

15 **Answer: 2** **Rationale:** These are classic symptoms of menopause. The first approach to management is implementing lifestyle changes, including following dietary and exercise plans. Reducing caffeine, salt, and sugar helps to reduce stimulation and water retention. With increased activity, more calories are burned, raising levels of endorphins for feelings of well-being and improving the glucose tolerance curve. Smaller meals are helpful so the client feels satisfied without overeating. This is not a psychiatric issue but a physiological adaptation to changing hormone levels; hormone therapy may be appropriate. There is no validity to increasing the amounts of red meat in the diet. This is a physiological adaptation to changing hormone levels; drugs for sedation or hypnotics are not necessary. There is no validity to increasing the amounts of dairy products in the diet. With increased activity, more calories are burned, raising levels of endorphins for feelings of well-being and improving the glucose tolerance curve. Asking the family to talk about the problem could help, but exercise is necessary to help overcome other symptoms. Resting too much only frustrates the client by leading to additional weight gain and/or decreased feelings of self-worth. **Cognitive Level:** Applying **Client Need:** Physiological Adaptation **Integrated Process:** Nursing Process: Planning **Content Area:** Foundational Sciences **Strategy:** Identify the age of the client and common problems associated with menopause. Then, use nursing knowledge and the process of elimination to choose the interventions that will be most helpful and that are within the scope of practice and teaching by the nurse.

16 **Answer: 4** **Rationale:** Older adults develop a slower metabolic rate and often decrease their activity at the same time. By reducing intake of refined carbohydrates, the calorie count meets the needs of the body. Low-fat dairy products are recommended to minimize complications of atherosclerosis and osteoporosis. Whole-grain products are recommended to minimize complications of constipation. Alternate proteins are recommended to minimize complications of atherosclerosis. **Cognitive Level:** Applying **Client Need:** Health Promotion and Maintenance **Integrated Process:** Nursing Process: Implementation **Content Area:** Foundational Sciences **Strategy:** The core concept of the question is to consider the physiological changes that occur with aging, which effect digestion and dietary impact. Select the food that is the least likely to promote health.

17 **Answer: 3** **Rationale:** Young adults as a group are at risk for improper eating habits and, if exercise is inadequate, this could lead to obesity. Obesity increases the risk of diseases such as atherosclerosis, hypertension, and heart disease. Heart disease occurs with greater frequency with increasing age; this is not the most appropriate prevention measure on which the nurse should focus with young adults. Hypoglycemia is not a common disorder among young adults. Cancer occurs with greater frequency with increasing age; this is not the most appropriate prevention measure on which the nurse should focus with this age group. **Cognitive Level:** Analyzing **Client Need:** Health Promotion and Maintenance **Integrated Process:** Nursing Process: Planning **Content Area:** Foundational Sciences **Strategy:** The core issue of the question is identification of health risks that are more likely to occur in young adults. Use nursing knowledge and the process of elimination to make a selection.

18 **Answer: 1, 2, 4** **Rationale:** Since elderly clients experience a decreased rate of drug excretion (and thus increased retention of drug), reduction of dosage would be appropriate. The decreased total body fluid proportion that accompanies physical aging increases the concentration of water-soluble drugs and requires lower dosing in older adults. Older adult clients experience a decreased rate of drug metabolism and thus a reduced dosage may be needed. Decreased efficiency in drug distribution would not correlate with a need to lower the dosage. Most older adults tend to lose weight as they age. **Cognitive Level:** Analyzing **Client Need:** Pharmacological and Parenteral Therapies **Integrated Process:** Nursing Process: Planning **Content Area:** Pharmacology **Strategy:** Select the options that would place the client at greatest risk and that correlate closest to the information in the question stem.

19 **Answer: 3** **Rationale:** Toddlers chew well, but may have difficulty swallowing large pieces of food. Young children cannot discard pits (such as from cherries). Foods like peanuts and hard candies are easily aspirated. Toddlers tolerate foods that are soft or easily chewed very well. Toddlers tolerate foods that are soft or easily chewed very well. Toddlers tolerate foods that are soft or easily chewed very well. **Cognitive Level:** Applying **Client Need:** Safety and Infection Control **Integrated Process:** Teaching and Learning **Content Area:** Child Health **Strategy:** Considering the normal activities of a child of this age will lead to the right answer.

20 **Answer: 18** **Rationale:** The anterior fontanel should be soft, flat, and pulsatile with the child in the sitting position and should completely close by age 12 to 18 months. If the fontanel is found to be open after 18 months, the child is referred for further evaluation. **Cognitive Level:** Applying **Client Need:** Health Promotion and Maintenance **Integrated Process:** Teaching and Learning **Content Area:** Child Health **Strategy:** Critical words are *6-month-old* and *concern that the anterior fontanel is still open*. Use knowledge of normal closure of anterior fontanel to choose the correct answer.

ANSWERS & RATIONALES

Key Terms to Review

cephalocaudal development p. 143
critical periods p. 143
differentiation p. 143
egocentricity p. 154
growth spurt p. 152
object permanence p. 150
proximodistal development p. 143
regression p. 153
ritualism p. 150
separation anxiety p. 153
therapeutic play p. 153

References

American Academy of Pediatrics (2011). *Car Safety Seats: Information for Families for 2011.* Retrieved July 14, 2011, from http://www.healthychildren.org/English/safety-prevention/on-the-go/pages/Car-Safety-Seats-Information-for-Families.aspx

Ball, J., Bindler, R., & Cowen, K. (2010). *Child nursing: Partnering with children and families* (2nd ed.). Upper Saddle River, NJ: Pearson Education, Inc.

D'Amico, D., & Barbarito, C. (2012). *Health & physical assessment in nursing.* (2nd ed.). Upper Saddle River, NJ: Pearson Education, Inc.

Jarvis, C. (2012). *Physical examination and health assessment* (6th ed.). St. Louis: Elsevier Science.

Hockenberry-Eaton, M., & Wilson, D. (2011). *Wong's nursing care of infants and children* (9th ed.). St. Louis: Elsevier Science.

Test Yourself

Are you ready for the NCLEX-PN® or course exams? Use the practice tests on the companion website to check.

Providing Immunizations 14

In this chapter

Cross Reference

Other chapters relevant to this content area are

Preventing and Controlling Infection **Chapter 7**
Uncomplicated Newborn Care **Chapter 12**
Lifespan Growth and Development **Chapter 13**
Promoting Healthy Lifestyle Choices **Chapter 16**
Maternal and Newborn Medications **Chapter 31**
Communicable or Infectious Diseases **Chapter 63**

I. OVERVIEW OF IMMUNIZATIONS

A. Overview

1. A **vaccine** is a suspension of live, usually **attenuated** or activated microorganisms (e.g., bacteria, viruses, or rickettsiae) or fractions of microorganisms administered to induce immunity and prevent infectious disease or sequelae
2. To produce immunity against various diseases in children and adults by introducing an antigen (a foreign substance that triggers an immune system response) into the body in the form of a vaccine
3. A vaccine produces **active immunity** in which antibody production is stimulated without causing clinical disease
4. **Passive immunity** can be conferred using immune globulins, in which antibodies to offending organism are already formed; it is also conferred via breast milk to breastfed infants

B. Information resources: Immunization schedules, vaccines, infectious and communicable diseases

NCLEX®

1. Recommended childhood, adolescent, and catch-up immunization schedules, United States, 2011 (see Figure 14–1)

Recommended Immunization Schedule for Persons Aged 0 Through 6 Years—United States • 2011

For those who fall behind or start late, see the catch-up schedule

Vaccine ▼ Age ►	Birth	1 month	2 months	4 months	6 months	12 months	15 months	18 months	19–23 months	2–3 years	4–6 years
Hepatitis B[1]	HepB	HepB			HepB						
Rotavirus[2]			RV	RV	RV[2]						
Diphtheria, Tetanus, Pertussis[3]			DTaP	DTaP	DTaP	see footnote[3]	DTaP				DTaP
Haemophilus influenzae type b[4]			Hib	Hib	Hib[4]	Hib					
Pneumococcal[5]			PCV	PCV	PCV	PCV				PPSV	
Inactivated Poliovirus[6]			IPV	IPV	IPV						IPV
Influenza[7]					Influenza (Yearly)						
Measles, Mumps, Rubella[8]						MMR			see footnote[8]		MMR
Varicella[9]						Varicella			see footnote[9]		Varicella
Hepatitis A[10]						HepA (2 doses)				HepA Series	
Meningococcal[11]										MCV4	

Range of recommended ages for all children

Range of recommended ages for certain high-risk groups

This schedule includes recommendations in effect as of December 21, 2010. Any dose not administered at the recommended age should be administered at a subsequent visit, when indicated and feasible. The use of a combination vaccine generally is preferred over separate injections of its equivalent component vaccines. Considerations should include provider assessment, patient preference, and the potential for adverse events. Providers should consult the relevant Advisory Committee on Immunization Practices statement for detailed recommendations: **http://www.cdc.gov/vaccines/pubs/acip-list.htm**. Clinically significant adverse events that follow immunization should be reported to the Vaccine Adverse Event Reporting System (VAERS) at **http://www.vaers.hhs.gov** or by telephone, **800-822-7967**. Use of trade names and commercial sources is for identification only and does not imply endorsement by the U.S. Department of Health and Human Services.

1. **Hepatitis B vaccine (HepB).** (Minimum age: birth)
   At birth:
   - Administer monovalent HepB to all newborns before hospital discharge.
   - If mother is hepatitis B surface antigen (HBsAg)-positive, administer HepB and 0.5 mL of hepatitis B immune globulin (HBIG) within 12 hours of birth.
   - If mother's HBsAg status is unknown, administer HepB within 12 hours of birth. Determine mother's HBsAg status as soon as possible and, if HBsAg-positive, administer HBIG (no later than age 1 week).

   Doses following the birth dose:
   - The second dose should be administered at age 1 or 2 months. Monovalent HepB should be used for doses administered before age 6 weeks.
   - Infants born to HBsAg-positive mothers should be tested for HBsAg and antibody to HBsAg 1 to 2 months after completion of at least 3 doses of the HepB series, at age 9 through 18 months (generally at the next well-child visit).
   - Administration of 4 doses of HepB to infants is permissible when a combination vaccine containing HepB is administered after the birth dose.
   - Infants who did not receive a birth dose should receive 3 doses of HepB on a schedule of 0, 1, and 6 months.
   - The final (3rd or 4th) dose in the HepB series should be administered no earlier than age 24 weeks.
2. **Rotavirus vaccine (RV).** (Minimum age: 6 weeks)
   - Administer the first dose at age 6 through 14 weeks (maximum age: 14 weeks 6 days). Vaccination should not be initiated for infants aged 15 weeks 0 days or older.
   - The maximum age for the final dose in the series is 8 months 0 days
   - If Rotarix is administered at ages 2 and 4 months, a dose at 6 months is not indicated.
3. **Diphtheria and tetanus toxoids and acellular pertussis vaccine (DTaP).** (Minimum age: 6 weeks)
   - The fourth dose may be administered as early as age 12 months, provided at least 6 months have elapsed since the third dose.
4. ***Haemophilus influenzae* type b conjugate vaccine (Hib).** (Minimum age: 6 weeks)
   - If PRP-OMP (PedvaxHIB or Comvax [HepB-Hib]) is administered at ages 2 and 4 months, a dose at age 6 months is not indicated.
   - Hiberix should not be used for doses at ages 2, 4, or 6 months for the primary series but can be used as the final dose in children aged 12 months through 4 years.
5. **Pneumococcal vaccine.** (Minimum age: 6 weeks for pneumococcal conjugate vaccine [PCV]; 2 years for pneumococcal polysaccharide vaccine [PPSV])
   - PCV is recommended for all children aged younger than 5 years. Administer 1 dose of PCV to all healthy children aged 24 through 59 months who are not completely vaccinated for their age.
   - A PCV series begun with 7-valent PCV (PCV7) should be completed with 13-valent PCV (PCV13).
   - A single supplemental dose of PCV13 is recommended for all children aged 14 through 59 months who have received an age-appropriate series of PCV7.
   - A single supplemental dose of PCV13 is recommended for all children aged 60 through 71 months with underlying medical conditions who have received an age-appropriate series of PCV7.
   - The supplemental dose of PCV13 should be administered at least 8 weeks after the previous dose of PCV7. See *MMWR* 2010:59(No. RR-11).
   - Administer PPSV at least 8 weeks after last dose of PCV to children aged 2 years or older with certain underlying medical conditions, including a cochlear implant.
6. **Inactivated poliovirus vaccine (IPV).** (Minimum age: 6 weeks)
   - If 4 or more doses are administered prior to age 4 years an additional dose should be administered at age 4 through 6 years.
   - The final dose in the series should be administered on or after the fourth birthday and at least 6 months following the previous dose.
7. **Influenza vaccine (seasonal).** (Minimum age: 6 months for trivalent inactivated influenza vaccine [TIV]; 2 years for live, attenuated influenza vaccine [LAIV])
   - For healthy children aged 2 years and older (i.e., those who do not have underlying medical conditions that predispose them to influenza complications), either LAIV or TIV may be used, except LAIV should not be given to children aged 2 through 4 years who have had wheezing in the past 12 months.
   - Administer 2 doses (separated by at least 4 weeks) to children aged 6 months through 8 years who are receiving seasonal influenza vaccine for the first time or who were vaccinated for the first time during the previous influenza season but only received 1 dose.
   - Children aged 6 months through 8 years who received no doses of monovalent 2009 H1N1 vaccine should receive 2 doses of 2010–2011 seasonal influenza vaccine. See *MMWR* 2010;59(No. RR-8):33–34.
8. **Measles, mumps, and rubella vaccine (MMR).** (Minimum age: 12 months)
   - The second dose may be administered before age 4 years, provided at least 4 weeks have elapsed since the first dose.
9. **Varicella vaccine.** (Minimum age: 12 months)
   - The second dose may be administered before age 4 years, provided at least 3 months have elapsed since the first dose.
   - For children aged 12 months through 12 years the recommended minimum interval between doses is 3 months. However, if the second dose was administered at least 4 weeks after the first dose, it can be accepted as valid.
10. **Hepatitis A vaccine (HepA).** (Minimum age: 12 months)
    - Administer 2 doses at least 6 months apart.
    - HepA is recommended for children aged older than 23 months who live in areas where vaccination programs target older children, who are at increased risk for infection, or for whom immunity against hepatitis A is desired.
11. **Meningococcal conjugate vaccine, quadrivalent (MCV4).** (Minimum age: 2 years)
    - Administer 2 doses of MCV4 at least 8 weeks apart to children aged 2 through 10 years with persistent complement component deficiency and anatomic or functional asplenia, and 1 dose every 5 years thereafter.
    - Persons with human immunodeficiency virus (HIV) infection who are vaccinated with MCV4 should receive 2 doses at least 8 weeks apart.
    - Administer 1 dose of MCV4 to children aged 2 through 10 years who travel to countries with highly endemic or epidemic disease and during outbreaks caused by a vaccine serogroup.
    - Administer MCV4 to children at continued risk for meningococcal disease who were previously vaccinated with MCV4 or meningococcal polysaccharide vaccine after 3 years if the first dose was administered at age 2 through 6 years.

The Recommended Immunization Schedules for Persons Aged 0 Through 18 Years are approved by the Advisory Committee on Immunization Practices (**http://www.cdc.gov/vaccines/recs/acip**), the American Academy of Pediatrics (**http://www.aap.org**), and the American Academy of Family Physicians (**http://www.aafp.org**).

Department of Health and Human Services • Centers for Disease Control and Prevention

Figure 14-1 Recommended Childhood, Adolescent, and Catch-up Immunization Schedules 2011.

Recommended Immunization Schedule for Persons Aged 7 Through 18 Years—United States • 2011

For those who fall behind or start late, see the schedule below and the catch-up schedule

Vaccine ▼ Age ▶	7–10 years	11–12 years	13–18 years
Tetanus, Diphtheria, Pertussis[1]		Tdap	Tdap
Human Papillomavirus[2]	see footnote [2]	HPV (3 doses)(females)	HPV Series
Meningococcal[3]	MCV4	MCV4	MCV4
Influenza[4]		Influenza (Yearly)	
Pneumococcal[5]		Pneumococcal	
Hepatitis A[6]		HepA Series	
Hepatitis B[7]		Hep B Series	
Inactivated Poliovirus[8]		IPV Series	
Measles, Mumps, Rubella[9]		MMR Series	
Varicella[10]		Varicella Series	

Range of recommended ages for all children

Range of recommended ages for catch-up immunization

Range of recommended ages for certain high-risk groups

This schedule includes recommendations in effect as of December 21, 2010. Any dose not administered at the recommended age should be administered at a subsequent visit, when indicated and feasible. The use of a combination vaccine generally is preferred over separate injections of its equivalent component vaccines. Considerations should include provider assessment, patient preference, and the potential for adverse events. Providers should consult the relevant Advisory Committee on Immunization Practices statement for detailed recommendations: **http://www.cdc.gov/vaccines/pubs/acip-list.htm**. Clinically significant adverse events that follow immunization should be reported to the Vaccine Adverse Event Reporting System (VAERS) at **http://www.vaers.hhs.gov** or by telephone, **800-822-7967**.

1. **Tetanus and diphtheria toxoids and acellular pertussis vaccine (Tdap).** (Minimum age: 10 years for Boostrix and 11 years for Adacel)
   - Persons aged 11 through 18 years who have not received Tdap should receive a dose followed by Td booster doses every 10 years thereafter.
   - Persons aged 7 through 10 years who are not fully immunized against pertussis (including those never vaccinated or with unknown pertussis vaccination status) should receive a single dose of Tdap. Refer to the catch-up schedule if additional doses of tetanus and diphtheria toxoid–containing vaccine are needed.
   - Tdap can be administered regardless of the interval since the last tetanus and diphtheria toxoid–containing vaccine.
2. **Human papillomavirus vaccine (HPV).** (Minimum age: 9 years)
   - Quadrivalent HPV vaccine (HPV4) or bivalent HPV vaccine (HPV2) is recommended for the prevention of cervical precancers and cancers in females.
   - HPV4 is recommended for prevention of cervical precancers, cancers, and genital warts in females.
   - HPV4 may be administered in a 3-dose series to males aged 9 through 18 years to reduce their likelihood of genital warts.
   - Administer the second dose 1 to 2 months after the first dose and the third dose 6 months after the first dose (at least 24 weeks after the first dose).
3. **Meningococcal conjugate vaccine, quadrivalent (MCV4).** (Minimum age: 2 years)
   - Administer MCV4 at age 11 through 12 years with a booster dose at age 16 years.
   - Administer 1 dose at age 13 through 18 years if not previously vaccinated.
   - Persons who received their first dose at age 13 through 15 years should receive a booster dose at age 16 through 18 years.
   - Administer 1 dose to previously unvaccinated college freshmen living in a dormitory.
   - Administer 2 doses at least 8 weeks apart to children aged 2 through 10 years with persistent complement component deficiency and anatomic or functional asplenia, and 1 dose every 5 years thereafter.
   - Persons with HIV infection who are vaccinated with MCV4 should receive 2 doses at least 8 weeks apart.
   - Administer 1 dose of MCV4 to children aged 2 through 10 years who travel to countries with highly endemic or epidemic disease and during outbreaks caused by a vaccine serogroup.
   - Administer MCV4 to children at continued risk for meningococcal disease who were previously vaccinated with MCV4 or meningococcal polysaccharide vaccine after 3 years (if first dose administered at age 2 through 6 years) or after 5 years (if first dose administered at age 7 years or older).
4. **Influenza vaccine (seasonal).**
   - For healthy nonpregnant persons aged 7 through 18 years (i.e., those who do not have underlying medical conditions that predispose them to influenza complications), either LAIV or TIV may be used.
   - Administer 2 doses (separated by at least 4 weeks) to children aged 6 months through 8 years who are receiving seasonal influenza vaccine for the first time or who were vaccinated for the first time during the previous influenza season but only received 1 dose.
   - Children 6 months through 8 years of age who received no doses of monovalent 2009 H1N1 vaccine should receive 2 doses of 2010-2011 seasonal influenza vaccine. See *MMWR* 2010;59(No. RR-8):33–34.
5. **Pneumococcal vaccines.**
   - A single dose of 13-valent pneumococcal conjugate vaccine (PCV13) may be administered to children aged 6 through 18 years who have functional or anatomic asplenia, HIV infection or other immunocompromising condition, cochlear implant or CSF leak. See *MMWR* 2010;59(No. RR-11).
   - The dose of PCV13 should be administered at least 8 weeks after the previous dose of PCV7.
   - Administer pneumococcal polysaccharide vaccine at least 8 weeks after the last dose of PCV to children aged 2 years or older with certain underlying medical conditions, including a cochlear implant. A single revaccination should be administered after 5 years to children with functional or anatomic asplenia or an immunocompromising condition.
6. **Hepatitis A vaccine (HepA).**
   - Administer 2 doses at least 6 months apart.
   - HepA is recommended for children aged older than 23 months who live in areas where vaccination programs target older children, or who are at increased risk for infection, or for whom immunity against hepatitis A is desired.
7. **Hepatitis B vaccine (HepB).**
   - Administer the 3-dose series to those not previously vaccinated. For those with incomplete vaccination, follow the catch-up schedule.
   - A 2-dose series (separated by at least 4 months) of adult formulation Recombivax HB is licensed for children aged 11 through 15 years.
8. **Inactivated poliovirus vaccine (IPV).**
   - The final dose in the series should be administered on or after the fourth birthday and at least 6 months following the previous dose.
   - If both OPV and IPV were administered as part of a series, a total of 4 doses should be administered, regardless of the child's current age.
9. **Measles, mumps, and rubella vaccine (MMR).**
   - The minimum interval between the 2 doses of MMR is 4 weeks.
10. **Varicella vaccine.**
    - For persons aged 7 through 18 years without evidence of immunity (see *MMWR* 2007;56[No. RR-4]), administer 2 doses if not previously vaccinated or the second dose if only 1 dose has been administered.
    - For persons aged 7 through 12 years, the recommended minimum interval between doses is 3 months. However, if the second dose was administered at least 4 weeks after the first dose, it can be accepted as valid.
    - For persons aged 13 years and older, the minimum interval between doses is 4 weeks.

The Recommended Immunization Schedules for Persons Aged 0 Through 18 Years are approved by the Advisory Committee on Immunization Practices (**http://www.cdc.gov/vaccines/recs/acip**), the American Academy of Pediatrics (**http://www.aap.org**), and the American Academy of Family Physicians (**http://www.aafp.org**).
Department of Health and Human Services • Centers for Disease Control and Prevention

Figure 14–1 Recommended Childhood, Adolescent, and Catch-up Immunization Schedules 2011 (continued).

Catch-up Immunization Schedule for Persons Aged 4 Months Through 18 Years Who Start Late or Who Are More Than 1 Month Behind—United States • 2011

The table below provides catch-up schedules and minimum intervals between doses for children whose vaccinations have been delayed. A vaccine series does not need to be restarted, regardless of the time that has elapsed between doses. Use the section appropriate for the child's age

Vaccine	Minimum Age for Dose 1	Minimum Interval Between Doses: Dose 1 to Dose 2	Dose 2 to Dose 3	Dose 3 to Dose 4	Dose 4 to Dose 5
PERSONS AGED 4 MONTHS THROUGH 6 YEARS					
Hepatitis B[1]	Birth	4 weeks	8 weeks (and at least 16 weeks after first dose)		
Rotavirus[2]	6 wks	4 weeks	4 weeks[2]		
Diphtheria, Tetanus, Pertussis[3]	6 wks	4 weeks	4 weeks	6 months	6 months[3]
Haemophilus influenzae type b[4]	6 wks	4 weeks if first dose administered at younger than age 12 months 8 weeks (as final dose) if first dose administered at age 12–14 months No further doses needed if first dose administered at age 15 months or older	4 weeks[4] if current age is younger than 12 months 8 weeks (as final dose)[4] if current age is 12 months or older and first dose administered at younger than age 12 months and second dose administered at younger than 15 months No further doses needed if previous dose administered at age 15 months or older	8 weeks (as final dose) This dose only necessary for children aged 12 months through 59 months who received 3 doses before age 12 months	
Pneumococcal[5]	6 wks	4 weeks if first dose administered at younger than age 12 months 8 weeks (as final dose for healthy children) if first dose administered at age 12 months or older or current age 24 through 59 months No further doses needed for healthy children if first dose administered at age 24 months or older	4 weeks if current age is younger than 12 months 8 weeks (as final dose for healthy children) if current age is 12 months or older No further doses needed for healthy children if previous dose administered at age 24 months or older	8 weeks (as final dose) This dose only necessary for children aged 12 months through 59 months who received 3 doses before age 12 months or for children at high risk who received 3 doses at any age	
Inactivated Poliovirus[6]	6 wks	4 weeks	4 weeks	6 months[6]	
Measles, Mumps, Rubella[7]	12 mos	4 weeks			
Varicella[8]	12 mos	3 months			
Hepatitis A[9]	12 mos	6 months			
PERSONS AGED 7 THROUGH 18 YEARS					
Tetanus, Diphtheria/ Tetanus, Diphtheria, Pertussis[10]	7 yrs[10]	4 weeks	4 weeks if first dose administered at younger than age 12 months 6 months if first dose administered at 12 months or older	6 months if first dose administered at younger than age 12 months	
Human Papillomavirus[11]	9 yrs	Routine dosing intervals are recommended (females)[11]			
Hepatitis A[9]	12 mos	6 months			
Hepatitis B[1]	Birth	4 weeks	8 weeks (and at least 16 weeks after first dose)		
Inactivated Poliovirus[6]	6 wks	4 weeks	4 weeks[6]	6 months[6]	
Measles, Mumps, Rubella[7]	12 mos	4 weeks			
Varicella[8]	12 mos	3 months if person is younger than age 13 years 4 weeks if person is aged 13 years or older			

1. **Hepatitis B vaccine (HepB).**
   - Administer the 3-dose series to those not previously vaccinated.
   - The minimum age for the third dose of HepB is 24 weeks.
   - A 2-dose series (separated by at least 4 months) of adult formulation Recombivax HB is licensed for children aged 11 through 15 years.
2. **Rotavirus vaccine (RV).**
   - The maximum age for the first dose is 14 weeks 6 days. Vaccination should not be initiated for infants aged 15 weeks 0 days or older.
   - The maximum age for the final dose in the series is 8 months 0 days.
   - If Rotarix was administered for the first and second doses, a third dose is not indicated.
3. **Diphtheria and tetanus toxoids and acellular pertussis vaccine (DTaP).**
   - The fifth dose is not necessary if the fourth dose was administered at age 4 years or older.
4. ***Haemophilus influenzae* type b conjugate vaccine (Hib).**
   - 1 dose of Hib vaccine should be considered for unvaccinated persons aged 5 years or older who have sickle cell disease, leukemia, or HIV infection, or who have had a splenectomy.
   - If the first 2 doses were PRP-OMP (PedvaxHIB or Comvax), and administered at age 11 months or younger, the third (and final) dose should be administered at age 12 through 15 months and at least 8 weeks after the second dose.
   - If the first dose was administered at age 7 through 11 months, administer the second dose at least 4 weeks later and a final dose at age 12 through 15 months.
5. **Pneumococcal vaccine.**
   - Administer 1 dose of 13-valent pneumococcal conjugate vaccine (PCV13) to all healthy children aged 24 through 59 months with any incomplete PCV schedule (PCV7 or PCV13).
   - For children aged 24 through 71 months with underlying medical conditions, administer 1 dose of PCV13 if 3 doses of PCV were received previously or administer 2 doses of PCV13 at least 8 weeks apart if fewer than 3 doses of PCV were received previously.
   - A single dose of PCV13 is recommended for certain children with underlying medical conditions through 18 years of age. See age-specific schedules for details.
   - Administer pneumococcal polysaccharide vaccine (PPSV) to children aged 2 years or older with certain underlying medical conditions, including a cochlear implant, at least 8 weeks after the last dose of PCV. A single revaccination should be administered after 5 years to children with functional or anatomic asplenia or an immunocompromising condition. See *MMWR* 2010;59(No. RR-11).
6. **Inactivated poliovirus vaccine (IPV).**
   - The final dose in the series should be administered on or after the fourth birthday and at least 6 months following the previous dose.
   - A fourth dose is not necessary if the third dose was administered at age 4 years or older and at least 6 months following the previous dose.
   - In the first 6 months of life, minimum age and minimum intervals are only recommended if the person is at risk for imminent exposure to circulating poliovirus (i.e., travel to a polio-endemic region or during an outbreak).
7. **Measles, mumps, and rubella vaccine (MMR).**
   - Administer the second dose routinely at age 4 through 6 years. The minimum interval between the 2 doses of MMR is 4 weeks.
8. **Varicella vaccine.**
   - Administer the second dose routinely at age 4 through 6 years.
   - If the second dose was administered at least 4 weeks after the first dose, it can be accepted as valid.
9. **Hepatitis A vaccine (HepA).**
   - HepA is recommended for children aged older than age 23 months who live in areas where vaccination programs target older children, or who are at increased risk for infection, or for whom immunity against hepatitis A is desired.
10. **Tetanus and diphtheria toxoids (Td) and tetanus and diphtheria toxoids and acellular pertussis vaccine (Tdap).**
    - Doses of DTaP are counted as part of the Td/Tdap series.
    - Tdap should be substituted for a single dose of Td in the catch-up series for children aged 7 through 10 years or as a booster for children aged 11 through 18 years; use Td for other doses.
11. **Human papillomavirus vaccine (HPV).**
    - Administer the series to females at age 13 through 18 years if not previously vaccinated or have not completed the vaccine series.
    - Quadrivalent HPV vaccine (HPV4) may be administered in a 3-dose series to males aged 9 through 18 years to reduce their likelihood of genital warts.
    - Use recommended routine dosing intervals for series catch-up (i.e., the second and third doses should be administered at 1 to 2 and 6 months after the first dose). The minimum interval between the first and second doses is 4 weeks. The minimum interval between the second and third doses is 12 weeks, and the third dose should be administered at least 24 weeks after the first dose.

Information about reporting reactions after immunization is available online at **http://www.vaers.hhs.gov** or by telephone, **800-822-7967**. Suspected cases of vaccine-preventable diseases should be reported to the state or local health department. Additional information, including precautions and contraindications for immunization, is available from the National Center for Immunization and Respiratory Diseases at **http://www.cdc.gov/vaccines** or telephone, **800-CDC-INFO** (800-232-4636).

Department of Health and Human Services • Centers for Disease Control and Prevention

Figure 14–1 Recommended Childhood, Adolescent, and Catch-up Immunization Schedules 2011 (continued).

2. American Academy of Pediatrics (AAP) Red Book: Report of the Committee of Infectious Diseases (updated each year)
3. Centers for Disease Control (CDC) website: http://www.cdc.gov/vaccines/
4. Advisory Committee on Immunization Priorities (ACIP)
5. CDC Morbidity and Mortality Weekly Report (MMWR)
6. *Journal of Pediatrics*

C. Potential nursing diagnoses associated with immunizations: see Box 14–1

D. General nursing considerations for vaccine administration

1. Provide a written vaccine information statement to client or caregiver and obtain written consent prior to administration
2. Strictly follow manufacturer's directions on storing, reconstituting, and administering any vaccine
3. *NCLEX®* Store vaccine in center shelf of body of refrigerator (not in door) at 2° to 8°C (35–46°F) to maintain stable temperature and maintain vaccine potency; do not freeze
4. Check manufacturer expiration date on single-dose or multidose vial or single-use ampule prior to administration; if a multidose vial is used, follow manufacturer's directions; some vials may be used for 30 days after initial use but must be relabeled with newer expiration date; follow agency policy and vaccine directions
5. *NCLEX®* If more than one vaccine is given at one time, draw up in different syringes and administer in different sites
6. *NCLEX®* Use age-appropriate techniques to reduce discomfort in a child receiving an immunization; see Box 14–2
7. *NCLEX®* Intramuscular (IM) vaccines are injected into vastus lateralis muscle (optimally) in newborns and in deltoid muscle of arm for children and older infants; avoid using dorsogluteal site
8. *NCLEX®* Document on immunization record the day, month, and year of administration; vaccine manufacturer, lot number, and expiration date; route and site of administration; and name, title, and work address of person who administered dose
9. If an adverse reaction to an immunization occurs, complete a Vaccine Adverse Event Report (VAER) form and report severe reactions to National Vaccine Injury Compensation Program, U.S. Department of Health and Human Services, in accordance with federal law

Box 14–1

Potential Nursing Diagnoses with Immunizations

- Risk for Ineffective Breathing Pattern related to possible laryngeal edema secondary to hypersensitivity to vaccine
- Impaired Comfort related to side or adverse effects of immunization
- Risk for Impaired Skin Integrity related to vaccine response
- Deficient Knowledge related to immunization schedules and recordkeeping
- Ineffective Health Maintenance related to cultural beliefs regarding routine immunization

Box 14–2

Reducing Discomfort from Immunizations

Reduce pain and anxiety associated with injections by using the following techniques:

- Determine feasibility of parent applying Emla cream to the site for an hour before the injection to numb the area
- Ensure use of correct needle size
- Distract child using age-appropriate measure (e.g., by blowing bubbles or spinning a pinwheel)
- Apply site pressure for 10 seconds before the injection
- Use a vapo coolant spray immediately before the injection
- Obtain the assistance of another provider and give two injections simultaneously in different extremities

Adapted from Ball, J., Bindler, R., & Cowen, K. (2010). *Child health nursing: Partnering with children & families* (2nd ed.). Upper Saddle River, NJ: Pearson Education, p. 634.

II. HEPATITIS B VACCINE

A. Hepatitis B virus (HBV)

1. Hepatitis B is a liver infection caused by HBV, which is transmitted in blood or body secretions
2. A series of three (3) injections prevent HBV infection

B. Administration technique (see Table 14–1)

1. Ask if there have been any previous immunization reactions
2. Vaccine will appear cloudy; shake prior to withdrawing; note strength and expiration date of vaccine prior to administering
3. NCLEX® An infant born from a HbsAg+ mother should also receive hepatitis B immune globulin (HBIG) at same time in a different site using new needle and syringe

C. Precautions

1. Give second dose at least 1 month after first dose
2. Give third dose at least 2 months after second dose and at least 4 months after first
3. Do not give third dose to infants younger than 6 months of age because this could reduce long-term protection
4. Reschedule dose to a later date if person is moderately or severely ill when scheduled to receive vaccine

NCLEX® **D. Contraindications**

1. People who have had a life-threatening allergic reaction to baker's yeast (yeast used for baking bread)
2. People who have had a serious reaction to a previous dose of hepatitis B vaccine including anaphylaxis
3. People who have liver abnormalities

Table 14–1 Hepatitis B Vaccine

Recommended Age	Dosage	Route
For infant whose mother is HbsAg + Within 12 hours of birth, 1–2 months, 6 months	0.5 mL	IM
For infant whose mother is HbsAg –		
Birth–2 months, 1–4 months, 6–18 months	0.5 mL	IM
or		
Birth–2 months, 1 month after first dose, 6 months after first dose	0.5 mL	IM
For older child, adolescent, or adult First dose anytime, second dose 1–2 months after first, third dose 4–6 months after first	≤ 19 yrs: 0.5 mL ≥ 20 yrs: 1.0 mL	IM
or		
Adolescents 11–15 years may only need two (2) doses separated by 4–6 months (consult health care provider)	1.0 mL	IM

Box 14–3 Actions to Take for Anaphylaxis

To be prepared for potential vaccine-induced anaphylaxis:

1. Keep epinephrine 1:1000 and resuscitation equipment immediately available
2. Administer once order obtained for epinephrine 0.01 mL/kg per dose
3. Repeat every 10 to 20 minutes up to 3 doses until symptoms subside or other emergency care interventions are initiated
4. Expect to use supportive measures such as oxygen, vasopressors, and other interventions as needed (American Academy of Pediatrics, 2009)

Adapted from Ball, J., Bindler, R., & Cowen, K. (2010). *Child health nursing: Partnering with children & families* (2nd ed.). Upper Saddle River, NJ: Pearson Education, p. 1209.

NCLEX® **E. Side effects/adverse reactions**

1. Common side effects include: pain or redness at injection site; headache; photophobia; elevated liver enzymes; fever
2. Rare serious side effects including anaphylaxis; see Box 14–3 for treatment

III. DIPHTHERIA, TETANUS, AND PERTUSSIS VACCINES

A. Diphtheria, tetanus, and pertussis

1. Diphtheria is an acute, contagious infection that can cause respiratory obstruction
2. Tetanus, referred to as lockjaw, can cause muscle spasms and rigidity over entire body; ultimately obstructs breathing; death occurs in 1 out of 10 cases
3. Pertussis, referred to as whooping cough, can lead to respiratory distress, pneumonia, seizures, brain damage, or death
4. Diphtheria, tetanus toxoids, and pertussis vaccines are examples of **inactivated vaccines**, (or **killed vaccines**), which confer a weaker response than a live virus and require regular booster injections
5. Current available vaccines include DTaP (tetanus, diphtheria, and acellular pertussis) for children receiving initial five-injection immunization series from ages 2 months to 4 to 6 years, Tdap (tetanus, diphtheria, and acellular pertussis) booster one time only for adolescents ages 11 through 18 years and adults 19 to 64 years, and Td (tetanus, diphtheria) booster every 10 years thereafter
6. Tdap booster was added because of rise in pertussis infections in adolescents, especially those who go to college and live in crowded conditions with exposure to large numbers of people; Tdap is also recommended for adults, especially those who work with infants less than 12 months of age (who are at high risk for pertussis-related complications and death)

B. Administration technique (see Table 14–2)

1. It may be given at same time as other vaccines
2. Encourage use of same brand for all doses; ask about previous reactions to immunizations
3. Vaccine will appear cloudy; shake prior to withdrawing; if clumps cannot be resuspended, do not use
4. Preferably administer in vastus lateralis muscle for nonwalking infants

C. Precautions

1. Anyone who is moderately or severely ill at time of vaccine should wait until they recover; people with minor illnesses, such as a cold, may be vaccinated
2. Aspirin-free pain reliever is recommended if fever or pain at injection site occurred after previous dose of DTaP; administer for a period of 24 hours according to package instructions or advice from health care provider
3. Delay for 1 month after immunosuppressive therapy
4. Delay if immune serum globulin has been administered within 90 days

NCLEX® **D. Contraindications**

1. Life-threatening reaction to a previous dose of DTaP
2. Seizure, inconsolable crying for 3 hours or more, or fever above 105°F after previous dose

NCLEX® **E. Side effects/adverse reactions**

1. Serious: anaphylaxis, seizure, inconsolable crying for 3 hours or more, fever greater than 105°F; decreased level of consciousness; and permanent brain damage (rare)
2. Common: redness, pain, swelling, and nodule at injection site; fever up to 101°F; drowsiness and fussiness; anorexia within two days of injection

Table 14-2 Diphtheria, Tetanus, and Pertussis Vaccines

Vaccine	Recommended Age	Dosage	Route
DTaP	2, 4, 6, and 15–18 months 4–6 years	0.5 mL	IM
Tdap	11–12 years 13–18 years for 1 dose if received Td at age 11–12 19–64 years for 1 dose if received Td for all previous boosters	0.5 mL	IM
Td	Every 10 years	0.5 mL	IM

IV. *HAEMOPHILUS INFLUENZAE* TYPE B (HIB) VACCINE

A. *Haemophilis influenzae*
1. *H. influenzae* type B was most common cause of meningitis in children over 1 month of age
2. Hib conjugate vaccine protects against a number of serious diseases such as meningitis, epiglottitis, pneumonia, sepsis, and septic arthritis

B. Administration technique (see Table 14–3)
1. It may be given at same time as other vaccines
2. Depending on what brand of Hib is used, child may not need a dose at 6 months of age; consult health care provider
3. Children older than 5 years of age generally do not need Hib vaccine; some children with special health needs such as sickle cell anemia, HIV/AIDS, cancer treatment, or bone marrow transplant may need vaccine
4. Encourage use of same brand for all doses (some brands require three doses while others require four doses)
5. Ask about previous reactions to immunizations
6. Preferably administer in vastus lateralis muscle

C. Precautions
1. Children with minor illnesses may receive immunization
2. Moderately or severely ill children should not be immunized until they recover from illness

NCLEX® **D. Contraindications: prior anaphylactic reaction or severe reaction to previous dose (rare)**

NCLEX® **E. Side effects/adverse reactions**
1. Serious: anaphylaxis (rare)
2. Common: pain, redness, or swelling at site

V. INACTIVATED POLIO VIRUS VACCINE (IPV)

A. Poliomyelitis
1. A disease caused by a virus that affects central nervous system (CNS); enters body through mouth; may not cause serious illness, but can cause paralysis, respiratory complications, and death
2. Live oral polio vaccine no longer recommended for use in United States
3. IPV is a trivalent vaccine that contains all three forms of polio; is given subcutaneously (SubQ)
4. IPV is an inactivated vaccine, or killed vaccine, which confers a weaker response than a live vaccine, necessitating frequent boosters

B. Administration (see Table 14–3): clear, colorless suspension; do not use if contains particulate matter, becomes cloudy, or changes colors

C. Precautions: prior to immunization, ask if child has allergies to neomycin, streptomycin, or polymyxin B

NCLEX® **D. Contraindications**
1. Anaphylactic reaction
2. Anyone who is moderately or severely ill at time of vaccination should wait until they recover; people with minor illnesses, such as a cold, may be vaccinated

NCLEX® **E. Side effects/adverse reactions**
1. Serious: anaphylaxis
2. Common: elevated temperature 1 to 2 weeks after immunization; redness or pain at injection site; noncontagious rash; joint pain; irritability

Table 14–3 Other Vaccines Started in Early Infancy

Vaccine	Recommended Age(s)	Dosage	Route
Haemophilus influenzae type B (Hib)	2, 4, 6, and 12–15 months	0.5 mL	IM
Inactivated polio vaccine (IPV)	2, 4, and 6–18 months, and 4–6 years	0.5 mL	SubQ
Measles, mumps, rubella (MMR) vaccine	12–15 months, and 4–6 years	0.5 mL	SubQ
Varicella vaccine (Varivax)	12–18 months	0.5 mL	SubQ
Pneumococcal conjugate vaccine (PCV)	2, 4, 6, and 12–15 months	0.5 mL	IM
Rotavirus Vaccine (RV)	2, 4 months (Rotarix) 2, 4, 6 months (RotaTeq)	1 mL 2 mL	Oral Oral

VI. MEASLES, MUMPS, RUBELLA (MMR) VACCINE

A. Measles (rubeola), mumps (parotitis), rubella (German measles)

1. Infectious and communicable diseases in children that are vaccine-preventable; rubella is generally a mild disease but presents a major risk of spontaneous abortion, stillbirth, fetal death, and other anomalies for fetus during first trimester of pregnancy
2. MMR vaccine is a **live, attenuated vaccine** created from a live organism grown under suboptimal conditions to produce a live vaccine with reduced virulence

B. Administration (see again Table 14–3)

1. Reconstituted solution is clear yellow; keep refrigerated and away from light; discard if unused within 8 hours; store diluent at room temperature or refrigerate
2. Table 14–3 lists recommended ages; however, second dose can be given at any age as long as it is at least 28 days after first dose
3. Those who have not received a second dose at 4 to 6 years of age should receive second MMR at scheduled visit at age 11 to 12 years

C. Precautions

1. College students are at greater risk due to increased exposure; ensure they have received a second MMR dose
2. *NCLEX®* Inform adolescent girls to avoid pregnancy for at least 3 months after immunization
3. MMR vaccine may be allowed for some infected with HIV; consult health care provider
4. Wait at least 3 to 11 months after administration of immune serum globulin or blood products before giving MMR vaccine
5. Thrombocytopenia or history of thrombocytopenic purpura

NCLEX® **D. Contraindications**

1. Allergy to neomycin, gelatin, or eggs
2. Severely impaired immune system due to malignancy, immune deficiency disease, immunosuppressive therapy
3. Avoid administering a live-virus immunization during pregnancy and in women likely to become pregnant within 3 months

NCLEX® **E. Side effects/adverse reactions**

1. Serious: anaphylaxis; encephalopathy; thrombocytopenic purpura; chronic arthritis
2. Common: elevated temperature 1 to 2 weeks after immunization; redness or pain at injection site; noncontagious rash; joint pain
3. Measles vaccine can cause a false-negative tine (TB) result

VII. VARICELLA VACCINE (VARIVAX)

A. Varicella (chicken pox)

1. A common childhood disease, usually mild, can lead to severe skin infection, scars, pneumonia, brain damage, or death
2. Varicella immunization is a live, attenuated vaccine used to stimulate immunity
3. The vaccine prevents chicken pox, or if the child has been vaccinated and gets the disease, it will be usually very mild, resulting in a faster recovery

B. Administration (see again Table 14–3)

1. Frozen at 5°F; store in center shelf of body of refrigerator at 2° to 8° (35–46°F) up to 72 hours before reconstitution; once reconstituted, must be used within 30 minutes or discarded; do not refreeze; keep diluent at room temperature
2. Individuals 13 years or older who have not had the disease require two doses 4 to 8 weeks apart
3. May use as postexposure if given within 3 to 5 days

C. Precautions

1. *NCLEX®* Instruct females of childbearing age to avoid pregnancy for 3 months after immunization
2. Varicella vaccine is *not* recommended for those infected with HIV
3. Wait at least 3 to 11 months after administration of immune serum globulin or blood products before giving varicella vaccine

NCLEX® **D. Contraindications**

1. Allergy to neomycin or gelatin
2. Active, untreated TB
3. Pregnancy
4. Immunodeficiency or receiving immunosuppression therapy
5. Moderate or severe febrile illness

NCLEX®

E. Side effects/adverse reactions

1. Serious: anaphylaxis
2. Common: pain or redness at injection site; fever up to 38.8°C (102°F) in children, up to 37.7°C (100°F) in adults, lasting for 1 week; varicella-like rash at injection site; irritability

VIII. PNEUMOCOCCAL CONJUGATE VACCINE (PCV)

A. Pneumoccocal infections

1. Pneumococcal infection caused by *Streptococcus pneumoniae* is a leading cause of bacterial meningitis in United States
2. Heptavalent pneumococcal conjugate vaccine (PCV) is recommended for all children 2 to 23 months of age

B. Administration (see again Table 14–3): is a clear, colorless, or slightly opalescent liquid

C. Precautions

1. It is highly recommended for children in day care
2. Also recommended for children with immunosuppression, pulmonary or cardiac illness, diabetes, sickle cell anemia, or asplenia

NCLEX®

D. Contraindications: hypersensitivity to diphtheria *toxoid* or severe illness and anaphylaxis to a previous dose

NCLEX®

E. Side effects/adverse reactions

1. Severe: anaphylaxis
2. Common: soreness, swelling, redness at injection site; mild to moderate fever; irritability; drowsiness; restlessness; sleep; decreased appetite; vomiting and diarrhea; rash or hives

IX. ROTAVIRUS VACCINE

A. Rotavirus infection

1. A leading cause of severe acute gastroenteritis (vomiting and diarrhea) among children worldwide; is often accompanied by fever
2. In clinical trials, rotavirus vaccine was found to prevent almost all (85–98%) severe rotavirus illness episodes and 74–87% of all rotavirus illness episodes (CDC)
3. Two rotavirus vaccines are approved for use in infants in United States (RotaTeq® [RV5] and Rotarix® [RV1])

B. Administration (see again Table 14–3): given as a liquid oral dose

C. Precautions

1. Delay dose for infant currently experiencing vomiting and/or diarrhea
2. Do not begin first dose before age 6 weeks and finish final dose by age 32 weeks
3. Safety or efficacy data are not available for infants who are potentially immunocompromised (e.g., HIV/AIDS), have a history of gastrointestinal or congenital abdominal disorders, chronic diarrhea, failure to thrive, abdominal surgery, and intussusception

D. Contraindications

1. Hypersensitivity to the vaccine or any component of the vaccine
2. History of severe combined immunodeficiency disease (SCID)

E. Side effects/adverse reactions

1. Severe: seizures, bronchiolitis, gastroenteritis, pneumonia, fever, urinary tract infection
2. Common: vomiting, diarrhea, irritability

X. HEPATITIS A (HEP A) VACCINE

A. Hepatitis A

1. Hepatitis A virus (HAV), which is found in stool of infected persons, causes serious liver disease; usually spread by close personal contact and sometimes eating food or drinking water contaminated by HAV
2. Hep A vaccine, an inactivated or killed vaccine, can be given for postexposure prophylaxis against hepatitis A
3. Immune globulin and Hep A vaccine can be given at same time in different sites

B. Administration (see Table 14–4)

1. Do not restart series no matter how long since previous dose
2. May give with all other vaccines
3. Can be combined with hepatitis B vaccine (Twinrix); follow package instructions

Table 14–4 Hepatitis A (Hep A) Vaccine

Recommended Age	Dosage	Route
2 doses given after age 12 months; second dose is given 6–12 months after first	≤ 18 yrs: 0.5 mL ≥ 19 yrs: 1.0 mL	IM

C. Precautions
1. Safety of hepatitis A vaccine for pregnant women is not yet known; risk is thought to be low

NCLEX®
2. Moderate to severe acute illness with or without fever warrants delay of vaccination

NCLEX®
D. Contraindications
1. Known hypersensitivity to any component of vaccine, including neomycin
2. Anaphylactic reaction to prior vaccine dose

NCLEX®
E. Side effects/adverse effects
1. Serious: anaphylaxis (rare)
2. Common: soreness at injection site, headache, loss of appetite, fatigue

XI. INFLUENZA TRIVALENT INACTIVATED VACCINE (TIV)

A. Influenza
1. Vaccine, also referred to as flu shot, provides protection against strains of influenza; protection begins 2 weeks after administration and lasts 1 year
2. Close contacts of healthy children aged 0 to 23 months should receive influenza
3. Injection is an inactivated or killed vaccine, but an intranasal form (live, attenuated vaccine) is acceptable for children ages 5 and older

B. Administration (see Table 14–5)
1. Administer in autumn and repeat yearly
2. Give two doses 4 weeks apart if first dose for children under age 12 years; one dose for those over 12 years

C. Precautions: is recommended for those undergoing immunosuppressive therapy or on chronic aspirin therapy (e.g., for rheumatoid arthritis or Kawasaki disease)

NCLEX®
D. Contraindications
1. Allergy to eggs
2. Anaphylaxis
3. Administration of live virus through intranasal route not appropriate for children with chronic illness (asthma, heart or renal disease, diabetes, immunosuppressed)

NCLEX®
E. Side effects/adverse reactions
1. Serious: allergic reaction (rare)
2. Common: redness, soreness, swelling at injection site; fever; aching

XII. MENINGOCOCCAL VACCINES

A. Meningococcal infection
1. A serious respiratory infection that can lead to critical illness such as meningitis, disseminated intravascular coagulopathy (DIC), shock, or death
2. This vaccine provides protection against *Neisseria meningitides*

B. Administration (see Table 14–6)
1. Recommended for children 2 years and older with terminal complement deficiencies and asplenia
2. Recommended for 11 to 12 year olds, unvaccinated high school freshmen and unvaccinated freshman college students, military recruits, and those traveling to certain countries where there is added risk for exposure

Table 14–5 Influenza Trivalent Inactivated Vaccine (TIV)

Recommended Age	Dosage	Route
6–23 months of age ≥ 24 months of age with risk factors ≥ 3 years	0.25 mL 0.5 mL	IM

Table 14-6 Meningococcal Vaccines

Vaccine	Recommended Age	Dosage	Route
Meningococcal polysaccharide vaccine or MPSV4 (Menomune)	2 years and older with asplenia	0.5 mL	SubQ
Meningococcal conjugate vaccine or MCV4 (Menactra)	11–12 years and unvaccinated adolescents at high school entry or college freshman	0.5 mL	IM

3. Administer subQ injection in anterolateral fat of thigh in young children or posterolateral fat of upper arm for older children and adults; administer IM injection in large muscle

C. Precautions: duration of protection is uncertain; safety in pregnancy not established

D. Contraindications: prior sensitivity to vaccine component; history of Guillain-Barré syndrome unless at high risk for meningococcal infection

E. Side effects/adverse reactions

1. Serious: anaphylaxis
2. Common: redness or tenderness at site

XIII. HUMAN PAPILLOMAVIRUS (HPV) VACCINE

A. Human papillomavirus infection

1. Clinical infection seen as clustered or single warts in genital area (on vulva, perineal area, vagina, or cervix in females; on penis, scrotal skin near base of penis or near anus in males)
2. Subclinical infection in females can be diagnosed on Papanicolaou (Pap) smear
3. Specific types of HPV infection are responsible for more than 99% of female cervical cancers
4. Quadrivalent vaccine (Gardisil) is recommended for females age 9–26 years to prevent genital warts (HPV types 6 and 11) and certain cervical, vaginal, and vulvar cancers caused by oncogenic HPV types 16 and 18; and for males age 9–26 years to prevent genital warts (HPV types 6 and 11) (effective October, 2009)
5. Bivalent vaccine (Cervarix) is recommended for females age 9–26 years to prevent certain cervical, vaginal, and vulvar cancers caused by oncogenic HPV types 16 and 18
6. Vaccine should be given before onset of sexual activity and offers protection against genital warts, but does not protect against other sexually transmitted infections

B. Administration (see Table 14–7): solution is white and cloudy; shake before use; protect vaccine from light to protect potency

C. Precautions

1. Delay dose if moderate to severe illness with or without fever; can give if mild acute illness present
2. Use cautiously in lactating women; unknown if vaccine is excreted in human milk

D. Contraindications

1. Severe allergic reaction to prior dose or hypersensitivity to any vaccine component (e.g., yeast)
2. Pregnancy or bleeding disorder

E. Side effects/adverse reactions

1. Severe: bronchospasm, asthma, arthritis and possibly headache or gastroenteritis, fainting or syncope
2. Common: pain, swelling, erythema at injection site, pruritus, fever

Table 14-7 Human Papillomavirus (HPV) Vaccine

Vaccine	Recommended Age(s)	Dosage	Route
Bivalent human papillomavirus vaccine (HPV2, Cervarix)	Females 11–12 years, second and third doses 2 and 6 months after first	0.5 mL	IM
Quadrivalent human papillomavirus vaccine (HPV4, Gardasil)	Males and females 11–12 years, second and third doses 2 and 6 months after first	0.5 mL	IM

Check Your NCLEX–PN® Exam I.Q.

You are ready for testing on this content if you can

- Determine a client's or family's knowledge of immunization schedules.
- Review client's or family's immunization status.
- Administer correctly prescribed immunizations.
- Reinforce teaching with a client or family about prescribed immunizations.
- Identify contraindications to immunizations and other precautions.
- Respond appropriately when a client experiences side effects, adverse effects, or allergy to an immunization.

PRACTICE TEST

1 A newly adopted 8-year-old child is brought to the pediatric immunization clinic to begin the hepatitis B immunization series. Before providing the immunization, the nurse inquires about any known history of allergy to which item?

1. Aminoglycoside antibiotics
2. Mold
3. Baker's yeast
4. Egg yolks

2 A mother brings her infant to the immunization clinic for the final hepatitis B vaccine. After picking up the vial of vaccine to draw up the dose, the nurse notes that it is cloudy. What action should the nurse take?

1. Warm the vaccine under running water.
2. Discard the vaccine and contact the supplier of the vaccine.
3. Agitate the vial gently and draw up the vaccine.
4. Calculate the pediatric dosage, since it is intended for adult use.

3 A nurse preparing to draw up a dose of vaccine notices that a vial of DTaP vaccine on the countertop does not have a date recorded for when it was opened. What action should the nurse take?

1. Use the vaccine but explain to the caregiver that the site may be quite tender.
2. Discard the vaccine according to agency's policy.
3. Contact the supervisor because this is reportable to the state Board of Public Health.
4. Use the vaccine just for the day and then discard it.

4 A parent brings a 3-year-old child to the immunization clinic for a DTaP vaccine. During the interview, the mother indicates the child is just finishing a tapered dose of prednisone for a chronic respiratory problem. Which action should the nurse take at this time?

1. Delay the vaccine administration for 1 month after the medication is completed.
2. Provide the child with the vaccine as scheduled.
3. Cleanse the injection site with sterile saline instead of alcohol and administer the vaccine.
4. Keep the child in the clinic for 30 minutes after administration to assess the child's response.

5 A child is brought to the pediatric ambulatory clinic with a runny nose and a low-grade fever. He is scheduled to receive the MMR (measles, mumps, and rubella) and DTaP (diphtheria, pertussis, and tetanus toxoid) vaccines. What should the nurse do at this time?

1. Get special permission from the physician to administer the vaccine.
2. Defer both vaccines until the child is well.
3. Administer the vaccines as scheduled.
4. Administer the DTaP vaccine but defer the MMR.

6 A pediatric client is scheduled to receive a dose of MMR (measles, mumps, rubella) vaccine. The nurse would question the order to give the dose at this time if which data was obtained during a short intake questionnaire?

1. Recent upper respiratory infection
2. Weight loss of 3 pounds during the last month
3. History of allergy to neomycin or gelatin
4. Local reaction to previous dose

PRACTICE TEST

7 The mother of a child who has been exposed to chicken pox telephones the pediatric clinic for advice. What would the nurse inquire about before relaying the question to the RN managing the office?

1. The child's exposure and immune status
2. Whether the child has had a rubella vaccination
3. The age, height, and weight of the child
4. The relationship of the person to whom the child was exposed

8 A 9-year-old client is brought to the pediatrician's office for a varicella virus vaccine. Before preparing the dose of the vaccine, the nurse would determine the child's status regarding which item?

1. Recent blood product transfusion
2. Allergy to milk
3. Allergy to penicillin
4. History of splenectomy

9 A child stepped on a rusty nail and is brought to the emergency department. The child's electronic health record indicates the child has not been adequately immunized against tetanus according to the immunization schedule. What would the nurse expect to be ordered for this child?

1. Diphtheria, tetanus, and pertussis vaccine
2. Tetanus immune globulin
3. A broad-spectrum antibiotic
4. Tetanus toxoid

10 A 2-month-old client is seen in the pediatric clinic for a well-baby checkup. The nurse anticipates that which routine immunizations will be administered at this time? Select all that apply.

1. Inactivated poliovirus vaccine (IPV)
2. Diphtheria, tetanus, and acellular pertussis (DTaP)
3. Haemophilus influenza B conjugate vaccine (Hib)
4. Measles, mumps, and rubella vaccine (MMR)
5. Varicella zoster vaccine (Varivax)

11 A nurse is preparing to draw up a dose of Haemophilus influenzae type B (Hib) vaccine for a pediatric client. The nurse concludes that the vial is acceptable to use after noting which expected coloration of the fluid in the vial?

1. Pale yellow
2. Light pink
3. Clear
4. Slightly brown tinged

12 The pediatric clinic nurse has just administered a dose of Haemophilus influenzae type B (Hib) vaccine to a child. The nurse reinforces an explanation to the parents that they can expect which type of local reaction following the injection?

1. Mild to moderate fever
2. Pain or redness at site
3. Irritability
4. Decreased appetite

13 The nurse has an order to give an infant a dose of inactivated poliovirus vaccine (IPV). The nurse would take which action before administering the medication to ensure the dose is safe and effective?

1. Take dose that has not expired from a box on the shelf in the medication room.
2. Inquire prior to dose for allergy to neomycin, streptomycin, or polymixin B.
3. Gently agitate the cloudy white solution before drawing up.
4. Select a proper size muscle for injection.

14 The nurse is reinforcing information about immunization schedules to the mother of a newborn infant. The nurse explains that the first dose of inactivated poliovirus vaccine (IPV) is given at what age?

1. 1 week
2. 1 month
3. 2 months
4. 4 months

15 A pediatric client has received a dose of heptavalent pneumococcal conjugate vaccine (PCV). The nurse recognizes that the parents understand postvaccination instructions if they state that which symptom is most important to report promptly to the health care provider?

1. Mild fever
2. Drowsiness
3. Decreased appetite
4. Rash with hives

16. A child with cardiac disease is recommended to receive the yearly influenza vaccine. The nurse would schedule the child to receive the vaccine at the routine visit scheduled in which month?
    1. January
    2. April
    3. July
    4. October

17. A 6-year-old child with asplenia is receiving the meningococcal vaccine. The nurse reinforces teaching to the child's mother that the vaccine should be effective for how many years?
    1. 1
    2. 2
    3. 5
    4. 10

18. A nurse working in an immunization clinic ensures at the beginning of each workday that which priority medication is available and within the expiration date?
    1. Lidocaine hydrochloride (Xylocaine)
    2. Epinephrine (adrenalin)
    3. Acetaminophen (Tylenol)
    4. Ibuprofen (Motrin)

19. The pediatric nurse is seeing a 2-month-old infant in the outpatient clinic for routine immunizations. The nurse should select which immunization teaching sheets to give to the mother before preparing the immunizations appropriate for this visit? Select all that apply.
    1. Varicella
    2. Diphtheria, tetanus, and acellular pertussis (DTaP)
    3. Measles, mumps, and rubella (MMR)
    4. Haemophilus influenzae type b (Hib)
    5. Inactivated polio (IPV)

20. What information should the nurse reinforce with a mother whose child is receiving the immunizations required at 1 year of age? Select all that apply.
    1. "You can give your child acetaminophen (Tylenol) if he develops a mild fever."
    2. "We give all these immunizations at the same time because they are more effective if given together."
    3. "If your child develops a mild fever, you need to call the physician."
    4. "You can expect your child to not feel well for a couple of days."
    5. "Some children develop itching or a rash after immunizations are given. This can be treated at home with an antihistamine."

21. The mother of a 15-month-old child is anxious about the immunizations her child is about to receive. What information should the nurse provide to the parents about immunizations? Select all that apply.
    1. Possible localized reactions to injection sites
    2. Administration of acetaminophen as needed after vaccine administration
    3. Need to sign either an informed consent or refusal form
    4. Administration of aspirin every four hours postvaccine administration
    5. Symptoms of anaphylaxis reaction with immediate access to emergency care

PRACTICE TEST

ANSWERS & RATIONALES

ANSWERS & RATIONALES

1. **Answer: 3 Rationale:** A history of an allergic reaction to baker's yeast would be a contraindication to receiving this series of immunizations. Aminoglycoside antibiotics, mold, and egg yolks do not pose any risk to the client for allergy to the vaccine. **Cognitive Level:** Analyzing **Client Need:** Health Promotion and Maintenance **Integrated Process:** Nursing Process: Data Collection **Content Area:** Pharmacology **Strategy:** Specific knowledge of contraindications to hepatitis B vaccine is needed to answer this question. Use the process of elimination, and review this content area if needed.

2. **Answer: 3 Rationale:** It is normal for the solution in the vial to appear cloudy. The nurse should gently agitate the vaccine and then draw it up for administration. It is unnecessary to discard it or to notify the manufacturer. Warming the solution will not affect the cloudiness. **Cognitive Level:** Applying **Client Need:** Health Promotion and Maintenance **Integrated**

Process: Nursing Process: Implementation **Content Area:** Pharmacology **Strategy:** Specific knowledge of the nursing considerations for hepatitis B vaccine is needed to answer this question. Use the process of elimination, and review this content area if needed.

3 **Answer: 2 Rationale:** The vial should be discarded according to agency policy. Administering the vaccine does not protect the safety of the client, and it is unnecessary to report this particular incident to the state Board of Public Health. **Cognitive Level:** Applying **Client Need:** Health Promotion and Maintenance **Integrated Process:** Nursing Process: Implementation **Content Area:** Pharmacology **Strategy:** The core issue of this question is safe handling of vaccinations. Use principles of general medication preparation to make a selection.

4 **Answer: 1 Rationale:** The dose should be delayed for 1 month following any type of immunosuppressive therapy, such as prednisone. The other actions do not protect the client or uphold safe administration procedures for immunizations. **Cognitive Level:** Applying **Client Need:** Health Promotion and Maintenance **Integrated Process:** Nursing Process: Implementation **Content Area:** Pharmacology **Strategy:** Use the process of elimination. Recall that immunizations affect the immune system and that steroids such as prednisone suppress the immune system to make the correct selection.

5 **Answer: 3 Rationale:** The immunizations should be administered as scheduled. They would be withheld for clients who are immunosuppressed or have moderate to severe febrile illnesses. The presence of a runny nose and low-grade fever is not a contraindication according to the literature. **Cognitive Level:** Applying **Client Need:** Health Promotion and Maintenance **Integrated Process:** Nursing Process: Implementation **Content Area:** Pharmacology **Strategy:** The core issue of the question is contraindications to administering scheduled immunizations. Use the process of elimination, and take time to review these immunizations as needed.

6 **Answer: 3 Rationale:** A contraindication to MMR vaccine is a history of allergic reaction to neomycin or gelatin. Minor illnesses and history of local reaction to a previous dose are not contraindications. Weight loss is irrelevant to the question. **Cognitive Level:** Applying **Client Need:** Health Promotion and Maintenance **Integrated Process:** Nursing Process: Implementation **Content Area:** Pharmacology **Strategy:** The core issue of the question is knowledge of contraindications to MMR vaccine. Use the process of elimination, keeping in mind that both neomycin and gelatin are reasons to withhold the dose.

7 **Answer: 1 Rationale:** The nurse would inquire about the nature of the exposure and the client's immune status. Chicken pox can be fatal in immunocompromised children, such as those who are undergoing steroid therapy, chemotherapy, and those with other illnesses. If warranted, the varicella zoster immune globulin can be given up to 4 days after exposure to those with no history of chicken pox or prior exposure. Exposure to rubella (a different disease), height and weight of the child, and the person to whom the child was exposed are irrelevant as priority items in protecting the health of this child. **Cognitive Level:** Analyzing **Client Need:** Health Promotion and Maintenance **Integrated Process:** Nursing Process: Data Collection **Content Area:** Pharmacology **Strategy:** The core issue of the question is knowledge of indications for use of varicella zoster immune globulin. Use the process of elimination and general concepts of immunity to answer the question.

8 **Answer: 1 Rationale:** Contraindications to varicella virus vaccine include allergy to neomycin or gelatin, immunosuppression, or administration of immune serum globulin or blood products in the last 3 to 11 months. A history of spleen removal and allergies to penicillin or milk are irrelevant to safe use of this vaccine. **Cognitive Level:** Applying **Client Need:** Health Promotion and Maintenance **Integrated Process:** Nursing Process: Data Collection **Content Area:** Pharmacology **Strategy:** The core issue of the question is knowledge of contraindications for use of varicella vaccine. Use the process of elimination and general concepts of immunity to make a selection.

9 **Answer: 2 Rationale:** When there is accidental exposure and inadequate vaccination, passive immunity with tetanus immune globulin is indicated for immediate protection from the bacterial spores in the nail. DTaP and tetanus toxoid provide active immunity and a broad-spectrum antibiotic is inadequate. **Cognitive Level:** Applying **Client Need:** Health Promotion and Maintenance **Integrated Process:** Nursing Process: Planning **Content Area:** Pharmacology **Strategy:** The core issue of the question is the ability to discriminate situations requiring active immunity and those requiring passive immunity. Use the process of elimination, and take time to review this information if needed.

10 **Answer: 1, 2, 3 Rationale:** The IPV, DTaP, Hib, and PCV vaccines are all scheduled to be given at 2 months of age. The MMR is given at 12 to 15 months, and again at 4 to 6 years. The varicella zoster vaccine is given at 12 to 18 months. **Cognitive Level:** Applying **Client Need:** Health Promotion and Maintenance **Integrated Process:** Nursing Process: Planning **Content Area:** Pharmacology **Strategy:** The core issue of the question is knowledge of routine immunization schedules for a 2-month-old infant. Use general knowledge of immunization schedules and the process of elimination to make your selections.

11 **Answer: 3 Rationale:** The solution used for Hib vaccine is clear and colorless. MMR and varicella vaccines are a clear yellow in color. No vaccines are pale pink or brown, although some are cloudy. **Cognitive Level:** Applying **Client Need:** Health Promotion and Maintenance **Integrated Process:** Nursing Process: Implementation **Content Area:** Pharmacology **Strategy:** The core issue of this question is the ability to determine safe appearance of vaccines before administration. Use nursing knowledge and the process of elimination to make a selection.

12 **Answer: 2 Rationale:** The parents should be taught to expect pain and redness at the site as possible local reactions to the Hib vaccine. Fever, irritability, and decreased appetite are common side effects of the heptavalent pneumococcal conjugate vaccine (PCV). **Cognitive Level:** Applying **Client Need:** Health Promotion and Maintenance **Integrated Process:** Teaching and Learning **Content Area:** Pharmacology **Strategy:** Use the process of elimination. One strategy to determine local reaction is to evaluate the options in terms of how confined they are to the site of injection. The incorrect responses are systemic in nature.

13 **Answer: 2 Rationale:** Before administering a dose of IPV, the nurse should check for allergy to neomycin, streptomycin, or polymixin B. The solution should be kept in the refrigerator and should be clear and colorless. The dose is administered by the subcutaneous route. **Cognitive Level:** Applying **Client Need:** Health Promotion and Maintenance **Integrated**

Process: Nursing Process: Implementation **Content Area:** Pharmacology **Strategy:** The core issue of this question is the ability to administer IPV safely. Use nursing knowledge and the process of elimination to make a selection.

14 **Answer: 3 Rationale:** The first dose of IPV is given at 2 months, with subsequent doses at 4 months, 12 to 18 months, and 4 to 6 years, for a total of four doses. The other timeframes do not match the time of the initial dose in the administration schedule for this vaccine. **Cognitive Level:** Applying **Client Need:** Health Promotion and Maintenance **Integrated Process:** Nursing Process: Implementation **Content Area:** Pharmacology **Strategy:** The core issue of this question is the ability to administer IPV safely according to its recommended schedule. Use nursing knowledge and the process of elimination to make a selection.

15 **Answer: 4 Rationale:** Although mild to moderate fever, drowsiness, and decreased appetite are some of the side effects of PCV, the most important one to report to the health care provider is rash with hives. This likely indicates an allergic reaction, which could progress to anaphylaxis if left untreated. **Cognitive Level:** Analyzing **Client Need:** Health Promotion and Maintenance **Integrated Process:** Nursing Process: Evaluation **Content Area:** Pharmacology **Strategy:** The core issue of this question is the highest priority teaching regarding PCV. The critical words in the question are *most important* and *promptly*, which tells you that one is more serious than the others. Use nursing knowledge, the ABCs, and the process of elimination to make a selection.

16 **Answer: 4 Rationale:** The influenza vaccine is administered annually in the autumn, especially during October, November, and into December. The other months do not correlate with administration times that would prevent development of influenza during the winter months. **Cognitive Level:** Applying **Client Need:** Health Promotion and Maintenance **Integrated Process:** Nursing Process: Planning **Content Area:** Pharmacology **Strategy:** The core issue of the question is the timing of the annual dosage of influenza vaccine. Use knowledge of the epidemiology of the disease to choose the month prior to when flu season occurs.

17 **Answer: 3 Rationale:** Meningococcal vaccine is indicated for children older than 2 years with asplenia. The vaccine duration is 5 years if the client is older than 4 years at the time of immunization. If the client is younger than 4 at the time of initial immunization, it should be repeated after 1 year. **Cognitive Level:** Applying **Client Need:** Health Promotion and Maintenance **Integrated Process:** Teaching and Learning **Content Area:** Pharmacology **Strategy:** Specific knowledge related to the meningococcal vaccine is needed to answer the question. Take time to review this material if needed, and use the process of elimination in making a selection.

18 **Answer: 2 Rationale:** Epinephrine is the priority medication to have on hand if a client should experience hypersensitivity reaction/anaphylaxis following a dose of an immunization. Lidocaine is given for cardiac dysrhythmias, while acetaminophen and ibuprofen are peripheral CNS analgesics. **Cognitive Level:** Analyzing **Client Need:** Health Promotion and Maintenance **Integrated Process:** Nursing Process: Planning **Content Area:** Pharmacology **Strategy:** The core issue of the question is knowledge that anaphylaxis is a potentially life-threatening consequence of immunization. Use the process of elimination, choosing the answer that is an emergency drug associated with reducing allergic response.

19 **Answer: 2, 4, 5 Rationale:** Diphtheria, tetanus, and acellular pertussis (DTaP), Haemophilus influenzae type b (Hib), inactivated polio vaccine (IPV), and the pneumococcal conjugate vaccine (PCV) are the routine immunizations scheduled for the 2-month well-child visit. The MMR is given first at 12 to 15 months, and the varicella can be given at or anytime after 12 months. **Cognitive Level:** Analyzing **Client Need:** Health Promotion and Maintenance **Integrated Process:** Nursing Process: Implementation **Content Area:** Pharmacology **Strategy:** The core issue of the question is knowledge of vaccinations that are due at a 2-month well-child visit. Use the process of elimination, recalling that MMR and varicella cannot be given before 12 months of age.

20 **Answer: 1, 4 Rationale:** A mild fever can be treated safely and effectively with acetaminophen (Tylenol). Sometimes children act as if they do not feel well because of mild discomfort after receiving immunizations. The immunizations are not given together. The physician does not need to be called unless the fever is high. Itching or rash is of concern because each could indicate hypersensitivity, and needs to be addressed rather than treated at home. **Cognitive Level:** Analyzing **Client Need:** Health Promotion and Maintenance **Integrated Process:** Communication and Documentation **Content Area:** Child Health **Strategy:** Differentiate between mild and severe adverse reactions to immunizations, and use the process of elimination to make the correct selections.

21 **Answer: 1, 2, 3, 5 Rationale:** The nurse should provide the current Vaccine Information Statement (VIS) to parents for each vaccine the child will receive, as required by the National Vaccine Injury Act of 1986 and 1993. The sheet will include information about the specific vaccine, side effects, how to manage them, and when to seek further care (such as with allergic reaction or anaphylaxis). A parent needs to sign to give informed consent for vaccines or a refusal form to document why they were not administered. Aspirin is contraindicated due to the risk of Reye's syndrome but acetaminophen (Tylenol) is acceptable for use as needed for discomfort. **Cognitive Level:** Applying **Client Need:** Safety and Infection Control **Integrated Process:** Nursing Process: Implementation **Content Area:** Child Health **Strategy:** Recall general information about immunizations, and use this information to recognize the common teaching points. Recall also that aspirin is contraindicated in children to prevent the risk of Reye's syndrome to eliminate this as a possible answer choice.

ANSWERS & RATIONALES

Key Terms to Review

active immunity p. 161
attenuate p. 161
inactivated vaccine p. 167
killed vaccine p. 167
live, attenuated vaccine p. 169
passive immunity p. 161
toxoid p. 170
vaccine p. 161

References

American Academy of Family Physicians. http://www.aafp.org

American Academy of Pediatrics. http://www.aap.org

Centers for Disease Control and Prevention (2011). *Recommended immunization schedule for persons aged 0 through 6 years—United States · 2011*. Retrieved July 2, 2011, from http://www.cdc.gov/vaccines/recs/schedules/downloads/child/0-6yrs-schedule-bw.pdf

Centers for Disease Control and Prevention (2011). *Recommended immunization schedule for persons aged 7 through 18 years—United States · 2011*. Retrieved July 2, 2011, from http://www.cdc.gov/vaccines/recs/schedules/downloads/child/7-18yrs-schedule-bw.pdf

Centers for Disease Control and Prevention (2011). *Catch-up immunization schedule for persons aged 4 months through 18 years who start late or who are more than 1 month behind—United States · 2011*. Retrieved July 2, 2011, from http://www.cdc.gov/vaccines/recs/schedules/downloads/child/catchup-schedule-bw.pdf

Centers for Disease Control and Prevention (2011). *Recommended adult immunization schedule—United States · 2011*. Retrieved July 2, 2011, from http://www.cdc.gov/vaccines/recs/schedules/downloads/adult/adult-schedule-bw.pdf

Centers for Disease Control and Prevention (n.d.). *Rotavirus vaccination*. Retrieved June 22, 2010, from http://www.cdc.gov/vaccines/vpd-vac/rotavirus/default.htm

Davidson, M., London, M., & Ladewig, P. (2012). *Olds' maternal newborn nursing and women's health across the lifespan* (9th ed.). Upper Saddle River, NJ: Pearson Education, Inc.

Ladewig, P., London, M., & Davidson, M. (2010). *Contemporary maternal-newborn nursing care* (7th ed.). Upper Saddle River, NJ: Pearson Education, Inc.

London, M., Ladewig, P., Ball, J., Bindler, R., & Cowen, K. (2011). *Maternal & child nursing care* (3rd ed.). Upper Saddle River, NJ: Pearson Education, Inc.

Perry, S., Hockenberry, M., Lowdermilk, D., & Wilson, D. (2010). *Maternal child nursing care* (4th ed.). St. Louis, MO: Elsevier.

Ward, S., & Hisley, S. (2009). *Maternal-child nursing care: Optimizing outcomes for mothers, children, and families*. Philadelphia, PA: F.A. Davis.

Test Yourself

Are you ready for the NCLEX-PN® or course exams? Use the practice tests on the companion website to check.

Credits

CREDITS AND COPYRIGHTS

The Authors and Publisher wish to thank the libraries, museums, galleries, and private collections for permitting the reproduction of works of art in their collections. Sources not included in the captions are gratefully acknowledged below. In addition, the Editors are grateful to the following correspondents: Barbara Nagelsmith, Paris; Elizabeth Meryman, New York; Achim Bednorz, Cologne; Carla Bertini, Rome; Angela Anderson, London; Kostas Kontos, Athens.

INTRODUCTION

I.1 The Newark Museum/Art Resource, NY; **I.2** V & A Images/Victoria & Albert Museum; **I.3** Digital Image © The Museum of Modern Art/Licensed by Scala/Art Resource, NY; **I.4** © Scala/Art Resource, NY; **I.5** Araldo De Luca/INDEX, Firenze; **I.6** © 2004 Board of Trustees, National Gallery of Art, Washington; **I.8** Peter Clayton; **I.9** Photograph © The Art Institute of Chicago; **I.10** AP Photo/Diane Bondareff; **I.11** Photograph by Lorene Emerson/Image © The Board of Trustees, National Gallery of Art, Washington; **I.12** Philippe Berthe © CMN, Paris; **I.13** © Scala/Art Resource, NY; **I.14** Photograph by Lynn Rosenthal, 1998; **I.15** Nimatallah/Art Resource, NY; **I.16** © John Bigelow Taylor/Art Resource, NY; **I.17** Courtesy Fraenkel Gallery, San Francisco; **I.18** Ikona

CHAPTER 1

1.1 Jean Vertut; **1.2** French Ministry of Culture and Communication, Regional Direction for Cultural Affairs-Rhone Alpes, Regional Department of Archaeology; **1.3** French Ministry of Culture and Communication, Regional Direction for Cultural Affairs-Rhone Alpes, Regional Department of Archaeology; **1.4** French Ministry of Culture and Communication, Regional Direction for Cultural Affairs-Rhone Alpes, Regional Department of Archaeology; **1.5** Jean Vertut; **1.6** Jean Vertut; **1.8** Jean Vertut; **1.9** Association Louis Begouen; **1.10** Philippe Berthe © CMN, Paris; **1.11** Thomas Stephan, copyright Ulmer Museum; **1.13** Photo by Max Begouen; **1.14** Jean Vertut; **1.15** © Reunion des Musees Nationaux/Art Resource, NY; **1.16** © Erich Lessing/Art Resource, NY; **1.17** © Erich Lessing/Art Resource, NY; **1.18** Folco Quilici; **1.19** R. Sheridan/Ancient Art & Architecture; **1.20** Cornucopia/Susanna Hickling; **1.22** Courtesy McDonald Institute for Achaeological Research; **1.23** © Erich Lessing/Art Resource, NY; **1.24** Yann Arthus-Bertrand/Altitude/Photo Researchers, Inc.; **1.25** Aerofilms Ltd., UK; **1. Unnumbered figure D,** Baffier - V. Feruglio/DRAC Rhone-Alpes

CHAPTER 2

2.1 © The Trustees of The British Museum; **2.3** Henri Frankfort, The Art and Architecture of the Ancient Orient, Yale University Press (1997), fig. 3.2; **2.5** Hirmer Fotoarchiv; **2.8** © The Trustees of The British Museum; **2.10** University of Pennsylvania Museum, Philadelphia (T4-29C); **2.11** Bildarchiv Preuussischer Kulturbesitz/Art Resource, NY; **2.12** © Erich Lessing/Art Resource, NY; **2.13** © Reunion des Musees Nationaux/Art Resource, NY; **2.14** The Ancient Art & Architecture Collection Ltd.; **2.15** Photograph © 2006, Museum of Fine Arts, Boston; **2.16** © Reunion des Musees Nationaux/Art Resource, NY; **2.17** Photo by Herve Lewandowski/Reunion des Musees Nationaux/Art Resource, NY; **2.18** Courtesy of the Oriental Institute Museum, The University of Chicago and Continuum International Publishing Group; **2.20** © The Trustees of the British Museum; **2.21** © The Trustees of the British Museum; **2.22** Bildarchiv Preussischer Kulturbesitz/Art Resource, NY; **2.23** The Art Archive/Dagli Orti; **2.24** © The Trustees of the British Museum; **2.25** Reunion des Musees Nationaux/Art Resource, NY; **2.27** © Scala/Art Resource, NY; **2.28** © Gerard Degeorge/Corbis; **2.29** © Erich Lessing/Art Resource, NY; **2.30** Ancient Art & Architecture Collection Ltd.; **2.31** © Corbis; **2.32** © Robert Harding World Imagery/Getty; **2.33** Photograph © 1995 The Metropolitan Museum of Art; **2. Unnumbered figure A,** John M. Russell; **2. Unnumbered figure B,** Penelope Davies; **2. Unnumbered figure C,** Penelope Davies

CHAPTER 3

3.1 Werner Forman/Art Resource, NY; **3.3** © The Image Works; **3.4** © Copyright the Trustees of The British Museum; **3.7** Free Agents Limited/Corbis; **3.9** Photo by Carl Andrews/© President and Fellows of Harvard College for the Semitic Museum; **3.10** Peter Clayton; **3.11** Araldo De Luca/INDEX, Firenze; **3.12** Photograph © 2004 Museum of Fine Arts, Boston; **3.13** Akg-images/Werner Forman; **3.14** © Andrea Jomolo/Ikona; **3.15** © Reunion des Musees Nationaux/Art Resource, NY; **3.16** The Art Archive/Egyptian Museum Cairo/Dagli Orti; **3.17** Jean Vertut; **3.18** Photograph © 1979 The Metropolitan Museum of Art; **3.19** Photograph © 2006, Museum of Fine Arts, Boston; **3.20** Jean Vertut; **3.21** © Graham Harrison; **3.22** Peter A. Clayton; **3.23** © The Trustees of The British Museum; **3.24** Robert Frerck/Woodfin Camp & Associates; **3.26** Photograph © 1986 The Metropolitan Museum of Art; **3.28** The Art Archive/Dagli Orti; **3.29** The Art Archive/Dagli Orti; **3.30** © G. Dagli Orti; **3.31** © Herve Champollion/Akg-images; **3.32** Bildarchiv Preussischer Kulturbesitz/Art Resource, NY; **3.33** © The Trustees of The British Museum; **3.34** Scala/Art Resource, NY; **3.35** © Araldo De Luca/Ikona; **3.36** Bildarchiv Preussischer Kulturbesitz/Art Resource, NY; **3.37** Bildarchiv Preussischer Kulturbesitz/Art Resource, NY; **3.38** Bildarchiv Preussischer Kulturbesitz/Art Resource, NY; **3.39** Boltin Picture Library/Bridgeman Art Library; **3.40** © The Trustees of The British Museum; **3. Unnumbered figure A,** Photo by D. Wildung; **3. Unnumbered figure B,** From Arnold Dieter, *Building in Egypt*, Oxford University Press, 1991, fig. 4.88; **3. Unnumbered figure C,** From Arnold Dieter, *Building in Egypt*, Oxford University Press, 1991, fig. 4.88

CHAPTER 4

4.1 © Studio Kontos/Photostock; **4.2** John Bigelow Taylor; **4.3** John Bigelow Taylor/Art Resource, NY; **4.4** From John Griffiths Pedley, *Greek Art and Archaeology*, 2/e, Prentice Hall, 1998, fig. 3.1, p. 65; **4.5** Courtesy McRae Books, Florence; **4.6** © Roger Wood/Corbis; **4.7** From Donald Preziosi and Louise A. Hitchcock, *Aegean Art and Architecture*, Oxford University Press, Oxford, 1999, fig. 54, p. 96; **4.8** © Studio Kontos/Photostock; **4.9** © Studio Kontos/Photostock; **4.10** Nimatallah/Art Resource, NY; **4.11** © Studio Kontos/Photostock; **4.12** © Scala/Art Resource, NY; **4.13** Nimatallah/Art Resource, NY; **4.14** © Studio Kontos/Photostock; **4.15** © Erich Lessing/Art Resource, NY; **4.16** Nimatallah/Art Resource, NY; **4.17** © Studio Kontos/Photostock; **4.18** © Studio Kontos/Photostock; **4.19** From John Griffiths Pedley, *Greek Art and Archaeology*, 2/e, Prentice Hall, 1998, fig. 3.40, p. 95; **4.20** Spectrum Colour Library, London; **4.21** Dartmouth Publishing; **4.22** © Studio Kontos/Photostock; **4.23** © Studio Kontos/Photostock; **4.24** © Vanni Archive/Corbis; **4.25** From John Griffiths Pedley, *Greek Art and Archaeology*, 2/e, Prentice Hall, 1998, Produced by Calmann and King Ltd., London, fig. 3.39, p. 93; **4.26** The Art Archive/Dagli Orti; **4.27** Hirmer Verlag, Munich; **4.28** © Studio Kontos/Photostock; **4. Unnumbered figure,** From Michael Kuepper, *Mykenische Archtiektur: Material Bearbeitungstechnik, Konstruktion und Erscheinungsbild* (1996), abb. 164 (Tiryns)

CHAPTER 5

5.2 Nimatallah/Art Resource, NY; **5.4** Photograph © 1996 The Metropolitan Museum of Art; **5.5** Photograph © 2006, Museum of Fine Arts, Boston; **5.6** Deutsches Archaeologisches Institut, Athens; **5.7** © The Trustees of The British Museum; **5.10** Marco Cristofori/Corbis; **5.11** John Heseltine/Corbis; **5.13** © The Trustees of The British Museum; **5.14** © Reunion des Musees Nationaux/Art Resource, NY; **5.15** Photograph © The Metropolitan Museum of Art; **5.16** Scala/Art Resource, NY; **5.17** © Studio Kontos/Photostock; **5.18** The Art Archive/Acropolis Museum Athens/Dagli Orti; **5.19** The Art Archive/Archaeological Museum Corfu/Dagli Orti; **5.22** © Studio Kontos/Photostock; **5.24** Staatliche Antikensammlungen und Glyptothek Munchen; **5.25** Staatliche Antikensammlungen und Glyptothek Munchen; **5.26** © Vatican Museums; **5.27** Staatliche Antikensammlungen und Glyptothek Munchen; **5.28** Giraudon/Art Resource, NY; **5.29** Nimatallah/Art Resource, NY; **5.30** © Pubbliphoto/Ikona; **5.32** Foto Vasari/INDEX, Firenze; **5.33** The Art Archive/Archeological Museum Naples/Dagli Orti; **5.34** Museo Nazionale, Reggio Italy/HIRMER; **5.35** © Studio Kontos/Photostock; **5.36** © Studio Kontos/Photostock; **5.37** © Studio Kontos/Photostock; **5.39** © Studio Kontos/Photostock; **5.42** © The Trustees of The British Museum; **5.43** © The Trustees of The British Museum; **5.44** © The Trustees of The British Museum; **5.45** © SEF/Art Resource, NY; **5.46** © Studio Kontos/Photostock; **5.47** © The Trustees of The British Museum; **5.48** © The Trustees of The British Museum; **5.49** © Studio Kontos/Photostock; **5.50** Nimatallah/Art Resource, NY; **5.51** © Studio Kontos/Photostock; **5.52** © Studio Kontos/Photostock; **5.53** Michael Holford Photography; **5.54** Ruggero Vanni/CORBIS; **5.56** From Howard Colvin, *Architecture and the After Life*, Yale University Press, 1991, fig. 31, p. 35; **5.57** From Howard Colvin, *Architecture and the After Life*, Yale University Press, 1991, fig. 31, p. 35; **5.58** © Studio Kontos/Photostock; **5.59** Hirmer Fotoarchiv; **5.60** © Vatican Museums; **5.61** © Studio Kontos/Photostock; **5.62** © Scala/Art Resource, NY; **5.63** © Reunion des Musees Nationaux/Art Resource, NY; **5.64** © Scala/Art Resource, NY; **5.65** From Jerome Pollitt, *Art in the Hellenistic Age,* Cambridge University Press, 1986, fig. 31, p. 35; **5.66** © Georg Gerster/Rapho; **5.67** From Jerome Pollitt, *Art in the Hellenistic Age*, Cambridge University Press, 1986, fig. 31, p. 35; **5.68** Bildarchiv Preussischer Kulturbesitz/Art Resource, NY; **5.69** From Renee Dreyfus and Ellen Schraudolph, *Pergamon: The Telephos Frieze from the Great Altar*, Volume 2, fig. 12, p. 36; **5.70** Erich Lessing/Art Resource, NY; **5.72** © Araldo De Luca/Ikona; **5.73** Bildarchiv Preussischer Kulturbesitz/Art Resource; **5.74** Bildarchiv Preussischer Kulturbesitz/Art Resource, NY; **5.75** © Reunion des Musees Nationaux/Art Resource, NY; **5.76** Nimatallah/Art Resource, NY; **5.77** Staatliche Antikensammlungen und Glyptothek Munchen; **5.78** © Studio Kontos/Photostock; **5.79** © Scala/Art Resource, NY; **5. Unnumbered figure A,** © Scala/Art Resource, NY; **5. Unnumbered figure B,** © Scala/Art Resource, NY

CHAPTER 6

6.1 © Vatican Museums; **6.2** Pubbli Aer Foto; **6.3** From Larissa Bonfante, ed., *Etruscan Life and the Afterlife: A Handbook of Etruscan Studies,* Wayne State University Press, fig. V-5, p. 177; **6.4** © Scala/Art Resource, NY; **6.5** © Soprintendenza Etruria Meridionale/Ikona; **6.6** © Scala/Art Resource, NY; **6.7** © Scala/Art Resource, NY; **6.8** Canali Photobank; **6.10** © Scala/Art Resource, NY; **6.11** © Orsi Battaglini/Ikona; **6.12** Photograph © 2006, Museum of Fine Arts, Boston; **6.13** Scala/Art Resource, NY; **6.14** From Larissa Bonfante, ed., *Etruscan Life and the Afterlife: A Handbook of Etruscan Studies*, Wayne State University Press, fig. V-33, p. 192; **6.15** Penelope Davies; **6.16** Canali Photobank; **6.17** © Erich Lessing/Art Resource, NY; **6.18** © Orsi Battaglini/Ikona; **6.19** Canali Photobank; **6.20** Canali Photobank; **6. Unnumbered figure,** © Reunion des Musees Nationaux/Art Resource, NY

CHAPTER 7

7.1 Anna Mura Sommella, from "La Grande Roma dei Tarquini," Alterne vicende di una felice intuizione." Bullcom (2000), fig. 7-26, p. 25; **7.2** Canali Photobank; **7.4** Reprinted from Frank Sear, *Roman Architecture*, Cornell University Press, © 1982 by Frank Sear, diagram 40, p. 74; **7.5** From Amanda Claridge, *An Archaeological Guide*, Oxford University Press, 1988, fig. 188, p. 389; **7.6** © Vanni/Art Resource, NY; **7.8** James Packer; **7.9** Foto Marburg/Art Resource, NY (top image) and Reunion des Musees Nationaux/Art Resource, NY (bottom image); **7.10** Araldo de Luca/Corbis; **7.11** Penelope Davies; **7.13** © Scala/Art Resource, NY; **7.14** Photograph © 2006, Museum of Fine Arts, Boston; **7.15** Canali Photobank; **7.16** Superstock; **7.18** © Soprintendenza di Roma/Ikona; **7.19** © Soprintendenza di Roma/Ikona; **7.21** Canali Photobank; **7.22** © Araldo de Luca/Corbis; **7.23** Canali Photobank; **7.24** Canali Photobank; **7.25** Canali Photobank; **7.26** Werner Forman/Art Resource, NY; **7.27** © Scala/Art Resource, NY; **7.28** Robert Frerck/Woodfin Camp & Associates; **7.29** © Scala/Art Resource, NY; **7.30** © Musei Vatico, M. Sarri; **7.31** Penelope Davies; **7.32** Photograph by Elke Estel; **7.34** © DAI, Roma/Ikona; **7.35** Gilbert Gorski, illustrator; **7.36** © Pubbli Aer Foto; **7.37** From Frank Sear, *Roman Architecture*, Cornell University Press, © 1982 by Frank Sear, diagram 78, p. 136; **7.38** Canali Photobank; **7.39** Canali Photobank; **7.40** From William L. McDonald, *Architecture of the Roman Empire, An Introductory Study*, Volume 1, Yale University Press, p. 96; **7.41** Hermera Technologies/Alamy; **7.44** © Scala/Art Resource; **7.45** Oronoz; **7.46** © Archivo Iconografico, S.A./Corbis; **7.47** Penelope Davies; **7.48** © Reunion des Musees Nationaux/Art Resource, NY; **7.49** © Trustees of the National Museum of Scotland; **7.50** Henri Stierlin/Bildarchiv Steffens; **7.51** From Mary Beard and John Henderson, *Classical Art: From Greece to Rome*, Oxford History of Art, Oxford University Press, 2001, p. 39; **7.52** © Soprintendenza Archeologica di Pompei/Ikona; **7.53** Canali Photobank; **7.54a** Photograph © 1986 The Metropolitan Museum of Art; **7.54b** Photograph © 1986 The Metropolitan Museum of Art; **7.55** Canali Photobank; **7.56** Photograph © 1987 The Metropolitan Museum of Art; **7.57** Canali Photobank; **7.58** Canali Photobank; **7.59** © Vatican Museums; **7.60** Alinari/Art Resource, NY; **7.61** Canali Photobank; **7.62** Canali Photobank; **7.63** © Araldo De Luca Archives, Rome; **7.64** From Jas Elsner, *Imperial Rome and Christian Triumph: The Art of the Roman Empire AD 100-400*, Oxford University Press, 1998, fig. 126, p. 188; **7.65** © Foto Vasari, Roma; **7.66** © Alinari Archives/Corbis; **7.68** Scala/Art Resource, NY; **7.70** © Peter M. Wilson/Corbis; **7.71** Akg-images; **7.72** © Foto Vasari, Roma; **7.73** From Jas Elsner, *Imperial Rome and Christian Triumph: The Art of the Roman Empire AD 100-400,* Oxford University Press, 1998, fig. 90, p. 131; **7.74** © Achim Bednorz, Koln; **7. Unnumbered figure A,** From Peter Rockwell, *The Art of Stoneworking*, Cambridge University Press, 1993, diagram 43; **7. Unnumbered figure B,** Photo by M. Sarri/Archivio Musei Vaticani

TEXT CREDITS

Page 25 Excerpts from *The Epic of Gilgamesh*, tr. by Maureen Gallery Kovacs with an introduction and notes. Copyright © 1985, 1989 by the Board of Trustees of the Leland Stanford Junior University. All rights reserved. Used with the permission of Stanford University Press, www.sup.org. **Page 32** From *The Art and Architecture of the Ancient Orient*, 4th ed. (1970) by Henri Frankfort is reprinted by permission of Yale University Press. Copyright © 1954, 1958, 1963, 1970 by Enriqueta Frankfort. **Page 56** "The Resurrection of King Unis" from *Ancient Egyptian Literature: An Anthology,* tr. by John L. Foster, copyright © 2001. By permission of the University of Texas Press. **Page 70** "Love Song" from *Love Songs of the New Kingdom*, tr. from the Ancient Egyptian by John L. Foster. Copyright © 1969, 1970, 1971, 1972, 1973, 1974 by John L. Foster. By permission of the University of Texas Press. **Page 127** From *The Politics*, Book VIII, by Aristotle, ed. by Stephen Everson (NY: Cambridge Univ. Press, 1988). Reprinted with the permission of Cambridge Univ. Press. **Page 198** From "The Jewish War" by Josephus from *The Art of Rome 753 BC to AD 337* by J.J. Pollitt. (NY: Cambridge Univ. Press, 1983). Reprinted with the permission of Cambridge Univ. Press. **Page 212** *Vitruvius.* From *Ten Books on Architecture*, tr. by Ingrid D. Rowland; commentary by Thomas Noble Howe (NY: Cambridge Univ. Press, 1999). Reprinted with the permission of Cambridge Univ. Press. **Page 230** From "A Hymn to Aten" from *The Ancient Near East* by Amelie Kuhrt Vol. 1 (London: Routledge, 1995). Used by permission of Taylor and Francis Group. **Page 231** From *The Aeneid of Virgil*, tr. Allen Mandelbaum, copyright © 1971 by Allen Mandelbaum. Used by permission of Bantam Books, a divison of Random House, Inc. **Page 232** *Vitruvius.* From *Ten Books on Architecture*, tr. by Ingrid D. Rowland; commentary by Thomas Noble Howe (NY: Cambridge Univ. Press, 1999). Reprinted with the permission of Cambridge Univ. Press.

Data Collection 15

In this chapter

Cross Reference

Another chapter relevant to this content area is
Lifespan Growth and Development Chapter 13

I. HEALTH HISTORY OF ADULT

A. Overview

1. A **health history** is a collection of data about client's present and past health status; using communication skills and interviewing techniques, it gathers **subjective data** while allowing opportunity to develop a therapeutic relationship with client
2. Sources of data
   a. Primary: client, who is best source of data unless confused, too young, or too ill to participate in interview
   b. Secondary: family members, caregivers, support people; old medical or other health records; and results of laboratory and diagnostic tests
3. Principles of history taking
   a. Provide privacy and maintain confidentiality
   b. If client is tired or ill, ask most critical questions first
   c. Immediately document data in chart; do not keep data on loose pieces of paper
   d. Plan an appropriate timeframe: may require up to 1 hour or longer; allot enough time to take health history to avoid missing pertinent data; pace interview so as not to overtire client
   e. Gain trust: approach client and family in a professional manner; explain rationale for interview; tell client to immediately report if he or she becomes ill during interview; use therapeutic communication skills
   NCLEX® f. Note nonverbal cues about client's demeanor, posture, and overall appearance: physical indicators include cleanliness, body odor, personal grooming, hygiene, client's eye contact; signs of physical discomfort include diaphoresis, tremors, grimaces, and continual changes in position; signs of client stress include tears, skin blotching, nervous movements, inability to concentrate, arms folded, diaphoresis; if client wants to end interview, respect this request
   g. Determine client's reliability: can use proper terminology or words that indicate an understanding of health status; offers pertinent information about health status; does not change data reported; refers to previous ailments and treatment associated with illness; is oriented to person, place, time, and event; family members present concur that data is accurate

h. Use an interpreter if there is a language barrier
i. Conduct interview in a logical, orderly manner; focus discussion by asking open-ended questions first regarding most important issues, then pertinent follow-up questions; use closed-ended questions (yielding yes-no responses) to clarify previous statements or to ask for specific additional information; clarify any discrepancies

B. Health history components

1. Format used may vary slightly depending on age of client and associated developmental considerations and reason for visit (routine care or an acute problem)
2. Biographical data includes name, address, telephone number, gender, marital status, religion, occupation, health insurance information, and possibly name and contact information for primary care physician and/or nurse practitioner
3. Chief complaint (current problem or reason for which client is seeking care)

NCLEX®

4. Symptom analysis, getting data about each of the following:
   a. Location: be as specific as possible regarding part(s) of body involved
   b. Quantity: sometimes referred to as *severity* or *intensity*; whenever possible, use a numerical rating scale (0 to 10) or some type of visual analog scale; examples of symptoms frequently assessed this way are pain and dyspnea
   c. Quality: description of symptoms using various adjectives such as *burning*, *stabbing*, *pressure*; some disorders tend to be described in similar ways by clients, which can aid in diagnosing problem
   d. Setting: location of client when symptom(s) began and a description of events going on at that time
   e. Timing or chronology: notation of when symptom first began; slow onset versus sudden; constant versus intermittent; whether symptom disturbs sleep
   f. Aggravating or alleviating factors: practices that make symptom worse or better (such as eating, resting, use of medication, among others)
   g. Associated factors: other symptoms that accompany primary symptom (such as diaphoresis or shortness of breath with chest pain)
5. Previous state of health and physical capabilities and how current symptoms have impacted physical, emotional, and psychosocial functioning

NCLEX®

6. History of present illness (useful if problem has occurred more than once)
   a. When symptoms originally started
   b. How frequently exacerbations occur and whether onset is gradual or sudden
   c. Medications and/or other therapies used to treat problem and their degree of success (or lack of success)
7. Past health history: sometimes called *past history* or *medical history*; includes the following:
   a. Other possible health problems; some agencies use a checklist to obtain this information; focused (more detailed) assessment can be done on areas that are still currently problematic; clients commonly seek treatment for one health problem while having an active history of others (called comorbidities) that require ongoing management

NCLEX®

   b. Childhood and adult immunizations and date of last tetanus prophylaxis; may also include influenzae vaccines
   c. Childhood illnesses such as measles, mumps, rubella (German measles), rubeola, chickenpox, rheumatic fever, scarlet fever, streptococcal infections, or other major illnesses
   d. Prior hospitalizations, including dates, reasons (includes accidents, injuries, and illnesses), surgical procedures, outcomes, and any complications experienced (such as reactions to anesthesia or blood products)

NCLEX®

   e. Allergies: medication (reaction and symptoms, includes prescription, over-the-counter, and herbal products), food, seasonal (and their treatment), allergy to dyes used in diagnostic procedures (often assessed by asking about allergy to iodine or shellfish)
   f. Pregnancy history and menstrual history as appropriate for female clients

NCLEX®

   g. Current medications: prescribed dose, rationale, and duration of drug therapy; date and time of last dose; over-the-counter medications; herbal remedies; home remedies; complementary or adjunctive health care (if so, have client explain remedies used and effects)
8. Family health history
   a. Identification of overall state of health of parents and relatives: any significant and chronic illnesses, cause of death, and age at time of death
   b. Family health history can highlight genetically transmitted traits or disorders; ethnic background also plays a role in risk of developing certain disorders

c. Establish any history of hereditary disorders such as coronary heart disease, diabetes mellitus, stroke, high blood pressure, cancer, obesity, arthritis, bleeding disorders, or mental health disorders

NCLEX® d. Helps to focus appropriate efforts on disease prevention and health promotion to lessen client's risk in an area; for example, cardiac health and healthy living

9. Personal/social history: includes social data and lifestyle assessment

NCLEX® a. Diet: foods eaten on a typical day; number of meals and snacks; who shops and cooks; food preferences and patterns based on culture and/or religion; usual fluid intake; intake of caffeine (such as coffee, tea, cola)

NCLEX® b. Activity and exercise: type, frequency, and duration of exercise; ability to perform activities of daily living (ADLs), including eating, bathing, elimination, dressing, grooming; ability to move about at will (locomotion)

c. Sleep and rest: usual number of hours of sleep, sleep problems, and effectiveness of any remedies used

NCLEX® d. Tobacco use: number of packs per day (cigarettes) and years of smoking; type, frequency, and duration of use for other tobacco products

e. Substance use: amount, frequency, and duration of alcohol or recreational drug use

f. Living arrangements: location, type of dwelling, number of stairs to climb, home safety information, ability to access neighborhood or community resources

g. Family relationships or friendships: who is/are support person(s) in times of need; effects of illness on client and family roles and relationships (dynamics); identification of next of kin

h. Psychological data: major lifestyle changes or stressors experienced and how client dealt with them; usual coping patterns; general communication style and ability; appropriateness of verbal and nonverbal behavior; whether client is seeing a mental health professional; significance of current illness to client; effect of current illness on self-esteem or body image

i. Occupation: presence of occupational hazards, such as exposure to carcinogens (e.g., asbestos, other chemicals); distance and length of time client commutes to work each day and associated concerns; amount of time missed from work due to illness; history of a need to change jobs because of illness

j. Travel: out of country, when and length of time; military service abroad

k. Current and past health resources used: physicians (primary and specialists), nurse practitioners, dentists, folk healers; satisfaction with and accessibility of care

10. LPN/LVNs assist with performing a review of systems (ROS): used to obtain subjective data in a medical model; health care agencies generally have a specific form to gather this data; forms may blend gathering of subjective data (history) and **objective data** (physical assessment or examination)

a. Skin: skin disease (eczema, psoriasis, hives), changes in moles, skin dryness or moisture, itching, bruising, rashes or other lesions, changes in hair or nails, sun exposure

b. Head: headaches, dizziness (vertigo) or fainting (syncope), head injury

c. Eyes: vision problems (blurring, blind spots, reduced acuity), double vision (diplopia), glaucoma, cataracts, eye pain, redness, discharge or watering, swelling, method of vision correction being used

d. Ears: hearing loss, hearing aid use, tinnitus, vertigo, earaches, infections, discharge, and characteristics

e. Nose/sinuses: frequency and severity of colds, sinus pain or obstruction, discharge, nosebleeds, allergies, reduced sense of smell

f. Mouth/throat: pain or lesions in mouth (or tongue), toothaches, change in taste, frequency of sore throats, bleeding gums, dysphagia, hoarseness, history of tonsillectomy, frequency of dental care and presence of any dental prostheses

g. Neck: pain, mobility, enlarged or tender lymph nodes, goiter, lumps or other swelling

NCLEX® h. Breasts: history of breast disease or surgery, pain, lumps, rashes, nipple discharge, knowledge and performance of breast self-examination (BSE); date of last mammogram

i. Axilla: rash, lumps, tenderness, or swelling

NCLEX® j. Respiratory: history of lung disease (tuberculosis, pneumonia, asthma, bronchitis, emphysema), shortness of breath (amount and triggering factors, such as activity level), wheezes/other noises associated with respiration, cough, sputum production (color, amount, and if relevant, timing), pain associated with breathing, hemoptysis, and exposure to pollutants or other inhaled toxins

NCLEX® k. Cardiovascular: history of heart disease, murmur, hypertension, or anemia; chest pain (precordial or retrosternal, radiation, and other pain characteristics); dyspnea on exertion (specify amount); orthopnea, paroxysmal nocturnal dyspnea (PND); edema, nocturia

l. Peripheral vascular: discoloration of extremities (especially feet and ankles; note whether associated with activity); coolness, numbness, or tingling of lower limbs (note relationship to activity and time of day); history of intermittent claudication, ulcerations, thrombophlebitis, or varicose veins

m. Gastrointestinal (GI): appetite, nausea and vomiting, constipation or diarrhea, frequency of bowel movements and whether any recent changes, tarry or bloody stools, history of rectal conditions (such as hemorrhoids), food intolerances, dysphagia, heartburn, pyrosis (upper-GI burning with sour eructation), indigestion, abdominal pain (with or without eating), history of GI disorder, antacid use, and prescribed diet

n. Urinary: frequency, urgency, or dysuria; nocturia; polyuria or oliguria; characteristics of stream (narrowed, hesitancy, straining); cloudy urine or hematuria; incontinence; history of urinary disorder (renal disease or calculi, urinary tract infections); pain in back, flank, suprapubic area, or groin

o. Male genital: lumps, hernia, penile lesions or discharge, pain in testicles or penis, knowledge and performance of testicular self-examination (TSE), sexual health practices (contraceptive method and prevention of sexually transmitted infections)

p. Female genital: menstrual history (age of menarche, last monthly period, duration of cycle, premenstrual pain, intermenstrual spotting or metrorrhagia, dysmenorrhea, amenorrhea, menorrhagia), vaginal itching or discharge, age at menopause, menopausal manifestations, postmenopausal bleeding, last Papanicolaou (Pap) test and gynecological exam, sexual health practices

q. Musculoskeletal: joint pain, stiffness, or swelling; history of arthritis or gout; limited movement, noise with joint movement, obvious deformity; muscle pain, weakness, or cramping; difficulty with gait or activities; back pain or stiffness, history of back pain or disease; use of mobility aids and satisfaction with ability to perform ADLs

NCLEX® **r.** Neurologic: weakness, tics or tremors, paralysis, problems with coordination, paresthesias (numbness and tingling), recent or distant memory disorder, nervousness, mood changes, history of depression or other mental health problem, hallucinations, history of stroke, fainting or blackouts, seizure disorder

s. Hematologic: easy bruising or bleeding, swollen lymph nodes, history of blood transfusion and reactions, exposure to radiation or other toxins

NCLEX® **t.** Endocrine: history of diabetes, thyroid disease, adrenal disease, abnormal hair distribution, change in skin (pigmentation, texture), excessive sweating, relationship between appetite and weight, hormone therapy

II. HEALTH HISTORY OF CHILD

A. Overview

1. Provides opportunity to observe parent–child interactions
2. Principles are same as for an adult health history

B. Demographic and biographical information: similar to adult with addition of child's nickname, ages of child, siblings, and parents

C. Reason for seeking care

1. Sometimes called *chief complaint*
2. May be wellness- or illness-oriented
3. Record in words of informant, parent, or child

D. History of present illness

NCLEX® 1. Symptom analysis as previously described for adult client

2. Parents' perceptions of illness versus child's perception, if applicable

E. Past medical history

1. Birth history
   - **a.** Length of pregnancy
   - **b.** Mother's health and access to prenatal care
   - **c.** Medications taken during pregnancy and any alcohol, tobacco, or street-drug use
   - **d.** Duration of labor and type of delivery
   - **e.** Apgar scores, if known
   - **f.** Birth weight, length, head circumference
   - **g.** Postnatal health problems
   - **h.** Feeding: formula, including type, or breastfed, including length of time
2. Past illnesses
3. Hospitalizations, injuries, accidents, or surgeries
4. *NCLEX®* Allergies: medication, food, or environmental
5. *NCLEX®* Immunizations including boosters

NCLEX®

6. Habits and behaviors: sleep; discipline; socialization; exercise or activity; behavior issues; wellness behaviors; use of alcohol, drugs, nicotine, or caffeine; sexuality issues
7. Medications taken regularly: prescription, over-the-counter, herbal, home, or folk remedies
8. Developmental data
   a. Age at which child achieved specific developmental milestones, including first held head erect, first rolled over, first sat unsupported, first steps, first used words appropriately, bowel and bladder control
   b. Current developmental performance measured by a screening tool such as Denver II, if known
   c. Academic performance if in school
9. Nutritional data
   a. Consider adequacy in terms of age
   b. Timing and frequency of meals and snacks (NCLEX®)
   c. Ethnic or cultural considerations in food choices
   d. Use a 24-hour diet recall or food frequency record to assess adequacy of diet
10. Family history
   a. Primarily to discover potential or actual hereditary diseases in child or parents (NCLEX®)
   b. Includes a **genogram** (pictorial representation of family tree) that includes hereditary diseases, ages and causes of death, and chronic conditions (see Figure 15–1)
   c. Family structure: immediate and extended members of family; previous marriages, divorces, separations, or deaths of spouses
   d. Home and community environment: type of dwelling, sleeping arrangements, safety features, relationships with neighbors
   e. Occupations and education of family members, including work schedules
   f. Cultural and religious traditions, including language spoken at home
   g. Family function: interactions and roles; power, decision making, and problem solving; communication; and expression of feelings and individuality
11. The LPN/LVN may assist with review of systems
   a. Includes a specific review of each body system
   b. Begin with a broad question about child's overall health
   c. Integument: pruritus, rashes (including location), acne, bruising, hair growth or loss, disorders or deformities of nails
   d. Head: headaches, dizziness, or injuries
   e. Eyes: visual problems (bumping into things, squinting, blurred vision, holding books close or sitting close to television or computer), rubbing eyes, eye infections, glasses or contact lenses
   f. Ears: earaches (frequency and treatment), evidence of hearing loss (needing to repeat requests, loud voice), previous hearing test results
   g. Nose: history of nosebleeds, constant or frequent runny or stuffy nose, problems with sense of smell
   h. Mouth: mouth breathing, dental visits, tooth-care habits (brushing, flossing), toothaches
   i. Throat: sore throats, difficulty swallowing, choking, hoarseness or voice problems
   j. Neck: stiffness or problems moving; difficulty in holding head erect
   k. Chest: breast enlargement or development, breast self-examination for adolescents

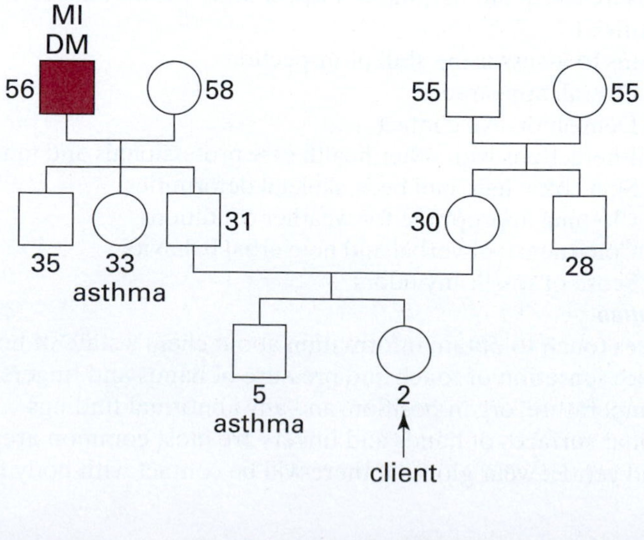

Figure 15–1

Sample genogram for a female child. The child's brother has asthma, a paternal aunt has asthma, and the paternal grandfather died having myocardial infarction (MI) and diabetes mellitus (DM).

l. Respiratory: frequency of colds, coughing or wheezing, difficulty breathing, sputum production, history of pneumonia or tuberculosis (TB), last TB test date

NCLEX® m. Cardiovascular: cyanosis or fatigue on exertion; history of heart murmurs, anemia, or rheumatic fever; blood type if known

NCLEX® n. Gastrointestinal: nausea or vomiting, jaundice, change in bowel habits, diarrhea, constipation

o. Genitourinary: pain on urination, unpleasant odor to urine, enuresis, testicular self-examination for adolescents, condom use if sexually active

p. Gynecological: date or age of menarche, date of last menstrual period, pain on menstruation, vaginal discharge, last Pap smear, and contraceptive use if sexually active

q. Musculoskeletal: weakness, clumsiness or lack of coordination, back or joint pain, muscle pain or cramps, abnormal gait or posturing or spasticity, history of fractures or sprains, usual activity level

r. Neurological: history of seizures, speech problems, nightmares or fears, dizziness or tremors, learning disabilities or problems with attention at home or school

NCLEX® 12. Review of psychosocial systems

a. Family composition: family members in home and relationship to child, marital status of parents, parents' educational level, persons participating in care of child, recent changes or crises in family

b. Financial resources: family members' employment status or occupation, health insurance coverage

c. Home environment: safe play area; well or community water supply; availability of heat, electricity, and so on; transportation; neighborhood safety issues

d. Child care arrangements: day-care resources needed/available, school attended

e. Daily living habits: peer relationships; sleep, rest, activity patterns; social activities; self-esteem and body image

f. Child's temperament

III. PREPARING FOR PHYSICAL EXAMINATION

A. Equipment needed

1. Basic equipment for a brief physical assessment includes blood pressure equipment, clean disposable gloves, drape, penlight, stethoscope, tape measure, thermometer, watch with a second hand, and weight scale
2. Additional equipment for a complete physical examination includes cotton ball, doppler, goniometer, lubricant, nasal speculum, near vision charts, neurologic hammer, ophthalmoscope, otoscope, reflex hammer, skin calipers, Snellen visual acuity chart, strabismoscope, tongue depressor/blade, tuning fork, tympanometer, and vaginal speculum; the LPN/LVN may not conduct these aspects of exam but may need to set up exam room

B. Promoting comfort during physical examination

1. Provide a comfortable room and minimize distractions
2. Ensure client privacy
3. Provide adequate lighting and normalize room temperature

IV. TECHNIQUES OF PHYSICAL EXAMINATION

A. *Inspection*

1. Uses observation to obtain information about client's state of health; also includes smell
2. Ensure adequate lighting to inspect body without distortions or shadows; lighting can be sunlight or artificial
3. Items to assess using skill of inspection

a. Overall appearance

b. Demeanor, eye contact

c. Interactions with other health care professionals and family

NCLEX® d. Skin color, hair, nail beds, skeletal deformities

e. Clothing appropriate for weather conditions

f. Congruence of verbal and nonverbal behavior

g. Sense of smell: any odors

B. *Palpation*

1. Uses touch to obtain information about client's state of health
2. Uses sensation of touch and pressure of hands and fingers to determine masses, elevations, temperature, organ position, and any abnormal findings

NCLEX® 3. Ulnar surfaces of hands and fingers are most common areas used for palpation; hands should be warm and gentle; wear gloves if there will be contact with body fluids, open skin areas, or mucosa

Table 15–1 Percussion Notes

Tone	Quality	Pitch	Example
Tympany	Drumlike	High	Gastric bubble
Resonance	Hollow	Low	Healthy lungs
Hyperresonance	Booming	Very loud	Emphysemic lung tissue
Flatness	Very dull	High	Muscle, bone
Dullness	Thudlike	Soft to moderate	Liver, spleen, heart

4. Can be light (1 cm in depth) or deep (4 cm in depth) depending on area being examined; nurse controls amount of pressure; deep palpation should occur after light palpation; most nurses use light palpation during physical exam, while deep palpation is used during a complete physical conducted by health care provider

C. *Percussion*

1. A skill in which finger of one hand touches or taps a finger of other hand to generate vibration, which in turn produces a specific, diagnostic sound; sound changes as practitioner moves from one area to next
2. Sounds can be classified as tympanic, hyperresonant, resonant, dull, or flat; further description and examples of percussion notes can be found in Table 15–1

D. *Auscultation*

NCLEX® 1. Place stethoscope over bare skin to eliminate change in sound caused by clothing
2. Listen to sound, duration, pitch, and intensity
NCLEX® 3. Must isolate sounds; if client has a large amount of chest or back hair, wet hair to flatten it and diminish extra sounds
4. Allot enough time to listen carefully to sounds; if in doubt, consult another health care professional for a second opinion

V. PHYSICAL EXAMINATION OF ADULT

A. Various purposes of physical examination

1. Full exam by health care provider as part of wellness screening (annually or as recommended)
2. Full history and physical assessment done at time of hospital admission by RN
3. Head-to-toe assessment at beginning of shift for hospitalized clients; is generally done by RN but LPN/LVN can contribute
4. Focused or body system–specific data collection that may be done frequently (more than once per shift, such as every 4 hours)

B. Vital signs

1. Temperature: average is 37°C or 98.6°F (normal range 35.8°C to 37.3°C or 96.4°F to 99.1°F); varies slightly depending on age, time of day, phase of menstrual cycle, exercise level, and method of measurement (rectal measures 1° higher than oral; axillary measures 1° lower than oral); measure using oral, rectal, axillary, or otic (tympanic membrane) route
2. Pulse: average is 68 to 78 beats per minute (bpm) in adult with a range of 60 to 100
   a. Radial: count rate and note rhythm and amplitude
   b. Apical: listen for a full minute and compare to radial pulse; place stethoscope on chest at fifth intercostal space, midclavicular line (5ICS, MCL)
   c. Rhythm should be regular; if pulse is irregular, assess whether rhythm is regularly irregular or irregularly irregular and alert health care provider
3. Respiration: normal rate in adult is 12 to 20 breaths/minute; count rate, rhythm, and depth of respiration; note comfort level as client breathes; normal respirations are relaxed, silent, automatic, and regular
4. Blood pressure (BP): normal range is 100/60 mm Hg to 130/85 mm Hg in adult; varies with age, gender, weight, exercise, emotion, stress, and diurnal rhythm (early morning low and late afternoon/early evening high)
   a. Have person sit or lie down with arm supported at heart level; allow a 5-minute rest period with no activity, smoking, eating, or drinking before measuring BP
   NCLEX® b. If there is a question about BP, wait 1 to 2 minutes before taking it again to avoid falsely high diastolic readings

c. If unable to hear BP, palpate BP by placing index finger over brachial artery, inflate cuff, deflate cuff while palpating, and note when pulsation disappears; only systolic pressure is noted and recorded as palpated
d. If client has poor circulation, BP may be faint; in this case or if BP cannot even be palpated, use a doppler to hear sounds; note systolic pressure only and record as a doppler BP

C. Height and weight

1. Height: using a balance scale, raise headpiece on measuring pole and align it with top of head while client is shoeless, standing erect, and looking forward
2. Weight: use platform scale if client can stand without assistance; special electronic scales and bed scales are also available if needed
3. *NCLEX®* Use professionally authorized charts to determine if client's height and weight fall within normal limits for age; also compare readings to client's own previous measurements

D. General appearance

1. Includes client's grooming and attire and personal hygiene
2. Includes gait and posture, general body build, and behavior

E. Mental status

1. A short mental status exam is often done during health history interview; assess client for overt signs of mental distress, crying, sullen demeanor, appropriate comments for situation
2. *NCLEX®* Four key areas of functioning (see Memory Aid)
a. Appearance: as noted in previous section
b. Behavior: level of consciousness (LOC), awake, alert, aware of and responding to internal and external stimuli; lethargic and drowsy, stuporous, or unresponsive (use Glasgow coma scale for additional information); facial expression, speech (quality, pace, articulation of words, word choice); aphasia (receptive/Wernicke's, motor/expressive/Broca's, global), mood and affect
c. Cognition: orientation (to time, place, person, and events), attention span, recent memory, remote memory, new learning (four unrelated words test), judgment
d. Thought processes: thought content (logical, consistent), client's perceptions (reality-based, congruent with others), and absence/presence of suicidal thoughts/ideation

Memory Aid

Remember the four key areas of mental status (appearance, behavior, cognition, and thought processes) by using the abbreviation ABCT.

e. The Mini-Mental State Exam (Folstein) may be used to gather this data; requires 5 to 10 minutes to administer; highest score is 30 (average people score 27)
f. A full mental status exam may be done if indicated, and other tests can be added if problems exist (brain lesions or cerebrovascular accident, aphasia, mental illness, memory changes, alcoholism, and others)

F. Integument

1. Skin provides first layer of protection for body, protecting against infection and trauma and preventing fluid loss; it also regulates body temperature, provides sensory perception, produces vitamin D, excretes sweat and impurities, and is a barometer of emotions
2. Inspection of skin
a. Note skin color; compare areas that are exposed to sun and those that are not
b. *NCLEX®* Daylight is best light to detect jaundice (yellowing of skin, sclera); use good lighting for best illumination; flashlights/penlights are also helpful for general inspection
c. Scan body for color, texture, tone, distribution of lesions, skin symmetry, differences between body areas, evidence of rashes or eruptions, hygiene
d. Observe moles (pigmented nevi) for defining features such as symmetry, elevation, color, and texture
e. Normal findings: range of skin color varies from person to person; color should be uniform; sun-exposed areas will be darker; calluses appear yellow; nevi (moles) can be normal findings
f. *NCLEX®* Abnormal findings: color changes in moles (could indicate cancerous changes); pale, shiny skin of the lower extremities (may indicate decreased peripheral circulation or diabetes mellitus); localized hemorrhages into skin (petechiae less than 0.5 cm in diameter or purpura more than 0.5 cm in diameter) that appear purple-red (could indicate injury, steroid use, or vasculitis)
3. Palpation of skin
a. Feel skin for moisture, temperature, texture, turgor, and mobility; gently pinch skin to test turgor; skin should immediately return to normal but will be delayed if edema or dehydration is present

b. Normal findings: skin should be cool to warm, dry, and smooth under normal conditions; in stressful situations, skin may feel cool and clammy; assess skin by touching bilaterally with dorsum of hands and comparing findings

NCLEX®

c. Abnormal findings: lesions (provide descriptions of size, shape, color, texture, elevation/depression, pedunculation, exudates, configuration, location, and distribution)

4. Inspection of nails
   a. Inspect for color, contour, texture, configuration, symmetry, and cleanliness
   b. Nails offer a quick assessment of individual; note whether they are clean and well-manicured, bitten down, yellow and tobacco-stained; color should be pink with a brisk capillary refill (less than 3 seconds) when depressed (blanch test)
   c. Normal findings: nail plate is smooth and flat or slightly convex; nail base angle is 160 degrees
   d. Abnormal findings: white bands can indicate melanoma; white spots can indicate cuticle manipulation or trauma; yellow can indicate psoriasis, fungal infections, and chronic respiratory diseases; diffuse darkening can indicate malaria medication, candidal infection, hyperbilirubinemia, or chronic trauma; a green-black color can indicate pseudomonas infection or nail bed trauma (subungual hematoma)
5. Palpation of nails: should be hard and smooth with uniform thickness
   a. Squeeze nail; if it separates from nail bed, can indicate psoriasis or trauma
   b. A clubbed boggy nail can indicate infection with candida or pseudomonas

G. Head and neck

1. Inspection
   a. Head should be erect and still with symmetrical facial features
   b. Note structure, conjunctiva, sclera, cornea, and iris of each eye
   c. Note position, alignment, skin condition, and external meatus of ear
   d. Inspect external nose
   e. Inspect inside of mouth and throat (mucosa, tongue, teeth and gums, floor of mouth, palate, uvula)
   f. Observe for tics, spasms, lesions, and facial paralysis
   g. Neck should be symmetrical without masses
2. Palpation: done by RN or health care provider, but includes assessment of cranium, scalp, and hair; salivary glands; temporal artery and temporomandibular joint; maxillary and frontal sinuses; tragus of ear (for tenderness); thyroid gland; and trachea (to check for midline position)
3. Inspect and palpate cervical lymph nodes
4. Special testing (by RN or health care provider)

NCLEX®

   a. Eyes: test visual fields (confrontation), extraocular movements, pupil size, equality, roundness, and response to light and accommodation (PERRLA); check ocular fundus (with an ophthalmoscope) for red reflex, condition of optic disc, blood vessels and background of retina; may be documented under neurological exam
   b. Ears: use an otoscope to inspect ear canal and tympanic membrane (should be movable, intact, and pearly white-gray in color); use tuning fork to do Rinne and Weber tests to check for bone and air conduction in hearing (see section on neurological exam for further information); may be documented under neurological exam
   c. Nose: use a nasal speculum to check nasal mucosa, septum, and turbinates

H. Breasts and axillae

1. With client in a sitting position, inspect breasts for symmetry, contour, and shape; should be rounded, generally symmetrical
2. Look for areas of discoloration, hyperpigmentation, dimpling or retraction, swelling or edema; should be uniform in color, smooth, and elastic
3. Detect any areas of retraction by asking client to do three maneuvers: raise arms above head, push hands together with elbows flexed, and press hands down on hips
4. Observe areola for size, shape, symmetry, color, general surface characteristics, lesions or masses; should be round or oval, and color may vary among individuals from light pink to dark brown
5. Inspect nipples for size, shape, position, color, and presence of any discharge or lesions; should be round, everted, and equal in size
6. Palpate axillary, subclavicular, and supraclavicular lymph nodes using palmar surface of fingertips in four areas: edge of greater pectoral muscle in anterior axillary line, thoracic wall in midaxilla, upper portion of humerus, and anterior edge of latissimus dorsi muscle in posterior axillary line

7. Palpate breast for masses and tenderness, using one of three patterns: hands-of-the-clock, spokes-on-a-wheel, concentric circles; there should be no masses or tenderness
8. Palpate areola and nipples for masses; there should be none

I. Chest

1. Lungs
    a. Use standard thoracic landmarks when performing respiratory assessment
    NCLEX®
    b. Inspection: note overall appearance, nutritional status (dyspnea can impair oral intake), ability to breathe, respirations (bradypnea, tachypnea, shortness of breath, dyspnea), contour and movement of chest (should be symmetrical); note presence of retractions (abnormal) and color of skin, nail beds, and lips
    c. Palpation (done by RN or health care provider): includes assessment of posterior aspect of chest (masses, bulges, muscle tone, subcutaneous emphysema or crepitus, and areas of tenderness), respiratory excursion, tactile **fremitus** (conduction of voice sounds through respiratory tract)
    d. Percussion (done by health care provider or RN): to determine percussion notes and lung excursion
    NCLEX®
    e. Auscultation: use flat diaphragm of stethoscope to listen systematically to chest; begin posteriorly and listen from apices (at C7 level) to bases (at about T10), and laterally from axilla to 7th or 8th rib; normal sounds include bronchial, bronchovesicular, and vesicular; compare findings side to side while working downward over posterior chest (see Table 15–2 for description of various adventitious breath sounds); note location, quality, and time of occurrence during respiratory cycle
    f. Other abnormal findings during auscultation include bronchophony (ask client to repeat words "ninety-nine"; if heard clearly, indicates lung density in that area); egophony (ask client to say "ee-ee-ee-ee" during auscultation; sound changes to a long "aaaa" sound in areas of consolidation or compression); whispered pectoriloquy (ask client to whisper "one-two-three" during auscultation; sound will be faint yet clear and distinct with small amounts of consolidation); pleural friction rub (grating, creaking, or groaning noise, often more noticeable on inspiration, and may be heard over inflamed areas of parietal and visceral pleura)
    g. Repeat entire assessment process with anterior chest

NCLEX®

2. Neck vessels
    a. Inspect carotid arteries for visible pulsation with head of exam table raised to 45 degrees
    b. Palpate carotid arteries *one at a time* in area medial to sternocleidomastoid muscle; avoid area higher in neck to prevent stimulating baroreceptors and triggering bradycardia from vagus nerve stimulation; note pulse contour and amplitude and compare findings side to side
    c. Auscultate over carotid arteries for bruits using bell of stethoscope; sound should be absent; if bruit present, note whether it sounds like a buzzing, swishing, or blowing sound; bruit indicates turbulent blood flow from obstruction (i.e., atherosclerotic narrowing of carotid vessel)
    d. Assess jugular vein distention (head elevated 45 degrees); turn head slightly away; highest pulsation should be no more than 1.5 inches above sternal notch
3. Heart
    a. Inspection: general appearance of client and color of skin and nail beds; observe for symmetry of movement, anatomical defects, retractions, pulsations, and heaves; locate point of maximal impulse (PMI) if visible (usually at the apex, 5ICS, MCL)
    b. Palpate PMI (not visible in all clients) with ball of hand, then fingertips; next assess for abnormal pulsations in sternoclavicular, aortic, pulmonic, tricuspid, and epigastric areas; palpate for thrills (over areas of turbulent blood flow)

Table 15–2 Adventitious Breath Sounds

Sound	Characteristics	Timing and Occurrence
Crackles (coarse)	Popping, frying sound; moist, low-pitched	Inspiration, some expiration
Crackles (medium)	Not as loud as coarse crackles	Middle of inspiration
Crackles (fine)	Noncontinuous, popping, high-pitched	End of inspiration
Rhonchi or gurgles	Continuous, low-pitched, prolonged	Expiration
Wheezes	Continuous, high-pitched, musical	Inspiration and/or expiration
Pleural friction rub	Low-pitched, dry, grating	Inspiration and/or expiration

Beazley, J. D. *Athenian Red Figure Vases: The Archaic Period: A Handbook*. The World of Art. New York: Thames & Hudson, 1991.
———. *Athenian Red Figure Vases: The Classical Period: A Handbook*. The World of Art. New York: Thames & Hudson, 1989.
———. *The Development of Attic Black-Figure*. Rev. ed. Berkeley: University of California Press, 1986.
———. *Greek Vases: Lectures*. Oxford and New York: Clarendon Press and Oxford University Press, 1989.
Boardman, J. *The Archaeology of Nostalgia: How the Greeks Recreated Their Mythical Past*. London: Thames & Hudson, 2002.
———. *Athenian Black Figure Vases: A Handbook*. Corrected ed. The World of Art. New York: Thames & Hudson, 1991.
———. *Early Greek Vase Painting: 11th–6th Centuries B.C.: A Handbook*. The World of Art. New York: Thames & Hudson, 1998.
———. *Greek Art*. 4th ed., rev. and expanded. The World of Art. New York: Thames & Hudson, 1996.
———. *Greek Sculpture: The Archaic Period: A Handbook*. Corrected ed. The World of Art. New York: Thames & Hudson, 1991.
———. *Greek Sculpture: The Classical Period: A Handbook*. Corrected ed. New York: Thames & Hudson, 1991.
———. *The History of Greek Vases: Potters, Painters, and Pictures*. New York: Thames & Hudson, 2001.
Burn, L. *Hellenistic Art: From Alexander the Great to Augustus*. London: The British Museum, 2004.
Carpenter, T. H. *Art and Myth in Ancient Greece: A Handbook*. The World of Art. New York: Thames & Hudson, 1991.
Carratelli, G. P., ed. *The Greek World: Art and Civilization in Magna Graecia and Sicily*. Exh. cat. New York: Rizzoli, 1996.
Fullerton, M. D. *Greek Art*. New York: Cambridge University Press, 2000.
Hampe, R., and E. Simon. *The Birth of Greek Art*. Oxford: Oxford University Press, 1981.
Haynes, D. E. L. *The Technique of Greek Bronze Statuary*. Mainz am Rhein: P. von Zabern, 1992.
Himmelmann, N. *Reading Greek Art: Essays*. Princeton, NJ: Princeton University Press, 1998.
Hurwit, J. M. *The Acropolis in the Age of Pericles*. New York: Cambridge University Press, 2004.
———. *The Art & Culture of Early Greece, 1100–480 B.C.* Ithaca, NY: Cornell University Press, 1985.
Lawrence, A. *Greek Architecture*. Rev. 5th ed. Pelican History of Art. New Haven: Yale University Press, 1996.
Osborne, R. *Archaic and Classical Greek Art*. New York: Oxford University Press, 1998.
Papaioannou, K. *The Art of Greece*. New York: Harry N. Abrams, 1989.
Pedley, J. *Greek Art and Archaeology*. 2d ed. New York: Harry N. Abrams, 1997.
Pollitt, J. *The Ancient View of Greek Art: Criticism, History, and Terminology*. New Haven: Yale University Press, 1974.
———. *Art in the Hellenistic Age*. New York: Cambridge University Press, 1986.
———., ed. *Art of Ancient Greece: Sources and Documents*. New York: Cambridge University Press, 1990.
Potts, A. *Flesh and the Ideal: Winckelmann and the Origins of Art History*. New Haven: Yale University Press, 1994.
Rhodes, R. *Architecture and Meaning on the Athenian Acropolis*. New York: Cambridge University Press, 1995.
Richter, G. M. A. *A Handbook of Greek Art*. 9th ed. New York: Da Capo, 1987.
———. *Portraits of the Greeks*. Ed. R. Smith. New York: Oxford University Press, 1984.
Ridgway, B. S. *Hellenistic Sculpture: Vol. 1, The Styles of ca. 331–200 B.C.* Bristol, England: Bristol Classical Press, 1990.
Robertson, M. *The Art of Vase Painting in Classical Athens*. New York: Cambridge University Press, 1992.
Rolley, C. *Greek Bronzes*. New York: Philip Wilson for Sotheby's Publications; Dist. by Harper & Row, 1986.
Schefold, K. *Gods and Heroes in Late Archaic Greek Art*. New York: Cambridge University Press, 1992.
Smith, R. *Hellenistic Sculpture*. The World of Art. New York: Thames & Hudson, 1991.
Spivey, N. *Greek Art*. London: Phaidon, 1997.
Stafford, E. *Life, Myth, and Art in Ancient Greece*. Los Angeles: J. Paul Getty Museum, 2004.
Stansbury-O'Donnell, M. *Pictorial Narrative in Ancient Greek Art*. New York: Cambridge University Press, 1999.
Stewart, A. F. *Greek Sculpture: An Exploration*. New Haven: Yale University Press, 1990.
Whitley, J. *The Archaeology of Ancient Greece*. New York: Cambridge University Press, 2001.

CHAPTER 6. ETRUSCAN ART

Boethius, A. *Etruscan and Early Roman Architecture*. 2d ed. Pelican History of Art. New Haven: Yale University Press, 1992.
Bonfante, L., ed. *Etruscan Life and Afterlife: A Handbook of Etruscan Studies*. Detroit, MI: Wayne State University, 1986.
Borrelli, F. *The Etruscans: Art, Architecture, and History*. Los Angeles: J. Paul Getty Museum, 2004.
Brendel, O. *Etruscan Art*. Pelican History of Art. New Haven: Yale University Press, 1995.
Hall, J. F., ed. *Etruscan Italy: Etruscan Influences on the Civilizations of Italy from Antiquity to the Modern Era*. Provo, UT: Museum of Art, Brigham Young University, 1996.
Haynes, Sybille. *Etruscan Civilization: A Cultural History*. Los Angeles: J. Paul Getty Museum, 2000.
Richardson, E. *The Etruscans: Their Art and Civilization*. Reprint of 1964 ed., with corrections. Chicago: University of Chicago Press, 1976.
Spivey, N. *Etruscan Art*. The World of Art. New York: Thames & Hudson, 1997.
Sprenger, M., G. Bartoloni, and M. Hirmer. *The Etruscans: Their History, Art, and Architecture*. New York: Harry N. Abrams, 1983.
Steingräber, S., ed. *Etruscan Painting: Catalogue Raisonné of Etruscan Wall Paintings*. New York: Johnson Reprint, 1986.
Torelli, M., ed. *The Etruscans*. Exh. cat. Milan: Bompiani, 2000.

CHAPTER 7. ROMAN ART

Allan, T. *Life, Myth and Art in Ancient Rome*. Los Angeles: J. Paul Getty Museum, 2005.
Andreae, B. *The Art of Rome*. New York: Harry N. Abrams, 1977.
Beard, M., and J. Henderson. *Classical Art: From Greece to Rome*. New York: Oxford University Press, 2001.
Bowe, P. *Gardens of the Roman World*. Los Angeles: J. Paul Getty Museum, 2004.
Brilliant, R. *Commentaries on Roman Art: Selected Studies*. London: Pindar Press, 1994.
———. *My Laocoon: Alternative Claims in the Interpretation of Artworks*. University of California Press, 2000.
Claridge, A. *Rome: An Oxford Archaeological Guide*. New York: Oxford University Press, 1998.
D'Ambra, E. *Roman Art*. New York: Cambridge University Press, 1998.
———., comp. *Roman Art in Context: An Anthology*. Englewood Cliffs, NJ: Prentice Hall, 1993.
Davies, P. *Death and the Emperor: Roman Imperial Funerary Monuments from Augustus to Marcus Aurelius*. Austin: University of Texas Press, 2004.
Dunbabin, K. M. D. *Mosaics of the Greek and Roman World*. New York: Cambridge University Press, 1999.
Elsner, J. *Imperial Rome and Christian Triumph: The Art of the Roman Empire, A.D. 100–450*. New York: Oxford University Press, 1998.
Gazda, E. K. *Roman Art in the Private Sphere: New Perspectives on the Architecture and Decor of the Domus, Villa, and Insula*. Ann Arbor: University of Michigan Press, 1991.
Jenkyns, R., ed. *The Legacy of Rome: A New Appraisal*. New York: Oxford University Press, 1992.
Kleiner, D. *Roman Sculpture*. New Haven: Yale University Press, 1992.
———., and S. B. Matheson, eds. *I, Claudia: Women in Ancient Rome*. New Haven: Yale University Art Gallery, 1996.
Ling, R. *Ancient Mosaics*. London: British Museum Press, 1998.
———. *Roman Painting*. New York: Cambridge University Press, 1991.
Nash, E. *Pictorial Dictionary of Ancient Rome*. 2 vols. Reprint of 1968 2d ed. New York: Hacker, 1981.
Pollitt, J. J. *The Art of Rome, c. 753 B.C.– A.D. 337: Sources and Documents*. New York: Cambridge University Press, 1983.
Ramage, N., and A. Ramage. *The Cambridge Illustrated History of Roman Art*. Cambridge: Cambridge University Press, 1991.
———. *Roman Art: Romulus to Constantine*. 4th ed. Upper Saddle River, NJ: Pearson Prentice Hall, 2005.
Richardson, L. *A New Topographical Dictionary of Ancient Rome*. Baltimore, MD: Johns Hopkins University Press, 1992.
Rockwell, P. *The Art of Stoneworking: A Reference Guide*. Cambridge: Cambridge University Press, 1993.
Strong, D. E. *Roman Art*. 2d ed. Pelican History of Art. New Haven: Yale University Press, 1992.
Vitruvius. *The Ten Books on Architecture*. Trans. I. Rowland. Cambridge: Cambridge University Press, 1999.
Ward-Perkins, J. B. *Roman Imperial Architecture*. Reprint of 1981 ed. Pelican History of Art. New York: Penguin, 1992.
Zanker, P. *The Power of Images in the Age of Augustus*. Ann Arbor: University of Michigan Press, 1988.

Index

Boldface names refer to artists. Pages in italics refer to illustrations.

NCLEX®

c. Auscultate in predetermined sequence (see Figure 15–2) for S_1, S_2, extra heart sounds (S_3 and S_4) and murmurs; see Table 15–3 for heart sounds; place client in three positions for complete assessment: lying on back with head of bed at 30 degrees, sitting up, and lying on left side; use diaphragm of stethoscope to detect higher pitched sounds and then bell to detect lower pitched sounds

Memory Aid

Moving from left to right and top to bottom (as when reading), remember location of valvular heart sounds with **A**ll **P**atients **T**ake **M**eds (**A**ortic, **P**ulmonic, **T**ricuspid, **M**itral). These sounds are best heard "downstream" from actual blood flow through valve, giving their unique auscultatory locations.

d. Percussion: not often done because chest x-ray determines cardiac size

J. Abdomen

1. Preparation: ask client to empty bladder before exam; position client supine with a small pillow under head; bend or place a pillow under client's knees; expose abdomen fully; place client's arms at sides or across chest (not over head because it tenses abdominal muscles); warm examiner's hands and stethoscope and ensure that fingernails are short; keep room warm to prevent chilling; use distraction techniques as needed
2. Inspection: observe four quadrants for contour, symmetry, bumps, bulges, or masses; note skin color (redness, jaundice) and condition (striae, scars), umbilicus, hair distribution, and any pulsations or movements of abdomen

NCLEX®

a. A bulge may indicate a distended bladder or hernia; look at shape and contour

b. Midline umbilicus: to assess for umbilical hernia, have client lift arms over head; if umbilicus protrudes, hernia may be present

c. Abdominal movements: slight, wavelike movements are normal, especially in a thin person; visible rippling waves may indicate obstruction

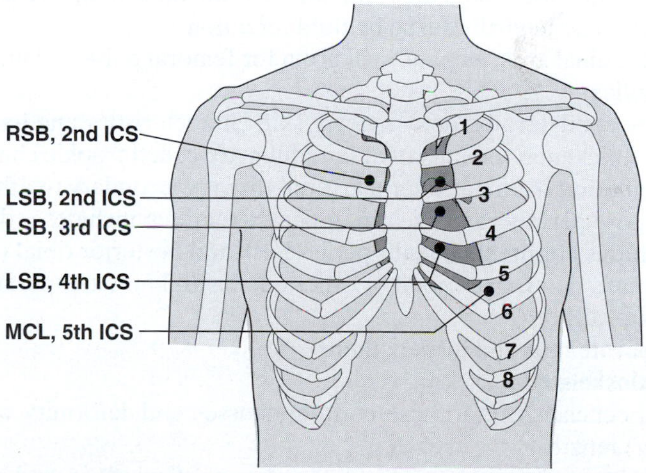

Figure 15–2

Sites for auscultation of the heart. Aortic valve area: right sternal border (RSB), 2nd ICS; pulmonic valve area: left sternal border (LSB), 2nd ICS; tricuspid valve area: left lateral sternal border (LLSB), 4th ICS; mitral valve area: left midclavicular line (MCL), 5th ICS.

Table 15–3 Heart Sounds

Sound	Location	Description	Character	Significance
S_1	Apex	Lub	Low-pitched and dull	Closure of mitral and tricuspid valves
S_2	Base	Dub	Shorter, more high-pitched than S_1	Closure of pulmonic and aortic valves
S_3	Apex	"Ken-tuck-y"	Low-pitched	Ventricles filling rapidly
S_4	Tricuspid or mitral areas	"Ten-ness-ee"	Occurs just before S_1 after atrial contraction	Increased resistance to ventricular filling
Pericardial friction rub	Left sternal border	Grating, leathery	Muffled, high-pitched, and transient	Pericardial inflammation

NCLEX® 3. Auscultation: must auscultate before palpation and percussion to avoid increasing frequency of bowel sounds
   a. Place diaphragm of stethoscope lightly against skin in right lower quadrant, where bowel sounds are most frequent (location of ileocecal valve)
   b. Listen in a clockwise fashion for at least 2 minutes
   c. Note character and quality; normal sounds are high-pitched and gurgling at a rate of 5 to 34 times per minute
   d. Sounds are classified as normal, hypoactive (heard infrequently), or hyperactive (loud, high-pitched, more frequent than normal)
   e. Use bell of stethoscope to hear vascular sounds over iliac, aortic, renal, and femoral arteries; listen for bruits, venous hums, and friction rubs

4. Percussion (usually done by RN or health care provider): do not percuss if abdominal aortic aneurysm is present or suspected
5. Palpation: with warm hands, palpate lightly (about 1 cm deep with four fingers positioned close together) using a rotary motion in all areas to assess skin surface and superficial musculature
   a. Light palpation helps detect superficial masses and fluid accumulation; a normal finding is a soft, nontender abdomen
   b. Deep palpation (to depth of 4 to 6 cm by RN or health care provider) can identify masses, tenderness, pulsations, organ enlargement (liver, spleen, kidneys); usually done by primary care provider or advanced practice nurse
   c. If a mass is found, note its location, size, shape, consistency (hard, firm, or soft), type of surface (smooth or nodular), mobility, pulsatility, and tenderness

NCLEX® d. If a mass is noted to be pulsatile, stop palpating in that area to avoid rupture

NCLEX® e. Identify rebound tenderness: if an area is tender to light palpation or if client reports pain in an area, move hand to an area away from painful site, and position hand perpendicular (at a 90-degree angle) in relation to abdomen; push down slowly and deeply and then lift up quickly; normally there is no pain or tenderness, but if present (often severe and accompanied by muscle rigidity), it indicates peritoneal inflammation, possibly appendicitis or peritonitis from another disorder

   f. Abdominal pain: indicates possible ulcers, intestinal obstruction, cholecystitis, peritonitis
   g. Ascites: use a tape measure at fullest site on abdomen, usually at or just above umbilicus, to determine changes in girth caused by fluid retention
   h. Inguinal area: palpate each groin for femoral pulse and inguinal nodes

K. Extremities

NCLEX® 1. Inspect bilaterally for symmetry, skin characteristics, and hair distribution; hair loss, thin shiny skin, and thickened toenails in older adults are called trophic changes and are often caused by decreased circulation from peripheral arterial disease secondary to atherosclerosis

2. Palpate peripheral pulses; in upper extremities, includes radial and ulnar pulses; in lower extremities, includes popliteal, dorsalis pedis (DP), and posterior tibial (PT) pulses

NCLEX® 3. Palpate skin for pretibial or other edema and note temperature of extremities; compare side-to-side bilaterally

4. Separate toes and inspect them

L. Musculoskeletal

1. Inspect each joint for size, contour, masses, and deformity; measure any discrepancies in extremity (leg) length
2. Palpate each joint for musculature, bony articulations, and crepitation; assess for heat, swelling, or tenderness
3. Test range of motion (ROM) of joints of upper extremities (shoulders, elbows, wrists, and fingers) and lower extremities (hips, knees, ankles, and toes); describe any physical limitations; if less than full ROM is present, a goniometer may be used during a full exam to measure joint angles more precisely
4. Note size, tone, and any involuntary movements of major muscle groups; compare findings bilaterally
5. Other musculoskeletal tests that can be done by RN or health care provider are to test strength of major muscle groups (grading scale 0 to 5), ROM in spine by having client bend forward and backward, and straight leg raising test (should not elicit pain unless problem with intervertebral disk)
6. Note any musculoskeletal pain present during assessment; pain description should be very specific
   a. Bone pain: pain unrelated to movement unless fracture is present, deep, aching, and continuous; it also causes insomnia
   b. Muscle pain: cramps or spasms with possible relationship to posture or movement; tremors, twitches, or weakness may be manifested; muscle tension may produce referred pain

c. Joint pain: joint may be tender to palpation; referred pain can be present; nerve root irritation may produce radiculitis (pain is distal); mechanical joint pain is worse with movement and worsens throughout day

M. Neurologic

1. Assist with examination of cranial nerves; see Table 15–4 for a summary of normal and abnormal findings
2. Assist with examination of motor system: inspect and palpate muscles as described in previous section
3. Assist with examination of cerebellar function by RN or health care provider: includes observing gait while walking, heel-to-toe walking, Romberg test (ability to stand without swaying while eyes closed), and miscellaneous cerebellar function tests (hopping on one leg, rapid alternating movements tests, finger-to-nose or finger-to-finger tests, heel-to-shin test)
4. Assist with examination of sensory system
   a. Requires client to be alert, cooperative, have an adequate attention span, and be in a comfortable position
   b. Test client's ability to discriminate between light pain (with a sharp object such as a pin) and touch (with a dull object such as a cotton wisp or pencil eraser), to detect temperature (warm water versus cold), vibration (placement of a vibrating tuning fork on various points of body), stereognosis (recognition of objects placed in hand while eyes are closed), graphesthesia (ability to determine a number traced on palm of hand) with eyes closed, two-point discrimination (ability to detect two separate

Table 15–4 Cranial Nerve Assessment

Cranial Nerve(s)	Assessment	Normal	Abnormal
CN I	Smell	Can identify common substances	Difficulty detecting common substances
CN II	Visual acuity	Able to read; visual fields intact	Visual field defects
CN III, IV, VI	Extraocular movements, elevation of eyelids, pupil constriction	Can elevate eyes, PERRLA, eyeball movement present	Drooping of the eye, ptosis, unequal pupils
CN V	Sensory: corneas, nasal and oral mucosa, facial skin Motor: jaw and chewing muscles	Sensory: able to detect both sharp and dull sensations when face touched with pointed or blunt object Motor: clenches teeth while palpating temporal and masseter muscles	Inability to feel or identify facial stimuli; muscle weakness Pertinent disorder: trigeminal neuralgia
CN VII	Sensory: taste on anterior portion of tongue Motor: facial muscles	Sensory: can discriminate sweet, sour, and salty tastes Motor: facial symmetry present at rest and when frowning and smiling	If neurological impairment, entire side of face could be immobile Pertinent disorders: Bell's palsy, stroke
CN VIII	Hearing and equilibrium	Cochlear (hearing): • Whisper test: client can repeat what was said • Weber test: sound lateralizes equally • Rinne test: sound heard normally twice as long by air conduction (AC) as bone conduction (BC) Vestibular (equilibrium): normal balance, absence of nystagmus	Whisper: sensorineural hearing loss Weber: Sound lateralizes to bad ear with conductive hearing loss or to good ear with sensorineural hearing loss Rinne: AC equal to or less than BC with conductive hearing loss; AC-to-BC ratio normal but reduced overall with sensorineural hearing loss Vestibular: problems with gait or balance; presence of nystagmus
CN IX, X	Swallowing, salivating, taste perception, voice quality	Client swallows; gag reflex present; with tongue depressor against posterior pharynx, client says *ahh;* movement of soft palate and uvula present	Soft palate does not rise; deviation of soft palate and uvula, no gag reflex, dysphagia, hoarseness, taste abnormalities
CN XI	Strength of sternocleidomastoid muscles and upper portion of trapezius	Client shrugs shoulders with equal strength bilaterally	Drooping shoulders, asymmetric muscle contraction
CN XII	Tongue movement in swallowing and speech	Tongue protrudes in midline; client pushes tongue into cheek against resistance from examiner	Tongue atrophy and fasciculation, deviation

stimuli, generally varies depending on area of body; fingertips are most sensitive at 2 to 8 mm; upper arms, thighs, and back are least sensitive at 40 to 75 mm)

5. Assist with examination of deep tendon reflexes using a reflex hammer
   a. Have limb relaxed and muscle partly stretched; strike reflex hammer on insertion tendon of biceps (C5 to C6), triceps (C7 to C8), brachioradialis (C5 to C6), quadriceps or "knee jerk" (L2 to L4), and Achilles or "ankle jerk" (S1 to S2)
   b. Reflexes are graded on a scale of 0 to 4 with 0 being absent and 4 being brisk or hyperactive; a rating of 2 is normal
6. Assist with examination of superficial reflexes
   a. Abdominal (upper T8 to T10; lower T10 to T12): stroke skin with a smooth object from one side of abdomen toward midline; abdominal muscle contracts on side of stimulus (ipsilateral response) and umbilicus deviates toward stroke; perform at both upper and lower end of abdomen
   b. Cremasteric reflex (L1 to L2): lightly stroke inner aspect of thigh of a male client with a reflex hammer or tongue blade and watch for elevation of ipsilateral testicle
   NCLEX® c. Plantar reflex or Babinski reflex (L4 to S2): use same object to stroke upward on lateral sole of foot and across ball of foot; normal (negative) response in adult is flexion of toes and possibly whole foot; an abnormal or positive response (which is normal in infants) is dorsiflexion of big toe and fanning of other toes

N. Genitals/rectum

1. Perianal region
   a. Don gloves and spread buttocks to visualize site
   b. Inspect for hemorrhoids, blood, fissures, scars, lesions, rectal prolapse, discharge
   c. Palpation: rectal exam is done by an experienced RN or advanced practice nurse; purpose is to palpate for rectal masses and assess stool for blood
2. Assist with examination of male genitalia
   a. Inspection: hair distribution in pubic region; penis (note presence of dorsal vein; urethral meatus appears slitlike; note bumps, blisters, redness, lesions, and masses; inspect underlying skin after moving pubic hair); scrotum should be loose, wrinkled, with deeply pigmented pouch at base of penis and each contains a testicle (oval, rubbery, suspended vertically and slightly forward in scrotum); may appear asymmetrical because left testicle has a longer spermatic cord
   b. Palpation: use thumb and first two fingers; area is sensitive to gentle compression; penis should feel smooth, semifirm, and nontender; testicles should feel smooth, rubbery, and moveable with no nodules, lumps, swelling, soreness, masses, or lesions
3. Assist with examination of female genitalia
   a. Inspection of external genitalia: mons pubis, labia majora, labia minora, clitoris, vagina, and urethra; with gloved hands, spread labia and assess urethral meatus; should be a pink, slitlike midline opening; labia majora and minora should be moist and free from swelling, lesions, discharge, and unusual odors
   b. Palpate external genitalia: spread labia and palpate; should feel smooth
   c. Internal genitalia examination and rectovaginal palpation are usually done by an advanced practice nurse or health care provider, not an LPN/LVN or RN nurse generalist

O. Postexamination responsibilities

1. Provide tissues or assist client to cleanse lubricant/secretions as needed
2. Remove drape
3. Allow client opportunity or assistance to get dressed
4. Leave client in comfortable position
5. NCLEX® Document data clearly and immediately; compare findings to established norms and to previous findings; note specimens obtained during exam
6. NCLEX® Handle collected specimens in a manner consistent with standard precautions; label specimens completely and send to laboratory with requisition attached according to agency policy

VI. PHYSICAL EXAMINATION OF CHILD

A. General considerations

1. Developmental level of child is most important consideration for a successful assessment (see Table 15–5)
2. NCLEX® Use terms understandable to and appropriate for child and parents; encourage active participation of all when possible; reassure child throughout exam
3. Allow child to become familiar with examiner prior to beginning exam
4. NCLEX® Save distressful or intrusive parts of exam for last

Table 15-5 Age-Specific Approaches to Physical Examination

Age	Approach
Infant	Child lying flat or held in parent's arms Use distraction with older infant Assess heart, pulse, lungs, respirations while quiet, then head to toe Eyes, ears, and mouth near end Check reflexes as body parts are examined Moro reflex last
Toddler	Minimal contact initially Allow to inspect equipment Assess heart and lungs while quiet, then head to toe Eyes, ears, and mouth last
Preschool	Allow to inspect equipment Head to toe if cooperative Same as toddler if uncooperative
School age	Respect privacy and explain procedures Head to toe with genitalia last
Adolescent	Explain proceedings and proceed as for school-age child

NCLEX® 5. Prepare child and parents for new or painful procedures
6. Examine child in a comfortable and secure position

NCLEX® **B. Methods of restraint**
1. May be necessary with infants, toddlers, or uncooperative children
2. When examining eyes, ears, nose, or throat, examiner may need to have a parent or other adult hold child supine with arms extended alongside head
3. "Hug" method has child sit on parent's lap with legs to one side and one arm tucked under parent's arm while parent holds other arm securely; child's legs may need to be held between parent's legs to prevent kicking
4. Ask another adult for assistance if parent is distressed and cannot help

C. Growth measurements
1. Plot results on growth charts; length/height to age, weight to age, length to weight

NCLEX® 2. Overall pattern of growth is more important than any single measurement
3. Use 5th and 95th percentiles to determine measurements outside normal limits

NCLEX® 4. Length/height
  a. Recumbent length (birth up to 36 months) with child supine and legs extended; use a horizontal measuring board; avoid using a tape measure because readings are often inaccurate; extend an infant's legs to obtain true length because infants tend to flex legs while at rest
  b. Use crown-to-heel measurement
  c. Children older than 2 or 3 years may stand shoeless as straight as possible
  d. A wall-mounted ruler can be used to measure height of small children if they have difficulty standing erect on a scale
5. Weight
  a. Weigh naked infant lying or sitting; measure infants on a platform-type balance scale; ensure calibration by noting that beam is balanced when weight is set to zero
  b. Weigh older children on upright scale dressed only in underpants or light gown
6. Head circumference

NCLEX®   a. Measure at every physical assessment for infants and toddlers under 2 years; always measure if neurological problem or developmental delay is suspected
  b. Is best indication of brain growth

c. Place measuring tape (paper or nonstretching tape) over most prominent part of occiput and just above supraorbital ridges
NCLEX® d. Make three measurements and take average as number to record
e. Percentiles should be comparable to child's height and weight
f. Head circumference exceeds chest circumference until between 1 and 2 years of age

7. Chest circumference
a. Is usually measured at birth and during early infancy
NCLEX® b. Place measuring tape at nipple level with child supine
c. Take measurement midway between inspiration and expiration
d. Head and chest circumference should be approximately equal between 1 and 2 years of age
e. During childhood, chest circumference exceeds head circumference by 2 to 3 inches

D. Vital signs (see Table 15–6)

1. Temperature
NCLEX® a. Rectal, axillary, skin, or tympanic when assessing infants
b. Oral route may be used in children over 4 years of age
NCLEX® c. Use rectal only when necessary because of discomfort and intrusiveness
d. May be altered by exercise, crying, stress, or environmental conditions

2. Pulse
a. Newborn average is 110–160 bpm (range of 100 to 180) and decreases with increasing age
NCLEX® b. Try to measure with child at rest, sleeping, or lying quietly
c. Take an apical pulse for children younger than 2 years and a radial pulse in children over 2 years of age
NCLEX® d. Count for one full minute
e. May be altered by anxiety, activity, pain, crying, medications, or disease
f. Record rate, rhythm, quality, and amplitude

3. Respirations
NCLEX® a. Try to measure while child is at rest, sleeping, or lying quietly
b. Measure in infants and young children by observing abdominal movements; measure in older children by observing rise and fall of chest
c. Record rate, rhythm, and quality
d. May be altered by anxiety, activity, medications, fever, or disease

4. Blood pressure
NCLEX® a. Measure annually in children over 3 years of age
b. Select cuff width that covers 75% of length of upper arm
c. Cuff should encircle arm circumference without overlapping
d. Use Doppler or electronic device for infants
e. May be altered by anxiety, activity, crying, medications, or disease

E. General appearance

1. Cumulative, subjective impression of a child's physical appearance, nutrition status, behavior, hygiene, personality, posture and body movement, interactions with parents and nurse, speech and development
2. Observe **facies** (facial expression and appearance) for clues about illness, pain, fear, and so on

Table 15-6 Normal Vital Signs for Infants and Children

Age	Pulse Rate Range	Respiratory Rate Range	Blood Pressure Range
Newborn	90–160	30–50	60–90/40–60
1–11 months	85–170	24–45	94–104/50–60
1–2 years	70–150	22–38	98–109/56–63
3–5 years	72–140	21–30	100–115/59–71
6–10 years	68–130	18–24	105–123/67–80
11–14 years	65–120	14–20	110–130/64–84
15 years and older	55–100	14–20	113–130/50–84

F. Skin, hair, and nails

1. Inspect and palpate
2. Skin: note color, texture, temperature, moisture, turgor, edema, rashes, or lesions
   a. **Mongolian spots**: bluish colored areas common on buttocks or lower back of dark-skinned infants; they disappear with age
   b. Storkbites, café au lait stains, or port-wine stains are common birthmarks
   NCLEX® c. Bruises in various stages or unusual locations or circular burn areas may indicate child abuse
   d. Acne vulgaris may be present in adolescents
3. Hair: observe for color, distribution, characteristics, quality, infestations, and texture
4. Nails: note color, texture, shape, and condition; clubbing frequently indicates pulmonary disease

G. Head, neck, and cervical lymph nodes

1. Inspect and palpate head, neck, and lymph nodes
2. Head: note shape and symmetry
   NCLEX® a. Anterior fontanel: closes by 12 to 18 months
   NCLEX® b. Posterior fontanel: closes by 2 months
   c. Infant should be able to hold head erect by 4 months of age
   d. Newborn skull may show molding from birth process or flattening from repeated lying in same position
   e. Note symmetry by having older child make faces
3. Neck and lymph nodes: note size, mobility, swelling, temperature, and tenderness
   a. Thyroid is difficult to palpate in infants because of thick neck
   b. Palpate submaxillary, sublingual, and parotid glands
   c. Observe trachea for midline placement
   d. Determine mobility of neck

H. Mouth, throat, nose, and sinuses

1. Inspect mouth, nose, and throat, and palpate sinuses
2. Mouth and throat
   a. Examine last in young children; is intrusive and may provoke fear
   b. Note tooth eruption, condition of gums, lips, teeth, palates, tonsils, tongue, and buccal mucosa
   NCLEX® c. Deciduous teeth erupt by about 6 months of age; all 20 appear by about 30 months
   NCLEX® d. Teeth begin to fall out at about 6 years when permanent teeth erupt; this progresses until all 32 teeth erupt by late adolescence
   e. Tonsils may normally be enlarged, atrophying to stable adult size by late adolescence
3. Nose and sinuses
   a. Inspect structure, patency of nares, discharge, tenderness, and any color or swelling of turbinates
   b. Percuss and palpate sinuses of children over age 3; sinuses of infants and young children not palpable

I. Eyes

1. Inspect external eye
   a. Note position, slant, epicanthal folds, eyelid placement, swelling, discharge, color of sclera and conjunctiva, redness, eyebrows, and lashes
   NCLEX® b. Epicanthal folds are normal in Asian children, suggestive of Down syndrome in others
   c. Outer canthus should be in line with tip of pinna
2. Visual acuity tests
   a. Include Snellen letter chart for school-age children, Snellen symbol chart (E chart) for preschool age, Faye symbol chart (pictures) for preschool age
   b. Visual acuity is difficult to assess in infants; test by observing infant's ability to fixate and follow objects
   c. Should be able to differentiate colors by 5 years
3. Extraocular muscle tests
   a. Cover-uncover test: cover one eye and have child look at object; observe uncovered eye for movement; remove cover and observe that eye for movement
   NCLEX® b. Eye movement during cover-uncover test may indicate **strabismus** (lack of eye muscle coordination), which can lead to **amblyopia** (blindness caused by weak eye muscle)
   c. Hirschberg test: shine light on cornea while child looks straight ahead; light should reflect symmetrically in center of both pupils
   d. Unequal reflection may indicate strabismus
4. Ophthalmoscopic examination
   a. Same procedure as for adults but save until last; may require restraint or distraction; done by primary care provider or advanced practice nurse

b. Expected finding: pupils equal, round, and reactive to light and accommodation (PERRLA); red reflex should be present

NCLEX® c. Permanent eye color by 9 months

J. Ears

1. Inspect and palpate external ear for placement, discharge, and lesions
2. Inspect internal ear with otoscope; done by advanced practice RN or health care provider
   a. Save until last; this usually requires restraint in infants and young children
   NCLEX® b. With infants, pull pinna down and back because canal is short and straight; with older child and adult, pull pinna upward and back
   c. Observe for **cerumen** (earwax), foreign bodies, or discharge
   d. Tympanic membrane should be pearly gray to light pink with landmarks visible
   NCLEX® e. Tympanic membranes redden during crying
   f. May assess mobility of tympanic membrane with pneumatic otoscope; tympanic membrane should move with pressure
3. Hearing acuity
   a. Tested in infants by noting reaction to loud noise
   b. Newborns exhibit Moro (startle) reflex and blink eyes
   c. Older children may be tested with whispered voice
   NCLEX® d. Audiometry testing of all children should be done before they enter school

K. Thorax and lungs

1. Inspect shape of thorax and respiratory rate, depth (deep or shallow), quality (effortless, difficult, or labored), and rhythm (regular or irregular)
2. Palpate and percuss lungs as described for adults; done by advanced practice RN or health care provider; hyperresonance is normal in infants and young children because of thin chest wall
3. Auscultate lungs
   NCLEX® a. Encourage deep breathing in children by having them blow a pinwheel, cotton ball, or other readily available object
   b. Breath sounds may seem louder or harsher because of thin chest wall
   c. Use bell and diaphragm of stethoscope to hear both low-and high-pitched sounds
   d. Evaluate breath sounds for noise, grunting, snoring, and so on
4. Inspect and palpate breasts
   a. Newborns may have enlarged or engorged breasts due to maternal hormones
   NCLEX® b. Breast exam and teaching of breast self-exam for adolescents

L. Heart

1. Inspect and palpate precordium for heaves and apical impulse
2. Perform early in exam because quiet child and environment are essential
   NCLEX® a. Apical pulse at 4th ICS until age 7; then apical pulse at 5th ICS after age 7
   b. Apical pulse to left of MCL until age 4; just lateral to left MCL from 4 to 6 years; and at left MCL by age 7
3. Auscultate heart sounds
   a. Rate (should be regular and same as radial pulse), rhythm (should be even and regular); note quality (should be clear, not muffled), and intensity (should not be heavy or pounding)
   NCLEX® b. Note that sinus arrhythmia (rate that speeds up with inspiration and slows with expiration) is common in children
   c. Evaluate for presence of murmurs
   d. Sounds are louder, higher pitched, and of shorter duration in infants and children

NCLEX® M. Abdomen

1. To promote relaxation and cooperation, have child place one hand beneath examiner's, use age-appropriate distraction, or use conversation focused on topic of interest to child; inspect shape
   a. Abdomen is prominent when standing and supine in infants and children until age 4; abdomen is somewhat prominent when standing but flat when supine after age 4
   b. Scaphoid abdomen indicates malnutrition or dehydration
   c. Umbilicus should be pink without redness or discharge
   d. Umbilical hernias fairly common, especially in African-American children
2. Auscultate bowel sounds in same manner as for adults
3. Palpate for masses or tenderness; principles are same as for adults; advanced practice nurses are more likely to do deep palpation to outine organs; palpate for inguinal or femoral hernias

N. Genitalia

1. May assist advanced practice RN or health care provider; always wear gloves during examination
2. Male
   a. Inspect penis and urinary meatus; foreskin should be retractable by 3 months
   b. Redness, discharge, or lacerations in young children may indicate abuse
   c. Inspect and palpate scrotum and testes to determine if both are descended
   d. In young children, testicle may withdraw into inguinal canal because of cremasteric reflex; block cremasteric reflex in infants by beginning palpation at inguinal ring and moving down to scrotum
   e. Check for inguinal hernias by having child blow or bear down
3. Female
   a. Inspect external genitalia for evidence of discharge or redness, which may indicate abuse in young children
   NCLEX® b. Internal examination for sexually active adolescents, or at age 16 to 18

O. Anus and rectum

1. Inspect for patency in infants
2. Skin should be smooth and free of lesions
3. Internal exam not done unless symptoms suggest a problem

P. Musculoskeletal

1. Inspect neck, extremities, hips, and spine for symmetry, increased or decreased mobility, and anatomical defects
   a. Extremities should be warm, mobile, with pulses strong and equal bilaterally
   NCLEX® b. Newborn's feet may be turned in but can be manipulated to normal position without resistance
   c. True deformities do not return to normal position with manipulation and include metatarsus varus (forefoot turned in), talipes varus (adduction of forefoot and inversion of entire foot), talipes equinovarus or clubfoot (adduction of forefoot, inversion of entire foot, and pointing downward of entire foot), medial tibial torsion (entire foot turned in while knee remains straight), medial femoral torsion (entire leg turned in with foot)
2. NCLEX® Examine for congenital hip dislocation until about 1 year of age
   a. Use Ortolani's maneuver (with infant supine, flex infant's knees while holding your thumbs on mid-thighs and fingers over greater trochanters; abduct legs, moving knees outward and down toward table); note click if dislocation present
   b. Use Barlow's maneuver (with infant supine, flex infant's knees while holding your thumbs on mid-thighs and fingers over greater trochanters; adduct legs until thumbs touch)
   c. Gluteal folds should be equal, hips abduct easily, and legs should be of same length
3. Examine spine and posture
   a. Newborn spine is flexible and rounded
   b. Cervical curve develops by 3–4 months; lumbar curve develops by 12–18 months
   c. Healthy toddler has **lordosis** (exaggerated curvature of lumbar spine)
   NCLEX® d. Check for **scoliosis** (lateral curvature of spine) in adolescent girls by looking at spine as child is bent over with knees straight
4. Examine gait, joints, and muscles
   a. Observe unobtrusively during history; joints should have full range of motion, and muscles should be equally strong bilaterally
   b. Toddlers have wide-based gait and are usually bowlegged
   c. Children ages 2 to 7 are often mildly knock-kneed
   NCLEX® d. Scissoring gait in which thighs cross over each other with each step is common in cerebral palsy

Q. Neurologic

1. Integrate into overall assessment as much as possible; assess child over 2 years the same as adult
2. Newborn and infant assessment
   a. Observe symmetry of spontaneous movements, appearance, positioning, posture, and responsiveness to parents and environment
   b. Observe level of consciousness, behavior, adaptation, and speech
3. Autonomic infant reflexes (see Table 15–7)
4. NCLEX® Presence of reflexes beyond expected times indicates CNS problem
5. Cranial nerves and deep tendon reflexes are same as for adults
6. NCLEX® Hand preference develops during preschool years

Table 15-7 Autonomic Infant Reflexes

Type of Reflex	Description
Rooting reflex	Touch infant's lip or cheek; infant should turn head toward stimulation and open mouth; should disappear by 3–4 months
Sucking reflex	Infant should suck vigorously when gloved finger inserted into mouth; disappears by 10–12 months
Palmar grasp reflex	Pressing fingers against palmar surface of infant's hand produces grasp strong enough to pull infant to sitting position; disappears by 3–4 months
Plantar grasp reflex	Touching ball of foot causes toes to curl downward tightly; disappears by 8–10 months
Tonic neck reflex	With infant supine, turn head to one side; arm and leg on side to which head is turned will extend and opposite extremities will flex; appears at about 2 months and disappears by 4–6 months
Moro (startle) reflex	Upon hearing a loud noise, infant flexes and abducts legs, laterally extends arms, forms a "C" with thumb and forefinger, and fans other fingers; is immediately followed by anterior flexion and adduction of arms; disappears by 3 months
Babinski reflex	While holding infant's foot, stroke up lateral edge across ball; positive reflex is fanning of toes; some infants have normal adult response of flexion of toes; either response should be symmetrical bilaterally; disappears within 2 years
Stepping reflex	Holding infant upright with support under arms, let feet touch a surface and infant appears to take steps in a walking motion; disappears by 2 months

7. Observe for "soft" neurologic signs, gray area between normal and abnormal, that may change with maturation
   a. Short attention span, easy distractibility
   b. Impulsiveness
   c. Poor coordination
   d. Language and articulation problems
   e. Problems with learning, especially reading, writing, and arithmetic

Check Your NCLEX-PN® Exam I.Q.

You are ready for testing on this content if you can

- Determine a client's perception of health.
- Describe expected physiological status based on age.
- Anticipate examiner's and age-related client's needs during a physical examination.
- Use critical thinking when interpreting data gathered during health history and physical examination.

PRACTICE TEST

1 While palpating a client's thorax, the nurse notes a crackling, popping noise under the skin. Upon auscultation, an additional finding is a sound similar to when hair is rubbed between the fingers. The nurse concludes that what problem is probably responsible for this finding?

1. Pneumocystis pneumonia
2. Pneumothorax
3. Hemothorax
4. Hemodilution

2 After checking the client's pupils with a penlight for reaction, roundness, symmetry, and accommodation, the nurse would document normal findings using which acceptable notation?

1. PARL
2. PERRLA
3. PRLE
4. PLRAE

3. The nurse would use which test to evaluate a client's motor ability and function as part of a neurological examination?
   1. Glasgow coma scale
   2. Abdominal reflex
   3. Babinski test
   4. Romberg test

4. The nurse notes unexpectedly during a routine screening examination that the client has a thready pulse. In what other way could this finding be documented?
   1. A 2+ pulse
   2. Pulse rate irregular and forceful
   3. Pulse difficult to palpate and easy to obliterate
   4. Pressure with the index finger causes pulsation

5. To assess the intensity of a client's pain during data collection, the nurse could ask the client to do which of the following?
   1. Identify the location.
   2. Rate the pain on a scale of 1 to 10.
   3. Identify the methods the client uses to control the pain.
   4. Disclose how long the pain has persisted.

6. The nurse would plan to do which of the following as a high priority during routine data collection regarding health?
   1. Reinforce client teaching about ways to maintain health and wellness.
   2. Identify all areas of pathology.
   3. Use humor if the client is anxious.
   4. Explore the client's family relationships.

7. When documenting data collection findings, the nurse should do which of the following?
   1. Wait until the client has left the area.
   2. Write the findings immediately on the appropriate form.
   3. Abbreviate the data whenever possible to save time.
   4. Ask the client to confirm that the documentation is accurate.

8. The nurse plans to do which of the following using the skill of inspection when performing data collection for an adult client?
   1. Use eyes, ears, and sense of smell to make observations.
   2. Look at one side of the body first, then the other.
   3. Leave all prepared supplies on a nearby table.
   4. Spend a significant amount of time completing this portion of the exam.

9. A client tells the nurse during the data collection, "I feel jumpy all over since using my new respiratory inhaler." Which question would be most appropriate for the nurse to ask next?
   1. "Do you also feel sweaty when this happens?"
   2. "Why are you using a respiratory inhaler?"
   3. "Can you tell me what you mean by jumpy?"
   4. "What helps you to get over this feeling?"

10. When asking a client newly admitted to the hospital about dietary habits, which question by the nurse would be most important?
    1. "What time of day do you eat each meal?"
    2. "Do you eat alone or with family members?"
    3. "How often do you eat meals at restaurants?"
    4. "Do you have any dietary restrictions?"

11. Which statement made during a client interview represents a value judgment by the nurse?
    1. "I think your weight loss of 50 pounds was beneficial to your health."
    2. "Why did you decide to stop taking your blood pressure pill?"
    3. "Can you tell me how many alcoholic drinks you have each night?"
    4. "How can you afford to smoke if you're currently unemployed?"

12. An older adult client has experienced Wernicke's aphasia following a cerebrovascular accident (CVA). The nurse performing data collection would expect the client to have difficulty with which activity?
    1. Reading the newspaper
    2. Reciting the alphabet
    3. Spelling his or her last name
    4. Chewing solid food

PRACTICE TEST

13 What information regarding the family history of an adult client is most important for the nurse to obtain during data collection?

1. Quality of emotional support provided by family
2. Dates of immunizations and vaccines received
3. Number and ages of client's siblings
4. Major diseases of close family members

14 When examining a preschool-age child's mouth, how many deciduous teeth should the nurse expect to find?

1. Up to 10
2. 11 to 15
3. 16 to 20
4. Up to 32

15 Which area is important for the nurse to examine in an infant that does not need to be examined in an older toddler?

1. Gag reflex
2. Nares
3. Head circumference
4. Tympanic membranes

16 When assisting in the examination of a child for strabismus, the nurse should expect which eye test will be used?

1. The Snellen eye chart
2. The cover-uncover test
3. An ophthalmoscope exam
4. Test of pupillary reaction

17 When interviewing a 7-year-old during a routine health visit, what question might the nurse ask the child that would help detect vision problems?

1. "How are you doing in school?"
2. "Do you have any problems seeing at night?"
3. "Do you have any problems with glare?"
4. "What color is your shirt?"

18 When listening to the apical pulse of a 10-year-old, the nurse notices that the heart rate varies with inspiration and expiration. The nurse concludes that which action is most appropriate?

1. Discuss a referral to a cardiologist for further workup.
2. Question the child about caffeine intake.
3. Do nothing, as this is a normal finding.
4. Schedule an electrocardiogram following the exam.

19 When preparing to measure the vital signs of an infant, the nurse should make a decision to use which sequence?

1. Measure temperature, pulse, and respirations at the end of the exam.
2. Measure respirations, pulse, and temperature in that order.
3. Measure vital signs after the infant becomes familiar with the nurse.
4. Measure blood pressure before other vital signs.

20 Which of the following would be of concern to the nurse when collecting data about the hearing of a 6-month-old?

1. Babbling quietly
2. Failure to say "da-da"
3. No response to interesting sounds
4. Absence of Moro reflex

21 When collecting data about a 1-month-old infant, the nurse finds a head circumference of 32 cm and a chest circumference of 30 cm. The nurse should draw which conclusion about this data?

1. Consider this normal.
2. Reevaluate the findings in 2 weeks.
3. Expect the chest circumference to be larger than the head circumference.
4. Report the finding to the physician.

22 When examining a 6-week-old infant, the nurse should plan on assessing the Moro reflex at what point in the examination?

1. At the very beginning of the exam
2. Before assessing vision
3. When the infant is sleeping
4. At the end of the exam

23 When inspecting the external auditory canal of a 2-year-old child, the nurse should pull the pinna in which direction? Select an arrow in the picture shown.

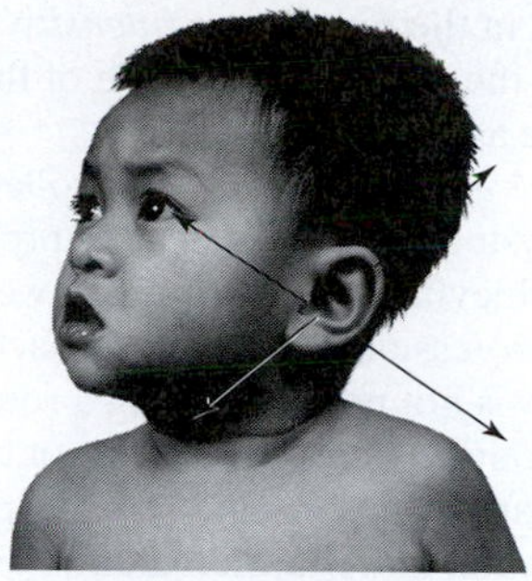

24 When preparing to examine a preschool child, the nurse should take which actions? Select all that apply.

1. Give detailed explanations to alleviate the child's anxiety.
2. Give reassurance and feedback to the child during the examination.
3. Suggest that the child act like "the big kids" when he or she is examined.
4. Say that the shirt is the only clothing that must be removed.
5. Ask if the child prefers to sit on the parent's lap to be examined.

25 The nurse is working in a well-child clinic and has been assigned to assist in data collection for five children ages 2 months, 3 years, 5 years, 8 years, and 13 years. Regardless of the child's age, which examination technique will the nurse always use first?

1. Palpation
2. Percussion
3. Auscultation
4. Inspection

ANSWERS & RATIONALES

1 **Answer: 2** **Rationale:** Subcutaneous emphysema or crepitus is caused by pneumothorax. This condition consists of air introduced into the tissue from another condition, such as pneumothorax. Pneumocystis pneumonia is an opportunistic infection often experienced by individuals who are HIV-positive; hemothorax refers to blood in the chest, and hemodilution is associated with fluid overload of the vascular system. **Cognitive Level:** Analyzing **Client Need:** Health Promotion and Maintenance **Integrated Process:** Nursing Process: Evaluation **Content Area:** Fundamentals **Strategy:** The core issue of the question is identification of subcutaneous emphysema and the ability to correlate this finding with common causes. Rely on knowledge of abnormal physical assessment findings and associated pathophysiological conditions to eliminate the incorrect options.

2 **Answer: 2** **Rationale:** The correct abbreviation for pupils that are equal, round, and responsive to light and accommodation is PERRLA. The other options represent incorrect abbreviations. It is important for nurses to document using agency-approved abbreviations to avoid misinterpretations and to enhance communication among caregivers. **Cognitive Level:** Applying **Client Need:** Health Promotion and Maintenance **Integrated Process:** Communication and Documentation **Content Area:** Fundamentals **Strategy:** Use knowledge of physical examination techniques of the eye to answer the question. Recall that the first observation is whether pupils are equal (symmetry), which will help you to choose the option that has an *E* near the beginning of the abbreviation.

3 **Answer: 4** **Rationale:** The Romberg test is done when the nurse asks the client to stand with eyes closed and feet together. There should be minimal swaying for up to 20 seconds. The Glasgow coma scale assesses the client's level of consciousness. The abdominal reflex, if absent, may indicate a disease of the upper and lower motor neurons. A positive Babinski test in adults indicates upper motor neuron disease of the pyramidal tract. **Cognitive Level:** Applying **Client Need:** Health Promotion and Maintenance **Integrated Process:** Nursing Process: Data Collection **Content Area:** Fundamentals **Strategy:** The core issue of the question is basic knowledge of physical examination techniques. Use this knowledge and the process of elimination to make a selection.

4 **Answer: 3** **Rationale:** A weak, thready pulse is one that is difficult to palpate and easily diminished by slight pressure. A 2+ pulse indicates one that is easily palpable and normal. A forceful pulse and a pulsation felt with pressure from the index finger may be labeled as *full* or *bounding*. **Cognitive Level:** Applying **Client Need:** Health Promotion and Maintenance **Integrated Process:** Nursing Process: Implementation **Content Area:** Fundamentals **Strategy:** The core issue of this question is knowledge of how to document an abnormal finding in a clear and objective manner. First eliminate +2 pulse, which is a normal finding. Use the process of elimination to select the option that most clearly matches the data in the question.

5 **Answer: 2** **Rationale:** The nurse seeks to identify the intensity of the pain by asking the client to rate the pain on a scale of 1 to 10, with 1 indicating a slight nagging pain and 10 indicating an excruciating pain. Some of the other components of data collection about pain would include the location, duration, and methods that the client has used to control the pain (also called alleviating factors). **Cognitive Level:** Applying **Client Need:** Health Promotion and Maintenance **Integrated Process:** Nursing Process: Data Collection **Content Area:** Fundamentals

Strategy: The critical word in the question is *intensity*. Correlate this word with the degree or strength of the pain to choose the rating scale as the answer.

6 **Answer: 1** **Rationale:** As the nurse performs data collection and focuses on various systems, time can be spent reinforcing information about achieving and maintaining wellness. The nurse should use a professional, caring approach. An in-depth focus on pathology is not needed during a routine screening. The focus of routine examinations is not to explore client–family relationships. **Cognitive Level:** Applying **Client Need:** Health Promotion and Maintenance **Integrated Process:** Nursing Process: Data Collection **Content Area:** Fundamentals **Strategy:** Note the critical words *high priority.* This means that some or all options may be partially or totally correct, and you must choose the most important item. Note also the critical word *routine*, which implies the client is healthy. With this in mind, the highest priority is to maintain and promote health and wellness.

7 **Answer: 2** **Rationale:** The information obtained during data collection should be documented in the client's medical record in a timely manner. If the nurse does not write the information down, the data could be forgotten or omitted from the record. The nurse should not wait until the client has left the area to document information unless there is an emergency. Standard abbreviations should be used in the chart in order to promote clarity and avoid errors when the information is accessed by others. Asking the client to review the documentation is not required; however, it is important to clarify the health assessment information as it is gathered. **Cognitive Level:** Applying **Client Need:** Health Promotion and Maintenance **Integrated Process:** Nursing Process: Data Collection **Content Area:** Fundamentals **Strategy:** The wording of the question tells you the correct answer is a true statement. Use the process of elimination, recalling that prompt documentation helps prevent omissions and errors at a later time.

8 **Answer: 1** **Rationale:** Inspection of a client can offer many clues about the overall state of health and can include all data gathered through the senses. The nurse should compare each side of the body for symmetry prior to inspecting the next system. Equipment such as a penlight or tape measure can be used during inspection but does not necessarily need to be prepared ahead of time. The time required depends on the client's condition and the nurse's skill level. **Cognitive Level:** Applying **Client Need:** Health Promotion and Maintenance **Integrated Process:** Nursing Process: Data Collection **Content Area:** Fundamentals **Strategy:** The core issue of the question is the skill of inspection. Choose the option that reflects principles of visual data collection.

9 **Answer: 3** **Rationale:** The nurse should use the communication technique of clarifying to fully understand the client's subjective complaint. After understanding the client's perception of this side effect, the other questions would be appropriate. **Cognitive Level:** Analyzing **Client Need:** Health Promotion and Maintenance **Integrated Process:** Communication and Documentation **Content Area:** Fundamentals **Strategy:** The core issue of this question is appropriate use of therapeutic communication techniques. Note the word *next* in the question that tells you that all questions may be asked, but one is more important to determine first. With this in mind, choose the option that obtains more information about the client's symptom.

10 **Answer: 4** **Rationale:** The client may have restrictions based on a medical condition (e.g., low-sodium for heart disease), food allergies (e.g., shellfish), or religious convictions (e.g., abstaining from pork if Jewish or Muslim). The nurse must note these restrictions and communicate with the nursing and dietary staff in order to avoid a potentially harmful occurrence. The other questions are pertinent for a dietary history but would not lead to a physiologic alteration if changed while hospitalized. **Cognitive Level:** Analyzing **Client Need:** Health Promotion and Maintenance **Integrated Process:** Nursing Process: Data Collection **Content Area:** Fundamentals **Strategy:** Note the critical words in the question are *dietary history* and *most important.* These tell you that the answer is the option that has a high priority, although some or all of the questions may be asked of the client. Select the option that impacts the diet the client will receive in the hospital. The others could be asked based on need or as the basis for later dietary teaching.

11 **Answer: 4** **Rationale:** How a client spends income, even on an unhealthy habit, is not necessary for the nurse to know in order to provide effective care; the statement represents a value judgment on the part of the nurse. It is considered appropriate in an interview for the nurse to provide acknowledgment and positive reinforcement for a lifestyle change that resulted in a potentially improved health status. Inquiring about a client's reason for discontinuing a medication regime would be common question to inquire about a client's behavior. Inquiring about a client's intake of alcoholic beverages would be common inquiry regarding a client's behavior. **Cognitive Level:** Analyzing **Client Need:** Health Promotion and Maintenance **Integrated Process:** Communication and Documentation **Content Area:** Fundamentals **Strategy:** The core issue of the question is communication techniques that force the nurse's values on the client and thus reduce the likelihood of open communication between client and nurse. Imagine you are the client and choose the option that is most likely to have an adverse effect on your willingness to communicate with the nurse.

12 **Answer: 1** **Rationale:** Wernicke's aphasia is the inability to understand verbal or written words. Impairment is located in the posterior speech cortex in the temporal and parietal lobes. Based on the information provided, the client should be able to speak, spell, and eat with this type of neurological deficit. **Cognitive Level:** Applying **Client Need:** Health Promotion and Maintenance **Integrated Process:** Nursing Process: Data Collection **Content Area:** Fundamentals **Strategy:** Specific knowledge of the types of aphasia is needed to answer this question. Use nursing knowledge and the process of elimination to make a selection.

13 **Answer: 4** **Rationale:** Major diseases such as diabetes, hypertension, arteriosclerosis, and cancer often have a genetic disposition and put the client at greater risk for developing them. The number and ages of siblings is a component of the family history, as well as inquiring about the client's support network. Vaccines and immunizations would be covered in the section known as past history. **Cognitive Level:** Applying **Client Need:** Health Promotion and Maintenance **Integrated Process:** Nursing Process: Data Collection **Content Area:** Fundamentals **Strategy:** Note the words *most important* in the question. This indicates that some or all options are data that you might wish to obtain but you must prioritize to choose the most essential piece of data. First eliminate immunization status because it does not relate to the family. Choose family history of diseases over emotional support and numbers and ages of family members because it has the greatest potential impact on physiological health status.

14 **Answer: 3** **Rationale:** Children get the first of 20 deciduous teeth between the ages of 6 months and 5 years. Permanent teeth begin to erupt about the age of 6 as deciduous teeth fall out. All 32 permanent teeth are usually erupted by late adolescence. **Cognitive Level:** Applying **Client Need:** Health Promotion and Maintenance **Integrated Process:** Nursing Process: Data Collection **Content Area:** Fundamentals **Strategy:** Specific knowledge of physical growth and development is needed to answer this question. Use nursing knowledge and the process of elimination to make a selection.

15 **Answer: 3** **Rationale:** The single most important measure of brain growth in infants is head circumference, so it should be measured at every health visit. It is equally important to assess the gag reflex in an infant and a toddler. Inspection of the nares should be performed, but it is not more important in an infant than in a toddler. It is equally important to examine the tympanic membranes of an infant and a toddler. **Cognitive Level:** Applying **Client Need:** Health Promotion and Maintenance **Integrated Process:** Nursing Process: Data Collection **Content Area:** Fundamentals **Strategy:** The core issue of the question is determining an assessment that discriminates between infants and older toddlers. Use specific knowledge of infant and toddler physical growth and development and the process of elimination to make a selection. Recall that in infants the anterior and posterior fontanels close at specific times. Then recall that while one or both fontanels are open, head circumference could increase beyond normal growth if there is a problem with cerebrospinal fluid production. Once closed (as with toddlers), this data is not useful for this purpose.

16 **Answer: 2** **Rationale:** The cover-uncover test assesses coordination of eye muscle movement. In strabismus, one muscle is weaker and the eye wanders rather than focusing forward. Undetected and untreated strabismus can lead to amblyopia. A Snellen eye chart is used to determine visual acuity. An ophthalmoscopic exam detects problems with interior structures of the eye. Pupillary reaction is the ability of the pupils to constrict in response to light. **Cognitive Level:** Applying **Client Need:** Health Promotion and Maintenance **Integrated Process:** Nursing Process: Data Collection **Content Area:** Fundamentals **Strategy:** The core issue of the question is assessment of strabismus. Use specific knowledge of physical examination procedures and the process of elimination to make a selection.

17 **Answer: 1** **Rationale:** By the time a child is 7 years old, the nurse can appropriately ask questions of the child. Problems in school could be a sign of vision issues and warrants a thorough visual assessment. A 7-year-old would not be expected to have problems with night vision. A 7-year-old would not be expected to have problems with a glare. A 7-year-old should know colors. **Cognitive Level:** Analyzing **Client Need:** Health Promotion and Maintenance **Integrated Process:** Nursing Process: Data Collection **Content Area:** Fundamentals **Strategy:** Note the critical words in the question are *vision problems*. Recall that children are more likely to have myopia (nearsightedness) than problems with night vision or glare. The child may be having problems in school due to a reduced ability to read a blackboard or other materials in the classroom.

18 **Answer: 3** **Rationale:** An irregular heart rate that increases with inspiration and decreases with expiration is a sinus arrhythmia, which is common in children. It requires no action on the part of the nurse. Further evaluation is not necessary, and an assessment of caffeine (such as in carbonated beverages) is not indicated. **Cognitive Level:** Analyzing **Client Need:** Health Promotion and Maintenance **Integrated Process:** Nursing Process: Implementation **Content Area:** Fundamentals **Strategy:** Note that a core issue of the question is the age of the child, which is 10 years. With this in mind, correlate the heart sounds described with normal growth and development findings. After determining that this is a normal finding, eliminate each of the incorrect options.

19 **Answer: 2** **Rationale:** Vital signs in an infant are best taken when the infant is quiet early in the exam. Counting respirations by observing the abdomen is least intrusive, followed by the heart rate and temperature. **Cognitive Level:** Analyzing **Client Need:** Health Promotion and Maintenance **Integrated Process:** Nursing Process: Data Collection **Content Area:** Fundamentals **Strategy:** Note that the client in the question is an infant. Recall that vital signs may be affected by activity such as crying. With this in mind, select the order or sequence that creates minimal disturbance for the infant.

20 **Answer: 3** **Rationale:** A 6-month-old should be able to babble as well as localize sounds by turning head toward sounds. Failure to turn toward sound is an indication that further hearing assessment is necessary. A 6-month-old should be able to babble; this is not an issue of concern. A 6-month-old should be able to babble, but an infant that young would not be forming words yet. The Moro reflex should not be present in a 6-month-old. **Cognitive Level:** Analyzing **Client Need:** Health Promotion and Maintenance **Integrated Process:** Nursing Process: Data Collection **Content Area:** Fundamentals **Strategy:** Note the key word *concern* in the question. This tells you the correct answer is an option that contains a questionable or abnormal finding. Use knowledge of growth and development and physical assessment techniques to make a selection.

21 **Answer: 1** **Rationale:** The normal head circumference of a full-term infant is 32 to 38 cm, about 2 cm greater than the chest circumference. In the toddler, both measures are about equal; after the age of 2, the chest circumference exceeds that of the head. **Cognitive Level:** Analyzing **Client Need:** Health Promotion and Maintenance **Integrated Process:** Nursing Process: Data Collection **Content Area:** Fundamentals **Strategy:** Use specific knowledge of growth and development of the infant to systematically eliminate incorrect options. Recall that the measurements "cross over" at about age 2 when the head becomes smaller in circumference than the chest.

22 **Answer: 4** **Rationale:** The Moro reflex is also known as the startle reflex, and it may cause the infant to cry. For this reason, it should be performed at the end of the exam. The Moro reflex is also known as the startle reflex and it may cause the infant to cry. This timing may make the remaining physical assessment difficult or impossible. The vision of an infant is assessed by the infant's ability to fixate on and follow a moving object; crying would interfere with data collection about vision. Startling a sleeping infant will cause the infant to cry and decrease the ability for the nurse to complete additional parts of the examination. **Cognitive Level:** Applying **Client Need:** Health Promotion and Maintenance **Integrated Process:** Nursing Process: Data Collection **Content Area:** Fundamentals **Strategy:** Use basic knowledge of infant responses and specific knowledge of the Moro reflex to systematically eliminate each of the incorrect options.

23 Answer:

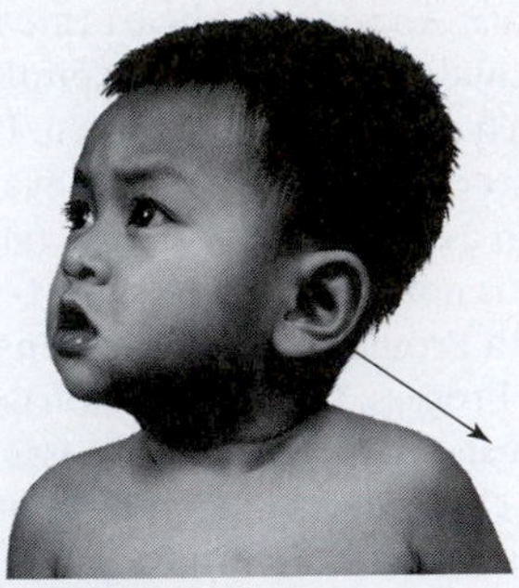

Rationale: The ear canal in infants and young children is shorter, wider, and more horizontally positioned than in older children. To adequately examine the external auditory canals of young children, the pinna must be pulled back and down. **Cognitive Level:** Applying **Client Need:** Health Promotion and Maintenance **Integrated Process:** Nursing Process: Data Collection **Content Area:** Child Health **Strategy:** Critical words are *external auditory canal* and *2-year-old.* Recall normal anatomy and physiology of the ear canal to answer the question correctly.

24 Answer: 2, 5 Rationale: Because the preschooler may be somewhat anxious, the nurse should give feedback and reassurance about what will be done. Younger children often prefer to sit on the parent's lap to be examined. Children do not need detailed explanations nor do they need to be told to act older than they are. Most children at this age are willing to remove clothing. **Cognitive Level:** Applying **Client Need:** Health Promotion and Maintenance **Integrated Process:** Nursing Process: Implementation **Content Area:** Child Health **Strategy:** Critical words are to *examine a preschool child.* Use knowledge of physical assessment of the preschooler to make a selection.

25 Answer: 4 Rationale: Inspection, or observation, is always done before proceeding with other techniques of physical assessment. It is the least intrusive method of assessment. Palpation is the most invasive method of assessment and should be performed last. Percussion is performed after inspection and auscultation; performing it earlier my result in auscultation findings related to physical stimulation. Percussion is not usually performed by licensed practical/vocational nurses (LPN/LVNs). Auscultation is the second step of physical assessment, following inspection. **Cognitive Level:** Applying **Client Need:** Health Promotion and Maintenance **Integrated Process:** Nursing Process: Data Collection **Content Area:** Child Health **Strategy:** The stem of the question indicates that all the techniques will be used. Recall that assessment will be easier if the child cooperates with the examiner. Therefore, consider which technique would be least intrusive to use first.

Key Terms to Review

amblyopia p. 195
auscultation p. 185
cerumen p. 196
facies p. 194
fremitus p. 188
genogram p. 183
health history p. 179
inspection p. 184
lordosis p. 197
Mongolian spots p. 195
objective data p. 181
palpation p. 184
percussion p. 185
scoliosis p. 197
strabismus p. 195
subjective data p. 179

References

Berman, A., & Snyder, S. (2012). *Kozier & Erb's fundamentals of nursing: Concepts, process, and practice* (9th ed.). Upper Saddle River, NJ: Pearson Education, Inc.

D'Amico, D., & Barbarito, C. (2012). *Health & physical assessment in nursing* (2nd ed.). Upper Saddle River, NJ: Pearson Education, Inc.

Jarvis, C. (2011). *Physical examination & health assessment* (6th ed). St. Louis, MO: Elsevier Science.

Test Yourself

Are you ready for the NCLEX-PN® or course exams? Use the practice tests on the companion website to check.

Promoting Healthy Lifestyle Choices

16

In this chapter

Cross Reference

Another chapter relevant to this content area is
Meeting Nutritional Needs Chapter 25

I. SUN EXPOSURE AND SKIN INTEGRITY

A. Sun exposure damages skin

NCLEX® 1. Most harmful ultraviolet rays occur between 10 a.m. and 4 p.m.
2. Whether sunny or overcast, daylight allows damaging rays to affect skin
3. Ultraviolet rays can penetrate loosely woven fabrics and harm skin
4. Individuals who are outside almost daily are particularly at risk for sun damage to skin: farmers, carpenters, fishermen, golfers
5. Exposure to chemicals may increase risk of skin damage: miners, asbestos and arsenic workers

B. Important points in health education to prevent skin cancer

1. Babies and children under age 6 and those with light complexion are at highest risk for skin damage
2. Immunosuppressed clients have increased risk for skin cancers
3. There is a genetic link to melanoma
4. Limit sun exposure during middle of day
NCLEX® 5. Use sunscreen with solar protection factor (SPF) of 15 and higher
NCLEX® 6. Apply sunscreen 30 minutes before sun exposure and reapply every 2 to 3 hours thereafter while outside
7. Daily use of sunscreen on exposed face, ears, and hands decreases risk
8. Wide-brimmed hats offer extra protection to head and neck
9. Apply sunscreen liberally to scarred skin, which is more vulnerable to damage
10. Preventing severe sunburns in early childhood is key to reducing risk of skin cancer later in life
11. Skin cancers can occur and recur in any age adult, so inspect bare skin, using two mirrors to inspect front and back of body to allow for early discovery

II. BREAST SELF-EXAMINATION

A. General concepts

1. Both men and women can get breast cancer
2. It is important to perform breast self-examination (BSE) monthly (both males and females)
3. Clients need to see health care provider for regular check-ups

NCLEX® 4. Women over age 40 need annual mammography testing
NCLEX® 5. Females should begin BSE at time of first gynecological exam, about age 18 or 20
6. Nurse's role is pivotal in educating females and males that BSE is important

NCLEX® **B. Procedure**

1. Focus on palpating consistency of breast tissue
2. Perform procedure 5 to 7 days after menses for female; for men and postmenopausal women, perform exam on same day of each month; associate it with a specific date, such as the first of month
3. Look at breasts in mirror, arms by side, over head, and on hips
4. Lie down and palpate each breast with opposite hand while other arm is under head, flattening out breast tissue
5. Palpate under axilla as well as nipple region (both males and females)
6. Feel breasts by pressing tissue firmly against chest wall, each region from outer to inner, with a circular or "corn-rows" approach
7. Once a baseline of "normal" is felt, each client will better understand changes to report to practitioner; report changes from personal baseline immediately for further evaluation
8. Menses, breastfeeding, and pregnancy enlarge the breast tissue naturally, and tissue feels more lobular
9. Clients who have cysts in breasts must carefully perform BSE to detect changes from personal baseline, which need to be reported

III. TESTICULAR SELF-EXAMINATION

A. General concepts

1. Males most at risk for testicular cancer are under age 40
2. Normal testicle is smooth and uniform in consistency
3. One testis is often larger and hangs lower in scrotum

NCLEX® **B. Procedure**

1. Once monthly, males should perform testicular self-examination (TSE), preferably during a warm shower when testicles are relaxed and may be soapy
2. Using one hand to displace penis, grasp testis with dominant hand, placing fingers beneath and thumb on top of testis to palpate it
3. Roll gently between thumb and fingers, feeling for any abnormality
4. Palpate testis, epididymis, and spermatic cord on each side
5. Report any nodules or lumps to health care provider as soon as possible
6. Report symptoms of testicular swelling, painless testicular swelling, or dragging sensation in scrotum (NCLEX®)

IV. EXERCISE

NCLEX® **A. Introduction**

1. Regular **aerobic exercise**, such as walking, jogging, or cycling, on most days of the week, is important to cardiovascular, respiratory, and musculoskeletal systems
2. Aerobic exercise is rhythmic, uses major muscle groups, and is maintained for 20 to 30 minutes or more

Memory Aid

Choose aerobic exercise over other forms when the goal is general health, because it increases circulation and respiration and burns calories for better weight control.

B. Client can monitor most appropriate level of exercise by monitoring pulse and speaking ability

1. Exercise is too vigorous if individual cannot speak without breathlessness
2. Exercising to specific target heart rates may be prescribed as part of a health-promoting exercise plan
3. To calculate target heart rate, first determine maximum heart rate by subtracting client's age from 220; then calculate target heart rate by subtracting client's resting heart rate from his or her maximum heart rate

C. Principles for instruction in exercise to promote good health and deter progressive complications of heart and musculoskeletal diseases

NCLEX® 1. Fast walking to target heart rate is an effective aerobic exercise that strengthens all muscles (including heart) and keeps bones strong, with less stress on knees than jogging
2. Inability to talk due to shortness of breath can mean excessively strenuous exercise
3. Current Centers for Disease Control and Prevention (CDC) 2008 Physical Activity Guidelines for Americans recommend for adults exercising with moderate intensity for 30 minutes or more five times

weekly (150 minutes); muscle strengthening activities (that work all major muscle groups) should also be done twice weekly

4. Whenever teaching parents of young children, stress importance of regular exercise as a lifelong habit
5. Children ages 6 to 17 should exercise for at least 60 minutes daily with most time being for aerobic activity; muscle strengthening (gymnastics, push-ups) and bone strengthening (jumping rope, running) activities should also be done three times per week as part of 60 minutes of activity
6. Walking or weight-bearing exercises help to prevent osteoporosis by increasing force exerted on long bones
7. *NCLEX®* Anyone with a chronic illness such as diabetes or hypertension should consult a health care provider before beginning a rigorous exercise routine
8. Cautions for clients with health problems should include: start slowly, monitor body's response to exercise, and take medication and fluids before exercise

V. NUTRITION

A. General concepts

1. Nutrition is an essential parameter of health and helps prevent some diseases and their complications
2. Nutritional intake is foundational for body's building up, growth, and all healing processes
3. A balanced diet for adults and children consists of protein, carbohydrates, and fruits and vegetables, with little fat

> **Memory Aid**
> To easily remember the components of a balanced diet, visualize a lunch plate divided into quadrants (fourths). Put fruits and vegetables in two, protein in one, and complex carbohydrates in one. Add milk and the meal is balanced!

4. *NCLEX®* 6 ounces of grains, 2.5 cups vegetables, 2 cups fruit, 3 cups milk products, and 5.5 ounces of meat and beans are recommended for adults daily in MyPyramid
5. Eating a variety of foods helps ensure all essential vitamins and nutrients in a balanced proportion
6. *NCLEX®* Sodium intake should be limited to 2 grams daily
   a. Cooking with other seasonings such as lemon, liquid smoke, pepper, and other spices helps to limit sodium intake
   b. Limit salt to what is naturally found in foods, especially for clients with hypertension or cardiac and renal disease
   c. Canned vegetables, soups, and tomato sauces may contain almost one gram sodium per serving
   d. Do not assume that salt substitutes are acceptable; these are often high in potassium, which could be contraindicated for clients with renal disease or who take potassium-sparing diuretics; clients should consult health care provider before using them
7. Fresh and frozen vegetables and fruit have more available nutrients than canned and highly processed foods
8. Color indicates freshness and usually more available nutrients, so recommend undercooking and retaining color, not overcooking vegetables
9. See also Chapter 25 for detailed information about nutritional needs of clients

B. Principles to guide nutrition instructions for disease prevention

1. *NCLEX®* Heart-healthy eating refers to consuming a low-fat, low-sugar, and balanced diet, which includes more than five fruits and vegetables daily and limits red meats
2. The ADA diet is recommended for clients with diabetes or with hypoglycemia because it controls insulin release by limiting glucose
3. Quickly accessible foods usually have more fat and sugar than adults can use in a day, and they add excess calories, which becomes fat
4. Sweets, like fats, should be limited in quantity for all ages; sugary foods provide ready glucose, increase insulin production, but do not sustain the body's energy
5. *NCLEX®* Vegetarians may choose to eat dairy products; strict vegetarians may not eat any eggs, cheese, or dairy products; alternative protein sources include soy milk, tofu, dry beans, and nuts; watch for vitamin B_{12} deficiency in those who avoid all meats
6. *NCLEX®* Many colorful orange and green vegetables have vitamins A, C, D, E, and K and serve as anti-aging antioxidants to body cells, especially skin
7. Eating leafy green vegetables interferes with anticoagulant therapy by increasing vitamins D or K

8. Eating more frequent and smaller meals or snacks, such as three meals and two snacks, is healthier for most adults than eating three large meals
9. NCLEX® Water is needed to move nutrients through and flush waste products from body; about 8 glasses daily promotes hydration, prevents constipation, and aids in digestion; as a general rule, drink 1 milliliter (mL) for each calorie consumed, so for a 2000 calorie diet, drink at least 2000 mL water daily
10. Folic acid is an important element to childbearing-aged female
11. NCLEX® Extra iron is needed during pregnancy and usually is added in a daily vitamin
12. NCLEX® Females need additional calcium after menopause
13. NCLEX® Daily calcium intake is important, especially for women and children; calcium is essential for bone growth; women who are prone to osteoporosis should supplement with 1500 milligrams daily, including vitamin D for uptake of calcium
14. Foods high in calcium include dairy products, green vegetables, salmon canned with bones, sardines, tofu, and molasses

C. See also Chapter 25 for additional information on meeting client's nutritional needs

VI. ALTERNATIVE HEALTH CARE PRACTICES

A. General concepts

1. Herbs should be used with medical supervision
2. Alternative and homeopathic health care practices can help relieve symptoms and aid healing with guidance from a trained nurse practitioner or holistic medical provider
3. Caution clients not to abandon traditional prescription medicines or replace medicines with herbs without guidance and monitoring of a physician or nurse practitioner
4. NCLEX® Individuals taking warfarin (Coumadin) or any other anticoagulants must avoid use of over-the-counter herbs such as garlic, ginseng, ginger, primrose oil, dong quai, and grape seed extract because of interactive effects
5. Certain vitamins—A, D, E, K—are fat-soluble and require healthy liver function to use; otherwise toxicity can result

B. Summary of specific key points

1. Echinacea is used to increase immunity and to treat colds and infections, but it is not intended or effective for daily use over long periods of time; persons with AIDS, lupus, arthritis, or any autoimmune disorders should not take echinacea
2. Individuals need to consult practitioners before adding herbal supplements such as St. John's wort to treat depression when already on prescription medications; such therapy is generally contraindicated
3. NCLEX® Ginseng and ginkgo are commonly taken by those who wish to improve cognition, and both cause drug interactions; monitor clients who take these herbs regularly for drug interactions, cross-toxicity, and altered bleeding times

VII. HEALTH SCREENING

A. Overview

1. Routine health screenings are recommended for early detection of disease; in addition, health screenings provide an opportunity to do health-related preventive teaching
2. NCLEX® General guidelines for health screenings for adults are presented in Table 16–1 and for children in Table 16–2

B. Specific points related to health screening

1. Children should be screened at least annually for first 6 years of life; nurses can monitor growth patterns, emotional and social skills, and motor and sensory (eye and ear) functions during routine physical exams and interactions with child and parent or caregiver
2. Premature infants need screening exams for deficits earlier and are more likely to experience developmental delays and motor and visual deficits
3. At age 4, arrange for child to begin 6-month dental checks and to have a baseline eye exam
4. The Denver Development Assessment is commonly used annually from infancy to age 6
5. NCLEX® Height and weight are charted annually and serve as screening for obesity
6. If muscle function, vision, or hearing is abnormal, exams may be done during infancy and several times yearly for follow-up and interventions
7. NCLEX® Hemoglobin assessment at any age is a common screening blood test for nutrition and general health
8. A complete blood count (CBC) gives information about development of all blood cells

Table 16–1 Unified Screening Recommendations for Adults*

Target Group	Type of Screening	Beginning Age	Frequency
Men and Women	Blood pressure measurement	20	Each regular health care visit, at least every 2 years
	Body mass index (BMI) measurement	20	Each regular health care visit
	Blood cholesterol test	20	At least every 5 years
	Blood glucose (sugar) test	45	Every 3 years
	Colorectal screening	50	Every 1 to 10 years depending on test used
Women	Clinical breast exam (CBE)	20	Every 3 years; yearly after age 40; may be modified by individual provider according to risk
	Mammography	40	Yearly
	Papanicolaou test	20	Yearly
		30	Every 1 to 3 years, depending on test used and individual risk
Men	Prostate-specific antigen (PSA) test and digital rectal exam	50	Variable according to individual risk and pros and cons of testing

*Developed collaboratively by the American Cancer Society, American Diabetes Association, and American Heart Association

Source: Adapted from information at http://www.everydaychoices.org/downloadables/pdf/screenings_acs_ada_aha.pdf

Table 16–2 Health Screening Recommendations for Children*

Type of Health Screening	Frequency
Well-child exam	Birth, 1, 2, 4, 6, 9, 12, and 15–18 months, age 2, 3, 4, 5, 6, 8, and annually age 10 to 21 years
Blood pressure	Age 3, 4, 5, 6, 8, and annually age 10 to 21 years
Vision	Age 3, 4, 5, 6, 8, 10, 12, 15 years
Hearing	Age 4, 5, 6, 8, 10, 12, 15 years
Hereditary metabolic screening	Birth to 1 month
Lead screening	As needed
Hemoglobin and hematocrit	12 months and as indicated; may be annually for females during adolescence
Urinalysis	Age 5, in adolescence, and when indicated

*Summary of recommendations from U.S. Preventative Services Task Force, American Academy of Pediatrics, American Academy of Family Physicians, and Centers for Disease Control and Prevention

9. Urinalysis and blood glucose testing is advised for obese children
10. Adolescents need to be screened for sexually transmitted infection if sexually active
11. Other health screening to include for adolescents: blood pressure (BP), heart murmurs, Pap smears for females who are sexually active, testicular exams for males, eyes, dental, hemoglobin testing
12. *NCLEX®* Height and weight should be documented annually for adolescents, and they should be monitored for obesity or anorexia
13. Chest x-rays may be necessary for smokers to establish lung function
14. Young adults who are college-bound (especially 20 to 30 years of age) need to continue with updating immunizations: tetanus, hepatitis, meningitis, tuberculosis and possibly pertussis; contact with larger numbers of people and possibly more crowded living conditions increases risk
15. Screenings for young adults include Pap smears for abnormal cell growth, height and weight to monitor for obesity, blood testing for normal blood cells and glucose, BP, chest x-rays, and female mammograms
16. *NCLEX®* Adults over age 40 need to have annual screenings or self-exams to detect heart disease, cancer, hypertension, or risks for other chronic diseases such as diabetes

17. If at higher than normal risk for breast or colon cancer, begin annual screening exams earlier than for general population and adhere to recommended frequency of exam
18. If at average risk and over 40, screen for cancer every 2 years with mammograms, and at every visit check feces for occult blood; consider a colon or sigmoid endoscopy exam every 5 years for polyps leading to colon cancer as recommended by health care provider
19. After age 60, screening should address changes related to aging: skin changes, bone density and osteoporosis, height (decreases due to bone loss), motor function and balance
20. Emotional well-being should be addressed as retirement and lifestyle changes occur
21. Health screening throughout life should include
    a. Hearing, vision, and all sensory functions
    b. Safety for living and functioning in home/work environment
    c. Emotional adjustments to life stage and world surroundings
    d. Nutritional status, excess or deficits
    e. Ability to seek help and manage health; independence

VIII. GENETIC COUNSELING

A. *Prenatal genetic counseling*

1. In prenatal clinics, a common reason for genetic counseling referrals is an abnormal alpha-fetoprotein (AFP) or quadruple screening
2. As a neural tube defect, spina bifida usually results from a multifactorial inheritance
3. Down syndrome can be diagnosed with true genetic testing and amniocentesis, and genetic links determined, as can cleft lip and palate
4. Marfan syndrome, sickle cell disease, and heart murmurs can be diagnosed and other family members tested, with follow-up counseling for future family planning

B. Nurses' role in genetic counseling

1. Consider total picture of health and well-being, not merely risks of a genetic disorder
2. Be aware that new information about genetic predispositions may be unwelcome or rejected at first
3. Ask for written permission to share and communicate information with spouse and other providers
4. Coordinate genetic health care with relevant community and national support resources
5. *NCLEX®* Offer support to clients and families throughout genetic counseling process

C. Role of heredity in child- and adult-onset health problems

1. Cancer, heart disease, and diabetes can be assessed as having familial or genetic tendencies
2. Certain eye diseases that lead to blindness and brain dementia can also be linked to genetic traits

Check Your NCLEX–PN® Exam I.Q. *You are ready for testing on this content if you can*

- Identify health-promotion activities for individuals relative to nutrition and exercise.
- Describe risks, screening, and prevention measures for skin cancer, breast cancer, and testicular cancer.
- Explain commonly used herbal remedies and alternative therapies.
- Utilize health education principles that guide client teaching about health management.

PRACTICE TEST

1 When discharging a client on oral anticoagulant therapy, the nurse would further reinforce teaching for the client who has a lifestyle that includes which of the following?

1. Growing green vegetables
2. Walking one mile a day
3. Living in a rural setting
4. Spending most of the time alone

2 The nurse is most concerned with reinforcing teaching for the client with diabetes who does which of the following?

1. Drinks orange juice each morning
2. Eats an apple and cheese before going to bed
3. Buys canned fruit instead of fresh because it is cheaper
4. Eats six meals per day

3 The nurse explains to a client who has had six teeth removed that he will likely be allowed to have which foods on the first postoperative day?

1. Sausage and biscuits
2. French toast and eggs
3. Milkshakes and cream of tomato soup
4. Gelatin and clear broth

4 When the nurse collects data about the intake of a vegetarian client's health and dietary patterns, which finding does the nurse conclude is most likely to negatively affect health status?

1. Use of vitamin B_{12} supplements
2. Intake of milk and dairy products
3. Genetic tendency toward lactose intolerance
4. Reports of problems with vision

5 Which of the following clients is most at risk for skin cancer?

1. An 80-year-old farmer who wears a cap when working
2. A 20-year-old lifeguard at the lake who wears sunscreen
3. A baby underneath a large beach umbrella
4. A teenager who wears a ski outfit when skiing

6 During a health fair at a public recreational park, the nurse providing cancer health risk information answers several questions for clients who use ultraviolet light tanning salons. Which piece of information is most important to include?

1. Tanning from ultraviolet light is safer than sunshine.
2. Skin damage from ultraviolet light is more likely than from indirect sunlight.
3. Using sunscreen will prevent skin cancers, even in tanning beds.
4. Using tanning beds without clothing contaminates skin and leads to infections.

7 When giving postoperative care to a 30-year-old male client, the nurse discusses cancer risks. The client states, "I have never heard of testicular exams." The nurse should include which priority intervention in the plan of care?

1. Explain that the client should see a physician for a yearly testicular examination.
2. Assist the client to set up a calendar of dates to perform self-testicular exams.
3. Allow the client to verbalize fears related to cancer risk.
4. Encourage a high-fiber diet to decrease the risk of testicular cancer.

8 When a client comes into the clinic reporting constipation and abdominal pain, the nurse should collect data regarding which common risk factors for constipation?

1. History of diverticulitis or diverticulosis
2. Dietary and exercise patterns
3. Nutritional intake of proteins and fatty acids
4. Level of nutrition understanding and laxative abuse

9 When reinforcing teaching with a 30-year-old male about testicular self-examination (TSE), the nurse recognizes more education is needed when the client makes which statement?

1. "I will perform TSE monthly and see my practitioner yearly."
2. "In the morning after a shower is the best time for TSE."
3. "The testicle and spermatic cords can be easily felt."
4. "One testicle may ride up into my lower abdomen during sleep, but I need to do TSE when it is descended."

10 The nurse is participating in a health promotion fair. When discussing aerobic exercise, the nurse should include which point?

1. Exercise should be done 7 days per week.
2. Fast walking is a good form of aerobic exercise.
3. If one cannot speak when exercising, then the appropriate level of energy is being used.
4. Each exercise session should last for at least 45 minutes, and preferably 60.

11 A postmenopausal client is just learning to do breast self-examination (BSE). To aid in remembering to perform the procedure, at which time should the nurse recommend that the client perform BSE?

1. Weekly just before grocery shopping
2. On a random day once each month according to convenience
3. Once a month on a standard day that the client can remember
4. Just prior to each 6-month check-up for another identified health problem

PRACTICE TEST

12. A nurse has finished reinforcing information about breast self-examination (BSE) with a client. The nurse concludes that the information was learned correctly when the client states to do the exam at which time?

1. Once per month when the client thinks she is ovulating
2. On the first day of each month
3. Seven days after menstruation begins
4. On the first day of the menstrual cycle

13. An older adult female client has osteoporosis. In reviewing with the client the best form of exercise, what exercise would the nurse recommend?

1. Swimming
2. Jogging
3. Cycling on a stationary bicycle
4. Walking

14. A 20-year-old female sees a health care provider for her first adult physical examination. The nurse anticipates that which screening measure will be done at this visit as a baseline for further reference? Select all that apply.

1. Body mass index (BMI) measurement
2. Blood glucose level
3. Clinical breast exam (CBE)
4. Mammography
5. Serum cholesterol level

15. A 4-year-old client is coming to the health care provider's office for a well-child visit. For which routine screenings does the nurse plan? Select all that apply.

1. Blood pressure
2. Vision
3. Urinalysis
4. Lead screening
5. Hearing

16. When reinforcing teaching with a male client about testicular cancer, which manifestations would the nurse include that are important? Select all that apply.

1. Painless swelling of scrotum
2. Dull pain in scrotum
3. Nodules in between testes and cord
4. Dragging sensation in scrotum
5. Reddened rash over affected testicle

17. When reinforcing teaching with a group of adults about health promotion practices, the nurse would include which of the following? Select all that apply.

1. Genetic screening is helpful in identification of cancer risks.
2. Annual medical exams uncover most tumors.
3. Men need to perform breast and testicle exams monthly.
4. Annual mammograms are recommended after a total mastectomy.
5. Colonoscopy is recommended after age 35.

18. The client with chronic renal failure stated on admission to the hospital, "I am a vegan type of vegetarian." What foods would the nurse consider most appropriate when filling out the client's dietary menu?

1. Canned vegetables and noodles
2. Steamed cabbage and sausage
3. Milk and tomato soup
4. Green salad with walnuts

19. The nurse would teach a male client, over age 50, that which health screenings should be done annually? Select all that apply.

1. Testicular self-examination
2. Prostate exam
3. Bone density test
4. Colonoscopy
5. Skin examination

20. The ambulatory pediatric nurse explains to the mother of a 4-year-old that a routine health screening would include which items? Select all that apply.

1. Reading an eye chart
2. Standing on one foot
3. Urinalysis
4. Measuring height and weight
5. Testing of all cranial nerves

ANSWERS & RATIONALES

1 **Answer: 1 Rationale:** The oral anticoagulant drug is sodium warfarin (Coumadin), and its action can be limited by excessive intake of foods containing vitamin K. Since green, leafy vegetables are high in vitamin K, the nurse needs to counsel this client about the possible antagonistic effect of these foods with the medication. Walking one mile a day would pose no particular risk to a client on Coumadin. Coumadin is an oral anticoagulant drug; cuts and injuries will bleed excessively when a client is on this therapy. The nurse should assess the client's knowledge contacting emergency assistance. However, living in a rural setting will not pose a significant risk to this client. Spending most of the time alone does not pose a significant risk to this client. It may be appropriate for the nurse to assess the adequacy of the client's social/support network. **Cognitive Level:** Analyzing **Client Need:** Health Promotion and Maintenance **Integrated Process:** Nursing Process: Planning **Content Area:** Pharmacology **Strategy:** The core issue of the question is oral anticoagulant therapy. With this in mind, review each option for an item that will have either an antagonistic or additive medication effect. Choose the *growing green vegetables* option because it could lead to antagonistic effect.

2 **Answer: 4 Rationale:** The client who has diabetes needs to have regular meals that are evenly spaced throughout the day and may need to supplement meals with snacks. Eating six meals per day is excessive and could lead to inadequate glucose control. Drinking orange juice and eating apples and cheese pose no risk as long as they are in the client's meal pattern. Canned fruit is acceptable as long as it is packed in 100% juice or water instead of syrup. **Cognitive Level:** Analyzing **Client Need:** Health Promotion and Maintenance **Integrated Process:** Nursing Process: Planning **Content Area:** Foundational Sciences **Strategy:** Use principles of general dietary planning and calorie control to answer the question. Remember not to "read in" information into the question or the options.

3 **Answer: 4 Rationale:** Gelatin and clear broth would be appropriate the day after surgery while the suture lines are still new and easily irritated. Sausage and biscuits both require chewing and will irritate the suture lines if eaten the day after surgery. Such foods will be allowed when the client can take a regular diet. French toast and eggs are part of a soft diet, but the client will not be able to tolerate a soft diet typically until the third postoperative day. Milkshakes and tomato soup are part of a full-liquid diet. The client should be allowed full liquids by the second postoperative day, although the tomato soup may be too acidic. **Cognitive Level:** Applying **Client Need:** Health Promotion and Maintenance **Integrated Process:** Nursing Process: Implementation **Content Area:** Foundational Sciences **Strategy:** Keep in mind principles of healing and principles of nutrition needed for healing to make a selection. The correct option is the one that combines appropriate nutrients and a soft form that can be tolerated by the client.

4 **Answer: 4 Rationale:** Problems with vision may be attributed to vitamin deficiency, especially vitamin A. This finding could adversely affect the client's health status and requires follow-up by the nurse. Vitamin B supplements and milk and dairy products will not adversely affect health status. Risk of lactose intolerance has a lesser chance of adversely affecting health status, since it is a familial risk and not a personally identified problem. **Cognitive Level:** Analyzing **Client Need:** Health Promotion and Maintenance **Integrated Process:** Nursing Process: Data Collection **Content Area:** Foundational Sciences **Strategy:** Use knowledge of components of a balanced diet to eliminate the options with vitamin supplements and dairy products. Choose vision problems over familial tendency toward lactose intolerance because actual problems take priority over potential problems.

5 **Answer: 1 Rationale:** The older adult client has more years of living to increase risk of skin cancer from exposure to the sun. In addition, the farmer wears a cap, but no mention is made of protectant sunscreens or long-sleeved shirts and pants. The clients in the remaining options have lesser risk because there are physical barriers to the sun identified in each option: sunscreen, umbrella, and ski outfit. **Cognitive Level:** Analyzing **Client Need:** Health Promotion and Maintenance **Integrated Process:** Nursing Process: Data Collection **Content Area:** Adult Health **Strategy:** First recall that exposure to ultraviolet light is a risk for skin cancer. Use the process of elimination while considering which option provides the least sufficient barrier to exposure to ultraviolet light to make your selection.

6 **Answer: 2 Rationale:** Ultraviolet light exposure greatly increases risk of skin cancer, both basal cell and melanoma types. While direct sunshine contains ultraviolet light, the amount is decreased in indirect light. The use of sunscreen can reduce the risk of cancer but not "prevent" it. Risk of infection from tanning beds may or may not be significant depending on the disinfectant methods used. **Cognitive Level:** Analyzing **Client Need:** Health Promotion and Maintenance **Integrated Process:** Nursing Process: Implementation **Content Area:** Adult Health **Strategy:** The core issue of the question is which option provides the most accurate and important information about ultraviolet light exposure. First eliminate statements that are not necessarily correct all of the time, then choose the true statement over the false statement because of the wording of the question.

7 **Answer: 2 Rationale:** The priority for this client is to learn and begin to perform testicular self-exam on a monthly basis. A yearly exam is insufficient in timeframe, and a physician does not need to perform the screening. A high-fiber diet and encouraging the client to verbalize fears are positive but general measures and do not target the immediate need of the client for information about detecting testicular cancer. **Cognitive Level:** Applying **Client Need:** Health Promotion and Maintenance **Integrated Process:** Nursing Process: Planning **Content Area:** Adult Health **Strategy:** Use the process of elimination and knowledge of cancer risk to make a selection. Note that the question and the options with physician and dates refer to testicular examination, which gives a clue that one of them may be correct. Choose correctly after noting the frequency and accuracy of the statement.

8 **Answer: 2 Rationale:** Two common and key factors that increase risk of constipation are a diet low in fiber and fluids and inadequate exercise to stimulate bowel motility, which could lead to impaction and abdominal pain. Diverticulitis is something to assess for but is not as frequently an etiology

ANSWERS & RATIONALES

as inadequate exercise and low-fiber diet. In addition, diverticulosis does not give rise to signs and symptoms. Intake of protein and fatty acids are irrelevant to the client's complaint. Nutrition intake and laxative abuse are too vague to be correct. **Cognitive Level:** Analyzing **Client Need:** Health Promotion and Maintenance **Integrated Process:** Nursing Process: Data Collection **Content Area:** Adult Health **Strategy:** Note the critical words *most significant* in the stem of the question. This tells you that more than one option is likely to be correct and that you must choose the best option, which in this case is the most frequent cause.

9 **Answer: 4 Rationale:** It is not normal to have one testicle that does not remain descended into the scrotal sac. The client needs to see a primary care provider for this health problem. Each of the other statements related to TSE is true. **Cognitive Level:** Analyzing **Client Need:** Health Promotion and Maintenance **Integrated Process:** Nursing Process: Evaluation **Content Area:** Adult Health **Strategy:** The critical words in the stem of the question are *more education is needed*, which tells you that the correct answer is an incorrect statement. Use the process of elimination and knowledge of TSE.

10 **Answer: 2 Rationale:** The latest recommendations indicate that clients should exercise most days of the week for a minimum of 30 minutes for best effectiveness of exercise. Fast walking is a good form of aerobic exercise. If one cannot speak when exercising, it is too strenuous and should be decreased in speed or amount. **Cognitive Level:** Applying **Client Need:** Health Promotion and Maintenance **Integrated Process:** Teaching and Learning **Content Area:** Adult Health **Strategy:** The core issue of the question is characteristics of effective aerobic exercise. Remember guidelines have changed to include most days of the week, to rule out some distractors. Then choose walking as an extremely effective exercise as the correct answer.

11 **Answer: 3 Rationale:** The client needs to perform BSE once per month, on the same day each month. The client is encouraged to associate performing BSE with another monthly activity, such as paying bills, or to do it on the same calendar date each month (such as the first). The other statements represent incorrect time frames. **Cognitive Level:** Applying **Client Need:** Health Promotion and Maintenance **Integrated Process:** Teaching and Learning **Content Area:** Adult Health **Strategy:** Use the process of elimination and note that the core issue of the question is frequency and timing of BSE. Because the client is postmenopausal, look for the monthly option that is not associated with menses (as none is in this question).

12 **Answer: 3 Rationale:** BSE should be performed once per month, 1 week after beginning menstruation. At this time, the breasts are least likely to be tender and/or swollen from the effects of hormones. At ovulation and menstruation, hormonal changes are likely to interfere with accurate palpation of breast tissue. Performing the exam on the first of the month is recommended for postmenopausal women who are not concerned with hormone level changes associated with the menstrual cycle. **Cognitive Level:** Analyzing **Client Need:** Health Promotion and Maintenance **Integrated Process:** Teaching and Learning **Content Area:** Adult Health **Strategy:** The core issue of the question is knowledge that accurate BSE results depend on the exam being done without the interference of hormonal factors that could alter the results or make the BSE difficult to perform. With this in mind, each of the incorrect options can be eliminated using the influence of hormones as a guide.

13 **Answer: 4 Rationale:** Although all exercises listed are aerobic and therefore beneficial, the older adult client with osteoporosis benefits from an exercise that has a weight-bearing component and does not stress the joints. Such an activity helps to retain calcium in bone and reduce the rate of bone loss. Walking is an aerobic exercise that does not stress the knee and ankle joints. Swimming and stationary cycling are not weight-bearing exercises. Jogging could harm the knee and ankle joints and is not a preferred method of exercise for this client. **Cognitive Level:** Applying **Client Need:** Health Promotion and Maintenance **Integrated Process:** Nursing Process: Implementation **Content Area:** Adult Health **Strategy:** The core issue of the question is the type of exercise that is appropriate for a client with osteoporosis and who is an older adult. With this in mind, eliminate swimming and stationary cycling as non-weight-bearing, and eliminate jogging as increasing stress on joints in the leg.

14 **Answer: 1, 3, 5 Rationale:** A body mass index (BMI) measurement is done at age 20 and at each health visit. Clinical breast exam is done starting at age 20 and may be done every 3 years or more frequently depending on risk. Serum cholesterol levels are started at age 20 and are recommended every 5 years. Blood glucose screening is recommended to begin at age 45 unless there is evidence of higher risk for diabetes. Mammography is done yearly starting at age 40. **Cognitive Level:** Analyzing **Client Need:** Health Promotion and Maintenance **Integrated Process:** Nursing Process: Planning **Content Area:** Adult Health **Strategy:** Specific knowledge of frequency of recommended health screenings is needed to answer the question. Use the process of elimination, and review this content area if needed.

15 **Answer: 1, 2, 5 Rationale:** Blood pressure screening is started at age 3 and continues with each visit. Vision screening is started at age 3 and continues with each visit. Hearing screening begins at age 4. Urinalysis is done at age 5, in adolescence, and otherwise only as indicated. Lead screening would only be done on an as-needed basis for a 4-year-old. **Cognitive Level:** Applying **Client Need:** Health Promotion and Maintenance **Integrated Process:** Nursing Process: Data Collection **Content Area:** Child Health **Strategy:** Specific knowledge of frequency of recommended health screenings is needed to answer the question. Use the process of elimination, and review this content area if needed.

16 **Answer: 1, 2, 3, 4 Rationale:** Painless swelling of scrotum, dull pain in scrotum, nodules between testes and cord, and dragging sensation in scrotum are signs of testicular cancer. A reddened rash in the area is not applicable to this diagnosis but should be followed up for general health reasons. **Cognitive Level:** Analyzing **Client Need:** Health Promotion and Maintenance **Integrated Process:** Nursing Process: Data Collection **Content Area:** Adult Health **Strategy:** Specific knowledge of manifestations of testicular cancer is needed to answer the question. Use the process of elimination and review this content area if needed.

17 **Answer: 1, 3 Rationale:** Genetic screening can identify markers for several types of cancer. One method of reminding men to perform self-checks for cancer is for them to mark on a calendar to do a monthly check for changes. Men and women both need to perform monthly breast exams. Self-exams as well as medical tests and exams uncover tumors. After a total mastectomy, women do not need mammograms. Colonoscopy is generally recommended once a client reaches age 50. **Cognitive Level:** Applying **Client Need:** Health Promotion and Maintenance **Integrated Process:** Teaching and

Learning **Content Area:** Adult Health **Strategy:** Begin by eliminating options that are unnecessary or statements that indicate inappropriate timeframes. Next look suspiciously at the phrase *most tumors*. Words such as *most* or *all* in options usually make them incorrect. When more than one option is correct, consider each option as a true/false statement.

18 **Answer: 4 Rationale:** A client who is a vegetarian of the vegan type does not eat meat, milk, or egg products. Steamed cabbage is appropriate, but it also contains meat (sausage). Canned vegetables and noodles, which may be acceptable in the diet, are high in sodium and inappropriate for a client with chronic renal failure. Depending on the preparation of the sausage, it may also be high in sodium. The most appropriate diet, therefore, is the green salad with walnuts, which contains only vegetables and nuts. **Cognitive Level:** Analyzing **Client Need:** Health Promotion and Maintenance **Integrated Process:** Nursing Process: Implementation **Content Area:** Foundational Sciences **Strategy:** The critical words in the question are *most appropriate*, which indicate that more than one option may be correct but that one is better than the others. Use knowledge of the vegan diet and the fact that processed foods are often high in sodium to make a selection.

19 **Answer: 2, 5 Rationale:** A prostate screening is recommended annually because of the incidence of prostate enlargement or cancer. With age the effects of sun exposure and the incidence of skin cancer become more common. Routine self-examination is important; however, a thorough annual examination is important to detect changes in areas difficult to self-assess. Testicular self-exams are performed monthly, not annually, although testicular cancer has higher frequency in late teens and in young adult males. If at risk for osteoporosis, or if symptoms present, a bone density test can be done for a baseline, but it is not indicated as a routine annual exam. Males and females over age 50 should have a baseline colonoscopy, but not annually. **Cognitive Level:** Analyzing **Client Need:** Health Promotion and Maintenance **Integrated Process:** Teaching and Learning **Content Area:** Adult Health **Strategy:** The core issue of the question is knowledge of the timetables for various health screenings. Use the process of elimination to make a selection, and review these recommendations if needed. When more than one option is correct, consider each option as a true/false statement.

20 **Answer: 1, 2, 4 Rationale:** A routine health screening for a child who is 4 years old would include routine assessment of growth and development and would screen for developmental delays, such as with the Denver II screening exam. A routine urinalysis could be done at age 5, but cranial nerve testing is unnecessary. **Cognitive Level:** Applying **Client Need:** Health Promotion and Maintenance **Integrated Process:** Teaching and Learning **Content Area:** Foundational Sciences **Strategy:** The critical word in the question is *routine*. Consider that an incorrect option would be more likely to be one that is excessively in-depth or one that is done to detect specific disorders.

ANSWERS & RATIONALES

Key Terms to Review

aerobic exercise p. 206

prenatal genetic counseling p. 210

References

American Cancer Society, American Diabetes Association, & American Heart Association (nd). *Recommended health screenings for people at average risk.* Retrieved July 14, 2011, from http://www.everydaychoices.org/downloadables/pdf/screenings_acs_ada_aha.pdf

Agency for Healthcare Research and Quality (2009). *The guide to clinical preventive services 2009. Recommendations of the U.S. Preventive Services Task Force.* Retrieved June 15, 2010, from http://www.ahrq.gov/clinic/pocketgd09/pocketgd09.pdf

Berman, A., & Snyder, S. (2012). *Kozier & Erb's Fundamentals of nursing: Concepts, process, and practice* (9th ed.). Upper Saddle River, NJ: Pearson Education, Inc.

Centers for Disease Control and Prevention (n.d.). *Physical activity for everyone.* Retrieved June 15, 2010, from http://www.cdc.gov/physicalactivity/everyone/guidelines/children.html

Craven, R., & Hirnle, C. (2009). *Fundamentals of nursing: Human health and function* (6th ed.). Philadelphia: Wolters-Kluwer.

Potter, P., & Perry, A. (2010). *Fundamentals of nursing enhanced multimedia edition package* (7th ed.). St. Louis, MO: Mosby.

The Skin Cancer Foundation (nd). *Skin cancer prevention guidelines.* Retrieved on June 15, 2010, from http://www.skincancer.org/Guidelines/References

Test Yourself

Are you ready for the NCLEX-PN® or course exams? Use the practice tests on the companion website to check.

17 Age-Related Care of Older Adults

In this chapter

Cross Reference

Other chapters relevant to this content area are

Lifespan Growth and Development Chapter 13
Promoting Healthy Lifestyle Choices Chapter 16

I. NEED FOR CARE

A. Older adults are the fastest growing population in the United States; subgroups of this age group have been identified

1. Young-old: 65–74 years
2. Old: 75–84 years
3. Old-old: 85–100 years
4. Elite old: over 100 years

B. As age increases, threats to health and need for assistance with daily care and health-related care increase

C. The majority of people 65 or older live in their own homes; only 5% of older adults live in a skilled nursing facility; retirement communities are changing the pattern of housing for older adults

D. Biological aging occurs at a loss of about 0.5% of maximum function per year, starting at age 35; most organ systems have large reserves, so detrimental effects are not noticed

E. Diseases that used to kill or disable middle-aged adults are reduced because of modern health practices and knowledge, with increase in degenerative diseases of old age; chronic illnesses occur frequently in older adults (see Box 17–1)

F. Disuse is a core problem; it is estimated that 2% of decline per year can be accounted for by simple disuse: "use it or lose it"

G. Preventative strategies related to health practices, nutritional intake, and exercise can slow aging process (see also Chapter 16)

NCLEX® **H. Health care practitioners need skill to assist clients in promoting healthy lifestyle choices and to differentiate between "normal aging" and indicators of underlying conditions/symptoms of disease**

Box 17–1

Most Frequently Occurring Conditions in Adults 65 Years and Older, 2006–2008

Hypertension: 38%	Cancer: 22%
Diagnosed arthritis: 50%	Sinusitis: 14%
Heart disease: 32%	Diabetes: 18%

From U.S. Department of Health and Human Services. Administration on Aging. *Profile of Older Americans 2010.*

II. AGE-RELATED PHYSIOLOGICAL CHANGES

A. Basic principles of physical aging

1. Rates between people vary; not year-specific
2. Each organ ages at a different rate within same person
3. Toxic compounds called free radicals damage cellular proteins and eventually cause cell mutation and senescence
4. Physical aging presents differently in different cultures and environments
5. Aging process can be slowed
6. Important to differentiate normal aging from illness

B. Specific system changes and related health promotion activity

1. Skin

NCLEX® a. Subcutaneous tissue loss and dermal thinning leads to a loss of moisture, wrinkles, sagging, decreased perspiration, increased risk of heat stroke, inability to respond to heat and cold rapidly, skin pallor, and slowed healing processes

b. Increase in **lentigines** (brown age spots)

c. Hair thins and loses pigment on the scalp, pubic, and ancillary areas but increases in male ears and female upper lip areas

d. Nail growth slows and nails may become thicker

NCLEX® e. Skin tissue is more fragile, with fewer elastic fibers, decreasing skin turgor and increasing vulnerability to tears and pressure ulcers; caution clients about effects of sun

NCLEX® f. Use mucous membranes to assess potential anemia and fluid volume deficit

g. Sebaceous glands secrete less sebum, causing dryness and itching

2. Sensory and perceptual changes

a. Visual acuity changes; ocular changes in cornea, pupil, and lens lead to farsightedness and inability of lens to accommodate (**presbyopia**); there is increased sensitivity to glare and decreased ability to adjust to light or darkness (slower constriction and dilation of pupils); it is also more difficult to differentiate colors because of changes in rods and cones

NCLEX® b. There is an increased need for light and use of glasses; night lights may be needed

NCLEX® c. Because decreased vision increases risk of falls, high-gloss wax should not be used on floors; safety strips should be placed at least on first and last steps

d. Cataracts may develop; eyelids lose elasticity

e. Arcus senilis often occurs because of deposits of calcium salts and cholesterol; appears as a gray-white ring or partial ring surrounding limbus or outer edge of iris

f. Dry eyes often develop because of inability of goblet cells in conjunctiva to secrete mucin

g. Clients need to have regular ophthalmic exams

NCLEX® h. Older adults may have difficulty driving in darkness

NCLEX® i. Auditory acuity changes; ear canal narrows with calcification of ossicles and increased cerumen, resulting in progressive hearing loss (**presbycusis**)

NCLEX® j. Older adults have particular difficulty hearing high-pitched tones and words that begin with consonants, especially *sh*, *th*, *wh*; they will not hear "Swish this around your mouth" accurately if they cannot see the speaker's face; shouting does not help clients to hear

k. Ears should be cleaned of cerumen; if hearing aids are used, check batteries and use regularly

NCLEX® l. Olfactory bulb decreases, leading to inability to smell and discriminate odors (**anosomia**); housing for older adults should include working smoke alarms to detect fires

NCLEX® m. Gustatory buds decrease on tongue, causing decline in ability to taste; sweet sensation is especially affected; avoid use of extra sugar and salt to satisfy desire; explore alternatives

NCLEX® n. Touch sensation changes with reduced ability to sense heat and cold; monitor temperature of liquids to avoid injuries, monitor extremities for wounds that may go unnoticed because of decreased sensation, and beware of myth that older adults do not experience pain

3. Neurological

a. Conduction speeds of neuron firing and transmission decrease; decreased sensation and slowed response time may impact safety, driving, and decision making

b. Actively participating in mind exercises (learning new things, crossword puzzles, reading) has been shown to slow changes; assist client to incorporate exercise into lifestyle

c. Memory retrieval is slower, and there is a decrease in vigilance, but intelligence and behavior does not change; older adults are capable of learning new health-related information, but may need more processing time

d. Sleep stage 2–4 will shorten, leading to a reduced deep sleep and less physiologic and psychological rejuvenation; monitor perception of sleep, immune system, and mood/cognition state; promote healthy sleep rituals (e.g., quiet restful environment, no stimulants before bedtime, go to bed only when tired)

NCLEX®
e. **Proprioception** (sensation about body's movement and position) decreases, so achieving balance or changing position may be difficult; demonstrate safe changes of position; incorporate safety devices and clear walkways in living spaces

4. Musculoskeletal
   a. Muscles **atrophy** (decrease in size and physiologic activity) leading to decreased strength and stamina; legs lose more strength than arms; encourage regular exercise
   b. Joints stiffen because of deterioration of joint cartilage

NCLEX®
   c. Intervertebral disks atrophy, resulting in a loss of height of 1 to 3 inches; bone demineralization may lead to **osteoporosis** and increased risk of fractures
   d. Encourage weight-bearing exercise, intake of calcium and vitamin D; walking is beneficial
   e. Monitor functional activity levels

5. Pulmonary
   a. Chest wall becomes rigid, thoracic muscles weaken, and ciliary activity decreases, so there is less efficient lung expansion, exchange of oxygen/carbon dioxide, effective coughing, and foreign body capture

NCLEX®
   b. Teach effective coughing and deep breathing
   c. Practice healthy hygiene because of increased susceptibility to infection; encourage appropriate vaccine administration; sputum specimen collection may require suction technique

NCLEX®
   d. Delivery and diffusion of oxygen to tissues decreases so that dyspnea can occur after moderate, stressful activity; teach pacing of activities between periods of rest and throughout day instead of clustered together

6. Cardiovascular
   a. Heart size remains same unless there is pathology

NCLEX®
   b. Cardiac output and stroke volume decrease, especially during time of increased demands, so there is a decreased stress response
   c. Shortness of breath on exertion and pooling of blood in extremities may occur
   d. Help client to incorporate pacing into activities of daily living (ADLs) and instrumental activities of daily living (IADLs)
   e. Valves stiffen so that murmurs may be heard; know baseline so that disease-related abnormalities can be detected
   f. Conductivity is altered, so there are more ectopic beats; assess apical heart rhythm and rate for a full minute

NCLEX®
   g. Vessels are less elastic, resulting in higher blood pressure; orthostatic hypotension may occur, and there is decreased perfusion to vital organs

NCLEX®
   h. Monitor client BP according to latest guidelines; monitor perfusion to and resulting function of vital organs
   i. Palpate peripheral pulses; use Doppler for measurement if needed
   j. Instruct not to make sudden position changes to avoid orthostatic hypotension because of altered physiology or effect of many medications taken for chronic health problems, such as hypertension

7. Renal
   a. Nephrons decrease in function because of aging and decreased arterial blood flow; monitor for output of at least 30 mL/hr (0.5 mg/kg/hr)
   b. Glomerular filtration rate (GFR) decreases, which may decrease rate of excretion of drug metabolites

NCLEX®
   c. Creatinine clearance decreases; monitor for nephrotoxic medication adverse effects
   d. Ability to concentrate urine and conserve water is decreased; urinary urgency and frequency may occur from enlarged prostate in men or decreased perineal muscle support and urinary sphincter strength in women
   e. Bladder capacity decreases

NCLEX®
   f. Incontinence is *not* part of normal aging; it occurs because of pathology
   g. Residual urine and nocturnal frequency may occur; teach client to credé bladder

NCLEX®
   h. Monitor for urinary infection (new-onset confusion may be sign in older adults) and for restful nights (lack of nocturia); refer for treatment if needed

8. Gastrointestinal (GI)
   NCLEX® a. Thirst sensation decreases; monitor intake to prevent fluid deficit, especially if taking diuretics or environment is hot
   b. GI system usually stays healthy overall but generates most complaints from older adults
   c. Swallowing time is delayed, and epiglottis does not completely cover trachea unless older adult is in a 90-degree position
   d. Monitor swallowing; have client sit upright when eating or drinking; gag reflex may diminish
   e. Gingivitis/periodontal disease often leads to loss of teeth and is caused by poor nutrition and inadequate oral care
   f. Saliva secretions lessen, so breakdown of carbohydrates may be decreased
   g. Intra-abdominal strength decreases; gastric acid and enzymes decrease, and absorption time is slower; monitor for reflux and vitamin deficiencies
   NCLEX® h. Intestinal walls weaken, and there is a slower neural transmission and resulting decrease in peristalsis; observe for constipation and incontinence; caution against inappropriate use of laxatives because of risk of dependence
9. Endocrine
   a. Thyroid stimulating hormone (TSH) and thyroxin are reduced; slowed basal metabolism, dry skin, and thin hair are characteristic of hypothyroidism in young adults but are normal age-related changes in older adults with no history of disease
   b. Insulin levels increase, but insulin sensitivity decreases; observe for hypoglycemia or hyperglycemia, depending on client condition
   c. Alteration in hormone regulation decreases ability to respond to stress
10. Genital
   NCLEX® a. Prostate enlarges in men (often benign); decreased sperm production occurs; encourage regular health checkups and prostate specific antigen (PSA) testing
   NCLEX® b. Vaginal changes in women occur because of diminished secretion of hormones; alkaline pH leads to vaginal dryness and atrophy; there may be a need for increased foreplay and use of a water-soluble lubricant; encourage regular gynecologic exams; monitor menopausal changes; estrogen is not routinely prescribed
   c. For both genders, collect data regarding sexual activity and safe sex practices
11. Immune
   a. Thymus has decrease in cell production with decreases in cell-mediated immunity and T-cell functioning
   NCLEX® b. Monitor for signs and symptoms of infection and/or altered cell production
   NCLEX® c. First sign of infection in an older adult may be a fall; temperature pattern may be lower than for younger adult with the same infection
   d. Autoimmune response may not be associated with disease; monitor for changes in soaps or detergents if older adult develops unknown allergic rash
   NCLEX® e. Outbreaks of shingles occur if varicella virus is reactivated during times when older adult's immune system is weakened, *not* if they come in contact with new cases of chicken pox

III. AGE-RELATED PSYCHOSOCIAL CHANGES

A. Role and relationship transitions occur; adaptation is critical to positive aging

NCLEX® **B. Maintain independence in as many activities as possible**

C. According to Erikson (1963), everyone has specific developmental stages and tasks to fulfill; in 8th (last) stage of life, older adults review their life to establish beliefs of integrity or despair

1. Erikson and Peck (1968) identified discrete tasks that must be addressed to establish integrity:
   a. Ego differentiation versus work role preoccupation; adults are no longer defined by work; satisfaction is found in other activities
   b. Body transcendence versus body preoccupation; adults care for themselves but do not spend all their energy caring for body; they see meaning in illness and death
   c. Ego transcendence versus ego preoccupation; adults focus on humanity outside of themselves; "I" is not as important; volunteerism for a greater good may be seen
2. Erickson's (1986) reframed work: ego integrity is tinged with some regrets, wisdom is balanced with frivolity, and letting go is balanced with hanging on; an adult comes to terms with life as it was lived and derives sustenance from past but is active in present and plans for future; reminiscence and life review are effective tools to encourage ego integrity

D. Other key changes

NCLEX® **1.** Balance is found in solitude and social interactions; adults who adapt develop a capacity for aloneness and ability to enjoy own company (not to exclusion of significant others but in preparation for loss and death); old and new friendships are still valued; communication problems (vision, hearing, and withdrawal) may detract from finding this balance

2. Grandparenting has become an important role; some grandparents are the primary caregivers; communication clarification is important

NCLEX® **3.** Retirement may be unattainable for some and undesirable for others; financial needs, resources, and loss of health insurance benefits may deter retirement, as may perceived loss of prestige, friends, and self-satisfaction; number of retirement years is increasing, so transition counseling or mentoring may be useful

4. Widowhood is more difficult for young-old during adaptation process; transitions for all include stages that span 5 years

- **a.** First stage (reactionary): early responses of disbelief, anger, inability to communicate, searching for mate; interventions: support, reduce expectations
- **b.** Second stage (withdrawal): occurs in first few months with depression, physiologic vulnerability, insomnia, unpredictable waves of grief; interventions: protect against suicide and involve in support groups
- **c.** Third stage (recuperation): occurs in second 6 months with periods of depression and feelings of personal control beginning to return; interventions: support usual lifestyle patterns while assisting to explore new possibilities
- **d.** Fourth stage (exploration): occurs in second year with new ventures but vulnerability during holidays, anniversaries, birthdays; interventions: prepare widow or widower for feelings during special times; support new roles
- **e.** Fifth stage (integration): occurs in fifth year with a healthy resolution of grief; interventions: assist individual to share own pattern of growth

E. Stressors of aging

NCLEX® **1.** Include loss of people or pets or driver license, abandonment, acute and chronic pain, sensory changes, medications, caregiving for spouse with dementia, illness, hospitalization, lack of protection when frail, fear of senility, abuse and neglect, housing and home maintenance, relocation, institutionalization, fear of loss of independence, and fear of death or dying alone

2. Encourage recognition of fears and reinforce positive coping methods; monitor for inappropriate coping: alcoholism, withdrawal, contemplation of suicide

3. Role transitions from worker to retiree/volunteer and spouse to widow(er) require looking at former roles differently; to the extent these are accepted and "at the right time," older adults can transition smoothly

F. Intimacy and sexuality

1. Continue to be critical at any age; touch is important to all; watch for touch deprivation; use of therapeutic touch and massage may enhance health

NCLEX® **2.** Sexually transmitted infections are not exclusively young people's diseases; safe sex practices should be followed

3. Sexual dysfunction counseling, if needed, is multidimensional; use of medications to promote erections requires education related to safety

4. Privacy is needed in residential settings for marital sexual relations; health care workers need to evaluate own feelings regarding sexuality in older adults

G. Many organizations promote positive aging adaptation, including American Association of Retired Persons (AARP), local senior centers, area councils/agencies on aging, churches, and groups such as Meals on Wheels

IV. MEDICATION CONSIDERATIONS

A. Issues with medications in older adults

1. Medication (drug) use is affected by finances, ability to acquire drugs, advertisements, and client's motivation and health

2. Fragmented care and lack of communication among prescribers can lead to **polypharmacy** (prescriptions for multiple drugs written by multiple prescribers and possibly filled at multiple pharmacies); this can lead to adverse drug interactions and possible toxicity

NCLEX® **3.** Nurse may be only caregiver who knows all prescribed and over-the-counter (OTC) drug and herbs used by client, making it critical for nurses to administer, educate, monitor for therapeutic effects and adverse effects, prevent and treat toxic effects, and advocate for appropriate and affordable medication use

B. Pharmacokinetics determines concentration of drug in body

1. Absorption: aging alone affects oral drug absorption minimally but may be reduced with intramuscular (IM) delivery
2. Distribution: decreased circulation to skin, muscles and fat results in slower and lower concentrations in these tissues; increased overall body fat and decreased lean body mass and water may also affect movement of drug; healthy older adults show little change in plasma binding proteins; however, the lowered albumin levels in disease states can result in increased normal and adverse effects; note that some disease states (cancer, arthritis) that elevate protein binding capacity decrease effectiveness of some drugs
3. Metabolism/biotransformation: liver size and hepatic blood flow decrease with advanced age so drugs that undergo a first-pass effect in liver are affected by age; drugs such as propranolol and lidocaine exhibit decreased metabolism and increased bioavailability, leading to risk of toxicity
4. Excretion: aging reduces renal drug excretion because of decreased glomerular filtration rate, renal plasma flow, tubular function and reabsorptive capacity; creatinine clearance rates are calculated and some drug dosages are calculated by lean body weight versus ideal body weight

C. Pharmacodynamics

1. Aging changes some receptor sites, which increases susceptibility to some adverse effects; older adults are very sensitive to anticholinergic side effects of drugs as well as orthostatic hypotension
2. Older adults tend to have more adverse effects related to a greater number of chronic problems and drugs taken

D. Medication usage

1. Older adults may require lower drug dosages especially when starting a drug regimen; therapeutic window narrows with age; "start low, go slow" is a common adage
2. Adverse effects are often atypical and may include falls, incontinence, **delirium** (acute onset confusion), depression, sedation, urinary retention
3. Use brown bag method to take adequate history of medications taken
4. Review whether medications are taken as prescribed
5. Confirm that clients can see what they are taking
6. Remind clients that pills should not be crushed if enteric coated
7. Antihypertensive should be taken as ordered even if blood pressure is within normal range
8. Diuretics should be taken during early waking hours so that effective sleep can occur
9. Drugs that have hypotensive or sedative effects may be best taken at bedtime, especially if single daily dose
10. Review all prescriptions if client takes more than five to eight drugs; primary prescriber reviews necessity of all drugs
11. Altered electrolytes such as potassium or sodium may exacerbate imbalance and adverse drug effects; if a client is taking spironolactone and a diet high in potassium, toxic potassium levels could occur
12. Mental status changes may be a drug side effect; diazepam, clonidine, digoxin, levodopa, and isoniazid cause delirium and confusion in many older adults
13. Monitor for oto- and nephrotoxicity; assess urine output and ringing in ears, especially in older adults receiving aminoglycosides or high doses of aspirin
14. Monitor for sexual changes; decreased sexual desire is seen with antipsychotics, SSRI type of antidepressants, ketoconazole; priapism (prolonged painful erection) is a surgical emergency associated with sildenafil, alprostadil, trazodone, and antipsychotics
15. Drug allergies may occur; take history especially of antibiotics (penicillin, cephalosporin, erythromycin, gentamicin, sulfa), nonsteroidal anti-inflammatory drugs, opiates, anesthetics, and contrast medias; monitor their usage and reactions
16. Changes in diet can impact medication; increased green vegetables counteract anticoagulant effects of warfarin; iron is not absorbed when calcium is taken at same time; decreased fluid intake, especially during hot weather, may lead to fluid volume deficit and increased sensitivity to orthostatic effects of beta blockers
17. Food–drug interactions must be reviewed; do not give dairy products with ciprofloxacin or tetracycline because drug will chelate with food; amiodarone, lovastatin, and buspirone levels increase dramatically when taken with grapefruit juice
18. Monitor where medications are stored; store nitrates in a dry, dark area; adhere to expiration dates

E. Common medications considered inappropriate for older adults

1. Analgesics: propoxyphene (Darvon) and combination products, meperidine (Demerol)
2. Hypnotics: diazepam (Valium), barbiturates except phenobarbital (Luminal)

3. Antiplatelet: dipyridamole (Persantine)
4. Anticoagulant: ticlopidine (Ticlid)
5. Antihypertensive: methyldopa (Aldomet)
6. Any medication with a highly anticholinergic profile
7. Garlic and ginkgo may increase risk of bleeding

V. OLDER ADULT ABUSE AND NEGLECT

A. Abuse is willful infliction of pain or injury physically, psychologically, financially, or socially

1. Examples include confinement, willful deprivation of services, verbal assaults, theft, mismanagement of belongings, demand to perform undesirable tasks, and physically injurious acts
2. Exploitation is illegal or improper use of an older adult's resources
3. NCLEX® Individuals at risk are those who are dependent because of health issues such as altered mental status, sensory deficits, or immobility
4. History of family violence and caregiver stress also increase risk of abuse

B. Neglect is lack of provision of services necessary for health

1. Self-neglect occurs when older adult chooses not to uses services that would promote health
2. If legally competent, an older adult has the right to refuse care

NCLEX® **C. Possible indicators of abuse and/or neglect**

1. Bruises, cuts, burns
2. Sprains, fractures, dislocations
3. Inconsistent history about injuries
4. Untreated medical problems
5. Improper use of medication
6. Malnutrition, dehydration, or both
7. Inappropriate dress, hygiene, drowsiness, or social interactions
8. Pulling away or expression of fear when touched
9. Excessive attachment to caregiver

D. Care includes

1. Continued observation
2. NCLEX® Reporting to appropriate agencies as mandated by each state
3. Involvement with protective services
4. Referral to appropriate resources and treatment for dysfunctional families

VI. COMMON PROBLEMS IN OLDER ADULTS

A. Nutrition

1. Data collection
   - a. Food patterns and preferences
   - b. Symbolism of food: sociability, security, and reward
   - c. Health screen for malnutrition
   - d. Dentition efficiency and oral hygiene
   - e. Taste and sensory changes influence choices; taste bud receptors decrease, especially for sweet and salt; olfactory receptors atrophy, decreasing taste ability further; visual changes affect presentation, while touch proprioception is altered also
   - f. Decreased thirst sensation and satiety
   - g. BMI, height and weight, ideal body weight; a BMI of 20 to 24.9 is considered healthy
   - h. Lab work: related to potassium levels, hemoglobin and hematocrit ranges, pre-albumin and albumin values
   - i. NCLEX® Disease and functional profile: any disease can cause poor food intake and weight loss for older adults; lactose intolerance is becoming more prevalent; arthritis may prevent use of regular forks, spoons, knives, and cups
   - j. Common nutritional problems include hypercholesterolemia, weight loss, protein malnutrition, osteoporosis (low bone density), obesity; see also Chapter 25
   - k. Income and food acquisition patterns may change
   - l. NCLEX® Clients at highest risk for decreased nutritional health: live alone, have many medications, have a history of dementia or depression, are institutionalized
2. Plan/implementation
   - a. Decrease total fats and saturated transfat
   - b. Control calories

c. Increase fluids to 30mL/kg body weight or up to 2 liters per day if not on fluid restriction
d. Increase whole grains and fiber intake

NCLEX®
e. Limit intake of sodium and sugar; 2300 mg or 1 teaspoon per day (current recommendation for sodium); canned and processed foods contain large amounts of sodium; use substitute flavor enhancers but beware of potassium content of salt substitutes if client takes potassium-sparing diuretics or has renal disease
f. Use supplements if vitamins or minerals are needed to get 100% of RDA if client has difficulty eating or illness that reduces absorption, is on a restricted diet, or takes medications that reduce appetite or nutrient absorption; assess calcium, iron, zinc, folic acid, and vitamins A, B_6, C, and E (frequently inadequate in older adult's diet)
g. Promote enjoyment of food by setting different table areas and eating with another; learn to savor foods; if alcohol is used, do so in moderation; include cultural preferences in diet

NCLEX®
h. Increase physical activity; walking is an efficient exercise, but increased exercise can be done in a chair too
i. Refer to a nutritionist if BMI is below 20 or above 25, food intake is limited in quality or quantity for prolonged time, or, there is a limited knowledge of and motivation to comply with diet
j. Refer to a nutritionist and specialist for disorders requiring nutritional intervention: elevated lipid profile, osteoporosis, malabsorption, uncontrolled diabetes, obesity, congestive heart failure and other cardiac conditions, advanced renal or liver disease, prolonged high doses of chemotherapy or radiation
k. Refer to Meals on Wheels if preparation and acquisition of food is not easily done

NCLEX®
l. Reinforce teaching about sources of nutrients (fat, protein, carbohydrate), and potassium (potato, banana, fortified orange juice) and reinforce with written or pictorial materials
m. Investigate food storage practices for hygienic safety; recommend nonperishable food items such as boxes of dry skim milk, peanut butter, canned tuna, dried fruit, fresh seasonal fruit, tea if refrigeration is limited
n. In health care settings, screen for nutritional risk, provide intervention and counseling, food and nutrition products, prescribed nutritional supplements, and monitor client response

B. Urinary incontinence

NCLEX®
1. Incontinence is not part of normal aging but a disease process or functional change
2. Prevalence is 40% of hospitalized clients, 60% of clients in long-term care facilities, 25% of older adults in community
3. Detection is critical so that treatment can be started

NCLEX®
4. Continence requires functional status in lower urinary tract, cognitive ability, dexterity in mobility, usable toileting environment, and motivation
5. Causes of transient incontinence include delirium; restricted mobility, retention; infection, inflammation, impaction; polyuria, pharmaceuticals; use the pneumonic DRIP to remember these causes (see Memory Aid)

Memory Aid

D—delirium
R—restricted mobility, retention
I—infection, inflammation, impaction
P—polyuria, pharmaceuticals

6. Adverse effects of urinary incontinence
   a. Physical: odor, discomfort, skin problems, urinary tract infections, falls
   b. Psychosocial: embarrassment, isolation, depression, need for nursing home care
   c. Economic: skilled nursing facility costs and national effect on Medicare and Medicaid
7. Types of persistent urinary incontinence include stress, urge, overflow, functional, and neurogenic
8. Treat according to cause and promote regular toileting schedules (such as every 2 hours), spacing fluids over day but not at night to avoid nocturia, and administering diuretics during early part of day

C. Constipation versus diarrhea

NCLEX®
1. Older adults are at risk for constipation if they excessively use laxatives

NCLEX®
2. A brown liquid ring on sheets may be a sign of impaction, not diarrhea

D. Vision and hearing

1. Visual problems associated with aging include presbyopia, dry eye, cataracts, glaucoma, diabetic retinopathy, and macular degeneration; see Chapter 59 for a discussion of these health problems
2. Hearing problems associated with aging include presbycusis, cerumen impaction, and possibly tinnitus; see Chapter 59 for a discussion of these health problems

E. Impaired skin integrity

1. Skin loses elasticity with aging process
2. Decreased mobility also increases risk of pressure ulcer development (see also Chapters 26 and 58 for skin-related health problems)

F. Impaired mobility

1. Can occur with chronic health problems such as arthritis, neuromuscular disorders, or osteoporosis leading to fractures, or because of acute illness, injury, or surgery (such as hip and knee replacement)
2. Can occur because client is afraid of falling; impaired mobility can lead to increased risk for falls; see Table 17–1 for risk factors for falls in older adults
3. May require use of assistive devices (mobility aids) such as a cane or walker

G. Dehydration

1. Monitoring is critical because older adults are at risk for dehydration
2. *NCLEX®* Mucous membranes provide indication of hydration
3. *NCLEX®* Use abdomen or forehead to note skin turgor; tenting is a normal, age-related change on hand and is not a reliable indicator of dehydration
4. Delirium (a reversible, acute confusional state that must be evaluated) is frequently caused by dehydration and may accompany urinary tract infection; it often goes undiagnosed in older adults, and client is labeled cognitively impaired
5. See Chapter 49 for a detailed discussion of dehydration or deficient fluid volume

H. Depression

1. *NCLEX®* Older adults are at risk for depression related to multiple losses in their lives
2. *NCLEX®* Differentiate between depression, delirium, and **dementia** (impairments in memory, abstract thinking, judgment, and personality); see Table 17–2
3. For detailed discussion, see Chapter 21 on mental health disorders

Table 17–1 Fall Risk Factors

Etiology of Risk	Examples of Type of Factor
Intrinsic Age-Related Changes	Gait (step length and height, symmetry and path); balance when sitting, standing or turning; stability; cognition
Intrinsic Disease-Related Changes	Orthostatic hypotension, dehydration, cardiac dysrhythmias and anemias, urinary tract and other infections, osteoporosis and fractures, hypoglycemia, seizures, transient ischemic attacks (TIAs), stroke, adverse effects of medication, delirium
Extrinsic Risk Factors	Clutter, high-heeled shoes, bathrooms without grab bars and shower seats, dim light or bright light with glare, curbing and other edges without contrasting colors, uneven steps, no hand rails, problems with floor surface (waxed, scatter rugs, tears in carpet)

Table 17–2 Comparisons of Delirium, Dementia, and Depression in Older Adults

	Delirium	Dementia	Depression
Onset	Acute	Gradual	Sudden or gradual
Duration	Brief, resolve underlying cause	Years	Weeks to years
State of Consciousness	Disoriented	Alert	Self-absorbed
Behavior	Difficulty with attention and concentration	Personality changes, labile, easily agitated	Apathetic, feelings of worthlessness, vague somatic complaints
Ability to Follow Instructions	Unable to do tasks	Tries hard to follow and do with gradual loss of abilities	Able to, but does not do tasks
Mental Ability	Fluctuations in memory and orientation, disorganized thinking	Impaired memory, gradual loss of knowledge, language, and judgment	Selective memory loss
Ability to cure	Reversible	Irreversible	Reversible

Check Your NCLEX-PN® Exam I.Q.

You are ready for testing on this content if you can

- State basic principles related to aging.
- List physical changes of aging and implied health promotion activities.
- Differentiate normal physical aging changes from indicators of illness.
- Discuss psychosocial issues of aging and how to promote healthy adaptation.
- Identify common problems, safety issues, and required health promotion teaching.

PRACTICE TEST

PRACTICE TEST

1 A nurse is reviewing information about aging with clients at a senior citizen center. The nurse concludes that a client needs further instruction if the client made which statement?

1. "Through nutrition and exercise, we can modify the rate of aging."
2. "Free radicals influence the quality of growing old."
3. "Some of the physical changes within our bodies are the result of disuse."
4. "Deterioration of body systems occurs at the same rate."

2 A nurse considers that information provided about normal physiologic changes of aging has been effective for a 70-year-old client if he makes which statement?

1. "I have more sweat gland activity."
2. "I have lost some of my social support systems."
3. "I have an increased need for sleep."
4. "I have less joint cartilage than I used to."

3 After assisting with a physical examination, the nurse would conclude that a 75-year-old client's ability to maintain personal safety would be most adversely affected by declining function in which body system?

1. Cardiovascular
2. Respiratory
3. Sensory
4. Integumentary

4 A 75-year-old woman with a pathological fracture of the arm asks, "How did I get a broken bone?" The nurse most appropriately responds by stating that which problem is most likely to be responsible for the fracture?

1. Decreased mobility
2. Osteoarthritis
3. Scoliosis
4. Osteoporosis

5 Which nursing intervention would be most appropriate to meet safety needs when caring for an older adult with sensory changes?

1. Assist in preparing a bath because the client may be less able to feel intensity of heat.
2. Use care when administering an injection because older adults experience more pain.
3. Massage with additional pressure because tactile perception of older adults is diminished.
4. Use minimal touch with an older adult because touch will feel uncomfortable.

6 When explaining the needs of older adults to children of aging parents, the nurse would include which element?

1. They require help with making important decisions.
2. They like an active family role and need to be with grandchildren often.
3. They should be supported when feasible in their desire to remain independent.
4. They must be protected from injury at all times.

7 After reviewing driving safety education principles with an older adult, a nurse should recognize which behavior as evidence of a favorable response by an older adult when driving?

1. Keeping car interior warm at all times because of loss of subcutaneous fat with decreased tolerance to cold
2. Not turning the head to look to the left or the right because the older adult's response time is slower
3. Driving at a speed that matches the flow of traffic to facilitate increased response time
4. Driving during the day to increase use of vision capabilities

8 A nurse reinforces teaching to an older adult client about misuse of medications. Which subsequent behavior by the client indicates that the instruction was effective?

1. Combining prescribed medications with over-the-counter ones
2. Having prescriptions from several physicians
3. Using someone else's medications
4. Taking medications on time and, if a dose is missed, taking the next one on time

9 Which instruction, if reinforced by the nurse while caring for an older adult who has "leaking urine," would be most effective in strengthening pelvic muscles?

1. When coughing, bear down in the standing position.
2. Percuss the lower abdomen for dull sounds, indicating a distended bladder.
3. Observe for bladder fullness immediately after voiding.
4. Stop the stream of urine during the middle of urination.

10 Which clinical manifestation would be most significant and require further investigation when inspecting the skin of an 85-year-old client?

1. Ecchymoses on both forearms
2. Cherry hemangiomas across the anterior and posterior trunk
3. Tenting of the skin on the back of the hands
4. Nevi on the neck and forehead

11 An older adult client is admitted to an extended care facility for continuing care after a total hip replacement. The nurse notes a BMI of 20, lackluster hair, and pallor. Which laboratory data will the nurse review to obtain the most sensitive information about the client's current nutritional status?

1. Serum albumin
2. Total cholesterol
3. Prealbumin
4. Complete blood cell count (CBC)

12 On admission, a 78-year-old client states that he uses laxatives three times a week for constipation. What is the nurse's best response?

1. "As people age, they need laxatives to stimulate defecation."
2. "Eat a balanced diet if you use laxatives."
3. "Long-term use of laxatives can actually lead to constipation."
4. "Please use laxatives two times a week at night."

13 Which finding in an older adult client obtained by medical record review and observation should alert the nurse to an increased risk of falls?

1. Decreased bone density
2. Increased bone prominence
3. Kyphotic posture
4. Cartilage deterioration

14 The nurse is irrigating the ears of an older adult man with a cerumen impaction. At what point would the nurse stop the procedure?

1. If the client became nauseated
2. If the irrigating fluid did not return
3. If the cerumen become softer
4. If the client says he cannot hear as well

15 An older adult client is receiving the third unit of packed red blood cells in the last 8 hours. One hour into the third transfusion, the nurse assisting with the client's care observes distended neck veins in the client. What action would the nurse take next?

1. Document the observation.
2. Measure the volume left in the bag.
3. Alert the registered nurse immediately to slow the rate of the infusion.
4. Measure the client's pulse and blood pressure.

16 The nurse explains to a group at a senior citizen center that older adults may be predisposed to fluid imbalances for which reasons? Select all that apply.

1. They might not pay attention to thirst or may experience less thirst.
2. They might fear too much fluid if they have a tendency for ankles to swell.
3. They might not drink fluids if it is difficult to go to the bathroom.
4. They eat only canned and prepackaged food.
5. They tend to dislike the taste of water.

17 A nurse is reinforcing instructions to an older adult client about cataract prevention. The nurse will instruct the client that which factors increase the incidence of cataract development? Select all that apply.

1. Ultraviolet light
2. Injury
3. Vitamin A
4. Viral infections
5. Eyestrain

18 An older adult client has fallen twice while getting up to go to the bathroom at night. The nurse implements which of the following to decrease the risk of further client falls?

1. Withhold all liquids after dinner.
2. Put all four side rails up at bedtime.
3. Leave the call bell within reach, and turn on the bathroom light.
4. Give the client a sleeping pill, so the client will sleep through the night.

19 A nurse has had a discussion with a group of senior citizens about age-related nutritional needs. The nurse knows the session was effective if a client states which of the following?

1. "I will eat oranges and carrots, and drink more low-fat milk."
2. "I will eat margarine at meals, and increase my calorie intake."
3. "I will reduce the amount of grains and uncooked vegetables in my meals."
4. "I will add canned vegetables to my dinner meals."

20 An older adult client with osteoarthritis is scheduled for discharge. The client says, "I don't know if I will be able to remember all that you have told me. I live alone and am not sure what pills to take or when to do the treatments." What is the next action the nurse would take?

1. Call the client's child to come home from college and care for the parent.
2. Ask the physician to delay the discharge so further teaching can be done in the hospital.
3. Ask the co-assigned RN to request the physician refer the client to a home health agency for nursing care.
4. Ask the pharmacist to call the client to reinforce taking the medicine appropriately.

ANSWERS & RATIONALES

1 **Answer: 4** **Rationale:** Each physiologic system of a person ages at a different rate. Proper diet and regular exercise can be beneficial in slowing the rate of the aging process. Free radicals do influence the aging process. Physical changes within the body can occur as a result of disuse. **Cognitive Level:** Applying **Client Need:** Health Promotion and Maintenance **Integrated Process:** Nursing Process: Implementation **Content Area:** Foundational Sciences **Strategy:** Note that the question has negative wording in the stem, which indicates the correct answer is an incorrect statement. Consider that tissues do not age at precisely the same rate to choose correctly.

2 **Answer: 4** **Rationale:** With normal aging, there is loss of cartilage and joint fluid. Overall wear and tear does occur. Sebaceous (sweat) glands are less active, and older adults sweat less. Social support may decrease with deaths and fewer resources but does not relate to the question of physiologic needs. There is a decreased need for sleep, with shorter REM and non-REM sleep cycles. **Cognitive Level:** Analyzing **Client Need:** Health Promotion and Maintenance **Integrated Process:** Nursing Process: Implementation **Content Area:** Foundational Sciences **Strategy:** Read all options and use concepts of the normal aging process to eliminate those that are incorrect.

3 **Answer: 3** **Rationale:** With normal aging changes, there is a decrease in vision, hearing, touch, smell, and taste. These changes can lead to falls and the inability to leave a situation when called to do so, distinguish temperature (with resulting burns), smell smoke in a fire, or taste contaminated food. These changes can have a major impact on the safety needs of an older adult. Age-related changes in the cardiovascular, respiratory or integumentary systems do not necessarily lead to safety issues. **Cognitive Level:** Analyzing **Client Need:** Safety and Infection Control **Integrated Process:** Nursing Process: Planning **Content Area:** Foundational Sciences **Strategy:** When answering questions related to development and aging, distinguish between normal development, which affects all, and illness, which affects some.

4 **Answer: 4** **Rationale:** Osteoporosis, a decrease in bone density, makes the older adult more prone to pathological fractures. Decreased mobility, osteoarthritis, and scoliosis do not cause pathological fractures. Scoliosis is a curvature of the spine, usually diagnosed in adolescents. **Cognitive Level:** Applying **Client Need:** Physiological Adaptation **Integrated Process:** Nursing Process: Implementation **Content Area:** Foundational Sciences **Strategy:** Consider the etiology of pathological fractures and correlate the best reason with the correct answer choice.

5 **Answer: 1** **Rationale:** Because of loss of skin receptors, the older adult has an increased threshold to pain, touch, and temperature. When feeding or bathing, remember that the older adult may be unable to distinguish hot or cold or to determine the intensity of heat. The older adult may feel less pain than younger adults and report only pressure or a minor sensation. The older adult, however, is the only one who can identify whether he or she has pain. An older client's sensory perception is less acute than that of younger adults, so when giving a massage, less pressure is needed. Everyone, and especially the older adult, needs touch. **Cognitive Level:** Analyzing **Client Need:** Safety and Infection Control **Integrated Process:** Nursing Process: Planning **Content Area:** Foundational Sciences **Strategy:** Imagine giving the stated care to assist in choosing the correct answer.

6 **Answer: 3** **Rationale:** Remaining independent is important for older adults. Older adults prefer to make their own decisions and do not appreciate others making decisions for them. Although some older adults cherish a family role, this is not necessarily the wish of every older adult. Excessive protection from injury is unnecessary and inappropriate. **Cognitive Level:** Applying **Client Need:** Psychosocial Integrity **Integrated Process:** Nursing Process: Implementation **Content Area:** Foundational Sciences **Strategy:** Recognize that usually the word *all* denotes an incorrect choice.

7 **Answer: 4** **Rationale:** Driving at night requires caution because accommodation of the eye to light is impaired and peripheral vision is diminished. Keeping the inside of the car warm at all times is not a significant issue when driving in warm climates or during warm seasons. Peripheral vision is diminished so it is important to look to the left and right. Reflexes are slowed for older adults; thus, caution regarding speed while driving should be emphasized. **Cognitive Level:** Analyzing **Client Need:** Health Promotion and Maintenance **Integrated Process:** Nursing Process: Evaluation **Content Area:** Foundational Sciences **Strategy:** The phrase *favorable response* cues you to look for the desired outcome.

8 **Answer: 4** **Rationale:** Proper self-administration of medications includes taking medications on time and, if a dose is missed, taking the next one on time. Misuse of medications by older adults includes behaviors such as combining prescribed and over-the-counter medications, having prescriptions from different physicians, failing to tell each doctor what has previously been prescribed and taking someone else's medications. **Cognitive Level:** Analyzing **Client Need:** Health Promotion and Maintenance **Integrated Process:** Nursing Process: Evaluation **Content Area:** Foundational Sciences **Strategy:** The phrase *indicates that the instruction was effective*, means the choices will have three incorrect outcomes and one desired outcome, which will be the correct choice.

9 **Answer: 4** **Rationale:** Interrupting the flow of urine assists the external urethra to contract and strengthens pelvic floor muscles. Coughing and bearing down will worsen urinary incontinence. Observing and percussing for bladder fullness after voiding represent data collection, not interventions. **Cognitive Level:** Applying **Client Need:** Physiological Adaptation **Integrated Process:** Nursing Process: Planning **Content Area:** Foundational Sciences **Strategy:** Distinguish between data collection and interventions, and then choose the intervention that will reduce urinary incontinence rather than worsen it.

10 **Answer: 1** **Rationale:** Ecchymoses are not the result of aging and should be investigated to determine whether the client is sustaining injury or taking anticoagulant therapy. Cherry hemangiomas do not require further investigation as to cause. Tenting of the skin is a normal, age-related change in an older adult. Nevi on the neck and forehead are not significant age-related findings. **Cognitive Level:** Applying **Client Need:** Health Promotion and Maintenance **Integrated Process:** Nursing Process: Data Collection **Content Area:** Foundational Sciences **Strategy:** The critical phrase *most significant* leads you to look for an option that is not an age-related change or a benign skin condition.

11 **Answer: 3** **Rationale:** Prealbumin is a sensitive indicator of changes in nutritional protein status and can also alert the nurse to clients at risk for pressure ulcer development. Serum albumin can provide data about visceral protein stores but has a relatively long half-life and may not accurately reflect recent protein losses. Total cholesterol would be assessed as a risk factor for cardiovascular disease. CBC is a hematology test commonly used for screening purposes although decreased red blood cell count would indicate anemia. **Cognitive Level:** Applying **Client Need:** Reduction of Risk Potential **Integrated Process:** Nursing Process: Data Collection **Content Area:** Foundational Sciences **Strategy:** Eliminate total cholesterol and CBC first as general screening measures, then choose prealbumin over albumin because the value changes more rapidly in response to nutritional intake.

12 **Answer: 3** **Rationale:** Prolonged use of laxatives can lead to dependence on them for stimulation of defecation and can actually lead to uncontrollable defecation. Laxatives are not necessarily required to stimulate defecation in older adults. A proper diet, adequate fluid intake, and sufficient activity will help to maintain normal bowel function during later years. A balanced diet is important even if not using laxatives. Laxatives should be used only as needed. **Cognitive Level:** Applying **Client Need:** Pharmacological and Parenteral Therapies **Integrated Process:** Nursing Process: Implementation **Content Area:** Foundational Sciences **Strategy:** Choose the

response that represents factual scientific information and teaches the client about risks associated with laxative use.

13 **Answer: 3 Rationale:** Posture changes shift the center of gravity in an older adult client and put the client at risk for falls. Bone and cartilage changes increase the risk of injury if a fall occurs but not the risk of falling. **Cognitive Level:** Applying **Client Need:** Safety and Infection Control **Integrated Process:** Nursing Process: Data Collection **Content Area:** Foundational Sciences **Strategy:** Read the question carefully and use similarities in the question stem and the answer to make a selection.

14 **Answer: 1 Rationale:** Motion receptors can be stimulated with instillation of large amounts of fluid. Nausea or vomiting can result and relief will occur if the irrigation procedure is stopped. If the irrigant did not return, the nurse should reposition the head. If the cerumen becomes softer, it indicates partial success of the procedure and the irrigation should continue. A temporary reduction in hearing is expected during the procedure in the affected ear and is not a cause for concern. **Cognitive Level:** Applying **Client Need:** Physiological Adaptation **Integrated Process:** Nursing Process: Implementation **Content Area:** Adult Health **Strategy:** The correct choice is the only answer that does not involve the ear or irrigation procedure directly.

15 **Answer: 3 Rationale:** Older adult clients are at risk for developing fluid overload during fluid and blood component therapy. The infusion rate should be slowed to prevent worsening of the problem. Documentation is a routine function that should be completed once the client has received care. Noting the volume remaining in the bag is a useful observation but is not the highest priority. The vital signs should be measured once an intervention is completed that will assist the client. **Cognitive Level:** Analyzing **Client Need:** Reduction of Risk Potential **Integrated Process:** Nursing Process: Implementation **Content Area:** Adult Health **Strategy:** Visualize care to determine first, second, third, and fourth action order.

16 **Answer: 1, 2, 3 Rationale:** Older adults may be at higher risk for fluid imbalances because of decreased thirst or oral intake, diagnosed health conditions that affect fluid balance, or if they have difficulty with mobility to use the bathroom. It is not necessarily true that older adults eat only canned or prepackaged foods, or that they dislike water. **Cognitive Level:** Analyzing **Client Need:** Physiological Adaptation **Integrated Process:** Nursing Process: Evaluation **Content Area:** Adult Health **Strategy:** Consider age-related changes (decreased thirst and mobility) and health problems that affect fluid balance (such as heart failure or renal insufficiency) to aid in making selections. Note the wording of the question indicates that more than one option is correct.

17 **Answer: 1, 2, 4 Rationale:** Ultraviolet light, injury, and viral infections increase the incidence of cataract development. The nurse recommends the use of sunglasses, eye protection, and safety throughout the lifespan. Vitamin A and eyestrain do not increase the risk of cataract development. **Cognitive Level:** Applying **Client Need:** Health Promotion and Maintenance **Integrated Process:** Nursing Process: Data Collection **Content Area:** Adult Health **Strategy:** Specific information is needed to answer the question. Consider that risk factors have the ability to cause damage to the eye.

18 **Answer: 3 Rationale:** Aging eyes require additional light and time to adapt to light to see effectively. Use of the call bell will provide assistance so that falls are prevented. Withholding all liquids after dinner does not assure that the client will not need to get up during the night to void. Depriving a client of fluids for this reason is unethical. Four side rails are considered a form of restraint and should not be used without a physician's order, and until other methods of keeping the client safe have failed. Chemical sedation is an inappropriate way to prevent a client from falling; some medications will lead to confusion. **Cognitive Level:** Analyzing **Client Need:** Safety and Infection Control **Integrated Process:** Nursing Process: Implementation **Content Area:** Fundamentals **Strategy:** Eliminate actions that increase the risk of client harm or violate legal rights of the client.

19 **Answer: 1 Rationale:** Older adults need increased fiber, calcium, and vitamins C and A. They also need to decrease the number of calories taken in. Margarine contains trans-fatty acids, which have been linked to heart disease and cancer. Older adults need increased fiber, calcium, and vitamins C and A. Canned foods and prepared package foods contain large amounts of sodium, which could adversely affect the cardiovascular, fluid-balance, and elimination systems. **Cognitive Level:** Analyzing **Client Need:** Health Promotion and Maintenance **Integrated Process:** Nursing Process: Evaluation **Content Area:** Foundational Sciences **Strategy:** It is important to read all of the components of each option. When picking the correct option, all the components of that option must be correct.

20 **Answer: 3 Rationale:** Appropriate use of the health care system allows needs to be met. Many clients might require direct care, or reinforcement of learning and application, in the home environment. Asking children or significant others to rearrange their lives might not be the first choice if home care is available and chosen by the client. Keeping clients in the hospital when home care is available is not an appropriate use of resources. Asking the pharmacist to call the client at home to take medicine is an inappropriate use of resources. **Cognitive Level:** Applying **Client Need:** Health Promotion and Maintenance **Integrated Process:** Nursing Process: Implementation **Content Area:** Adult Health **Strategy:** Application of development and knowledge of the health care system can help you to select the best answer.

Key Terms to Review

anosomia p. 217
atrophy p. 218
delirium p. 221
dementia p. 224
lentigines p. 217
osteoporosis p. 218
polypharmacy p. 220
presbycusis p. 217
presbyopia p. 217
proprioception p. 218

References

Berman, A., & Snyder, S. (2012). *Kozier & Erb's fundamentals of nursing: Concepts, process, and practice* (9th ed.). Upper Saddle River, NJ: Pearson Education, Inc.

Touhy, T. & Jett, K. (2011). *Ebersole & Hess' toward healthy aging: Human needs and nursing response* (8th ed.). St. Louis, MO: Elsevier.

Lehne, R. (2010). *Pharmacology for nursing care* (7th ed.). St. Louis, MO: Elsevier.

U.S. Dept. of Health and Human Services, Administration on Aging (2010). *A profile of older Americans: 2010*. Retrieved July 2, 2011, from http://www.aoa.gov/aoaroot/aging_statistics/Profile/2010/docs/2010profile.pdf

Test Yourself

Are you ready for the NCLEX-PN® or course exams? Use the practice tests on the companion website to check.

Therapeutic Communication and Environment 18

In this chapter

Cross Reference

Another chapter relevant to this content area is

Cultural Awareness **Chapter 19**

I. OVERVIEW OF COMMUNICATION

A. Characteristics of effective *communication*

1. An exchange of information, ideas, attitudes, and emotions occurs; effective communication occurs when message intended is message received
2. A basic skill in providing health care to clients; occurs between nurse and clients and between nurse and other health care providers

B. Elements of communication (see Box 18–1): can either promote or inhibit flow of accurate communication

C. Levels of communication

1. Intrapersonal: occurs within oneself and happens constantly; involves thinking about a message before it is sent, interpreting it, and evaluating it (self-talk)
2. Interpersonal: occurs between people and involves sending and receiving a message and **feedback**
3. Public communication: involves sending a message to a group of people for dissemination of information; it generally does not require feedback

D. Forms of communication

1. Communication occurs both verbally and nonverbally in a therapeutic relationship; purposeful communication between nurse and client is often termed **therapeutic communication**
2. *NCLEX®* Be aware of communication chosen to ensure message sent is message received; be aware of own nonverbal body language and physical boundaries, such as client's personal space
3. *NCLEX®* **Verbal communication**: use of spoken or written words
   a. Therapeutic rapport: verbal communication is facilitated by a trusting nurse–client relationship (client believes nurse cares about client's well-being and wants to assist in meeting health-related client goals)
   b. Pacing: rhythm and speed with which verbal message is sent; pace of a message may indicate interest, disinterest, or anxiety, among other emotions
   c. Intonation: pattern of pauses and accents or stresses when sending a message can reflect an underlying mood of sender, such as anger, boredom, excitement
   d. Clarity and brevity: clear, brief messages are more likely to be interpreted correctly than vague and lengthy messages; clarity is influenced by congruence between verbal and nonverbal behavior
   e. Timing and relevance: messages should contain content of interest to client and be delivered when client is interested in receiving it

Box 18–1

Elements of Communication

1. Sender: initiates communication to convey information, thoughts, ideas, or feelings to another; encodes information by selecting signs and symbols used (language, word selection, voice intonations, gestures, etc.)
2. Message: information to be communicated; includes codings (vocabulary, tone of voice, body language, and way the message is transmitted); effective communication occurs when message intended is message received
3. Channel: vehicle used to convey message using any of five senses; for example, written documentation (sight), oral communication (hearing), and therapeutic touch; use correct medium to send message, such as writing a message for a hearing-impaired client to ensure message intended is message received
4. Receiver: person or group that message is intended for, also called *decoder* of message; perceives or interprets message
5. Environment: physical, cultural, and social conditions in which information is transmitted; sometimes called *context* of communication
6. Feedback: sometimes called *response*; requires that receiver respond to message communicated by sender; may be verbal or nonverbal and helps to determine whether communication was effective or ineffective

NCLEX®

4. **Nonverbal communication**: occurs without words; often called body language
   a. Facial expression: can either convey or mask emotions; cautiously interpret eye and facial movements and validate impressions with further assessment; some facial expressions are universal, such as a smile for happiness and a frown for displeasure
   b. Eye contact: can be influenced by cultural norms; avoiding eye contact may be culturally appropriate or can indicate other feelings, such as embarrassment or lack of interest in communicating
   c. Gestures: can convey urgency of message or be a coping response when client cannot express an urgent message quickly enough using words; some gestures (such as a hand wave) have almost universal meanings, while others are culture-specific; can also be used as signals when unable to communicate with words
   d. Posture and gait: can indicate physical well-being, self-concept, and mood; an erect posture and a steady purposeful gait generally indicate a sense of well-being; slouching or a shuffling, slow gait may indicate depressed mood, presence of Parkinson's disease, or being tired or uncomfortable; validate with client any impressions gained from observing posture and gait
   e. Territoriality and personal space: all people have a physical zone around body considered to be an extension of self that should not be entered by others; size of space can vary considerably among cultures and individuals; type of relationship also affects desired personal space; body language is often used to signal when someone has violated personal space (such as taking a step back)
   f. Personal appearance: can be a general indicator of self-esteem, social status, emotional status, culture or other group association; selection of clothing is often highly personal; hygiene may be influenced by physical ability, emotional status, mental illness, energy level, and time; be careful not to judge clients based on personal appearance

NCLEX®

E. **Effective communication techniques (see Box 18–2)**
   1. Maintain appropriate boundaries as part of therapeutic communication
   2. Understand that one cannot always know how others perceive or misperceive messages sent; developing a sense of self-awareness and checking client's understanding of messages is critical to good communication

NCLEX®

F. **Communication techniques (blocks) to avoid (see Box 18–3)**
   1. Avoid statements that discourage further communication from client to nurse and/or place client's feelings on hold
   2. Such communications are disruptive to nurse–client relationship

G. **Communicating with clients who have special needs (see Box 18–4)**

Box 18–2

Effective Communication Techniques

Acknowledging: gives nonjudgmental recognition to a client for a certain behavior or contribution, or indicates attention to and care of client

Clarifying: asks for additional information to ensure understanding of message sent; a statement like "Would you tell me more about what you have just said?" conveys client's message is important to the nurse

Focusing: focuses client on pertinent information and helps client expand on that information; directs client toward information that is important

Giving information: provides specific information to a client either with or without client's request

Offering self: offers nurse's presence without attaching any expectations or conditions on client's behavior during that time

Restating or paraphrasing: ensures nurse understands message sent; utilizing this technique, nurse repeats main thought of message sent

Reflecting: redirects content of a client's message back to client for further thought or consideration

Summarizing: may be used at end of an interaction to identify material discussed; helps to sort out relevant from irrelevant information

Using silence: allows for quiet time without conversation for several seconds or minutes to allow for reflection about discussion that just occurred, to reduce tension, or to gather thoughts about how to proceed

Box 18–3

Communication Blocks to Avoid

Self-disclosure: communicates personal experience to client that focuses relationship on nurse instead of client; is not client-centered or goal-directed

Inattentive listening: blocks communication by indicating that client's needs are not important

Overuse of medical jargon: confuses client and indicates nurse is not interested in ensuring health care information is understood

Giving personal opinions (approval, disapproval) or offering advice: may give impression that a person is closed to new ideas or to open discussion

Prying or probing techniques: if not used to seek specific health-related information or to clarify a client's statement, this is a nontherapeutic technique; in such instances, client may provide information to satisfy nurse's curiosity and nurse's questions are inappropriate and may violate client's right to privacy

Changing the subject: blocks therapeutic communication by indicating that client should not continue to talk about previous topic; leads conversation to only those areas that nurse wants to discuss

Challenging the client or being defensive: creates a power struggle between client and nurse and does not foster open and honest communication (asking "why?")

Providing false reassurance: does not contribute to open and honest communication and can break bond of trust between client and nurse

Memory Aid

The answers to communication questions are those that utilize therapeutic communication techniques while avoiding the use of communication blocks.

Box 18-4

Communication with Clients with Special Needs

Difficulty hearing

- To ensure that effective communication occurs with a client who is hearing impaired, stand or sit near client and speak clearly and slowly using a low-pitched voice.
- Ensure environment has adequate lighting and is quiet and free from distractions.
- Use therapeutic communication techniques to ensure that message sent is message received.
- Use writing, if necessary, to enhance communication with a client who is hearing impaired.
- Avoid using a loud voice when speaking to a client who is hearing impaired.

Difficulty seeing

- Ensure environment has adequate light.
- Ensure that quality of spoken word matches message communicated.
- Remember a visually impaired person may not be able to use nonverbal cues to help interpret message.

Mute or unable to speak clearly

- When communicating with a client who is unable to speak clearly, has an artificial airway, or is mute, encourage client to write a response or utilize word boards or pictures to ensure effective communication.
- Utilize therapeutic technique of clarification or paraphrasing as needed to assist in communication.

Cognitively impaired

- Ensure language is simple, concise, and spoken slowly and calmly.
- Allow adequate time for client to process information.
- Use environmental cues to convey message to client; for instance, hold a toothbrush in view while asking if client would like to brush teeth.

Unresponsive

- Use touch along with spoken word and try to elicit a response from client.
- Ask a closed question such as "Can you hear me?" and observe for nonverbal cues that may indicate client has received message to try to obtain a response.
- Speak to client in a manner that assumes client can hear every spoken word; avoid having conversations about client's status or that are irrelevant to client at the bedside.

Non-English-speaking clients

- Seek an interpreter fluent in client's primary language if client does not speak English; until an interpreter is available, communication must take place through nonverbal means.
- Use pictures, environmental cues, and body language to communicate with a client who speaks a different language.

II. THERAPEUTIC NURSE–CLIENT RELATIONSHIPS

A. A *therapeutic relationship* is a nurse–client interaction that focuses on client needs and is goal-specific, theory-based, and open to observation or scrutiny by other health care team members

B. Phases of therapeutic relationship

1. Pre-interaction phase
   - **a.** Occurs prior to initial contact with a person and is similar to planning stage before an interview
   - **b.** Any information that nurse has related to client is organized and analyzed prior to contact with client; during this phase, nurse prepares for initial contact

NCLEX®

2. Orientation phase
   - **a.** May also be called introductory phase or pre-helping phase
   - **b.** Nurse and client get to know one another and develop a degree of trust
   - **c.** Three processes occur during this phase: opening the relationship, clarifying the problem, and structuring and formulating the contract for what will be accomplished during relationship

NCLEX®

3. Working phase
   - **a.** Includes exploring and understanding thoughts and feelings, along with facilitating client's work and taking action
   - **b.** Skills required during this phase are empathetic listening and understanding, respect, genuineness, concreteness, and confrontation
   - **c.** Client **transference**, an unconscious process of displacing feelings for significant people in past onto nurse in present relationship, can occur in this phase; **countertransference** is nurse's emotional reaction to clients based on feelings for significant people in past
   - **d.** At completion of this phase, client makes decisions and takes action, while nurse provides information and collaborates with and supports client

NCLEX®

4. Termination phase
   - **a.** Primary goal of termination phase of therapeutic relationship is to review client's progress and plans for immediate future after reaching goals
   - **b.** May be difficult for both nurse and client; to reduce feelings of loss and ambivalence, it may be helpful for nurse to summarize relationship and make follow-up phone calls to help client transition to independence
   - **c.** Nurse should prepare client for termination phase early in relationship

C. Components of a therapeutic relationship

1. Physical component of relationship includes all procedures and technical skills that nurses provide for clients
2. Psychosocial component involves qualities such as positive regard, nonjudgmental attitude, acceptance, warmth, empathy, and authenticity
3. Spiritual component is feeling of connectedness with clients and respect for diversity of spiritual needs among clients
4. Power component includes beliefs about external and internal locus of control
   - **a.** A client with a strong internal locus of control tends to believe that he or she is able to make own decisions and can influence own health; this client may experience more positive health outcomes
   - **b.** A client with a strong external locus of control tends to believe that other people and events heavily affect his or her health and related decisions, and may perceive self as somewhat powerless; this client may have less positive health outcomes unless appropriate support people and services are in place

D. Nurse's responsibilities in a therapeutic relationship

1. Deliver care that is holistic and comprehensive of current client needs and priorities
2. Respect client's uniqueness, with consideration given to cultural and spiritual beliefs, values, and practices that provide comfort, support, and hope during illness
3. Foster open and honest communication that focuses on client's needs and feelings
4. Value empathy, respect, and genuineness in interactions with client
5. Set limits when necessary to foster client progress and growth
6. Promote client independence by assisting client to utilize internal resources (such as personal strengths, problem-solving skills) and community resources

III. TEACHING AND LEARNING AS THERAPEUTIC COMMUNICATION

A. Purposes of client teaching

1. Maintenance and promotion of health and prevention of illness
   - **a.** Examples include providing information about immunization requirements, nutrition, and exercise; offering parenting and prenatal classes
   - **b.** Generally these programs are aimed toward groups of people with a health care need and disseminate information and skills needed for clients to develop positive health practices
2. Restoration of health
   - **a.** Teaching is intended for clients with an active health problem and focus on cause, condition, and treatment
   - **b.** An example of this type of client teaching is insulin administration for a client who has new onset type 1 diabetes mellitus
3. Coping with impaired functioning
   - **a.** Teaching centers around providing instruction to a client who has not made or cannot make a complete recovery
   - **b.** An example is a client who modifies activities of daily living because of a lower limb amputation

B. Domains of learning

1. Cognitive learning involves acquiring and using knowledge; for example, when teaching a parenting class, nurse provides information on developmental stages of children; when applying that knowledge to toilet training child, parent is learning in **cognitive domain**
2. Affective learning occurs when a client changes unhealthy attitudes or feelings and values; a parent who accepts and understands that children have specific developmental stages and may not become toilet trained until after age 2 is learning in **affective domain**
3. Psychomotor: learning to complete a physical act is learning in **psychomotor domain**; for example, nurse may role-play with a parent an appropriate dialogue to use if a toddler refuses to use toilet or appropriate assistance and supervision to provide while child is using toilet

C. Factors that influence client learning

1. Motivation: desire to learn
   a. Important to learning is that client recognizes need to learn a new behavior
   b. Nurses can assist a client in solving problems and identifying needs that may increase desire to learn

NCLEX®
2. Health beliefs
   a. Must be assessed to develop beneficial teaching plan; client's health beliefs may or may not be congruent with information to be taught
   b. Assist a client by showing a cause-and-effect relationship between positive and negative health practices; for example, if cardiac client does not believe that smoking will affect cardiac status, individual is unlikely to change behavior
   c. Understand that a client's health care beliefs may not change, despite concentrated efforts, because of multiple psychological, cultural, and environmental factors
3. Psychosocial adaptation to illness
   a. Describes transition from a healthy, independent state to an illness state
   b. Successful adaptation or acculturation to illness depends on client's emotional makeup

NCLEX®
   c. Understand that a client is unlikely to learn new health-related behaviors if not ready or motivated to learn or is experiencing problems unrelated to health
   d. Regularly assess how a client is adapting
4. Active participation
   a. Active participation by client in teaching and learning process makes learning more meaningful

NCLEX®
   b. Assess a client's learning needs and involve client in learning process to encourage active participation
5. Literacy level and educational level: ability of client to read materials provided and understand spoken word
6. Developmental level affects ability to understand health problem and learn information needed for self-management
7. Individual learning style: learning is enhanced when nurse uses instructional methods that match client's preferred learning style

D. Basic teaching principles

NCLEX®
1. Set priorities: rank client's learning needs according to importance; involve client in ranking needs because learning is more likely to occur when client's perceived needs are met

NCLEX®
2. Use appropriate timing; for example, a client with diabetes is more likely to successfully self-administer insulin immediately after watching a video than waiting until next morning
3. Organize materials: learning occurs from simple to complex; organize material in this manner to allow learner to assimilate information more readily
4. Promote and maintain learner attention and participation: keep environment physically comfortable and free from distractions; involve client actively in learning process; ensure that information is personally relevant to client; provide opportunity for client feedback
5. Build on existing knowledge: assess client's knowledge of subject before teaching to make material more personal to client and enhance learner's confidence in material
6. Select appropriate teaching methods
   a. Discussion: one-on-one formal or informal instruction allows client to set pace of learning and engage in verbal exchange with nurse; promotes customized learning
   b. Question and answer: meets needs of clients for specific pieces of information as requested by client; often beneficial as a follow-up to other teaching methods
   c. Role-play, discovery: allows client to simulate real-life situations and apply new knowledge or skills in an artificial or "safe" setting; helps to build client's confidence in newly acquired knowledge and skills once feelings of shyness, embarrassment, or awkwardness are worked through

d. Computerized instruction: can include CAI (computer-assisted instruction) or interactive computer programs (using touch-screen technology); allows client to regulate pace of instruction and possibly direct nature of material presented next (interactive programs)

7. Use appropriate teaching aids: are useful supplements to instruction if well-selected according to content and client's learning style; may include visual aids (drawings, charts, models, printed materials), audiotapes, films or videotapes, programmed instruction, games, and others

8. Provide content of teaching related to developmental level

NCLEX®
a. Infant: immunizations, infant safety, nutrition, rest/sleep patterns, and sensory stimulation; assess parents' learning needs and provide instruction accordingly; complete client teaching when infant is calm and happy to minimize parents' distraction

NCLEX®
b. Toddler: accident prevention, toilet training, dental hygiene, and appropriate play activities; toddlers fear pain and separation from parents; parent teaching for a hospitalized toddler includes participation in care, purpose of care plans, and developmental regression that can occur because of hospitalization

NCLEX®
c. Preschooler: accident prevention, dental health, nutrition, cognitive stimulation, and sleep patterns; assist hospitalized preschooler by using visual, tactile, and auditory images to decrease fear of procedures; therapeutic play or using dolls or puppets to demonstrate procedures before they are done is also helpful

NCLEX®
d. School-age child: dental hygiene, safety measures, promotion of physical fitness, and hygiene measures to prevent spread of infection; provide concrete examples and explanations of procedures to help child understand health care; encourage child to identify own learning needs; therapeutic play may assist child to learn

NCLEX®
e. Adolescent: effects of drugs and alcohol, sexually transmitted infections, reducing risk of injury (e.g., motor vehicle accidents, sports), and nutrition information; actively involve adolescent in learning to aid assimilation of information provided; client contracting and peer education also promote learning

NCLEX®
f. Young to middle-aged adult: importance of routine health tests and screening, sun protection measures, nutrition (especially adequate protein and calcium intake), and exercise to maintain health; evaluate client's learning needs and determine those that client believes are important to maintaining health

NCLEX®
g. Older adult: importance of exercise in maintaining joint mobility, nutrition (including caloric and fluid requirements), and fall prevention information; ensure there is adequate lighting and use large print if necessary for visually impaired client; for hearing impaired client, use written teaching materials and visual aids

IV. THERAPEUTIC ENVIRONMENTS

A. Overview

1. A therapeutic environment is one that is manipulated or created to help restore or promote physical and mental health
2. See Box 18–5 for practice settings in which therapeutic environments are integral to care
3. Physical space may be designed with attention to color, layout (such as circular halls for clients with Alzheimer's disease), and aesthetic appeal, including artwork
4. Aids to memory or cognition, such as clock and white boards in room identifying names of caregivers for day, may be used in hospital or long-term care environments

Box 18–5

Practice Settings That Utilize a Therapeutic Environment

- Psychiatric hospitals
- Community mental health centers
- General hospitals
- Community health agencies (e.g., home health, primary-care centers, homeless clinics)
- Outpatient services
- Senior centers and daycare centers
- Schools
- Prisons
- Emergency and crisis centers

B. Nursing interventions commonly used during care in a therapeutic environment
1. Health promotion and maintenance
2. Assessment and evaluation
3. Case management
4. Provision of a therapeutic milieu
5. Client education about factors that influence mental health and mental illness
6. Promotion of self-care and independence
7. Administration and monitoring of psychobiological treatment regimens
8. Crisis intervention and counseling
9. Engaging in social and community mental health efforts

C. *Milieu* therapy
1. Provides a therapeutic and safe environment in which client is free to express thoughts and feelings; this is particularly employed in mental health settings (see also Chapter 21)
2. Clients interact, share frustrations, and learn to relate to others in honest and constructive ways under supervision and assistance of mental health professionals
3. There are norms for client behavior on unit to foster safety of all clients and staff and are shared with clients; when client behavior violates these norms, such as being verbally or physically aggressive with other clients or staff, staff sets limits with client and may enforce sanctions that are discussed in advance
4. Individual client growth is often achieved through group meetings in which focus may be learning social skills, problem solving, goal setting, or otherwise effecting positive self-change
5. A prime tenet of group therapy is that all group members are valued and contribute to overall functioning of group

Check Your NCLEX-PN® Exam I.Q. *You are ready for testing on this content if you can*

- Utilize communication techniques appropriately and effectively.
- Determine accurately the components of a therapeutic relationship and how to maintain one.
- Create an environment conducive to client teaching, including preparation of the teaching plan.

PRACTICE TEST

1 The nurse has explained a therapeutic diet to a client. To ensure that learning has occurred, the nurse should take which follow-up action?

1. Repeat details of the diet once or twice more.
2. Listen to comments from client.
3. Ask another nurse to verify client understands the diet.
4. Refer client to a nutritionist.

2 A nurse is trying to establish whether a client who appears unconscious can communicate. What would be the best approach for the nurse to use?

1. Ask open-ended questions.
2. Ask client to blink once or twice in response to questions.
3. Observe for facial grimaces during verbal stimuli from the nurse.
4. Observe for response to painful stimuli.

3 A client who is legally blind has been admitted to the cardiac unit. Which action by the nurse would be best to promote adjustment to the environment?

1. Speak slowly and in a low-pitched voice while facing the client.
2. Post a sign on the door indicating the client is blind.
3. Explain unit noises and physical surroundings.
4. Give clear, concise, simple instructions to the client.

4 The nurse has asked the client to demonstrate self-injection technique. In doing so, the nurse is primarily attempting to determine which of the following?

1. Number of postdischarge home visits that will be required.
2. Other support services the client will need after discharge.
3. Quality of the client teaching plan.
4. Client's ability to perform the skill.

5 Which of the following would be the most appropriate time for a nurse to use confrontation as a therapeutic technique in communication with an assigned client?

1. When a good relationship exists and client's anxiety level is low.
2. During periods when client is noncompliant.
3. After client has had time to reflect on his or her behavior.
4. Immediately after a negative behavior has occurred.

6 Which teaching strategy should the nurse choose as being most likely to be effective when reinforcing health instruction to an adolescent client?

1. Lecture format
2. Professionally made videos
3. Client contracting
4. Role play

7 A nurse is observing a client's ability to change the surgical dressing before discharge. During the demonstration, the nurse notices the client has not performed the procedure correctly. What is the most appropriate action of the nurse at this time?

1. Immediately change dressing again to demonstrate correct technique.
2. Praise client for aspects of the procedure done accurately and correct the client's mistakes.
3. Praise client for steps completed correctly and refer the client to home care for follow up.
4. Explain kindly that the procedure was performed incorrectly and have client repeat the procedure.

8 When beginning to reinforce information about heart disease to a client newly diagnosed with heart disease, what is most important for the nurse to do first?

1. Find out what client knows or has heard about the disorder.
2. Consult with physician to determine content based on individual severity of disease.
3. Have a family member or significant other present who can reinforce diet and exercise tips.
4. Proceed from simple to complex concepts when discussing pathophysiology.

9 When caring for an older adult female client, the nurse would enhance communication by taking which action?

1. Speaking loudly and using many gestures
2. Interviewing client quickly to conserve the client's energy
3. Interviewing client with family present to verify responses to questions
4. Restating terms or phrases in different ways if the client does not understand

10 Which statement by the nurse best encourages a client to express feelings and allows the nurse to genuinely respond to those feelings?

1. "You mentioned that you broke your leg last year. Can you tell me more about how that happened?"
2. "You shared with me much information about your history of depression. It sounds as if medication alone may not be controlling your symptoms as you hoped."
3. "You said your back pain has not gone away since surgery. How difficult has it been to adapt to having pain during everyday activities?"
4. "You said you have had asthma since you were 11 years old and that medication therapy requires adjustment every 8 to 10 months or so. Is that right?"

11 What would be the best approach for a nurse to use to encourage a client with psychological distress to develop an awareness of feelings and express them effectively?

1. Challenge the client.
2. Offer reassurance.
3. Suggest coping strategies.
4. Offer empathy.

12 While talking with the nurse, a client says, "You are just like my mother; you don't trust me or like me. You and she wish I were dead." The nurse interprets this statement as indicating which process?

1. Psychosis
2. Countertransference
3. Transference
4. Projection

PRACTICE TEST

13. The nurse is preparing to explain an upcoming procedure to a 72-year-old, English-speaking Latino client. The nurse determines that which approach is best to verbally communicate with this client?

1. Speak quickly and avoid eye contact which could be perceived as threatening.
2. Speak slowly and provide brief and simple explanations.
3. Get an interpreter or family member to interpret for the nurse as needed.
4. Give very complete explanations of all information.

14. The nurse observes a client who is fidgeting, wringing the hands, and has body tenseness and a wrinkled brow. What is the best response to the client by the nurse?

1. "You look tense. Can you tell me if something is making you afraid or nervous?"
2. "You look upset. Would you like some medication to help you become calmer?"
3. Say, "You look worried. Is something bothering you?"
4. "Why are you so nervous and jumpy?"

15. A nurse floating to the nursing unit learns during inter-shift report that a client suffered disfiguring injuries in an accident a week ago. What is the best way for the nurse to prepare for the first encounter with this client?

1. Learn about client's support systems (family, friends, religion).
2. Obtain specifics of the disfigurement to better control first reactions by the nurse.
3. Review all medications and treatment procedures prior to meeting the client.
4. Have all supplies and equipment ready to be able to provide efficient care.

16. The nurse enters a client's room to speak to the client, moves the chair to the top of the bed by the client's head, and sits down to better hear the client. The client draws back and moves to the opposite side of the bed. What is the best response by the nurse?

1. Move the chair a foot or two away from the bed and observe the client's response.
2. Say, "I will come back later when you are ready to talk to me."
3. Ignore the behavior and continue with the interview, observing the client for depression.
4. Lean over and touch the client to convey reassurance.

17. The nurse, who has a heavy work assignment for the shift due to high client census, sees that a client is crying. What would be the best way for the nurse to convey a willingness to be with the client for support?

1. State, "Let's talk while I change your colostomy bag."
2. Ask, "Would you like to talk?" from the doorway, and go in if the client says yes.
3. Pull up a chair, sit down, and state, "I see something is bothering you. Do you want to talk?"
4. State, "I'll be back later and we can talk about what is troubling you at the moment."

18. A client asks about a new diagnostic test with which the nurse is unfamiliar. What is the best response by the nurse?

1. "I don't know much about that procedure, but I will find out and bring you information about it."
2. "The technicians in the radiology department will explain the procedure to you when you go for the test."
3. "It is your doctor's responsibility to explain that procedure to you. Would you like me to telephone the doctor?"
4. "I can't explain that now, but I'll get back to you later after all the morning medications are distributed."

19. A client can understand only minimal English, and no interpreter is available. What alternative measures can the nurse use to enhance communication?

1. Speak loudly to the client.
2. Provide a paper and pencil to write questions and information.
3. Use pictures and non-verbal cues to communicate.
4. Speak more slowly and face the client.

20 A client has been on the nursing unit for a few weeks because of surgical complications requiring extensive wound care. During the last dressing change before discharge to home with home health services, the client becomes angry with the nurse and says, "You don't have to be so careful. I'm being sent home anyway!" Which response by the nurse would be therapeutic? Select all that apply.

1. "I hear frustration or perhaps anger in your voice. Can you tell me more about how you are feeling right now?"
2. "Many people who have been in the hospital for an extended period have mixed feelings about going home. Can you tell me how you are feeling about discharge?"
3. "It sounds as though you are nervous about going home, but the wound care nurse who will see you also uses excellent technique. I'm sure your wound will continue to heal."
4. "Just because you are going home doesn't mean that your wound doesn't still require strict technique during a dressing change. Do you have any questions about your wound care after discharge?"
5. "Do you have any concerns about what will happen after discharge that you would like to talk about?"

ANSWERS & RATIONALES

1 **Answer: 2** **Rationale:** It is important for the nurse to listen to the feedback given by the client to ensure the message sent was the message received. Repetition is important in the teaching process but does not evaluate clients' understanding. Asking another nurse to verify teaching or referral to a nutritionist are not necessary as part of evaluation of nursing instruction. **Cognitive Level:** Applying **Client Need:** Psychosocial Integrity **Integrated Process:** Communication and Documentation **Content Area:** Fundamentals **Strategy:** The core issue of the question is determining the client response to teaching. In evaluation questions such as these, the correct option is likely to be one that focuses directly on the client.

2 **Answer: 2** **Rationale:** To evaluate an unresponsive client's ability to communicate, it is best for the nurse to ask questions that will elicit a single act or response by the client. Asking open-ended questions is not appropriate for the client's condition. Facial grimacing and response to pain may be noted during neurological assessment but do not relate to communication. **Cognitive Level:** Analyzing **Client Need:** Psychosocial Integrity **Integrated Process:** Communication and Documentation **Content Area:** Fundamentals **Strategy:** In communication questions such as these, the correct option is one that is client-focused and relates directly to communication. With this in mind, eliminate facial grimaces and painful stimuli immediately, and choose the option to blink because of its simplicity.

3 **Answer: 3** **Rationale:** A client who is blind does not have the benefit of nonverbal cues to facilitate communication and understanding of the environment. It is important for the nurse to explain physical surroundings and noises because the client cannot determine these without the added benefit of sight. Speaking slowly while facing the client and giving simple explanations are approaches that are useful with a client who is hearing impaired. Placing a sign on the client's door encroaches on confidentiality. **Cognitive Level:** Analyzing **Client Need:** Psychosocial Integrity **Integrated Process:** Communication and Documentation **Content Area:** Fundamentals **Strategy:** In communication questions with a client who has loss of vision, the correct option is one that supplements vision impairment with verbal communication. Note the critical word *best* in the stem of the question, which indicates more than one response may be partially or totally correct.

4 **Answer: 4** **Rationale:** A return demonstration specifically identifies the client's ability to perform a skill. The client's skill level may provide incidental information related to the quality of the teaching plan, number of home visits needed, or additional support services needed, but they are not the primary reasons for asking the client to demonstrate a skill. **Cognitive Level:** Analyzing **Client Need:** Psychosocial Integrity **Integrated Process:** Communication and Documentation **Content Area:** Fundamentals **Strategy:** Recall that to evaluate learning of a skill, which is in the psychomotor domain, the best option is the one that utilizes return demonstration. In this way, the nurse can verify that the client can perform the skill and also has an opportunity to provide additional feedback.

5 **Answer: 1** **Rationale:** Confrontation should not be used as a therapeutic communication technique unless trust has been established in the nurse–client relationship. Because confrontation can be uncomfortable for the client, it is important for the nurse and client to have a trusting relationship as a foundation. The other options represent situations in which the nurse might like to use confrontation but that are not appropriate for this communication technique. **Cognitive Level:** Applying **Client Need:** Psychosocial Integrity **Integrated Process:** Communication and Documentation **Content Area:** Fundamentals **Strategy:** Note the critical words *most appropriate* in the stem of the question. This tells you that more than one option will be plausible and that you must choose one over the others based on what is most therapeutic for the client.

6 **Answer: 3** **Rationale:** Client contracting provides adolescents with the ability to be involved in their care. Adolescents should be involved in planning and decision making regarding their need for information about their own health issues. Lecture, viewing a video, and role play would not provide opportunity for feedback. **Cognitive Level:** Analyzing **Client Need:** Psychosocial Integrity **Integrated Process:** Communication and Documentation **Content Area:** Fundamentals **Strategy:** In teaching and learning questions in which communication is key, choose the option that provides for two-way communication between the client and nurse. Note the critical words *most likely to be effective* in the stem of the question, which tells you that more than one

option is plausible and that you must choose based on knowledge of communication theory.

7 **Answer: 2** **Rationale:** Praising the client for steps performed correctly provides positive reinforcement. In addition, explaining the client's mistakes reinforces the correct way to perform the procedure. Redoing the dressing decreases the client's confidence and is not useful. Praising the client without correcting the mistakes gives feedback that the procedure was done correctly. Having the client repeat the procedure and stating it was done correctly without further guidance does not reinforce or assist learning. **Cognitive Level:** Analyzing **Client Need:** Psychosocial Integrity **Integrated Process:** Communication and Documentation **Content Area:** Fundamentals **Strategy:** Note the critical words *most appropriate* in the stem of the question. This tells you that more than one option is plausible and that you must choose based on knowledge of communication theory.

8 **Answer: 1** **Rationale:** When presenting information to a client, it is important that the nurse find out what the client already knows, and then build on existing knowledge. It is not necessary to consult with a physician. It may be helpful to have family members present, but it is not the priority at the time of initial teaching. It is important when teaching to begin with basic concepts and progress to the complex after determining current client knowledge. **Cognitive Level:** Analyzing **Client Need:** Psychosocial Integrity **Integrated Process:** Communication and Documentation **Content Area:** Fundamentals **Strategy:** Focus on the critical word *first* in the stem of the question. This indicates that more than one option may be correct and that a time sequence is involved. Recalling that assessment is the first step of the nursing process, choose an option that assesses the client's current level of knowledge before beginning instruction.

9 **Answer: 4** **Rationale:** Restating the information using different words or phrases as needed may assist the older adult client's understanding. Increasing speech volume is unnecessary and the use of gestures is helpful only if the client has a hearing deficit. Older adults do better with a slower paced interview with frequent breaks to decrease fatigue. Relying on family to verify responses is not respectful of the older adult's autonomy. **Cognitive Level:** Applying **Client Need:** Psychosocial Integrity **Integrated Process:** Communication and Documentation **Content Area:** Fundamentals **Strategy:** The core issue of the question is how to communicate most effectively with an older adult client. The correct option is the one that focuses on the client, incorporates age-related needs, and does not incorporate ageism into the response.

10 **Answer: 3** **Rationale:** The communication technique of reflection occurs when the nurse directs feelings and questions back to the client to encourage elaboration. The nurse uses the technique of focusing by asking questions to help the client focus on a specific area of concern. With the use of summarizing, the nurse highlights important points of the conversation. The nurse uses restating by repeating back to clients the main points or content of the conversation. **Cognitive Level:** Analyzing **Client Need:** Psychosocial Integrity **Integrated Process:** Communication and Documentation **Content Area:** Fundamentals **Strategy:** The core issue of the question is knowledge of various types of therapeutic techniques, specifically one that utilizes reflection as a means of encouraging continued communication. Use this knowledge and the process of elimination to make a selection.

11 **Answer: 4** **Rationale:** Empathy is the ability of the nurse to see the client's perception of the world, which aids in therapeutic communication and the nurse–client relationship. Challenging clients is not helpful and often triggers them to defend themselves from what appears to be an attack by the nurse. False reassurance can be seen as a way to encourage clients how to feel and ignores their distress. Advising occurs when the nurse tells clients what to do, preventing them from exploring problems and using the problem-solving process to find solutions. **Cognitive Level:** Applying **Client Need:** Psychosocial Integrity **Integrated Process:** Communication and Documentation **Content Area:** Fundamentals **Strategy:** The core issue of the question is knowledge of the purpose and use of therapeutic communication techniques. Use this knowledge and the process of elimination to make a selection.

12 **Answer: 3** **Rationale:** Transference is the unconscious process of displaying feelings for significant people in the client's past onto the nurse in the present relationship. Psychosis is a state in which a client is unable to comprehend reality and has difficulty relating to others. Countertransference is the nurse's emotional reaction to clients based on feelings for significant people in the nurse's past. Projection is a defense mechanism in which blame for unacceptable desires, thoughts, shortcomings, and mistakes is attached to others in the environment. **Cognitive Level:** Analyzing **Client Need:** Psychosocial Integrity **Integrated Process:** Communication and Documentation **Content Area:** Fundamentals **Strategy:** The core issue of the question is knowledge of various processes that can occur during therapeutic communication. Eliminate psychosis (a disorder) and projection (a defense mechanism) first. Choose transference over countertransferance because it is the client who has made the transference, not the nurse.

13 **Answer: 2** **Rationale:** Taking into account the age and ethnicity of the client, it is helpful to speak slowly and provide short and simple explanations. Speaking quickly does not help the client understand the information presented. Eye contact is acceptable. There is no need for an interpreter based on the information in the question. Simple explanations are more effective than lengthy ones. **Cognitive Level:** Applying **Client Need:** Psychosocial Integrity **Integrated Process:** Communication and Documentation **Content Area:** Fundamentals **Strategy:** Note that some options have more than one part to them. In such questions, all parts must be correct for the option to be correct. Eliminate incorrect options using principles of therapeutic communication and information presented in the question.

14 **Answer: 1** **Rationale:** After noting the client's nonverbal behavior, the best response is one that will elicit further data from the client, which is accomplished by providing a broad opening for the client. Asking whether the client would like medication to become calm places a judgment on the client's behavior. By asking, "Is something bothering you?" after acknowledging the client's feelings, the nurse risks placing the client on the defensive. Asking a question using the word "why" is a block to communication and will likely make the client defensive. **Cognitive Level:** Analyzing **Client Need:** Psychosocial Integrity **Integrated Process:** Communication and Documentation **Content Area:** Fundamentals **Strategy:** The core

issue of the question is how to apply general principles of therapeutic communication. In this question, the correct option is the one that is nonjudgmental, uses therapeutic communication techniques, and avoids communication blocks.

15 **Answer: 2 Rationale:** The nurse is more likely to exhibit therapeutic verbal and nonverbal communication by being aware of the extent of the client's disfiguring injuries. This will reduce the likelihood of surprise that can be seen in nonverbal behavior. The remaining options are also items that the nurse will do, but they are general to all clients and not particular to the client in the question. **Cognitive Level:** Analyzing **Client Need:** Psychosocial Integrity **Integrated Process:** Communication and Documentation **Content Area:** Fundamentals **Strategy:** The critical phrases in the stem of the question are *best way* and *first encounter*. The phrase *best way* indicates that more than one option is a true statement and more than one option may compete for priority. The phrase *first encounter* assists you to focus on the real core issue of the question, which relates to communication.

16 **Answer: 1 Rationale:** The client may have a need for increased personal space, which may account for moving to the other side of the bed. However, cultural considerations cannot be ruled out by the information in this stem. Thus, the correct action is to validate the reason for the client's behavior. This is what moving the chair represents, an attempt to determine whether increased need for personal space is the reason for the behavior. Leaving the client alone punishes the client for the behavior. Ignoring the behavior is inappropriate because it does not acknowledge an unspoken need by the client. Touching the client would further invade personal space and is inappropriate until further data is gathered. **Cognitive Level:** Analyzing **Client Need:** Psychosocial Integrity **Integrated Process:** Communication and Documentation **Content Area:** Fundamentals **Strategy:** The core issue of the question is how to respond to a client's nonverbal behavior in a therapeutic manner. Eliminate options that are nontherapeutic or that could worsen the situation.

17 **Answer: 1 Rationale:** The nurse has two competing priorities: the need to accomplish work on a busy shift and the need to address the psychosocial needs of a client in distress. Talking while working takes into consideration both of these factors. Asking a question from the doorway creates psychological as well as physical distance between the nurse and the client because the question is asked from the doorway. Immediately sitting down ignores the other workload of the nurse. Stating the nurse will come back later puts the client's feelings on hold. **Cognitive Level:** Analyzing **Client Need:** Psychosocial Integrity **Integrated Process:** Communication and Documentation **Content Area:** Fundamentals **Strategy:** The core issue of the question is the most therapeutic response to a client in distress. Note that the question also contains the critical words *best way*, which implies that the options will have greater or lesser degrees of correctness and that you must choose between them. Use the process of elimination and choose the option that takes into account all of the relevant information in the stem of the question.

18 **Answer: 1 Rationale:** Stating a lack of knowledge and intent to find out demonstrates honesty and openness between the client and the nurse. It also addresses the client's need for information. The other options are incorrect because they put the client's information needs on hold and do not represent a candid response by the nurse. The correct answer to communication questions is the one that best acknowledges the client and utilizes therapeutic communication techniques. **Cognitive Level:** Analyzing **Client Need:** Psychosocial Integrity **Integrated Process:** Communication and Documentation **Content Area:** Fundamentals **Strategy:** First eliminate options that are similar by putting the client's request on hold and divert the responsibility to someone else. Next eliminate the option that is not a totally candid response. Alternatively, choose correctly by selecting the response that incorporates all the information in the question regarding the nurse's level of knowledge and the client's need to know.

19 **Answer: 3 Rationale:** Because the client does not speak English, the nurse must utilize non-verbal communication. With this in mind, the one use of pictures and non-verbal cues takes this need into account. Speaking loudly or more slowly while facing the client is helpful when the nurse is working with a client who is hearing impaired. Using paper and pencil would be useful for the aphasic client who has use of the dominant hand, such as after a CVA. **Cognitive Level:** Applying **Client Need:** Psychosocial Integrity **Integrated Process:** Communication and Documentation **Content Area:** Fundamentals **Strategy:** The core issue of the question is the best method for communicating with a client when there is a language barrier. Eliminate the options that are similar with respect to the spoken word. Eliminate the option that also relies on words that may not be in the client's vocabulary.

20 **Answer: 1, 2, 5 Rationale:** The correct answers to communication questions are those that utilize therapeutic communication techniques and avoid communication blocks. Options that focus on the client's feelings utilize these techniques, while the incorrect options use communication blocks of false reassurance and challenging the client. **Cognitive Level:** Analyzing **Client Need:** Psychosocial Integrity **Integrated Process:** Communication and Documentation **Content Area:** Fundamentals **Strategy:** Analyze each statement in terms of being a communication enhancer or blocker. Choose the ones that incorporate therapeutic communication techniques without having any components of communication blocks.

ANSWERS & RATIONALES

Key Terms to Review

References

Berman, A., & Snyder, S. (2012). *Kozier & Erb's fundamentals of nursing: Concepts, process, and practice* (9th ed.). Upper Saddle River, NJ: Pearson Education, Inc..

Craven, R., & Hirnle, C. (2009). *Fundamentals of nursing: Human health and function* (6th ed.). Philadelphia: Wolters-Kluwer.

Potter, P., & Perry, A. (2010). *Fundamentals of nursing enhanced multimedia edition package* (7th ed.). St. Louis, MO: Mosby, Inc.

Test Yourself

Are you ready for the NCLEX-PN® or course exams? Use the practice tests on the companion website to check.

Cultural Awareness 19

In this chapter

Cross Reference

Other chapters relevant to this content area are
Reproduction, Family Planning, and Infertility Chapter 8
Uncomplicated Antenatal Care Chapter 9
Uncomplicated Postpartum Care Chapter 11

I. CULTURALLY COMPETENT CARE OVERVIEW

A. *Culture* defined

1. A complex whole, encompassing knowledge, beliefs, values, practices, customs, and any habits acquired by members of society
2. Represents ways of perceiving, behaving, and evaluating world

B. Culture and nursing care

1. Leininger's Theory of Culture Care Diversity and Universality includes concepts of culture care delineated as preservation/maintenance, accommodation/negotiation, and repatterning/restructuring
2. *Health Traditions Model* explores what one does to maintain, protect, and restore health (physical, mental, and spiritual) within a framework of one's ethnoreligious cultural heritage
3. *National Standards for Culturally and Linguistically Appropriate Services (CLAS) in Health Care* can be used by accreditation and credentialing agencies to assess delivery of culturally competent services and assure quality care for diverse populations; these standards must be met by most health care–regulated agencies
4. Cultural phenomena that can affect health include environmental control (health practices and remedies), biological (physical and genetic) variations, social organization (holidays, special events such as births and funerals), communication (greetings, gestures, smiling, eye contact), personal space (body language and distance), and time orientation (punctuality, announced versus surprise visits from family and friends)
5. Prerequisites to delivering culturally competent care are understanding one's personal cultural values and health beliefs, being respectful and understanding of client's culture, and becoming familiar with health beliefs and practices held by commonly encountered groups in health care agency's service area
6. Purposeful strategies can be used to aid communication with clients of various cultures
   a. Assess fluency in English and make arrangements for an interpreter if needed; speak directly to client even if using an interpreter

b. Use language that is free of slang or currently popular jargon; use simple, straightforward sentences or questions and rephrase if client does not understand
c. Be attentive to body language that might offend client
d. Learn and follow how client wishes to be addressed
e. Provide an environment for communication that respects habits regarding eye contact and amount of personal space
f. Prior to giving written health teaching materials, even if written in client's primary language, assess reading ability; health literacy can affect ability to learn health information regardless of cultural background

7. Religious laws may influence dietary practices, which in turn may influence nursing care during illness (see Table 19–1); common restrictions include pork and alcohol; fasting may be done on certain religious holidays; children, pregnant women, and those who are ill are usually exempt from fasting
8. Religious beliefs may also influence views on health-related issues and events (see Table 19–2)
9. Culturally based dietary preferences are lifelong habits and can significantly influence health as well as compliance with medically recommended dietary changes (see Table 19–3)
10. Cultural beliefs about maintaining or restoring health may clash with those of health care provider; remain nonjudgmental and work with client to incorporate client's cultural health practices while assisting client to meet health goals
11. Avoid generalizing and **stereotyping** (an expectation that all people within same ethnic or cultural group are alike and share same beliefs and attitudes)

Table 19–1 Dietary Practices of Selected Religions

Religion	Dietary Restrictions or Practices
Orthodox Judaism	Kosher dietary laws allow fish that have scales and fins, cloven-hoofed animals, and animals that eat vegetables or are slaughtered in a ritualistic manner. Milk and meat may not be combined in any way. Fasting during Yom Kippur (24 hours).
Roman Catholicism	Meat is prohibited on Ash Wednesday, and Fridays during Lent, including Good Friday. Fasting is done on Ash Wednesday and Good Friday, is optional during rest of Lent.
Russian Orthodox	Meat and dairy products are prohibited on Wednesdays, Fridays, and during Lent. Fasting occurs during Advent.
Buddhism	Vegetarianism for some sects. Alcohol and drug use is not favored.
Hinduism	Vegetarianism for some with beef and veal prohibited for all. Fasting rituals vary depending on god worshiped.
Islam	Prohibited meats include pork and meats not slaughtered as part of ritual. Drug and alcohol use prohibited.
Jehovah's Witness	Meats that are allowed have been drained of blood; no foods to which blood has been added are allowed.

Table 19–2 Religious Influence on Common Health Issues and Events

Religion	Abortion	Autopsy	Birth Control	Blood/Blood Products	Medication Use	Organ Donation
Baha'i	Not allowed	Allowed with medical or legal need	Allowed	Allowed	Narcotics with prescription; vaccines allowed	Allowed
Buddist	Mother's condition determines	Allowed	Allowed	Allowed	Allowed	Act of mercy
Roman Catholic	Not allowed	Allowed	Natural means only	Allowed	Use if benefits outweigh risks	Allowed

Table 19–2 Religious Influence on Common Health Issues and Events *(continued)*

Religion	Abortion	Autopsy	Birth Control	Blood/Blood Products	Medication Use	Organ Donation
Christian Science	Not allowed	Not usual, family decides	Allowed	Usually not used	None except vaccines to comply with law	Individual choice
Hindu	No policy	Allowed	Allowed	Allowed	Allowed	Allowed
Islam	Not allowed	Allowed with medical or legal need	Allowed	Allowed	Allowed	Controversial; discuss with family
Jehovah's Witness	Not allowed	Allowed with legal need	Allowed except for sterilization	Forbidden	Allowed unless derived from blood products	Forbidden
Judaism	Therapeutic allowed, otherwise varies within groups	Allowed under some conditions; all body parts buried together	Allowed except for Orthodox Jews	Allowed	Allowed	Complex issue; consult rabbi
Mennonite	Therapeutic only	Allowed	Allowed	Allowed	Allowed	Allowed
Mormon	Not allowed	Allowed with next of kin consent	Incompatible with beliefs	Allowed	Allowed	Allowed
Seventh-day Adventist	Therapeutic only	Allowed	Allowed	Allowed	Allowed	Allowed
Unitarian/ Universalist	Allowed	Recommended	Allowed	Allowed	Allowed	Allowed

Table 19–3 Preferred Foods of Various Cultures

Cultural Group	Preferred Foods
Mexican Americans	Corn, dried beans, and chili peppers are basic foods. Tortillas are used for bread (corn, sometimes wheat). Relatively small amounts of meat are used. Fruits such as papaya and mango are used in varying amounts (based on availability and price).
Hispanic/Latino Americans	Similar food pattern to Mexican diet. Rice and beans are basic foods. Dried codfish is a staple, but meat, milk, green and yellow vegetables are used less often. Viandas (starchy vegetables and fruits such as plantains and green bananas) are used, but other fruits are used in limited amounts.
Native American and Alaska Natives	Variable depending on region and local crops or game. Fish (Alaskan) and meat (Navajo), including game, chicken, pork, and mutton, are daily staples. Other staples are bread (tortillas or fry bread, blue corn bread, corn meal mush), eggs, vegetables (corn, potatoes, green beans, tomatoes), and some fruit.
African Americans	Breads and cereals include biscuits, cornmeal mush or muffins or cornbread, cooked cereals with corn and oats. Eggs and cheese are used, but milk is not as popular (perhaps because lactose intolerance has greater prevalence). Preferred vegetables include leafy greens, okra, sweet potatoes, potatoes, corn, and a variety of beans, often served with rice. Pork, poultry, fish, and organ meats are often more popular than beef. Fried foods are popular.
Asian Americans	Varies to some extent based on region. Chinese: rice, vegetables cooked in wok, eggs, soybean products (tofu), small amounts of meat, green tea. Japanese: rice, soy products, and green tea (similar to Chinese); seafood, sushi, steamed vegetables, fresh fruit. Southeast Asian: rice, fresh fruits and vegetables, seafood, chicken, duck, pork, nuts, and legumes.
European Americans	Varies somewhat by country of origin but tends to include more red meat and carbohydrates as well as vegetables and fruits.

II. CULTURAL CONSIDERATIONS FOR BLACK/ AFRICAN AMERICANS

NCLEX®

A. Communication

1. English is primary language; may be called African American Vernacular English, or AAVE
2. Direct eye contact may be considered inappropriate
3. May use oculistics (eye rolling) in response to communications deemed inappropriate
4. May use silence in response to a question deemed inappropriate
5. Verbal and nonverbal communication is integral in communication process

B. Time orientation

1. Tend to be present rather than future oriented; thus, preventive health care may be difficult to implement or maintain; however, time orientation varies with age, subculture, and socioeconomic status
2. May not be punctual for appointments if needs of family or friends require immediate attention

C. Social roles

1. Extended family is important; tend to have large family support systems
2. Strong sense of obligation to relatives
3. Value friendships
4. Many single-parent families, typically headed by females
5. Religious affiliation common

NCLEX®

D. Views of health and illness

1. Body, mind, and spirit are integrated
2. Good health is result of good luck; thus individual has little impact on health status
3. Illness may be a punishment from God or related to one's harmony with nature
4. Emotional or personal problems can be resolved through use of a spiritualist who is called by God to heal
5. Voodoo may be considered a powerful cultural healer
6. Practitioners who use roots, herbs, oils, candles, and ointments may be used in healing process

E. Health risks

1. Lactose intolerance and lactase deficiency
2. Hypertension and coronary artery disease
3. Sickle cell anemia
4. Cancers, including breast, colorectal, esophageal, stomach, cervical, uterine, and prostate
5. Coccidioidomycosis
6. Diabetes mellitus

NCLEX®

F. Nursing considerations

1. Include family in medical care if desired by client
2. Allow for flexibility in scheduling appointments
3. Facilitate and encourage use of folk healers and spiritualists
4. Encourage family to bring traditional diet if medically acceptable

III. CULTURAL CONSIDERATIONS FOR ASIAN AMERICANS

NCLEX®

A. Communication

1. Primary languages include Chinese, Japanese, Vietnamese, Korean, and English
2. May use silence to demonstrate respect for elders
3. If direct eye contact is considered impolite or aggressive, may look away as nurse attempts to make direct eye contact
4. Unlikely to criticize or disagree with others verbally
5. Consider word "no" to be disrespectful
6. Nodding head or smiling does not always mean agreement with what was said

B. Time orientation: tend to be present oriented while highly regarding past

C. Social roles

1. Respect aging members of society
2. Family bonds are important; large extended family networks exist with devotion to tradition
3. Daughters and daughters-in-law may be expected to care for older family members as their health declines
4. Structured and hierarchical family unit, with men and elders being greatly respected; women are expected to be subservient to men
5. Loyalty to family members is expected and highly regarded

6. Education is highly valued
7. Religious affiliation common, including Taoism, Islam, Buddhism, and Christianity

NCLEX®

D. Views of health and illness

1. Chinese concept of yin and yang is a metaphor for forces of nature being balanced to produce harmony
2. Illness is a state of disharmony or imbalance of yin and yang
3. Foods are associated with concept of yin and yang; for example, yin foods are cold, whereas yang foods are hot; cold foods and beverages are consumed for hot illnesses, and hot food and beverages are consumed for cold illnesses
4. Illnesses may be attributed to overexertion or to prolonged sitting or lying

E. Health risks

1. Thalassemia
2. Lactase deficiency
3. G6PD deficiency
4. Hypertension
5. Cancer, with stomach and liver more common sites
6. Coccidioidomycosis

NCLEX®

F. Nursing considerations

1. Clients are likely to be quiet and compliant during illness, thus placing them at risk for not having needs met
2. Clients may wish to take medications with certain foods or beverages believed to promote correct balance for health
3. Clients often do not trust health care providers and wish to include traditional healers along with Western medicine practices
4. Clients may expect health care providers to be authoritative
5. Limit eye contact and physical touching; touch a client's head only with permission from client or parent
6. Encourage and facilitate family involvement in care
7. Clients of Chinese descent may expect nurse to intuitively know their disease process
8. Alternative therapies such as acupuncture and herbal remedies are widely used

IV. CULTURAL CONSIDERATIONS FOR LATINO/ HISPANIC AMERICANS

NCLEX®

A. Communication

1. Primary languages include Spanish and Portuguese
2. May utilize code switching, a systematic mixing of English and Spanish languages
3. Simpatia, a desire for smooth or harmonious interpersonal relationships, should be considered; it is characterized by courtesy, respect, and absence of critical or confrontational behavior; confrontational interaction is avoided
4. Eye contact reflects respect; in nurse–client relationship, eye contact may be expected of nurse, although it may not be reciprocated by client
5. Tend to be verbally expressive
6. May engage in "small talk" or general conversation as a method of establishing rapport
7. Nonverbal communication plays important role in client assessment and interaction

B. Time orientation: tend to be present oriented, but varies according to age, subculture, and socioeconomic status

C. Social roles

1. Family is most valued institution and is a primary source of personal identification
2. While nuclear families are common, extended families may also exist
3. Father is likely to assume head of household role and may make decisions for family
4. Collective achievement tends to be valued more than individual achievement
5. Religion is important; Catholicism is prevalent

NCLEX®

D. Views of health and illness

1. *Mal de ojo* (evil eye) is a childhood disease characterized by fitful sleep, crying, and diarrhea; a common belief among Latinos is that *mal de ojo* is caused by unconscious energy of an adult flowing into child when adult simply looks at child
2. Health is thought to be the will of God

3. *Curanderos,* folk healers, may be consulted
4. Health may represent a state of equilibrium in world, which is characterized by balance of hot, cold, wet, and dry; when an imbalance exists, treatment focuses on application of opposite quality

E. Health risks

1. Diabetes mellitus
2. Hypertension
3. Pernicious anemia
4. Childhood obesity

NCLEX®

F. Nursing considerations

1. Clients may seek guidance from within family network rather than from health care providers; include family members in health care education when appropriate
2. Male family member may be decision maker for client
3. Modesty is important, and measures should be taken to protect client's privacy at all times; clients may prefer to have a health care provider of same gender
4. Use of alternative therapies is prevalent and should be explored when client enters health care system; if possible, facilitate continuation of such services
5. Encourage family to bring traditional diet if medically acceptable

V. CULTURAL CONSIDERATIONS FOR NATIVE AMERICANS

NCLEX®

A. Communication

1. Native American group includes American Indians and Alaskan natives (Eskimos/Aleuts); languages primarily include Navajo and English
2. Language involves tonal speech, with pitch being important
3. When shaking hands, Navajos tend to extend a hand and lightly touch hand of person they are greeting
4. May appear silent and reserved upon meeting strangers
5. As a sign of honor to ancestors, Navajos may state their clan and location of their home

B. Time orientation

1. Time exists in a three-point range, including past, present, and future
2. Viewed as being primarily present oriented, with some members being both past and present oriented

C. Social roles

1. Family oriented, with biological family being central social organization
2. Family includes all members of extended family
3. Family members work collaboratively to assure success of family unit
4. Male family members may be given greatest respect and may make decisions for family
5. Extended family may care for hospitalized relative for duration of hospital stay
6. Religion guided by sacred myths and legends

NCLEX®

D. Views of health and illness

1. Desire to be in harmony with environment and family
2. Health is not limited to body; includes harmony with family, environment, livestock, supernatural forces, and community
3. Health and religion are considered to be connected; healing ceremonies are common; magic, religion, and folk medicine may all be used for healing; healers may be men or women
4. The Blessingway ceremony is practiced to remove ill health through stories, songs, rituals, prayers, sand paintings, and symbols
5. Navajo medicine men and women may be utilized, including diagnosticians (to diagnose illness), singers (to perform healing ceremonies), and herbalists (to use herbs to treat ailments)

E. Health risks

1. Alcoholism and chronic liver disease
2. Accidents
3. Arthritis
4. Chronic lower respiratory diseases and tuberculosis
5. Diabetes mellitus
6. Heart disease, including hypertension and myocardial infarction
7. HIV and AIDS
8. Influenza

9. Malignant neoplasms
10. Malnutrition caused by high rates of poverty
11. Maternal and infant deaths
12. Obesity
13. Suicide

NCLEX® **F. Nursing considerations**

1. When possible, accommodate client's request to attend healing ceremonies held outside of hospital
2. Respect client's desire to be in harmony with environment whenever possible
3. Incorporate all medically acceptable practices into client's plan of care
4. Following birth, umbilical cord may be buried near a place or an object that symbolizes parents' hope for child's future
5. Encourage active participation of family in client's care

VI. CULTURAL CONSIDERATIONS FOR WHITE/ EUROPEAN AMERICANS

A. Communication

1. English is primary language
2. Eye contact is valued and shows interest and respect
3. Body language is important in communication process
4. Facial expression tends to be utilized as part of communication process
5. Handshake is utilized for formal greetings
6. Personal space tends to be required during communication

B. Time orientation

1. Considered to be future oriented
2. Adhere to schedules and timeframes

C. Social roles

1. Nuclear family is predominant although extended family plays important role
2. Religion is important, with a variety of denominations existing
3. Encourage children to develop their personal sense of identity
4. Subscribe to Protestant work ethic values, which stress importance of planning for future
5. Individual goals may take precedence over those of family

D. Views of health and illness: health is considered absence of disease or illness; utilize Western health care system

E. Health risks

1. Cardiovascular disease
2. Obesity
3. Diabetes mellitus
4. A variety of cancers
5. Thalassemia

F. Nursing considerations

1. Respect client's need for autonomy and personal space
2. Maintain eye contact with client
3. Include family members in health care decisions when appropriate and with client's approval
4. Respect a resurgence in interest in homeopathic medicine

Check Your NCLEX-PN® Exam I.Q.

You are ready for testing on this content if you can

- Be respectful, interested in, and understanding of other cultures without being judgmental.
- Consider the impact of clients' culture or ethnicity when planning, implementing, and evaluating nursing care.
- Determine level of fluency in English and need for interpreter to aid in planning care effectively for clients with a language barrier.
- Consider client's culture when providing client teaching.
- Demonstrate cultural sensitivity when communicating with clients.
- Evaluate client understanding and acceptance of health-related recommendations.

PRACTICE TEST

1 While examining an infant, a nurse notices that the infant is wearing a soiled piece of braided yarn around the neck. Which action by the nurse is most appropriate?

1. Leave the yarn in place but wash it with a cloth and mild soap.
2. Ask about its significance and suggest that it be placed more safely on the body.
3. Explain that the yarn offers no benefit and ask the parents to remove it.
4. Remove the yarn because it is soiled and could lead to strangulation.

2 A Native American client who has a low-grade fever tells the nurse on the reservation that he will only use a sweat lodge to treat his illness. Which approach by the nurse would be most therapeutic?

1. Explain to the client that the sweat lodge is likely to worsen the fever.
2. Alert the physician and ask him or her to talk to the medicine man of the tribe.
3. Continue to monitor the client's status.
4. Ask the client's family to convince him not to use the sweat lodge.

3 A male nurse needs to check the vital signs and oxygen saturation level of a female client from a different culture. As the nurse approaches, the client moves to the other side of the bed and draws up the blanket. What is the best nursing action at this time?

1. Invite a family member to be present and to assist with the oxygen saturation reading.
2. Ask a female nurse to perform the procedures.
3. Perform the assessments without acknowledging her reaction because she will adjust over time to hospital procedures.
4. Before touching the client, explain the procedure and ask for permission to continue.

4 A nurse in a small Appalachian community is caring for a terminally ill client who wishes to die at home and is an active member of the community church. As death nears, the minister and several members of the congregation come together in the home for a "death watch." Which action by the nurse is most therapeutic?

1. Ask the minister to have church members come in scheduled time blocks to avoid overcrowding.
2. Observe client's religious beliefs and allow family and minister unlimited access to the client.
3. Allow family and three other visitors at a time to stay with the client, but keep everyone else in the next room.
4. Explain that the watch will not be a problem as long as it does not conflict with medical care.

5 The nurse is checking the dietary trays that have been delivered to the nursing unit. A client of Orthodox Jewish faith has received a tray containing a chicken dinner with vegetables, tea, and a carton of 2% milk. What action by the nurse is best?

1. Instruct nursing assistant to deliver the meal tray after removing the tea.
2. Remove the chicken from the dietary tray.
3. Have dietary department replace the entire meal tray.
4. Ask client if lactose-free milk would be preferred.

6 A nurse is working with a group of postpartum women. Using culturally based practices as a guide, which of the following clients is at greatest risk for postpartum depression?

1. Chinese client
2. Hispanic client
3. Hindu client
4. American client

7 The nurse is caring for a Native American woman who has given birth. The nurse anticipates that the couple will make which request regarding the umbilical cord?

1. Have it burned
2. Have the blood drained from it
3. Take it home
4. Inspect it

PRACTICE TEST

8 The nurse has taken a position in an ambulatory clinic in a Hispanic neighborhood. The nurse would use knowledge of which practices to provide culturally sensitive care to this population? Select all that apply.

1. Herbal medicines are believed to be as important as Western medicines in treating illness.
2. Mourners are likely to be hired by a family to demonstrate grief after a death.
3. Staring at a client who is a child will help to prevent or ward off the "evil eye."
4. Depending on the specific illness, hot or cold foods would be used in treatment.
5. The client may want a caregiver of the same gender to enhance privacy.

9 The nurse has accepted a nursing position in an urban facility that serves clients of many different cultures. Which of the following is a prerequisite for the nurse, who wishes to provide culturally competent care?

1. Acceptance of cultural diversity
2. Awareness of one's personal biases
3. Appreciation of cultural diversity
4. Sensitivity to culturally diverse populations

10 A Chinese client with cancer is likely to prefer consuming which of the following food items? Select all that apply.

1. Fried foods
2. Green vegetables
3. Cold foods
4. Spicy foods
5. Bland foods

11 A Latino client presents to the emergency department with a complaint of severe abdominal pain and cramping. The client's family expresses concern that food has stuck to the client's intestines. Which of the following culture-bound syndromes would be consistent with the presenting symptoms?

1. Hysteria
2. *Empacho*
3. *Mal ojo*
4. Bulimia

12 A Mexican-American infant presents to the emergency department with *caida de la mollera*, or fallen fontanel. Which of the following would the client identify as a potential cause of this condition? Select all that apply.

1. Failure of midwife to press on the palate after delivery
2. Falling on the head
3. Slow removal of the nipple from the infant's mouth after feedings
4. Failure to place a cap on the infant's head
5. Too much intake of fluids

13 An Islamic client is hospitalized for minor elective surgery during Ramadan. The nurse anticipates that the client might desire which intervention?

1. Offer to arrange meals to be served after dusk and before dawn.
2. Serve meatless meals according to the hospital's schedule.
3. Provide total parenteral nutrition (TPN) throughout Ramadan.
4. Notify physician that the client will not have any by-mouth intake.

14 The nurse working with a client who emigrated from Mexico would consider during care that which cultural characteristics are typically associated with Mexican American culture? Select all that apply.

1. Value extended family
2. Have patriarchal outlook
3. Value independence and autonomy
4. Respect authority
5. Oppose the status quo

15 An Asian client presents to the emergency department with a report of recurrent body aches. Upon examination, the nurse identifies numerous circular, flat, ecchymotic burns. The burns appear to be approximately 2 inches in diameter, and are symmetrical. What is the likely cause of the condition?

1. Abuse
2. Cigarette burns
3. Coining
4. Cupping

16. While realizing that all clients are unique, the nurse would tend to associate which cultural values with clients of African-American descent? Select all that apply.

1. Extended family
2. Religion
3. Long-term goals
4. Interdependence
5. Seclusion

ANSWERS & RATIONALES

1. **Answer: 2 Rationale:** The action that demonstrates cultural sensitivity is the one that inquires about the significance of the braided necklace while taking into account issues of client safety (in this case risk of strangulation). Washing it addresses risk of infection but not safety, while options that remove it fail to demonstrate any cultural sensitivity. **Cognitive Level:** Applying **Client Need:** Psychosocial Integrity **Integrated Process:** Communication and Documentation **Content Area:** Fundamentals **Strategy:** Use the process of elimination and basic principles of culturally sensitive communication to make a selection. Eliminate options that remove the yarn as least respectful, and choose the correct option because it addresses the priority need of safety.

2. **Answer: 3 Rationale:** The nurse should continue to monitor the client's status because the fever is low grade and considering that treatment consistent with the client's beliefs will probably be the most successful. The other options fail to show cultural sensitivity in respecting the client's culturally based beliefs about health. **Cognitive Level:** Applying **Client Need:** Psychosocial Integrity **Integrated Process:** Communication and Documentation **Content Area:** Fundamentals **Strategy:** Use basic principles of therapeutic communication, client autonomy, and cultural sensitivity to make a selection. The critical words in the stem are *low-grade fever*, which tells you that the situation is not life threatening or even an emergency. Avoid alerting the physician because it does not keep the responsibility with the nurse and engaging the family because this action would violate a client's right to self-determination.

3. **Answer: 4 Rationale:** The response that shows cultural sensitivity is one that respects the personal boundaries of the client and asks permission to engage in care activities. There is no need for family or a female nurse to assist in these non-invasive procedures at this time without assessing first what the client's issues may be. The nurse should also not ignore the non-verbal communication being sent by the client; this would not be therapeutic. **Cognitive Level:** Applying **Client Need:** Psychosocial Integrity **Integrated Process:** Communication and Documentation **Content Area:** Fundamentals **Strategy:** Use basic principles of therapeutic communication, client autonomy, and cultural sensitivity to make a selection. First note that the nature of the nursing care activities involved indicate that this is not a situation that requires assistance from family or other nurses. Choose an option that focuses directly on the client.

4. **Answer: 2 Rationale:** Cultural practices near the time of death are important for clients and their families. The nurse should respect the client and family wishes, since medical care is ineffective at this point in time. Time blocks and limiting visitors do not fully respect the needs of the client and those who are important in his life. **Cognitive Level:** Applying **Client Need:** Psychosocial Integrity **Integrated Process:** Communication and Documentation **Content Area:** Fundamentals **Strategy:** Recall that practices related to birth and death are highly culturally influenced. With this in mind, select the option that provides the greatest respect for the client and significant people in his life.

5. **Answer: 3 Rationale:** The Jewish religion prohibits the ingestion of meat and dairy products during the same meal. The nurse should ask that the entire meal tray be replaced by the dietary department. Removing the tea does not address the culturally-based dietary issue. Removing the chicken from the dietary tray is not sufficient because Kosher law says meat and dairy cannot be combined in any way, which would include being on the same meal tray. The use of lactose-free milk will not resolve the dietary issue. **Cognitive Level:** Applying **Client Need:** Psychosocial Integrity **Integrated Process:** Nursing Process: Implementation **Content Area:** Fundamentals **Strategy:** The core issue of this question is that milk and meat products cannot be consumed during the same meal or combined in any way for clients of the Orthodox Jewish faith. Use knowledge of culturally based dietary practices to make a selection.

6. **Answer: 4 Rationale:** Many non-Western cultures will have family involvement in the care of the mother and infant for up to 50 days after delivery. This prolonged support helps to prevent the new mother from feeling overwhelmed with new responsibilities or feeling abandoned; the Chinese, Hispanic, and Hindu clients are at low risk for postpartum depression. **Cognitive Level:** Analyzing **Client Need:** Psychosocial Integrity **Integrated Process:** Nursing Process: Planning **Content Area:** Fundamentals **Strategy:** Use the process of elimination and knowledge of the social roles and support of various cultural groups to make a selection. Recall that American society generally tends to value autonomy and independence, which affects the nature of relationships in the postpartum period.

7. **Answer: 3 Rationale:** Following birth, the umbilical cord may be buried near a place or an object that symbolizes the parents' hope for the child's future. For this reason, the parents of the newborn are likely to request to take it home. The other options do not represent the cultural beliefs of Native Americans regarding the significance of the umbilical cord after birth. **Cognitive Level:** Analyzing **Client Need:** Psychosocial Integrity **Integrated Process:** Nursing Process: Planning **Content Area:** Fundamentals **Strategy:** Use the process of elimination and knowledge of the cultural practices surrounding childbirth to make a selection. If needed, take time to review key cultural practices of Native American clients.

8. **Answer: 1, 4, 5 Rationale:** In the Latino culture, herbal medicines are just as important as Western medicines in treating illness. Cold foods would be used to treat an illness that is considered hot, while hot foods would be used to treat an

illness that is considered to be cold. Depending on the client, a caregiver of the same gender may be preferred to enhance privacy. Mourners would not be hired by a family to demonstrate grief after a death (that practice could occur in Korean culture). Staring at a child could cause the "evil eye" because of his or her inexperienced and vulnerable spirit. **Cognitive Level:** Applying **Client Need:** Psychosocial Integrity **Integrated Process:** Nursing Process: Planning **Content Area:** Fundamentals **Strategy:** The wording of the question tells you that the correct options will also be correct statements about the Latino American culture. Use knowledge of specific Hispanic cultural practices to make a selection.

9 **Answer: 2 Rationale:** When providing culturally competent care, it is essential as a first step for the nurse to be aware of personal biases. While appreciation of, sensitivity toward, and acceptance of diverse cultures is desired, these will not be accomplished until the nurse first considers his or her own biases. **Cognitive Level:** Applying **Client Need:** Psychosocial Integrity **Integrated Process:** Nursing Process: Planning **Content Area:** Fundamentals **Strategy:** The key to answering the question correctly is identifying the quality that is essential first step to providing culturally competent care.

10 **Answer: 1, 4 Rationale:** Cancer is a disease associated with excessive yin forces. Diseases with yin forces are treated with foods with yang qualities. Yin is associated with cold, while yang is associated with warmth. Yang foods, such as fried foods and spicy foods, are associated with warmth, whereas green vegetables and cold foods are associated with cold. **Cognitive Level:** Applying **Client Need:** Health Promotion and Maintenance **Integrated Process:** Nursing Process: Planning **Content Area:** Foundational Sciences **Strategy:** An understanding of the concept of yin and yang is necessary for the learner to correctly answer the question.

11 **Answer: 2 Rationale:** *Empacho* is a culture-bound syndrome associated with Latino culture that occurs when food forms into a ball and clings to the stomach or intestines, resulting in pain or cramping. Hysteria is a Greek culture–bound syndrome associated with the belief that the uterus has left the pelvis for another part of the body. *Mal ojo*, or the evil eye, is a Latino culture–bound syndrome believed to be caused by an individual excessively admiring a child. Bulimia is a white culture–bound syndrome associated with overeating followed by vomiting. **Cognitive Level:** Applying **Client Need:** Psychosocial Integrity **Integrated Process:** Nursing Process: Data Collection **Content Area:** Fundamentals **Strategy:** An understanding of specific culture-bound syndromes is necessary for correctly answering the question.

12 **Answer: 1, 2, 4 Rationale:** Fallen fontanel, a Mexican American culture–bound syndrome, is associated with this behavior. Fallen fontanel, a Mexican American culture–bound syndrome, is associated with this event. Fallen fontanel, a Mexican American culture–bound syndrome, is associated with this behavior. Fallen fontanel, a Mexican American culture–bound syndrome, is not associated with slow removal of the nipple after feeding. Rather, it is associated with abrupt removal of the nipple during feeding. Fallen fontanel, a Mexican American culture–bound syndrome, is not associated with excess fluids. **Cognitive Level:** Applying **Client Need:** Psychosocial Integrity **Integrated Process:** Nursing Process: Planning **Content Area:** Fundamentals **Strategy:** An understanding of culture-bound syndromes, including the etiology of the condition, is essential for answering this question correctly.

13 **Answer: 1 Rationale:** During the 28-day period of Ramadan, Islamic adults refrain from food and drink from dawn until sunset. Regardless of their content, meals are not accepted during the daylight. Total parenteral nutrition would not be indicated for all clients who are fasting. While the physician should be made aware that oral medications may not be taken until night hours, it would not be correct to identify the client as having no oral intake. **Cognitive Level:** Applying **Client Need:** Psychosocial Integrity **Integrated Process:** Nursing Process: Planning **Content Area:** Fundamentals **Strategy:** An understanding of Islamic culture, including Ramadan, is necessary for the correct answering of the question.

14 **Answer: 1, 2, 4 Rationale:** Mexican American culture is associated with placing a high value on extended family relationships. Mexican American culture is associated with being patriarchal (machismo). Mexican American culture does not value independence and autonomy. Rather, interdependence is valued. Mexican American culture is associated with having respect for authority. Mexican American culture is not associated with defying the status quo. **Cognitive Level:** Applying **Client Need:** Psychosocial Integrity **Integrated Process:** Nursing Process: Planning **Content Area:** Fundamentals **Strategy:** Recall more common characteristics of Mexican American culture to correctly answer the question. Note the wording of the question suggests that more than one option is likely to be correct.

15 **Answer: 4 Rationale:** Cupping occurs when a vacuum is created inside a cup by igniting cotton soaked in alcohol sitting within the cup. When the flame is extinguished, the cup is placed onto the skin at the painful site. The cup remains in place until the suction is released. The symmetrical burns would not be associated with abuse or cigarette burns. The burns described are too large to be from cigarettes; cigarette burns would lack symmetry. Coining occurs when the edge of a coin is rubbed over a painful area; the areas are not circular or symmetrical. **Cognitive Level:** Applying **Client Need:** Psychosocial Integrity **Integrated Process:** Nursing Process: Data Collection **Content Area:** Fundamentals **Strategy:** An understanding of Southeast Asian folk healing processes is necessary for correctly identifying the best response.

16 **Answer: 1, 2, 4 Rationale:** African-American culture typically values extended family, religion, and interdependence. Long-term goals and seclusion are not typically associated with African-American culture. **Cognitive Level:** Applying **Client Need:** Psychosocial Integrity **Integrated Process:** Nursing Process: Planning **Content Area:** Fundamentals **Strategy:** Recall characteristics that are commonly associated with African-American culture to identify the correct responses. The wording of the question indicates more than one option is likely to be correct.

Key Terms to Review

culture p. 245

stereotyping p. 246

References

Andrews, M., & Boyle, J. (2008). *Transcultural concepts in nursing care* (5th ed.). Philadelphia: Lippincott, Williams & Wilkins.

Berman, A., & Snyder, S. (2012). *Kozier & Erb's fundamentals of nursing: Concepts, process, and practice* (9th ed.). Upper Saddle River, NJ: Pearson Education, Inc.

Potter, P., & Perry, A. (2010). *Fundamentals of nursing* (7th ed.). St. Louis, MO: Mosby.

Purnell, L. (2008). *Transcultural health care: A culturally competent approach* (3rd ed.). Philadelphia: F.A. Davis.

Spector, R. (2009). *Cultural diversity in health and illness* (7th ed.). Upper Saddle River, NJ: Pearson Education, Inc.

Test Yourself

Are you ready for the NCLEX-PN® or course exams? Use the practice tests on the companion website to check.

Coping with Stressors 20

In this chapter

Cross Reference

Other chapters relevant to this content area are

I. COPING AND DEFENSE MECHANISMS

A. Coping behaviors

1. Influence a client's response to a stressful event
2. **Coping** (cognitive, physical, or emotional attempts to manage stress) implies that client is trying to reduce tension to manage situation effectively; both adaptive and maladaptive coping behaviors are typically manifested
3. **Adaptive coping** behaviors: ability to mobilize internal/external resources and sustain general homeostasis
4. **Maladaptive coping** behaviors: inability to mobilize internal/external resources; disorganization occurs; ineffective and destructive behaviors appear; general homeostasis is not preserved

NCLEX® **B. Defense mechanisms (see Table 20–1)**

1. Strategies that assist client to protect own ego and reduce anxiety
2. Support appropriate use of defense mechanisms
3. *NCLEX®* Do not attempt to break down inappropriate defense mechanisms until other coping strategies are learned

Memory Aid

All clients exhibit coping behaviors. The nurse's key role is to determine whether they are healthy (adaptive) or unhealthy (maladaptive) behaviors and to support healthy ones.

Table 20–1 Common Defense Mechanisms

Defense Mechanism	Description
Compensation	Making up for real or imagined weaknesses in one area
Denial	Refusing to acknowledge thoughts or impulses that are unacceptable to self
Displacement	Directing feelings about a person who is threatening to self to another person who is less threatening to self
Identification	Attempting to change oneself unconsciously for the purpose of resembling someone who is admired
Intellectualization	Using excessive reasoning ability to minimize or avoid feelings associated with distressing events or occurrences
Introjection	Incorporating the values and characteristics of another into oneself
Minimization	Refusing to acknowledge importance or significance of one's behavior
Projection	Transferring unacceptable desires, thoughts, or internal feelings to another
Rationalization	Justifying unacceptable feelings or behavior by using faulty logic or applying false but socially acceptable motives to behavior
Reaction formation	Behaving or displaying attitudes that are exactly opposite of those that are felt
Regression	Reverting back to an earlier, less well-developed stage of functioning to deal with an uncomfortable reality
Repression	Using an unconscious process to block threatening or unacceptable thoughts, feelings, or desires to keep them from becoming conscious
Sublimation	Displacing energy associated with unacceptable needs or drives into more socially acceptable activities
Substitution	Replacing a highly valued but unobtainable or unacceptable object with a less satisfying but acceptable and available one
Undoing	Using words or actions to cancel out previous unacceptable thoughts or behaviors in an attempt to relieve guilt by making reparation

II. COPING WITH ABUSE OR NEGLECT

A. Victims
1. Often present with depression and tend to have low self-esteem
2. Describe feelings of powerlessness, dependency, or a sense of being trapped
3. Often do not recognize that they are victims
4. *NCLEX®* Frequently believe they are to blame for abuse and that it would stop if client could do "better"

B. Abusers/perpetrators
1. Also have low self-esteem
2. May have been abused themselves during childhood
3. Depersonalize victims so as to feel entitled to engage in abuse
4. Tend to be self-absorbed, suspicious, and highly dependent on victim

C. Types of abuse/violence
1. Partner: cycle of physical or emotional threats and assaults by abuser followed by abuser remorse or attempts to make peace
2. Child: physical, emotional, or sexual
3. Elder: physical, emotional, sexual, or financial (lack of knowledge of finances and inability to pay bills while cognitively intact)
4. Abuse versus neglect: neglect is passive in nature, while abuse is active and purposeful

NCLEX® **D. Data collection**
1. Neglect: intentional or unintentional failure to care for victim (see Table 20–2)
2. Abuse (see Table 20–3)

E. Collaborative management (see also Chapter 6)
1. *NCLEX®* Report suspected abuse cases; this is part of mandatory reporting laws
2. Support client during physical assessment and treatment of physical injuries
3. Provide safe, nonthreatening environment for care; interview client without abuser present whenever possible
4. *NCLEX®* Document data and client-reported events in an objective manner
5. *NCLEX®* Do not leave victim alone with abuser
6. Support coping mechanisms of victim

Table 20–2 Signs of Neglect

Child	Poor hygiene, presence of chronic hunger and inadequate weight gain, chronic fatigue, excessive school absences, and inadequate or lack of supervision
Elder	Poor hygiene and unkempt appearance, inadequate dress, absence of necessary physical aids (dentures, glasses, hearing aids), malnutrition, dehydration, skin tears

Table 20–3 Signs of Abuse

Type of Abuse	Child	Elder
Physical	Unexplained physical or thermal injuries Unusual apprehension, aggression, or withdrawal Withdraws from or is fearful of parents Does not cry when approached by strangers/caregivers	Skin tears Bruises that are multiple or in patterns (finger or hand prints) Burn injuries Lacerations or punctures Bone fractures
Emotional	Presence of repetitive motion habits such as sucking or rocking Psychoneurotic reactions Disorders of speech Difficulty with concentration or learning Suicidal behavior	Confusion Fear and apprehension Agitation Withdrawal from social activities Loss of interest in self Decreased appetite and weight
Sexual	Difficulty in sitting or walking Torn, stained, or bloody undergarments Pain, swelling, bruising, or bleeding in area of genitalia Change in usual routine, such as disruptive behavior or disrupted sleep Changes in school behavior, such as withdrawal from peers, truancy, or refusal to undress/change clothes for physical education classes	Difficulty in sitting or walking New onset genital infection Pain or bleeding in area of genitalia Torn, stained, or bloody undergarments

7. Encourage therapy for abuser, victim, and appropriate others (family)

NCLEX®

8. Monitor support systems of victim and abuser
9. Refer to appropriate community agencies for support
10. Assist with legal procedures as appropriate (police reports, restraining order/order of protection)

Memory Aid Safety is always a key concern for victims of abuse.

NCLEX®

11. Child-specific interventions
    a. Avoid loud noises
    b. Position self to be at eye level with child when speaking
    c. Make no sudden movements
    d. Reassure child that he or she is a good person and is not to blame for abusive behavior

NCLEX®

12. Elder-specific interventions
    a. Explore alternative housing that provides greatest freedom to client and least amount of disruption to routine
    b. Assist with exploring protection of finances

III. OVERVIEW OF PSYCHOLOGICAL ASPECTS OF MEDICAL ILLNESS

A. **Factors influencing response to medical illness include developmental level, personality type/behaviors, coping behaviors, precipitating stressors, support systems, and nature of illness**

NCLEX®

B. **Developmental/lifespan issues**: developmental stage at time of diagnosis of medical illness influences client's response to illness; in addition, illness can affect client mastery of a developmental level, which further affects how client responds to illness

1. Early to middle adulthood
   a. Medical illnesses during early to middle adulthood can interfere with intimacy, sexuality, and career goals
   b. An adolescent with a chronic illness is at high risk, and this may result in severe emotional stress, depression, anxiety, and possible suicidal ideation (see also Chapter 21)
2. Late adulthood: medical illnesses that occur during late adulthood can interfere with self-care and daily functioning, which may result in severe emotional stress

C. **Personality traits**: predictable pattern of response to events; can be used to predict how client may respond to medical diagnosis, which then assists with planning care
1. Type A personality trait behaviors: might increase unhealthy responses to medical illness; these traits include rapid speech, irritability, rapid movements, time consciousness, difficulty relaxing, internalization of feelings, excessive dependence on approval of others, and low self-esteem
2. Type B personality trait behaviors: may contribute to healthy responses to medical illness and include easygoing manner, and relaxed and goal-directed behaviors
3. Behaviors that increase likelihood of occurrence of medical illness include pessimism, repression, limited/guarded social interactions, hostility, and despair
4. Behaviors that decrease likelihood of occurrence of medical illness include behaviors that are self-healing, energetic, questioning, humorous, inspirational, and that demonstrate good interpersonal skills

D. ***Precipitating stressors***
1. Defined as events occurring prior to a medical illness that initiated a stress response consisting of physiological and psychological alterations
2. These can influence a client's response to medical illness because client may already be in an emotionally compromised state prior to diagnosis of medical illness

E. **Support systems**: presence or absence of strong support systems influences response to medical illness; strong family, friend, and community support systems can result in positive or negative responses

F. **Nature of illness**: response to medical illness can depend on whether illness is an acute (or short-lasting), chronic (long-lasting), or terminal, life-ending type
1. Acute illness: sudden onset, may be caused by injury or fast onset illness
   a. Often results in crisis for client and family; **crisis** refers to an event in which client's regular coping mechanisms are inadequate
   NCLEX® b. Client may demonstrate a short attention span and a tendency to be unproductive and impulsive
NCLEX® 2. Chronic illness: client must cope with illness that may be long-standing and debilitating in nature; often results in ongoing stress for client and family; client often feels frustrated, hopeless, and fatigued
3. Terminal illness: may place client and family in a crisis mode
   a. Is extremely disruptive to client and family functioning
   NCLEX® b. Client often exhibits signs of anger, hopelessness/helplessness, and despair

IV. ASSOCIATED COMMON PSYCHOLOGICAL SYMPTOMS

A. **Anger**
1. Clients with medical illness may demonstrate behaviors indicative of anger
2. These behaviors reflect feelings of helplessness and frustration about illness and effects it has on daily functioning
NCLEX® 3. Common behaviors include demanding types of action, loud verbalization, slamming of items, and social withdrawal

B. **Depression**
1. Clients with medical illness may demonstrate symptoms of depression related to disruption of daily functioning
2. Signs of depression include feelings of helplessness/hopelessness, flat affect, poor eye contact, disrupted eating/sleeping patterns, absence of motivation and compliance, and a decreased energy level

C. **Anxiety**
1. Clients with medical illness may demonstrate feelings and behaviors of anxiety
2. Anxious behavior reflects feelings of real or imagined threat to body image
NCLEX® 3. Anxiety results in autonomic nervous system stimulation with increased heart rate, increased respirations, increased visual acuity, diaphoresis, shortness of breath, and restlessness

D. **Helplessness/hopelessness**
1. Clients with medical diagnoses may demonstrate feelings of helplessness/hopelessness

NCLEX®
2. Helplessness relates to feelings of powerlessness associated with being unable to change what is happening, while hopelessness relates to feelings of despondency and loss of optimism
3. This is reflected in feelings of loss of **control** (feeling that an event can be managed), loss of individuality, and increased dependency on others

V. MEDICAL CONDITIONS CONTRIBUTING TO PSYCHOLOGICAL SYMPTOMS

A. **Critical/acute illness**: may occur without warning and immediately affect a client's daily functioning; clients typically experience feelings of loss of control, anxiety, helplessness, and anger
  1. Cardiovascular illnesses
     a. Have been linked to occurrence of stress
     b. Include myocardial infarction, cerebrovascular accident, and hypertension
     c. Stress levels can influence course and/or outcomes of medical illness
  2. Trauma
     a. May result from an accident or crime
     b. Behavioral and physiological responses occur and are demonstrated in client through social isolation, agitation, nightmares, and numbness
     c. Client typically struggles to control episodes of anxiety related to traumatic event
  3. Surgery performed because of a critical or an acute medical condition may be disfiguring or incapacitating; surgical procedures can result in changes in client daily functioning and self-image
  4. Pain can accompany many acute illnesses; client's response is based on a need to protect oneself from harm

B. **Chronic illness**: produces long-term effects that client must cope with for a longer time; can be unpredictable in nature and require ongoing use of adaptive coping behaviors; lower socioeconomic status increases risks of multiple ongoing health problems, reduced access to health care, and insufficient finances to adhere to treatment plans
  1. Pulmonary diseases
     a. Include disorders such as chronic obstructive pulmonary disease (COPD) and asthma

NCLEX®
     b. Higher stress levels lead to increased secretions and airway spasms and result in more frequent episodes of breathing difficulties
  2. Gastrointestinal (GI) diseases
     a. Irritable bowel syndrome, peptic ulcer, and ulcerative colitis are stress-influenced illnesses
     b. GI tract and autonomic nervous system are involved; increased acid and increased parasympathetic stimulation of lower bowel occurs and exacerbates symptoms when stress levels increase

NCLEX®
  3. Medical illnesses that result in chronic pain can have profound effect on clients and their adaptive and maladaptive coping behaviors; clients respond to pain in a psychological and physiological manner that requires them to continually attempt to adapt

C. **Life-ending illnesses (see also Chapter 24)**
  1. HIV/AIDS: human immunodeficiency virus (HIV) and acquired immunodeficiency syndrome (AIDS) result simultaneously in a compromised immune system and occurrence of a psychiatric disorder; this further compromises health and well-being of client

NCLEX®
     a. Monitoring of clients with HIV disease is crucial because of occurrence of psychiatric symptoms/illness and enormous losses that client and family endure
     b. Psychosocial factors influencing occurrence of psychiatric symptoms/illness include fear that diagnosis will be shared with others, concern about stigma related to diagnosis, intimacy and sexual disruptions, and employment/insurance issues

NCLEX®
     c. Symptoms of HIV and psychiatric illness overlap, especially with symptoms of depression and anxiety; these include fatigue, hopelessness/helplessness, weight loss, aching muscles, and diarrhea; other psychiatric symptoms specifically related to HIV/AIDS diagnosis include irritability, paranoia, psychosis, substance abuse, and suicidal ideation
     d. Cognitive changes related to HIV/AIDS diagnoses include dementia (chronic irreversible brain disorder associated with memory difficulties, impaired judgment, personality changes, and decline in physical appearance) and delirium (acute reversible brain disorder associated with inability to be attentive, cloudy consciousness, apathy, and bizarre behaviors)
     e. Interventions for clients with HIV/AIDS should include those that relate to AIDS dementia/delirium, changes in body image/self-esteem, imminent death, support of family/significant others, and management of pain

2. Other life-ending illnesses
   a. Dying client experiences feelings of helplessness and possibly hopelessness
   b. In addition, feelings of depression, anger, and hostility may be experienced
   c. Client's response to a life-ending diagnosis is affected by coping skills, developmental level, and spiritual, cultural, biological, and psychosocial factors
   d. Interventions include use of empathy and compassion; a focus on positive aspects of client's life; spirituality assessment and reinforcement; support of family and significant others; allowing client dignity and control; and managing pain

VI. ASSOCIATED PSYCHIATRIC SYMPTOMS

A. Psychosis is a disorder of organic or emotional origin characterized by gross impairment in reality testing

B. Psychotic symptoms that may be demonstrated in clients with selected medical illness diagnoses include evidence of delusions and hallucinations, thought process disruption, and difficulty in caring for oneself (see also Chapter 21)

1. Delusions may be persistent and recurrent; they are beliefs that are false but cannot be altered by reason or evidence
2. Hallucinations may be persistent and recurrent; they are defined as occurrences of a sight, sound, smell, taste, or touch when there is no external stimulus to corresponding sensory organ

VII. DATA COLLECTION

A. Use various resources to collect psychological, biological, and social data

B. Consider subjective and objective symptoms, family/significant other reports, and diagnostic reports

C. Psychological data collection

1. Elicits client's emotional reaction to medical illness diagnosis, coping abilities, and support resources
2. Perform a stress appraisal to identify source, number, and duration of stressors
3. Complete a full mental status exam if client exhibits severe symptoms induced by stress
4. *NCLEX®* Complete a depression symptom assessment, noting time of initial symptoms, duration of symptoms, and physical appearance
5. *NCLEX®* Identify coping behaviors, including adaptive and maladaptive behaviors that reflect client's ability to identify problems and analyze feelings
6. Determine substance abuse/dependence, which is crucial because it can contribute to symptoms of depression, anxiety, hopelessness, helplessness, and eating/sleeping disruptions
7. Theoretical emotional stages of medical illness include the following (individual clients may move forward and backward through these stages to some degree):
   a. Denial of medical illness and associated limitations
   b. Anger at loss of control and associated limitations
   c. Bargaining, with a plea for another chance and seeking new answers/treatments
   d. Depression when grieving occurs due to loss or anticipated loss
   e. Acceptance/adaptation when conflicts are resolved and client participates in care
8. Identify emotional stage of medical illness; plan interventions accordingly

D. Biologic data collection

1. Helps in understanding how stress might alter a client's internal body functioning
2. Biological changes can assist nurse with determining severity of an illness
3. Question for recent and past health conditions that may contribute to current level of physical and psychological functioning; recent and chronic illnesses alter client's immune system and raise susceptibility to additional health problems
4. Assist with complete physical exam to reveal any physical conditions contributing to psychological symptoms; some medical illnesses can cause client to exhibit psychological symptoms that may be misdiagnosed as a mental health disorder
5. Assist with a thorough neurological status exam to reveal current neurological state and any changes; findings will provide baseline level of functioning and may alert nurse to medical problems
6. Analyze laboratory results, which can provide insight into occurrence of psychological symptoms
7. *NCLEX®* Note client's current abilities with physical functioning, activities, and exercise to identify baseline information from which to develop plan of care
8. *NCLEX®* Investigate sleep patterns, noting disruptions such as inability to fall asleep, stay asleep, or a desire to sleep constantly; sleep disruptions may indicate either physiological or psychological problems

NCLEX® 9. Determine eating patterns, noting disruptions such as lack of appetite, failure to enjoy previously enjoyable food, and overeating; eating disruptions can indicate either physiological or psychological stress

NCLEX® 10. Note current medications that could account for level of physical and psychological functioning

E. Social history

1. Explore family history, client lifestyle, life-changing events, and social support systems (either negative or positive)
2. Explore recent life-changing events that may impact adaptation to current illness
3. Discuss client's lifestyle patterns and potential impact of lifestyle choices on development and progression of disease

NCLEX® 4. Note cultural practices for unique aspects that may indicate specific responses or need for special interventions

NCLEX® 5. Observe family communication patterns, level of cohesion, flexibility, functioning, and general support

6. Explore community and support resources for availability of home services, mental health services, and other related services
7. Question spiritual concerns; note traditional patterns or rituals, and inquire about other forms of spirituality that may be important to the client
8. Determine whether client can continue in current occupation, either at present time or in future
9. Determine economic status, specifically whether finances will support current and future expenses

VIII. EMPOWERING STRATEGIES

A. Interventions

1. Collaborate with client and family to develop a plan of care in which client response can be monitored; counseling and possibly psychotherapy may be appropriate
2. Interventions serve as foundation for all client care and are subject to change as client's condition changes

NCLEX® 3. Specific interventions that exemplify empowering strategies
   a. Increase client control; provide opportunities for client decision making regarding care
   b. Engage in therapeutic interactions—empathetic listening
   c. Assist with stress management—teach relaxation methods, imagery, biofeedback, exercise
   d. Reinforce current positive, adaptive coping behaviors
   e. Promote comfort and healing
   f. Utilize spiritual resources—provide opportunities for client to engage in spiritual traditions or rituals; offer resources related to complementary medicine if desired

B. Differential interventions for critical/acute versus chronic illnesses

NCLEX® 1. Critical/acute illnesses typically result in abrupt interruption of a client's usual daily activities; this can precipitate a crisis stage if client perceives events as a threat to safety, self-esteem, or self-image
   a. Seek immediate ways to increase client's control
   b. Engage in therapeutic interactions with client and family; encourage verbalization of feelings
   c. Assist with immediate anxiety reduction through use of relaxation techniques
   d. Use firm, direct limit-setting to assist client with staying focused

NCLEX® 2. Chronic illnesses typically require ongoing adaptation because long-term effects are unpredictable; chronic illnesses often deplete energy levels, support systems, coping reserves, and economic abilities, and may lead to suicidal ideation
   a. Increase self-care responsibilities as appropriate to preserve or facilitate functioning, self-esteem, and self-image
   b. Reward positive adaptive coping behaviors
   c. Reinforce existing support network and assist client with creating new links to support; identify support groups, self-help groups, and special interest groups

IX. EVALUATION/OUTCOMES

A. Preservation of healthy physiological function

B. Disease process reduction/cessation: client learns about illness and ways to decrease disease process, such as diet, exercise, and stress reduction activities

C. Development/reinforcement/strengthening of adaptive coping behaviors: this includes ability to express feelings about medical diagnosis and effects of illness; it also includes productive interdependence of client with ongoing support systems, such as family and friends

D. Participation in treatment/rehabilitation process

E. Optimal level of functioning and independence in self-care

F. Development of functional support systems

G. Decreased anxiety

H. Evidence of an *internal locus of control*

1. Clients who believe they are able to decrease likelihood of illness or effects of illness have an internal locus of control and are less likely to experience symptoms of distress
2. In contrast, clients who have an external locus of control, who believe that forces outside them determine their lives, are less likely to believe they can control illness or manage stressors

Check Your NCLEX–PN® Exam I.Q.

You are ready for testing on this content if you can

- Identify clients experiencing stress.
- Support appropriate use of coping strategies and defense mechanisms for clients experiencing stress.
- Assist with providing care to the abused client and family.
- Identify common clinical symptoms of psychotic disorders due to medical illness.
- Differentiate intervention strategies for clients experiencing critical/acute illness and chronic illness.

PRACTICE TEST

1 A client diagnosed with a terminal illness states, "What's left for me? I feel hopeless." The nurse determines that which of the following would be the best response?

1. "It makes me feel sad that you feel hopeless."
2. "Sometimes people in your situation get depressed, which makes them feel hopeless."
3. "It must be difficult feeling as though there is no hope."
4. "Can you think of one or two reasons to not feel so bad?"

2 The nurse observes that a client hospitalized with newly diagnosed heart disease is frequently crying and stays in the room. The nurse should interpret these actions to be examples of what type of behaviors? Select all that apply.

1. Inappropriate
2. Psychiatric
3. Psychotic
4. Coping
5. Expected

3 A client with a terminal illness states, "If I could only live until I can walk my daughter down the aisle at her wedding, I will donate all of my money to research." The nurse reports that the client is in which phase of the grief process?

1. Denial
2. Seeking
3. Bargaining
4. Acceptance

4 A client diagnosed with a medical illness states, "I don't enjoy my food anymore." The nurse notes that this statement indicates what kind of nutritional pattern?

1. Eating disruption
2. Eating disorder
3. Bulimia
4. Compulsive disorder

5 As part of the admission process, the nurse is assisting in gathering data to be included in a social assessment of a client. The nurse should ask which question for this purpose?

1. "What medications are you currently taking?"
2. "Can you tell me what illnesses you have had in the past?"
3. "Do you have any culturally based practices that you would like continued in the hospital?"
4. "Do your brothers or sisters have any chronic illnesses?"

6 A client who has a diagnosis of a chronic illness states, "I'm so tired. I can't keep on like this every day." The nurse interprets that the feeling the client is expressing can be described as which of the following?

1. Atypical
2. Expected
3. Pathological
4. Resentful

7 The client hospitalized for 5 days with a medical illness says loudly, "Bring me my pain pills now!" The nurse makes which initial interpretation of the client's statement?

1. This is a common response to feeling lack of situational control.
2. This response by the client is inappropriate.
3. This indicates a problem with care delivery to the client.
4. This response reflects the client's feeling of anger at the self.

8 To determine susceptibility to additional health problems in a client who has a medical illness, the nurse should ask about which of the following during data collection as part of the biological assessment? Select all that apply.

1. Past medications
2. Recent illnesses
3. Spiritual needs
4. Cultural background
5. Functional abilities

9 A client with a recent onset of multiple sclerosis is observed taking part in self-care. The nurse interprets this behavior to be consistent with which stage of adaptation?

1. Acceptance
2. Denial
3. Compensation
4. Indulgence

10 A client who underwent surgery for removal of a bowel tumor is exhibiting new onset of verbal outbursts and speaks aloud when no one is in the room. What should the nurse conclude that the client would benefit from next?

1. Psychiatric workup
2. Physical exam
3. Counseling session
4. Teaching session about the illness

11 The nurse is collecting data about a client's coping behaviors when assisting with a psychological assessment and wishes to address factors that can contribute to depression. The nurse would ask the client about which priority items? Select all that apply.

1. Occupation
2. Substance abuse
3. Number of siblings
4. Level of income
5. Recent losses

12 In a client newly diagnosed with amyotrophic lateral sclerosis, an illness that leads to progressive loss of ability to perform activities of daily living, the nurse should anticipate that the client may react to the diagnosis using which initial coping strategy?

1. Denial
2. Gambling
3. Exercise
4. Verbal abuse

13 The nurse observes a client and family interaction. Observed behaviors include anger, rigidity, and lack of support for one another. The nurse should consider this interaction as an example of which family characteristic?

1. Recent life-changing events
2. Communication patterns
3. Lifestyle patterns
4. Community resources

14 A client with inflammatory bowel disease has exacerbations when job responsibilities become heavy or when family conflicts occur at home. The nurse determines that this client would benefit from instruction that focuses on which of the following?

1. How to keep feelings inside
2. Communication strategies
3. How to ignore stress
4. Stress management techniques

15 A client with chronic obstructive pulmonary disease (COPD) has given up smoking and spaces out activities over the course of the day. The nurse should respond by doing which of the following?

1. Say nothing about the behavior to avoid refocusing the client on the disease process.
2. Ignore the maladaptive behaviors.
3. Reward the adaptive coping behaviors.
4. Tell the client that adjustment was bound to occur over time.

16 A client who has experienced a recent heart attack makes a change in work schedule in order to make work less stressful. The nurse concludes that the client is demonstrating what kind of behavior?

1. Anxiety-provoking
2. Anger-releasing
3. Being hopeful
4. Adaptive coping

17 A client recently injured in a severe automobile accident states, "All I remember is that before the accident I was upset about a situation at work." What conclusion should the nurse draw about the client from this statement?

1. There are inadequate coping skills.
2. This is a maladaptive response.
3. The client has pre-existing stressors.
4. The client's work situation is not supportive.

18 A hospitalized client states, "I just want to sleep all of the time." The nurse recognizes that this sleep pattern is most clearly indicative of which of the following?

1. Emotional problems
2. Physical illnesses
3. Attempt to escape from stressors
4. Sleep disruptions

19 The nurse anticipates that a client's ability to adapt to a significant medical illness is most influenced by the presence or absence of which of the following? Select all that apply.

1. Support systems
2. Ability to describe involved anatomical parts
3. Number of siblings
4. Nurse–client ratio
5. Feelings of self-efficacy

20 A client with chronic hypertension has recently been having difficulty with blood pressure readings being higher than usual. The priority intervention by the nurse is to explore which of the following?

1. Personality type
2. Family dynamics
3. Stress levels
4. Number of supportive friends

21 The client was involved in a severe automobile accident and had emergency surgery 2 days ago. At this time, the nurse should anticipate the need to assist the client to adapt to change or loss in which areas? Select all that apply.

1. Verbal communication ability
2. Cognitive patterns
3. Body image
4. Personal autonomy
5. Family relationships

ANSWERS & RATIONALES

1 **Answer: 3 Rationale:** Use of empathy communicates understanding to the client and allows him or her to explore inner feelings of hopelessness. The incorrect options ignore or explain the client's feelings, or focus on the nurse instead of the client. These responses would not encourage the client to further explore feelings with the nurse. **Cognitive Level:** Applying **Client Need:** Psychosocial Integrity **Integrated Process:** Communication and Documentation **Content Area:** Mental Health **Strategy:** For questions involving nurse–client communication, choose the answer that provides the broadest opening in promoting further communication and sharing of client's feelings.

2 **Answer: 4, 5 Rationale:** Crying indicates the client is attempting to cope with the situation in some way and is an expected behavior. The descriptions inappropriate, psychiatric, and psychotic do not reflect accurate or helpful interpretations of the client's behavior. **Cognitive Level:** Applying **Client Need:** Psychosocial Integrity **Integrated Process:** Nursing Process: Data Collection **Content Area:** Mental Health **Strategy:** Consider that the client has just learned about diagnosis of a chronic illness. Reason that the client may engage in any number of behaviors, such as crying, to cope with the initial diagnosis.

3 **Answer: 3 Rationale:** Bargaining is the stage in which the client attempts to bargain for more time. Denial indicates the stage in which the client denies that he or she is terminally ill. Seeking reflects the stage in which a client seeks more answers and cures. Acceptance is the stage in which the client has come to terms with the illness. **Cognitive Level:** Applying **Client Need:** Psychosocial Integrity **Integrated Process:** Communication and Documentation **Content Area:** Mental Health **Strategy:** The core issue of the question is ability to analyze a stage of grief by interpreting client comments. Use nursing knowledge and the process of elimination to make a selection.

4 **Answer: 1 Rationale:** The client's statement indicates an eating disruption in that the client's normal eating pattern has been disturbed in some way. An eating disorder is a specific, possibly severe disruption in eating pattern, and is a specific diagnosis. Bulimia is a more severe, true eating disorder characterized by binge eating and vomiting and is not merely a lack of enjoyment of food. A compulsive disorder would be one in which the client feels the need to carry out certain behaviors. **Cognitive Level:** Analyzing **Client Need:** Psychosocial Integrity **Integrated Process:** Nursing Process: Data Collection **Content Area:** Mental Health **Strategy:** The core issue of the question is the ability to associate medical illness with the appropriate alteration in eating pattern. Use the process of elimination and nursing knowledge to make a selection.

5 **Answer: 3 Rationale:** Culturally based practices are part of a social assessment and provide information about how a client might respond to the illness based on cultural background.

Medications, history of medical illness, and family history of illness are biological assessments. **Cognitive Level:** Analyzing **Client Need:** Psychosocial Integrity **Integrated Process:** Nursing Process: Data Collection **Content Area:** Mental Health **Strategy:** The core issue of the question is knowledge of the components of a social assessment. Use the process of elimination and focus on the option that takes into account the social habits or expectations of a client.

6 **Answer: 2 Rationale:** It is typical of clients with a chronic illness to become tired and feel as though they cannot continue on in this way. Atypical is the opposite of expected (typical), and pathological and resentful are incorrect labels for the feelings expressed by the client. **Cognitive Level:** Analyzing **Client Need:** Psychosocial Integrity **Integrated Process:** Nursing Process: Planning **Content Area:** Mental Health **Strategy:** The core issue of the question is the nurse's ability to draw accurate conclusions about client statements in terms of coping with chronic illness. Use nursing knowledge and the process of elimination to make a selection.

7 **Answer: 1 Rationale:** Hospitalized clients often feel that things are out of their control and their frustration rises. Although the behavior may not be appropriate if it is disruptive, the nurse should first recognize that it is a common response. There is not enough data to support the other options. **Cognitive Level:** Analyzing **Client Need:** Psychosocial Integrity **Integrated Process:** Nursing Process: Data Collection **Content Area:** Mental Health **Strategy:** The core issue of the question is the recognition that clients who are hospitalized may feel out of control and may express this feeling in ways that are not socially acceptable. Note the critical word *initially*, which indicates that more than one option may be partially correct but that one conclusion is more appropriate to draw first.

8 **Answer: 2, 5 Rationale:** Recent illnesses should be considered when assisting with a biological assessment to determine impact on current illness. Functional abilities (ability to perform activities of daily living) may impact the client's ability to adhere to therapy for the current illness. Past medications are not a primary concern related to biological assessment, although current medications would be. Spiritual needs and cultural background are a part of social assessment. **Cognitive Level:** Analyzing **Client Need:** Psychosocial Integrity **Integrated Process:** Nursing Process: Data Collection **Content Area:** Mental Health **Strategy:** The core issue of the question is the ability to determine what elements to include in a biological assessment of a client. Use nursing knowledge and the process of elimination to make a selection.

9 **Answer: 1 Rationale:** Acceptance indicates that the client is accepting limitations imposed by the illness and is attempting to help self as much as possible. A client would not be helping self if the stage was denial because there would be no awareness of need in the denial stage. Compensation and indulgence are not stages related to helping the self in medical illness. **Cognitive Level:** Analyzing **Client Need:** Psychosocial Integrity **Integrated Process:** Nursing Process: Evaluation **Content Area:** Mental Health **Strategy:** The core issue of the question is the ability to determine the client's stage of adaptation to a chronic illness. Use nursing knowledge and the process of elimination to make a selection.

10 **Answer: 2 Rationale:** Physical illnesses can create psychiatric symptoms and a physical examination would help to identify or rule out a physiological basis for the symptoms. A psychiatric workup or counseling session represents a conclusion that the origin of the client's symptoms is psychiatric in nature, which is premature. Teaching when the client is in distress may not be appropriate as it may not lead to retention of information. **Cognitive Level:** Applying **Client Need:** Psychosocial Integrity **Integrated Process:** Nursing Process: Planning **Content Area:** Mental Health **Strategy:** The core issue of the question is recognition that psychiatric symptoms may have a medical basis in a hospitalized client. Note the critical word *first*, which indicates that one action should be taken before some others.

11 **Answer: 2, 5 Rationale:** Substance abuse is of primary interest as a maladaptive coping strategy and is also associated with depression. One or more recent losses can also increase the client's risk for developing depression. Number of siblings, income level, and occupation are general factors related to lifestyle but do not directly relate to risk of developing depression. **Cognitive Level:** Analyzing **Client Need:** Psychosocial Integrity **Integrated Process:** Nursing Process: Data Collection **Content Area:** Mental Health **Strategy:** Note the critical word *depression* in the question. The wording of the question indicates that more than one option may be correct. Review each option and choose those that correlate best with depression, which are substance abuse and recent losses.

12 **Answer: 1 Rationale:** Denial is most accurate because it is a typical and initial stage of grief related to loss. Gambling, exercise, and verbal abuse are isolated responses that could possibly occur but would be based on individual client characteristics rather than anticipated general patterns of response. **Cognitive Level:** Analyzing **Client Need:** Psychosocial Integrity **Integrated Process:** Nursing Process: Planning **Content Area:** Mental Health **Strategy:** Note that the correct answer is a more comprehensive and global option, while the others refer to specific behaviors. This makes the correct option different from the others, and also recalls that a global option is often correct.

13 **Answer: 2 Rationale:** Communication patterns within the family should be assessed for flexibility and support. Recent life-changing events, lifestyle patterns, and community resources would not directly relate to this observed pattern of family interaction. **Cognitive Level:** Analyzing **Client Need:** Psychosocial Integrity **Integrated Process:** Nursing Process: Data Collection **Content Area:** Mental Health **Strategy:** The core issue of the question is the nurse's ability to observe family behavior and interpret it correctly. Note the critical word *interaction* in the stem of the question and the word *communication* in the correct response.

14 **Answer: 4 Rationale:** Stress management techniques assist the client with ways to effectively cope with stress, which may limit exacerbations of the disease. Keeping feelings inside is not a healthy way to cope with stress. Focusing on communication strategies is not indicated based on the information provided. Ignoring stress is not a healthy way to cope with stress. **Cognitive Level:** Applying **Client Need:** Psychosocial Integrity **Integrated Process:** Nursing Process: Planning **Content Area:** Mental Health **Strategy:** The core issue of the question is the ability to recognize the association between client stressors and exacerbation of the disease. First eliminate ignoring stress and keeping feelings inside as inappropriate, then choose stress management techniques because of the association between client stressors in the stem and the words stress reduction in the correct option.

15 **Answer: 3 Rationale:** A client's appropriate behavior should be acknowledged and reinforced. Saying nothing is incorrect

ANSWERS & RATIONALES

because the client is already living with the disease process and an attempt to avoid drawing attention to it is not reasonable. The client's adjustment is not maladaptive. Saying the adjustment was bound to occur over time is incorrect because it patronizes the client. **Cognitive Level:** Applying **Client Need:** Psychosocial Integrity **Integrated Process:** Communication and Documentation **Content Area:** Mental Health **Strategy:** Use principles of communication to answer the question. The core issue of the question is recognition that the client has made an adaptation to medical illness and that this adaptation should be positively reinforced with the client.

16 **Answer: 4 Rationale:** The client is attempting to cope or deal with the situation by making life style changes. The client is not trying to provoke anxiety, but rather is trying to relieve it. This type of behavior is not demonstrated by the client as described. However, the client's changing of pre-existing behaviors could lead to reduced anxiety anger, as well as increased hopefulness. **Cognitive Level:** Applying **Client Need:** Psychosocial Integrity **Integrated Process:** Nursing Process: Evaluation **Content Area:** Mental Health **Strategy:** Notice that the client is accommodating to having had the physical illness, a major stressor.

17 **Answer: 3 Rationale:** The client described stressful circumstances that existed prior to the accident. There is no data in the question to support this conclusion. There is insufficient data in the question to support this conclusion. **Cognitive Level:** Applying **Client Need:** Psychosocial Integrity **Integrated Process:** Nursing Process: Data Collection **Content Area:** Mental Health **Strategy:** Look for an answer that is fully supportable by the data given.

18 **Answer: 4 Rationale:** Sleep disruptions can take a number of forms, including hypersomnolence and impaired sleep efficiency. To reach the conclusion that the client is experiencing emotional problems, the nurse would require more data. To reach the conclusion that the client is experiencing physical problems, the nurse would require more data. To reach the conclusion that the client is trying to escape from stressors, the nurse would require more data. **Cognitive Level:** Applying **Client Need:** Basic Care and Comfort **Integrated Process:** Nursing Process: Data Collection **Content Area:** Mental Health **Strategy:** Select the option that is the broadest and least judgmental.

19 **Answer: 1, 5 Rationale:** Support systems can provide emotional sustenance that can help reduce stress, diminish feelings of isolation, and positively influence the ability to cope and adapt. Self-efficacy is the belief that personal abilities and efforts affect the events in our lives. Having a sense of control allows an individual to believe that personal behavior can make a difference. Accordingly, this client is most likely to take action and cope more effectively. A specific anatomical understanding is not necessarily imperative for the person to adapt to the diagnosis. The number of siblings may or may not be helpful. What is more important is whether the siblings are able to be support systems for the client. An appropriate nurse–client ratio would provide more time for the nurse to interact with the client; this alone is not sufficient to ensure adequate coping. **Cognitive Level:** Analyzing **Client Need:** Psychosocial Integrity **Integrated Process:** Nursing Process: Planning **Content Area:** Mental Health **Strategy:** Look carefully at the stem of the question to understand fully what it is asking. Paraphrase the question if that would help to understand it better.

20 **Answer: 3 Rationale:** Hypertension has a strong psychophysiologic component and is highly correlated with increased stress levels. Personality type addresses psychodynamic factors that may have an impact on emotions which affects biochemical functioning such as blood pressure. However, there is a stronger and more direct link between hypertension and poorly managed stress. Family dynamics address psychodynamic factors that may have an impact on emotions which affects biochemical functioning such as blood pressure. Data about friends addresses psychodynamic factors that may have an impact on emotions, which affects biochemical functioning such as blood pressure. **Cognitive Level:** Applying **Client Need:** Physiological Adaptation **Integrated Process:** Nursing Process: Planning **Content Area:** Mental Health **Strategy:** Apply basic concepts of stress adaptation and psychophysiologic disorders.

21 **Answer: 3, 4 Rationale:** Since the client has experienced both injury and surgery to the body, changes in body image should be anticipated. Having experienced an accident, this client is now in a situation (acute illness and hospitalization) that is expected to limit the client's personal autonomy. There is inadequate information to suggest that changes in verbal communication ability may occur. There is inadequate information to suggest that changes in cognitive patterns may occur. There is inadequate information to suggest that changes in family relationships may occur. **Cognitive Level:** Analyzing **Client Need:** Psychosocial Integrity **Integrated Process:** Caring **Content Area:** Mental Health **Strategy:** Look for what is expected to be universally true of clients in this type of situation.

Key Terms to Review

adaptive coping p. 257
control p. 261
coping p. 257
crisis p. 260
internal locus of control p. 264
maladaptive coping p. 257
precipitating stressors p. 260

ANSWERS & RATIONALES

References

Fontaine, K. (2009). *Mental health nursing* (6th ed.). Upper Saddle River, NJ: Pearson Education.

Keltner, N., Bostrom, C., & McGuinness, T. (2011). *Psychiatric nursing* (6th ed.). St. Louis, MO: Mosby.

Kniesl, C., Wilson, H., & Trigoboff, E. (2009). *Contemporary psychiatric-mental health nursing* (2nd ed.). Upper Saddle River, NJ: Pearson Education.

Stuart, G., & Laraia, M. (2009). *Principles and practice of psychiatric nursing* (9th ed.). St. Louis: Elsevier Science.

Townsend, M. (2010). *Essentials of psychiatric mental health nursing: Concepts of care in evidence-based practice* (5th ed.). Philadelphia: F.A. Davis.

Varcarolis, E. (2010). *Foundations of psychiatric mental health nursing: A clinical approach* (6th ed.). Philadelphia: Saunders.

Test Yourself

Are you ready for the NCLEX-PN® or course exams? Use the practice tests on the companion website to check.

21 Mental Health Disorders

In this chapter

Cross Reference

Other chapters relevant to this content area are

Therapeutic Communication and Environment	Chapter 18
Coping with Stressors	Chapter 20
Dependency and Addiction	Chapter 22
Crisis Intervention and Suicide	Chapter 23
Psychiatric Medications	Chapter 32

I. OVERVIEW OF MENTAL HEALTH CONCEPTS

NCLEX® **A. Data collection**

1. Appearance, behavior, and mood: grooming, relaxed state, confidence
2. Level of consciousness/sensorium: oriented to time, place, person; memory intact; able to think abstractly
3. Speech, content/thought processes, insight and judgment, self-perception
4. Stage of growth and development
5. Satisfaction of Maslow's hierarchy of needs (see Figure 21–1)
6. Interactions with others: satisfying interpersonal relationships, ability to cope with stress, ability to trust
7. Risk factors for mental health problems: family history of mental illness, stressful life events, hormonal influence, weak or ineffective mental defense mechanisms
8. Poor support systems

B. Therapeutic management

1. Therapeutic communication techniques (see Chapter 18)
2. NCLEX® Therapeutic milieu and treatment modalities (see Table 21–1)

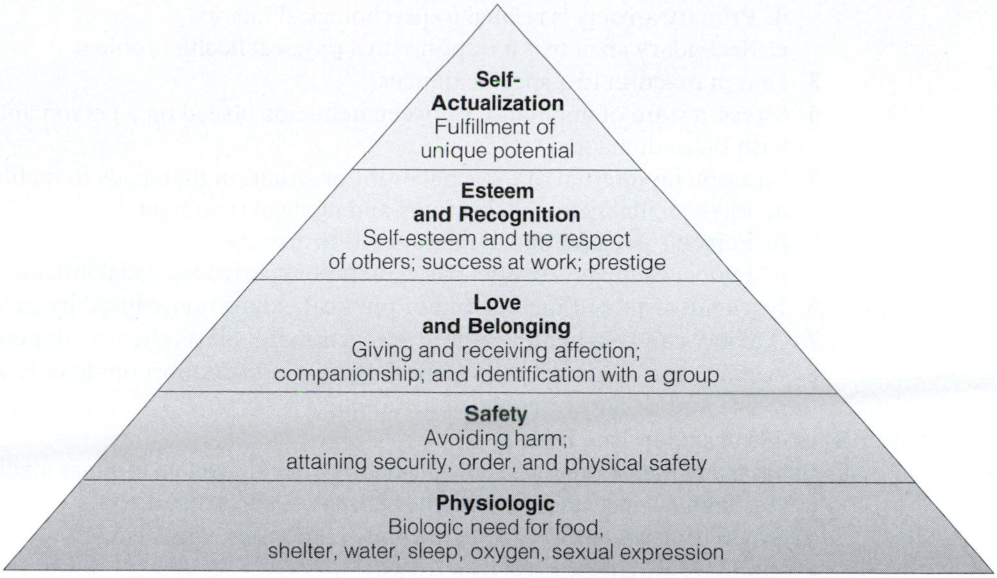

Figure 21–1

Maslow's hierarchy of needs.

Source: Maslow, A. (1962). *Motivation and personality* (3rd ed.). Upper Saddle River, NJ: Pearson Education (as reproduced in Kniesl, C., Wilson, H., & Trigoboff, E. (2004), p. 36. *Contemporary psychiatric-mental health nursing.* Reprinted by permission from Pearson Education, Upper Saddle River, NJ.

Table 21–1 Therapies and Treatment Modalities in Mental Illness

Type of Therapy	Underlying Assumptions	Summary of Treatment
Behavior modification therapy	Mental health problems are learned and can be corrected through relearning	Aimed at changing undesirable behaviors; operant conditioning (rewarding positive behavior to reinforce it); desensitization for phobias
Biologically based therapies	Mental health problems are illnesses that may be inherited and/or caused by chemical imbalances	A variety of medications; electroconvulsive therapy (ECT)
Cognitive therapies	Distorted conceptualizations and dysfunctional beliefs lead to mental health problems	Reality testing; correcting distorted conceptualizations and dysfunctional beliefs by reinterpreting them
Activity therapy	A group task can set the stage to allow important group interactions to occur	Organized group activities that promote socialization and increase self-esteem
Family therapy	A person's emotional symptoms or problems are an expression of family's emotional symptoms or problems	Unit of therapy is entire family; develop a sense of self for each member; members learn new insights and coping behaviors and ways of interacting and behaving
Group therapy	Relationships with others can be recreated and worked on with group members	Regular meetings are held with a leader to form a stable group; members learn new behaviors and coping skills during group work
Milieu therapy	A therapeutic environment helps increase self-awareness of feelings and promotes acquisition of adaptive coping, interaction, and relationship skills	Possible open wards, self-medication programs, token programs; client-planned group and social interactions
Play therapy	Children can express in play thoughts and feelings they cannot verbalize; child reflects his/her situation in family using toys, colors, activities (drawing)	A variety of toys are provided to facilitate interaction; play is observed; child is helped to work through problems through play
Psychoanalytical	Conflicts between id and ego lead to anxiety; ineffective or inappropriate defense mechanisms form to reduce anxiety	Interactions with therapist assist client to recognize unconscious thoughts, feelings, anxieties, and defenses

II. ANXIETY DISORDERS

A. Overview of Anxiety

1. **Anxiety**: a state of apprehension, dread, uneasiness, or fear of the unknown
2. Anxiety is an emotional, subjective response
   - **a.** Anxiety is commonly experienced by all human beings
   - **b.** Acute anxiety is also known as state anxiety
   - **c.** Chronic anxiety is also known as trait anxiety

   d. Primary anxiety is related to psychological factors
   e. Secondary anxiety is a response to a physical health problem
3. Fear: a reaction to a specific danger
4. Stress: a state of imbalance between demands placed on a person and his/her ability to deal with these demands
5. Stressor: an internal or external event or situation that leads to feelings of anxiety
   a. Physical illness, hospitalizations, and medical treatment
   b. Person's perception of stressor leads to anxiety
   c. People evaluate stressors based on past experiences, social influences, and current resources
6. Burnout: a state of mental and/or physical exhaustion, caused by excessive, prolonged stress
7. Anxiety can be a healthy adaptive reaction if it alerts client to impending threats
8. Anxiety is considered pathological when it is disproportionate to risks, continues after threat no longer exists, and/or interferes with functioning

NCLEX®

B. Levels of anxiety (see Table 21–2)

C. General adaptation syndrome: an automatic physical reaction to stress mediated by sympathetic nervous system (SNS); three distinct stages are alarm, resistance, and exhaustion

1. Stress is viewed as a nonspecific body response to any demand
2. Alarm is initial response to a stressor
   a. Hormonal activity triggers a fight-or-flight reaction (an automatic psychological state of high anxiety mediated by SNS), causing increased alertness that is focused on immediate task or threat
   b. Level of anxiety is mild to moderate
3. Resistance occurs when body mobilizes resources to combat stress
   a. Body stabilizes and adapts to stress but functions below optimal level
   b. Coping (efforts to manage specific demands that are appraised as threatening) and defense mechanisms (unconscious psychological responses designed to diminish or delay anxiety and protect client) are used
   c. Psychosomatic symptoms begin to develop
   d. Level of anxiety is moderate to severe
4. Exhaustion occurs when adaptational resources are depleted
   a. Results from inability to cope with overwhelming or long-lasting stress
   b. Thinking becomes disorganized and illogical; may experience sensory misperceptions, delusions, hallucinations, and/or reduced orientation to reality
   c. Level of anxiety is severe to panic
   d. Physical illness and even death can occur if period of exhaustion is prolonged

D. Data collection

1. Because anxiety can contribute to organic illness, and organic illness can lead to anxiety, include physical assessment when assessing anxious individuals
2. Shame and fear may prevent individuals from disclosing anxiety
3. Determine anxiety using direct and specific questions (consider cognitive ability, level of education, and language)

NCLEX®

4. Note physical, affective, cognitive, social, and spiritual symptoms of anxiety (see Table 21–3)

Table 21–2 Response to Varying Levels of Anxiety

	Mild	Moderate	Severe	Panic
Cognitive and perceptual response	Alert, increased perceptual field, learning is facilitated	Perceptual field is narrowed, focus is on immediate concerns	Perceptual field greatly reduced, learning cannot occur, behavior directed toward relief of anxiety	Details are exaggerated, personality disorganization occurs, person fails to function
Physiological response	Normal physiological responses	Low-level sympathetic nervous system arousal occurs	Sympathetic nervous system is aroused	Physiological arousal interferes with motor activities
Emotional response	Positive affect	Tension and fear are experienced	Severe emotional distress is experienced	Dread and terror, possible regression to primitive or childish behaviors

E. Therapeutic management

1. Assist in developing mental coping strategies
   a. Include breathing exercises, guided imagery, meditation, listening to music, progressive muscle relaxation, recreational activities, crying, exercising, laughing, sleeping, diet and fluid intake, time management

NCLEX®
   b. Problem-focused coping is task oriented and consists of assessing facts, developing a goal, determining alternatives for coping, identifying risks and benefits of each alternative, selecting an alternative, implementing alternative, evaluating outcome, and modifying actions based on evaluation
   c. Emotional-focused coping requires client to reinterpret meaning of situation and explore defense mechanisms (see Chapter 20)
2. Psychopharmacology
   a. Common anti-anxiety agents (also called anxiolytics) used to treat anxiety are listed in Table 21–4 and discussed in Chapter 32
   b. Benzodiazepines are commonly used, but prolonged use can lead to dependency
   c. Nonbenzodiazepine sedative-hypnotics are newer class of drugs used for short-term treatment of insomnia associated with anxiety
   d. Buspirone (Buspar) is a serotonin and dopamine agonist used in short-term treatment of anxiety
   e. Beta blockers have a calming effect on central nervous system (CNS): propranolol (Inderal) is a beta blocker sometimes used to treat physical symptoms of anxiety, such as tremors and tachycardia
   f. Antidepressants may be used to treat coexisting depression and insomnia associated with anxiety
3. Individual and **group therapy** (see again Table 21–1)
   a. Helps clients to discuss feelings and problems with empathetic listeners
   b. Helps anxious individuals develop insight and rationales for feelings of anxiety

NCLEX®
   c. See Box 21–1 for intervention strategies to assist anxious clients
   d. Client education is an important intervention for anxious clients
4. Other useful therapies
   a. Cognitive-behavior therapy helps clients learn to identify stressors and plan responses to stressors

NCLEX®
   b. In cognitive restructuring, clients are encouraged to examine involuntary negative thoughts and to replace negative self-talk with more positive thoughts
   c. Response prevention is a form of behavior modification used to teach clients with obsessive-compulsive disorder how to prevent compulsive behaviors associated with obsessive thoughts

Table 21–3 Manifestations of Anxiety

Category	Specific Manifestations
Physical signs	↑ blood pressure, respiration, and heart rate; diaphoresis; dilated pupils; dyspnea or hyperventilation; vertigo or lightheadedness; blurred vision; urinary frequency; headache; sleep disturbance; muscle weakness or tension; anorexia, nausea and vomiting
Affective symptoms	Depression; irritability; apathy; crying; hypercriticism; feelings of guilt, grief, anger, worthlessness, apprehension, and helplessness
Cognitive symptoms	Inability to concentrate, indecisiveness, inability to think and reason, lack of interest, and forgetfulness
Social symptoms	Refusal to communicate or excessive communication, self-isolation, social withdrawal, and possibly suicidal ideation
Spiritual symptoms	Feelings of hopelessness and despair, fear of death, and inability to find life meaningful

Table 21–4 Medications Used to Treat Anxiety

Class	Specific Medications
Benzodiazepine	Alprazolam (Xanax), chlordiazepoxide (Librium), clonazepam (Klonopin), clorazepate (Tranxene), diazepam (Valium), lorazepam (Ativan), oxazepam (Serax)
Nonbenzodiazepine Anxiolytics	Buspirone (Buspar), eszopirlone (Lunesta), ramelteon (Rozerem), zaleplon (Sonata), zolpidem (Ambien)
Antidepressants (approved for anxiety and insomnia)	Duloxetine (Cymbalta), escitoprolam (Lexapro), fluoxetine (Prozac), fluvoxamine (Luvox), paroxetine (Paxil), sertraline (Zoloft), venlafaxine (Effexor)

Box 21-1

Therapeutic Nursing Interventions to Assist Anxious Clients

- Use a quiet, calm approach to reduce interpersonal transmission of anxiety.
- Establish a trusting relationship; protect and reassure client.
- Structure environment to eliminate stressors; stay with client who has high anxiety level (panic) and place in a smaller, less stimulating environment.
- Provide ongoing assessment of client's anxiety.
- Assess client's use of caffeine, nicotine, and other stimulants.
- Assess client for signs of depression and suicidal ideations.
- Help client to identify stressors, express feelings, and explore sources of feelings.
- Help client to examine cognitive processes and encourage positive self-talk.
- Help client to maintain hope and find meaning in life.
- Support use of effective coping mechanisms.
- Teach new coping behaviors and provide opportunities for client to practice them.
- Teach client relaxation techniques and provide opportunity to practice them.
- Encourage appropriate grooming, sleep, diet, recreational activity, and exercise.
- Facilitate client's interactions with supportive significant others.
- Use role-playing to help client rehearse appropriate reactions to stressors.
- Refer client to community resources as indicated.

d. Systematic desensitization is a form of behavior modification used to treat anxiety
e. Flooding, also known as implosion therapy, exposes client to imaginary or real-life stress-provoking stimuli for an extended period of time, and session is terminated when client's anxiety decreases
f. Thought-stopping involves such techniques as instructing client to shout "Stop!" or snap a rubber band placed on wrist when unwelcome thoughts occur
g. Other behavior modification techniques used to treat anxiety include modeling, shaping, token economy, role-playing, social skill training, aversion therapy, response prevention, and contingency contracting

F. Phobic disorders

1. A **phobia** (persistent, irrational fear of specific object or situation) develops when an unconscious conflict is displaced onto an external object or situation related symbolically to conflict
2. Diagnosis is often made when avoidance of feared stimuli drastically interferes with routine activities
3. Phobias
   a. **Agoraphobia** (fear of being in a public place where escape might not be possible or help might not be available) without panic attacks commonly involves fear of situations such as crowds, standing in line, being on a bridge, and traveling in a plane, bus, train, or car
   b. Social phobia is excessive fear of embarrassment and humiliation in public settings
   c. Specific phobia involves unrealistic fear of a particular object or situation
4. Treatments include cognitive therapy and graduated exposure or desensitization; anti-anxiety medications may provide short-term relief of phobic anxiety
5. *NCLEX®* Nursing care includes accepting but not supporting phobia, exploring client's perceptions of threats, discussing feelings that may contribute to irrational fears, and identifying strategies for change

G. Generalized anxiety disorder (GAD)

1. Characterized by pervasive, persistent anxiety of at least 6 months duration without panic attacks, phobias, or obsessions and compulsions
2. Anxiety leads to symptoms such as restlessness, irritability, fatigue, depression, difficulty concentrating, muscle tension, sleep disturbance, and feeling helpless
3. Symptoms interfere with normal daily activities
4. In an attempt to control symptoms, clients sometimes become dependent on alcohol or other substances
5. GAD has been successfully treated by combined cognitive therapy and relaxation training
6. *NCLEX®* Encourage clients with GAD to rethink perceptions of stressor, recognize that some anxiety is a normal part of life, and learn new coping mechanisms
7. Benzodiazepines and buspirone are sometimes used to treat GAD

H. Panic disorder

1. Characterized by recurrent panic attacks; between panic attacks, client may have little or no debilitating anxiety or may have chronic worry about future panic attacks
2. Onset of a panic attack is sudden, and source of anxiety may not be identifiable; clients frequently associate their symptoms with physical illness and are concerned about death
3. NCLEX® Symptoms of panic attacks include a desire to escape, chest pain, chills or hot flashes, choking sensations, depersonalization, dizziness, nausea, palpitations, shortness of breath, sweating, trembling, and fear of loss of control and mental illness
4. Feelings of hopelessness, helplessness, and despair may lead to suicidal ideations
5. NCLEX® Agoraphobia is frequently associated with panic disorder
6. NCLEX® During panic attacks, remain calm, stay with client, offer reassurance, use short clear sentences, and reduce environmental stimuli
7. When level of anxiety is mild or moderate, explore possible causes of anxiety, teach signs and symptoms of escalating anxiety, and teach and reinforce appropriate coping mechanisms and strategies
8. Benzodiazepines and antidepressants treat panic disorders

I. Obsessive-compulsive disorder (OCD)

1. Characterized by recurrent irrational obsessive thoughts and uncontrollable compulsive behaviors; control of self, others, and environment is an important issue
2. Common **obsessions** (unwanted, persistent thoughts that cannot be removed from consciousness without anxiety or distress) include thoughts about specific objects, contamination, questions, order, sex, aggressive feelings, and unacceptable impulses
3. Common **compulsions** (persistent unwanted urges to perform acts to relieve severe tension) include such behaviors as counting, handwashing, repeating words, checking doors or locks, and dressing and undressing rituals
4. NCLEX® Anxiety increases if obsessive thoughts and compulsive behaviors are interrupted
5. Depression and/or substance abuse may occur as a complication
6. Treatments include relaxation and cognitive-behavioral techniques such as flooding and thought stopping
7. NCLEX® Assist clients to identify situations that increase anxiety, explore meaning and purpose of thoughts and behavior, and support client attempts to decrease obsessions and compulsions
8. NCLEX® Conduct teaching immediately after completion of a ritual when client is least anxious
9. Selective serotonin reuptake inhibitors (SSRIs) are most effective somatic treatment for OCD; electroconvulsive therapy (ECT) has been used to treat depressive symptoms associated with OCD

J. Posttraumatic stress disorder (PTSD)

1. Associated with exposure to an extremely traumatic, menacing event such as military combat, rape, assault, kidnapping, torture, incarceration, disasters, and life-threatening illnesses
2. NCLEX® Symptoms
   a. Apathy, social withdrawal and isolation, loss of interest in activities, and possible depression and hopelessness
   b. Restlessness, irritability, intrusive and unwanted memories of traumatic event, amnesia for certain aspects of trauma, nightmares, flashbacks, and occasional outburst of anger and rage
3. Denial, repression, and suppression are used as coping mechanisms
4. NCLEX® Provide a nonthreatening environment; encourage client to discuss traumatic event and associated feelings; assess and acknowledge feelings of guilt, grief, and shame
5. NCLEX® Encourage and reinforce appropriate coping strategies, teach new coping strategies, and assist client in resuming regular activities
6. SSRIs, especially sertraline (Zoloft), seem to have some effect in treating PTSD

III. MOOD DISORDERS

A. Overview

1. **Mood**: a prolonged emotional state that affects a person's life and personality
2. Change of mood is a normal and expected life occurrence; each person feels a range of emotions, such as joy, happiness, sadness, depression, anger, and fear
3. **Affect**: a person's present feelings and moods with verbal and nonverbal behavioral cues
4. *Mood disorders* are characterized by changes in mood that range from depression to elation
   a. **Major depression** (also called **unipolar disorder**): a loss of interest in life and a mood that transforms from mild to severe and lasts at least 2 weeks; if uncontrolled, results in disturbances in eating, sleeping, and functioning at work, home, and/or school; withdrawal and decreased sociability;

possible delusions and/or hallucinations with psychotic features if disorder progresses to severe depression; 15% of clients die by suicide

b. **Dysthymic disorder**: a chronic disorder in which depressed mood fluctuates with normal mood; symptoms are less severe than in major depression

c. **Bipolar disorder** (also called manic-depressive disorder): alternation of depression and elation; categorized as bipolar I disorder (one or more manic episodes and one or more depressive episodes) or bipolar II disorder (less severe, has one or more *hypomanic* or mild manic episodes and one or more depressive episodes)

d. **Cyclothymic disorder**: mood changes between moderate depression and hypomania; lasts for at least 2 years; usually no sign of a normal range

e. **Seasonal affective disorder (SAD)**: depressed mood occurs during fall and winter; there is a direct correlation with light and production of melatonin

f. **Schizoaffective disorder**: a combination of manifestations of schizophrenia and mood disorders; delusions, hallucinations, disorganized speech and behavior, communication difficulties, poor abstractions, passive social withdrawal, poor grooming and hygiene, poor rapport, and major depressive or manic symptoms or mixed symptoms, and possibly other physical or psychological disorders

B. Data collection

NCLEX®

1. Assist with intake assessment in 15- to 20-minute segments at one time
   a. Clients with mood disorders do not have enough energy to talk or focus attention for extended periods of time
   b. Clients with mania may not be able to sit still and concentrate because of elevated mood and flight of ideas
2. Bipolar disorders
   a. Characterized by moods alternating between episodes of depression and episodes of mania or hypomania
   b. Manic episodes are periods of elation during which there is an abnormally and persistently elevated, expansive, or irritable mood for at least 1 week and also includes at least three of the following: inflated self-esteem, decreased need for sleep, more than usual talkativeness, racing thoughts, distractibility, increase in goal-directed activity, and excessive involvement in pleasurable activities
   c. Hypomania is described as an elevation in mood with increases in activity but not as severe elation as in mania
3. Major depression
   a. Loss of interest in life and a depressed mood, which moves from mild to severe and lasts at least 2 weeks
   b. Depressed mood is present for most of day, nearly every day, as indicated by subjective (client reports) or objective (facial expression, appears tearful) data
   c. Markedly diminished interest or pleasure in all or almost all activities most of day, nearly every day (as indicated by subjective or objective data)
   d. Significant weight loss or gain
   e. Insomnia or hypersomnia
   f. Psychomotor agitation or retardation nearly every day
   g. Fatigue or loss of energy nearly every day
   h. Diminished ability to think or concentrate, or indecisiveness nearly every day
   i. Social withdrawal
   j. Recurrent thoughts of death; suicidal ideation with or without a specific plan or a suicide attempt
4. Dysthymic disorder differs from major depression in that it is a chronic, low-level depression; must have depressed mood and at least three of these symptoms for most of the day, nearly every day, for at least 2 years: poor appetite or overeating; insomnia or hypersomnia; low energy; low self-esteem; poor concentration and difficulty making decisions; and feelings of hopelessness
5. Key characteristic differences between depressive disorder and bipolar disorders are noted in Table 21–5

C. Therapeutic management

1. Risk for Violence, Self-directed related to depressed mood, feelings of worthlessness, hopelessness, and suicide ideation or plan
   a. Client's safety is nurse's first priority

NCLEX®

   b. Danger for self-harm is more prominent as client begins to regain strength and hope; frequently assess for levels of hopefulness or hopelessness and self-esteem, and be alert for signs of thoughts or plan for suicide
   c. History of violence is *always* important in determining seriousness of client's present risk for self-harm

Table 21-5 Findings in Major Depression and Mania

	Major Depression	Mania
Behavior	Progression from a decreased desire to engage in social, work, and school activities to an absence of participation in common ADLs; progressive loss of self-esteem, feelings of incompetence, decreased motivation; statements such as, "Why bother, I can't anyway" are common	Initially high energy and productivity with positive reinforcement from others; reduced ability to concentrate, make judgments, or engage in activities; increasing frustration and irritability, shortened attention span, unrealistic self-confidence, and poor judgment (spending sprees, foolish financial investments, high-risk lifestyle changes)
Relationships	Withdrawal from personal and social activities and events	Unable to set boundaries; incessant talkativeness and gregarious behaviors that are often an embarrassment upon return to normal range of mood
Affective characteristics	Sense of sadness that becomes increasingly pronounced; guilt that may be expressed as a vague concern or a specific issue: "I have so much to be thankful for, I shouldn't feel this way"; loss of emotional attachment evidenced by expressions of indifference toward family and friends; anhedonia, or a lack of pleasure	Mood ranges between cheerful and euphoric; if there is an external negative stimulus, can become irritable, argumentative, hostile, and combative, then return to euphoria when stimulus is removed; absent sense of guilt; responds to others' feelings of hurt or anger with anger, laughter, or indifference; tries to participate in every available activity or event
Cognitive characteristics	Personal worth: presents self as a failure and incompetent; personalizes comments by others; is self-critical and perfectionistic; anticipates disapproval; while in a depressed state: • Exhibits a decreased ability or even an inability for decision making • Has decrease in rate and number of thoughts • Perceives self as unattractive • Has somatic delusions • Has hallucinations (15–25% of cases)	Personal worth: very grandiose belief about self; exhibits unwarranted positive expectations, is unable to see potential negative outcomes, and is irate if criticized by others; while in manic state: • Presents as easily distractible and impulsive • Has flight of ideas • Believes self to be very attractive • Exhibits delusions of grandeur • Exhibits hallucinations in approximately 15–25% of cases
Sociocultural characteristics	Loss of desire in sexual activities	Increase in sexual activity, even to promiscuity
Physiological characteristics	Increased or decreased appetite; when severely depressed, a decrease in appetite usually occurs; increased or decreased sleep in mild to moderate depression; sleep is usually decreased in severe depression; constipation	Difficulty eating because of the inability to physically slow down or sit still; sleeps only 1 or 2 hours per night and is usually hyperactive when engaged in activities; constipation
Physical appearance	Unkempt appearance with little to no attention to hygiene	Bright clothes, frequent clothing changes, exaggerated presentation of physical self

d. Client often displays ambivalence or expresses sadness, dejection, hopelessness, or loss of pleasure or purpose in life

e. Client makes overt attempts to harm self (e.g., hoards medications, performs self-mutilation, attempts to hang self)

NCLEX® **f.** Assess for overt signs of hopelessness: refusal to eat, withdrawal from milieu, resistance to or refusal of medications; inability to see future for self; sudden giving away of possessions; refusal to sign a no self-harm contract

2. Risk for Violence Directed at Others related to poor impulse control and labile affect

NCLEX® **a.** Safety is nurse's first priority; provide a safe environment, removing objects and barriers to prevent accidental or purposeful injury to self or others

b. Help client identify alternative behaviors that are acceptable to client and staff

c. Encourage client, during calm moments, to recognize and identify factors leading to agitation and loss of control

d. Give realistic and positive feedback and encouragement to client

NCLEX® **e.** Decrease environmental stimuli when client is agitated; gradually increase environmental stimulation after agitation subsides

f. Monitor client's ability to tolerate frustration and/or individual situations

g. Offer alternatives when available (e.g., "There is no coffee available; how about a glass of juice?")

h. Communicate with respect and a nonjudgmental tone

3. Ineffective Individual Coping related to lack of energy, inability to concentrate or make decisions
   a. Maintain activities of daily living (ADLs)
   b. Use a problem-solving approach
   c. Maintain a safe environment; observe client closely
   d. Encourage client to focus on strengths rather than weaknesses and identify people and systems that can support client
   e. Help client to learn strategies that will effect more positive thinking (cognitive, behavioral, imagery)
   f. NCLEX® Encourage client to express feelings and needs
   g. Inform family and friends that client may direct anger toward them but that client is learning more effective coping skills to deal with feelings
   h. NCLEX® Help client to gradually become involved with activities on unit and to socialize as tolerated with staff, other clients on unit, and family members in a structured environment
4. Imbalanced Nutrition, Less/More Than Body Requirements related to inappropriate nutritional intake to meet metabolic needs; lack of interest in eating/food or choosing nutritional foods; aversion to eating; dysfunctional eating pattern (e.g., eating in response to internal cues other than hunger)
   a. Client may have an aversion to eating because of paranoid thoughts, such as that food is contaminated or someone is trying to poison him or her
   b. NCLEX® Note common findings in manic states, including weight loss; easy distraction from eating; inability to sit through routine meals; wary or frightened appearance when offered food; physical signs of poor nutrition, dehydration, and electrolyte imbalances; hyperactive bowel sounds
   c. NCLEX® Offer small frequent feedings and carbohydrate- and protein-rich snacks
   d. NCLEX® Offer nutritious finger foods and sandwiches and easy-to-carry drinks that are high in vitamins, minerals, and electrolytes
   e. NCLEX® Monitor fluid and electrolyte status, especially sodium, potassium, and lithium levels
   f. Monitor and record daily intake and output; monitor body weight
   g. Monitor daily bowel movements for frequency and consistency
   h. Note abdominal pain or discomfort
   i. NCLEX® Administer high-fiber foods unless contraindicated
   j. Clients with depression may have a nutritional pattern that relates more to their depressed mood, including disinterest in eating, poor or no appetite, aversion to food, dysfunctional eating patterns, poor food choices, recent weight loss or gain, poor muscle tone, pale conjunctivae and mucous membranes
   k. Explain to client importance of maintaining adequate intake of food and fluids to prevent malnutrition
   l. NCLEX® Determine client's daily caloric intake needs
   m. Monitor laboratory studies (such as serum prealbumin, albumin, glucose, electrolytes, nitrogen balance)
5. Disturbed Sleep Pattern related to biochemical alterations (decreased serotonin) or psychological stress, lack of recognition of fatigue or need to sleep, hyperactivity
   a. In clients with mania, assess sleep disturbances by denial of need for sleep, changes in behavior and performance, increasing irritability, restlessness, and dark circles under eyes
   b. Identify environmental factors that might prevent or interrupt sleep
   c. NCLEX® Identify nature of sleep disturbance and variations from usual pattern (difficulty falling asleep, remaining asleep, or waking early and unable to return to sleep)
   d. Restrict intake of caffeine
   e. Offer small snack or warm milk at bedtime or when client is awake during night
   f. NCLEX® Encourage activities in morning and early afternoon, and restrict activities during evening and prior to bedtime
   g. Encourage routine bedtime relaxation techniques; identify previously effective nighttime rituals and reestablish when possible
   h. Administer medications as indicated
   i. Restrict evening fluids, and have client void before retiring
6. Spiritual Distress related to a sense of no purpose or joy in life; lack of connectedness to others; misperceived shame and guilt
   a. NCLEX® Allow client to express feelings and thoughts about religious doubt or fears of abandonment
   b. Explore with client alternative or past effective religious or spiritual practice or ritual as an illness-prevention measure
   c. Eliminate or reduce causative and contributing factors of illness if possible
   d. Encourage client to discuss thoughts and feelings with clergy or chaplain when possible

7. ECT as treatment
   a. Useful for clients with severe depression who resist other types of treatment modalities, including medications such as TCAs and MAOIs
   b. Involves application of pulses of electrical energy to forehead and temporal area of scalp, sufficient to cause a brief convulsion or seizure; usually carried out under anesthesia
   c. A series of ECT treatments is usually carried out over a short period of time
   d. Effects of ECT are usually very positive for treatment of depression
   NCLEX® e. Side effects are low and seem to be limited to short-term, temporary memory deficits; infrequent deaths have been reported in clients who undergo ECT; risks related to anesthesia are present
   NCLEX® f. Nursing care involves same principles as those used for client undergoing surgery or moderate (conscious) sedation; protect client's airway and provide for safety; monitor vital signs and provide explanations to client as needed
8. Medication therapy includes TCAs, SSRIs, MAOIs, atypical antidepressants, and mood stabilizers (see Chapter 32 for full discussion of medications to treat depression and mania)
9. Group and individual therapies may help, including cognitive therapy, behavioral therapy, and interpersonal therapy for mild to moderate depression
10. Phototherapy
    a. A treatment that has been used effectively to lessen symptoms of recurrent SAD, because possibly exposure to *morning light* causes a circadian rhythm shift that regulates normal relationships between sleep and circadian rhythms
    b. Phototherapy treatment consists of a minimum of 2500 lux of light usually administered on waking in morning; clients can be exposed for 30 minutes to several hours, depending on strength of light source
    NCLEX® c. An antidepressant effect is usually seen within 2 to 4 days and is complete after 2 weeks
    d. Maintenance treatment usually consists of 30 minutes of exposure each day; side effects are usually minimal
11. Note achievement of short- and long-term goals for clients with mood disorders
    a. Remain safe and free from harm
    b. Verbalize suicidal ideations and contract not to harm self or others
    c. Verbalize absence of suicidal or homicidal intent or plan
    d. Establish a pattern of rest, activity, and sleep that enables fulfillment of role and self-care demands
    e. Describe information about disorder, including triggers for relapse, preventive measures in place for relapse prevention, and medications to control symptoms

IV. SCHIZOPHRENIA AND OTHER PSYCHOTIC DISORDERS

A. ***Schizophrenia***: a syndrome characterized by difficulty in thinking clearly, knowing what is real, managing feelings, making decisions, or relating to others
   NCLEX® 1. Positive symptoms of schizophrenia are added behaviors not normally seen, such as delusions, hallucinations, disorganized speech, and disorganized behavior (pacing, touching objects) or catatonic behavior
   NCLEX® 2. Negative symptoms of schizophrenia are an absence of healthy behaviors; may include flat affect, apathy, anhedonia (inability to experience pleasure), avolition (inability to pursue goal-directed behavior), alogia (poverty of speech), minimal self-care, ineffective social skills with social withdrawal, and isolation and concrete thinking
   3. Delusions are false beliefs that cannot be changed by logical reasoning or evidence; they may represent dysfunction in information-processing circuits between hemispheres of brain
   4. Neurobiological factors of schizophrenia include genetic defects, abnormal brain development, neurodegeneration, disordered neurotransmission, and abnormal brain structures
   5. Psychiatric rehabilitation emphasizes development of skills and supports; considers client to be in control; and promotes choices, self-determination, and individual responsibility

B. **Schizoaffective disorder**: having clinical manifestations characteristic of both schizophrenia and a mood disorder, such as depression, mania, or a mixed episode
   1. Client experiences symptoms of a mood disorder with one or more of the following: delusions, hallucinations, disorganized speech or behavior, and negative characteristics
   2. Clients often have difficulty maintaining a job or functioning in school, experience problems with self-care, are socially isolated, and often experience suicidal ideation

C. **Schizophreniform disorder**: essential features of schizophrenia are present with the exception that duration is at least 1 month but less than 6 months

D. Other psychotic disorders

1. Delusional disorder: presence of nonbizarre delusions (delusions that could possibly occur in reality) that persist for at least 1 month with no other manifestations of psychosis
2. Brief psychotic disorder: presence of at least one positive symptom of schizophrenia with duration between 1 day and 1 month; existence or absence of any stressor should be noted
3. Shared psychotic disorder (*folie a deux*): a delusional system develops in context of a close relationship between two people who share a similar delusion
4. Substance-induced psychotic disorder: presence of hallucinations and delusions are a direct result of physiological effects of a substance
5. Psychotic disorder due to a general medical condition: presence of hallucinations and delusions are a direct result of general medical condition

E. Overview and classification of schizophrenia

1. Schizophrenia is one of a cluster of related psychotic brain disorders of unknown etiology
2. Schizophrenia is a combination of disordered thinking, perceptual disturbances, behavioral abnormalities, affective disruptions, and impaired social competency
3. NCLEX® Symptoms of schizophrenia
   - a. **Delusional ideation**: a false belief occurring without appropriate external stimulation and inconsistent with client's knowledge and experience
   - b. **Hallucinations**: false sensory perceptions that may involve any of five senses (auditory, visual, tactile, olfactory, and gustatory)
   - c. Disorganized speech patterns
   - d. Bizarre behaviors
4. At least two symptoms must be present for a significant portion of time during a 1-month period
5. NCLEX® Generally, client exhibits normal behavior early in life, has subtle changes after puberty, and severe symptoms in late teens to mid-thirties
6. Most clients develop disorder in early twenties (men) or late twenties (women), with only 10% first diagnosed after age 45
7. Etiology of schizophrenia is still uncertain; several types of factors have been identified as being highly correlated or associated with development of schizophrenia:
   - a. Brain structure and functioning: structure, physiology, and neurotransmitters
   - b. Genetic factors: increased risk if first-degree relatives also have disorder
   - c. Psychological factors (stress does not cause but exacerbates disorder)
   - d. Environmental factors: viruses and complications at labor and delivery

F. Critical essential features of each subtype of schizophrenia (see Table 21–6)

G. Data collection

1. Positive symptoms indicate a distortion or excess of normal functioning; they often occur as initial symptoms of schizophrenia and precipitate need for hospitalization
2. Delusions—fixed false beliefs or ideas
   - a. Paranoid type: client believes others are out to get him or her; may be hostile, suspicious, and aggressive
   - b. Grandiose type: client has excessive feelings of importance and power over others
   - c. Religious type: client has delusions that focus on a religious context
   - d. Somatic type: client has delusions fixed on an irrational belief about his or her body

Table 21–6 Essential Features of Subtypes of Schizophrenia

Subtype	Features
Paranoid	Auditory hallucinations, preoccupation with one or more delusions usually of a persecutory nature, may appear hostile or angry
Catatonic	Stupor (state of daze or unconsciousness) or extreme motor agitation, excessive negativism, inappropriate or bizarre body postures, echolalia (an involuntary, parrotlike repetition of words spoken by others) or echopraxia (a meaningless imitation of motions made by others)
Residual	Absence of prominent psychotic symptoms, social withdrawal and inappropriate affect, eccentric behavior, past history of at least one episode of schizophrenia
Disorganized	Disorganized speech or behavior, inappropriate or flat affect
Undifferentiated	Disorganized behaviors, psychotic symptoms (including delusions and hallucinations)

e. Nihilistic: client has delusions of nonexistence
f. Persecutory: client has delusions that others are out to get or are plotting against him or her
g. **Thought broadcasting**: client believes that others can hear his or her thoughts
h. **Thought insertion**: client believes that others have ability to put thoughts in his or her mind against client's will
i. **Thought control**: client believes that others can control his or her thoughts against client's will

3. Hallucinations are usually auditory; visual is second-most common type
4. **Psychosis**: a disorderly mental state in which client has difficulty distinguishing reality from his or her own internal perceptions
5. **Illusions**: inaccurate perception or misinterpretation of sensory impressions
6. Agitation or hostility
7. Bizarre behaviors (catatonic, etc.)
8. Association disturbances
   a. Echolalia or echopraxia
   b. **Clang associations**: rhyming words in a sentence that makes no sense
   c. Illogical thinking patterns
   d. **Neologisms**: inventing new words, which are meaningful only to that person
   e. **Word salad**: combining in a sentence words that have no connection and make no sense
9. Negative symptoms indicate a loss or lack of healthy functioning; they develop over time and hinder client's ability to endure life tasks; include anhedonia (diminished ability to experience pleasure or intimacy), alogia (poverty of speech), anergia (lack of energy), avolition (lack of motivation and goals), ambivalence (inability to make a decision because of conflicting emotions), affect disturbances (blunted, flat, or inappropriate behavior, restricted emotion), ineffective social skills and social withdrawal, dependency, and lack of self-care
10. Lack of ego boundaries
11. Concrete thought processes
12. Sleep disturbance

H. Psychopharmacology (see Chapter 32)

1. Typical antipsychotics (traditional)
2. Atypical antipsychotics
3. Anti-parkinsonian agents (anticholinergics)

I. Individual and group interventions

NCLEX® 1. Management of delusions and hallucinations
   a. Establish a trusting, therapeutic relationship with client by being honest, supportive, and consistent
   b. Encourage expression of feelings and thoughts
   c. Monitor for signs of delusions or hallucinations
   d. Communicate with client using clear, direct statements
   e. Provide an environment with a low degree of stimulation
   f. Express understanding of client's belief about delusion or hallucination but do not share in it; do not argue with client
   g. Provide reality testing and focus on reality
   h. If client has visual hallucinations, provide a room with adequate lighting

2. General nursing considerations and interventions
   a. Provide an environment that is safe for client and others
   NCLEX® b. Avoid any physical contact or touching of client
   NCLEX® c. Encourage client to verbalize feelings and thoughts openly
   d. Utilize therapeutic communication techniques with client
   e. Identify support systems for client
   NCLEX® f. Observe for self-destructive behaviors and provide needed precautions
   g. Provide for ADLs when client is not able to meet those needs
   h. Provide opportunities for client that promote socialization and decrease isolation
   i. Involve client in setting realistic goals in treatment plan
   j. Provide daily living skills groups for client to participate in

J. *Milieu therapy*: a method of psychotherapy that controls client's environment to provide interpersonal contacts in order to develop trust, assurance, and personal autonomy

NCLEX® 1. Provide for client's safety and safety of others in milieu
2. Provide a supportive, structured, and predictable environment

3. Collaborate with multidisciplinary team, client, and family regarding client's plan of care
4. Encourage client to participate in milieu groups and activities that promote socialization
5. Assist client with ADLs as needed, but encourage independence as client progresses

K. Family therapy

1. Involve family to determine use of appropriate community resources
2. Reinforce explanations of chronic nature of schizophrenia, implications, early signs and symptoms of relapse, disease management, medication management, and community support systems available
3. Provide an outlet for family to discuss their feelings and explore alternative effective coping skills

NCLEX® **L. Evaluation of client outcomes**

1. Remains free of harm and demonstrates absence of violence toward others
2. Reports cessation of hallucinations or delusional thought processes
3. Demonstrates increased socialization skills and decreased isolative behavior
4. Demonstrates appropriate affect and improved thought processes
5. Demonstrates improved speech patterns and congruent communication
6. Adheres to medication schedule as prescribed without adverse medication effects
7. Demonstrates effective coping patterns, including use of community resources

M. Evaluation of family outcomes: can identify early signs and symptoms of disease exacerbation, implications of schizophrenia as a chronic illness, medication regimen, and how and when to access emergency services

V. PERSONALITY DISORDERS

A. Overview

1. Personality is composed of enduring patterns or traits that determine how individuals perceive, relate to, and think about environment and themselves; **personality traits** or patterns are reflected in how people cope with feelings and impulses, see themselves and others, respond to their surroundings, and find meaning in relationships
2. **Personality disorders** are diagnosed when personality patterns or traits are inflexible, enduring, pervasive, maladaptive, and cause significant functional impairment or subjective distress
   a. Reflect patterns of inner experience and behavior that differ from cultural expectations
   b. Result in problems in living rather than in clinical symptoms
   c. Clients frequently experience their personality patterns as natural or comfortable (**egosyntonic**) rather than painful or uncomfortable (**egodystonic**)
   d. With egosyntonic personality patterns, clients rarely seek treatment because they tend to externalize cause of any functional impairment or subjective distress
   e. With egodystonic personality patterns, clients are more likely to seek treatment to ease their distress
   f. Are coded under axis II disorders (personality disorders or mental retardation) using American Psychiatric Association's *Diagnostic and Statistical Manual of Mental Disorders, Fourth Edition Text Revision* (*DSM-IV-TR*) diagnostic criteria
   g. Frequently overlap: clients may exhibit patterns or traits associated with more than one personality disorder
   h. Develop before or during adolescence and persist throughout life; symptoms may become less obvious by middle or old age
   i. May coexist with clinical disorders coded as axis I disorders (mood and thought disorders) using *DSM-IV-TR*
   j. Are organized into three diagnostic clusters (see Table 21–7)
3. Manifestations of personality disorders occur in four areas
   a. Behavioral: patterns of day-to-day behavior and impulse control
   b. Affective: range, intensity, lability, and appropriateness of emotional response
   c. Cognitive: how self, others, and events are interpreted
   d. Sociocultural: interpersonal functioning
4. May result from limbic system dysregulation and CNS irritability, decreased levels of serotonin (5-HT), elevated levels of norepinephrine (NE) or abnormal levels of dopamine (DA); genetic factors may play a role
5. Other possible etiologies vary widely and include hostility toward self, trying to live up to perfectionistic standards, underdeveloped superego rules, inadequate parenting and unsatisfied basic needs, anxiety, social oppression, a changing societal value system, inability to manage family conflict, growing up in a multigenerational enmeshed family system and failure to individuate self, a chaotic and abusive environment, and possibly rigid gender-role stereotyping

B. Data collection guidelines

1. Since client probably does not perceive that a problem exists or believes that problem is related to behavior of others, maintain sensitivity during interview process so client does not become guarded or defensive
2. Use professional judgment to protect client rights and maintain confidentiality
3. *NCLEX®* Note client's level of function in areas of affect, cognition, behavior (including impulse control), and sociocultural adaptation (interpersonal relationships)

C. Basic principles of nursing intervention

1. Recognize and accept that clients change or do not change; if patterns of behavior are egosyntonic, clients may lack motivation required to effect change
2. *NCLEX®* Help clients to see how behavior affects their lives to motivate them to develop a more adaptive lifestyle
3. Remember that personality traits are too ingrained to expect radical, long-term behavioral change; interventions should be based on short-term goals and focus on small steps designed to improve role functioning and decrease distress
4. Maintain hope for each client's improvement; all clients have potential for change
5. *NCLEX®* Identify own emotional responses when caring for clients diagnosed with a personality disorder because power struggles between staff members related to best treatment approach create staff divisiveness and a chaotic rather than structured milieu

D. Specific nursing management strategies: cluster-specific nursing interventions can be individualized for each client

1. *NCLEX®* Cluster A personality disorders (paranoid, schizoid, and schizotypal)
   - **a.** Approach client in a gentle, interested, but nonintrusive manner
   - **b.** Respect client's needs for distance and privacy
   - **c.** Be mindful of own nonverbal communication because a client may perceive others as threatening
   - **d.** Gradually encourage interaction with others, if appropriate
2. *NCLEX®* Cluster B personality disorders (antisocial, borderline, histrionic, narcissistic)
   - **a.** Be patient when client displays emotional and erratic behavior
   - **b.** Provide a consistent and structured milieu to avoid manipulation and power struggles
   - **c.** Safety is always first priority of care—protect clients from suicide and self-mutilation until they can protect themselves
   - **d.** Set limits as necessary to help client maintain impulse control to protect client and others from injury
   - **e.** Engage in frequent staff conferences to prevent client's ability to play one staff member against another
   - **f.** Help client recognize and discuss fear of abandonment
   - **g.** Help client recognize presence of dichotomous thinking or splitting, in which self and others are perceived as all good or all bad

Table 21-7 Personality Disorders Organized by *DSM-IV* Diagnostic Criteria Clusters

Cluster	Specific Type of Personality Disorder
Cluster A disorders: characterized by odd or eccentric behavior	*Paranoid:* distrust and suspiciousness in which others' motives are interpreted as malevolent *Schizoid:* detachment from social relationships and a restricted range of emotions *Schizotypal:* acute discomfort in close relationships, cognitive or perceptual distortions, and eccentricities of behavior
Cluster B disorders: characterized by dramatic and erratic behavior	*Antisocial:* disregard for and violation of rights of others *Borderline:* instability in interpersonal relationships, self-image, and affect, and marked impulsivity *Histrionic:* excessive emotionality and attention seeking *Narcissistic:* grandiosity, need for admiration, lack of empathy
Cluster C disorders: characterized by anxious and fearful behavior	*Avoidant:* social inhibition, feelings of inadequacy, and hypersensitivity to negative evaluation *Dependent:* submissive and clinging behavior related to a need to be taken care of *Obsessive-compulsive:* preoccupation with orderliness, control, and perfectionism

h. Encourage direct communication to minimize attention seeking through use of dramatic, seductive behavior
i. Help client who displays a sense of entitlement to acknowledge needs of others

NCLEX®

3. Cluster C personality disorders (avoidant, dependent, and obsessive-compulsive)
    a. Point out avoidance behaviors and related losses and secondary gains
    b. Provide problem-solving and assertiveness training to increase self-confidence and independence
    c. Encourage expression of feelings to decrease rigidity and need for control
    d. Help client recognize any impairment or distress related to need for perfection and control
    e. Help client acknowledge and discuss sense of inadequacy and fear of rejection

E. Psychopharmacology

1. Antipsychotic agents may be prescribed on a short-term basis to alleviate psychotic symptoms associated with schizotypal or borderline personality disorders
2. SSRIs may be prescribed to diminish rapid mood swings and impulsive, aggressive, self-destructive behavior associated with borderline personality disorder
3. SSRIs may be prescribed to treat obsessive rumination associated with certain personality disorders (see Chapter 32)

F. Individual and group therapy

1. A decision for participation in individual or group therapy or both is based on a client's level of function and specific needs
2. Self-help groups may increase clients' self-awareness and assist them in coping with problems in living

G. Behavioral therapy

1. Impulse-control training is designed to support client safety by decreasing risk of suicide or self-mutilation through use of antiharm contracts, staff and client (self) monitoring, identifying triggers and patterns related to self-destructive behavior, and identifying alternative coping strategies

NCLEX®

2. Setting limits discourages tendency to test and manipulate others
    a. Involves establishing a structured environment with clear ground rules
    b. Setting limits reflects three principles: limits must be clearly stated, necessary, and enforceable
3. Behavioral modification: social skills for clients who are helpless and dependent; goal is to increase coping skills and independent functioning
    a. Assist clients to acknowledge feelings of helplessness and fear of becoming more independent
    b. Explore clients' dichotomous thinking or tendency to see themselves as totally dependent or totally independent
    c. Help clients identify what they would gain and lose by becoming less helpless
    d. Engage clients in problem-solving exercises to increase their self-confidence
    e. Provide assertiveness training
    f. Take care not to be seen as a rescuer
4. Behavioral modification: social skills for clients who are socially isolative related to a fear of rejection; goal is to increase self-confidence
    a. Help clients acknowledge their fear of criticism and rejection
    b. Help clients identify what they would gain and lose by risking criticism and rejection
    c. Help clients identify interpersonal effects of social isolation and feelings associated with it
    d. Engage clients in problem-solving exercises to increase their self-confidence
    e. Provide assertiveness training
5. For clients who are socially isolated related to suspicion and mistrust of others, respect their need to be isolative while gradually encouraging interaction with others; if appropriate, help clients identify interpersonal effects of social isolation and feelings associated with them
6. For clients who seek out relationships with others through behavior that is attention seeking (dramatic, seductive) but superficial, help them to interact in a more direct fashion; help clients identify what they would gain and lose by communicating more directly
7. For clients whose relationships are based on manipulation, focus on their attempts at manipulation and help them to identify ways to interact in a more collaborative and less power-based manner; help clients identify what they would gain and lose by becoming less manipulative

H. Psychological comfort promotion—anxiety reduction

1. Encourage decision making to support a sense of competence and an internal locus of control; point out that an imperfect decision may be better than no decision and that many decisions can be remade
2. Some clients become perfectionistic to guard against anxiety of feeling inferior; explore their fear
3. Anxiety prevents some clients from asking for help because they fear rejection; help clients identify what they would gain and lose by asking for help

I. Evaluation and client outcomes

1. Be aware that realistic goals must reflect small steps to improve function and decrease subjective distress
2. Note effectiveness of nursing interventions in relation to stated outcomes

VI. DISSOCIATIVE DISORDERS

A. Overview

1. Usually consciousness, memory, identity, and perception are integrated functions
2. In dissociative disorders, there is a sudden disruption in client's consciousness, identity, or memory
3. Defense mechanisms of dissociation and repression are used
   a. May experience considerable anxiety caused by expressed or fantasized forbidden wishes, often of sexual or aggressive nature
   b. May have considerable anxiety related to stressors or traumatic events
   c. Person does not consciously "decide" to dissociate
4. Physiological origins of "trance states" or dissociation
   a. Childhood trauma resulting in neurotransmitter and anatomical changes in brain
   b. Genetic predisposition to dissociate is hypothesized
5. Possible etiologies include traumatic experience (commonly accidents, natural disasters, assault) or severe physical, sexual, or emotional abuse; more easily induced if using psychoactive drugs (hallucinogens or cannabis)

B. Specific dissociative disorders

1. **Dissociative amnesia**: client cannot remember important personal information, and memory loss cannot be accounted for by ordinary forgetfulness
   a. Client suddenly cannot recall memories: *localized amnesia* is loss of memory of a short time period (hours) after a disturbing event; *selective amnesia* is loss of memory of some, but not all, events; *generalized amnesia* is loss of memory of a whole lifetime of experiences (very rare); *continuous amnesia* is inability to remember successive events as they occur
   b. Client with amnesia can recall other information, learn, and function coherently
   c. Most common during wars and natural disasters
   d. **Primary gain**: symbolic resolution of unconscious conflict that decreases anxiety and keeps conflict from awareness
   e. **Secondary gain**: receipt of extra support and caring when experiencing an illness
   f. Usually terminates abruptly
   g. Special interventions: survivor support groups; gradual reconstruction of events through talking, listening, and reading others' accounts of the trauma
2. **Dissociative fugue**: client suddenly leaves his or her usual place with no memory of some or all of past
   a. Travels from usual environment
   b. Unable to recall important aspects of identity and assumes new identity; old and new identities do not alternate; incomplete new identity; does not know information is forgotten
   c. Usually lasts from hours to days, rarely months; considerable confusion when client returns to prefugue state
   d. Often is a response to psychological stressors (war, family, marital)
   e. Client has no memory of events during fugue after returning to prefugue state
   f. Special interventions: hypnosis, drug-facilitated interviews, support groups
3. **Dissociative identity disorder (DID)**: presence of two or more distinct personalities or identities (alters) in one person
   a. An alter is a personality state or identity that recurrently takes over behavior of a person with DID; alters are personalities with different influences and power over one another; may represent different ages or genders
   b. Each alter has relatively enduring pattern of perceiving, relating to, and thinking about self and environment
   c. Alters each have different physiological responses and disorders (one alter may be myopic, while another is not)
   d. Alters communicate with one another through "executive" alter
   e. Some alters share "co-consciousness," aware of each other's experience and behavior; others are aware only of their own existence
   f. "Switching" occurs by dissociating from one alter to another
   g. **Host personality**: primary identity that holds person's name; is typically unaware of alters (anxiety-provoking aspects of personality), but alters are typically aware of host personality

h. Client "loses time" when alternate personality is present for a period of time: usually client is unable to give full account of childhood (few memories) because of dissociation; may appear forgetful and is often accused of lying
i. Mental status variations: marked variation in appearance from time to time; blinking, eye rolls, headaches, covering or hiding face, and twitches may occur when "switching" from one alter to another; marked variation in speech in brief periods of time; impaired insight, may appear anxious or depressed
j. Can be associated with severe physical or sexual abuse during childhood and may be accompanied by many posttrauma symptoms (nightmares, flashbacks, hypervigilance), self-mutilation, suicidal or aggressive behavior

NCLEX®

k. Special interventions: institute no-harm contract and environmental safety if client is suicidal or is self-mutilating; meet and recognize alters and their unique experiences and needs; "map" personality system, noting characteristics of alters and co-consciousness; create emotionally safe environment for all alters; individual therapy with therapist skilled in working through trauma leading to integration (moving together of aspects of all identities); development of new coping skills; family therapy with partners and children; hypnosis or drug-facilitated interviews (use is controversial because of possibility of remembering "too much, too soon" and being overwhelmed with anxiety)

4. Depersonalization disorder
   a. **Depersonalization**: feeling of detachment or separation from one's self, as if in a dreamlike state
   b. Client describes self as "detached from my body" or "being in a dream"; feels strange or unreal but is able to function during experience
   c. Client may report distress about experiences and become depressed and anxious; often fears being "crazy"; feelings may be accompanied by **derealization**, a feeling that external world is unreal or strange
   d. Precipitated by stress and anxiety
   e. Most common in teenagers and young adults

NCLEX®

   f. Special interventions: problem solving to reduce stress in general; stress-management techniques; "grounding" or focus on external environment

C. Data collection and observation

1. Recounts trauma and/or severe stress
   a. Client acknowledges history of childhood abuse but often does not recall trauma
   b. Symptoms appear in adulthood after stressful event(s)
   c. Symptoms appear immediately or may be delayed for years
2. Extent of symptoms of dissociation or amnesia varies widely with different dissociative disorders
   a. **Dissociation** is a defense mechanism in which experiences are blocked from consciousness so that affect, behavior, identity, memories, and/or thoughts are not integrated
   b. **Repression** is a defense mechanism in which thoughts and feelings are kept from consciousness
3. May report symptoms of depression or anxiety
4. Physical symptoms: headaches common with DID, but other dissociative disorders have no associated physical symptoms

NCLEX®

5. Mental status examination
   a. Appearance: facial expressions and mannerisms may vary widely within one session or appearance may vary widely from day to day (DID)
   b. Mood: anxious, depressed; some clients have little mood change
   c. Memory: amnesia for events (variable extent)
   d. Perception: feelings of detachment from self or environment, feeling of physical change in body
   e. Insight: impaired, unaware of memory impairment

NCLEX®

D. Nursing intervention strategies

1. Create safe, calm environment; prevent stressors that could elicit dissociation; mutually develop plan of care
2. Teach stress management and coping techniques
   a. Progressive muscle relaxation
   b. Physical exercise
   c. "Grounding," or focus on external environment (what client can see and hear) rather than on internal feelings, thoughts, or sensations that can lead to "spacing out" (a lay term indicating lack of awareness of immediate environment)
   d. Problem-solving strategies
   e. Distraction

3. Discuss and explore traumatic event
4. Reconstruct memories through client's account and those of others
5. Reinforce education to client, family, and significant others about specific dissociative disorder and relationship between anxiety and dissociation
6. Help staff and other clients to understand disorder (especially DID)
7. Plan for use of leisure time (anxiety often increases when alone without activities)

E. Psychopharmacology

1. Drug-facilitated interviews using thiopental sodium (Pentothal) to recover memory
2. Anti-anxiety agents
3. Antidepressants for depression and antipsychotics for extreme agitation (if those symptoms are present)

F. Individual and group therapy

1. Hypnosis therapy to recover memories
2. Focus on emotional responses to trauma or stressors
3. Work through unacceptable impulses or behavior verbally
4. Refer to support groups, such as parenting or occupational support groups, or "survivor" groups, particularly for natural disasters or abuse

G. Behavior modification

1. Reinforce cognitive techniques to promote positive self-statements
2. Reinforce stress management and coping strategies rather than dissociation

H. Evaluation and client outcomes

1. Client explains relationship between trauma, stress, anxiety, and dissociation, and can recall stressors and traumatic events with congruency
2. Client employs stress-management and positive coping behaviors, and actively seeks to solve problems
3. Client assumes or resumes social and occupational roles and uses leisure time constructively

VII. SOMATOFORM DISORDERS

A. Overview

1. **Somatoform disorders** are psychophysiological responses with amplified awareness of somatic stimuli caused by impaired CNS inhibitory function
2. Deficient communication between hemispheres of brain may impair ability to express emotions directly
3. Disorder is a defense against anxiety
   a. A person expresses conflict and resultant anxiety through physical symptoms because being physically ill is socially acceptable, and client receives help and nurturance and has dependency needs met
   b. Conflict does not have to be acknowledged
   c. May consciously seek relief from physical symptoms or may unconsciously not want to give up symptoms because they decrease anxiety
4. Family dynamics
   a. Family rules may prevent direct expression of conflict
   b. Family may view physical illness as an acceptable way to avoid meeting otherwise required developmental tasks and role demands
   c. Family may provide secondary gain
   d. Symptoms may serve to control others or to stabilize relationships
5. *NCLEX®* Physical symptoms have no *organic basis*; that is, objective diagnostic tests usually do not reveal structural or functional changes
6. Somatoform disorders, in which there is no organic basis for physical symptoms, may or may not begin after a physical illness or injury
7. Culture influences physical expressions
   a. In some cultures, distress may be manifested in bodily symptoms, with psychological distress viewed as unacceptable
   b. Somatization is defined as a disorder primarily in Western societies
   c. Many culture-bound illnesses have little influence on role performance
8. Somatization disorders, characterized by multiple complaints of multiple body systems, are more prevalent in women than in men

B. Specific disorders

1. Somatization disorder
   a. Onset prior to age 30 with symptoms of several years duration
   b. Multiple physical complaints; must include four pain symptoms, two GI symptoms, sexual symptoms, and symptoms suggesting neurological disorders

c. New symptoms often arise with increased emotional distress
d. Lifestyle changes are evoked by physical illness, affecting occupational, family, and community relationships and self-care, and resulting in disability and inability to work, thereby leading to financial struggles
e. Client seeks treatment for physical symptoms, occasionally for psychosocial complaints
f. Special interventions: long-term medical management; treat physical symptoms conservatively, "matter-of-fact" approach; antidepressants if depressive symptoms present but no drug therapy for anxiety symptoms

2. **Conversion disorder**
a. A somatoform disorder in which a motor, sensory, or visceral function is lost and about which client is usually indifferent
b. Symptoms do not have an underlying organic cause
c. Motor symptoms: mutism, paralysis, tremors
d. Sensory symptoms: blindness, deafness, numbness
e. Visceral symptoms: urinary retention, breathing difficulties, headaches
f. Medically naïve clients have more implausible symptoms, which correspond to client's ideas of the problem but do not follow neurological pathways
g. Clear, identifiable psychological factors (stress, conflict) are related to onset or exacerbation of symptoms
h. Client's mood may be inappropriate for symptoms, and he or she may display little concern for symptoms (*la belle indifference*)
i. Symptoms are often symbolically related to primary gain, such as glove anesthesia that prevents a student about to take comprehensive examination from being able to write or bilateral paralysis of lower extremities of man about to get married, preventing him from "walking down the aisle"
NCLEX® j. Special interventions: nurse must treat symptom as "real" because client experiences it; use problem-solving approaches for dealing with conflicts and stressors

3. Pain disorder
a. A somatoform disorder characterized by pain as dominant physical symptom
b. Client seeks medical attention for severe, prolonged pain with no organic basis for pain
c. Preoccupation with pain that is not controlled by analgesics
d. Manifestations vary: low back pain, headache, chronic pelvic pain
e. Historical relationship between stress, conflict, and initiation or exacerbation of pain; often follows physical trauma or injury; client usually refuses to consider psychological origin; diagnosis difficult because of personal and cultural differences in definition and expression of pain
f. Commonly accompanied by depression, hopelessness, helplessness, anger, or irritability
NCLEX® g. Special interventions: teach client about stress-tension-pain cycle; acupuncture, biofeedback training, transcutaneous electrical nerve stimulation (TENS); specific exercise programs, physical therapy; visualization and relaxation training; pain management techniques (note: analgesics and anti-anxiety agents may be ineffective for pain, and addiction is possible)

4. **Hypochondriasis**
a. A disorder in which a physical symptom is interpreted as severe or life threatening, resulting in exaggerated worry and preoccupation with symptom
b. Physical symptoms may begin with sensitivity to vague physical sensations or mild physical symptoms that most people would not notice
c. History of multiple visits to multiple practitioners, and concern persists despite negative findings and clinician reassurances
d. Accompanied by significant anxiety
NCLEX® e. Special interventions: teach rational interpretation of body sensations; assist resolution of family conflict about medical treatment and client distress; nonpharmacological treatment of anxiety

5. **Body dysmorphic disorder**
a. A somatoform disorder characterized by preoccupation with or excessive concern about an imagined or minor defect in appearance
b. Causes significant distress or impairment in role function
c. Varies from flaws of face or head (complexion, hair thinning, asymmetry) to abdomen, extremities, or body shape/size
d. Client embarrassed about defects so may express them vaguely ("ugly," for example)
e. May frequently check defects, avoid reminders (removing mirrors), seek reassurances from others, or attempt to improve defect (exercise, surgery, cosmetics)
f. Often leads to social isolation

g. Disorder is persistent; client has repeated surgeries, dental work, or dermatological treatment for defects
h. Emotional distress may be severe enough to lead to depression and suicidal ideation
NCLEX® i. Special interventions: respect preoccupation; avoid challenging validity of client perceptions; focus on coping techniques; contract with client to increase social activities and relationships

C. Data collection

1. Onset is variable, depending upon disorder
2. Client has seen multiple care providers without relief of symptoms
3. Client sees problem as "physical" and denies psychological influences on symptoms
4. Primary gain: illness allows reprieval from responsibilities
5. Secondary gain: sick role allows for dependency needs to be met
6. Over time, client is increasingly socially isolated and physically inactive
7. Family may insist on client seeking assistance due to altered role performance
8. Mental status variations
   a. Depends upon type of disorder
   b. Appearance: ranges from deeply anguished to indifferent; may assume antalgic position
   c. Mood: depressed, anxious, or unaffected, or labile
   d. Thought: usually preoccupied with symptoms
   e. Insight: highly impaired, usually denying any stressors or minimizing reactions to stressful events; not "psychologically minded"
9. Physical symptoms
   a. Monitor physical symptoms respectfully, thoroughly, and objectively
   b. Common organ system responses: see Table 21–8 for specific symptoms
   c. Thorough health assessment including laboratory studies is necessary to rule out physical illness with organic basis or other mental disorders

D. Specific nursing intervention strategies

NCLEX® 1. Establish trusting, therapeutic relationship
   a. Avoid describing physical symptoms as "in client's head"
   b. Note that symptoms are not an attempt to get attention
   c. Recall that client does not create symptoms consciously or purposefully
   d. Accept reality of symptoms as client presents them, avoiding dispute

NCLEX® 2. Client education
   a. Explain symptoms on a physiological level, using simple and acceptable language
   b. Present current knowledge of mind–body interaction, emphasizing how stress and anxiety affect physiological functioning
   c. Reinforce methods to reduce physiological arousal, including relaxation techniques, visual imagery, self-talk strategies, and physical exercise (see Box 21–2)
3. Encourage verbalization of thoughts and feelings, life events, and stressors
4. Assist in problem solving specific conflicts or situations
5. Self-care strategies
   a. Modify exercise/activity plan to fit client's physical status
   b. Promote sleep and rest
   c. Promote healthy nutritional practices
   d. Reinforce day-to-day client management of symptoms
6. Encourage client to gradually resume expected work, family, and community roles commensurate with physical capabilities

Table 21–8 Specific Symptoms in Somatoform Disorders

Organ System	Specific Symptom
Cardiovascular	Fainting, hypertension, migraine headache, tachycardia
Musculoskeletal	Back pain, fatigue, tension headache, tremor
Respiratory	Bronchospasm, dyspnea, hyperventilation
Integumentary	Pruritis
Genitourinary	Difficulties in micturation, menstrual disturbances, sexual dysfunction

E. Psychopharmacology

1. No specific psychotropic medications for somatoform disorders
2. Some evidence for use of antidepressants with pain and somatization disorders
3. Comorbid anxiety or depression treated symptomatically with anxiolytics and antidepressants
4. Medication for physical symptoms
   a. Give medications according to presentation of physical symptoms
   b. Encourage client to express thoughts and feelings at time of discomfort
   c. Reinforce teaching about medication use, emphasizing provider–client collaboration to reduce self-adjustment of dosages

F. Individual and group treatment

1. Cognitive-behavioral approaches
   a. Identify self-statements and assumptions about stress, anxiety, and sick role
   b. Challenge irrational beliefs and self-statements regarding seriousness of illness, inability to cope, and/or mind–body relationships
   c. Provide accurate data to counter misinformation
   d. Encourage positive, self-coping statements
2. Groups for clients and families
   a. Discuss mind–body relationships
   b. Provide forum for discussion and encourage client to talk out problems as a deterrent to physical symptoms
   c. Correct misinformation about origin of somatoform disorders
   d. Provide support for families and/or clients as roles shift during recovery
3. Supportive approaches
   a. Convey empathy: "This must be very trying for you"
   b. Convey respect: "I am impressed by how you have been able to do as much as you have, given how you feel"
   c. Explore with client ways to decrease isolation, improve role performance, and enhance self-esteem
   d. Focus on verbally expressing feelings and coping techniques rather than symptoms
   e. Keep discussion of symptoms brief and matter-of-fact, but without dismissal
4. Behavior modification
   a. In addition to cognitive behavioral approaches, engage client in self-modification to reward for engagement in treatment plan
   b. Assist family members to reinforce verbalization of stressors and life difficulties rather than symptoms

G. Evaluation and client outcomes

1. Identifies interaction of mind and body and effects of stress
2. Increases ability to verbalize thoughts and feelings, and conflicts and/or problems in situations and relationships
3. Employs self-help strategies: challenges irrational thoughts; corrects own misinformation; uses positive coping statements; engages in physical activity on regular basis; employs relaxation techniques or visual imagery; demonstrates sound nutritional practices, and resumes appropriate roles

Box 21-2

Tips for Teaching Relaxation Training

- Emphasize the relationship between stress and physiological arousal/symptoms.
- Note that relaxation techniques work by focusing attention to relaxation task, thus interrupting the preoccupation with symptoms, and decreasing physiological arousal, which negates physical symptoms of anxiety.
- To promote a sense of control, remind the client that he or she (not the technique) effects the change.
- Promote a daily return to physiological and psychological baseline to calm the mind and body through relaxation techniques, thus keeping general arousal low.
- Note that daily practice rather than episodic use builds skill level.
- Suggest additional techniques for use when client anticipates a stressful situation or finds himself or herself becoming anxious.
- Explain and teach a variety of techniques so that client can choose a technique that is acceptable and can be used in specific client environments.

VIII. COGNITIVE IMPAIRMENT DISORDERS

A. Overview

1. **Delirium**: an acute, abrupt-onset confusional state characterized by disorientation, disturbed perception, vivid dreams, frightening hallucinations, agitated behavior, inability to sleep at night with daytime napping, and emotional disturbances
   NCLEX® a. Develops over a short period of time (usually hours to days) and tends to fluctuate during course of day
   b. Evidence from history, physical examination, or laboratory findings suggests that disturbance is caused by direct physiological consequences of a general medical condition, substance intoxication, substance withdrawal, or multiple etiologies
2. **Dementia**: a chronic, irreversible brain disorder characterized by impairments in memory, cognition (abstract thinking, judgment, insight, affect and spatial orientation) as well as personality changes
   a. **Aphasia**: inability to understand or use language
   b. **Apraxia**: inability to carry out skilled and purposeful movement; inability to use objects properly
   c. **Agnosia**: inability to recognize familiar situations, people, or stimuli; not related to impairment in sensory organs
   d. Disturbance in executive functioning (i.e., planning, organizing, sequencing, abstracting)
   NCLEX® e. Course is insidious and progressive, characterized by gradual onset and continuing cognitive decline
   f. Cognitive deficits cause significant impairment in social or occupational functioning and represent a significant decline from previous level of functioning
   g. Can be classified as Alzheimer's type (DAT), vascular dementia (formerly multi-infarct dementia), dementia due to other general medical conditions, substance-induced persisting dementia, or multiple etiologies
3. Amnestic disorder
   a. Development of memory impairment characterized by inability to learn new information or inability to recall previously learned information
   b. Can be transient (lasts 1 month or less) or chronic (lasts more than 1 month); can result from a general medical condition, substance abuse, or other cause
   c. Causes significant impairment in social or occupational functioning and represents a significant decline from a previous level of functioning
4. Other cognitive disorders: mild neurocognitive disorder or postconcussional disorder

B. Etiologies

1. Regardless of specific cause, delirium, dementia, and other cognitive disorders result from an interference with cerebral blood flow and delivery of nutrients (e.g., oxygen, glucose, vitamins)
2. Associated medical conditions leading to reduced cerebral blood flow include cardiovascular and respiratory conditions, vitamin deficiencies, infections, endocrine and metabolic disorders, hepatic and renal failure, and trauma or tumors
3. Substances causing toxicity to the brain either by exposure to, high doses of, or withdrawal from substance can lead to cognitive disorders; these include a variety of prescribed medications and illegal drugs
4. Genetic or viral diseases can cause pathological changes or biochemical imbalances in the brain that interfere with cerebral blood flow (dementia of Alzheimer's type, Parkinson's disease, Huntington's disease, Pick's disease, Creutzfeldt-Jakob disease)

C. Data collection

1. Delirium has a sudden onset and an identifiable cause
   a. A thorough medical evaluation reveals abnormal lab results
   b. An electroencephalogram (EEG) confirms cerebral dysfunction
   c. More than one examination at different times of day detects fluctuations in level of consciousness
   d. Identify underlying cause and rule out other reasons for delirium (depression, anxiety, dementia, or personality disorder)
2. *NCLEX®* Presenting signs and symptoms of delirium
   a. Cyclic alternating periods of coherence with periods of confusion, specifically with disorientation that worsens at end of day, usually referred to as **sundown syndrome**
   b. Alternating patterns of hyperactivity (typical of drug withdrawal) to hypoactivity (typical of metabolic imbalance)
   c. Hyperactive behaviors: rambling, bizarre, incoherent, rapid, pressured, or loud speech; restlessness, picking at clothes or bed linen, irritability, euphoria; calling out for help, striking out at others, bizarre and destructive behavior, combativeness, anger, profanity

d. Hypoactive behaviors: limited, dull patterns of speech; lethargy, apathy, withdrawn behavior; reduced alertness or awareness of environment
e. Cognitive changes: disorganized thinking; diminished ability to focus attention, easily distracted; disorientation to time and place; impairment in recent and remote memory; visual or auditory hallucinations, frightening delusions
f. Sleep pattern disturbances, including vivid and terrifying dreams or nightmares
g. Predominant emotion is fear with a high level of anxiety

3. Dementia is a progressive disease and symptoms can be divided into three stages (Box 21–3)

D. Screening tools

1. Folstein Mini-Mental State Examination: an organic screening tool useful for differentiating dementia from functional states
   a. Total score of 30 points
   b. Score of 9–12 indicates a high likelihood of organic illness
2. Cognitive Performance Scale: a subscale from nursing home Minimum Data Set (MDS)
   a. Ranges from 0 (cognitively intact) to 6 (very severe cognitive impairment)

Box 21–3

Stages of Alzheimer's Disease

Stage 1 (2–4 Years)

- Decline in short-term memory leads to client losing things, and difficulty with completing complex tasks such as selecting appropriate clothing and dressing.
- Decreases in cognitive function are seen as decreased ability to make accurate judgments or plan effectively, poor driving skills, reduced concentration (with increased distractibility), and decline in verbal skills and time orientation (memory of people still intact).
- Client experiences gaps in memory, which leads to confabulation (filling in memory gaps with imaginary information) in an attempt to hide the deficit.
- Client compensates by using memory aids such as developing routines and using lists.
- Client is concerned and aware of problem; may be frightened by confusion.
- Client may become depressed, which worsens symptoms and may experience anxiety, frustration, helplessness, and shame.

Stage 2 (Several Years)

- Disorientation occurs in three spheres of person, place, and time.
- Progressive recent and remote memory loss are characteristic.
- Client exhibits lack of spontaneity in verbal and nonverbal communication, which declines over time to aphasia.
- Client exhibits poor impulse control with frequent outbursts and tantrums, labile emotions, catastrophic reactions, or overreactions to minor stresses.
- Client loses ability to carry out ADLs in a typical order: bathing, grooming, choosing clothes, dressing, toileting.
- Client loses ability to carry out instrumental ADLs such as cooking, housekeeping, transportation, legal affairs, and money management.
- Client may exhibit wandering behavior.
- Misidentification syndrome occurs (familiar people are seen as unfamiliar, and strangers are seen as people known to client).

Stage 3 (1–2 Years)

- Hyperorality, the need to taste, chew, and examine any object small enough to be placed in the mouth.
- Hyperetamorphosis, the need to compulsively touch and examine every object in the environment.
- Progressive motor deterioration, including inability to walk, sit up, or even smile.
- Progressive decrease in response to environmental stimuli leading to total nonresponsiveness or vegetative state.
- Severe decline in cognitive function, losing ability to recognize others or even self.

b. Items assessed on MDS include comatose status, short-term memory, decision-making ability, making self understood, eating self-performance

3. Geriatric Depression Screening Scale (GDSS)
   a. Useful screening tool specifically developed for older adults to screen for possible depression (which can mimic dementia)
   b. A 15- or 30-item questionnaire with dichotomous yes or no answers; easy to administer in approximately 15 to 20 minutes; certain items are reverse-scored for more accurate assessment
   c. Results indicate absence of or mild depression (0 to 10), moderate depression (11 to 20), or severe depression (21 to 30) using the 30-item questionnaire

E. Differentiating between delirium and dementia

1. Delirium may coexist with dementia, making accurate assessment and appropriate treatment difficult; Table 21–9 compares delirium and dementia
2. Most prevalent primary dementia is Alzheimer's type, (occurs in 50% of older adults); vascular dementia resulting from narrowing of arteries affects 20–50% of older adults; less common forms of dementia stem from degenerative nervous system disorders (e.g., Parkinson's disease) and other pathological processes (e.g., AIDS dementia complex)

F. *Pseudodementia*: reversible disorder that frequently mimics dementia

1. Depression (most common pseudodementia) is frequently misdiagnosed or overlooked in older adult; Table 21–10 compares dementia and depression
2. Other causes include drug toxicity, metabolic disorders, infections, nutritional deficiencies, and chronic lung or heart disease

G. *Pseudodelirium*: symptoms of delirium without any identifiable organic cause

1. Symptoms may occur from psychosocial stress, sensory deprivation, or sensory overload (e.g., ICU psychosis)
2. A preexisting biochemical imbalance such as mood disorder, anxiety, schizophrenia, or dementia can make persons vulnerable to pseudodelirium

H. Specific treatment modalities

NCLEX® 1. Psychopharmacology
   a. Cholinesterase inhibitors such as tacrine (Cognex) or donepezil (Aricept) can slow rate of decline in mild to moderate dementia
   b. NMDA receptor antagonist memantine (Nemanda) improves abnormal glutamate activity that may contribute to Alzheimer's disease
   c. Anti-anxiety agents: lorazepam (Ativan), trazodone (Desyrel), buspirone (Buspar)
   d. SSRIs, which are better tolerated than TCAs in older adults; include fluoxetine (Prozac), paroxetine (Paxil), sertraline (Zoloft), nefazodone (Serzone)
   e. Atypical antipsychotic agents such as olanzapine (Zyprexa), quetiapine (Seroquel), and risperidone (Risperdal); use of haloperidol (Haldol), a potent neuroleptic, is controversial and has caused tardive dyskinesia in older adults; small doses (0.5 mg) may help to regulate sleep

NCLEX® 2. Behavior modification
   a. Use physical restraints carefully and as a last resort; use sensor devices for client safety that alert staff when a client is out of bed or going outside
   b. Use reality orientation (large-print calendars and clocks); discuss client's significant life events, family, work, or hobbies; avoid arguing about actual reality; communicate in a calm, quiet voice with simple, clear instructions

3. Group and individual therapies
   a. "Review of life" therapy: discuss specific life transitions such as childhood, adolescence, marriage, childbearing, grandparenthood, and retirement; pets, music, and special foods can be used to evoke memories from client's past; share positive and negative feelings
   b. Validation therapy: interact with clients on a topic they initiate, in a place and time where they feel most secure; reflect underlying feelings of concern (e.g., "You miss your husband. You must be feeling lonely here"); reality orientation is geared to person and place rather than to time

4. Milieu therapy (see Box 21–4)
   a. Special care units (SCU): environmentally designed and specifically programmed to serve needs of residents with Alzheimer's disease and related dementias
   NCLEX® b. Design components of SCU: safe, secure, specially adapted physical environment to accommodate wandering behavior inside and outside (circular design, secure walkway and patio); personalized rooms with own furniture and familiar belongings; clean, well-maintained, well-lit environment with windows; stimuli from birdcage, fish aquarium, or other pets; location adjacent to child daycare programs so that multigenerational interaction occurs

Table 21-9 Comparisons between Delirium and Dementia

Delirium	Dementia
Onset is usually sudden (acute)	Onset is insidious and progressive (chronic)
Temporary, reversible disturbance in brain function	Irreversible alteration of brain function
Duration: hours to days	Duration: months to years
EEG: diffuse slowing of fast cycles related to state of excitement	EEG: normal or mildly slow
Disturbed attention, learning, and thinking, poor perception	Disorientation, impairments in judgment, abstract thinking, and learning
Impaired memory, both recent and remote	Impaired memory (recent affected before remote)
Orientation: fluctuates throughout day; periods of lucidity; sundown syndrome (worsens at night)	Progressively loses orientation to time, then place, then person; sundown syndrome
Hallucinations, delusions, illusions	Change in personality; normal peculiarities are exaggerated: suspicious—paranoid, compulsive—rigid, orderliness
Labile affect	Labile affect; prone to apathy, depression, withdrawal, stubbornness in attempt to cope with surroundings and decreased abilities

Table 21-10 Comparisons between Dementia and Depression

Dementia	Depression
Onset slow and progressive, difficult to pinpoint onset	Onset relatively rapid, can be traced to distressing event or situation
Recent memory is impaired; attempts to hide cognitive losses with confabulation	Readily admits to memory loss; other cognitive impairments possible; recalls recent events
Affect is shallow and labile	Depressed mood is pervasive
Attention and concentration may be impaired	Attention and concentration usually intact
Unable to recognize familiar people and places, may get lost easily, disoriented to time	Oriented to person, place, and time
Approximate "near miss" answers are common; tries to answer	"Don't know" answers are common; refuses to participate in activities; prefers to be left alone
Changes in personality (from cheerful and easygoing to angry to suspicious)	Personality remains stable
Struggles to perform ADLs; is frustrated as a result	Apathetic to ADLs, loses interest in appearance
Appetite and sleep patterns may not be affected	Changes in appetite, weight, and sleep pattern

c. Structured programs and activities that provide quality interaction between staff, residents, and families
d. Caring staff: special training programs leading to certification for all levels of education (RN, LPN, CNA); consistent staffing pattern with stable personnel assignments

I. Evaluation and client outcomes

1. Client remains free of injury (no falls, fractures, bruises, contusions, burns)
2. Client participates in self-care with appropriate supervision and guidance
3. Client communicates basic needs using visual and verbal clues as necessary, and has minimal level of response to frustrating situations
4. Client sleeps 5 to 7 hours per night and naps 1 to 2 hours per day, and maintains stable vital signs and weight
5. Caregivers demonstrate adaptive coping strategies for caregiver role stress

IX. EATING DISORDERS

A. Overview of eating disorders

1. Eating disorders are manifested by gross disturbance in a client's eating patterns
2. People with anorexia lose weight by dramatically decreasing food intake and sharply increasing amount of physical exercise

3. People with bulimia nervosa remain at near-normal weight and develop a cycle of minimal food intake, followed by binge-eating, and then purging
4. These disorders have many features in common, and a person can alternate between disorders

B. Anorexia nervosa

1. Overview
   a. Life-threatening health problem because of fluid and electrolyte imbalance or starvation
   b. Client is preoccupied with food intake, fears obesity, and has a disturbed body image and self-concept
   c. Client eats minimal amounts of food, often in a rigid and regimented manner, such as eating only 3 bites of carrots or 2 mouthfuls of cereal; denies hunger
   d. Onset is often in teens and frequently associated with a major stressful life event
   e. Client is often an overachiever, seeks perfection, and experiences feelings of lack of control

NCLEX®

2. Data collection findings
   a. Weight loss
   b. Electrolyte imbalances
   c. Vital signs: decreased body temperature, pulse, and blood pressure; cyanosis of extremities
   d. Gastrointestinal (GI): constipation, tooth and gum degeneration
   e. Skin: dry, scaly
   f. Neuromuscular/skeletal: numbness of extremities, bone deterioration
   g. Amenorrhea for at least 3 cycles
   h. Reports of sleep disturbances

C. Bulimia nervosa

1. Overview
   a. Client is preoccupied with food intake and body size, appearance
   b. Associated with low self-esteem and poor relationships with others
   c. Client engages in cycles of eating large amounts of low-nutrient food (binges), which may be done in secret, followed by purging through vomiting, laxatives, enemas, diuretics, or amphetamines
   d. Client experiences conflict between perceived loss of control and need for control, as well as guilt from binge–purge cycles; may exhibit mood swings
   e. Client is at risk for self-mutilating behavior and may have suicidal ideation or suicide attempts

NCLEX®

2. Data collection findings
   a. Weight is often normal or near-normal
   b. Electrolyte imbalances
   c. Cardiovascular: cardiac disease, hypertension
   d. GI: tooth decay with loss of enamel (from vomiting), stomach ulcers, rectal bleeding, esophageal varices (vomiting), and possible rectal bleeding

Box 21–4

Nursing Interventions for Clients with Cognitive Impairment

Incorporate the following interventions into the care of confused clients:

- Provide simple, clear instructions focusing on one task at a time.
- Break tasks into very small steps.
- Speak slowly and face-to-face when communicating with clients who have hearing loss; shouting causes distortion of high-pitched sounds and can frighten the client.
- Allow the client to have familiar objects to maintain reality orientation and enhance self-worth and dignity.
- Discuss topics that are meaningful to the client, such as significant life events, family, work, hobbies, and pets.
- Refrain from arguing or convincing client that delusions are not real.
- Provide a simple, structured environment with consistent personnel to minimize confusion and provide a sense of security and stability in the client's environment.
- Encourage reminiscence and discussion of life review by sharing picture albums.
- Discuss family traditions and holidays, memories of school, courtship, dating rituals, favorite pets, and other past events.
- Encourage family/caregivers to express feelings, particularly frustration and anger.
- Provide a list of community resources and support groups available to assist in decreasing stress and role strain for the family/caregiver.

NCLEX®

D. Specific nursing intervention strategies

1. Clients with anorexia nervosa are typically treated in an eating disorders unit
2. Develop therapeutic, nonjudgmental relationship with client to foster sharing of precipitating factors to eating disorder and feelings about it
3. Support client during behavior modification, psychotherapy, support groups; encourage client to take any prescribed medications, such as antidepressants
4. Perform baseline and periodic assessments of nutritional status, including fluid and electrolyte balance and daily intake of food
5. With severe malnutrition, refeeding protocols and tube feedings may be used
6. Form a contract with client regarding daily intake of food
7. Set a time limit for meals
8. Provide a pleasant environment for meals and observe client at meal times and following meals
9. Provide positive feedback for appropriate eating behaviors and goal attainment; token economy rewards system may be used
10. Record intake and output and daily weight (postvoid, same clothing, same time, same scale)
11. Monitor elimination patterns
12. Monitor and limit activity level (anorexia and bulimia)
13. Assess risk of suicide and implement suicide precautions as necessary

E. Evaluation and client outcomes

1. Client has normal or near normal nutritional status, gaining weight at rate of 1 to 2 pounds per week (anorexia nervosa), using newly learned eating behaviors regularly
2. Client is free of fluid and electrolyte imbalance and other complications of eating disorder
3. Client identifies and utilizes available support programs or services

Check Your NCLEX–PN® Exam I.Q. *You are ready for testing on this content if you can*

- Explain alteration in mood, judgment, and cognition in clients with a mental health problem.
- List signs and symptoms of specific mental health problems.
- Discuss the client's and family's reaction to diagnosis of an acute or chronic mental health problem.
- Help a client to adhere to the treatment plan for a mental health problem.
- Describe changes in a client's mental status and impaired cognition.
- Assist in planning care for a client with an acute or chronic mental health problem.
- Provide client and family with information about an acute or chronic mental health problem.
- Provide appropriate nursing care to a client undergoing electroconvulsive therapy.

PRACTICE TEST

1 A nurse has been told that a client's anxiety is at the panic level. The nurse would observe the client for which manifestations expected at this level of anxiety?

1. Dizziness, palpitations, and nausea
2. Feelings of "butterflies" in the stomach
3. Feelings of fatigue and inability to remain awake
4. Obsessive thoughts and compulsive behavior

2 A nurse asks a client, "Have you ever felt a sudden, intense fear for no apparent reason?" When the client responds "yes," the nurse monitors the client for other symptoms compatible with which problem?

1. Agoraphobia
2. Obsessive-compulsive disorder
3. Panic disorder
4. Posttraumatic stress disorder

3 A client has just been told that a second operation must be performed to correct a physical health problem. The client begins to cry and says, "I just can't take it anymore. Everything has gone wrong. I can't even think straight anymore." The nurse interprets that the client is in which stage of anxiety?

1. Alarm
2. Exhaustion
3. Fight-or-flight
4. Resistance

4 A counselor working with an extremely anxious client reports feeling short of breath, tense, restless, apprehensive, and nervous. The nurse would most appropriately draw which conclusion?

1. The client's anxious feelings have been transmitted to the counselor.
2. The client is probably becoming angry with the counselor.
3. The client should be reassigned to a different counselor.
4. The counselor probably is new to the position.

5 The nurse concludes that which living environment would be safest for a client who inflicted harm on a family member earlier in the day? Select all that apply.

1. In a local respite home
2. In a locked unit
3. In an open-door seclusion room
4. In a closed-door seclusion room
5. With a family member in another state

6 The nurse is working with a client diagnosed with bipolar disorder in the out-patient clinic following discharge 2 weeks ago from an inpatient unit. The nurse observes the client for which behaviors that are expected at this time?

1. Euphoric and talkative presentation with nurse
2. Gregarious interactions with significant others
3. Quiet and evasive presentation
4. Calm, focused exchange of self-care information with nurse

7 A client with schizophrenia is exhibiting delusions, hallucinations, minimal self-care, and hyperactive behavior. Which of these observations would the nurse document as a negative symptom of schizophrenia?

1. Minimal self-care
2. Delusions
3. Hallucinations
4. Inappropriate affect

8 A client living in an assisted living facility is taking conventional antipsychotic medications. One evening the nurse notices that the client is experiencing muscle rigidity, confusion, delirium, and has a temperature of 104° F. The nurse recognizes these as symptoms of which adverse drug effect?

1. Dystonia
2. Akathisia
3. Neuroleptic malignant syndrome
4. Tardive dyskinesia

9 A client states that he is able to receive radio waves from aliens because they placed a computer chip in his brain. The nurse would document this behavior as which of the following in the medical record?

1. A hallucination
2. Reality oriented
3. An illusion
4. A delusion

10 A client reports depersonalization experiences that have been frightening to him. Which response by the nurse would be therapeutic? Select all that apply.

1. "It must be very scary for you to have these experiences."
2. "Don't worry; you will always come back together."
3. "Being in the hospital must be very frightening."
4. "Let's focus on the stressors in your life."
5. "Can you tell me more about how these experiences occur?"

11 A client with amnesia is hospitalized. What might the nurse expect to find during the initial data collection?

1. Confabulation of historical information
2. Gradual loss of memory over months
3. Disheveled appearance
4. History of severe stress

12 The nurse would look for which characteristics in the behavior of a client diagnosed with obsessive-compulsive disorder (OCD)? Select all that apply.

1. Dramatic
2. Eccentric
3. Anxious
4. Ritualistic
5. Erratic

PRACTICE TEST

13 The nurse looks for which characteristic that is expected in a client diagnosed with a personality disorder?

1. Flexibility and adaptability to stress
2. A tendency to evoke some form of interpersonal conflict
3. A concurrent physical disorder
4. A desire for interpersonal relationships

14 The nurse monitoring a client with obsessive-compulsive personality disorder (OCD) anticipates that most of the client's cognitive content will be centered around which of the following?

1. The importance of rules and regulations
2. Global approaches to problem solving
3. Relationships with others
4. Preferred leisure activities

15 A female client with hypochondriasis discloses she may leave the psychiatric facility without completing her treatment and seek exploratory surgery. What is the nurse's *best* response to the client?

1. "If you decide to leave now, you will be committed against your will."
2. "You should not go until your doctor releases you. She knows what you need."
3. "Tell me more about your decision."
4. "Your surgery will probably prove useless. Please stay."

16 Which of the following approaches would be best for the nurse who is communicating with the cognitively impaired client? Select all that apply.

1. Loud
2. Concise
3. Clear
4. Non-verbal
5. Unhurried

17 A client with suspected Alzheimer's disease is undergoing diagnostic workup. When the family asks the nurse the reasons for the "tests," the nurse responds that the diagnosis of Alzheimer's disease is usually based on which of the following?

1. Laboratory test findings
2. A definitive CT scan
3. Physiological findings
4. Ruling out other causes for symptoms

18 Which intervention would the nurse perform to support optimal memory function for a client with dementia?

1. Develop stimulating and meaningful therapeutic activities.
2. Remind the client of forgotten events.
3. Orient the client to reality.
4. Restrain the client when agitated.

19 The nurse would conclude that a client with schizophrenia is exhibiting positive symptoms of the disorder after noting that the client does which of the following? Select all that apply.

1. Exhibits lack of energy
2. States he is a king
3. Repeats words the nurse says
4. Has a flat affect
5. Withdraws from other people

20 When the nurse informs an adolescent client that a scheduled parental visit will not occur, the client throws a cup at the nurse. In order to best respond to this behavior, the nurse should conclude that the client is displaying which defense mechanism?

1. Reaction formation
2. Displacement
3. Projection
4. Denial

21 The parents of a 10-year-old take the child to the mental health clinic. The nurse establishes rapport and credibility with the child by asking the child about which of the following?

1. Behavioral symptoms
2. Hobbies and interests
3. Relationships with friends and family members
4. Medical problems in the past

22 When collecting data for depression from an adolescent client, what is most important for the nurse to recognize regarding depression in adolescents?

1. Adolescent depression is similar in presentation to depression in adult clients.
2. Adolescent depression is masked by aggressive behaviors.
3. Adolescent depression is situational and not as serious as depression in adults.
4. Adolescent depression is an indication of family dysfunction.

23 The client diagnosed with bipolar I disorder is in an inpatient locked unit. The client begins to yell loudly at another client who is also sitting in the dayroom. In order to provide a safe environment for both clients, the nurse should take which action?

1. Turn on the television in the dayroom to distract the client.
2. Redirect the client in a calm, firm, nondefensive manner.
3. Call the physician for a prn medication order for the client who is escalating.
4. Escort the client to the seclusion room.

24 The client is being discharged after a suicide attempt. Discharge plans include medications and participation in a day treatment program, as well as returning to live with family members. When the family members tell the nurse that they are concerned about the client's safety, what is the most appropriate response by the nurse?

1. Listen to the family members and ask them how the nurse can make them feel less concerned.
2. Reassure the family that the day hospital program will provide the client with emergency telephone numbers.
3. Allow the family members to voice concerns and teach them the indications of possible relapse.
4. Recommend developing a planned schedule so that a family member is always with the client.

25 The nurse is preparing to take a client to the electroconvulsive therapy (ECT) treatment suite. The nurse must ensure that which pretreatment process is completed before the treatment can be administered?

1. The client's spouse has signed the consent form.
2. The client is wearing snug-fitting clothing.
3. The client is NPO.
4. The client has been given a light meal before the procedure.

26 The nurse observes that a client is pacing in the hallway, talking rapidly, and gesturing dramatically. The nurse concludes that the client is beginning to demonstrate what kind of behavior?

1. Psychomotor retardation
2. Anxiety
3. Psychomotor agitation
4. Depression

27 A client in an inpatient unit is awake at 1 a.m. and tells the nurse, "I can't sleep because of the light in the hall and the noise from the kitchen. I need to have another sleeping pill." What is the most appropriate nursing intervention?

1. Administer a prn sedative.
2. Move the client to a quieter room.
3. Close the door to the client's room.
4. Allow the client to watch television for 1 hour.

28 The client is being admitted to the inpatient psychiatric unit with a diagnosis of major depression. During data collection, the nurse anticipates that the client will report which symptoms? Select all that apply.

1. Suicidal thoughts or plans of suicide over at least the past 2 weeks
2. History of one depressive episode within the past 2 years
3. Loss of appetite for approximately 3 days
4. Loss of interest in previously enjoyed activities
5. Presence of hallucinations for at least 3 days

29 Which question would be most appropriate for the nurse to ask when monitoring a client for signs of generalized anxiety disorder?

1. "Are you more anxious at home or in a crowd?"
2. "Do you experience sudden, intense fear for no reason?"
3. "Do you find yourself worrying frequently about a number of different things?"
4. "Have you ever had a 'flashback' or a nightmare about a traumatic event?"

ANSWERS & RATIONALES

1 **Answer: 1** **Rationale:** Subjective complaints of panic level of anxiety include choking or smothering sensation, dizziness, chest pain or pressure, and fear of loss of control and death. Feelings of stomach "butterflies" are seen in the fight-or-flight response. Feelings of fatigue and inability to remain awake may be seen in the exhaustion stage of the general adaptation syndrome. Obsessive thoughts and compulsive behaviors are common in obsessive-compulsive disorder. **Cognitive Level:** Applying **Client Need:** Psychosocial Integrity **Integrated Process:** Nursing Process: Data Collection **Content Area:** Mental Health **Strategy:** The core issue of the question is an ability to identify signs of panic in a client with anxiety. Use nursing knowledge and the process of elimination to make a selection.

2 **Answer: 3** **Rationale:** The onset of a panic attack is sudden, and the client may not be aware of the source of the anxiety. The nurse should collect data for other associated symptoms of panic disorder that would occur at the onset of the fear. Agoraphobia is fear of being incapacitated by being trapped in an unbearable situation from which there is no escape. Obsessive-compulsive disorder is characterized by obsessive thoughts and compulsive behaviors. Posttraumatic stress disorder is associated with exposure to an extremely traumatic, menacing event. **Cognitive Level:** Applying **Client Need:** Psychosocial Integrity **Integrated Process:** Nursing Process: Data Collection **Content Area:** Mental Health **Strategy:** The core issue of the question is an ability to identify signs of panic disorder. Use nursing knowledge and the process of elimination to make a selection.

3 **Answer: 2** **Rationale:** Because coping resources are depleted, the client can no longer deal with stressors and is in the stage of exhaustion. The stage of alarm is characterized by the fight-or-flight response, and increased alertness is focused on the immediate task or threat. The stage of resistance occurs when the body mobilizes resources to combat stress. **Cognitive Level:** Applying **Client Need:** Psychosocial Integrity **Integrated Process:** Nursing Process: Data Collection **Content Area:** Mental Health **Strategy:** The core issue of the question is an ability to differentiate stages of anxiety based on client presentation. Use nursing knowledge and the process of elimination to make a selection.

4 **Answer: 1** **Rationale:** Anxiety in a client may be empathetically experienced by the counselor. It is imperative that these symptoms be recognized. There is not enough data to support the client being angry. Reassigning the client may not be therapeutic. Even those with work experience may develop anxiety empathetically. **Cognitive Level:** Analyzing **Client Need:** Psychosocial Integrity **Integrated Process:** Nursing Process: Data Collection **Content Area:** Mental Health **Strategy:** The core issue of the question is the ability to determine the effect that an anxious client can have on health care workers. Use nursing knowledge and the process of elimination to make a selection.

5 **Answer: 2, 4** **Rationale:** Admission to a locked unit would be a safe option for this client. The client would be safe in a closed-door seclusion room. The client would not have the necessary continuous monitored care if he were in a respite home. In an open-door seclusion room, the client could leave the area and harm others if there were distractions to the staff on the unit. The client would have less safety or care in the home of a relative in another state than is needed at this time. **Cognitive Level:** Analyzing **Client Need:** Psychosocial Integrity **Integrated Process:** Nursing Process: Planning **Content Area:** Mental Health **Strategy:** The core issue of the question is placement of a client who has harmed another. Use nursing knowledge and the process of elimination to make a selection. Keep in mind that the safety of the client and others around him or her is the first priority.

6 **Answer: 4** **Rationale:** A client who demonstrates a calm, focused exchange of information and self-care information would demonstrate control of the disorder, which is expected following discharge from an inpatient setting. A client in a manic state would present with euphoric, talkative, and gregarious behaviors, while a client with depression would be more likely to have a quiet and evasive presentation. **Cognitive Level:** Applying **Client Need:** Psychosocial Integrity **Integrated Process:** Nursing Process: Data Collection **Content Area:** Mental Health **Strategy:** The core issue of the question is appropriate behavior exhibited by a client with bipolar disorder after treatment. Use nursing knowledge and the process of elimination to make a selection.

7 **Answer: 1** **Rationale:** Minimal self-care is a behavioral negative symptom of schizophrenia. A delusion is a cognitive positive symptom; a hallucination is a perceptual positive symptom; and an inappropriate affect is an affective positive symptom. **Cognitive Level:** Applying **Client Need:** Psychosocial Integrity **Integrated Process:** Communication and Documentation **Content Area:** Mental Health **Strategy:** The core issue of the question is an ability to discriminate between positive and negative signs of schizophrenia. Use nursing knowledge and the process of elimination to make a selection.

8 **Answer: 3** **Rationale:** Neuroleptic malignant syndrome is a potentially fatal extrapyramidal symptom characterized by muscle rigidity, respiratory problems, and hyperpyrexia. Dystonia is an extrapyramidal symptom characterized by involuntary movements and prolonged muscle contraction, resulting in twisting body motions, possible tremors, and abnormal posture. Akathisia is an extrapyramidal symptom characterized by restlessness and an inability to sit still. Tardive dyskinesia symptoms include frowning, blinking, grimacing, puckering, blowing, smacking, licking, chewing, tongue protrusion, and spastic facial distortions, which can be socially disfiguring. **Cognitive Level:** Analyzing **Client Need:** Psychosocial Integrity **Integrated Process:** Nursing Process: Data Collection **Content Area:** Mental Health **Strategy:** The core issue of the question is an ability to identify signs of adverse medication effects in a client being treated for psychosis. Use nursing knowledge and the process of elimination to make a selection.

9 **Answer: 4** **Rationale:** A delusion is a false belief that cannot be changed by logical reasoning or evidence. A hallucination is the occurrence of a sight, sound, touch, smell, or taste without any external stimulus to the corresponding sensory organ; however, it is real to the client. The client is not exhibiting reality orientation. An illusion is a sensory misperception of environmental stimuli. **Cognitive Level:** Applying **Client Need:** Psychosocial Integrity **Integrated Process:** Communication and Documentation **Content Area:** Mental Health **Strategy:** The core issue of the question is an ability to correctly identify the types of thought patterns expressed in a client's communications. Use nursing knowledge and the process of elimination to make a selection.

10 **Answer: 1, 5** **Rationale:** The two correct responses demonstrate empathy or encourage the client to elaborate further about his experience. Telling the client not to worry dismisses the affective component of the client's communication. Focusing on being in the hospital misses the point of the client's communication because it is the depersonalization that is frightening to the client. Focusing on stressors is ultimately helpful, but is not timely in response to the client's current concern. **Cognitive Level:** Applying **Client Need:** Psychosocial Integrity **Integrated Process:** Communication and Documentation **Content Area:** Mental Health **Strategy:** The core issue of the question is selection of therapeutic responses to a client who is experiencing depersonalizing events. Use nursing knowledge of therapeutic communication skills and use the process of elimination, noting that more than one option is likely to be correct.

11 **Answer: 4** **Rationale:** Amnesia is precipitated by stress related to trauma or conflict. The amnesia occurs abruptly and there is no attempt to cover the memory loss. Confabulation to fill in memory gaps, gradual loss of memory, and disheveled appearance are common in clients experiencing dementia. **Cognitive Level:** Analyzing **Client Need:** Psychosocial Integrity **Integrated Process:** Nursing Process: Data Collection **Content Area:** Mental Health **Strategy:** The core issue of the question is knowledge of expected findings in a client with amnesia. Use nursing knowledge and the process of elimination to make a selection.

12 **Answer: 3, 4** **Rationale:** A client with OCD, a Cluster C personality disorder, experiences anxiety and uses ritualistic compulsive behaviors to reduce this anxiety. Individuals with a Cluster A personality disorder appear odd or eccentric. Clients with a Cluster B personality disorder appear dramatic or erratic. **Cognitive Level:** Applying **Client Need:** Psychosocial Integrity **Integrated Process:** Nursing Process: Data Collection **Content Area:** Mental Health **Strategy:** The core issue of the question is knowledge of expected behaviors that would be exhibited by a client with OCD. Recall that a client with this type of diagnosis is anxious and uses ritualistic behaviors to cope with anxiety. Note that the wording of the question indicates more than one option is likely to be correct.

13 **Answer: 2** **Rationale:** Individuals diagnosed with personality disorders display either functional impairment or subjective distress. Frequently these problems in living are reflected in impaired interpersonal relationships. Flexibility and adaptability to stress are incongruent with a diagnosis of a personality disorder. The presence of a physical disorder has no relation to the diagnosis of a personality disorder. Individuals diagnosed with personality disorders may or may not desire interpersonal relationships. **Cognitive Level:** Applying **Client Need:** Psychosocial Integrity **Integrated Process:** Nursing Process: Data Collection **Content Area:** Mental Health **Strategy:** The core issue of the question is knowledge of expected assessment findings regarding behavior style in a client with a personality disorder. Note that the type of disorder is not specified, so the answer is a global or general pattern. Use nursing knowledge and the process of elimination to make a selection.

14 **Answer: 1** **Rationale:** Individuals diagnosed with obsessive-compulsive personality disorder become overly involved in details such as rules and regulations related to a need to be perfect. As a result, they fail to see the "big picture." Their relationships with others and participation in leisure activities are less important than their devotion to work and productivity. **Cognitive Level:** Applying **Client Need:** Psychosocial Integrity **Integrated Process:** Nursing Process: Data Collection **Content Area:** Mental Health **Strategy:** The core issue of the question is knowledge of expected behavior styles in a client with OCD. Use nursing knowledge and the process of elimination to make a selection.

15 **Answer: 3** **Rationale:** The best response is nonjudgmental and affirms the client's personal power in the decision-making process. It also would help the client understand connections in her own decision-making process. The best responses would not threaten, judge, or disempower the client. **Cognitive Level:** Applying **Client Need:** Psychosocial Integrity **Integrated Process:** Caring **Content Area:** Mental Health **Strategy:** The core issue of the question is a therapeutic communication to a client with hypochondriasis. Use nursing knowledge of therapeutic communication skills and the process of elimination to make a selection.

16 **Answer: 2, 3, 5** **Rationale:** Verbal communication should be clear, concise, and unhurried. Loud communication (or shouting) may be interpreted as anger; therefore, a pleasant, calm, supportive tone of voice should be used. The use of mostly non-verbal gestures would be frustrating to the client who may not understand what is being said. **Cognitive Level:** Applying **Client Need:** Psychosocial Integrity **Integrated Process:** Caring **Content Area:** Mental Health **Strategy:** The core issue of the question is a therapeutic communication to a client with a cognitive impairment. Use nursing knowledge of therapeutic communication skills and the process of elimination to make a selection.

17 **Answer: 4** **Rationale:** Alzheimer's disease is diagnosed by ruling out causes for the client's symptoms. Reviewing laboratory findings, CT scan results, and noting physiological findings all assist in ruling out other causes of the client's symptoms. **Cognitive Level:** Analyzing **Client Need:** Psychosocial Integrity **Integrated Process:** Nursing Process: Data Collection **Content Area:** Mental Health **Strategy:** The core issue of the question is methods of diagnosis for Alzheimer's disease. Use nursing knowledge and the process of elimination to make a selection.

18 **Answer: 1** **Rationale:** Cognitive function is supported by participation in meaningful activities that the client enjoys. Stimulating activities also promote self-esteem and encourage the client to attain the highest level of cognitive function possible. Reminding the client of forgotten events may be helpful momentarily but could also lead to frustration. Reorienting the client to reality will not support sustained memory function and while it might be helpful momentarily, it could also lead to frustration. Restraining a client who is agitated could increase agitation rather than decrease it. **Cognitive Level:** Applying **Client Need:** Psychosocial Integrity **Integrated Process:** Nursing Process: Implementation **Content Area:** Mental Health **Strategy:** The core issue of the question is planning for a client with dementia that supports remaining memory function. Use nursing knowledge and the process of elimination to make a selection.

19 **Answer: 2, 3** **Rationale:** Positive symptoms of schizophrenia are those behaviors that a client would not usually exhibit in everyday life, including echolalia or a delusion of being a king. Negative symptoms of schizophrenia are those that reflect the absence of what is normally seen in a person's behavior. These would include energy, flat affect, and social

withdrawal. **Cognitive Level:** Applying **Client Need:** Psychosocial Integrity **Integrated Process:** Nursing Process: Data Collection **Content Area:** Mental Health **Strategy:** The core issue of the question is the ability to discriminate between positive and negative symptoms of schizophrenia. Use nursing knowledge of these manifestations and the process of elimination to make a selection.

20 **Answer: 2 Rationale:** Displacement is the transfer of emotional reactions from one object or person to another object or person. Like other defense mechanisms of the ego, displacement is an unconsciously determined behavior that attempts to reduce anxiety. The client is exhibiting displacement behavior. Reaction formation is a mechanism that causes a person to act exactly opposite to the way he or she feels. Projection is a process in which blame is attached to others or the environment. Denial is an attempt to screen or ignore unacceptable realities by refusing to acknowledge them. **Cognitive Level:** Applying **Client Need:** Psychosocial Integrity **Integrated Process:** Nursing Process: Data Collection **Content Area:** Mental Health **Strategy:** Recall definitions of defense mechanisms of the ego and reasons why they are employed.

21 **Answer: 2 Rationale:** Children at age 10 are egocentric and concerned with themselves; discussing hobbies and interests will be helpful in establishing rapport and credibility with the client. Focusing on behavioral symptoms could lead to an adversarial relationship. Children often are uncomfortable talking about friends and family until they get to know a person better; pursuit of this topic will block the establishment of rapport and credibility for the nurse. Most children are unconcerned about past medical problems; they are focused on the "here and now." **Cognitive Level:** Applying **Client Need:** Psychosocial Integrity **Integrated Process:** Communication and Documentation **Content Area:** Mental Health **Strategy:** Think of 10-year-olds you know. How do they respond to adults? Use this knowledge to select the correct answer.

22 **Answer: 2 Rationale:** Depression in adolescents is often masked by aggressive and/or behavioral problems, including intense mood swings, academic difficulties, asocial behavior, and hypersomnia. While the *DSM-IV-TR* criteria for depression are the same for adults, children, and adolescents, the clinical presentation may be different in the different age groups. Depression in adolescents can have the same consequences as in adults and should be treated seriously. Family dysfunction may or may not be present when the adolescent client is depressed. As with adults who are depressed, there is evidence that depression in adolescence is highly associated with psychobiologic changes, especially in neuroendocrine functioning. **Cognitive Level:** Applying **Client Need:** Psychosocial Integrity **Integrated Process:** Nursing Process: Data Collection **Content Area:** Mental Health **Strategy:** Consider normal or expected adolescent behavior. Ask yourself what relationship exists between this developmental level and the way in which the adolescent experiences depression.

23 **Answer: 2 Rationale:** Redirecting the client in a calm, firm, nondefensive manner is the most appropriate action to begin de-escalation. This client will be distractible but irritable, so it is important that the nurse's approach is one of quiet, matter-of-fact calmness. Turning on the television is not an appropriate approach because it is not likely to distract the client. If the client with bipolar disorder is in a locked unit, prn orders should already be in place. At this time, the client's behavior requires the nurse's personal attention and intervention, not medication. If medication is given before other less restrictive interventions are used, this is a legal issue, since medication is a form of chemical restraint. The client's behavior is not sufficiently out of control to warrant the use of seclusion. In addition, the nurse should be aware that before seclusion can be legally justified; all other less restrictive techniques should be attempted. **Cognitive Level:** Analyzing **Client Need:** Safety and Infection Control **Integrated Process:** Nursing Process: Implementation **Content Area:** Mental Health **Strategy:** Recall that persons with elevated mood are distractible, as well as irritable and hostile. This will help to choose an option that shows elements of being calm yet firm.

24 **Answer: 3 Rationale:** The family members need the nurse to listen and support them. Reinforcing signs and symptoms of relapse will help the family members decrease their anxiety, knowing they have a clear role in the recovery and ongoing care of the client without being totally responsible for the client. The family members need to express their concerns, not be asked to identify what will make them feel better. This option does not address the family members' concerns and attempts to give them false reassurance. Having a family member always with the client is an unreasonable recommendation that would place undue pressure on the family. The family and the client should be assisted to formulate safety plans that will allow all to carry out usual responsibilities. **Cognitive Level:** Analyzing **Client Need:** Psychosocial Integrity **Integrated Process:** Nursing Process: Implementation **Content Area:** Mental Health **Strategy:** Recognize that both survivors of suicidal attempts and their family members should be provided assistance and support. Remember also that once a person has made a suicide attempt, they are statistically at increased risk for suicide at all points in the future.

25 **Answer: 3 Rationale:** The client should be NPO before the procedure in order to be given anesthesia for the procedure. The client, not the spouse, should sign the consent form. The client should be wearing loose-fitting clothing that would not restrict movements of breathing. The client should be NPO before the procedure, not being given a light lunch, in order to be given anesthesia. **Cognitive Level:** Applying **Client Need:** Reduction of Risk Potential **Integrated Process:** Nursing Process: Planning **Content Area:** Mental Health **Strategy:** Recall the similarity between the pre-surgical and pre-ECT procedures.

26 **Answer: 3 Rationale:** Psychomotor agitation is recognized when a person's behavior involves increased physical activity, restlessness, and/or aggression. The behavioral manifestations will be accompanied by strong affects, such as anxiety and speeding of physiologic processes. When psychomotor agitation is present, the client and others are at risk for injury. Psychomotor retardation is a term that refers to slowing of physical activities and bodily processes. It is the opposite of what is described in this situation. Anxiety is a feeling, not a behavior. The behavior of the client may indeed be related to anxiety, but there are other possible reasons for the behavior. Depression is a mood state, not a behavior. The behavior of the client indeed may be related to depressed mood, but there are other possible reasons for the behavior. **Cognitive Level:** Applying **Client Need:** Psychosocial Integrity **Integrated Process:** Nursing Process: Data Collection **Content Area:** Mental Health **Strategy:** The critical word in the question is *behavior*. Select an option that reflects a behavior rather than an emotion.

27 **Answer: 3 Rationale:** Because the client has indicated that environmental noise and activity are preventing sleep, the nurse should first attempt to minimize environmental stimuli. Simply closing the client's door is a non-invasive,

nonstimulating strategy that may work, as long as it does not pose a safety hazard for the client. Before administering a prn sedative, the nurse should attempt other nonpharmacological options. It is not necessary to move the client if another less extreme alternative is available. Turning on the television will increase the amount of noise in the environment and could further stimulate the client and/or others. **Cognitive Level:** Analyzing **Client Need:** Safety and Infection Control **Integrated Process:** Nursing Process: Implementation **Content Area:** Mental Health **Strategy:** Pay attention to the client's words. They define the exact nature of the problem.

28 **Answer: 1, 4** **Rationale:** The nurse should understand that in order for a client to be diagnosed with major depression, *DSM-IV-TR* specifies that symptoms consistent with at least 5 of 9 criteria must have been present for at least 2 weeks. Suicidal ideations and plans are included in one criterion. The nurse should understand that in order for a client to be diagnosed with major depression, *DSM-IV-TR* specifies that symptoms consistent with at least 5 of 9 criteria must have been present for at least 2 weeks. One criterion for major depression involves markedly diminished interest or pleasure in all, or almost all, activities. Major depressive symptoms represent a more recent change in functioning, not a single episode within 2 years. While persons with major depression often have changes in weight and appetite, the relevant *DSM-IV-TR* criterion for major depression does not involve a 3-day period. It also allows for either increases or decreases in appetite to have occurred. Hallucinations may occur in psychotic levels of major depression, but they are not part of the diagnostic criteria in *DSM-IV-TR*. **Cognitive Level:** Analyzing **Client Need:** Psychosocial Integrity **Integrated Process:** Nursing Process: Data Collection **Content Area:** Mental Health **Strategy:** Compare and contrast usual presenting symptoms and *DSM-IV-TR* criteria for dysthymia and major depression.

29 **Answer: 3** **Rationale:** Generalized anxiety disorder is characterized by chronic, unrealistic, and excessive anxiety concerning a number of different stressors. Agoraphobia involves anxiety and fear of places or situations, such as crowds. Panic attacks are characterized by sudden anxiety that may not be identifiable. Posttraumatic stress disorder is characterized by "flashbacks" and/or nightmares about a traumatic event. **Cognitive Level:** Applying **Client Need:** Psychosocial Integrity **Integrated Process:** Nursing Process: Data Collection **Content Area:** Mental Health **Strategy:** Recall the basic definition of generalized anxiety disorder. Look for a response that fits with that definition.

Key Terms to Review

References

American Psychiatric Association. (2000). *Diagnostic and statistical manual of mental disorders* (revised 4th ed.). Washington, DC: Author.

Fontaine, K. (2009). *Mental health nursing* (6th ed.). Upper Saddle River, NJ: Pearson Education.

Kniesl, C.,Wilson, H., & Trigoboff, E. (2009). *Contemporary psychiatric-mental health nursing* (2nd ed.). Upper Saddle River, NJ: Pearson Education.

Stuart, G. (2009). *Principles and practice of psychiatric nursing* (9th ed.). St. Louis: Elsevier Science.

Townsend, M. (2010). *Essentials of psychiatric mental health nursing: Concepts of care in evidence-based practice* (5th ed.). Philadelphia: F.A. Davis.

Varcarolis, E. & Halter, M. (2010). *Foundations of psychiatric mental health nursing: A clinical approach* (6th ed.). Philadelphia: Saunders.

Test Yourself

Are you ready for the NCLEX-PN® or course exams? Use the practice tests on the companion website to check.

22 Dependency and Addiction

In this chapter

Cross Reference

Other chapters relevant to this content area are

Coping with Stressors	Chapter 20
Mental Health Disorders	Chapter 21
Psychiatric Medications	Chapter 32

I. OVERVIEW OF DEPENDENCY AND ADDICTION

A. Commonly used terms

NCLEX® 1. **Substance abuse**: purposeful but maladaptive substance use pattern evidenced by recurring and significant adverse consequences to self or others of repeated use

2. **Substance dependence**: drug use is no longer under control and continues despite adverse effects; client develops tolerance and experiences withdrawal symptoms if use stops

NCLEX® 3. Treatment focus is **abstinence** (voluntarily going without drugs), medications as appropriate, education, lifestyle change, and increasing self-awareness and personal growth

B. Types and various diagnoses of addiction

1. Substance abuse disorder and **process addiction** syndrome are characterized by preoccupation with and compulsion to engage in an activity
   - a. Substances: depressants (opiate, opioids, sedatives, hypnotics), stimulants (cocaine, amphetamines), cannabinoids and hallucinogens, inhalants
   - b. Processes: eating disorders, compulsive gambling or shopping/spending, compulsive sexual disorders, compulsive Internet use or use of video games
2. Definitions associated with substance use disorders
   - NCLEX® a. *Diagnostic and Statistical Manual of Mental Disorders, Fourth Edition Text Revision* (*DSM-IV-TR*) clinical syndromes: intoxication, withdrawal, abuse, dependence
   - b. Substance dependence: a maladaptive pattern of substance use leading to clinically significant impairment or distress; characterized by compulsive use, unsuccessful attempts to decrease amount and frequency of use, continued use despite adverse effects, **tolerance** (needing increased amounts of substance to achieve desired effect), and **withdrawal** (uncomfortable and maladaptive physiological, cognitive, and behavior changes associated with lowered levels of substance in blood or tissues)
   - NCLEX® c. Addiction: an illness characterized by compulsion, loss of control, and continued pattern of abuse despite perceived negative consequences; obsession with a dysfunctional habit; dysfunctional patterns include patterns of alcoholism, drug abuse, misuse of tobacco, eating disorders, excessive gambling or spending, and certain compulsive sexual disorders (American Nurses Association and National Nurses Society on Addictions)

II. ETIOLOGY

NCLEX® **A. Addiction is a chronic brain disease evidenced by abnormalities in neuronal activities of brain reward system (BRS)**

B. Process of BRS activation

1. All drugs affect cells in some way (increasing or decreasing some cellular activities)
2. Use of CNS-altering substances or engaging in addictive behaviors increases availability of dopamine, serotonin, and opioid peptides, and facilitates dysregulation of other neurotransmitters (gamma-aminobutyric acid, glutamate, acetylcholine)
3. Short-term euphoric response is generated by this activity, which eventually leads to symptoms of addictive thinking, denial, and impaired control
4. NCLEX® Euphoric response engenders immediate and profound desire for readministration (**cravings** that are like psychological "hunger," triggers, and urges)
5. Positive, immediate short-term euphoria overshadows any long-term consequences associated with engaging in addictive behaviors
6. Continued use leads to development of tolerance, which leads to increased dose and frequency of use
7. Physical and psychological dependence and withdrawal syndrome may develop

C. Genetic/biologic risk

1. No one specific marker is responsible for addictions—the more risk factors, the greater the risk for developing disease
2. NCLEX® Genetics: clients who have biological relatives with substance problems are at increased risk; drug use negatively affects egg and sperm health
3. Biology: changes in limbic area of brain occur with substance abuse; genes may affect function of different biochemical systems

D. Psychosocial risk

1. Personality traits: client with certain personality traits may be susceptible to reinforcing effects of engaging in addictive behaviors
   a. Dominant and critical with underlying self-doubts; personal insecurity with low self-esteem and self-criticism
   b. Problems with sexual identification, difficulty with intimacy
   c. Rebellious toward authority, escapist or sensation-seeking tendencies, marked narcissistic tendencies, difficulty with impulse control, lack of a strong and efficient superego
2. Developmental failures: clients who have lived with painful experiences are at risk to self-medicate or misuse medication
   a. Abuse survivors—may experience disturbances in sense of self
   b. Lack of nurturance in childhood—may lead to an inability to self-soothe
   c. Coping skills deficit; sufficient positive coping skills not learned in person's family of origin; learning positive coping skills was inhibited because of positive reinforcing euphoric effect of addictive drug or behavior to cope with feelings

E. Dual disorders risk

1. Some clients with a psychiatric disorder also have addiction
   a. Client with psychiatric disorder is at risk for addictive disorders
   b. NCLEX® Initially drugs and alcohol may be used to compensate for lack of coping skills if client experiences depressive symptoms, anxiety, or recurrence of painful memories; with continued use, addiction develops for client at risk
2. Client with addiction may have or is at risk for developing a psychiatric disorder
   a. Substance use can induce development of psychiatric illness by affecting nucleus accumbens and ventral tegmental area (cognition, motivation, and learning) and neurotransmitter system (mood regulation)
   b. Any one of a number of psychiatric disorders can develop
3. Clients with addictive disorders may be misdiagnosed because some disorders, such as anxiety disorders, depression, and chronic pain, mask addiction

Memory Aid

When a client has a problem with substance abuse or addiction, carefully collect data about other mental health disorders as well, which may be comorbidities.

4. NCLEX® Clients with dual diagnoses and who are intoxicated are at increased risk of suicide
5. Treatment for dual diagnoses is more successful if both are treated concurrently

F. Environmental risk

1. Social learning theory: use of addictive substances is a learned behavior
   a. Normalized behavior: engaging in addictive behavior is influenced by exposure to peer pressure, role models, societal norms
   b. Culture: engaging in addictive behaviors is influenced by culture; alcohol is widely used in Western culture; marijuana use is more prominent in Muslim countries because alcohol is forbidden; opium is widely used in China and other Eastern countries; native herbs and chemicals are more widely used in India and Africa; Native Americans tend to use alcohol and peyote (a cactus button with hallucinogenic properties) more often
2. Profession: health care professionals (HCPs) are at risk to develop addictive disorders because of high-stress, high-pressure jobs and exposure to substances
   NCLEX® a. Nursing practice is impaired when nurse is unable to uphold professional code of ethics and standards of practice because nurse's cognitive, interpersonal, or psychomotor skills have been affected by condition (psychiatric illness, excessive alcohol or drug use or addiction) in interaction
   b. Risk factors for vulnerability: access to drugs, long hours, tremendous responsibility, job-related stress, family history of chemical dependence or mental disorder
   NCLEX® c. Signs and symptoms: increased irritability with clients and colleagues; mood swings; withdrawn or isolated and often wants to work night shift; avoids informal staff get-togethers; purposely waits until alone to sign out narcotics; late for work, misses work, offers elaborate excuses for missing work; work quality decreases; charting is illegible; signs out more narcotics than other nurses on unit
   d. System response: intervention and immunity from prosecution; in most states, there is opportunity for supportive intervention rather than loss of licensure if impaired nurse seeks treatment and strictly follows treatment and monitoring recommendations from Board of Nursing; if noncompliant, may lose nursing license

III. DATA COLLECTION

A. Screening and assessment tools

1. CAGE: a positive answer for two of these screening questions indicates need for further assessment
   a. Have you ever attempted to *Cut back* on your alcohol?
   b. Have you ever been *Annoyed* by comments made about your drinking?
   c. Have you ever felt *Guilty* about your drinking?
   d. Have you ever had an *Eye-opener* in the morning to calm your nerves?

Memory Aid

Use the initials of the CAGE questionnaire to trigger the memory of what each question refers to.

2. Michigan Alcoholism Screening Test (MAST)
3. Addiction Severity Index (ASI)

B. Nursing admission assessment data that focuses on use of mood-altering chemicals

1. Physical data collection/systems review
   a. Blackout or lost consciousness: can be related to use of alcohol or other substances
   NCLEX® b. Changes in bowel movement: changes range from diarrhea caused by drinking to constipation caused by pain medications; withdrawal from narcotics can cause diarrhea
   c. Liver problems: include manifestations of Wernicke's encephalopathy or Korsakoff's psychosis
   NCLEX® d. Weight loss or weight gain: regular alcohol or drug use may lead to weight loss or gain and/or poor nutritional balance
   e. Stress: stressful situations can lead to increased drinking; stress can also result from drinking or using drugs regularly
   NCLEX® f. Sleep disturbances: alcohol and/or drug use can lead to a variety of sleep disturbances; client may start using alcohol to promote sleep, but once tolerance develops, sleep is more difficult
   g. Chronic pain: may lead to use of drugs and/or alcohol to self-medicate
   NCLEX® h. Concern over substance use: if friends and relatives worry about substance use, it is generally because a genuine problem exists
   i. Cutting down on alcohol consumption (or drug use, prescription medication use, gambling, or addictive behavior): if client feels a need to cut down, it is usually because there are problems

Memory Aid

It is just as important to screen for psychosocial data as for physical assessment data during admission for treatment for addiction.

2. Personal family history: persons with positive family history are at risk for developing an addictive disorder

NCLEX®

3. Substance use data collection: key elements
   a. Identify type of substance used
   b. Identify type of compulsive behavior
   c. Pattern and frequency of substance use
   d. Amount
   e. Age at onset
   f. Age of regular use
   g. Changes in use patterns
   h. Periods of abstinence in history
   i. Previous withdrawal symptoms
   j. Date of last substance use/compulsive behavior
   k. Ask about each substance or behavior separately
   l. Illicit drugs can be ingested into body in numerous ways; remember that alcohol users may also use another substance

NCLEX®

4. Medication history
   a. Ask about pain relief medications, laxatives, cold medications, and medications to induce sleep, help client stay awake, and/or control anxiety
   b. Prescribed dose is now not enough to control pain or anxiety even though it helped at first
   c. Runs out of medication early and needs a refill early
   d. Pain medication intended for physical pain is now used for emotional pain
   e. Medication is used for dealing with "stress" or stressful events
   f. More medication was taken than intended
   g. Laxatives are used regularly because pain medications cause constipation or because client has difficulty having bowel movements without laxative use
   h. Cold tablets or cough syrup are taken more frequently than expected
5. Over-the-counter (OTC) or nutritional supplement history: use of any herbal, vitamin, or OTC products to help with sleep, weight loss, staying awake, increasing energy, stabilizing and/or improving mood, or making client feel a certain way
6. Social history data collection: clients experiencing physical, sexual, or emotional abuse may medicate internal distress by using mood-altering substances
7. Laboratory data collection: laboratory values that may be elevated in substance abusers:
   a. Gamma glutamyl transferase (GGT)
   b. Aspartate aminotransferase (formerly SGOT) and alanine aminotransferase (formerly SGPT)
   c. Alkaline phosphatase (AK)
   d. Lactate dehydrogenase (LD)
   e. Total bilirubin
   f. Cholesterol and triglycerides
   g. Mean corpuscular volume (MCV)
   h. Urine toxicology and blood screen for drugs of abuse

IV. PLANNING AND IMPLEMENTATION

A. Care of client while intoxicated

1. Focus is on safety
2. Monitor signs and symptoms of intoxication (see Table 22–1)

NCLEX®

3. Interventions
   a. Maintain safe environment
   b. Orient to time, place, and person
   c. Maintain adequate nutrition and fluid balance
   d. Monitor for beginning of withdrawal signs and symptoms; note that, in general, drugs that depress the CNS lead to signs of CNS excitation during withdrawal, and drugs that are CNS stimulants lead to CNS depression during withdrawal
4. Outcome: client remains safe during periods of intoxication

Table 22–1 Signs of Substance Intoxication and Withdrawal with Treatments

Type of Substance	Signs of Intoxication	Signs of Withdrawal	Treatment of Withdrawal
CNS Depressants (alcohol, benzodiazepines, barbiturates)	Impaired memory, attention, judgment, or general functioning; drowsiness, slurred speech, irritability, hypotension	Nausea, vomiting, tachycardia, diaphoresis, abdominal cramping, insomnia, irritability, delirium, tremors, seizures	Seizure precautions Alcohol: chlordiazepoxide (Librium), thiamine (vitamin B_1), antiepileptics Benzodiazepines: flumazenil (Romazicon) IV Barbiturates: phenobarbital or long-acting benzodiazepine
CNS Stimulants (amphetamines, cocaine, crack)	Ataxia, fever, respiratory distress, seizures, coma, cerebrovascular accident, myocardial infarction, death	Apathy, extreme fatigue, lethargy, disorientation, anxiety, insomnia, agitation, depression, drug craving	Primarily supportive treatment Drug therapy: antidepressants, bromocriptine (Parlodel), a dopamine agonist as off label use
Opioids (codeine, morphine, opium, heroin, meperidine, hydromorphone, methadone, fentanyl, oxycodone)	Euphoria, drowsiness, constricted pupils, hypotension, slurred speech, decreased respirations, and impaired movements, memory, attention, and judgment	Excessive sweating, restlessness, agitation, dilated pupils, piloerection, tremors, yawning, tachycardia, hypertension, abdominal cramps, muscle spasms	Methadone/buprenorphine Clonidine/lofexidine to reduce severity of withdrawal Oxazepam (muscle spasms and insomnia) Antiemetics (nausea and vomiting)
Hallucinogens (lysergic acid diethylamide [LSD]), mescaline (peyote), psilocybin (mushrooms), phencyclidine (PCP)	Agitation, bizarre or violent behavior, dilated pupils, blank stare, piloerection, tachycardia and hypertension, incoordination, muscle rigidity with jerking, paranoia, hallucinations, tremors or seizures	Depends on specific drug; possible anxiety, mental depression, lethargy, insomnia, paranoid delusions, panic attacks	Supportive care with low environmental stimuli Gastric lavage or acidification of urine with vitamin C or ammonium chloride to speed drug clearance (PCP)
Marijuana (cannabis sativa)	Relaxation, euphoria, detachment, more talkative, slowed perception of time, possible anxiety or paranoia	Irritability, restlessness, insomnia, tremors, chills, weight loss	Supportive care; no specific medications

B. Care of client experiencing withdrawal from psychoactive substances: focus is safe withdrawal process

1. Maintain safe environment
2. Create a low-stimulation environment
3. *NCLEX®* Monitor vital signs (especially increased blood pressure) and withdrawal symptoms, such as nausea/vomiting, tremor, paroxysmal sweats, anxiety, agitation, tactile/auditory/visual disturbances, headache or fullness in head, disorientation, and sensorium changes (see again Table 22–1)
4. Methadone is used to manage some clients who are opiate-dependent; may be initially prescribed for withdrawal but then client is maintained on certain daily dose; contrary to popular belief, many people who are maintained on methadone do well in recovery
5. Be careful in observing client with chronic pain for withdrawal because some pain experienced is related to chronic pain and is not an acute withdrawal symptom
6. *NCLEX®* Even if female clients were initially screened for pregnancy, screen again later in episode of care to ensure that use of any substance potentially harmful to fetus is eliminated or minimized; alcohol is most harmful drug of all to fetus
7. Monitor for alcohol withdrawal delirium (formerly delirium tremens), psychotic symptoms, suicide risk, and seizure risk
8. *NCLEX®* Administer withdrawal medication: antiepileptics, benzodiazepines, sedatives, vitamins, or other medications as ordered; thiamine helps to prevent confusion (Wernicke's psychosis) and other mental status changes (see again Table 22–1)
9. *NCLEX®* Maintain adequate nutrition and fluid intake
10. Maintain normal comfort measures
11. Monitor for covert substance use during detoxification period
12. Provide emotional support and reassurance to client and family
13. Provide reality orientation and address hallucinations in a therapeutic manner
14. Advise client of depressive uneasy feelings and fatigue that usually occur during withdrawal
15. Begin to educate client about disease of addiction and initial treatment goal of abstinence

NCLEX® 16. Outcomes are safe withdrawal from drugs and alcohol, client is oriented to reality and begins to develop motivation for and commitment to abstinence and **recovery** (abstinence plus working a program of personal growth and self-discovery)

C. Nursing care during rehabilitative stages of abuse

1. Focus is on teaching about disease and recovery process and building on client's motivation for abstinence, lifestyle change, and recovery
2. NCLEX® Assist client to complete detoxification from all psychoactive substances; monitor for suicide and/or seizure risk
3. Promote abstinence from all psychoactive substances
4. Administer medications to enhance abstinence or treat mood, anxiety, and/or thought disorders as applicable
5. Assist client in putting structure and discipline back into life
6. Facilitate hope
7. Reinforce teaching about disease and recovery dynamics
8. Reinforce teaching about how disease has impacted roles and functions for individual and family
9. NCLEX® Provide therapeutic interaction/group counseling to
   a. Process losses (i.e., loss of independence)
   b. Discuss memories and flashback
   c. Address shame and guilt
   d. Reinforce information about disease/recovery
   e. Facilitate acceptance of illness
10. NCLEX® Reinforce and encourage practice of recovery skills
    a. Encourage daily commitment to sobriety and recovery
    b. Build and utilize sober support networks (i.e., Alcoholics Anonymous or other 12-step groups)
    c. Reinforce importance of honesty and making amends
    d. Encourage daily prayer or meditation
    e. Reinforce drink refusal skills and managing cravings
    f. Enhance coping, communication, and problem-solving skills
    g. Practice asking for help
    h. NCLEX® Recognize signs of impending **relapse** (return to addictive behavior): being hungry, angry, lonely, or tired (acronym HALT); having thoughts about using but not telling anyone, slipping back into using old defensive mechanisms instead of honesty and openness
11. NCLEX® Help client to develop an emergency plan (list of things client can do and people to call if he or she has urge to use or actually uses)

Memory Aid

Development of an emergency plan is high priority before discharge to home so that the client is better empowered to act on own behalf when the urge to abuse occurs.

12. Demonstrate how to use affirmations, slogans, and serenity prayer
13. Assist with random breathalyzers and urine drug screens to determine sobriety/substance use
    a. Breathalyzers are an inexpensive way to randomly check if clients are sober coming into program; because many clients have high tolerance, it is difficult to determine if they have been drinking
    b. Random urine drug screen test provides client with objective evidence of sobriety or use (urine collection procedure: instruct client not to turn on water or flush toilet until specimen is given to nurse)
14. NCLEX® Clients with anorexia nervosa or bulimia need to work with dietitian and primary care provider about increasing or decreasing (as indicated) caloric intake and discontinuing laxative use; they will need to increase daily water and fiber intake
15. Clients with multiple relapses who seem to have severe addiction may not have a goal of immediate total abstinence; their goals may be to increase number of sober days within a specific period of time or reduce number of drinks ingested or money gambled at one sitting (harm reduction model; while not an ideal goal, it decreases risk of more serious consequences if someone is using lesser amounts of substances)

D. Treatment modalities and nursing interventions

1. Medical model: teach disease and recovery dynamics
2. Assist client in complying with treatment recommendations
3. Assist with dual diagnosis treatment

4. Detoxification, abstinence medications
   NCLEX® a. Disulfiram (Antabuse): prevents breakdown of alcohol; person who drinks alcohol becomes very sick (flushing, weakness, nausea/vomiting, dizziness, tachycardia, and hypotension); teach about avoiding alcohol in any form (cough or cold products, mouthwash); can elevate liver enzymes
   NCLEX® b. Naltrexone (ReVia): prevents or diminishes cravings for substance use; can elevate liver enzymes
   NCLEX® c. Antidepressant/antianxiety medications: enhance and stabilize mood and diminish anxiety; teach about decreased effectiveness of medication with use of psychoactive substances; medication should be discontinued gradually to prevent rebound effect or seizures
5. NCLEX® The 12-step model
   a. Reinforce teaching that there is no effective cure for addiction
   b. Encourage 12-step involvement
   c. Regular attendance at meetings diminishes ambivalence and promotes acceptance about never engaging in addictive behaviors again
   d. Key elements of 12-step framework are acceptance, surrender, processing grief, higher power, and power of group
6. Cognitive behavioral model
   a. Help client to develop and use positive coping skills
   NCLEX® b. Reinforce specific skill training: assertiveness, drink refusal, problem solving, cognitive restructuring, mood management, anger problems, social skills, listening and communication skills
   c. Identify and change behaviors associated with addictive behaviors (i.e., going into liquor store to buy soft drinks)
7. Relapse prevention model
   a. Identify situations and factors that contribute to relapse
   NCLEX® b. Increase positive self-efficacy expectations about ability to achieve abstinence
   c. Identify euphoric recall about engaging in addictive behavior, which can serve to keep someone actively engaging in addiction
8. Motivational enhancement and stages of change
   NCLEX® a. Use various types of reflective listening and other specialized communication strategies to help build client's commitment to change
   b. Express empathy; ambivalence is a normal part of change process
   NCLEX® c. Help clients develop discrepancy between how they see themselves and how they really are
   d. Avoid getting into arguments over things, especially labels
   e. Change strategies if resistance is encountered
   NCLEX® f. Support client's self-efficacy
9. Assist in monitoring client's stage of change and apply nursing interventions accordingly
   a. Precontemplation: "We are blind to our problems"
   b. Contemplation: "We are not ready to change"
   c. Determination and preparation: "We are getting ready to change"
   d. Action: "We are learning how to change; we are doing it"
   e. Maintenance: "We make changes stick"

V. EVALUATION/OUTCOMES

A. Completes withdrawal process safely
B. Makes a commitment to sobriety, participates in treatment process
C. Identifies consequences of substance use or addictive behaviors
D. Begins to practice some recovery behaviors while in treatment and identifies coping behaviors to address cravings, thoughts, and triggers to use or engage in addictive behaviors
E. Begins to accept having an addictive disorder and never being able to use safely or engage in addictive behavior again

VI. DUAL DISORDER ISSUES

A. Focus is on teaching that each disorder is an illness that requires treatment and builds on client's motivation for abstinence, remissions of mental illness, lifestyle change, and recovery process
B. Additional interventions
1. Discuss physiological aspects of mental illness, substance abuse, and interaction effects
2. Reinforce teaching that psychiatric medications are nonaddictive and can enhance recovery
3. Medication teaching includes emphasizing that drinking or drug use will interfere with efficacy of psychiatric medication and not to mix medication with other substances

VII. FAMILY ISSUES

- **A. Anger and alienation of substance dependent person**
- **B. Teach disease dynamics**
  1. Family rules and communication
  2. Family members' dysfunctional behaviors and denial about addiction of family member
- **C. Problematic coping skills**
- **D. Mood adjustment problems**
- *NCLEX®* **E. Codependency and low self-esteem**
- **F. Learn and practice recovery dynamics and skills**
  1. Include self-love and self-care
  2. Utilize support groups (i.e., Al-Anon)
  3. Establish healthy relationships and boundaries
  4. Engage in daily prayer or meditation
  5. *NCLEX®* Improve coping and problem-solving skills
  6. *NCLEX®* Ask for help
  7. Confront dysfunctional beliefs and learn how to change them
  8. Use affirmations, slogans, serenity prayer
- **G. Processing anger, losses, and memories**
  1. Confront substance abuser about consequences of use and effect on family
  2. Process emotional distance between family members
  3. *NCLEX®* Process loss of "helper/competent" role now that recovering family member is taking back some of his or her lost family roles

Check Your NCLEX-PN® Exam I.Q.

You are ready for testing on this content if you can

- Assist in data collection regarding dependency or addiction.
- Explain reactions of clients and families to a diagnosis related to dependency or addiction.
- Communicate with clients who have a substance-related disorder.
- Participate in providing therapy to a client with a disorder of dependency or addiction.
- Identify factors that could interfere with the recovery of a client from a substance-related disorder.
- Reinforce teaching about treatments, including support groups, for disorders of dependency or addiction.
- Assist with providing care to a client undergoing substance withdrawal or drug toxicity.

PRACTICE TEST

1 A client is transitioning to a less intensive level of outpatient treatment for addiction. The nurse concludes the client is most at risk for relapse after the client makes a statement reflecting which theme?

1. Dreaming about gambling or engaging in compulsive sex
2. Not feeling happy
3. Feeling hungry or tired
4. Keeping thoughts of using opioids a secret

2 What statement made by the mother of a recovering compulsive Internet user would indicate the need for further reinforcement of teaching?

1. "My son is not going to enough 12-step meetings, he doesn't do his daily readings, and I don't think he is taking this seriously enough."
2. "My daughter and I are going to go to Al-Anon for the first time because we realize we have been affected by my son's addiction."
3. "I need to sign up for a meditation class for me because I get too preoccupied with what my son is or is not doing."
4. "I still have a lot of anger about the relationship problems that occurred between my son and me as a result of his addiction."

3 The nurse observes a family visit on the unit and recognizes that the family is suffering with effects of addiction and codependence. What long-lasting interpersonal problems might the nurse expect family members to manifest?

1. Lowered self-esteem
2. Impatience
3. Frustration tolerance
4. Being argumentative

4 A mother brings her daughter to the emergency department. The daughter was at a party and danced for the last few hours, but now she is sweating and does not look well. Data collection reveals temperature of 103°F, weight loss, and that the client is grinding the teeth. What should the nurse be most concerned about?

1. Poor nutrition from excessive alcohol consumption
2. Possible eating disorder
3. Dehydration and electrolyte imbalance
4. Influenza with accompanying high fever

5 The nurse is assisting with an admission for a client with alcohol dependence. During the admission process, the client acknowledges occasional sexual performance problems but says, "It's nothing a little alcohol can't fix." The nurse explains that regular alcohol use can have which effect on sexual functioning?

1. Increased desire and performance ability
2. Headaches and the "too tired syndrome"
3. Hyperarousal and premature ejaculation for men and anorgasmia for women
4. Decreased desire and ability to perform

6 A physician just wrote a prescription for a client to take naltrexone (ReVia). What would be the greatest concern of the nurse while getting ready to administer this medication?

1. The medication blocks the euphoric feeling from narcotics and alcohol
2. Whether the physician provided good medication teaching
3. The medication can precipitate withdrawal if the client is not completely detoxified
4. The client will not be able to experience pleasurable sensations

7 The nurse is conducting routine data collection on a client with gambling and alcohol addictions who is in the outpatient addiction program. Which client statement reflects a need for more teaching?

1. "I am going to have a night out with some friends at an area night club."
2. "I felt like drinking, so I cleaned the house instead."
3. "It is hard for me to make phone calls if I feel like using, but I did it last night."
4. "I told my brother that I couldn't help him as much as I have in the past."

8 After completing a family session about addiction, a woman approaches the nurse and shares that as a mother, she will always have to bear the suffering of having a chemically dependent daughter who could relapse at any time. What important information should the nurse share about family recovery from addiction?

1. Family recovery can begin when the addictive behavior ceases.
2. Family recovery can begin even if active use continues.
3. Family recovery will fail if the recovering addicted client relapses.
4. Family recovery will be enhanced if the recovering addict attends several Alcoholics Anonymous meetings.

9 A married client with marijuana dependence has difficulty keeping her house clean because she spends a lot of time playing an entertaining game on the Internet. She also says that she waits until everyone goes to bed to start writing messages with sexual content online with another man. What is the nurse's greatest concern?

1. The Internet usage may lead to an extramarital affair.
2. Her children will stop bringing friends home because the house is messy.
3. She seems preoccupied with the Internet and is using poor judgment.
4. She is depressed and may find her marriage unfulfilling.

10 A new mother who bottle-feeds her infant comes in for a 6-week postpartum visit and discusses being depressed and is prescribed an antidepressant. The nurse reinforcing medication instruction collects data regarding the client's alcohol-use patterns, and learns the client has 1–2 drinks once or twice a week. What explanation should the nurse provide for not using alcohol or drugs in this situation?

1. It will cause nausea and vomiting.
2. It will lead to excessive antidepressant effects.
3. It will decrease the effectiveness of the antidepressant.
4. It will cause increased blood pressure.

11 A cocaine-dependent client in recovery shares with the nurse that she has been using an over-the-counter (OTC) medication to help her get to sleep each night for the past 3 weeks. She becomes defensive when the nurse raises concerns, stating emphatically that it is not addictive. How should the nurse respond to the client? Select all that apply.

1. Validate how difficult it is to have trouble sleeping.
2. Acknowledge to the client that because the medication cannot be abused, it is not addictive.
3. Confront her firmly because there is increased risk for addiction if she uses this medication too often.
4. Suggest an herbal sleep aid such as valerian or melatonin, which cannot activate the brain reward system.
5. Explain that nonaddictive medication can be abused if taken in larger doses or more frequency than recommended.

12 The mental health nurse explains to clients who are learning about cross-addiction that there is a synergistic or addictive effect from using various kinds of chemicals together. The nurse illustrates this point using which example of items that create this combined additive effect?

1. Drinking beer and smoking cigarettes
2. Drinking coffee and eating donuts
3. Drinking wine and taking a benzodiazepine
4. Drinking wine and coffee

13 A male client is saying he is "wired," feels like he is on "pins and needles," and is irritable. He says he stopped using alcohol abruptly. What is the nurse's next intervention in caring for this client?

1. Observe whether other symptoms occur in the next few hours and then report them to the physician.
2. Note the time of his last drink and observe for signs and symptoms of alcohol withdrawal.
3. Collect data for all current substance-use patterns, including time of last use, and begin to assess for withdrawal.
4. Request an order for a stimulant medication to help prevent alcohol withdrawal delirium.

14 A booth at a church parish health fair addresses safe driving. The nurse at this booth explains that coordination and mental alertness are affected at a blood alcohol level of 0.04, even though many states have a legal limit of intoxication of 0.08. When asked how many drinks per hour the average person needs to be close to the 0.08 intoxication level, the nurse would make which reply?

1. A 4-ounce glass of wine if the individual has eaten recently
2. A 4-ounce glass of wine on an empty stomach
3. Three to five 4-ounce glasses of wine, depending on how recently food was consumed
4. Seven to eight 4-ounce glasses of wine, depending on how recently food was consumed

15 A nurse working in the addictions unit is stopped by a co-worker who states she is upset about something the nurse told to a client. The client understands that the nurse said, "If your drinking has created any problems for you, then you have addiction." The nurse clarifies that the statement was, "If you have the hallmark symptom of drinking, you have addiction." The nurse goes on to share which of the following as the *hallmark*?

1. Use despite negative consequences
2. Impaired control of use
3. Withdrawal
4. Tolerance

16 The nurse is co-teaching a drug prevention class at the local high school to teens, who do not believe cigarettes should be labeled as a drug. The nurse explains that when dealing with addiction, the word "drug" has which meaning?

1. An illegal substance that activates the pleasure center
2. A substance that activates the pleasure center in the brain
3. A chemical that is limited to a pharmacological action when ingested.
4. Any kind of pill that is broken down in the stomach by digestive action

17 The nurse is assisting in conducting an education session about alcoholism. Which statement should the nurse include when explaining the concept of alcohol dependence? Select all that apply.

1. Continuing to drink despite critical alcohol-related problems
2. Drinking larger amounts or over a longer time than was intended
3. Drinking to the point of drunkenness at least once per week
4. Experiencing a diminished effect with continued use of the same amount of alcohol
5. Using confabulation as a defense mechanism

PRACTICE TEST

18 Which comment by a substance-dependent client should lead the nurse to conclude that the client is vulnerable for relapse? Select all that apply.

1. "I like being able to have a lot of free time."
2. "Going to a football game makes me want to use again."
3. "I've been sober for 2 years. I've got this problem under control."
4. "No one else seems to work as hard as I do."
5. "It's easy. I can go to a club and just drink soft drinks."

19 As part of data collection activities to determine if the client is alcohol dependent, the nurse needs to conduct a CAGE assessment with the client. Which question asked by the nurse would be consistent with the structure of CAGE? Select all that apply.

1. "Have you ever felt that you needed to cut down on your drinking?"
2. "Have you ever been annoyed by comments made about your drinking?"
3. "Have you ever found yourself gulping drinks before going out?"
4. "Have you ever had a morning 'eye-opener' to calm your nerves?"
5. "Have you ever been embarrassed about your drinking?

ANSWERS & RATIONALES

1 **Answer: 4** **Rationale:** The problem with thoughts of using is keeping them a secret. When keeping things secret, the client is not telling the whole truth and is manipulating something. Engaging in secrets is reminiscent of using behaviors and can trigger addiction behaviors. It is natural to feel sad, hungry, or tired, and to have thoughts of engaging in the addictive behavior. **Cognitive Level:** Applying **Client Need:** Psychosocial Integrity **Integrated Process:** Nursing Process: Evaluation **Content Area:** Mental Health **Strategy:** Use the process of elimination and nursing knowledge to answer the question. The wording of the question tells you that one answer is better than the others because it contains the key critical word *best*.

2 **Answer: 1** **Rationale:** Checking on the compliance of a family member is an example of codependent behavior. The nurse would focus the teaching on helping the mother detach from her son and his recovery program and focus on her own well-being. Learning meditation and expressing anger would indicate that she is trying to identify and deal with her feelings. Attending Al-Anon is an obvious healthy behavior. **Cognitive Level:** Applying **Client Need:** Psychosocial Integrity **Integrated Process:** Nursing Process: Evaluation **Content Area:** Mental Health **Strategy:** The wording of the question tells you that only one answer is correct. Use knowledge of codependency to differentiate the problematic behavior from the other expected behaviors.

3 **Answer: 1** **Rationale:** Three communication rules are learned in families in which addiction is present: don't talk, don't trust, don't feel. While these experiences cause anger, anxiety, or maladaptive coping, they can also contribute to development of shame, depression, and low self-esteem. Without family healing, these problems can create much pain and suffering for all involved. Impatience, frustration tolerance, and being argumentative are not hallmarks or features of long-term family interpersonal problems. **Cognitive Level:** Applying **Client Need:** Psychosocial Integrity **Integrated Process:** Nursing Process: Planning **Content Area:** Mental Health **Strategy:** The core issue of the question is underlying consequences to families when addiction is present. Use nursing knowledge and the process of elimination to make a selection.

4 **Answer: 3** **Rationale:** The client most likely has used one of the "club drugs" or "rave drugs" (which are often are a cross between a stimulant and a hallucinogen). The stimulant effect of the drug causes users to grind their teeth. The combination of drug, dancing, and dehydration leads to a dangerous body temperature increase, which must be addressed immediately. The weight loss might also be related to an eating disorder, but that would not be the nurse's primary concern. Poor nutrition due to alcohol consumption and flu are not issues of concern at this time. **Cognitive Level:** Applying **Client Need:** Psychosocial Integrity **Integrated Process:** Nursing Process: Data Collection **Content Area:** Mental Health **Strategy:** Note the stem of the question contains the critical words *most concerned*. This tells you that more than one option may be partially correct and that you must prioritize an answer. Correlate elevated body temperature and weight loss with fluid balance to choose dehydration and electrolyte imbalance as correct.

5 **Answer: 4** **Rationale:** While most individuals believe that drugs of abuse enhance their sexual experience, the opposite is mostly true. The four types of sexual problems that commonly occur as the result of chemical use are anxiety about one's sexual performance; decrease or absence of sexual arousal; difficulties in reaching orgasm; and decrease or absence of pleasure in and/or intensity of orgasm. **Cognitive Level:** Analyzing **Client Need:** Psychosocial Integrity **Integrated Process:** Teaching and Learning **Content Area:** Mental Health **Strategy:** The core issue of the question is the relationship between chronic substance abuse and sexual performance. Use the process of elimination and nursing knowledge to answer the question. The wording of the question tells you that only one option is correct.

6 **Answer: 3** **Rationale:** If the client is not completely detoxified from opiates, the use of naltrexone can precipitate withdrawal. Clients should be opiate-free for 7–10 days before starting this medication. Naltrexone is an excellent medication to treat alcohol or opiate dependence. It helps to prevent cravings and triggers to use, and blocks the euphoric response if alcohol or opioids are ingested as an expected drug effect. The nurse should routinely evaluate the client's current knowledge level and provide education as needed but this is not the greatest concern at the onset of use of this drug. Naltrexone does not interfere with the client being able to experience pleasurable sensations in general. **Cognitive Level:** Analyzing **Client Need:** Psychosocial Integrity **Integrated Process:** Nursing Process: Planning **Content Area:** Mental Health **Strategy:** Note the critical words *greatest concern* in the question. This tells you that more than one option could be partially correct and that you must prioritize an answer. Use nursing knowledge of this medication to choose the option in which the client is at greatest risk.

7 **Answer: 1 Rationale:** Recovering clients may underestimate how difficult it will be to stay sober if they visit with friends who are still using or visit old "hangout" places where they used to engage in addictive behaviors. In early recovery, clients are encouraged to detach from people, places, and things associated with their addiction. As they gain sobriety and recovery, they may be able to re-engage, on a limited basis, with certain activities, such as being with friends who drink or celebrating an occasion at a bar. Physical activity, use of support systems, and limiting demands of others demonstrates positive coping measures and good management of potential triggers. **Cognitive Level:** Analyzing **Client Need:** Psychosocial Integrity **Integrated Process:** Nursing Process: Data Collection **Content Area:** Mental Health **Strategy:** The wording of the question indicates the correct option is a statement that contains either a false statement or one that indicates the client is at risk. Choose the correct option over the others because it puts the client in an area where temptation is likely.

8 **Answer: 2 Rationale:** Addiction affects the entire family system: communication roles and boundaries. Family members may experience low self-esteem, guilt, shame, insecurity, and preoccupation with the chemically dependent family member. Families need treatment to facilitate their own healing. Programs such as a treatment facility–operated family program, a spiritually centered family recovery program, or any of the family 12-step programs, may help active healing to take place whether the addicted family member is using or not. **Cognitive Level:** Analyzing **Client Need:** Psychosocial Integrity **Integrated Process:** Teaching and Learning **Content Area:** Mental Health **Strategy:** The core issue of the question is the family dynamics and impact on the family of a substance-using family member. Use nursing knowledge and the process of elimination to make a selection. The wording of the question indicates that only one answer is correct.

9 **Answer: 3 Rationale:** The client is spending excessive time on the Internet, which seems to be interfering with her parental relationships but also the time spent with her husband. If the client does not stop using marijuana and start practicing recovery, and if her Internet problems are not addressed, they are unlikely to resolve spontaneously and the secondary problems (online encounters, messy house, status of marriage) may get worse. There is not enough data to determine if the client is depressed. **Cognitive Level:** Applying **Client Need:** Psychosocial Integrity **Integrated Process:** Nursing Process: Planning **Content Area:** Mental Health **Strategy:** Use the process of elimination and critical thinking skills to answer the question. The correct answer is one that is most comprehensive of all aspects of the problem described and does not place judgment on the client.

10 **Answer: 3 Rationale:** Antidepressants regulate dysfunction in the neurotransmitter system, which results in mood equilibrium. Alcohol has depressant effects in the neurotransmitter system, which can cause depression and/or anxiety, and decrease the effectiveness of the antidepressant drug. Use of alcohol or other mood-altering drugs while taking antidepressants is contraindicated. Combining alcohol or drugs with an antidepressant will not raise blood pressure, cause nausea or vomiting, or lead to excessive antidepressant effects. **Cognitive Level:** Analyzing **Client Need:** Pharmacological and Parenteral Therapies **Integrated Process:** Teaching and Learning **Content Area:** Mental Health **Strategy:** The core issue of the question is the interaction of a prescribed antidepressant with alcohol use. Recall that alcohol is a CNS depressant, which has an opposite effect of antidepressants. Use the process of elimination and general knowledge of drug interactions to make a selection.

11 **Answer: 1, 5 Rationale:** Sleep difficulties are often a problem for people in early recovery. Clients can experience tolerance or tolerancelike symptoms in response to taking certain OTC medications. OTC sleep medications or psychoactive sleep medications are meant for short-term use, no longer than 1 week consecutively. Because the FDA does not regulate herbal products, it is difficult to know what dose to recommend or how the product might interact with the client. An initial approach that is educational rather than confrontational is more likely to be effective. **Cognitive Level:** Applying **Client Need:** Psychosocial Integrity **Integrated Process:** Communication and Documentation **Content Area:** Mental Health **Strategy:** Use the process of elimination and nursing knowledge to answer the question. Eliminate incorrect options because of the presence of "red flag" words *cannot* in two options and *firmly* and persistently in another.

12 **Answer: 3 Rationale:** Alcohol and benzodiazepines are both depressants. Persons often use two drugs within the same class to enhance their effects. The capacity of other psychoactive substances within the same class of drugs to enhance the effect of the primary drug is called cross-tolerance. Cigarettes are a stimulant while beer is a depressant, which have opposite effects rather than synergistic ones. Coffee is a stimulant while donuts have no direct effect on the central nervous system. Coffee is a stimulant while wine is a depressant, which have opposite effects rather than synergistic ones. **Cognitive Level:** Applying **Client Need:** Psychosocial Integrity **Integrated Process:** Nursing Process: Planning **Content Area:** Mental Health **Strategy:** The core issue of the question is knowledge that cross-addiction occurs between drugs in the same class. Use the process of elimination and knowledge of the categories of the chemicals in the options to make a selection.

13 **Answer: 3 Rationale:** Tactile disturbances are a symptom of alcohol dependence, and if the client reports stopping alcohol use abruptly, he or she may be starting to experience withdrawal symptoms. However, the client may also have used and stopped other substances abruptly as well. The nurse must assess for other substances used. Multiple drug use is the rule more than the exception. Waiting to take action by only observing the client places the client at risk, and stimulants are not indicated. **Cognitive Level:** Applying **Client Need:** Psychosocial Integrity **Integrated Process:** Nursing Process: Implementation **Content Area:** Mental Health **Strategy:** The wording indicates that the core issue of the question is possible withdrawal. Choose the option that is most comprehensive in nature and takes into account the possibility of multiple drug use and cessation.

14 **Answer: 3 Rationale:** It takes the average person 1 hour to metabolize 1 ounce of alcohol or a 4-ounce glass of wine. If three to five glasses of wine are consumed within an hour,

the average person reaches the legal intoxication level. A 4-ounce glass of wine (with or without food) is insufficient, while 7 to 8 glasses of wine would far exceed the legal intoxication level. **Cognitive Level:** Analyzing **Client Need:** Psychosocial Integrity **Integrated Process:** Teaching and Learning **Content Area:** Mental Health **Strategy:** Use the process of elimination to answer the question. Recognize that the question has the critical words *average person* and *be close to.* First eliminate the options that have 4 ounces of wine, since there is no room for individual variation, and then choose the option that has 3–5 glass of wine, since it is more moderate in amount than the option with 7–8 glasses.

15 **Answer: 2 Rationale:** Impaired control is the defining symptom that moves someone's use or abuse category to the dependence category. The symptom of "use despite negative consequences" fits in both the abuse and dependence category. Withdrawal may or may not be present for someone who has dependence. Tolerance may or may not be present for someone who has dependence. **Cognitive Level:** Analyzing **Client Need:** Psychosocial Integrity **Integrated Process:** Communication and Documentation **Content Area:** Mental Health **Strategy:** The core issue of the question is knowledge of hallmarks of alcohol abuse. Use the process of elimination and nursing knowledge to make a selection.

16 **Answer: 2 Rationale:** Any substance, legal or illegal, that activates the pleasure center in the brain has the potential to cause dependence. Any substance, legal or illegal, that activates the pleasure center in the brain has the potential to cause dependence. Nicotine causes a physical pharmacological action and also leads to physical and psychological dependence. Cigarettes are not broken down in the stomach by digestive action; the smoke is inhaled. **Cognitive Level:** Analyzing **Client Need:** Psychosocial Integrity **Integrated Process:** Teaching and Learning **Content Area:** Mental Health **Strategy:** Use the process of elimination and basic knowledge of addiction to make a selection. The wording of the question indicates that only one option contains a correct statement.

17 **Answer: 1, 2, 4 Rationale:** Continuing to drink despite critical alcohol-related problems, drinking larger amounts or over a longer time than intended, and experiencing a diminished effect from the same amount of alcohol are three *DSM IV-TR* criteria for alcohol dependence. The *DSM IV-TR* specifies that substance dependency can be diagnosed if client behaviors over the past 12-month period are consistent with three or more of seven specific criteria. Drinking to the point of drunkenness at least once weekly is not included in the *DSM IV-TR* criteria, which recognize that alcohol dependency can follow many different patterns, including episodic drinking to excess. The only time frame mentioned in the criteria is one year, and this is because persistent patterns of use are necessary to establish the diagnosis of alcohol dependency. Using confabulation as a defense mechanism is not included in the *DSM IV-TR* criteria. Also, the characteristic defense mechanisms used by an alcohol dependent individual are denial, rationalization and projection, not confabulation. **Cognitive Level:** Analyzing **Client Need:** Psychosocial Integrity **Integrated Process:** Teaching and Learning **Content Area:** Mental Health **Strategy:** Review *DSM IV-TR* criteria for substance dependency. Specific information is needed to answer this question. Note the wording of the question indicates more than one option is likely to be correct.

18 **Answer: 1, 3, 4, 5 Rationale:** Substance dependence clients should be taught to have structure and routine in their lives, as well as to avoid boredom and loneliness, to reduce the risk of relapse. Stating the problem is under control suggests that the client feels overly confident, which can be lead to unwise behaviors that test the recovery. Stating that no one else seems to work as hard as the client indicates dissatisfaction and impatience with others and can lead the client to feel justified in returning to the "solace" of using a substance. An intention to go to a club but only buy soft drinks indicates that the client is putting him- or herself into a situation of high risk to return to alcohol use. Also, the client is showing complacency rather than cautiousness. Verbalizing knowledge of high-risk situations that could lead to relapse is healthy. After developing awareness, the client can make a conscious decision as to how to cope with the situation without using a substance. **Cognitive Level:** Analyzing **Client Need:** Psychosocial Integrity **Integrated Process:** Nursing Process: Evaluation **Content Area:** Mental Health **Strategy:** Look for options that clearly indicate that the client is in a situation of risk. Notice that only one option shows insight, while the question is looking for risk of relapse.

19 **Answer: 1, 2, 4 Rationale:** The *C* in the CAGE mnemonic represents the need to *cut* down or reduce alcohol intake. The *A* in the CAGE mnemonic represents being *annoyed* at what others say about the drinking. The *E* in CAGE represents having an early morning drink to open the *eyes* and calm the nerves. The *G* in the CAGE mnemonic represents *guilt*, not gulping drinks. The *E* in CAGE does not represent embarrassed. **Cognitive Level:** Applying **Client Need:** Psychosocial Integrity **Integrated Process:** Nursing Process: Data Collection **Content Area:** Mental Health **Strategy:** Notice the word *consistent* in the stem of this question, which indicates the correct answer will also be a true statement about what the CAGE questionnaire represents. The wording of the question indicates that more than one option is correct.

Key Terms to Review

abstinence p. 304
craving p. 305
process addiction p. 304
recovery p. 309
relapse p. 309
substance abuse p. 304
substance dependence p. 304
tolerance p. 304
withdrawal p. 304

References

American Psychiatric Association. (2000). *Diagnostic and statistical manual of mental disorders* (revised 4th ed.). Washington, DC: Author.

Fontaine, K. (2009). *Mental health nursing* (6th ed.). Upper Saddle River, NJ: Pearson Education.

Kniesl, C.,Wilson, H., & Trigoboff, E. (2009). *Contemporary psychiatric-mental health nursing* (2nd ed.). Upper Saddle River, NJ: Pearson Education.

Stuart, G. (2009). *Principles and practice of psychiatric nursing* (9th ed.). St. Louis: Elsevier Science.

Townsend, M. (2010). *Essentials of psychiatric mental health nursing: Concepts of care in evidence-based practice* (5th ed.). Philadelphia: F.A. Davis.

Varcarolis, E. & Halter, M. (2010). *Foundations of psychiatric mental health nursing: A clinical approach* (6th ed.). Philadelphia: Saunders.

Test Yourself

Are you ready for the NCLEX-PN® or course exams? Use the practice tests on the companion website to check.

23 Crisis Intervention and Suicide

In this chapter

Cross Reference

Other chapters relevant to this content area are

Coping with Stressors	**Chapter 20**
Mental Health Disorders	**Chapter 21**
Psychiatric Medications	**Chapter 32**

I. OVERVIEW OF CRISIS

A. Definition of *crisis*: experience of being confronted by a stressor with which client is unable to cope and cannot resolve

1. Change or loss threatens client's **equilibrium** (state of balance; a condition in which contending forces are equal)
2. Accompanying anxiety and tension make coping with this experience more difficult
3. Feelings of hopelessness and helplessness result in cognitive disorganization in which previous experience and coping fail to aid problem solving; **coping** is a conscious attempt to manage stress and anxiety; may be physical, cognitive, or affective
4. **Hopelessness**: a subjective state in which client sees limited or no alternatives or personal choices available and is unable to mobilize energy on own behalf
5. **Helplessness**: a state that may arise when client has a condition causing dependency on outside sources for life support
6. Loss of equilibrium ensues
7. *NCLEX®* Crises are generally time limited, lasting from 4 to 6 weeks; during this time there is potential for either increased psychological vulnerability or personal growth

Memory Aid A crisis cannot go on for extended periods; it lasts generally for 4 to 6 weeks.

NCLEX® **B. Developmental phases of crisis**

1. Initial increase in tension as stimulus continues and further discomfort is experienced
2. Failure to succeed in coping with stimulus while continuing to experience distress

3. Additional tension forces mobilization of internal and external resources directed at emergency problem-solving efforts; problem may be redefined or client may give up certain aspects of a goal perceived to be unattainable
4. If problem remains unresolved and cannot be ignored, tension builds and major disorganization results

C. **Characteristics of crisis**
1. Stimulus is beyond client's usual experience
2. Previously developed coping mechanisms are ineffective
3. Anxiety, tension, and cognitive disorganization ensue
4. Client perceives threat to own integrity or established goals

NCLEX®
5. Maturational crises involve normal life transitions that evoke changes in client's self-perception in role, status, and integrity

Memory Aid

Associate the term *maturational* with a crisis event that occurs as the client gets older.

NCLEX®
6. Situational crises involve an external event that disturbs client's equilibrium (loss, change) and threatens consistency between self-behaviors and values or beliefs

Memory Aid

Associate the term *situational* with a crisis event that occurs unexpectedly to a single client.

NCLEX®
7. Adventitious crises involve external events (natural disasters or other catastrophic events) that are unpredictable and often engender fear, confusion, and loss of consistency with internalized beliefs or values and behavior; these may also be called community crises
8. Cultural crises accompany culture shock experienced by people adapting to a new culture or returning to own culture after being assimilated into another culture

D. **Balancing factors determining client's response to crisis**
1. Client's perception of event
2. Past experience in coping with stress and established coping strategies
3. Availability of support persons and other resources

Memory Aid

The better a client's coping strategies are in general, the better the client will be prepared to cope with a crisis.

E. **Client goals for treatment**
1. Remain free of self-harm
2. Identify specific problem and verbalize feelings related to event
3. Analyze event or problem and express perceptions of it
4. Identify and seek help from support systems
5. Explore alternatives for coping with crisis
6. Participate in choosing an action plan and implement plan
7. Experience less anxiety and tension and verbalize enhanced self-esteem

II. NURSING PROCESS DURING CRISIS

A. **Data collection**
1. Identify history of presenting problem

NCLEX®
a. Focus on immediate problem, not on past history

NCLEX®
b. Determine client's perception of problem: how threatened is he or she?

c. Monitor client's cognitive appraisal; identify any faulty thinking

2. Identify current feelings
   a. Help client express current feelings
   b. Validate current feelings and help client to accept them
   c. Acknowledge that client ultimately makes own decisions
3. Identify coping mechanisms
4. Identify client's support systems
   a. Identify available resources in whom client trusts
   b. Identify spiritual and religious beliefs

NCLEX®
5. Determine potential for self-harm
   a. Ask directly if client has had any thoughts of hurting or killing himself or herself; some clients engage in self-mutilation and do not want to die but do inflict self-harm, such as with razor blades or glass
   b. Use questions such as "Do you have thoughts of killing yourself?" and "Do you have thoughts of hurting yourself?"
   c. If client has thoughts of self-harm, determine if client has made specific plans to accomplish this, which is a danger signal—the more specific the plan, the more likely it is that the client will carry it out
   d. Determine if client has means to harm or kill self (guns in house, access to medications with potential for overdose)
   e. Determine if client can contract with nurse to maintain safety; work with client to identify an action plan if suicidal ideation increases or client feels he or she will act on ideas to harm self

B. Planning and implementation for clients in crisis

1. Specific treatment modalities
   a. Mutual goal planning; often nurse must use a directive approach
   b. Goals are set based on assessment and nursing diagnoses
   c. Overarching goals include establishing relationship with client, identifying problem, identifying and reducing client's perceptual distortions, enhancing self-esteem, alleviating anxiety, promoting use of support systems (family and friends), reinforcing healthy coping, and validating problem-solving ability

NCLEX®
   d. Examine client's feelings that may block ability to cope adaptively

NCLEX®
   e. Reinforce client teaching about how to ask for help from others
   f. Identify previously acquired adaptive coping strategies and help client modify and expand these coping strategies to new stress

NCLEX®
   g. Encourage use of expression of feelings, comfort strategies, and self-care activities

NCLEX®
   h. Focus on problem resolution in a step-by-step, concrete way, first focusing on alternatives and then selecting and acting on appropriate ones

Memory Aid

Clients in crisis tend to be disorganized in their thinking. Use simple words and sentences, and give concrete, step-by-step instructions to facilitate effective communication.

   i. Consider involving client in a crisis group, which helps clients feel less isolated and engage in group problem solving to identify alternatives
   j. Involve family in crisis intervention because other family members often experience crisis

C. Evaluation and outcomes for clients in crisis

NCLEX®
1. Client remains free of self-harm and clearly identifies problem
2. Perceptual distortions are identified and resolved
3. Client verbalizes a stable sense of self-esteem and ability to work on problem
4. Anxiety is reduced by identifying and implementing effective coping strategies; unhealthy coping mechanisms are identified and explored if client is willing
5. Client acknowledges need for help and asks for help; identifies and verbalizes feelings
6. Client demonstrates self-care behaviors
7. Client verbalizes an action plan and begins to implement action plan

D. Potential for growth

1. Client identifies and practices new coping skills that may be useful in future in dealing with stressful and potentially traumatic events
2. Client verbalizes a renewed or enhanced sense of self-worth

III. PSYCHOPHARMACOLOGY AS TREATMENT DURING CRISIS

A. General principles

NCLEX® 1. Drug therapy should not interfere with crisis intervention strategies; rather, they target symptoms that interfere with ability to function

2. A crisis is not a psychiatric illness nor a prolonged condition; therefore, pharmacologic interventions are not interventions of choice

B. Medications useful during crisis

1. Anxiolytics such as alprazolam (Xanax), clonazepam (Klonopin), diazepam (Valium), and lorazepam (Ativan), may be used to treat anxiety, panic, and sleep disturbances that accompany a crisis; short-term use is encouraged because of risk of dependence
2. Other agents, such as zolpidem (Ambien) and zaleplon (Sonata), may be used to manage insomnia
3. Neuroleptic medications: the atypicals, such as olanzapine (Zyprexa), risperidone (Risperdal), quetiapine (Seroquel), and typical agents such as haloperidol (Haldol), may be used to treat psychotic symptoms that emerge; however, psychosis does not commonly follow experience of a crisis unless client has a pre-existing psychotic disorder

IV. ANGER AND AGGRESSION

A. Data collection regarding other-directed violence

NCLEX® 1. Violence is frequently, although not always, preceded by specific behaviors
   a. Increased activity or hyperactivity such as restlessness or pacing behaviors
   b. Verbal abuse, instigation of arguments, and use of profanity
   c. Change in amount of eye contact (greater or lesser)
   d. Visible signs of tension such as clenched fists or jaws, rigid facial expression or posture, talking or muttering to self
   e. Change in voice such as louder or softer, and possibly either faster or slower rate of speech

2. Key risk factors: client history of violent behavior and impulsivity
3. Precipitating events for violence in in-patient settings often include staff factors such as inexperience, controlling behavior, inability to set effective limits, and indiscrimate removal of unit privileges

B. Planning and implementation to de-escalate violent client

1. Remain calm
2. Maintain client dignity and self-esteem
3. Identify client stressors and indications of stress presented by client
4. Determine what client considers to be his or her need

NCLEX® 5. Use calm and clear tone of voice and nonaggressive body posture

NCLEX® 6. Keep large personal space between self and client and assess for personal safety; always stay positioned facing client with an escape route to the back

NCLEX® 7. Provide several options to client

8. Remain goal oriented and avoid arguing with client
9. Use stepwise progression of interventions from least restrictive to more restrictive, according to client's behavior

NCLEX® 10. Use time-outs when appropriate

NCLEX® 11. Use seclusion and restraints as a last option when other interventions have failed; use least amount of restraint that is effective; if physical restraints are used, check circulation every 30 minutes and release one at a time every 2 hours and provide range of motion

12. Administer medications according to order or protocol
13. Provide debriefing session for staff to ventilate feelings immediately after event in which violence has occurred

C. Evaluation

1. Client is able to control own behavior
2. Safety of client, other clients, and staff is maintained

V. OVERVIEW OF SUICIDE

A. *Suicide*: intentionally and voluntarily taking one's life

B. Statistics on suicide (National Institute of Mental Health, 2009)

1. Suicide is 11th leading cause of death among all age groups and third leading cause of death in those age 15 through 24 in United States

2. Native Americans and non-Hispanic whites are more likely than Hispanics, blacks, and Asian/Pacific Islanders to die from suicide
3. Men are three to four times more likely than women to commit suicide, and older adults are at higher risk than younger adults

C. Risk factors and warning signs for suicide

1. Risk factors include depression and other mental disorders, a substance-abuse disorder in combination with other mental disorder, prior suicide attempt, family history of mental disorder, substance abuse or suicide, family violence (including physical or sexual abuse), firearms in home, incarceration, exposure to suicidal behavior of family members, peers, or media figures
2. *NCLEX®* Clients contemplating suicide often perceive themselves as isolated through physical distance or interpersonal discord; they often experience feelings of helplessness, loss of self-esteem with feelings of worthlessness and hopelessness, the latter being most predictive of suicide
3. Often a desire to be free from pain or to be dead is accompanied by depression and anger
4. *NCLEX®* Warning signs that may indicate risk for suicidal ideations and self-injurious behavior include changes in personal habits such as appetite, sleep patterns, personal appearance, personality, use of alcohol and other drugs, as well as bodily complaints, self-deprecating comments, making wills, and giving away personal belongings
5. *NCLEX®* Academic and occupational warning signs include truancy and absenteeism, decline in academic or occupational performance, boredom, apathy, disruptive classroom or work behavior, and anger and hostility toward authority figures
6. *NCLEX®* Family and social relationship warning signs include decreased interactions with peers and friends; a change in people with whom client spends time, and a decrease in or absence of romantic relationships

Memory Aid

Do not ignore warning signs of suicide; take action to collect data and assist in determining risk of suicide immediately, seeking help from other health care professionals.

7. *NCLEX®* The single-most predictive psychiatric disorder for suicide is presence of a mood disorder

D. Common myths of suicide

1. People who talk about suicide won't actually commit suicide
2. People who are serious about suicide will show warning signs or give clues
3. Young children do not commit suicide
4. An improvement in mood means risk for suicide is over
5. Only people who are depressed commit suicide
6. A written/verbal safety contract guarantees that client will not commit suicide

E. Conscious and unconscious suicidal intention

1. Conscious suicidal ideations include an awareness of potential outcomes or results of suicidal behavior, awareness of others' response to suicidal threats or attempts, awareness of lethality index of a chosen method, and awareness of rescue possibilities
2. Unconscious suicidal ideation may be more difficult to assess
   a. The desire to cause self-harm or self-destruction may be beyond client's conscious awareness
   b. Client may engage in high-risk behaviors as a way of acting out unconscious desire for self-harm (e.g., drinking and driving and engaging in potentially lethal activity)
   c. Careful attention must be paid to direct and indirect ways in which client may be communicating unconscious suicidal ideations

VI. NURSING PROCESS FOR SUICIDAL CLIENTS

A. Determining risk for suicide

1. *NCLEX®* During initial data collection, question client about any thoughts or feelings related to harming or killing himself or herself; determine suicidal ideations, how client has sought help, what kind of plan client has made and client's mental status, available support systems, and lifestyle
   a. Ask questions like, "Have you had any thoughts about life not being worth living?"
   b. Move from general to specific questions like, "Have you had any ideas about killing yourself?"
   c. It is a false assumption that client will volunteer this information without being asked
   d. Be comfortable asking these questions directly and in a matter-of-fact way

e. If client answers yes, ask client, "Have you thought of, or made any plans for, how you might harm or kill yourself?" (passive suicidal ideation is presence of suicidal thoughts without a plan, in contrast to suicidal ideation with a plan)
f. Gauge level of lethality further by asking about access to means for self-harm, (e.g., do you have a gun in your home? Do you know how to use it?) and evaluating lethality of means (e.g., guns vs. pills)
g. Take a careful history of previous self-harming behaviors by asking client such questions as, "Have you ever tried to harm or kill yourself in the past?"
h. Question also use of alcohol, drugs, and level of impulsivity
i. Complete a mental status assessment to determine alterations in thought process, impulsiveness, perceptual distortions, insight, and judgment
j. Inquire about currently available support systems

2. Many people experience ambivalence about committing suicide; assessment of these ambivalent feelings is important
3. Initially, clients may lack emotional or psychic energy to act on suicidal ideations because of some negative or neurovegetative symptoms they experience

NCLEX®

4. Be aware that a sudden sense of peace or wellness reported by client may indicate that client has sufficient psychic energy to carry out a suicidal act; this risk increases as client stabilizes on antidepressant medications

B. Goals for clients at risk for suicide

1. Remain safe and free of self-harm
2. Verbalize suicidal ideations and discuss these with nursing staff
3. Develop a safety plan with nursing staff and other members of treatment team that identifies steps to keep self safe, and ask for help before acting out a suicidal or self-harm thought
4. Verbalize a decrease in or absence of suicidal ideations
5. Verbalize a desire to live and reasons for living

NCLEX®

6. Identify an aftercare plan following discharge from hospital that includes a commitment to follow up with psychotherapy and adherence to psychopharmacologic interventions
7. Identify a support system outside hospital

C. Nursing interventions to reduce risk of suicide (self-directed violence)

1. Inpatient treatment is indicated if client is assessed as high risk for self-directed or other-directed violence
2. Inpatient interventions include providing a safe milieu in which client's ability to act out on suicidal ideations or other-directed violence is minimized

a. While client may be admitted to milieu voluntarily, unit is self-contained and doors are commonly locked; nursing staff regulate flow of traffic on and off unit

NCLEX®

b. Depending on degree of suicidal ideation and lethality assessed, place client on constant observation for first 24 hours or until degree of suicidal risk is lessened according to agency policy

NCLEX®

c. Place client on every-15-minute checks or every-30-minute thereafter, depending on agency policy
d. Maintain an awareness of client's whereabouts constantly
e. Develop rapport and foster a therapeutic relationship with client
f. On admission to unit, assess client's personal belongings and remove items that could be used by client to harm self or others (drugs, potentially sharp objects, cords, shoelaces, belts, neck ties, lighters) and keep them in a safe place

NCLEX®

g. Keep unit free of materials that can be readily used by clients to harm themselves or others (e.g., metal or glass objects that may be altered to create a sharp edge, shoelaces, belts, electrical or call bell cords); keep windows locked and count silverware; check gifts and other items brought in by family members or friends for safety before they are given to client; let family members place belongings in locker before entering unit; scan all visitors with a metal detector prior to entering unit

Memory Aid

When a client is at risk for self-directed or other-directed violence, act to protect the safety of all: the client, other clients, and staff.

h. Work with client to develop a safety plan, and assess client frequently
i. Meet one on one with client to explore client's feelings and help client work toward reengagement with significant others and fulfilling life activities

NCLEX®
j. Give suicidal client a roommate to reduce opportunity for solitude
k. Make sure that client swallows oral medications and is not holding medication in oral cavity (cheeking) to hoard for a later overdose
l. Work with client's participation to identify an aftercare plan that includes a commitment on client's part to attend aftercare appointments, maintain contact with social support systems, and identify a safety plan with emergency contact numbers and an action plan should suicidal ideations return
m. Realize that despite precautions, a client may still take own life after hospitalization (if unable to do so during); an ultimate decision to live rests with client
n. Initiate debriefing session for staff members after client's suicide or any violent behavior to provide forum for staff to ventilate feelings

NCLEX®
D. Evaluation and outcomes for clients comtemplating suicide; the client will
1. Remain safe and free from self-directed violence
2. Verbalize absence or decreased intensity and severity of suicidal ideations, with absence of plan and intent
3. Verbalize a desire to live and state several reasons for living
4. Agree to maintain a no-self-harm contract with nursing staff and other treatment staff for specified periods of time
5. Identify a safety plan that provides for asking for help before acting out should suicidal ideations worsen, intent reemerge, or unsafe feelings occur
6. Meet other goals in treatment plan relative to other problems identified

VII. PSYCHOPHARMACOLOGY AS TREATMENT TO PREVENT SUICIDE

A. Description
1. Pharmacologic interventions used in presence of suicidal ideations are aimed at treating underlying mood disorder, other psychiatric disorder, or coexisting psychiatric disorders; see Chapter 32 for detailed information on these medications
2. Since a high correlation exists between mood disorders and suicide, adequate treatment of a mood disorder is essential in overall treatment of client at risk for suicide

NCLEX®
B. Depressive disorders are treated with antidepressants
1. Because of relatively low risk of lethal overdose and relatively low side-effect profiles with use of selective serotonin reuptake inhibitors (SSRIs), these agents are often first-line drugs to treat depression that could lead to suicide (see Table 23–1)

NCLEX®
2. While effective in treatment of depression, tricyclic antidepressants can be highly lethal in overdose and are not a first-line agent; when used, quantity dispensed at any one time should be kept to a minimum and may need to be managed by a family member (see again Table 23–1)
3. Other agents such as tetracyclics and atypical antidepressants are also helpful in treating depressive disorders (see again Table 23–1)

NCLEX®
4. Monoamine oxidase inhibitors (MAOIs) are useful occasionally in treating depressive disorders; however, serious drug and food interactions make these agents particularly challenging; they can be used if clients will comply with a tyramine-free diet (noncompliance can lead to hypertensive crisis); see again Table 23–1

Table 23–1 Antidepressants Useful in Treating Depression That Could Lead to Suicide

Type of Antidepressant	Specific Drug Names
Selective serotonin reuptake inhibitors	Citalopram (Celexa), paroxetine (Paxil), fluoxetine (Prozac), sertraline (Zoloft), escitalopram (Lexapro)
Tricyclic antidepressants	Amitriptyline (Elavil), clomipramine (Anafranil), desipramine (Norpramin), doxepin (Sinequan), imipramine (Tofranil), nortriptyline (Pamelor), trimipramine (Surmontil)
Tetracyclic and atypical antidepressants	Bupropion (Wellbutrin), nefazadone (Serzone), trazadone (Desyrel), venlafaxine (Effexor), mirtazipine (Remeron), duloxetine (Cymbalta)
Monoamine oxidase inhibitors	Tranylcypromine (Parnate), phenelzine (Nardil), isocarboxazid (Marplan)

C. Bipolar disorders: characterized by cycling of moods with episodes of mania and depression and are also associated with suicide; treated with a class of drugs known as mood stabilizers:

1. Lithium
2. Valproic acid (Depakote)
3. Carbamazepine (Tegretol), lamotrigine (Lamictal), gabapentin (Neurontin), and topiramate (Topamax) as antiepileptic drugs
4. Olanzapine (Zyprexa), an atypical antipsychotic, which is associated with increased risk of metabolic syndrome

D. Clients with other psychiatric disorders are also at risk for suicide and may be treated with anxiolytics, neuroleptics, and other psychotropic agents

1. Any psychotropic medication can be dangerous in overdose, so a careful assessment must be made with proper client and family teaching about each drug (see Section III, Psychopharmacology as Treatment during Crisis)
2. *NCLEX®* Clients may be at increased risk of suicide once medication takes effect and client has sufficient energy to act on suicide plan; assess client carefully and provide protective measures as needed

Check Your NCLEX-PN® Exam I.Q.

You are ready for testing on this content if you can

- Assist with determining a client's coping mechanisms.
- Help a client to use and enhance coping mechanisms.
- Assist in monitoring a client experiencing a crisis.
- Help a client to process the experience of a crisis.
- Explore social supports to aid a client in recovery from a crisis.
- Collect data regarding a client's risk of self-harm.
- Provide care to reduce a client's risk of harm to self or others.

PRACTICE TEST

1 When collecting data from a client admitted to the mental health unit to determine the potential for violent or aggressive behavior, what important communication strategy should the nurse use?

1. Reassure the client that everything will be all right, and the staff will make sure nothing untoward happens.
2. Reinforce that the client is solely responsible for his or her own actions and will experience the consequences of acting out.
3. Explain that violence is not acceptable, and the staff will not allow the client to act out.
4. Reassure the client that limited acting out will be allowed but only in a controlled setting.

2 When responding to a client who displays the potential for violence, the nurse would use which intervention as the most restrictive technique?

1. Meeting in a quiet room to reduce stimulation
2. Administering a PRN medication to reduce anxiety
3. Providing physical interventions, such as two-person escort out of a program area
4. Using restraints, such as a four-point restraint

3 What is the most important intervention by the nurse when a client does not respond to less restrictive interventions and is rapidly escalating toward violence?

1. Cease negotiation with client and implement plan of intervention to control client and provide safety.
2. Bargain with client to determine what can be done to prevent assaultive behavior.
3. Offer a PRN medication to reduce anxiety.
4. Ask client to move to a less stimulating, private area and spend some time alone.

4 After a staff member has been involved in a particularly violent episode with a client, when should the nurse expect debriefing to occur?

1. After the staff has had an opportunity to become calm
2. Immediately, so as to facilitate the processing of feelings
3. Not until the staff requests such an intervention
4. After a 3-day time-off period

PRACTICE TEST

5 The nurse is working with a client in psychological distress. Which event experienced by the client would the nurse document as a situational crisis?

1. Approaching the age of retirement
2. Recently being involved in a severe motor vehicle accident
3. Being a survivor of a flood following a hurricane
4. Recently returning home from military duty after an armed conflict

6 A nurse is carrying out planned interventions for a client in crisis who witnessed a violent crime. What key component of crisis intervention should the nurse implement at this time?

1. Identify the client's maladaptive coping mechanisms.
2. Identify and support the client's coping patterns.
3. Assist the client in forgetting the crisis situation.
4. Teach the client to handle future crises.

7 The nurse carrying out a plan of care for a client using crisis management principles understands that interventions are based on which primary tasks of crisis management? Select all that apply.

1. Provide support.
2. Relieve anxiety.
3. Provide encouragement.
4. Foster independence.
5. Provide guidance.

8 An adult client is having difficulty coping with a new diagnosis of colon cancer. The nurse telephones the physician for an order for a medication to assist the client during this crisis situation. The nurse anticipates an order for which medication?

1. Haloperidol (Haldol)
2. Amitriptyline (Elavil)
3. Lorazepam (Ativan)
4. Valproic acid (Depakote)

9 The family of a client with suicidal ideations asks the nurse if the medication the client is taking will prevent suicide. What would be the best response by the nurse?

1. "Clients who take their medication as prescribed are at decreased risk for suicide."
2. "Medication helps to treat an underlying mood disorder associated with suicidal thinking and therefore prevents suicide."
3. "Medication helps decrease the frequency and intensity of suicidal thoughts."
4. "The client has said that she would never try to hurt herself again. There is no need to worry."

10 A suicidal client with low self-esteem seems less lethargic today and agrees to participate in an occupational therapy program. To help make the session successful, the nurse should take which action?

1. Introduce the client to wood carving; show him how to safely use the carving and burning tools.
2. Stay away from the client in occupational therapy so that he is free to express himself.
3. Teach the client to macramé a plant hanger from jute rope and encourage him to work on it later in his room.
4. Structure his activity to help him complete one simple task, such as painting a picture.

11 A client has recently been admitted for depression and suicidal ideations with a plan to hang himself. The nurse monitors the client most carefully for risk for attempting suicide at which time?

1. When the client is silent and unlikely to tell anyone
2. When the client is ready to go home and afraid of leaving the hospital
3. When the client's family goes on vacation
4. When the client begins to demonstrate clinical improvement

12 A client states that voices are telling him to hang himself. The nurse documents that the client is at risk for suicide on the basis of which of the following?

1. An intractable sense of hopelessness
2. Intolerable emotional pain
3. Delusions of grandeur
4. Command hallucinations

13 Which statement made by a client would indicate the highest risk for suicide?

1. "I know you've been worried about me. You won't have to worry too much longer."
2. "I think I've found a solution to my problem. I'm going to check it out with my doctor."
3. "I'm looking forward to the holiday season and the kids coming home from school. They will be a good distraction."
4. "Over the past week I have been hearing the voices that tell me to hurt myself less often."

14 A client who became violent on the psychiatric unit had restraints applied at 0800. The nurse makes a note to release the restraints at no later than what time per protocol? Record your answer as a number using military time.

Fill in your answer below:

Answer: ______________

15 A female client has been admitted to the psychiatric unit after spending 24 hours in the intensive care unit. Before the client's admission, she overdosed on 12 sertraline (Zoloft) tablets. Of the following nursing interventions, which would be a priority on admission?

1. Assuring the client that someone is concerned about her
2. Protecting the client until she can protect herself
3. Teaching the client how to solve problems
4. Discussing the meaning of death

16 When interviewing a potentially violent or aggressive client, which environmental factor is most important for the nurse to consider?

1. The interview should take place in a calm and quiet area to reduce stimuli.
2. Care should be taken to make sure that other staff does not interrupt.
3. Restraint devices should be in full view of the client to reinforce consequences for violent behavior.
4. The client should be told that violent behavior will not be tolerated.

17 A 19-year-old female client, recently admitted after attempting suicide, becomes very dejected and states that life has no meaning and no one cares what happens to her. What is the nurse's best response?

1. "Of course people care. Your parents stayed with you in the ICU."
2. "Let's not talk about sad things. Why don't we go for a walk?"
3. "Can you write down a list of who does not care for you?"
4. "I care about you, and I am concerned that you feel so down."

18 When the nurse is interviewing a potentially violent or aggressive client, which factor is most important?

1. Initiate the interview with a firm handshake.
2. Conduct the interview in a large public area of the unit.
3. Conduct the interview in a calm quiet area.
4. Precede the interview with a statement that violent behavior will not be tolerated.

19 The client is hospitalized following an unsuccessful suicidal attempt by drug overdose. When offered a no-harm contract by the nurse, the client says, "I don't think I can agree to that." Which nursing intervention is most appropriate?

1. Visual observation of the client every 15 minutes, during both day and night
2. Constant visual observation of the client, including when in the bathroom
3. Constant visual observation of the client, remaining at arm's length at all times
4. Constant visual observation at all times during waking hours

ANSWERS & RATIONALES

1 **Answer: 2** **Rationale:** Clients need to have communicated to them that they are in control of their own behaviors and that "acting out" will result in consequences. Reassuring the client that the staff will make sure nothing happens takes away responsibility from the client. Just explaining that violence is unacceptable without explaining to the client that he or she is in control is nontherapeutic. Acting out is usually not allowed because of the risks to the safety of the client and others. **Cognitive Level:** Applying **Client Need:** Psychosocial Integrity **Integrated Process:** Nursing Process: Implementation **Content Area:** Mental Health **Strategy:** The core issue of the question is effective communication with a client at risk for acting out. Use the process of elimination and choose the option that provides accurate information to the client and holds the client accountable for his or her actions.

2 **Answer: 4** **Rationale:** Preventing a client from free mobility, such as the use of restraints, is the most restrictive technique. Meeting in a quiet room is the least restrictive and most therapeutic. Chemical restraint with medication is restrictive but less so than full four-point restraints. Escorting a client is restrictive but less so than full four-point restraints. **Cognitive Level:** Analyzing **Client Need:** Psychosocial Integrity **Integrated Process:** Nursing Process: Implementation **Content Area:** Mental Health **Strategy:** Note the critical word *most* in the stem of the question. This tells you that ordering the interventions presented from least restrictive to most restrictive will assist you to choose correctly.

3 **Answer: 1** **Rationale:** Once a client has escalated beyond least restrictive interventions, the nurse should plan for the next step. Bargaining with a client is counterproductive and positively reinforces behavior. Offering a PRN medication to reduce anxiety would occur after negotiation for least restrictive interventions is complete. Asking a client to take a time out is a least restrictive intervention to which the client is not responding. **Cognitive Level:** Applying **Client Need:** Psychosocial Integrity **Integrated Process:** Nursing Process: Implementation **Content Area:** Mental Health **Strategy:** The wording of the question tells you that more than one option may be partially or totally correct and that you must prioritize your answer. Choose the option that best protects the safety of all people in the environment, including other clients and staff.

4 **Answer: 2** **Rationale:** Debriefing allows the staff an opportunity to ventilate feelings and to calm down. It should always occur, and should be done as soon as possible after the client and all others are safe. All staff should be encouraged to participate. **Cognitive Level:** Applying **Client Need:** Psychosocial Integrity **Integrated Process:** Nursing Process: Evaluation **Content Area:** Mental Health **Strategy:** The core issue of the question is the need for staff to process personal feelings after an episode of violence occurs with a client. Use the process of elimination and knowledge that staff can be traumatized by these events to choose the correct option.

5 **Answer: 2** **Rationale:** A situational crisis is one that occurs from external life events, such as being involved in a severe motor vehicle accident. An event involving normal stages of development (such as aging) is a maturational crisis. A natural disaster such as a flood is an example of a community crisis. An armed conflict is an example of a community crisis. **Cognitive Level:** Analyzing **Client Need:** Psychosocial Integrity **Integrated Process:** Nursing Process: Data Collection **Content Area:** Mental Health **Strategy:** Use the process of elimination. The core issue of the question is the ability to differentiate among various types of crises (maturational, situational, and community) and to document them appropriately.

6 **Answer: 2** **Rationale:** Assisting the client to identify coping patterns and then supporting them is essential to managing a crisis. Identifying the client's maladaptive coping mechanisms may be beneficial after identifying the client's strengths. Assisting the client to forget is not a therapeutic intervention for crisis management. Teaching a client to handle future crises is more appropriate once the current crisis has abated. **Cognitive Level:** Applying **Client Need:** Psychosocial Integrity **Integrated Process:** Nursing Process: Implementation **Content Area:** Mental Health **Strategy:** The critical words in the question are *at this time*. This tells you that more than one option may be correct, but one of them is timelier than the others. Use nursing knowledge and the process of elimination to make a selection.

7 **Answer: 1, 5** **Rationale:** Providing support and guidance are the primary objectives of crisis management. The client's anxiety may be needed in order for him or her to be energized to cope with the crisis; the goal is to achieve a manageable level of anxiety. Providing encouragement and fostering independence are important and may occur during crisis intervention, but they are not the primary tasks of crisis management. **Cognitive Level:** Understanding **Client Need:** Psychosocial Integrity **Integrated Process:** Nursing Process: Planning **Content Area:** Mental Health **Strategy:** The critical word in the question is *primary*. This tells you that more than one option may be correct, but some of them are more important than the others. Use nursing knowledge and the process of elimination to make a selection.

8 **Answer: 3** **Rationale:** A short-acting anti-anxiety agent such as lorazepam is most useful in helping a client to achieve an effective reduction in level of anxiety. Antipsychotics such as haloperidol are not helpful and should be avoided. An antidepressant such as amitriptyline requires some time to achieve therapeutic levels and is not useful in a crisis situation. Mood stabilizers such as valproic acid are not indicated. **Cognitive Level:** Applying **Client Need:** Psychosocial Integrity **Integrated Process:** Nursing Process: Planning **Content Area:** Mental Health **Strategy:** The critical words in the question are *crisis situation*, which tell you that the correct answer is a medication that has a rapid onset of action and will be effective in treating the client's reaction to the diagnosis. Use nursing knowledge and the process of elimination to make a selection.

9 **Answer: 3** **Rationale:** Medications will help decrease the frequency and intensity of suicidal thoughts. Medication does not prevent suicide; in fact, many times when clients regain their energy from medications, they are at an increased risk for completing suicide. Medication may treat the underlying cause of the suicidal ideation but does not necessarily reduce the risk for completing suicide. A client may not be currently suicidal according to self-reports, but medications do not assure that they will not be suicidal in the future. **Cognitive Level:** Applying **Client Need:** Psychosocial Integrity

Integrated Process: Communication and Documentation **Content Area:** Mental Health **Strategy:** The critical word in the question is *best*. This tells you that more than one option may be partially correct, but one of them is better than the others. Use nursing knowledge and the process of elimination to make a selection.

10 **Answer: 4 Rationale:** A client who is just regaining his or her energy should be encouraged to do simple tasks, which will also promote the client's self-esteem. Suicidal clients are most at danger when they are feeling better and regaining their energy. Introducing the client to wood carving places the client at risk for self-harm. The nurse should encourage the client participate in the occupational therapy for self-expression. Teaching the client how to make a plant hanger from jute rope places the client at risk for self-harm. **Cognitive Level:** Analyzing **Client Need:** Psychosocial Integrity **Integrated Process:** Nursing Process: Implementation **Content Area:** Mental Health **Strategy:** The core issue of the question is a safe activity for a client who is suicidal. The correct answer is the option that does not pose risk to the client or provide the client with the means to engage in self-harm.

11 **Answer: 4 Rationale:** Suicidal clients are at most risk when they begin to demonstrate improvement and have the energy to carry out suicide. A silent client who is not willing to share with others is at risk for suicide but may be placed on constant observation. Being afraid to go home may be a positive sign that the client is aware of the danger he or she may pose to him- or herself. Vacation is a stressful time, and being left alone would place the client at risk; however, it is well documented that clients are at greatest risk when showing signs of improvement. **Cognitive Level:** Applying **Client Need:** Psychosocial Integrity **Integrated Process:** Nursing Process: Planning **Content Area:** Mental Health **Strategy:** The core issue of the question is recognition that the risk of suicide increases when a client begins to feel better, since the client now may have the energy to carry out a suicide attempt. Use the process of elimination and this knowledge to make a selection. The wording of the question tells you that only one answer is correct.

12 **Answer: 4 Rationale:** Voices telling a client to hurt himself or others are called *command hallucinations*. There is not enough data to support hopelessness, emotional pain, or delusions of grandeur. **Cognitive Level:** Applying **Client Need:** Psychosocial Integrity **Integrated Process:** Communication and Documentation **Content Area:** Mental Health **Strategy:** The core issue of the question is correct interpretation of a client's symptoms. The wording of the question tells you only one answer is correct. Use nursing knowledge and the process of elimination to make a selection.

13 **Answer: 1 Rationale:** The client is communicating that he or she may not be around for the nurse to worry about. Being able to find a solution, expressing hope for the future and making plans, and decreasing frequency of voices indicate that the client is experiencing a reduction in the risk for suicide. **Cognitive Level:** Analyzing **Client Need:** Psychosocial Integrity **Integrated Process:** Nursing Process: Evaluation **Content Area:** Mental Health **Strategy:** The critical words in the stem of the question are *highest risk*. This tells you that more than one option may indicate risk, but one is stronger than the others. Use nursing knowledge and the process of elimination to make a selection.

14 **Answer: 1000 Rationale:** Releasing restraints at least every 2 hours is a standard of care to prevent physical harm. In addition to this intervention, the client's circulation should be checked at least every 30 minutes. Ensuring the client's safety and well-being is of high priority. **Cognitive Level:** Applying **Client Need:** Safety and Infection Control **Integrated Process:** Nursing Process: Planning **Content Area:** Mental Health **Strategy:** The core issue of the question is knowledge of safe care for a client who is in restraints. Use nursing knowledge to formulate an answer, recalling that 2-hour release times are a standard of care.

15 **Answer: 2 Rationale:** Safety of the client is always a priority for clients who have recently attempted suicide. The remaining goals are appropriate after safety has been assured. **Cognitive Level:** Analyzing **Client Need:** Psychosocial Integrity **Integrated Process:** Nursing Process: Planning **Content Area:** Mental Health **Strategy:** The critical word in the stem of the question is *priority*. This indicates that more than one or all options may be correct actions for the client, but one is more important than the others. To aid in making a selection, recall that safety needs are high priority for clients following a suicide attempt.

16 **Answer: 1 Rationale:** The nurse should ensure that the interview be conducted in a quiet environment. Interruption should be kept to a minimum, but may not be possible to prevent. Intimidation of the client either verbally or visually with restraints is inappropriate. **Cognitive Level:** Applying **Client Need:** Psychosocial Integrity **Integrated Process:** Nursing Process: Implementation **Content Area:** Mental Health **Strategy:** The critical words in the stem of the question are *most important.* This is a clue that more than one option may be partially or totally correct, but one is more important than the others. Use nursing knowledge and the process of elimination to make a selection.

17 **Answer: 4 Rationale:** Stating "I care about you..." provides the client with information that the nurse is concerned about her, which may ease her emotional pain. Telling the client, "Of course people care" is false reassurance. Telling the client not to talk about sad things invalidates and ignores the client's feelings. Asking the client to write information may be seeking clarification but may also cause the client to feel she has to defend her position. **Cognitive Level:** Analyzing **Client Need:** Psychosocial Integrity **Integrated Process:** Communication and Documentation **Content Area:** Mental Health **Strategy:** The core issue of the question is a therapeutic communication technique to use with a client who attempted suicide and is experiencing emotional pain. Use knowledge of therapeutic communication techniques and the process of elimination to make a selection.

18 **Answer: 3 Rationale:** The interview should be conducted in a nonpublic, quiet area in order to reduce stimuli. A potentially aggressive client is hypervigilant, distractible, and over reactive. At the same time, the nurse needs to be aware of own safety as well. The potentially violent person is likely to perceive an extended hand, or the touch associated with it, as a threatening gesture and/or act of aggression. Touch of any type should be avoided or used very cautiously with aggression prone clients. Large public areas of a unit are designed for use by groups of clients and staff. In such a setting, people come and go freely, and these kinds of interruptions and distractions are likely to further agitate the client. This client, who is hyperresponsive and suspicious of the motives of others, is likely to interpret this as a statement of threat. **Cognitive Level:** Applying **Client Need:** Safety and Infection Control **Integrated Process:** Nursing

Process: Planning **Content Area:** Mental Health **Strategy:** Remember that agitated and potentially violent persons are hyperresponsive to the environment and will respond aggressively to events that others would not notice or would not consider bothersome.

19 **Answer: 2 Rationale:** Providing safety and preventing violence on an inpatient unit involves one-to-one supervision for the client as warranted, based on an assessment of current lethality level. This client did not make a commitment to the no-harm contract, so the nurse should consider that the risk for self-harm is still present. (The nurse should be aware of the suicide protocol in the employing agency. In some situations, this client might be placed on a different level of suicidal precautions.) **Cognitive Level:** Analyzing **Client Need:** Safety and Infection Control **Integrated Process:** Nursing Process: Implementation **Content Area:** Mental Health **Strategy:** Notice the client's hesitance and indefiniteness in not contracting. Recognize that as an indicator of continuing suicidal risk.

Key Terms to Review

coping p. 318
crisis p. 318
equilibrium p. 318
helplessness p. 318
hopelessness p. 318
suicide p. 321

References

Fontaine, K. (2009). *Mental health nursing* (6th ed.). Upper Saddle River, NJ: Pearson Education.

Kniesl, C., Wilson, H., & Trigoboff, E. (2009). *Contemporary psychiatric-mental health nursing* (2nd ed.). Upper Saddle River, NJ: Pearson Education.

Stuart, G. (2009). *Principles and practice of psychiatric nursing* (9th ed.). St. Louis: Elsevier Science.

Townsend, M. (2010). *Essentials of psychiatric mental health nursing: Concepts of care in evidence-based practice* (5th ed.). Philadelphia: F.A. Davis.

Varcarolis, E., & Halter, M. (2010). *Foundations of psychiatric mental health nursing: A clinical approach* (6th ed.). Philadelphia: Saunders.

Test Yourself

Are you ready for the NCLEX-PN® or course exams? Use the practice tests on the companion website to check.

End-of-Life Care 24

In this chapter

Cross Reference

Other chapters related to this content are

Coping with Stressors Chapter 20

I. GENERAL NEEDS NEAR END OF LIFE

A. There is no typical death

B. Quality end of life

1. Positive experience for client and family with accomplishment of personal goals, even with suffering and loss
2. Caregiver-led client advocacy with a meaningful and dignified death

NCLEX®

C. Core principles guiding clinical policy and professional practice for end-of-life care

1. Respect dignity of both client and caregivers
2. Be sensitive to and respectful of client's and family's wishes
3. Use most appropriate measures that are consistent with client's choices
4. Make alleviation of pain and other physical symptoms (palliation) a high priority
5. Assist with management of psychological, social, and spiritual or religious problems
6. Offer continuity (client should be able to continue to be cared for, if so desired, by his or her primary care and specialist providers)
7. Provide access to any therapy that may realistically be expected to improve client's quality of life, including alternative or nontraditional treatments; ensure clients are not abandoned because of their choice
8. Provide access to palliative care and hospice care
9. Respect right to refuse treatment, as expressed by client or authorized surrogate
10. Respect health care provider's professional judgment and recommendations with consideration for both client and family preferences
11. Recognize that dying is a profoundly personal experience and part of life cycle
12. Encourage health care professionals to help ensure that care environment provides quality care and accountability for performance

D. Issues of policy, ethics, and law

1. Ethical issues are influenced by personal values, religion, and culture
2. Principles of autonomy, privacy, and **veracity** (truthfulness) are foundational to nursing practice
3. **Beneficence**, **nonmaleficence**, and **justice** are basic ethical principles for end-of-life care; beneficence is ethical principle of doing good; nonmaleficence means "first, do no harm"; and justice is being fair
4. Client preferences or **advance directives (AD)** are based on the 1990 Patient Self-Determination Act that directs agencies receiving Medicare and Medicaid to provide information about ADs; ADs allow clients to make decisions in advance about end-of-life care should they become unable to communicate their desires

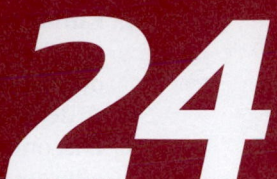

5. **Euthanasia** is a controversial intervention that offers a deliberate end to life for persons with a terminal illness or intolerable suffering; the Code for Nurses and American Nurses Association's position statements indicate nurses should not participate in euthanasia
6. A decision to withdraw food and fluids allows disease to progress to its natural end
7. Discontinuing life support is a difficult decision for health care providers because they have been educated to support life in all situations
8. Professional standards and guidelines have been developed and approved by American Nurses Association, the Hospice and Palliative Nurses Association, and National Hospice and Palliative Care Organization to guide end-of-life practices
9. Confidentiality allows client to feel secure in safely discussing sensitive matters regarding health care without fearing disclosure

II. PHYSIOLOGICAL CARE NEAR END OF LIFE

A. *Palliative care* focuses on assessing and treating symptoms while evaluating whether to deal with cause; palliative care is care of client whose disease is no longer responsive to curative treatment

B. Symptom management is important at end of life; nurses should focus on interventions that promote client advocacy, assess client needs, provide pharmacologic and nonpharmacologic treatments, and educate client and family

NCLEX®
1. Fatigue
   a. A subjective symptom that may be disease related or may be psychological and/or treatment related
   b. Treatment of disease-related causes, such as anemia, may alleviate fatigue
   c. Fatigue may not be relieved by frequent rest periods, though an exercise program may decrease its severity

NCLEX®
2. Pain
   a. American Nurses Association (2010) upholds nurses' obligation to promote comfort, relief of pain, and provide support for patients, families, and their surrogates when a decision has been made to withhold further life-sustaining treatments
   b. Become comfortable with decision not to limit use of opioids and to provide pain relief without fear of respiratory depression
   c. The usual course of death is for clients to become sleepy but this may not occur in small cohort of clients who experience intractable pain; for these clients, sedation may be only option
   d. Non-verbal signs of pain include grimaces, moans, irritability or withdrawal; carefully monitor for these in noncommunicative clients
3. Depression
   a. Is frequently associated with a terminal illness; may be disease related, treatment related, psychological in origin, or associated with other symptoms such as pain
   b. Include questions to rule out suicide intentions in data collection
   c. Early diagnosis and intervention allow client to accomplish goals associated with a quality end of life
   d. Interventions can include medication therapy

   NCLEX®
   e. Nonpharmacological approaches include life review, grief or psychiatric counseling as appropriate, and encouraging client to draw on previous successful coping mechanisms, such as use of faith
4. Delirium
   a. An acute state of disorientation without drowsiness; commonly accompanied by agitation
   b. Pharmacological treatments may diminish agitation
   c. Minimize stimulation by family or staff and intervene with relaxation or massage therapy
   d. Hydration may also be effective
5. Dyspnea
   a. Occurs frequently

   NCLEX®
   b. Elevate head of bed, provide oxygen as ordered, and teach pursed lip breathing (to keep airways open longer) to possibly alleviate dyspnea
6. Nausea and vomiting
   a. Goal is immediate treatment
   b. Identify underlying cause to adequately control this frustrating symptom dyad

   NCLEX®
   c. Use nonpharmacological measures such as serving meals at room temperature, distraction, and avoiding strong odors

7. Anorexia and cachexia
   a. Anorexia is a loss of appetite; cachexia is a general wasting and lack of nutrition seen with most terminal illnesses
   b. Causes can include symptoms of pain, nausea and vomiting, constipation, and other gastrointestinal (GI) disruptions; metabolic changes due to inflammation and cytokine activity may be contributing factors
   c. Depression and anxiety are also associated with loss of appetite
   d. Treatments such as chemotherapy can cause taste alterations
   e. Pharmacological interventions include appetite stimulants or antiemetics
   f. Alcohol before meals can be a helpful nonpharmacological approach

NCLEX®

   g. If odors are a problem, moving client away from kitchen at mealtimes might stimulate appetite
8. GI alterations
   a. To prevent constipation, encourage client to follow personal bowel regimen; encourage high-fiber intake with adequate fluids and stool softeners
   b. Differentiate between diarrhea caused by fecal impaction (rapid onset) and anal incontinence (twice a day)
   c. Malabsorption is associated with foul-smelling, fatty, pale stools

NCLEX®

   d. Problems with skin integrity occur as circulation to periphery diminishes; encourage very gentle massage with emollients and position change at regular intervals

C. Prognosis

1. Exact time of death cannot be predicted
2. Some individuals instinctively know when it is time to die
3. The type and stage of disease, client's will to live, and wish to wait for a special event, person, or attainment of a goal can extend life
4. Suggested signs and symptoms of dying are a guideline and may occur out of order or may never occur
5. Process of dying is natural with a decline of physical processes and mental abilities; changes can occur in a few minutes or hours or may develop over days or weeks prior to actual death

NCLEX®

D. Physical symptoms of nearing death

1. Changes in neurological function with alteration in level of consciousness, confusion, disorientation, and/or delirium
2. Weakness and fatigue, which are enhanced by decline in food and fluid intake
3. Increased drowsiness and sleeping with diminished reaction
4. Decreased oral intake; it is rare for client to report hunger as death approaches; dehydration can promote comfort of dying client because of these effects:
   a. Increased ketone production, causing sleepiness, euphoria, and decrease in pain with accompanied decreased urinary output
   b. Diminished GI secretions and stimulation, resulting in less nausea and vomiting, abdominal distention, and hunger
   c. Decreased generalized edema and possible shrinkage of edematous layer around tumor if tumor is present
   d. Increased opioid peptide production, causing elevated endorphin levels, producing "natural" analgesia
5. Dehydration, which can also result in concerns for client comfort because of potential for "dry mouth"; feeding (including provision of fluids) is symbolic of nurturing; withholding intake suggests abandonment of client; provision of nutrition and fluid is considered "basic" care
6. Hypernatremia and uremia, resulting in clouding of consciousness
7. Smaller quantities of lung secretions
8. Decreased or lack of swallow reflex
9. Surges of energy
10. Terminal restlessness and/or agitation, which may be due to metabolic alterations near end of life; these need to be distinguished from behavior change caused by untreated symptoms
11. Fever
12. Change in bowel elimination ranging from constipation to diarrhea
13. Incontinence of stool and/or urine

E. Imminent death

1. Monitor for signs and symptoms of imminent death
2. Teach family signs and symptoms so they understand client's impending death (see Box 24–1)

F. Postmortem care of body (see Box 24–2)

Box 24–1

Signs/Symptoms of Imminent Death

- Decreased urine output with darkening and/or colorations such as brown or red
- Drop in body temperature, with cold and mottled extremities
- Vital sign changes, including systolic blood pressure below 70 and diastolic below 50; pulse is weak and difficult to locate
- Respiratory congestion, including respiratory bubbling with breathing pattern changes, with very rapid respirations and/or Cheyne-Stokes respirations
- Glassy eyes that are tearing and half open

Box 24–2

Care of the Body Postmortem

- Close eyes and place dentures in mouth.
- Clean body of mucus, wound drainage, urine, and feces released at time of death.
- Remove external tubing and drains.
- Bathe body and pad any drainage areas.
- Pack anal orifice with gauze.
- Align body with hands folded across chest or lap.
- Pull a sheet up to neck to cover body for viewing and then shroud after family leaves.
- Keep ID band in place; attach two more to toe and outside shroud.
- Document time of death, and deposition of body and belongings.

III. PSYCHOSOCIAL SUPPORT NEAR END OF LIFE

A. Communication with dying clients and families

1. Goals of communication focus on individualized needs of client and family, keeping communication lines open, and ensuring nurse clearly understands expectations of clients, family, and plan developed by partners in care
2. *NCLEX®* Sensitive listening is a communication tool that encompasses mental, emotional, and physical presence of individuals
3. Physical limitations due to age, disease treatment, or progression need to be addressed with sensitivity
4. *NCLEX®* Fear of a variety of death-related issues can create communication barriers at end of life; can be due to lack of experience with topic, unresolved loss, concern about showing emotion or not knowing answers, and even worry that family/caregivers would be held responsible for client's death
5. Truthfulness is an important element when reinforcing bad news previously given by physician; building rapport, planning what to say in understandable terms, and continuously identifying what client wants and needs to know are important nursing activities
6. *NCLEX®* Changes in roles of family members at end of life can cause altered family dynamics; family members may require assistance to work through these issues
7. *NCLEX®* Beliefs about spirituality and organized religions are not necessarily the same; sensitivity to culture, ethnic values, and religion is important when discussing palliative care options or decisions with clients and family members (see Table 24–1)
8. Communication within interdisciplinary team promotes accurate implementation of client's desires and end-of-life goals for care; accomplish this through well-documented medical records and daily communication among multiple team members

B. The dying child

1. End-of-life care provided by pediatric nurse includes working with dying child as well as with siblings, parents, and extended family and friends
2. Some families prefer not to tell a child that she or he has a terminal illness; however, children are often aware even if it is not openly discussed; they are sensitive to subtle changes in how staff and family members interact with them both interpersonally and during physical care
3. *NCLEX®* Respect parents' choices and decision making while assessing opportunities to encourage open communication between parents and child
4. Provide support and caring to client and family without taking away realistic need for hope
5. Be available to listen and talk, even if child chooses not to talk about disease
6. Consider child's developmental and educational level and interact accordingly

Table 24–1 Comparison of Diverse Religious Practices and Beliefs

	Hinduism	Islam	Judaism	Christianity	American Indian	Buddhism
Terminal Care		Do not prolong	Do not prolong	Varies	Traditional healers	
Drugs or blood	May refuse pain meds	Allowed	Allowed	Allowed; Jehovah Witnesses refuse blood	Allowed	May refuse pain meds
DNR/advanced directives	Yes/varies	No/varies	Allowed	Allowed/varies	No/varies	Allowed
Autopsies		Restricted	Restricted		Restricted	
Organ donation			Restricted		Restricted	
Upon death		Family handles body	Burial society prepares body; body not left alone			
Bereavement	Reincarnation	Grief counseling may be intrusive	Active mourning supported	Public grieving	Grief counseling may be intrusive	Restrained
Burial	Cremation	No embalming	No embalming	Cremation or burial	Cremation or burial	Cremation or burial

Adapted from Sheehan, O. K. & Forman, W. B. (2003). *Hospice and palliative care: Concepts and practice.* Sudbury, MA: Jones & Bartlett Publishers, p. 192.

NCLEX®

7. Be aware that a child may let nurse know he or she no longer wants to talk about a topic by walking away, changing subject, shifting posture, or with other verbal or non-verbal cues
8. Understand that nurse's presence can be meaningful to a child and/or parents
9. Encourage all family members to care for child

NCLEX®

10. Siblings often feel left out as parents focus on dying child
    - **a.** Monitor all children in family for acting out, negative behavior, or "perfect child" behavior
    - **b.** Encourage parents to find resources and support people to take siblings to their extracurricular activities
    - **c.** Allow siblings to verbalize feelings in a safe place without feeling as though they are making parents feel worse
11. Encourage a life review by getting family members and friends to discuss meaningful events (birthdays, vacations, anniversaries, and special events)
12. Provide support to other family members, including grandparents, extended families through divorce and remarriage, and classmates

C. The dying older adult

NCLEX®

1. Determine whether client has examined his or her own mortality before learning of impending death; elders may or may not easily accept idea of own death
2. Elders generally have less death anxiety with advancing age
3. Elders may find it easier to face their mortality if they
    - **a.** Philosophically accept what their life had to offer
    - **b.** Have numerous experiences with death, including parents, friends, spouse, or children
    - **c.** Learn to cope with personal losses
    - **d.** Are able to recover emotionally between multiple deaths
    - **e.** Believe death is a part of living
    - **f.** Find support in religious beliefs and concept of life after death
4. Cultural aspects
    - **a.** Many cultures view death and dying differently from the open and blunt Euro-American approach

NCLEX®

    - **b.** From a cultural perspective, it is important to talk with client and family about a designated decision maker, management of pain, and care of body after death (see again Table 24–1)

IV. FAMILY SUPPORT NEAR END OF LIFE

A. Theoretical tasks of grief

1. Models that assist nurses to work with clients and families who are grieving
    - **a.** Psychodynamic models (e.g., Freud) address factors that can complicate grief, such as quality of relationship with deceased or mental health of any affected individuals
    - **b.** Task models (e.g., Lindemann, et al.) identify steps individual must complete to deal with grief

Table 24–2 Theoretical Tasks of Grief

Kubler-Ross (1969)	Parkes (1987)	Bowlby (1980)	Wordon's Tasks (1991)	Rando's Process of Bereavement (1993)
1. Denial 2. Anger 3. Bargaining 4. Depression 5. Acceptance	1. Alarm 2. Searching 3. Mitigation 4. Anger and guilt 5. Gaining a new identity	1. Numbing 2. Searching and longing 3. Disorganization and despair 4. Reorganization	1. Accept reality of the loss 2. Experience the pain of grief 3. Adjust to an environment without the deceased 4. Withdraw emotional energy and reinvest in another relationship	1. Recognize the loss and death 2. React to, experience, and express the separation and pain 3. Reminisce 4. Relinquish old attachments 5. Readjust and adapt to the new role while maintaining memories, and form a new identity 6. Reinvest

Source: Adapted with permission of Oncology Nursing Society from Brown-Satlzman, K. (1998). *Transforming the grief process.* In R. Carroll-Johnson, L. Gorman, and N. J. Bush (Eds.), *Psychosocial nursing care: Along the cancer continuum.* Pittsburgh, PA: Oncology Nursing Press.

c. Stage models (Kubler-Ross) and family function models (Kissanne, et al.) suggest grief occurs within individuals and their families

d. Table 24–2 summarizes additional models of grief work

NCLEX®

B. Data collection regarding grief

1. Distinguish between **loss**, **grief**, **mourning**, and **bereavement** and relevant social, cultural, and religious characteristics; loss is absence of a possession or future possession; grief is emotional response to loss; mourning is external behaviors, rituals, and traditions; bereavement is a combination of grief and mourning
2. Differentiate between anticipatory, normal, complicated, and disenfranchised grief
3. Identify grief reactions, including stage, task, and factors affecting grieving process
4. Perform careful review of caregiver survivor to determine if he or she is maintaining nutritional status and self-care, sleeping, able to work, and sustaining family roles and social networks

C. Interventions and resources

1. Working with dying clients may require nurse to move through five stages of adaptation: intellectualization, emotional survival, depression, emotional arrival, and deep compassion
2. Education in end-of-life care provides nurse with tools to deliver competent and nurturing care to dying client and his or her family
3. Formal support systems need to be available to nurse for safe expression of feelings; these can include postclinical debriefing and ceremonies or programs that enable acknowledgment and expression of grief

D. Diagnosis of staff grief

1. Multiple losses within a brief period of time put staff at risk for "bereavement overload" and dysfunctional grieving
2. Focusing on only physical needs and care of clients, avoiding emotion-laden conversations, or talking only about topics of comfort are indications a nurse may be experiencing **death anxiety** (being overcome with fears about death)
3. Awareness of feelings, responses, and reactions to death allows a nurse to provide sensitive care to clients and families

Check Your NCLEX–PN® I.Q. *You are ready for testing on this content if you can*

- Monitor the physiological status of a dying client.
- Provide effective physical, psychological, and spiritual support; teaching; and nursing care to a dying client and his or her family members.
- Identify how culture impacts end-of-life care.
- Differentiate between the needs of the dying child and the dying adult.

PRACTICE TEST

1 While the nurse is discussing a client's likely death with family members, one of the adult children asks, "We plan on taking turns being here for now, but we all want to be here at the time of mother's death. Is there any way we can tell when that time is close?" What is the nurse's best response?

1. "Often, people become lucid for about 15 minutes during the last hour before death. Watch for your mother to become more alert with clearer eyes, focus on faces, and clear her throat. Call the others in at that time."
2. "I wish I could tell you that there was a way to know. It could be minutes from now or another 3 days. One just never knows."
3. "The arms and legs become more bluish in color and are cool to touch. Breathing becomes irregular and shallow and will change speed. Call me if you hear mucus in the throat. The pulse and blood pressure will decrease."
4. "You can expect muscles to become rigid, with staring eyes and mouth closed. The head is pulled back with neck rigidity. Don't be alarmed when you hear a death rattle in the throat."

2 A 90-year-old client expresses a wish to die at home after being told that an esophageal stricture prevents swallowing. The client refuses a feeding tube. The family fully supports this decision. What would be the most appropriate resource for the nurse to call?

1. Hospice care
2. The rabbi
3. An attorney
4. The medical examiner's office

3 The nurse is providing postmortem care for a client. Which intervention would be appropriate prior to allowing the family to visit? Select all that apply.

1. Prepare the body to look as clean and natural as possible.
2. Keep the sheet over the client's face until the family is comfortably seated in the room.
3. Wear sterile gloves to pack the anal canal with gauze.
4. Remove the external tubes and drains.
5. Call the physician to verify the time of death before taking the body to the morgue.

4 A dying client's spouse is afraid to leave the client's room to eat in the cafeteria for fear the client will die while she is gone. No other family members or visitors are present. The client is nonresponsive, his pulse is irregular and bradycardic, and he has Cheyne-Stokes respirations. What is the best course of action for the nurse?

1. Encourage the spouse to take a break and go eat in the cafeteria. The client is nonresponsive and will not know she is gone.
2. Make arrangements for the spouse to receive a meal in the client's room.
3. Tell the spouse she will be called if any changes occur and ask a nurse aide to sit with the client while the wife is out of the room.
4. Do not interfere with the spouse's decision.

5 The family of a client diagnosed with terminal cancer has been informed the client is not expected to live more than 2 months. Which statement made by a family member indicates to the nurse that the family understands the client's prognosis?

1. "Hospice nurses are going to help care for him at home until he gets better."
2. "Hospice nurses are going to help care for him until we learn how to provide the care."
3. "Hospice nurses are going to help care for him until he can take care of himself."
4. "Hospice nurses are going to help care for him to make him more comfortable."

6 The nurse anticipates that which client newly diagnosed with a terminal illness is least likely to have difficulty facing his or her mortality?

1. A 71-year-old female whose grandson, sister, and best friend died over the past 6 months
2. A 59-year-old male who never married, is an only child, and lives with his parents, both of whom are healthy
3. A 70-year-old male who has planned his funeral and enjoys riding his motorcycle at high speeds in rural areas
4. A 68-year-old female who is an atheist

PRACTICE TEST

7 A client with terminal lung cancer is receiving total brain radiation therapy to control hand tremors due to multiple metastatic lesions. As the nurse assists him to his wheelchair he says, "I'm hoping this treatment will let me see my first tomatoes on the Fourth of July. It makes me want to cry to think I won't make it 'til then." According to Kübler-Ross, this statement contains elements of which stage of death and dying? Select all that apply.

1. Denial
2. Bargaining
3. Anger
4. Depression
5. Acceptance

8 The licensed practical/vocational nurse (LPN/LVN) would intervene after hearing an unlicensed assistant make which statement regarding a client with severe arthritis who is also newly diagnosed as being terminally ill with a rapidly growing colorectal cancer?

1. "Even though it hurts a bit, your arthritic joints will become less stiff with gentle exercise."
2. "If we give more pain medication, will it stop his breathing?"
3. "He has a living will that says he does not want to be resuscitated."
4. "You have on a diaper so it's OK if you do not make it to the bathroom."

9 The nurse is speaking with a client who is grieving his father's death. Based on Rando's process of bereavement, in what order would the nurse expect a client to make the following statements as he moves through the bereavement process? Place the options in the correct order. All options must be used.

1. "This is the second anniversary of my father's death."
2. "My father was an alcoholic, so every Christmas I make certain that local AA groups have coffee and chocolates to help the members through the holidays."
3. "It was so much fun to rummage through the antique stores together."
4. "It's too difficult to be around his stepfamily, so I visit friends on vacation."
5. "The homestead has run down since his death. It was hard to drive past and see the lack of care in his vegetable garden."

10 A 46-year-old female client with a history of head and neck cancer was recently told she has multiple metastatic sites in her lung. The nurse is discussing the situation with the client and her sister. Which statement during the conversation reflects the ethical principle of justice?

1. "The staff will do everything possible to make your sister comfortable while she is in hospice."
2. "She told the doctor she didn't want to lose her hair. It is not right that he coerced her into taking experimental chemotherapy. Now she is bald and dying."
3. "Why did I have to get this terrible disease? I just want my life back."
4. "We've made arrangements for her care at home. Now the doctor says she needs more tests to see if cancer is also in her liver. Why? We know she's dying."

11 A 22-year-old hospitalized client with a recent diagnosis of acquired immunodeficiency syndrome (AIDS) says to the nurse, "The food on this breakfast tray is terrible. Why can't you people do even simple things well?" What is the nurse's best response?

1. "I know you are angry, but I cannot let you make me the object of your anger. I will send up the dietitian."
2. "This is not about breakfast. Tell me what you are really angry about."
3. "I understand you are angry. I'll shut the door and let you cool off."
4. "I hear a lot of anger in your voice that is quite normal and healthy. Do you want a new breakfast or do you want something else?"

12 While talking to adult children of a dying male client, the nurse finds them tearful, with ambivalent feelings toward the client. The client often expresses beliefs of a wasted life. The children say that their father often showed love but followed it with criticism, anger, and emotional abuse. The nurse would suggest which intervention as most likely to be helpful at this time?

1. Listen to relaxation tapes before visiting each other. If negative feelings arise, listen to the tapes together.
2. Have a nurse stay in the room when a family member visits the client so the nurse can intervene with conflict resolution if problems arise.
3. Assure the client and children that what matters is the present and the future, not the past. Encourage the children to spend more time with their father.
4. Videotape each adult child speaking of a time when their father showed love, while the client tells of a special love for each child. Plan a time for them to watch the tape together.

13 A terminally ill client questions the nurse about the difference between a living will and power of attorney. What is the nurse's best response?

1. "A living will allows you to indicate treatments to be omitted, while durable power of attorney legally appoints another to make those decisions on your behalf."
2. "A lawyer carries out a living will, while a designated family member or friend carries out advanced directives."
3. "In a living will, you specify treatments to be carried out if you become unable to make decisions. A durable power of attorney allows you to include both treatments to be carried out and those to be omitted."
4. "The living will indicates when you wish life support to be discontinued, while a durable power of attorney gives that power to someone else."

14 The nurse working with a terminally ill client wishes to support the client's decisions concerning end-of-life care. To do this appropriately, the nurse should do plan to which of the following?

1. Be comfortable in assisting the client with euthanasia when requested to do so.
2. Ask another nurse to provide care if the client has a belief system that differs from own belief system.
3. Respect the client's wishes about death to the extent possible by law.
4. Encourage the client to request a do-not-resuscitate order because of terminal illness.

15 The terminally ill client asks the nurse for information about hospice care. What response by the nurse would be best?

1. "Hospice care is home nursing care provided to terminal cancer clients."
2. "The client qualifies for hospice care at the time of diagnosis with a terminal illness."
3. "The main focus of hospice is to educate the client concerning treatment options and alternatives."
4. "Hospice regards dying as a normal part of life and provides support for a dignified and peaceful death."

16 The nurse recognizes that which behaviors indicate grief resolution in a bereaved client whose husband died a year ago? Select all that apply.

1. Becoming future-oriented when discussing details of everyday life
2. Considering the opinions of the deceased prior to making decisions about everyday life
3. Experiencing occasional waves of grief triggered by pictures or events
4. Sharing stories of good times that the client and her husband shared over the years
5. Being unable to visit places that hold happy memories of times spent with her husband.

17 A client is dying, is in great pain, and refuses anything for relief that alters his sensorium. The nurse checks the psychosocial data part of the medical record, expecting that which religion is likely to be practiced by the client? Select all that apply.

1. Islam
2. Judaism
3. Buddhism
4. Catholicism
5. Hindu

18 Which manifestation indicates to the nurse that the pain of a terminally ill nonverbal client is not well-managed?

1. Crackles in the lungs
2. Hyperactive bowel sounds
3. Unwillingness to eat without assistance
4. Constant restlessness and leg movement

19 The family members of a client dying from heart failure are concerned about making certain their mother is comfortable as she goes through the dying process. Which statement indicates to the nurse that the family understands that lack of fluid and nutrition can promote comfort as a client dies? Select all that apply.

1. "There will be less nausea and vomiting, since gastrointestinal secretions will be decreased."
2. "Natural analgesia from the body's endorphin production will help with pain control."
3. "A dry mouth will not be a problem, even without fluid."
4. "Coughing and mucus production will continue, even after the fluids are discontinued."
5. "Swelling and edema might decrease once we stop giving fluids."

20 Before speaking with a mother who recently placed her newborn baby up for adoption, it is important for the nurse to deal with personal feelings about adoption, grief, and loss. This self-awareness would have which benefit?

1. Prevent the nurse from being personally affected by the client's choice in adoption
2. Prevent the nurse from sharing any personal feelings with the client
3. Assist the nurse to avoid discussing unpleasant feelings with the client
4. Assist the nurse to help the client express grief fully

ANSWERS & RATIONALES

1 **Answer: 3 Rationale:** Peripheral circulation decreases and shifts to vital organs. The vascular system collapses, causing decreasing pulse and blood pressure. The gag reflex is lost, and mucus accumulates in the back of the throat. Respirations decrease in rate and become irregular. Vision is blurred near the time of death. A lucid moment is not a pattern in death. It is difficult to pinpoint the exact time when death will occur, but the imminence of clinical death can be detected. Muscle rigidity typically occurs after death. **Cognitive Level:** Applying **Client Need:** Psychosocial Integrity **Integrated Process:** Teaching and Learning **Content Area:** Mental Health **Strategy:** Note the issue of the question, which is knowledge of impending signs of death. The words *best response* in the question tell you it is a true statement and will be a priority in client care. Choose the option in which all information stated is true.

2 **Answer: 1 Rationale:** Hospice specializes in end-of-life care. A rabbi is an important person during the end of life, but there is not an immediate need to make this call. An attorney or medical examiner is not necessary at this time. **Cognitive Level:** Applying **Client Need:** Psychosocial Integrity **Integrated Process:** Nursing Process: Planning **Content Area:** Mental Health **Strategy:** The core issue is that the client wishes to die at home. Recall that hospice care can be provided in the home at all times. The other options (the attorney, rabbi, or medical examiner) do not address the client's issue, which is 24-hour care in the home at the end of life.

3 **Answer: 1, 4 Rationale:** The body is to be handled with dignity. The body is cleaned and linens are freshened. All external tubes and drains are removed. A sheet is pulled up to cover the client's shoulders. While gloves should be worn during postmortem care, sterility is not an issue. State laws and policies differ regarding the nurse's ability to declare death. Even if a physician is required to declare death, verification of time of death is not required prior to the family being allowed to view the client after death. **Cognitive Level:** Applying **Client Need:** Psychosocial Integrity **Integrated Process:** Nursing Process: Implementation **Content Area:** Fundamentals **Strategy:** Use the process of elimination to identify the options that contain inaccurate information. Recall that if an option contains only partially correct information, then that option is then incorrect.

4 **Answer: 2 Rationale:** Obtaining a meal for the client's spouse while she remains at the bedside demonstrates knowledge of the dying process in addition to compassion and concern for the client and spouse. The signs and symptoms listed indicate death will occur soon and encouraging the spouse to go to the cafeteria to eat does not address the spouse's fear of leaving the client alone. Changes have already occurred that indicate the client is dying and if further changes occur, there may not be time to reach the wife in the cafeteria

before death occurs. Allowing the spouse to stay in the room without assisting in providing nourishment for the spouse demonstrates an absence of caring or compassion. **Cognitive Level:** Applying **Client Need:** Psychosocial Integrity **Integrated Process:** Nursing Process: Implementation **Content Area:** Mental Health **Strategy:** The focus of the question is the signs and symptoms of imminent death of the client and the spouse's desire to be with the client at the time of death. Choose the option that minimizes the spouse's anxiety and also shows support for the spouse.

5 **Answer: 4 Rationale:** Hospice care is provided to those clients who have 6 months or less to live. Hospice nurses are skilled in pain and symptom management as well as in emotional support for dying clients and their families. A client in need of hospice services cannot be expected to "get better." Hospice care does not terminate once families learn to provide care. A client in need of hospice services cannot be expected to resume self-care. **Cognitive Level:** Applying **Client Need:** Psychosocial Integrity **Integrated Process:** Nursing Process: Evaluation **Content Area:** Mental Health **Strategy:** The core issue of the question is knowledge of the purpose and goals of hospice care. The incorrect options indicate that the family expects improvement in the client's condition, which is not realistic.

6 **Answer: 3 Rationale:** People cope better when they accept what their life has had to offer, have previously coped with personal losses, have the time and ability to recover emotionally between multiple deaths, believe that death is a part of living, and have religious beliefs. The 70-year old client who has planned for the future demonstrates the belief that death is part of living. The 71-year old client who lost 3 people in the last 6 months may not cope with terminal illness as well because this client has not had time to recover from multiple losses. The 59-year-old male client shows dependence, having never moved out of the home of his parents, and has not had to cope with the personal loss of parents. The client who is an atheist may have difficulty facing his or her own mortality because individuals with religious beliefs are found to cope better. **Cognitive Level:** Applying **Client Need:** Psychosocial Integrity **Integrated Process:** Nursing Process: Data Collection **Content Area:** Mental Health **Strategy:** The focus of this question is knowledge of how older adults cope with a diagnosis of a life-threatening illness. Using the criteria outlined in the rationale, use the process of elimination to make the correct choice.

7 **Answer: 2, 4 Rationale:** During bargaining, clients "negotiate" to meet a life goal, such as going through radiation to see one more crop of tomatoes bloom. Feelings of sadness evidenced by wanting to cry are consistent with the stage of depression. Denial would be evidenced by a refusal to accept the diagnosis of terminal cancer. There is no evidence in the client's words that he is feeling anger. Acceptance would be shown when the client has come to terms with the illness and anticipated death. **Cognitive Level:** Applying **Client Need:** Psychosocial Integrity **Integrated Process:** Communication and Documentation **Content Area:** Mental Health **Strategy:** This question focuses on Kübler-Ross's five stages of death and dying. Evaluate the content of the client's statements and match them to the stages of death and dying. Note that the wording of the question indicates that more than one option is likely to be correct.

8 **Answer: 4 Rationale:** The statement about wearing a diaper does not treat the client with respect and sensitivity and therefore is an example of maleficence. The RN should intervene after hearing this communication. The statement about joints becoming less stiff with gentle exercise is therapeutic and does not require intervention by the RN. Being worried about the effects of analgesics on respirations shows client advocacy, and does not require the RN to intervene. The statement about the living will indicates client advocacy and does not require the RN to intervene. **Cognitive Level:** Applying **Client Need:** Psychosocial Integrity **Integrated Process:** Caring **Content Area:** Fundamentals **Strategy:** The critical word in the stem of the question is *intervene*, making the correct option the one that is physically or emotionally harmful. Eliminate the helpful options that are therapeutic or demonstrate client advocacy.

9 **Answer: 1, 5, 3, 4, 2 Rationale:** Rando's process of bereavement is to (1) recognize the loss and death, (2) react to experience and express the separation and pain, (3) reminisce, (4) relinquish old attachments, (5) readjust and adapt to the new role while maintaining memories and form a new identity, and (6) reinvest. **Cognitive Level:** Analyzing **Client Need:** Psychosocial Integrity **Integrated Process:** Nursing Process: Evaluation **Content Area:** Mental Health **Strategy:** Remember the Six R's of Rando: recognize, react, reminisce, relinquish, readjust, and reinvest. They all begin with *re* and then the letters *CAMLAI*. A helpful memory aid could be Chocolate Always Makes Lads Act Icky.

10 **Answer: 1 Rationale:** The definition for the ethical principle of justice is "fairness." The statement that the staff will do everything possible to maintain comfort is just and fair. The statement about coercion reflects anger on the part of the family. The statement about getting "this terrible disease" reflects anger on the part of the client. The statement about knowing the client is dying demonstrates a concern that the client will not benefit from such tests, and thus further testing does not uphold beneficence. **Cognitive Level:** Applying **Client Need:** Psychosocial Integrity **Integrated Process:** Communication and Documentation **Content Area:** Fundamentals **Strategy:** The core issue of the question is the ethical principle of justice. Evaluate each statement and eliminate all options that do not reflect a sense of "fairness."

11 **Answer: 4 Rationale:** Anger is a common element to all the theories of grief and stages of dying. It is important to acknowledge the client's anger, help him or her identify the source of the anger, and offer choices or control when possible. It is important to be nonconfrontational, not to take the anger personally, and not to ignore the client's issue. **Cognitive Level:** Applying **Client Need:** Psychosocial Integrity **Integrated Process:** Nursing Process: Implementation **Content Area:** Mental Health **Strategy:** Use the principles of therapeutic communication to answer the question. The correct option is the one that acknowledges the client's anger and helps the client to deal with it, while offering the client choices to maintain some control.

12 **Answer: 4 Rationale:** Open communication with concrete evidence of emotional attachments assists in coping at the end of life. A videotape provides concrete assurance in the presence of the loved ones. Relaxation tapes help with stress reduction but do not help with resolution of problems experienced by the family. Staffing patterns do not permit a nurse to be with one client continually, and families require privacy as well. Assurance that the past no longer matters is an assurance lacking concrete properties. **Cognitive Level:** Applying **Client Need:** Psychosocial Integrity **Integrated Process:** Caring **Content Area:** Mental Health **Strategy:**

Use the process of elimination and address the client in the question. In this case, both the client and the adult children are the affected clients, so the correct option is one that benefits all of them.

13 **Answer: 1 Rationale:** A living will is written by the client and includes desires for use of different types of treatment in case of a life-threatening illness. A durable power of attorney is a legal document designating an individual to make legal decisions if the client is unable to make choices independently. **Cognitive Level:** Applying **Client Need:** Psychosocial Integrity **Integrated Process:** Teaching and Learning **Content Area:** Fundamentals **Strategy:** The core issue of the question is knowledge of a living will. The wording of the question indicates that the correct answer is a true statement. Systematically eliminate options containing incorrect statements.

14 **Answer: 3 Rationale:** To uphold client autonomy, the nurse needs to consider the client's wishes while also acting within the law. Euthanasia constitutes illegal nursing practice in the United States at this time. To act ethically, the nurse should provide care to clients according to need, regardless of belief systems. Clients who are diagnosed with terminal illness may or may not be ready for do-not-resuscitate orders, depending on anticipated life expectancy, quality of current life, and psychosocial variables. **Cognitive Level:** Applying **Client Need:** Psychosocial Integrity **Integrated Process:** Nursing Process: Implementation **Content Area:** Fundamentals **Strategy:** Eliminate options that are illegal, fail to provide unbiased care, or may not consider the client's preference at this time.

15 **Answer: 4 Rationale:** The focus of hospice is improving the quality of life and preserving dignity for the client in death. Hospice care may be provided by nurses, volunteers, or other members of the health care team in a variety of settings. It is available to any client who has a terminal illness with a life expectancy of 6 months or less. **Cognitive Level:** Applying **Client Need:** Psychosocial Integrity **Integrated Process:** Teaching and Learning **Content Area:** Fundamentals **Strategy:** Eliminate incorrect options because they are either less sensitively stated or represent incorrect definitions of hospice and do not accurately reflect the care provided.

16 **Answer: 1, 3, 4 Rationale:** Grief resolution requires letting go of the past and looking forward to the future. The client needs to be able to put the loss in perspective and engage fully and effectively in daily life as an independent person. Having occasional grief triggered by pictures or events is consistent with healthy grief resolution. Being able to share stories of good times indicates healthy grief resolution. If decisions are made in the present only through memories of preferences of the deceased, the client has not let go of the past and grief is not resolving. To be unable to visit one year later places that used to be enjoyed with her spouse indicate inadequate resolution of grief. **Cognitive Level:** Applying **Client Need:** Psychosocial Integrity **Integrated Process:** Nursing Process: Evaluation **Content Area:** Mental Health **Strategy:** The focus of the question is on grief resolution, so eliminate options that do not show resolution one year later. The wording of the question indicates that more than one option is likely to be correct.

17 **Answer: 3, 5 Rationale:** The Hindu and Buddhist religions require that believers are alert and mindful as they leave the life on earth and transcend to their next life. This requirement is not found in Islam, Judaism, or Catholicism. **Cognitive Level:** Applying **Client Need:** Psychosocial Integrity **Integrated Process:** Nursing Process: Planning **Content Area:** Fundamentals **Strategy:** Use the process of elimination. Select the religions that require a state of being *mindful* and *alert* as their faithful transcend from life into death. The wording of the question indicates there is more than one correct answer.

18 **Answer: 4 Rationale:** Constant restlessness and leg movement can be physiological indicators of pain. Crackles in the lungs indicate fluid overload or ineffective pumping action of the heart, but not pain. Hyperactive bowel sounds are more likely a reflection of gastrointestinal status than pain. Unwillingness to eat without assistance could indicate weakness, loneliness, or other factors but is not a manifestation of pain. **Cognitive Level:** Applying **Client Need:** Psychosocial Integrity **Integrated Process:** Nursing Process: Data Collection **Content Area:** Fundamentals **Strategy:** First eliminate lung crackles and bowel sounds, which directly reflect functioning of the cardiopulmonary and gastrointestinal systems, respectively. Choose restlessness and leg movements over unwillingness to eat without assistance, because unwillingness to eat could have psychosocial as well as physiological etiologies.

19 **Answer: 1, 2, 5 Rationale:** Lack of fluids can promote comfort in the dying client by decreasing gastrointestinal and respiratory secretions, reducing fluid accumulation in the peripheral tissues, and stimulating endorphin production. Lack of fluids, however, would contribute to the client's sense of dry mouth. **Cognitive Level:** Applying **Client Need:** Basic Care and Comfort **Integrated Process:** Teaching and Learning **Content Area:** Fundamentals **Strategy:** Consider the possible physiological benefits of lack of fluids to a dying client. Note that the question indicates that more than one option is likely to be correct.

20 **Answer: 4 Rationale:** Self-awareness is a key component of any nurse—client experience. The nurse must be able to examine personal feelings, actions, and reactions to better assist the client in fully expressing his or her own feelings and thoughts and to enhance empathy toward the client. A firm understanding and acceptance of self allows the nurse to acknowledge a client's differences and uniqueness. Trying not be personally affected does not focus on self-awareness. Refraining from sharing feelings not focused on self-awareness. Avoiding discussion of unpleasant feelings does not focus on self-awareness. **Cognitive Level:** Understanding **Client Need:** Health Promotion and Maintenance **Integrated Process:** Caring **Content Area:** Mental Health **Strategy:** Look at what the question is asking, which is, *In what way can self-awareness benefit the nurse?*

Key Terms to Review

advance directives (AD) p. 331
beneficence p. 331
bereavement p. 336
death anxiety p. 336
euthanasia p. 332
grief p. 336
justice p. 331
loss p. 336
mourning p. 336
nonmaleficence p. 331
palliative care p. 332
veracity p. 331

ANSWERS & RATIONALES

References

American Nurses Association. (1994). *Ethics and human rights statement: Active euthanasia.* Retrieved June 24, 2010, from http://www.nursingworld.org/position/ethics/euthanasia.aspx.

Bednash, G., & Ferrell, B. (2000). *End-of-Life Nursing Education Consortium (ELNEC): Faculty Guide; Module 1, Nursing Care at End of Life.* American Association of Colleges of Nursing and City of Hope National Medical Center.

Bednash, G., & Ferrell, B. (2000). *End-of-Life Nursing Education Consortium (ELNEC): Faculty Guide; Module 2, Pain.* American Association of Colleges of Nursing and City of Hope National Medical Center.

Bednash, G., & Ferrell, B. (2000). *End-of-Life Nursing Education Consortium (ELNEC): Faculty Guide; Module 3, Symptom Management.* American Association of Colleges of Nursing and City of Hope National Medical Center.

Bednash, G., & Ferrell, B. (2000). *End-of-Life Nursing Education Consortium (ELNEC): Faculty Guide; Module 4, Ethical/Legal Issues.* American Association of Colleges of Nursing and City of Hope National Medical Center.

Bednash, G., & Ferrell, B. (2000). *End-of-Life Nursing Education Consortium (ELNEC): Faculty Guide; Module 5, Culture.* American Association of Colleges of Nursing and City of Hope National Medical Center.

Bednash, G., & Ferrell, B. (2000). *End-of-Life Nursing Education Consortium (ELNEC): Faculty Guide; Module 9, Preparation and Care for the Time of Death.* American Association of Colleges of Nursing and City of Hope National Medical Center.

Guido, G. (2010). *Nursing care at the end of life.* Upper Saddle River, NJ: Pearson Education, Inc.

Karnes, B. (1986). *Gone from my sight: The dying experience.* New York: Dutton.

Kubler-Ross, E. (1969). *On death and dying.* New York: MacMillan.

Test Yourself

Are you ready for the NCLEX-PN® or course exams? Use the practice tests on the companion website to check.

25 Meeting Nutritional Needs

In this chapter

Cross Reference

Another chapter relevant to this content area is

Common Laboratory Tests **Chapter 42**

I. OVERVIEW OF NUTRIENTS

A. Proteins (macronutrients)

1. Composed of amino acids; required for proper growth and development; provide 4 calories/gram
2. Proteins may be complete, incomplete, or complementary depending on composition of amino acids
3. Essential amino acids cannot by synthesized by body and must be obtained in diet
4. High-quality proteins are found in meat, fish, poultry, eggs, and dairy products
5. Protein is needed for energy, growth, bodily repair, maintenance of fluid and electrolyte balance, and production of enzymes, hormones, and antibodies
6. Adult recommended daily allowance (RDA) for protein is 0.8 grams/kg/day, which correlates to roughly 10% of total calories; additional protein may be needed by infants, children, and pregnant or lactating women
7. Insufficient protein intake can lead to protein energy malnutrition, which is characterized by atrophy and wasting of muscle tissue

B. Carbohydrates (macronutrients)

1. Include starches, sugars (fructose, glucose, lactose, sucrose), and cellulose
2. Provide 4 calories/gram and are a key source of energy
3. Found in fruits, vegetables, milk, and grains
4. Promote normal metabolism, including fat metabolism, and prevent protein from being used for energy (protein sparing)
5. Insufficient intake results in protein and fat being used for energy

C. Fats (macronutrients)

1. Concentrated sources of energy, providing 9 calories/gram
2. Needed for proper absorption of fat-soluble vitamins

3. Stored in body to maintain body warmth and cushion or protect internal organs
4. Sources include animal products, egg yolks, organ meats (including liver), butter, cheeses, and various oils
5. Can be described according to cholesterol content and as saturated, monounsaturated, or polyunsaturated; in general, the more solid the fat, the higher the saturated fat content
6. Can lead to obesity, heart disease, and some cancers if taken in excess of bodily needs
7. Insufficient intake can result in increased risk of infection, skin lesions, amenorrhea, and cold sensitivity (insufficient fat stores)

D. Minerals (micronutrients)

1. Part of bones, cells, and hormones
2. Enhance cellular function and catalyze various bodily processes
3. Widely abundant in foods
4. Major minerals include calcium, sodium, potassium, magnesium, chloride, and phosphorus
5. Trace elements that are also needed include iron, iodine, copper, zinc, selenium, manganese, fluoride, chromium, and molybdenum
6. Mineral intake can also be supplemented, often as part of a multivitamin

E. Vitamins (micronutrients)

1. Classified as water soluble (B and C vitamins), which are easily excreted from body, or fat soluble (vitamins A, D, E, K), which can be stored and cause toxicity if taken to excess
2. Used as catalysts of body functions, coenzymes in metabolic processes, for growth, collagen production, wound healing, hormone synthesis, and vision
3. See Table 25–1 for summary of vitamin functions, food sources, and signs of deficiency or excess states
4. Vitamins can be obtained by diet alone or by supplemented, either with or without minerals

Table 25–1 Overview of Fat- and Water-Soluble Vitamins

Vitamin	Function	Food Sources	Deficiency	Excess
Thiamin (B_1)	Coenzyme	Pork, wheat germ, fortified cereals	Beriberi, Wernicke-Korsakoff syndrome	
Riboflavin (B_2)	Coenzyme	Milk, enriched grains	Ariboflavinosis	
Niacin (B_3)	Coenzyme	Peanuts, legumes, enriched grains	Pellagra (3 Ds: dermatitis, diarrhea, dementia)	Flushing, abnormal blood glucose and liver function
Pantothenic acid (B_5)	Coenzyme	Meat, whole grains	Rash, fatigue	
Pyridoxine (B_6)	Coenzyme	Pork, organ meats, whole grains, wheat germ	Nutritional anemia	
Cobalamin (B_{12})	Coenzyme	Animal protein	Pernicious anemia	
Folic acid	Coenzyme	Orange juice, meat, leafy green vegetables	Nutritional anemia, neural tube defects	
Biotin	Coenzyme	Egg yolks, liver	Dermatitis	
Ascorbic acid (vitamin C)	Antioxidant, wound healing, hormone synthesis	Citrus fruits	Scurvy, bleeding gums	
Vitamin A	Vision, bone and tissue growth, immune and reproductive function	Animal foods, fruits, vegetables, fortified milk	Night blindness, xerophthalmia	Toxicity can result
Vitamin D	Calcium and phosphorus metabolism, PTH, kidney	Dairy products, fortified food sources	Rickets, osteomalacia	Toxicity can result
Vitamin E	Antioxidant, immune function	Vegetable oil, peanuts, margarine	Hemolysis of RBCs	May interfere with vitamin K activity
Vitamin K	Blood clotting	Liver, and through intestinal synthesis	Hemorrhagic disease of the newborn, hemorrhage	Toxicity can result

II. GENERAL DIETARY GUIDELINES

NCLEX®

A. Characteristics of healthy diet (U.S. Department of Agriculture [USDA] and U.S. Department of Health and Human Services [USDHHS])

1. Emphasizes fruits, vegetables, whole grains, and fat-free or low-fat milk and milk products
2. Includes lean meats, poultry, fish, beans, eggs, and nuts
3. Is low in saturated fats, *trans* fats, cholesterol, salt (sodium), and added sugars

B. Individualized food guidance system: MyPyramid Plan (USDA)

1. A computer-generated, individualized daily food intake plan that considers age, gender, and physical activity (< 30 minutes, 30–60 minutes, or > 60 minutes/day); see Figure 25–1
2. Components
   a. Grains: all foods made from wheat, rice, oats, cornmeal, and barley, such as bread, pasta, oatmeal, breakfast cereal, tortillas, and grits
   b. Vegetables: all fresh, frozen, dried, or canned vegetables or vegetable juices
   c. Fruits: all fresh, frozen, dried, or canned fruits or fruit juices
   d. Milk: all fluid milk products and foods made from milk that retain calcium content (yogurt and cheese, but not cream cheese, cream, or butter, which do not have significant calcium content)
   e. Meats and beans: lean meat, poultry, fish, eggs, peanut butter, beans, nuts, and seeds

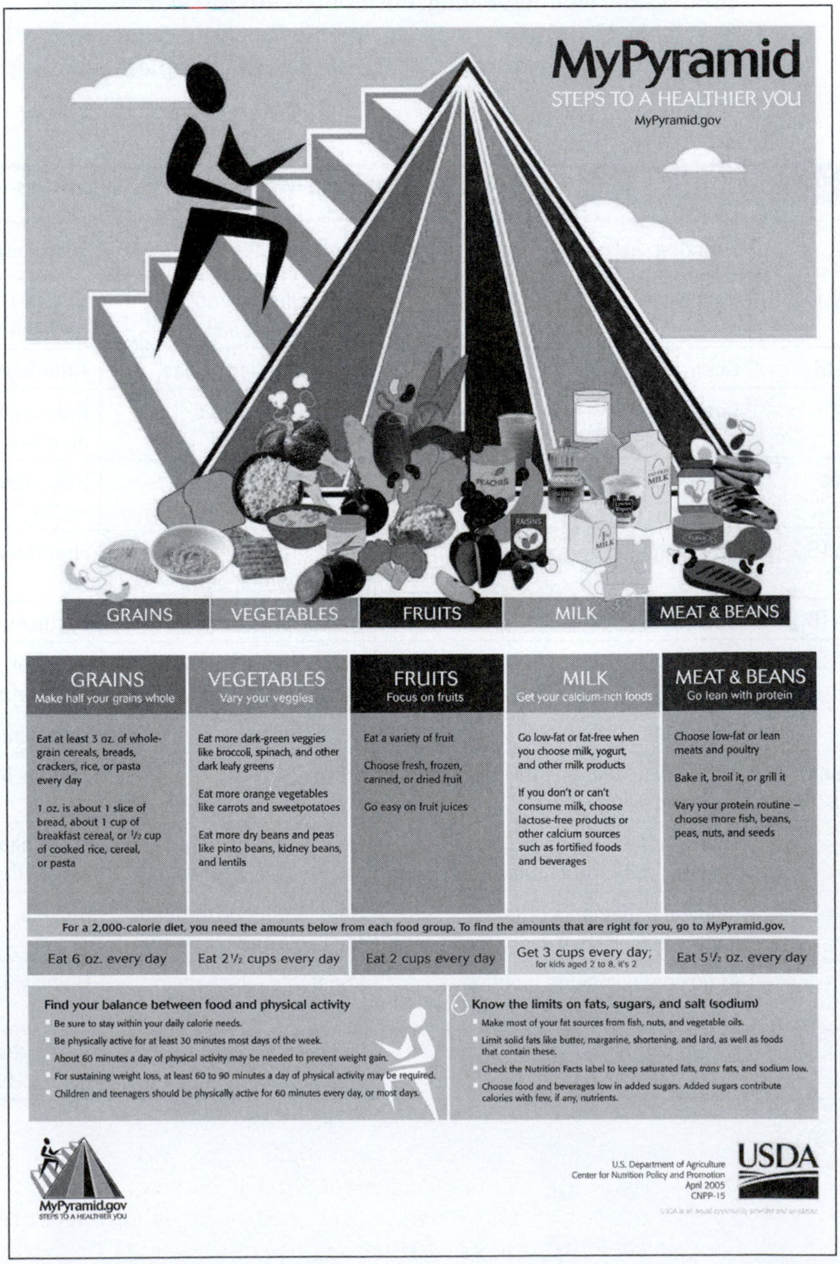

Figure 25–1

MyPyramid Plan replaces the Food Guide Pyramid for diet selection. Color bands from left to right indicate grains, vegetables, fruits, fats, milk, and meat and beans. Staircase emphasizes role of physical activity in health.

Source: USDA. Online: http://www.mypyramid.gov. Accessed 01/12/11.

C. Key recommendations for general public from *Dietary Guidelines for Americans 2010* (USDA & USDHHS, www.health.gov/dietaryguidelines/dga2010/DietaryGuidelines2010.pdf)

1. Adequate nutrients within calorie needs
   - **a.** Consume a variety of nutrient-dense foods and beverages from basic food groups while limiting intake of saturated and trans fats, cholesterol, added sugars, salt, and alcohol
   - **b.** Choose foods providing more potassium, dietary fiber, calcium, and vitamin D (nutrients of concern in American diets); such foods include vegetables, fruits, whole grains, and milk and milk products
   - **c.** Adopt a balanced eating pattern, such as the USDA MyPyramid or the Dietary Approaches to Stop Hypertension (DASH) eating plan

NCLEX®

2. Weight management
   - **a.** Control total calorie intake to manage body weight
   - **b.** Increase physical activity and reduce time spent in sedentary behaviors

NCLEX®

3. Food groups to encourage
   - **a.** Increase fruits and vegetables while staying within energy needs (e.g., 2 cups of fruit and 2½ cups of vegetables daily are recommended for a reference 2000-calorie intake, adjusting to higher or lower amounts as needed)
   - **b.** Eat a variety of fruits and vegetables (especially dark-green, red, and orange vegetables, as well as beans and peas)
   - **c.** Eat three or more ounce-equivalents of whole-grain products per day; at least one-half of grains should come from whole grains by replacing refined grains with whole grains
   - **d.** Choose a variety of protein foods (seafood, lean meat and poultry, eggs, beans and peas, soy products, unsalted nuts and seeds)
   - **e.** Increase amount and variety of seafood consumed by choosing seafood in place of some meat and poultry
   - **f.** Drink 3 cups daily of fat-free or low-fat milk or equivalent milk products, such as yogurt, cheese, or fortified soy beverages
4. Fats
   - *NCLEX®* **a.** Consume less than 10% of calories from saturated fat and less than 300 mg/day of cholesterol, and keep trans fatty acid consumption as low as possible by limiting foods containing synthetic sources of trans fats, such as partially hydrogenated oils, and by limiting other solid fats
   - *NCLEX®* **b.** Keep total fat intake 20–35% of calories, with most fats coming from polyunsaturated and monounsaturated fatty acids, such as in fish, nuts, and vegetable oils
   - **c.** When selecting and preparing meat, poultry, dry beans, and milk or milk products, make choices that are lean, low-fat, or fat-free
5. Carbohydrates (CHOs)
   - **a.** Eat fiber-rich fruits, vegetables, and whole grains often
   - **b.** Add little sugar or caloric sweetener to food and beverages, such as amounts suggested by USDA MyPyramid and DASH eating plan
   - **c.** Practice good oral hygiene and eat sugar- and starch-containing foods and beverages less frequently to reduce risk of dental caries
6. Sodium and potassium
   - **a.** Take in less than 2,300 mg of sodium (about 1 teaspoon of salt) per day and only 1,500 mg daily for those age 51 and older, African Americans of any age, or those with hypertension, diabetes, or chronic kidney disease
   - *NCLEX®* **b.** Choose and prepare foods with little salt, while increasing potassium-rich foods, such as fruits and vegetables (provided no contraindication to potassium in diet, such as in renal failure)

III. ASSISTING WITH DETERMINATION OF NUTRITIONAL STATUS

A. Documented history

1. Food record: client records ingestion of all foods and beverages over several days (often a 1-week period); this record is then analyzed for nutrient content
2. Diet recall (24-hour recall): dietary intake recording tool in which all foods, liquids, and dietary supplements consumed in last 24 hours are recalled either verbally or in writing (includes time and location of intake, portion sizes, preparation methods, whether foods are fortified); is greatly affected by changes in usual eating patterns and routines
3. Food frequency questionnaire: documents intake of foods and food groups by day, week, or month; is useful in capturing intake of nutrients that are not eaten daily
4. Review of systems: reviews each body system for symptoms of nutrition problems related to excess or deficiency (example: constipation as a result of low fiber and water intake)

5. Nutritional screening initiatives (NSIs) can be performed for special populations, such as pregnant women or elderly
6. After diet history is completed, nutrient content can be determined by comparing data collected with food composition tables or using a computerized diet analysis program

B. Anthropometric measurements

1. Height and weight are measured and recorded; a history of weight gain or loss is also assessed
2. BMI: assesses relative weight for height; calculated by dividing weight in kilograms (2.2 pounds = 1 kg) by the square of height in meters (2.54 cm = 1 inch), or Weight ÷ $(\text{Height})^2$ = BMI; charts or nomograms may be used to calculate BMI (see Figure 25–2)

NCLEX®

   a. Provides a range to evaluate a healthy body weight ("healthy" range 18.5 – 24.9) and underweight, overweight, and obese status (see Table 25–2)
   b. BMI in children ages 2 to 20 years is tracked using growth charts that outline BMI-for-age in percentiles, with less than 5th percentile as risk for underweight and greater than 95th percentile as risk for overweight
   c. BMI does not reflect body composition, and individuals with greater muscle mass may appear to be overweight and yet not have increased body fat
   d. High or low BMIs may correlate with clinical or disease pathology
3. Basal metabolic rate (BMR): measures oxygen consumption and rate of calories burned during basic activities—a higher BMR indicates client can consume more calories without weight gain
   a. Lean muscle tissue mass most directly affects BMR; BMR decreases about 2% during each decade after maximum at age 30
   b. BMR increases with activity, stress, temperature, pregnancy, smoking, caffeine, stress, and during growth spurts
   c. BMR decreases with sleep, fasting, or starvation states and undernutrition

NCLEX®

   d. Identification of BMR and typical activities/lifestyle is necessary to determine exact caloric requirements

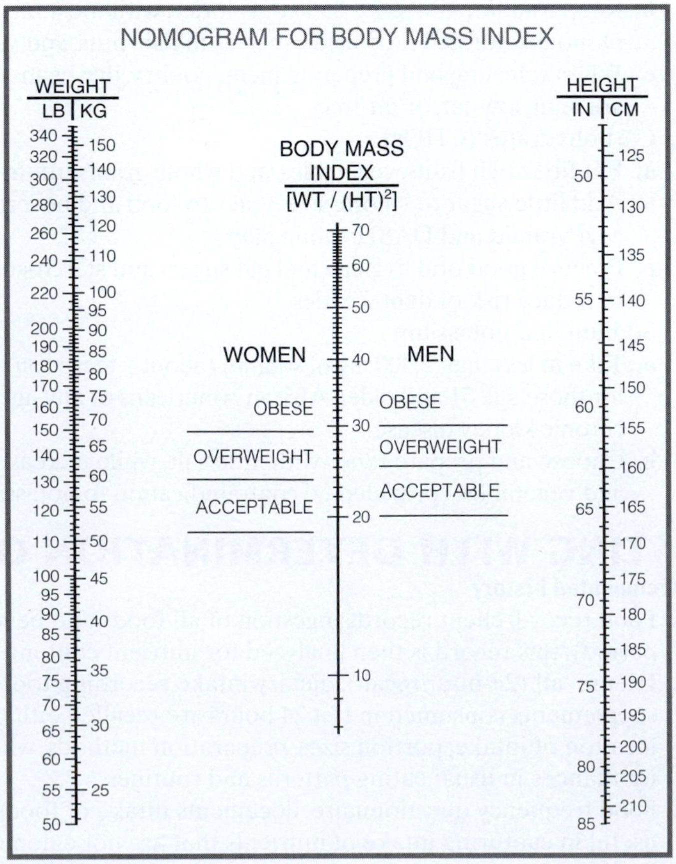

Figure 25–2

Body mass index nomogram plots height against weight to identify the BMI and determine weight status.

Source: Nutrition Screening Initiative, a project of the American Academy of Family Physicians, American Dietetic Association, and the National Council on Aging, Inc. Accessed 11/01/03 @ www.aafp.org/

Table 25–2 Classifications of Body Mass Index for Adults

Classification	BMI Measurement
Severe malnutrition	Less than 16
Moderate malnutrition	16 to 16.99
Mild malnutrition	17 to 18.49
Normal	18.5 to 24.9
Overweight	25 to 29.9
Obese class 1	30 to 34.9
Obese class 2	35 to 39.9
Obese class 3	40 or higher

Sources: National Heart, Lung and Blood Institute and World Health Organization.

Table 25–3 Serum Albumin Levels

Category	Serum Albumin Level
Normal	3.5–5.5 grams/dl
Mild depletion	2.8–3.4 grams/dl
Moderate depletion	2.1–2.7 grams/dl
Severe depletion	less than 2.1 grams/dl

NCLEX® 4. Distribution of body fat aids assessment of health risk potential
   a. Central (truncal) **obesity** represents increased intra-abdominal fat and is associated with increased risk of disease
   b. Determination of waist circumference and/or hip–waist ratio correlates with "apple" versus "pear" body type and reflects risk pattern for disease ("apple" types are at greater risk than "pear" types)

5. Skin fold measurements using calipers are an objective measure of body fat stores and nutritional status
   a. Triceps skin fold (TSF) is most commonly performed measurement using subscapular and suprailiac skin folds
   b. Mid-arm circumference (MAC) provides information about muscle and fat stores; is used to calculate mid-arm muscle circumference (MAMC), which provides information about skeletal muscle mass and distinguishes differences in muscle and body fat

C. Laboratory and diagnostic measurements

NCLEX® 1. Albumin levels: good overall indicator of nutritional status because of long half life (18–20 days); body can store and maintain normal levels until chronic malnutrition occurs (refer to Table 25–3)
   NCLEX® a. Prealbumin levels are a more sensitive indicator of nutritional status because of shorter half life and thus faster response to short-term changes in protein stores
   NCLEX® b. Transferrin levels identify iron stores, which reflects visceral body protein
   NCLEX® c. Albumin, prealbumin, and transferrin levels are used to evaluate clinical response of clients to total parenteral nutrition (TPN) and overall nutritional status in other clients

2. Total lymphocyte count (TLC) decreases as protein stores become depleted, which can negatively affect immune system function

NCLEX® 3. Screening for specific nutrient deficiencies: hemoglobin levels reflect iron intake; transferrin transports iron from intestine into serum and drops more rapidly than albumin

IV. KEY NUTRITIONAL CONCERNS ACROSS THE LIFESPAN

A. Culture and religion influence food choices in times of health and illness; see Table 25–4

B. Pregnancy and lactation

NCLEX® 1. Calorie needs increase during pregnancy by about 300 cal/day and during lactation by 500 cal/day

2. Intake of a balanced diet is important, with adequate intake of protein, folic acid, magnesium, iron, calcium, vitamin C, and B complex vitamins (especially folic acid to prevent neural tube defects)

Table 25-4 Influences of Culture and Religion on Nutritional Status

Cultural or Religious Group	Practices and/or Issues*
African American	Traditional foods high in fat, cholesterol, and sodium and low in calcium. Frying and adding fat to food is common. Obesity, cardiovascular disease, and diabetes are common.
Asian	Traditional diet is plant-based: low in fat, saturated fat, and cholesterol; rich in fiber and nutrients; may be high in sodium. High risk for osteoporosis.
Native American	Diet varies with region. Some use corn and other cultivated crop staples; many attempt to live off land. Widespread poverty and use of food assistance programs (food stamps, food distribution on reservations) exist in this group. Diabetes and obesity are common.
Hispanic (Mexican origin)	Traditional diet is vegetarian, high in complex carbohydrates, such as corn, beans, and squash. High levels of calories, saturated fats, and sugar are eaten. Food preparation commonly uses fat. Obesity, diabetes, and high triglyceride levels are common.
Islam	No pork, birds of prey, alcohol, tea, or coffee are consumed. Fasting is common during certain religious events.
Christianity	Catholics eat no meat on Ash Wednesday or Fridays during Lent; fasting is common on some religious days. Eastern Orthodox practice some fasting. Mormons consume no coffee, tea, alcohol, or tobacco. Seventh Day Adventists generally are lacto-ovovegetarians. No coffee, tea, alcohol, or strong seasonings are consumed. Meals are at least 4 to 5 hours apart with no snacking between meals.
Judaism (those following strict dietary rules)	Only kosher meat and poultry (no pork, shellfish, or fishlike mammals) are eaten. Consuming milk or dairy at same meal with meat or poultry is forbidden. Separate utensils are required for preparing and serving meat and dairy.

*Although identified by a specific ethnic or religious group, practices vary with area of origin and sect. Not all individuals within these groups follow these practices or have these issues.

NCLEX® 3. Weight gain during pregnancy is based on prepregnant weight using BMI as a reference point (note variation in underweight classification from nonpregnant state)
   a. Underweight clients (BMI < 19.8) should gain 28 to 40 pounds
   b. Healthy weight clients (BMI 19.8–24.9) should gain 25 to 35 pounds
   c. Overweight clients (BMI 25–29) should gain 15 to 25 pounds
   d. Obese clients (BMI > 29) should gain 15 pounds or less

NCLEX® 4. Common symptoms that may affect nutrition
   a. Nausea and vomiting: consume CHOs before getting out of bed in morning; eat small, frequent meals; avoid foods with offensive odors; do not drink fluids with meals; avoid coffee, tea, and spicy foods; limit high-fat foods
   b. Heartburn: interventions are similar to above; wait at least 1 hour before reclining after a meal
   c. Cravings and aversions: avoid nonnutritive substances (pica) that replace essential nutrients or interfere with their absorption; aversions are often self-limiting
   d. Constipation: caused by iron intake, enlarging uterus, decreased physical activity, and possibly inadequate fiber and fluid; consume at least 8 glasses of water daily and increase fiber in diet

C. Infancy

1. Infants may be breast- or bottle-fed according to maternal preference; breastfeeding is accepted as preferred nutrition whenever possible

NCLEX® 2. Weight doubles in first 6 months of life and triples by 1 year

NCLEX® 3. Avoid giving cow's milk during first year (deficient in essential fatty acids, iron, zinc, vitamin E, and vitamin C); could lead to decrease in hemoglobin and hematocrit and possible intestinal bleeding

4. Fluoride supplements are generally prescribed for infants 6 months of age and older if water supply has less than 0.3 parts per million (ppm) fluoride
5. Do not add cereal to bottle because of risk of aspiration with stronger suck reflex needed
6. Do not give bottle containing milk, juice, or sweetened beverage before sleep to avoid nursing bottle syndrome (dental caries)

NCLEX® 7. Start solid foods at 4 to 6 months of age to reduce risk of food allergies and because of immaturity of GI tract

NCLEX® 8. Introduce one new food no more frequently than every 4 to 7 days to detect allergy; give only 1 to 2 teaspoons initially and increase over time

NCLEX® 9. Cook foods well and cut or grind into tiny pieces to reduce risk of choking; supervise during meals and avoid giving hard round foods such as grapes, peanuts, popcorn, hotdogs, and others

10. Avoid using honey because of risk of infant botulism

D. Childhood

1. Dietary needs differ among toddlers, preschoolers, and school-age children; total energy needs increase with age, but calories per kilogram of weight decrease

NCLEX® 2. Toddlers and preschoolers may have erratic and ritualistic eating patterns and strong food preferences, including food jags (preferring one or a few types of foods over all others); these place child at risk for nutritional deficiencies; provide a balanced diet over time if not at each meal

NCLEX® 3. Facilitate nutrient intake in young children by not forcing child to eat, maintaining relaxed mealtimes, offering one new food with a favorite food, using child-sized portions, serving foods with mild flavors, and providing finger-foods

4. Encourage school-age children not to skip breakfast; encourage regular meal patterns; nutrient stores for puberty are laid during this time

5. Encourage healthy after-school snacks rather than high-calorie and high-fat items found in fast foods; choose popcorn, fresh fruits and vegetables, peanut butter, cheese, nuts, eggs, and yogurt

6. Encourage adequate physical activity to reduce risk of childhood obesity

7. Daily intake of a multivitamin may reduce risk of vitamin deficiency from occasional erratic dietary patterns (such as from after-school and sports schedules)

E. Adolescence

1. Need for macro- and micronutrients significantly increases during this time

2. Male adolescent growth spurt begins at 12 to 13 years, peaks at 14, and continues until approximately 19 years

3. Female adolescent growth spurt begins at 10 to 11 years, peaks at 12, and continues until approximately 15 years

4. Adolescents frequently consume inadequate amounts of vitamin A, C, B_6, iron, calcium, zinc, and magnesium

NCLEX® 5. Adolescents frequently engage in dieting; follow fad or restrictive diets; skip meals; snack on high-calorie, high-fat, or high-sugar foods; and eat more meals outside home (including fast foods); these eating patterns increase risk of calorie and/or nutrient deficiencies

NCLEX® 6. Diet should be well-balanced with sufficient calories but eliminating empty (nonnutritive) calories and high fat foods; vitamin supplements may be helpful

7. Eating disorders (anorexia nervosa, bulimia nervosa) or obesity may be of concern; see Chapter 21 for discussion of eating disorders

F. Adulthood (age 18–64 years)

1. Dietary needs include balanced intake and maintaining ideal body weight

2. There is significant variation in metabolic needs based on age, weight, height, and physical activity; overall energy needs decrease during adulthood, although needs for selected nutrients may increase

3. Stress (which affects metabolic processes) and occupational influences (such as travel) may affect meal patterns and dietary intake

4. Poor nutritional habits during a lifetime increase risk of cardiovascular disease, diabetes mellitus, cancer, and obesity

5. Take multivitamin and mineral supplements as needed and follow balanced meal plan and possibly therapeutic diet based on identified health problem(s)

6. Lose weight if indicated to reduce further health risks

G. Older adulthood (age 65 and older)

1. Caloric requirements continue to decrease

2. Nutrient absorption may be adversely affected because of chewing difficulties (periodontal disease, loss of teeth, dysphagia due to stroke or other neuromuscular disease), decreased peristalsis, and reduced secretion of digestive enzymes

3. Therapeutic diets may affect intake of calories and specific nutrients

NCLEX® 4. Clients who have dysphagia from cerebrovascular accident (CVA) (stroke) will have dysphagia staged using videofluoroscopy and evaluated by speech and language therapist; diet will be prescribed as (1) pureed foods, (2) ground/minced meat, (3) soft/easy-to-chew foods, or (4) modified general diet; commercial thickeners for liquids will also be used

5. Prescribed medications may interact with specific foods or may cause side effects (nausea, vomiting, diarrhea, constipation, inactivation of nutrients) that affect nutritional health

6. Loss of family or friends may reduce socialization at mealtimes and provide for fewer opportunities for social eating
7. Those who have insufficient finances or rely on others to shop for food or prepare food are at risk for nutritional deficiencies

NCLEX®

8. Thirst response declines with age and can lead to dehydration and electrolyte imbalances
9. Common nutrient deficiencies in older adults include protein, fiber, total calories, iron, calcium, magnesium, and vitamins D, B_{12}, and B_6

V. PHYTOCHEMICALS, DIETARY SUPPLEMENTS, AND HERBS

A. *Phytochemicals*

1. Nonnutrient chemical substances found in plants that may correlate with health benefits in disease treatment and prevention

NCLEX®

2. *Functional foods* are food items (nutrients) that correlate with health benefits; this newer term is being used to assess therapeutic effects of foods that contain phytochemicals
3. Phytochemicals are found in plant sources (fruits and vegetables), whole grains, tea and soy products; many foods contain several phytochemicals and therefore can exert multiple effects on many body systems (see Table 25–5)

NCLEX®

4. Health applications
   a. Antioxidant function and cancer prevention ability of phytochemicals have led to great interest and continued research; they may be part of therapeutic treatment for clients with cancer, CAD, and hypercholesterolemia
   b. Dietitians can assist in selecting food products that contain phytochemicals

B. Dietary supplements

1. Must follow FDA guidelines to be labeled as such, and are products that contain vitamins, minerals, herbs, botanicals, amino acids, enzymes, extracts, or combinations of these
2. Available in several forms including pills, liquids, powders, or being incorporated into foods (such as power bars or energy beverages)

Table 25–5 Types of Phytochemicals

Phytochemical	General Information
Carotenoids	Found in colorful fruits and vegetables (green, orange, red, and yellow) Chemical classification includes beta-carotene and lycopene (found in tomato products, sauces, and ketchup); function as both pro-oxidant and antioxidant Health benefit claims include retinal protection; decreased risk of CAD, lung, prostate, and breast cancers; enhanced immune effects in older adults
Indoles	Found in vegetables such as broccoli, cauliflower, cabbage, and kale Chemical classification includes organosulphur compounds; are members of cruciferous vegetable family Health benefit claims include hormone stimulation to make estrogen less effective (decreasing risk of non–hormone-dependent breast cancer) and influencing DNA enzyme activity to protect against cancer
Isoflavones	Found in soy foods (tofu, soy milk, and soybean products) and black and green tea Chemical composition includes phenylpropanoids that include flavonoid group (also found in nuts, wine, and oregano) Health benefit claims include inhibiting cancer cell growth (breast, prostate, and endometrial), alleviating menopausal symptoms, and preventing osteoporosis by increasing bone density
Phenolic Acids	Found in coffee beans, fruits and vegetables, green tea, wine, and soybeans Chemical structure includes phenylpropanoids, which act as antioxidants and bind metals to promote excretion of carcinogenic substances Health benefit claims include decreased risk of certain cancers (skin, lung, and stomach) and controlling blood glucose
Terpones	Found in the oil of citrus peel and menthol Chemical structure includes isoprenoid Health benefit claims include protection against carcinogens
Phytoestrogens	Found in vegetables, plants, soybean, and whole-grain fruits and berries Chemical structure falls under phenylpropanoids; includes isoflavones and lignans Health benefit claims include protection against cardiac disease, cancer (breast and prostate), and osteoporosis
Catechins	Found in teas Chemical structure includes phenylpropanoids; are rich in phenolic acid Health benefit claims include possible antioxidant activity, prevention of cancer, and antihypertensive effects

3. Also included in this category are **ergonomic aids** that include a variety of items used to enhance body performance and promote muscle growth
   a. Amino acids are often used to promote anabolism and maintain strength in the form of glutamine and branch chain amino acids (BCAA); protein is increased often to the level of 1.3 to 2 grams/day
   b. CHO loading (glycogen loading) consists of high glucose ingestion before intense exercise in order to increase glycogen stores and delay onset of fatigue
   c. Metabolic end products are often used as ergonomic aids (creatine and steroids) in body

NCLEX® 4. Although many products claim to be ergonomic aids, clinical research does not support all claims; clients should consider each product's potential harm and/or available benefit prior to use

NCLEX® 5. Indications for use
   a. Nutritional supplements are used to decrease risk of disease, support increased needs during growth and periods of stress, and improve overall functioning
   b. Nutritional supplements may be useful for selected clients who are in at-risk categories due to life cycle concerns (pregnancy, lactation, or children), underlying disease states (illness, stress, or malabsorption), inadequate intake of nutrients (strict vegans or constant dieters), and/or clinical intervention that requires therapy

C. Herbal therapy

1. The Dietary Supplement Health and Education Act (DSHEA) of 1994 defines herbs as dietary supplements; because they are not defined as medicines, herbs cannot be promoted with therapeutic claims but only with information about how they affect bodily structure and function
2. The Food and Drug Administration (FDA) does not regulate use of herbs in United States but approves certain herbs for their action on body (how they affect structure and function); does not monitor herbs for quality, composition, or preparation; formulations vary in their potency and recommended dosage, with frequent lack of consensus on dosing

NCLEX® 3. Not intended for acute illness episodes or long-term therapy; may be appropriate as adjunct to conventional Western therapies

NCLEX® 4. Therapeutic effectiveness is slower than prescription medications; may take as long as several weeks, depending on herb; client should start with one herb at a time, at lower than recommended doses, and closely monitor response

5. Many herbs are sold in multiple forms, such as teas, extracts, tinctures, and capsules or tablets containing powdered or freeze dried forms of herb

NCLEX® 6. Safe use in pregnancy and lactation is either contraindicated or unknown and may dry up breast milk during lactation; ginger may be an exception

NCLEX® 7. Many herbs interact with other herbs, food, and prescription medications; become familiar with herb–herb, herb–drug, and herb–food interactions

NCLEX® 8. Report use of all herbs to health care provider

9. See Table 25–6 for common herbs and their uses, interactions, and contraindications

VI. THERAPEUTIC DIETS WITH ALTERED CONSISTENCY

A. Clear liquid diet

1. Provides adequate fluid/water, 500–1000 kcal of simple sugars and electrolytes but is fiber free
2. Requires minimal digestion because there is no residue or fiber
3. Recommended for short-term use (1–2 days); can be used before and after surgery or diagnostic procedures, during acute stages of illness, or as initial diet after significant period of GI inactivity/bowel rest
4. Consists of clear foods that are liquid at body temperature: gelatin, bouillon, clear broth, popsicles, apple or cranberry juice, clear carbonated beverages, tea or coffee with no added milk or milk product

B. Full liquid diet

1. Provides water, calories, protein, vitamins and minerals, and dairy products (contains lactose) and is considered to be low in residue
2. Indicated for some clients who have difficulty chewing or swallowing, but not indicated for a client following a CVA (stroke)
3. Can be a transition diet (temporary diet as client progresses postoperatively or postprocedure from clear liquids to solids); is deficient in many nutrients and calories
4. Consists of all foods found on a clear liquid diet and opaque liquids (milk, juices, pudding, ice cream, strained soups, yogurts, any prepared liquid formulas) and all foods that are liquid at body temperature
5. Clients who are lactose intolerant may require lactose-free supplements to prevent clinical symptoms

Table 25-6 Uses, Interactions, Contraindications/Side Effects of Common Herbs

Name	Uses	Interactions	Contraindications/Side Effects
Bilberry	Simple diarrhea Eye disorders: diabetic retinopathy, night blindness, glaucoma, cataracts Antioxidant	Use cautiously with aspirin, anticoagulants, vitamin E, fish oils, feverfew, garlic, ginger, ginkgo	May prolong coagulation time Iron absorption is ↓ when taken internally Contraindicated in lactation as well as pregnancy
Black cohosh	Menopause Dysmenorrhea Premenstrual syndrome	Potentiates hormone replacement medications (do not use together)	Dizziness, nausea, slowed pulse, increased sweating
Chondroitin sulfate	Helps slow cartilage degradation in osteoarthritis	May ↑ risk of bleeding with aspirin, anticoagulants, antiplatelet and nonsteroidal anti-inflammatory drugs	Headache, indigestion Contraindicated in pregnancy and lactation
Echinacea	Antimicrobial for colds and influenza Boosts immune system and ↑ resistance to infection (upper respiratory and urinary) Treat herpes simplex and Candida infection Topically: improves wound healing, provides antioxidant protection from UV A and B rays	May ↓ effectiveness of immunosuppressants (including corticosteroids) Use with antifungals (which ↑ liver enzymes) can cause liver damage Do not use with other hepatotoxicants (such as anabolic steroids, amiodarone, methotrexate, ketoconazole) Many tinctures contain large amounts of alcohol	Do not use in presence of autoimmune disease (e.g., HIV/AIDS, collagen disease, multiple sclerosis, tuberculosis), severe illness, or allergy to sunflower/daisy family Use longer than 8 weeks may cause hepatotoxicity and immunosuppression May influence fertility by spermatozoa enzyme interference Contraindicated in alcoholism, children, pregnancy, and lactation Risk of allergic reaction and anaphylaxis
Feverfew	Principle uses: prevention of recurrent migraine headaches, treatment of arthritis Relief of menstrual pain Asthma Dermatitis, psoriasis Antipyretic (promotes diaphoresis)	Do not use while taking prescription drugs for headache May interfere with blood clotting mechanism; do not use with aspirin or anticoagulants such as warfarin (Coumadin), or with bilberry, garlic, ginger, ginkgo	Cross-allergy to ragweed Adverse effects: lip and tongue swelling, mouth ulcers and ↓ taste from chewing leaves, abdominal colic, palpitations, ↑ menstrual flow, rebound headaches Sudden withdrawal may cause post-feverfew syndrome (muscle aches, pain, and stiffness); taper off to discontinue Avoid use in pregnancy, lactation, ↓ age 2
Garlic	Principle uses: ↓ cholesterol (triglycerides and low-density lipoproteins); ↑ high-density lipoproteins ↓ BP in mild hypertension (use should be monitored by health care provider [HCP]) Anticoagulant, antibacterial, antiviral, antifungal	↑ anticoagulant effect of anticoagulants, aspirin, and herbs that affect coagulation (bilberry, feverfew, ginger, ginkgo) Further ↓ blood glucose with hypoglycemic agents for diabetes May ↑ or ↓ effectiveness of drugs for HIV	Adverse effects: contact dermatitis, vertigo, garlic breath, hypothyroidism, GI irritation, nausea, vomiting (N/V) with large doses Enteric-coated tablets containing powdered form may reduce bad breath but are not as potent as raw garlic Contraindicated in pregnancy, GI (peptic ulcer and GERD) and bleeding disorders Chronic use may lower hemoglobin levels
Ginger	Principle use: antiemetic; ↑ appetite, digestion aid; alleviates dyspepsia Anti-inflammatory in treatment of rheumatoid arthritis and osteoarthritis Relieves muscle pain May ↓ motion sickness and relieve vertigo	May ↑ anticoagulant effects of bilberry, feverfew, garlic, ginkgo, or other anticoagulants such as aspirin or warfarin (Coumadin)	Adverse effects: headache, anxiety, insomnia, ↑ blood pressure, tachycardia, asthma attack, postmenopausal bleeding Contraindicated for postoperative nausea in clients with ↑ risk of bleeding and for treatment of hyperemesis gravidarum Severe overdose: possible CNS depression and dysrhythmias Conflicting data regarding safe use in pregnancy (FDA: relatively safe)
Ginkgo	Improves attention and memory, headaches Macular degeneration Intermittent claudication Erectile dysfunction Tinnitus	May ↑ anticoagulant effects of bilberry, feverfew, garlic, ginkgo, or aspirin or other anticoagulants such as warfarin (Coumadin)	Side effects: mild GI upset, ↑ risk bleeding Large doses may cause restlessness, headache, N/V, diarrhea, dizziness, or palpitations Avoid use of unprocessed leaves (contain allergens related to urushiol [chemical responsible for itch in poison ivy]) Avoid use in pregnancy, lactation, and children

Table 25-6 Uses, Interactions, Contraindications/Side Effects of Common Herbs *(continued)*

Name	Uses	Interactions	Contraindications/Side Effects
Ginseng	Counteracts physical and mental fatigue and ↑ stamina and concentration ↑ body's ability to resist stress and disease; ↑ vitality Regulates blood pressure May ↓ mood swings Regulates blood glucose levels in type 2 diabetes mellitus	↑ potency of estrogen in oral contraceptives leading to weight gain, breast pain, and vaginal bleeding May cause mania with MAOIs May cause irritability with caffeine May ↓ effectiveness of glaucoma medications	Most side effects reported are related to excessive or inappropriate use Avoid concurrent use with stimulants, such as coffee, tea, cola May potentiate MAOI actions Adverse effects: insomnia, palpitations, pruritus, nervousness, euphoria Do not use when acutely ill with cold or flu or if diagnosed with hypoglycemia
Glucosamine	↓ pain and ↑ movement on osteoarthritis, ↓ TMJ pain	↑ dose of glucosamine may be needed if taking diuretics	May ↑ glucose and cause mild GI upset Use of nonsulfated forms may not have beneficial effect
Hawthorn	Treats mild hypertension, athero- and arteriosclerosis, early heart failure Treats (prevents) chronic angina (not intended for acute angina)	May interfere with digoxin pharmacodynamics and monitoring Contraindicated with concomitant use of prescription antihypertensives or nitrates	Supervision of health care provider needed for those with existing cardiac disease Adverse effects: nausea, fatigue, perspiration and cutaneous eruption of hands, increased CNS depression and sedation Contraindicated in pregnancy and lactation
Milk thistle	Adjunct antioxidant therapy in liver disease close monitoring by HCP needed Treats overdose of death cap mushroom ↓ hepatotoxicity of psychoactive drugs such as phenothiazines	↓ effectiveness of oral contraceptives	May trigger menstruation Insoluble in water, do not take in tea form Avoid alcohol-based extract in decompensated cirrhosis Cross-allergy to ragweed Adverse effects: loose stools, diarrhea in high doses Contraindicated in pregnancy and lactation
Saw palmetto	Treat symptoms of BPH with HCP supervision Helps initiate urine stream; ↓ urinary frequency, residual volumes, nocturia, dysuria	May potentiate finasteride (Proscar) resulting in overdose May interfere with iron absorption	Insoluble in water; do not take in tea form Adverse effects: nausea, abdominal pain, ↑ BP, headache, diarrhea with large doses Contraindicated in pregnancy and lactation
St. John's wort	Treats mild to moderate depression Not intended to treat suicidal ideation, psychotic behavior, or severe depression Possible antibacterial, antiviral, wound healing properties	Do not use concurrently with prescription antidepressants, especially SSRIs or MAOIs Do not use concurrently with opioids, amphetamines, or OTC cold and flu preparations May inhibit absorption of iron May decrease digoxin levels	Avoid foods containing tyramine (aged cheese, smoked meats, liver, figs, dried or cured fish, yeast, beer, Chianti wine) Adverse effects (may last 2–4 weeks): GI distress, fatigue, pruritus, weight gain, headache, dizziness, restlessness May cause photosensitivity; avoid sun exposure, especially if fair skinned Contraindicated in pregnancy, lactation, and in children
Valerian root	Sedative for insomnia, reduction of anxiety Muscle pain Menstrual and intestinal cramps Benzodiazepine withdrawal	Do not use concurrently with other sedatives, anxiolytics, or antidepressants Do not use with alcohol or disulfiram (Antabuse)	May be used safely while operating machinery or car, but monitor CNS effects Adverse effects: headache; upset stomach; others with long-term use or overdose (2.5 grams): excitability, insomnia, cardiac dysfunction, blurred vision, hepatotoxicity May cause hepatotoxicity; monitor liver function and avoid use in liver disease Extract contains 40% to 60% alcohol; avoid use in clients with alcoholism Contraindicated in pregnancy and lactation

C. Pureed diet

1. Provides essential nutrients in a chopped, ground, or pureed form for clients who are unable to chew or swallow
2. Can be used as a long-term diet—preparation of food items is deciding factor
3. Use of seasoning depends on individual client preferences
4. Uses a blender or food processor to change foods into pureed or blended form
5. Certain foods such as raw eggs, nuts, whole breads, raw fruits and vegetables, and foods containing seeds are not allowed

D. Dysphagia diet

1. Uses thickened liquids provided to clients who have swallowing problems and are at risk for aspiration (such as post-CVA)
2. Thickening agents can also be added to foods to maximize texture and aid swallowing process
3. Dysphagia diet is a modification of soft diet with increased attention to liquid component to avoid possible aspiration
4. Foods to avoid because of risk of aspiration include stringy, raw, dry, and fried foods, and those that are small in size or hand held, such as popcorn, nuts, and small candies
5. *NCLEX®* Position client to at least 30 to 45 degrees head elevation, use chin tuck (head and neck slightly flexed), and monitor feedings to decrease risk of aspiration and evaluate client's attempts at eating

E. Soft diet

1. Used for clients who have problems with chewing (dental problems, oral lesions, difficulty chewing or swallowing)
2. Includes food items that contain small amounts of seasoning and moderate fiber content but are easy to chew, digest, and absorb
3. Avoid highly seasoned, fried, and high-fiber foods; nuts; coconuts; and foods that contain seeds because they could cause GI upset
4. Can be used as a progressive or transition diet and is a modification of regular diet

F. Mechanical soft diet

1. Includes all foods and seasonings in a form that is easily handled by client
2. Soft-textured, tender, and chopped foods are included in diet, while tough foods (seeds, nuts, and fruits with pits) are not
3. Can be used as a long-term diet or a transition diet
4. Is a modification of regular diet with attention to texture

G. Bland diet

1. Consists of foods that do not irritate GI tract, reduce gas formation, and reduce gastric acid stimulation
2. Avoids spicy or fried foods, pepper, alcohol, and caffeine-containing beverages
3. Is used for a wide variety of GI disorders, such as esophagitis, gastritis, inflammatory bowel disease

H. High-residue/high-fiber diet

1. Includes intake of 20 to 25 grams of fiber daily to add bulk to stool and speed rate of passage through GI tract
2. Used for clients with constipation, asymptomatic diverticular disease, and to treat alternating constipation and diarrhea of irritable bowel syndrome; stimulates peristalsis, promotes regularity, and maintains normal bowel function and elimination patterns
3. Fruits, vegetables, legumes, and whole grains are eaten in larger quantities or proportions
4. Additional benefits are reduced serum cholesterol and blood glucose, which is useful to clients with heart disease and diabetes mellitus

I. Low-residue/low-fiber diet

1. Includes foods such as white bread, cereals, and pasta (high CHO)
2. Avoids raw vegetables, fruits (bananas allowed), whole grains, plant fiber, and seeds; limits intake of dairy products to 2 servings daily
3. Fried foods, pepper, alcohol, and heavily seasoned foods are restricted because of possible GI upset
4. Used for conditions in which GI inflammation or scarring has narrowed bowel lumen and food intake could contribute to obstruction, such as inflammatory bowel disease, partial bowel obstruction, enteritis, and diarrhea

VII. RESTRICTED OR ENHANCED DIETS

A. Carbohydrate-controlled diet

1. Assists in regulating serum glucose levels in conditions in which they rise and fall, such as in diabetes mellitus, hypoglycemia, dumping syndrome, galactosemia, and obesity

2. Utilizes a dietary exchange system that groups foods according to protein, CHO, and fat content per specified food serving
3. Includes complex CHOs for 55–60%, proteins for 10–20%, and saturated fats for less than 10% of total daily calories; also includes recommended fiber intake of 20 to 35 grams/day
4. Gestational diabetes diet encourages adequate calories based on prepregnant weight status, frequent small feedings, and snacks during day to normalize postprandial glucose levels, maintain euglycemia during pregnancy, and prevent ketosis
5. *NCLEX®* Hypoglycemic diet consists of small feedings at frequent intervals to help normalize blood glucose levels; when episodes of hypoglycemia occur, ingest 15 gram CHO snack, recheck glucose in 15 minutes, and repeat if necessary (15/15 rule)
6. Carbohydrate counting is a means of controlling CHO intake over a 24-hour period

B. Gastric bypass diet

1. *NCLEX®* Consists of eating small nutrient-dense meals several times a day, drinking liquids between meals, instead of with meals, and taking multivitamin supplements
2. Diet is low in fat and high in protein, with restrictions on carbonated beverages, simple CHOs, and foods high in fiber and residue

C. Fat-controlled diet

1. Used to manage malabsorption, chronic pancreatitis, and gallbladder disease
2. Medium chain triglycerides (MCT) are used in diet because they are easily digested along with high intake of CHOs and protein
3. High-fat foods are limited or omitted (such as red meats and dairy products) and no additional fat is used in cooking process
4. Enzyme replacements and fat-soluble vitamin and mineral supplements may be needed
5. Foods that are high in oxalates (spinach, rhubarb, sweet potato, beet greens, nuts, wheat bran, tea, and chocolate) are limited to prevent risk of kidney stone formation
6. Clients with hyperlipidemia (high cholesterol and/or triglyceride levels) should eat on a low-saturated-fat diet (increased monounsaturated fats and small amounts of polyunsaturated fatty acids) with restricted sodium and hydrogenated food products
7. Clients who have cardiovascular disease, heart failure, or are posttransplant will control dietary fat as a life-long dietary pattern

D. Protein-controlled diet

1. *NCLEX®* Used for clients with renal disease (renal failure, end-stage renal disease, dialysis, and transplant) or liver disease (liver failure, hepatic encephalopathy, cirrhosis, transplant, and hepatitis) because they are unable to handle protein load
2. Provides protein needed to maintain nutritional status without causing excess wastes or metabolites of protein breakdown (usually 40–60 grams protein daily or 0.8 grams/kg of dry weight)
3. Depending on client's clinical condition, protein levels may be increased to account for metabolic response to dialysis and regeneration of liver tissue (1.5–2.0 grams/kg/day)
4. A minimum level of CHOs must be present in the diet (50–100 grams/day) in order to spare protein; protein intake must be high quality
5. Vitamin and mineral supplements may be ordered for clients who have liver failure
6. *NCLEX®* Restricts foods such as meat, fish, poultry, and dairy products; other foods need to be evaluated individually for protein content

E. Food allergy diet

1. Many foods, such as cow's milk, eggs, fish, shellfish, nuts, soybean, and wheat, have allergic potential
2. Primary therapy is avoidance of the particular food item
3. Egg-free diet is used for clients who have a known sensitivity to eggs and restricts use of eggs and egg products
4. Children often present with food allergies and certain diets (allergy I and allergy II) are used in sequence to identify potential food allergens by eliminating their intake in a controlled manner; these diets are used for a limited time frame because they are not nutritionally complete

Box 25–1

Gluten-Restricted Diet

- Foods included: cornmeal, corn flakes, popcorn, hominy, and potato chips
- Food substitutions: corn, potato, rice, soybean flour, and low-gluten wheat flour
- Foods to avoid: processed (commercially prepared) foods with wheat flour extenders, additives, or stabilizers; root beer, beer, and all products that contain identified grain sources (wheat, rye, barley, buckwheat, oats and malt)

Box 25–2

Lactose-Restricted Diet

- Foods included: aged cheese (hard) rather than soft cheese because hard cheese is lower in lactose due to aging process.
- Yogurt can be included because of its bacterial action, and frozen yogurt may have even less lactose due to bacterial action and freezing process.
- OTC products such as Lactaid are specific formulations for those with identified lactase deficiency; these products are usually available in liquid or tablet form.
- Special milk products formulated with Lactaid are available for use by lactose-intolerant clients (these products are usually sweeter than regular milk products).
- Individual tolerance varies, and client is best judge of how little or how much "lactose" can be ingested without onset of clinical symptoms.
- Check food labels for milk, milk solids, casein, and whey, which are sometimes used as additives and stabilizers in processed food products.
- Check medication ingredients because lactose can be used as binders or fillers in certain formulations.
- Lactose-restricted diets are often low in calcium, vitamin B_2 (riboflavin), and vitamin D, so additional nutrient supplements may be needed.

Box 25–3

Foods High in Sodium

Condiments: pickles, olives, nuts, meat tenderizers, commercial salad dressings, ketchup, soy sauce, Worcestershire and other sauces, monosodium glutamate (MSG), commercial mustard, table salt, and seasoned or buttered salts

Breads: commercial breads with salt added, salted crackers, potato chips, popcorn, pretzels, other salted snacks

Meats: smoked, cured, or processed meats (ham, bacon, hot dogs, luncheon meat, canned meats); all cheeses except cottage cheese and low-sodium cheese

Soups: canned or dehydrated soups, bouillon

Vegetables: sauerkraut, pork and beans, canned tomato or vegetable juices, hominy

Beverages: commercial milk, instant drink mixes

5. Gluten-restricted diet (gluten gliaden–free diet) is used for clients who have celiac disease (malabsorption syndrome); see Box 25–1
   a. Clinical manifestations caused by inability to handle gluten protein are steatorrhea, diarrhea, weight loss, anemia, and edema formation caused by loss of nutrients
   b. Lactose-intolerant clients must follow additional diet restrictions
6. Lactose-restricted diet is used for clients who have lactose intolerance (lactase enzyme deficiency) and may require lactase enzymes in diet to tolerate dairy products (see Box 25–2)
   a. Primary lactose intolerance is more common among certain ethnic groups (African Americans, Asian, Hispanic, and Native Americans)
   b. Secondary lactose intolerance is caused by another established disease process (such as infection) or medication (chemo agents that inhibit cell growth) that affect GI tract's ability to produce lactase
   c. Clinical symptoms affect GI tract, resulting in gas, bloating, and diarrhea
7. Restriction and/or avoidance therapy is used to minimize food allergies

F. Purine-controlled diet

1. Indicated for clients who have gout, tumor lysis syndrome, or multiple myeloma, all of which cause elevated uric acid levels
2. Excessive purine accumulation leads to an increase in uric acid, which is a normal end product of purine catabolism; this excess can lead to uric acid deposits in joints and tissues, and can lead also to development of uric acid renal stones
3. *NCLEX®* Includes use of dairy products and restricts organ meats, anchovies, alcohol, and seafood

G. Sodium-controlled diet

1. Indicated for clients with hypertension, cardiovascular disease, heart failure, and conditions in which fluid restriction is beneficial (renal failure, cirrhosis, or liver failure)
2. Restriction ranges from mild (3000–4000 mg/day) to severe (500 mg/day)

Box 25–4

Foods High in Potassium

Apricots	Dried beans or peas	Potatoes (white or sweet)
Avocado	Dried fruits	Prune juice
Bananas	Melons	Spinach
Cantaloupe	Oranges and orange juice	Tomatoes and tomato products
Raw carrots	Peanuts	Winter squash

NCLEX® 3. It is important to evaluate food labels (sodium is a common preservative), medications, and restaurant dietary intake pattern for hidden sources of sodium
4. Clients using salt substitutes may be at risk for elevated potassium levels and should be evaluated for risk of hyperkalemia, especially if taking potassium-sparing diuretics, such as triamterene (Dyrenium)

NCLEX® 5. Avoid table salt and using salt in cooking; meat and dairy products have physiological saline, while fruits tend to be lowest overall in sodium
6. See Box 25–3 for examples of high-sodium foods to avoid

H. Tyramine- and dopamine-restricted diet

1. Indicated for clients taking monoamine oxidase inhibitor (MAOI) antidepressants; foods containing tyramine affect drug action by blocking enzyme pathways, which leads to norepinephrine release and hypertensive crisis
2. Tyramine is an intermediate product of amino acid metabolism formed in conversion of tyrosine to epinephrine and is found in many food items
3. Other amines, such as dopamine, are also restricted because excess accumulation can lead to similar hypertensive effects

NCLEX® 4. Diet restrictions include aged cheese, chocolate, smoked fish, processed meats such as bologna, bananas, liver, fava beans, and large amounts of soy sauce
5. Foods that can be eaten are unfermented cheese (ricotta and cottage cheese) and small amounts of certain foods such as sour cream

I. Low-potassium diet

1. Used for clients who have renal failure or take potassium-sparing diuretics
2. Potassium is found in many foods, but avoid high-potassium foods in Box 25–4
3. Reduce potassium content of vegetables by cooking and then draining cooking water; however, this method also reduces vitamin content of foods
4. Avoid use of salt substitutes, which are high in potassium

J. High-calcium diet

1. Indicated for client disease states that promote calcium loss and lead to bone demineralization (osteoporosis, osteopenia), endocrine abnormalities, and kidney failure

NCLEX® 2. Good sources of calcium include milk and other dairy products; green, leafy vegetables are adequate sources

K. High-protein diet

1. The use of a high-protein diet has been indicated for burns, liver disease, and for athletes (1.2–1.6 grams/kg/day) to maximize endurance, according to current research evidence

NCLEX® 2. Includes meat, fish, poultry, and dairy products and protein supplements

L. High-calorie diet

1. Indicated for clients with debilitating disease or need for tissue repair, including cancer, burns, stress, acquired immunodeficiency disease (AIDS), and others
2. Should include added protein to preserve muscle mass
3. Includes nutritious snacks (milkshakes, puddings) between meals and added use of sugars and possibly fats to increase overall calories

M. High-iron diet

1. Indicated for clients with anemia

NCLEX® 2. Includes added sources of iron, such as meat (especially organ meats), egg yolks, leafy vegetables, whole wheat breads and products, legumes, and dried fruits

N. Vegetarian diets

1. Vegan (strict vegetarian): includes plant-based foods with no meat, fish, poultry, dairy products, or eggs
2. Ovovegetarian: no meat, fish, or poultry and no dairy products; eggs are allowed
3. Lactovegetarian: no meat, fish, poultry, or eggs; diary products are allowed
4. Ovolactovegetarian: no meat, fish, or poultry; diary products and eggs are allowed

VIII. ENTERAL NUTRITION

A. Overview

1. **Enteral nutrition** is a method of feeding clients who have a functioning GI tract but have chewing or swallowing difficulty or impaired upper GI tract function, leading to poor nutrient digestion, transport, and absorption
2. Liquid feedings can be administered for short-term use via nasogastric tubes or oral route, while clients requiring long-term use have an enterostomy placed surgically or percutaneously

B. Administration

1. Continuous feedings are given over a 24-hour period at a prescribed flow rate and a set total volume using an infusion pump
2. Intermittent feedings are given over 30 minutes or more (to mimic usual eating pattern) with a prescribed set total volume ranging from 250 to 400 mL using an infusion pump or gravity
3. **Cyclic feeding** occurs over a period of several hours (prescribed flow rate and a set total volume using an infusion pump), usually at night as a transitional approach to healthy GI functioning
4. **Bolus feeding** occurs when there is a rapid delivery of a large amount of formula in a short time frame (preset volume 250–300 mL in a preset time of 10 minutes or less)

C. Collaborative management

1. Formula selection
   - a. Characteristics of formula include protein classification, nutrient density, and amounts of residue and fiber; different osmolality of formulas are available (isotonic and hypertonic)
   - b. Client's underlying clinical condition influences selection of formula
   - c. Elderly clients and newborns may be unable to tolerate large volume feedings and may need modified treatment regimens to meet nutritional needs

NCLEX® 2. Monitoring response to treatment
   - a. Document weight status; note trends and communicate to health care team
   - b. Monitor for expected weight gain and stabilization of visceral protein measurements (albumin, prealbumin, and transferrin), TLC, BUN, creatinine, and other pertinent serum chemistries during therapy
   - c. Dietitian will evaluate requirements for macronutrients and fluid requirements based on body weight calculations

D. Nursing responsibilities

NCLEX® 1. Record baseline weight and then daily weights to evaluate response to therapy

2. Inspect tube insertion site for signs of potential irritation or infection

NCLEX® 3. Check tube placement prior to administering any feeding regimen or medications
   - a. Aspirate to check for gastric contents and measure pH of gastric aspirant
   - b. Use stethoscope to auscultate for "whoosh" caused by air placement in stomach if agency does not provide pH testing strips

Box 25-5

Interventions for Enteral Tube Feedings

- Inspect formula for particulate matter and unusual appearance that might suggest chemical breakdown.
- Do not hang more formula than is allowed per shift according to hospital protocol to prevent bacterial overgrowth and chemical breakdown.
- Change solution and tubing per hospital protocol to prevent risk of infection.
- Check tube placement prior to any feeding, flush, or medication to ensure patency.
- Flush tube with water per hospital protocol to prevent dehydration that can occur if formula feedings are used as the sole fluid replacement.
- Include flush or irrigation used in the client's I&O.
- Position client to ensure patency and maintain head of bed at 30 degrees prior to and during feeding.
- Monitor pertinent labs per hospital protocol and document daily weights.
- Work with health care team members (dietitian and enterostomal therapist) to maintain nutritional balance and skin integrity.
- Address altered nutritional status and body image when developing plan of care.

Box 25-6

Complications of Tube Feedings

- Mechanical complications include clogged tube, tube dislodgment, and malfunctioning infusion pump.
- Metabolic complications include dehydration, electrolyte imbalances, and altered blood glucose levels (usually hyperglycemia).
- Complications related to formula selection and client tolerance include diarrhea, cramps, abdominal distention, constipation, nausea, and vomiting.
- If client is experiencing diarrhea from enteral feedings, a decreased rate and volume of solution may be indicated; the feeding interval may need to be lengthened to allow client to digest and absorb feedings.
- Check serum albumin levels because changes in colloid oncotic pressure can cause fluid shifting (greater amount of water in the bowel), which also can lead to diarrhea; low serum albumin levels also represent a malnourished state with decreased intestinal enzyme action that can increase incidence of diarrhea.
- Formula may have to be switched to an isotonic formula or a less hypertonic formula to minimize risk of diarrhea from dumping syndrome.
- Dermatologic complications include irritation at feeding tube site (enterostomy) caused by leakage of formula or in response to skin applications or dressings at site.
- Potential complications from medication instillation via tube include clogging of tube from incorrect medication form or formula-drug interactions.
- Monitor amount of feeding and fluid replacement (water) specified per shift and 24-hour totals to minimize risk of dehydration and maintain hydration.
- Clients who have nasogastric tube feedings may be at risk for aspiration due to positioning or decreased gastric emptying; maintain adequate client position by elevating head of bed during feedings and check residuals.

NCLEX® 4. Check for residual on all tube feedings (based on rate per hour) to prevent complications, and document response to therapy
   a. Residuals are often checked every 4 hours during continuous feedings
   b. When feedings are intermittent, check residual prior to instituting next feeding
5. If residual amount is greater than expected, feeding will be withheld or rate will be decreased to prevent overload complications caused by inadequate digestion
   a. In a continuous feeding checked every 4 hours, if residual is greater than or equal to the 1 hour rate, then feeding should be withheld and residual rechecked in 1 hour to determine if client is now able to tolerate feeding
   b. If feeding is not on a continuous schedule, then if half of volume from previous feeding is remaining, then feeding should be withheld and residual rechecked in 1 hour as with a continuous feeding
   c. Adjustment of volume and/or method of feeding (bolus, continuous, cyclic, or intermittent) may be needed based on residual volume measured
   d. Follow agency or provider guidelines if different from those listed above
6. Check pertinent labs, daily weight, and I&O to monitor response to clinical therapy
7. Communicate with other health team members to meet specific client goals

NCLEX® 8. Refer to Box 25–5 for nursing interventions specific to enteral tube feedings

NCLEX® 9. Be aware of potential complications of tube feedings (Box 25–6)

IX. PROBLEMS WITH WEIGHT CONTROL

A. Overview of obesity

1. Obesity: weight that is more than 20% above ideal body weight (IBW)
2. Caused by an excess of body fat; can exist in a person of normal weight
   a. Men: greater than 22% body fat in young men and greater than 25% body fat in older men
   b. Women: greater than 35% body fat
   c. Morbid obesity is generally more than 100% above ideal body weight and having an adverse effect on a person's health
3. Uncommon causes of obesity include genetic factors (Prader-Willi syndrome)
4. Neuroendocrine causes of obesity include Cushing's syndrome, polycystic ovarian syndrome, hypogonadism, insulinoma, and growth hormone insufficiency

5. Most common cause is dietary; associated with high-fat diet and sedentary lifestyle
6. Some drugs promote obesity, such as estrogens, corticosteroids, antidepressants, antiepileptics, antihypertensives, nonsteroidal anti-inflammatory drugs (NSAIDs), and phenothiazines
7. Social factors such as loneliness, stress, depression, guilt, and boredom, as well as cultural views of obesity as desirable and a sign of prosperity, influence eating habits and development of obesity
8. NCLEX® Complications of obesity include hypertension, hiatal hernia, diabetes mellitus, hyperlipidemia, coronary artery disease, sleep apnea, cholelithiasis, osteoarthritis, back pain, and increased susceptibility to infection

B. Assisting with nursing assessment of obesity

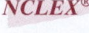

1. Measure height and weight and determine BMI; refer back to Table 25–2 for interpretation of BMI
2. Assess fat distribution profile: "apple" (intra-abdominal/truncal obesity) and "pear" (hips and thighs) waist-to-hip ratio (greater than 1.0 in males and 0.8 in females) can help establish a diagnosis of obesity
3. Examine body type: endomorph (stocky), ectomorph (tall), and mesomorph (middle range), along with upper body (android) and lower body (gynecoid) categories
4. Calculate body weight as a percentage of IBW, usual weight, and recent weight changes to assist in clinical diagnosis
5. Detect complications of obesity or comorbid conditions by measuring serum glucose, serum cholesterol and lipid profile, and by electrocardiogram (ECG)
6. NCLEX® Obtain history of eating habits, duration of obesity, medications, cultural factors, 24-hour food recall, usual physical activity, and situations that trigger eating behavior
7. Assess methods used for previous attempts at weight loss

C. Therapeutic management of obesity

1. Diet therapy
   a. Developed collaboratively with client, health care provider, and dietitian
   b. Safe weight loss rate is 1 to 2 pounds per week; results may be higher at first and then slow over time; FDA indicates weight loss is effective if maintained for 2 years
   c. Goals of diet therapy are aimed at decreasing weight to a healthy level based on client's BMI, activity status, and basal energy expenditure (BEE)
2. Behavioral therapy: helps client to change daily eating habits and includes keeping a food diary, establishing exercise patterns, controlling external cues to eating behavior, and switching focus from physical appearance to health
3. Surgery is an option for obese individuals who do not respond to other methods of weight loss and have a BMI above 35 with additional health risks, or for anyone with a BMI above 40; operative procedures include gastroplasty (most common), intestinal bypass, maxillomandibular fixation, and esophageal banding; pre- and postoperative care is similar to that for other gastric surgeries
4. NCLEX® Exercise enhances weight loss and should be part of daily schedule; recommendations for a healthy lifestyle include at least 30 minutes aerobic activity per day; walking is recommended; plan activity appropriate for client considering physical and environmental limitations
5. Provide information about support groups such as Overeaters Anonymous and Weight Watchers
6. Medication/pharmacological intervention
   a. Drug treatment is controversial and is usually only suggested with BMI above 30 (or >27 with comorbidities) and in conjunction with diet modifications and exercise
   b. Anorexic medications may be used to suppress appetite so client eats less and loses weight slowly over time; they are contraindicated during pregnancy and lactation and in clients with cardiac, hepatic, or renal disease
   c. Amphetamines and antidepressants are controversial because of reported cases of toxicity and dependency

D. Client teaching related to obesity

1. Prescribed diet therapy and exercise
2. New food pyramid (MyPyramid, see Figure 25-1) and portion sizes (e.g., a serving of meat is 3 oz and is about size of a deck of cards; a serving of dry breakfast cereal is 1 oz or 1 cup)
3. Symptoms of possible adverse effects of weight loss medications, such as chest pain, shortness of breath, insomnia, and nervousness

E. Overview of underweight status

1. An **underweight** client has a BMI below 18.5 with subsequent ill effects on health
2. Physical conditions caused by disease or medical treatments can lead to underweight status
3. Failure to thrive (FTT) infants do not meet expected growth curves and developmental milestones and are clinically malnourished; weight and height are below expected percentile; these infants start out underweight and become more underweight over time

Box 25–7

Realistic Eating Plans for Underweight Client

- Do not skip meals; it is important to start an eating pattern based on eating all scheduled meals.
- Increase portion sizes and add nutrient-dense foods to eating plan; now is the time to add new foods, taste new foods, and sample old foods.
- Drink fluids and make sure to include them as sources of energy by using fruit juices and milkshakes to add to dietary intake.
- Incorporate physical activity to maintain muscle tone, gain strength, and promote endurance.
- Supplemental feedings may be required via enteral or parenteral route to realize dietary goals.
- Be aware of reasonable weight gain expectations and note that weight gained over time is more likely to stay on than weight gained through daily forced feeding.
- Medications may be prescribed to boost appetite and stimulate weight gain; if nausea or other GI symptoms occur, additional medications may be prescribed to minimize these symptoms and promote an adequate eating pattern.

4. Psychological conditions (anorexia, bulimia, and depression) can lead to decreased intake, poor nutrition, and underweight status
5. Loss of visceral protein stores (body storage) results in negative nitrogen balance
6. Underweight clients may have adverse health effects if further compromised by stress, injury, or infection

NCLEX®

F. Therapeutic management of underweight status

1. Increase calories and reestablish regular meal pattern to promote weight gain
2. Increase intake of foods with high nutrient density (highest kcal/food)
3. Calculate ongoing nutrient needs based on BEE and evaluation of pertinent lab work (albumin, pre-albumin, transferrin levels, and TLC) in collaboration with dietitian and health care provider
4. Refer to Box 25–7 for realistic eating plan to promote weight gain
5. Medication therapy: megestrol acetate (Megace) and dronabinol (Marinol) as appetite stimulants (useful in clients with cancer, HIV, and AIDS)

G. Overview of malnutrition

1. State of poor nutrition from either undernutrition or overnutrition
2. Includes protein-calorie malnutrition (PCM) or protein-energy malnutrition (PEM)
3. Healing is adversely affected because of loss of protein stores and essential and nonessential nutrients that are coenzymes in metabolic processes
4. Immune function is compromised because of insufficient nutrients
5. Fluid shifts due to low protein levels can lead to third spacing (ascites as in Kwashiorkor) and edema states (dependent and/or periorbital) because of electrolyte imbalances
6. Dermatologic changes include brittle hair that can fall out, nail changes (brittle with ridges), pruritus, and poor healing
7. Hormonal imbalances can develop, affecting neurological status (irritability, paresthesias, decreased reflex response), musculoskeletal status (decreased muscle tone, cramping, deformities), and cardiac status (altered blood pressure, murmurs, possible cardiac enlargement)
8. Clinical evidence of malnutrition: mouth sores, oral cavity changes, and decreased hydration status

NCLEX®

H. Therapeutic management of malnutrition

1. Nutrient calculation by dietitian uses BEE, BMI, activity level, and lab results
2. A significant increase in caloric intake is required to effect weight gain (3500 calories per week for a 1-pound weight gain requires additional 500 calories per day)
3. Supervised program is needed to work toward achieving individual client goals
4. Supplemental feeding may be required via enteral or parenteral routes
5. Frequent feeding regimen may be utilized to prevent hypoglycemia and hypothermia, which can cause further tissue catabolism
6. Controlled regimen for children (not less than 80 calories/kg/day up to 100 or more) and for adults (30–40 kcal/kg/day) may be used to meet nutritional goals
7. Document and trend pertinent labs and weight status and correlate with client's underlying medical condition

PRACTICE TEST

l. Weight cycling

1. "Yo-yo" effect is a weight loss/weight gain pattern that can lead to a higher weight than when diet therapy was started; this usually occurs with unrealistic weight goals and/or altered dietary patterns without benefit of activity or lifestyle changes

NCLEX®

2. For weight control to be effective, a combination of dietary, lifestyle, behavioral, and activity changes (not merely changes in food intake) are necessary

Check Your NCLEX-PN® Exam I.Q.

You are ready for testing on this content if you can

- Apply knowledge of nursing procedures to the care of a client with nutritional needs.
- Collect data regarding nutritional status of client, including a diet history.
- Determine impact of illness on nutritional status.
- Provide a special diet based on health problem and nutritional needs of a client.
- Provide dietary teaching according to client need.
- Provide nutritional supplements to clients as needed.
- Promote independence in eating.
- Check placement and patency of a feeding tube.
- Describe side effects of enteral nutrition.
- Collect data regarding effectiveness of diet therapy on weight and overall nutritional status.

PRACTICE TEST

1 The nurse has read the admission assessment of a Hispanic client and notes that some cultural food practices place the client at risk for cardiovascular disease. Which suggestion by the nurse is appropriate for this client?

1. "Try to stop eating so many complex carbohydrates."
2. "Try to bake some foods instead of frying them."
3. "Lean meats should replace the beans and nuts in your diet."
4. "Do not stop stewing meat and vegetables together; it is a healthy cooking method."

2 Which dietary recommendation should the nurse reinforce in the discharge instructions of a client diagnosed with coronary artery disease?

1. Limit intake of whole grains.
2. Limit intake of tuna.
3. Limit intake of soybean products.
4. Limit intake of egg yolks.

3 The nurse is reinforcing discharge teaching for the client with gastroesophageal reflux disease (GERD). What dietary modification should be included?

1. Eat three meals and a bedtime snack daily.
2. Avoid intake of caffeine and alcoholic beverages.
3. Drink 12–16 ounces of water with each meal.
4. Lie down for 15–20 minutes after eating.

4 The nurse interprets that which client behavior matches the restriction of a 2-gram sodium-restricted diet?

1. Using the two packets of salt found on the meal tray
2. Limiting milk to 1 cup per day
3. Avoiding use of salt in cooking
4. Using salt-free butter with meals

5 The nurse determines that a hypertensive client understands the DASH diet (Dietary Approaches to Stop Hypertension) when the client chooses which items from a sample menu used in dietary teaching?

1. Caesar salad, bread sticks, frozen yogurt
2. Grilled chicken sandwich, strawberries, and lettuce salad
3. Grilled cheese sandwich, canned pineapple, brownie
4. Chicken and vegetable stir-fry, rice, egg roll

6 A client who is recovering from partial- and full-thickness burns has been advanced to a general diet. Which foods should the nurse encourage the client to eat most often?

1. Meats, citrus fruits, milk
2. Vegetables, cheese, pasta
3. Milkshakes, salads, soups
4. Breads, cereals, yogurt

7. Which client comment indicates to the nurse that more reinforcement of teaching is needed for the client experiencing dumping syndrome after gastric surgery? Select all that apply.

1. "I should eat six small meals per day."
2. "I should not drink fluids with my meals."
3. "I should use honey or jelly instead of butter."
4. "I should lie down for 30–60 minutes after eating."

8. Which statement would the nurse make during dietary teaching to a client who has renal calculi?

1. "The presence of renal calculi is directly correlated to dietary intake."
2. "Decreasing calcium intake will prevent the formation of renal calculi."
3. "An increase in dietary protein can increase the likelihood of renal calculi."
4. "Reducing dietary intake of complex carbohydrates decreases formation of renal calculi."

9. A client with chronic obstructive pulmonary disease (COPD), who has been consuming more than 3000 calories/day to gain weight, now reports increased breathing difficulty. The client states, "I thought that if I gained weight by eating more, I would feel better." How would the nurse respond to the client's concern?

1. "The increase in calories is not as important as an increase in the fat percentage in the diet."
2. "It is not necessary to increase caloric intake because medication therapy can be given to help with desired weight gain."
3. "An increase in both calories and carbohydrates can lead to increased respiratory effort and clinical symptoms that you are having."
4. "An increase in high-quality proteins will help correct the respiratory symptoms."

10. Which snack selection would be most appropriate for the nurse to make for a client with cancer who has stomatitis?

1. Peanut butter sandwich
2. Soft pretzels with salt
3. Tomato soup
4. Yogurt

11. A client who is lactose intolerant is recovering from a surgical procedure. What impact does the nurse expect this to have on progression of diet as tolerated?

1. The client will be able to progress from a clear to full liquid diet easily once bowel sounds and gag reflex return.
2. There is no impact with regard to diet progression because of lactose intolerance.
3. The client's diet can be progressed following a bowel movement indicating return of bowel activity.
4. The client's full liquid diet may have to be altered because this diet contains milk products.

12. A client is placed on enteral feedings via nasogastric tube to meet nutritional goals. Which intervention should the nurse carry out in the plan of care to help maintain fluid balance?

1. Observe the skin area around the tube site.
2. Weigh the client every other day.
3. Maintain strict I&O and flush the tube once a day to ensure patency.
4. Irrigate the tube with water as ordered and include this fluid in total I&O.

13. Which of the following points would the nurse make when reinforcing dietary teaching with a client placed on a fat-restricted diet because of significant cardiac history?

1. "This diet will be used temporarily to reduce saturated fat intake and cholesterol levels."
2. "All forms of fat should be restricted because of your significant cardiac history."
3. "No additional fat should be utilized when cooking or preparing foods."
4. "Ice cream can be included in the diet, although fat from butter and meat is excluded."

14 A client's mother wants to know why she should have her daughter follow an allergy I and II diet. How would the nurse reply to this mother's concern?

1. "This is a short-term therapy diet and it will be over before you know it."
2. "This diet needs to be followed until your daughter grows out of her allergy phase."
3. "This diet sequence helps to both identify and eliminate potential allergens, making future diet selection choices easier."
4. "Allergy testing usually accompanies this type of diet pattern and you should see an immunologist."

15 Which food item should the nurse encourage in the diet of a client diagnosed with celiac disease?

1. Oatmeal
2. Whole wheat toast
3. Beef barley soup
4. Cornflakes

16 Which of the following foods would the nurse suggest as an item from the lunch menu for a client taking a monoamine oxidase (MAO) inhibitor?

1. Smoked fish
2. Bologna sandwich
3. Cottage cheese
4. Salad with bleu cheese dressing

17 The client states, "I am always dieting, but I never seem to lose weight." How would the nurse best respond to the client?

1. "Weight loss is only maintained if you really want to lose the weight."
2. "Dieting is a way of life, and compliance is required to maintain weight loss."
3. "By saying you are always dieting, it sounds like you need some assistance in attaining your weight-loss goals."
4. "I need to know which type of the diet you are on because it may not be effective."

18 The nurse would encourage the client wishing to reduce risk of cancer to maintain adequate intake of which foods?

1. Meat and dairy products
2. Fruits and vegetables
3. Rice and beans
4. Milk and cheese

19 An athletic client states that he is thinking of using carbohydrate (CHO) loading to increase his performance. How should the nurse respond to this client?

1. Suggest the use of alternative ergonomic aids such as creatine or creatinine because they provide better results.
2. Discuss foods that are high in CHOs to assist the client in meeting his desired goal.
3. Ask the client what type of sport activity he is doing to see if this method would help.
4. Refer the client to a sports/nutritional specialist or trainer so that he can be properly supervised.

20 The nurse would consult with the physician about either advancing the diet or instituting parenteral nutrition if the client has been on a clear-liquid diet for the maximum ________ days? Provide a numerical answer.

Fill in your answer below:

________ days

21 The nurse is instructing a client who wants to begin following a vegetarian diet about foods that provide protein. The nurse explains that which food choices would be appropriate for this client? Select all that apply.

1. Soy
2. Beans
3. Nuts
4. Turkey
5. Wheat germ

ANSWERS & RATIONALES

1 **Answer: 2** **Rationale:** One characteristic of Hispanic diets is the high-fat preparation method, such as frying, used in cooking. Suggesting a new preparation method for a familiar food item would best help the client to begin changing cooking habits. Complex carbohydrates should not be eliminated because they are components of a healthy diet. The Hispanic client would probably be unwilling to relinquish beans and nuts in the diet because these are considered staple food products. Stewing is considered a high-fat method of cooking because the fat from the meat does not drain off. **Cognitive Level:** Applying **Client Need:** Basic Care and Comfort **Integrated Process:** Nursing Process: Implementation **Content Area:** Foundational Sciences **Strategy:** The core issue of the question is knowledge of methods of reducing fat in the diet. Use nutrition knowledge and the process of elimination to make a selection.

2 **Answer: 4** **Rationale:** Egg yolks are high in cholesterol and should be limited to two or three per week. Dietary fiber is necessary in the body to promote regulation of elimination patterns and to help lower blood lipids. Tuna is an excellent source of omega-3 fatty acids, which are helpful in protecting cardiac function and decreasing clot formation. Soybean products are a source of phytoestrogens and have been shown to be cardioprotective. **Cognitive Level:** Applying **Client Need:** Basic Care and Comfort **Integrated Process:** Nursing Process: Implementation **Content Area:** Foundational Sciences **Strategy:** The core issue of the question is knowledge of the components of a low-fat diet and that this is the diet required by clients with heart disease. Use nutrition knowledge and the process of elimination to make a selection.

3 **Answer: 2** **Rationale:** Foods that decrease lower esophageal sphincter (LES) pressure should be avoided to reduce reflux symptoms; these include caffeine, alcohol, and chocolate. Clients should also avoid eating large meals, drinking fluids with meals, and eating at bedtime; they should remain upright for 1–2 hours after eating. **Cognitive Level:** Applying **Client Need:** Basic Care and Comfort **Integrated Process:** Teaching and Learning **Content Area:** Foundational Sciences **Strategy:** The core issue of the question is knowledge of foods that lower LES pressure and increase risk of reflux in GERD. Use nutrition knowledge and the process of elimination to make a selection.

4 **Answer: 3** **Rationale:** A 2-gram sodium-restricted diet requires use of no salt in cooking, no salt added at the table, avoiding high-sodium foods, and limiting milk to 2 cups per day. No salt can be added in this restricted diet. One cup of milk per day and the use of salt-free butter are requirements of a 1-gram sodium-restricted diet. **Cognitive Level:** Applying **Client Need:** Basic Care and Comfort **Integrated Process:** Nursing Process: Evaluation **Content Area:** Foundational Sciences **Strategy:** The core issue of the question is knowledge of the various degrees of sodium restriction in the diet. Use nutrition knowledge and the process of elimination to make a selection.

5 **Answer: 2** **Rationale:** The DASH diet increases daily servings of vegetables and fruits, and recommends low-fat dairy foods and reduced intake of saturated fats and cholesterol. A menu consisting of grilled chicken, strawberries, and lettuce salad meets the DASH diet requirements. A menu consisting of Caesar salad, bread sticks, and frozen yogurt reflects increased fats. A menu consisting of a grilled cheese sandwich, canned pineapple, and a brownie represents increased fat, cholesterol, and sugar. A menu consisting of chicken and vegetable stir-fry, rice, and egg roll reflects increased sodium content. **Cognitive Level:** Applying **Client Need:** Basic Care and Comfort **Integrated Process:** Nursing Process: Evaluation **Content Area:** Foundational Sciences **Strategy:** The core issue of the question is knowledge that hypertensive clients should lose weight if necessary and restrict dietary intake of sodium. Use nutrition knowledge and the process of elimination to make a selection.

6 **Answer: 1** **Rationale:** The client with burns needs increased amounts of protein and vitamins C and D until the wounds are completely healed. The meal with meat, fruit, and milk reflects high-protein sources, an antioxidant source, and fortified milk that includes vitamin D and calcium. The other options do not reflect the necessary protein, vitamins, and mineral sources needed for the care of clients recovering from burns. **Cognitive Level:** Applying **Client Need:** Basic Care and Comfort **Integrated Process:** Nursing Process: Implementation **Content Area:** Foundational Sciences **Strategy:** The core issue of the question is knowledge that increased protein and vitamins are needed for wound healing. Use nutrition knowledge about food sources of protein and vitamins and the process of elimination to make a selection.

7 **Answer: 2, 3, 4** **Rationale:** Simple sugars and carbohydrates, including honey and jelly, increase the osmolality of the gastric contents and enhance movement of food out of the stomach. Therefore, these should be avoided by the client at risk for dumping syndrome. Six small meals per day, avoiding fluids with meals, and lying down for 30–60 minutes after meals will help reduce the risk of dumping syndrome. **Cognitive Level:** Analyzing **Client Need:** Basic Care and Comfort **Integrated Process:** Nursing Process: Evaluation **Content Area:** Foundational Sciences **Strategy:** The stem of the question has a negative wording, which tells you that the correct answer is an incorrect statement. Recall that sugars and concentrated carbohydrates should be avoided to help choose the statement that is incorrect.

8 **Answer: 3** **Rationale:** Increased dietary protein can lead to increased uric acid formation, which in turn lowers urinary pH and causes precipitation of uric acid stones. Clients should not exceed protein intake of 100 grams per day and should monitor purine content of foods. Factors other than dietary intake can cause the formation of renal calculi, specifically alterations in urinary pH and the presence of metabolic disease. There is no clinical evidence to suggest that decreasing calcium intake will prevent the formation of renal calculi; rather, research shows that a high-calcium diet offers protection against stone formation. Even though most renal calculi are composed of calcium oxalate, it is the oxalate component that appears to cause the formation of stones. Foods that are high in absorbable oxalate include spinach, beets, rhubarb, nuts, chocolate, tea, and wheat bran.

Increasing intake of complex carbohydrates is recommended to prevent renal calculi formation. **Cognitive Level:** Applying **Client Need:** Basic Care and Comfort **Integrated Process:** Nursing Process: Implementation **Content Area:** Foundational Sciences **Strategy:** The core issue of the question is knowledge that protein sources can lead to uric acid formation and subsequent stone formation. Use nutrition knowledge and the process of elimination to make a selection.

9 **Answer: 3 Rationale:** Clients with COPD who overeat, in addition to consuming excess carbohydrates, have increasing difficulty with breathing because of excessive CO2 levels that place additional stress on the lungs. The client should eat a proper diet and correct percentages of macronutrients to maintain adequate weight. Chronic COPD is associated with PEM (protein-energy malnutrition), infection, and unintentional weight loss. Increased calories alone can lead to increased work of breathing. The percentage of fat in the diet may also pose a problem if the client is experiencing contributory disease or malabsorption. Merely providing medication therapy to stimulate weight gain does not address the problem of the obvious excess of calories that the client is consuming or that the client is experiencing difficulty breathing. An increase in high-quality proteins will not help to correct the clinical symptoms. **Cognitive Level:** Analyzing **Client Need:** Basic Care and Comfort **Integrated Process:** Teaching and Learning **Content Area:** Foundational Sciences **Strategy:** The core issue of the question is knowledge that excessive carbohydrate intake results in excess carbon dioxide production, which can be harmful to the client with COPD. Use nutrition knowledge and the process of elimination to make a selection.

10 **Answer: 4 Rationale:** A client who has stomatitis will have pain upon ingestion of food caused by the inflammatory process. Cool foods are often tolerated better than hot foods, as are soft, creamy products, such as yogurt. Peanut butter is a thick, dense food that may irritate the mouth by sticking on mucous membranes and requiring more effort to swallow. Pretzels are high in salt, which may cause further irritation to the oral cavity. Tomatoes are high in ascorbic acid; even though they are in the form of a soup, they may cause irritation. **Cognitive Level:** Applying **Client Need:** Basic Care and Comfort **Integrated Process:** Nursing Process: Implementation **Content Area:** Foundational Sciences **Strategy:** The core issue of the question is knowledge that clients with stomatitis need foods that are soft, nonirritating, and not hot. Use nutrition knowledge and the process of elimination to make a selection.

11 **Answer: 4 Rationale:** A client who is lactose intolerant has difficulty handling milk and dairy products because of deficient lactase enzyme. Full-liquid diets are based on milk and dairy products. The diet of a lactose-intolerant client will have to be adjusted to reflect lactose-reduced or lactose-free products to prevent GI irritation. Focusing on bowel sounds and return of gag reflex does not address the added clinical condition of lactose intolerance but merely refers to progression of diet. Lactose intolerance does have an impact on dietary patterns and progression. While the client's diet can be progressed following a bowel movement, this does not address lactose intolerance. **Cognitive Level:** Analyzing **Client Need:** Basic Care and Comfort **Integrated Process:** Nursing Process: Planning **Content Area:** Foundational Sciences **Strategy:** The core issue of the question is knowledge of concepts related to lactose intolerance. Use nutrition knowledge and the process of elimination to make a selection.

12 **Answer: 4 Rationale:** A client who is receiving enteral feedings via nasogastric tube can be at risk for dehydration caused by inadequate fluid intake. It is important to irrigate the tube with water as ordered (before and after feedings or medication administration) and include these irrigations in the client's total I&O measurements. Although inspection of the skin surrounding the tube is necessary, it does not relate specifically to fluid balance. Clients are often weighed daily, not every other day. Feeding tubes are flushed at least once per shift, not only once a day. **Cognitive Level:** Applying **Client Need:** Basic Care and Comfort **Integrated Process:** Nursing Process: Planning **Content Area:** Foundational Sciences **Strategy:** The core issue of the question is knowledge that a client receiving enteral feedings is at risk for dehydration if there are no sources of free water provided. Use nutrition knowledge and the process of elimination to make a selection.

13 **Answer: 3 Rationale:** A client with a significant cardiac history on a fat-restricted diet should not use additional fat during the cooking or preparation process. This client will require some form of fat control or restriction as part of a dietary pattern for the rest of his or her life. Fat is a necessary nutrient for the body. To deprive a client of all fat sources can lead to a clinical deficiency of essential fatty acids that can cause further problems for the client. Ice cream is considered a high-fat product. The client could have low-fat ice cream, yogurt, or sherbet to satisfy dietary needs. **Cognitive Level:** Applying **Client Need:** Basic Care and Comfort **Integrated Process:** Teaching and Learning **Content Area:** Foundational Sciences **Strategy:** The core issue of the question is knowledge of aspects of a low-fat diet and that the diet needs to be lifelong. Use nutrition knowledge and the process of elimination to make a selection.

14 **Answer: 3 Rationale:** Allergy I and II diets are used in sequence to identify and eliminate potential food allergens. Even though this diet pattern is used over a short time period, this response does not address why it is necessary to follow the diet pattern. A client will not "grow out" of a true allergy. Referral to an immunologist for allergy testing is not a required accompaniment to this dietary pattern. Referral to an immunologist for allergy testing may eventually be indicated if the client is found to have a multiple allergy profile. **Cognitive Level:** Applying **Client Need:** Basic Care and Comfort **Integrated Process:** Communication and Documentation **Content Area:** Foundational Sciences **Strategy:** The core issue of the question is knowledge regarding the purposes of allergy I and II diets. Use nutrition knowledge and the process of elimination to make a selection.

15 **Answer: 4 Rationale:** Foods that contain gluten (wheat, oats, rye, and barley) are restricted for a client with celiac disease because of an inability to handle gluten protein. All of the other choices reflect items that cannot be used in a gluten-restricted diet. **Cognitive Level:** Applying **Client Need:** Basic Care and Comfort **Integrated Process:** Nursing Process: Implementation **Content Area:** Foundational Sciences **Strategy:** The core issue of the question is knowledge that a foods containing wheat, rye, oats, and barley are restricted in celiac disease. Use nutrition knowledge about foods containing these grains and the process of elimination to make a selection.

16 **Answer: 3 Rationale:** A client taking MAO inhibitors has to avoid foods that are high in tyramine because it can lead to significant complications resulting in hypertensive crisis. Cottage

cheese is an unfermented cheese that can be used in the diet. Smoked fish, bologna sandwich, and bleu cheese dressing are high in tyramine and are not allowed in the diet. **Cognitive Level:** Analyzing **Client Need:** Basic Care and Comfort **Integrated Process:** Nursing Process: Planning **Content Area:** Foundational Sciences **Strategy:** The core issue of the question is knowledge that clients taking MAOIs require a low-tyramine diet. Use nutrition knowledge of low-tyramine foods and the process of elimination to make a selection.

17 **Answer: 3** **Rationale:** The perception of being in a state of "always dieting" can be problematic in terms of compliance and goal attainment because it can be viewed either as a restriction or as a form of punishment. Wanting to lose weight is not the only factor to consider; many other variables affect weight loss. Focusing on compliance does not explore the difficulty the client is having with weight management. While it is important to find out the type of the diet the client is on (or has been on), this knowledge does not address the main concern of the client regarding "always dieting" and yo-yo effect (weight cycling). **Cognitive Level:** Applying **Client Need:** Basic Care and Comfort **Integrated Process:** Communication and Documentation **Content Area:** Foundational Sciences **Strategy:** The core issue of the question is identification of a client's need for assistance with weight control. Use nutrition knowledge and the process of elimination to make a selection.

18 **Answer: 2** **Rationale:** Diets that are rich in fruits and vegetables have been proven to be effective in decreasing the risk of developing cancer because these foods contain phytochemicals. None of the other food groupings have been shown to decrease the risk of cancer. **Cognitive Level:** Applying **Client Need:** Basic Care and Comfort **Integrated Process:** Nursing Process: Implementation **Content Area:** Foundational Sciences **Strategy:** The core issue of the question is knowledge of foods that contain protective chemicals against cancer development. Use nutrition knowledge and the process of elimination to make a selection.

19 **Answer: 4** **Rationale:** When an athletic client is considering utilizing any ergonomic aid or supplement, trainers and/or nutritional specialists can monitor the client closely to establish a client baseline, provide education, and prevent potential complications related to therapy. The nurse should not suggest an alternative ergonomic aid. The client needs a proper referral to an expert in the field. Discussing foods that are high in CHO does not address the priority need—to make the referral. Although it is important to note what type of exercise the client practices, it is still more important to refer the client to the proper specialist who can assist in supervising an athletic treatment regimen. **Cognitive Level:** Applying **Client Need:** Coordinated Care **Integrated Process:** Nursing Process: Implementation **Content Area:** Foundational Sciences **Strategy:** The core issue of the question is appropriate anticipatory guidance to a client seeking to use nontraditional methods of nutrition for supplemental use. Use knowledge that this client requires special monitoring and the process of elimination to make a selection.

20 **Answer: 2** **Rationale:** A clear-liquid diet is recommended for short-term use (1–2 days). Therefore, the maximum is 2 days. It can be used both before and after surgery or diagnostic procedures, during acute stages of illness, or as an initial diet after a significant period of GI inactivity or bowel rest. **Cognitive Level:** Applying **Client Need:** Basic Care and Comfort **Integrated Process:** Nursing Process: Implementation **Content Area:** Foundational Sciences **Strategy:** The core issue of the question is the length of time a clear-liquid diet is appropriate. Use knowledge of clear-liquid diet as a therapeutic diet to answer.

21 **Answer: 1, 2, 3** **Rationale:** Soy belongs to the protein group and is often used in the vegetarian diet. Beans are part of the protein group and would be appropriate for a vegetarian. Nuts contain good amounts of protein and are appropriate for use by a vegetarian client. Vegetarians do not eat animal meat; most vegetarians (other than vegans) will consume eggs, legumes, and dairy products. Wheat germ may be acceptable in the vegetarian diet but it is a grain rather than a good source of protein. **Cognitive Level:** Applying **Client Need:** Health Promotion and Maintenance **Integrated Process:** Teaching and Learning **Content Area:** Foundational Sciences **Strategy:** Notice that the client is vegetarian; eliminate the option that is of animal origin. Then recall knowledge of protein-containing foods and eliminate the option that is a grain.

Key Terms to Review

bolus feeding p. 360
cyclic feeding p. 360
enteral nutrition p. 360
ergonomic aids p. 353
obesity p. 349
phytochemicals p. 352
underweight p. 362

References

Ball, J., & Bindler, R. & Cowen, K. (2010). *Child health nursing: Partnering with children and families.* (2nd ed.). Upper Saddle River, NJ: Pearson Education., Inc.

Berman, A., & Snyder, S. (2012). *Kozier & Erb's fundamentals of nursing: Concepts, process, and practice* (9th ed.). Upper Saddle River, NJ: Pearson Education, Inc.

Lutz, S. & Przytulski, K. (2011). *Nutrition & diet therapy* (5th ed.). Philadelphia: F.A. Davis.

National Heart, Lung, and Blood Institute (NLHBI) (n.d.). *Guidelines on the identification, evaluation and treatment of overweight and obesity in adults: The evidence report.* Retrieved July 27, 2010, from http://www.nhlbi.nih.gov/guidelines/obesity/ob_gdlns.pdf

Nix, S. (2009). *Williams' basic nutrition and diet therapy* (13th ed.). St. Louis, MO: Elsevier Mosby.

Test Yourself

Are you ready for the NCLEX-PN® or course exams? Use the practice tests on the companion website to check.

Smith, S., Duell, D., & Martin, B. (2012). *Clinical nursing skills: Basic to advanced skills* (8th ed.). Upper Saddle River, NJ: Pearson Education.

Tucker, S. & Dauffenbach, V. (2011). *Nutrition and diet therapy for nurses*. Upper Saddle River, NJ: Pearson Education, Inc.

U.S. Department of Agriculture & U.S. Department of Health and Human Services (2010). *Dietary guidelines for Americans 2010* (7th ed.). Washington, DC: U.S Government Printing Office. Retrieved July 2, 2011, from http://www.health.gov/dietaryguidelines/dga2010/DietaryGuidelines2010.pdf

U.S. Department of Agriculture (USDA), Center for Nutrition Policy and Promotion (2005). *MyPyramid food guidance system*. Washington, DC: Author. Retrieved July 27, 2010, from www.mypyramid.gov

World Health Organization (WHO) (1999). *Management of malnutrition: A manual for physicians and other senior healthcare workers*. Retrieved July 27, 2010, from http://whqlibdoc.who.int/hq/1999/a57361.pdf

Meeting Basic Human Needs 26

In this chapter

Cross Reference

Other chapters relevant to this content area are

Meeting Nutritional Needs	Chapter 25
Maintaining Function of Tubes and Drains	Chapter 27

I. MEETING HYGIENE NEEDS

A. Functions of skin

1. Protection: body's first line of defense against microorganisms
2. Sensation: pain, temperature, and pressure
3. Temperature regulation
4. Excretion and secretion: of sweat (water, chloride, potassium, glucose, and urea) and sebum (an oily substance); acid pH of skin secretions inhibits bacterial growth

B. Skin care

1. Developmental changes: age and ability influence skin care practices
   a. A newborn requires only sponge baths, not tub baths; dry newborn immediately and wrap to prevent heat loss; shivering in newborns starts at a lower body temperature than in adults, and infants have greater body surface area for heat loss compared to adults
   b. A toddler depends on caregiver to provide care but may want to perform tasks (such as brushing teeth) independently
   c. An older adult who is frail may be dependent but may still be able to identify skin care preferences; excessive bathing can contribute to dry skin
2. Cultural considerations
   a. Hygiene practices vary considerably among different cultures; in some cultures, daily bathing is a ritual, while in others, a weekly routine is acceptable; other differences may be use of deodorants and preference for tub or shower
   b. Some cultures are concerned with hot/cold imbalances as a cause of illness
   c. Bathing may be avoided with some body conditions; for instance, some cultures avoid bathing during menstruation and childbirth

NCLEX®

3. Common skin problems requiring care
   a. Dryness: flaky, rough skin may crack; pruritus (itching) may occur
   b. Abrasions: epidermis (superficial layer of skin) rubbed or scraped off
   c. Ammonia dermatitis (diaper rash): reddened skin that may be excoriated, caused by skin bacteria reacting to urea in urine

Box 26–1

Care of an Eye Prosthesis

- Using gloves, exert slight pressure below eyelid and remove artificial eye.
- Clean eye socket and periorbital tissues with moistened washcloth.
- Clean artificial eye with warm normal saline and rinse.
- To reinsert prosthetic eye
  - retract eyelids and exert pressure on supraorbital and infraorbital bones.
  - hold prosthetic eye with index finger and thumb of other hand and slip it gently into socket.

d. Contact dermatitis: reddened skin accompanied by pruritus that may result in infection if scratched
e. Erythema: redness of skin associated with rashes, infections, and allergies
f. **Pressure ulcer**: an open skin lesion, often over bony prominences, caused by decreased circulation

C. Specific hygiene measures

1. Partial bed bath: client may do certain portions of bath as desired or as condition permits; includes only parts that may cause discomfort or odor if not washed
2. Complete bed bath: nurse washes client's entire body
3. Perineal care to genitalia and rectal area
4. Nail and foot care
5. *NCLEX®* Document observations such as general skin condition, reddened areas over bony prominences, irritation, and inflammation
6. Oral care: brushing and flossing teeth and denture care; document abnormalities such as irritated mucous membranes and ill-fitting dentures
7. Hair and scalp care: includes brushing and shampooing hair; personal habits and cultural influences affect hair care practices; clean hair limits microbe count, and groomed hair can increase general comfort level
8. Care of eyes, ears, and nose
   a. *NCLEX®* Eye care: wipe loosened secretions from inner to outer canthus; for unconscious client, use artificial tears every 2 hours or as ordered to reduce corneal injury
   b. Ear care: if cerumen (earwax) is visible, loosen it by retracting auricles downward, then remove with a damp washcloth
9. Care of removable prosthetic (artificial) eye: see Box 26–1
10. Promote client independence as much as possible during care
11. *NCLEX®* Document ability to bathe, feed, groom, and toilet self as indicators of functional ability; communicate this information to discharge planners, long-term or rehabilitation care centers, and home health nurses

D. Care of client's room environment

1. *NCLEX®* Keep area clutter-free
   a. Arrange furniture to avoid accidents; for example, no furniture in middle of room
   b. Remove unnecessary objects; keep obstacles out of walkways
2. Keep objects needed by client nearby; put necessary objects for daily hygiene and activities of daily living within reach (e.g., client's eyeglasses, cane, fluids, and call bell)
3. Control odors
   a. Provide good ventilation
   b. Remove and dispose of offensive waste products appropriately
   c. Use room deodorizers as necessary

II. MEETING OXYGENATION NEEDS

A. Summary of physiology of cardiovascular and respiratory systems

1. Heart serves as a system pump, moving blood through blood vessels to tissues and transports blood containing oxygen and nutrients to cells; wastes are collected for elimination
2. Respiratory system
   a. Pulmonary ventilation, or breathing: inspiration (inhalation)—air flows into lungs; expiration (exhalation)—air moves out of lungs
   b. Alveolar gas exchange: after alveoli are ventilated, diffusion of oxygen occurs from alveoli into pulmonary blood vessels
   c. Transport of oxygen (O_2) and carbon dioxide (CO_2): O_2 is transported from lungs to tissues, and CO_2 is transported from tissues back to lungs; O_2 combines with hemoglobin in red blood cells (RBCs) and is then carried to tissues as oxyhemoglobin

B. Factors affecting oxygenation

1. Environment
   - **a.** Altitude: higher altitude increases respiratory and heart rate (HR) and respiratory depth
   - **b.** Heat: causes peripheral vessel dilation, increased blood flow to skin, and decreased resistance to blood flow; cardiac output (CO) increases, raising blood pressure (BP); rate and depth of breathing also increase
   - **c.** Cold: vasoconstriction occurs and BP elevates, decreasing cardiac action because of reduced need for oxygen
   - **d.** Air pollution: causes symptoms such as coughing, choking, and difficulty breathing
   - **e.** Health status: healthy clients have sufficient O_2 to meet body's demands; in cardiovascular disease, O_2 transport is compromised; in respiratory disease, oxygenation of blood is affected
   - *NCLEX®* **f.** Narcotics: opioids such as morphine decrease respiratory rate and depth by depressing respiratory center of medulla
2. Developmental factors
   - *NCLEX®* **a.** Premature infants: inadequate respiratory status is caused by immature lungs; respiratory center of brain is immature; gag and cough reflexes are weak
   - *NCLEX®* **b.** Infants and toddlers have smaller airway passages, which contributes to obstruction by foreign objects such as peanuts, coins, and small toys; diseases such as cystic fibrosis and asthma lead to difficulty breathing and affect oxygenation
   - **c.** Because of exposure to infectious agents at school and play, upper respiratory problems are common in school-age children
   - **d.** At puberty, heart and lungs increase considerably in size and heart rate drops
   - **e.** Starting at age 35–40, aerobic capacity (ability to provide O_2 to body's organs) and CO show age-related changes during work or exercise; loss of blood vessel elasticity may contribute to hypertension, which affects oxygenation; atherosclerosis (plaque buildup in arterial walls) decreases blood flow
   - **f.** In older adults, chest wall becomes more rigid and lungs are less elastic, so more air is retained in lungs at expiration; cough effectiveness decreases; protective cilia are less effective, increasing risk of upper respiratory infections; decreased respiratory reserve reduces exercise tolerance; blood flow may be impaired by hypertension, atherosclerosis, and obstructive lung disease
3. Lifestyle factors
   - **a.** Nutrition: high fat and salt intake may increase risk for heart disease, and inadequate diet can lead to anemia (insufficient RBCs)
   - **b.** Physical exercise: increases rate and depth of respirations and HR, thus increasing supply of oxygen in body
   - *NCLEX®* **c.** Smoking: nicotine increases HR, BP, and peripheral resistance; vasoconstriction occurs and decreases oxygenation to tissues
   - **d.** Substance abuse: alcohol is a respiratory depressant and slows respirations; long-term use increases BP and tendency for malnutrition and anemia
   - *NCLEX®* **e.** Anxiety: when moderate or severe, client hyperventilates and arterial O_2 pressure rises and CO_2 pressure falls; client often reports lightheadedness, numbness of fingers and toes; epinephrine and norepinephrine released under stress increase BP and HR

C. Alterations in respiratory functioning

1. **Hyperventilation**: reduced rate and depth of respirations
   - **a.** Causes: stress, increased CO_2 retention; metabolic acidosis may cause Kussmaul breathing, a type of hyperventilation
   - **b.** Manifestations: increased rate and depth of respiration
2. **Hypoventilation**: inadequate alveolar ventilation
   - **a.** Causes: alveolar collapse, airway obstruction, or side effect of some drugs
   - **b.** Manifestations: inadequate alveolar ventilation; CO_2 retained in bloodstream; can lead to hypoxia
3. Hypoxia: inadequate amount of O_2 transported to tissues
   - **a.** Causes: anemia, pulmonary edema, heart failure; drugs such as anesthetics
   - **b.** Manifestations: rapid HR, rapid shallow respirations, **dyspnea** (difficulty breathing progressing to air hunger), flaring of nostrils, restlessness, substernal or intercostal retractions, and cyanosis; in chronic hypoxia, client may have fatigue, lethargy, and clubbing of digits

Memory Aid

Early respiratory symptoms are mild in nature, such as increasing respiratory rate and mild dyspnea; later signs are more extreme, such as severe dyspnea and air hunger.

4. Cyanosis
   a. Causes: severe anemia, respiratory tract obstruction, heart disease, cold environment; a very late indicator of hypoxia
   b. Manifestations: bluish discoloration of skin, nail beds, mucous membranes
5. Pain: chest pain can impair breathing patterns and respiratory functioning
   a. Causes: respiratory diseases such as pneumonia, pulmonary embolism, advanced bronchogenic carcinoma; and heart conditions, such as coronary artery disease and angina
   b. Manifestations: reports of pain that may be dull, aching, persistent or localized and radiating; pallor; rapid or slowed breathing; anxiety; rapid HR

Memory Aid

Cyanosis is always a late sign, regardless of what the health problem is!

6. **Orthopnea**: (positional breathing discomfort associated with lying down)
   a. Causes: respiratory and cardiac diseases, airway obstruction
   b. Manifestations: inability to breathe except when sitting or standing upright; dyspnea when in a reclining position
7. Wheezing
   a. Causes: severely narrowed bronchus
   b. Manifestations: high-pitched, continuous musical, rasping, or whistling sounds heard during inspiration or expiration; does not clear with coughing
8. Cough: natural lung clearance mechanism to remove secretions
   a. Causes: excessive sputum production; allergies; pulmonary diseases
   b. Manifestations: forced exhalation and clearing of airway passages
9. Hemoptysis
   a. Causes: lung infection, cancer of lungs, heart or blood vessel abnormalities
   b. Manifestations: bright red, frothy blood mixed with sputum; initial symptoms include tickling in throat, salty taste, burning or bubbling sensation in chest

D. Nursing interventions to promote oxygenation

1. Positioning: Fowler's position allows maximum chest expansion that eases respirations in clients with dyspnea; turn clients from side to side every 1 to 2 hours so alternate sides of chest can expand
2. Decrease anxiety: promote relaxation techniques, alleviate pain by using distraction or guided imagery
3. Deep breathing and coughing: helps to clear fluid from lungs and promote oxygenation
   a. Assume a comfortable position: sitting or lying position with knees flexed
   b. Place one hand on abdomen just below ribs
   c. With mouth closed, breathe in deeply through nose to count of three; concentrate on feeling abdomen rise
   d. Purse lips and breathe out slowly and gently; concentrate on feeling abdomen fall and tightening abdominal muscles; count to seven during exhalation
   e. Repeat several times (about 10 times initially) and gradually increase to 5 to 10 minutes, 4 times per day
   f. For coughing: inhale deeply and hold breath for a few seconds, lean forward and cough rapidly, using abdominal, thigh, and buttock muscles (coughing is contraindicated in postoperative eye, ear, neck, or brain surgery or in other clients at risk for increased intracranial pressure)
4. Suctioning: oro/nasopharyngeal, tracheal
   a. See Box 26–2 for procedure
   b. *NCLEX®* Limit suctioning time to 10–15 seconds because no O_2 exchange occurs during this time; provide rest periods between suctioning to allow client to inhale oxygen

Memory Aid

Airway and *breathing* are the A and B of ABCs. Assessments and interventions to promote these are high priority using Maslow's hierarchy of needs theory for prioritizing care.

NCLEX®

c. Assess for dysrhythmias or cyanosis as grave indicators of inadequate oxygenation; hyperoxygenate before suctioning, between attempts, and when suctioning is complete

5. Chest physiotherapy: percussion, vibration, postural drainage (often done by respiratory therapist unless nurse is authorized and competent to perform); see Box 26–3

NCLEX®

6. Oxygen therapy: when oxygen therapy is used, follow safety precautions (see Box 26–4)
   a. Check physician's orders and assess client's respiratory and cardiovascular status
   b. Explain procedure and place client in a semi-sitting position
   c. Set up O_2 equipment: attach flow meter to wall outlet or portable oxygen cylinder; fill humidifier with water and attach to base of flow meter

Box 26–2

Summary of Key Points for Suctioning

- Prepare equipment: portable or wall suction with tubing and collection container; sterile normal saline or water; sterile gloves; water-soluble lubricant; Y-connector; sterile gauzes; disposal bag
- Select appropriate sterile suction catheters, usually #12 to #18 for adults, #8 to #10 for children, and #5 to #8 for infants
- Set pressure on suction gauge
  - Wall unit: adults: 100–120 mm Hg; children: 95–110; infants: 50 to 95
  - Portable unit: adults: 10 to 15 mm Hg; children: 5 to 10; infants: 2 to 5
- Explain procedure to client; position a conscious client in a semi-Fowler's or an unconscious client in a lateral position with head turned toward nurse
- Apply sterile gloves, maintain sterility of the dominant hand, and connect sterile catheter to suction tubing
- Measure distance between client's nose and earlobe (approximately 13 cm or 5 in. for adult) and mark position with fingers of sterile gloved hand; test pressure and patency by placing nondominant thumb or finger on port or open branch of Y-connector
- Hyperoxygenate client with deep breaths or bag-valve-mask device (Ambu bag)
- Lubricate catheter tip with sterile water or saline (or for nasopharyngeal suctioning, may use lubricant)
- Insert catheter
  - For oropharyngeal suctioning: pull tongue forward with gauze; introduce and advance catheter along one side of mouth into oropharynx
  - For nasopharyngeal suctioning: introduce catheter through nostril (naris) and advance to recommended distance
  - For tracheal suctioning: insert during inhalation because epiglottis is open; continue to advance catheter to approximately 20 cm or until resistance is met; pull back slightly (expect client to cough during insertion)
- Do not apply suction while inserting catheter
- Apply nondominant gloved thumb or finger to port to start suction and gently rotate catheter; apply suction intermittently and release while catheter is being withdrawn; allow 20- to 30-second intervals between each suction and limit each suctioning to 10–15 seconds maximum
- Oxygenate client between suction attempts and at completion of procedure
- For oropharyngeal suctioning, it may be necessary to suction secretions that collect in buccal cavity
- Clean catheter by wiping off secretions with sterile gauze; flush catheter with sterile water; relubricate and repeat suctioning until air passage is clear; alternate nares for repeat suctioning; encourage client to breathe deeply and cough between suctions
- Provide nasal or oral hygiene; dispose of equipment
- Assess effectiveness of suctioning: observe respiratory rate, skin color, dyspnea, and level of anxiety; document relevant information

Box 26-3

Performing Chest Physiotherapy

Percussion or Clapping

1. Explain procedure to client.
2. Encourage client to breathe slowly and deeply.
3. Place client in comfortable sitting or side-lying position.
4. Cover area with a gown or towel.
5. Cup hands, alternately flex and extend wrists rapidly to percuss affected lung segments for 1 to 2 minutes.

Vibration (vigorous or high-frequency quivering over chest wall used alternately with or after percussion)

1. Explain procedure to client and position comfortably.
2. Encourage client to breathe slowly and deeply.
3. Place hands one on top of other with palms down.
4. During exhalation, tense hand and arm and, using mostly heel of hand, vibrate or shake hands against client's chest.
5. Stop vibrating when client inhales.
6. After each vibration, encourage client to cough and expectorate mucus.
7. Vibrate five times over each lung segment.

Postural Drainage (use of gravity to drain secretions from respiratory tract)

1. Explain procedure to client.
2. Position client so that head is lower than chest (in prone or side-lying position).
3. Place sputum container and wipes within client's reach.
4. Do percussion and vibration for 5 minutes and allow 5 minutes for drainage.
5. Encourage client to cough and expectorate mucus.
6. Instruct client to turn to other side as appropriate, then to supine position, and repeat procedure.
7. Assist client to a sitting position and offer mouth care.
8. Document observations.

Box 26-4

Safety Precautions During Oxygen Therapy

- Place cautionary signs reading, "No Smoking: Oxygen in Use" on client's door, at head or foot of bed, and on oxygen equipment.
- Instruct client and visitors about danger of smoking when oxygen is in use; if necessary, remove matches, lighters, and ashtrays.
- If oxygen therapy is used at home, instruct family members or caregivers to smoke only outside; if smoking is permitted, teach visitors to use smoking room.
- Avoid materials that generate static electricity, such as woolen blankets and synthetic fabrics; use cotton fabrics instead.
- Avoid use of volatile, flammable substances such as acetone in nail polish removers, alcohol, ether, and oils near clients using oxygen.
- Remove any friction type or battery-operated gadgets, devices, or toys.
- Make sure electric devices such as radios, razors, and televisions are in good working order to prevent short-circuit sparks.
- Ensure that electric monitoring equipment and suction machines are properly grounded; disconnect any ungrounded equipment.
- Know location of fire extinguishers and be able to use them properly; know location of oxygen meter turn-off valve.

d. Attach delivery system and tubing to flow meter; turn on O_2 at prescribed rate; see Table 26–1 for types of O_2 delivery systems
e. Monitor client's respiratory and cardiovascular status regularly; check client's nares for irritation if cannula is used, facial skin if face mask is used; document observations
f. Check flow of O_2 and level of water in humidifier regularly

7. Incentive spirometer
a. Check physician's orders; assist client to a sitting or Fowler's position and explain procedure
b. Assemble equipment; set marker at recommended volume goal
c. Instruct client to place mouth tightly around mouthpiece
d. Instruct client to inhale slowly and maintain a steady flow, like pulling through a straw; encourage client to raise and maintain flow rate indicator
e. Instruct client to remove mouthpiece but hold breath for 2 to 3 seconds and then exhale slowly through pursed lips
f. Have client repeat procedure a few times and then cough; encourage to use 5 to 10 times hourly; keep spirometer within reach of client

Table 26–1 Types of Oxygen Delivery Systems

Nasal cannula	Has either single or double short prongs inserted into nostrils. Often uses flow of 1 to 6 L/min of a 23–42% O_2 concentration.
Oxygen mask	Most effective means of delivering O_2. Must fit well over the nose and mouth. Use only clean and uncontaminated plastic or other nonlatex masks to avoid hospital-acquired infection. May deliver either low or high concentrations of O_2, up to 100%.
Simple face mask	Useful for short-term therapy (i.e., early postoperative period or when intermittent O_2 therapy is required). Flow rate is only 6 to 8 L/min at a low-O_2 concentration of 40–60%. Because mask is loose fitting and can leak, it is suitable for those with CO_2 retention. Also indicated for clients who cannot use a nasal cannula, such as those who have a nasal obstruction.
Partial rebreathing mask	A disposable, lightweight plastic face mask with a reservoir bag and a partial rebreathing valve. A concentration of 50–75% O_2 can be delivered at a flow rate of 8 to 11 L/min. Commonly used by individuals who require O_2. On expiration, conserves approximately one-third of exhaled air; because this air comes from trachea and bronchi (does not participate in gas exchange), it is rich in O_2. To prevent rebreathing of CO_2, reservoir bag should deflate only slightly on inhalation.
Nonrebreathing mask	Fits tightly over face. Usually made of rubber with a reservoir bag and a nonrebreathing valve. On inhalation, O_2 flows into bag and mask, and one-way valve prevents exhaled air from flowing back into bag. Expired air escapes through one-way flap valve in mask. Oxygen concentration is 80–100%, with flow adjusted to keep bag fully inflated. Used for short-term therapy, such as counteracting smoke inhalation. Prolonged use can cause discomfort because mask becomes warm and sticky.
Oxygen tent	Used rarely, but may be useful during infancy. Disadvantage is need to open canopy to monitor vital signs and provide care. Flow rate is 20 L/min at an O_2 concentration of 60% but is hard to control with intermittent opening by staff.
Plastic hoods	May be used to deliver O_2 to infants. Clear plastic head hood allows maintenance of either low or high concentrations of O_2 even during nursing care. A rate of 4 to 5 L/min is required to maintain O_2 concentration and remove exhaled CO_2.
Ventimask (Mix-O-Mask)	Originated from Venturi mask. Used for clients with chronic alveolar hypoventilation and CO_2 retention. Delivers exact low-flow concentrations of O_2. Provides an air–oxygen mixture with the desired O_2 concentration. Size of opening in mask determines concentration of O_2—24% or 28%, 31%, 35%, and 40% with flow rates of 4, 6, 8, and 10 L/min, respectively. A thin elastic band holds Ventimask in position and tends to press into skin behind the ears; gauze padding under each side of elastic band alleviates pressure. Must be removed when client eats and may give client a feeling of being smothered.

III. MEETING CLIENT'S NEED FOR SLEEP

A. Physiology of sleep

1. Circadian rhythm: rhythmic repetition of patterns each 24 hours; sleep is a complex biologic rhythm; if a person's biological clock coincides with sleep–wake patterns, the person is in **circadian synchronization**
2. Sleep regulation: centers in lower portion of brain actively inhibit wakefulness, causing sleep
3. NREM (non–rapid eye movement): deep and restful sleep characterized by decrease in physiologic functions: BP and HR decrease, skeletal muscles relax, basal metabolic rate (BMR) decreases, brain waves become slower; there are four stages of NREM
   - **a.** Stage I: very light sleep; sleeper is relaxed and drowsy and feels a floating sensation; eyes roll from side to side; lasts only a few minutes
   - **b.** Stage II: light sleep; sleeper is easily roused; HR and respirations decrease slightly; lasts 10 to 15 minutes
   - **c.** Stage III: medium-depth sleep; sleeper is less easily aroused; HR, respirations, and other physiologic functions such as BP and temperature continue to fall; skeletal muscles are relaxed, reflexes diminished; snoring may occur
   - **d.** Stage IV: called delta sleep; deepest stage; sleeper is difficult to rouse and rarely moves; muscles are completely relaxed; dreaming may occur; may last about 30 minutes
4. REM (rapid eye movement) sleep: usually occurs every 90 minutes and lasts 5 to 30 minutes; active dreaming occurs and dreams are remembered; brain is highly active, and sleeper is difficult to rouse or may wake up spontaneously; REM and irregular muscle movements occur; muscle tone is depressed; heart and respiratory rates are irregular

B. Normal sleep requirements and patterns

1. Neonates: newborns sleep, on average, 16–18 hours per day, divided into about 7 sleep periods; most NREM sleep is spent in stages III and IV, and nearly 50% is in REM sleep
2. Infants: range of sleep is 12–22 hours; periods of wakefulness increase with age; by 4 months, infants sleep through night and nap during day; at end of first year, they sleep about 14 of every 24 hours; half of time, infants have light sleep, and 20–30% is REM sleep
3. *NCLEX®* Toddlers: normal sleep–wake cycle established by 2 to 3 years; generally sleep for 10–12 hours, still require a midafternoon nap, but morning nap needs decrease; still 20–30% is REM sleep
4. Preschoolers: need 11–12 hours sleep but may fluctuate because of activity and growth spurts; older preschoolers do not need a nap; continue to have 20–30% REM sleep
5. School-age: most school-age children sleep 8–12 hours without daytime naps; REM sleep decreases to about 20%
6. Adolescents: amount of sleep time declines, but adolescents still need 8–10 hours of sleep; changes in pattern occur for adolescents who need daytime napping
7. Young adults: generally, young adults require 7–8 hours, but because of lifestyle changes, they may have erratic sleep patterns
8. Middle-aged adults: sleep pattern established earlier is maintained, and middle-aged adult sleeps 6–8 hours/night; about 20% is REM sleep; duration of stage IV NREM sleep decreases
9. *NCLEX®* Older adults: sleep about 6 hours a night with about 20–25% REM and a marked decrease in stage IV NREM sleep; they awaken more frequently and have difficulty returning to sleep, so they experience less restorative sleep

C. Factors affecting sleep

1. Illness: increases sleep requirement; however, illness may cause pain, breathing difficulty, or discomfort with movement that interferes with sleep; elevated body temperature can reduce stages III and IV NREM and REM sleep
2. Drugs and substances
   - **a.** Excessive alcohol disrupts REM sleep, although it may accelerate onset of sleep; individuals with tolerance to alcohol may have difficulty with sleep, and when drug effects wear off, may have nightmares
   - **b.** *NCLEX®* Caffeine and amphetamines are stimulants and interfere with sleep
   - **c.** Nicotine has stimulating effect, and smokers have more difficulty falling asleep
3. Lifestyle: shift work may interfere with ability to adjust sleeping patterns; inactivity or boredom may contribute to sleep problems
4. Usual sleep patterns and excessive daytime sleepiness: individuals commonly refer to themselves as morning or night people; these are their sleep patterns; excessive daytime sleepiness may be caused by nighttime sleep deprivation
5. Emotional stress: anxiety makes it difficult to fall asleep; depression may cause difficulty in falling asleep or premature awakening

6. Environment: any change in noise level may inhibit sleep—people are habituated to certain noises; ventilation and environmental temperature can affect sleep

NCLEX®

7. Various prescribed drugs: decongestants, narcotics, sedatives, beta-blockers, and antidepressants may cause drowsiness and may disrupt REM sleep
8. Exercise and fatigue: moderate exercise is conducive to sleep but, if excessive, may delay sleep; moderate fatigue may lead to a restful sleep
9. Food/calorie intake: weight loss may be associated with reduced quantity of sleep, broken sleep, and earlier awakening; weight gain may be associated with increased total sleep time, less broken sleep, and later waking

D. Overview of sleep disorders

1. Insomnia: inability to obtain an adequate amount or quality of sleep
   a. Can be initial (difficulty falling asleep), middle or intermittent (difficulty maintaining sleep because of frequent or prolonged waking), or terminal (early or premature awakening), which may be associated with depression

NCLEX®

   b. Treatment usually involves developing new sleep-inducing and sleep-maintaining behaviors such as modifying environment or relaxation techniques
2. Sleep apnea: periodic cessation of breathing during sleep; episode lasts from 10 seconds to 2 minutes, and incidence may range from 50 to 600 per night
   a. Suspected when person snores loudly, has frequent nocturnal awakening, and experiences excessive daytime sleepiness, fatigue, irritability, and personality changes caused by disrupted sleep
   b. Incidence of sleep apnea is high in older adult men
   c. Apnea is also common among obese clients
   d. Complications of prolonged sleep apnea may be increased BP, cardiac dysrhythmias, and left-sided heart failure
   e. Treatment is directed at cause: if obstructive, enlarged tonsils or adenoids may be removed
   f. Use of a nasal continuous positive airway pressure (CPAP) device may be effective
3. Narcolepsy: overwhelming daytime sleepiness caused by lack of chemical (hypocretin) that regulates sleep; client may doze while involved in activities; treated with stimulants, such as amphetamines
4. Parasomnias: abnormal behavioral or physiologic events associated with stages of sleep and that interfere with sleep; treatment consists of relaxation technique and sleep hygiene practices
   a. Somnambulism: sleepwalking that occurs in stages III and IV NREM sleep; it is episodic and occurs 1–2 hours after falling asleep; sleepwalker does not notice dangers such as stairs and requires protection from injury
   b. Sleeptalking: talking occurs during NREM sleep, before REM sleep
   c. Nocturnal enuresis: bedwetting, more common in male children over 3 years old; often occurs 1 to 2 hours after falling asleep, when rousing from stage III and IV of NREM sleep
   d. Bruxism: clenching and grinding teeth during stage II NREM sleep
5. Sleep deprivation: syndrome in which client's prolonged disturbance results in a decrease in amount, quality, and consistency of sleep
   a. REM sleep deprivation can be caused by alcohol, shift work, jet lag, or extended ICU hospitalization and can result in excitability, confusion, and emotional lability; delay procedures or medications when possible to avoid waking a client during REM sleep
   b. NREM sleep deprivation can be caused by same factors as REM deprivation, as well as hypothyroidism, depression, sleep apnea, and age (common in elderly), and can result in withdrawal, excessive sleepiness, and hyporesponsiveness

NCLEX®

   c. A client with both REM and NREM sleep deprivation may have marked fatigue, perceptual distortions, and difficulty with concentration, judgment, and attention

E. Health promotion to improve sleep

1. Environmental controls: ensure appropriate lighting, ventilation, and temperature; keep noise level to a minimum
2. Promote bedtime routines: respect client's customary rituals or routines to promote relaxation and encourage sleep; provide hygiene such as washing face, brushing teeth, and voiding; allow listening to music or praying, children's bedtime stories, or adults' conversations with caregivers or family members if possible

NCLEX®

3. Promote comfort: provide backrubs, change of linen/clothing, position for comfort; administer medications for pain to promote and help maintain sleep; listen to client's concerns to alleviate emotional stress and promote relaxation; avoid heavy meal 3 hours before bedtime, decrease fluid intake 2 hours before sleep, and avoid alcohol, caffeine, and heavily spiced foods

4. Promote activity: encourage adequate exercise during day to reduce stress, and a nonstrenuous activity prior to sleep

NCLEX®

5. Pharmacological aids (sedatives and hypnotics) should be used as a last resort and be taken prn (as necessary); clients need to know desired and adverse effects of medications (they vary in onset and duration); regular use may lead to drug tolerance and possibly rebound insomnia

IV. MEETING URINARY ELIMINATION NEEDS

A. Healthy urinary function

1. Normal output of urine is 60 mL/hr or 1500 mL/day; should remain 30 mL/hr (0.5 mL/kg/hr) or higher to ensure continued healthy kidney function
2. Urine usually consists of 96% water
3. Solutes found in urine
   a. Organic: urea, ammonia, uric acid, and creatinine
   b. Inorganic: sodium, chloride, potassium, sulfate, magnesium, and phophorus
4. Table 26–2 describes characteristics of healthy urine and possible abnormal findings

B. Common abnormal assessment findings

1. Urgency: strong desire to void may be caused by inflammation or infection in bladder or urethra
2. Dysuria: painful or difficult voiding

Table 26–2 Characteristics of Normal and Abnormal Urine

Characteristic	Normal	Abnormal	Nursing Considerations
Amount in 24 hours (adult)	1200–1500 mL	Under 1200 mL Over 1500 mL	Urinary output normally is approximately equal to fluid intake. Report output less than 30 mL/hr, which may indicate decreased blood flow to kidneys.
Color, clarity	Straw, amber; transparent	Dark amber Cloudy Dark orange Red or dark brown Mucus plugs, viscid, thick	Concentrated urine is darker, while dilute urine is almost clear, or pale yellow. Some foods and drugs discolor urine. Red blood cells in urine (hematuria) may be seen as pink, bright red, or rusty brown urine. Menstrual bleeding can color urine but should not be confused with hematuria. White blood cells, bacteria, pus, prostatic fluid, sperm, or vaginal drainage may cause cloudy urine.
Odor	Faint, aromatic	Offensive	Some foods (e.g., asparagus) cause a musty odor; infected urine can have a fetid odor; urine high in glucose has a sweet odor.
Sterility	No microorganisms present	Microorganisms present	Urine specimens may be contaminated by bacteria from the perineum during collection.
pH	4.5–8	Under 4.5 Over 8	Freshly voided urine should be somewhat acidic. Alkaline urine may indicate alkalosis, urinary tract infection, or a diet high in fruits and vegetables. More acidic urine (low pH) is found in acidosis, starvation, diarrhea, or with a diet high in proteins or cranberries.
Specific gravity (SG)	1.010–1.025	Under 1.010 Over 1.025	Concentrated urine has a higher SG; dilute urine has a lower SG.
Glucose	Not present	Present	Glucosuria indicates high blood glucose levels (>180 mg/dL) and may indicate undiagnosed or uncontrolled diabetes mellitus, or gestational diabetes mellitus.
Ketone bodies	Not present	Present	Ketones (end products of fatty acid breakdown) are not normally present in urine. They may be present with uncontrolled diabetes mellitus, starvation, or excessive aspirin ingestion.
Blood	Not present	Occult (microscopic) Bright red	Hematuria may indicate urinary tract infection, kidney disease, or bleeding from urinary tract.
Protein	Not present	Present	Proteinuria can occur with damage to glomerular membrane of kidney.

Adapted from Berman, A., & Snyder, S., Kozier, B., & Erb, G., (2008). *Fundamentals of nursing: Concepts, process, and practice* (8th ed.). Upper Saddle River, NJ: Prentice Hall, p. 1293.

3. Frequency: voiding that occurs more than usual when compared with client's regular pattern or generally accepted norm of voiding once every 3 to 6 hours
4. Hesitancy: undue delay and difficulty in initiating voiding
5. Polyuria: a large volume of urine voided at any given time
6. Oliguria: a small volume of urine or output between 100 and 500 mL/24 hr
7. Nocturia: excessive urination at night, interrupting sleep
8. Hematuria: RBCs in urine

C. Common urinary elimination problems

1. Urinary retention: bladder emptying is impaired, urine accumulates, and bladder becomes overdistended; causes include prostatic hyperplasia, surgery, medications such as anticholinergics, antidepressants, antipsychotics, antiparkinsonian agents, antihypertensives
2. Urinary tract infections (UTI): infectious process leads to inflammation (*-itis*) in any portion of urinary tract
   a. Lower UTI: urethritis affects urethra; cystitis affects urinary bladder (and is most common UTI); prostatitis affects prostate gland
   b. Upper UTI: pyelonephritis affects renal pelvis and parenchyma (functional portion of kidney tissue)
3. Incontinence: involuntary urination
   a. Stress incontinence: involuntary loss of urine of less than 50 mL occurring with increased abdominal pressure through coughing, laughing, or lifting
   b. Reflex incontinence: involuntary loss of urine at predictable intervals when bladder reaches a specific volume
   c. Urge incontinence: involuntary loss of urine soon after a strong urge to void
   d. Functional incontinence: involuntary, unpredictable passage of urine
   e. Total incontinence: continuous and unpredictable involuntary loss of urine

D. Urinary diversion devices: ureterostomy is a surgical rerouting of urine from kidneys to a site other than bladder, usually when bladder is removed or diseased

1. Cutaneous ureterostomy: ureter is brought directly to skin surface to form a small stoma; disadvantages include that stomas provide direct access to microorganisms from skin to kidneys, small stomas may present difficulty in fitting pouches, stenosis of stomas may occur as a complication
2. Ileal conduit: a segment of ileum is separated from small intestine and formed into a pouch with open end brought out through abdominal wall to form a stoma; ureter is implanted into ileal pouch (see Figure 26–1)

E. Common urinary tests

NCLEX®

1. Urinalysis: macroscopic and microscopic analysis of urine to determine physical and chemical characteristics (see again Table 26–2)
2. Urine culture/sensitivity: a clean-catch specimen or catheterized specimen is needed to identify infecting organism and most effective antibiotic; culture requires 24–72 hours for organism growth and identification
3. Intravenous pyelogram (IVP) or intravenous urogram (IVU): IV injection of a radiopaque contrast medium concentrates in urine to aid visualization of kidneys, ureters, and bladder
4. Renal scan: IV injection of radiotraces or isotopes evaluates renal size, shape, position, function or blood flow to kidneys; is recorded by a scintillation camera
5. Ultrasound: high-frequency sound waves are used to create images of urinary system

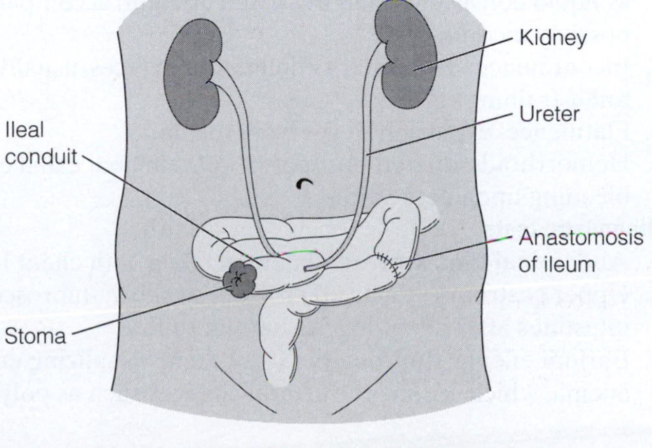

Figure 26–1
Ileal conduit as it is connected to abdominal organs.

6. Cystoscopy: directly visualizes urethra and bladder with a cystoscope that is a self-contained optical lens system and provides a magnified illuminated view of bladder

NCLEX®
7. Bladder scan at bedside: detects amount of urine in bladder to help determine need for voiding or straight catheterization; may be done by nurses or other personnel trained to use portable device

F. Health promotion for urinary elimination

NCLEX®
1. Adequate hydration: daily intake of 1500 mL of measurable fluids recommended; if prone to development of stones or infections, increase to 2000–3000 mL per day; if experiencing abnormal fluid losses, additional fluids are necessary
2. Personal hygiene: teach client to wash perineum with soap and water daily and wipe after defecation; instruct female clients to wipe from front to back (urinary meatus toward anus) after voiding and discard after each wipe; for recurrent infections, avoid tub baths
3. Empty bladder completely: regular exercise increases muscle tone that helps maintain ability to contract bladder's detrusor muscle for complete emptying; abdominal muscle contraction assists in bladder emptying; teach **Kegel exercises**—contract perineal muscles and hold for a count of 3–5 seconds and relax; do 10 contractions five times daily

NCLEX®
4. Infection prevention measures
   a. Drink eight 8-ounce glasses of water daily
   b. Empty bladder at least every 2 to 4 hours while awake, avoiding voluntary retention; if client is incontinent, instruct to void according to a timetable rather than urge to void (bladder training), void at regular intervals (habit training), or supplement habit training by reminding client to void (prompted voiding); instruct client to practice deep, slow breathing until urge to void diminishes
   c. For women: wear cotton briefs; cleanse perineal area from front to back after voiding and defecating; void before and after sexual intercourse; avoid bubble baths, feminine hygiene sprays, and douches
   d. Unless contraindicated: teach client to maintain acidity in urine by drinking at least two glasses of cranberry juice per day and avoiding excess milk products and sodium bicarbonate; vitamin C acidifies urine also
   e. Describe symptoms and prevention measures of UTI and importance of reporting symptoms promptly

V. MEETING BOWEL ELIMINATION NEEDS

NCLEX®
A. Factors that influence bowel elimination (see Table 26–3)

B. Characteristics of normal stool

1. Color: varies from light to dark brown; foods and medications may affect color
2. Odor: aromatic, affected by ingested food and person's bacterial flora
3. Consistency: formed, soft, semisolid; moist
4. Frequency: varies with diet; once a day is a common pattern
5. Amount: varies with diet (about 100 to 400 grams/day)
6. Constituents: small amounts of undigested roughage, sloughed dead bacteria and epithelial cells, fat, protein, dried constituents of digestive juices (bile pigments), inorganic matter (calcium, phosphates)

NCLEX®
C. Common bowel elimination problems

1. Constipation: abnormal infrequency of defecation and abnormal hardening of stools
2. Impaction: accumulated mass of dry feces that cannot be expelled
3. Diarrhea: increased frequency of bowel movements (more than 3 times a day) as well as liquid consistency and increased amount; accompanied by urgency, discomfort, and possibly incontinence
4. Incontinence: involuntary elimination of feces, usually indicates a health problem at any age after toilet-training
5. Flatulence: expulsion of gas from rectum
6. Hemorrhoids: dilated portions of veins in anal canal causing itching and pain and possible bright red bleeding upon defecation

D. Diagnostic tests

1. Abdominal film: x-ray of abdomen taken with client in flat and upright positions
2. Upper gastrointestinal (GI) barium swallow: fluoroscopic x-ray exam of esophagus, stomach, and small intestines after client ingests barium sulfate
3. Barium enema: fluoroscopic x-ray exam visualizing entire large intestine after client is given a barium enema, which outlines structural changes such as polyps and diverticulitis

Table 26–3 Factors That Influence Bowel Elimination

Factor	Effect on Bowel Elimination
Age	Infants and toddlers: have immature control of bowel elimination; daytime control is achieved by age 2½ with toilet training School-age and adolescents: have similar bowel habits as adults; however, school-age children involved in play may delay elimination Older adults: prone to constipation because of slowing of GI motility and decreased food intake and activity
Diet	Sufficient bulk is needed to provide fecal volume Low-residue or low-fiber diet may provide insufficient volume to stimulate reflex for defecation Irregular eating can interfere with regular elimination Diarrhea can be caused by spicy or overly sweet foods Gas-producing foods include cabbage, onions, beans, and cauliflower A laxative effect is exerted by bran, prunes, figs, and alcohol Constipating foods include cheese, eggs, pasta, and lean meat
Fluid Intake	Healthy elimination requires an intake of 2000 to 3000 mL/day Inadequate fluid intake or excessive fluid loss may lead to hard feces
Activity	Stimulates peristalsis; immobility, weak muscles from lack of exercise, or impaired neurologic functioning can lead to constipation
Personal habits	Repeatedly ignoring urge to defecate allows continued water absorption from bowel and feces to harden; reflexes tend to be progressively weakened and may be lost
Positioning	Normal bowel elimination is facilitated by thigh flexion (increases intraabdominal pressure) and a sitting position, which increases downward pressure on rectum Using a bedpan while in a supine position is uncomfortable and does not facilitate defecation, so place client in a semi-sitting position
Psychological	Anxiety or anger can increase peristalsis and lead to diarrhea Depression slows intestinal activity, resulting in constipation
Pain	Pain or discomfort during defecation, may lead client to suppress urge to defecate, causing constipation
Medications	Many drugs have a constipating effect, including antidepressants, antipsychotic and antiparkinsonian agents, morphine, and codeine
Surgery	General anesthetics may cause a slowing of intestinal movement resulting in constipation Surgery in abdominal area that involves handling of intestines may cause cessation of intestinal movement (paralytic ileus) that lasts for 24 to 48 hours
Pregnancy	There is decreased intestinal secretion and colon is displaced upward, laterally, and posteriorly Peristaltic activity is decreased, causing constipation Venous pressure increases, causing hemorrhoids later in pregnancy

4. Endoscopy: use of a flexible tube (fiberoptic endoscope) to visualize GI tract; images produced are transmitted to a video screen
5. Upper endoscopy: a telescopic eyepiece is inserted through mouth; EGD—esophagogastroduodenoscopy
6. Lower endoscopy: a telescopic eyepiece is inserted through rectum—proctosigmoidoscopy

E. Health promotion for elimination problems

NCLEX® 1. Constipation: increase fluid intake; instruct client to drink liquids, fruit juices (especially prune juice) and to eat foods high in roughage or fiber, such as raw fruits and vegetables, bran products, whole-grain cereals and bread

NCLEX® 2. Diarrhea: encourage oral intake of fluids and bland foods; avoid spicy and fatty foods, alcohol, beverages with caffeine, and high-fiber foods

3. Flatulence: limit chewing gum, carbonated drinks, use of drinking straws, and gas-producing foods such as cabbage, cauliflower, beans, and onions

F. Bowel diversion ostomies: an ostomy is a surgical opening in abdominal wall for elimination of feces or urine; bowel diversion ostomies are classified according to status (temporary or permanent), anatomic location, and construction of stoma

1. Permanence: colostomies can be temporary (for traumatic injuries or inflammatory conditions) or permanent (birth defect or disease such as cancer)
2. Anatomic location (see Figure 26–2): identifies site in small or large bowel from which ostomy empties

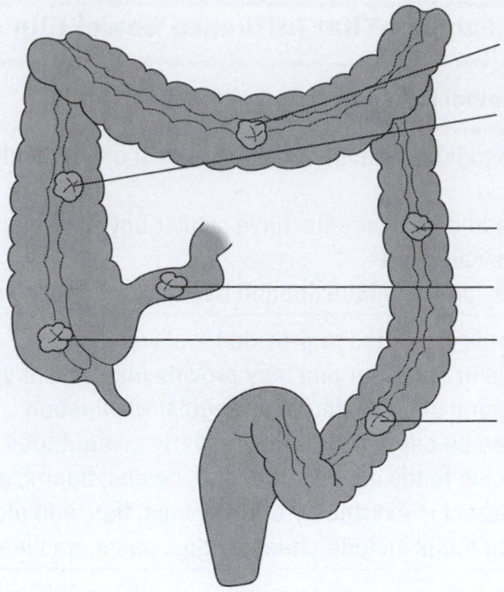

Figure 26–2

Locations of various bowel diversion ostomies.

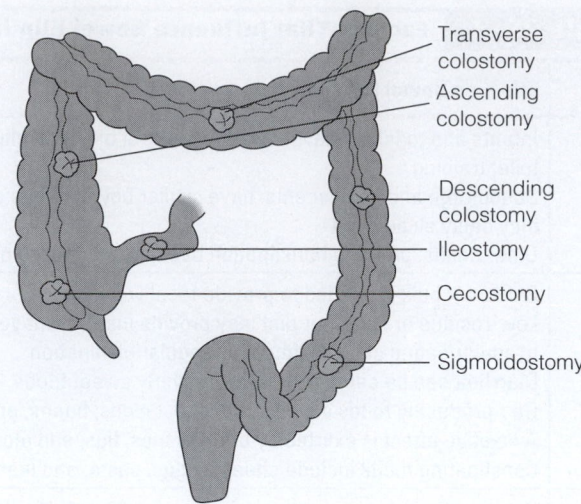

3. Construction of stoma
   a. Single: one end of bowel as opening
   b. Loop: a loop of bowel brought out into abdominal wall and supported by a glass rod or a plastic bridge; has two openings—proximal, or active, and distal, or inactive; usually performed as an emergency procedure and situated often in right transverse colon
   c. Divided: two separated stomas; opening from digestive end is colostomy and distal end is mucus fistula (bowel continues to secrete mucus)
   d. Double-barreled: proximal and distal loops are sutured together and both ends are brought out through the abdominal wall

G. Health promotion for clients with ostomies

NCLEX®
1. For a client with a colostomy, dietary teaching needs to include information about
   a. Foods that cause stool odor: asparagus, beans, eggs, fish, onions, garlic
   b. Foods that increase gas: cabbage, onions, beans, and cauliflower
   c. Foods that thicken stool: applesauce, bananas, rice, tapioca, cheese, yogurt
   d. Foods that loosen stool: chocolate, dried beans, fried foods, highly spiced foods, leafy green vegetables, raw fruits and vegetables

NCLEX®
2. For a client with ileostomy, teaching to relieve food blockage should include
   a. Drink warm fluids or grape juice if not vomiting
   b. Take a warm shower
   c. Assume a knee-chest position
   d. Massage peristomal area
   e. Remove pouch if stoma is swollen and apply one with a larger opening
   f. Eat a low-residue diet initially; avoid foods that cause blockage such as popcorn, nuts, cucumbers, celery, fresh tomatoes, figs, blackberries, and caraway seeds
   g. Limit high-fiber foods and chew them well if eaten

   NCLEX®
   h. Know signs of blockage: abdominal cramping, swelling of stoma, and absence of ileostomy output for 4 to 6 hours

VI. MEETING SENSORY AND PERCEPTUAL NEEDS

A. Factors affecting sensation and perception

1. Are numerous and include illness, developmental stage, medications, stress, and lifestyle
2. Illness may result in hospitalization; this change of environment may affect mentation, especially for older clients; in some cases, mental status changes result from an underlying disease process
3. Developmental stage affects sensory perception
   a. Infants have adequate sensory organs but have no mental concepts to understand sensory input
   b. As development occurs, person develops understanding of sensory input
   c. Adults have many learned responses to sensory cues; with aging, sensory input diminishes because of decreased sense organ functioning

NCLEX®
4. Medications can affect both sensory function and awareness; many drugs decrease level of consciousness (LOC); others contribute to mental confusion; in older adults, polypharmacy may lead to drug interactions that cause decreased sensory functioning

5. Stress can be described as eustress (optimal level of stress that stimulates enhanced functioning and response to stressor) or distress (excessive stress that depresses ability to function and may limit amount of sensory input client can manage)
   a. Illness and hospitalization can both cause distress
   b. Today, hospitals try to create aesthetic environments more conducive to healing, such as with bright and cheerful walls with beautiful pictures, carpeted floors, and an overall attempt to create a pleasant, "homelike" environment
6. Lifestyle influences sensory perception; one client may thrive in a stimulating environment that may overwhelm others

B. Sensory and perceptual alterations

1. Three factors known to contribute to alterations in client behavior include (but are not limited to) sensory deprivation, sensory overload, and sensory deficits
2. **Sensory deprivation**: a lack of meaningful stimuli; reduced amount of incoming stimuli because of either decreased environmental stimuli or impairment in one or more of client's senses; can lead to disorientation over time
   a. Risk factors that may lead to sensory deprivation include dysfunction of senses (vision or hearing impairment, impaired sensation because of neurological problem), medications, immobility, isolation, and language barriers
   NCLEX® b. See Box 26–5 for clinical signs and symptoms of sensory deprivation
   c. Hospital rooms have clocks, calendars, and sometimes boards that identify names of work shift caregivers, all of which provide meaningful stimuli to hospitalized clients and promote orientation to surroundings
3. **Sensory overload**: an increase in intensity of stimuli to levels beyond normal; generally occurs when client is unable to process amount or intensity of stimuli or when exposed to numerous stimuli that are not meaningful
   a. Increased internal stimuli (such as anxiety) and increased external stimuli (noise, equipment, multiple health care personnel, which are familiar to staff but unfamiliar to client) can lead to sensory overload
   b. Sensory overload leads to sleep deprivation, which reduces individual coping abilities; when overloaded with sensory stimuli, client may feel out of control
   NCLEX® c. Contributing factors to overload could be pain, anxiety, and lack of sleep; incidence is increased in clients in intensive care units after 2 to 3 days
   d. Refer again to Box 26–5 for clinical signs and symptoms of sensory overload
4. **Sensory deficit**: impairment of both reception and perception of one or more senses; when loss is gradual, individual can compensate; for instance, clients with impaired vision may decrease area in which they travel alone

Box 26–5

Signs of Sensory Deprivation and Sensory Overload

Sensory Deprivation

- Excessive yawning, drowsiness, sleeping
- Decreased attention span, difficulty concentrating, decreased problem solving
- Impaired memory
- Periodic disorientation, general or nocturnal confusion
- Preoccupation with somatic complaints, such as palpitations
- Hallucinations or delusions
- Crying, annoyance over small matters, depression
- Apathy, emotional liability

Sensory Overload

- Increased muscle tension
- Fatigue and inability to sleep
- Irritability and restlessness
- Inability to concentrate
- Decreased problem-solving performance

C. Common sensory deficits

1. Visual: vision is important in aiding clients to interact with environment
   a. Clients with visual impairment may wear glasses or contact lenses to correct refraction errors of lens
   b. Refraction errors include myopia (nearsightedness), hyperopia (farsightedness), and presbyopia (loss of lens elasticity that reduces ability to focus on close objects; occurs with aging, around age 45, and requires corrective lenses—"reading" glasses or bifocals)
   c. Cataracts: often seen after age 65; lens opacity blocks light rays and distorts and impairs visual field; surgical removal is often required as cataract progresses; see also Chapter 59
   d. Glaucoma: a painless blockage in circulation of aqueous fluid in eye that leads to an increase in intraocular pressure and possibly blindness; see also Chapter 59
   e. Diabetic retinopathy: leading cause of blindness among adults age 20 to 70; proliferative retinopathy or neurovascular disease occurs when ischemic retinal blood vessels (BVs) bleed, causing vitreous hemorrhage, which can be repetitive and may lead to permanent visual loss
   f. Macular degeneration: degenerative changes in BVs in macular area of retina; macular BVs leak and damage macula; scarring occurs and visual loss results; symptoms are blurring and distortion of visual images; see also Chapter 59
2. Hearing: difficulty with hearing may make client feel isolated, interfere with health teaching, and even increase client's risk of injury
   a. Conductive hearing loss results from interrupted transmission of sound waves through outer and middle ear; possible causes are a tear in eardrum (tympanic membrane); obstruction in auditory canal caused by swelling or other factors; degeneration of hammer, anvil, and stirrup from infection; or continuous low-sensory input
   b. Sensorineural hearing loss results from damage to inner ear, auditory nerve, or hearing center in brain from viral infection or ototoxic medications (whose names often end with *mycin*)
   c. **Presbycusis** is age-related gradual loss of hearing ability; is more common in men than in women
3. Balance: a gradual reduction of power and contraction of muscles occurs with aging, especially after age 50; often balance is impaired with this process as well; degenerative joint changes may occur, making movement more restricted
4. Taste: decreased ability to taste can reduce appetite and contribute to poor nutrition; if a corresponding loss of smell occurs, client's appetite will fail to be stimulated by aroma of food
5. Smell: in addition to its effect on client's appetite, loss of smell can be a safety issue; with decrease in smell, client will not be aware of a gas leak, for example
6. Touch: tactile deprivation can occur from disease or an injury that causes destruction or damage to nerve cells
   a. Children born with myelomeningocele have damage to nerves below level of pathology; injuries that destroy nerves will have same effect; loss of tactile ability may contribute to safety issues, such as risk for burns if cannot feel heat
   b. Peripheral neuropathy interferes with innervation of peripheral nerves; with aging, diabetes, or arteriosclerosis, overall effectiveness of BVs decreases; superficial BVs constrict to divert blood to larger BVs; with constriction of peripheral BVs, peripheral nerve endings in constricted area have decreased blood flow and neuropathy develops
   c. Multisensory deficit conditions: some conditions, such as stroke, cause damage to more than one sense and lead to ischemia in affected area of brain; results may be decreased sensation and/or paresis or paralysis of extremities, as well as aphasia, blindness or other visual impairment, or impaired swallowing

NCLEX®

D. Promoting self-care

1. Screening and prevention: early detection of sensory deprivation is an important health-screening function
   a. Routine auditory testing is done at birth and during early school years
   b. Periodic vision screening of all school-age children is done
   c. Health fairs often provide a means to screen many healthy people
   d. Be aware of disease processes that can lead to sensory deprivation, and screen for symptoms to detect sensory problems early
   e. Reinforce measures to protect sensory organs; encourage protective eye and ear gear; emphasize, especially to teenagers, risk of ear damage from loud noises or music

f. Reinforce general health measures such as regular eye and ear exams

g. The Occupational Safety and Health Administration (OSHA) provides regulations and guidelines to limit hazards affecting senses to individuals in workplace; OSHA guidelines are carefully followed in health care settings also

2. Assistive aids: encourage use of specific aids to support sensory function, promote use of other senses, communicate effectively, and work to ensure client's safety

NCLEX®

a. Visual and hearing aids: give eyeglasses to clients upon awakening and assist in storage at bedtime; ensure that hearing aid is in place and functioning during daytime and prior to any explanations about care or treatment; see Box 26-6 for information on possible visual and auditory aids

b. For clients with smell and taste deficits, supply diets that include a variety of flavors, temperatures, and textures to stimulate taste buds

c. Evaluate each client who has a sensory deficit to determine appropriate assistive device

3. Communication

a. Client with a sensory deficit is at risk for not accurately interpreting information shared during communication

b. Convey respect to client and enhance his or her self-esteem

c. A person with a hearing deficit needs to concentrate at all times during a conversation

d. A client with visual deficits might misinterpret non-verbal clues during conversation

e. See Box 26–7 for tips on communicating with clients who have visual or hearing deficits

VII. SKIN INTEGRITY AND WOUND CARE

A. Healthy skin integrity

1. Layers of skin

a. Epidermis: outermost layer (stratified squamous epithelial cells); subdivided into five layers; innermost layer is basal-cell layer responsible for replacing sloughed and damaged cells

b. Dermis: second layer composed of connective tissue that gives elasticity to skin; has BVs, nerve fibers, glands, and hair follicles

c. Subcutaneous tissue: made of adipose tissue; provides support and blood flow to dermis

Box 26–6

Aids for Clients with Visual and Auditory Deficits

For Clients with Visual Deficits

- Prescription eyeglasses
- Proper lighting in rooms, including night lights
- Shades on windows to reduce glare
- Large-print, recorded, or Braille books
- Magnifying glass
- Contrasting colors in environment
- Large numbers on clocks, watches, and phone
- Seeing-eye dog
- Red-tipped cane or laser cane

For Clients with Auditory Deficits

- Hearing aids
- Closed caption service for television
- Telephone with amplifiers
- Flashing alarm clocks, smoke detectors, doorbells, and phone
- Cochlear implants
- Service dogs
- TDD phone
- Wireless page, phone, and e-mail service

Box 26-7

Communicating with Clients Who Have a Visual or Hearing Deficit

Visual Deficit

- Always announce presence and identify self by name when entering client's room.
- Stay in client's field of vision if vision loss is partial.
- Speak in a warm and pleasant tone of voice, but not with excessive loudness.
- Always explain what you will do before touching client.
- Explain sounds in environment.
- Indicate when conversation has ended and you are leaving the room.

Hearing Deficit

- Before initiating a conversation, move to a position where you can be seen or gently touch client.
- Decrease background noises (e.g., radio) before speaking.
- Talk at a moderate rate and in a normal tone of voice; shouting does not make voice more distinct and could make understanding more difficult.
- Address client directly; do not turn away during a remark or story; make sure client can see your face easily and that it is well-lighted.
- Avoid talking with chewing gum or other substances in your mouth; avoid covering your mouth with your hand.
- Keep voice at about the same volume throughout each sentence, without dropping the voice at the end of each sentence.
- Always speak as clearly and accurately as possible; articulate consonants with particular care.
- Do not "overarticulate"; mouthing or overdoing articulation is just as troublesome as mumbling; pantomime or write ideas, or use sign language or finger spelling when appropriate.
- Use longer phrases, which tend to be easier to understand than short ones; also, word choice is important: "Fifteen cents" and "fifty cents" may be confused, but "half a dollar" is clear.
- Pronounce names with care; add a reference to name for easier understanding—for example, "Joan, the girl from the office" or "Talbots, the big store at the mall."
- Change to a new subject at a slower rate, ensuring that client follows the change; a key word or two at the beginning of a new topic is a good indicator.

Adapted from Berman, A., Snyder, S., Kozier, B., & Erb, G. (2008). *Fundamentals of nursing: Concepts, process, and practice* (6th ed.). Upper Saddle River, NJ: Prentice Hall, p. 990.

2. Skin glands: sebaceous glands, soporiferous glands, and cerumenous glands
   a. Sebaceous glands (within dermis) secrete an oily substance called sebum that protects hair from drying, forms a protective film to prevent excessive water evaporation, and inhibits growth of certain bacteria on skin
   b. Soporiferous (sweat) glands produce a watery secretion and have two types: apocrine (primarily found in skin of axilla and pubic regions; produce odor when decomposed by bacteria) and eccrine (chiefly found on palms of hands, soles of feet, and forehead; produce a watery discharge to cool body through evaporation)
   c. Ceruminous glands secrete a thick, oily substance called cerumen, a waxy secretion of external ear (also known as earwax)

3. Skin alterations related to aging: overall health status, age, nutritional status, and energy and activity level play a role in maintaining client's skin condition; skin alterations in older adults include
   a. Epidermis thins and has a lower water content, leading to dry skin
   b. Elasticity and some of fatty cushion are lost, resulting in wrinkles and fragile skin
   c. BVs in skin also become more fragile, leading to easy bruising

B. Classification of wounds: a wound is a break in skin or mucous membrane resulting from physical means; may be superficial (affecting skin surface only) or deep (involving blood vessels, nerves, muscle, fascia, tendons, ligaments, and bones)

1. Wounds are classified according to continuity of surface they cover (tissue involved)
    a. Open wound: break in skin that can be superficial or deep; examples are an abrasion, laceration, or puncture
    b. Closed wound: injury with no break in skin; examples are contusion and ecchymosis; may be caused by a blow or other type of trauma
2. Superficial, partial, and full thickness refer to depth of injury and are used most often to describe burns
    a. Superficial thickness involves epidermal layer only, such as a mild sunburn or burn from contact with hot object
    b. Partial thickness involves entire epidermis, part of dermis; sweat glands and hair follicles are intact
    c. Full thickness involves epidermis and dermis, extending to subcutaneous tissue and possibly even to muscle and bone
3. Noninfected and infected wounds
    a. A noninfected or clean wound has not been invaded by pathogenic microorganisms and heals without infection
    b. An infected wound or septic wound has been invaded by pathogenic microorganisms; clinical signs and symptoms of infection develop
4. Surgical wound: an intentional wound made by a surgeon for therapeutic purposes using a sharp cutting instrument; it is a clean wound that heals without infection
5. Pressure ulcers: lesions caused by unrelieved pressure, which also damages underlying tissues; see Table 26–4 for staging of pressure ulcers
    a. Contributing factors include immobility, fragile skin in older adults, moisture, malnutrition, shearing, and friction
    b. *NCLEX®* Assess individual client's relative risk using scales such as Braden scale or Norton scale (see Table 26–5)
    c. Assess existing pressure ulcers for healing using a tool such as Pressure Ulcer Scale for Healing (PUSH), which evaluates wound size, exudate amount, and type of tissue present in wound bed

C. Wound healing

1. Three phases
    a. Inflammatory: fibrin network of protein fibers forms in wound; blood flow increases to area; damaged tissue then heals; drying of fibrin and protein form a scab that seals skin in 3 to 4 days
    b. Proliferative phase: fibroblasts grow to form granulation tissue (4 to 21 days), which is very friable, soft, and pinkish red in color because of new capillaries; epithelial cells grow from edges; connective tissue fills area forming a scar that is stronger than granulation tissue; a large wound requiring excessive granulation tissue for closure can lead to formation of a **keloid**, a large, uneven scar
    c. Maturation or remodeling phase (healing of scar): often occurs by weeks 3 to 4, but can extend for 2 years after injury; reorganization of collagen fibers, wound remodeling, and tissue maturation occurs; a fully healed wound has tensile strength of up to 80% of preinjury state (more susceptible to future injury)

Table 26–4 Staging of Pressure Ulcers

Stage	Description
I	Skin is intact, erythema noted but does not blanche Client may report tingling or burning Darker-skinned clients may have skin discoloration, warmth, edema, and induration as indicators
II	Superficial partial-thickness skin loss with blister or abrasion-like appearance May also look like a shallow crater
III	Full-thickness skin loss Necrotic tissue is seen in subcutaneous layer that extends down to (but not through) underlying fascia Ulcer will appear as a deeper crater with or without undermining of surrounding tissue
IV	Continuation of stage III with damage to muscle, bone, and possibly tendons or joint capsule Undermining of tissue and sinus tracts may also be present

Table 26-5 Pressure Ulcer Risk Assessment Scales

Norton Scale

Physical Condition		Mental Condition		Activity		Mobility		Continence	
Good	4	Alert	4	Walks	4	Full	4	Good	4
Fair	3	Apathetic	3	Walks with help	3	Slightly limited	3	Occasional incontinence	3
Poor	2	Confused	2	Sits in chair	2	Very limited	2	Frequent incontinence	2
Very poor	1	Stuporous	1	Remains in bed	1	Immobile	1	Urine and fecal incontinence	1
Total	___	Total	___	Total	___	Total	___	Total	
Grand total = _____									

A score of 14 or less indicates a risk of pressure ulcer; a score under 12 indicates a high risk.

Braden Scale

Sensory Perception		Moisture		Activity		Mobility		Nutrition		Friction and Shear	
No impairment	4	Rarely moist	4	Walks frequently	4	No limitations	4	Excellent	4		
Slightly limited	3	Occasionally moist	3	Walks occasionally	3	Slightly limited	3	Adequate	3	No apparent Problems	3
Very limited	2	Moist	2	Chairfast	2	Very limited	2	Probably inadequate	2	Potential problem	2
Completely limited	1	Constantly moist	1	Bedfast	1	Immobile	1	Very poor	1	Problem	1
Total	___	Total	___	Total	___	Total	___	Total	___	Total	___
Grand total = _____											

Assign a score of 1 to 4 in each category. Total the score; no risk: 19–23; at risk: 15–18; moderate risk: 13–14; high risk: 10–12; very high risk: 9 or below.

Source: Smith, S., Duell, D., & Martin, B. *Clinical nursing skills: Basic to advanced skills* (7th ed.), p. 918, © 2008. Reprinted by permission of Pearson Education, Inc., Upper Saddle River, NJ 07458.

2. Factors affecting wound healing

NCLEX®

a. Age: healthy children and adults heal faster than older clients; factors that inhibit healing in older adults include age-related vascular changes, cardiovascular disease or diabetes (which reduce blood flow to area), immune system changes, possible nutritional deficiencies, and slower rate of cell renewal

NCLEX®

b. Nutrition: protein helps build new tissue; vitamin C aids maturation of fibrous tissue and protein synthesis; undernutrition results in inadequate nutrient stores, while obesity tends to decrease blood flow to tissue and increase risk of infection

c. Condition of tissues: wound contamination and infection slow healing process; organisms present in wound will compete with body cells for O_2 and nutrition

d. Efficiency of circulation: factors that restrict local blood supply to a wound (damaged arteries, edema of tissues, and dehydration) interfere with healing; anemia and blood dyscrasias may interfere with oxygen delivery; conditions such as diabetes and liver dysfunction can delay healing; regular exercise promotes circulation and faster healing; smoking may limit O_2 supply to tissues

Memory Aid

Remember that foods containing protein or vitamin C are good choices for clients who have healing wounds.

e. Rest, anxiety, and stress: adequate rest of injured part will aid wound closure; anxiety and stress can stimulate release of hormones that slow healing

NCLEX®

f. Medications: anti-inflammatory drugs such as steroids and hormones slow formation of fibrous tissue and therefore impair healing

3. Wound closures
   a. **Primary intention**: wound edges are well approximated and wound heals without infection; tissues return to a healthy state with minimal inflammation and little to no scarring
   b. **Secondary intention**: healing occurs by granulation when wound is extensive and edges cannot or should not be approximated; healing time is prolonged; carries greater risk for infection and results in deeper, more extensive scarring
   c. Surgical interventions: sutures, staples, and clips are devices used to approximate wound edges; some sutures absorb and others must be removed; staples and clips are alternatives to suturing and are usually made of silver; these require removal in approximately 7 to 10 days
4. Complications that affect wound healing
   a. Hemorrhage: assess internal hemorrhage by distention in area of wound; external hemorrhage is noted by blood on dressing or leaking from dressing; if bleeding is severe, client may exhibit signs of shock; risk of hemorrhage is greater within first 48 hours; if pressure dressings do not successfully stop bleeding, surgical intervention may be needed
   b. Infection: noted by redness, swelling, heat, and pain at site; purulent exudate may be noted; client may be anorexic, nauseous, febrile, and have chills; health care provider will order a wound culture, and antibiotics will be administered after culture is obtained
   c. **Dehiscence**: accidental reopening of suture line (usually abdominal, but could occur with any wound) with tissue separation under wound; results from infected suture line or factors that impede wound healing; clients often "feel something giving way"; place client in bed with head of bed low to eliminate gravity and with knees bent to decrease pull on suture line; cover wound with large, sterile, wet saline dressings; notify surgeon immediately because repair of surgical site is necessary
   NCLEX® d. **Evisceration**: internal organs (viscera) protrude through incisional edges after dehiscence; contributing factors include infection, poor nutrition, failure of suture material, dehydration, and excessive coughing; treated in a manner similar to dehiscence

D. Wound data collection and management

1. Inspect wound and gently palpate surrounding area regularly
2. Note whether wound edges are approximated; a healing ridge may be noted during healing
3. *NCLEX®* Note presence and characteristics of wound drainage; outline drainage on dressing, noting date and time
4. *NCLEX®* Observe for signs of infection: redness, swelling, increased tenderness, or disruption of wound edges; note body temperature and white blood cell count as other indicators
5. Purposes for dressing a wound
   a. Absorb drainage
   b. Splint or immobilize wound to provide rest
   c. Protect wound from mechanical injury
   d. Promote hemostasis
   e. Prevent contamination
   f. Provide mental and physical comfort for client
6. Purposes for maintaining a wound undressed
   a. Eliminate conditions that favor growth of microorganisms
   b. Allow for better wound observation and assessment
   c. Facilitate bathing and hygiene
   d. Avoid adhesive tape reaction
   e. Avoid friction and irritation that destroy new epithelial cells
7. Wound irrigation: may be needed to cleanse or flush wound to enhance healing; normal saline and antibiotic solutions are most commonly used

E. Wound management products

1. *NCLEX®* Wound cleansers: all wounds should be cleansed appropriately; in clean wounds where tissue is granulating, minimize disruption of wound bed; clean wound gently and rinse away debris with normal saline (see Box 26–8 for wound cleansing guidelines)
2. Enzymatic debriding agent: an enzyme paste or solution, such as Elase, that is applied to necrotic tissue; enzyme digests necrotic tissue
3. Dressings: a variety of dressing materials are available, each with different purposes; some are designed to provide barrier protection from contamination; some may be impregnated with antibiotics; others are moist and aid in liquefying necrotic tissue; see Table 26–6
4. Bandages are strips of cloth used to wrap a body part
   a. Made of gauze, (light and porous) or an elasticized material (which provides pressure to area)
   b. Widths vary from 1 to 4 inches and are determined by body part to be wrapped

Box 26–8

Clinical Guidelines for Cleaning Wounds

- Use isotonic saline or wound cleansers to clean or irrigate wounds; if antimicrobial solutions are used, make sure they are well diluted.
- When possible, warm solution to body temperature before use.
- If a wound is grossly contaminated by foreign material, bacteria, slough, or necrotic tissue, clean wound at every dressing change.
- If a wound is clean, has little exudate, and reveals healthy granulation tissue, avoid repeated cleaning.
- Use gauze squares; avoid using cotton balls and other products that shed fibers onto wound surface and can act as foci for infection or stimulate foreign body reactions, delaying the healing process.
- To retain wound moisture, avoid drying a wound after cleaning it.
- Hold cleaning sponges with forceps or a sterile gloved hand.
- Clean wound in an outward direction.

Adapted from Berman, A., Snyder, S. Kozier, B., & Erb, G. (2008). *Fundamentals of nursing: Concepts, process, and practice* (8th ed.). Upper Saddle River, NJ: Pearson Education, Inc., p. 925.

Table 26–6 Types of Dressings

Dressing Type	Description
Gauze	Plain or impregnated with an antimicrobial Packs and fills wound; absorbs drainage Used for full- and partial-thickness wounds with drainage May be applied dry, wet-to-moist, and wet-to-wet
Transparent	Adhesive plastic membrane that allows oxygen into wound but is impermeable to liquids and bacteria Protects wound from contamination and friction, prevents fluid evaporation from wound, and aids wound assessment Op-Site, Bioclusive, and Tegaderm are examples
Impregnated nonadherent	Cotton or synthetic material is impregnated with saline, zinc-saline, antimicrobials, petrolatum, or others Protects partial- and full-thickness wounds that do not have exudate Require secondary dressings to keep them in place, hold in moisture, and protect wound
Hydrocolloid	Contains adhesive wafer, paste, or powder Protects wound from contamination Eliminates risk of maceration of surrounding skin Inner layer absorbs exudates and forms hydrated gel over wound, while outer film provides occlusive seal Can be worn up to 7 days; Duo-Derm and Tegasorb are examples
Hydrogel	Water or glycerin is primary component of jelly-like sheet, granules, or gels Maintains moist wound bed and helps liquefy necrotic tissue or slough Permeable to oxygen and can fill dead spaces in a wound Secondary occlusive dressing is required
Alginate (exudate absorbers)	Nonadherent dressings of powder, beads, granules, ropes, sheets, or paste Purpose is to absorb up tp 20 times their weight in drainage Secondary dressing is required Examples are Kaltostat and Algiderm
Polyurethane foam	Nonadherent hydrocolloid dressing that absorb large amounts of exudate absorbers while keeping wound moist Requires secondary dressing for an occlusive environment, or tape around edges to secure it Skin around area needs protection from maceration
Clear absorbent acrylic	Transparent absorbent wafer for 5–7 day use Acrylic layer absorbs exudates and evaporates moisture through transparent membrane Aids in wound assessment while protecting from bacteria and shearing forces Tegaderm is an example

c. Purposes are to anchor dressings, immobilize or provide support to a body part, or promote venous return
d. Apply bandage with body part in normal position
e. Pad bony prominences
f. Bandage from distal to proximal area to support blood return
NCLEX® g. Use even pressure while applying bandage, especially when using elastic bandages that could impair circulation
NCLEX® h. Inspect and palpate the area regularly—more frequently on a fresher wound, less frequently on an older wound; note neurovascular status of extremity (temperature, blanching, and sensation) and pain (evaluate for its cause)

VIII. MEETING NEEDS FOR MOBILITY

A. Common causes of immobility

1. Pain: reduces spontaneous movement may inhibit client from participating in care activities, including coughing and deep breathing
2. Motor and nervous system impairment: disorders of musculoskeletal system (such as arthritis or amputation) and nervous system (such as multiple sclerosis or Parkinson's disease) can limit mobility; certain neurological diseases can cause muscles to become stiff or lose function (such as stroke)
3. Functional problems: some chronic conditions that limit supply of O_2 and nutrients or increase cardiac work affect activity tolerance, such as chronic obstructive lung disease, congestive heart failure, angina, and obesity
4. Generalized weakness: from age-related loss of muscle tone, flexibility and reaction time, decreased bone density, or chronic illness
5. Psychological problems: emotional disorders such as depression or stress can reduce motivation and energy to participate in activities
6. Medically induced immobility
   a. Clients may be placed on bedrest or have activity restrictions to allow healing of body parts
   b. Orthopedic devices (traction, casts, splints, braces) can also cause immobility

NCLEX® **B. Major complications of immobility**

1. Psychological effects: powerlessness and possible reduced self-esteem
2. Atrophy and contractures
3. Disuse osteoporosis
4. Pressure ulcers
5. Orthostatic intolerance (postural or orthostatic hypotension)
6. Deep vein thrombosis
7. Pneumonia
8. Decrease in peristalsis (paralytic ileus)
9. Kidney stones

C. Nursing interventions for impaired mobility

1. Explain benefits of exercise
   a. Improves tone and strength of muscles, joint flexibility and range of motion (ROM)
   b. Promotes good pulmonary ventilation, which prevents pooling of secretions in lungs and reduces risk of pneumonia
   c. Improves GI motility and tone, thereby improving digestion and elimination
   d. Decreases bone loss of calcium, which helps maintain acidic urine to decrease risk for renal calculi
2. Types of exercise
   a. Isometric: muscle tension or resistance is produced without a change in muscle length; strengthen muscle groups that will be used later in ambulation; teach client to push or pull against a stationary object; muscles exercised are abdominal, gluteus, and quadriceps
   b. Isotonic: exercises that shorten muscle to produce contraction and active movement with no significant change in resistance, so force of contraction stays stable; increase muscle tone and maintain joint flexibility; examples are using a trapeze to lift body or pushing body into a sitting position
   c. Passive ROM: accomplished with assistance of a caregiver who supports client's body part while moving it
   d. Active ROM: isotonic exercises of each joint in body that are performed by client; can maintain or improve muscle strength; prevent deterioration of joint movement and subsequent contractures

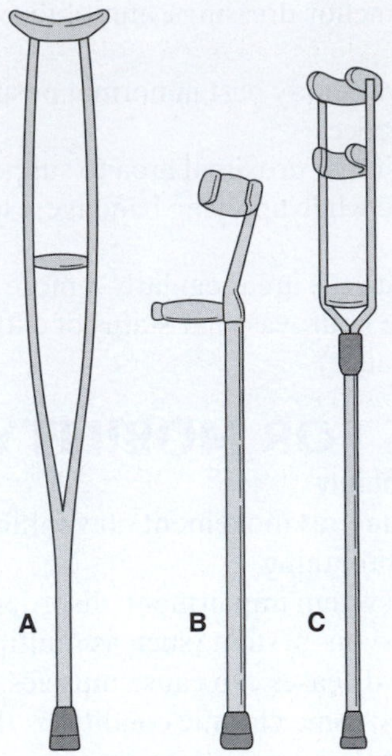

Figure 26–3

Three types of crutches: *A.* axillary crutch; *B.* Lofstrand crutch; *C.* Canadian or elbow extension crutch.

D. Assistive ambulation device: crutches

NCLEX®

1. Assist client in moving and ambulating; require rubber tips to prevent slipping on floors; various types of crutches are available (see Figure 26–3)
   - **a.** An axillary crutch is most frequently used type of crutch
   - **b.** A Lofstrand or forearm crutch is used as a substitute for a cane; consists of a single tube of aluminum with a handle and a cuff for forearm; allows user to release hand bar because metal cuff maintains placement of crutch and prevents it from falling
   - **c.** Canadian or elbow extensor crutch is used for client whose forearm extensor muscles are weak; it allows upper arm to provide stability to crutch
2. Measuring for crutches
   - **a.** Measure client who is lying supine from anterior fold of axilla to heel of foot and add 1 inch (2.5 cm)
   - **b.** Also measure placement of hand on crutch while client stands and adjust crutch so that it maintains elbow at a 30-degree angle
   - **c.** With client standing erect, ensure that shoulder rest of crutch is 3 fingerwidths (2.5 to 5 cm, or 1 to 2 inches) below axilla

NCLEX®

3. Safety with crutches
   - **a.** Place rubber tip on end of crutch
   - **b.** Teach client appropriate gait
   - **c.** Prior to gait training, assist client in preparing for crutch walking by encouraging client to push body off the bed with hands and arms
   - **d.** While using crutches, have client bear weight on arms, not axillae, to avoid nerve damage to axillae caused by continued pressure
4. Gaits used for crutch walking: client's ability to bear weight and maintain balance determines choice of five gaits; client alternates body weight between one or both legs and crutches; see Box 26–9

E. Cane: assists a client to walk with greater balance and support

1. Three types of canes
   - **a.** Quad cane has four feet
   - **b.** Tripod has three feet
   - **c.** Straight cane
2. Canes are adjustable; length should allow elbow to bend slightly
3. Canes allow clients to ambulate faster and with less fatigue
4. Clients may use one or two canes; a single cane is used on unaffected side
5. A rubber cap is fitted at tip of cane to prevent slipping

F. Walker: provides more support than a cane

1. Used for clients who have poor balance, cardiac problems, or cannot use crutches
2. Standard walker has four legs with rubber tips on feet and plastic grips for hands

Box 26-9

Crutch Walking Gaits

Four-Point Gait: Partial Weight-Bearing

1. The client must be able to bear weight on both legs.
2. It is the safest gait and provides three points of support at all times.
3. It requires constant shifting of weight and coordination of movement of legs and crutches.

Three-Point Gait: Requires One Leg to Be Able to Bear Weight of Entire Body

1. Non-weight-bearing on affected leg.
2. Alternates between good leg and affected leg with both crutches.

Two-Point Gait: Requires Partial Weight-Bearing on Both Legs

1. Client can move at a faster gait than with the four-point gait.
2. Two points are used to support the body at all times.
3. Crutch movement is similar to the swinging of the arms while walking.

Swing-Through Gait: Weight-Bearing Gait that Requires Strength and Coordination

1. Client moves both crutches forward together.
2. Then the client lifts his or her body weight and swings through.

Swing-To Gait: Weight-Bearing on Both Legs

1. Similar to swing-through gait except body motion is only to level of crutches.
2. Useful for clients with paralysis of legs and hips.

3. Client must be partial weight-bearing and have strength in wrists and arms
4. Client uses upper body to propel walker forward
5. Two- or four-wheeled walker is useful for client who is too weak or not stable enough to move a walker by lifting it; some walkers have an attached seat to allow client to sit and rest as needed during walk
6. Walkers are height-adjustable

G. Other assistive devices

1. Hydraulic lift used for clients who are unable to stand and too heavy for health care workers to lift safely
2. Lift has three parts: sling, arm, and base; a pressure release valve is on base
3. Place sling under client: arm of device has a hook that attaches to sling; lift is raised to elevate client
4. Lift is then moved and aligned with chair; pressure release valve is released, and client is lowered to chair
5. Sling can be removed from hooks but left under client to facilitate returning client to bed

Check Your NCLEX-PN® Exam I.Q.

You are ready for testing on this content if you can

- Assist a client with personal hygiene needs.
- Monitor a client's ability to perform activities of daily living.
- Plan nursing care to promote rest and sleep.
- Identify the elimination needs of a client.
- Provide care to a client to assist with urinary and bowel elimination.
- Take action to prevent complications of immobility.
- Observe a client's wound-healing status.
- Implement nursing measures to promote wound healing.
- Determine a client's need for assistive devices.
- Implement care for a client using an assistive device.

PRACTICE TEST

PRACTICE TEST

1 A 92-year-old client who is very hard of hearing has been admitted to the skilled nursing facility. Which action is appropriate for the nurse when collecting data from the client?

1. Use a cotton swab to clean cerumen in the client's ear before the interview.
2. Speak louder into the client's ear determined to have better hearing.
3. Lower the pitch of the voice and face the client during conversation.
4. Put new batteries in the hearing aid to ensure proper functioning.

2 A 72-year-old client has been in the ICU for the past 2 days. Which intervention would be the most appropriate in decreasing the risk for sensory deprivation? Select all that apply.

1. Remove equipment from the room.
2. Explain procedures and routines to the client upon admission.
3. Provide a clock and calendar in the client's room.
4. Maintain a balance of activity and rest periods.
5. Maintain constant conversation when in the client's room.

3 The nurse must apply an elastic bandage to provide support to a client's sprained ankle. Which action should the nurse take during this procedure?

1. Moderately stretch the bandage and wrap it from distal extremity to proximal.
2. Wrap the extremity loosely enough to insert two fingers beneath the bandage.
3. Maintain a tight stretch with each wrap of the bandage.
4. Start proximal to the injury site and work distally.

4 All of the following clients appear in the emergency room during one shift. For which clients should the nurse expect the health care provider to order an antibiotic? Select all that apply.

1. Cat bite to the hand of an elderly client
2. Laceration from broken glass in a 6-year-old client
3. Stab wound in the arm of a 37-year-old client
4. Closed fracture to the ankle of a 40-year-old soccer player
5. A wrist sprain in a 17-year-old who was playing basketball

5 An 80-year-old client has been admitted to the nursing unit with Parkinson's disease. Which of the following activities would be most appropriate in preventing disuse syndrome?

1. Providing for the nutritional needs of the client
2. Promoting weight-bearing exercises
3. Encouraging 8 glasses of fluid in 24 hours
4. Turning and positioning every 2 hours

6 A female client can move her right arm and leg but has hemiplegia on the left. What should the nurse instruct the nursing assistant to do on the client's left side during care?

1. Active range of motion
2. Passive range of motion
3. Isotonic exercises
4. Isometric exercises

7 A client has weakness of the lower extremities and uses crutches for mobility. What client behavior should indicate to the nurse that the client needs further reinforcement of teaching about using crutches?

1. Uses the swing-to gait
2. Uses axillary crutches
3. Bears weight on the armpits
4. Replaces rubber tips on the crutches

8 A male client suffered numerous types of wounds when he lost control of his motorcycle and was thrown onto the pavement. The client asks the nurse which wounds will scar more. The nurse's reply will be based on analysis that which wound would generally be least likely to scar?

1. A wound that heals by primary intention
2. A wound that heals by secondary intention
3. A wound that becomes infected
4. A wound to an extremity

9. A postoperative client tells the nurse that he developed dehiscence after his last surgery and wants to make sure it doesn't happen this time. Which nursing intervention is most effective for attempting to prevent dehiscence in a postoperative client?

1. Helping the client lose weight
2. Preventing vomiting
3. Administering antibiotics
4. Keeping the wound dry

10. An elderly postoperative client's abdominal wound is still healing weeks after the surgery. The client asks the clinic nurse why the wound is healing so slowly. Which factor should the nurse identify that negatively affects healing in the elderly?

1. Vascular changes decrease blood flow to the wound.
2. Most elderly clients are overweight.
3. Decreased activity levels prevent blood from reaching the area.
4. Keloid formation prevents healing.

11. A client, admitted to the hospital for gallbladder surgery, is diagnosed as having a vitamin C deficiency. The nurse places high priority on monitoring this client for which development postoperatively?

1. Unusual muscle weakness
2. Mental confusion
3. Delayed wound healing
4. Ataxia upon ambulating

12. The nurse is working with a client who has a mobility problem and needs an appropriate assistance device. The client's lower extremities have no paralysis, but are very weak. Upper-body strength is also reduced. The nurse should anticipate which device will be prescribed for this client?

1. Cane
2. Four-wheeled walker
3. Canadian or elbow extension crutch
4. Lofstrand crutch

13. The nurse is monitoring a client using a cane. Which observation made by the nurse would indicate that the client is using the cane appropriately?

1. Client holds the cane with the hand on the stronger side.
2. Client holds the cane with the hand on the affected side.
3. Client moves the cane and the affected leg together.
4. The cane tip is made of aluminum to prevent slippage.

14. A client is at risk for developing a pressure ulcer and is placed on a repositioning regimen. The client does not like to lie on his side and complains about the need to turn. Which explanations by the nurse will most effectively enhance compliance? Select all that apply.

1. "Turning helps maintain skin integrity by alternating area pressure."
2. "Excess pressure interferes with skin absorption of vitamin D."
3. "Staying in one position prevents proper heat loss from that area of the body."
4. "Changing position prevents tissue breakdown that could ultimately become infected."
5. "A repositioning schedule is a standard part of hospital policy."

15. The nurse is changing the abdominal dressing of a client who is 4 days postoperative. The nurse notes a moderate amount of serosanguineous drainage, wound edges not approximated, and puffy tissue protruding through the wound. What condition should the nurse suspect from theses manifestations?

1. Hemorrhage
2. Normal healing by primary intention
3. Normal healing by secondary intention
4. Evisceration

16. The nurse is speaking with a 74-year-old client who is hearing impaired. What should the nurse do to enhance the client's ability to hear? Select all that apply.

1. Position self to be within the client's line of vision.
2. Dim the lights in the room.
3. Over-articulate words.
4. Turn down the television in the room.
5. Talk at a moderate rate and with the same tone for all words.

PRACTICE TEST

17 A middle-aged client reports to the nurse that sleep patterns are different than when the client was younger. Which of the following suggests a normal developmental pattern?

1. Client sleeps about 6 hours per night with about 20–25 percent of REM sleep and a marked decrease in Stage IV NREM sleep.
2. Client sleeps 6–8 hours per night with about 20 percent REM sleep and the amount of Stage IV NREM sleep decreases.
3. Client sleeps erratically because of work schedules with about 30 percent of REM sleep and no marked decrease in Stage IV NREM sleep.
4. Client has light sleep with equal amounts of REM sleep and NREM sleep.

18 The nurse assigns an unlicensed assistive person (UAP) to a client who needs total hygiene care. In what order should the nurse expect the UAP to perform this assignment? Place the options in the correct order. All options must be used.

1. Makes a bath mitt with the washcloth
2. Washes, rinses, and dries leg from ankle to knee to thigh
3. Positions the bed at a working height and lowers closest side rail
4. Provide the client with hair and mouth care
5. Cleans the client's eyes from inner to outer canthus

ANSWERS & RATIONALES

1 **Answer: 3 Rationale:** Hearing loss, especially of upper-range tones, is common in the elderly. Speaking to the client slowly and in a lower-pitched voice while facing the client is the best means of communication. Cleaning cerumen from the client's ears will not overcome age-related hearing loss. Depending on the level of hearing loss, speaking louder into the ear with the better hearing may still not be an effective action. The question states that the client is hard of hearing without reference to a hearing aid. If a hearing aid is used, changing the batteries may not be an effective action. **Cognitive Level:** Applying **Client Need:** Basic Care and Comfort **Integrated Process:** Communication and Documentation **Content Area:** Fundamentals **Strategy:** Apply knowledge related to communicating with a client who is hearing impaired. Remember that if the age of the client is included in the stem, it is important in determining the correct option. Consider the question as it is written and do not make assumptions.

2 **Answer: 3, 4 Rationale:** Providing the client with a clock and calendar helps the client to be oriented to time and date. These would be meaningful stimuli for the client and decrease the chance for sensory deprivation. Activities and rest periods should be spaced and planned to balance high and low levels of sensory stimuli. It may not be realistic in an ICU to remove equipment from the room. Explaining all procedures and routines would increase the risk of information overload. Continuous conversation is not therapeutic; and could place the client at risk for sensory overload as a different problem. **Cognitive Level:** Applying **Client Need:** Basic Care and Comfort **Integrated Process:** Nursing Process: Implementation **Content Area:** Fundamentals **Strategy:** The core issue of the question is nursing actions that can prevent the client from experiencing sensory deprivation. Use knowledge of basic nursing measures to help a client stay oriented to time, place, and person.

3 **Answer: 1 Rationale:** To prevent vascular impairment, proper application of elastic bandages is required. Wrapping distal to proximal is compatible with the flow of venous return. Wrapping the bandage evenly while stretching it moderately ensures that there will be even tension applied to the extremity while not occluding circulation. Wrapping the bandage loosely enough to be able to insert two fingers will not secure the bandage in place or provide adequate support for the injury. Excessive tension when applying an elastic bandage would cause circulation to be compromised. Wrapping distal to proximal is compatible with the flow of venous return. **Cognitive Level:** Applying **Client Need:** Basic Care and Comfort **Integrated Process:** Nursing Process: Implementation **Content Area:** Fundamentals **Strategy:** The core issue of the question is knowledge of basic wound care procedures. Use nursing knowledge of these procedures and concepts related to blood flow to make your selection.

4 **Answer: 1, 2, 3 Rationale:** A closed fracture or a sprain has no break in the skin. A cat bite, a laceration, and a stab wound all impair skin integrity, which could lead to infection and thus may require prophylactic use of an antibiotic. **Cognitive Level:** Analyzing **Client Need:** Basic Care and Comfort **Integrated Process:** Nursing Process: Implementation **Content Area:** Fundamentals **Strategy:** The core issue of the question is appropriate use of antibiotic therapy. Restate this question in the following way: "Which client is *not* at risk for infection?" Use the process of elimination and nursing knowledge to make selections that pose little risk of infection.

5 **Answer: 2 Rationale:** Weight-bearing exercise is the best approach to preventing disuse syndrome. Disuse syndrome occurs because the stresses of weight bearing are absent and the bone releases calcium. Providing for nutritional needs is a general nursing intervention that is not specific to weight bearing. Encouraging fluids is a general nursing intervention that is not specific to weight bearing. Turning and repositioning is a general nursing intervention that is not specific to weight bearing. **Cognitive Level:** Applying **Client Need:** Basic Care and Comfort **Integrated Process:** Nursing Process: Implementation **Content Area:** Fundamentals **Strategy:** The core issues of the question are the cause of disuse syndrome and

nursing approaches that will minimize it. Use concepts of basic nursing care to answer the question.

6 **Answer: 2** **Rationale:** Passive range of motion is most appropriate because the client is unable to move that side of the body on her own. Active range of motion requires resistance on the part of the muscles on the left side and the client is unable to do that. Isotonic exercises require resistance on the part of the muscles on the left side and the client is unable to do that. Isometric exercises require resistance on the part of the muscles on the left side and the client is unable to do that. **Cognitive Level:** Applying **Client Need:** Basic Care and Comfort **Integrated Process:** Nursing Process: Implementation **Content Area:** Fundamentals **Strategy:** The critical words in the question are *unable to move*. This indicates that the client has hemiplegia and is unable to actively participate in exercising the joints. The wording of the question tells you that there is only one correct answer.

7 **Answer: 3** **Rationale:** The weight of the body should be borne on the arms, not the axillae. When clients allow the axillae to bear the weight of the body, they are at risk of developing crutch palsy, nerve damage. This behavior would require additional client teaching. The ability to perform the swing-to gait represents correct use of crutches; therefore no further teaching is needed on those points. Axillary crutches are crutches that are appropriately positioned beneath the axillae of the body. If a client is able to use axillary crutches without bearing weight on the armpits, no further teaching is needed. Placing new rubber tips on the crutches indicates an awareness of equipment safety that requires no further teaching. Worn crutch tips can cause a client to slip or fall. **Cognitive Level:** Analyzing **Client Need:** Reduction of Risk Potential **Integrated Process:** Nursing Process: Evaluation **Content Area:** Fundamentals **Strategy:** The core issue of the question is proper use of crutches. Keep in mind that this question has a negative stem and the correct answer is the option that reflects incorrect information.

8 **Answer: 1** **Rationale:** Primary intention healing occurs when the wound edges are well approximated. Wounds that heal by secondary intention have edges that cannot be approximated. Scarring is greater for wounds that heal by secondary intention. Scarring is greater for wounds that become infected. The location of a wound has little to do with scarring. **Cognitive Level:** Applying **Client Need:** Basic Care and Comfort **Integrated Process:** Nursing Process: Evaluation **Content Area:** Fundamentals **Strategy:** The core issue of this question is knowledge of physiological wound healing. Use nursing knowledge and the process of elimination to make a selection.

9 **Answer: 2** **Rationale:** Activities that are likely to lead to dehiscence include vomiting and coughing because they increase intra-abdominal pressure. Clients who are obese and those with poor nutrition are candidates for dehiscence. Since the client is already postoperative, encouraging weight loss at this time would not affect risk for dehiscence, and there is no indication that the client is overweight. Administering antibiotics is effective in preventing or treating infection. Antibiotic therapy alone cannot prevent dehiscence. Keeping a wound dry will promote healing and prevent infection; however, this action alone will not prevent dehiscence. **Cognitive Level:** Analyzing **Client Need:** Basic Care and Comfort **Integrated Process:** Nursing Process: Planning **Content Area:** Fundamentals **Strategy:** The core issue of the question is knowledge of risk factors for dehiscence. Recall that dehiscence is most likely to occur when there is some type of stress on the incision line. Consider that vomiting puts sudden tension on the suture line to select it as the option that is most likely to be harmful to the client.

10 **Answer: 1** **Rationale:** Vascular changes, such as atherosclerosis and atrophy of capillaries, impair blood flow to the wound. Older adults are not necessarily overweight, although weight gain does tend to occur with increasing age. Decreased activity levels with aging do not diminish local blood supply to a healing wound. Keloid formation is an abnormal type of healing of a wound. **Cognitive Level:** Analyzing **Client Need:** Basic Care and Comfort **Integrated Process:** Nursing Process: Evaluation **Content Area:** Fundamentals **Strategy:** The core issue of the question is age-related changes that have a negative impact on wound healing. Use nursing knowledge and the process of elimination to make a selection.

11 **Answer: 3** **Rationale:** Protein and vitamin C are necessary for building and maintaining tissues. A deficiency of vitamin C would prolong wound healing. The other options are not manifestations of a vitamin C deficiency. **Cognitive Level:** Understanding **Client Need:** Basic Care and Comfort **Integrated Process:** Nursing Process: Planning **Content Area:** Fundamentals **Strategy:** The core issue of this question is the role of vitamin C in wound healing. Use nursing knowledge and the process of elimination to make a selection.

12 **Answer: 2** **Rationale:** The client has bilateral weakness of the lower extremities, and the proper assistive device is one that will provide bilateral support. In this case, a four-wheeled walker provides the most support and does not require the client to lift the walker as steps are taken. A cane would provide unilateral support, while this client has bilateral weakness. A Canadian or elbow crutch provides unilateral support only and requires upper limb strength to use. A Lofstrand crutch provides unilateral support and the client has bilateral weakness. **Cognitive Level:** Analyzing **Client Need:** Safety and Infection Control **Integrated Process:** Nursing Process: Planning **Content Area:** Fundamentals **Strategy:** The core issue of the question is the assistive device that will provide the safest support to the client. The critical word *legs* in the stem of the question guides you to look for an option that provides bilateral support.

13 **Answer: 1** **Rationale:** To provide maximum support and appropriate body alignment while walking, the cane is held in the hand on the stronger side. The client moves the cane and the unaffected leg together. The tip of the cane should have rubber to prevent slippage. **Cognitive Level:** Applying **Client Need:** Safety and Infection Control **Integrated Process:** Nursing Process: Data Collection **Content Area:** Fundamentals **Strategy:** The core issue of the question is the proper use of a cane as an assistive aid. Use the process of elimination and basic nursing knowledge to make a selection.

14 **Answer: 1, 4** **Rationale:** Relieving pressure increases allows capillaries to stay open to maintain circulation to the affected area. A loss of skin integrity places the client at risk for bacterial invasion and subsequent infection. Unless the skin loss is extensive, the skin will continue to absorb vitamin D. Unless the skin loss is extensive, the skin will continue to prevent the loss of heat from the body. Referring to policy does not promote client understanding or compliance. **Cognitive Level:** Applying **Client Need:** Basic Care and Comfort **Integrated Process:** Teaching and Learning

Content Area: Fundamentals **Strategy:** The core issue of the question is knowledge of the functions of the skin and how pressure ulcers interfere with normal skin function. Use the process of elimination and basic nursing knowledge to make selections. Note the question indicates that more than one option may be correct.

15 **Answer: 4 Rationale:** Evisceration occurs when internal viscera protrude from an incision that is dehiscing. In this situation, the nurse notes changes in wound appearance such as increased serosanguineous drainage, edges lacking approximation, and the protruding viscera. The nurse notes a moderate amount of serosanguineous drainage, which should be nearly diminished by the 4th day postoperative. However, this description does not fit hemorrhage. Healing by primary intention includes well-approximated incision edges and no signs of infection or complication. Secondary healing is when the wound is extensive and the edges cannot or should not be approximated; healing time is prolonged. **Cognitive Level:** Analyzing **Client Need:** Basic Care and Comfort **Integrated Process:** Nursing Process: Evaluation **Content Area:** Fundamentals **Strategy:** The core issue of this question is the ability to draw accurate conclusions about the status of a surgical wound. Use the process of elimination and basic nursing knowledge to make a selection.

16 **Answer: 1, 4, 5 Rationale:** The nurse should select a position within the client's line of vision to enable the client to read lips during the conversation. It is good to decrease background noises that interfere with the client's ability to hear the nurse. It is helpful to speak at a moderate rate and use the same voice tone throughout each sentence, not dropping the tone at the end of a sentence. The lighting should not be dimmed because doing so would interfere with the client's ability to see the nurse clearly in order to read lips. Words should not be over articulated; exaggerated, unnatural movement of the lips can distort words for the client who relies on lip reading to compensate for hearing loss. **Cognitive Level:** Applying **Client Need:** Basic Care and Comfort **Integrated Process:** Communication and Documentation **Content Area:** Fundamentals **Strategy:** The core issue of the question is effective communication strategies with a client whose hearing is impaired. Remember that correct answers to questions such as these focus on enhancing the client's vision during communication and are moderate in overall approach (i.e., not excessive or insufficient).

17 **Answer: 2 Rationale:** Middle-aged adults have a decrease in deep sleep, Stage IV NREM. This is an expected pattern in older adults. This is expected in young adults. This pattern is expected in neonates. **Cognitive Level:** Analyzing **Client Need:** Physiological Adaptation **Integrated Process:** Nursing Process: Data Collection **Content Area:** Foundational Sciences **Strategy:** Select the option that describes the sleep change most closely matched with the middle-aged group, gradual reduction in quality sleep.

18 **Answer: 3, 1, 5, 2, 4 Rationale:** Positioning the bed first helps avoid undue reaching and straining, promotes good body mechanics, and increases client safety. Making a bath mitt from the washcloth as the second action retains water and heat better than a loosely held washcloth; it also keeps wet ends from trailing across the client's body. Third, cleaning the eyes from inner to outer canthus prevents secretions from entering the nasolacrimal ducts and begins the bath while working from cleaner to dirtier areas. Washing from the distal to proximal promotes circulation by stimulating venous blood return, and is done fourth to continue working from cleaner to dirtier areas. While some clients may want or need mouth care prior to the bath, most frequently these activities are performed at the end of bathing, and, therefore, are last. **Cognitive Level:** Applying **Client Need:** Basic Care and Comfort **Integrated Process:** Nursing Process: Implementation **Content Area:** Fundamentals **Strategy:** The core concept of the question is recognizing the correct order in which total hygiene is provided for the client. Use mental images to put the options in the correct order.

ANSWERS & RATIONALES

Key Terms to Review

References

Berman, A., & Snyder, S. (2012). *Kozier & Erb's fundamentals of nursing: Concepts, process, and practice* (9th ed.). Upper Saddle River, NJ: Pearson Education., Inc.

Craven, R., & Hirnle, C. (2009). *Fundamentals of nursing* (6th ed.). Philadelphia: Lippincott Williams & Wilkins.

Potter, P., & Perry, A. (2010). *Fundamentals of nursing enhanced multimedia edition package* (7th ed.). St. Louis, MO: Mosby.

Smith, S., Duell, D., & Martin, B. (2012). *Clinical nursing skills: Basic to advanced skills* (8th ed.). Upper Saddle River, NJ: Pearson Education, Inc.

Test Yourself

Are you ready for the NCLEX-PN® or course exams? Use the practice tests on the companion website to check.

Maintaining Function of Tubes and Drains 27

In this chapter

Cross Reference

Other chapters relevant to this content area are

Meeting Nutritional Needs	Chapter 25
Perioperative Care	Chapter 44
Respiratory Disorders	Chapter 51
Renal and Genitourinary Disorders	Chapter 54
Gastrointestinal Disorders	Chapter 55

I. RESPIRATORY TUBES

A. Tracheostomy tube

1. Overview
   a. Tracheotomy is a surgical procedure that creates an opening in trachea to establish a patent airway
   b. A **tracheostomy** is an opening (stoma) that is surgically created
   c. A variety of tubes can be inserted into a tracheostomy, depending on length of anticipated use, whether temporary or permanent, on whether mechanical ventilation will be used, and on need to be able to speak while in place (see Figure 27–1)
   NCLEX® d. Variations in tubes include double-lumen or single-lumen (inner cannula or no inner cannula), cuffed or cuffless, fenestrated or nonfenestrated, and talking tracheostomy tube (for client on long-term mechanical ventilation) (see Table 27–1)
   e. Clients who have permanent tracheostomies often use metal trach tubes, which are cuffless and have an inner cannula; can be used long term with regular cleaning (examples: Jackson and Tucker tubes)
2. Therapeutic management
   a. Maintain head of bed elevated at least 30 degrees
   NCLEX® b. Ensure that a manual resuscitation (Ambu) bag is at bedside at all times
   NCLEX® c. Keep spare tracheostomy (trach) set of same size, obturator, and clamps at bedside for use if trach is accidentally removed
   d. Ensure that air and oxygen (O_2) flowing into airway is humidified; notify respiratory therapy if water bottle attached to O_2 flowmeter runs low

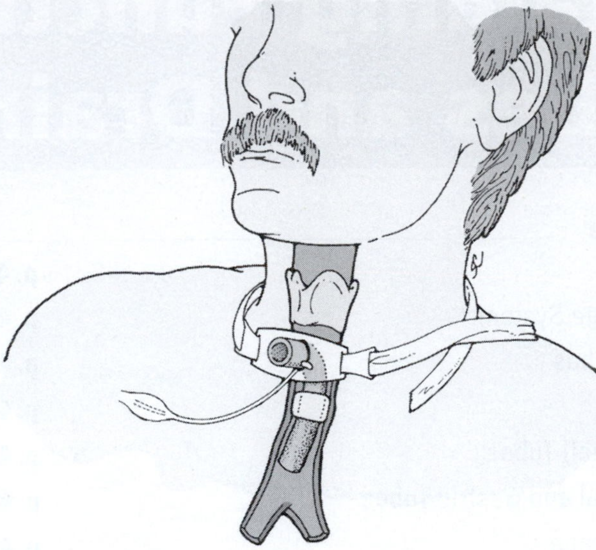

Figure 27–1
Tracheostomy tube in place.

Table 27–1 Comparison of Features of Tracheostomy Tubes

Feature	Present	Absent
Inner cannula (a removable inner tube within an outer tracheostomy tube)	Double-lumen tubes have both inner and outer cannulas (e.g., Shiley); inner one can be removed for easy cleaning, especially with heavy secretions, and may be reusable or disposable.	Single-lumen tubes have no inner cannula (e.g., Portex) and may be used short term or in clients not anticipated to have copious respiratory secretions.
Cuff (a balloon that seals airway)	Cuffed tube prevents air loss during mechanical ventilation and prevents aspiration of saliva, gastric contents, or tube feedings; is inflated with air using syringe attached to pilot balloon.	Cuffless tube is often selected for long-term use in clients who do not need mechanical ventilation and are at low risk of aspiration.
Fenestration (holes to allow air flow between larynx and trachea)	Fenestrated trach is used frequently during weaning so client regains ability to breathe naturally; it allows client to speak.	Nonfenestrated trachs have no holes and are ideal for clients on mechanical ventilation or who cannot speak.

e. Teach coughing and deep breathing to reduce risk of atelectasis and pneumonia
f. Perform respiratory assessments, including breath sounds, at regular intervals, minimally every 4 hours
g. Monitor and document O_2 saturation and/or arterial blood gas results and note trends
NCLEX® **h.** Suction client as indicated by results of assessment (cough, noisy respirations, or adventitious breath sounds); hyperoxygenate client before and after, suction for no more than 10 seconds at one time; assess nature of secretions (purulent secretions indicate infection)
NCLEX® **i.** Assess stoma for redness or signs of infection; assess for and report subcutaneous emphysema (subcutaneous air, also called crepitus)
j. Perform trach care every 8 hours; use normal saline for cleansing site and inner cannula unless agency policy is different
k. Change trach ties daily or more often if soiled; have assistant hold trach in place so client cannot cough it out; if assistance is unavailable, place new ties before cutting and removing old ones to prevent client from coughing out tube
l. Monitor cuff pressures (if inflated) at least every 8 hours per agency policy (should not exceed 20 mm Hg); see endotracheal tube section that follows for cuff inflation techniques
NCLEX® **m.** Provide for alternate means of communication (word or picture board, writing pad) if client cannot talk because of cuff inflation
n. If client has order for oral intake while trach is in place, inflate cuff to reduce risk of aspiration and sit client upright during meals and for 1 hour afterward as ordered
NCLEX® **o.** Before capping with Passey-Muir valve or plugging trach as final stage of weaning before trach removal, ensure that fenestrated trach is in use (necessary for plugging and is preferred for capping) and that cuff, if present, is deflated; note that cuff inflation during capping and plugging will occlude client's airway, leading to respiratory distress and arrest

NCLEX® **3.** Complications (see Table 27–2)

4. Planned removal

NCLEX® **a.** Suction trachea and oropharyngeal area to remove any secretions

b. Ensure that cuff is deflated

c. Physician cuts sutures that hold tracheostomy in place and withdraws tube during exhalation

d. Place dry sterile dressing over stoma and tape gently in place

e. Stoma closes over next few days and leaves small scar

B. *Endotracheal tube* (ETT) (see Figure 27–2)

1. Overview

a. An artificial airway that maintains airway patency and allows for mechanical ventilation; intended for short-term use, up to 10 to 14 days

b. Consists of a long tube with a universal adapter at proximal end for attachment to oxygen source or ventilator, inflatable cuff at distal end, and pilot balloon at proximal end for cuff inflation

Table 27–2 Complications of Tracheostomy

Complication	Prevention and Therapeutic Management
Short term	
Tube dislodgment (accidental removal)	Secure tube properly. Prevent traction on tube and avoid excessive tube movement. Do not allow client to pull at tube. Keep spare tube of same size at bedside. Follow agency policy if tube displacement occurs. If dislodged in first 72 hours after surgical tube placement, manually ventilate client with bag-valve-mask unit while an assistant calls resuscitation team. If dislodged after 72 hours following surgical tube placement, extend neck and separate tissues of stoma to restore airway; use retention sutures and/or tracheal dilator (curved clamp) to hold stoma open; insert obturator into trach tube, insert tube into trachea, remove obturator, ventilate with bag-valve-mask unit, and assess air exchange and respiratory status; if unsuccessful or ineffective, call for resuscitation team.
Tube obstruction	Assess client for respiratory difficulty, audible noisy respirations, thick and viscous tracheal secretions, and newly increased peak pressure on mechanical ventilator. Humidify oxygen. Suction client as needed. Encourage client to cough and deep breathe. Keep inner cannula clean by doing trach care regularly as scheduled. Prepare for rapid tube replacement if obstruction is caused by cuff prolapse over distal end of tube.
Long term	
Tracheomalacia (tracheal dilation and erosion from high cuff pressures)	Note whether trach tube has low pressure cuff for prevention. Monitor air volumes needed to keep cuff inflated and cuff pressures as per policy; identify and report increases. Assess for air leaks around cuff or lost tidal volume if mechanical ventilation is being used. Assess for aspiration of food or fluids if client is allowed oral intake. Monitor for and report onset of bleeding caused by pressure. Progress client to use of uncuffed tube at earliest opportunity.
Tracheoesophageal fistula (abnormal connection between posterior tracheal wall and esophagus from high cuff pressure)	Similar to tracheomalacia above. Use soft-feeding feeding tube instead of nasogastric (NG) tube for feeding as possible prevention. Assess for coughing or respiratory distress while taking food or fluids. Administer supplemental oxygen by mask to treat hypoxemia. Prepare client for possible insertion of gastric or jejunostomy tube for feedings if pressure of NG tube in esophagus was contributing factor.
Tracheal stenosis (tracheal lumen narrowing from scar formation secondary to cuff irritation)	Prevent by avoiding high cuff pressures and avoiding traction or pulling on tube, keeping properly secured and using correct cuff pressures. Observe for respiratory difficulty, increased coughing, inability to manage secretions, or difficulty in speaking after cuff deflation or trach tube removal. Prepare client for surgical dilation of trachea for definitive treatment as needed.
Tracheal-innominate artery fistula (erosion of lateral wall of trachea into artery caused by pressure from distal end of tube)	Prevent by keeping tube in midline position and avoiding traction on tube from any cause. Assess for pulsation of trach tube with each client heartbeat and notify physician immediately if it occurs. Note fresh bleeding at or through stoma and report immediately. Physician may remove trach tube immediately and apply direct pressure to blood vessel at stoma site. Prepare client for immediate life-saving surgical repair.

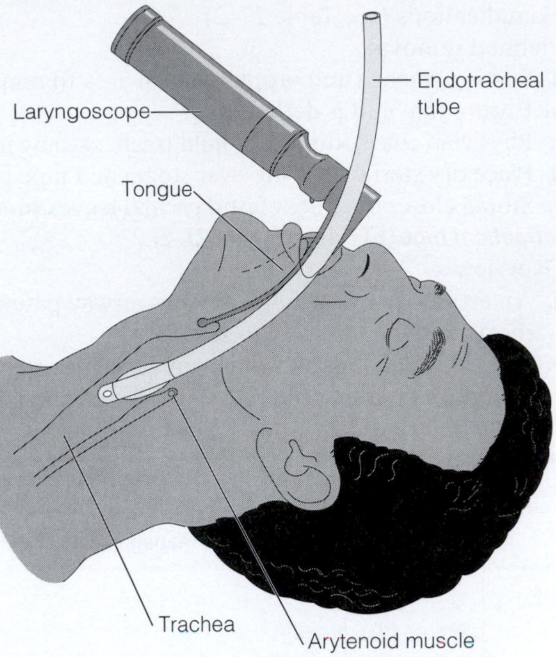

Figure 27–2

Endotracheal tube insertion assisted by laryngoscope.

2. Routes of insertion
   a. Orotracheal insertion route allows for use of larger tube, rapidly restores airway, and reduces respiratory effort; disadvantages are discomfort to client, possible displacement by tongue movement, and occlusion from biting on tube; oral airway may need to be used
   b. Nasotracheal route allows for use of smaller tube, prevents dislodgement by tongue, but increases respiratory effort; contraindicated with bleeding disorders, epistaxis, or nasal obstruction
3. Therapeutic management
   NCLEX® a. To check placement after insertion, ventilate with manual resuscitation bag, assess that both left and right sides of chest rise and fall, and auscultate for bilateral breath sounds; if only right-sided chest movement and breath sounds are present, tube needs to be pulled back slightly from placement in right mainstem bronchus until bilateral chest movements are seen
   b. Auscultate over epigastric area to ensure esophageal intubation did not occur; if it did, ventilation sounds will be louder over stomach than chest, and abdomen will rise and fall with ventilations; tube is removed immediately if this occurs
   c. A carbon dioxide (CO_2) analyzer is frequently used to check proper placement in trachea using advanced cardiac life support (ACLS) protocols
   NCLEX® d. Confirm placement by portable chest x-ray; distal tip of tube should be 1 to 2 cm above carina (point of bifurcation of right and left mainstem bronchi)
   e. Note position of tube by noting centimeter marking at lip line and then tape tube in place or use other securing device; monitor placement at least every 8 hours
   f. Ensure manual resuscitation bag is kept at bedside at all times
   NCLEX® g. Perform respiratory assessments every 4 hours and as needed; suction client as indicated by results of assessment as with tracheostomy
   h. Check cuff pressure every 8 hours or per agency policy; ensure it does not exceed 20 mm Hg by anaeroid manometer using either minimal occluding volume or minimal leak technique
   i. Inflate cuff using minimal occluding volume technique by injecting air into pilot balloon just until no air leakage sounds can be heard during inspiration with stethoscope placed over trachea
   j. Inflate cuff using minimal leak technique by injecting air into pilot balloon until sealed and then deflating slightly so that no harsh sounds can be heard during inspiration but slight leak is heard at peak of inspiration
   k. Insert oral airway if orotracheal route is used to prevent client from biting tube or displacing tube with tongue movement
   l. Reposition orotracheal tube from one side of mouth to other daily with assistance of one other person; assess oral cavity for ulceration or necrosis
   m. Provide oral care every 2 hours to prevent drying and cracking of lips and mucous membranes
   NCLEX® n. Provide for alternative means of communication (word or picture board, writing pad)

4. Removal (extubation)
   a. Hyperoxygenate; suction endotracheal tube well; then suction oropharyngeal area
   b. Elevate head of bed to semi-Fowler's or high-Fowler's position as tolerated
   c. Cuff is deflated and client is asked to inhale; at peak inspiration, tube is removed
   d. Encourage client to cough and deep breathe to clear any residual secretions in pharyngeal area
   e. Apply oxygen as ordered
   f. Monitor client closely for first 30 minutes after extubation and continue to monitor frequently thereafter; notify physician if respiratory rate or effort show steady increase, oxygen saturation decreases, or respiratory distress occurs
   g. Explain that sore throat and hoarse voice are common and to limit talking; monitor status and report hoarseness that does not improve over time, which may indicate damage to vocal cords

II. CLOSED CHEST DRAINAGE SYSTEMS

A. Overview

1. A **chest tube** is used to drain air (pneumothorax), blood (hemothorax), or large amounts of fluid (pleural effusion) from pleural cavity
2. Restores negative pressure to intrapleural space

B. Design

1. Most systems in use today have 3 chambers: collection, water seal, and suction (Figure 27–3)

NCLEX® 2. Collection chamber is on right under point of connection between tube and system and consists of marked columns (generally three) that indicate amount of drainage collected

NCLEX® 3. Water seal chamber (middle chamber) is filled to 2-cm marking during system setup; water allows air to escape system but not to reenter; water moves up and down in a tube in this chamber with inhalation and exhalation (called tidaling) to indicate patency

NCLEX® 4. Suction control chamber allows use of suction to provide negative pressure to chest, which aids in reinflating lung more quickly by removing air, blood, pus, or effusion; some systems use "dry" suction, controlled by adjusting suction knob to appropriate level; both types are connected to low wall suction using a connecting tube

C. Therapeutic management

1. Maintain occlusive dressing at chest tube insertion site; dressing is secured with large strips of wide tape or Elastoplast and may be reinforced as needed but not changed

NCLEX® 2. Secure all chest tube and suction tubing connections with tape

NCLEX® 3. Keep collection apparatus 12 inches below chest level to allow gravity to promote chest drainage; keep tubing straight to prevent dependent loops or obstructions

NCLEX® 4. Milk chest tube to maintain tube patency *only if ordered*; milking chest tube can cause tissue damage; this is done by alternately folding or squeezing and then releasing drainage tubing; chest tube stripping by nurses is generally contraindicated in hospital policy because it causes pressure changes within tubing and pleural space

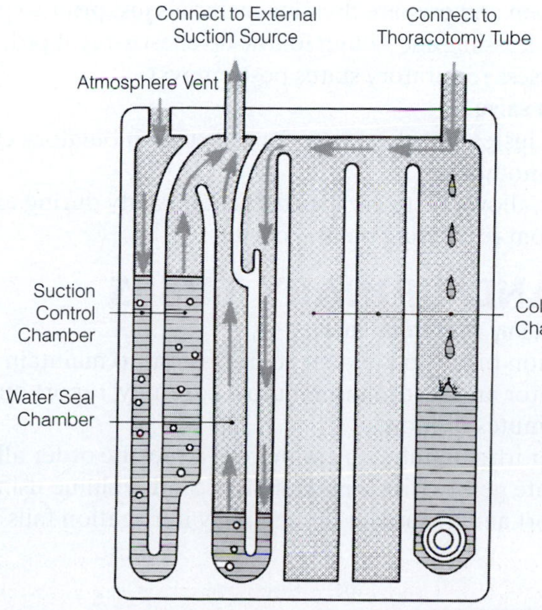

Figure 27–3
Disposable closed chest drainage system with three chambers: collection, water seal, and suction.

NCLEX®
5. Do not clamp chest tube when client is mobile and never clamp tube without a physician order; keep a clamp at bedside for use by surgeon if needed and according to agency policy

NCLEX®
6. Monitor chest tube drainage at 1- to 4-hour intervals; report and document bright red blood, sudden increase in drainage, or consistent drainage greater than 100 mL/hour (physician may also specify volume to report)
7. Maintain 2-cm water level in water seal chamber; low water volume creates higher suction than may be desired, contributing to pleural tissue damage

NCLEX®
8. Observe for fluctuation in water seal chamber, which indicates tube is patent; lack of fluctuation may indicate tube obstruction, loop, or kink (requires correction) or may indicate full lung reexpansion (indicating tube is ready for removal); check client condition and timeframe to aid in interpretation

NCLEX®
9. Observe for bubbling in water seal chamber
   a. Continuous bubbling indicates an air leak in system and needs to be corrected; if leak is not found, notify surgeon
   b. Intermittent bubbling with inspiration indicates drainage of air (pneumothorax) from pleural space and proper function of chest tube; continue to monitor
10. Monitor suction control chamber for correct amount of suction by either dial (dry system) or water level (fluid system); add sterile water if level is low (excessive wall suction speeds evaporation); remove excessive water by aspirating from rubber seal in chamber
11. Suction control chamber in system that uses water should have gentle, continuous bubbling as sign of proper function; vigorous bubbling will evaporate water but not increase suction, and lack of continuous bubbling will not harm client but will not provide suction to help clear pneumothorax or hemothorax
12. Monitor respiratory status, breath sounds, oxygen saturation, and comfort level every 4 hours or as indicated; assess that dressing is intact and check for and report subcutaneous emphysema
13. Change client position every 2 hours and encourage coughing and deep breathing
14. Anticipate that client may have frequent (up to daily) portable chest x-rays to monitor lung reexpansion

NCLEX®
15. Keep occlusive dressing materials (petrolatum gauze, dry sterile gauze, wide adhesive tape) and sterile water at bedside for emergency use

NCLEX®
16. If drainage system becomes damaged or broken, insert chest tube into sterile water to reestablish underwater seal and replace with new system

NCLEX®
17. If chest tube is accidentally pulled out of chest, pinch skin together, apply occlusive dressing using materials noted above, and notify surgeon immediately
18. Chest tube removal
   a. Indicated when fluctuation stops in water seal chamber, chest x-ray shows full lung expansion, and client has returned to normal or baseline respiratory status

   NCLEX®
   b. Obtain suture removal set, petrolatum gauze, dry sterile gauze or Telfa gauze, and wide adhesive tape; premedicate client with oral medication 30 minutes prior to removal if possible
   c. Instruct client to take deep breath, hold breath (Valsalva) or exhale according to surgeon preference just prior to tube removal
   d. Open and prepare dressing materials just prior to physician's removal of tube; assist with application of dressing, and obtain follow-up chest x-ray if ordered
   e. Assess respiratory status postremoval

D. Heimlich valve

1. Used instead of chest tube for selected ambulatory clients who have pneumothorax or to treat tension pneumothorax
2. Valve allows air to escape from chest cavity during exhalation but closes during inhalation to prevent air from reentering pleural cavity

III. RENAL AND URINARY TUBES

A. Nephrostomy or ureteral tube

1. Position tube (no kinks or compression) to maintain patency; do not clamp
2. Monitor and record urine output carefully; report output of less than 30 mL/hr or no drainage for 15 minutes or more
3. Never irrigate tube unless there is a specific order allowing it

NCLEX®
4. Irrigate gently with a maximum of 5 mL volume using strict surgical aseptic technique
5. Report and document immediately if irrigation fails to restore tube patency

B. Urinary catheters

1. Types include straight catheter (for intermittent catheterization), indwelling urinary catheter (inflated balloon keeps catheter in bladder), and triple lumen or 3-way catheter (allows for balloon inflation, urinary drainage, and inflow of bladder irrigation)
2. Insert using sterile technique; measure and record initial outflow amount and characteristics of urine
3. Properly position drainage bag below level of bladder (if indwelling) and secure catheter to thigh to prevent traction of balloon against urethra and bladder neck
4. Measure and record outputs accurately
5. Provide catheter care with soap and warm water using standard precautions
6. Wash front to back for females; in males retract foreskin if present, and return to original position after cleansing
7. Explain procedure to client just prior to removal; empty and record drainage, deflate balloon, and withdraw catheter while client exhales to reduce discomfort

IV. NASOGASTRIC TUBES

A. Overview

1. Inserted via naris to stomach to decompress stomach, reduce risk of aspiration, administer enteral feedings or medications, or irrigate stomach
2. Commonly used is Salem sump, a double-lumen tube with air vent that allows for continuous (rather than intermittent) suction for gastric decompression; keep air vent above level of stomach and do not clamp; 30 mL air can be instilled through vent as needed to promote drainage through drainage lumen
3. Much less commonly used tube is Levin tube, a single-lumen tube that requires use of intermittent suction (lack of air vent causes tube to collapse if continuous suction is used)

B. Insertion procedure

1. Sit client upright (high-Fowler's position)
2. *NCLEX®* Place distal end of tube at tip of nose and measure to earlobe and then to xiphoid process to determine distance for tube insertion; apply tape to tube to indicate point at which to stop insertion
3. Lubricate distal 2–3 inches of tube with lidocaine gel or water-soluble gel according to policy (not oil-based lubricant, which could cause pneumonia if tube enters trachea)
4. Ask client to tilt head downward (to close epiglottis so tube will enter esophagus)
5. Insert tube into naris and advance upward and backward until meeting resistance at back of nose; rotate catheter gently and advance into nasopharynx
6. *NCLEX®* Ask client to take sips of water if able while tube advanced gently into stomach
7. Stop tube insertion and pull back on tube if client coughs or chokes during procedure; when client's respiratory status returns to normal, continue insertion
8. Stop advancing tube once tape reaches naris; check placement as outlined below
9. Tape tube in place
10. Place tube to low continuous (Salem sump) or intermittent (Levin) suction for gastric decompression
11. Do not begin enteral feedings by nasogastric tube (see Chapter 25) until placement confirmed by x-ray

C. Therapeutic management

1. Assess placement
   a. *NCLEX®* Chest x-ray is most reliable method of assessing tube placement
   b. *NCLEX®* Aspirate gastric contents using piston syringe and apply to strip of pH test paper (pH of 4 or less is consistent with gastric placement and pH of 6 or greater indicates intestinal placement); note that enteral feedings could alter pH and make this method less reliable
   c. Insert 5 to 10 mL air into tube while listening over epigastric area with stethoscope for "whooshing" or popping sound as air enters stomach; this method is less reliable than x-ray or gastric pH measurement
   d. *NCLEX®* Check placement every 4 hours after insertion
2. Measure residual prior to and regularly during enteral feedings (see Chapter 25)
3. Irrigate tube with 30 to 50 mL water or saline as ordered to check tube patency; instill fluid using piston syringe and aspirate contents back; repeat if tube is difficult to irrigate or sluggish; document fluid instilled and aspirated back on intake and output record
4. Inspect naris for ulceration from pressure when changing tape daily; provide nose care by removing any crusted areas with moist swabs
5. Provide mouth care every 2 hours; presence of tube in nose leads to mouth breathing and dryness

6. Tube removal
   a. Check order and apply gloves
   b. Remove tape securing tube to nose
   c. Ask client to hold breath
   d. Withdraw tube smoothly over 3–6 seconds; coil tube around hand for control
   e. Provide comfort care and document procedure

V. NASOENTERIC (INTESTINAL) TUBES

A. Overview

1. Andersen tube is inserted nasally into stomach and passed into intestine via peristalsis assisted by tungsten weight at lower end of tube; older intestinal tubes (Miller-Abbott and Cantor) had mercury weights; a general name for these tubes is **nasoenteric (intestinal) tubes**
2. Tube moves from stomach into intestines and is secured to nose once final placement is reached and verified by serial abdominal x-rays
3. Suction applied to tube allows for bowel decompression and removal of accumulated intestinal secretions

B. Therapeutic management

1. Check physician order and institutional policy regarding tube advancement and removal
2. NCLEX® After tube insertion into stomach, maintain client position on right side initially to facilitate tube passage through pyloric sphincter of stomach into small intestine; then reposition client side to side every 2 hours to faciliate migration of tube to area of obstruction
3. NCLEX® Wait until tube has reached final placement, as verified by x-ray (may take several hours), before securing to nose with tape
4. NCLEX® Perform routine abdominal assessments and measure abdominal girth
5. Monitor and record amount and characteristics of tube drainage; if tube becomes blocked, notify physician; a small amount of air may be prescribed to help clear lumen
6. Remove tube according to institutional policy and procedure
   a. Aspirate tungsten and air using 5 mL syringe
   b. Withdraw tube approximately 6 inches each hour or as prescribed
   c. Dispose of tungsten as per agency policy

VI. COMBINED ESOPHAGEAL AND GASTRIC TUBES

A. Overview

1. Exert pressure against or provide tamponade to bleeding esophageal varices
2. Contraindicated with history of esophageal surgery or ulceration or necrosis of esophageal area
3. Airway management is an ongoing priority concern
4. NCLEX® **Sengstaken-Blakemore tube** has three lumens; one gastric lumen provides low intermittent gastric suction while round gastric balloon (in area of lower esophageal sphincter) and tubular esophageal balloon apply pressure against bleeding blood vessels
   a. Gastric balloon is inflated first, and then esophageal balloon is inflated (25 to 45 mm Hg pressure) if gastric balloon is insufficient to stop bleeding
   b. Traction on tube is needed to maintain position of inflated balloons
   c. Check placement of tube by x-ray of chest and upper abdomen
   d. Prepare to insert NG tube in opposite naris to suction secretions that accumulate above esophageal balloon in esophagopharyngeal area to prevent aspiration
5. Minnesota tube is similar to Sengstaken-Blakemore tube but has additional (fourth) lumen to drain secretions from esophagopharyngeal area, eliminating need for separate NG tube placement in this area

B. Therapeutic management

1. Position client upright for insertion
2. Check all balloons prior to insertion and label each lumen
3. Double clamp lumens to avoid air leaks
4. NCLEX® Keep head of bed raised after insertion
5. Obtain chest and upper abdominal x-ray to verify placement
6. Release esophageal balloon pressure intermittently per agency policy to prevent esophageal injury from ulceration or necrosis
7. NCLEX® Keep scissors at bedside to cut tube to rapidly deflate balloons if respiratory distress occurs
8. Monitor for complications

a. Continued bleeding: steady or increased bloody drainage from gastric suction port; notify health care provider

NCLEX® b. Esophageal rupture: upper abdominal and back pain, hypotension, tachycardia; report immediately: this is medical emergency

VII. TUBES FOR GASTRIC LAVAGE

A. Overview

NCLEX® 1. Used to remove toxins from stomach due to drug or chemical poisoning or overdose
2. An **Ewald tube** is a large, reusable tube with a single lumen used for one-time rapid irrigation followed by aspiration of stomach contents
3. A Lavacuator tube has a lavage/vent lumen for irrigation and another lumen to provide continuous suction so that irrigation and suction can occur simultaneously

B. Therapeutic management

1. Determine that the poison is appropriate for removal by lavage prior to procedure
2. Substances that have probably already been absorbed or substances that must be dialyzed out would contraindicate the need for irrigation

NCLEX® 3. Airway management is a priority because of risk of aspiration, especially with possible decreased level of consciousness depending on poison or substance overdosed

VIII. WOUND AND MISCELLANEOUS DRAINS

A. Closed wound drainage system

1. Consists of wound drain connected to electric suction apparatus or portable drainage suction (such as Jackson-Pratt drain or Hemovac drain)
2. Tube is sutured into place in surgery and attached to drainage reservoir

NCLEX® 3. Measure and record drainage every shift; notify physician if drainage stops or increases suddenly or is brighter red in color; drainage should decrease over time

NCLEX® 4. Wear gloves when emptying reservoir; avoid touching drainage port to prevent infection while uncapping port and draining fluid into collection device

NCLEX® 5. Reestablish suction after emptying by compressing device with one hand while cleansing drainage port with alcohol swab and then closing cap or plug before releasing pressure; check device every 4 hours to be sure system is still compressed (which provides suction)

6. Often removed between 3 and 5 days postop, so prepare to teach some clients how to empty and maintain system at home

B. Penrose wound drain

1. A surgical drain less commonly used but may be optimal when excessive serosanguineous or purulent drainage is expected from wound
2. Usually inserted via a stab wound a few inches away from original incision to keep incision dry; drain is often 0.5 to 1.5 inches in diameter and up to 10 to 14 inches long
3. Advantage is preventing formation of abscesses because of excessive drainage
4. Drain may be drawn out or shortened by 1 to 2 inches each day as drainage lessens
5. Thick dressings, need for frequent dressing changes, and careful assessment of underlying skin are all priorities based on nature of drainage
6. Use of sterile technique is essential to prevent infection

C. T-tube

1. A T-shaped device inserted into common bile duct to maintain duct patency and allow drainage following cholecystectomy with bile duct exploration until surgical edema decreases
2. Keep T-tube below level of surgical wound and attached to sterile drainage device
3. Monitor drainage for color and consistency; up to 500 mL is expected in first 24 hours postop, decreasing to less than 200 mL in 2 or 3 days, and minimal after that; color is blood tinged at first and changes to brown-green
4. Assess for bile leakage during dressing changes and ensure tubing is properly secured after dressing change to prevent traction or pulling on tube
5. Blockage of tube is noted by absence of drainage from tube, jaundice, and pale-colored stools
6. Follow clamping schedule before and after meals when ordered
7. If client will be discharged with T-tube (may be left in for 7–10 days), teach client care of T-tube, how to clamp, and signs of infection to report

PRACTICE TEST

Check Your NCLEX–PN® Exam I.Q.

You are ready for testing on this content if you can

- Use critical-thinking skills and scientific principles when caring for a client with a therapeutic tube or drain.
- Determine for patency and function of a therapeutic tube or drain.
- Monitor the progress of a client who has a therapeutic tube or drain.
- Reinforce to client and family pertinent information about a therapeutic tube or drain.
- Reinforce to client or family self-care of a therapeutic tube or drain as appropriate.

PRACTICE TEST

1 A client has returned to the nursing unit following a tracheostomy. The nurse would place highest priority on monitoring which of the following?

1. Respiratory rate and breath sounds
2. Amount of oxygen ordered to be delivered
3. Time when client last received pain medication
4. Status of tracheostomy dressing

2 The nurse is providing care to a client who is 2 weeks postoperative for a tracheostomy. The nurse sees the tracheostomy tube come out when the client coughs. What should be the nurse's first action?

1. Call aloud for help.
2. Suction the stoma to remove residual secretions.
3. Grasp and spread the retention sutures to open the stoma.
4. Attempt to reinsert a new tracheostomy tube.

3 The client has just had emergency intubation for respiratory distress. Immediately following insertion of the endotracheal tube, what action by the nurse is most appropriate?

1. Tape the tube securely in place.
2. Assess for bilateral breath sounds.
3. Call for a chest x-ray to determine placement.
4. Assure the client that alternative communication means will be provided.

4 Which of the following respiratory findings is of greatest concern to the nurse following endotracheal tube extubation?

1. Increased respiratory rate from 16 to 20 bpm
2. Scattered bilateral rhonchi
3. Expectoration of whitish yellow secretions
4. A harsh or crowing sound with inspiration

5 A client with a closed chest drainage system tries to get out of bed alone and disconnects the chest tube from the drainage system, which falls on the floor. Which action should the nurse take first upon entering the client's room?

1. Submerge the tube in sterile water or saline.
2. Set up and attach a new closed chest drainage system.
3. Check the client's respiratory status.
4. Check the client's pulse and blood pressure.

6 During routine data collection on a client's chest tube, the nurse notes the presence of continuous bubbling in the water seal chamber of the closed chest drainage system. The nurse suspects that which of the following has most likely occurred?

1. The client has developed a sudden new pneumothorax.
2. There is an air leak in the system.
3. The wall suction unit has been set to intermediate or high level instead of low suction.
4. The drainage tube connections are taped too tightly.

7 The client is scheduled for removal of a chest tube at 0900. At approximately 0830, what action should the nurse take?

1. Call the radiology department for a telephone report of the morning chest x-ray findings.
2. Premedicate the client with an analgesic, if ordered.
3. Ensure that a suture-removal set and dressing materials are available.
4. Explain to the client the upcoming removal procedure.

8 The nurse has received an order to irrigate a nephrostomy tube after the tube stopped draining. The nurse plans to use no more than how many milliliters to carry out this procedure safely?

1. 2 mL
2. 5 mL
3. 10 mL
4. 20 mL

9 The nurse should perform which action when caring for a client with a nephrostomy tube?

1. Maintain patency with hourly irrigations.
2. Keep a clamp at the bedside.
3. Ensure the tubing is free of kinks.
4. Tape the drainage bag to the bedrail.

10 A nurse is assigned to a client with a nasogastric tube and is checking gastric pH to verify correct tube placement. Which pH reading should the nurse expect if the tube is properly positioned?

1. 4
2. 6
3. 7
4. 8

11 A client with a partial bowel obstruction will have a nasoenteric tube placed by the physician later in the day. The nurse should explain that which client position will be utilized, after the tube is placed, to promote tube migration to the intended area?

1. Flat and on the left side
2. Flat and on the right side
3. Head of bed elevated and on the left side
4. Head of bed elevated and on the right side

12 A client underwent insertion of a nasoenteric tube for partial bowel obstruction the previous evening. The nurse notes that the tube is not taped at the nose. Which of the following actions is most appropriate at this time?

1. Call the physician immediately.
2. Tape the tube in place.
3. Note the finding on the client's flowsheet.
4. Call the radiology department to see if an abdominal x-ray has been done.

13 The nurse is about to receive an inter-shift report on a client who has a Sengstaken-Blakemore tube in place. The nurse expects that the client has which problem documented as the primary reason for tube placement?

1. Cirrhosis of the liver
2. Esophageal varices
3. Portal hypertension
4. Abdominal ascites

14 The nurse has just assisted with insertion of a Sengstaken-Blakemore tube. Before leaving the client's room, the nurse ensures that which piece of equipment is at the bedside in case of tube dislodgement?

1. Suction machine
2. Oxygen mask
3. Scissors
4. Laryngoscope

15 The nurse working in the emergency department learns that a client will be arriving who took an overdose of acetaminophen (Tylenol) a short while ago. The nurse should anticipate that which tube will be used to evacuate the client's stomach upon arrival?

1. Minnesota
2. Sengstaken-Blakemore
3. Ewald
4. Miller-Abbott

16 A client who took an overdose of a prescribed medication was treated with gastric lavage. The nurse monitors which of the following as a priority to detect possible complications of treatment?

1. Respiratory status and breath sounds
2. Heart rate and blood pressure
3. Skin color and body temperature
4. Urine output and peripheral edema

17 The nurse has emptied a Jackson-Pratt wound drainage device and needs to reestablish suction to the tube. Which action should the nurse take to accomplish this objective?

1. Ensure the tubing has no kinks.
2. Squeeze the collection chamber.
3. Wipe the port with alcohol.
4. Close the cap on the device.

18 A client, who underwent pelvic surgery the previous day, has a Penrose drain placed in the lower abdomen. The nurse should take which action in the care of this wound drain? Select all that apply.

1. Ensure that the drain stays in the original position placed by the surgeon.
2. Place only a few gauze dressings around the tube to allow for easier assessment.
3. Assess the abdominal skin for irritation or breakdown with dressing changes.
4. Notify the physician for moderate amount of drainage.
5. Use aseptic technique with dressing changes.

19 The nurse monitors the functioning of a client's Salem sump nasogastric suction following abdominal surgery. Which option indicates that a problem exists with the suctioning?

1. A pH of 3.0 on the aspirated gastric contents when tested
2. Suction regulator set at 100 mm Hg intermittent suction
3. Suction tubing connected to the air vent tube
4. Gastric secretions that are yellow/green in color

20 When assisting in orienting a newly hired nurse, which action by the new nurse indicates a need for additional skill development when performing nasotracheal suctioning?

1. Waits 2–3 minutes before suctioning again
2. Hyperventilates the lungs prior to suctioning
3. Hyperoxygenates before and after suctioning
4. Rotates the suction catheter only during catheter withdrawal when suctioning

21 When a drainage tube is located at the site of a radical neck dissection, and edema is noted, what should the nurse do? Select all that apply.

1. Monitor the airway, gag reflex, and the ability to talk.
2. Check for negative pressure, to make sure suction is present in the drainage tube.
3. Wait 2 hours to see if the edema increases in size or location.
4. Release the suture before it ruptures the incision.
5. Check quickly for edema of the feet and sacrum.

ANSWERS & RATIONALES

1 **Answer: 1 Rationale:** The status of the client's airway and breathing is of highest concern. Once the nurse has observed the airway and breathing, then the amount of oxygen and dressing status can be checked. The time lapse since any analgesic medication can be determined last after all data pertaining directly to airway have been obtained. **Cognitive Level:** Analyzing **Client Need:** Basic Care and Comfort **Integrated Process:** Nursing Process: Planning **Content Area:** Adult Health **Strategy:** Remember the ABCs: *airway*, *breathing*, and *circulation.* In questions asking for a priority action, all options may be correct, and you need to select the option that is most important or timely. Remembering this sequence may help with questions that relate to respiratory or circulatory disorders or procedures.

2 **Answer: 3 Rationale:** The priority action of the nurse restores a patent airway. With this in mind, the nurse spreads the retention sutures to reopen the stomal area. After reestablishing a patent airway, the nurse quickly calls aloud for help as the second action so assistance will arrive to aid in tube reinsertion. The nurse is not likely to suction the area at this time, which would remove air and oxygen from the airway at a critical time. The nurse would reinsert a new tracheostomy tube only if allowed by agency policy, since the tube has been in place for more than 72 hours. **Cognitive Level:** Analyzing **Client Need:** Basic Care and Comfort **Integrated Process:** Nursing Process: Implementation **Content Area:** Adult Health **Strategy:** Remember the ABCs: *airway*, *breathing*, and *circulation*. The correct answer is one that directly affects the client's airway, which is opening the stoma. The other options are incorrect because they either are not the first action or may not be done at all.

3 **Answer: 2 Rationale:** The first action by the nurse is to auscultates for bilateral breath sounds as an initial indication of correct tube placement. After the nurse auscultates for bilateral breath sounds as an initial indication of correct tube placement, the tube should be securely taped in place to prevent dislodgement. The nurse would call for chest x-ray to confirm tube placement after determining placement and securing the tube. Once the client's airway and breathing have been attended to, then the nurse can assure the client about alternative communication means. **Cognitive Level:** Analyzing **Client Need:** Basic Care and Comfort **Integrated Process:** Nursing Process: Implementation **Content Area:** Adult Health **Strategy:** Remember the ABCs: *airway*, *breathing*, and *circulation*. The correct answer is one that directly affects the client's airway, which is assessing for bilateral breath sounds. Because the question asks for the priority action of the nurse, the other actions must be systematically eliminated.

4 **Answer: 4 Rationale:** A harsh or crowing sound with inspiration indicates stridor, which is consistent with airway narrowing and edema following endotracheal tube removal. This is of greatest concern because it could lead to upper respiratory obstruction. The nurse needs to notify the physician. An increase in respiratory rate from 16 to 20 bears watching for trends but is still with normal limits. Clients may be expected to have some rhonchi immediately after tube removal. Clients may be expected to have secretions immediately after tube removal. **Cognitive Level:** Analyzing **Client Need:** Basic Care and Comfort **Integrated Process:** Nursing Process: Data Collection **Content Area:** Adult Health **Strategy:** Note the critical words *of greatest concern*. This indicates the correct option is the finding that is most abnormal. Use the process of elimination and knowledge of normal and abnormal physical assessment data to make a selection.

5 **Answer: 1** **Rationale:** The priority action of the nurse is to submerge the tube in sterile water or saline to reestablish the underwater seal. This will prevent the client from sucking air through the chest tube into the pleural space during inspiration, thereby causing pneumothorax. The nurse would set up a new system third after submerging the tube and checking respiratory status. After reestablishing an underwater seal, the nurse would check the client's respiratory status second. The nurse would check the client's full vital signs last in preparation for reporting the incident to the physician. **Cognitive Level:** Analyzing **Client Need:** Basic Care and Comfort **Integrated Process:** Nursing Process: Implementation **Content Area:** Adult Health **Strategy:** Note the critical word *first* in the question. This tells you that more than one option may be technically correct but one is better than the others based on the client's status or the needs of the situation. Recall that an underwater seal is critical to chest tube functioning to select the correct option.

6 **Answer: 2** **Rationale:** Continuous bubbling in the water seal chamber most often indicates a leak or loose connection in the system, and air is being sucked continuously into the closed chest drainage system. If the client experienced a new large pneumothorax, there could be rapid bubbling, but this is not the most likely explanation. The client would also likely exhibit new onset respiratory symptoms, which are not evident. Turning up the suction on the wall unit would increase the bubbling in the suction control chamber, not the water seal chamber. Taping the connections too tightly is not a concern. **Cognitive Level:** Analyzing **Client Need:** Basic Care and Comfort **Integrated Process:** Nursing Process: Evaluation **Content Area:** Adult Health **Strategy:** The core issue of the question is the significance of finding continuous bubbling in the water seal chamber. Use the process of elimination and knowledge of closed chest drainage systems to make a selection.

7 **Answer: 2** **Rationale:** The client should be premedicated approximately 30 minutes before chest tube removal if the client has an analgesic order. It is the physician's responsibility to determine the results of the daily chest x-ray. Obtaining equipment for removal can be done earlier or later than the timeframe indicated. Explaining the procedure to the client can be done earlier or later than the timeframe indicated. **Cognitive Level:** Analyzing **Client Need:** Basic Care and Comfort **Integrated Process:** Nursing Process: Planning **Content Area:** Adult Health **Strategy:** The core issue of the question is what action is timely *30 minutes* before chest tube removal. Analyze each option to determine whether each needs to occur at that time. Recall that analgesics are usually given about 30 minutes prior to a painful procedure to select the correct option.

8 **Answer: 2** **Rationale:** The maximum amount of fluid that should be used to irrigate a nephrostomy tube is 5 mL. The nurse should also use strict aseptic technique to prevent infection of the renal pelvis as a result of the procedure. **Cognitive Level:** Applying **Client Need:** Basic Care and Comfort **Integrated Process:** Nursing Process: Planning **Content Area:** Adult Health **Strategy:** The core issue of the question is knowledge of appropriate volumes of fluid that should be used to irrigate tubes such as a nephrostomy tube. Eliminate the smallest and largest numbers as being least plausible. Choose 5 mL over 10 mL after visualizing the amount in the syringe and estimating the size of the renal pelvis. Memorize this number if the question was difficult.

9 **Answer: 3** **Rationale:** The nurse should ensure that the tubing is free of kinks or other obstructions to urine flow. The tube is irrigated according to physician order only. The tube should never be clamped. Taping the drainage bag to the bedrail is dangerous because it could cause traction when the client moves in bed and could become dislodged. **Cognitive Level:** Applying **Client Need:** Basic Care and Comfort **Integrated Process:** Nursing Process: Implementation **Content Area:** Adult Health **Strategy:** Use general principles of tube management to answer the question. Eliminate taping the tube to the bed rail first as being hazardous. Eliminate hourly irrigation next as being excessive. Choose correctly from the remaining two options knowing that the tubing should be kept free of kinks and that these tubes should not be clamped.

10 **Answer: 1** **Rationale:** Gastric pH is acidic and readings should be 4 or less if the tube is placed properly in the stomach. Other readings indicate placement in the intestine or higher up in the esophagus, since normal body pH is 7.35 to 7.45. **Cognitive Level:** Analyzing **Client Need:** Basic Care and Comfort **Integrated Process:** Nursing Process: Evaluation **Content Area:** Adult Health **Strategy:** The core issue of the question is knowledge of pH readings that are consistent with placement of a nasogastric tube in the stomach. Use specific nursing knowledge and the process of elimination to make a selection.

11 **Answer: 4** **Rationale:** In order for the tube to migrate to the area of intestinal blockage, the tube must pass through the pyloric sphincter of the stomach. Recall that this tube has a weighted tip and thus gravity will affect its movement, as will peristalsis. Positioning the client with head elevated and on the right side will utilize gravity to help the tube migrate into the intestines. The other responses will lead to less effective tube movement. **Cognitive Level:** Analyzing **Client Need:** Basic Care and Comfort **Integrated Process:** Teaching and Learning **Content Area:** Adult Health **Strategy:** The core issue of the question is knowledge of proper client position following nasoenteric tube placement. Visualize tube movement using laws of gravity to aid in making a selection. Gravity should be a prime consideration as a possible influence whenever answering questions related to tube placement.

12 **Answer: 3** **Rationale:** The nurse should note the assessment finding on the medical record. The nurse does not need to call the physician. Nasoenteric tubes are not taped in place until they have migrated to proper position and been confirmed by x-ray. It is unnecessary to immediately determine when x-rays have been scheduled. **Cognitive Level:** Analyzing **Client Need:** Basic Care and Comfort **Integrated Process:** Nursing Process: Implementation **Content Area:** Adult Health **Strategy:** The core issue of the question is knowledge that nasoenteric tubes are not taped until they have reached final position. Use specific nursing knowledge and the process of elimination to answer this question.

13 **Answer: 2 Rationale:** A Sengstaken-Blakemore tube is inserted to control upper GI bleeding from esophageal varices, which is the primary problem of concern with use of this tube. Cirrhosis of the liver is the original problem that led to a series of complications, which ultimately resulted in tube placement. Portal hypertension is a complication of cirrhosis of the liver that can lead to esophageal varices. Abdominal ascites may accompany cirrhosis but is not a reason for placing this tube. **Cognitive Level:** Analyzing **Client Need:** Basic Care and Comfort **Integrated Process:** Nursing Process: Evaluation **Content Area:** Adult Health **Strategy:** The core issue of the question is knowledge of the rationale for placement of a Sengstaken-Blakemore tube. Use knowledge of pathophysiology and the process of elimination to make a selection.

14 **Answer: 3 Rationale:** Scissors need to be kept at the bedside of a client who has a Sengstaken-Blakemore tube. If the tube becomes dislodged and the client cannot breathe, the nurse cuts the tube to allow the balloons to deflate rapidly and restore a patent airway. A suction machine is generally helpful as an airway adjunct, but it is not the priority bedside equipment needed in this situation. An oxygen mask is a generally helpful airway adjunct, but does not apply to this situation. A laryngoscope is used to insert an endotracheal tube. **Cognitive Level:** Analyzing **Client Need:** Basic Care and Comfort **Integrated Process:** Nursing Process: Planning **Content Area:** Adult Health **Strategy:** The core issue of the question is knowledge that tube dislodgement can block the airway and that scissors are needed for rapid balloon deflation if this occurs. Use nursing knowledge and the process of elimination to make a selection.

15 **Answer: 3 Rationale:** An Ewald tube is a large-bore tube used to evacuate stomach contents rapidly following poisoning or overdose. A Minnesota tube is used for clients with bleeding esophageal varices. A Sengstaken-Blakemore tube is used for clients with bleeding esophageal varices. A Miller-Abbot tube is a nasoenteric tube used to decompress the bowel with small bowel obstruction. **Cognitive Level:** Applying **Client Need:** Basic Care and Comfort **Integrated Process:** Nursing Process: Planning **Content Area:** Adult Health **Strategy:** The core issue of the question is knowledge of the use of various types of drainage tubes. Use nursing knowledge and the process of elimination to make a selection.

16 **Answer: 1 Rationale:** The risk of aspiration with gastric lavage is of concern to the nurse. For this reason, assessment of respiratory status, including respiratory rate and breath sounds, is of great concern. Other vital signs, such as heart rate and blood pressure, are important as a measure of general condition but are not focused on detection of complications of this procedure. Skin color and temperature are measures of general condition but are not focused on detection of complications of this procedure. Urine output is of general concern, but peripheral edema is not a priority. **Cognitive Level:** Analyzing **Client Need:** Basic Care and Comfort **Integrated Process:** Nursing Process: Data Collection **Content Area:** Adult Health **Strategy:** The core issue of the question is knowledge that gastric lavage can lead to aspiration as a complication. Use nursing knowledge and the process of elimination to make a selection.

17 **Answer: 2 Rationale:** The nurse should squeeze the collecting chamber to reestablish negative pressure and suction to the device. The tubing should always be free of kinks to prevent obstruction. The nurse wipes the port with alcohol before closing the cap to reduce the risk of infection. The cap is closed after negative pressure or suction has been reestablished. **Cognitive Level:** Analyzing **Client Need:** Basic Care and Comfort **Integrated Process:** Nursing Process: Implementation **Content Area:** Adult Health **Strategy:** The core issue of the question is the action by the nurse that will reestablish suction to a Jackson-Pratt wound-drainage device. Use nursing knowledge and the process of elimination to make a selection.

18 **Answer: 3, 5 Rationale:** The nurse should monitor the skin for irritation and breakdown from contact with abdominal skin because the drainage flows from the drain to the gauze, and could macerate the skin if drainage is extensive, if dressing is not changed on time, or if an insufficient number of gauze dressings are used around the drain. Because the drain goes into the abdominal cavity, it is especially important to use aseptic technique during dressing changes. The drain may be advanced over several days for gradual removal. Thick layers of gauze dressings are placed around the drain when moderate to large amounts of drainage are expected, as with extensive abdominal surgeries. The surgeon does not need to be notified of moderate amounts of drainage because it is expected. **Cognitive Level:** Applying **Client Need:** Basic Care and Comfort **Integrated Process:** Nursing Process: Planning **Content Area:** Adult Health **Strategy:** The core issue of the question is knowledge that this type of drain can cause skin irritation by nature of the volume of drainage. Use nursing knowledge and the process of elimination to make a selection.

19 **Answer: 3 Rationale:** The air vent opening should remain open, to allow air to decompress the stomach, and suction is connected to the larger, primary opening of the double-lumen tube. Connecting the suction tubing to the air vent tubing will pull secretions from the stomach through the smaller tubing canal, and probably clog the tubing. Only air should be pushed through the air vent tubing, to maintain the integrity of the system. Normal pH of stomach contents is strongly acidic (0–4). If the tube passed into the intestines, the secretions will yield a pH of 6–8. Accidental placement of the tube in the pulmonary tree would yield a 6–7 pH range. Suction for nasogastric tubing is to be in the low range of 30–40 mm Hg for continuous suction or high, intermittent suction up to 120 mm Hg. Normal gastric secretions are yellow greenish to tan or off-white. Duodenal samples can be deep yellow. Pulmonary secretions are clear to light yellow. **Cognitive Level:** Analyzing **Client Need:** Reduction of Risk Potential **Integrated Process:** Nursing Process: Data Collection **Content Area:** Adult Health **Strategy:** The critical word in the question is *problem*. This indicates the correct option is an incorrect finding. Use the process of elimination and basic knowledge of gastric tubes to choose correctly.

20 **Answer: 2 Rationale:** Hyperventilation is giving too much volume of air into the lungs, and is not recommended, due to the risk of rupture of lung tissue. This action is recommended to minimize the loss of oxygen when suctioning the client. Maintaining maximum oxygenation should always be the focus when suctioning the client who has a compromised respiratory function. This action is recommended to minimize the loss of oxygen when suctioning the client. **Cognitive Level:** Applying **Client Need:** Reduction of Risk Potential **Integrated Process:** Nursing Process: Planning **Content Area:** Adult Health **Strategy:** Recall the steps of the suction procedure and choose the option that represents an incorrect statement, based on the critical words *need for additional skill development* in the question.

21 **Answer: 1, 2 Rationale:** The issue of the question is proper interpretation and action after noting edema after radical neck dissection. Consider that this could threaten the airway to make proper selections. Note that the wording of the question indicates more than one option is likely to be correct. **Cognitive Level:** Applying **Client Need:** Reduction of Risk Potential **Integrated Process:** Nursing Process: Data Collection **Content Area:** Adult Health **Strategy:** Swelling often indicates that the drain is occluded or the suction has been lost. A leak in the tubing or displacement of the tube should also be assessed. Waiting for the edema to change can be life-threatening if it cuts off the airway or ruptures the incision, causing bleeding. Opening up a suture for release of pressure on an incision is a medical management decision, and should not be a decision of the professional nurse. Opening the incision still does not guarantee an open airway. An airway must be maintained at all times for maximum O_2/CO_2 exchange for life to continue.

Key Terms to Review

chest tube p. 405
endotracheal tube p. 403
Ewald tube p. 409
nasoenteric (intestinal) tube p. 408
Sengstaken-Blakemore tube p. 408
tracheostomy p. 401

References

Berman, A., & Snyder, S. (2012). *Kozier & Erb's fundamentals of nursing: Concepts, process, and practice* (9th ed.). Upper Saddle River, NJ: Pearson Education, Inc.

LeMone, P., Burke, K., & Bauldoff, G. (2012). *Medical-surgical nursing: Critical thinking in patient care* (5th ed.). Upper Saddle River, NJ: Pearson Education, Inc.

Lewis, S., Dirksen, S., Heitkemper, M., & Bucher, L. (2011). *Medical-surgical nursing: Assessment and management of clinical problems* (8th ed.). St. Louis, MO: Elsevier Science.

Smeltzer, S., Bare, B., Hinkle, J., & Cheever, K. (2010). *Textbook of medical-surgical nursing* (12th ed.). Philadelphia: Lippincott Williams & Wilkins.

Smith, S., Duell, D., & Martin, B. (2012). *Clinical nursing skills: Basic to advanced skills* (8th ed.). Upper Saddle River, NJ: Pearson Education, Inc.

Test Yourself

Are you ready for the NCLEX-PN® or course exams? Use the practice tests on the companion website to check.

28 Dosage Calculation and Medication Administration

In this chapter

Cross Reference

Other chapters relevant to this content area are

Pediatric Dosage Calculation and Medication Administration Chapter 29
Intravenous Therapy Chapter 30

I. GENERAL PRINCIPLES OF MEDICATION ADMINISTRATION

A. Medication names

1. **Generic name**: a name that reflects chemical family of a drug and does not change according to manufacturer; an example is hydromorphone
2. **Brand name** or **trade name**: a proprietary name given to a generic drug by its manufacturer, resulting in various names for same drug; for example, Dilaudid is trade name for generic drug hydromorphone

B. Medication order components

1. Include drug name, dose, route, frequency, and special parameters (such as blood pressure [BP] or pulse) for administering or withholding dose; each order must be dated and timed
2. Medication order must include client's name and be signed by prescriber
3. *NCLEX®* Call prescriber immediately if order is difficult to read or for any questions about order; do not administer a medication that has an unclear order
4. *NCLEX®* Under law, nurses are responsible for their own actions (e.g., if a drug order is written incorrectly, nurse who administers incorrect order is also responsible for error)
5. Telephone orders written by nurses are done as agency policy allows, must include all elements noted above, and must be cosigned by prescriber as soon as possible and within time frame of agency policy (usually 24 hours)
6. Verbal orders are generally discouraged and are usually used during emergency or near emergency situations; these orders are written as soon as possible and appropriately signed

C. Essential concepts of pharmacology

1. **Pharmacokinetics**: study of how body absorbs, distributes, metabolizes or biotransforms, and excretes medication (four processes)

2. **Absorption**: process by which a drug moves from administration site into bloodstream; drugs are absorbed through gastrointestinal (GI) tract, respiratory tract, or skin, and absorption depends upon correct drug form or preparation being administered by correct route
3. **Distribution**: movement of drug from site of absorption to site of action; depends upon vascularity for speed of onset and upon chemical and physical drug properties to attract drug to a certain area of body where it will exert its effect
4. **Metabolism/biotransformation**: conversion of a drug by enzymatic action of liver into a less active substance that is easily excreted through renal or biliary systems; can be affected by a variety of factors, including disease states
5. **Excretion**: elimination of drug and metabolites from body, primarily through kidneys but also through feces, respiration, perspiration, saliva, and breast milk
6. Prescriber determines frequency of drug dosing according to drug's **half-life** (time it takes for total amount of drug to diminish by one-half); a drug's half-life provides information about its accumulation in body with repeated doses

D. Principles and process of medication administration

1. Determine completeness and accuracy of order
2. *NCLEX®* Check client allergies to ordered medication and to any of its ingredients
3. Assess client condition related to why medication is being ordered
4. *NCLEX®* Check ordered medication against other ordered medications for interactions; be aware of **side effects** (mild), **adverse effects** (more severe), and **toxic effects** (most harmful), associated with high doses
5. *NCLEX®* Calculate dose properly, using any conversions needed (see next section)
6. Do not use any medication for which expiration date has passed
7. Label all drawn up or reconstituted medications with drug name, dose, date, time, and initials
8. Discard any partially used single-dose containers; label multiuse vials with date, time, and initials when opened or apply expiration date stickers used by some agencies (many expire 30 days after initial use; see product literature and agency policy)
9. Complete six rights when administering medications: right drug, dose, route, time, client, and documentation (date, time, initials and/or signature, site if parenteral, any parameters such as BP, pulse, or blood glucose)
10. *NCLEX®* Address any client concerns about medication; do not administer a medication that client questions until order and dose are rechecked
11. Follow universal principles of medication administration and complete client teaching related to medication therapy (see Box 28–1)

Box 28–1

Universal Principles for Medication Administration and Related Client Teaching

Administration Principles

1. Assess current medications (including OTC drugs and herbal products) and history of allergies to identify any potential risks to client.
2. Administer doses on time to maintain therapeutic blood levels.
3. Do not break, crush, or allow client to chew sustained release or enteric coated preparations.
4. Be aware of side effects and adverse effects of medications and monitor client to maintain client safety.
5. Provide both verbal and written instructions to client, and provide phone number to call if questions arise or problems occur.

Client Teaching

1. Understand medication actions, side effects, signs of toxicity, importance of follow-up with prescriber and complying with follow-up laboratory tests, and how to self-administer.
2. Do not take any over-the-counter (OTC) drugs or herbal products without first consulting prescriber.
3. Take exactly as prescribed and do not miss or double doses.
4. Report adverse effects promptly.
5. Do not discontinue drug without consulting prescriber's knowledge.
6. Do not drink alcohol while taking prescription medications.

II. MEASUREMENT AND CONVERSION SYSTEMS

A. Medication measurement systems

1. **Metric system**: a decimal system of measurement based upon units of 10; gram is a unit of weight, and liter is a unit of liquid volume
2. **Apothecary system**: oldest system of pharmacologic measurement, expressed in roman numerals and special symbols; a unit of liquid measure is a minim, and unit for weight is a grain
3. Household: a less accurate system of measurement based upon drops, teaspoons, tablespoons, cups, and glasses

B. Conversions

1. When a medication order is written in one system and medication label utilizes another system, one system must be converted to equivalent measure in other
2. See Table 28–1 for approximate weight equivalents and Table 28–2 for volume equivalents of various systems
3. When converting within metric system, move decimal point 3 places to right to convert from a larger unit of measure to a smaller unit of measure (e.g., 2.5 grams converts to 2500 milligrams) and 3 places to left to convert from a smaller unit of measure to a larger unit of measure (e.g., 3000 milliliters converts to 3 liters)
4. Apothecary system is not often used for volumes less than one ounce
5. All conversions must be done before dosage can be calculated

Table 28–1 Approximate Weight Equivalents

Metric System	Apothecary System
1 milligram (mg)	1/60 grain
60 mg	1 grain
1000 mg = 1 gram	15 grains
1000 grams or 1 kilogram	2.2 lb (pounds)

Table 28–2 Approximate Volume Equivalents

Metric	Apothecary	Household
1 mL (milliliter)	15 m (minim)	15 gtt (drop)
5 mL	60 m = 1 dram	60 gtt = 1 tsp (teaspoon)
15 mL	4 dram	3 tsp = 1 tbsp (tablespoon)
30 mL	1 ounce	2 tbsp
240 mL	8 ounces	1 cup
500 mL	16 ounces	1 pint
1000 mL	2 pints	1 quart
4000 mL	4 quarts	1 gallon

III. DOSAGE CALCULATIONS

A. Medications are prescribed in a specific amount or weight per volume; for instance, if a single tablet has 100 mg of medication, the volume of that tablet is 1; a medication that comes in 80 mg per 2 mL of liquid has a volume of 2

B. A few liquid medications are prescribed by volume alone because they are available in only one strength, such as a dose of 30 mL of a liquid antacid

C. Common formulas for calculating medications are ratio and proportion, "desired over have," and dimensional analysis (see Box 28–2)

Memory Aid

No single drug calculation formula is better than any other. Choose one that works for you and use it consistently.

Box 28–2

Calculating Medication Dosages

Formula 1 "Desired over Have"

$$\frac{\text{Dose ordered (desired)}}{\text{Dose on hand (have)}} \times \text{Amount available (quantity)} = \text{amount to give}$$

Example: Lasix 60 mg IV is ordered and medication is labeled as 80 mg per 2 mL.

$$\frac{60 \text{ mg}}{80 \text{ mg}} \times 2 \text{ mL} = 1.5 \text{ mL}$$

Formula 2 Ratio and Proportion

Dose ordered is to (:) dose on hand as (::) *x* quantity is to (:) quantity available.
Multiply the two outer values by the inner value and *x* to solve.
Example: Lasix 60 mg IV is ordered and medication is labeled as 80 mg per 2 mL.

60 mg : 80 mg :: × : 2
80x = 120; x = 1.5 mL

Formula 3 Dimensional Analysis

Uses a set of rules to set up problems for solving.

Rule 1: Multiplying one side of an equation by a conversion factor will not change the value of the equation.

Rule 2: Set up the problem in fractions called factors so that all labels cancel from the numerator and denominator except the label desired in the answer.
Example: Lasix 60 mg IV is ordered and medication is labeled as 80 mg per 2 mL.

$$\text{mL} = \frac{2 \text{ mL}}{80 \text{ mg}} \times 60 \text{ mg}$$

$$\text{mL} = \frac{120}{80} = 1.5$$

D. **When giving liquid medications for injection,** round amounts greater than 1 mL to nearest tenth (0.1) to coincide with calibrations on syringe (see next section)

E. **When giving liquid medications for injection,** round amounts less than 1 mL to nearest hundredth (0.01) to coincide with calibrations on syringe (see next section)

F. **Rules for rounding generally require carrying out decimals to one place further than needed** and then rounding back only once at very end of calculation

IV. ORAL MEDICATIONS

A. **Tablets may be divided into partial dosages** (e.g., half) only when scored (marked in half with indented line)

B. **Extended-release and enteric-coated medications**

NCLEX® 1. Do not break or crush enteric-coated medications, which are designed for release and absorption in small intestine

NCLEX® 2. As a rule, do not break or crush extended-release medications; some scored formulations can be broken without affecting release mechanism; some mixed-release capsules can be opened and contents sprinkled on food; read product literature carefully

3. Abbreviations used in brand names identifying drugs as extended-release include CR (controlled release), CRT (controlled-release tablet), LA (long acting), SA (sustained action), SR (sustained release), TR (time release), and XL or XR (extended length or release)

C. **Liquid doses**

1. Use medicine cup to pour liquid volumes of 5 mL or greater; hold cup at eye level and measure to middle of meniscus
2. Use syringe with needle removed to draw up liquid volumes less than 5 mL
3. If a calibrated dropper is supplied with medication, it may be used

V. ENTERAL MEDICATIONS

A. **Perform hand hygiene and place client in semi-Fowler's position**

B. **Determine correct tube placement**

1. It may not be possible to reliably determine placement of small-bore enteral tubes by any technique other than radiography, which is most reliable

2. Nasogastric tube: aspirate stomach contents and check pH of 4 or less, or auscultate air insufflation (less reliable); secretions should be greenish tan to clear
3. Nasointestinal tubes: aspirate stomach contents and check pH higher than 6; duodenal secretions should be deep yellow
4. Percutaneous endoscopic gastrostomy (PEG) and percutaneous endoscopic jejunostomy (PEJ) tubes do not require placement verification prior to each medication administration

C. **Flush enteral tube with approximately 30 mL water prior to administering medication**

D. **Administer medication in solution or elixir forms when available;** crush tablets to a fine powder and mix in warm water to make a solution or suspension; do not mix medications—administer each medication separately; flush well between medications

NCLEX® E. **If client is receiving enteral feeding, ensure compatibility of medication and feeding; if they are not compatible, turn off tube feeding for 30 to 60 minutes before and after medication administration**

F. **Flush enteral tube with approximately 30 mL of water following each medication**

NCLEX® G. **If enteral tube is connected to suction, disconnect from suction for at least 30 minutes after administering medication**

H. **Maintain client in semi-Fowler's position for at least 30 minutes following administration of medication**

VI. INJECTIONS

A. **See Box 28–3 for withdrawing medications from a vial**

B. **See Box 28–4 for withdrawing medications from an ampule**

C **Maintain sterility while assembling syringe and needle;** select appropriate size needle and syringe based on volume and type of medication, desired site, client's size, and viscosity of medication

NCLEX® D. **See Table 28–3 for a summary of syringes, needles, and uses;** see Figure 28–1 for examples of 3 mL, insulin, and tuberculin syringes, with illustration of various calibrations

E. **Using anatomical landmarks,** select site of injection appropriate for type of injection and medication (e.g., intramuscular, intradermal, or subcutaneous); see Box 28–5 (p. 422) for a summary of injection sites

F. **Perform hand hygiene and put on gloves**

G. **Cleanse area with alcohol swab and wait for it to dry (usually 30 seconds)**

Box 28–3

Withdrawing Medications from a Vial

1. Remove vial cap.
2. Cleanse rubber top of vial with alcohol.
3. Tighten needle on syringe or use needleless syringe.
4. Fill plunger with amount of air equal to amount of solution to be withdrawn.
5. Inject air into vacant area of vial, keeping needle above surface of medication.
6. Invert vial, touching only syringe barrel and plunger tip. Withdraw medication.
7. While syringe remains attached to vial, expel any air bubbles from syringe by tapping side of syringe sharply.
8. Recheck amount of medication in syringe.
9. Remove syringe from vial and recap needle, if appropriate, using scoop technique.

Box 28–4

Withdrawing Medications from an Ampule

1. Tap neck of ampule to move solution to body of ampule.
2. Using a pad, break ampule away from you.
3. Use a filter needle to withdraw solution. Solution can be withdrawn from either an upright or inverted position—insert needle, without touching sides of neck, with bevel down and touching bottom of ampule (it is not necessary to add air).
4. Return ampule to upright position.
5. Tap barrel below bubbles to dislodge air in syringe.
6. Eject air with syringe in upright position.
7. Recheck amount of medication in syringe.
8. Remove filter needle and replace with appropriate needle.

Table 28-3 Summary of Syringes, Needles, and Uses

Use/Purpose	Site	Maximum Volume	Syringe	Needle Size	Needle Angle
Insulin Slow absorption to produce a sustained effect	Abdomen, lateral and posterior areas of upper arm or thigh, scapular area, upper ventro-dorsal gluteal areas	1 mL	Insulin—calibrated on 100 unit scale	Non-removable ⅜ in. 29 gauge	45° or 90°
Intradermal or intracutaneous Antigens and skin testing, slow absorption	Inner lower arm or scapular area, upper chest	0.1 mL	1 mL tuberculin syringe	⅜ in. 25–27 gauge	10–15° just under epidermis; bevel of needle up
Subcutaneous Absorbed slowly for sustained effect	Abdomen, lateral and posterior aspects of upper arm or thigh, scapular area, upper ventro- and dorsogluteal areas	1 mL	0.5–3 mL syringe	⅜–⅝ in. 25 gauge	⅝ in.–45° when 1 in. of tissue can be grasped ⅜ in.–90° when 2 in. of tissue can be grasped
Intramuscular Rapid absorption *Ventrogluteal*—preferred for adults *Vastus lateralis*—preferred for infant < 7 months of age	Ventrogluteal, dorsogluteal, vastus lateralis, deltoid	*Adult deltoid* 0.5–1 mL *Adult gluteus medius* 1–4 mL	1–5 mL syringe	*Deltoid* ⅝–1 in. 23–25 gauge *Vastus lateralis, ventrogluteal, and dorsogluteal* 1½ in.	90°

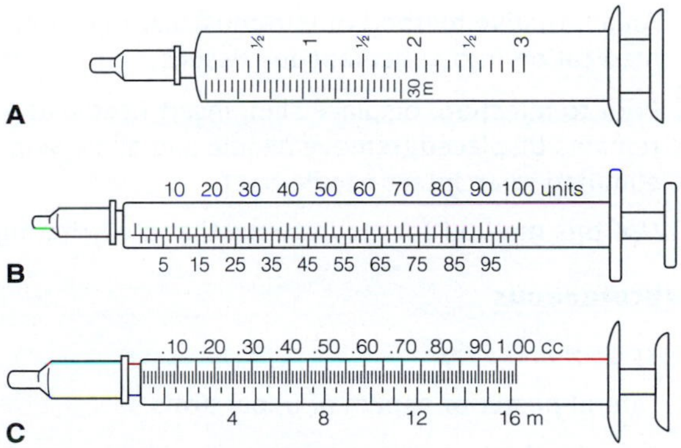

Figure 28-1

Three kinds of syringes for injection, *A.* 3 milliliter (mL) hypodermic syringe is calibrated in tenths (0.1) mL and minims. *B.* Insulin syringe is calibrated in 100 units for use with U100 insulin. *C.* Tuberculin syringe is calibrated in tenths and hundredths (0.01) of an mL and in minims.

H. Inject medication

I. Discard syringe and needle into a sharps container

J. Specific information appropriate to injection sites

1. **Intradermal (ID)**: gently pull skin taut; do not aspirate; inject medication slowly and observe for wheal formation and blanching at site
2. **Subcutaneous (SubQ)**: grasp SQ tissue; hold syringe like a dart (between thumb and forefinger) and insert needle; release SQ tissue; aspirate (except with heparin or insulin) and inject medication slowly if no blood appears (if blood returns, withdraw needle, discard, and prepare a new injection); with insulin administration, rotate injection sites systematically to minimize tissue damage (**lipodystrophy**, atrophy, or hypertrophy of SQ tissue), which affects absorption
3. **Intramuscular (IM)**: hold syringe like a dart; spread skin taught or grasp skin in geriatric client; use quick, darting motion to insert needle; aspirate and inject medication slowly unless blood returns (if blood returns, withdraw needle, discard, and prepare new injection); Z-track technique prevents "tracking" and is used to administer medications irritating to SQ tissue (e.g., hydroxyzine)—pull skin approximately 1 inch laterally away from injection site, inject medication, withdraw needle, then release tissue

Box 28–5

Summary of Injection Sites

Intramuscular

Ventrogluteal

- Place client in side-lying position.
- Use right hand for left anterior hip and left hand for right anterior hip.
- Place palm over greater trochanter and point index finger toward client's anterior-superior iliac spine; spread out index finger from other 3 fingers to form a V area.
- Inject at a 90-degree angle within V area.

Dorsogluteal

- Place client either in prone position with toes pointed inward or in side-lying position with upper knee flexed and in front of lower leg.
- Draw imaginary line between greater trochanter and postero-superior spine (prominence) of iliac crest.
- Inject at 90-degree angle lateral and superior to imaginary line.

Vastus Lateralis

- Place client in supine position.
- Inject at a 90-degree angle using anterior-lateral middle third of thigh between greater trochanter and lateral femoral condyle.

Deltoid

- Palpate lower edge of acromion and midpoint of lateral aspect of arm. Inject at 90-degree angle 2 inches below acromion process within triangle between boundaries.
- Alternate method—place four fingers across deltoid muscle with first finger on acromion process; site is three finger breadths below acromion process.

Z-Track Injection

- An alternative method of intramuscular injection designed to reduce seepage of medication into subcutaneous tissues.
- Prior to injection, displace skin, insert needle at 90-degree angle while skin remains displaced; remove needle and allow skin to return to neutral position, eliminating an intact needle tract.
- Use this method for medications that are irritating to subcutaneous tissues.

Subcutaneous

Most Common Sites

- Lateral posterior aspect of upper arms
- Anterior thighs
- Lower quadrants of abdomen (outside 2-inch radius of umbilicus): preferred site for heparin

Other Sites

- Scapular areas
- Dorsogluteal

Intradermal

- Forearms
- Upper back beneath scapulae
- Upper chest

VII. *INTRAVENOUS (IV)* MEDICATIONS

A. Mixtures of medications within large volumes of IV fluids help to maintain constant therapeutic blood levels of medication; examples are potassium (e.g., 20 mEq added to 1 liter of IV solution) or heparin (25,000 units added to 250 mL solution)

B. To add medication to an IV solution, prepare medication from a vial or ampule and draw into syringe

C. To add medication to a new IV container

1. Clean injection port with alcohol swab and allow to dry for 30 seconds
2. Remove needle cap from syringe, insert needle through center of injection port, and inject medication into IV solution
3. Mix medication and solution by gently rotating bag
4. Complete and attach medication label to IV solution; include name and dose of medication, date and time, and nurse's initials
5. Proceed with setting up IV for administration

D. To add medication to an existing infusion

1. Ensure there is sufficient IV solution in container to properly dilute medication
2. Proceed as with adding a medication to a new IV container
3. Piggyback infusion without interrupting existing IV

NCLEX®

   a. Ensure compatibility of piggyback medication with any other currently infusing IV solutions and any ingredients (such as potassium) or currently infusing medications; if incompatible, discontinue primary infusion temporarily if safe to do so or start a second IV line; set up secondary set following procedure for setting up an IV
   b. Hang existing infusion set lower than piggyback secondary set
   c. Cleanse uppermost infusion port with alcohol swab and let dry for 30 seconds
   d. Connect secondary set to primary set using needleless access device above existing IV roller clamp
   e. Maintain existing IV roller clamp position and regulate piggyback rate using roller clamp on secondary tubing or programming secondary rate and volume into infusion pump; piggyback solution will infuse first, and existing IV will resume at original rate when complete
   f. When intermittent solution is in a syringe pump, connect syringe to secondary access port on pump; follow protocols for specific pump to administer intermittent medication as either a continuous infusion or an infusion that interrupts existing IV

Memory Aid

Look up in a drug handbook or other standard reference the infusion rate of IV piggyback medications. They vary in length, but many are given over 30 minutes or longer.

VIII. *TOPICAL* MEDICATIONS

A. Medications applied to skin

NCLEX®

1. After performing hand hygiene, apply gloves to prevent drug absorption through fingertips
2. Remove prior applications remaining on client's skin unless otherwise specified
3. Remove ointments and creams from their containers and apply to skin with tongue depressors in thin layers unless otherwise specified
4. For transdermal patch or premeasured paper, read package insert for application directions
   a. Remove previously applied patch or paper and cleanse skin
   b. Record date and time of application and initials directly onto transdermal patch, and remove protective covering
   c. Place prescribed amount of medication directly on premeasured paper and apply immediately; secure paper with tape

NCLEX®

   d. Alternate application areas to prevent skin irritation and apply to clean, dry, intact, and hairless skin

B. Nasal medications

1. Apply gloves after performing hand hygiene
2. Ask client to blow nose and tilt client's head back
3. Nasal spray: occlude one nostril with gloved finger and have client inhale through nose while squeezing medication bottle; client may self-medicate if able

4. Bottle with dropper: fill dropper with prescribed amount of medication, place dropper just inside nare and instill correct number of drops
5. Wipe excess medication with tissue
6. Repeat with other nostril if appropriate
7. *NCLEX®* Instruct client not to sneeze or blow nose and to keep head tilted back for 5 minutes until medication is absorbed

C. *Ophthalmic* (eye) medications

1. Ophthalmic drops
   a. Tilt client's head slightly backward and ask client to look up
   b. Supply tissue so that client can wipe off excess medication
   c. Hold eyedropper ½ to ¾ inch above eyeball
   d. Expose lower conjunctival sac by pulling down on cheek, creating a "cup"
   e. *NCLEX®* Drop prescribed number of drops into center of lower conjunctival sac while applying pressure to inner canthus to reduce systemic absorption of medication
   f. Instruct client to close eyelids and move eyes; gently massage closed lid
   g. Remove excess medication with tissue
2. Ophthalmic ointment
   a. Supply tissue so that client can wipe off excess medication
   b. Put on gloves
   c. Gently separate eyelids with two fingers, grasping lower lid immediately below lashes; exert pressure downward over bony prominence of cheek to form a trough
   d. Instruct client to look upward
   e. *NCLEX®* Apply ointment along inside edge of entire lower eyelid, from inner canthus to outer canthus
   f. Instruct client to close eyelids and move eyes to spread ointment under lids and over eye surface
   g. Remove excess medication with tissue
   h. Instruct client that vision may be blurred temporarily following administration of an ointment

D. Otic (ear) medications

1. Position client on side with ear to be treated facing up
2. Fill medication dropper with prescribed amount of medication
3. Put on gloves
4. Straighten ear canal; for an infant or young child, pull pinna of ear gently downward and backward; in an adult, pull pinna gently upward and backward
5. Instill medication drops, holding medication slightly above ear
6. Insert cotton loosely into ear canal, if ordered
7. Instruct client to remain on side for 5 to 10 minutes

E. Vaginal medications

1. Position client in dorsal recumbent or Sims' position
2. Perform hand hygiene and put on gloves
3. Suppository: remove foil wrapper and insert suppository into applicator
4. Cream: attach medication tube to applicator and squeeze tube to fill applicator with prescribed dose; remove tube
5. Insert applicator into vaginal canal 3 to 4 inches, push plunger until all medication is released, and remove applicator
6. Instruct client to lie quietly for 15 minutes until medication is absorbed; vaginal medications may be ordered at bedtime to aid retention
7. Wash applicator and return to appropriate storage area

F. Rectal medications

1. Place client in Sims' (left lateral) position
2. Perform hand hygiene and put on gloves
3. Remove foil wrapper from suppository
4. Apply small amount of water-soluble lubricant to suppository
5. With index finger, insert suppository flat end first approximately 10 cm or 4 inches in adults beyond internal sphincter to ensure retention (studies indicate that inserting flat end first promotes better retention than inserting tapered end first)
6. Instruct client to lie quietly for 15 minutes while medication is absorbed

IX. *INHALATION* MEDICATIONS

A. Metered-dose inhaled (MDI) medication

1. Shake canister before each puff to mix medication and propellant
2. Instruct client to
   a. Hold inhaler 2 inches away from mouth
   b. Exhale through pursed lips
   c. Depress inhalation device, inhaling slowly and deeply through mouth
   d. Hold breath for 10 seconds and slowly exhale through pursed lips
   e. Wait 2 to 5 minutes (as drug literature recommends) between puffs (*NCLEX®*)
3. Clean device according to manufacturer's instructions

B. Spacer with MDI

1. Insert MDI mouthpiece into spacer
2. Remove mouthpiece cover from spacer
3. Shake MDI with spacer
4. Hold MDI and spacer with drug canister upright
5. Instruct client to inhale, exhale slowly through pursed lips, then close lips around spacer mouthpiece
6. Activate MDI canister by pushing it further down into plastic adapter while client inhales slowly and deeply
7. Instruct client to hold breath for 10 seconds, then exhale and relax
8. Wipe mouthpiece after use
9. Remove rubber end of spacer, rinse with warm water, and dry thoroughly

Check Your NCLEX–PN® Exam I.Q.

You are ready for testing on this content if you can

- Determine the medication schedule of a client.
- Calculate medication dosages with accuracy.
- Reconstitute or mix medications appropriately.
- Verify dosage calculations before administering medications.
- Identify proper procedures for medication administration.
- Utilize the "six rights" of medication administration.
- Dispose of unused medications properly.

PRACTICE TEST

1 The nurse is administering an intradermal tuberculin skin test to a client. The nurse should use which angle of needle entry for the injection?

1. 10–15 degrees
2. 30–40 degrees
3. 45 degrees
4. 90 degrees

2 The nurse is preparing to administer a watery medication via an intramuscular injection into the deltoid muscle of a 160-pound male. What is the preferred needle size for the medication, muscle, and weight of the client?

1. 1.5 inch, 20-gauge
2. 1 inch, 20-gauge
3. 1.5 inch, 25-gauge
4. 1 inch, 25-gauge

3 A client is postoperative with an IV in place. During assessment, the client rates pain at being 6 on a 1–10 scale. The nurse notes an order in the client's chart for morphine sulfate 6–8 mg every 4 hours as needed for pain. Given the order and the client's condition, what action should the nurse take?

1. Administer 8 mg morphine sulfate intramuscularly (IM)
2. Administer 6 mg morphine sultate through the IV
3. Withhold the pain medication and contact the physician
4. Give one 10 mg dose of morphine sulfate to regain pain control.

PRACTICE TEST

4. A client has a history of renal impairment. The nurse is administering a medication known to be excreted through the kidneys. What should the nurse monitor to detect adverse reactions to the medication?

1. Serum blood urea nitrogen (BUN) and creatinine
2. Color and odor of the urine
3. Urine sugar and acetone levels
4. Serum hemoglobin

5. The nurse is preparing to administer an oral medication to a client. Upon entering the client's room, the nurse finds that the client has developed vomiting and diarrhea, is confused, and has a fever. What should the nurse do next? Select all that apply.

1. Administer the medication IM.
2. Give the medication as ordered.
3. Withhold the medication.
4. Omit this dose of medication.
5. Call the physician.

6. The nurse has prepared an IM injection for a preoperative client. Suddenly, another client becomes entangled in IV tubing and yells for help. As the nurse rushes to assist, the surgery orderly arrives for the preoperative client. The nurse asks a second nurse to give the injection to the preoperative client. What is the best response by the second nurse?

1. Offer to assist the second client.
2. Give the client the preoperative medication.
3. Prepare a new syringe for the preoperative client.
4. Explain that the nurse should give the prepared medication.

7. A client is in the bathroom. When the nurse enters the room to give medications, the client asks the nurse to leave the pills on the bedside table. What is the best nursing action?

1. Leave the medication on the bedside table.
2. Wait in the room until the client comes out of the bathroom.
3. Go into the bathroom and give the client the pills.
4. Inform the client that you will return later with the medication.

8. The client has an order for dexamethasone (Decadron) 6 mg as an oral liquid dose. Available is a vial of dexamethasone containing 4 mg/mL. The nurse draws _____ milliliters into the syringe for the dose. Record your answer rounding to one decimal place.

Fill in your answer below:
_________ mL

9. The client has an order for glyburide (DiaBeta) 1.25 mg before breakfast and dinner. Available are 2.5 mg tablets. The nurse should plan to administer ____ tablet(s). Record your answer rounding to one decimal place.

Fill in your answer below:
_________ tablet(s)

10. The client has an order for lorazepam (Ativan) 0.5 mg. Available is a vial containing 2mg/mL. The nurse should draw up ____ milliliters of solution. Record your answer rounding to one decimal place.

Fill in your answer below:
_________ mL

11. A client has a temperature of 101.2°F. There is an order for acetaminophen (Tylenol) 650 mg PO for fever, and 325 mg tablets are available. The nurse should give ____ tablets. Record your answer rounding to the nearest whole number.

Fill in your answer below:
_________ tablet(s)

12. A client has an order for a dose of digoxin (Lanoxin) 0.25 mg. Available are 0.125 mg tablets. The nurse should take ____ tablets to administer the dose. Record your answer rounding to the nearest whole number.

Fill in your answer below:
_________ tablet(s)

13. The client has an order to receive methylprednisolone (SoluMedrol) 120 mg. Available are tablets labeled 40 mg. The nurse should administer_____ tablets. Record your answer rounding to the nearest whole number.

Fill in your answer below:
_________ tablet(s)

14 The client has an order to receive 40 mg prednisone (Deltasone) by mouth daily. Available are 10 mg tablets. The nurse should prepare to give ____ tablets. Record your answer rounding to the nearest whole number.

Fill in your answer below:

________ tablet(s)

15 While the nurse is administering a client's dose of nitroglycerin sublingual, the client asks why it is administered sublingually rather than orally. What is the best response by the nurse?

1. "It is absorbed more rapidly sublingually than when swallowed."
2. "It is absorbed more rapidly when swallowed than sublingually."
3. "The absorptions are the same so it really doesn't matter."
4. "Sublingual provides a sustained release of the medication."

16 The nurse is to administer 25 mg of promethazine (Phenergan) IM to a 150-pound client. The nurse prepares to inject the dose into which site?

1. Deltoid
2. Dorsogluteal
3. Vastus lateralis
4. Ventrolgluteal

17 The nurse is to administer 10 grains of aspirin, which comes 325 mg per tablet. The nurse would give _____ tablets to administer 10 grains? Record your answer rounding to the nearest whole number.

Fill in your answer below:

________ tablet(s)

18 The nurse is preparing to administer a less viscous (i.e., watery) IM injection into the deltoid muscle of a 160-pound male. What would be the preferred size needle for the medication, muscle, and size of the client?

1. 1½-inch, 20-gauge
2. 1-inch, 20-gauge
3. 1½-inch, 25-gauge
4. 1-inch, 25-gauge

19 In what order should the nurse implement the steps to administer an ophthalmic medication to a client? Place the options in the correct order. All options must be used.

1. Use finger on non-dominate hand to expose conjunctival sac.
2. Check the client's allergy status.
3. Clean the eyelid and lashes from inner to outer canthus.
4. Apply firm pressure to nasolacrimal duct for 30 seconds.
5. Instruct the client to look up toward the ceiling.

20 A nurse giving an intramuscular injection places the heel of the hand on the client's greater trochanter, with the fingers pointing toward the client's head. The nurse places the index finger on the client's anterior superior iliac spine, while the middle finger is stretched dorsally, palpating the iliac crest. After giving the injection in the triangle formed, the nurse documents the injection as being given in which intramuscular injection site?

1. Vastus lateralis
2. Ventrogluteal
3. Dorsogluteal
4. Rectus femoris

ANSWERS & RATIONALES

1 **Answer: 1** **Rationale:** For an intradermal injection, the needle enters the skin at a 10- to 15- degree angle and the medication forms a bleb under the epidermis. The other options would permit the medication to be deposited too deeply into either subcutaneous or muscle tissue, depending on needle length and size of client. **Cognitive Level:** Applying **Client Need:** Pharmacological and Parenteral Therapies **Integrated Process:** Nursing Process: Implementation **Content Area:** Pharmacology **Strategy:** The core issue is knowledge of the correct needle angle to achieve the appropriate depth of penetration. The option that has the smallest angle, which will keep the injection from going too deeply, should be selected for an intradermal injection.

2 **Answer: 4** **Rationale:** Several factors indicate the size and length of the needle to be used: the muscle, the type of solution, the amount of adipose tissue covering the muscle, and the age of the client. A smaller needle such as a 23- to 25-gauge needle that is 1 inch long is commonly used for the deltoid muscle. A 1.5 inch, 20 gauge needle is appropriate for an injection of a viscous medication into a larger muscle, well-covered by adipose tissue. Commonly, a smaller 23- to 25-gauge needle that is 1 inch long is appropriate for an injection of watery medication into the deltoid muscle. A 1 inch long needle is usually appropriate for an injection into the deltoid muscle. More viscous solutions require a larger gauge (e.g., 20- gauge). A smaller 23- to 25-gauge needle is appropriate for an injection of watery medication into the deltoid muscle. However, a 1.5 inch needle is appropriate for an injection into a larger muscle, well-covered by adipose tissue. **Cognitive Level:** Analyzing **Client Need:** Pharmacological and Parenteral Therapies **Integrated Process:** Nursing Process: Implementation **Content Area:** Pharmacology **Strategy:** The critical concepts in the question are that the deltoid muscle commonly requires the use of a shorter needle and a watery solution allows the use of a smaller gauge needle. Use the process of elimination to choose the option that combines these concepts.

3 **Answer: 3 Rationale:** The essential parts of a drug that must be present in order to implement the order are name of the drug, date and time the order was written, dosage, route, frequency, and signature of the person writing the order. This client's order is missing a route and the physician must be contacted for clarification. Nurses may not independently administer a medication without all of the essential parts of the order. Administering medication in amounts greater than the physician orders constitutes practicing medicine without a license. **Cognitive Level:** Analyzing **Client Need:** Pharmacological and Parenteral Therapies **Integrated Process:** Nursing Process: Implementation **Content Area:** Pharmacology **Strategy:** The core issue of the question is recognizing and understanding that medication cannot be given with an incomplete order. Apply knowledge about medication administration to select the correct answer.

4 **Answer: 1 Rationale:** Blood levels of two metabolically produced substances, urea and creatinine, are routinely used to evaluate renal function. Both are normally eliminated by the kidneys and are measured as serum BUN and creatinine. The color and odor of the urine are general observations and are not specific to detect adverse renal reactions. Sugar and acetone in urine are found in diabetes mellitus with ketoacidosis and are not indicators of kidney function. Serum hemoglobin is a measure of the RBC count but does not reflect kidney function. **Cognitive Level:** Applying **Client Need:** Pharmacological and Parenteral Therapies **Integrated Process:** Nursing Process: Evaluation **Content Area:** Fundamentals **Strategy:** The core issue of the question is knowledge of what to assess to determine kidney function as an indicator for the clearance of medications. Use the process of elimination and basic nursing knowledge to make a selection.

5 **Answer: 3, 5 Rationale:** The correct action should be to withhold the medication and call the physician. The physician should be called regarding the client's change of condition and the inability to administer the prescribed medication. The nurse cannot change the route that a medication is to be given without a physician's order. Oral medications should not be administered to clients who are vomiting, which could interfere with the ability to absorb the medication and possibly initiate further vomiting. The nurse should not just omit the dose without notifying the physician of the client's change in condition. **Cognitive Level:** Applying **Client Need:** Pharmacological and Parenteral Therapies **Integrated Process:** Nursing Process: Implementation **Content Area:** Fundamentals **Strategy:** Use the process of elimination and general measures for administering medications safely to make a selection. When there is more than one correct answer for a question, consider each option as a true/false statement.

6 **Answer: 1 Rationale:** It would be prudent for the second nurse to assist the second client so that the first nurse may continue medication administration. The nurse who prepares the medication must be the nurse to give the medication. Preparation of a new syringe by the second nurse is acceptable but requires wasting of the original medication, additional time for the preparation, and unnecessary expense; therefore, this is not the best action. The explanation is appropriate, but does not resolve the issue of the preoperative client. **Cognitive Level:** Analyzing **Client Need:** Pharmacological and Parenteral Therapies **Integrated Process:** Nursing Process: Implementation **Content Area:** Fundamentals **Strategy:** The core issue of the question is the principle that nurses may not administer medications prepared by another nurse. Look at each option carefully with consideration given to client needs, time constraints, and expenses.

7 **Answer: 4 Rationale:** Informing the client that the nurse will return with the medication meets the principles of medication administration and the client's needs. Medications should not be left at the bedside, with certain exceptions that are ordered in advance (e.g., nitroglycerin and cough syrup). Waiting in the room for the client is an example of poor time management by the nurse. Going into the bathroom to give the client medication is an unnecessary invasion of the client's privacy. **Cognitive Level:** Applying **Client Need:** Pharmacological and Parenteral Therapies **Integrated Process:** Nursing Process: Implementation **Content Area:** Fundamentals **Strategy:** Use the process of elimination. There is one correct answer utilizing basic principles of medication administration.

8 **Answer: 1.5 Rationale:** Use the following formula to solve the problem:

$$\frac{6 \text{ mg}}{x \text{ mL}} = \frac{4 \text{ mg}}{1 \text{ mL}}$$

Cross-multiply 6 by x and 4 by 1 to yield $4x = 6$. Divide 6 by 4 to yield 1.5 mL. **Cognitive Level:** Applying **Client Need:** Pharmacological and Parenteral Therapies **Integrated Process:** Nursing Process: Implementation **Content Area:** Fundamentals **Strategy:** Use knowledge of basic pharmacological math to set-up the question. Carefully review your work and double-check placement of decimals for accuracy.

9 **Answer: 0.5 Rationale:** The following is one way to set up the calculation: Cross-multiply 2.5 by x and 1.25 by 1 to yield $2.5x = 1.25$. Divide 1.25 by 2.5 to yield 0.5 tablet. **Cognitive Level:** Applying **Client Need:** Pharmacological and Parenteral Therapies **Integrated Process:** Nursing Process: Implementation **Content Area:** Fundamentals **Strategy:** Use knowledge of basic pharmacological math procedures to set up the question. Check your work carefully and double check placement of decimals for accuracy.

10 **Answer: 0.25 Rationale:** The following is one way to set up the calculation: Cross-multiply 2.0 by x and 0.5 by 1 to yield $2x = 0.5$. Divide 0.5 by 2 to yield 0.25 mL. **Cognitive Level:** Applying **Client Need:** Pharmacological and Parenteral Therapies **Integrated Process:** Nursing Process: Implementation **Content Area:** Fundamentals **Strategy:** Use knowledge of basic pharmacological math procedures to set up the question. Carefully review your work and double-check placement of decimals for accuracy.

11 **Answer: 2 Rationale:** The following is one way to set up the calculation: Cross-multiply 325 by x and multiply 650 by 1 to yield $325x = 650$. Divide 650 by 325 to yield 2 tablets. **Cognitive Level:** Applying **Client Need:** Pharmacological and Parenteral Therapies **Integrated Process:** Nursing Process: Implementation **Content Area:** Fundamentals **Strategy:** Use knowledge of basic pharmacological math procedures to set up the question. Check your work carefully.

12 **Answer: 2 Rationale:** The following is one way to set up the calculation: Cross-multiply 0.125 by x and 0.25 by 1 to yield

ANSWERS & RATIONALES

$0.125x = 0.25$. Divide 0.25 by 0.125 to yield 2 tablets. **Cognitive Level:** Applying **Client Need:** Pharmacological and Parenteral Therapies **Integrated Process:** Nursing Process: Implementation **Content Area:** Fundamentals **Strategy:** Use knowledge of basic pharmacological math to set up the question. Carefully review your work and double-check placement of decimals for accuracy.

13 **Answer: 3** **Rationale:** The following is one way to set up the calculation: Cross-multiply 40 by x and 120 by 1 to yield $40x = 120$. Divide 120 by 40 to yield 3 tablets. **Cognitive Level:** Applying **Client Need:** Pharmacological and Parenteral Therapies **Integrated Process:** Nursing Process: Implementation **Content Area:** Fundamentals **Strategy:** Use knowledge of basic pharmacological math procedures to set up the question. Check your work carefully for accuracy.

14 **Answer: 4** **Rationale:** The following is one way to set up the calculation: Cross-multiply 10 by x and 40 by 1 to yield $10x = 40$. Divide 40 by 10 to yield 4 tablets. **Cognitive Level:** Applying **Client Need:** Pharmacological and Parenteral Therapies **Integrated Process:** Nursing Process: Implementation **Content Area:** Fundamentals **Strategy:** Use knowledge of basic pharmacological math to set up the question. Check your work carefully for accuracy.

15 **Answer: 1** **Rationale:** The thin layer of epithelium and the vast network of capillaries under the tongue enhance sublingual absorption. This medication dissolves rapidly and is absorbed immediately. The dose is not absorbed more rapidly when swallowed. The sublingual route leads to rapid absorption through the mucous membranes of the mouth. The sublingual route leads to faster absorption than the oral route. It is the form of the medication, not the route that determines whether it is sustained-release. **Cognitive Level:** Applying **Client Need:** Pharmacological and Parenteral Therapies **Integrated Process:** Nursing Process: Implementation **Content Area:** Pharmacology **Strategy:** Note that two options are opposites. When opposites are offered, one of the opposites may have a greater chance of being correct.

16 **Answer: 4** **Rationale:** For an adult with well-developed muscle mass, the preferred intramuscular (IM) injection site for medications requiring a large muscle mass is the ventrogluteal. Promethazine should be given into a site that has a large muscle mass. The deltoid muscle does not have a large mass. For an adult with well-developed muscle mass, the preferred intramuscular (IM) injection site for medications requiring a large muscle mass is the ventrogluteal. The vastus lateralis is the preferred IM injection site for children under 7 months of age. The dorsogluteal muscle is not a preferred site. The vastus lateralis is the preferred IM injection site for children under 7 months of age. **Cognitive Level:** Applying **Client Need:** Pharmacological and Parenteral Therapies **Integrated Process:** Nursing Process: Planning **Content Area:** Fundamentals **Strategy:** Use the process of elimination to narrow options. Dorsogluteal is not recommended for anyone. Vastus lateralis is recommended for injection in children who are very young and cannot yet walk. Ventrogluteal is larger and better developed in most adults than the deltoid.

17 **Answer: 2** **Rationale:** In the apothecary system, 1 grain equals 60–65 mg. 10 grains equal 600–650 mg. Therefore, 2 tablets would be needed at 325 mg each to reach the needed dose. **Cognitive Level:** Applying **Client Need:** Pharmacological and Parenteral Therapies **Integrated Process:** Nursing Process: Implementation **Content Area:** Pharmacology **Strategy:** Use knowledge of the apothecary system and simple dosage calculation.

18 **Answer: 4** **Rationale:** Several factors indicate the size and length of the needle to be used: the muscle, the type of solution, the amount of adipose tissue covering the muscle, and the age of the client. A smaller needle such as an inch-long, 23–25-gauge needle is commonly used for the deltoid muscle. More viscous solutions require a larger gauge (e.g., 20-gauge) needle. **Cognitive Level:** Applying **Client Need:** Pharmacological and Parenteral Therapies **Integrated Process:** Nursing Process: Implementation **Content Area:** Pharmacology **Strategy:** Select the combination of shortest length and smallest gauge.

19 **Answer: 2, 3, 5, 1, 4** **Rationale:** The client's allergy status should be checked routinely before administering medications. Cleaning the lid and lashes prevents material from being washed into the eye during administration. Cleaning from the inner to the outer canthus prevents microorganisms from entering the lacrimal duct. Instructing the client to look up toward the ceiling reduces the possibility of the client blinking. Exposing the conjunctival sac will decrease the possibility of squinting or blinking and forms an appropriate reservoir for the medication. Pressing on the nasolacrimal duct prevents medication from running down the duct and being systemically absorbed. **Cognitive Level:** Applying **Client Need:** Basic Care and Comfort **Integrated Process:** Nursing Process: Implementation **Content Area:** Fundamentals **Strategy:** The core concept of the question is the administration of eye medication. Mentally visualize the process and apply nursing knowledge to select the correct order of administration.

20 **Answer: 2** **Rationale:** The ventrogluteal site is in the gluteus medius muscle with the greater trochanter, the anterior superior iliac spine, and the iliac crest as the landmarks. The vastus lateralis is located on the thigh. The dorsogluteal is located on the buttocks. The rectus femoris is located on the thigh. **Cognitive Level:** Analyzing **Client Need:** Pharmacological and Parenteral Therapies **Integrated Process:** Communication and Documentation **Content Area:** Pharmacology **Strategy:** Basic knowledge of injection sites and landmarks is necessary to answer this question. Utilize knowledge of anatomy and physiology to select the option that matches the description given in the question. Visualize the description.

Key Terms to Review

absorption p. 417
adverse effects p. 417
apothecary system p. 418
biotransformation p. 417
brand name p. 416
distribution p. 417
excretion p. 417
generic name p. 416
half-life p. 417
inhalation p. 425
intradermal (ID) p. 421
intramuscular (IM) p. 421
intravenous p. 423
lipodystrophy p. 421
metabolism p. 417
metric system p. 418
ophthalmic p. 424
pharmacokinetics p. 416
side effects p. 417
subcutaneous (SubQ) p. 421
topical p. 423
toxic effects p. 417
trade name p. 416

References

Berman, A., Snyder, S. (2012). *Kozier & Erb's fundamentals of nursing: Concepts, process, and practice* (9th ed.). Upper Saddle River, NJ: Pearson Education.

Giangrasso, A. & Shrimpton, D. (2010). *Ratio & proportion dosage calculations*. Upper Saddle River, NJ: Pearson Education, Inc.

Olsen, J., Giangrasso, A., & Shrimpton, D. (2012). *Medical dosage calculations: A dimensional analysis approach* (10th ed.). Upper Saddle River, NJ: Pearson Education, Inc.

Pickar, G., & Abernethy, A. (2011). *Dosage calculations: A ratio-proportion approach* (3rd ed.). Clifton Park, NY: Delmar Learning.

Smith, R., Duell, D., & Martin, B. (2012). *Clinical nursing skills: Basic to advanced skills* (8th ed.). Upper Saddle River, NJ: Prentice Hall.

Test Yourself

Are you ready for the NCLEX-PN® or course exams? Use the practice tests on the companion website to check.

Pediatric Dosage Calculation and Medication Administration

29

In this chapter

Cross Reference

Other chapters relevant to this content area are

Dosage Calculation and Medication Administration	Chapter 28
Intravenous Therapy	Chapter 30

I. DOSAGE CALCULATION USING BODY WEIGHT

A. Consists of two steps:

1. Calculate body weight (often in kilograms)
2. Calculate actual drug dosage

B. Converting body weight between pounds (lb) and kilograms (kg): see Box 29–1

C. Calculating pediatric drug dosages: see Box 29–2

1. Drugs are often ordered in mg/kg/day (total daily dose) or mg/kg/dose (actual single dose or divided daily dose)
2. Occasionally a pediatric drug may be ordered in mg/lb/day
3. Most pediatric drugs are given in divided doses rather than a single daily dose
4. *NCLEX®* It is critical to check ordered dose against safe dosage range to ensure that dose is within recommended range
5. *NCLEX®* Question an order for a drug that does not fall within safe dosage range

Box 29–1

Converting Body Weight between Pounds and Kilograms

Recall that 2.2 pounds (lb) = 1 kilogram (kg).

To convert from pounds to kilograms, divide the pounds by 2.2.

To convert from kilograms to pounds, multiply the kilograms by 2.2.

Express either pounds or kilograms to the nearest tenth (e.g., 20.6 kg or 45.3 lb).

Box 29–2

Calculating Pediatric Drug Dosages Using Body Weight

Calculating a Single Pediatric Dose by Body Weight

1. Multiply child's weight in kilograms by dosage ordered per kilogram.
   Example: A pediatrician orders a dose of 15 mg of a drug per kilogram of body weight (15 mg/kg).

   $$20 \text{ kg weight} \times \frac{15 \text{ mg of drug}}{1 \text{ kg}} = 300 \text{ mg of drug should be given as the dose}$$

2. Calculate volume (tablets, solution) using a standard pharmaceutical math calculation (such as "desired over have multiplied by quantity" or ratio and proportion; see Chapter 30)

Calculating a Single Pediatric Dose from a Total Daily Dose Using Body Weight

1. Multiply child's weight in kilograms by daily dosage ordered per kilogram.
   Example: A pediatrician orders a dose of 45 mg of a drug per kilogram of body weight per day (45 mg/kg/day).

   $$20 \text{ kg weight} \times \frac{45 \text{ mg of drug per day}}{1 \text{ kg}} = 900 \text{ mg of drug should be given per day}$$

2. Divide total daily dose by number of doses per day to calculate single dose.
   Example (continued from above): 900 mg of drug per day divided by 3 doses per day = 300 mg per dose.

II. DOSAGE CALCULATION USING BODY SURFACE AREA (BSA)

A. ***Body surface area* is a measurement of surface area of body;** is possibly a more important factor than weight for calculating precise medication dosages for infants and children in selected circumstances

B. **A pediatric client's BSA can be estimated using a *nomogram* as shown in Figure 29–1;** a nomogram is a chart that contains graphs for height, BSA, and weight

C. **Use simple multiplication** when dose is ordered based on either milligrams or micrograms (mcg) of drug per meters squared (m^2) (see Box 29–3)

D. **Use a formula** to calculate a pediatric drug dose when dosage is specified only for adults (see Box 29–3)

III. ORAL MEDICATIONS

A. **Children under 5 years old** often have difficulty swallowing tablets and capsules

B. **Most medications for pediatric use** are available in both solid dose forms (pill, tablet) and liquid forms (suspension, elixir, syrup)

C. **If a pill or tablet must be administered** to a child who cannot swallow it easily, dose may need to be crushed

NCLEX® D. **Do not crush** enteric-coated, time-released, or extended-release medications

E. **If oral medications are crushed,** disguise taste by mixing with a small amount of flavored substance such as applesauce or juice

NCLEX® F. **Check child's mouth** to ensure that oral pills or tablets are swallowed if given whole

G. **Pour liquid medications using a syringe or calibrated medicine cup or dropper,** especially if volumes are 5 mL or fewer

H. **Measure medication dose accurately**

NCLEX® I. **Mix suspensions well before pouring** and administer immediately so dose does not precipitate out of suspension

J. **If it is necessary to disguise taste of a liquid dose,** mix in 30 mL or less of a flavored liquid such as juice

K. **Wear clean gloves when administering medications** to avoid coming in contact with child's saliva

NCLEX® L. **To administer dose to an infant,** place small amounts of liquid along inside of mouth slowly and allow time for infant to swallow before giving more (to prevent aspiration and reduce likelihood of spitting out dose)

M. **To administer dose to a small child,** sit child sideways in own lap or in parent/caregiver's lap; place child's closest arm under adult's arm and behind back; gently hold child's other arm near elbow, use dominant hand to give dose

IV. INJECTIONS

A. **Subcutaneous (SubQ)**

1. Site depends on age; for older children, use same sites as adults, but newborns, infants, and toddlers often require use of dorsum of upper arm or anterior thigh
2. Syringe size and needle length also depend on size of child, but infants and children often require 25- to 26-gauge needles that are ⅜- to ⅝-inch long

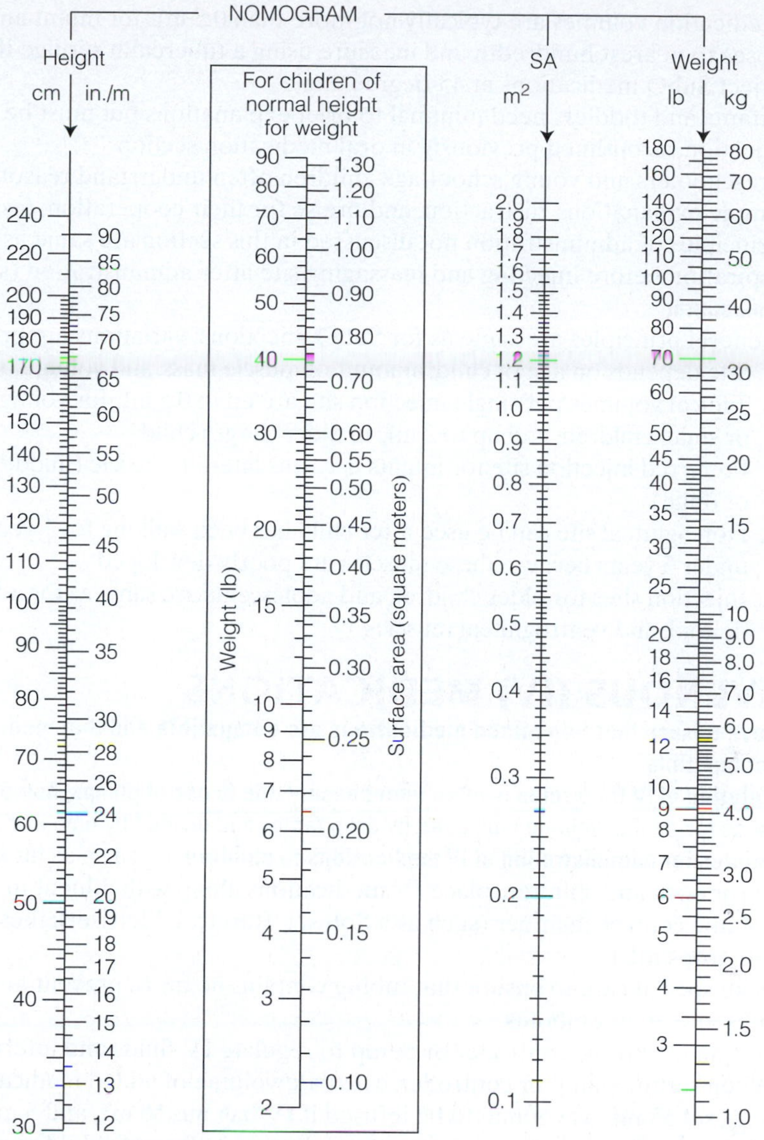

Figure 29–1

West nomogram for infants and children. Obtain child's height and weight and note those points on the nomogram. Draw a connecting line between these two points; the point where the line intersects the BSA column indicates the body surface area in square meters (m^2).

Box 29–3

Calculating Pediatric Drug Dosages Using Body Surface Area

Calculating a Single Pediatric Dose Ordered by Body Surface Area

1. Multiply recommended dosage (in milligrams or micrograms per m^2) by body surface area (m^2).
   Example: 2.5 (mg per m^2) × 0.8 (m^2) = 2 mg dose
2. Calculate the volume (tablets, solution) using a standard pharmaceutical math calculation (such as "desired over have multiplied by quantity" or ratio and proportion; see Chapter 28).

Calculating a Single Pediatric Dose From an Adult Dose Using Body Surface Area

1. Divide child's body surface area (m^2) by 1.73 (m^2) and then multiply it by adult dose.
   Example:

$$\frac{0.8\ m^2}{1.73\ m^2} \times 25\ \text{mg (adult dose)} = 11.56\ \text{mg (child's dose)}$$

2. Calculate volume (tablets, solution) using a standard pharmaceutical math calculation (such as "desired over have multiplied by quantity" or ratio and proportion; see Chapter 28).

NCLEX® 3. Medication volumes are typically not more than 0.5 mL for infant and 2 mL for large child; calculate doses to nearest hundredth and measure using a tuberculin syringe if less than 1 mL
4. Inject SubQ medications at 45-degree angle
5. Infants and toddlers need minimal to brief explanations but must be held securely for medication injection, as outlined previously in oral medication section
6. Preschoolers and young school-age children often understand reason for injection and benefit from simple explanations, distraction, and praise for their cooperation; restraint is on an as-needed basis

NCLEX® 7. Principles of administration not discussed in this section are same as for adult, including guidelines for aspiration before injecting and massaging site after administration (see Chapter 28)

B. Intramuscular

1. General principles are same as for SubQ injections; variations are presented here
   a. Site depends on age of child, amount of muscle mass, and volume of medication to be injected
   NCLEX® b. Typical volumes per single injection site are up to 0.5 mL for young infant, up to 1 mL for older infant or small children, and up to 2 mL in older (large) child
   NCLEX® c. Preferred injection site for infants is vastus lateralis muscle (middle third of anterior-lateral aspect of thigh)
   d. Dorsogluteal site can be used after child has been walking for 1 year, but it is not ideal for children under 5 years because these muscles are poorly developed
   e. Injection sites for older children and adolescents are same as for adult and include vastus lateralis, deltoid, and ventrogluteal muscles

V. INTRAVENOUS (IV) MEDICATIONS

NCLEX® A. **Always ensure that two mixed medications are compatible** and that medications and IV solutions are compatible

B. **Calculation of IV flow rates is often unnecessary due to use of pumps;** however, formula for calculation is same as for adults (volume multiplied by drop factor and divided by time in minutes)

C. **Principles for administration of IV medications to children** are same as for adults but with special considerations

1. For infants and children, place IV medications along with diluent in an IV administration set with a volume control chamber (such as a Soluset, Buretrol, Metriset); these sets have a small drop factor (60 drops/mL)
2. Take special care to ensure that tubing contains no air to prevent air injection into child's vein and subsequent air embolus

NCLEX® 3. Use an electronic controller or pump to regulate IV fluids and intermittent IV medications
4. When setting pump or controller, calculate volume of added medications into total volume (e.g., set 55 mL as volume to be infused if IV bag has 50 mL and 5 mL of medication has been added)
5. For intermittent medication infusions, select port close to child (ensures medication is delivered at proper time; with slowly running IVs, medication could take some time to travel from distal port to child's vein)

NCLEX® 6. Check on IV medication and site several times during administration to ensure that client is not experiencing side effects and that IV is patent with no infiltration

VI. PEDIATRIC CONSIDERATIONS FOR OTHER ROUTES

A. Ophthalmic

1. Young children fear anything being placed in eyes; communicate in a manner to reduce anxiety and promote cooperation during procedure
2. Take care to maintain sterility in a child who is less than cooperative
3. Apply ointment or drops as for adults and close eyelids to prevent leakage

NCLEX® 4. Encourage child not to squeeze eyes shut and have child lie quietly for 30 seconds

B. Otic

1. Use sterile technique if tympanic membrane is ruptured and draining

NCLEX® 2. For children under 3 years of age, pull pinna straight back and slightly downward to straighten ear canal

NCLEX® 3. For older children, pull pinna back and upward as for an adult

C. Nasal

1. Saline drops are commonly given to infants with nasal congestion
2. Because nasal medications drain into back of throat, they may cause tickling, bad taste, and occasional difficulty breathing

NCLEX® 3. Check child for choking or vomiting after instillation of drops

4. Keep child in same position for 5 minutes after administration to allow medication to contact nasal mucosa

D. Aerosol: as per adults

E. Rectal

1. If suppository needs to be cut in half, do so lengthwise
2. Obtain assistance if needed to keep child in side-lying position (or prone in parent's lap if small enough)
3. After lubricating, insert gently into rectum just beyond internal sphincter *NCLEX®*
4. Hold buttocks together until urge to expel medication has passed (5 to 10 minutes)

Check Your NCLEX–PN® Exam I.Q.

You are ready for testing on this content if you can

- Calculate pediatric medication dosages with accuracy.
- Verify dosage calculations before administering medications.
- Apply principles of medication administration to pediatric clients.

PRACTICE TEST

1 A 4-month-old client has an order for D_5 ½ NS IV to run at a rate of 40 mL/hr. While the unlicensed assistant obtains an infusion pump, the nurse sets the drip rate at____ drops/minute, using a Soluset with microdrip tubing that has a drop factor of 60 gtts/mL? Provide a numerical answer. Record your answer rounding to the nearest whole number.

Fill in your answer below:

________ drops/min

2 A 3½-month-old infant has an order for acetaminophen (Tylenol) suspension 45 mg by mouth q4h prn. The product label lists a concentration of 500mg/5mL. After determining that the dosage is safe, the nurse should administer____ mL? Record your answer rounding two decimal places.

Fill in your answer below:

________ mL

3 A 4-year-old client's medication order reads cefotaxime (Claforan) 1380 mg every 8 hours. The client weighs 13.8 kg. Which nursing action is appropriate if the safe dosage range for a child from 1 month to 12 years of age is listed as 100–200 mg/kg/day given in divided doses?

1. Give the dose as scheduled and document it appropriately.
2. Question the order for the excessively high dose.
3. Administer the slightly high dose but give it at half the recommended rate.
4. Withhold the dose and question the prescriber, since it is below the recommended range.

4 A 5-year-old client has an order for baclofen (Lioresal), one-half of a 10 mg tablet by mouth three times per day. The safe dose range for a 2–7-year-old child is 10–15 mg/day in divided doses. Which nursing action is most appropriate?

1. Question the total daily dose ordered.
2. Question the single dose ordered.
3. Refuse to give the dose because the child's weight is not factored into the dose.
4. Administer the dose as ordered.

5 A 3-year-old client has an order for 120 mg acetaminophen (Tylenol) every 4–6 hours prn for pain. The maximum total dose is 2.6 grams/day for a child of 2–3 years. The nurse could legally administer____ doses per 24-hour period? Record your answer rounding to the nearest whole number.

Fill in your answer below:

________ doses/24 hours

PRACTICE TEST

6 The 6-year-old client has an order for fexofenadine (Allegra) one half of a 60 mg tab by mouth twice daily. The nurse calculates the child's total daily dose as ____ milligrams? Record your answer rounding to the nearest whole number.

Fill in your answer below:

________ mg

7 The nurse is reviewing insulin administration techniques with a 13-year-old client with uncontrolled diabetes. The nurse evaluates that the client is using proper procedure after noting that the client performs which action during self-injection?

1. Aspirates before injection but does not massage the site following injection
2. Uses a 45-degree injection angle and aspirates before injection
3. Uses a 90-degree angle and massages the site following injection
4. Uses a 90-degree injection angle and does not massage the site following injection

8 A 15-year-old client admitted with dehydration has an order for a bolus infusion of 0.9% sodium chloride (normal saline, NS) 500 mL IV for 1 hour. An infusion device is available that counts the number of drops per minute delivered. The IV tubing has a drop factor of 10 drops/mL. If the bolus is to infuse on time, the nurse should set the drip rate to ____ drops per minute. Record your answer rounding to the nearest whole number.

Fill in your answer below:

________ drops/minute

9 A 6-year-old postoperative client has a medication order for cefazolin (Ancef) 500 mg every 6 hours. The client weighs 44 pounds. The safe dose range of cefazolin for a child is 25–100 mg/kg/day in 3 to 4 divided doses. The total daily dose that this client will receive is ____ mg/kg/day? Record your answer rounding to the nearest whole number.

Fill in your answer below:

________ mg/kg/day

10 A client has a medication order for ceftazidime (Fortaz) 250 mg every 8 hours. The client weighs 55 pounds. The safe dose range of ceftazidime for a child is 30–50 mg/kg/day in three divided doses. The total daily dose ordered for this client is ____ mg/kg/day? Record your answer rounding to the nearest whole number.

Fill in your answer below:

________ mg/kg/day

11 A child has an order to receive a bolus 0.9% sodium chloride (normal saline, NS) 400 mL IV. To infuse this volume over 90 minutes, the nurse should set the infusion pump at ____ mL/hour. Record your answer rounding to the nearest whole number.

Fill in your answer below:

________ mL/hr

12 The nurse is about to administer a dose of acetaminophen (Tylenol) 200 mg via nasogastric tube to a child. Available is a suspension with a concentration of 80 mg per 5 mL. The nurse should administer ____ mL to give the dose? Record your answer rounding to one decimal place.

Fill in your answer below:

________ mL

13 A pediatric client has been diagnosed with conjunctivitis. The nurse is to administer eye drops four times a day. The nurse should administer the medication by gently dropping the medication onto which area?

1. Center of the cornea
2. Sclera by the inner canthus
3. Sclera by the outer canthus
4. Lower conjunctival sac

14 A mother is to be taught to administer ear drops to her 4-month-old infant. The important concept in teaching would be to do which of the following?

1. Wear gloves when administering the ear drops.
2. Do not contaminate the bottle by touching the nozzle to the ear.
3. Turn the baby on its back after administration to avoid the risk of SIDS.
4. Pull the pinna gently downward and backward.

15 A 3-year-old client weighing 33 pounds is to receive liquid Advil (ibuprofen) 150 mg PO q6 hours prn for temperature above 101 degrees F. The nurse should administer ____ mL to the client from a bottle labeled 100 mg/5 mL? Record your answer rounding to one decimal place.

Fill in your answer below:

________ mL

ANSWERS & RATIONALES

1 **Answer: 40** **Rationale:** Use the following formula to calculate the rate of IV solutions:

$$\frac{\text{Volume} \times \text{drop factor}}{\text{Time (in minutes)}}$$

Set up the problem as follows:

$$\frac{40 \times 60}{60}$$

Multiply 40 by 60 to yield 2400 and divide 2400 by 60 (or cancel out the 60s) to yield 40 drops/minute. **Cognitive Level:** Applying **Client Need:** Pharmacological and Parenteral Therapies **Integrated Process:** Nursing Process: Implementation **Content Area:** Pharmacology **Strategy:** Use knowledge of basic IV calculation to set up the question. Calculate the problem carefully and double-check your answer for accuracy.

2 **Answer: .45** **Rationale:** The problem can be set up using the following formula:

$$\frac{45\,\text{mg (dose desired)}}{500\,\text{mg (available)}} \times \frac{x\text{(unknown)}}{5\text{ mL (quantity)}}$$

Multiply 500 by x and multiply 45 by 5 to yield $500x = 225$. Divide 225 by 500 to yield 0.45 mL **Cognitive Level:** Applying **Client Need:** Pharmacological and Parenteral Therapies **Integrated Process:** Nursing Process: Implementation **Content Area:** Pharmacology **Strategy:** Use knowledge of basic dosage calculation to set up the question. Calculate the problem carefully and double check your answer for accuracy.

3 **Answer: 2** **Rationale:** First calculate the daily dose of the medication by dividing the number of mg (1380) by the client's weight in kg (13.8) to yield a single dose of 100 mg/kg. Because there are three doses ordered during a 24-hour period, multiply 100 by 3 to yield 300 mg/kg/day. Since the dose range is 100 to 200 mg/kg/day, the dosage is excessively high and the nurse should question the order as part of safe nursing practice. **Cognitive Level:** Analyzing **Client Need:** Pharmacological and Parenteral Therapies **Integrated Process:** Nursing Process: Implementation **Content Area:** Pharmacology **Strategy:** Use knowledge of basic pediatric dosage calculation to set up the question. Calculate the problem carefully and double check your answer for accuracy. Remember that any dose that falls outside the safe dosage range needs to be questioned.

4 **Answer: 4** **Rationale:** The dose can be administered as ordered. The order for half of a 10 mg tab means that the child is receiving 5 mg per dose. If there are three doses per day, then the total daily dose is 15 mg, which is within the safe dosage range. The total daily dosage does not need to be questioned. The amount of the single dose does not need to be questioned. The drug does not require weight to be factored when determining the safe dose range. **Cognitive Level:** Analyzing **Client Need:** Pharmacological and Parenteral Therapies **Integrated Process:** Nursing Process: Implementation **Content Area:** Pharmacology **Strategy:** Use knowledge of basic pediatric dosage calculation to set up the question. Calculate the problem carefully and double check your answer for accuracy. Recall that any dose that falls within the safe dosage range may be administered.

5 **Answer: 6** **Rationale:** Convert 2.6 grams to 2600 mg. Since a single dose is only 120 mg, the client could theoretically receive this dose 21 times (2600 divided by 120 = 21.66) within a 24-hour period without exceeding the top of the dosage range. However, since the medication is ordered only every 4–6 hours, the nurse can legally administer the medication only six times maximum (every 4 hours). **Cognitive Level:** Analyzing **Client Need:** Pharmacological and Parenteral Therapies **Integrated Process:** Nursing Process: Planning **Content Area:** Pharmacology **Strategy:** Use knowledge of basic math calculations to determine your answer. If the drug can be given no more frequently than every 4 hours, it cannot exceed six doses, since 24 divided by 4 is 6.

6 **Answer: 60** **Rationale:** One half of a 60 mg tablet is 30 mg. Because the dose is ordered twice a day, the total daily dose is 30 multiplied by 2, or 60 mg. **Cognitive Level:** Analyzing **Client Need:** Pharmacological and Parenteral Therapies **Integrated Process:** Nursing Process: Implementation **Content Area:** Pharmacology **Strategy:** Use knowledge of basic math calculation to set up the problem. Calculate carefully and double check your answer for accuracy.

7 **Answer: 4** **Rationale:** Correct administration technique is to use a 90-degree angle (insulin syringes have a short, half-inch needle), avoiding aspiration before injection (e.g., to avoid tissue complications over time), and avoiding massaging the area after injection (which would enhance quicker absorption of the dose). **Cognitive Level:** Analyzing **Client Need:** Pharmacological and Parenteral Therapies **Integrated Process:** Nursing Process: Evaluation **Content Area:** Pharmacology **Strategy:** The core issue of the question is knowledge of subcutaneous injection techniques. Use the process of elimination and nursing knowledge to answer the question. To help eliminate incorrect answers, recall that insulin and heparin should not be massaged and that a 90-degree angle is used for injection.

8 **Answer: 83** **Rationale:** Since the infusion device delivers fluid in drops/min, the nurse must calculate the number at which to set the machine. The formula to use is:

$$\frac{\text{Volume} \times \text{drop factor}}{\text{Time in minutes}}$$

Thus, the problem should be set up as follows:

$$\frac{500 \times 10}{60}$$

Multiply 500 by 10 to yield 5000 and divide it by 60 to obtain a flow rate of 83.33 gtts/min, which rounds down to 83 drops/minute. **Cognitive Level:** Analyzing **Client Need:** Pharmacological and Parenteral Therapies **Integrated Process:** Nursing Process: Implementation **Content Area:** Pharmacology **Strategy:** Use knowledge of basic IV calculation procedures to set up the question. Calculate the problem carefully and double check your answer for accuracy.

9 **Answer: 100** **Rationale:** First convert the client's weight to kg by dividing 44 by 2.2 to yield a weight of 20 kg. Then calculate the daily dose of the medication by dividing the number of mg (500) by the client's weight in kg (20) to yield a single dose of 25 mg/kg. Because there are four doses (every 6 hours) ordered during a 24-hour period, multiply 25 by 4 to yield a total daily dose of 100 mg/kg/day. **Cognitive Level:** Analyzing **Client Need:** Pharmacological and Parenteral Therapies **Integrated Process:** Nursing Process: Implementation **Content Area:** Pharmacology **Strategy:** Use knowledge of basic dosage calculation to set up the question. Calculate the problem carefully and double-check your answer for accuracy.

10 **Answer: 30** **Rationale:** First convert the child's weight to kg by dividing 55 by 2.2 to yield a weight of 25 kg. Then calculate the daily dose of the medication by dividing the mg (250) by the client's weight in kg (25) to yield a single dose of 10 mg/kg. Because there are three doses (every 8 hours) ordered during a 24-hour period, multiply 10 by 3 to yield a total daily dose of 30 mg/kg/day. **Cognitive Level:** Analyzing **Client Need:** Pharmacological and Parenteral Therapies **Integrated Process:** Nursing Process: Implementation **Content Area:** Pharmacology **Strategy:** Use knowledge of basic pediatric dosage calculation to set up the question. Calculate the problem carefully and double check your answer for accuracy.

11 **Answer: 267** **Rationale:** Since the infusion pump delivers fluid in mL/hour, the nurse must calculate the equivalent hourly rate when infusing the 400 mL over 90 minutes. The problem can be set up as follows to cancel out the labels and end up with mL/hour:

$$\frac{400\text{ mL (volume)}}{90\text{ minutes (time)}} \times \frac{60\text{ minutes}}{1\text{ hours}}$$

Multiply 400 by 60 to yield 24,000 and divide it by 90 (90 × 1) to obtain an equivalent hourly flow rate of 266.66 or 267 mL/hr. **Cognitive Level:** Analyzing **Client Need:** Pharmacological and Parenteral Therapies **Integrated Process:** Nursing Process: Implementation **Content Area:** Pharmacology **Strategy:** Use knowledge of basic math calculation to set up the question. Read the question carefully, noting that the time needs to convert from minutes to hours in order to have the correct labeling. Calculate the problem carefully and double-check your answer for accuracy.

12 **Answer: 12.5** **Rationale:** The problem can be set up using ratio and proportion as follows:

$$\frac{200\text{ mg (dose desired)}}{80\text{ mg (available)}} = \frac{x\text{(unknown)}}{5\text{ mL (quantity)}}$$

Multiply 80 by x and multiply 200 by 5 to yield $80x = 1000$. Divide 1,000 by 80 to yield 12.5 mL **Cognitive Level:** Analyzing **Client Need:** Pharmacological and Parenteral Therapies **Integrated Process:** Nursing Process: Implementation **Content Area:** Pharmacology **Strategy:** Use knowledge of basic pediatric dosage calculation to set up the question. Calculate the problem carefully and double check your answer for accuracy.

13 **Answer: 4** **Rationale:** Eye drops are placed in the lower conjunctival sac to prevent damage to the cornea and to facilitate coating the eye with the medication. Eye drops are not placed in the center of the cornea. Eye drops are not placed in the sclera by the inner canthus. Eye drops are not placed in the sclera by the outer canthus. **Cognitive Level:** Applying **Client Need:** Pharmacological and Parenteral Therapies **Integrated Process:** Nursing Process: Implementation **Content Area:** Pharmacology **Strategy:** The correct option describes the area of the eye that will allow the medication to remain in contact with the infected area.

14 **Answer: 4** **Rationale:** Pulling the ear pinna down and back straightens the ear canal allowing the drops to enter the ear. It is unnecessary to wear gloves. The ear canal is not sterile so this is not as important as ear position. Turning the baby on the back is not as important for medication administration as technique. **Cognitive Level:** Analyzing **Client Need:** Pharmacological and Parenteral Therapies **Integrated Process:** Nursing Process: Implementation **Content Area:** Pharmacology **Strategy:** Note that the correct option has the most direct relationship to the actual teaching needed to accomplish the task.

15 **Answer: 7.5** **Rationale:** Use the following formula to calculate:

$$\frac{100\text{ mg}}{5\text{ mL}} = \frac{150\text{ mg}}{x\text{ mL}}$$

$$100x = 750$$

$$x = 7.5\text{ mL}$$

Cognitive Level: Analyzing **Client Need:** Pharmacological and Parenteral Therapies **Integrated Process:** Nursing Process: Planning **Content Area:** Pharmacology **Strategy:** Use ratio and proportion or dimensional analysis to solve the problem.

ANSWERS & RATIONALES

Key Terms to Review

body surface area (BSA) p. 432 **nomogram** p. 432

References

Giangrasso, A., & Shrimpton, D. (2010). *Ratio & proportion dosage calculations.* Upper Saddle River, NJ: Pearson Education, Inc.

Olson, J., Giangrasso, A. & Shrimpton, D. (2012). *Medical dosage calculations: A dimensional analysis approach* (10th ed.). Upper Saddle River, NJ: Pearson Education, Inc.

Pickar, G. & Abernethy, A. (2008). *Dosage calculations: A ratio-proportion approach* (3rd ed.). Clifton Park, NY: Delmar Learning.

Smith, R., Duell, D., & Martin, B. (2012). *Clinical nursing skills: Basic to advanced skills* (8th ed.). Upper Saddle River, NJ: Prentice Hall.

Test Yourself

Are you ready for the NCLEX-PN® or course exams? Use the practice tests on the companion website to check.

30 Intravenous Therapy

In this chapter

Cross Reference

Another chapter relevant to this content area is
Fluid and Electrolyte Imbalances **Chapter 49**

I. OVERVIEW OF INTRAVENOUS (IV) THERAPY

A. Indications

1. Replaces fluid and electrolytes for clients unable to have oral intake (such as NPO status for diagnostic or surgical procedures or problems related to swallowing or GI tract)
2. Provides a route for peripheral parenteral nutrition (PPN) in peripheral veins or total parenteral nutrition (TPN) in central veins for clients with increased caloric needs, such as with severe burns or other conditions requiring increased caloric needs above what can be taken orally
3. IV route can be used to give medications that would be destroyed by GI tract or are too irritating to be given by another route, to avoid discomfort of frequent intramuscular (IM) injections, or to maintain a constant blood level of a medication
4. In life-threatening situations, it provides rapid access to administer medications and fluids directly into bloodstream, ensuring prompt onset of action and most complete absorption

B. Types of fluids provided by IV route

1. Hydrating solutions (see Table 30–1)
2. Total parenteral nutrition (TPN)

C. Equipment needed for IV therapy

1. Catheters and needles
   a. Over-the-needle catheters: 16- to 26-gauge plastic catheter fits over a needle that pierces skin and vein; once in vein, needle is withdrawn and discarded, leaving catheter in place; available in a variety of lengths and gauges; use smallest appropriate length and gauge of catheter
   b. Winged needle or butterfly: steel needle with plastic flaps (wings) attached to shaft to facilitate venipuncture; commonly used to obtain some blood samples or for short-term therapy
   c. These devices come in protected needle styles designed to protect health care workers from accidental needlesticks and blood exposure

Table 30–1 Hydrating Solutions

Solution	Uses	Nursing Implications
Isotonic 0.9% sodium chloride (normal saline or NS) Lactated Ringer's (LR) 5% dextrose in water (D_5W)	Has same concentration of solutes as plasma, so it remains in vascular compartment, expanding vascular volume NS and LR are crystalloid solutions that ↑ fluid volume in both intravascular and interstitial spaces with minimal fluid volume expansion NS is the only solution to be administered with blood products D_5W is isotonic on initial administration but provides free water when metabolized, expanding intra- and extracellular fluid volumes	Assess for signs of hypervolemia • Bounding pulse • Shortness of breath • Distended neck veins Assess for signs of hypovolemia • Urine output < 30 mL/hr • Weak, thready pulse • Subnormal temperature • Flat neck veins
Hypotonic 0.45% sodium chloride (½ NS) 0.225% sodium chloride (¼ NS)	Has lesser concentration of solutes than plasma, so treats cellular dehydration through fluid shifting out of blood vessels into cells; promotes elimination by kidneys	Do not administer to clients at risk for third-space fluid shift or fluid sequestration in a body space (results in circulating volume loss and ↑ risk for organ failure or ↑ intracranial pressure)
Hypertonic 5% dextrose in normal saline (D_5NS) 5% dextrose in 0.45% sodium chloride (D_5½NS) 5% dextrose in lactated Ringer's (D_5LR) 10% dextrose in water ($D_{10}W$) 20% dextrose in water ($D_{20}W$) 50% dextrose in water ($D_{50}W$)	Has higher concentration of solutes than plasma, thus causing fluid to shift from cells into vascular compartment, expanding vascular volume 10% dextrose—stand-by solution for clients receiving TPN 50% dextrose—used for hypoglycemia	Do not administer to clients with kidney or heart disease or clients who are dehydrated; monitor for signs of hypervolemia
Volume Expanders (colloid solutions) Albumin 5% (Buminate 5%) Albumin 25% (Buminate 25%) Dextran 40 (Gentran 40) Hetastarch (Hespan [HESI]) Plasma protein fraction (Plasmanate, others)	Colloid solutions contain substances that cannot diffuse through capillary walls, resulting in ↑ plasma volume and ↑ osmotic pressure, causing fluids to move into vascular compartment; used to treat hypovolemic shock	Establish baseline vital signs, lung and heart sounds, and central venous pressure; repeat per agency protocols Administer with a large-gauge (18–19 gauge) needle Monitor intake and output Monitor for signs of hypervolemia
Nutrient 5% dextrose (D_5W) 5% dextrose in 0.45% sodium chloride (D_5½NS)	Contain some form of carbohydrate (e.g., dextrose, glucose) and water D_5W provides 170 calories per liter	Useful in preventing dehydration but does not provide sufficient calories to promote wound healing, weight gain, or normal growth in children
Electrolyte 0.9% sodium chloride (NS) Ringer's solution (has sodium, chloride, potassium, calcium) 5% dextrose in 0.45% sodium chloride (D_5 ½NS)	Saline and electrolytes restore vascular volume and replace electrolytes LR is also an alkalinizing solution that treats metabolic acidosis (D_5½NS) is an acidifying solution to treat metabolic alkalosis	Monitor fluid and electrolytes Monitor arterial blood gases Monitor intake and output

2. Infusion pumps and electronic delivery devices (EDDs)
   a. Deliver fluids by exerting positive pressure on tubing or fluid to maintain fluid flow despite increased venous resistance
   b. Regulate rate at preset limits; alarms are triggered when fluid level is low, air is in line, or an occlusion is present
   c. Must be used when volume needs to be carefully controlled, and is commonly used on all IV infusions per agency policy
3. Regulators, controllers, and mechanical infusion devices
   a. Devices designed to aid in monitoring IV flow rates
   b. Regulators are in-line devices in which flow rate is set by a dial instead of relying on gravity flow drip counting
   c. Controllers sense drops that flow from bag of fluid into drip chamber

d. Mechanical infusion devices include elastomeric balloon and spring-coil piston devices; these disposable devices control speed of infusion by size of tubing; often used with home infusions to simplify medication administration
e. These devices are convenience devices and should not be used when flow rate must be carefully regulated

4. Tubing: may be vented or nonvented
   a. Vented tubing is used with glass bottles; nonvented is used with plastic bags
   b. When infusions flow by gravity, drip chamber of tubing determines size of drop
   c. Drip chambers commonly are rated at 10, 12, 15, or 20 drops per mL; pediatric sets usually are rated at 60 drops per mL
5. Filters: devices that may be part of infusion set or an addition to infusion line; filters remove contaminants (air, bacteria, or particulate matter); not all medications or solutions can or must be filtered
   a. *NCLEX®* TPN requires a filter change every 24 hours when tubing is changed
   b. *NCLEX®* Some medications, such as phenytoin (Dilantin) and pantoprazole (Protonix), require a filter change with each dose
   c. *NCLEX®* A filter must be used whenever blood is transfused; many blood administration sets have an in-line filter, but be sure one is used
   d. To prime a filter, point filter downward so proximal half fills with fluid first, then invert to complete priming

II. TYPES OF INTRAVENOUS INFUSIONS

A. Peripheral *intravenous* infusion

1. IV device with an internal tip that terminates in a peripheral vein
2. In adults, internal tip lies between fingertips and shoulder
3. Some fluids and medications cannot be administered by peripheral line because of fluid characteristics
4. Peripheral devices are usually rotated every 3 to 4 days, according to agency policy and current evidence-based practice

B. Central intravenous infusion

1. IV device with an internal tip that lies in central venous system; these can include such catheters as central venous catheter (CVC) or peripherally inserted central catheter (PICC line)
2. Internal tip most commonly ends at superior vena cava
3. These devices can remain in place for long periods of time
4. Any fluid or medication that can be given IV can be given via a central line
5. *NCLEX®* Most central lines require sterile dressings to reduce risk of contamination; agency policy and type of dressing determine frequency of dressing changes

C. Continuous infusion: an uninterrupted infusion that runs 24 hours a day

D. Intermittent infusion

1. An infusion designed for clients who do not require IV fluid replacement therapy but require an IV access
2. An intermittent infusion device (saline lock or prn adapter) is fitted to end of IV catheter providing a connection for intermittent solution or medication administration
3. These devices require a saline flush at least once every 8 hours and before and after medication administration
4. Some central lines require saline flush be followed by a heparin flush (10 units/mL or 100 units/mL solutions) per agency policy to maintain patency of device

III. PROCEDURES AND SKILLS FOR INTRAVENOUS THERAPY

A. Preparing for IV therapy

1. Verify allergies, such as latex
2. Gather equipment (IV catheter, tourniquet, alcohol and cleansing wipes, sterile tape, gauze or semipermeable transparent membrane dressing materials, IV fluid and appropriate tubing, filter if indicated, pump and regulator device as appropriate, and gloves)
3. Wash hands
4. Verify type and amount of solution with physician's order; note expiration date
5. Prepare equipment
   a. Obtain needleless adapter to connect to venous access device if device does not include one
   b. Remove outer wrappers from tubing, connect tubing and filter device, and close tubing roller clamp

NCLEX®
c. Remove outer wrapper around IV bag; inspect bag for leaks (small amount of condensation is normal), tears, discoloration, cloudiness, or particulate matter; do not use bag if any of these conditions are present
d. Hang IV bag on pole
e. Using aseptic technique, remove port cap on IV bag and plastic protector from IV tubing spike (end with drip chamber) and insert spike into IV bag
f. Squeeze drip chamber until it is partially full
g. Remove protective cap on tubing if it is not an air-vented cap, open roller clamp on tubing to prime tubing and filter; invert and tap Y injection sites to remove air during priming, replace protective tubing cap
h. If solution to be hung is in a glass bottle (such as to administer medication that would absorb into plastic IV bag), use vented tubing, or solution will not infuse

B. Inserting an IV line

1. Follow agency policy when starting and maintaining an IV
2. NCLEX® Wear gloves for protection from blood-borne pathogens
3. Prepare client for infusion, explain procedure, and obtain client's permission for procedure
4. Identify appropriate vein for cannulation
   a. In adults, peripheral IVs are inserted in arm or hand from proximal metacarpals to shoulder depending on age
   b. Peripheral IVs in children can also include scalp and leg veins
   c. Avoid sites where veins are sclerotic, inflamed, or have decreased blood flow (common in adults following a stroke or mastectomy on that side)
5. Use tourniquet to distend vessel
   a. NCLEX® Verify absence of latex allergy before applying
   b. In absence of a tourniquet, a blood pressure cuff may be used
   c. Some older adult clients may be accessed without a tourniquet
   d. Place tourniquet 4 to 6 inches above proposed site tightly enough to obstruct venous circulation but not arterial circulation (use light stroking, gravity, and/or topical heat application to aid vein distention)
6. Prepare skin; clean site with alcohol followed by cleansing agent such as povidone-iodine or chlorhexidine wipe; clean skin in a circular manner, starting at inside and moving outward, to remove bacteria from insertion site; allow cleansing agent to dry on skin for up to 2 minutes
7. Introduce needle at a 10- to 30-degree angle with bevel up; once blood return occurs, hold needle still and advance catheter by pushing it forward off needle until hub is in contact with insertion site
8. Release tourniquet and remove needle from catheter
9. Connect catheter to IV tubing and apply sterile dressing to insertion site (tape is no longer recommended to secure catheter first); apply label to dressing that identifies length and gauge of catheter, date and time of insertion, and nurse's initials
10. Complete and apply date sticker to IV tubing
11. Initiate prescribed flow rate: gravity flow tubing is regulated by drops per minute, and drops delivered per mL of solution vary with different brands and types of infusion sets (drop factor) from 10 to 20 drops/mL; microdrip sets are always 60 drops/mL; to administer 1000 mL in 8 hours with a drop factor of 15 drops/mL, calculate as follows:

$$\frac{\text{Total infusion volume} \times \text{drop factor}}{\text{Total time of infusion in minutes}} = \text{drops} > \text{minute}$$

$$\frac{1000\text{ mL} \times 15}{8 \times 60\text{ min (480 min)}} = 31.25\text{ drops} > \text{min (31 drops} > \text{minute)}$$

12. Dispose of sharps in rigid sharps disposal container
13. Document date, time, solution, amount, infusion device, rate, site location, and condition of site and dressing

C. Maintaining an IV infusion

1. Ensure that correct solution is infusing
2. Check rate of flow hourly or more often per policy for selected situations
3. Inspect patency of IV tubing and needle
4. Maintain solution container 3 feet above IV site for gravity infusion devices; keep bag higher than IV pump when using a pump

5. Inspect tubing for kinks or obstructions; ensure tubing is not hanging below IV site
6. Check for blood return by lowering solution container below IV site and observe for blood return, or use a sterile syringe to withdraw fluid from port nearest venipuncture site, causing blood to flow into tubing
7. Splint a joint if IV is positional (movement of arm impedes flow of solution)
8. Ensure tight connections to prevent leakage
9. Discontinue solution and remove IV access device if there is no blood return and acceptable drip rate cannot be established
10. *NCLEX®* Inspect insertion site for fluid infiltration (IV access device becomes dislodged from vessel, causing fluid to flow into interstitial tissues and other complications); see Table 30–2 for list of complications and associated nursing care
11. Instruct client to notify the nurse of these conditions:
    a. Flow rate changes or solution stops dripping
    b. Solution container is nearly empty
    c. There is blood in IV tubing or at insertion site
    d. There is discomfort or swelling at insertion site
12. At least every 8 hours, document solution, amount, infusion device, rate, site location, and condition of site and dressing

Table 30–2 Complications of IV Therapy

Complication	Nursing Implications
Infection (catheter-related) (sepsis)—common occurrence with TPN solutions that have high glucose concentration that invites bacteria; characterized by fever, chills, erythema, or drainage at insertion site, elevated white blood count, and possibly septic shock	Use strict aseptic technique when working with IVs. Change IV solutions at least every 24 hours. Change IV tubing and dressings per agency protocols (TPN tubing every day). When discontinuing central line, remove catheter and apply an occlusive dressing. Monitor site for 48 hours; catheter tip may be sent to lab for culture if sepsis is suspected.
Air embolism—air is introduced into IV line during catheter insertion, tubing change, or administration of solutions and medications; characterized by respiratory distress, chest pain, dyspnea, hypotension, and weak and rapid pulse	When changing tubing or reflux valves on CVADs without Groshong valves or catheters, instruct client to perform Valsalva maneuver (forcefully exhale with glottis, nose, and mouth closed). Ensure all catheter connections are tight. Ensure all connections on central lines are luer lock, not slip lock. During insertion of a percutaneous CVC, position client in head down position with head turned in opposite direction of insertion site. If an air embolism is suspected, clamp the catheter, position the client in left Trendelenburg's position, administer oxygen, and contact physician.
Hypersensitivity reaction—sensitivity to medication; characterized by flushing, itching, and urticaria	Check client allergies prior to administering medications. Stop the infusion and check vital signs. Notify the physician and continue to monitor client.
Circulatory overload—also called speed shock; fluids are administered faster than circulation can accommodate; characterized by cough, dyspnea, crackles, distended neck veins, tachycardia, hypertension, S_3 heart sounds, and cardiac rhythm	Use IV pumps or controllers to regulate infusion rate. Do not "catch up" with IV solutions that fall behind schedule. Carefully monitor fluid volumes when administering multiple concurrent IV solutions or medications. Check client's IV infusion rates at least hourly per agency protocols. Avoid selecting an IV container with a larger volume than volume ordered. Monitor client's vital signs, intake and output, breath and heart sounds. For signs and symptoms of fluid volume overload: slow or stop infusion rate per order, place client in high Fowler's position, administer oxygen and diuretics per order, and notify physician.
Infiltration—localized swelling, coolness, pallor, and discomfort at IV site	Stop IV and remove venous access device. Apply a warm compress to infiltration site and elevate arm on a pillow. Restart infusion at another site.

Table 30-2 Complications of IV Therapy *(continued)*

Complication	Nursing Implications
Phlebitis—inflammation of a vein; characterized by warmth, swelling, red streak at vein site, pain along course of the vein, and localized warmth	Inspect and palpate IV site at least every 8 hours for redness; if phlebitis is detected, discontinue infusion and remove venous access device. A medical order is not required to remove and replace a peripheral catheter that shows symptoms of phlebitis. Apply warm compresses to venipuncture site. Select a large vein when administering irritating solutions or medications. Dilute irritating medications (e.g., promethazine [Phenergan]) and administer over prescribed amount of time on an infusion pump; if client reports pain at site, further dilute medication and slow the flow rate.
Hypoglycemia—↓ blood glucose (BG) level related to TPN being abruptly discontinued or excessive insulin administration; characterized by BG less than 70 mg/dL, hunger, diaphoresis, weakness, anxiety	Monitor blood glucose per agency protocols (at least every day). Gradually decrease infusion when discontinuing TPN. Have 10% dextrose available as stand-by (medical order required for prn use).
Hyperglycemia—↑ BG related to TPN administration or use of excessive solutions in diabetic clients; characterized by BG greater than 200 mg/dL, excessive thirst, fatigue, restlessness, confusion, weakness, and diuresis	Monitor blood glucose per agency protocols (at least every day). Check medications affecting blood glucose levels (e.g., steroids). Begin infusion at a slow rate (40 mL/hr) and gradually increase. Do not "catch up" if infusion rate falls behind.

IV. CENTRAL VENOUS ACCESS DEVICES (CVADS)

A. A CVAD enters a central vein that empties into superior vena cava; placement can occur in numerous settings but all placements must be verified by x-ray

1. Percutaneous (nontunneled) catheter: a single or multiple lumen catheter is inserted by physician at client's bedside
2. Tunneled catheter
   a. Terminates in a central vein
   b. Remainder of catheter passes through a subcutaneous tract and exits on chest or abdominal wall
   c. Dacron cuff triggers scar formation that prevents ascending tract infection
   d. Does not require a sterile dressing once subcutaneous tract has healed
3. PICC
   a. Inserted into basilic or cephalic vein just above or below antecubital space of right arm by a physician or specially trained IV therapy nurse
   b. Used for longer term inpatient or outpatient therapy
   c. Although insertion site is in periphery, catheter terminates in superior vena cava
4. Implantable venous access devices or ports
   a. Surgically implanted into small subcutaneous pocket, usually on upper chest using local anesthesia
   b. Port is attached to catheter that terminates in a central vein
   c. Most subcutaneous ports are accessed with a Huber needle to prolong life of port's septum
5. Mid-line venous access device
   a. Is a shorter version of a PICC, with catheter terminating in axilla
   b. Used for two weeks or fewer and cannot be used for medications or fluids that are irritants or vesicants
6. Peripheral access system (PAS) ports are similar to a subcutaneous port except port itself is implanted in antecubital area

B. Internal tips: internal tip of catheter comes in two versions

1. Open-tipped: end of catheter opens directly into bloodstream; if flushing techniques are not performed correctly, blood can back up into catheter causing occlusion; there are two types of open-tipped catheters; they must be flushed with saline followed by heparin flush solution to maintain patency when not in use
   a. Hickman: adult form of open-tipped catheter
   b. Broviac: pediatric version, which usually means smaller lumen size
2. Closed-tip catheter or Groshong: has a valve on its internal tip that prevents backflow of blood; Groshong catheters are routinely flushed with double volumes of saline but do not require heparin flush solution; advantages are
   a. Decreased risk of air emboli or bleeding
   b. Elimination of heparin flush

c. Elimination of catheter clamping
d. Reduced flushing protocols between use

C. **Lumens: central catheters may have a single, double, triple, or quadruple lumen;** each lumen corresponds to a separate catheter and has a separate exit point
1. Multiple lumens allow for administration of incompatible drugs
2. Blood drawn from one lumen will not be contaminated by drugs administered through another lumen of catheter
3. Each lumen is treated as a separate catheter and is flushed according to agency policy

D. **Indications for use of CVAD**
1. Long-term IV therapy
2. Obtaining frequent blood specimens
3. Central venous pressure (CVP) monitoring
4. Administration of TPN and medications that are irritating to veins, thus requiring a high-flow vein for rapid dilution
5. Sclerosed peripheral veins
6. Limited peripheral venous access

E. **Nursing care**

NCLEX®
1. Take special precautions with all CVADs to ensure asepsis and catheter patency; refer again to Table 30–2 for complications
2. Site care: subclavian, jugular, and PICC sites
a. Require air occlusive dressings: dressings should be changed when soiled or loose

NCLEX®
b. Follow agency protocol for frequency of dressing changes—usually every 2 to 7 days; gauze dressings must be changed at least every 48 hours; semipermeable transparent membrane dressings may remain in place for up to 1 week
c. Follow agency protocol for cleaning solution and types of dressing; isopropyl alcohol followed by an antiseptic are often used to clean insertion site
d. Using surgical asepsis and a mask, clean area 2 inches in diameter around site using alcohol swab; use a circular motion starting at center and work outward; allow to dry, clean with approved antiseptic; allow to dry, then apply air occlusive dressing over entire insertion site

NCLEX®
e. Monitor site for redness, swelling, tenderness, or drainage, and compare length of external portion of catheter with its documented length to assess for displacement
f. Document date, condition of site, and dressing
3. Site care: implantable devices
a. Follow agency protocols for cleaning solutions and types of dressings; isopropyl alcohol and approved antiseptic are often used to clean insertion site

NCLEX®
b. Monitor site for redness, swelling, tenderness, or drainage
4. Client teaching: reinforce these instructions:
a. Do not allow anyone to measure BP on arm with a PICC or mid-line catheter or PAS port
b. Wear a Medic-Alert bracelet if device will be implanted for a long time
c. PICC, midline catheters, and nonimplanted CVADs: there is no activity restriction but do not immerse site in water
d. Implanted CVADs: no restriction of activities is necessary; there are no restrictions regarding bathing or swimming when device is not accessed

V. INTRAVENOUS MEDICATION ADMINISTRATION

A. **Mixtures of medications within large volumes of IV fluids** provide and maintain a constant, well-diluted level of a medication in bloodstream

B. **To add medication to an IV solution,** prepare medication from a vial or ampule and draw into a syringe

C. **To add medication to a new IV container**
1. Clean injection port with an alcohol swab and let dry for 30 seconds
2. Remove needle cap from syringe, insert needle through center of injection port, and inject medication into IV solution
3. Mix medication and solution by gently rotating bag
4. Complete and attach a medication label to IV solution, with drug name and dose, date and time, and nurse's initials
5. Proceed with setting up IV for administration

D. **To add medication to an existing infusion**
1. Ensure there is sufficient IV solution to properly dilute medication
2. Proceed as with adding a medication to a new IV container

E. Tandem infusion (not often used)

1. An intermittent method of administering medications through an existing IV
2. Ensure that existing IV solution and intermittent infusion are compatible and client's condition, vein, and gauge of access device can tolerate volume of fluid
3. Medication will be administered in a second bag of fluid, usually 50 to 100 mL, by secondary line into Y port of a continuously running infusion; attach a needleless adapter to tubing of secondary set
4. Cleanse Y port of continuous infusion line with an alcohol swab and let dry for 30 seconds
5. Hang secondary infusion and existing infusion at same level
6. Maintain existing IV rate and regulate piggyback rate using roller clamp on secondary tubing; primary and secondary solutions will run concurrently at their respective rates

F. Piggyback infusion

1. To administer intermittent infusion without disconnecting existing IV
   a. Set up secondary set following procedure for setting up an IV
   b. Hang existing infusion set lower than piggyback secondary set
   c. Cleanse upper infusion port with alcohol swab and let dry for 30 seconds
   d. Connect secondary set to primary set using a needleless adapter placed above existing IV roller clamp
   e. Maintain existing IV roller clamp position, and regulate piggyback rate using roller clamp on secondary tubing; piggyback solution will infuse first, and when complete, existing IV will resume at original rate
2. To administer an intermittent infusion using an infusion pump that is regulating existing IV:
   a. When intermittent solution is in an IV bag, set up secondary administration set following procedure for setting up an IV; connect infusion tubing to secondary access port on pump; follow protocols for specific pump for administering intermittent medication as either a continuous infusion or an infusion interrupting existing IV
   b. When intermittent solution is in a syringe, connect syringe to secondary access port on pump; follow protocols for specific pump for administering intermittent medication as either a continuous infusion or an infusion interrupting existing IV

VI. SPECIAL CONSIDERATIONS IN IV THERAPY

A. IV lines increase risk of bacteremia and sepsis by breaking skin as a line of defense

B. Various preparations (such as Emla cream or intradermal lidocaine) may be used to numb site before IV insertion, but these are considered to be drugs and must be ordered by a health care provider

C. Solutions and medications administered by IV route act within seconds to minutes and cannot be retrieved once infused or injected

D. It is a critical nursing responsibility to ensure that medications and IV solutions are compatible before administration; this includes any additives (such as potassium) to an IV line, not only primary solution and intermittent medication

E. The young and old are at greater risk of circulatory overload as a speed-related complication of IV infusion

F. Clients who have cardiac, renal, respiratory, or liver disease may also be at greater risk of circulatory overload as a speed-related complication of IV infusion

NCLEX®

G. Certain IV additives should be avoided in specific disease states

1. Clients with diabetes mellitus should not receive dextrose
2. Clients with heart failure or otherwise at risk for excess fluid volume should not receive sodium in IV fluids; if sodium-containing solutions are necessary, they should be infused cautiously and with use of an IV pump
3. Clients with liver disease should not receive lactated Ringer's because of possible lack of ability to convert lactate to bicarbonate
4. Clients with renal failure should not receive potassium additives in IV solutions because they cannot excrete it

VII. MONITORING BLOOD TRANSFUSIONS

A. General blood transfusion principles

1. LPN/LVNs may assist in blood transfusion therapy according to state law, usually participating in monitoring of client status; an RN prepares and administers transfusions
2. Common blood products include packed red blood cells (RBCs), fresh frozen plasma, platelets, and albumin; client's blood is typed and cross-matched to ensure compatible blood product is transfused

3. All agencies have policies and procedures related to blood product procurement and use; unlicensed personnel may sign blood out of blood bank if allowed by agency policy
4. IV catheter must be 20-gauge or larger to accommodate red blood cell transfusion without hemolyzing red blood cells
5. No medications may be added to blood product; only 0.9% sodium chloride (isotonic or "normal" saline) IV solution may be used to hang blood or blood product
6. A filter is used for every blood transfusion; this is standardly built into blood administration tubing
7. Blood products should be started within 30 minutes of receipt from blood bank, infused within specified time period (usually within 2 hours for packed RBCs, but not longer than 4 hours for a single unit)

B. Transfusion reactions

1. Monitor client for transfusion reaction: types of reaction are hypersensitivity, hemolytic, febrile, and bacterial reactions (see Table 30-3)
2. Prescreen clients for risk by asking whether they have ever had a transfusion, a reaction to it, and what the symptoms were
3. Management of transfusion reaction
   a. Stop transfusion of blood or blood product
   b. Maintain IV access with infusion of normal saline (0.9% sodium chloride)
   c. Monitor client and measure vital signs as often as every 5 minutes; do not leave client unattended
   d. Ensure that RN, blood bank, and health care provider are notified
   e. Provide supportive care and be ready to administer medications according to type of reaction; see Table 30–3
   f. Blood sample may be drawn from client per policy for culture, retyping, and/or Hgb/Hct levels; a urine specimen may be obtained for Hgb measurement; observe voidings for hematuria
   g. Return blood product bag, tubing, labels, and transfusion record to blood bank

C. Other complications

1. Circulatory overload (formerly called speed shock)
   a. Results from excessively rapid infusion of blood product beyond what client's circulatory system can tolerate
   b. Data collection: signs of fluid overload, including tachycardia and bounding pulse, hypertension, distended neck veins, crackles upon lung auscultation, dyspnea, and possibly cough
   c. Management: slow infusion rate; elevate head of bed to upright with feet dependent; note irregular pulse or cardiac dysrhythmias; notify RN; supportive care includes orders for oxygen and diuretics; morphine sulfate may be prescribed for vasodilating effect

Table 30–3 Blood Transfusion Reactions

Type and Cause	Assessment	Management
Hypersensitivity (antibodies in donor blood)	Fever Urticaria Anaphylactic shock	Airway management/oxygen Supportive care including treatment of shock state Diphenhydramine (Benadryl)
Febrile (nonspecific and most common)		Premedication with acetaminophen (Tylenol) or aspirin Airway management/oxygen Supportive care
Hemolytic (blood incompatibility)	Nausea and vomiting Lower back pain Tachycardia Hypotension Hematuria and ↓ urine output	Airway management/oxygen Supportive care Diphenhydramine (Benadryl)
Bacterial (septicemia from contaminated blood product)	Fever and chills Tachycardia Hypotension/shock	Blood culture Antibiotic therapy Fluid resuscitation Vasopressors Corticosteroids

2. Electrolyte imbalances
   a. Hyperkalemia can occur when potassium is released from hemolyzed cells in stored blood; monitor serum potassium level and signs of hyperkalemia (see Chapter 49); if noted, slow transfusion rate, notify RN or health care provider, and monitor cardiac status
   b. Hypocalcemia can occur when calcium binds with citrate in banked blood and is excreted; clients receiving multiple transfusions are at greater risk; monitor serum calcium level and for signs of hypocalcemia (see Chapter 49); if noted, slow transfusion rate, notify RN or health care provider, and assess client if signs of hypocalcemia occur (such as twitching of cheek, called Chvostek's sign)
   c. Iron overload can occur with repeated transfusions; is considered a delayed complication; findings include nausea and vomiting, hypotension, and elevated serum iron level; treated with desferoxamine (Desferal) subQ or IV to clear iron via kidneys; urine will appear red during excretion of iron

VIII. DISCONTINUING AN IV

A. Indications

1. Client is able to take fluids orally
2. IV medication is no longer needed
3. Access route for emergency fluid and drug administration is no longer needed

B. Procedure

1. Gather equipment: (2 × 2 gauze, clean gloves, and tape)
2. Explain procedure to client
3. Turn off IV infusion
4. Apply gloves and loosen dressing and tape by peeling edges back; stabilize catheter to prevent vein injury
5. Fold sterile gauze in half or quarters and hold steadily over insertion site while withdrawing IV catheter flush to skin; apply pressure when catheter is completely removed from vein
6. *NCLEX®* Hold pressure for 2 minutes or until bleeding stops; assess site for bleeding, redness, or hematoma formation; apply clean gauze and tape in place
7. Inspect catheter tip to be sure it is intact
8. *NCLEX®* Document procedure and volume of IV fluid infused
9. Recheck site in 15 minutes for redness, swelling, or hematoma formation

Check Your NCLEX–PN® Exam I.Q.

You are ready for testing on this content if you can

- Use nursing knowledge and skills in caring for a client receiving IV therapy via peripheral or central vein.
- Monitor a client receiving IV therapy, including an infusion pump.
- Initiate, maintain, and discontinue a client's IV using appropriate technique.
- Document accurately a peripheral or central IV infusion.
- Monitor a client for complications of IV therapy.
- Provide care to a client with a central venous access device.
- Provide client teaching about IV therapy.

PRACTICE TEST

1 A client has a continuously running peripheral infusion. The physician orders an antibiotic as a piggyback infusion four times per day. In order to administer the antibiotic, the nurse should do which of the following? Select all that apply.

1. Avoid compatibility issues by starting an additional IV access.
2. Start a new IV access to eliminate the problem of too much volume for one site.
3. Flush the IV line before and after infusion of an incompatible drug.
4. Check to see if the antibiotic is compatible with the continuous infusion.
5. Change the flow rate to facilitate the administration of the antibiotic.

PRACTICE TEST

2 A client rings the call bell to report that the electronic infusion pump is alarming. What should the nurse anticipate as the cause of the infusion pump alarming? Select all that apply.

1. The client's pulse and blood pressure are falling.
2. The client is experiencing a reaction to the medication.
3. The prescribed infusion is complete.
4. There is an incompatibility with the medications.
5. An occlusion has interrupted the infusion.

3 The client is to receive vancomycin (Vancocin) by IV piggyback. To prevent adverse reactions from rapid infusion, by what method should the nurse plan to administer this drug?

1. Using gravity
2. With a regulator
3. Electronic infusion pump
4. Elastomeric pump

4 The physician is going to order a hypotonic intravenous solution for a client with cellular dehydration. The nurse would expect which fluid to be administered?

1. 0.9% normal saline
2. 5% dextrose in normal saline
3. Lactated Ringer's solution
4. 0.45% sodium chloride

5 The client is receiving 5% dextrose in 0.45% sodium chloride. The physician has ordered the client receive one unit of packed cells. Which IV solution would the nurse obtain from the supply area that will be used by the RN to prime the blood tubing?

1. 5% dextrose
2. Lactated Ringer's
3. 0.9% sodium chloride
4. 5% dextrose in 0.45% sodium chloride

6 While assessing a client's intravenous (IV) line, the nurse notes that the area is swollen, cool, pale, and causes the client discomfort. What complication should the nurse document?

1. Infiltration
2. Phlebitis
3. Infection
4. Air embolism

7 The client is receiving 5% dextrose and 0.45% sodium chloride intravenously and is complaining of pain at the IV site. The nurse assesses the site and notes erythema and edema. What is the appropriate action for the nurse to take? Select all that apply.

1. Slow the infusion to a keep-open rate.
2. Discontinue the IV and apply a warm compress to the IV site.
3. Apply antibiotic ointment to the IV site.
4. Gently pull back on the IV catheter to attempt repositioning.
5. Relocate the IV site and document the event.

8 A client with dry skin and mucous membranes is weak, has orthostatic blood pressure changes, and has decreased urine output. The client's serum osmolality, however, is normal. Which of the following IV fluids would the nurse anticipate being prescribed for this client?

1. 5% Dextrose in Water
2. 0.45% Sodium Chloride
3. 10% Dextrose in Water
4. 0.9% Sodium Chloride

9 A client with gastrointestinal (GI) bleeding suddenly develops diaphoresis with a rapid and thready pulse, and the nurse finds it difficult to hear a blood pressure. Which IV fluid does the nurse anticipate the physician will order stat?

1. Dextrose in water (D_5W)
2. 0.9% sodium chloride (normal saline)
3. 0.45% sodium chloride (½ normal saline)
4. Dextrose 5% in 0.45% sodium chloride (D_5½NS)

10 The physician is going to order a hypotonic intravenous solution for a client with cellular dehydration. The nurse would expect which fluid to be administered?

1. 0.9% Sodium Chloride (normal saline, NS)
2. 5% Dextrose in Normal Saline
3. Lactated Ringer's
4. 0.45% Sodium Chloride (½NS)

11 The client receiving 5% dextrose and 0.45% sodium chloride intravenously reports pain at the IV site. The nurse assesses the site and notes erythema and edema. Recognizing these as signs of phlebitis, what would be the appropriate nursing action?

1. Slow the infusion rate.
2. Discontinue the IV and apply a warm compress to the IV site.
3. Apply antibiotic ointment to the IV site.
4. Gently pull back the IV access device to reposition within the vein.

12 A client has a continuously running peripheral infusion. The physician orders the addition of an antibiotic as a piggyback infusion four times per day. What action should the nurse take first to administer the antibiotic?

1. Start a new IV access to administer the antibiotic so that there will not be compatibility issues.
2. Start a new IV access to eliminate the problem of too much volume for one site.
3. Increase the flow rate of the continuous infusion to facilitate the administration of the antibiotic.
4. Check to see if the antibiotic is compatible with the continuous infusion.

13 The nurse is preparing to hang an intravenous piggy-back (IVPB) medication for a client with a continuous intravenous infusion (IV). Into which port should the nurse connect the IVPB? Draw an "X" on the correct area on the image shown.

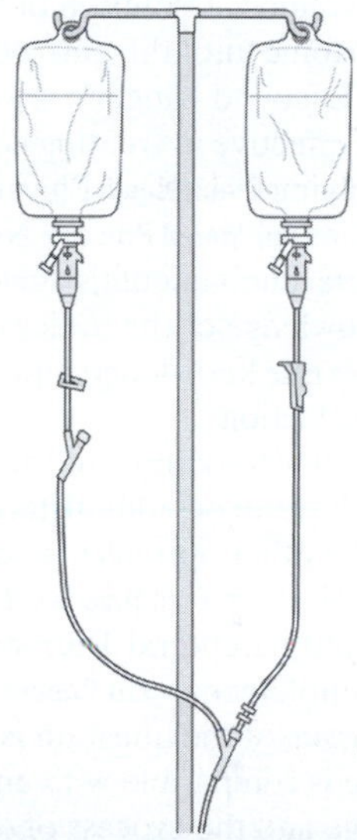

ANSWERS & RATIONALES

1 **Answer: 3, 4, 5 Rationale:** If the drug and infusion were incompatible, the nurse would stop the infusion during the period of antibiotic administration and flush the line carefully before and after the antibiotic. Before making a decision about how to infuse the antibiotic, the nurse should check compatibility of the antibiotic with the continuous IV solution. The flow rate of the IVPB antibiotic may need to be adjusted to accommodate the physician's ordered rate of delivery. A determination of drug compatibility with the IV solution needs to be made first. Starting a second IV site should be avoided if possible. The continuous IV fluid is paused while the antibiotic infusion is occurring. It is inadvisable to start a second IV site unless absolutely necessary. **Cognitive Level:** Analyzing **Client Need:** Pharmacological and Parenteral Therapies **Integrated Process:** Nursing Process: Implementation **Content Area:** Fundamentals **Strategy:** The core issue of the question is the knowledge regarding the administration of IVPB medications when a continuous IV infusion exists. It is critical to check for compatibilities when infusing IV solutions through the same line. With multiple correct answers, approach each option as a true/false statement.

2 **Answer: 3, 5 Rationale:** Alarms sound on electronic infusion devices when the infusion is interrupted by an occlusion or when it is complete. A fall in the client's pulse and blood pressure, the client experiencing a medication reaction, or incompatibility with the prescribed medications would not cause the alarm on an electronic infusion device to activate. **Cognitive Level:** Analyzing **Client Need:** Pharmacological and Parenteral Therapies **Integrated Process:** Nursing Process: Evaluation **Content Area:** Fundamentals **Strategy:** The core issue of this question is the ability to interpret the significance of an alarm on an infusion pump. Use knowledge of pump function in general. When there is more than one correct answer, consider each option as a true/false statement.

3 **Answer: 3 Rationale:** The device that provides the most accurate infusion rate is the electronic infusion pump. Gravity IV infusions can be difficult to control, even with a roller clamp, because the rate can be impacted by a change in height of the

infusion, the position of the intravenous catheter, and the client's activities. The roller clamp is subject to tampering. A regulator is an in-line device where the flow rate is set by a dial rather than relying on gravity. An elastromeric device is a mechanical device used to control the rate of infusion by tubing size; used with home infusions to simplify medication administration. **Cognitive Level:** Analyzing **Client Need:** Pharmacological and Parenteral Therapies **Integrated Process:** Nursing Process: Planning **Content Area:** Fundamentals **Strategy:** The core issue of the question is the best method to prevent speed-related adverse reactions from a drug infused intravenously. Use knowledge of IV infusion devices and the process of elimination to make a selection.

4 **Answer: 4 Rationale:** 0.45% sodium chloride (one-half normal saline) is a hypotonic solution that draws fluid from the vascular compartment into the cells. Normal saline is an isotonic solution that remains in the vascular compartment and expands vascular volume. A solution of 5% dextrose in normal saline is hypertonic until the glucose is metabolized, then it is isotonic. Lactated Ringer's is an isotonic solution that would not be effective in treating cellular dehydration. **Cognitive Level:** Applying **Client Need:** Pharmacological and Parenteral Therapies **Integrated Process:** Nursing Process: Planning **Content Area:** Fundamentals **Strategy:** The core issue of the question is knowledge of the tonicity of various intravenous solutions. Use this knowledge and the process of elimination to make a selection.

5 **Answer: 3 Rationale:** 0.9% sodium chloride (normal saline) is the only solution that can be administered with blood or blood products. The other options may cause the blood cells to clump or cause clotting. **Cognitive Level:** Applying **Client Need:** Pharmacological and Parenteral Therapies **Integrated Process:** Nursing Process: Implementation **Content Area:** Fundamentals **Strategy:** The core issue of the question is the knowledge that only normal saline is compatible with any blood product. Use this knowledge and the process of elimination to make a selection.

6 **Answer: 1 Rationale:** Infiltration is leakage of fluids into the surrounding tissues, resulting in edema around the insertion site, blanching, and coolness of skin around the site. Phlebitis is inflammation to the lumen of a vein manifested by warmth, swelling, a red streak and pain along the course of the vein, and localized warmth. Infection is characterized by fever, chills, erythema, or drainage at the IV insertion site. An air embolism occurs when air is introduced into an IV line; characterized by respiratory distress, chest pain, dyspnea, hypotension, and a weak and rapid pulse. **Cognitive Level:** Analyzing **Client Need:** Pharmacological and Parenteral Therapies **Integrated Process:** Communication and Documentation **Content Area:** Fundamentals **Strategy:** The core issue of the question is the ability to accurately interpret an IV complication. Use knowledge of various IV complications and the process of elimination to make a selection.

7 **Answer: 2, 5 Rationale:** The IV is discontinued and restarted at a new site. Applying a warm compress to an area of phlebitis dilates the vessel, improving circulation, and reduces the resistance to blood flow from within the vein reducing the pain. The site of the IV will need to be changed in order to prevent further damage of the current site. The event will need to be documented; however, the physician does not need to be contacted unless a change in the IV order is necessary. The client is exhibiting signs of phlebitis; continuing the infusion at that site and at any rate would only increase the phlebitis. The nurse cannot change the infusion rate without a physician's order. Applying antibiotic ointment to the IV site will not affect the development of phlebitis. Repositioning the IV catheter will not affect the development of phlebitis. **Cognitive Level:** Applying **Client Need:** Pharmacological and Parenteral Therapies **Integrated Process:** Nursing Process: Implementation **Content Area:** Fundamentals **Strategy:** The core issue of the question is the ability to accurately interpret an IV complication and initiate the correct nursing action. When there is more than one correct answer to a question, look at each option as a true/false statement.

8 **Answer: 4 Rationale:** The client is manifesting signs and symptoms of dehydration. Since the serum remains isotonic, this is isotonic dehydration or hypovolemia. Appropriate treatment is with an isotonic fluid to replace fluid volume. These solutions are hypotonic and would cause fluid shifting leading to cellular edema (i.e., client's cells are normal size and free water is not needed for cells). **Cognitive Level:** Analyzing **Client Need:** Pharmacological and Parenteral Therapies **Integrated Process:** Nursing Process: Evaluation **Content Area:** Adult Health **Strategy:** Critical words are *normal osmolality*, indicating the fluid replacement will need to maintain the normal osmolality. Recognize the need to restore fluid balance with use of an isotonic solution to direct you to the correct option.

9 **Answer: 2 Rationale:** Normal saline solution is an isotonic solution that will replace lost vascular volume and promote perfusion. In addition, when blood is available, it can be hung with the normal saline. D_5W is hypotonic in the bloodstream, providing free water that moves into interstitial space and cells. Administration can cause further fluid shifting, which will not help to replace lost volume or promote perfusion. In addition, when blood is available, dextrose will cause lysis of red blood cells. Half normal saline is hypotonic, providing free water that moves into the interstitial space and cells. Administration can cause further fluid shifting, which will not help to replace lost volume or promote perfusion. D_5½NS acts as a hypotonic solution in the bloodstream once dextrose is metabolized, providing free water that moves into the interstitial space and cells. Administration can cause further fluid shifting, which will not help to replace lost volume or promote perfusion. **Cognitive Level:** Analyzing **Client Need:** Pharmacological and Parenteral Therapies **Integrated Process:** Nursing Process: Evaluation **Content Area:** Adult Health **Strategy:** Recall tonicities of various IV solutions. Recognize the need for replacement with an isotonic fluid to direct you to the correct option.

10 **Answer: 4 Rationale:** ½NS is a hypotonic solution that draws fluid from the vascular compartment into the cells. NS is an isotonic solution; however, a hypotonic solution would be better for this client. A hypotonic solution is needed, while D_5NS is hypertonic until dextrose is metabolized, and then it is isotonic. Lactated Ringers is a balanced salt solution while a hypotonic solution is required. **Cognitive Level:** Understanding

Client Need: Pharmacological and Parenteral Therapies **Integrated Process:** Nursing Process: Planning **Content Area:** Pharmacology **Strategy:** Recall that 0.45% sodium chloride is referred to as half normal saline. Then identify that normal saline is isotonic while half normal would be hypotonic.

11 **Answer: 2** **Rationale:** Continuing the infusion at that site would only increase the phlebitis. The IV is discontinued and restarted at a new site. Applying a warm compress to an area of phlebitis dilates the vessel, improving circulation, and reduces the resistance to blood flow from within the vein reducing the pain. Continuing the infusion at that site would only increase the phlebitis. Applying antibiotic ointment would not be useful. Pulling back on the IV is insufficient. It must be discontinued and restarted at a new site. **Cognitive Level:** Applying **Client Need:** Pharmacological and Parenteral Therapies **Integrated Process:** Nursing Process: Implementation **Content Area:** Pharmacology **Strategy:** Discontinuing the IV is usually the best option when site problems are described.

12 **Answer: 4** **Rationale:** Before making a decision about how to infuse the antibiotic, the nurse should check compatibility of the antibiotic with the continuous IV solution. If the drug and the infusion were compatible, they would be run at the same time. If the drug and infusion were incompatible, the nurse would stop the infusion during the period of antibiotic administration and flush the line carefully before and after the antibiotic. It is inadvisable to start a second IV site unless absolutely necessary. Increasing the flow rate would not address the issue of incompatibility if the antibiotic and current IV solution were not compatible. **Cognitive Level:** Applying **Client Need:** Pharmacological and Parenteral Therapies **Integrated Process:** Nursing Process: Implementation **Content Area:** Pharmacology **Strategy:** Omit two options as they are similar by requiring another mildly invasive procedure to insert another IV line. Omit next the option that addresses the flow rate rather than focusing on compatibility.

13 **Answer:**

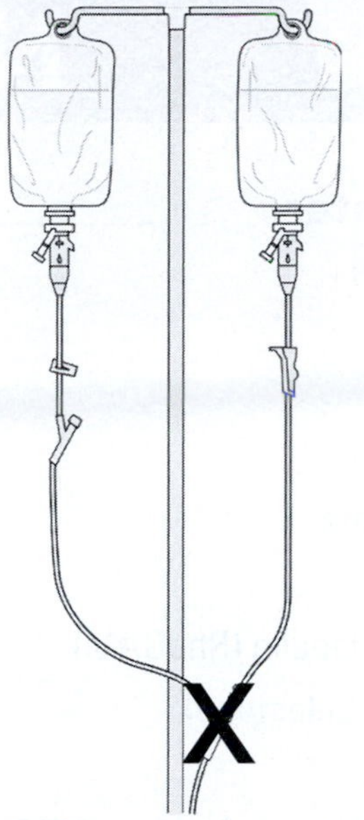

Rationale: An IVPB medication is infused intermittently. The IVPB tubing does not have an infusion control clamp; therefore, the rate of infusion is controlled by the roller clamp on the primary tubing. The IVPB port is used for intermittent infusions only. **Cognitive Level:** Applying **Client Need:** Pharmacological and Parenteral Therapies **Integrated Process:** Nursing Process: Implementation **Content Area:** Pharmacology **Strategy:** The core concept of the question is identifying the correct port on primary IV tubing in which to connect an IVPB infusion. Use nursing knowledge to select the correct answer.

Key Terms to Review

intravenous p. 442

References

Ball, J., & Bindler, R., & Cowen, K. (2010). *Child health nursing: Partnering with children and families* (2nd ed.). Upper Saddle River, NJ: Pearson Education, Inc.

Berman, A., & Snyder, S. (2012). *Kozier & Erb's fundamentals of nursing: Concepts, process, and practice* (9th ed.). Upper Saddle River, NJ: Pearson Education, Inc.

LeMone, P., Burke, K., & Bauldoff, G. (2012). *Medical surgical nursing: Critical thinking in patient care* (5th ed.). Upper Saddle River, NJ: Pearson Education, Inc.

Lewis, S., Heitkemper, M., Dirksen, S. & Bucher, L. (2011). *Medical surgical nursing: Assessment and management of clinical problems* (8th ed.). St. Louis, MO: Elsevier Science.

Smeltzer, S., Bare, B., Hinkle, J., & Cheever, K. (2010). *Brunner & Suddarth's textbook of medical surgical nursing:* (12th ed.). Philadelphia: Lippincott Williams & Wilkins.

Smith, S., Duell, D., & Martin, B. (2012). *Clinical nursing skills: Basic to advanced skills* (8th ed.). Upper Saddle River, NJ: Pearson Education, Inc.

Test Yourself

Are you ready for the NCLEX-PN® or course exams? Use the practice tests on the companion website to check.

31 Maternal and Newborn Medications

In this chapter

Cross Reference

Other chapters relevant to this content area are

Reproduction, Family Planning, and Infertility	Chapter 8
Uncomplicated Antenatal Care	Chapter 9
Uncomplicated Labor and Delivery	Chapter 10
Uncomplicated Postpartum Care	Chapter 11
Uncomplicated Newborn Care	Chapter 12
Complicated Antenatal Care	Chapter 45
Complicated Labor and Delivery Care	Chapter 46
Complicated Postpartum Care	Chapter 47
Complicated Newborn Care	Chapter 48

I. OXYTOCIN (PITOCIN)

A. Overview

1. A uterine stimulant that increases frequency and force of uterine contractions or stimulates contractions with uterine inertia
2. Helps to progress labor in clients who are at term and induce labor in clients with maternal diabetes, preeclampsia, eclampsia, and erythroblastosis fetalis
3. Should be used only in final stages of labor after cervix has dilated, membranes have rutptured, and presentation of fetus has occurred
4. Stimulates letdown reflex in breastfeeding mother and relieves pain from breast engorgement
5. Controls postpartum hemorrhage and promotes postpartum uterine involution

B. Administration considerations

1. Dilute as ordered in IV solution and hang as a titratable IV drip, using an IV pump
2. Use normal saline as a primary line, with medication piggybacked at secondary port or stopcock
3. Monitor effects on contractions while titrating dosage
4. Nasal spray may be used to promote milk ejection
5. NCLEX® Keep magnesium sulfate (antidote) on hand for use if needed to relax uterus
6. NCLEX® Do not confuse Pitocin (oxytocin) with Pitressin (vasopressin)

C. Side/adverse effects

1. Maternal: rare and with IV use, causes more rapid, painful contractions from effects on uterine smooth muscle; also hypersensitivity, cardiac dysrhythmias, hypotension, hypertension if given following use of vasopressors, water intoxication (hyponatremia and hypochloremia), nausea and vomiting (N/V)
2. Fetal: tachycardia; rare adverse effects include dysrhythmias, intracranial hemorrhage, hypoxia

D. Nursing considerations

1. Use flowsheet to record baseline maternal BP and other vital signs, weight, intake and output (I&O), contractions (frequency, duration, strength), and fetal heart rate (FHR) and tones
2. Continue to monitor maternal pulse and BP, FHR, contractions, and resting uterine tone at least every 15 minutes
3. Record time medication was initiated and any changes in dosage
4. NCLEX® Monitor for hypertonic contractions (less than 2 minutes apart, greater than 90 seconds long, and about 50 mm Hg in strength), and shut off IV drip if uterine hyperstimulation or nonreassuring FHR occurs; turn client onto left side, increase rate of normal saline IV, and apply oxygen via facemask as appropriate
5. Effects of drug will diminish 2 to 3 minutes after discontinuing medication
6. Watch for hypertensive crisis in clients also receiving local or regional anesthesia (caudal, spinal); signs include sudden onset of intense occipital headache, palpitations, hypertension, stiff neck, N/V, fever and sweating, photophobia and dilated pupils, constricting chest pain, and bradycardia or tachycardia
7. NCLEX® Monitor I&O; report signs of water intoxication (drowsiness, headache, confusion, anuria, weight gain); report decreasing urine output with adequate intake
8. Keep emergency resuscitation equipment available

E. Client teaching

1. Purpose and effect of medication
2. Importance of reporting sudden, severe headache immediately

II. ERGOT ALKALOIDS

A. Overview

1. Used to control postpartum hemorrhage; should not be used before delivery of placenta
2. Cause clonic contractions of uterus
3. Produce arterial vasoconstriction and possible vasospasm of coronary arteries
4. Common medications (Box 31–1)

B. Administration considerations: causes rebound uterine relaxation

C. Side/adverse effects

1. NCLEX® Contraindicated in pregnancy or hypersensitivity to ergot, hypertension
2. Should be used cautiously in unstable angina and recent myocardial infarction
3. Significant increase in systolic and diastolic BP, cardiac dysrhythmias
4. Uterine cramping
5. Decreased milk production
6. NCLEX® **Ergotism** or overdose: N/V, weakness, muscle pain, insensitivity to cold, paresthesia of extremities

Box 31–1 Ergot Alkaloids	
	Ergonovine (Ergotrate)
	Methylergonovine (Methergine)

D. Nursing considerations

1. Closely monitor BP after administration; if hypertension noted, withhold dose and notify prescriber
2. Monitor lochia after administation and uterine contractions (strength, duration, and frequency)
3. *NCLEX®* Observe for and report as indicated hypertension, chest pain, ergotism, or hypersensitivity (shortness of breath, itching)
4. Administer analgesics as needed to control pain of uterine contractions caused by ergot

E. Client teaching

1. Indication for administration
2. Route of administration (oral, IM, possible IV in emergency) and possible side effects, such as cramping
3. Report increased blood loss, increased temperature, or foul-smelling lochia
4. *NCLEX®* Perform pad count to monitor bleeding
5. Do not smoke because of increased/additive vasoconstriction with ergonovine use

III. PROSTAGLANDINS

A. Overview

1. **Prostaglandins** terminate pregnancy from 12th week through second trimester (Table 31–1); can also be used to stimulate myometrium to promote delivery
2. Dinoprostone (Prepidil, Cervidil) has FDA approval only for cervical ripening prior to labor induction; available as a gel
3. Carboprost tromethamine (Hemabate) has FDA approval for control of postpartum bleeding unresponsive to oxytocin and induce abortion at 13–20 weeks' gestation
4. Misoprostol (Cytotec) is a synthetic analog of prostaglandin E1 that is used off-label for pharmacologic abortion, cervical ripening, and control of postpartum bleeding

B. Administration considerations

1. *NCLEX®* Client should remain supine for 20 to 30 minutes after receiving dinoprostone
2. Before dinoprostone, client should receive antiemetic and antidiarrheal medications

C. Side/adverse effects

1. *NCLEX®* Diarrhea, N/V, possible increase in BP
2. Uterine cramping and possible uterine rupture
3. Tension headache
4. Flushing, cardiac dysrhythmias, hypertension
5. Uterine tetany may develop with prelabor or intrapartum administration
6. Contraindicated with acute pelvic inflammatory disease and history of pelvic surgery; use cautiously in hypertension and with history of asthma

D. Nursing considerations

1. *NCLEX®* Prenatal: follow manufacturer's instructions for placement of medication; client must lie down for 20–30 minutes after administration and have fetal monitoring during this time
2. *NCLEX®* Postpartum: monitor lochia and BP, be prepared for client to develop diarrhea

E. Client teaching

1. Prenatal: report long or continuous contractions, as uterine tetany may develop; count fetal movement as an indicator of fetal well-being
2. Postpartum: prepare client for route of administration and possible side effects

Table 31–1 Common Prostaglandins

Category	Generic (Trade Name)	Route	Indications for Use
Prostaglandin E2	Dinoprostone (Prepidil, Cervidil)	Prepidil intracervical gel Cervidil vaginal insert	Ripen cervix prior to induction of labor or abort fetus that has died
Prostaglandin F2	Carboprost tromethamine (Hemabate)	Hemabate: IM	Postpartum hemorrhage

Table 31–2 Common Uterine Relaxant Medications

Generic (Trade Name)	Notes
Terbutaline sulfate (Brethine)	Not FDA-approved for preterm labor but most commonly used medication
Ritodrine (Yutopar)	FDA-approved for preterm labor, but no longer available in United States; increased incidence of pulmonary edema
Nifedipine (Procardia)	Not FDA-approved for preterm labor but commonly used; may cause oligohydramnios

IV. UTERINE RELAXANTS

A. Overview

1. Inhibit contractions and arrest preterm labor for 24–72 hours so that corticosteroids (betamethasone) can be given to facilitate fetal lung maturity
2. Used to stop contractions to allow intrauterine fetal resuscitation when uterine hyperstimulation is present
3. Common medications (Table 31–2)

B. Administration considerations

1. Start at lowest possible dose and increase as indicated until contractions cease
2. Be certain about recommended dose
3. If GI symptoms occur, advise client to take medication with food
4. Dilute IV terbutaline by adding each 5 mg to 1000 mL D_5W or NS to yield a concentration of 5 micrograms/mL
5. Infuse medication via microdrip using an infusion pump

C. Side/adverse effects

NCLEX® 1. Beta-adrenergics: maternal and fetal tachycardia, palpitations, tremors, jitteriness and anxiety, pulmonary edema
2. May cause or exacerbate constipation
3. Nausea and vomiting
4. Nifedipine (Procardia) can cause oligohydramnios

D. Nursing considerations

1. Beta-adrenergics: if client delivers after receiving uterine relaxant medications, be prepared with oxytocic if needed to treat postpartum hemorrhage
2. Monitor vital signs and I&O
3. Nifedipine (Procardia): avoid grapefruit juice during administration (interferes with effect)
4. If mother uses terbutaline during pregnancy, monitor neonate for hypoglycemia

E. Client teaching

1. Possible side effects and coping strategies
2. Use and dose of oral medications and importance of taking them on time
NCLEX® 3. Nifedipine (Procardia): encourage client to change position slowly due to possible orthostatic hypotension
4. How to self-monitor pulse
5. Importance of consulting physician prior to taking over-the-counter (OTC) medications

V. MAGNESIUM SULFATE

A. Overview

1. When given parenterally, acts as central nervous system (CNS) depressant and also depresses smooth, skeletal, and cardiac muscle function
2. Used to arrest preterm labor (common off-label use) and to prevent or to treat seizures with preeclampsia and eclampsia

B. Administration considerations

1. Use in conjunction with beta-adrenergics increases risk of pulmonary edema
2. A loading dose is often given over 20–30 minutes via infusion pump

C. Side/adverse effects

1. Flushed warm feeling, drowsiness or sedation
NCLEX® 2. Decreased or absent deep tendon reflexes

3. Decreased strength or absence of hand grasp; muscle weakness
4. Fluid and electrolyte imbalance, hyponatremia, thirst
5. Nausea and vomiting
6. NCLEX® Respiratory depression leading to respiratory arrest
7. Contraindicated in fetal anomaly incompatible with life, pulmonary edema or CHF, anuria, renal failure, and organic CNS disease

D. Nursing considerations
1. NCLEX® Check patellar reflex prior to initial dose and any subsequent doses; depressed reflex could indicate risk for respiratory arrest
2. NCLEX® Monitor hand grasps and deep tendon reflexes hourly for signs of toxicity
3. Monitor vital signs every 30–60 minutes, especially respiratory rate (needs to be 16/min or greater for additional doses to be safe)
4. NCLEX® Call prescriber for respiratory depression if respirations less than 12/minute
5. NCLEX® Ensure that calcium gluconate (antidote) is available at bedside
6. NCLEX® IV infusion flow rate is generally adjusted to maintain urine flow of at least 30 to 50 mL/hour, monitor I&O carefully; be certain to use infusion pump
7. Monitor IV site closely to avoid extravasation
8. Monitor serum magnesium levels for target range of 4 to 7 mEq/L and call prescriber if greater than 7 mEq
9. Take accurate daily weight

E. Client teaching
1. Side effects of medication
2. Report signs of preeclampsia, including headache, epigastric pain, and visual disturbance
3. Report any signs of confusion

VI. ANALGESICS

A. Overview (Box 31–2)
1. Used to manage moderate to severe pain of labor
2. Common opioid agonist analgesic is fentanyl (Sublimaze); less common is meperidine (Demerol)
3. Common opioid agonist-antagonists are butorphanol tartrate (Stadol) and nalbuphine (Nubain)
4. Epidural or intrathecal opioid agents commonly include fentanyl (Sublimaze) and sufentanil (Sufenta); sufentanil should be used in combination with low-dose bupivacaine if by epidural
5. NCLEX® Antidote to opioids is naloxone (Narcan)

B. Administration considerations
1. Do not administer in early labor because it could slow labor
2. Birth should occur more than 4 hours or less than 1 hour after dose of meperidine to minimize neonatal CNS depression
3. Agonist-antagonists provide adequate analgesia, less respiratory depression and N/V, but equal or greater sedation when compared to meperidine
4. NCLEX® Do not use agonist-antagonists for women with opioid dependence because antagonist activity could precipitate withdrawal (abstinence) symptoms in mother and neonate (irritability, hyperactive reflexes, tremors, seizures, yawning, sneezing, vomiting and diarrhea; and excessive crying in neonate)

C. Side/adverse effects
1. Meperidine, fentanyl, and sufentanil: N/V, sedation, drowsiness or confusion, tachycardia or bradycardia, hypotension, dry mouth, urinary retention, pruritis, respiratory depression
2. Butorphanol or nalbuphine: confusion, sedation, N/V, sweating; respiratory depression less likely to occur

Box 31–2 Analgesics During Labor

Opioid Agonists	Opioid Agonist-Antagonists
Meperidine (Demerol)	Butorphanol (Stadol)
Fentanyl (Sublimaze)	Nalbuphine (Nubain)
Sufentanil (Sufenta)	

D. Nursing considerations

1. Meperidine, fentanyl, and sufentanil
   - a. Monitor FHR and uterine contractions
   - b. Monitor for respiratory depression less than 12 breaths/minute
   - NCLEX® c. Monitor newborn for respiratory depression if born in 1 to 4 hours of dose
   - d. Keep naloxone available as antidote
   - e. Keep siderails raised for safety
   - f. Supplement pain relief using nonpharmacologic methods, such as deep breathing, and imagery
2. Butorphanol or nalbuphine
   - a. Similar to opioid analgesics
   - b. Watch for withdrawal symptoms if administered to opioid-dependent women and neonates

E. Client teaching

1. Purpose and expected effects of medication
2. Use of nonpharmacological pain relief measures

VII. RH_0(D) IMMUNE GLOBULIN (RHOGAM)

A. Overview

1. Prevents anti-Rh_0(D) antibody formation (isoimmunization) in Rh-negative women
2. Used when there is potential or actual exposure to Rh-positive blood: pregnancy, labor and delivery, amniocentesis, chorionic villus sampling, termination of pregnancy, abdominal trauma, or transfusion

B. Administration considerations

1. NCLEX® Administer within 72 hours of potential or actual exposure to Rh-positive blood
2. NCLEX® Readminister with each subsequent possible or actual exposure
3. Do not administer if client has developed positive antibody titer to Rh antigen
4. NCLEX® In typical pregnancy, administer at 28 weeks' gestation and within 72 hours of delivery
5. Do not administer to newborn infant

C. Side/adverse effects

1. Tenderness at injection site
2. Slight elevation in temperature
3. NCLEX® Contraindicated with hypersensitivity to human immunoglobulins and in Rh-positive women

D. Nursing considerations: administer as described previously

E. Client teaching: purpose and effects of medication and need for repeat injections with subsequent pregnancies

VIII. BETAMETHASONE (CELESTONE)

A. Overview

1. Synthetic glucocorticoid (corticosteroid)
2. NCLEX® Prevention of neonatal respiratory distress syndrome (RDS) as an unlabeled use
3. Enhances production of surfactant

B. Administration considerations

1. Administered to a client in preterm labor between 28 and 32 weeks' gestation
2. NCLEX® Used if client and fetus can safely tolerate inhibition of labor for 48 hours
3. Administer as once-daily dose by the intramuscular (IM) route

C. Side/adverse effects

1. Contraindicated during lactation
2. Similar to other corticosteroids, with risk of infection and delayed wound healing being notable

D. Nursing considerations

1. Monitor maternal vital signs and fetal well-being
2. Monitor for increased temperature and WBC as general indicators of infection

E. Client teaching: purpose and intended effects of medication to parents

IX. LUNG SURFACTANTS

A. Overview (Box 31–3)

1. **Surfactant** lowers surface tension on alveolar surfaces during respiration, which improves gas exchange
2. Stabilizes alveoli against collapse at resting pressures
3. NCLEX® Prevents or treats respiratory distress syndrome (RDS) in premature infants

Box 31–3 Lung Surfactants	
	Beractant (Survanta)
	Calfactant (Infasurf)

B. Administration considerations
1. Given by intratracheal route into endotracheal tube (using #5 French catheter with end hole) every 4–6 hours until condition improves
2. Do not suction within 1 hour after dose unless significant airway obstruction occurs

C. Side/adverse effects
1. Oxygen desaturation
2. Transient bradycardia
3. Crackles and moist breath sounds occur transiently after dose; does not necessarily indicate suctioning is needed

D. Nursing considerations
1. Ensure proper endotracheal tube placement prior to dosing
2. Monitor heart rate, chest expansion, facial expression during administration
3. Monitor oxygen saturation and periodically assess arterial or transcutaneous oxygen and CO_2 levels

E. Client teaching: purpose and intended effects of medication to parents

X. PHYTONADIONE OR VITAMIN K_1 (AQUAMEPHYTON)

A. Overview
1. Fat-soluble vitamin that aids synthesis of clotting factors II, VII, IX, and X in immature newborn liver
2. Prevents and treats hemorrhagic disease of newborn until neonate has intestinal flora to absorb vitamin K from GI tract

B. Administration considerations
1. NCLEX® Give IM in vastus lateralis thigh muscle, usually within 1 hour of birth but may be delayed until after first breastfeeding in birthing area
2. Protect from light
3. Be sure to give prior to circumcision procedure

C. Side/adverse effects: hyperbilirubinemia, bleeding on second or third day

D. Nursing considerations
1. Monitor for signs of bleeding, such as bruising at injection site, bleeding from umbilical cord, nose, or GI tract
2. NCLEX® Observe for jaundice and monitor results of bilirubin levels to detect hyperbilirubinemia

E. Client teaching: purpose and intended effects of medication to parents

XI. NEONATAL EYE PROPHYLAXIS

A. Overview
1. Mandated by law for prophylaxis against *Neisseria gonorrhoeae* and *Chlamydia trachomatis*, which could be transmitted to neonate during birth
2. Common agents include erythromycin ophthalmic ointment (Ilotycin Ophthalmic) and tetracycline ophthalmic ointment or solution

B. Administration considerations
1. NCLEX® Apply up to but within 1 hour of delivery (allow time for eye contact that promotes parent–infant bonding)
2. Cleanse eyes before application of dose
3. Administer 1 cm ribbon of ointment along each lower conjunctival sac, from inner canthus to outer canthus
4. Gently close eye and manipulate to ensure spread of ointment
5. Do not rinse eyes following dose, but may wipe away excess after 1 minute with sterile cotton
6. Use a new tube of ointment for each neonate

C. Side/adverse effects: blurring of vision possible after application of ointment, sensitivity reaction may cause edema and inflammation of eyes, which subsides in 24–48 hours

D. Nursing considerations: as noted previously

E. Client teaching: purpose and effects of medication to parents

Check Your NCLEX-PN® Exam I.Q. *You are ready for testing on this content if you can*

- Apply knowledge of expected actions and effects of maternal and newborn medications to client care.
- Correctly administer maternal and newborn medications to clients.
- Monitor for side effects and adverse effects of maternal and newborn medications.
- Take appropriate action if a client has an unexpected response to a maternal or newborn medication.
- Monitor a client for expected outcomes or effects of treatment with maternal or newborn medications.

PRACTICE TEST

1 What should the nurse anticipate being included in the therapeutic plan of care for a postpartum client with subinvolution?

1. Oral methylergonovine maleate (Methergine)
2. Oxytocin (Pitocin) IV infusion for 8 hours
3. Oral fluids to 3000 mL per day
4. Blood replacement

2 In which postpartum client would the nurse consider that methylergonovine maleate (Methergine) is contraindicated?

1. A client with a blood pressure of 120/60
2. A client with a heart rate of 60
3. A client with a blood pressure of 140/100
4. A client with a respiratory rate of 12

3 A postpartum client has an epidural catheter in place following delivery of an infant via cesarean section. The nurse determines that which medication is a priority to have on hand for use if needed?

1. Meperidine hydrochloride (Demerol)
2. Betamethasone (Celestone)
3. Carboprost (Hemabate)
4. Naloxone (Narcan)

4 The nurse is assisting in monitoring a client in labor who is receiving oxytocin (Pitocin) as a continuous infusion to augment labor. What observations of the client would indicate to the nurse that the infusion needs to be stopped? Select all that apply.

1. Contractions lasting 120 seconds
2. Maternal blood pressure increase from 124/82 to 130/86
3. Early fetal heart rate decelerations on the fetal monitor
4. The mother squeezing her eyes shut during each contraction
5. Development of nausea and vomiting

5 The nurse is collecting data regarding the status of a pregnant client receiving magnesium sulfate. What manifestation should indicate to the nurse that the medication is having the intended effect?

1. BP has stabilized at 128/76.
2. Serum magnesium level reaches 2.2 mEq/L.
3. Contractions are steady at a frequency of every 4 minutes.
4. There is an absence of seizure activity.

6 The nurse notes that the client is Rh-negative and her baby is Rh-positive. Which maternal laboratory result would be important to interpret next in determining if the client is a candidate for RhoGAM?

1. Hemoglobin level
2. Direct Coombs' test
3. Indirect Coombs' test
4. Bilirubin level

7 In addition to routine data collection and care, nursing care of the client who is receiving terbutaline (Brethine) to prevent premature labor should include monitoring for what indicator of an adverse drug effect?

1. Oral temperature every 2 hours
2. Fetal heart tones every 30 minutes
3. Breath sounds every 4 hours
4. Deep-tendon reflexes every 4 hours

PRACTICE TEST

8 A client in premature labor is scheduled to receive a dose of betamethasone (Celestone). In reinforcing information about this medication, how should the nurse explain the purpose and expected action of the medication?

1. Stops uterine contractions
2. Prevents infection
3. Hastens fetal lung maturity
4. Prevents cervical dilatation

9 The nurse is preparing to administer an intramuscular injection of phytonadione (AquaMEPHYTON) to a healthy newborn. What is the best explanation for the nurse to reinforce to the neonate's mother regarding the medication?

1. "This medication is specifically used to treat hemorrhagic disease of the newborn."
2. "This medication supplies vitamin K, which the newborn cannot produce in the first 5–8 days of life."
3. "This medication is a multivitamin that has many effects, including helping to produce prothrombin in the blood."
4. "This medication is also known as vitamin K, and it is a water-soluble vitamin that is deficient in newborns."

10 The nurse is caring for a newborn 30 minutes after birth. What should the nurse do when administering a prescribed dose of ophthalmic erythromycin? Select all that apply.

1. Withhold the dose for 2 hours to allow for parent–infant bonding.
2. Administer the dose across each lower conjunctival sac.
3. Irrigate the eyes after the dose to flush out microorganisms.
4. Use a new tube of ointment for the prescribed dose.
5. Explain to the mother that the medication will cause infant eye irritation.

11 A breastfeeding mother and her newborn are to be discharged from the postpartum unit. The client has no immunity to rubella, and has orders to receive rubella vaccine on the day of discharge. What is the most important instruction for the nurse to reinforce to the client? Select all that apply.

1. Utilize a reliable method of contraception.
2. Continue to breastfeed the newborn.
3. Avoid public outings for 2 weeks due to contagious period.
4. Have the infant screened for active rubella virus at the 2-month checkup.
5. Avoid becoming pregnant for at least 6 months.

12 A primigravida with blood type A-negative is at 28 weeks' gestation. Today, the client is to receive an ordered RhoGAM injection. Which statement by the client demonstrates to the nurse that more reinforcement of teaching is needed related to this therapy?

1. "I'm getting this shot so that my baby won't develop antibodies against my blood, right?"
2. "I understand that if my baby is Rh-positive, I'll be getting another one of these injections."
3. "This shot will prevent me from becoming sensitized to Rh-positive blood."
4. "This shot should help to protect me in future pregnancies if this baby is Rh-positive like my husband."

13 A pregnant woman is having an exacerbation of asthma. What factor is most important for the nurse to consider in delivering aerosol medication?

1. Aerosol medication is used instead of postural drainage.
2. The droplets produced should be large enough to dilate the bronchioles.
3. The aerosol delivers medication to the lower respiratory tract.
4. Aerosol medications are contraindicated in pregnancy.

14 What explanation should the nurse give to a new nurse about the reason that phytonadione (AquaMEPHYTON) is administered to the neonate? Select all that apply.

1. It prevents the neonate from acquiring maternal gonorrhea.
2. It inhibits the production of prothrombin by the liver.
3. The neonate lacks the intestinal flora for vitamin K production.
4. The neonate cannot absorb vitamin K from the gastrointestinal tract.
5. Administration of phytonadione to a neonate is state law.

15 A pregnant client is receiving magnesium sulfate. What should the nurse recognize as a sign of toxicity of the drug?

1. Development of seizures
2. Disappearance of the knee-jerk reflex
3. Increase in respiratory rate
4. Increase in blood pressure

16 After receiving magnesium sulfate, a client develops signs of toxicity. What should the nurse expect to be administered?

1. Oxygen
2. Epinephrine
3. Potassium chloride
4. Calcium gluconate

17 The LPN/LVN is assisting the RN in the maternal-newborn unit. Before the RN administers IV magnesium sulfate therapy to a client with preeclampsia, which parameters should the nurse assisting the RN recognize as the highest priority for data collection?

1. Urinary glucose, acetone, and specific gravity
2. Temperature, blood pressure, and respirations
3. Urinary output, respirations, and patellar reflexes
4. Level of consciousness, funduscopic appearance, and knee reflex

18 A client with preeclampsia is receiving magnesium sulfate. For what adverse effect should the nurse observe the client during administration of the drug?

1. Dry, pale skin
2. Hyporeflexia
3. Agitation
4. Increased respirations

19 A client in active labor is to have an epidural block. While this is being administered, which of the following nursing actions takes priority?

1. Checking the uterine contractions for an increase in strength
2. Positioning the mother flat in bed to avoid postspinal headache
3. Telling the mother she will feel the need to void more frequently
4. Monitoring the maternal blood pressure for possible hypotension

20 A client is receiving magnesium sulfate for severe preeclampsia. What nursing actions are appropriate interventions? Select all that apply.

1. Limit fluid intake to 1000 mL/24 hours.
2. Prepare for the possibility of a precipitate delivery.
3. Restrict visitors and keep the room darkened and quiet.
4. Obtain calcium gluconate for use as an antagonist if necessary.
5. Note the results of assessment of patellar reflexes.

PRACTICE TEST

ANSWERS & RATIONALES

1 **Answer: 1** **Rationale:** Methergine provides long-sustained contraction of the uterus. It is commonly used to treat late postpartum hemorrhage (subinvolution). Oxytocin and prostaglandin are more frequently used to treat early postpartum hemorrhage caused by uterine atony. Increased fluid intake is a general, helpful measure for any client who has lost body fluid volume, but it is not a specific therapy. When blood products are used, they are generally ordered for early postpartum hemorrhage. **Cognitive Level:** Applying **Client Need:** Pharmacological and Parenteral Therapies **Integrated Process:** Nursing Process: Planning **Content Area:** Maternal-Newborn **Strategy:** Specific knowledge of ergonovine maleate (Methergine) is needed to answer this question. Use medication knowledge and the process of elimination to make your selection.

2 **Answer: 3** **Rationale:** Methergine has a side effect of raising the blood pressure. A woman with hypertension or gestational hypertension would not be a good candidate for use of Methergine. This client has a normal blood pressure, which is not a contraindication for prescribing Methergine. A pulse of 60 is not a contraindication to use of Methergine. A respiratory rate of 12 is not a contraindication to use of Methergine. **Cognitive Level:** Analyzing **Client Need:** Pharmacological and Parenteral Therapies

ANSWERS & RATIONALES

Integrated Process: Nursing Process: Planning **Content Area:** Pharmacology **Strategy:** Specific knowledge of ergonovine maleate (Methergine) is needed to answer this question. Use nursing knowledge and the process of elimination to make your selection.

3 **Answer: 4 Rationale:** Naloxone is the antidote to the opioid analgesics that are used with epidural analgesia. If respiratory depression occurs, this medication needs to be readily available for use. Meperidine is an opioid analgesic, but is not used for epidural analgesia. Betamethasone is a glucocorticoid used to enhance fetal lung maturity before premature delivery. Carboprost is an abortifacient. **Cognitive Level:** Analyzing **Client Need:** Pharmacological and Parenteral Therapies **Integrated Process:** Nursing Process: Planning **Content Area:** Pharmacology **Strategy:** The core issue of the question is a priority medication to have on hand during epidural analgesia. Use the process of elimination to select the antidote needed for respiratory depression, a priority adverse effect of epidural analgesia.

4 **Answer: 1, 5 Rationale:** Contractions lasting longer than 90 seconds indicate uterine hyperstimulation, which is a reason to stop the oxytocin infusion. Nausea and vomiting is an adverse effect related to the use of Pitocin, and a reason to stop the administration of the medication. The increase in blood pressure is not significant enough to be of concern. Early decelerations of fetal heart rate do not indicate fetal distress; rather, they are a reassuring sign. Squeezing the eyes shut during contractions could have variable meanings, including coping with the contraction, and needs to be correlated with other client data for proper interpretation. **Cognitive Level:** Analyzing **Client Need:** Pharmacological and Parenteral Therapies **Integrated Process:** Nursing Process: Data Collection **Content Area:** Pharmacology **Strategy:** The core issues of the question are knowledge of adverse effects of oxytocin and how to recognize them in the woman in labor. When there is more than one correct answer to a question, consider each option as a true/false statement.

5 **Answer: 4 Rationale:** The danger of preeclampsia is that it can progress to eclampsia, characterized by seizure activity. Magnesium sulfate is given to prevent seizures. Magnesium is not given to stabilize BP or to regulate magnesium level or uterine contractions. **Cognitive Level:** Analyzing **Client Need:** Pharmacological and Parenteral Therapies **Integrated Process:** Nursing Process: Evaluation **Content Area:** Pharmacology **Strategy:** The core issue of the question is the action of magnesium sulfate in a client with preeclampsia. Use drug knowledge and the process of elimination to make a selection.

6 **Answer: 3 Rationale:** An indirect Coombs' test assesses for the presence of Rh antibodies in the maternal blood, an indication that the mother is a candidate for RhoGAM. Hemoglobin is not a determinant for the administration of RhoGAM. Direct Coombs' test and bilirubin tests are conducted on the newborn. **Cognitive Level:** Analyzing **Client Need:** Pharmacological and Parenteral Therapies **Integrated Process:** Nursing Process: Data Collection **Content Area:** Pharmacology **Strategy:** The core issue of the question is the laboratory indicator that signals the need for administration of RhoGAM. Specific knowledge of this drug is needed to answer this question. Use the process of elimination.

7 **Answer: 3 Rationale:** Terbutaline, a beta-adrenergic agent, has many maternal and fetal side effects, including tachycardia, cardiac dysrhythmias, and pulmonary edema. In addition to taking routine vital signs, the nurse should monitor for pulmonary edema. The frequency of measurement of fetal heart tones and oral temperature depends on the intensity and length of the drug therapy, as well as surrounding circumstances. Deep-tendon reflex monitoring is not indicated. **Cognitive Level:** Analyzing **Client Need:** Pharmacological and Parenteral Therapies **Integrated Process:** Nursing Process: Data Collection **Content Area:** Pharmacology **Strategy:** The core issue of the question is knowledge that terbutaline is a beta-adrenergic drug that can lead to adverse effects, including pulmonary edema. Use the ABCs to help focus on breathing and respiratory assessment.

8 **Answer: 3 Rationale:** Corticosteroids such as betamethasone have been shown to enhance fetal lung maturity and prevent respiratory distress. Betamethasone does not stop labor. A side effect of betamethasone is an increased risk of infection. Betamethasone does not stop cervical changes. **Cognitive Level:** Applying **Client Need:** Pharmacological and Parenteral Therapies **Integrated Process:** Nursing Process: Implementation **Content Area:** Pharmacology **Strategy:** Specific medication knowledge is needed to answer the question. Recall that a drug ending in *-sone* is likely to be a steroid, and this hastens lung maturity in the fetus at risk for premature delivery.

9 **Answer: 2 Rationale:** Phytonadione is given to supply vitamin K, which the newborn cannot produce in the early days of life because of lack of the intestinal flora needed to synthesize it. Although phytonadione does treat hemorrhagic disease of the newborn, its use in the healthy infant is prophylactic. Phytonadione is given to supply vitamin K only; the medication is not a multivitamin. Phytonadione is not water-soluble, it is fat soluble. **Cognitive Level:** Analyzing **Client Need:** Pharmacological and Parenteral Therapies **Integrated Process:** Communication and Documentation **Content Area:** Pharmacology **Strategy:** Note the critical word *best* in the stem of the question, which tells you that more than one or all answers might be factually correct. Note also the critical word *healthy*, which eliminates the option pertaining to disease.

10 **Answer: 2, 4 Rationale:** The nurse would give the ophthalmic dose by applying a 0.5–1 cm ribbon of ointment into each lower conjunctival sac. To prevent a possible contamination, a new tube is used for each newborn. The dose can be delayed up to an hour after birth, but not 2 hours. The eyes are not cleansed or irrigated after the dose. Ophthalmic erythromycin does not cause eye irritation; the previously used silver nitrate (1%) solution caused eye irritation in the neonate. **Cognitive Level:** Applying **Client Need:** Pharmacological and Parenteral Therapies **Integrated Process:** Nursing Process: Implementation **Content Area:** Pharmacology **Strategy:** Use the process of elimination, keeping in mind the principles of aseptic technique and standard procedure for administration of eye medications. When more than one answer is correct, consider each option as a true/false statement.

11 **Answer: 1, 2 Rationale:** The rubella vaccine is prepared with a live virus; therefore, it is not appropriate to administer during pregnancy. Clients are counseled to avoid pregnancy for three months after immunization. It is not necessary for the mother to stop breastfeeding the newborn after receiving a rubella vaccine. Rubella vaccine does not cause the recipient to become contagious; this is an unnecessary action. Rubella vaccine, given to the mother, does not place the infant at risk for acquiring the disease. After receiving a rubella vaccine, pregnancy should be avoided for 2–3 months. **Cognitive Level:** Analyzing **Client Need:** Pharmacological and Parenteral Therapies **Integrated Process:** Nursing Process: Planning

Content Area: Pharmacology **Strategy:** Knowledge of immunizations is critical to planning care for clients. Rubella vaccine is a live-virus vaccine, and therefore pregnancy should be avoided while immunity is formed. When there is more than one correct answer, consider each option as a true/false statement.

12 **Answer: 1 Rationale:** This client statement indicates that she does not understand the fundamental indications for treatment of this potential blood incompatibility. If the infant is found to be Rh-positive, the client will be given RhoGAM within 72 hours of delivery to block any antigen–antibody formation. If an Rh-negative client is carrying an Rh-positive infant, the potential for mixing of fetal blood into the maternal system could occur at mid-pregnancy and at delivery of the placenta. This client statement indicates that she does understand the fundamental indications for treatment of this potential blood incompatibility and the need to block any antigen–antibody formation. **Cognitive Level:** Analyzing **Client Need:** Pharmacological and Parenteral Therapies **Integrated Process:** Nursing Process: Evaluation **Content Area:** Pharmacology **Strategy:** Mapping out the case management of a client with Rh-negative blood is helpful in choosing potential interventions throughout pregnancy.

13 **Answer: 3 Rationale:** Aerosol medications are delivered via a liquid mist, which delivers medication to the lower respiratory tract. Postural drainage would be done if indicated. The droplets of the aerosol medication need to be small, not large. Drugs are always administered during pregnancy after evaluating both the benefit to the mother and the risks to the fetus. **Cognitive Level:** Analyzing **Client Need:** Pharmacological and Parenteral Therapies **Integrated Process:** Nursing Process: Planning **Content Area:** Pharmacology **Strategy:** Remember that the underlying principle of respiratory care entails postural drainage, mist oxygen that delivers medication to the lower respiratory tract, and oral medications to decrease viscous secretions. The pregnant client actually breathes in more volume than the nonpregnant client. The nurse would be wise to monitor the fetal effects of the medications given to the mother; in this case, beta-adrenergic agents cause fetal tachycardia.

14 **Answer: 3, 4 Rationale:** The neonate intestinal tract is sterile at birth. Colonization of bacteria in the gut necessary for vitamin K synthesis takes approximately a week to occur. The neonate cannot absorb vitamin K from the gastrointestinal tract due to a lack of intestinal flora. Phytonadione is vitamin K and does not prevent neonate contamination from maternal gonorrhea. Vitamin K is a fat-soluble vitamin that aids the synthesis of clotting factors in the immature liver of the neonate. The administration of phytonadione to a neonate is not mandated by state law. **Cognitive Level:** Analyzing **Client Need:** Pharmacological and Parenteral Therapies **Integrated Process:** Communication and Documentation **Content Area:** Pharmacology **Strategy:** Vitamin K is critical to normal clotting; careful attention to the subtle differences in the available answers will support better scores. When more than one answer is correct, consider each option as a true/false statement.

15 **Answer: 2 Rationale:** Magnesium sulfate is a CNS depressant; therefore, disappearance of the patellar or knee-jerk reflex would indicate serious CNS depression. It is given to prevent seizures, relaxes smooth muscles resulting in a decrease in blood pressure, and would not cause an increase in respiratory rate. **Cognitive Level:** Analyzing **Client Need:** Pharmacological and Parenteral Therapies **Integrated Process:** Nursing Process: Evaluation **Content Area:** Pharmacology **Strategy:** Remember your CNS assessments and that the patellar reflex is a specific indicator of CNS integrity. In a client receiving magnesium sulfate, you would expect the patellar reflex to be decreased or absent.

16 **Answer: 4 Rationale:** The antidote for magnesium sulfate is calcium gluconate. Oxygen, epinephrine, and potassium chloride will not reverse the effects of magnesium sulfate toxicity. **Cognitive Level:** Remembering **Client Need:** Pharmacological and Parenteral Therapies **Integrated Process:** Nursing Process: Implementation **Content Area:** Pharmacology **Strategy:** Calcium gluconate is an antidote for excessive magnesium sulfate, and safe practice indicates that this drug should be available at the bedside.

17 **Answer: 3 Rationale:** Excretion of magnesium sulfate is primarily accomplished through the renal system. Critical assessments prior to administration of the drug would be focused on the body's ability to excrete the medication and the status of the CNS. Both assessments should be within normal limits, or the prescribing health care provider should be notified. Urinary glucose, acetone, and specific gravity may be important data but they are not of highest priority for this client. Vital signs are important data, but they are not a high priority specific to a client receiving magnesium sulfate therapy. A funduscopic exam of the eyes would not be performed prior to starting magnesium sulfate therapy. **Cognitive Level:** Analyzing **Client Need:** Pharmacological and Parenteral Therapies **Integrated Process:** Nursing Process: Data Collection **Content Area:** Pharmacology **Strategy:** The key to correctly answering this question is to focus on indications for stopping the drug; if these signs are present prior to administration, they must be reported to the prescriber and recorded as baseline data.

18 **Answer: 2 Rationale:** Magnesium sulfate is an antiepileptic medication given to pregnant women with preeclampsia to diminish the risk of seizures. The drug is a CNS depressant and therefore acts to reduce central nervous system activity. Agitation, dry, pale skin, and increased respirations would not be expected effects. **Cognitive Level:** Understanding **Client Need:** Pharmacological and Parenteral Therapies **Integrated Process:** Nursing Process: Data Collection **Content Area:** Pharmacology **Strategy:** Understanding the actions of CNS depressants is essential in finding the correct answer. Remember that CNS depressants should diminish reflex activity, not stop it altogether, or the client will cease respiratory and cardiac function.

19 **Answer: 4 Rationale:** Epidural medications cause vasodilatation, which can lead to hypotension. This is the primary risk factor the nurse needs to monitor after placement. Strength of uterine contractions can be considered once the client's ABCs are stable. Positioning can be considered once the client's ABCs are stable. Teaching can be considered once the client's ABCs are stable. **Cognitive Level:** Analyzing **Client Need:** Pharmacological and Parenteral Therapies **Integrated Process:** Nursing Process: Implementation **Content Area:** Pharmacology **Strategy:** Remember that many local anesthetics cause vasodilatation.

20 **Answer: 3, 4, 5 Rationale:** It is important to keep the room quiet; too much stimulation may trigger seizures. The most critical incident that could occur in a client receiving magnesium sulfate is toxic CNS depression, which could affect respiratory and cardiac function. Therefore, the antidote should be available at the bedside. The nurse should

assess for patellar reflexes to detect excessive dosing. It is notnecessary to severely limit fluid intake. It is not necessary to prepare for precipitous birth. **Cognitive Level:** Analyzing **Client Need:** Pharmacological and Parenteral Therapies **Integrated Process:** Nursing Process: Implementation **Content Area:** Pharmacology **Strategy:** The critical word in the stem of the question is *appropriate*, which tells you that the correct options are also correct interventions. Use knowledge of magnesium sulfate and the process of elimination to make a selection.

Key Terms to Review

ergotism p. 455 **prostaglandins** p. 456 **surfactant** p. 459

References

Adams, M., Holland, L., & Urban, C. (2011). *Pharmacology for nurses: A pathophysiologic approach.* (3rd ed.). Upper Saddle River, NJ: Pearson Education, Inc.

Adams, M., & Koch, R. (2010). *Pharmacology: Connections to nursing practice.* Upper Saddle River, NJ: Pearson Education, Inc.

Davidson, M., London, M., & Ladewig, P. (2012). *Olds' maternal newborn nursing and women's health across the lifespan* (9th ed.). Upper Saddle River, NJ: Pearson Education, Inc.

Ladewig, P., London, M., & Davidson, M. (2010). *Contemporary maternal-newborn nursing care* (7th ed.). Upper Saddle River, NJ: Pearson Education, Inc.

London, M., Ladewig, P., Ball, J., Bindler, R., & Cowen, K. (2011). *Maternal & child nursing care* (3rd ed.). Upper Saddle River, NJ: Pearson Education, Inc.

Wilson, B., Shannon, M., & Shields, K. (2012). *Pearson nurse's drug guide 2012.* Upper Saddle River, NJ: Pearson Education, Inc.

Test Yourself

Are you ready for the NCLEX-PN® or course exams? Use the practice tests on the companion website to check.

ANSWERS & RATIONALES

Psychiatric Medications 32

In this chapter

Cross Reference

Other chapters relevant to this content area are

Mental Health Disorders **Chapter 21**
Dependency and Addiction **Chapter 22**
Crisis Intervention and Suicide **Chapter 23**

I. GENERAL GUIDELINES FOR PSYCHIATRIC MEDICATIONS (SEE BOX 32–1)

II. ANTIPSYCHOTICS

A. Phenothiazines

1. Are **neuroleptics** (drugs used to treat psychosis); also called typical (traditional) antipsychotic agents (Box 32–2)
2. Assist in improving thought processes and positive symptoms in schizophrenia and other psychoses; are less effective in treating negative symptoms
3. Typical antipsychotics are predominantly dopamine **antagonists** (DA), which block postsynaptic D_2 receptors in several DA tracts in brain
4. Selected agents are also used as antiemetics and antihistamines; chlorpromazine is also used for intractable hiccups
5. **Tolerance** to antipsychotic medications is very uncommon; they are the most toxic drugs used in psychiatry

NCLEX® 6. Medication effects can usually be seen in 1–2 days, but substantial improvement usually takes 2–4 weeks and full effects may not occur for several months

7. Initially, a thorough baseline evaluation is needed, including laboratory tests such as white blood cell (WBC) count and electrocardiogram (ECG)
8. Side/adverse effects
   a. Gynecomastia, galactorrhea, amenorrhea (occasionally), and weight gain
   b. Sedation and orthostatic hypotension
   NCLEX® c. **Anticholinergic effects** (dry mouth, blurred vision, urinary retention, photophobia, constipation, tachycardia)
   NCLEX® d. **Akathisia** (an uncontrollable need to move)
   NCLEX® e. **Parkinsonism** (a set of symptoms that resembles Parkinson's disease)

Box 32–1

General Guidelines for Psychiatric Medications

Administration Principles

1. Review current medications (including OTC drugs and herbal products) and history of any allergies to identify potential risks to client.
2. Administer doses on time to maintain therapeutic blood levels.
3. Do not break or allow client to chew sustained release or enteric-coated preparations.
4. Many drugs cause CNS depression, so monitor for adverse effects and maintain a safe environment.
5. Provide both verbal and written instructions to client, and provide phone number to call if questions arise or problems occur.
6. When risk of suicide is of concern, do not allow access to large quantities of medication; ensure that doses are swallowed and not "cheeked."

Client Teaching

1. Understand medication actions, side/adverse effects, signs of toxicity, importance of follow-up with prescriber and follow-up laboratory tests, and how to self-administer.
2. Do not take any OTC or herbal preparations without first consulting prescriber.
3. Take exactly as prescribed and do not miss or double doses.
4. Report adverse or toxic effects promptly.
5. Many psychiatric medications cause CNS depression; do not drive, use hazardous equipment, or engage in other activities requiring alertness until individual effects are known.
6. Do not drink alcohol or take other OTC medications that cause drowsiness to avoid interactive effects.
7. Do not discontinue without consulting with prescriber.

f. **Agranulocytosis** is rare, marked by a severe deficit or lack of granulocytic WBCs (neutrophils, basophils, eosinophils)

NCLEX® g. **Neuroleptic malignant syndrome (NMS)**, characterized by catatonia, rigidity, stupor, unstable blood pressure (BP), hyperthermia, profuse sweating, dyspnea, and incontinence; treated with bromocriptine (Parlodel) and dantrolene (Dantrium) if usual treatment for hyperthermia is ineffective; drug must be changed

NCLEX® h. **Tardive dyskinesia**: (inability to perform voluntary movement; "tardive" indicates late onset); a serious side effect of antipsychotic agents

NCLEX® i. Overdoses are not usually fatal; treatment is supportive (e.g., gastric lavage to empty the stomach); can cause severe central nervous system (CNS) depression (somnolence to coma, hypotension),

Box 32–2

Typical and Atypical Antipsychotic Drugs

Typical Antipsychotics	Atypical Antipsychotics
Phenothiazine	Aripiprazole (Abilify)
Chlorpromazine (Thorazine)	Clozapine (Clozaril)
Fluphenazine (Prolixin)	Olanzapine (Zyprexa)
Perphenazine (Trilafon)	Paliperidone (Invega)
Thioridazine (Mellaril)	Quetiapine (Seroquel)
Trifluoperazine (Stelazine)	Risperidone (Risperdal)
Nonphenothiazine	Ziprasidone (Geodon)
Haloperidol (Haldol)	
Loxapine (Loxitane)	
Molindone (Moban)	
Pimozide (Orap)	
Thiothixene (Navane)	

extrapyramidal side effects or ESPEs (parkinsonism, dystonia, akathisia, tardive dyskinesia) and restlessness or agitation, seizures, hyperthermia, increased anticholinergic symptoms, and dysrhythmias

j. Low-potency drugs are more likely to cause sedation and hypotension, while high-potency drugs cause more EPSEs

9. Nursing considerations

NCLEX® **a.** Observe client taking medication in an inpatient setting to ensure medications are swallowed and not "cheeked"

b. Monitor vital signs and urine output

NCLEX® **c.** Monitor and manage side effects, as appropriate (see Table 32–1)

Table 32–1 Interventions for Side Effects of Antipsychotic Drugs

Side Effects	Nursing Interventions
Peripheral Nervous System Effects	
Constipation	Increase fluid intake and dietary fiber intake; provide laxatives as needed
Dry mouth	Advise client to use sugarless hard candy or gum and take sips of water often
Nasal congestion	Suggest OTC nasal decongestants that are safe for use with antipsychotic agents
Blurred vision	Ask client to avoid dangerous tasks (symptom usually lasts only a short time at beginning of treatment; eye drops should be used for short-term need)
Mydriasis	Advise client to report any eye pain immediately
Photophobia	Advise client to wear sunglasses when in sunlight
Orthostatic hypotension	Advise client to get out of chair or bed slowly, to sit before standing, and to rise slowly; observe to see if change to another antipsychotic is advisable
Tachycardia	This is usually a reflex response to hypotension; with effective treatment of hypotension, reflex tachycardia usually decreases; with clozapine, withhold dose if pulse rate is over 140
Urinary retention	Encourage client to void when urge is present and to void frequently; catheterize for residual urine; client should closely monitor output; older men with benign prostatic hyperplasia are particularly susceptible
Urinary hesitation	Provide privacy; encourage client to take time to void, run water in sink, or pour warm water over perineum
Sedation	Help client to get up, get dressed, and begin the day early
Weight gain	Advise client to maintain appropriate diet
Agranulocytosis	Monitor WBC counts weekly; there is a high incidence of agranulocytosis for clients who are taking clozapine If WBC is less than 3500 cells/mm^3 prior to therapy, no treatment should begin After treatment has begun, a WBC under 3000 cells/mm^3 and a granulocyte count under 1500 cells/mm^3 warrant interruption of treatment to monitor for infection; if WBC is under 2000 cells/mm^3 and granulocyte count is less than 1000 cells/mm^3, halt therapy and do not begin treatment with drug again; if infection develops, antibiotics should be prescribed
Central Nervous System Effects	
Akathisia	Usually develops within the first 2 months Client experiences an uncontrollable need to move; occurs most often with high potency antipsychotics Treatment is usually with beta-blockers, benzodiazepines, and anticholinergic drugs; antipsychotic agent should be changed to a lower potency one Distinguish between akathisia and exacerbation of psychosis; if akathisia is confused with anxiety or psychotic agitation, antipsychotic dosage may be increased, making akathisia more intense
Dystonias	Acute: Often occur early in treatment and are dangerous and severe; oculogyric crisis or torticollis are most common Immediate treatment includes antiparkinson drug or antihistamine; reassure client Obtain order for IM administration when client begins treatment with antipsychotics, or if in acute state of dystonia, call physician immediately For less acute dystonias, notify physician when an order for an antiparkinson drug is warranted
Drug-induced parkinsonism	A chronic disease characterized by a fine, slowly spreading tremor, muscular parkinsonism weakness and rigidity, and a peculiar gait induced by some antipsychotic drugs; monitor for three major symptoms: tremors, rigidity, and bradykinesia; report to physician immediately; antiparkinson drugs will be indicated

(continued)

Table 32–1 Interventions for Side Effects of Antipsychotic Drugs *(continued)*

Side Effects	Nursing Interventions
Tardive dyskinesia (TD)	Develops in 15% to 20% of clients during long-term therapy; risk is related to dyskinesia (TD) duration of treatment and dose; often symptoms are irreversible; monitor for signs using Abnormal Involuntary Movement Scale (AIMS); anticholinergic agents will worsen TD, so use is contraindicated
Neuroleptic malignant syndrome	This is a fatal side effect of antipsychotic drugs; routinely take client's temperature and encourage adequate water intake; monitor for rigidity, tremor, and similar symptoms
Seizures	Occur in approximately 1% of clients taking antipsychotic medications; clozapine causes an even higher rate, up to 5% of clients taking 600–900 mg/day For dosages of clozapine greater than 600 mg/day, an EEG should be performed; if a seizure occurs, it may be necessary to discontinue clozapine

NCLEX® **d.** Consider long-acting depot injections such as haloperidol and fluphenazine for long-term therapy of schizophrenia; usually reduces rate of relapse

NCLEX® **e.** Monitor results of periodic WBC counts and other laboratory studies

10. Client teaching

a. Take medication as prescribed; discontinuing therapy is a major relapse factor for clients with schizophrenia

b. Take oral doses with food, milk, or a full glass of water to decrease gastric irritation

c. Dilute most concentrates in 120 mL of distilled or acidified tap water or fruit juice just before use; avoid skin contact with liquid to prevent contact dermatitis

NCLEX® **d.** Use sunscreen and protective clothing such as long sleeves, pants, and hats when outdoors to prevent photosensitivity

Memory Aid

Many drugs cause photosensitivity as a side effect; when protection from the sun is an option, consider carefully whether this could be the correct answer.

e. Expect observable response after 7–10 days, but full effects take 3–6 weeks

NCLEX® **f.** Expect urine color to change from yellow to pinkish or red-brown; this is an expected change and is not harmful

NCLEX® **g.** Change position slowly to avoid orthostatic hypotension

NCLEX® **h.** Report fever, malaise, and other signs of infection such as sore throat; these may indicate agranulocytosis

i. Follow-up WBC count and liver function studies are needed

j. Avoid sudden withdrawal of drug, which may lead to return of psychotic symptoms

k. Learn about other drugs that may be used for ESPEs (see Box 32–3)

B. Atypical antipsychotic drugs

1. Exert both dopamine receptor subtype 2 (D_2) and serotonin receptor subtype 2 ($5HT_2$) receptor-blocking action (are DA and 5HT antagonists)
2. Blockage of serotonin receptors is thought to liberate dopamine in cortex and may explain some reduction in negative symptoms
3. Atypical agents cause few or no EPSEs
4. NCLEX® Used to treat positive and negative symptoms of schizophrenia and other disorders with psychotic features and to treat mood symptoms, hostility, violence, suicidal behavior, and cognitive impairment seen in schizophrenia

Memory Aid

Remember that typical drugs are effective against positive symptoms of schizophrenia, while atypical antipsychotics are effective against both positive and negative symptoms.

Box 32–3

Medications Used to Treat Extrapyramidal Side Effects

Anticholinergic: Benztropine (Cogentin)

Antihistamine: Diphenhydramine (Benadryl)

Dopamine Agonist: Amantadine (Symmetrel)

5. Are especially useful for clients experiencing first psychotic episode and are not responding well to typical antipsychotics or have had dose-limiting side effects from traditional neuroleptics
6. Refer back to Box 32–2 for listing of drugs in this category
7. Side/adverse effects

NCLEX®
   a. Clozapine (Clozaril): agranulocytosis, requiring weekly WBC count and a limit of not more than a 1-week supply of drug to enforce compliance with weekly labwork; NMS and seizures are also of concern

Memory Aid

Remember that clozapine begins with *c* and associate that with *CBC* to help you remember that white blood cell counts can drop with this medication, requiring close monitoring.

   b. Risperidone (Risperdal): orthostatic hypotension, insomnia, agitation, headache, anxiety, rhinitis, NMS
   c. Olanzapine (Zyprexa): few incidents of EPSEs, but NMS and seizures are possible
   d. Aripiprazole is similar to others but with increased risk of suicidal tendency

NCLEX®
   e. In general, side effects of atypical antipsychotics include weight gain, anticholinergic effects, sedation and cardiac effects, with a low incidence of EPSEs
8. Nursing considerations
   a. Clozapine is usually given 1–2 times daily
   b. Risperidone is usually administered PO in 1–2 daily doses; for debilitated or elderly clients or for those with renal or hepatic impairment, dosage should be reduced

NCLEX®
   c. Because of risk of fatal agranulocytosis, clozapine is reserved for clients with severe schizophrenia who have not responded to traditional antipsychotic drugs
9. Client teaching: as per Box 32–1

III. ANTIDEPRESSANTS

A. Tricyclic antidepressants (TCAs)

1. TCAs block monoamine reuptake, elevate mood, increase activity and alertness, decrease client's preoccupation with morbidity, improve appetite, and regulate sleep patterns

NCLEX®
2. Therapeutic effect occurs in 1–3 weeks, with maximum effect in 6–8 weeks
3. Other uses include treatment of chronic insomnia, attention-deficit hyperactivity disorder (ADHD) and panic disorder
4. Common medications are listed in Table 32–2
   a. TCAs are equally effective; major differences are in side effects; for example, doxepin has sedative effects and is more useful in clients with insomnia
   b. Older adults and those with glaucoma, constipation, or prostatic hyperplasia can be especially sensitive to anticholinergic effects of TCAs; therefore, a TCA such as desipramine with weak anticholinergic effects would be more appropriate with such clients
5. Administration considerations
   a. Dosing with TCAs is individualized and based on clinical response or plasma drug levels (must be above 225 ng/mL for antidepressant effects to occur)
   b. TCAs have long half-lives, so may be taken daily in a single dose
   c. Once-a-day dosing at bedtime is more easily incorporated into daily routine, promotes sleep (sedative effect), and reduces intensity of daytime side effects
   d. For clients at risk for suicide, do not allow access to large quantity of medication; keep hospitalized until risk of suicide has been ruled out
6. Significant drug interactions

NCLEX®
   a. TCAs taken with a monoamine oxidase inhibitor (MAOI) can lead to severe hypertension from excessive adrenergic stimulation of heart and blood vessels

Table 32–2 Medications Commonly Used to Treat Depression

Drug Class and Name: Generic (Trade)	Nursing Responsibilities
Tricyclic Antidepressants (TCAs)	
Amitriptyline (Elavil) Clomipramine (Anafranil) Desipramine (Norpramin) Doxepin (Sinequan) Imipramine (Tofranil) Nortriptyline (Pamelor) Protriptyline (Vivactil) Trimipramine (Surmontil)	• Educate client early about potential side effects • Inform client that side effects will diminish with time and, if needed, management alternatives can be implemented • Advise that response will take time and continued use is essential • Inform client that first-time treatment for major depression should continue for 6 to 12 months • Warn client of a possible significant weight gain • Monitor for improvement; if no change or minimum change after 2–4 weeks, it may be necessary to change medication
Second-Generation Tetracyclics	
Amoxapine (Asendin) Maprotiline (Ludiomil) Mirtazepine (Remeron)	• General considerations are same as for tricyclics
Selective Serotonin Reuptake Inhibitors (SSRIs)	
Citalopram (Celexa) Escitalopram (Lexapro) Fluoxetine (Prozac) Fluvoxamine (Luvox) Paroxetine (Paxil) Sertraline (Zoloft)	• Inform client to take medication as prescribed; abrupt discontinuation of drug is contraindicated • Continuously monitor client for side/adverse effects, particularly in area of sexual dysfunction; client may be reluctant to discuss
Monoamine Oxidase Inhibitors (MAOIs)	
Isocarboxazid (Marplan) Phenelzine (Nardil) Selegiline (Emsam) Tranylcypromine (Parnate)	• Educate client concerning a tyramine-restricted diet • Caution client about side effects and adverse effects of MAOIs • Educate client about careful use of OTC or other prescription drug and be sure client understands seriousness of effects • Monitor efficacy of drugs and continuously re-educate client to avoid abruptly discontinuing medication or not taking it as prescribed
Atypical Antidepressants	
Amoxapine (Asendin) Bupropion (Wellbutrin) Desvenlafaxine (Pristiq) Duloxetine (Cymbalta) Mirtazapine (Remeron) Nefazodone (Serzone) Trazodone (Desyrel) Venlafaxine (Effexor)	• Instruct client about adverse or side effect of medication, especially seizure risks at higher drug doses • Instruct client about importance of taking this and all medication as prescribed • Instruct client to take medication as prescribed and monitor for any adverse or side effects • Instruct client to report any signs of sexual dysfunction, especially priapism, immediately

b. TCAs potentiate responses to direct-acting sympathomimetics (e.g., epinephrine and norepinephrine) by blocking uptake of these drugs into adrenergic terminals, prolonging their presence in synaptic space

c. TCAs decrease responses to indirect-acting sympathomimetics (e.g., ephedrine and amphetamine) by blocking uptake of these drugs into adrenergic nerves, preventing them from reaching their site of action in nerve terminal

NCLEX® **d.** TCAs exert anticholinergic actions of their own; thus, they intensify effects of other medications with anticholinergic actions (antihistamines and OTC sleep aids); avoid these products while taking TCAs

e. CNS depression caused by TCAs adds to CNS depression caused by other drugs; avoid use of CNS depressants, including alcohol, antihistamines, opioids, and barbiturates

7. Side/adverse effects

NCLEX® **a.** Most common are orthostatic hypotension, sedation, and anticholinergic effects

b. Most serious is cardiac toxicity; clients over age 40 and those with heart disease should have baseline ECG and then every 6 months

NCLEX® **c.** Adverse effects of each drug are more fully described in Table 32–3

Table 32–3 Most Common Adverse Effects from Antidepressant Medications

Effect	Manifestations
Orthostatic hypotension	Major decrease in BP with body position changes
Anticholinergic	Blockade of muscarinic cholinergic receptors, which produces dry mouth, blurred vision, photophobia, constipation, urinary hesitancy, tachycardia
Sedation	Sleepiness and difficulty maintaining arousal (caused by blockade of histamine receptors in CNS)
Cardiac toxicity	Decreased vagal influence (secondary to muscarinic blockade) and acting directly on bundle of His to slow conduction
Seizures	Lower seizure threshold
Hypomania	Mild mania can occur
Sexual dysfunction	Anorgasm, delayed ejaculation, decreased libido
Hypertensive crisis from dietary tyramine	Although MAOIs normally produce hypotension, can also cause severe hypertension if client eats tyramine-rich foods

8. Nursing considerations
   a. Advise clients of possible side effects and that therapeutic response takes some weeks to achieve; clients and families often become impatient when client is experiencing drug side effects while still having original symptoms
   b. Refer back to Table 32–2 for nursing responsibilities with TCAs, and see Table 32–3 for manifestations of common adverse effects
9. Client teaching
   a. Side effects diminish with time, and symptoms will lessen as medication regime is followed
   b. Encourage client and family to utilize other available therapies as well
   c. Refer back to Box 32–1 and Tables 32–2 and 32–3 for specific points to include in teaching

B. MAOIs

1. Because of potentially fatal food and drug interactions, MAOIs are not a first choice to treat depression unless client has atypical depression
2. Monoamine oxidase (MAO) is an enzyme present in liver, intestinal wall, and terminals of monoamine-containing neurons; it converts monoamine transmitters (norepinephrine, serotonin, and dopamine) into inactive products; in liver and intestine, MAO inactivates tyramine and other biogenic amines in food
3. MAOIs decrease amount of MAO in liver that breaks down amino acids tyramine and tryptophan
4. MAOIs have been used with some success to treat bulimia, obsessive-compulsive disorder, and panic disorder
5. Common medications: refer again to Table 32–2
6. Contraindications: clients over age 60 or those with pheochromocytoma, heart failure, liver disease, severe renal impairment, cerebrovascular defect, cardiovascular disease, or hypertension
7. Significant drug interactions
   NCLEX® a. Taking SSRIs with MAOIs can cause **serotonin syndrome** (agitation, sweating, confusion, fever, hyperreflexia, tachycardia, hypotension, muscle rigidity, ataxia); avoid this combination
   NCLEX® b. Antihypertensive drugs potentiate hypotensive effects of MAOIs
   c. Meperidine can produce hyperthermia in clients taking MAOIs and should be avoided
8. NCLEX® Significant food interactions
   a. Dietary tyramine, some other dietary constituents, and indirect-acting sympathomimetics (e.g., amphetamine, methylphenidate, ephedrine, cocaine) can precipitate a hypertensive crisis in clients taking MAOIs
   b. See Box 32–4 for lists of foods to avoid or use cautiously while taking an MAOI
9. NCLEX® Side/adverse effects
   a. Orthostatic hypotension
   b. Edema, weight gain
   c. Reports of insomnia, anxiety, agitation, hypomania, and even mania
   d. Sexual dysfunction
10. Nursing considerations
    a. Monitor client for ability to adhere to strict dietary regime
    NCLEX® b. Consult with primary physician about changes in vital signs to avoid potentially fatal hypertensive crisis
11. Client teaching
    a. Explain symptoms of orthostatic hypotension and to avoid injury by rising from bed or chair slowly
    NCLEX® b. Provide dietary teaching to avoid hypertensive crisis (include written list of foods to avoid)

Box 32–4

Foods to Avoid with Monoamine Oxidase Inhibitors

Foods to Avoid

- Dairy: aged cheeses such as Roquefort, blue, brie, and camembert; sour cream, yogurt, all cheeses except those noted below
- Meats and fish: aged/cured such as hot dogs, bologna, pepperoni, salami, sausage
- Fruits and vegetables: canned figs, papaya products (including meat tenderizers), raisins, broad bean pods, tofu, soybean extracts
- Alcohol: draft beer, Chianti red wine
- Other: sauerkraut, soy sauce, yeast extracts, soups (especially miso) that have protein extract, and Brewer's yeast or extracts
- Drugs: other antidepressant drugs, nasal and sinus decongestants, allergy, hay fever and asthma remedies, narcotics (especially meperidine), epinephrine, stimulants, cocaine, amphetamines

Consume with Caution

- Cheeses: mozzarella, cottage, ricotta, cream, processed
- Meats and fish: beef and chicken liver, meats, herring
- Fruits and vegetables: raspberries, bananas, small amounts only of avocado, spinach
- Alcohol: wine
- Other: monosodium glutamate, pizza, small amounts only of chocolate, caffeine, nuts, dairy products
- Drugs: insulin, oral antidiabetics, oral anticoagulants, thiazide diuretics, anticholinergic agents, muscle relaxants

C. SSRIs

1. Block reuptake of serotonin and intensify transmission at serotonergic synapses; effects are often seen after 1–3 weeks and similar to TCA effects
2. SSRIs have the same efficacy as TCAs, exhibit fewer side effects than either TCAs or MAOIs, and have shorter time between initial dose and beginning of reduced signs and symptoms of depression
3. All SSRIs are effective in treatment of obsessive-compulsive disorder (OCD), panic disorder, and bulimia nervosa
4. Common medications (refer again to Table 32–2)
5. Administration considerations
   a. Most SSRIs should not be prescribed for clients with a hypersensitivity to drug or severe hepatic or renal disease
   NCLEX® b. Lowered drug doses or longer dosing interval may be needed with impaired hepatic function, multiple drug therapy, or older adult clients
   NCLEX® c. To prevent serotonin syndrome, SSRIs should not be administered with MAOIs
   d. If a client is on an MAOI and is transferred to fluoxetine, at least 5 weeks should elapse before beginning the fluoxetine; to transfer from fluoxetine to MAOIs, at least 2 weeks should elapse before beginning MAOI
   e. In a client taking fluoxetine and warfarin, monitor coagulation closely because fluoxetine is highly bound to plasma proteins and may displace other highly bound drugs such as warfarin
   NCLEX® f. Monitor complete blood count (CBC) for decreased red blood cells (RBCs), WBCs, and platelets, and monitor bleeding time for increase
6. Side/adverse effects
   NCLEX® a. Common initial side effects include nausea, drowsiness, dizziness, headache, sweating, anxiety, insomnia, anorexia, and nervousness; are generally milder and better tolerated than TCAs
   b. Sexual dysfunction is experienced by 20–40% of clients, and must be discussed with client
7. Nursing considerations
   a. Monitor mood changes; notify physician if client demonstrates an increase in anxiety, nervousness, or insomnia
   NCLEX® b. Monitor for suicidal tendencies, especially during early drug therapy when client begins to have increased energy and can act on suicidal thoughts
   NCLEX® c. Restrict amount of drug available to client to prevent overdose
   d. Monitor appetite, nutritional intake, and weight

8. Client teaching: as per Box 32–1 and notify prescriber if a rash occurs, which may indicate hypersensitivity

D. Atypical antidepressants

1. Serotonin-norepinephrine reuptake inhibitors (SNRIs): desvenlafaxine (Pristiq), venlafaxine (Effexor), and duloxetine (Cymbalta)
2. Norepinephrine and dopamine reuptake inhibitors (NDRIs): bupropion (Wellbutrin)
3. Combined reuptake inhibitor and receptor blocker: trazodone (Desyrel), nefazodone (Serzone), and mirtazapine (Remeron)
4. Administration considerations: bupropion can cause dose-related seizures, but does not have cardiotoxic, anticholinergic, and antiadrenergic side effects; dosage should be reduced in older adults or those with severe hepatic or renal disease
5. Side/adverse effects
   a. Most common side effects of bupropion are agitation and insomnia
   b. Common side effects of trazodone are sedation, orthostatic hypotension, nausea, and vomiting; in contrast to tricyclic agents, it lacks anticholinergic actions and is not cardiotoxic; it may cause priapism (sustained erection)
   c. Most common side effect of venlafaxine (Effexor) is nausea, but can also cause either CNS stimulation (nervousness, insomnia) or sedation
   d. Major adverse effect of bupropion is seizure activity
   e. Adverse effects of trazodone frequently include CNS changes
   f. Side effects among drugs may vary as they inhibit reuptake of different neurotransmitters (serotonin, norepinephrine, dopamine) and may also act as a receptor blocker (trazodone, nefazodone, and mirtazapine)
   g. Some common side effects include insomnia, dry mouth, constipation, elevated BP and pulse, dizziness, sweating, blurred vision, headache, drowsiness, increased appetite and increased blood glucose (duloxetine)
6. Nursing considerations
   a. Monitor clients with a history of bipolar disorder taking bupropion for symptoms of mania
   b. Monitor BP and pulse rate before and during initial therapy; clients with pre existing cardiac disease should have ECG monitored before and periodically during therapy to detect dysrhythmias
   NCLEX®
   c. Check for mental status and mood changes frequently; monitor for suicidal tendencies, especially during early therapy; restrict amount of drug available to client
7. Client teaching: as per Box 32–1

IV. MOOD STABILIZERS

A. Lithium

1. Used to control manic episodes in bipolar disorder and for long-term prophylaxis against recurrent mania and depression
2. Alters many neurotransmitter functions, possibly correcting an ion exchange abnormality or normalizing neurotransmission of norepinephrine, serotonin, dopamine, and acetylcholine
3. Common medications (see Box 32–5)
4. Administration considerations
   a. Precise dosing is based on serum lithium levels
   NCLEX®
   b. Mood stabilizing effects are usually seen in 5–7 days after initial doses, but full effect usually takes 2–3 weeks
   c. Adjunctive therapy with a benzodiazepine can provide the sedation clients need
   NCLEX®
   d. Contraindicated with sensitivity to drug; use cautiously in debilitated, dehydrated, or older adult clients; those with cardiac, renal, or thyroid disease or diabetes mellitus
   e. Should be used only where therapy (including blood levels) may be closely monitored (every 1–2 months and as needed based on client behaviors)

Box 32–5

Commonly Used Mood-Stabilizing Drugs

Lithium carbonate (Eskalith, Lithobid, lithium citrate, etc.)
Carbamazepine (Tegretol)
Lamotrigine (Lamictal)
Divalproex (Valproic Acid, Depakote ER)

NCLEX® f. Large changes in sodium intake may alter renal elimination of lithium; increasing sodium intake will increase renal excretion; conditions leading to loss of sodium (such as dehydration, sweating, diuretics, diarrhea) may lead to toxicity

NCLEX® g. Therapeutic level and the toxic levels are very close; therapeutic range is 0.8 to 1.4 mEq/L, while the toxic dose is 1.5 mEq/L or greater

h. It is essential to monitor serum lithium levels frequently because of risk of toxicity

5. Side/adverse effects
   a. Fatigue, headache, lethargy
   b. Abdominal pain, anorexia, bloating, diarrhea, nausea, dry mouth, metallic taste in mouth
   c. Polyuria, glycosuria, nephrogenic diabetes insipidus, and renal toxicity
   d. Also reported are weight gain, muscle weakness, hyperirritability, rigidity, and tremors
   e. Toxic effects classified as mild, moderate, or severe

NCLEX® f. Mild toxicity (1.5 mEq/L) leads to mild CNS changes: lethargy, decreased concentration, slight muscle weakness, coarse hand tremors, and mild ataxia

NCLEX® g. Moderate toxicity (1.5–2.5 mEq/L) leads to GI symptoms (nausea, vomiting [N/V], severe diarrhea), blurred vision, tinnitus, muscle tremors/twitching, slurred speech, worsening ataxia/incoordination

NCLEX® h. Severe toxicity (higher than 2.5 mEq/L) leads to nystagmus, hyperreflexia, impaired level of consciousness (LOC), hallucinations, muscle twitching/fasciculations, seizures, or renal shutdown; coma and death may result

6. Nursing considerations
   a. Note mood, ideation, and behaviors frequently; initiate suicide precautions if indicated

NCLEX® b. Monitor intake and output ratios; report significant changes in totals

NCLEX® c. Unless contraindicated, provide fluid intake of at least 2000 to 3000 mL/day

d. Monitor weight at least every 3 months

NCLEX® e. Observe client for signs of lithium toxicity (vomiting, diarrhea, slurred speech, decreased coordination, drowsiness, muscle weakness, or twitching); if these occur, report before administration of next dose

7. Client teaching
   a. Take medication even if feeling well; take a missed dose as soon as remembered unless within 2 hours of next dose (6 hours if extended release)

NCLEX® b. May cause dizziness or drowsiness: avoid driving, operating heavy machinery, and other activities requiring alertness until response to medication is known

NCLEX® c. Low sodium levels may lead to toxicity: drink 2000 to 3000 mL fluid each day and eat a diet with consistent and moderate sodium intake

NCLEX® d. Avoid excessive amounts of coffee, tea, and cola (because of diuretic effect); avoid activities that cause excess sodium loss; notify prescriber of fever, vomiting, and diarrhea, which also cause sodium loss

e. Weight gain may occur: follow principles of a low-calorie diet

f. Consult with prescriber before taking any OTC medications, before use of contraception, or if pregnancy is suspected

g. For clients with cardiovascular disease or over 40 years of age: understand need for ECG evaluation before and periodically during therapy; report any irregular pulse, difficulty breathing, or fainting

B. Other mood stabilizer medications

1. A variety of antiepileptic drugs demonstrate beneficial effects in bipolar disorder when lithium is ineffective, although they are not FDA approved for this use
2. Carbamazepine (Tegretol) and divalproex (e.g., Valproic Acid, Depakote; active chemical is valproic acid) have acute antimanic and long-term mood-stabilizing effects in bipolar disorder; are better than lithium in treating mixed or dysphoric bipolar states and in clients who are rapid cyclers
3. Lamotrigine is used for long-term maintenance therapy to prevent or delay relapses
4. Contraindications
   a. Carbamazepine: hypersensitivity or bone marrow depression; pregnancy unless potential benefits outweigh fetal risks; use cautiously in clients with cardiac or hepatic disease, prostatic hyperplasia, or increased intraocular pressure
   b. Divalproex: hypersensitivity or hepatic impairment; avoid use with products containing tartrazine; use cautiously with bleeding disorders, liver disease, organic brain disease, bone marrow depression, renal impairment, and in children (increased risk of hepatotoxicity); safe use in pregnancy not established

NCLEX® 5. Side/adverse effects
   a. Side effects generally include dizziness, ataxia, sedation, headache, N/V, double or blurred vision, prolonged bleeding time, transient leukopenia
   b. Adverse effects tend to include heart block, bone marrow depression, respiratory depression, exfoliative dermatitis, Stevens-Johnson syndrome, liver failure, pancreatitis

6. Nursing considerations
   a. Observe frequently for seizure activity when taking carbamazepine and monitor for facial pain because of possibility of trigeminal neuralgia
   NCLEX® b. Perform liver function tests, urinalysis, and blood urea nitrogen (BUN) routinely; measure serum ionized calcium levels at least every 6 months
   NCLEX® c. Check results of routine CBC and serum iron weekly during first 2 months and yearly thereafter for potentially fatal blood cell abnormalities; drug should be stopped if bone marrow depression occurs
7. Client teaching
   a. Take around the clock, exactly as directed
   NCLEX® b. Immediately report fever, sore throat, mouth ulcers, easy bruising, petechiae, unusual bleeding, abdominal pain, chills, rash, pale stools, dark urine, or jaundice
   c. Use sunscreen and protective clothing to prevent photosensitivity reactions with carbamazepine
   d. For female clients: use a nonhormonal form of contraception while taking carbamazepine
   e. Carry information, such as a Medic-Alert tag/bracelet, describing disease and medication regimen at all times
   f. Understand importance of follow-up monitoring
   NCLEX® g. For divalproex, be sure to take medication exactly as directed; abrupt withdrawal may lead to seizures in a susceptible client

V. SEDATIVE-HYPNOTICS AND ANXIOLYTICS

A. Benzodiazepines (BZs)

1. BZ molecules and GABA bind to each other at GABA receptor sites, resulting in *inhibition* of neurotransmission that results in a clinical decrease in anxiety level
2. **Metabolites** (result of drug biotransformation) are pharmacologically active, so drug effects persist long after parent drug is gone from plasma
3. Major indications for use are anxiety, insomnia (sedative-hypnotic effect), and seizure disorders
4. Other uses include alcohol withdrawal, skeletal muscle relaxation, substance-induced (except for amphetamines) and psychotic agitation in crisis situations
5. Common medications are listed in Box 32–6

Memory Aid

Remember that a drug that ends with the suffix *-zepam* is a benzodiazepine.

Box 32–6

Sedative-Hypnotic and Anxiolytic Medications*

Barbiturates
- Butabarbital (Butisol)
- Pentobarbital (Nembutal)
- Phenobarbital (Luminal)
- Secobarbital (Seconal)

Benzodiazepines
- Alprazolam (Xanax)
- Chlordiazepoxide (Librium)
- Clonazepam (Klonopin)
- Clorazepate (Tranxene)
- Diazepam (Valium)
- Estazolam (ProSom)**
- Flurazepam (Dalmane)**
- Lorazepam (Ativan)
- Oxazepam (Serax)
- Temazepam (Restoril)**
- Triazolam (Halcion)**

Nondiazepine Anxiolytics/ Miscellaneous
- Buspirone (Buspar)
- Eszopiclone (Lunesta)**
- Ramelteon (Rozerem)**
- Zaleplon (Sonata)**
- Zolpidem (Ambien)**

Benzodiazepine Antagonist
- Flumazenil (Romazicon)

*Drug class and name: Generic (Trade)

**Used to treat insomnia

6. Administration considerations
   NCLEX® a. BZs should be started at low doses and gradually increased to achieve desired clinical response
   b. For treatment of anxiety, BZs are usually dosed at bedtime or twice daily; only occasionally are 3 doses/day required
   c. Treatment for insomnia should be no longer than 7–10 days to avoid rebound insomnia; use sleep hygiene techniques also to establish regular sleep pattern
   NCLEX® d. BZs are contraindicated with drug sensitivity or during pregnancy or lactation (cross blood–brain barrier and enter breast milk with ease and develop quickly to toxic levels)
   e. BZs should not be used with clients who have pre existing CNS depression, severe uncontrolled pain, or narrow-angle glaucoma
   f. Because liver is site of drug biotransformation, drugs that interfere with liver metabolism (e.g., alcohol) dangerously compound BZ effects

NCLEX® 7. Side/adverse effects
   a. Hypotension
   b. Dry mouth, ataxia, dizziness, drowsiness, nausea
   c. Withdrawal symptoms (increased anxiety, flu-like symptoms, tremors)

8. Nursing considerations
   a. Note degree and manifestation of anxiety before client begins therapy
   NCLEX® b. Check client for drowsiness, light-headedness, and dizziness periodically during treatment; these usually disappear as therapy progresses
   c. Monitor BP, pulse, and respirations, and provide supportive care as needed
   NCLEX® d. Prolonged therapy may lead to psychological or physical dependence; risk is greater with larger drug doses; restrict amount of drug available to client

9. Client teaching
   a. As per Box 32–1
   b. If dose is missed, take within 1 hour or skip dose and return to regular schedule
   c. If medication is less effective after a few weeks, check with prescriber; do not increase dose
   NCLEX® d. Abrupt withdrawal of drug may cause sweating, vomiting, muscle cramps, tremors, and seizure

B. Benzodiazepine antagonist

NCLEX® 1. Flumazenil (Romazicon) is a BZ antagonist that selectively blocks BZ receptors but does not block adrenergic or cholinergic receptors

NCLEX® 2. Can reverse *sedative* effects of BZs but may not reverse BZ-induced *respiratory depression*

3. Because it does not stimulate CNS or block other receptors, it can be given for suspected BZ overdose and to reverse effects of BZs following general anesthesia

4. Works within 30 to 60 seconds of IV administration

5. Contraindicated with hypersensitivity; if receiving BZs for life-threatening medical problems, including status epilepticus or increased intracranial pressure; and for clients with serious TCA overdose

NCLEX® 6. Side effects: dizziness, agitation, confusion, N/V, hiccups, paresthesia, rigors, and shivering; principle adverse effect is seizures (occur most often with epilepsy or physical dependence on BZs)

7. Nursing considerations
   a. Monitor LOC and respiratory status before and throughout therapy
   b. Establish that client has patent airway before administration
   NCLEX® c. Institute seizure precautions
   NCLEX® d. For suspected BZ overdose: if no effects are seen after giving flumazenil, consider other causes of decreased LOC (alcohol, barbiturates, opioid analgesics)
   e. Observe client for at least 2 hours after last dose for resedation; hypoventilation may occur

8. Client teaching
   a. Client may appear alert at time of discharge but sedative effects of BZ may reoccur; avoid driving or other activities requiring alertness for at least 24 hours after discharge
   NCLEX® b. Do not take *any* alcohol or nonprescription drugs for at least 18–24 hours after discharge
   c. Resume usual activities only when no residual effects of BZs remain

C. Barbiturates

1. Cause relatively nonselective CNS depression and are prototypes of general CNS depressants; used for daytime sedation, induction of sleep, suppression of seizures, and general anesthesia

2. Can cause tolerance and dependence, have a high abuse potential, and are subject to multiple drug interactions; are powerful respiratory depressants

3. Common medications (see again Box 32–4)
4. Administration considerations
   a. Avoid intramuscular (IM) route; barbiturate solutions are highly alkaline and can cause pain and necrosis when injected IM
   NCLEX® b. As dosage is increased, response progresses from *sedation* to *sleep* to *general anesthesia*
   NCLEX® c. At hypnotic doses, barbiturates may reduce BP and heart rate; in contrast, toxic doses can cause profound hypotension and shock (from direct depressant effects on both myocardium and vascular smooth muscle)
   NCLEX® d. Tolerance to sedative and hypnotic effects and to other effects that underlie barbiturate abuse develops with repeated drug use
5. Side/adverse effects
   a. Long half-lives can produce residual effects (hangover) when taken to treat insomnia; can manifest as sedation, impaired judgment, reduced motor skills
   b. Paradoxical excitement (especially in older adult or debilitated clients)
   c. Barbiturates can intensify sensitivity to pain and may cause pain directly; their use has produced muscle pain, joint pain, and pain along nerves
   NCLEX® d. Acute barbiturate overdose produces a classic triad of symptoms: *respiratory depression*, *coma*, and *pinpoint pupils*, frequently accompanied by *hypotension* and *hypothermia*
6. Nursing considerations
   NCLEX® a. Monitor respiratory status, pulse, and BP frequently
   NCLEX® b. Prolonged therapy may lead to psychological or physical dependence; restrict amount of drug available, especially if client is depressed, suicidal, or has a history of addiction
   c. Monitor client for safety, alertness, and assist as needed with ambulation or self-care
7. Client teaching
   a. As per Box 32–1
   b. For female using oral contraceptives: use additional nonhormonal contraceptive during therapy

D. Nonbenzodiazepine anxiolytics and miscellaneous agents

1. Buspirone: used to manage anxiety; binds to serotonin and dopamine receptors and increases norepinephrine metabolism in brain
2. Buspirone's major advantages are that it is nonsedative, has no abuse potential, and does not enhance CNS depression caused by BZs, alcohol, barbiturates, and related drugs; major disadvantage is delayed onset of anxiolytic effects
3. Zolpidem, eszopiclone, and zaleplon are used for short-term treatment of insomnia; produce CNS depression; have no analgesic properties but produce sedation and induction of sleep; ramelteon treats chronic insomnia in those who have difficulty falling asleep
4. Administration considerations
   a. Giving buspirone with food delays absorption but enhances bioavailability (by reducing first-pass metabolism in liver)
   b. Zolpidem, eszopiclone, ramelteon, and zaleplon are usually given just before bedtime because of rapid onset of action
5. Side effects
   a. Most common reactions are dizziness, nausea, headache, daytime drowsiness, dream disturbances, and unpleasant taste (eszopiclone, ramelteon)
   b. Adverse effects include paradoxical excitation, mood changes, tachycardia, burred vision, confusion, myalgia
6. Nursing considerations
   NCLEX® a. Note degree and manifestations of anxiety before and periodically during therapy with buspirone
   NCLEX® b. Clients changing from other anti-anxiety agents should receive gradually decreasing doses; buspirone will not prevent withdrawal symptoms
   NCLEX® c. With zolpidem, there may be a potential for physical or psychological dependence if used longer than 7 to 10 days; limit the amount of drug available to client
   d. With zolpidem, check alertness at time of peak effect; notify prescriber if desired sedation does not occur
7. Client teaching
   a. As per Box 32–1
   NCLEX® b. With buspirone, report any chronic abnormal movements such as **dystonia** (muscle rigidity), motor restlessness, involuntary movements of facial or cervical muscles, or if pregnancy is suspected
   NCLEX® c. With drugs used for insomnia, go to bed immediately after taking dose because of rapid onset of action

VI. SUBSTANCE MISUSE

A. Alcohol abuse and disulfiram (Antabuse) therapy

1. Alcohol is a CNS depressant that causes general (relatively nonselective) depression of CNS function, primarily by enhancing GABA
2. Effect of alcohol on CNS is dose-dependent; low dosage primarily affects cortical brain function (thought processes, self-restraint, motor function); as dosage increases, CNS depression deepens, reflexes diminish greatly, and LOC is impaired
3. Management of withdrawal (outpatient versus inpatient) depends on degree of alcohol dependence
4. Most medical treatment for withdrawal includes use of BZs—chlordiazepoxide (Librium), diazepam (Valium), and lorazepam (Ativan); a regime of atenolol (a beta-adrenergic blocking agent) used in conjunction with BZs decreases amount of BZs necessary for safe detoxification
5. Disulfiram inhibits enzyme *alcohol dehydrogenase*, which catalyzes a major step in breakdown of alcohol

NCLEX®

6. When enzyme is inhibited and an individual drinks alcohol, blood concentrations of toxic metabolite *acetaldehyde* increase significantly, producing unpleasant symptoms of flushing, tachycardia, nausea, vomiting, and hypotension
7. Administration considerations
   a. Disulfiram is used only with highly selected individuals in good physical health
   b. At least 12 hours should elapse from last alcohol intake and initial dose
   c. Relatively long half-life of disulfiram ensures that several days must elapse between stopping medication and safely drinking alcohol; this probably decreases impulsive relapse
8. Adverse effects/toxicity: acetaldehyde syndrome (from ingesting alcohol and disulfiram) is noted by marked respiratory depression, cardiovascular collapse, cardiac dysrhythmias, myocardial infarction, acute heart failure, convulsions, and death
9. Nursing considerations
   a. Simultaneous use with alcohol can precipitate acetaldehyde syndrome
   b. Disulfiram effects may persist for about 2 weeks after last dose
10. Client teaching
    a. Avoid all forms of alcohol, including alcohol in sauces, cough and cold syrups, aftershave lotions, colognes, and liniments
    b. Adhere to all forms of self-help groups, both individual and group therapies, while using disulfiram therapy to establish a recovery program

B. Opioids

1. Opioids (e.g., morphine, heroin) are major drugs of abuse; are usually Schedule II substances
2. Opioid toxicity produces a classic triad of symptoms: respiratory depression, coma, and pinpoint pupils
3. Naloxone (Narcan), an opioid antagonist, rapidly reverses opioid poisoning
4. Naloxone dosage must be titrated carefully; too much naloxone reverses client from intoxicated state to withdrawal
5. Because of short half-life, naloxone must be given every few hours until opioid has dropped to a nontoxic level
6. Nalmefene (Revex), a long-acting opioid antagonist, is an alternative to naloxone; because of its long half-life, nalmefene does not require repeated dosing; however, if dose is excessive in an opioid-dependent person, it will lead to prolonged withdrawal
7. Methadone, a long acting oral opioid, is commonly used to ease opioid withdrawal and prevent abstinence syndrome; once stabilized on methadone, withdrawal is accomplished by administering it in gradually smaller doses
8. With methadone withdrawal, abstinence syndrome is mild, with symptoms resembling those of moderate influenza; entire process of methadone substitution and withdrawal takes about 10 days
9. Objective of maintenance methadone therapy is to avoid withdrawal and need to procure illicit drugs; methadone maintenance is most effective in conjunction with nondrug measures directed at altering patterns of drug use

C. Cocaine

1. Is a fine, white, odorless powder extracted from coca plant; it passes blood–brain barrier readily and causes an instant high; when taken IV (mainlining), it is rapidly metabolized by liver, so "rush" does not last long
2. Exerts both CNS and peripheral nervous system (PNS) effects because it blocks norepinephrine and dopamine reuptake into presynaptic neurons; it depletes these neurotransmitters
3. Is highly addictive and produces mild physical withdrawal but severe psychological withdrawal

4. Treatment is aimed at restoring depleted neurotransmitters; three approaches include use of amino acid catecholamine precursors (such as tyrosine and phenylalanine), TCAs, and dopamine agonist bromocriptine

D. Cannabis (marijuana/hashish)

1. Marijuana is derived from the Indian hemp plant *Cannabis sativa*; major psychoactive substance is delta-9-tetrahydrocannabinol (THC), an oily chemical with high lipid solubility
2. Produces three main subjective effects: euphoria, sedation, and hallucinations
3. Common effects of low-dose THC include euphoria and relaxation; an increased sensitivity to visual and auditory stimuli; enhanced sense of touch, taste, and smell; increased appetite and more intense perceived flavor of food; distortion of time (seems to move more slowly)
4. Cannabinoids are sometimes used to treat N/V (more effectively than traditional antiemetics) caused by cancer chemotherapy; THC is approved for stimulating appetite in clients with AIDS

Check Your NCLEX–PN® Exam I.Q.

You are ready for testing on this content if you can

- Apply knowledge of expected actions and effects of psychiatric medications to client care.
- Correctly administer psychiatric medications to clients.
- Monitor for side effects and adverse effects of psychiatric medications.
- Take appropriate action if a client has an unexpected response to a psychiatric medication.
- Monitor a client for expected outcomes or effects of treatment with psychiatric medications.

PRACTICE TEST

1 The client is reporting vague dread. She is pacing and hyperventilating. Her jaw is clenched, and she is wringing her hands. What type of medication should the nurse conclude that this client needs?

1. A barbiturate
2. An anxiolytic
3. An antipsychotic
4. A CNS stimulant

2 A client has an order for 30 mg of flurazepam (Dalmane). The nurse determines that the client understands the effects of this medication by which client statement?

1. "After I take my medication at bedtime, I can watch the TV boxing match and then go to sleep."
2. "Once I take my medicine, I should be able to go to bed and read for a short time."
3. "I will take my medicine, go straight to bed, and go to sleep."
4. "I will take my medicine before preparing for bed and the next day's work."

3 The nurse is reinforcing medication teaching with a client about clozapine (Clozaril). The nurse should include information about what weekly intervention?

1. Physical exam by a psychiatrist
2. Weekly blood test
3. Follow-up visits with a physician
4. Urinalysis

4 A client is taking sertraline (Zoloft). The nurse explains to the client that how much time will pass before the onset of the medication occurs?

1. 5–7 days
2. 1–4 weeks
3. 4–6 weeks
4. 4–8 weeks

5 A client is taking phenelzine (Nardil). The visiting nurse is monitoring for client safety. What should the nurse reinforce as a priority regarding client teaching?

1. Limiting daily intake of salt
2. Encouraging a fluid intake of at least 2000 mL
3. Encouraging the client to have scheduled blood tests on time
4. Eliminating foods containing tyramine

PRACTICE TEST

6 The client is diaphoretic, disoriented, and has a temperature of 100°F. Additionally, the client reports insomnia, feeling anxious, and an inability to sit still. What should the nurse suspect regarding this client? Select all that apply.

1. Withdrawing from alcohol use
2. Demonstrating flu symptoms
3. Withdrawing from an antipsychotic medication
4. Abruptly discontinuing lithium carbonate
5. Withdrawing from CNS depressants

7 Immediately after taking alprazolam (Xanax) the client says, "I know I shouldn't feel this guilty, but I don't want to take medicine that makes me feel this way." What would be the most appropriate response by the nurse?

1. "You can't worry what people say about the medicine you take."
2. "Once the medication begins to work, you'll feel differently about taking it."
3. "Let's talk about how you're feeling about taking Xanax."
4. "Your long-term mental health will benefit from taking this medication."

8 The client is taking carbamazepine (Tegretol) for treatment of mania. For what weekly laboratory testing should the nurse remind the client?

1. Neuroleptic malignant syndrome
2. Agranulocytosis
3. Thrombocytopenia
4. Anemia

9 A client with schizophrenia has been taking haloperidol (Haldol) for three weeks with good effect. Today, he comes to group, but reports feeling like his legs are on fire. The nurse notes that he is moving continuously and leaves group early. The nurse should document and report that the client is experiencing which medication side effect?

1. Anticholinergic effects
2. Gustatory hallucinations
3. Akathisia
4. Oculogyric crisis

10 A client is taking trazodone (Desyrel). The nurse recognizes the client understands the desired effects and major side effects of the drug by making which statement? Select all that apply.

1. "I can go downstairs to the bathroom during the night if I have a nightlight."
2. "I am drinking more fluids so the medication will work effectively."
3. "I should not worry about becoming addicted to this medication."
4. "I have been prescribed this medication to treat my insomnia."
5. "If I have a problem with priapism, I will notify my doctor immediately."

11 The client is hospitalized because of a suicide attempt while in a manic phase. The client has now been taking chlordiazepoxide (Librium) for 2 days. What is the most important safety measure for the nurse to implement with this client?

1. Frequently remind the client to remain visible to the nurses at all times.
2. Elicit the client's promise to tell someone about any suicidal feelings.
3. Make a contract for safety.
4. Enforce the client's promise to eat all meals in the dining room.

12 If an overdose of benzodiazepines is suspected, the nurse should anticipate what medication order to reverse that drug's effects?

1. Diazepam (Valium)
2. Triazolam (Halcion)
3. Fluvoxamine (Luvox)
4. Flumazenil (Romazicon)

13 The nurse is assigned to care for a client who is prescribed fluphenazine (Prolixin) 1 mg daily at bedtime. The nurse will implement which intervention because of side effects of the medication?

1. Remind the client to rise slowly when getting out of bed or a chair.
2. Assess for dizziness or lightheadedness frequently during the day.
3. Make sugarless hard candy, gum, and water available during the day.
4. Monitor the client frequently for manifestations of confusion.

14 A client who is receiving thioridazine (Mellaril) 100 mg t.i.d. comes to the clinic with the chief complaint of a "dry mouth." To what should the nurse conclude this side effect is related?

1. High anticholinergic effects of thioridazine
2. Extrapyramidal side effects (EPSE)
3. Weight loss effect from the medication
4. Neuroleptic malignant syndrome (NMS) side effect

15 A client asks the nurse if it is true that marijuana is not just a street drug but has legitimate uses. What therapeutic uses should the nurse relate to the client regarding marijuana? Select all that apply.

1. Stimulates appetite
2. Promotes organization and motivation
3. Heightens auditory sensitivity
4. Acts as an antibacterial agent
5. Promotes relaxation

16 A client has been diagnosed with anxiety related to a recent attack and robbery in his apartment. He reports having episodes of immobilizing apprehension. A short-term anxiolytic has been prescribed. What is the primary nursing priority for this client?

1. Help client learn alternative responses to the anxiety.
2. Promote client's involvement in group or community support activities.
3. Provide for physical safety.
4. Assist with desensitization to phobic place (apartment).

17 A client, admitted to the inpatient unit with a diagnosis of paranoid schizophrenia, is prescribed risperidone (Risperdal). After 5 days of treatment, the client reports feeling dizzy. What should the nurse explain to the client is associated with this manifestation?

1. The desired effect of sedation
2. The side effect of loss of appetite
3. Anticholinergic side effect of this agent
4. The side effect of orthostatic hypotension

18 What should be the nurse's highest priority when caring for a client who, after withdrawing from alcohol, is beginning to use disulfiram (Antabuse)?

1. Becoming socially reintegrated
2. Learning about the disease process
3. Remaining abstinent
4. Remaining in the rehabilitation unit

19 The psychiatrist is prescribing chlorpromazine (Thorazine) 50 mg IM as an initial dose for a client hospitalized with psychosis. The nurse's initial concern is to monitor which of the following?

1. Blood pressure and pulse
2. A decrease in psychotic symptoms
3. The client's ability to walk
4. The client's ability to eat lunch

20 After observing the client taking phenelzine sulfate (Nardil), eating a lunch of yogurt, sliced bananas, and chocolate milk, the nurse should take which action?

1. Monitor client's body temperature for elevation above normal
2. Observe client for dyspnea
3. Test a urine specimen for glucose and ketones
4. Monitor client for elevated blood pressure

ANSWERS & RATIONALES

1 **Answer: 2 Rationale:** This client is suffering from anxiety and the appropriate type of medication is an anxiolytic. Barbiturates are sedative-hypnotics, which would not be prescribed. The client is not suffering from psychosis or hallucinations, so an antipsychotic is inappropriate. A CNS stimulant is inappropriate for the signs and symptoms described. **Cognitive Level:** Analyzing **Client Need:** Pharmacological and Parenteral Therapies **Integrated Process:** Nursing Process: Evaluation **Content Area:** Pharmacology **Strategy:** This question requires you to interpret the client's symptoms as being representative of anxiety, and to choose the drug category that is effective against it. Focus on the client manifestations to eliminate each of the incorrect options.

2 **Answer: 2 Rationale:** The medication normally works within 30 minutes to one hour after administration; the medication will not work instantly. The client should not take a sedative and then stay active for an extended period of time. Watching stimulating shows on television at bedtime is not conducive to sleep. **Cognitive Level:** Analyzing **Client Need:** Pharmacological and Parenteral Therapies **Integrated Process:** Nursing Process: Evaluation **Content Area:** Pharmacology **Strategy:** The word *understands* in the stem of the question tells you the correct answer is also a true statement. Recall that the medication is used to enhance sleep, and utilize principles of good sleep hygiene to eliminate each of the incorrect options.

3 **Answer: 2 Rationale:** In order to safely monitor clozapine, a weekly blood test is mandatory. If the client does not have the hematologic exam, the medication is not given for the following week. This is to monitor for agranulocytosis (decreased white blood cells), the drug's major adverse effect. A weekly physical exam is unnecessary. Follow-up visits are done periodically, but might not be needed weekly with the physician. Weekly urinalysis is unnecessary when taking clozapine. **Cognitive Level:** Applying **Client Need:** Pharmacological and Parenteral Therapies **Integrated Process:** Nursing Process: Data Collection **Content Area:** Pharmacology **Strategy:** The core issue of the question is knowledge of possible adverse effects of clozapine. Recall that the drug can cause bone marrow depression and agranulocytosis to choose the correct monitoring technique.

4 **Answer: 2 Rationale:** Sertraline is an antidepressant of the SSRI type. These agents work within 1–4 weeks. **Cognitive Level:** Remembering **Client Need:** Pharmacological and Parenteral Therapies **Integrated Process:** Nursing Process: Implementation **Content Area:** Pharmacology **Strategy:** Specific knowledge of the time frame in which SSRIs exert an effect is needed to answer this question. Use medication knowledge and the process of elimination to make a selection.

5 **Answer: 4 Rationale:** With an MAOI, such as phenelzine, the client must eliminate foods that contain tyramine. Intake of tyramine-containing foods could lead to severe hypertension and other complications. The other options are not major teaching considerations for MAOIs. **Cognitive Level:** Applying **Client Need:** Pharmacological and Parenteral Therapies **Integrated Process:** Teaching and Learning **Content Area:** Pharmacology **Strategy:** The core issue of the question is knowledge regarding priority teaching for a client taking phenelzine (Nardil), which is an MAOI. From there, recall that foods high in tyramine need to be avoided to make the correct selection.

6 **Answer: 1, 5 Rationale:** These symptoms are the commonly seen symptoms of withdrawal from alcohol. The symptoms are commonly seen during withdrawal from CNS depressants. A client would usually not be complaining of disorientation or insomnia with flu-like symptoms. Individuals do not usually have withdrawal symptoms from antipsychotic medications. These are not signs of lithium carbonate being discontinued. **Cognitive Level:** Analyzing **Client Need:** Pharmacological and Parenteral Therapies **Integrated Process:** Nursing Process: Evaluation **Content Area:** Pharmacology **Strategy:** Clients withdrawing from a substance are likely to experience the opposite effects of the original drug. With this in mind, review the client's symptoms, and note that they represent excitation of the CNS. You can deduce that the original substance was some type of CNS depressant, leading you to the correct answer. When there is more than one correct answer, consider each option as a true/false statement.

7 **Answer: 3 Rationale:** In the correct response, the nurse acknowledges the client's feelings, and asks the client to discuss his or her feelings and thoughts. An open and trusting nurse-client relationship helps support the client in decisions related to medication therapy. The nurse is not addressing the client's comment by talking about other people. The comment about when it starts to work dismisses the client's feelings; there is no way to determine how the client will feel over time. The statement about long-term mental health may or may not be a correct statement; however, it does not address the client's feelings or concern. **Cognitive Level:** Applying **Client Need:** Psychosocial Integrity **Integrated Process:** Communication and Documentation **Content Area:** Mental Health **Strategy:** The correct answer is one that is the most therapeutic response by the nurse. Use knowledge of communication techniques and the process of elimination to make a selection.

8 **Answer: 2 Rationale:** The most serious side effect of carbamazepine is agranulocytosis (low WBC count). Neuroleptic malignant syndrome is not common with carbamazepine and there is no laboratory test for it. There is no need for weekly monitoring for low platelet count while taking carbamazepine. There is no need for weekly monitoring for anemia while taking carbamazepine. **Cognitive Level:** Applying **Client Need:** Pharmacological and Parenteral Therapies **Integrated Process:** Nursing Process: Implementation **Content Area:** Pharmacology **Strategy:** The core issue of the question is that an adverse effect of carbamazepine is agranulocytosis. With this in mind, eliminate each of the incorrect responses that do not address this concern.

9 **Answer: 3 Rationale:** Akathisia is an uncontrollable need to move; a common extrapyramidal side effect after long-term use of haloperidol. Anticholinergic effects would include dry mouth, urinary hesitance, constipation, mydriasis, tachycardia, and diminished lacrimation. Gustatory hallucination is tasting something that is not present. Oculogyric crisis involves painful twisting and turning of the head and neck. **Cognitive Level:** Analyzing **Client Need:** Pharmacological and Parenteral Therapies **Integrated Process:** Nursing Process: Data Collection **Content Area:** Pharmacology **Strategy:** The

core issue of the question is correct identification of side effects of haloperidol. Knowledge of terminology will help identify the connection between *gustatory* referring to taste and *oculo-* referring to eyes; also, the word *akathisia* is consistent with the client's presentation, while the word *anticholinergic* is not.

10 **Answer: 3, 4, 5** **Rationale:** The abuse potential for trazodone is minimal. Trazadone is an atypical antidepressant that is used more for insomnia than for depression. Priapism is a penile erection that occurs without stimulation, and is an adverse side effect to trazadone; the doctor should be notified. For safety reasons, it is not a good practice when taking trazodone as a sleep aid to ambulate in low lighting because the drug produces a profound sedative effect. Taking more fluids will not increase the effectiveness of the medication. **Cognitive Level:** Analyzing **Client Need:** Pharmacological and Parenteral Therapies **Integrated Process:** Nursing Process: Evaluation **Content Area:** Pharmacology **Strategy:** First, recall that trazodone is often used as a sleep aid. Knowledge regarding the adverse effects of this drug will be helpful in finding the correct answer. When there is more than one correct answer to a question, consider each option as a true/false statement.

11 **Answer: 3** **Rationale:** The client needs to make an agreement with the nurse to remain safe, or to report to the nurse if not feeling safe. The agreement to remain visible to the nurses at all times is too vague, and does not give specific responsibility to the nurse or the client. The promise to tell is vague, and does not make the client specifically accountable to the health care professionals. Eating all meals in the dining room does not keep the client safe for 24 hours, only during meals. **Cognitive Level:** Applying **Client Need:** Pharmacological and Parenteral Therapies **Integrated Process:** Nursing Process: Implementation **Content Area:** Pharmacology **Strategy:** Note that the question contains a key phrase: *most important safety measure*. This tells you that more than one option might be partially or totally correct. Keep in mind that medication therapy alone is not sufficient in treating this client and select another appropriate intervention.

12 **Answer: 4** **Rationale:** Flumazenil is the only drug available that acts as an antagonist to the benzodiazepines. Diazepam and triazolam are benzodiazepines and would not be ordered to counteract the overdose of a drug from the same classification. Fluvoxamine is a selective serotonin reuptake inhibitor (SSRI) type of antidepressant. **Cognitive Level:** Applying **Client Need:** Pharmacological and Parenteral Therapies **Integrated Process:** Nursing Process: Planning **Content Area:** Pharmacology **Strategy:** Specific knowledge of the antidote to benzodiazepines is needed to answer this question. It might help to remember that the antidote to benzodiazepines is a generic drug name that contains the letters *ze*, and is not a benzodiazepene itself.

13 **Answer: 3** **Rationale:** Dry mouth occurs from the anticholinergic effects seen with fluphenazine. Orthostatic hypotension is not a major side effect of fluphenazine. Dizziness or lightheadedness is a sign of orthostatic hypotension, which is not a major side effect of fluphenazine. Confusion is not a side effect of fluphenazine. **Cognitive Level:** Applying **Client Need:** Pharmacological and Parenteral Therapies **Integrated Process:** Nursing Process: Implementation **Content Area:** Pharmacology **Strategy:** First, eliminate options that are similar in referring to orthostatic hypotension. Select between the remaining options by choosing the anticholinergic effects, which are of concern.

14 **Answer: 1** **Rationale:** With thioridazine, the anticholinergic side effects of dry mouth, constipation, urinary retention, and blurred vision are usually severe. Dry mouth is not associated with extrapyramidal side effects or neuroleptic malignant syndrome. There is usually not a weight loss as a side effect of thioridazine; there is usually a weight gain. **Cognitive Level:** Analyzing **Client Need:** Pharmacological and Parenteral Therapies **Integrated Process:** Nursing Process: Evaluation **Content Area:** Pharmacology **Strategy:** Specific knowledge of the intended effects and side effects of thioridozine is needed to answer the question. Use the process of elimination to make your selection.

15 **Answer: 1, 3, 5** **Rationale:** Marijuana has been used for individuals with AIDS and on chemotherapy for cancer by enhancing the client's sense of taste and smell, which increases their appetite. A common effect of low doses of marijuana is an increased sensitivity to auditory stimuli. Low doses of marijuana do produce a state of relaxation. Marijuana does not promote organization and motivation. Marijuana does not have antibacterial properties. **Cognitive Level:** Applying **Client Need:** Pharmacological and Parenteral Therapies **Integrated Process:** Nursing Process: Implementation **Content Area:** Pharmacology **Strategy:** The core issue of the question is legitimate uses for marijuana. To aid in making the correct selection, keep in mind that an effect of the drug is to stimulate appetite and the senses, and promote relaxation. When there is more than one correct answer to a question, consider each option as a true/false statement.

16 **Answer: 3** **Rationale:** The need for physical safety is the primary nursing priority for the client at this time. Teaching alternative responses to anxiety is an appropriate nursing intervention, but should be addressed once physical safety is established. Involvement in group or community support activities is appropriate; however, the need for physical safety is the primary nursing priority for the client at this time. Helping to desensitize the client to phobic reaction related to place is an appropriate nursing intervention. This need should be addressed once physical safety is established. **Cognitive Level:** Analyzing **Client Need:** Pharmacological and Parenteral Therapies **Integrated Process:** Nursing Process: Planning **Content Area:** Pharmacology **Strategy:** Note that the drug prescribed is an anxiolytic. Next, relate the cause of the anxiety to the need for the medication. Choose the option that targets the best concern of the client and is congruent with the need for the medication.

17 **Answer: 4** **Rationale:** Risperidone has very few side effects; they include orthostatic hypotension and insomnia, agitation, headache, anxiety, and rhinitis. The effect of dizziness is not a desired effect of risperidone. There is no information in the question that indicates that the client has a loss of appetite. Risperidone does not cause sedation. **Cognitive Level:** Analyzing **Client Need:** Pharmacological and Parenteral Therapies **Integrated Process:** Nursing Process: Evaluation **Content Area:** Pharmacology **Strategy:** The core issue of this question is recognition of dizziness as a sign of orthostatic hypotension. With this concept in mind, eliminate each of the other options, because they do not relate to this concern.

18 **Answer: 3** **Rationale:** The principle of remaining abstinent is one of the three most important goals of treatment for alcoholism. It is also critical when taking disulfiram, in order to avoid adverse effects from the interaction of the medication and alcohol. The other two goals of treatment are amelioration of concurrent psychiatric conditions and long-term

prevention of relapse. The other options are important but not the priority. **Cognitive Level:** Applying **Client Need:** Pharmacological and Parenteral Therapies **Integrated Process:** Nursing Process: Planning **Content Area:** Pharmacology **Strategy:** The core issue of the question is the interactive effect of disulfiram and alcohol. With this in mind, eliminate each of the incorrect options because they do not address this critical concern.

19 Answer: 2 Rationale: Because the client is hospitalized and is receiving an IM dose of Thorazine, the primary concern should be to monitor for a decrease in the psychosis. Blood pressure and pulse should be monitored as a general measure for initial treatment with Thorazine, whether IM or PO. Ability to walk is not significant to the issue of initial concern. Ability to eat lunch is not significant to the issue of initial concern. **Cognitive Level:** Analyzing **Client Need:** Physiological Adaptation **Integrated Process:** Nursing Process: Data Collection **Content Area:** Mental Health **Strategy:** Note the key word *initial*, and focus on the diagnosis of psychosis. Recall strong knowledge base of disease process of psychosis and usual mode of treatment to select the correct answer.

20 Answer: 4 Rationale: The foods are high in tyramine, a chemical that can result in a hypertensive crisis if ingested while taking MAOIs such as phenelzine. The central nervous system side effects involve mental alterations such confusion and anxiety rather than physical changes such as temperature elevation. Respiratory depression is more likely to occur than dyspnea. Diabetes mellitus is not associated with the drug. **Cognitive Level:** Applying **Client Need:** Pharmacological and Parenteral Therapies **Integrated Process:** Nursing Process: Data Collection **Content Area:** Pharmacology **Strategy:** Associate negative reactions between MAOIs and foods containing tyramine.

Key Terms to Review

agranulocytosis p. 468
akathisia p. 467
antagonists p. 467
anticholinergic effects p. 467
dystonia p. 479
extrapyramidal side effects (EPSE) p. 469
metabolite p. 477
neuroleptic malignant syndrome (NMS) p. 468
neuroleptic p. 467
parkinsonism p. 467
serotonin syndrome p. 473
tardive dyskinesia (TD) p. 468
tolerance p. 467

References

Adams, M., Holland, L., & Urban, C. (2011). *Pharmacology for nurses: A pathophysiological approach* (3rd ed.). Upper Saddle River, NJ: Pearson Education, Inc.

Adams, M., & Koch, R. (2010). *Pharmacology: Connections to nursing practice.* Upper Saddle River, NJ: Pearson Education, Inc.

American Psychiatric Association. (2000). *Diagnostic and statistical manual of mental disorders.* (revised 4th ed.). Washington, DC: Author.

Deglin, J. H. & Vallerand, A. H. (2011). *Davis's drug guide for nurses* (12th ed.). Philadelphia: F. A. Davis.

Kniesl, C., Wilson, H., & Trigoboff, E. (2009). *Contemporary psychiatric-mental health nursing* (2nd ed.). Upper Saddle River, NJ: Pearson Education.

Lehne, R. (2010). *Pharmacology for nursing care* (7th ed.). St. Louis, MO: Saunders.

Wilson, B., Shannon, M., & Shields, K. (2012). *Pearson nurse's drug guide 2012.* Upper Saddle River, NJ: Pearson Education.

Test Yourself

Are you ready for the NCLEX-PN® or course exams? Use the practice tests on the companion website to check.

Respiratory Medications

33

In this chapter

Cross Reference

Other chapters relevant to this content area are

Dosage Calculation and Medication Administration **Chapter 28**
Immunological and Anti-Infective Medications **Chapter 41**
Respiratory Disorders **Chapter 51**

I. BRONCHODILATORS

A. Beta-agonists (sympathomimetics)

1. Sympathetic nervous system (SNS) **adrenergic agonists** raise intracellular levels of cAMP (cyclic adenosine monophosphate) to dilate constricted bronchi and bronchioles by relaxing smooth muscle
2. Used during an **acute asthma attack**, characterized by bronchospasm with shortness of breath and wheezing, for quick airway dilation and relief of bronchospasm; used also for emphysema and acute and chronic bronchitis
3. **Sympathomimetics** can have $beta_1$ or $beta_2$ activity; $beta_1$ adrenergic receptors increase heart rate and force of myocardial contraction
4. Beta-adrenergic agents can be classified as **catecholamines** released from adrenal medulla in response to SNS stimulation or **noncatecholamines**, which are not released by SNS; all beta-adrenergic agents stimulate $beta_2$ receptors; catecholamines affect both alpha and beta receptors and cause cardiovascular effects
5. Selective $beta_2$ agonists are preferred for bronchial smooth muscle dilation because they produce fewer cardiac side effects
6. Common medications are listed in Box 33–1

Memory Aid If a medication ends in *-terol* or *-terenol*, it is a sympathomimetic type of bronchodilator.

7. Administration considerations

NCLEX® a. Adverse effects may occur with albuterol, levalbuterol, and pirbuterol if used too frequently because they lose $beta_2$–specific actions at larger doses ($beta_1$ receptors are stimulated, leading to elevated heart rate [HR], nausea, anxiety, palpitations, and tremors)

NCLEX® b. Use with caution in young children and monitor for tremors, restlessness, hallucinations, dizziness, palpitations, tachycardia, and gastrointestinal (GI) difficulties

Box 33–1

Common Bronchodilators

Beta Agonists/Sympathomimetics

Albuterol (Proventil)

Arformoterol (Brovan)

Formoterol fumarate (Foradil)

Levalbuterol hydrochloride (Xopenex)

Metaproterenol sulfate (Alupent)

Pirbuterol acetate (Maxair)

Salmeterol (Serevent)

Terbutaline sulfate (Brethine)

Methylxanthines

Aminophylline (Truphylline)

Theophylline (Theo-Dur, others)

Anticholinergic

Ipratropium (Atrovent, Combivent)

Tiotropium (Spiriva)

c. Salmeterol is not used in an acute asthma attack because of slow onset of action (20 minutes); do not dose more often than every 12 hours because of the 12-hour duration of action

NCLEX® d. Contraindicated with hypersensitivity to sympathomimetics or with tachydysrhythmias

e. Use with caution in clients with cardiovascular disease because of potential for increasing myocardial oxygen demand

f. Use with caution in clients with hypertension, diabetes mellitus, seizures, and hypothyroidism

NCLEX® g. Children under 12 should not use inhalations of albuterol and terbutaline

NCLEX® h. Concurrent use of monoamine oxidase inhibitors (MAOIs) may lead to hypertensive crisis

8. Side/adverse effects

NCLEX® a. May cause nervousness, tremors, increased HR, and increased blood pressure (BP) when beta_1 receptors are stimulated

b. With alpha- and beta-adrenergic stimulation, may lead to insomnia, restlessness, anorexia, tremors, cardiac stimulation, anginal pain, and vascular headache

c. Additional side effects may include hypokalemia, hyperglycemia, nausea, vomiting (N/V), chest pain, and dysrhythmias

NCLEX® d. Paradoxic bronchospasm and urinary retention may also occur

9. Nursing considerations

a. Monitor elderly clients carefully

NCLEX® b. Monitor vital signs, especially HR and BP, when administering beta-agonists (because of cardiovascular effects)

NCLEX® c. Proper use of metered dose inhaler (MDI) is essential for maximum benefit (see Box 33–2 for client teaching about use and care of inhalers)

d. At times, use of multiple drugs is effective and dosages of each can be reduced

NCLEX® e. Note amount, color, and character of sputum

Box 33–2

Client Education about the Use and Care of Metered Dose Inhalers

- Insert medication firmly into inhaler.
- Remove cap and hold inhaler upright.
- Shake inhaler for 3 to 5 seconds to ensure even mixing of medication in propellant.
- Tilt head back slightly and hold inhaler upright.
- Position inhaler 1 to 2 inches away from open mouth or attach it to spacer/holding chamber; if a medicine chamber is used, seal lips around mouthpiece.
- Press on inhaler while beginning to breathe in slowly through mouth.
- Breathe in slowly and deeply for 3 to 5 seconds.
- Hold breath for 8 to 10 seconds as able to allow medication to move down into airways.
- Wait 1 to 3 minutes per product directions before next inhalation if another is ordered.
- Rinse mouth with water and blow nose.
- Use mild soap and water to clean mouthpiece; allow to air dry.
- Store inhaler at room temperature.

f. Monitor baseline and periodic pulmonary function tests during therapy
g. Administer oral medications with meals to decrease GI irritation
h. Solutions may remain diluted for 24 to 48 hours
NCLEX® i. Monitor blood glucose (BG) levels closely in diabetic clients because some medications may elevate BG; an adjustment in maintenance doses of antidiabetic drugs may be indicated

10. Client teaching
a. If diabetic, monitor BG level closely
NCLEX® b. Report chest pain, palpitations, seizures, headaches, hallucinations, or blurred vision to physician
c. Do not take more than prescribed dose because of risk for hypertension, tachycardia, dysrhythmias, and angina
d. Record prn use of these drugs, noting date, time, symptoms, and effectiveness
NCLEX® e. Wait 1–3 minutes (some references suggest 3–5 minutes) between inhalations of aerosol medications
f. Avoid eye contact with inhaler spray
g. Avoid contact with allergens and avoid contact with smoke and other irritants, such as aerosol hair spray, perfumes, and cleaning products
h. Increase fluid intake if not contraindicated by other diseases
i. Explain early symptoms of respiratory difficulty (activity intolerance and waking at night with asthma symptoms) for early intervention
NCLEX® j. Avoid caffeine, which may increase nervousness and insomnia from bronchodilating drugs
NCLEX® k. An inhaled bronchodilator is treatment of choice in an acute asthma attack
l. Nervousness and tremors may occur when a medication is newly administered, but they frequently decrease over time
m. Use inhaled preparations properly (have client demonstrate proper use)
NCLEX® n. Understand care of nebulizer and/or inhaler: wash daily in warm water and dry; use white vinegar to rinse the nebulizer tubing; read and follow manufacturer's instructions about use, storage, and cleaning of equipment
o. Anticipated response to use of nebulizer or inhaler is absence of wheezing and dyspnea

B. *Xanthines*

1. Inhibit phosphodiesterase (PDE), which leads to increased levels of cAMP and bronchial dilation due to smooth muscle relaxation
2. Can also increase catecholamine levels, inhibit calcium ion movement into smooth muscle, inhibit prostaglandin synthesis, and inhibit release of bronchoconstrictive substances from leukocytes and **mast cells** (which contain histamine, prostaglandins, and thromboxanes)
3. By bronchodilation, they increase ability of cilia to clear mucus from airways
4. Used to treat bronchoconstriction associated with chronic obstructive pulmonary disease (COPD, including chronic bronchitis, asthma, and emphysema) and other chronic respiratory disorders
5. Have a slow onset of action, so they are used to prevent rather than treat asthma attacks; can be used during an asthma attack if it is mild to moderate
6. Can be used as an additional treatment in pulmonary edema by decreasing vascular permeability and paroxysmal nocturnal dyspnea (PND)
7. NCLEX® Used to treat **status asthmaticus**, a bout of severe asthma that cannot be controlled with typical medications (use IV theophylline if no response to faster-acting beta agonist)
8. Common medications: see again Box 33–1

Memory Aid If a medication ends in *-phylline*, it is a xanthine type of bronchodilator.

9. Administration considerations
a. Use cautiously in older adults because of risk for increased sensitivity
NCLEX® b. Carefully monitor serum drug levels and therapeutic response to avoid potential toxicity; therapeutic range of theophylline is 10 to 20 mcg/mL

Memory Aid Remember 10–20 mcg/mL as the therapeutic serum range for aminophylline.

c. Xanthines have a stimulating effect on CNS, which may be enhanced in children

NCLEX® d. Use cautiously in clients with cardiovascular disorders

e. Theophylline doses should be based on lean body weight because it does not enter adipose tissue

f. Theophylline can enter breast milk and cross placenta

NCLEX® g. Aminophylline is administered slowly by intravenous (IV) route because of risk for cardiovascular collapse

h. Dosages are often started low and titrated up as needed for relief of symptoms

i. Children and adults who smoke cigarettes metabolize these drugs more quickly and thus may need higher doses for therapeutic effects

j. Theophylline levels may be increased in liver disease, congestive heart failure (CHF), and acute viral infections because of impaired biotransformation

k. Avoid with known hypersensitivity to xanthines; tachydysrhythmias; hyperthyroidism (exacerbates disease); history of seizure disorders unless unresponsive to other drugs (can cause seizures); peptic ulcer disease, acute gastritis, or other GI disorders because of increased gastric acid secretion

NCLEX® l. Avoid caffeinated drinks and foods, which have additive effects with xanthines

NCLEX® 10. Side/adverse effects

a. N/V, anorexia, and gastroesophageal reflux during sleep

b. Sinus tachycardia, chest pain, palpitations, and ventricular dysrhythmias

c. Hyperglycemia and transient increased urination

d. Tremors, dizziness, hallucinations, restlessness, agitation, headache, and insomnia

11. Nursing considerations

NCLEX® a. Monitor for toxicity (restlessness, insomnia, irritability, tremors, N/V)

NCLEX® b. Observe client for hypoxia if restlessness occurs to differentiate cause

c. Refrigerate suppository forms

NCLEX® d. Children may exhibit hyperactive behavior while taking theophylline because of CNS stimulation

12. Client teaching

a. Refrigerate suppository forms

b. Notify prescriber if suppositories cause rectal burning, itching, or irritation

NCLEX® c. Notify prescriber if palpitations, N/V, weakness, dizziness, chest pain, or seizure occur

d. Comply with monitoring blood levels periodically

NCLEX® e. Avoid use of caffeine, which could lead to an additive effect with xanthines

NCLEX® f. Avoid contact with allergens if possible; avoid contact with smoke and other respiratory irritants such as aerosol hair spray, perfumes, and cleaning products

g. Increase fluid intake if no contraindication because of other disease process

h. Take medications even when there are no symptoms of asthma

i. Take medications with food if GI symptoms develop

II. INHALED CORTICOSTEROIDS

A. Overview

1. Decrease airway inflammation by inhibiting inflammatory mediators, such as **histamine**, leukotriene, cytokines, and prostaglandins
2. Decreased inflammation also reduces mucosal edema, secretions, and bronchoconstriction
3. May aid in increasing responsiveness of bronchial smooth muscle to beta-agonists
4. Appear to help inhibit movement of fluid and protein into tissues as well as inhibit production of prostaglandins, **leukotrienes** (substances released after exposure to an allergen), and **interleukins** (plasma proteins that increase during inflammatory process)
5. Promote mobilization of mucus by increasing mucociliary action
6. Used in chronic asthma to decrease inflammation and therefore decrease airway obstruction, and are used prophylactically, not during acute attack
7. Treats bronchospastic disorders when bronchodilators are not completely effective
8. Used to treat chronic bronchitis, COPD, and cystic fibrosis
9. Common inhaled drugs are listed in Box 33–3; oral corticosteroids such as prednisone (Deltasone) and methylprednisolone (Medrol) may also be used

Memory Aid

Many corticosteroids contain *-cort* or *-sone* in either the generic or trade name.

Box 33-3 Inhaled Corticosteroid Medications

Beclomethasone (Beconase AQ)	Fluticasone (Flovent)
Budesonide (Pulmicort)	Mometasone (Asmanex)
Flunisolide (AeroBid)	Triamcinolone (Azmacort)

B. Administration considerations

NCLEX® 1. Proper technique is essential when administering medications via inhalation

2. Beclomethasone has greater anti-inflammatory action and causes fewer side effects than dexamethasone

NCLEX® 3. If client is also taking a systemic corticosteroid, that dose may need to be decreased with addition of inhaled corticosteroids

4. Beclomethasone, flunisolide, and fluticasone are available as nasal solutions for treatment of allergic rhinitis

5. Monitor for impaired bone growth in children receiving inhaled corticosteroids

NCLEX® 6. Contraindicted with known allergy, psychosis, fungal infection, acquired immunodeficiency syndrome (AIDS), tuberculosis, idiopathic thrombocytopenia, and in children under age 2 years

7. Use cautiously in clients with diabetes, glaucoma, osteoporosis, ulcers, renal disease, CHF, myasthenia gravis, seizure disorders, inflammatory bowel disease, hypertension, thromboembolic disorders, esophagitis, and infections (due to risk for suppressed immune system)

NCLEX® 8. Because of possible decreased response to skin test antigens, postpone skin testing if possible until after corticosteroid therapy

C. Side/adverse effects

1. Pharyngeal irritation, sore throat, and **rhinitis** (inflamed nasal mucous membranes)
2. Coughing or dry mouth
3. Oral fungal infections
4. Increased susceptibility to infection, dermatologic effects, and osteoporosis
5. Diarrhea, N/V, and stomach upset
6. Headache, fever, dizziness, angioedema, rash, urticaria, and paradoxical bronchospasm
7. Menstrual disturbances
8. Palpitations
9. Adrenocortical insufficiency, fluid and electrolyte disturbances, nervous system effects, and endocrine effects if absorbed systemically

D. Nursing considerations

1. Observe sputum color and viscosity for signs of infection
2. Children may need prescriber's order to keep an inhaler with them at school

E. Client teaching

1. Keep equipment clean and in working order per manufacturer's guidelines

NCLEX® 2. Rinse mouth after use of inhalation devices such as **inhaler** or **nebulizer**

NCLEX® 3. Do not abruptly stop taking this medication; taper dose slowly over a 2-week period under direction of prescriber

4. Wear a bracelet or necklace to identify self as a steroid user

NCLEX® 5. Learn symptoms of steroid use, including moon face, acne, increased fat pads, increased edema; notify prescriber if these symptoms arise

6. Report signs of decreased steroid levels, including nausea, dyspnea, joint pain, weakness, and fatigue

NCLEX® 7. Report weight gain of more than 5 pounds per week

8. Avoid contact with allergen responsible for producing allergic response if possible

9. Recognize early signs of respiratory difficulty so treatment can begin promptly

10. Take drug at approximately same time each day for maximal effectiveness

NCLEX® 11. Use inhaled corticosteroids as maintenance drugs; they are ineffective in acute bronchospasm

III. INHALED MAST CELL STABILIZERS

A. Overview

1. Stabilize mast cells to prevent release of bronchoconstrictive and inflammatory substances when stimulated by allergen; therefore, inflammation is limited
2. Used to prevent and treat inflammation of airways, and decrease mucosal edema, mucous secretions, and bronchoconstriction

3. Used for prophylaxis of acute asthma attacks and to prevent and treat allergic rhinitis
4. Common medications
   a. Cromolyn (Intal): oral spray or nebulizer solution for oral inhalation
   b. Nedocromil (Tilade): given by inhalation

B. Administration considerations

NCLEX® 1. Bronchodilator and corticosteroid doses may be decreased with use of these drugs
NCLEX® 2. Use cautiously with impaired hepatic or renal function; lower doses may be needed
3. Administer using proper inhalation technique
4. It may take 3 weeks of daily dosing to see therapeutic effects
NCLEX® 5. Do not use in clients with acute bronchospasm, status asthmaticus, or hypersensitivity to drug

C. Side/adverse effects

1. Headache
2. Dry mouth and unpleasant taste
NCLEX® 3. Cough and irritation of throat and trachea, bronchospasm
NCLEX® 4. Erythema, rash, urticaria

D. Nursing considerations

NCLEX® 1. Use cautiously in clients with coronary artery disease (CAD) and/or dysrhythmias, which may be aggravated by propellants in aerosols
2. Pulmonary function testing may be ordered prior to therapy

E. Client teaching

1. Use inhaler properly to ensure maximal drug effectiveness; use spacer as appropriate
2. Record frequency and severity of asthma attacks
NCLEX® 3. Allow 2 to 4 weeks for full medication effectiveness
NCLEX® 4. Rinse mouth after taking medication to avoid dry mouth
5. Do not take during an acute attack because symptoms may be aggravated
NCLEX® 6. Optimally, take bronchodilator 20 to 30 minutes prior to taking cromolyn or according to product literature; wait a minimum of 3 to 5 minutes between inhalations

IV. LEUKOTRIENE MODIFIERS

A. Overview

1. Leukotrienes are substances released during an allergic response; they cause inflammation, bronchoconstriction, and mucus production that leads to coughing, sneezing, and shortness of breath
2. Leukotriene modifiers reduce airway inflammation by either blocking leukotriene receptors or blocking an enzyme that controls leukotriene synthesis
3. Provide relief of inflammatory symptoms of asthma
4. Used for prophylaxis and chronic treatment of asthma in adults and children over 12; they are not used in managing an acute asthma attack
5. Common medications are listed in Box 33–4

Memory Aid If a medication ends in *-lukast*, it is a leukotriene modifier.

B. Administration considerations

1. Leukotriene modifiers are oral drugs used in adults and children 12 and older
NCLEX® 2. Therapeutic effects may take up to a week
3. They have localized effects in lungs
NCLEX® 4. They are used alone or in combination with corticosteroids

C. Side/adverse effects

1. Headaches may occur with all drugs
2. Zileuton may also cause dyspepsia, nausea, dizziness, insomnia, and hepatotoxicity
3. Zafirlukast may cause nausea and diarrhea
4. Monitor clients over age 55 for infection

Box 33–4 Leukotriene Modifiers

Zileuton (Zyflo)	Montelukast (Singulair)
Zafirlukast (Accolate)	

D. **Nursing considerations**

1. Be sure drug is prescribed for chronic, not acute, treatment of asthma

NCLEX® 2. Monitor liver enzymes during zileuton therapy and discontinue drug if elevated to five times normal value or if liver dysfunction develops

E. **Client teaching**

NCLEX® 1. Expect drugs to take a week before therapeutic effects are seen

NCLEX® 2. Follow-up liver function studies may be needed

NCLEX® 3. Drugs prevent some asthma symptoms but are not to be used for acute attacks

4. Avoid contact with specific allergen if possible
5. Increase fluid intake if not contraindicated because of other disease processes
6. Take zafirlukast 1 hour before or 2 hours after meals
7. Montelukast and zileuton may be taken with or without food

V. ANTIHISTAMINES

A. **Overview**

1. **Antihistamines** are used to treat allergies, allergic rhinitis (hay fever), allergic conjunctivitis, allergic contact dermatitis, vertigo, motion sickness, insomnia, allergic reactions, cough, and sneezing and runny nose from common cold
2. Compete with histamine for receptor sites and thereby block action of histamine following its release; work best early in response because they do not displace histamine from receptors
3. Cause bronchial smooth muscle relaxation and reduce bronchial, salivary, gastric, nasal, and **lacrimal** (tear) secretions
4. Reduce itching (urticaria) and are used to treat anaphylactic shock
5. Can be used to prevent or treat allergic reactions to medications
6. Common medications are listed in Box 33–5

B. **Administration considerations**

NCLEX® 1. Treat symptoms but not the cause of a problem

2. Should not be used to treat acute asthma attack or lower respiratory disorder
3. Most antihistamines are tolerated better when taken with meals
4. Hydroxyzine is effective with pruritis
5. Azelastine is topically applied to nasal mucosa and action peaks in 2 to 3 hours; it does not tend to cause drowsiness but does leave an unpleasant taste in mouth

NCLEX® 6. Antihistamines may be used as premedication before administering blood products to decrease risk of allergic reactions

7. Oral antihistamines act in 15 to 60 minutes and last 4 to 6 hours; sustained-release medications last 8 to 12 hours
8. Use a rapid acting agent with an acute allergic reaction
9. Longer-acting agents give more consistent relief with chronic allergic conditions

Box 33–5

Antihistamines

Second-Generation or Nonsedating Antihistamine

cetirizine (Zyrtec)
desloratadine (Clarinex)
fexofenadine (Allegra)
levocetirizine (Xyzal)
loratidine (Claritin)
triprolidine (Zymine)

First-Generation or Traditional Antihistamines

azelastine (Astelin)
diphenhydramine (Benadryl)
brompheniramine (Dimetane)
chlorpheniramine (Chlor-Trimeton)
clemastine (Tavist)
cyproheptadine
dexbrompheniramine (Drixoral)
dexchlorpheniramine (Polaramine)
dimenhydrinate (Dramamine)
doxylamine (Unisom)
hydroxyzine (Vistaril, Atarax)
meclizine (Antivert)
promethazine (Phenergan)

10. Should be used cautiously with history of increased intraocular pressure, cardiac or renal disease, hypertension, bronchial asthma, stenosing peptic ulcer disease, prostatic hyperplasia, convulsive disorders, or during pregnancy

NCLEX® 11. Can mask positive skin test results; discontinue use for 3 days (72 hours) before allergy skin testing

C. Side/adverse effects

NCLEX® 1. Drowsiness is main side effect; children can experience paradoxical excitement

NCLEX® 2. **Anticholinergic** side effects include dry mouth and nose, changes in vision, difficulty urinating, and constipation

3. Sedation from drowsiness to deep sleep, dizziness, syncope, muscular weakness, unsteady gait, paradoxical excitement (especially in older adults), restlessness, insomnia, and nervousness
4. Anorexia, N/V, diarrhea, constipation, and jaundice

NCLEX® 5. Urinary retention, impotence, vertigo, visual disturbances, blurred vision, tinnitus, hypotension, syncope, and headache

6. Hemolytic anemia, leukopenia, thrombocytopenia, and pancytopenia

D. Nursing considerations

1. Cetirizine, loratadine, and fexofenadine may be used in children over age of 6
2. Help client determine precipitating factors and symptoms of allergic reactions

NCLEX® 3. Monitor for drowsiness and dizziness, especially during first few days of therapy

4. Encourage fluid intake of 2000–3000 mL/day to loosen secretions unless contraindicated by another condition
5. Give antihistamines prior to contact with allergen if possible

NCLEX® 6. Administer at bedtime to reduce side effect of drowsiness

7. Administer intramuscular antihistamines deep into large muscles
8. Intravenous injection should be over a few minutes; see product literature

E. Client teaching

1. Take with meals to decrease stomach upset
2. Avoid contact with allergen if possible; if unable, take medication prior to exposure
3. Do not take more than one medication at a time

NCLEX® 4. Contact prescriber if excessive sedation, confusion, or hypotension occur

5. Use hard, sugarless candy to relieve dry mouth
6. Antihistamines may dry and thicken respiratory tract secretions and make them difficult to expectorate: increase fluid intake
7. Take loratadine on an empty stomach to increase absorption
8. Avoid prolonged exposure to sunlight because of potential for sunburn
9. Take medication at bedtime to reduce drowsiness, which should become less significant after repeated doses

NCLEX® 10. Do not take antihistamines for 72 hours prior to allergen skin testing to reduce likelihood of false negative results

VI. MEDICATIONS TO CONTROL BRONCHIAL SECRETIONS

A. Nasal *decongestants*

1. Relieve nasal stuffiness by shrinking swollen nasal mucous membranes
2. Adrenergic agents (sympathomimetics) cause vasoconstriction, decreasing blood flow to nasal mucosa and thereby reducing swelling
3. Nasal steroids suppress inflammatory response
4. Used to relieve nasal congestion and nasal discharge caused by acute or chronic rhinitis (common cold), sinusitis, hay fever, and other allergies
5. May be used to decrease local blood flow prior to nasal surgery or as an aid to visualizing nasal mucosa during diagnostic exams
6. Common medications are listed in Box 33–6

Memory Aid

A medication that ends in *-zoline* is a nasal decongestant, although not all nasal decongestants end in *-zoline*.

Box 33-6

Medications That Control Bronchial Secretions

Nasal Decongestants

Ephedrine (Pretz-D)

Naphazoline (Privine)

Oxymetazoline (Afrin)

Phenylephrine (Neo-Synephrine)

Pseudoephedrine (Sudafed)

Tetrahydrozoline (Tyzine)

Xylometazoline (Otrivin)

Expectorants

Guaifenesin (Robitussin, others)

Antitussives

Nonopioid type

Benzonatate (Tessalon Perles)

Dextromethorphan (Robitussin DM, others)

Opioid type

Codeine (several products)

Hydrocodone with homatropine (Hycodan)

Mucolytics

Sodium chloride solution by nebulization

Acetylcysteine (Mucomyst) (nebulizer)

Dornase alfa (rhDNAse; Pulmozyme—a proteolytic enzyme for clients with cystic fibrosis only)

7. Administration considerations
   a. Can be used topically (with sprays or drops) or orally
   b. NCLEX® Sustained use of topical drugs (longer than 3 days or in excessive amounts) can cause rebound congestion; therefore, oral agents should be used if needed for longer than 3 days
   c. Topical drugs are potent decongestants with prompt onset of action
   d. Topical drugs are preferred if client has cardiovascular disease because of decreased risk of cardiovascular side effects
8. Side/adverse effects
   a. Local nasal mucosal irritation and dryness
   b. Rebound congestion is common
   c. Nervousness, insomnia, palpitations, and tremor (with systemic absorption) are rare
9. Nursing considerations
   a. NCLEX® Review other medical history to determine risk for side effects; older adults with significant cardiac disease should avoid nasal decongestants because of high risk for hypertension, dysrhythmias, nervousness, and insomnia
   b. To administer nose drops, have client lie down or sit with neck hyperextended
   c. Wash medication droppers after each use to prevent contamination
   d. Client should sit and squeeze nasal spray container once and avoid touching nares with spray dispenser; tip of dispenser should be rinsed after each use
   e. Observe client for intended decrease in nasal congestion
   f. NCLEX® Monitor for tachycardia, hypertension, and cardiac dysrhythmias; also observe for rebound nasal congestion, chronic rhinitis, and ulceration of the nasal mucosa
10. Client teaching
    a. NCLEX® Avoid concurrent use of caffeine, which can cause nervousness, tremors, and insomnia
    b. Avoid smoking because it increases secretions and decreases ciliary action
    c. Avoid exposure to crowds to minimize spread of disease
    d. NCLEX® Increase fluid intake to 2000–3000 mL/day unless contraindicated by another medical condition
    e. NCLEX® Nasal congestion in infants can decrease ability to suck effectively: apply nasal solution prior to feeding to increase infant's ability to feed
    f. Avoid eating or drinking for 30 minutes after medication administration
    g. Practice good hand hygiene
    h. NCLEX® Rinse droppers and spray bottles after each use to avoid contamination

B. *Expectorants*

1. Expectorants reduce viscosity of secretions and increase mucus flow in respiratory tract to aid removal by cough reflex and ciliary action
2. Used to relieve nonproductive cough associated with common cold, bronchitis, laryngitis, and influenza
3. Common medications are listed in see Box 33–6

NCLEX® 4. Administration considerations: use with caution in older adults or debilitated clients, or those with asthma and respiratory insufficiency
5. Side/adverse effects
   a. N/V and gastric irritation
   b. Rash, dizziness, and headache
6. Nursing considerations: none specific to this group
7. Client teaching
   NCLEX® a. Report a fever or cough to physician if it lasts longer than a week
   NCLEX® b. Increase fluid intake if not contraindicated by other disease processes
   c. Avoid smoking because it increases secretions and decreases ciliary action
   d. Avoid drinking fluids for 30 minutes after taking this medication

C. ***Antitussives***
1. **Opioid** (narcotic) and nonopioid antitussives suppress cough reflex by directly affecting cough center; nonopioid antitussives do so without CNS suppression
2. Peripherally acting agents (glycerin, ammonium chloride) have local anesthetic effects to decrease irritation of pharyngeal mucosa; they are available in gargles, lozenges, and syrups; lozenges increase saliva flow and therefore suppress cough
3. Used to stop a nonproductive cough or a dry, hacking, nonproductive cough that interferes with rest and sleep
4. Common medications are listed in Box 33–6
5. Administration considerations
   NCLEX® a. There is risk for addiction and CNS and respiratory depression with opioids
   b. Most are given as liquid or as oral tablets; syrup form may soothe irritated mucosa in pharynx
   c. Dextromethorphan is preferred over codeine because it provides desired effect without use of opioids; is available in many OTC products and does not require a prescription
   d. Dextromethorphan is contraindicated with asthma, emphysema, chronic headaches, or hypersensitivity
   NCLEX® e. Codeine preparations are contraindicated with respiratory depression, increased intracranial pressure, severe liver or renal disease, hypothyroidism, adrenal insufficiency, or seizure disorders
6. Side/adverse effects
   a. Dizziness, headache, drowsiness or sedation, N/V, constipation, pruritus, nasal congestion, dry mouth, blurred vision, and sweating
   NCLEX® b. Dependence and respiratory depression with codeine
   c. Dry mouth, palpitations, thickened respiratory mucus, anorexia, urinary retention or frequency, diarrhea, photosensitivity, and dysuria with nonopioids
   d. Nasal congestion and burning of the eyes with benzonatate
7. Nursing considerations
   a. Monitor for inability to cough effectively from excessive cough suppression
   b. Observe for listed side effects and potential drug dependence
   NCLEX® c. Cough may be a useful diagnostic tool and protective measure for client; use antitussives cautiously for irritating, nonproductive, ineffective cough
8. Client teaching
   NCLEX® a. Notify physician if cough lasts longer than a week or if persistent headache, fever, or rash occurs
   b. Do not drink liquids for 30–35 minutes after taking a chewable tablet or a lozenge
   c. Avoid smoking because it increases secretions and decreases ciliary action
   d. For excessive respiratory secretions, understand benefits of coughing, deep breathing, and ambulation
   NCLEX® e. Liquefy secretions with increased oral intake up to 2000–3000 mL/day unless contraindicated

D. ***Mucolytics***
1. Are administered by inhalation to liquefy (thin) mucus in respiratory tract and aid in removal of viscous secretions
2. Used with sinusitis and common cold
3. An oral form of acetylcysteine (Mucomyst) can be used to treat acetaminophen overdose
4. Common medications are listed in Box 33–6
5. Administration considerations
   a. No longer commonly used because of questionable effectiveness
   NCLEX® b. These drugs are nebulized using a face mask or a mouth piece; can be instilled into a tracheostomy
   c. Acetylcysteine is effective 1 minute after inhalation or immediately after direct instillation; maximal effect is in 5 to 10 minutes
   NCLEX® d. Activated charcoal limits effectiveness of acetylcysteine when used as antidote to acetaminophen overdose

6. Side/adverse effects
   a. Oral irritation and sore throat
   b. Cough and bronchospasm
   c. Nausea and vomiting, headaches
7. Nursing considerations
   NCLEX® a. May cause bronchospasm and are usually given with bronchodilators
   b. Suction client if cough is ineffective
   c. Rinse mouth after therapy to decrease oropharyngeal irritation
   NCLEX® d. Discard unused medication after 4 days
8. Client teaching
   NCLEX® a. Increase fluid intake unless contraindicated by other disease processes
   b. Avoid smoking because it increases secretions and decreases ciliary action

VII. OXYGEN

A. Indications

1. **Hypoxia**, deficiency of oxygen (O_2) in cells and tissues, and **hypoxemia**, deficiency of O_2 in arterial blood
2. Conditions associated with decreased arterial oxygen (PO_2) levels (pulmonary edema), decreased cardiac output (myocardial infarction), decreased blood oxygen–carrying capacity (anemia), increased O_2 demand (sepsis, sustained fever), and others

B. Types of delivery systems

1. Nasal cannula (nasal prongs): most common form of O_2 delivery
   a. Go into nostrils and tubing attaches to oxygen source and flowmeter
   b. Client can eat and talk with a nasal cannula
   NCLEX® c. Oxygen can be administered at a rate ranging from 1 L/min to 6 L/min
   d. Dryness of mucous membranes can occur
2. Nasal catheter: inserted into throat through a nostril, change to other nostril every 8 hours; not used frequently because of client discomfort; gastric distention sometimes occurs
3. Oxymizer: a nasal cannula with a reservoir that can deliver higher concentrations of O_2 than a regular cannula (approximately twice) without use of a mask
NCLEX® 4. Face mask: a mask that fits over client's mouth and nose
   a. Simple face mask: flow rate is 5–10 L/min with O_2 delivery capabilities of 40–60%
   b. Partial rebreather mask: consists of a face mask with a reservoir bag; some exhaled air goes into reservoir bag and is mixed with 100% O_2 for next inhalation; permits conservation of O_2 and can deliver 70–90% O_2 at rates of 6–15 L/min
   c. Nonrebreather mask: delivers highest concentration of O_2 by mask; no exhaled air goes into reservoir bag; reservoir bag contains O_2, which client breathes in with inspiration; exhaled air goes out through side vents and can deliver 60–100% O_2 at flow rates of 6–15 L/min
   d. Venturi mask: percentage of O_2 is adjusted by a dial at end of mask; amount of air pulled into system varies with needed amount of O_2 and gives precise oxygen concentrations

C. Oxygen toxicity

NCLEX® 1. Lung tissue can be damaged from prolonged exposure to high O_2 concentrations
2. Exact amount of O_2 and length of time required to cause O_2 toxicity varies depending on degree of underlying lung disease; some sources say lung damage can occur with O_2 delivery of greater than 50% for more than 24–48 hours
NCLEX® 3. **Atelectasis**, or alveolar collapse, can result with O_2 administration at rates of 60% for more than 36 hours or 90% for more than 6 hours
4. Adult respiratory distress syndrome (ARDS) can result from breathing 80–100% oxygen for more than 24 hours
5. Symptoms of O_2 toxicity begin as a nonproductive cough, substernal chest pain, GI upset, and dyspnea; as it worsens, client develops decreased vital capacity, lung compliance, and hypoxemia; atelectasis, pulmonary edema, and pulmonary hemorrhage can result if not reversed
NCLEX® 6. Oxygen should be weaned as soon as possible according to O_2 saturation (SaO_2) level

D. Nursing considerations (see also Chapter 26)

1. Oxygen therapy can be anxiety-provoking; provide sufficient explanation and allow client to express anxieties
2. Flow rate is measured in liters per minute (L/min); it is a measure of O_2 delivered but is not completely accurate because there is loss of O_2 content with leaking and mixing with room air

3. Oxygen analyzers are available to measure percentage of O_2 client inhales; this is recommended every 4 hours
4. NCLEX® Clients with COPD should not receive O_2 at more than 2 L/min by nasal cannula because higher levels of O_2 in bloodstream can cause hypoventilation; a COPD client's drive to breathe is from low levels of O_2 tension
5. NCLEX® Check O_2 delivery system frequently to ensure proper functioning
6. Oxygen should be humidified when client is receiving rates higher than 2 L/min
7. A face mask should fit client's face to avoid unnecessary leakage; if mask is too snug, skin irritation can occur
8. Masks can be changed to a nasal cannula during meals with physician order
9. NCLEX® The reservoir bag on a partial rebreather should deflate slightly with inspiration
10. Provide reassurance if client becomes claustrophobic
11. NCLEX® Flaps on side of nonrebreather mask should open during exhalation and close during inhalation
12. NCLEX® Monitor SaO_2 with pulse oximeter during O_2 therapy; with physician order, O_2 may be titrated to achieve desired SaO_2 level
13. Monitor for signs of hypoxia and respiratory distress, changes in vital signs and color changes (pallor, dusky, cyanosis)
14. Monitor arterial blood gases (ABGs) per physician order
15. Normal arterial O_2 levels decrease with age
16. NCLEX® Provide oral care for comfort because of potential drying of mucous membranes
17. Identify clients at high risk for developing O_2 toxicity

E. **Client teaching**

1. Expect noise with flow of O_2
2. NCLEX® Avoid open flames with O_2 administration because it is flammable
3. NCLEX® Ensure there are no frayed electrical cords near O_2 so there are no sparks causing combustion
4. NCLEX® Do not smoke when O_2 therapy is being utilized
5. Expect delivery to cause dryness of mouth and nasal mucosa
6. NCLEX® Remove O_2 when using an electric razor
7. Continue O_2 therapy at home as prescribed by physician
8. NCLEX® Keep O_2 tank in holder and away from direct sunlight to reduce effects of heat
9. Understand signs of hypoxia and report them to physician

Check Your NCLEX–PN® Exam I.Q.

You are ready for testing on this content if you can

- Apply knowledge of expected actions and effects of respiratory medications to client care.
- Correctly administer respiratory medications to clients.
- Monitor for side effects and adverse effects of respiratory medications.
- Take appropriate action if a client has an unexpected response to a respiratory medication.
- Monitor a client for expected outcomes or effects of treatment with respiratory medications.

PRACTICE TEST

1 A client with congestive heart failure is taking digoxin (Lanoxin) and furosemide (Lasix). A new diagnosis of acute bronchitis is made, and albuterol (Proventil) via inhalation is started. For what complication should the nurse conclude that this client is at risk?

1. Hyperkalemia
2. Hypernatremia
3. Hypocalcemia
4. Hypokalemia

2 A client with asthma has started to take a beta-adrenergic agent. The client also takes a monoamine oxidase inhibitor (MAOI). For what complication should the nurse monitor the client?

1. Hypotension
2. Hypertension
3. Tachycardia
4. Bradycardia

3. A diabetic client, admitted to the emergency department with acute bronchospasm, is given epinephrine (Bronkaid). Which finding noted during data collection should indicate to the nurse that the client is experiencing a side effect of this medication?

1. Blood glucose level 156 mg/dL
2. Blood glucose level 77 mg/dL
3. Potassium level 5.4 mEq/L
4. Potassium level 3.1 mEq/L

4. The nurse is reinforcing instructions to a client with chronic obstructive pulmonary disease (COPD) about how to administer multiple medications by inhalation. Which statement by the client indicates an understanding of the instruction? Select all that apply.

1. "If my symptoms get worse, I can double my dosage."
2. "I will wait at least 1 minute between use of my different inhalers."
3. "I should consult my physician before using over-the-counter medications."
4. "I cannot rinse my inhaler equipment, because it is not supposed to get wet."
5. "I should store my inhaler in the refrigerator door between uses."

5. A client reports that a newly prescribed beta-adrenergic agent is causing nervousness and tremors. Which reply by the nurse is most appropriate?

1. "The symptoms are common at first, but decrease over time."
2. "Stop taking the medicine, because the symptoms will only get worse."
3. "Drinking coffee or tea will help decrease the symptoms."
4. "Those symptoms indicate a worsening of the disease process."

6. The nurse has reinforced teaching to the client about home administration of theophylline (Theo-Dur). Which statement to the nurse is reflective of appropriate learning?

1. "I can crush the sustained-release forms so they are easier to swallow."
2. "If a dose is omitted, I can take a double dose the next time."
3. "I should take the medication as soon as symptoms occur."
4. "Taking the medication with food will prevent stomach upset."

7. A client who takes theophylline (Theo-Dur) reports restlessness. Which is the most appropriate action for the nurse to take first?

1. Monitor the client for hypoxia.
2. Explain that this is a toxic reaction, and call the physician.
3. Observe the client for other signs and symptoms of theophylline toxicity.
4. Call the physician to obtain an order for a theophylline level.

8. A client asks the nurse why the physician ordered beclomethasone (Beclovent) for his chronic obstructive pulmonary disease (COPD). Which statement by the nurse is most appropriate?

1. "Beclovent prevents airway dilation."
2. "Beclovent decreases inflammation, and makes it easier to breathe."
3. "Beclovent suppresses the immune response."
4. "Beclovent decreases responsiveness to medications that dilate the airway."

9. The nurse is teaching a client about cromolyn (Intal). Which statement should the nurse make about the mechanism of action for cromolyn?

1. Relaxes bronchial smooth muscle to assist with bronchodilation
2. Limits inflammation and bronchoconstriction with exposure to allergens
3. Helps to liquefy respiratory secretions to promote expectoration
4. Promotes bronchoconstriction of overly dilated airways

10. The nurse is monitoring the client who takes cromolyn (Intal). Which symptom indicates to the nurse that the client is experiencing a potential side effect? Select all that apply.

1. Vomiting
2. Dry mouth
3. Tachycardia
4. Headache
5. Throat irritation

PRACTICE TEST

11 A client beginning medication therapy with montelukast (Singulair) asks the nurse how the medication is helping the symptoms. Which is the nurse's best response?

1. "Singulair decreases inflammation and mucus secretion."
2. "Singulair increases mucus secretion and bronchodilation."
3. "Singulair prevents smooth muscle contraction by nervous system stimulation."
4. "Singulair protects the airway from the effects of allergen exposure."

12 The client asks the nurse about self-care related to newly ordered zafirlukast (Accolate). What is an appropriate response by the nurse?

1. Renal function tests should be monitored.
2. Liver function tests should be monitored.
3. Fluid intake should be decreased.
4. The medication should be taken with meals.

13 A client asks the nurse if there is a benefit to taking second-generation antihistamines instead of first-generation antihistamines. The nurse responds that second-generation antihistamines have a reduced incidence of which side effect?

1. Nausea
2. Anxiety
3. Drowsiness
4. Euphoria

14 A client asks the nurse about drug interactions with diphenhydramine (Benadryl). The nurse informs the client that which substances will increase the effects of Benadryl? Select all that apply.

1. Alcohol
2. Opiates
3. Caffeine
4. Antianxiety agents
5. Tricyclic antidepressants

15 The nurse is reinforcing teaching to a client about proper technique for administration of nasal sprays. Which explanation should the nurse use in order to provide accurate information?

1. "Squeeze the bottle twice in each nostril for an adequate dose."
2. "Inhale while holding your finger over the other nostril."
3. "Rinsing the tip of the spray bottle can contaminate the medication."
4. "Lying down for administration assures the medication is instilled."

16 The nurse is assisting in developing a teaching plan for a client using nasal decongestant. What instruction should the nurse include in the teaching plan?

1. "Be sure to stay on the medication for at least 7 days."
2. "Decrease fluid intake to 1L/day to decrease nasal secretions."
3. "Avoid eating or drinking for 30 minutes after medication administration."
4. "Decrease smoking activity while using this medication."

17 The nurse is reinforcing important information related to self-administration of guaifenesin (Robitussin) to a client. What information should the nurse include?

1. Side effects include nausea, vomiting, and rash.
2. Report a cough to the physician if it lasts longer than 2 weeks.
3. Take the medication with meals.
4. If the medication is not effective, double the dose.

18 The nurse is monitoring a client for side effects of an opioid antitussive. Which side effect is the most significant if noted during data collection?

1. Dry, cracked lips
2. Reports of blurred vision
3. Inability to stay awake
4. Respirations of 10/min

19 Which statement by the client taking a mucolytic indicates a need for further teaching?

1. "I will drink at least 2–3 liters of fluid each day."
2. "I will avoid smoking."
3. "I will rinse my mouth after I take my medicine."
4. "I should discard what I do not use of the medicine after a week."

20 The nurse has an order to administer 50% oxygen to a client with pulmonary edema. Which oxygen administration system should the nurse select that allows that percentage of oxygen to be delivered?

1. Nasal cannula
2. Nonrebreather mask
3. Partial rebreather mask
4. Venturi mask

ANSWERS & RATIONALES

1 **Answer: 4 Rationale:** Risk of hypokalemia is worsened by the concurrent use of a potassium-wasting diuretic (Lasix) and a beta-agonist (albuterol) medication. Furthermore, the risk of cardiac glycoside toxicity is worse in the presence of hypokalemia. The other options are not a concern with this drug regimen. **Cognitive Level:** Analyzing **Client Need:** Pharmacological and Parenteral Therapies **Integrated Process:** Nursing Process: Evaluation **Content Area:** Pharmacology **Strategy:** The core issue of this question is the effect of taking a potassium-losing diuretic with other cardiac or respiratory medications, which helps you to focus on hypokalemia. Note also that two options are opposites, so there is a greater chance that one of these is the correct answer.

2 **Answer: 2 Rationale:** Concurrent use of an MAOI and a beta-agonist can lead to hypertensive crisis. Hypotension is not of concern with this combination of medications; the client is at risk for a hypertensive crisis. The beta-agonist could lead to tachycardia, but since no specific agent is listed, the nurse should consider the potential interaction of the MAOI and the beta-agonist first. Bradycardia is not of concern with this combination of medications; it is more likely that the client will experience tachycardia. **Cognitive Level:** Analyzing **Client Need:** Pharmacological and Parenteral Therapies **Integrated Process:** Nursing Process: Data Collection **Content Area:** Pharmacology **Strategy:** The core issue of the question is the interactive effects of beta-agonists and MAOIs. Use the process of elimination, and recall that an agonist type of drug enhances the action of a system, in this case the beta-adrenergic system. Then recall that these effects include increased pulse and blood pressure. Note also that two of these options are opposites, making it more likely that one of them is the correct answer.

3 **Answer: 1 Rationale:** Epinephrine is a beta-adrenergic agent used to dilate bronchial airways. It can cause an increased blood glucose level, which is especially an issue for a client with diabetes mellitus. Diabetic clients should be instructed to monitor blood glucose levels because an adjustment in maintenance doses of hypoglycemic agents could be indicated. The other options are not expected effects of the medication on diabetic clients. **Cognitive Level:** Analyzing **Client Need:** Pharmacological and Parenteral Therapies **Integrated Process:** Nursing Process: Data Collection **Content Area:** Pharmacology **Strategy:** The core issue of the question is the knowledge that beta-adrenergic medications stimulate the sympathetic nervous system, and that one of the end effects of the stimulation is increased blood glucose. Correlate this knowledge with the client in the question, who has diabetes, to make a correct selection relative to hyperglycemia.

4 **Answer: 2, 3 Rationale:** The client should wait at least one minute between inhalations. OTC products should not be added without consulting the physician. Dosages should be taken exactly as prescribed. Inhaler equipment should be cleaned with mild soap, rinsed, and dried daily. The inhaler should be stored at room temperature. **Cognitive Level:** Applying **Client Need:** Pharmacological and Parenteral Therapies **Integrated Process:** Nursing Process: Evaluation **Content Area:** Pharmacology **Strategy:** The core issue of the question is correct administration procedure for inhaled medications. The wording of the question tells you the correct answers are options phrased as true statements. When more than one answer is correct, consider each option as a true/false statement.

5 **Answer: 1 Rationale:** Nervousness and tremors might be experienced when medication is newly administered, but they frequently decrease over time. Clients should not terminate medication use without consulting the prescriber. Caffeine would exacerbate the problem. The symptoms are likely related to the medication, and not to the disease process. **Cognitive Level:** Analyzing **Client Need:** Pharmacological and Parenteral Therapies **Integrated Process:** Communication and Documentation **Content Area:** Pharmacology **Strategy:** Knowledge of the side effects with a beta-adrenergic agent will be helpful in answering the question. Combine information about the drug with the principles of therapeutic communication to select the correct answer.

6 **Answer: 4 Rationale:** Taking the medication with food can decrease GI symptoms. Sustained-release forms should not be crushed or chewed, because doing so irritates the gastric mucosa and changes the absorption of the medication. Medications should be taken as prescribed, without omissions or doubled doses. Theophylline should be taken at all times and as ordered, not just when the client is symptomatic. **Cognitive Level:** Applying **Client Need:** Pharmacological and Parenteral Therapies **Integrated Process:** Teaching and Learning **Content Area:** Pharmacology **Strategy:** The core issues of the question are general medication knowledge and instructions for use of theophylline. Eliminate the options that are not consistent with the general principles for self-administration of medication.

7 **Answer: 1 Rationale:** Restlessness is a sign of theophylline toxicity, but often is a first indicator of hypoxia. The first and best action is to monitor for hypoxia. The nurse needs to perform additional data collection before calling the physician and reporting a toxic reaction. After ruling out hypoxia, the client should be observed for other possible signs and symptoms of toxicity (insomnia, irritability, nausea/vomiting, tremors), before contacting the physician. Obtaining an order for a theophylline level is appropriate after ruling out hypoxia and performing additional data collection. **Cognitive Level:** Analyzing **Client Need:** Pharmacological and Parenteral Therapies **Integrated Process:** Nursing Process: Planning **Content Area:** Pharmacology **Strategy:** The question contains the word *first*, which indicates that more than one option might be technically correct, but one is best. All the incorrect options

refer to the theme of toxicity. If options are very similar, none of them can be correct. Use the integrated principles of data collection and ABCs to help determine the correct answer.

8 **Answer: 2 Rationale:** Beclovent is an inhaled corticosteroid that is thought to decrease inflammation and dilate the airway. Preventing airway dilation is undesirable for this client, and the exact opposite action of Beclovent. The exact mechanism of action is unknown. Beclovent, like any other corticosteroid, does suppress the immune response, but this is not the rationale for administration of the medication. Inhaled corticosteroids are thought to increase responsiveness of bronchial smooth muscle to beta-agonist drugs. **Cognitive Level:** Applying **Client Need:** Pharmacological and Parenteral Therapies **Integrated Process:** Teaching and Learning **Content Area:** Pharmacology **Strategy:** Use medication knowledge and the process of elimination to make a selection. Knowledge about the pathology of COPD will be helpful in identifying the correct answer.

9 **Answer: 2 Rationale:** Cromolyn is a nonsteroidal agent that stabilizes mast cells so bronchoconstrictive and inflammatory substances are not released when stimulated with an allergen. It is used to treat inflammation of the airway. Cromolyn is a nonsteroidal agent; not a bronchodilator. Cromolyn is a nonsteroidal agent; not an expectorant. Cromolyn is used to treat inflammation of the airway. It does not cause bronchoconstriction. **Cognitive Level:** Applying **Client Need:** Pharmacological and Parenteral Therapies **Integrated Process:** Teaching and Learning **Content Area:** Pharmacology **Strategy:** Use medication knowledge in conjunction with knowledge of the pathophysiology of COPD to select the correct answer.

10 **Answer: 2, 4, 5 Rationale:** Side effects of cromolyn include dry mouth, headaches, and throat irritation. Vomiting and tachycardia are not side effects of cromolyn. **Cognitive Level:** Applying **Client Need:** Pharmacological and Parenteral Therapies **Integrated Process:** Nursing Process: Data Collection **Content Area:** Pharmacology **Strategy:** Specific medication knowledge is needed to answer this question. Use the process of elimination to make a selection.

11 **Answer: 1 Rationale:** Leukotriene modifiers such as montelukast block the action of leukotrienes, and therefore decrease mucous secretion and reduce inflammation, preventing bronchoconstriction. Montelukast blocks the action of leukotrienes and decreases mucous secretion. Leukotriene modifiers such as montelukast do not prevent smooth muscle contraction; they decrease mucous secretion and reduce inflammation. Leukotrienes are released when a client is exposed to an allergen. Leukotriene modifiers such as montelukast do not protect the airway from the effects of allergen exposure. **Cognitive Level:** Applying **Client Need:** Pharmacological and Parenteral Therapies **Integrated Process:** Teaching and Learning **Content Area:** Pharmacology **Strategy:** Specific medication knowledge is needed to answer this question. Use the process of elimination to make a selection.

12 **Answer: 2 Rationale:** Liver function tests should be monitored with leukotriene modifiers because of the potential for liver dysfunction with this type of medication. Renal studies are unnecessary in relation to this medication. Fluid intake should be increased unless contraindicated by another condition, in order to thin secretions and assist in their mobilization. The medication should be taken one hour before or two hours after meals. **Cognitive Level:** Applying **Client Need:** Pharmacological and Parenteral Therapies **Integrated Process:** Teaching and Learning **Content Area:** Pharmacology **Strategy:** Recall that metabolism and excretion of many drugs occurs in either the hepatic or renal systems. This provides a clue that two of the options may be correct. Associate the letter *l* in *leukotrienes* with the letter *l* for *liver*.

13 **Answer: 3 Rationale:** Second-generation antihistamines cause less sedation than do first-generation medications, so the client experiences less drowsiness. They are selective for peripheral H1 histamine receptors, and do not cross the blood–brain barrier. The other options are unrelated as comparison points between first- and second-generation antihistamines. **Cognitive Level:** Applying **Client Need:** Pharmacological and Parenteral Therapies **Integrated Process:** Teaching and Learning **Content Area:** Pharmacology **Strategy:** Recall that second-generation drugs generally have some type of improvement over first-generation drugs. In this case, since antihistamines often cause drowsiness, it is easy to reason that this side effect would be decreased in second-generation medications in this category.

14 **Answer: 1, 2, 4, 5 Rationale:** The effects of first-generation antihistamines, such as Benadryl, are increased with alcohol, opioid analgesics, antianxiety agents, and tricyclic antidepressants. The consumption of caffeine, a stimulant, would not have an additive effect when taking Benadryl. **Cognitive Level:** Analyzing **Client Need:** Pharmacological and Parenteral Therapies **Integrated Process:** Teaching and Learning **Content Area:** Pharmacology **Strategy:** Recall first that first-generation antihistamines cause drowsiness, and look for an option that would have an additive effect. Eliminate any choice that acts as a stimulant. When there is more than one correct answer, consider each option as a true/false statement.

15 **Answer: 2 Rationale:** The proper application of nasal spray decongestants is with the client sitting and squeezing the bottle once, holding a finger over the other nostril, and inhaling. Unless otherwise specified, administering more than a one-squeeze application would increase the dose. The applicator should be rinsed after each use to prevent contamination. The proper application of nasal spray decongestants is with the client in a sitting position. **Cognitive Level:** Applying **Client Need:** Pharmacological and Parenteral Therapies **Integrated Process:** Teaching and Learning **Content Area:** Pharmacology **Strategy:** A critical word in the question is *accurate*. The core issue of the question is the instruction that is a true statement. Use the process of elimination and knowledge of basic medication administration procedures to make a selection.

16 **Answer: 3 Rationale:** Avoidance of eating or drinking for 30 minutes after medication administration allows the medication time to work. Nasal spray decongestants should not be taken for more than 3 days, because they can cause rebound congestion. Fluid intake should be increased to 2–3 L/day, not decreased, to liquefy secretions. Smoking should be avoided, not merely reduced, because it increases secretions and decreases ciliary action. **Cognitive Level:** Applying **Client Need:** Pharmacological and Parenteral Therapies **Integrated Process:** Teaching and Learning **Content Area:** Pharmacology **Strategy:** The wording of the question tells you the correct answer is also a true statement. Eliminate the options that are least likely to be true. Choose the correct option using knowledge about the side effects of decongestants.

17 **Answer: 1 Rationale:** It is important to teach clients side effects of medications. The side effects of expectorants include nausea, vomiting, gastric irritation, and rash. If a

cough lasts longer than a week it should be reported to the physician. The client should avoid eating or drinking for 30 minutes after medication administration to allow the medication to work. The medication should be taken as directed, and doses should not be doubled. **Cognitive Level:** Applying **Client Need:** Pharmacological and Parenteral Therapies **Integrated Process:** Nursing Process: Implementation **Content Area:** Pharmacology **Strategy:** Use the process of elimination and general medication knowledge to answer the question. Eliminate options with excessive time frames, those that hinder medication absorption, and any option that does not support standard medication teaching.

18 **Answer: 4** **Rationale:** The most significant side effect is respiratory depression, evidenced by a respiratory rate of 10, when normal is 12–20 breaths/minute. The other options are potential side effects of opioid antitussives; however, the most significant side effect is respiratory depression. **Cognitive Level:** Analyzing **Client Need:** Pharmacological and Parenteral Therapies **Integrated Process:** Nursing Process: Data Collection **Content Area:** Pharmacology **Strategy:** The key words *most significant* tell you that more than one option might be technically correct, and that you must select the most important option. Use the ABCs (airway, breathing, and circulation) to make your selection.

19 **Answer: 4** **Rationale:** Unused medication should be discarded after four days, not seven. This statement indicates that the client needs additional teaching. Increasing fluids assists with thinning secretions; this statement does not indicate a need for additional teaching. The client does not need further teaching if there is an understanding that avoidance of smoking is necessary; smoking increases secretions and decreases ciliary action. Rinsing the mouth after administration is an appropriate action because this action decreases oropharyngeal irritation. **Cognitive Level:** Applying **Client Need:** Pharmacological and Parenteral Therapies **Integrated Process:** Nursing Process: Evaluation **Content Area:** Pharmacology **Strategy:** The phrase *further teaching* tells you the correct answer is an incorrect or false statement. Eliminate options that indicate that the client is expressing an understanding of appropriate actions.

20 **Answer: 4** **Rationale:** The Venturi mask has a dial to set the percentage of oxygen, and can administer 50% oxygen. The nasal cannula can administer up to 6 L/min, which is approximately 44% oxygen. The nonrebreather mask administers 60–100% oxygen. The partial rebreather mask administers 70–90% oxygen. **Cognitive Level:** Applying **Client Need:** Pharmacological and Parenteral Therapies **Integrated Process:** Nursing Process: Implementation **Content Area:** Pharmacology **Strategy:** Specific knowledge of the various concepts related to oxygen therapy is needed to answer this question. Use the process of elimination to make a selection, and remember that Venturi masks deliver precise oxygen concentrations.

Key Terms to Review

References

Adams, M., Holland, L., & Urban, C. (2011). *Pharmacology for nurses: A pathophysiological approach* (3rd ed.). Upper Saddle River, NJ: Pearson Education, Inc.

Adams, M., & Koch, R. (2010). *Pharmacology: Connections to nursing practice.* Upper Saddle River, NJ: Pearson Education, Inc.

Berman, A., & Snyder, S. (2012). *Kozier & Erb's fundamentals of nursing: Concepts, process, and practice* (9th ed.). Upper Saddle River, NJ: Pearson Education, Inc.

Deglin, J., & Vallerand, A. (2011). *Davis's drug guide for nurses* (12th ed.). Philadelphia: F. A. Davis.

Lehne, R. (2010). *Pharmacology for nursing care* (7th ed.). St. Louis, MO: Mosby.

LeMone, P., Burke, K., & Bauldoff, G. (2012). *Medical surgical nursing: Critical thinking in patient care* (5th ed.). Upper Saddle River, NJ: Pearson Education, Inc.

Smeltzer, S., & Bare, B. (2011). *Textbook of medical-surgical nursing* (12th ed.). Philadelphia: Lippincott, William & Wilkins.

Wilson, B., Shannon, M., & Shields, K. (2012). *Pearson nurse's drug guide 2012.* Upper Saddle River, NJ: Pearson Education.

Test Yourself

Are you ready for the NCLEX-PN® or course exams? Use the practice tests on the companion website to check.

34 Cardiovascular Medications

In this chapter

Cross Reference

Other chapters relevant to this content area are

Dosage Calculation and Medication Administration	Chapter 28
Cardiovascular Disorders	Chapter 52

I. NITRATES

A. **Increase oxygenated blood flow to myocardium** by dilating coronary and systemic blood vessels (BVs)

B. **Dilation of systemic vascular bed** leads to pooling of blood in peripheral BVs and reduced **preload** (volume in left ventricle just prior to contraction) and **afterload** (resistance to blood being ejected by left ventricle) and myocardial oxygen (O_2) demand

C. **Common medications are listed in Box 34–1**

Memory Aid

Remember that drugs that are nitrates have the letters *nitro-* or *nitr-* in them.

D. **Administration considerations**

1. Ensure oral mucous membranes are moist when giving sublingual (SL) nitroglycerin (NTG) tablets
2. For a hospitalized client, keep NTG tablets at bedside with a physician order if policy allows; instruct client to report all chest pain episodes; count tablets daily if kept at bedside

Box 34–1

Nitrates and Nitrites

Nitroglycerin (Nitrostat, Nitrodur, others)

Isosorbide mononitrate (Ismo, Monoket, Imdur)

Isosorbide dinitrate (Isordil Iso-Bid, others)

3. Administer intravenous (IV) NTG as a continuous or intermittent infusion (not IV push) using an infusion pump
4. *NCLEX®* IV NTG must be diluted in 5% dextrose or 0.9% sodium chloride (normal saline) solution, mixed in glass bottles and infused only through manufacturer-supplied IV tubing; regular polyvinylchloride IV tubing can absorb 40–80% of NTG
5. Nitroglycerin IV drips are often **titrated** (dose adjusted according to a predetermined parameter, such as chest pain)
6. *NCLEX®* Monitor blood pressure (BP) and heart rate (HR) every 15 minutes when using IV form of NTG and titrating medication; be prepared to treat hypotension by decreasing or stopping NTG infusion
7. *NCLEX®* Use gloves or an applicator to spread NTG paste or ointment evenly and avoid absorption of medication into nurse's skin
8. *NCLEX®* Rotate location of NTG paste or patch to reduce skin irritation and enhance absorption; place on hairless areas and avoid scar tissue or lesions; appropriate areas include chest, upper abdomen, anterior thigh, or upper arm
9. NTG dosing regimen should allow for an 8- to 10-hour nitrate-free period to prevent development of tolerance; apply NTG patch in morning and remove at bedtime
10. *NCLEX®* Do not administer any nitrate to a client who has hypersensitivity to nitrates, is hypotensive, has severe bradycardia or tachycardia, or has used erectile dysfunction medications such as sildenafil (Viagra) within 24 hours (causes profound hypotension)

E. Side/adverse effects

1. *NCLEX®* Headache (50%), postural or orthostatic hypotension, flushing, blurred vision, dry mouth
2. Weakness, dizziness, vertigo, and faintness
3. Severe postural hypotension
4. Nausea and vomiting (N/V), fecal and urinary incontinence, abdominal pain

F. Nursing considerations

1. *NCLEX®* Ensure client is sitting or lying down when taking NTG to prevent dizziness or fainting
2. Allow SL tablet to dissolve naturally under tongue; if mouth is dry, instruct client to take a sip of water before placing tablet under tongue
3. *NCLEX®* Give no more than 3 tablets total, one every 5 minutes; notify physician or emergency services if pain is unrelieved after third dose
4. *NCLEX®* Remove paste or patch each day at designated time before applying next dose
5. Store ointment in a cool, dry place with cap attached tightly
6. *NCLEX®* Monitor BP and HR frequently during titration (may be as often as every 5 to 10 minutes)
7. Check infusion concentration carefully because different dilutions are possible

G. Client teaching

1. All forms of NTG may cause dizziness and headache; rest for at least 15 minutes after taking SL medication to avoid dizziness
2. Report to health care provider if symptoms become worse or increase in frequency
3. Sit down next to a phone when taking sublingual (SL) NTG tablets in case it becomes necessary to call for help
4. *NCLEX®* If pain persists after three NTG tablets (or sprays) at 5-minute intervals, notify physician or emergency medical services because persistent pain could indicate an impending myocardial infarction (MI)
5. *NCLEX®* NTG degrades in heat, light, or moisture; store medication in original container in a cool, dry place
6. *NCLEX®* Replace NTG tablets every 3 to 6 months after opening; each tablet should cause a slight stinging or tingling sensation when placed under tongue if fresh
7. Write down emergency numbers and place them next to phone with home address and exact directions
8. Take a SL or spray NTG before an event that might cause angina, such as stair climbing, exercise, or sexual intercourse
9. Keep a written record for prescriber of times, dates, amount of medication required for relief of each attack, and possible precipitating factors
10. Shake aerosol spray well prior to use

11. If wearing an NTG patch or paste and experiencing an anginal attack, an NTG tablet may be taken SL following safety measures outlined above
12. Swimming or bathing with an NTG patch in place is acceptable
13. Frequent and prolonged use of NTG may reduce efficacy, requiring a medication adjustment

II. BETA-ADRENERGIC BLOCKERS

A. Block beta$_1$ adrenergic receptors found chiefly in cardiac muscle, and in higher doses, may cause blocking of beta$_2$ adrenergic receptors in airways, leading to increased airway resistance, especially in clients with asthma or chronic obstructive pulmonary disease (COPD)

Memory Aid

Use the number to remember the organs affected by beta-adrenergic receptors. Remember β_1—you have 1 heart, and β_2—you have 2 lungs.

B. Used therapeutically to manage hypertension, angina pectoris, acute MI, and supraventricular tachycardia

NCLEX® **C. Block cardiac effects of beta-adrenergic stimulation, resulting in**

1. Reductions in HR, myocardial **irritability** (cardiac muscle response to a variety of external stimuli such as hypoxia), and force of contraction
2. A negative **inotropic** (force of contraction) and **chronotropic** (heart rate) effect
3. Depression of **automaticity** (heart's ability to initiate impulses on its own without external stimulation) of sinus node
4. Reduction in atrioventricular (AV) node and intraventricular **dromotropic** (conduction velocity) effect

D. Also useful in controlling panic attacks and stage fright in some clients

E. Common medications are listed in Box 34–2

Memory Aid

Recognize beta-adrenergic blockers because they end in *-olol* or *-lol.*

F. Administration considerations

1. Monitor client before, during, and after initial dose
2. NCLEX® Monitor BP, apical pulse, and cardiac rhythm frequently during initial administration; if given orally, check client 30 minutes before and 60 minutes after initial dose
3. Prior to next dose, reevaluate BP, HR, and cardiac rhythm
4. Give drug at consistent times with or without meals; recommended before meals and at bedtime
5. NCLEX® Use of beta-adrenergic blockers with calcium channel blockers (see section to follow) may increase adverse response, including bradycardia and hypotension
6. Tablets may be crushed as needed (prn) before administration and taken with fluid of choice
7. NCLEX® Do not discontinue therapy abruptly; dosage is reduced gradually over 1–2 weeks, observe client for paradoxical reactions such as hypertension and tachycardia
8. NCLEX® Contraindicated with first-degree heart block (PR interval greater than 0.2 second), heart failure, bradycardia, shock, significant aortic or mitral valve disease, hyperactive airway syndrome (asthma or bronchospasm), severe seasonal allergies (allergic rhinitis during pollen season), concurrent use of psychotropic that augments adrenergic system or within 2 weeks of an monoamine oxidase inhibitor (MAOI)
9. Use cautiously before and after major surgery, with renal or hepatic impairment, diabetes mellitus, myasthenia gravis, or Wolff-Parkinson-White (WPW) syndrome, and systemic allergies to insect stings

Box 34–2

Common Beta-Adrenergic Blocker Medications

Acebutolol (Sectral)	Nadolol (Corgard)
Atenolol (Tenormin)	Pindolol (Visken)
Betaxolol (Kerlone)	Propranolol (Inderal)
Bisoprolol (Zebeta)	Timolol (Blocadren)
Metoprolol (Lopressor)	

G. Side/adverse effects

1. Dizziness, sleep disturbances, depression, confusion, agitation, or psychosis
2. Hypotension, bradycardia, heart block, acute heart failure, and peripheral paresthesias resembling Raynaud's phenomenon (NCLEX®)
3. Laryngospasm or bronchospasm
4. Dry eyes with a gritty sensation, blurred vision, tinnitus, or hearing loss
5. Dry mouth, N/V, heartburn, diarrhea, constipation, abdominal cramps, and flatulence
6. Agranulocytosis, hypo- or hyperglycemia, and hypocalcemia in clients with hyperthyroidism

H. Nursing considerations

1. Take apical pulse and BP before administering; evaluate for fluid volume overload as sign of heart failure (NCLEX®)
2. Monitor intake and output (I&O) and daily weight
3. Withhold dose if HR is less than 60 beats per minute (bpm) or if systolic BP is less than 90 mm Hg (NCLEX®)

Memory Aid

Many cardiovascular drugs that have antihypertensive and vasodilating effects cause orthostatic hypotension and dizziness, so assist client to arise slowly from lying to sitting, and from sitting to standing positions; provide a safe environment to decrease injury in case of falls.

4. Determine history of asthma, allergies, or COPD; realize beta-blockers may lead to bronchospasm in clients with no previously documented history of pulmonary disease (NCLEX®)
5. Monitor HR, BP, and respiratory status carefully during periods of dosage adjustment; maintain effective communication with prescriber
6. Restrict dietary sodium as ordered to prevent fluid volume overload; check with prescriber regarding sodium restriction or concurrent use of a diuretic
7. Fasting longer than 12 hours may induce hypoglycemia, which is worsened by beta-blocker therapy because signs are masked
8. Review results of periodic renal, hepatic, cardiac, and hematologic studies
9. Beta-blockers may induce false-negative exercise tolerance electrocardiogram (ECG) results (NCLEX®)

I. Client teaching

1. How to check pulse and BP and their desired ranges, how to record daily measurements, and when to call prescriber
2. Abrupt withdrawal can lead to severe paradoxical or rebound reactions, including sweating, tremulousness, severe headache, malaise, palpitations, hypertension, MI, and life-threatening heart rhythm disturbances (NCLEX®)
3. Establish a routine for taking medication and strive to comply with plan for results; write out a daily schedule for medication
4. Notify prescriber if any dizziness or lightheadedness occurs; avoid driving or operating machinery until these symptoms are relieved (NCLEX®)

Memory Aid

Teach clients taking antihypertensive or vasodilating drugs to take measures to reduce risk of injury from orthostatic hypotension; avoid use hot baths and hot tubs and limit amount of time spent out of doors in hot weather to minimize risk of orthostatic blood pressure changes.

5. Stop smoking because smoking might offset desired outcomes of controlled HR, BP, and prevention of angina; smoking also increases hepatic metabolism of beta-blocker medication, leading to unpredictable or diminished drug effects (NCLEX®)
6. Avoid OTC medications and herbal supplements without consulting prescriber
7. Inform all health care providers, including ophthalmologist or optometrist of medication; beta-blockers may lower intraocular pressure
8. Reduce salt intake while taking medication

III. CALCIUM CHANNEL BLOCKERS

A. Are class IV antiarrhythmic drugs that inhibit calcium ion influx through slow channels into cells of myocardial and arterial smooth muscle (cardiac and peripheral BV)

1. Intracellular calcium remains below levels needed to stimulate cell
2. Dilate coronary arteries and arterioles and prevent coronary artery spasm
3. Increase myocardial O_2 delivery to prevent angina
4. Slow conduction through sinoatrial (SA) node and AV node, lowering HR and decreasing strength of cardiac contraction (negative inotropic effect)
5. Decrease automaticity and **conductivity** (amount of force and pressure to pump blood out of ventricles) by blocking flow of calcium into cell
6. Decrease systemic vascular resistance (SVR) and thus afterload by dilating peripheral arterioles
7. Reduce arterial BP (antihypertensive effect) and HR

B. Used for vasospastic angina (Prinzmetal's variant or angina at rest), chronic stable (classic and activity-induced) angina, and essential hypertension; IV form is useful in atrial fibrillation, atrial flutter, and supraventricular tachycardia

C. Common medications are listed in Box 34–3

Memory Aid

Recognize many calcium channel blockers by noting the suffix *-dipine*. This is not true for all, however; exceptions are verapamil and diltiazem.

D. Administration considerations

1. Administer oral diltiazem before meals and at bedtime and oral verapamil with food to reduce gastric irritation
2. Evaluate BP and ECG before initiation of therapy
3. Monitor for headache; an analgesic may be required
4. Give IV forms of verapamil and diltiazem using infusion pump and carefully following package directions
5. *NCLEX®* Withhold dose if BP is less than 90/60
6. Contraindicated with known hypersensitivity to drug, sick sinus syndrome (without artificial pacemaker), second- or third-degree heart blocks
7. Does not alter serum calcium levels

E. Adverse effects and toxicity

1. Headache, dizziness, nervousness, insomnia, confusion, tremor, and gait disturbance
2. *NCLEX®* Postural hypotension, heart block and profound bradycardia, heart failure, possible syncope, palpitations, and fluid volume overload
3. N/V, constipation, and impaired taste
4. Skin rash

F. Nursing considerations

1. Evaluate BP and ECG prior to treatment and monitor closely during dose adjustment; monitor for orthostatic changes
2. Monitor hepatic and renal lab test results
3. May induce hyperglycemia; monitor diabetic clients closely
4. Can cause constipation; increase fiber and fluids as tolerated
5. Monitor for signs of CHF (dyspnea, crackles, frothy pink-tinged sputum)

Box 34–3

Common Calcium Channel Blockers

Selective for Blood Vessels	*Nonselective: Both Heart and Blood Vessels*
Amlodipine (Norvasc)	Diltiazem (Cardizem, others)
Felodipine (Plendil)	Verapamil (Calan, Isoptin)
Isradipine (Dynacirc)	
Nicardipine (Cardene)	
Nifedipine (Procardia, others)	
Nisoldipine (Nisocor)	

G. Client teaching

NCLEX® 1. Take radial pulse before each dose (especially verapamil); report an irregular pulse or if slower than identified parameter (such as 50 or 60)

NCLEX® 2. Change position slowly to prevent postural hypotension

3. Avoid driving if dizziness or faintness is noted; report these symptoms immediately

NCLEX® 4. Report gradual weight gain and evidence of edema; may indicate onset of CHF

NCLEX® 5. Avoid grapefruit and grapefruit juice when taking verapamil

6. Use typical measures to prevent constipation (fluids, fiber, activity)

IV. ANGIOTENSIN-CONVERTING ENZYME (ACE) INHIBITORS

A. Inhibit renin-angiotensin-aldosterone mechanism by blocking conversion of angiotensin I to angiotensin II, which prevents peripheral vasoconstriction and reduces blood volume by inhibiting secretion of aldosterone

NCLEX® **B. Used to treat hypertension; preferred for hypertensive clients with diabetic nephropathy**

C. Common medications are listed in Box 34–4

Memory Aid Generic names of ACE inhibitors can be recognized because they end in *-pril.*

D. Administration considerations

1. Discontinue with prescriber supervision if pregnancy is detected
2. Give moexipril and captopril on empty stomach due to decreased absorption with food
3. Contraindicated with hypersensitivity to ACE inhibitors
4. Avoid use with potassium supplements and potassium-sparing diuretics
5. When initiating therapy, watch for first dose effect (profound hypotension with syncope); prevent by giving while sitting or lying down

E. Side/adverse effects

1. Headache, dizziness, anxiety, fatigue, insomnia, nervousness

NCLEX® 2. Hypotension and palpitations

3. N/V, abdominal pain, constipation
4. Persistent, dry, nonproductive cough, dyspnea
5. Rash, arthralgia, impotence, and dysgeusia (altered taste)

NCLEX® 6. Angioedema, leukopenia, agranulocytosis, pancytopenia, thrombocytopenia

7. Cerebrovascular accident (CVA), MI, and hypertensive crisis

F. Nursing considerations

1. Administer 1 hour before meals to increase absorption; may crush tablets
2. Do not administer to pregnant or lactating women

NCLEX® 3. Monitor labs for increased potassium, liver enzymes, bilirubin, BUN and creatinine, and decreased sodium levels and WBC count

NCLEX® 4. Take BP before giving dose and monitor regularly

NCLEX® 5. Monitor for rashes or hives and for peripheral edema

6. Monitor urine protein in renal disease regularly by dipstick method
7. Discontinue diuretics 2 to 3 days before ACE inhibitor therapy

G. Client teaching

1. Report peripheral edema, signs of infection, facial swelling, loss of taste, or difficulty breathing
2. Do not skip doses or stop taking drug; it may cause serious rebound increase in BP

NCLEX® 3. Persistent, dry cough is a side effect and does not indicate respiratory disease or infection

Box 34–4

Common ACE Inhibitors

Benazepril (Lotensin)	Moexipril (Univasc)
Captopril (Capoten)	Perindopril (Aceon)
Enalapril (Vasotec)	Quinapril (Accupril)
Fosinopril (Monopril)	Ramipril (Altace)
Lisinopril (Prinivil, Zestril)	Trandolapril (Mavik)

4. Take antacids 2 hours before or after dose of fosinopril and captopril
NCLEX® 5. Avoid potassium-containing salt substitutes to prevent hyperkalemia
6. Monitor for bruising, petechiae, or bleeding with captopril
7. Taste of food may be diminished during the first month of therapy
8. Take captopril 20 minutes to 1 hour before a meal

V. ANGIOTENSIN II RECEPTOR BLOCKERS (ARBS)

A. Act as antagonists at angiotensin II receptor of vascular smooth muscle, blocking vasoconstriction and aldosterone-secreting effects and lowering BP
B. Common medications are listed in Box 34–5

Memory Aid
ARBs are easily recognized because they end in the suffix *-sartan*.

C. Administration considerations
1. Discontinue immediately if pregnancy is detected
NCLEX® 2. Use cautiously in clients with renal or hepatic disease

D. Side/adverse effects
1. Hypotension and dizziness, tachycardia or bradycardia
2. Cough, GI upset, insomnia, nasal congestion, and myalgia
NCLEX® 3. Neutropenia and hyperkalemia

E. Nursing considerations
NCLEX® 1. Monitor client taking diuretics for additive hypotension
NCLEX® 2. Regularly monitor renal function, potassium level, and WBC with differential
3. Do not administer to pregnant or lactating women
NCLEX® 4. Monitor BP and apical pulse regularly

F. Client teaching
1. Do not discontinue medication abruptly
NCLEX® 2. Avoid salt substitutes because of potassium content
3. Notify physician immediately if pregnancy is suspected
4. If using oral contraceptives, use alternate birth control methods
5. Maintain adequate hydration

Box 34–5
Common Angiotensin II Receptor Blockers (ARBs)

Candesartan (Atacand)	Olmesartan (Benicar)
Eprosartan (Tevetan)	Telmisartan (Micardis)
Irbesartan (Avapro)	Valsartan (Diovan)
Losartan (Cozaar)	

VI. DIRECT-ACTING VASODILATORS

A. Potent antihypertensive agents that act directly on arterial smooth muscles
B. Produce peripheral vasodilation, resulting in lowered arterial BP, increased HR, and increased cardiac output (CO)
C. Some may also be used as an adjunct in treating heart failure or to treat Raynaud's disease by increasing blood flow to extremities
D. Common medications are listed in Box 34–6
E. Administration considerations
1. Take oral forms with food to increase bioavailability
NCLEX® 2. IV hydralazine may be given undiluted via direct IV push at a rate of 10 mg/min

Box 34–6
Direct-Acting Vasodilators

Diazoxide (Hyperstat)	Minoxidil (Loniten)
Hydralazine (Apresoline)	Nitroprusside (Nipride)

NCLEX® 3. IV sodium nitroprusside is diluted to 50 mg in 250 mL D_5W (200 mcg/mL); infuse cautiously through an IV pump; when mixed, it appears orange and must be covered in a foil pouch to avoid exposure to light during infusion
4. Do not mix with other IV solutions
5. Discontinue all vasodilators slowly to avoid paradoxical hypertensive effects
6. Store medication in light-resistant container
7. Monitor HR and BP closely during administration to prevent sudden hypotension
8. Contraindicated in compensatory hypertension (arteriovenous shunt or coarctation of aorta), inadequate cerebral perfusion leading to a decreased cerebral perfusion pressure (CPP), or hypovolemia

NCLEX® 9. During administration of sodium nitroprusside, monitor serum thiocyanate levels after 48–72 hours or in clients with impaired renal function

F. Side/adverse effects
1. Headache, dizziness, tremors, apprehension, and muscle twitching

NCLEX® 2. Angina, palpitations, tachycardia or bradycardia, flushing, paradoxical pressor response (sudden rise in BP), ECG changes, profound hypotension, shock, and dysrhythmias
3. Systemic lupus erythematosus (SLE)–like syndrome (with hydralazine), edema
4. Anorexia, N/V, constipation or diarrhea, abdominal pain, and paralytic ileus
5. Difficulty urinating and glomerulonephritis
6. Decreased hematocrit and hemoglobin, anemia, agranulocytosis (rare)
7. Rash, irritation at IV site, urticaria, pruritus, fever, chills, arthralgia, eosinophilia, and cholangitis; excessive hair growth with minoxidil
8. With sodium nitroprusside, thiocyanate toxicity is noted by profound hypotension, tinnitus, fatigue, pink skin color, metabolic acidosis, and loss of consciousness

G. Nursing considerations
1. Monitor carefully baseline HR, BP, cardiac rhythm, ECG, and neurological status

NCLEX® 2. When administering IV vasodilators
   a. Establish a large, stable IV site because infusions are irritating to tissue; administer with an IV infusion pump
   b. Monitor BP every 5–15 minutes with an automatic external BP machine or arterial line during initial infusion and medication adjustment
   c. Monitor I&O
   d. If hypotension occurs, decrease infusion and monitor client closely; if sudden, severe hypotension occurs, discontinue medication; maintain airway, breathing and circulation (ABCs); establish IV site; contact physician, and initiate emergency protocols as necessary
3. Check BP, heart rate, and cardiac rhythm before each oral dose

H. Client teaching

NCLEX® 1. How to self-monitor pulse and BP
2. Possibility of headache and palpitations within 2 to 4 hours after first PO dose
3. Write down questions to ask provider on each follow-up visit
4. Stop smoking as this negates positive effects of medication
5. Monitor weight daily and report edema

NCLEX® 6. Avoid hot tubs and baths that might induce profound vasodilation and hypotension

VII. ALPHA ADRENERGIC ANTAGONISTS (CENTRAL AND PERIPHERAL)

A. Centrally acting sympatholytics
1. Stimulate $alpha_2$ receptors in CNS to inhibit sympathetic cardio-accelerator and vasoconstrictor centers
2. Decrease sympathetic outflow from CNS, resulting in decreased arterial pressure

B. Peripheral anti-adrenergics
1. Deplete catecholamine stores in peripheral nervous system (PNS); some act in CNS
2. Decrease total peripheral resistance, HR, and CO

C. Common medications are listed in Box 34–7

D. Administration considerations

NCLEX® 1. Do not discontinue abruptly; may result in rebound hypertension
2. Guanabenz: allow 1 to 2 weeks before adjusting dose
3. Guanfacine: give at bedtime to decrease daytime sleepiness; allow 3 to 4 weeks before adjusting dose

Box 34–7
Alpha₁ and Alpha₂ Blockers

Alpha$_1$ blockers
Doxazosin (Cardura)
Prazosin (Minipress)
Terazosin (Hytrin)

Alpha$_2$ blockers
Clonidine (Catapres)
Methyldopa (Aldomet)

Alpha and Beta Blockers (Centrally Acting)
Carvedilol (Coreg)
Labetalol (Trandane)

Adrenergic Neuron Blockers (Peripherally Acting)
Reserpine (Serpasil)
Guanethidine (Ismelin)
Guanabenz acetate
Guanfacine (Intuniv)

4. Methyldopa: allow 2 days for maximum response before adjusting dose
5. Contraindicated in hypersensitivity, active hepatitis or cirrhosis, co-administration with MAOIs (methyldopa), heart failure (methyldopa), history of mental depression, active peptic ulcer disease, ulcerative colitis, asthma, and bronchitis (reserpine)

E. Side/adverse effects
1. Sedation, headache, weakness, dizziness, and decreased mental acuity
2. Involuntary choreoathetoid movements, parkinsonism, depression, nightmares
3. Bradycardia, orthostatic hypotension, aggravation of angina, edema
4. GI disturbance, rash, gynecomastia, galactorrhea, amenorrhea, impotence, dry mouth, weight gain
5. Myocarditis, hemolytic anemia, thrombocytopenia
6. Hepatic necrosis
7. Severe rebound hypertension

F. Nursing considerations
1. Administer orally; tablets may be crushed and do not need to be given with food unless GI upset occurs
2. IV methyldopa should be given over 30–60 minutes; do not give subcutaneously or IM
3. *NCLEX®* Apply transdermal systems (Clonidine) to dry, hairless skin of chest or upper arm; monitor areas for rash
4. *NCLEX®* Monitor labs for elevated liver enzymes, alkaline phosphatase, bilirubin, BUN, creatinine, potassium, sodium, and uric acid
5. May prolong prothrombin times
6. *NCLEX®* Obtain baseline BP and apical pulse, and monitor weight regularly
7. *NCLEX®* Monitor client for peripheral edema
8. Dry mouth may contribute to development of dental caries, periodontal disease, oral candidiasis, and discomfort

G. Client teaching
1. *NCLEX®* Possible need for sodium restriction and weight reduction; report weight gain of more than 5 lb per week
2. Relieve dry mouth by sipping water or chewing sugarless gum
3. Treat nausea by eating unsalted crackers, noncola beverages, or dry toast
4. Report mental acuity changes to health care provider
5. Some drugs cause urine to become darker
6. *NCLEX®* Do not drive a car or perform hazardous activities if drowsiness occurs
7. *NCLEX®* Take medication as prescribed; do not stop abruptly to avoid rebound hypertension

VIII. CARDIAC GLYCOSIDES

A. Used primarily to treat heart failure but also used to treat atrial *dysrhythmia* (abnormality in electrical activity of heart)
B. Increase *contractility* (force of contraction) and efficiency of myocardial contraction
C. Is a positive inotrope that increases force of myocardial contraction
D. Is a negative dromotrope that decreases conduction velocity through AV node
E. Common medication: digoxin (Lanoxin)

F. Administration considerations

1. May be given with or without food
2. Tablet may be crushed and mixed with fluid or food; pediatric elixir is available
3. NCLEX® IV push digoxin may be administered undiluted or diluted in 4 mL of sterile water, 5% dextrose, or NS; administer each direct IV dose over 5 minutes; client may receive a loading dose (digitalization) to achieve adequate serum drug levels
4. Never administer digoxin IM because it would cause tissue irritation and great variation in bioavailability
5. Infiltration into subcutaneous tissue can cause local irritation and tissue sloughing
6. Contraindicated in clients with known hypersensitivity to digitalis or digoxin toxicity
7. Full digitalizing dose should not be given if client has received digoxin during previous week
8. NCLEX® Use cautiously with following conditions: renal insufficiency, hypokalemia, advanced heart disease, acute MI, heart block, cor pulmonale, hypothyroidism, and lung disease
9. Use cautiously in pregnant or nursing mothers, children, premature infants, and older adults

NCLEX® **G. Side/adverse effects**

1. Fatigue, muscle weakness, headache, facial neuralgia, depression, paresthesias, hallucinations, confusion, drowsiness, agitation, dizziness, and malaise
2. Dysrhythmias, hypotension, A-V heart block, and diaphoresis
3. Anorexia, N/V, diarrhea, and dysphagia
4. Visual disturbances (blurred, green or yellow vision, photophobia, or halo effect)
5. Digoxin toxicity may be unrecognized because it may present same early manifestations as a flu, such as anorexia, N/V, diarrhea, or visual disturbances

H. Nursing considerations

1. Obtain baseline data and perform ongoing physical assessments, including neurological status, HR, BP, and cardiac rhythm
2. Check baseline serum digoxin level prior to initiating digoxin therapy
   a. Blood level is 0 if client has not taken digoxin before
   b. NCLEX® Therapeutic levels are 0.5 to 2.0 ng/mL (ranges vary slightly among texts)
   c. NCLEX® Toxic levels are greater than 2 ng/mL
3. Note baseline and ongoing serum electrolytes, creatinine clearance, magnesium, and calcium
4. Monitor older clients taking digoxin and a diuretic to treat CHF or atrial fibrillation for digoxin toxicity
5. NCLEX® Take apical pulse for 1 full minute prior to dose, noting rate, rhythm, and quality; if changes are noted, withhold dose and notify prescriber; an ECG will likely be ordered
6. NCLEX® Withhold dose if client has symptoms of digoxin toxicity (anorexia, N/V, diarrhea, or visual disturbances)
7. In children, early signs of toxicity include cardiac dysrhythmias; children rarely demonstrate anorexia, N/V, diarrhea, or visual disturbances
8. NCLEX® Provide foods high in potassium, such as oranges, bananas, fruit juices, vegetables, and potatoes if client is taking loop diuretics
9. NCLEX® Monitor I&O and daily weight, especially with impaired renal failure; auscultate breath sounds for crackles
10. NCLEX® Antidote: digoxin immune Fab (Digibind) is used in extreme toxicity
11. NCLEX® Observe extremities for edema as indicator of fluid volume overload
12. Concurrent antibiotic-digoxin therapy can precipitate toxicity because of altered intestinal flora
13. Monitor client closely when changing from one drug form to another; often a dose adjustment is required (if tablet form is replaced by elixir, potential for toxicity increases)

I. Client teaching

1. NCLEX® Check pulse for 1 full minute prior to taking dose; contact prescriber before taking dose if pulse is below 60 bpm or above 110 or if skipped beats are present
2. Suspect toxicity with N/V, anorexia, diarrhea, or visual disturbances such as halos or green or yellow vision; withhold dose and notify prescriber
3. NCLEX® Weigh self daily with same clothes and at same time; report weight gain greater than 2 lb/day
4. Take as ordered; do not to skip or add additional dose if experiencing chest discomfort (a common report from clients admitted with digoxin toxicity is that they take digoxin as a "heart pill" when experiencing chest pain)
5. Insist on original brand of digoxin ordered by prescriber to avoid errors in dosing

IX. ANTIDYSRHYTHMICS

A. Class IA (note all Class I drugs are fast sodium channel blockers)

1. Used to treat both atrial and ventricular dysrhythmias; prevent recurrence of premature ventricular contractions (PVCs) and ventricular tachycardia (VT) that are not severe enough to require cardioversion
2. Depress myocardial contractility and excitability and prolong **refractory period** (making cells able to respond only to strong stimulus)
3. Reduce rate of spontaneous diastolic depolarization in pacemaker cells, thereby suppressing ectopic focal activity
4. Disopyramide shortens sinus node recovery time and increases atrial and ventricular effective refractory period
5. Quinidine is classified as a chemical cardioversion agent used to convert atrial fibrillation to normal sinus rhythm
6. Common medications are listed in Box 34–8
7. Administration considerations
   - **a.** Give first dose of disopyramide 6 to 12 hours after last quinidine dose and 3 to 6 hours after last procainamide dose
   - **b.** Do not administer controlled-release capsules as loading dose when a rapid control is required or when creatinine clearance is less than 40 mL/min
   - **c.** Do not crush or open controlled-release capsules (may deliver potentially toxic dose of medication)
   - **d.** Start controlled-release form of capsule 6 hours after last dose of conventional capsule when switching between these forms
   - **e.** Contraindicated in cardiogenic shock, second- or third-degree heart block, severe heart failure, and hypotension
   - **f.** Use caution when administering disopyramide in the presence of delayed cardiac conduction, hepatic or renal impairment, benign prostatic hyperplasia, myasthenia gravis, and angle-closure (narrow-angle) glaucoma
   - **g.** Monitor blood glucose levels and serum potassium levels because hyperkalemia worsens toxic effects; correct hypokalemia and other electrolyte imbalances before initiating therapy
   - **h.** Follow ECG results closely; notify physician of conduction delays (prolonged QT interval, widening of QRS greater than 25%), HR less than 60 or greater than 120, unusual change in pulse rate, rhythm, or quality
8. Adverse effects/toxicity
   - **a.** Blurred vision, dizziness, headache, fatigue, muscle weakness, convulsions, paresthesias, nervousness, acute psychosis, and peripheral neuropathy
   - NCLEX® **b.** Hypotension, chest pain, edema, dyspnea, syncope, bradycardia, tachycardia, increased dysrhythmias, CHF, cardiogenic shock, and heart block
   - **c.** N/V, epigastric and abdominal pain, jaundice, dry mouth, constipation

Box 34–8

Common Antidysrhythmic Drugs

Class I drugs: Sodium Channel Blockers

Class IA drugs

Disopyramide (Norpace)

Procainamide (Pronestyl)

Quinidine gluconate

Quinidine sulfate (Quinidex)

Class IB drugs

Lidocaine (Xylocaine)

Mexiletine (Mexitil)

Phenytoin (Dilantin)

Class IC drugs

Flecainide (Tambocor)

Propafenone (Rhythmol)

Class II Drugs

Beta-Adrenergic Blockers

Class III drugs: Potassium Channel Blockers

Bretylium tosylate (generic)

Amiodarone (Cordarone)

Dofetilide (Tikosyn)

Ibutilide (Corvert)

Sotalol (Betapace)

Class IV Drugs

Calcium Channel Blockers

d. Urinary retention, frequency, urgency, and renal insufficiency
e. Pruritis, urticaria, rash, photosensitivity, and laryngospasm
f. Drying of nose, throat, and bronchial secretions
g. Uterine contraction during pregnancy, precipitation of myasthenia gravis, agranulocytosis (decreased granulocytes), and thrombocytopenia

9. Nursing considerations
NCLEX® a. Check apical pulse before administering the medication
NCLEX® b. Monitor ECG and report any changes to physician immediately
c. Monitor BP, especially during dosage adjustment and with high doses
d. Monitor I&O especially in older adults and those with impaired renal function, prostatic hyperplasia, and urinary retention/hesitancy
e. Monitor lab results as appropriate
f. Monitor for peripheral neuritis

10. Client teaching
a. Weigh self daily and report gain of more than 2 to 4 lb/week
b. Inspect ankles and tibia daily for edema
NCLEX® c. Avoid prolonged standing, and lie down if feeling lightheaded; avoid driving and other hazardous activities if dizzy or lightheaded
d. Be sure to avoid use of nasal decongestants without contacting prescriber
e. Avoid exposure to sunlight or ultraviolet radiation
f. Notify all other health care providers of medication and have regular eye exams for glaucoma

B. Class IB

1. Decrease refractory period and raise electrical stimulation threshold of ventricle during diastole
2. Suppress automaticity in the bundle of His–Purkinje system
3. Treat or prevent ventricular dysrhythmias
4. Common medications are listed in Box 34–8
5. Administration considerations
a. Bolus dose of lidocaine may be given undiluted IVP at a rate of 25 to 50 mg/min; be sure to use lidocaine manufactured specifically for IV use
b. Add 1 gram lidocaine to 250 to 500 mL of D_5W for infusion; flow rate should not be more than 4 mg/mL
NCLEX® c. Use microdrip tubing and infusion pump for an infusion
d. Discontinue IV infusion as soon as client's basic cardiac rhythm stabilizes
e. Contraindicated in hypersenstivity to amide-type anesthetics, Stokes-Adams syndrome, untreated sinus bradycardia, and severe SA, AV, and intraventricular heart block
NCLEX® f. Use cautiously with hepatic or renal disease, heart failure, hypovolemia or shock, myasthenia gravis, debilitated clients or elderly, and family history of malignant hyperthermia
6. Side/adverse effects
a. Drowsiness or restlessness, confusion, disorientation, irritability, apprehension, euphoria, wild excitement, numbness of lips, tongue, and other paresthesias, chest heaviness, and difficulty speaking
b. Dyspnea and difficulty swallowing, muscular twitching, tremors, psychosis, convulsions, and respiratory depression with high doses
NCLEX® c. Hypotension, lightheadedness, bradycardia, heart block, cardiovascular collapse, and cardiac arrest
d. Tinnitus and decreased hearing
e. Severe blurred vision, double vision, and impaired color perception
f. Anorexia, N/V, and excessive perspiration
g. Urticaria, rash, edema, and anaphylactoid reactions
7. Nursing considerations
a. Monitor ECG for prolonged PR interval, widened QRS, aggravation of dysrhythmias, and heart block
b. Monitor BP frequently
c. Monitor CNS status at baseline and frequently during infusions
d. Administer via infusion pump and observe rate carefully
NCLEX® e. Auscultate breath sounds for crackles and monitor respiratory rate
NCLEX® f. Review results of serum drug levels and creatinine levels
8. Notify prescriber if adverse effects occur; see previous section

C. Class IC

1. Decrease automaticity and conductivity through AV node and ventricles
2. Used to treat life-threatening ventricular dysrhythmias

3. Common medications are listed in Box 34–8
4. Administration considerations
   a. Medications are available in oral forms
   b. Do not increase dosages more frequently than every 4 days, especially with older adults or those with previous extensive myocardial damage
   c. Dosage reduction should be considered in severe liver dysfunction and with significant QRS widening
   d. Contraindicated with drug hypersensitivity, severe degrees of heart block or intraventricular block, cardiogenic shock, or hepatic failure
5. Side/adverse effects
   a. Headache, dizziness, prolonged lightheadedness, unsteadiness, paresthesias, fatigue, and fever
   NCLEX® b. Worsening dysrhythmias, chest pain, CHF, edema, and dyspnea
   c. Prolonged blurred vision and spots before eyes
   d. Nausea, constipation, and changes in taste perception
6. Nursing considerations
   NCLEX® a. Review laboratory data and treat hypokalemia/hyperkalemia before initiating therapy
   NCLEX® b. Monitor ECG rhythm for adverse changes; client may need Holter monitoring for ambulatory assessment
   c. Determine threshold levels of pacemaker before initiating medication and at regular intervals thereafter
7. Client teaching: report any visual changes

D. Class II (beta-blockers): see previous section

E. Class III (potassium channel blockers)

1. Prolong repolarization and refractory period
2. Decrease intraventricular conduction
3. Used to treat ventricular tachycardia (VT) and ventricular fibrillation (VF)
4. May also be used to treat supraventricular tachycardias
5. Common medications are listed in Box 34–8
6. Administration considerations
   a. Gastroenteritis symptoms may occur with high oral dose therapy and loading dose
   b. May be given by IV route
   c. Contraindicated with hypersensitivity to amiodarone, cardiogenic shock, severe sinus bradycardia or heart block, and hepatic disease
   d. Use cautiously in hyper- or hypothyroidism, heart failure, electrolyte imbalance, preexisting pulmonary disease, cardiac surgery, and sensitivity to iodine
7. Side/adverse effects
   a. Peripheral neuropathy, muscle wasting, weakness, fatigue, abnormal gait, dyskinesia, dizziness, paresthesias, and headache
   NCLEX® b. Bradycardia, hypotension, sinus arrest, cardiogenic shock, CHF, worsening dysrhythmias, and heart block
   NCLEX® c. Corneal microdeposits, blurred vision, optic neuritis, optic neuropathy, permanent blindness, corneal degeneration, macular degeneration, and photosensitivity
   d. Alveolitis, pneumonitis, and interstitial pulmonary fibrosis
   e. Slate-blue pigmentation to skin and rash; reverses slowly after drug is discontinued
   f. Anorexia, N/V, and constipation
   g. Angioedema, hyperthyroidism or hypothyroidism, and hepatotoxicity
8. Nursing considerations
   NCLEX® a. Monitor BP during IV infusion; titrate to prevent hypotension or bradycardia
   NCLEX® b. Monitor client continually due to unusually long drug half-life (10–55 days)
   c. Check laboratory and other reports for liver, lung, thyroid, GI, and neurological dysfunction
   NCLEX® d. Baseline and regular ophthalmic examinations with a slit-lamp are recommended throughout therapy
   e. Report adverse reactions promptly
   f. Be alert to signs of pulmonary toxicity: dyspnea, fatigue, cough, pleuritic pain, or fever; auscultate breath sounds for adventitious sounds
   NCLEX® g. Monitor for CNS changes, which often develop within a week after amiodarone therapy begins; muscle weakness and tremors are a potential safety risk
   h. Observe client already receiving other antiarrhythmic therapy for adverse effects, especially heart block and worsening dysrhythmias

9. Client teaching
NCLEX®
   a. Monitor pulse daily and report HR less than 60 bpm
   b. Have regular ophthalmic examinations every 6 months to 1 year
NCLEX®
   c. Photophobia may be eased by wearing darkened glasses, but some clients should avoid daylight entirely
   d. Erythema and pruritus may develop when exposed to ultraviolet radiation; avoid sunlight, tanning beds, and sunlamps
   e. Wear protective clothing and a barrier-type sunblock to avoid exposure to sun (zinc-oxide or titanium-oxide preparations)
NCLEX®
   f. Blue-gray skin pigmentation (found after 1 year) may slowly disappear after medication is stopped

F. Class IV (calcium channel blockers): see previous section

G. Miscellaneous antidysrhythmic: Adenosine (Adenocard, Adenoscan)

1. Slows conduction through SA and AV nodes; interrupts reentry pathways through AV node
2. Depresses left ventricular function (very temporary)
NCLEX®
3. Treats supraventricular dysrhythmias
4. Administration considerations
NCLEX®
   a. Rapid IV bolus: administer IV push over 1–2 seconds and follow with a rapid normal saline flush
   b. Solution contains no preservatives so it must be clear; discard any unused portion
   c. Expect sudden slowing of the HR or even asystole for a brief period of time; do not repeat dose if high grade AV heart block develops after first dose
   d. Store at room temperature to avoid crystallization; if crystals appear, dissolve by warming to room temperature
   e. Contraindicated in severe heart block, sick sinus syndrome (without a pacemaker), atrial fibrillation or atrial flutter, VT
   f. Use cautiously with asthma, pregnancy, hepatic failure, and renal failure
5. Side/adverse effects
   a. During conversion to sinus rhythm, many dysrhythmias can occur
   b. Facial flushing, transient dyspnea, or headache
NCLEX®
6. Nursing considerations
   a. Monitor ECG continuously and HR and BP every 15 minutes until stable
   b. Monitor carefully for bronchospasm, especially in clients with asthma
7. Client teaching: monitoring will be done during drug administration, and transient facial flushing may occur

X. ANTIHYPOTENSIVES (SYMPATHOMIMETICS)

A Mimic fight-or-flight response of sympathetic nervous system (SNS), selectively stimulating alpha-adrenergic and beta-adrenergic receptors

B. Stimulation of alpha-adrenergic receptors results in vasoconstriction and increased systemic BP

C. Stimulation of beta-adrenergic receptors increases force and rate of myocardial contraction

D. Used to treat shock

E. Common medications are listed in Box 34–9

F. Administration considerations

1. Drug must be diluted before administration; use infusion pump to control dose
2. Client should be attended constantly during drug administration
3. Contraindicated in uncorrected dysrhythmias, mesenteric or vascular thrombosis, profound hypoxia, hypercapnia, hypotension due to hypovolemia
4. Use with caution in those receiving MAOIs or imipramine-type antidepressants

G. Side/adverse effects

1. Anxiety, weakness, dizziness, tremor, restlessness
2. Bradycardia, tachycardia, palpitations
3. N/V, flushing, diaphoresis, sloughing upon extravasation
4. Azotemia, shortness of breath, and bronchospasm

Box 34–9 Antihypotensives (Sympathomimetics)

Norepinephrine (Levophed)	Dobutamine (Dobutrex)
Metaraminol bitartrate	Isoproterenol (Isuprel)
Dopamine (Intropin)	Phenylephrine (Neo-synephrine)

NCLEX® 5. Severe hypertension, anaphylaxis

NCLEX® 6. Arrhythmias, cardiac arrest, ventricular tachycardia

7. Seizures, asthmatic episodes

H. Nursing considerations

1. Reevaluate if 3 to 5 treatments in 6 to 12 hours provide minimal to no relief

NCLEX® 2. Carefully monitor vital signs, ECG, and I&O

3. Monitor for rebound hypertension
4. Correct blood volume depletion first
5. Monitor infusion site frequently; stay with client constantly during administration

NCLEX® 6. Antidote for extravasation: phentolamine mesylate (Regitine) diluted in normal saline injected at site of IV infiltration

7. Protect solution from light
8. Sympathomimetics are incompatible with sodium bicarbonate

I. Client teaching

1. Report adverse reactions and side effects immediately
2. Vital signs will be monitored frequently
3. Report anginal pain while on dobutamine

XI. ANTICOAGULANTS

A. Oral medication; sodium warfarin (Coumadin and its derivatives); see Box 34–10

1. Oral **anticoagulants** prevent or delay blood coagulation and are used to treat and prevent thromboembolic disorders in clients at risk
2. Warfarins prevent conversion of vitamin K, thereby decreasing its production in liver and subsequently reducing several clotting factors (II, VII, IX, and X)
3. Vitamin K plays an active role in **extrinsic pathway** (forms fibrin and acts within seconds) in **clotting cascade** (a coagulation pathway)
4. Warfarin is bound to plasma proteins (especially albumin), metabolized in liver
5. Used to treat deep vein thrombosis (DVT), pulmonary embolism (PE), acute MI, heart valve replacement (bioprosthetic and mechanical), atrial fibrillation, and antiphospholipid syndrome
6. Administration considerations
   a. Warfarin is given orally at a usual dose of 1 to 15 mg daily
   b. Requires close monitoring because of a narrow therapeutic range, frequent need for dose adjustments, and high risk for food and drug interactions that can lead to either ineffective therapy or toxicity

   NCLEX® c. Full anticoagulant effect is not seen until after approximately 1 week; thus drug may be started during heparin therapy and overlap while heparin is tapered

   NCLEX® d. **Prothrombin time (PT)**, a laboratory test that measures extrinsic clotting response, and **international normalized ratio (INR)**, a standard reference range for reporting PT levels, are both used to monitor client response and determine ongoing dose

   e. Desired range of PT and INR vary based on indication for use; PT levels are usually maintained at 1.5 to 2.5 times control value; INR levels range from a usual 2.0 to 3.0 range to a higher level of 3.0 to 4.5 range for specific prosthetics
   f. Warfarin is usually given in evening based on laboratory test results from earlier in day
   g. Therapy can last from several months to lifelong depending on specific need
   h. Refer to specific hospital protocol and prescriber's order for dose adjustments and monitoring of PT and INR levels
   i. Vitamin K is antidote for warfarin (Coumadin)

Box 34–10

Anticoagulants

Oral Anticoagulant

Sodium warfarin (Coumadin)

Heparin

Heparin sodium (Liquaemin)

Low Molecular Weight Heparins

Dalteparin (Fragmin)

Enoxaparin (Lovenox)

Tinzaparin (Innohep)

Fondaparinux (Arixtra) (synthetic)

Direct Thrombin Inhibitors

Argatroban (Acova)

Bivalirudan (Angiomax)

Desirudin (Iprivask)

Lepirudin (Refludan)

NCLEX®
j. Foods high in vitamin K such as liver, cheese, egg yolk, leafy vegetables (broccoli, cabbage, spinach, and kale), and oils (peanut, corn, olive, or soybean) should be avoided or used sparingly during therapy; refer to dietitian for teaching

k. Contraindicated in pregnancy (may be given if needed during lactation), hemorrhage or bleeding tendencies, clients with malignant hypertension, and those with history of allergic reaction

7. Side/adverse effects

NCLEX®
a. Bleeding is the major adverse effect and is usually seen at higher dosage levels; also thrombocytopenia may occur

b. Nausea, diarrhea, intestinal obstruction, anorexia, abdominal cramping

c. Rash, urticaria, and purple toe syndrome (due to decreased perfusion from release of microemboli)

d. Increased serum transaminase levels, hepatitis, jaundice

e. Burning sensation in feet

f. Transient hair loss

NCLEX®
8. Nursing considerations

a. Monitor baseline and ongoing PT and INR; report high or low abnormal values (ineffective therapy versus toxicity)

b. Review drug and dietary history for potential drug and food interactions; be sure to include nutritional and herbal supplements

NCLEX®
c. Institute bleeding precautions (see Box 34–11)

d. If client experiences adverse effects or toxicity, withhold Coumadin dose; depending on INR or client manifestations, administration of phytonadione (vitamin K) may be indicated

e. For significant bleeding, prescriber may order transfusion of fresh frozen plasma (FFP) or prothrombin concentrate

NCLEX®
9. Client education

a. Bleeding precautions (Box 34–11)

b. Stress need for frequent (weekly to monthly) follow-up blood tests to ensure safe therapy

c. Point-of-care (POC) testing is available for self-monitoring PT and INR; prescriber may establish a home protocol to help manage care and necessary dose adjustments

d. Take dose daily; do not stop therapy unless prescriber orders a dose to be withheld (pending PT and INR results) or client experiences a bleeding episode

e. Avoid intake of foods high in vitamin K (see previous section)

B. Heparin and related medications (see Box 34–10)

1. Heparin plays an active role in the **intrinsic pathway** (where fibrin formation occurs) of clotting cascade; inhibits conversion of fibrinogen to fibrin, prevents formation of a fibrin clot, and inhibits thrombin
2. Molecular weight of heparin varies depending on whether drug is unfractionated heparin (UFH) or **low molecular weight heparin (LMWH)**
3. Has immediate effect and is treatment of choice for DVT, PE, and embolism resulting from atrial fibrillation
4. Also used as a prophylaxis for clients at risk for thrombi following surgery
5. Also used in a weak concentration as a flush solution to maintain access and prevent thrombus formation in vascular access devices

Box 34–11

Bleeding Precautions for Clients Taking Anticoagulant and Fibrinolytic (Thrombolytic) Drugs

1. Use a soft toothbrush and ensure gentle mouth care to minimize even mild trauma that could lead to bleeding.
2. Use an electric razor rather than a straight razor for shaving.
3. Use work gloves, do not go barefoot, and take other ordinary precautions as appropriate to avoid minor trauma to skin.
4. Observe for and report to prescriber evidence of bleeding, including bleeding gums, epistaxis (nosebleed), ecchymosis (bruising), petechiae, tarry stools, hematuria, and hematemesis.
5. Notify health care providers, including dentists, about use of medications that cause bleeding, especially prior to any procedures or surgery.
6. Avoid use of OTC drugs that could increase risk of bleeding, such as acetylsalicylic acid (ASA or aspirin), nonsteroidal anti-inflammatory drugs (NSAIDs).

6. LMWH is a newer class of heparin molecule consisting of heparin fragments, with enoxaprin (Lovenox) being most commonly used
7. Heparin (Liquaemin) sodium is most commonly used anticoagulant for treatment and prevention of recurrent thromboembolic episodes
8. Administration considerations
   a. Heparin can be administered by IV or subcutaneously
   b. LMWH has a higher bioavailability when compared to standard UFH
   c. NCLEX® **Activated partial thromboplastin time (APTT)** is used to monitor heparin therapy; results are trended over time to determine client response
   d. Low-dose UFH therapy: used as a prophylactic treatment for DVT; dosage ranges from 5000 units subcutaneously every 8 to 12 hours or 3 doses in the immediate postoperative period depending on protocol; enoxaparin or Lovenox (an LMWH) comes in prefilled syringes ready for individual use
   e. High-dose UFH therapy achieves a therapeutic APTT; normal APTT value is 25 to 40 seconds, and therapeutic values are often 1.5 to 2.0 times control
   f. NCLEX® Use an infusion pump for IV administration; use a dedicated infusion line because of its incompatibility profile
   g. Be sure to carefully identify strength on product label; several concentrations of IV heparin are available; some are used only as flushes for IV lines
   h. NCLEX® **Protamine sulfate** is antidote that reverses action of heparin; dose depends on amount of heparin given and time period following its administration; however, do not give more than 50 mg IVP in a 10-minute period
   i. Hypersensitivity reaction can be seen in clients receiving heparin, so epinephrine 1:1000 should be readily available if a reaction develops
   j. Contraindicated with uncontrolled bleeding, known hypersensitivity, and thrombocytopenia
   k. NCLEX® Should not be given with aspirin (acetylsalicylic acid, or ASA) and nonsteroidal anti-inflammatory drugs (NSAIDs), which increase risk of bleeding
9. NCLEX® Side/adverse effects
   a. Hemorrhage, hematuria, epistaxis, bleeding gums
   b. Thrombocytopenia **heparin-induced platelet aggregation (HITT)**, a more serious form of thrombocytopenia with platelet count less than 100,000/mm^3; also called white clot syndrome; can be fatal if not treated aggressively; begins 3 to 12 days following start of heparin therapy
   c. Clients who are on heparin therapy longer than 6 months are prone to develop osteoporosis
10. Nursing considerations
    a. Monitor client's baseline labs according to heparin protocol (specifically APTT); commonly measured every 6 hours; when level is critically high, infusion may be stopped for 1 or more hours and APTT measured in 2 to 3 hours
    b. Obtain daily weight for client on weight-based heparin protocol
    c. NCLEX® Institute bleeding precautions, hemocult all stools, and evaluate pertinent labs
    d. Verify with pharmacy or another RN the correct dosage of heparin before administering or adjusting heparin infusion
    e. NCLEX® Evaluate dosage for safety and therapeutic range (normal adult dosage range of 20,000 to 40,000 units/24 hr); heparin is usually infused in units per hour
    f. NCLEX® Have antidote available (protamine sulfate)
    g. NCLEX® Subcutaneous (SubQ) administration of heparin requires rotation of sites; *do not aspirate or rub injection site*
    h. NCLEX® When administering heparin SubQ, inject into abdomen using a small (5/8-inch, 25- to 27-gauge) needle at a *90-degree angle*
11. Client teaching
    a. Heparin administration if used after discharge
    b. Frequent blood work monitoring is required to ensure effective anticoagulation
    c. As per Box 34–11

C. Direct thrombin inhibitors (see Box 34–10)

1. Bind reversibly to thrombin to prevent fibrin formation
2. Exhibit same anticoagulant actions and have same indications as heparin and LMWHs
3. Are given by IV route except for desirudin, which is given SubQ
4. A common adverse effect is bleeding and less common adverse effect is allergic reaction
5. Nursing considerations and client teaching is similar to other anticoagulants

XII. ANTIPLATELET AGENTS

A. Prevent or disrupt aggregation of platelets needed to form a clot

B. Often used as adjuncts to other anticoagulants such as warfarin (Coumadin)

C. Used often for clients with history of MI, stroke, and cardiac surgery

D. Inhibit or block certain enzyme pathways to prevent clot formation

E. Common medications

1. ASA: most common antiplatelet medication; other therapeutic properties include analgesic, anti-inflammatory, and antipyretic action
2. Ticlopidine (Ticlid): can be used by clients who cannot take aspirin
3. Dipyridamole (Persantine): used for antiplatelet effect and in cardiac stress testing
4. Clopidrogrel bisulfate (Plavix) is used as a form of secondary prevention for clients who have had MI, stroke, and peripheral arterial disease
5. Glycoprotein inhibitors prevent platelet activation and thrombus formation with recent MI, CVA, and percutaneous coronary intervention; a disadvantage is that they are expensive
6. Antiplatelet medications are listed in Box 34–12

F. Administration considerations

1. ASA is administered in dosages ranging from 81 to 325 mg/day (baby ASA to adult strength); it can also be given as an enteric-coated preparation to minimize GI upset
2. Dipyridamole (Persantine) has a better profile when used with clients who have prosthetic mechanical heart valves; is contraindicated in pregnant or lactating clients
3. Ticlopidine (Ticlid) has been used effectively as a preventive measure in clients at risk for MI
4. Glycoprotein inhibitors are administered by the IV route and effect is maintained by continuous IV infusion administered via the parenteral route, and client can receive a bolus dose as well as a constant infusion
5. NCLEX® ASA is contraindicated with known hypersensitivity to salicylates, bleeding disorders, asthma, or GI bleeding; do not give to pediatric clients because of risk for developing Reye's syndrome
6. Antiplatelet agents are generally contraindicated with conditions that increase risk of bleeding

G. Side/adverse effects

1. NCLEX® ASA: blood dyscrasias, hemorrhage, GI symptoms, increased bleeding tendencies, hemorrhage, N/V, dizziness, confusion, tinnitus, and ototoxicity
2. Persantine: GI complaints, N/V, CNS alterations, headache, and dizziness
3. Ticlopidine: serious blood dyscrasias such as agranulocytosis and neutropenia; GI symptoms, such as nausea, vomiting, and jaundice
4. Clopidrogrel: flu-like symptoms, chest pain, edema, and hypertension
5. Glycoprotein receptor antagonists: dyspepsia, dizziness, pain at injection site, hypotension, bradycardia
6. NCLEX® In general: bruising, hematuria, tarry stools, other signs of bleeding

H. Nursing considerations

1. Perform baseline hematological labs on admission; monitor coagulation studies
2. Monitor vital signs and for bleeding

Box 34-12

Antiplatelet Drugs

Aspirin (ASA, acetylsalicylic acid)

Dipyridamole (Persantine)

Adenosine Diphosphate (ADP) Receptor Blockers

Clopidogrel (Plavix)

Ticlopidine (Ticlid)

Glycoprotein IIb/IIIa Receptor Antagonists

Abciximab (Reopro)

Eptifibatide (Integrillin)

Tirofiban (Aggrastat)

Agents for Intermittent Claudication

Cilostazol (Pletal)

Pentoxyphylline (Trental)

3. Antiplatelet agents should be stopped at least 7 days prior to a planned surgery

NCLEX® 4. Older adult clients may require closer monitoring to avoid toxicity because tinnitus and ototoxicity may be harder to determine if baseline hearing is already diminished

NCLEX® 5. Lifespan concerns: children, pregnant women, and lactating women should not take antiplatelet medications

I. Client teaching

1. Carry a Medic-Alert bracelet

NCLEX® 2. Monitor for and report side effects related to bleeding; may use bleeding precautions (Box 34–11) on advice of prescriber

3. Adults should not self-treat pain with aspirin for more than 5 days without consulting prescriber
4. Maintain adequate fluid intake to prevent salicylate crystalluria
5. Prolonged use of ASA can lead to iron-deficiency anemia (especially important for females of childbearing age)

XIII. THROMBOLYTICS

A. *Thrombolytics* are substances that dissolve or break down a thrombus or blood clot to reestablish blood flow and increase perfusion to an ischemic area

B. Activate *fibrinolytic system* that breaks down thrombus or blood clot

C. Conversion of plasminogen to plasmin helps break down clot by digesting fibrin and degrading fibrinogen and other procoagulant proteins into soluble fragments

D. Indicated for clients at risk for developing thrombus with resultant ischemia, such as acute MI, arterial thrombosis, DVT, pulmonary embolism, and occlusion of catheters or shunts

E. Primarily used in emergency and critical care settings

F. Common medications are listed in see Box 34–13

Memory Aid

Remember that the suffix *-ase* often indicates a fibrinolytic/thrombolytic drug if it is given IV.

G. Administration considerations

1. Record baseline vital signs and obtain baseline coagulation studies
2. Give IV according to specific protocols; monitor IV sites for signs of infiltration and/or phlebitis; change IV site to opposite extremity if any problems are noted with IV

NCLEX® 3. Place client on cardiac monitor during administration

NCLEX® 4. Antidote to streptokinase is aminocaproic acid (Amicar)

5. Contraindicated in clients who are actively bleeding or have a recent history of CVA, severe uncontrolled hypertension, recent trauma, neoplasm, or are pregnant

H. Side/adverse effects (dose-related)

NCLEX® 1. Hemorrhage

NCLEX® 2. Hypersensitivity reactions

3. N/V and hypotension
4. Cardiac dysrhythmias; reperfusion dysrhythmias may pose further problems for acutely ill client

I. Nursing considerations

1. Monitor coagulation studies and continue to monitor client during therapy

NCLEX® 2. Monitor for vital sign changes, because drug may cause variations in pulse, BP, and temperature

3. Maintain adequate IV site for administration; observe closely for infiltration

NCLEX® 4. Institute bleeding precautions and limit invasive procedures and injections to reduce risk of bleeding

NCLEX® 5. If bleeding occurs, medication should be stopped; fresh frozen plasma (FFP) and packed red blood cells (PRBCs) may be ordered

6. Monitor client closely for development of dysrhythmias

Box 34–13

Thrombolytics

Alteplase (Activase)	Streptokinase (Kabikinase, Streptase)
Reteplase (Retavase)	Tenecteplase (TNKase)

7. Maintain aseptic technique to prevent infection
8. Provide adequate nutrition and rest to support client

J. **Client teaching**

1. Treatment methods and medication administration; measurable signs of clinical response may not occur for 6 to 8 hours after therapy is started
2. *NCLEX®* Bleeding precautions as per Box 34–11
3. Lifestyle changes may be needed to prevent further abnormal clotting
4. Discontinue medication if bleeding occurs, and notify physician

XIV. ANTIHYPERLIPIDEMICS

A. **HMG-CoenzymeA reductase inhibitors**

1. Also called *statins;* reduce LDL cholesterol levels when diet therapy has not been effective
2. Have a dose-dependent effect on HDL cholesterol; lipoprotein levels are not affected by statins
3. Common medications are listed in Box 34–14

Memory Aid

The suffix *-statin* indicates the cholesterol-lowering drugs known as HMG CoenzymeA reductase inhibitors.

4. Usually administered at night to increase effectiveness because cholesterol synthesis normally occurs during evening hours
5. Contraindicated with active liver disease, abnormal serum transaminase levels, and during pregnancy and lactation
6. Monitor for elevation of liver function tests
7. Side/adverse effects
   a. *NCLEX®* GI upset, dyspepsia, flatulence, pain and myalgias
   b. Headache, rash, dizziness, sinusitis
8 Nursing considerations
   a. *NCLEX®* Monitor lipid levels within 2–4 weeks after initiation of therapy
   b. May be given without regard to food
9. Client education
   a. *NCLEX®* Take dose with evening meal to coincide with body's timing of cholesterol production
   b. Required lab monitoring for compliance and client response
   c. *NCLEX®* Report immediately any unexplained muscle pain, tenderness, yellowing of skin or eyes, or loss of appetite (liver toxicity)
   d. Avoid or minimize alcohol intake

B. **Bile acid sequestrants**

1. Work in GI tract to bind with bile acids; liver cells respond by sending cholesterol to maintain bile acid synthesis, lowering plasma levels of LDL cholesterol
2. Indicated for use with elevated cholesterol levels with or without high triglyceride levels
3. Common medications: cholestyramine (Questran), colesevelam (WelChol), and colestipol (Colestid)
   a. Colestipol and colesevelam are available as a tablet or powder, given in 2–4 doses before meals and at bedtime
   b. Cholestyramine is available as a powder, given 2–4 times daily before meals and at bedtime
4. Administration considerations
   a. *NCLEX®* Do not crush, chew, or cut colestipol tablets; they should be given with adequate fluids
   b. *NCLEX®* Mix powdered drug forms at bedside to prevent overthickening and esophageal obstruction; they may be plain or have flavoring; cholestyramine powder contains phenylalanine and should not be used in clients with phenylketonuria (PKU)

Box 34–14

HMG-Coenzyme A Reductase Inhibitors ("Statins")

Atorvastatin (Lipitor)	Pravastatin (Pravachol)
Fluvastatin (Lescol)	Rosuvastatin (Crestor)
Lovastatin (Mevacor)	Simvastatin (Zocor)

c. Administer bile acids alone to avoid binding with other medications; give other drugs 1–2 hours before or 4–6 hours after bile acid administration
d. Mix contents of one packet with at least 120–180 mL of water or other preferred liquid; dissolve before administration because drug is irritating to mucous membranes

5. Side/adverse effects
NCLEX® a. Abdominal pain, dyspepsia, bloating, reflux, and constipation
NCLEX® b. Associated fat-soluble vitamin deficiencies (A, D, K) and decreased erythrocyte folate levels

6. Nursing considerations
a. Not often used as first-line therapy because of poor compliance
b. Vitamin deficiencies may require supplementation, if not discontinuation of bile acids, to restore normal levels
c. Increase fluids and fiber to counteract constipation as tolerated
d. If client develops GI complaints, dosage reduction may be needed to maintain client compliance
e. Serum cholesterol levels are reduced within 24–48 hours after starting therapy
NCLEX® f. Monitor baseline cholesterol and triglyceride levels; trend results to determine client response
g. Decreased levels of LDL cholesterol should be seen within 1 month of therapy
h. Long-term use of cholestyramine can increase bleeding tendency

NCLEX® 7. Client teaching
a. Proper administration and scheduling of medication to maximize effect
b. Be alert for signs and symptoms indicating side effects of these agents
c. Follow-up serum cholesterol levels are necessary
d. Increase high-bulk diet with adequate fluid intake; report constipation immediately

C. Fibric acid agents

1. Act on very low lipid–density lipoproteins (VLDL) and chlyomicrons to reduce triglyceride levels
2. HDL cholesterol levels are increased but this is not primary effect; also has variable effect on LDL
3. Indicated for use with elevated triglyceride and cholesterol levels resistant to dietary management
4. Common medications are listed in Box 34–15
5. Administration considerations
a. Usually given in divided doses, 30 minutes prior to morning and evening meals
b. Contraindicated in clients with gallbladder disease, renal problems, liver or biliary cirrhosis, and in pregnant or lactating women

6. Side/adverse effects
NCLEX® a. Abdominal or epigastric pain
b. Jaundice, blurred vision, headache, and depression
c. Rash, dermatitis, pruritus with gemfibrozil
d. Back pain, muscle cramps, myalgia, and swollen joints
NCLEX® e. Client may develop gallbladder disease and acute appendicitis
f. Eosinophilia and/or hypokalemia

7. Nursing considerations
NCLEX® a. Obtain baseline lipid levels, monitor periodically
b. If there is no response to therapy or if liver function tests are persistently abnormal after 3 months, then therapy should be discontinued
c. Hypokalemia may be seen in response to therapy
d. Decreased hemoglobin, hematocrit, and WBC count may be seen with the use of gemfibrozil
e. Monitor client for potential side effects and adverse effects
NCLEX® f. Monitor closely for right upper quadrant (RUQ) abdominal pain or vomiting

NCLEX® 8. Client teaching
a. Need for periodic lab work to evaluate response
b. Immediately report unexplained bleeding or any serious side effects such as acute appendicitis or gallbladder disease
c. Restrict fat and alcohol intake

Box 34–15 Fibric Acid Derivatives		
	Clofibrate (Abitrate, Atromid-S)	Gemfibrozil (Lopid)
	Fenofibrate (Tricor)	

D. Nicotinic acid (niacin, vitamin B_3)

1. Water-soluble vitamin that lowers most lipoprotein levels (total cholesterol, LDL, triglyceride, and lipoproteins) and increases HDL levels
2. Indications for use are high cholesterol levels and as adjunctive therapy when dietary management is ineffective
3. Causes peripheral vasodilation and can be used for clients with peripheral vascular disease
4. Pellagra (dermatitis, diarrhea, and dementia) is a clinical deficiency state associated with niacin deficiency
5. NCLEX® Dosage to lower cholesterol is higher (greater than 3 grams/day) than normal vitamin dose (500 mg/day in adults)
6. Administration considerations
   - a. Tablets should be taken whole; do not crush or divide the pill
   - b. Can be taken with meals to prevent GI upset
   - c. NCLEX® Flushing is a common side effect caused by niacin's vasodilator properties; usually subsides after an hour
   - d. Oral nicotinic acid should be taken with cold water
   - e. Contraindicated with liver disease and/or unexplained elevated serum transaminases and with active peptic ulcer disease
   - f. Contraindicated in clients with severe hypotension
   - g. Leads to increases in blood glucose, uric acid, and serum transaminase levels
7. Side/adverse effects
   - a. NCLEX® Flushing, postural hypotension, vasovagal attacks
   - b. Pruritus, increased sebaceous gland activity
   - c. Dyspepsia, epigastric pain, and nausea
   - d. Dark-colored urine
   - e. Megadose therapy has been associated with liver damage, hyperglycemia, hyperuricemia, and cardiac dysrhythmias
8. NCLEX® Nursing considerations
   - a. Dosing of nicotinic acid varies depending on whether prescribed to reduce cholesterol levels or merely as a vitamin supplement; be aware of specific dosing levels
   - b. Expect side effect of flushing when administering medication
   - c. Evaluate client for food sources high in niacin (dairy, meats, tuna, and egg) and monitor dietary intake
9. Client teaching
   - a. NCLEX® Change position slowly to avoid sudden BP drop
   - b. Avoid direct exposure to sunlight
   - c. NCLEX® Flushing in face, neck, and ears may occur within 2 hours after oral ingestion and immediately after IV administration and may last several hours; alcohol and niacin cause increased flushing
   - d. Follow-up lab work will be done periodically to determine response to therapy
   - e. Do not self-medicate with additional sources of niacin, which can lead to overdose

XV. HEMOSTATICS

A. Systemic hemostatics

1. Systemic **hemostatics** are substances that inhibit bleeding after an injury
2. Common medications
   - a. Aminocaproic acid (Amicar) and tranexamic acid (Cyklokapron) both impede **fibrinolysis**
   - b. NCLEX® Aminocaproic acid is used to treat hyperfibrinolysis-induced hemorrhage after surgery, aplastic anemia, hepatic cirrhosis, and some neoplastic disease states; it is also an antidote to thrombolytic drugs
   - c. Tranexamic acid is used 1 day before and 2–8 days after dental or other surgery in clients with hemophilia
   - d. NCLEX® Phytonadione, vitamin K_1 (Aquamephyton), is antidote to warfarin and is fat soluble; used to reverse excess effects of oral anticoagulants
   - e. Menadiol sodium diphosphate, vitamin K_4 (Synkayvite), is a water-soluble compound
   - f. Vitamin K is also used as mandatory treatment to prevent hemorrhagic disease of newborn
3. Nursing considerations
   - a. Monitor client's baseline labs for renal and liver function
   - b. NCLEX® Monitor PT levels and response to therapy for vitamin K administration

NCLEX® c. Monitor client's coagulation profile as antifibrinolytics can cause **hypercoagulation** or rapid coagulation of blood
d. Rotate injection sites for vitamin K; monitor for signs of local irritation
e. Monitor client closely for signs of hypersensitivity and allergic reaction
f. Monitor client closely during parenteral infusion because of risk for volume overload and adverse reactions
g. Use an infusion pump for IV administration

4. Client teaching
a. Dietary sources of vitamin K
b. Periodic PT levels will be drawn to monitor response to therapy
c. Monitor for signs and symptoms of bleeding
d. Use of yogurt and buttermilk products in diet can help restore normal intestinal flora that aid in synthesis of vitamin K; clients who are on antibiotic therapy or who have intestinal problems may benefit from this supportive therapy
e. Report difficulty urinating or reddish brown urine (caused by myoglobinuria) while taking aminocaproic acid
f. Report chest pain, arm or leg pain, or difficulty breathing

B. Topical thrombin

1. Used to stop oozing of blood or minor bleeding from capillaries
2. Common medications: topical thrombin (Evithron, Recothrom, Thrombinar)
3. Administration considerations
a. Available as a spray or gelatin sponge
b. Irrigation with normal saline may be needed to prevent further tissue destruction with removal
4. Nursing considerations
a. Monitor local site for signs of hypersensitivity and document findings; antihistamine such as diphenhydramine (Benadryl) may be given to either prevent or treat allergic reaction
NCLEX® b. Remove topical hemostatics as indicated by product guidelines; irrigate site with normal saline if necessary to prevent further tissue destruction with removal; document site assessment

XVI. ANTIANEMIC AGENTS

A. Iron salts

1. Iron is an essential trace element that aids oxygen transport, tissue respiration, and enzyme reactions
2. Iron is stored as ferritin; ferritin levels reflect visceral iron stores that are available to body; transferrin levels reflect how iron is transported in body
3. Common medications are listed in Box 34–16
4. Administration considerations
NCLEX® a. Oral iron is given with meals to decrease gastric upset
NCLEX® b. Iron dextran is administered by Z-track technique to minimize discomfort, prevent tissue discoloration, and ensure absorption
c. There is risk of anaphylaxis following iron dextran administration; a test dose may be ordered to determine client response
d. Monitor client for intake of dietary sources of iron to avoid potential overdosing and toxicity
NCLEX® e. Liquid (elixir) iron is administered by straw to avoid discoloration of tooth enamel
f. Contraindicated in clients with ulcerative colitis, peptic ulcer disease, cirrhosis, hemolytic anemia, and iron overload syndromes (hemosiderosis and hemochromatosis)
NCLEX® g. Vitamin C can increase absorption of oral iron
5. Side/adverse effects
a. Upset stomach, N/V, diarrhea, and constipation
NCLEX® b. Dark and tarry stools
c. Discoloration of skin and pain upon injection
d. **Pica** (ingestion of nonfood items) can interfere with iron levels and cause anemia; pregnant women are most likely to be affected

Box 34–16 Iron Salts

Ferrous fumarate (Feostat)	Ferrous sulfate (Feosol)
Ferrous gluconate (Fergon)	Iron dextran injection (DexFerrum)

e. Iron can accumulate in body, leading to potentially toxic levels
f. Chelation therapy removes iron from body; additional supportive measures include airway maintenance, correction of acidosis, and administration of IV fluids

6. Nursing considerations
   a. Monitor client for expected side effects, such as tarry stools
   b. Since anemia is often a symptom of a disease, monitor for underlying cause
   c. If client does not show a clinical response to iron therapy, notify prescriber
   d. Refer to dietitian as needed for instruction on foods rich in iron
   e. Evaluate client for pica if there is a high index of suspicion
   f. (NCLEX®) Monitor reticulocyte count, which will increase if RBC production is increasing
   g. (NCLEX®) If hemoglobin and hematocrit levels do not rise following iron therapy, additional testing may be required to determine type of anemia
7. Client education
   a. Proper self-administration of oral iron medications
   b. (NCLEX®) Importance of adequate food sources to maintain iron levels; these include lean meats, liver, egg yolks, dried beans, green vegetables (e.g., spinach)
   c. (NCLEX®) Expected changes in characteristics of stool (black, tarry)

B. Vitamin B_{12} (cyanocobalamin)

1. Is a water-soluble vitamin used in many coenzyme reactions during metabolism of carbohydrate, protein, and fat
2. (NCLEX®) Is found primarily in foods of animal origin (liver, meat, shellfish, and dairy food items)
3. Deficiency of vitamin B_{12} affects neurological, hematological, and GI systems
4. Vitamin B_{12} is considered an extrinsic factor, whereas intrinsic factor is released by parietal cells in stomach
5. (NCLEX®) Clients with GI surgeries with partial or complete removal and/or anastomosis of stomach cannot produce intrinsic factor and will require weekly and then monthly vitamin B_{12} injections for life; a nasal form (Nascobal) is now available as well
6. **Pernicious anemia** is name of anemia that results from vitamin B_{12} deficiency; is classified as a megaloblastic macrocytic anemia
7. Atrophic gastritis is associated with vitamin B_{12} deficiency
8. Because B-complex vitamins work together, it is likely that more than one deficiency exists, making assessment and treatment of other anemias (such as folic acid deficiency) necessary

Check Your NCLEX-PN® Exam I.Q. *You are ready for testing on this content if you can*

- Apply knowledge of expected actions and effects of cardiovascular medications to client care.
- Correctly administer cardiovascular medications to clients.
- Monitor for side effects and adverse effects of cardiovascular medications.
- Take appropriate action if a client has an unexpected response to a cardiovascular medication.
- Monitor a client for expected outcomes or effects of treatment with cardiovascular medications.

PRACTICE TEST

1 A client with angina pectoris received nitroglycerin tablets sublingually for chest pain. The client reports a severe headache shortly after the medication is administered. What interpretation should the nurse make based on the client's statement?

1. This is a common, but unhealthy response to the medication.
2. This common response will diminish as tolerance to the medication develops.
3. This is a response caused by cerebral hypoxia induced by the medication.
4. This adverse reaction should be reported to the physician immediately.

PRACTICE TEST

2 A diabetic client newly diagnosed with hypertension also smokes. The nurse would question an order for which antihypertensive medication?

1. Diltiazem (Cardizem)
2. Propranolol (Inderal)
3. Prazosin (Minipress)
4. Furosemide (Lasix)

3 Diltiazem (Cardizem) is prescribed for a client with chronic, stable angina. Which statement by the client indicates to the clinic nurse that the client needs additional medication information?

1. "I will call the physician if shortness of breath occurs."
2. "I will rise slowly when getting out of bed."
3. "I will take the medication after meals."
4. "I may notice changes in mental alertness until my dose is regulated."

4 The nurse has given medication instructions to the client receiving nicardipine (Cardene) for angina. What statement by the client would indicate to the nurse that the teaching needs to be reinforced?

1. "I will keep track of angina episodes, and report them if they increase."
2. "Edema and weight gain are expected side effects of the medication."
3. "I will report a pulse rate of fewer than 50 beats per minute."
4. "I will take any missed dose as soon as remembered, unless it is almost time for the next dose."

5 A client with hypertension has been given a prescription to treat the disorder. The nurse should explain that cough and loss of taste are side effects if which antihypertensive agent has been prescribed?

1. Lisinopril (Prinivil)
2. Propranolol (Inderal)
3. Diltiazem (Cardizem)
4. Furosemide (Lasix)

6 The health care provider prescribes losartan (Cozaar) for a client with hypertension. The nurse carrying out the order reinforces to the client that this medication promotes vasodilation by which action?

1. Preventing calcium from going into the cells
2. Promoting epinephrine and norepinephrine
3. Promoting release of aldosterone
4. Inhibiting conversion of a substance that would cause vasoconstriction

7 A client with hypertension monitors his blood pressure daily, and is ordered on verapamil (Calan SR) 240 mg daily and hydrochlorothiazide (HCTZ) 12.5 mg daily. The client states that if his systolic BP reading is lower than 140, he skips his medication for the day. What would be an appropriate response by the nurse? Select all that apply.

1. "As long as the systolic is lower than 140, it is OK to skip the dose."
2. "You should not skip doses unless instructed by the ordering physician."
3. "Maybe you won't even need your BP medications in a few more months."
4. "Your doctor may want to stop the HCTZ and have you take only the Calan."
5. "Your lower systolic blood pressure is a response to the medication."

8 The ambulatory clinic nurse would be concerned that a client is experiencing digoxin toxicity after noting which manifestations during a routine visit? Select all that apply.

1. Palpitations, elevated blood pressure, and shortness of breath
2. Anorexia, nausea, and reports of yellow vision
3. Chest pain, fatigue, and decreased blood pressure
4. Taste alterations, dry mouth, and constipation
5. Visual disturbances, vomiting, and diarrhea

9 Which medication does the nurse anticipate will be used for a pregnant client who requires anticoagulation therapy?

1. Low-molecular-weight heparin (LMWH)
2. Epoetin (Procrit)
3. Heparin (Liquaemin)
4. Enoxaparin (Lovenox)

10 A client is taking warfarin (Coumadin) for atrial fibrillation. The nurse would include in a teaching plan that the client will need to remain on drug therapy for what period of time?

1. 6 months
2. 2–3 months
3. Indefinite, or long-term
4. 1 year

11 A client is placed on ticlopidine (Ticlid) following a stroke. What follow-up blood work is indicated in managing the client?

1. Frequent CBC monitoring to evaluate for blood dyscrasias
2. Monthly PT and INR levels to evaluate for clotting problems
3. ABGs to evaluate respiratory status
4. Serum chemistries to monitor for potential electrolyte imbalances

12 A client is receiving thrombolytic therapy. The nurse monitors the client for which potential problems? Select all that apply.

1. Headache
2. Bruising
3. Hematuria
4. Bone pain
5. Hypotension

13 The nurse would monitor a client who is receiving thrombolytic therapy for which manifestation?

1. Dry mouth
2. Decreased urine output
3. Decreased clotting times
4. Cardiac dysrhythmias

14 The nurse should remind a client taking folic acid (Folvite) for anemia to expect which side effect during therapy?

1. Dark-yellow urine
2. Dark-green or black stools
3. Mild temperature elevations
4. Slightly increased pulse rate

15 Which measures should the nurse utilize when administering ferrous sulfate (Feosol) elixir? Select all that apply.

1. Mix the medication with milk to decrease GI effects.
2. Administer the oral form of the medication with food.
3. Administer the medication through a straw.
4. Mix the medication with carbonated beverages to minimize gastric upset.
5. Increase dietary intake of vitamin C to promote absorption.

16 A client has an order to receive 5,000 units of heparin subcutaneously. Available is a vial labeled "Heparin 10,000 units per mL." The nurse should administer _____ mL of heparin solution. Record your answer rounding to one decimal place.

Fill in your answer below:

_____ mL

17 A client diagnosed with iron deficiency anemia (IDA) who is also taking an iron supplement wants to know what foods would help to achieve adequate iron levels in the body. Which diet information would be beneficial for the nurse to reinforce that will help the client achieve increased iron levels?

1. Maintain a strict vegetarian diet.
2. Eat ice cubes that are present in beverages.
3. Increase tea and cereal in the diet.
4. Use adequate sources of vitamin C in the diet.

18 A client is taking anti-platelet medication for several weeks, and presents with a noticeable bruise on the arm. What information should the nurse determine first to see if this skin manifestation is related to drug therapy?

1. Whether the bruising is a result of a specific injury and therefore not caused by drug therapy.
2. Whether the client has taken the medication for the last several days.
3. Whether the client self-monitors for skin manifestations.
4. Whether the client has bruising and discoloration on other areas of the body.

19 A client is taking epoetin alfa (Epogen) for treatment of anemia related to chronic renal disease. What clinical finding reveals to the nurse that this medication is working effectively?

1. The client is not experiencing any related bone pain when the medication is being administered.
2. The client's hemoglobin and hematocrit levels are rising rapidly based on the latest two daily blood draws.
3. The client's hematocrit is in the established target range at 33%.
4. The client is afebrile.

20 A client is being discharged with a diagnosis of angina. What client teaching should the nurse reinforce related to the use of nitroglycerine (NTG) tablets for chest pain?

1. "Keep NTG tablets in your pants pocket next to your body to keep them handy at all times. Take two NTG tablets with a glass of water, and then go back to your activities."
2. "Stop your activity and sit down near a telephone if possible, and place 1 NTG under your tongue. Take no more than 3 tablets total, 1 every five minutes. If the pain is not relieved after 3 tablets, call for help."
3. "Stop your activities, take 2 NTG tablets, and drive immediately to your doctor's office."
4. "Continue your activities slowly. Take 3 NTG tablets every 5 minutes until your chest pain is gone."

ANSWERS & RATIONALES

1 **Answer: 2** **Rationale:** The incidence of headache decreases over time as the client develops tolerance to the medication. Headache is a common side effect (not adverse reaction) related to the vasodilation properties of nitroglycerin. Headache is not an indication of cerebral hypoxia induced by nitroglycerine; the medication has vasodilation properties. The client should be encouraged to continue to use nitroglycerine as needed; acetaminophen or aspirin can be taken for the headache, according to the preference of the physician. **Cognitive Level:** Analyzing **Client Need:** Pharmacological and Parenteral Therapies **Integrated Process:** Nursing Process: Data Collection **Content Area:** Pharmacology **Strategy:** The core issue of the question is knowledge of common adverse effects of nitroglycerin therapy. Use nursing knowledge related to pharmacology and the process of elimination to make a selection.

2 **Answer: 2** **Rationale:** Adverse effects of beta-adrenergic blockers such as propranolol include their potential to cause bronchospasm and to mask hypoglycemia attacks. Therefore, the clients who are at risk for these conditions should not utilize beta-blockers as antihypertensive medications. Diltiazem is a calcium channel blocker, which would not directly affect the client's conditions. Alpha blockers such as prazosin do not directly increase the risk of side effects of possible concern when the client smokes. Furosemide is a diuretic, which is not an antihypertensive, although reducing fluid in the body aids in reducing blood pressure in some clients.. **Cognitive Level:** Applying **Client Need:** Pharmacological and Parenteral Therapies **Integrated Process:** Nursing Process: Implementation **Content Area:** Pharmacology **Strategy:** The core issue of the question is knowledge of contraindications for beta-adrenergic blockers, such as propranolol. Use nursing knowledge related to pharmacology and the process of elimination to make a selection.

3 **Answer: 3** **Rationale:** Diltiazem (Cardizem) is usually administered before meals and at bedtime to increase the absorption of medication. The client should notify the physician if shortness of breath, irregular heartbeat, pronounced dizziness, nausea, or constipation develops. Postural hypotension can occur, so the client must be instructed to rise slowly to avoid dizziness and falling. The medication can cause a decrease in mental alertness until the body adjusts and the proper dosage is established. **Cognitive Level:** Analyzing **Client Need:** Pharmacological and Parenteral Therapies **Integrated Process:** Nursing Process: Evaluation **Content Area:** Pharmacology **Strategy:** The wording of the question tells you that the correct answer is an incorrect statement. Recall information about calcium channel blockers and use the process of elimination to make a selection.

4 **Answer: 2** **Rationale:** Nicardipine (Cardene) is a calcium channel blocker. Weight gain and edema are potential signs of heart failure, and must be reported to the physician. The client taking this medication should keep track of angina episodes, and report any increase in the episodes or change in the pattern. The client should be taught to check his pulse, note the rate, and report if the heart rate is lower than 50 beats per minute. The client may take a missed dose of medication if not too close to the next dose; otherwise, the dose should be omitted. **Cognitive Level:** Analyzing **Client Need:** Pharmacological and Parenteral Therapies **Integrated Process:** Nursing Process: Evaluation **Content Area:** Pharmacology **Strategy:** The core issue of the question is knowledge of teaching points regarding calcium channel blockers, such as nicardipine. The wording of the question tells you that the correct answer is an incorrect statement. Use nursing knowledge related to pharmacology and the process of elimination to make a selection.

5 **Answer: 1** **Rationale:** Cough and loss of taste are common side effects of angiotensin-converting enzyme (ACE) inhibitors such as lisinopril. They disappear with discontinuation of the medication. Cough and loss of taste are not common side effects of Inderal, which is a beta-adrenergic blocker. Cardizem, a calcium channel blocker, does not cause the side effects of cough and loss of taste. Lasix, a diuretic, will not cause the client to develop a cough or loss of taste as side effects.

Cognitive Level: Analyzing **Client Need:** Pharmacological and Parenteral Therapies **Integrated Process:** Teaching and Learning **Content Area:** Pharmacology **Strategy:** The core issue of the question is knowledge that ACE inhibitors lead to cough and loss of taste perception. From there, you must be able to identify which drug is an ACE inhibitor. Recall that these drugs end in *-pril* to help make a selection.

6 **Answer: 4 Rationale:** Losartan is an angiotensin II antagonist that inhibits the conversion of angiotensin I to angiotensin II. Because angiotensin II is a powerful vasoconstrictor, this inhibition results in vasodilation and normalizing blood pressure. The client should be assessed for dizziness, cough, and diarrhea while taking this medication. Calcium channel blockers prevent calcium from entering cells, but do not promote vasodilation. Epinephrine and norepinephrine are sympathomimetic antihypotensives, which promote vasoconstriction. The primary effect of aldosterone is sodium reabsorption, which would cause an elevation in blood pressure and not be prescribed for a client with hypertension. **Cognitive Level:** Applying **Client Need:** Pharmacological and Parenteral Therapies **Integrated Process:** Teaching and Learning **Content Area:** Pharmacology **Strategy:** The core issue of the question is knowledge of the mechanism of action of angiotensin-receptor blockers. To reach the correct answer, it is necessary to recognize that the drug is in this class. Use nursing knowledge related to pharmacology and the process of elimination to make a selection.

7 **Answer: 2, 5 Rationale:** Lack of adherence to pharmacologic treatment strategies prevents the client from establishing good control of the disease, and ultimately places him at risk for developing long-term complications of hypertension. Noncompliance with the therapeutic program is a significant problem in people with hypertension. It is an important nursing activity to reinforce the need for the client to adhere to the medication as prescribed. The client should not skip doses of medications without consulting the physician. The comment about not needing medications is inappropriate; the client may require long-term treatment for hypertension. The physician is responsible for adjusting the client's medication regimen; to state HCTZ may be stopped is not appropriate. **Cognitive Level:** Applying **Client Need:** Pharmacological and Parenteral Therapies **Integrated Process:** Communication and Documentation **Content Area:** Pharmacology **Strategy:** The core issue of the question is knowledge that antihypertensive medications need to be taken as scheduled without missing or skipping doses. Use nursing knowledge related to pharmacology and the process of elimination to make a selection. When more than one answer is correct, consider each option as a true/false statement.

8 **Answer: 2, 5 Rationale:** Anorexia, nausea, and yellow vision, visual disturbances, vomiting, and diarrhea are signs of digoxin toxicity. The other options are not signs of digoxin toxicity. **Cognitive Level:** Analyzing **Client Need:** Pharmacological and Parenteral Therapies **Integrated Process:** Nursing Process: Data Collection **Content Area:** Pharmacology **Strategy:** The core issue of the question is knowledge of the signs of digoxin toxicity. Recall that early signs are usually more subtle than are later signs. Use nursing knowledge related to pharmacology and the process of elimination to make a selection. When more than one answer is correct, consider each option as a true/false statement.

9 **Answer: 3 Rationale:** Heparin is the drug of choice in pregnancy. Low-molecular-weight heparins are not recommended for use during pregnancy. Epoetin alfa (Procrit) is a colony-stimulating growth factor to increase production of red blood cells and is not used for anticoagulation. Low-molecular-weight heparins, of which enoxaparin is an example, are not recommended for use during pregnancy. **Cognitive Level:** Applying **Client Need:** Pharmacological and Parenteral Therapies **Integrated Process:** Nursing Process: Planning **Content Area:** Pharmacology **Strategy:** The core issue of the question is knowledge of the anticoagulant that is safe to use during pregnancy. Use nursing knowledge related to pharmacology and the process of elimination to make a selection.

10 **Answer: 3 Rationale:** Clients who have atrial fibrillation are at risk to develop emboli. Therapy with Coumadin is considered to be ongoing in nature, in order to prevent such an occurrence. Timeframes of 2–3 months, 6 months, and even 1 year are insufficient because the anticoagulation effect stops shortly after drug therapy is terminated. **Cognitive Level:** Applying **Client Need:** Pharmacological and Parenteral Therapies **Integrated Process:** Nursing Process: Planning **Content Area:** Pharmacology **Strategy:** The core issue of the question is knowledge that treatment for prevention of blood clot formation from atrial fibrillation is indefinite. Use nursing knowledge related to pharmacology and the process of elimination to make a selection.

11 **Answer: 1 Rationale:** A client taking ticlopidine should be monitored for potential blood dyscrasias that can occur with this drug. Monthly PT and INR levels are not indicated as follow-up for ticlopidine, but are used in conjunction with Coumadin therapy. ABGs are not indicated in the management of clients who are taking ticlopidine. There are no reported electrolyte imbalances with the use of ticlopidine. **Cognitive Level:** Applying **Client Need:** Pharmacological and Parenteral Therapies **Integrated Process:** Nursing Process: Planning **Content Area:** Pharmacology **Strategy:** The core issue of the question is knowledge of adverse effects of ticlopidine that can be detected using laboratory monitoring. Use nursing knowledge related to pharmacology and the process of elimination to make a selection.

12 **Answer: 2, 3, 5 Rationale:** The client on thrombolytic therapy should be monitored closely for skin bruising, which can be an indication of bleeding. Urine should be monitored for the presence of occult or obvious blood, which are indications of hemorrhage or bleeding. When on thrombolytic therapy, the client's blood pressure should be monitored for dose-related or hemorrhage-related hypotension. Headache should not occur with thrombolytic therapy. Bone pain is not directly related to thrombolytic therapy. **Cognitive Level:** Analyzing **Client Need:** Pharmacological and Parenteral Therapies **Integrated Process:** Nursing Process: Data Collection **Content Area:** Pharmacology **Strategy:** The core issue of the question is knowledge that thrombolytics can lead to bleeding. With this in mind, recall the various ways that bleeding can manifest in a client taking drugs that interfere with clotting. Use nursing knowledge related to pharmacology and the process of elimination to make a selection. When there is more than one correct answer, consider each option as a true/false statement.

13 **Answer: 4 Rationale:** The use of thrombolytic agents can cause cardiac irritation and lead to reperfusion dysrhythmias that can be life-threatening. The nurse must be aware of the serious likelihood that treatment can cause further cardiac compromise. The other options are not seen with thrombolytic therapy. **Cognitive Level:** Applying **Client Need:** Pharmacological and Parenteral Therapies **Integrated Process:** Nursing Process: Data Collection **Content Area:** Pharmacology **Strategy:** The core

issue of the question is knowledge that thrombolytic drugs can cause reperfusion dysrhythmias as a result of clot lysis. Use nursing knowledge related to pharmacology and the process of elimination to make a selection.

14 **Answer: 1 Rationale:** Folic acid (in large doses) can cause the urine to become discolored and turn to a darker-yellow color. Dark-green or black stools are more commonly associated with iron therapy. Temperature elevations and increased pulse rate are not associated with folic acid. **Cognitive Level:** Applying **Client Need:** Pharmacological and Parenteral Therapies **Integrated Process:** Nursing Process: Evaluation **Content Area:** Pharmacology **Strategy:** The core issue of the question is knowledge of expected side effects of folic acid. Recall that B complex vitamins can turn the urine a darker yellow as an aid to answering the question. Use nursing knowledge related to pharmacology and the process of elimination to make a selection.

15 **Answer: 2, 3, 5 Rationale:** The oral form of ferrous sulfate is usually taken with food to minimize GI upset. Liquid iron preparations can cause staining of teeth. It is important for the nurse to be aware of proper administration methods, which include drinking the mixture through a straw. Vitamin C promotes the absorption of ferrous sulfate when the medication is taken orally. Mixing ferrous sulfate with milk will decrease its absorption. Mixing medication with carbonated beverages will decrease its absorption. **Cognitive Level:** Analyzing **Client Need:** Pharmacological and Parenteral Therapies **Integrated Process:** Nursing Process: Implementation **Content Area:** Pharmacology **Strategy:** The core issue of the question is knowledge of the administration considerations that should be made when giving ferrous sulfate. Keeping other administration principles in mind helps you to eliminate the incorrect options. When more than one answer is correct, consider each option as a true/false statement.

16 **Answer: 0.5 Rationale:** To calculate the dose, divide the desired dose (5,000) by the dose on hand (10,000 units) and multiply that by the quantity (1 mL). The result is 0.5 mL. **Cognitive Level:** Applying **Client Need:** Pharmacological and Parenteral Therapies **Integrated Process:** Nursing Process: Implementation **Content Area:** Pharmacology **Strategy:** The core issue of the question is the ability to calculate a drug dose. If necessary, memorize this basic formula for use in solving many medication questions.

17 **Answer: 4 Rationale:** Vitamin C helps to enhance the absorption of iron in the diet, and is an easy step in diet management towards improving iron levels in the body. A strict vegetarian diet focuses on non-heme sources of iron that are not as readily absorbable as heme sources. Eating ice cubes is an example of pica, which is ingestion of a non-food substance. Tea contains tannic acid, and cereals contain phytates and fibers, both of which lead to decreased iron absorption in the diet. **Cognitive Level:** Applying **Client Need:** Health Promotion and Maintenance **Integrated Process:** Nursing Process: Planning **Content Area:** Foundational Sciences **Strategy:** Note that the question is referring to maintaining iron levels, which should lead to thinking about how iron can best be absorbed. Knowledge of the need to consume vitamin C with iron will lead you to the only correct option.

18 **Answer: 4 Rationale:** Inspection of the client's skin is necessary to check for additional areas of bruising or discoloration of which the client might not be aware. It is important to review current findings and compare them with baseline findings, as this might provide data to support a potential response to drug therapy. Asking the client if the bruising is related to a particular incident is helpful; however, it does not rule out the possibility that drug therapy has made the individual more susceptible to bruising or bleeding tendencies. If the client has not taken the medication as ordered, it would be unlikely that the bruise would be a consequence of drug therapy. It is important for the client to continue to self-monitor during drug therapy, but that choice by itself does not answer the question. **Cognitive Level:** Applying **Client Need:** Physiological Adaptation **Integrated Process:** Nursing Process: Data Collection **Content Area:** Adult Health **Strategy:** The question is asking about data collection, the first part of the nursing process. Inspection of the client's body for other bruising and discolorations should be the first part of care. The other options are all subjective data and can be gathered as a unit after inspecting the client's body.

19 **Answer: 3 Rationale:** The target range for hematocrit with epoetin alfa therapy is 30–36%. A client who is taking Epogen must be monitored closely, to prevent adverse side effects that can occur because of either a rapid increase or high-level hematocrit. Bone pain is seen in response to administration, and is not an indicator of effective drug management. Rapid or increased hematocrit levels can cause the client to develop seizures and hypertension. Fever is seen in response to administration, and is not an indicator of effective drug management. **Cognitive Level:** Analyzing **Client Need:** Pharmacological and Parenteral Therapies **Integrated Process:** Nursing Process: Evaluation **Content Area:** Adult Health **Strategy:** Recall knowledge of client responses to the medication to choose correctly. If this was difficult, review the acceptable client responses to the medication.

20 **Answer: 2 Rationale:** Teach the client that the activity in which he is engaged might be causing the chest pain. Instruct the client in the exact method of taking NTG to avoid dizziness. NTG becomes unstable when exposed to heat, light, and moisture. The client can take up to 3 tablets, one at a time every 5 minutes, and shouldn't drive for safety reasons. The frequency of the medication must be accurate and specific to prevent overdose, as could happen with these instructions. **Cognitive Level:** Applying **Client Need:** Pharmacological and Parenteral Therapies **Integrated Process:** Nursing Process: Implementation **Content Area:** Adult Health **Strategy:** The question is referring to safe and effective administration of the medication. The options are all interventions, so in order to select the correct answer, recall knowledge of the correct administration of the medication.

Key Terms to Review

activated partial thromboplastin time (APTT) p. 520
afterload p. 504
anticoagulants p. 518
automaticity p. 506
chronotropic p. 506
clotting cascade p. 518
conductivity p. 508
contractility p. 512
dromotropic p. 506
dysrhythmia p. 512
extrinsic pathway p. 518
fibrinolysis p. 525
fibrinolytic system p. 522
hemostatics p. 525
heparin-induced platelet aggregation (HITT) p. 520
hypercoagulation p. 526
inotropic p. 506
international normalized ratio (INR) p. 518
intrinsic pathway p. 519
irritability p. 506
low molecular weight heparin (LMWH) p. 519
pernicious anemia p. 527
pica p. 526
preload p. 504
protamine sulfate p. 520
prothrombin time (PT) p. 518
refractory period p. 514
thrombolytics p. 522
titrate p. 505

References

Adams, M., Holland, L., & Urban, C. (2011). *Pharmacology for nurses: A pathophysiological approach* (3rd ed.). Upper Saddle River, NJ: Pearson Education, Inc.

Adams, M., & Koch, R. (2010). *Pharmacology: Connections to nursing practice.* Upper Saddle River, NJ: Pearson Education, Inc.

Berman, A., & Snyder, S. (2012). *Kozier & Erb's fundamentals of nursing: Concepts, process, and practice* (9th ed.). Upper Saddle River, NJ: Pearson Education, Inc.

Deglin, J. H., & Vallerand, A. H. (2011). *Davis's drug guide for nurses* (12th ed.). Philadelphia: F. A. Davis.

Lehne, R. (2010). *Pharmacology for nursing care* (7th ed.). Philadelphia: W. B. Saunders.

Wilson, B., Shannon, M., & Shields, K. (2012). *Pearson nurse's drug guide 2012.* Upper Saddle River, NJ: Pearson Education.

Test Yourself

Are you ready for the NCLEX-PN® or course exams? Use the practice tests on the companion website to check.

35 Neurological and Musculoskeletal Medications

In this chapter

Cross Reference

Other chapters relevant to this content area are

Dosage Calculation and Medication Administration	Chapter 28
Psychiatric Medications	Chapter 32
Neurological Disorders	Chapter 53
Musculoskeletal Disorders	Chapter 57

I. ANALGESICS

A. Opioids

1. Used to relieve severe acute and chronic pain
2. Produce effects by binding to opioid receptors in CNS and peripheral tissues
3. Are labeled controlled substances by Food and Drug Administration (FDA)
4. Cross blood–brain and placental barriers and also into breast milk
5. Common medications are listed in Table 35–1
6. Administration considerations

NCLEX®

a. Use caution because of possibility of dependence

b. Determine client's pattern of use if long term; be aware that some opioids are used as street drugs

c. May increase intracranial pressure (ICP)

d. Closely monitor clients with severe heart, liver, or kidney disease or respiratory or seizure disorders

e. Decrease dosages for older adults or debilitated clients

NCLEX®

f. Additional CNS depression can occur if used with barbiturates, other narcotics, hypnotics, antipsychotics, or alcohol

7. Side/adverse effects

a. Nausea and vomiting (N/V), anorexia

NCLEX®

b. Sedation, respiratory or circulatory depression

Memory Aid

Remember that opioid analgesics are CNS depressants; watch for sedation as an early sign and respiratory rate decrease as a later sign of CNS depression.

c. Constipation, gastrointestinal (GI) cramps, urinary retention, oliguria
d. Pruritis, light-headedness, dizziness, increased ICP

8. Nursing considerations
NCLEX® a. Determine pain type, intensity (pain scale), and location prior to administration
NCLEX® b. Note respiratory rate, depth, and rhythm; if less than 12, withhold medication
c. Monitor for CNS changes, including changes in level of consciousness (LOC); monitor vital signs (VS) regularly
NCLEX® d. Check for allergic reaction such as rash or urticaria
e. Administer opioids for pain and antiemetics for N/V
f. Monitor therapeutic response and maintain comfort

NCLEX® 9. Client teaching
a. Avoid other CNS depressants while using opioids
b. Use caution in ambulation, and avoid smoking, driving, and strenuous activities without assistance until drug response is known
c. Report any CNS changes, allergic reactions, or shortness of breath
d. If using medication on a long-term basis, be aware of withdrawal symptoms, including N/V, cramps, fever, faintness, and anorexia

B. Opioid antagonists

1. Include naloxone (Narcan) and naltrexone (ReVia)
2. Compete with opioids at opiate receptor sites, blocking opioid effects
NCLEX® 3. Reverse respiratory depression induced by overdose of opioids, pentazocine, and propoxyphene
4. Onset of effect is 1 to 2 minutes, duration is 45 minutes; assess client because CNS depression could recur when drug wears off
5. Side/adverse effects
NCLEX® a. Reversal of analgesia
b. Increased or decreased blood pressure (BP), tachycardia, hyperpnea, N/V
c. Tremors, drowsiness, nervousness, convulsions
d. Ventricular tachycardia and fibrillation, pulmonary edema
6. Nursing considerations
NCLEX® a. Measure VS every 3 to 5 minutes, and cardiac status (tachycardia, hypertension)
b. Monitor arterial blood gases (ABGs) and respiratory function (rate, rhythm)
c. Monitor electrocardiogram (ECG)
NCLEX® d. Administer only with resuscitative equipment nearby
e. Monitor therapeutic response, LOC, and need to reverse respiratory depression

Table 35–1 Common Opioid Analgesics

Type	Generic/Trade Names
Pure agonists (no ceiling effect, increase in analgesia with increase in dose)	Codeine (Paveral) Hydrocodone bitartrate (Vicodin) Oxycodone (Oxycontin) Morphine sulfate (generic, Duramorph) Fentanyl (Sublimaze) Oxymorphone (Opana) Hydromorphone (Dilaudid) Meperidine (Demerol) Methadone (Dolophine) Levorphanal tartrate (Levo-dromoran)
Mixed agonists-antagonists (have ceiling effect)	Pentazocine hydrochloride (Talwin) Butorphanol tartrate (Stadol) Buprenorphine (Buprenex) Nalbuphine hydrochloride (Nubain)

C. Nonopioids

1. Acetylsalicylic acid (ASA), or aspirin
   a. Inhibits prostaglandins involved in producing inflammation, pain, and fever
   b. Blocks pain impulses in CNS and provides relief of mild to moderate pain
   c. Antipyretic action results from vasodilation of peripheral vessels
   d. Powerfully inhibits platelet aggregation
   NCLEX® e. Check for allergy to salicylates prior to administration
   f. Decrease gastric irritation by administering with full glass of water, milk, food, or antacid, or by using an enteric-coated preparation
   NCLEX® g. Side/adverse effects include visual changes, tinnitus, hepatotoxicity, allergic reactions and bleeding; instruct client to report these
   h. Instruct client not to combine with other OTC medications that also contain ASA and avoid alcohol ingestion to decrease risk of GI bleeding
   NCLEX® i. Warn client that ASA should not be given to children or teens with flu-like or chickenpox symptoms (can lead to Reye's syndrome, characterized by encephalopathy and fatty liver degeneration)
2. Acetaminophen (Tylenol)
   a. Used for mild to moderate pain or fever, especially when ASA or nonsteroidal anti-inflammatory drugs (NSAIDs) are not tolerated; blocks pain impulses peripherally
   b. Antipyretic action occurs by inhibiting prostaglandins in CNS, resulting in peripheral vasodilation, sweating, and dissipation of heat
   NCLEX® c. Do not use if allergic to acetaminophen or phenacetin
   d. Avoid use in anemia or hepatic diseases, including alcoholism, malnutrition, or thrombocytopenia
   NCLEX® e. May cause **hepatotoxicity** at doses greater than 4 grams/day with chronic use; assess for dark urine, clay-colored stools, yellowing of skin or sclera, itching, abdominal pain, fever, and diarrhea, especially if on long-term therapy
   NCLEX® f. Prepare to administer acetylcysteine (Mucomyst) as antidote for acetaminophen poisoning
   g. Monitor client for therapeutic response, such as decreased pain or fever
3. NSAIDs
   a. Decrease prostaglandin synthesis by inhibiting an enzyme needed for biosynthesis
   b. Used for mild to moderate pain, osteo- or rheumatoid arthritis, and dysmenorrhea
   c. Common medications are listed in Box 35–1
   d. Decrease gastric irritation by administering with full glass of water or milk or with food
   e. Give dose at least 30 minutes prior to planned activity to minimize discomfort
   NCLEX® f. Contraindicated with asthma, severe renal or hepatic disease, GI bleeding, bleeding disorders, peptic ulcer disease, anemia, or anticoagulant therapy
   NCLEX® g. Instruct client to report blurred vision, ringing or roaring in ears; may indicate toxicity
   h. Monitor for therapeutic response, including decreased pain, stiffness in joints, decreased swelling in joints, ability to move more easily; may take up to 1 month

D. Medications to treat headaches

1. Aimed at prevention with prophylactic therapy and acute symptomatic treatment during attack
   a. Ergot alkaloids and triptans are serotonin receptor agonists; triptans are thought to act by constricting certain intracranial blood vessels and are used first; ergot alkaloids are used for migraine headaches unresponsive to triptans; ergot dose should be separated from triptan dose by at least 24 hours

Box 35–1

Common Nonsteroidal Anti-Inflammatory Agents

Celecoxib (Celebrex)	Meclofenate (generic)
Diclofenac (Voltaren)	Mefenemic acid (Ponstel)
Diflunisal (Dolobid)	Meloxicam (Mobic)
Etodolac (Lodine)	Nabumetone (Relafen)
Fenoprofen (Nalfon)	Naproxen (Naprosyn)
Flurbiprofen (Ansaid)	Oxaprozin (Daypro)
Ibuprofen (Advil, others)	Piroxicam (Feldene)
Indomethacin (Indocin)	Sulindac (Clinoril)
Ketoprofen (Actron)	Tolmetin (Tolectin)
Ketorolac (Toradol)	

b. Prophylaxis for migraine headaches includes beta-adrenergic blockers and antiepileptics
c. Mild analgesics and muscle relaxants are first-line medications for tension-type headaches; antidepressants may be used with counseling; ASA, acetaminophen, and ibuprofen are used for pain; amitriptyline (Elavil) is helpful for muscle contraction pain
d. Preventative therapies for cluster headaches may include high-dose calcium channel blockers, lithium, methysergide, or corticosteroids

2. Common medications are listed in Box 35–2

NCLEX®
3. Administration considerations
 a. For abortive treatment medications, take early in headache to be effective
 b. Start with dose that was effective on last headache at start of this headache
 c. Contraindicated with hypersensitivity to ergot alkaloids, pregnancy, cardiovascular disease, coronary artery disease, hypertension, sepsis, or severe pruritus

4. Nursing considerations
 a. Carefully assess history, including past treatments that were effective
 NCLEX® b. Monitor for medication-specific side effects as well as efficacy of treatment
 c. Provide a quiet and low-light environment
 d. Obtain accurate dietary history to determine if onset of headache is associated with certain foods
 e. Avoid prolonged medication use
 NCLEX® f. Beware of ergotamine rebound or an increase in frequency and duration of headache

5. Client teaching
 NCLEX® a. Identify triggers for headaches and how to ameliorate them
 b. Keep a headache diary
 c. Use stress reduction, stress management, lifestyle changes, including diet, to minimize headaches
 d. Do not eat, drink, or smoke while tablet is dissolving (if using sublingual tablet)
 e. Avoid prolonged exposure to cold weather (may increase adverse reactions to medication)
 f. Do not increase dose without consulting prescriber
 NCLEX® g. Use comfort measures during attack, such as lying in darkened, quiet room with cold compresses applied to head

Box 35–2

Medications Used to Treat Headaches

Ergot Alkaloids	Frovatriptan (Frova)
Dihydroergotamine (Migranal)	Naratriptan (Amerge)
Ergotamine (Ergostat)	Rizatriptan (Maxalt)
Triptans	Sumatriptan (Imitrex)
Almotriptan (Axert)	Zolmitriptan (Zomig)
Eletriptan (Relpax)	

II. ANTIEPILEPTICS

A. Hydantoins

1. Inhibit spread of seizure activity in motor cortex
2. Used in general **tonic-clonic seizures** (grand mal seizures), **status epilepticus seizures** (seizures that last longer than 4 minutes), and **psychomotor seizures** (complex focal seizures)
3. Common medications are listed in Table 35–2
4. Administration considerations
 a. Fosphenytoin should only be given IV for status epilepticus in emergency department or critical care area; monitor respiratory rate, BP, and ECG
 b. Do not interchange chewable phenytoin products with capsules
 NCLEX® c. Phenytoin readily binds with protein, so do not give with gastric feedings, which inhibit uptake
 d. Do not crush tablets or capsules of valproate sodium; take whole
 e. Contraindicated with hypersensitivity, pregnancy, bradycardia, SA and AV node block, Stokes-Adams syndrome, hepatic failure
5. Side/adverse effects
 NCLEX® a. Drowsiness, dizziness, insomnia, **paresthesias** (abnormal sensations), depression, suicidal tendencies, aggression, headache, confusion, slurred speech
 NCLEX® b. **Nystagmus** (involuntary oscillation of eye), **diplopia** (double vision), blurred vision

Table 35–2 Antiepileptics

Type	Generic (Trade) Names
Hydantoins	Fosphenytoin sodium (Cerebyx), phenytoin (Dilantin)
Iminostilbenes	Carbamazepine (Tegretol), oxcarbazepine (Trileptal)
Succinimides	Ethosuximide (Zarontin), methsuximide (Celontin), phensuximide (Milontin)
Benzodiazepines	Clonazepam (Klonopin), clorazepate (Tranxene), diazepam (Valium), lorazepam (Ativan), midazolam (Versed)
Barbiturates	Amobarbital (Amytal), mephobarbital (Mebaral), phenobarbital (Luminal), primidone (Mysoline)
Miscellaneous	Felbamate (Felbatol), gabapentin (Neurontin), lamotrigine (Lamictal), levetiracetam (Keppra), pregabalin (Lyrica), tiagabine (Gabitril), valproic acid (Depakene), zonisamide (Zonegran)

NCLEX®
c. Constipation, anorexia, N/V, weight loss, hepatitis, jaundice, **gingival hyperplasia** (increased growth of gum tissue)
d. Urine discoloration
e. Rash, hirsutism, lupus erythematosus, **Stevens-Johnson syndrome** (an acute inflammatory skin disorder)
f. Toxicity: bone marrow suppression (agranulocytosis, leukopenia, aplastic anemia, thrombocytopenia), N/V, ataxia, diplopia, cardiovascular collapse, slurred speech, confusion

6. Nursing considerations

NCLEX®
a. Observe for seizure activity, including type, location, duration, and character; provide seizure precautions
b. Monitor cardiovascular status; monitor CBC with differential, platelet count, liver function tests, and calcium and magnesium levels
c. Monitor respiratory status for depression, rate, depth, and character of respirations

NCLEX®
d. Review complete blood count (CBC) for blood dyscrasias; also note any fever, sore throat, bruising, rash, and jaundice
e. Monitor client for therapeutic responses such as decreases in severity and number of seizures or decreased ventricular dysrhythmias
f. Monitor blood glucose (BG) with diabetes; phenytoin can cause loss of glycemic control

NCLEX®
g. Monitor results of serum drug levels to ensure they are in therapeutic range

Memory Aid

Therapeutic serum phenytoin levels are 10 to 20 mg/dL. Memorize this value because it is an important one to know in practice and in test situations.

7. Client teaching
a. Carry Medic-Alert bracelet stating medication use
b. Urine may turn pink or red-brown but this is expected

NCLEX®
c. Perform proper brushing of teeth with soft toothbrush and proper flossing to prevent gingival hyperplasia; maintain routine or more frequent dental exams
d. Do not change brands of medication once seizure activity has stabilized; bioavailability differs among formulations

B. Barbiturates

1. Decrease impulse transmission to cerebral cortex
2. Can be used in all forms of **epilepsy**, a chronic disorder characterized by recurring seizures; however, they have been largely replaced by newer drugs as first-line agents because of CNS depressant effects
3. Common medications are listed in Table 35–2
4. Administration considerations
a. If ordered by intramuscular (IM) route, inject into large muscle mass to prevent tissue sloughing; use less than 5 mL/site
b. When ordered IV, give slowly (after dilution) at a rate of 65 mg or less per minute
5. Contraindicated with hypersensitivity, pregnancy, porphyria, and liver disease

6. Side/adverse effects
   NCLEX® a. Paradoxical excitement (older adults), drowsiness, lethargy, hangover headache, flushing, hallucinations
   b. Diarrhea, constipation, N/V
   c. Rash, urticaria, local pain or swelling or necrosis, Stevens-Johnson syndrome, angioedema, thrombophlebitis
7. Nursing considerations
   NCLEX® a. Monitor mental status for changes in mood, sensorium, affect, and memory (long and short term)
   b. Observe for respiratory depression
   c. Monitor for blood dyscrasias, fever, sore throat, bruising, rash, and jaundice
   NCLEX® d. Observe for seizure activity, including type, duration, and precipitating factors
   e. Obtain routine blood studies and liver function tests during long-term treatment
   f. Evaluate for therapeutic responses such as decreased seizures or increased sedation
8. Client teaching
   NCLEX® a. Avoid use of other CNS depressants; carry Medic-Alert bracelet stating medication use
   NCLEX® b. Avoid hazardous activities until stabilized on drug; drowsiness may occur
   c. Therapeutic effects may not be seen for 2 to 3 weeks

C. Succinimides

1. Inhibit spike and wave formation in absence seizures (petit mal), although recent research questions actual mechanism of action; may be used as one element of drug therapy for other types of seizures
2. Common medications are listed in Table 35–2
3. Administration considerations: give with food or milk to decrease GI symptoms; contraindicated with hypersensitivity
4. Side/adverse effects
   NCLEX® a. Drowsiness, dizziness, fatigue, euphoria, lethargy
   b. Anorexia, N/V, diarrhea, and abdominal pain
   NCLEX® c. Pink urine
   d. Urticaria, pruritic erythema, Stevens-Johnson syndrome
   e. Myopia, blurred vision
   NCLEX® f. Toxicity: bone marrow depression, ataxia, diplopia, and cardiovascular collapse
5. Nursing considerations
   a. Monitor mental status for changes in mood, sensorium, affect, and behavior
   NCLEX® b. Monitor periodically renal studies (urinalysis, blood urea nitrogen [BUN], creatinine), CBC, and liver function test
   c. Monitor for eye problems; may need regular ophthalmic exams
   d. Check for allergic reactions such as red, raised rash or exfoliative dermatitis
   NCLEX® e. Monitor for fever, sore throat, bruising, rash, or jaundice
6. Client teaching
   a. Carry ID card or Medic-Alert bracelet with medication, client's name, physician's name, and phone number
   NCLEX® b. Avoid driving and other activities that require alertness; avoid alcohol ingestion and other CNS depressants because they may increase sedation

D. Benzodiazepines

1. Enhance inhibitory neurotransmitter gamma-aminobutyric acid (GABA) to decrease anxiety and only as an adjunct for seizure activity
2. Used to treat delirium tremens; diazepam and lorazepam are used to treat status epilepticus; clonazepam, clorazepate, and midazolam are used for specific types of seizures when other drugs are not effective
3. Common medications are listed in Table 35–2
4. Administration considerations
   a. Give with food or milk to reduce GI symptoms; give IV injection into large vein
   NCLEX® b. Can lead to dependency; monitor client's use
5. Contraindicated with hypersensitivity, acute narrow-angle glaucoma or psychosis, children younger than 6 months, liver disease (clonazepam), or during lactation (diazepam)
6. Side/adverse effects
   NCLEX® a. Dizziness, drowsiness, confusion, headache, fatigue, blurred vision
   NCLEX® b. Orthostatic hypotension, ECG changes, tachycardia, respiratory depression
   c. Constipation, dry mouth, rash, itching, neutropenia

7. Nursing considerations
   NCLEX® a. Measure BP (lying, standing), pulse; if systolic BP drops 20 mm Hg, withhold drug, notify physician because of orthostatic hypotension
   b. Monitor hepatic and renal function (AST, ALT, bilirubin, creatinine, high density lipoprotein), alkaline phosphatase
   c. Monitor mental status for changes in mood, sensorium, affect, memory (long and short term)
   d. Observe respiratory status for depression, rate, rhythm, depth
   e. Monitor for seizure activity, including type, duration, and precipitating factors
   f. Evaluate client for therapeutic responses such as reduced or absent seizure activity, anxiety
8. NCLEX® Client teaching: avoid other CNS depressants, including alcohol; avoid hazardous activities until stabilized on drug; drowsiness may occur

E. Iminostilbenes and miscellaneous drugs

1. Iminostilbenes consist of carbamazepine and oxcarbamazepine (see Table 35–2)
   a. Inhibit nerve impulses by limiting influx of sodium ions across cell membrane in motor cortex; have other actions not explained by this mechanism, including analgesic, anticholinergic, antidysrhythmic, antidepressant and sedative effects
   b. Used in tonic-clonic, complex-partial, and mixed seizures
   NCLEX® c. Give oral forms with food or milk to reduce GI symptoms
   d. When administered via NG tube, must be mixed with D_5W or NS and flushed with at least 100 mL solution afterwards
   e. Contraindicated with hypersensitivity to carbamazepine or tricyclic antidepressants (TCAs), bone marrow depression, and concurrent use of MAOIs
   NCLEX® f. Side/adverse effects are many and include drowsiness, dizziness, confusion, N/V, constipation, diarrhea, tinnitis, dry mouth, blurred vision, nystagmus, thrombocytopenia, agranulocytosis, neutropenia, paralysis, worsening of seizures, Stevens-Johnson syndrome, and possible fatal reaction with MAOIs
   g. Observe for seizure activity, including type, duration, and precipitating factors
   h. Monitor blood, hepatic, and renal studies
   i. Monitor mental status for changes in mood, sensorium, affect, and memory (long and short term)
   NCLEX® j. Check for eye problems; may need regular ophthalmic exams
   NCLEX® k. Monitor for blood dyscrasias, fever, sore throat, bruising, rash, or jaundice
   l. Monitor client for therapeutic response such as decreased or absent seizure activity
   NCLEX® m. Instruct client to avoid other CNS depressants and activities that cause additive drowsiness
   n. Inform client that urine may turn pink to brown
2. Valproic acid (miscellaneous agent)
   a. Increases levels of gamma-aminobutyric acid (GABA) in brain, which decreases seizure activity
   b. Used in simple (petit mal), complex (petit mal), absence, or mixed seizures; manic episodes associated with bipolar disorder and migraine headaches
   c. Do not crush tablets or capsules; take them whole; may give with food or milk to decrease GI symptoms
   d. Contraindicated with hypersensitivity, during pregnancy, and with hepatic disease
   e. Side/adverse effects include sedation, drowsiness, N/V, constipation, diarrhea, thrombocytopenia, leukopenia, lymphocytosis, hepatic failure, pancreatitis, toxic hepatitis
   f. Observe for seizure activity, including type, duration, and precipitating factors
   NCLEX® g. Monitor blood, hepatic, and renal function
   h. Monitor mental status for changes in mood, sensorium, affect, and memory (long and short term)
   i. Observe respiratory status for depression, (rate, rhythm, and depth)
   j. Monitor client for therapeutic response, such as decreased seizure activity
   NCLEX® k. Inform client that physical dependency may result from extended use
   NCLEX® l. Advise client to report visual disturbances, rash, diarrhea, light-colored stools, jaundice, or protracted vomiting to provider

III. CENTRAL NERVOUS SYSTEM (CNS) STIMULANTS

A. Anorexiants

1. Most act similarly to amphetamines, as indirect sympathomimetic amines with alpha- and beta-adrenergic activity
2. Used for **narcolepsy** (inability to stay awake during day), **attention deficit disorder** (ADD), **attention deficit/hyperactivity disorder** (ADHD), and in short-term adjunct to control obesity
3. Common medications are listed in Table 35–3

4. Administration considerations
NCLEX® a. Anorexiant effects are temporary
b. To avoid insomnia, take 6 hours prior to bedtime
NCLEX® c. Do not abruptly discontinue medication
5. Contraindicated with hypersensitivity, angle-closure glaucoma, advanced cardiac disease, hyperthyroidism, agitated states, history of drug abuse, and children under 12 years
6. Side/adverse effects
a. Restlessness, insomnia, decrease in seizure threshold in epilepsy
b. Palpitations and tachycardia
c. Dysmenorrhea
NCLEX® 7. Nursing considerations
a. Monitor BP and pulse during treatment
b. Current dosage of antihypertensives and antidiabetics may need to be adjusted
c. Evaluate client for therapeutic response such as decrease in weight over time
8. Client teaching
a. Discuss all current medications (including OTC) with provider; serious or fatal interactions can occur
b. Avoid driving or other hazardous activities until drug effect is determined

B. Amphetamines

1. Increase release of norepinephrine and dopamine in cerebral cortex to reticular activating system
2. Used in treating narcolepsy, exogenous obesity, ADD
3. Common medications are listed in Table 35–3
4. Administration considerations
NCLEX® a. Give first dose on awakening and last dose no closer than 6 hours before bedtime
b. Administer on empty stomach 30 to 60 minutes before meal
5. Contraindicated with hypersensitivity, hyperthyroidism, hypertension, glaucoma, severe arteriosclerosis, drug abuse, cardiovascular disease, anxiety, and lactation
NCLEX® 6. Side/adverse effects
a. Hyperactivity, insomnia, restlessness, talkativeness
b. Dry mouth, N/V, impotence, change in libido, palpitations, tachycardia
7. Nursing considerations
NCLEX® a. Monitor VS, especially BP, since anorexiants may reverse antihypertensive medication action
b. Monitor CBC, urinalysis, and in diabetics, BG; changes in insulin may be required
c. Monitor mental status for mood, sensorium, and affect; stimulation, insomnia, or aggressiveness may occur
d. Observe for withdrawal symptoms: headache, N/V, muscle pain, weakness
NCLEX® e. Monitor client for therapeutic responses such as decreased activity in ADHD, absence of sleeping during day in narcolepsy, decrease in weight

Table 35–3 CNS Stimulants and Other Drugs for Narcolepsy and Attention Deficit Hyperactivity Disorder (ADHD)

Type	Generic (Trade) Names	Use
Amphetamines and amphetamine-like drugs	Benzphetamine (Didrex)	Weight loss
	Diethylpropion (Propion)	Weight loss
	Amphetamine sulfate (Adderall)	Narcolepsy, weight loss
	Methylphenidate (Ritalin)	Narcolepsy, ADHD
	Dexmethylphenidate (Focalin)	ADHD
	Dextroamphetamine (Dexadrine)	Narcolepsy, ADHD
	Lisdexamphetamine (Vyvanse)	ADHD
Non-stimulant for ADHD	Atomoxetine (Strattera)	ADHD
Other drugs for narcolepsy	Armadafinil (Nuvagil)	Narcolepsy
	Modafinil (Provigil)	Narcolepsy
	Sodium oxybate (Xyrem)	Narcolepsy

8. Client teaching
    a. Understand the importance of rest
    b. Avoid or decrease caffeine intake (coffee, tea, cola, chocolate); may increase irritability or stimulation

NCLEX®

C. Medications to treat narcolepsy and ADHD

1. Affect norepinephrine and dopamine have varying mechanisms of action to exert intended effects
2. Administer medication at least 6 hours before bedtime (NCLEX®)
3. Common medications are listed in Table 35–3
4. Many are contraindicated with hypersensitivity, anxiety, history of Tourette's syndrome, children under 6 years, and glaucoma
5. Increased stimulation and increased amine effect occurs with caffeine
6. Side/adverse effects vary but commonly include irritability, headache, dizziness, drowsiness, insomnia, nausea (NCLEX®)
7. Nursing considerations
    a. Measure VS, especially BP, since reversal of antihypertensive drug effects may occur
    b. Monitor CBC, urinalysis, and in diabetics, monitor closely BG; changes in insulin may be required
    c. Monitor mental status for changes in mood, sensorium, and affect; stimulation, insomnia, and aggressiveness may occur
    d. Observe for withdrawal symptoms: headache, N/V, muscle pain, weakness
    e. Monitor client for changes in appetite, sleep, speech patterns (NCLEX®)
    f. Observe client for increased attention span and decreased hyperactivity (NCLEX®)
    g. Monitor client for therapeutic responses such as decreased activity in ADHD, absence of sleeping during day in narcolepsy, or decrease in weight
8. Client education (NCLEX®)
    a. Avoid or decrease caffeine intake (coffee, tea, cola, chocolate); may increase irritability or stimulation
    b. Avoid hazardous activities until stabilized on drug; drowsiness may occur
    c. Seizure threshold is decreased in clients with seizure disorders

Memory Aid

Foods or beverages containing caffeine or theobromine (coffee, tea, cola, chocolate), which are CNS stimulants, are often contraindicated with medications that affect the CNS.

IV. ANTIPARKINSONIAN MEDICATIONS

A. Anticholinergics

1. Block or compete at central acetylcholine receptor sites in autonomic nervous system (ANS)
2. Used to decrease involuntary movements in parkinsonism
3. Common medications are listed in Table 35–4
4. Administration considerations
    a. Parenteral dose of trihexyphenidyl is given with client in recumbent position to prevent postural hypotension; oral form is given with or after food to prevent GI upset; may give with fluids other than water
    b. Parenteral dose of benztropine is given slowly; keep client at rest at least 1 hour after administering medication and monitor VS
    c. Monitor drug dosage carefully; even slight overdose can lead to toxicity (NCLEX®)
5. Contraindicated for clients with narrow-angle glaucoma, myasthenia gravis, or GI obstruction
6. Side/adverse effects: dry mouth, constipation, paralytic ileus, urinary retention or hesitancy, headache or dizziness
7. Nursing considerations (NCLEX®)
    a. Monitor intake and output (I&O); retention may cause decreased urine output; assess for urinary hesitancy and retention; palpate bladder if retention occurs
    b. Monitor for constipation; increase fluids, bulk, and exercise to counteract this
    c. If tolerance occurs during long-term therapy, dose may need to be increased or changed
    d. Assess mental status for affect, mood, CNS depression, worsening of mental symptoms during early therapy
    e. Evaluate client for therapeutic responses such as decreased tremors, secretions, absence of N/V
8. Client education: avoid driving, other hazardous activities or use of OTC cough and preparations with alcohol or antihistamines; drowsiness may occur (NCLEX®)

B. Medications affecting amount of dopamine in brain

1. Include levodopa, dopamine agonists, amantadine, and MAO type B inhibitors (see Table 35–4)
   a. L-dopa is the immediate, natural precursor of dopamine; replacement therapy with levodopa is most effective therapy for treating Parkinson's disease
   b. Catecholamine O-methyl transferase (COMT) inhibitors prevent destruction of levodopa in peripheral tissues, with same side effects as levodopa
   c. Amantadine (an antiviral) promotes the synthesis and release of dopamine
   d. Dopamine agonists (DA) directly stimulate specific subclasses of dopamine receptors
   e. MAO type B inhibitors (MAOBI) increase dopamine activity by an incompletely understood mechanism
   NCLEX® f. DAs and MAOBIs are used to enhance the effects of L-dopa
   g. All increase availability of dopamine, which reduces symptoms of Parkinson's disease
2. NCLEX® Administration considerations
   a. Administer dose after meals for better absorption and to decrease GI symptoms
   b. Give levodopa and selegiline with a low-protein snack or meal
3. Contraindicated with hypersensitivity, narrow-angle glaucoma, and undiagnosed skin lesions
4. Significant food interactions
   a. Decreased levodopa and selegiline absorption with high-protein foods
   NCLEX® b. With selegiline, tyramine-containing foods may increase hypertensive reactions
5. Side/adverse effects
   a. Dry mouth, N/V, and constipation
   b. Dizziness, headache, depression, and cough
   c. Cardiac dysrhythmias and orthostatic hypotension
   NCLEX® d. Sleep disturbance, "on-off" phenomenon
   NCLEX® e. Amantadine: seizures, congestive heart failure (CHF), leukopenia
   f. Levodopa: hemolytic anemia, leukopenia, agranulocytosis
   g. DAs: seizures, shock
   h. MAOBIs: tachycardia or sinus bradycardia
   NCLEX® i. Levodopa toxicity: mental or personality changes, increased twitching, grimacing, tongue protrusion
6. Nursing considerations
   a. Measure BP and respirations
   b. Observe mental status for affect, mood, behavioral changes, depression; complete a suicide assessment
   NCLEX® c. Monitor for involuntary movement, akinesia, tremors, staggering gait, muscle rigidity, and drooling
   NCLEX® d. Monitor for therapeutic responses such as decreased akathisia and increased mood
7. Client education
   NCLEX® a. Change positions slowly to prevent orthostatic hypotension
   b. Report side effects such as twitching and eye spasm; may indicate overdose
   NCLEX® c. Never discontinue drugs abruptly because this may precipitate parkinsonian crisis
   NCLEX® d. Do not take medication with foods high in protein

V. MEDICATIONS TO TREAT ALZHEIMER'S DISEASE

A. Action and use: reversible cholinesterase inhibitors raise acetylcholine level in cerebral cortex by slowing degradation of acetylcholine released in cholinergic neurons; memantine is an N–methyl–O–aspartate receptor antagonist

B. Common medications are listed in Box 35–3

Table 35–4 Medications Used to Treat Parkinson's Disease

Type	Generic (Trade) Names
Anticholinergics	Trihexyphenidyl hydrochloride (generic), benztropine mesylate (Cogentin)
Dopamine replacement drugs	Levodopa/carbidopa (Sinemet), levodopa (L-dopa, Larodopa)
Dopamine agonists	Apomorphine (generic), bromocriptine (Parlodel), pramipexole (Mirapex), ropinirole (Requip), rotigotine (Neupro)
COMT inhibitors	Entacapone (Comtan), tolcapone (Tasmar)
Miscellaneous drugs	Amantadine (Symmetrel), seligeline (Eldepryl)

C. Administration considerations

NCLEX® 1. Administer dose between meals; may give with meal to reduce GI symptoms
2. Adjust dosage to response no more frequently than every 6 weeks

D. Contraindications: hypersensitivity to drug or development of jaundice when taking drug

E. Side/adverse effects

NCLEX® 1. Insomnia, headache, dizziness, confusion, ataxia, anxiety, depression, hostility, and abnormal thinking
2. Constipation, diarrhea, N/V, and abdominal pain
3. Urinary frequency and incontinence
4. Rhinitis or cough; rash; seizures or hepatotoxicity

F. Nursing considerations

NCLEX® 1. Monitor BP for hypotension or hypertension
2. Monitor mental status for affect, mood, behavioral changes, depression, hallucinations, confusion; complete a suicide assessment
3. Monitor GI status for side effects; monitor liver function test results
4. Monitor client for urinary frequency and incontinence
5. Monitor for therapeutic responses such as decreased confusion, improved mood

G. Client teaching

NCLEX® 1. Report side effects such as twitching, nausea, vomiting, sweating; they might indicate overdose
2. Dose may be taken with food to decrease GI upset
NCLEX® 3. Medication is not a cure; it only relieves symptoms

Box 35–3

Medications Used to Treat Alzheimer's Disease

Donepezil hydrochloride (Aricept)	Rivastigmine (Exelon)
Galantamine (Razadyne)	Tacrine (Cognex)
Memantine (Namenda)	

VI. MEDICATIONS TO TREAT MYASTHENIA GRAVIS (MG)

A. Actions and use

1. Inhibit breakdown of acetylcholine (Ach) at myoneural junction via acetylcholinesterase (AchE); used to treat muscle weakness associated with MG
NCLEX® 2. Edrophonium (Tensilon) is used to diagnose MG
3. As symptoms worsen over time, AchE inhibitors alone may not be effective and corticosteroids may be added (for immunosuppressant effect)

B. Common medications are listed in Box 35–4

C. Administration considerations

1. Administer prior to mealtimes for optimal absorption
NCLEX® 2. Administer doses on time to prevent muscle weakness from impairing ability to chew food and swallow medications

NCLEX® **D. Use of edrophonium (Tensilon) as diagnostic aid**

1. Tensilon test consists of giving a dose by IV injection
2. Aids in diagnosis of MG in an undiagnosed client or myasthenic crisis (undermedication) in a diagnosed client; positive findings noted when muscle tone improves within 30–60 seconds following dose, and improved muscle strength lasts 4–5 minutes (positive Tensilon test)
3. Diagnosis of cholinergic crisis (often caused by overmedication) in a diagnosed client is made when muscle strength does not improve after Tensilon injection, and symptoms may worsen (negative Tensilon test)
NCLEX® 4. Keep atropine sulfate on hand as antidote

E. Contraindications: bowel obstruction or other conditions with GI motility, or urinary tract obstruction

Box 35–4

Medications Used to Treat Myasthenia Gravis

Edrophonium (Tensilon, Enlon)	Pyridostigmine (Mestinon)
Neostigmine (Prostigmin)	Ambenonium chloride (Mytelase)

NCLEX® **F. Side/adverse effects**

1. Increased bronchial secretions, sweating, drooling, and urge to urinate
2. Pinpoint pupils and eye watering, N/V, diarrhea

G. Nursing considerations

NCLEX® 1. Keep atropine sulfate on hand as antidote

NCLEX® 2. Keep equipment for respiratory support on hand; muscles of head, neck, and respiratory system are affected before muscles in the lower body

3. Observe client for weakness; if it begins 1 hour after drug dose, overdose or cholinergic crisis may be occurring; if it begins 3 or more hours after dose, myasthenic crisis (undermedication) may be occurring

NCLEX® 4. Observe for subtle changes in speech and facial expression, ptosis, and decreased ability to swallow as indicators that additional medication is needed

5. Monitor general neuromuscular strength, including gait and reflexes
6. Monitor VS, especially respirations, pulse, and BP

H. Client teaching

1. Report side effects such as twitching, N/V, sweating; they might indicate overdose
2. Do not increase or abruptly decrease dose; serious consequences may result

NCLEX® 3. Medication is not a cure; it only relieves symptoms

VII. SKELETAL MUSCLE RELAXANTS

A. Direct acting skeletal muscle relaxants are often used to treat *spasticity* in conjunction with physical therapy; dantrolene (Dantrium) is only drug in its class used for this purpose; others are botulinum type A and B for cervical dystonia and type A only for wrinkles

1. Decrease synaptic responses at neurotransmitters to decrease frequency, severity of **spasms** (involuntary contractions of large muscles), and pain in musculoskeletal conditions
2. Reduce spasticity after spinal cord injury, stroke, and in cerebral palsy, multiple sclerosis; dantrolene is also used to treat malignant hyperthermia
3. Commonly used direct-acting drug is dantrolene (Dantrium), although centrally acting drugs such as baclofen (Lioresal) and tizanidine (Zanaflex) are also effective in treating spasticity (see Box 35–5)
4. Contraindicated in hypersensitivity and active hepatic disease, and should be used cautiously with impaired respiratory and cardiac function
5. Side/adverse effects
   a. Dizziness, weakness, fatigue, drowsiness
   b. Photosensitivity, tachycardia and erratic BP, urinary retention
   c. Hepatotoxicity
6. Nursing considerations

NCLEX® a. Monitor BP, weight, and hepatic function

   b. Measure I&O; check for urinary retention, or hesitancy
   c. Monitor for severe weakness or numbness in extremities

NCLEX® d. Observe for CNS depression, dizziness, drowsiness, or psychiatric symptoms

   e. Review results of liver and renal function studies

NCLEX® f. Monitor for therapeutic responses such as decreased pain or spasticity

NCLEX® 7. Client teaching

   a. Do not discontinue medication quickly; spasticity, tachycardia will occur; it should be tapered off gradually by prescriber
   b. Notify prescriber of abdominal pain, jaundiced sclera, clay-colored stools, or change in color of urine
   c. Do not break, crush, or chew capsules

Box 35–5

Skeletal Muscle Relaxants

Direct Acting Skeletal Muscle Relaxant

Dantrolene sodium (Dantrium)

Centrally Acting Skeletal Muscle Relaxants

Baclofen (Lioresal)

Carisoprodol (Soma)

Chlorzoxazone (Paraflex)

Cyclobenzaprine (Flexeril)

Metaxalone (Skelaxin)

Methocarbamol (Robaxin)

Orphenadrine (Banflex)

Tizanidine (Zanaflex)

B. Centrally acting skeletal muscle relaxants are often used to treat muscle spasms associated with inflammation and injury

1. Depress multisynaptic pathways in spinal cord, causing skeletal muscle relaxation and/or sedation; have no effect neuromuscular junction or muscle tissue
2. Used for adjunct relief of spasms in acute musculoskeletal conditions not associated with CNS disease
3. Common medications are listed in Box 35–5
4. NCLEX® Contraindicated in hypersensitivity, children under 12, intermittent porphyria, and use cautiously in thyroid disease and cardiac disease including myocardial infarction (MI), heart block, and CHF
5. Side/adverse effects
   - a. NCLEX® Dizziness, weakness, drowsiness, xerostomia
   - b. Edema of tongue and face with sweating, myalgia
   - c. Unpleasant taste, coated tongue with discoloration, vomiting, anorexia, diarrhea with flatulence
   - d. Angioedema, anaphylaxis
   - e. Orthostatic hypotension, tachycardia, syncope, palpitations, vasodilation
6. Nursing considerations
   - a. Periodically monitor results of blood studies (including CBC, WBC with differentials) and liver studies (including AST, ALT, alkaline phosphatase)
   - b. Monitor results of EEG in clients with seizures
   - c. NCLEX® Monitor for allergic reactions, including idiosyncratic reaction, anaphylaxis, rash, fever, and respiratory distress
   - d. Monitor for severe weakness or numbness in extremities
   - e. NCLEX® Observe for CNS depression, dizziness, drowsiness, and psychiatric symptoms
   - f. Monitor for therapeutic responses such as decreased pain, spasm, and spasticity
7. NCLEX® Client teaching
   - a. Do not discontinue medication abruptly; insomnia, nausea, headache, spasticity, tachycardia will occur
   - b. Avoid hazardous activities if drowsiness or dizziness occurs

Check Your NCLEX–PN® Exam I.Q.

You are ready for testing on this content if you can

- Apply knowledge of expected actions and effects of neurological and musculoskeletal medications to client care.
- Correctly administer neurological and musculoskeletal medications to clients.
- Monitor for side effects and adverse effects of neurological and musculoskeletal medications.
- Take appropriate action if a client has an unexpected response to a neurological or musculoskeletal medication.
- Monitor a client for expected outcomes or effects of treatment with neurological and musculoskeletal medications.

PRACTICE TEST

1 A client is receiving phenytoin (Dilantin) to control seizures. What statement by the client to the nurse indicates an understanding regarding administration of this medication?

1. "I need to take more of my Dilantin when I am having a stressful day."
2. "I will be able to stop taking this medicine in about a year."
3. "I will probably need to take this medicine all my life."
4. "I will never have another seizure if I take this medicine."

2 A client with a history of seizures is admitted with a partial occlusion of the left common carotid artery. The client has taken phenytoin (Dilantin) for 10 years. What is the most important nursing consideration when assisting with care planning for this client?

1. Obtain a history of seizure incidence.
2. Place an airway, suction, and restraints at the bedside.
3. Ask the client to remove any dentures.
4. Observe the client for increased restlessness and agitation.

3 A client with a history of seizures is scheduled for an arteriogram at 10:00 a.m., and is to have nothing by mouth before the test. The client is scheduled to receive a daily prescribed dose of phenytoin (Dilantin) at 9:00 a.m. What action should the nurse should take regarding this situation?

1. Omit the 9:00 a.m. dose.
2. Give the same dosage of the drug rectally.
3. Ask the physician if the drug can be given by another route.
4. Administer the drug with 30 mL of water at 9:00 a.m.

4 The nurse is monitoring a client with Parkinson's disease to determine the results of medication therapy. The nurse would determine that the medication is not working optimally if the client is demonstrating which characteristic?

1. A flattened affect
2. Tonic-clonic seizures
3. Decreased intelligence
4. Changes in pain tolerance

5 The client with Parkinson's disease asks the nurse, "How will levodopa treat this disease?" What action of levodopa should the nurse incorporate into a response?

1. Improves myelination of neurons
2. Increases acetylcholine production
3. Replaces dopamine in the brain cells
4. Causes regeneration of injured thalamic cells

6 A female client who takes medications for seizures has been placed on warfarin (Coumadin) for thrombophlebitis. After the weekly prothrombin time, the client mentions that she is out of her barbiturate sleeping pill and needs a refill. What is the most important reason that the nurse should instruct the client to obtain the refill immediately?

1. The client is at risk of developing withdrawal symptoms.
2. The absence of sleep could precipitate seizures.
3. Discontinuance of the drug can affect the prothrombin level.
4. Seizure control depends on the combined action of the medications.

7 A client is brought to the emergency department in the midst of a persistent tonic-clonic seizure. Diazepam (Valium) is administered intravenously. The nurse assisting in this client's care anticipates that in addition to decreasing central neuronal activity, what other effect of diazepam will be occurring?

1. Slowing of cardiac contractions
2. Relaxation of peripheral muscles
3. Dilation of tracheobronchial structures
4. Promoting amnesia of the seizure episode

8 The nurse would monitor for which symptoms of morphine overdose in a client receiving patient-controlled analgesia? Select all that apply.

1. A decrease in blood pressure and respiration rate
2. Dilated pupils and restlessness
3. Profuse sweating and a state of deep sleep
4. Constricted pupils and sedation
5. Lethargy and depressed reflexes

9 Levodopa is prescribed for a client with Parkinson's disease. What information should the nurse reinforce in the teaching plan for the client about levodopa?

1. It is poorly absorbed if given with meals.
2. It must be monitored by weekly laboratory tests.
3. It causes an initial euphoria, followed by depression.
4. It can cause a side effect of orthostatic hypotension.

10 When caring for the client who is receiving phenytoin (Dilantin), the nurse emphasizes meticulous oral hygiene to the client. This nursing intervention is based on the nurse's knowledge that phenytoin has what effect on oral tissue?

1. It causes hyperplasia of the gums.
2. It increases alkalinity of the oral secretions.
3. It erodes and destroys tooth enamel.
4. It promotes bacterial growth at the gum lines.

11 The physician prescribes phenobarbital sodium (Luminal) for a client who has had a tonic-clonic seizure. What statement indicates to the nurse that the client understands the side effects of phenobarbital? Select all that apply.

1. "I can expect a loss of appetite or persistent fatigue."
2. "I might feel lightheaded or off balance."
3. "Diarrhea accompanied by an anal itch is common."
4. "Decreased tolerance to common foods can occur."
5. "I should be aware of becoming depressed."

PRACTICE TEST

12. The nurse administering methylphenidate (Ritalin) is monitoring the client for side effects associated with this medication. Which finding would the nurse disregard as unrelated to this medication?

1. Insomnia
2. Fever
3. Rash
4. Palpitations

13. The nurse is reinforcing medication information to a client taking benztropine (Cogentin) for Parkinson's disease. Which client statement would indicate the need for additional instruction regarding this medication?

1. "I may crush the tablets to make them easier to take."
2. "I should not drive until I know how this medication will affect me."
3. "I can take OTC medications for a cough or cold."
4. "I should never discontinue the medication abruptly."

14. The nurse should include which item in data collection for the client with Alzheimer's disease who is receiving tacrine (Cognex)?

1. Blood pressure (BP), mental status, and gastrointestinal (GI) status
2. Hemoglobin (Hgb), white blood cells (WBCs), and liver function tests
3. Hgb, red blood cells (RBCs), and mental status
4. BP, electrolytes, and edema in legs

15. The client has migraine headaches. The provider has prescribed amitriptyline hydrochloride (Elavil) as prophylaxis for the headaches. The nurse would warn the client about what over-the-counter (OTC) medication, which might intensify the actions of Elavil?

1. Acetaminophen (Tylenol)
2. Aspirin (ASA)
3. Nonsteroidal anti-inflammatory drugs (NSAIDs)
4. Cimetidine (Tagamet HB)

16. When administering anticholinergic medications for Parkinson's disease, what finding should be of least concern to the nurse in regard to the medication?

1. Dry mouth
2. Constipation
3. Fever
4. Urinary retention or hesitancy

17. The client has been diagnosed with narcolepsy. The provider is considering prescribing methylphenidate (Ritalin). The nurse notes that the client has a history of which prior medical condition that would be a contraindication to using this medication?

1. Congestive heart failure (CHF)
2. Diabetes mellitus
3. Glaucoma
4. Hyperthyroidism

18. The client has just been diagnosed with a seizure disorder. The medication regimen has controlled the seizures for several days. Prior to discharge, the nurse should place highest priority on sharing which of the following information with the client?

1. Seizure disorders will often eventually stop on their own.
2. Adherence to medication therapy is essential to avoid recurrence of seizures.
3. Urine will turn pink or brown from the medication.
4. The client can never drive a vehicle again.

19. The client with a history of cluster headaches should be taught what information regarding use of ergotamine tartrate (Gynergen)?

1. "Take the medication every 4 hours."
2. "Take the medication with plenty of water."
3. "You will feel energetic and warm after taking the medication."
4. "Lie down in a darkened room after taking the medication."

20. The client is experiencing spasticity related to a spinal cord injury. The nurse anticipates that which medication will most likely be added to the client's medication list?

1. Dexamethasone (Decadron)
2. Dantrolene (Dantrium)
3. Dichlorphenamide (Daranide)
4. Dobutamine (Dobutrex)

21 The nurse is reinforcing information about anti-inflammatory medications, including aspirin, acetaminophen, and non-steroidal anti-inflammatory drugs (NSAIDs). The nurse should include which precautions in this discussion?

1. Take radial pulse and temperature prior to taking a dose of medication.
2. Consult a health care provider before taking over-the-counter (OTC) medications, since many are combinations that can include more of the prescribed medication than is safe.
3. Cholesterol levels must be measured prior to treatment with medication.
4. Do not discontinue use of medication abruptly; discontinuation must be tapered over a week.

22 The client is prescribed carbamazepine (Tegretol) for a seizure disorder. The nurse cautions the client to avoid taking which type of medications that could cause a fatal reaction with this medication?

1. Nonsteroidal anti-inflammatory drugs (NSAIDs)
2. Opioid analgesics
3. Skeletal muscle relaxants
4. Monoamine oxidase inhibitors (MAOIs)

23 The nurse is transcribing medication orders for a client taking selegiline (Eldepryl). The nurse makes it a priority to telephone the prescriber after noting an order for which type of medication?

1. Monoamine oxidase inhibitor (MAOI)
2. Opioid analgesic
3. Skeletal muscle relaxant
4. Anticholinergic

ANSWERS & RATIONALES

1 **Answer: 3** **Rationale:** Clients with seizure disorders rarely are able to stop taking the anticonvulsants. Extra doses of Dilantin are not taken in response to real or anticipated stress. There is no indication in this question whether medication therapy could be terminated near the one-year mark. The goal of taking Dilantin is to eliminate and/or control seizure activity; the use of the word *never* indicates a lack of understanding. **Cognitive Level:** Analyzing **Client Need:** Pharmacological and Parenteral Therapies **Integrated Process:** Nursing Process: Evaluation **Content Area:** Pharmacology **Strategy:** The wording of the question tells you that the correct answer is also a true statement. Use the process of elimination and medication knowledge to make a selection. Avoid selecting options that contain definitive terms such as *never*.

2 **Answer: 1** **Rationale:** Phenytoin (Dilantin) is an anti-epileptic most effective in controlling tonic-clonic seizures. Data collection before planning nursing care for a client with a seizure disorder should always include a history of seizure incidence. Putting an airway in place or restraining a client during a seizure could cause physical harm. Removal of dentures might be indicated during a seizure, but not at this time. Restlessness and agitation might be a prodromal phase in some clients, but a history of incidence is more important data. **Cognitive Level:** Analyzing **Client Need:** Pharmacological and Parenteral Therapies **Integrated Process:** Nursing Process: Planning **Content Area:** Pharmacology **Strategy:** The words *most important* in the stem of the question tell you that more than one, perhaps all options, might be correct and that you must choose the best option. Use medication knowledge as well as knowledge of how to manage a client during a seizure to eliminate any of the incorrect options.

3 **Answer: 3** **Rationale:** The therapeutic blood levels of the anti-epileptic need to be maintained. The nurse should question the physician about alternate routes of administration. Omission of a dose is not prudent; the nurse should contact the physician. Changing the route of medication is not appropriate without a physician order. Administering the drug is a violation of the physician's order related to the client's test; the physician should be contacted for alternative orders. **Cognitive Level:** Applying **Client Need:** Pharmacological and Parenteral Therapies **Integrated Process:** Nursing Process: Implementation **Content Area:** Pharmacology **Strategy:** The core issue of the question is how to maintain the client in a seizure-free state while NPO. Analyze each of the options to determine the method that will best protect the client from seizure activity and not violate the principles of medication administration.

4 **Answer: 1** **Rationale:** Destruction of the neurons of the basal ganglia in Parkinson's disease results in decreased muscle tone. This gives the face a masklike appearance, and causes a monotone speech pattern that can be interpreted as flat. If medication therapy was ineffective, the client would still exhibit symptoms of the disorder, such as flattened affect. Tonic-clonic seizures and decreased intelligence are not a common manifestation of Parkinson's disease. Clients with Parkinson's do not experience changes in their ability to tolerate pain. **Cognitive Level:** Applying **Client Need:** Pharmacological and Parenteral Therapies **Integrated Process:** Nursing Process: Data Collection **Content Area:** Pharmacology **Strategy:** The core issue of the question is the symptom that should be abolished

by medication therapy. Use medication knowledge and the process of elimination to make a selection.

5 **Answer: 3 Rationale:** Levodopa is the precursor of dopamine. It is converted to dopamine in the brain cells until needed as a neurotransmitter. The other options cannot be attributed to levodopa. **Cognitive Level:** Applying **Client Need:** Pharmacological and Parenteral Therapies **Integrated Process:** Communication and Documentation **Content Area:** Pharmacology **Strategy:** The wording of the question tells you that the correct option is also a true statement. Use medication knowledge and the process of elimination to make a selection.

6 **Answer: 3 Rationale:** Barbiturates decrease the body's response to warfarin (Coumadin). As a result, there is less suppression of prothrombin; when inhibition caused by barbiturates disappears, hemorrhage could result. Withdrawal symptoms are not a priority concern if the client just takes the barbiturate for sleep. Absence of sleep is not likely to result in seizure activity. Control of seizure activity is not dependent on combined use of phenytoin and the barbiturate sleep aid. **Cognitive Level:** Analyzing **Client Need:** Pharmacological and Parenteral Therapies **Integrated Process:** Nursing Process: Implementation **Content Area:** Pharmacology **Strategy:** The words *most important* in the stem of the question tell you that more than one or perhaps all options might be partially or totally correct, and that you must choose the most important option. The core issue of the question is knowledge of the interactive effects of barbiturates and warfarin.

7 **Answer: 2 Rationale:** Diazepam is a benzodiazepene tranquilizer and an anticonvulsant used to relax smooth muscles during seizures. Diazepam does not slow cardiac contractions. Diazepam does not dilate tracheobronchial structures. Diazepam does not promote amnesia of seizure activity. **Cognitive Level:** Applying **Client Need:** Pharmacological and Parenteral Therapies **Integrated Process:** Nursing Process: Planning **Content Area:** Pharmacology **Strategy:** The wording of the question tells you that the correct option is also a true effect of the medication. Use medication knowledge and the process of elimination to make a selection.

8 **Answer: 1, 4, 5 Rationale:** Morphine could lower blood pressure; its major adverse effect is respiratory depression. Morphine can cause pupillary constriction and sedation. Morphine can lead to lethargy and depressed reflexes. Morphine can lead to lethargy and pupillary constriction. Morphine does not produce profuse sweating; the state of sedation caused by morphine should not be confused with deep sleep. **Cognitive Level:** Analyzing **Client Need:** Pharmacological and Parenteral Therapies **Integrated Process:** Nursing Process: Evaluation **Content Area:** Pharmacology **Strategy:** Use specific medication knowledge and the process of elimination to make a selection. When there is more than one correct answer, consider each option as a true/false statement.

9 **Answer: 4 Rationale:** Levodopa is the precursor of dopamine. It reduces sympathetic outflow by limiting vasoconstriction, which can result in orthostatic hypotension. Levodopa should be administered with food to minimize gastric irritation. Levodopa is not monitored by weekly laboratory tests. Levodopa does not cause initial euphoria followed by depression. **Cognitive Level:** Applying **Client Need:** Pharmacological and Parenteral Therapies **Integrated Process:** Nursing Process: Planning **Content Area:** Pharmacology **Strategy:** The wording of the question indicates the correct option is also a true statement that would be included in client teaching. Use medication knowledge and the process of elimination to make a selection.

10 **Answer: 1 Rationale:** Gingival hyperplasia (over growth of gum tissue) is an adverse effect of long-term phenytoin (Dilantin) therapy. The other options are not side effects of phenytoin (Dilantin). **Cognitive Level:** Applying **Client Need:** Pharmacological and Parenteral Therapies **Integrated Process:** Nursing Process: Implementation **Content Area:** Pharmacology **Strategy:** The wording of the question tells you that the correct option is also a true statement that would be included in client teaching. Use medication knowledge and the process of elimination to make a selection.

11 **Answer: 1, 2, 5 Rationale:** Phenobarbital depresses the CNS, particularly the motor cortex, producing side effects such as lethargy and loss of appetite, and vertigo. It also depresses the CNS, particularly the motor cortex, producing side effects such as depression. Phenobarbital does not cause diarrhea or anal itching, nor does it cause a decreased tolerance to common foods or constipation. **Cognitive Level:** Applying **Client Need:** Pharmacological and Parenteral Therapies **Integrated Process:** Nursing Process: Evaluation **Content Area:** Pharmacology **Strategy:** Use medication knowledge and the process of elimination to make a selection. When there is more than one correct answer, consider each option as a true/false statement.

12 **Answer: 2 Rationale:** Fever is not a side effect of methylphenidate. The other options are possible side effects of methylphenidate. **Cognitive Level:** Applying **Client Need:** Pharmacological and Parenteral Therapies **Integrated Process:** Nursing Process: Data Collection **Content Area:** Pharmacology **Strategy:** Note that the stem of the question contains the word *not*, which indicates that the correct option is not an actual manifestation of the drug. Use knowledge of side/adverse medication effects to make a selection.

13 **Answer: 3 Rationale:** Many OTC cough and cold medications contain alcohol; medications with alcohol (another CNS depressant) should be avoided unless specifically directed by the provider. Cogentin may be crushed before administering the medication. Cogentin is a CNS depressant and the client should avoid activities such as driving until the effects of the medication are known. Cogentin should not be discontinued abruptly; it may precipitate a parkinsonian crisis. **Cognitive Level:** Analyzing **Client Need:** Pharmacological and Parenteral Therapies **Integrated Process:** Teaching and Learning **Content Area:** Pharmacology **Strategy:** Note that the question contains the words *more instruction*, which indicates that the correct answer option contains incorrect information. Use medication knowledge and the process of elimination to make a selection.

14 **Answer: 1 Rationale:** Tacrine (Cognex) increases the available acetylcholine in the brain; therefore, the parasympathetic system is stimulated. Blood pressure, mental status, and GI status would be affected. Hemoglobin, white blood cell count, and liver function do not relate to this medication. Hemoglobin and red blood cell count do not relate to this medication; however, mental status should be monitored. Blood pressure is an appropriate data collection item, but electrocyte balance and edema in legs do not relate to this medication. **Cognitive Level:** Applying **Client Need:** Pharmacological and Parenteral

Therapies **Integrated Process:** Nursing Process: Data Collection **Content Area:** Pharmacology **Strategy:** The wording of the question tells you that the correct option is also a true statement that would be included in client teaching. Use medication knowledge and the process of elimination to make a selection.

15 **Answer: 4** **Rationale:** Tagamet can increase the levels of Elavil in the blood, causing seizures, tachycardia, hypertension, or toxicity. The other options do not intensify the effect of Elavil. **Cognitive Level:** Applying **Client Need:** Pharmacological and Parenteral Therapies **Integrated Process:** Teaching and Learning **Content Area:** Pharmacology **Strategy:** Options that are similar are not likely to be correct. All of the incorrect options relate to analgesia, and so must be eliminated.

16 **Answer: 3** **Rationale:** Fever is not a side effect of anticholinergic medications; the presence of fever should be a concern, but it is not connected to the medication. The other options are possible side effects and should be noted by the nurse. **Cognitive Level:** Analyzing **Client Need:** Pharmacological and Parenteral Therapies **Integrated Process:** Nursing Process: Data Collection **Content Area:** Pharmacology **Strategy:** The critical words in the stem of the question are *least concerned*. This tells you that the correct answer is an option that is not characteristic of this medication. Use medication knowledge and the process of elimination to make a selection.

17 **Answer: 3** **Rationale:** Methylphenidate is a central nervous system stimulant. It increases the release of norepinephrine and dopamine in cerebral cortex to the reticular activating system. Ritalin is contraindicated in clients with glaucoma. Congestive heart failure does not represent a contraindication to the use of methylphenidate. Diabetes mellitus does not represent a contraindication to the use of methylphenidate. Hyperthyroidism does not represent a contraindication to the use of methylphenidate. **Cognitive Level:** Applying **Client Need:** Pharmacological and Parenteral Therapies **Integrated Process:** Nursing Process: Planning **Content Area:** Pharmacology **Strategy:** In order to select the correct answer to this question, recall knowledge of the contraindications for the medication. If this is difficult, review Ritalin and the contraindications for the medication.

18 **Answer: 2** **Rationale:** Medication must be taken to maintain therapeutic blood levels, even if there is no seizure activity. Seizures do not stop on their own; treatment must be continued. The urine might turn pink or brown, but that is not the most important item to teach. After 6 months with no seizures, a client can often drive again. **Cognitive Level:** Analyzing **Client Need:** Health Promotion and Maintenance **Integrated Process:** Nursing Process: Implementation **Content Area:** Adult Health **Strategy:** Note that the question asks for selection of the highest priority teaching option. The highest priority in teaching about medication is to adhere to the medication protocol.

19 **Answer: 4** **Rationale:** The client needs to give the medication the opportunity to work without aggravating the headache. Ergotamine should be given orally 1–2 mg, followed by 1–2 mg every 30 minutes until the headache abates or until the maximum dose of 6 mg/24 hours. It is unnecessary to drink large amounts of fluids. Increased warmth and energy are not associated with this medication. **Cognitive Level:** Applying **Client Need:** Pharmacological and Parenteral Therapies **Integrated Process:** Nursing Process: Implementation **Content Area:** Pharmacology **Strategy:** In looking at the stem, note that the client has cluster headaches. Understanding the disease process and usual treatment regimen, or knowing that a quiet darkened room will help clients obtain pain relief from cluster headaches, will lead to the correct answer.

20 **Answer: 2** **Rationale:** Dantrolene is a central-acting skeletal muscle relaxant. This medication may be used to control spasticity after spinal cord injury. Dexamethasone is a corticosteroid used to decrease swelling, especially cerebral edema. Dichlorphenamide is a carbonic anhydrase inhibitor used to treat glaucoma by decreasing production of aqueous humor, thereby lowering intraocular pressure. Dobutamine is a medication used to treat hypotension by increasing cardiac output. **Cognitive Level:** Applying **Client Need:** Pharmacological and Parenteral Therapies **Integrated Process:** Nursing Process: Implementation **Content Area:** Pharmacology **Strategy:** In order to select the correct option for this question, first know the classification of each of the medications. Note that the correct option is the only medication that will work as a muscle relaxant.

21 **Answer: 2** **Rationale:** Clients might take more aspirin, acetaminophen, and NSAIDs than prescribed by their providers if they are not aware that many OTC medications are combined with these medications. An anti-inflammatory drug may reduce fever but would have no effect on radial pulse. Cholesterol monitoring would be important with lipid-lowering agents. Anti-inflammatory use does not need to be tapered. **Cognitive Level:** Applying **Client Need:** Pharmacological and Parenteral Therapies **Integrated Process:** Nursing Process: Implementation **Content Area:** Pharmacology **Strategy:** Part of any teaching plan is to caution people to consult with their practitioner prior to taking over-the-counter medications when they take prescribed medications. The other options are incorrect, as these instructions are usually given with a variety of prescribed medications.

22 **Answer: 4** **Rationale:** Tegretol is contraindicated within 14 days of taking MAOIs, to help prevent a fatal reaction. The other drug classes listed do not have this interactive effect with carbamazepine. NSAIDs are used to treat inflammation and pain. Opioid analgesics exert an effect on the central nervous system. Skeletal muscle relaxants exert an effect on the central nervous system. **Cognitive Level:** Applying **Client Need:** Pharmacological and Parenteral Therapies **Integrated Process:** Nursing Process: Implementation **Content Area:** Pharmacology **Strategy:** Recall knowledge of the contraindications for the medication. There is only one correct option for this question. If this was difficult, review Tegretol and the contraindications for the medication.

23 **Answer: 2** **Rationale:** Potentially fatal interactions occur between selegiline and opioids, especially meperidine (Demerol). Therefore, nurses should be aware of all analgesics that a client routinely takes when selegiline is ordered concurrently. MAOIs, skeletal muscle relaxants, and anticholinergics could have interactions with selegiline, but none are potentially fatal. **Cognitive Level:** Analyzing **Client Need:** Pharmacological and Parenteral Therapies **Integrated Process:** Nursing Process: Implementation **Content Area:** Pharmacology **Strategy:** In order to select the correct answer to this question, recall knowledge of the contraindications for the medication. There is only one correct option for this question. If this was difficult, review selegiline (Eldepryl) and the contraindications for the medication.

Key Terms to Review

attention deficit disorder p. 540
attention deficit/hyperactivity disorder p. 540
diplopia p. 537
epilepsy p. 538
gingival hyperplasia p. 538
hepatotoxicity p. 536
narcolepsy p. 540
nystagmus p. 537
paresthesias p. 537
psychomotor seizures p. 537
spasms p. 545
spasticity p. 545
status epilepticus seizures p. 537
Stevens-Johnson syndrome p. 538
tonic-clonic seizures p. 537

References

Adams, M., Holland, L., & Urban, C. (2011). *Pharmacology for nurses: A pathophysiological approach* (3rd ed.). Upper Saddle River, NJ: Pearson Education, Inc.

Adams, M., & Koch, R. (2010). *Pharmacology: Connections to nursing practice.* Upper Saddle River, NJ: Pearson Education, Inc.

Berman, A., & Snyder, S. (2012). *Kozier & Erb's fundamentals of nursing: Concepts, process, and practice* (9th ed.). Upper Saddle River, NJ: Pearson Education, Inc.

Deglin, J. H., & Vallerand, A. H. (2011). *Davis's drug guide for nurses* (12th ed.). Philadelphia: F. A. Davis.

Lehne, R. (2010). *Pharmacology for nursing care* (7th ed.). Philadelphia: W. B. Saunders.

Wilson, B., Shannon, M., & Shields, K. (2012). *Pearson nurse's drug guide 2012.* Upper Saddle River, NJ: Pearson Education.

Test Yourself

Are you ready for the NCLEX-PN® or course exams? Use the practice tests on the companion website to check.

Renal Medications 36

In this chapter

Cross Reference

Other chapters relevant to this content area are

Age-Related Care of Older Adults Chapter 17
Dosage Calculation and Medication Administration Chapter 28
Renal and Genitourinary Disorders Chapter 54

I. DIURETICS

A. Loop diuretics

1. **Diuretics** (agents that increase amount of urine excreted) inhibit electrolyte reabsorption in thick ascending loop of Henle, promoting excretion of sodium, water, chloride, and potassium
2. Mechanism of action involves renal vasodilation, to provide a temporary increase in glomerular filtration rate (GFR) and decrease in peripheral vascular resistance
3. Loop diuretics are more potent than thiazide diuretics, causing rapid diuresis and reducing vascular fluid volume, cardiac output, and blood pressure (BP)
4. Used in clients with low GFR and hypertensive emergencies
5. Also used in clients with edema, pulmonary edema, congestive heart failure (CHF), chronic renal failure (CRF), and hepatic cirrhosis
6. May be used as treatment in drug overdose to increase renal elimination
7. Common medications (Box 36–1)
8. Administration considerations

NCLEX®

   a. Take early in day to avoid nocturia
   b. Give IV doses slowly per drug literature; rapid injection may cause hypotension
   c. For IV infusion, dilute in 5% dextrose in water, 0.9% NaCl, or lactated Ringer's; use infusion fluids within 24 hours
   d. Administer IV furosemide (Lasix) slowly (20 mg/minute or less), as hearing loss can occur if injected rapidly

Box 36–1

Common Loop Diuretics

Bumetanide (Bumex)	Ethacrynic acid (Edecrin)
Furosemide (Lasix)	Torsemide (Demadex)

Memory Aid

Remember that loop diuretics such as furosemide (Lasix) can cause ototoxicity, so be sure to monitor hearing and avoid exceeding recommended injection rates.

9. Side/adverse effects
   - NCLEX® **a.** Contraindicated with **anuria** (urine output less than 400 mL daily), electrolyte depletion
   - **b.** CNS: dizziness, headache, orthostatic hypotension, weakness
   - **c.** GI: nausea or vomiting (N/V), abdominal pain, elevated lipids with decreased high-density lipoprotein (HDL), pancreatitis, anorexia, constipation
   - **d.** GU: excessive urination, nocturia, urinary bladder spasms
   - NCLEX® **e.** Photosensitivity, sulfonamide allergy, and ototoxicity (tinnitus, hearing impairment, deafness, vertigo, and sense of fullness in ears)
   - **f.** Skin: dermatitis, urticaria, pruritis, and muscle spasm
   - **g.** Severe watery diarrhea is a side effect of ethacrynic acid (Edecrin)
   - **h.** Electrolyte imbalances: hyponatremia, hypochloremia, hypokalemia, hypomagnesemia, hypocalcemia, and hypouricemia
   - **i.** Thrombocytopenia, systemic vasculitis, interstitial nephritis, thrombophlebitis, agranulocytosis, and aplastic anemia
10. Nursing considerations
    - NCLEX® **a.** Monitor vital signs (VS) for hypotension and tachycardia
    - NCLEX® **b.** Monitor serum electrolytes (especially potassium, as well as sodium and calcium) and uric acid levels
    - NCLEX® **c.** Measure body weight at regular intervals at same time of day and with same scale
    - **d.** Monitor intake and output (I&O)
    - **e.** Observe for indicators of dehydration: thirst, poor skin turgor, coated tongue
    - **f.** Monitor for inadequate tissue perfusion and weakness, decreased muscle strength, restlessness, anxiety and agitation
    - **g.** Monitor hemoglobin and hematocrit, which may increase due to hemoconcentration
    - **h.** Monitor for blood dyscrasias and liver or kidney damage
11. Client education
    - NCLEX® **a.** Eat foods high in potassium to prevent hypokalemia (such as bananas, cantaloupe)
    - **b.** Restrict sodium intake; do not use salt substitutes if taking potassium supplement
    - **c.** Avoid dehydration by avoiding beverages with alcohol or caffeine and replacing fluids during exercise or hot weather
    - **d.** Avoid exposure to intense heat as with baths, showers, and electric blankets
    - **e.** Take small, frequent amounts of ice chips or clear liquids if vomiting
    - **f.** During episodes of diarrhea, replace fluids with fruit juice or bouillon
    - **g.** Diuretics increase amount and frequency of urination; therefore, take medication in morning (daily) and afternoon (twice-daily dosing) to avoid nighttime urination (nocturia)
    - **h.** Photosensitivity can occur while taking a loop diuretic
    - NCLEX® **i.** Change position slowly to avoid dizziness and **orthostatic hypotension** (a fall of more than 10 to 15 mm Hg of systolic blood pressure [SBP] or a fall of more than 10 mm Hg of diastolic blood pressure [DBP] and a 10–20% increase in heart rate)
    - **j.** Weigh self daily and report sudden weight gains or losses
    - NCLEX® **k.** Report ringing in ears immediately; this indicates ototoxicity
    - **l.** Loop diuretics should not be used while breastfeeding

B. Thiazide and thiazide-like diuretics

1. Increase urinary excretion of sodium and water by inhibiting sodium reabsorption in cortical diluting tubule of kidney
2. Hypotensive effect may be caused by direct arteriolar vasodilation and decreased total peripheral resistance
3. Used for edema and hypertension (SBP above 140 mm Hg and DBP above 90 mm Hg)
4. Not effective for immediate diuresis
5. Common medications (Box 36–2)
6. Administration considerations
   - NCLEX® **a.** Give medication early in the day to avoid nocturia
   - **b.** Thiazide diuretics are ineffective if creatinine clearance level is less than 30 mL/min

Box 36–2

Common Thiazide Diuretics

Short Acting	Long Acting
Chlorothiazide (Diuril)	Chlorthalidone (Hygroton)
Hydrochlorothiazide (HydroDIURIL, HCTZ)	Indapamide (Lozol)
	Methyclothiazide (Enduron)
Intermediate Acting	
Bendroflumethiazide and nadolol (Corzide)	
Metolazone (Zaroxylin)	

c. Allow 2 to 4 weeks for maximum antihypertensive effect
d. Metolazone (Zaroxylin) is not recommended in children because safety has not been established

7. Side/adverse effects
NCLEX® a. Dizziness, vertigo, headache, and weakness
NCLEX® b. Fatigue, dehydration, orthostatic hypotension, hyperglycemia, and frequent urination
NCLEX® c. Electrolyte imbalance, (hyponatremia, hypokalemia, hypomagnesemia, hypochloremia) jaundice, muscle cramps, photosensitivity, impotence, and hyperuricemia
NCLEX® d. Contraindicated with hypersensitivity to thiazide diuretics or sulfonamide derivatives, anuria, severely impaired renal or hepatic function, pregnancy or lactation
e. Renal failure, aplastic anemia, agranulocytosis, thrombocytopenia, and anaphylactic reaction

8. Nursing considerations
NCLEX® a. Monitor VS for hypotension and tachycardia
NCLEX® b. Monitor serum electrolytes (especially potassium), calcium, and uric acid levels
NCLEX® c. Measure body weight at regular intervals at same time of day and on same scale
NCLEX® d. Monitor I&O
e. Observe for indicators of dehydration: thirst, poor skin turgor, coated tongue
f. Monitor for inadequate tissue perfusion and weakness, decreased muscle strength, restlessness, anxiety and agitation

9. Client education
NCLEX® a. Eat foods high in potassium to prevent hypokalemia
NCLEX® b. Restrict sodium intake; instruct client not to use salt substitutes if taking a potassium supplement
c. Avoid dehydration by avoiding alcohol and caffeine-containing beverages and replacing fluids during exercise or hot weather
d. Avoid exposure to intense heat as with baths, showers, and electric blankets
e. Take small, frequent amounts of ice chips or clear liquids if vomiting
f. During episodes of diarrhea, replace fluids with fruit juice or bouillion
NCLEX® g. Diuretics increase amount and frequency of urination; therefore, take medication in morning and afternoon to avoid nocturia
NCLEX® h. Change position slowly to avoid dizziness and orthostatic hypotension
NCLEX® i. Weigh self daily and report sudden weight gains or losses
j. Diabetic clients should check blood glucose as recommmended

C. Potassium-sparing diuretics

1. Act in distal convoluted tubule to increase sodium excretion and decrease potassium secretion
2. Used for hypertension and edema associated with heart failure
3. Spironolactone is also used for cirrhosis of liver, primary hyperaldosteronism, hirsutism, and premenstrual syndrome
4. Common medications (Box 36–3)
5. Administration considerations
a. Take with food or milk
NCLEX® b. Avoid salt substitutes, which are high in potassium
NCLEX® c. Avoid excessive ingestion of foods high in potassium
d. When administering spironolactone to children, crush tablet and mix in flavored syrup as oral suspension

Box 36–3

Potassium-Sparing Diuretics

Sodium channel inhibitors	*Aldosterone antagonists*
Amiloride (Midamor)	Eplerenone (Inspra)
Triamterene (Dyrenium)	Spironolactone (Aldactone)

6. Side/adverse effects
   a. CNS: headache, weakness, dizziness, and orthostatic hypotension
   b. GI: N/V, diarrhea, and constipation
   c. Impotence, muscle cramps, urticaria, gynecomastia, and breast soreness
   d. Dry mouth, photosensitivity, transient elevated blood urea nitrogen (BUN) and creatinine
   e. Aplastic anemia and thrombocytopenia
   NCLEX® f. Hyperkalemia (potassium greater than 5.1 mEq/L)
   NCLEX® g. Contraindicated with serum potassium levels greater than 5.5 mEq/mL, concurrent use with other potassium-sparing diuretics, fluid and electrolyte imbalances, anuria, acute and chronic renal insufficiency, diabetic nephropathy, hypersensitivity, and impaired hepatic function
7. NCLEX® Nursing considerations
   a. Monitor VS and urine output
   b. Discontinue potassium supplements
   c. Observe closely older and debilitated clients for drug-induced diuresis and hyperkalemia
   d. Monitor for dehydration and electrolyte imbalance
   e. Monitor periodic serum electrolytes such as BUN and creatinine
8. Client education
   a. Take medication with food to avoid GI upset except with triamterene
   b. Avoid eating large quantities of foods high in potassium
   c. Report any mental confusion or lethargy immediately
   NCLEX® d. Monitor for symptoms of hyperkalemia such as nausea, diarrhea, abdominal cramps, and tachycardia followed by bradycardia
   e. Side effects usually disappear after drug is stopped, but gynecomastia may persist
   f. With spironolactone, maximal diuresis may not occur until day 3 of therapy and diuresis may continue 2 to 3 days after the drug is stopped
   g. Triamterene may turn urine blue
   NCLEX® h. Avoid salt substitutes because they contain potassium
   NCLEX® i. Avoid exposure to direct sunlight to prevent photosensitivity reaction

D. Carbonic anhydrase inhibitors

1. Achieve noncompetitive reversible inhibition of enzyme carbonic anhydrase, which promotes excretion of bicarbonate, sodium, potassium, and water
2. Used to treat edema caused by CHF, to decrease intraocular pressure in open-angle glaucoma, and to treat epilepsy and metabolic alkalosis
3. Common medications (Box 36–4)
4. Administration considerations
   a. Increasing dose does not appear to increase diuresis
   b. Do not administer with high-dose aspirin
   c. Intramuscular administration is not recommended
5. Side/adverse effects
   a. Confusion, drowsiness, and paresthesias
   b. Hearing dysfunction, GI upset, polyuria, and transient myopia
   c. Electrolyte imbalance, fever, rash, renal calculus, and photosensitivity
   d. Metabolic acidosis
   e. Anaphylaxis

Box 36–4

Carbonic Anhydrase Inhibitors

Acetazolamide (Diamox)
Methazolamide (Neptazane)

f. Bone marrow depression (thrombocytopenia purpura, hemolytic anemia, leukopenia, pancytopenia, and agranulocytosis)
g. Severe reactions to sulfonamides, including Stevens-Johnson syndrome, toxic epidermal necrolysis, fulminant hepatic necrosis, coma, and death
NCLEX® h. Contraindicated in narrow-angle or acute glaucoma, any situation with decreased sodium and/or potassium levels, marked kidney or liver dysfunction; use cautiously with chronic obstructive pulmonary disease (COPD)

6. Nursing considerations
   a. Monitor for signs and symptoms of dehydration
   b. Observe for alterations in skin integrity and for edema
   NCLEX® c. Measure VS, daily weight, and I&O
   d. Monitor cardiovascular and respiratory status
   e. Observe for changes in level of consciousness and activity level
   f. Monitor dietary intake for foods high in salt
   g. Maintain fluid restriction as ordered
7. Client education
   NCLEX® a. Do not take aspirin or aspirin-containing medications
   b. Report symptoms of anorexia, lethargy, or tachypnea
   NCLEX® c. Use caution while driving or performing tasks that require alertness, coordination, or physical dexterity because these drugs can cause drowsiness
   d. Monitor for signs of renal calculi
   e. Follow-up with scheduled lab tests is important
   NCLEX® f. Weigh self daily at same time of day and report acute weight gain or loss (more than 2–3 lb/day)
   g. Avoid foods and beverages containing high amounts of sodium

E. Osmotic diuretics

1. Increase osmotic pressure of glomerular filtrate in proximal tubule and loop of Henle inhibiting reabsorption of water and electrolytes, thus promoting diuresis
2. Used to prevent and manage acute renal failure (ARF) and oliguria
3. NCLEX® Used to decrease intracranial or intraocular pressure
4. Mannitol is used with chemotherapy to induce diuresis
5. Common medications (Box 36–5)
6. Administration considerations
   a. Medications are administered IV by slow infusion
   b. Urea turns to ammonia if left standing
   c. Do not infuse with blood or blood products
   NCLEX® d. Mannitol crystallizes at low temperatures
7. Side/adverse effects
   a. Headache, syncope, and hypotension
   b. Dry mouth, N/V, urine retention, electrolyte imbalance, and urticaria
   c. Seizures
   d. Thrombophlebitis, CHF cardiovascular collapse
   e. Contraindicated with severely impaired renal function, marked dehydration, breastfeeding, hepatic failure, active intracranial bleed, anuria, severe pulmonary congestion, and severe CHF
8. Nursing considerations
   NCLEX® a. Maintain adequate hydration
   NCLEX® b. Monitor fluid and electrolyte balance, daily weight
   c. Indwelling catheter should be used in comatose clients for accurate I&O
   NCLEX® d. Monitor I&O and VS hourly while on Mannitol
   e. Monitor renal function, (BUN, creatinine) fluid balance, serum and urinary sodium and potassium levels
   NCLEX® f. Observe for signs of decreasing intracranial pressure if appropriate
   g. Monitor lung and heart sounds for signs of pulmonary edema

Box 36–5	
Common Osmotic Diuretics	Mannitol (Osmitrol) Urea (Ureaphil)

9. Client education
   a. Monitor weight
   b. Report immediately pain in chest or legs, shortness of breath, or apnea
   c. Change position slowly to prevent dizziness or orthostatic hypotension
   d. Drink only fluids ordered if on a fluid restriction also
   e. Use sugarless hard candies to reduce dry mouth

II. URINARY ANTI-INFECTIVES

A. Overview

1. Act as **bacteriostatic** (inhibition of the growth of bacterial without destruction) and **bactericidal** (destroying bacteria) agents
2. Act as disinfectants within urinary tract
3. Used to treat urinary tract infections
4. Common medications (Box 36–6)

B. Administration considerations

1. May take with food or milk to decrease GI upset
2. Check renal and hepatic function before administering
3. NCLEX® Oral suspension of nitrofurantoin may stain teeth; instruct client to rinse mouth following dose
4. NCLEX® Complete full course of therapy to prevent reinfection or overgrowth of resistant organisms

C. Side/adverse effects

1. Drowsiness, weakness, headache, dizziness
2. NCLEX® Sensitivity to light, blurred vision
3. GI distress, pruritis, rash, arthralgia
4. Seizures, increased intracranial pressure
5. Leukopenia, thrombocytopenia, angioedema
6. NCLEX® Contraindicated with hypersensitivity, megaloblastic anemia and folate deficiency, renal insufficiency, severe hepatic insufficiency, severe dehydration, anuria, oliguria, and seizure disorder

D. Nursing considerations

1. Drugs work best if client is well (but not overly) hydrated
2. Administer with meals to decrease GI distress
3. Monitor renal and liver function
4. Check urine pH before administration because some drugs work best in acidic urine
5. Cranberry juice or vitamin C may be added to acidify urine
6. Monitor CNS side effects
7. Ingestion of large amount of fluid while taking methenamine will reduce antibacterial effects by diluting medication and raising urinary pH

E. Client education

1. Long-term therapy is common even if feeling fine
2. NCLEX® Drink at least 8 glasses of water daily
3. Take medications with meals to decrease GI distress
4. NCLEX® Avoid alkalizing fluids such as milk, fruit juices, or sodium bicarbonate
5. Notify prescriber of any new medications
6. NCLEX® Use sunscreen and avoid excessive exposure to sunlight
7. Notify physician of any CNS side effects
8. NCLEX® Nitrofurantoin may discolor urine brown; this is not harmful and will disappear after drug is discontinued

Box 36–6

Common Urinary Tract Anti-Infectives

Sulfonamides	*Urinary antiseptics and other drugs for urinary tract infection*
Sulfadiazine	Fosfomycin (Monurol)
Sulfadiazine-pyrimethamine (Fandisar)	Methenamine hippurate (Hiprex)
Sulfisoxazole (Gantrisin)	Methenamine mandelate (Mandelamine)
Trimethoprim-sulfamethoxazole (Bactrim, Septra)	Nalidixic acid (NegGram)
	Nitrofurantoin (Furadantin)

III. URINARY ANTISPASMODICS

A. Overview

1. Muscarinic antagonists (anticholinergics) that relax smooth muscles of the urinary tract to decrease bladder and detrusor muscle spasms
2. Used to manage lower urinary tract symptoms associated with hypermotility: dysuria, urgency, nocturia, suprapubic pain, frequency, and incontinence
3. Common medications (Box 36–7)

B. Administration considerations: administer 1 hour before antacids or antidiarrheals

C. Side/adverse effects

1. Headache, insomnia, drowsiness, dizziness, confusion, excitement, palpitations
2. Blurred vision, dry mouth, GI distress, urinary hesitancy, urine retention, urticaria, leukopenia
3. *NCLEX®* Contraindicated in glaucoma, obstructive breathing, obstructive GI disease, severe ulcerative colitis, and myasthenia gravis, hypersensitivity to anticholinergics, paralytic ileus, unstable cardiovascular status, urinary tract obstruction

D. Nursing considerations

1. *NCLEX®* Monitor effect of medication and any CNS manifestations
2. Monitor I&O

E. Client education

1. *NCLEX®* Drowsiness and blurred vision may occur; use caution with driving or operating machinery; avoid alcohol, which increases drowsiness
2. *NCLEX®* Use hard, sugarless candy for dry mouth
3. Swallow pill whole and do not chew or crush
4. The shell of medication may appear in stool
5. Inform client of side effects and to report them to prescriber

IV. CHOLINERGIC AGENT

A. Overview

1. Direct-acting cholinergic agent is indicated for use with neurogenic bladder and urinary retention from nonobstructive causes
2. *NCLEX®* Contracts detrusor muscle of urinary bladder, which increases bladder tone and ability to initiate micturition (voiding)
3. Common medication: bethanechol chloride (Urecholine)

B. Administration considerations

1. Give oral dose on empty stomach to reduce N/V (1 hour before or 2 hours after meals)
2. Alternate route is subcutaneous; do not give by IM or IV route to avoid life-threatening symptoms of cholinergic stimulation
3. *NCLEX®* Keep atropine sulfate available as an antidote

NCLEX® **C. Side/adverse effects**

1. Headache and malaise, flushing and increased sweating
2. Hypotension with dizziness and faintness; dyspnea or acute asthmatic attack
3. Blurred vision and lacrimation; urgency with urination or defecation
4. N/V, diarrhea, and abdominal cramps
5. Contraindications of cholinergic drugs include mechanical obstruction of GI or urinary tracts, peptic ulcer disease, COPD, bradycardia, parkinsonism, hypotension, and AV blocks

D. Nursing considerations

1. *NCLEX®* Monitor for 1 hour after subcutaneous dose for early signs of overdosage: salivation, sweating, flushing, abdominal cramps, and nausea
2. *NCLEX®* Use atropine as ordered for antidote
3. Monitor I&O to determine effectiveness
4. Monitor client's ambulation as needed according to response to drug

Box 36–7 Common Antispasmodic Medications

Hyoscyamine (Cystospaz)	Flavoxate (Urispas)
Tolterodine tartrate (Detrol)	Propantheline (Pro-Banthine)
Oxybutynin chloride (Ditropan)	

E. Client education

NCLEX®
1. Change postions slowly, especially from lying to standing
2. Do not stand in place for long periods, and lie down at first sign of faintness
3. Use caution in activities to maintain safety because of risk of blurred vision

V. DOPAMINE FOR RENAL PERFUSION

A. Action and use

NCLEX®
1. Primary focus of low-dose dopamine is to restore and maintain renal perfusion in shock states and to eliminate drugs that are directly nephrotoxic
2. Stimulation of dopaminergic receptors causes vasodilation in renal, mesenteric, coronary, and intracerebral vascular beds

NCLEX®
3. Used to increase urine flow beyond minimum 30 mL/hr or 0.5 mg/kg/hr

B. Dosage: dopamine (Intropin) 2 to 5 mcg/kg/min IV to increase renal perfusion; may increase to 50 mcg/kg/min IV to raise blood pressure

C. Administration considerations

NCLEX®
1. Use an IV infusion device to control rate of flow
2. Administered into a large vein to prevent possibility of extravasation

NCLEX®
3. Correct hypovolemia before initiation of dopamine therapy
4. Decrease dose as soon as hemodynamic condition is stabilized
5. Do not mix with other medications
6. Discard solution after 24 hours and replace with new solution

D. Side/adverse effects

NCLEX®
1. Headache, tachycardia, angina, palpitations, hypotension, bradycardia, vasoconstriction, widening of QRS complex on electrocardiogram
2. N/V, piloerection, azotemia
3. Anaphylaxis asthmatic episodes; severe hypertension

NCLEX®
4. Contraindicated in uncorrected tachydysrhythmias, pheochromocytoma, or ventricular fibrillation; use cautiously with occlusive vascular disease, cold injuries, diabetic endarteritis, and arterial embolism

E. Nursing considerations

NCLEX®
1. Carefully monitor I&O, VS, cardiac output, and EKG

NCLEX®
2. Inspect infusion site frequently for extravasation; possibly use phentolamine mesylate (Regitine) diluted in normal saline and injected into site of extravasation as an antidote
3. Monitor for side effects

F. Client education: purpose and effects of medication; report side effects

VI. HEMATOPOIETIC GROWTH FACTOR

A. Action and use

NCLEX®
1. Used to stimulate red blood cell (RBC) production to raise hematocrit (Hct)
2. Reverses anemia associated with chronic renal failure (CRF), HIV infection, and chemotherapy used to treat nonmyeloid malignancies

B. Common medication: epoetin (Epogen, Procrit) dosed 3 times/wk

C. Administration considerations

NCLEX®
1. Do not shake solution

NCLEX®
2. Use only one dose per vial, and do not reenter vial
3. Inspect solution for particulate matter prior to use
4. IV administration: may be given undiluted by direct IV as a bolus dose or during hemodialysis
5. Rotate injection sites if given subcutaneously to minimize irritation

D. Side/adverse effects

NCLEX®
1. Hypertension; headache, seizure
2. Iron deficiency, sweating, bone pain, arthralgias
3. Thrombocytosis, clotting of AV fistula
4. Contraindicated in uncontrolled hypertension, known hypersensitivity to mammalian cell-derived products, and albumin

E. Nursing considerations
1. Evaluate serum ferritin and transferrin levels prior to beginning therapy

NCLEX®
2. BP may rise during early therapy as Hct increases; notify prescriber of a rapid rise in Hct greater than 4 points in 2 weeks

3. Do not give with any other drug solution
4. Initial effects can be seen within 1 to 2 weeks
5. Hct reaches satisfactory levels (30–36%) in 2 to 3 months NCLEX®
6. Monitor for hypertensive encephalopathy in clients with CRF during period of increasing Hct
7. Client may require additional heparin during dialysis to prevent clotting of vascular access

F. Client education

1. Self-monitor VS, especially BP NCLEX®
2. Headache is a common adverse effect; it should be reported if severe
3. Avoid driving and other hazardous activity because of possible seizure, especially during first 90 days of therapy NCLEX®
4. Keep all follow-up appointments

Check Your NCLEX–PN® Exam I.Q. *You are ready for testing on this content if you can*

- Apply knowledge of expected actions and effects of renal medications to client care.
- Correctly administer renal medications to clients.
- Monitor for side effects and adverse effects of renal medications.
- Take appropriate action if a client has an unexpected response to a renal medication.
- Monitor a client for expected outcomes or effects of treatment with renal medications.

PRACTICE TEST

PRACTICE TEST

1 A client is taking nalidixic acid (NegGram) for treatment of a urinary problem. The nurse explains to the client that the medication is best described as what type of drug?

1. An antispasmodic
2. A uricosuric
3. An anti-infective
4. An analgesic

2 The client with congestive heart failure (CHF) is eating a 1-gram-sodium diet, and will be having a potassium-sparing diuretic added to the medication regimen. The nurse prepares to reinforce teaching about which medication that is likely to be prescribed?

1. Hydrochlorothiazide (HCTZ)
2. Spironolactone (Aldactone)
3. Furosemide (Lasix)
4. Atenolol (Tenormin)

3 The nurse is assigned to the care of an older adult client who is taking furosemide (Lasix) twice daily. Which client statements indicate the need for further reinforcement of medication information? Select all that apply.

1. "I will take my medication in the morning and before bedtime."
2. "I will change my position slowly, so that I don't fall."
3. "I will notify my physician if my ankles swell."
4. "I can drink coffee and tea in an effort to get enough fluid."
5. "I should expect to experience some ringing in my ears."

4 The nurse is reviewing the medication administration record for a client newly admitted for congestive heart failure. The client is receiving hydrochlorothiazide (HydroDiuril). Which conditions should concern the nurse in relation to administration of this medication? Select all that apply.

1. Hypokalemia, hyperglycemia, and sulfa allergy
2. Hyperkalemia, hypoglycemia, and penicillin allergy
3. Hypouricemia and hyperglycemia
4. Hyponatremia and hypocalcemia
5. Hypercalcemia, hyperuricemia, and hyperglycemia

5 A client is being prescribed oxybutynin (Ditropan) for a neurogenic bladder. The nurse determines that the client is possibly experiencing toxic effects of this medication after noting which manifestation?

1. Restlessness
2. Drowsiness
3. Pallor
4. Bradycardia

PRACTICE TEST

6 The nurse is admitting a client with a hypertensive emergency and a history of renal insufficiency. The nurse should ensure that which diuretic is readily available for use if ordered?

1. Furosemide (Lasix)
2. Hydrochlorothiazide (HCTZ)
3. Chlorthalidone (Hygroton)
4. Spironolactone (Aldactone)

7 A client being discharged from the hospital is beginning medication therapy with bumetanide (Bumex). The nurse reminds the client to contact the prescriber if which contraindication for use develops?

1. Increase in peripheral edema
2. Absence of urine output
3. Shortness of breath
4. Increase in blood pressure

8 The nurse notes while reading an admission history that a client is taking acetazolamide (Diamox). The nurse next looks for documentation of a history of which medical condition?

1. Hypertensive crisis
2. Congestive heart failure (CHF)
3. Open-angle glaucoma
4. Peripheral vascular disease

9 A client is in the neurological unit following a serious closed head injury. Medication is administered to decrease developing intracranial pressure. What is the priority manifestation the nurse should monitor for after the drug is given?

1. Hypotension
2. Cardiovascular collapse
3. Seizures
4. Electrolyte imbalance

10 A client who has been taking bethanechol chloride (Urecholine) for three days begins to complain of abdominal pain and difficulty breathing. After assigning another staff member to remain with the client, the nurse checks to see that which medication is available on the nursing unit?

1. Phytonadione (AquaMEPHYTON)
2. Atropine sulfate (generic)
3. Oxybutynin (Ditropan)
4. Epinephrine (Adrenalin)

11 A client who requires diuretic therapy has a creatinine clearance less than 30 mL/min. The nurse checks the physician order sheet, expecting to find a prescription for which type of medication?

1. Mannitol (Osmitrol)
2. Spironolactone (Aldactone)
3. Chlorothiazide (Diuril)
4. Furosemide (Lasix)

12 The nurse practitioner has prescribed oxybutynin (Ditropan) for a 65-year-old female with urinary frequency and urgency. The nurse who is reinforcing information about medication side effects should explain that which manifestations are associated with this medication? Select all that apply.

1. Dizziness
2. Increased bruising
3. Diarrhea
4. Dry mouth
5. Blurred vision

13 Phenazopyridine (Pyridium) is prescribed to a client with dysuria. The nurse explains that the client should expect which urine characteristic while taking phenazopyridine?

1. Decrease in volume
2. Odor that is foul
3. Increase in volume
4. Color that is orange or red

14 A client who is taking spironolactone (Aldactone) at home arrives in the clinic reporting unrelieved edema in the legs. The nurse shares what data with the physician that indicates a need to withhold the medication?

1. Blood glucose level of 170
2. Blood pressure of 110/70
3. Sodium level of 146 mEq/L
4. Potassium of 5.9 mEq/L

15 A client is admitted to an acute care facility due to anemia related to HIV infection. Based on the nurse's knowledge about hematopoietic growth factor (Procrit) administration, which action is not appropriate?

1. Gently shaking the medication for adequate mixing
2. Discarding the medication vial after the first dose
3. Giving undiluted medication as an IV bolus dose
4. Closely inspecting solution for particulate matter

16 The client beginning medication therapy with sulfisoxazole (Gantrisin) needs instructions for its use. What client teaching should the nurse reinforce about the medication?

1. Call the prescriber if the urine turns dark brown.
2. Maintain a high fluid intake.
3. Restrict salt intake.
4. Decrease the dosage when symptoms are improving.

17 The nurse has an order to administer a first dose of epoetin (Epogen) to a client with chronic renal failure. The nurse would make note of which laboratory test results to establish a baseline? Select all that apply.

1. Hemoglobin of 9%
2. Hematocrit of 26%
3. White blood cell count 3000/mm^3
4. Creatinine 3.2 mEq/L
5. Blood urea nitrogen 56 mg/dL

18 The nurse provides instructions to the client who has been prescribed a diuretic. The nurse informs the client that which diuretic causes a persistent gynecomastia?

1. Hydrochlorothiazide (HCTZ)
2. Furosemide (Lasix)
3. Spironolactone (Aldactone)
4. Indapamide (Lozol)

19 A client was just prescribed hydrochlorothiazide (HCTZ) for hypertension. The client asks the nurse how this medication works in the body. The nurse explains that thiazide diuretics aid excretion of sodium and water in which part of the kidney?

1. Loop of Henle
2. Cortical diluting tubule
3. Collecting ducts
4. Distal convoluted tubule

20 The nurse taking care of a client with benign prostatic hyperplasia (BPH) explains to the client that what category of antihypertensive drug can also be prescribed for BPH?

1. Beta blocker
2. Calcium channel blocker
3. Alpha-adrenergic blocker
4. Vasodilator

ANSWERS & RATIONALES

1 **Answer: 3** **Rationale:** Nalidixic acid is bactericidal, and inhibits microbial synthesis of DNA. The spectrum includes most Gram-negative organisms except Pseudomonas. The other categories are incorrect. **Cognitive Level:** Remembering **Client Need:** Pharmacological and Parenteral Therapies **Integrated Process:** Nursing Process: Planning **Content Area:** Pharmacology **Strategy:** The core issue of the question is knowledge of basic information about nalidixic acid and its uses. Use the process of elimination and nursing knowledge to make a selection.

2 **Answer: 2** **Rationale:** Spironolactone is a potassium-sparing diuretic that promotes sodium excretion while conserving potassium. Hydrochlorothiazide and furosemide are diuretics, but are not potassium-sparing. Atenolol is not a diuretic; it is an antihypertensive of the beta-blocker type. **Cognitive Level:** Applying **Client Need:** Pharmacological and Parenteral Therapies **Integrated Process:** Nursing Process: Planning **Content Area:** Pharmacology **Strategy:** The core issue of the question is knowledge of drugs that are potassium-sparing diuretics. Use the process of elimination and nursing knowledge to make a selection.

3 **Answer: 1, 4, 5** **Rationale:** Taking medication at the same time each day improves compliance. In addition, morning and *early* evening are the best times to take Lasix, so as not to interrupt sleep. Tea and coffee are poor choices for hydration. They are mild diuretics, and can cause severe dehydration if used concurrently with diuretics. Tinnitus is an indication of ototoxicity when taking furosemide; this is an adverse effect and should be reported to the physician; the client needs additional teaching. A common side effect to furosemide is orthostatic hypotension; the client should be advised to rise slowly to prevent falls. Notifying the physician when edema is noticed is important, and should be emphasized by the nurse. **Cognitive Level:** Analyzing **Client Need:** Pharmacological and Parenteral Therapies **Integrated Process:** Nursing Process: Evaluation **Content Area:** Pharmacology **Strategy:** The critical words in the stem of the question are *need for further teaching*. This tells you that the correct answers are incorrect statements on the part of the client. Use the process of elimination and knowledge of diuretic therapy to narrow the selection to the one that utilizes additional diuretic substances. When more than one answer is correct, consider each option as a true/false statement.

4 **Answer: 1, 5** **Rationale:** Thiazide diuretics are sulfa-based medications; therefore, a client with a sulfa allergy is at risk for an allergic reaction. The side effects of hydrochlorothiazide are hypokalemia and hyperglycemia. Hypercalcemia, hyperuricemia, and hyperglycemia are all conditions of concern when administering hydrochlorothiazide.

Hyperkalemia, hypoglycemia, and penicillin allergy are not conditions of concern when administering hydrochlorothiazide. Hyperglycemia is a concern when administering hydrochlorothiazide; hypouricemia is not a concern. Hyponatremia is not a concern when administering hydrochlorothiazide. **Cognitive Level:** Analyzing **Client Need:** Pharmacological and Parenteral Therapies **Integrated Process:** Nursing Process: Data Collection **Content Area:** Pharmacology **Strategy:** Remember that in order for an option to be correct, all of the parts of the option must be correct. Options to which this strategy applies will include the word *and*. Recall that diuretics generally can cause hypokalemia or hyperkalemia as adverse effects. Recall that sulfa rather than penicillin is of concern in order to choose the correct option. When there is more than one correct answer, consider each option as a true/false statement.

5 **Answer: 1 Rationale:** Excessive dosing of oxybutynin produces nervousness, hallucinations, restlessness, tachycardia, confusion, flushed or red face, and signs of respiratory depression. The other options are the opposite of what the nurse should expect. **Cognitive Level:** Analyzing **Client Need:** Pharmacological and Parenteral Therapies **Integrated Process:** Nursing Process: Data Collection **Content Area:** Pharmacology **Strategy:** Note that when two options are opposite, one of them likely is correct. Use this strategy to eliminate two of the options first. Use the process of elimination and medication knowledge to choose the correct answer.

6 **Answer: 1 Rationale:** Furosemide is a loop diuretic. The antihypertensive action involves renal and peripheral vasodilation, a temporary increase in glomerular filtration rate (GFR), and decreased peripheral vascular resistance. For this reason, it is the drug of choice for clients with low GFR as a result of renal insufficiency. The other options are not associated with use in clients with low GFR. **Cognitive Level:** Applying **Client Need:** Pharmacological and Parenteral Therapies **Integrated Process:** Nursing Process: Planning **Content Area:** Pharmacology **Strategy:** Specific knowledge of the benefits of furosemide as a loop diuretic and as the diuretic of choice with renal insufficiency is needed to answer this question. Take time to learn about this common medication if you had difficulty with this question.

7 **Answer: 2 Rationale:** Anuria is the absence of urine formation, and is a contraindication for using this medication. An increase in peripheral edema is not a contraindication for the use of Bumex. Diuretics such as bumetanide are used to increase the amount of urine excreted in clients with pulmonary edema, which may be characterized by shortness of breath and increased blood pressure. **Cognitive Level:** Applying **Client Need:** Pharmacological and Parenteral Therapies **Integrated Process:** Nursing Process: Implementation **Content Area:** Pharmacology **Strategy:** The core issue of the question is knowledge of expected effects and adverse effects of loop diuretics such as bumetanide. Knowing that diuretics help to relieve the symptoms in three of the options will help you to eliminate each of them.

8 **Answer: 3 Rationale:** Acetazolamide is a carbonic anhydrase inhibitor. Inhibition of carbonic anhydrase decreases the rate of formation of aqueous humor, and thereby reduces intraocular pressure. Acetazolamide may be used for treatment of edema caused by CHF, but it is not a first-line therapy. Acetazolamide does not have a therapeutic effect on hypertensive crisis or peripheral vascular disease. **Cognitive Level:** Analyzing **Client Need:** Pharmacological and Parenteral Therapies **Integrated Process:** Nursing Process: Data Collection **Content Area:** Pharmacology **Strategy:** The critical word in the stem of the question is *next,* which tells you that more than one follow-up question might be appropriate, but you must select the most important one. Eliminate the options that are not targeted by this type of therapy. Use knowledge regarding the uses of the drug to select the correct answer.

9 **Answer: 2 Rationale:** The drug of choice will be an osmotic diuretic and cardiovascular collapse can occur due to the amount of fluid that can be lost; this life-threatening, adverse effect should be the nurse's priority concern. Hypotension is an expected side effect, and seizure activity is possible as is electrolyte imbalance so the client should be monitored; however, they are not the priority concern. **Cognitive Level:** Analyzing **Client Need:** Pharmacological and Parenteral Therapies **Integrated Process:** Nursing Process: Data Collection **Content Area:** Pharmacology **Strategy:** The core issue in this question is being able to identify the type of drug that is appropriate for treatment of increasing intracranial pressure. Knowledge regarding the effects of the drug, and which manifestation is the highest priority will assist in selecting the correct answer.

10 **Answer: 2 Rationale:** The client is exhibiting signs of cholinergic toxicity, and atropine is the antidote. Phytonadione or vitamin K is the antidote to warfarin (Coumadin). Oxybutinin is indicated for use as a urinary antispasmodic. Epinephrine is used to treat severe hypersensitivity reactions (anaphylaxis). **Cognitive Level:** Analyzing **Client Need:** Pharmacological and Parenteral Therapies **Integrated Process:** Nursing Process: Implementation **Content Area:** Pharmacology **Strategy:** Use the process of elimination, focusing on the critical words *abdominal pain* and *difficulty breathing*. After determining that the client is experiencing adverse or toxic effects of the medication, choose the option that is an anticholinergic drug, which will treat the cholinergic symptoms.

11 **Answer: 4 Rationale:** Loop diuretics have the disadvantage of requiring more frequent dosing, but are advantageous in clients with creatinine clearance less than 30 mL/min. The other options are not as helpful when the client has a decreased creatinine clearance level. **Cognitive Level:** Analyzing **Client Need:** Pharmacological and Parenteral Therapies **Integrated Process:** Nursing Process: Implementation **Content Area:** Pharmacology **Strategy:** The core issue of the question is knowledge that loop diuretics are the most beneficial type of diuretic for clients with low creatinine clearance levels. Specific knowledge of this drug category and the ability to recognize drugs from each diuretic class are needed to answer this question.

12 **Answer: 1, 4, 5 Rationale:** Oxybutynin (Ditropan) is an antispasmodic medication used to restore normal voiding patterns in clients with spasms of smooth muscle of the urinary bladder. It produces anticholinergic side effects such as dizziness, blurred vision, and dry mouth. Periodic interruptions in therapy are recommended to determine continued need for this medication. It does not cause increased bruising or diarrhea. **Cognitive Level:** Applying **Client Need:** Pharmacological and Parenteral Therapies **Integrated Process:** Teaching and Learning **Content Area:** Pharmacology **Strategy:** Use the process of elimination. The core issue of this question is knowledge of side and adverse effects of this medication. Choose the

options that indicate anticholinergic effects. When there is more than one correct answer, consider each option as a true/false statement.

13 **Answer: 4 Rationale:** Phenazopyridine is a urinary analgesic with a local anesthetic effect on the urinary tract mucosa, and relieves pain during urinary tract infection. It causes the urine to have an orange-to-red color. Phenazopyridine has no effect on volume of urine. Foul odor to the urine can be caused by urinary tract infection. Phenazopyridine is a urinary analgesic with a local anesthetic effect; has no effect on volume of urine. **Cognitive Level:** Applying **Client Need:** Pharmacological and Parenteral Therapies **Integrated Process:** Teaching and Learning **Content Area:** Pharmacology **Strategy:** The core issue of the question is knowledge of the effects of phenazopyridine on the urine. A critical word in the stem of the question is *dysuria*, which should remind you that the medication is a urinary analgesic, and as the only drug of its type, it causes orange-to-red discoloration in body fluids, including urine.

14 **Answer: 4 Rationale:** Aldactone is a potassium-sparing diuretic that increases sodium excretion and decreases potassium secretion in the distal convoluted tubule. Potassium levels higher than 5.5 mEq/L are contraindicated with spironolactone, due to increased risk of hyperkalemia. Elevated blood glucose is not a priority issue related to this medication. A blood pressure of 110/70 is within normal limits, and does not warrant withholding the medication. An elevated sodium level could be alleviated by the medication, and thus it is not a reason to withhold the dose of medication. **Cognitive Level:** Analyzing **Client Need:** Pharmacological and Parenteral Therapies **Integrated Process:** Nursing Process: Data Collection **Content Area:** Pharmacology **Strategy:** The core issue of the question is the need to monitor potassium levels in a client taking potassium-sparing diuretics. Use knowledge of expected effects of diuretics to eliminate the incorrect options.

15 **Answer: 1 Rationale:** The nurse should not shake hematopoietic growth factor medications. After the first dose of a hematopoietic growth factor is drawn from the vial, the vial should not be reentered; the vial should be discarded. Hematopoietic growth factor can be given undiluted as a direct IV bolus. Hematopoietic growth factor should be inspected for particulate matter before administration and discarded if it is present. **Cognitive Level:** Applying **Client Need:** Pharmacological and Parenteral Therapies **Integrated Process:** Nursing Process: Implementation **Content Area:** Pharmacology **Strategy:** The core issue of the question is knowledge related to the administration of hematopoietic growth factor. The stem of the question is worded so that an incorrect option is the correct answer. Knowledge related to this medication is necessary to answer correctly.

16 **Answer: 2 Rationale:** Each dose of this medication should be administered with a full glass of water, and the client should be encouraged to maintain a high fluid intake. Sulfisoxazole does not discolor urine brown (although nitrofurantoin does), and it is not harmful. It is not necessary to restrict salt intake when taking sulfisoxazole. Prescribed medication should be taken as directed and until complete; the dose should not be decreased even if symptoms improve. **Cognitive Level:** Applying **Client Need:** Pharmacological and Parenteral Therapies **Integrated Process:** Teaching and Learning **Content Area:** Pharmacology **Strategy:** Specific drug knowledge is needed to answer the question; however, recalling that fluid intake should be increased with urinary infections should help to eliminate the incorrect options.

17 **Answer: 1, 2 Rationale:** Epoetin is given to stimulate red blood cell production in the client with chronic renal failure. For this reason, the nurse should look at the hemoglobin and hematocrit as baseline measurements. A white blood cell stimulant such as filgrastim (Neupogen) would be given to raise white blood cell counts; a baseline for white blood cells is not necessary. Epoetin alfa will not treat creatinine or BUN levels; the client would be receiving dialysis to control these values. **Cognitive Level:** Analyzing **Client Need:** Pharmacological and Parenteral Therapies **Integrated Process:** Nursing Process: Data Collection **Content Area:** Pharmacology **Strategy:** Use the process of elimination and knowledge of drug therapy. Recall that dialysis is needed to treat renal failure, and options that require dialysis can be eliminated first. Recall that clients in renal failure are anemic because of impaired ability to produce erythropoietin to eliminate the white blood cell count. When there is more than one correct answer; consider each option as a true/false statement.

18 **Answer: 3 Rationale:** Spironolactone is a potassium-sparing diuretic used to treat hypertension. Gynecomastia is one of its adverse reactions. HCTZ does not cause a persistent gynecomastia. Furosemide does not cause a persistent gynecomastia. Indipamide does not cause a persistent gynecomastia. **Cognitive Level:** Applying **Client Need:** Physiological Adaptation **Integrated Process:** Nursing Process: Implementation **Content Area:** Pharmacology **Strategy:** There is only one correct answer to this question. Having knowledge of the adverse reactions to the medication will lead to the correct answer. If this was difficult, review the side effects of the medications.

19 **Answer: 2 Rationale:** Thiazide diuretics increase urinary excretion of sodium and water by inhibiting sodium reabsorption in the cortical diluting tubule of the nephron, thus relieving edema. The loop diuretics inhibit electrolyte reabsorption in the thick, ascending loop of Henle, thereby promoting the excretion of sodium, water, and potassium. The collecting ducts are not the site of action for diuretics as they are too distal in the nephron. Potassium-sparing diuretics directly increase sodium excretion and decrease potassium secretion in the distal convoluted tubule. **Cognitive Level:** Understanding **Client Need:** Pharmacological and Parenteral Therapies **Integrated Process:** Nursing Process: Data Collection **Content Area:** Pharmacology **Strategy:** Having knowledge of pathophysiological processes of diuretics will assist in selecting the correct answer. If this was difficult, review the glomerular filtration system, and its functioning with diuretics.

20 **Answer: 3 Rationale:** Alpha-adrenergic blockers are used for peripheral vascular disorders, hypertension, and BPH. Beta blockers are not used as part of drug treatment for BPH. Calcium channel blockers do not play a role in treatment for BPH. Vasodilators would serve no benefit for the client with symptoms of BPH. **Cognitive Level:** Applying **Client Need:** Pharmacological and Parenteral Therapies **Integrated Process:** Nursing Process: Implementation **Content Area:** Pharmacology **Strategy:** There is only one correct answer to this question. While all the listed options are classifications of antihypertensive options, review the purposes of each classification in order to select the correct option.

Key Words to Review

anuria p. 554
bactericidal p. 558
bacteriostatic p. 558
diuretic p. 553
orthostatic hypotension p. 554

References

Adams, M., Holland, L., & Urban, C. (2011). *Pharmacology for nurses: A pathophysiological approach* (3rd ed.). Upper Saddle River, NJ: Pearson Education, Inc.

Adams, M., & Koch, R. (2010). *Pharmacology: Connections to nursing practice.* Upper Saddle River, NJ: Pearson Education, Inc.

Berman, A., & Snyder, S. (2012). *Kozier & Erb's fundamentals of nursing: Concepts, process and practice* (9th ed.). Upper Saddle River, NJ: Pearson Education, Inc.

Deglin, J. H., & Vallerand, A. H. (2011). *Davis's drug guide for nurses* (12th ed.). Philadelphia: F. A. Davis.

Lehne, R. (2010). *Pharmacology for nursing care* (7th ed.). Philadelphia: W. B. Saunders.

Wilson, B., Shannon, M., & Shields, K. (2012). *Pearson nurse's drug guide 2012.* Upper Saddle River, NJ: Pearson Education, Inc.

Test Yourself

Are you ready for the NCLEX-PN® or course exams? Use the practice tests on the companion website to check.

Gastrointestinal Medications

37

In this chapter

Cross Reference

Other chapters relevant to this content area are

Dosage Calculation and Medication Administration	Chapter 28
Gastrointestinal Disorders	Chapter 55

I. GASTROINTESTINAL ANTISPASMODIC AND ANTI-INFLAMMATORY DRUGS

A. Overview

1. **Antispasmodics** are muscarinic antagonists (**anticholinergics**) that antagonize action of acetylcholine (Ach) at cholinergic receptor sites and slow intestinal motility
2. Antispasmodics are used to treat spasms of gastrointestinal (GI) tract, such as pylorospasm, ileitis, and reduce cramping and diarrhea with irritable bowel syndrome (IBS)
3. GI anti-inflammatory drugs (5-aminosalicylic acid agents) are useful for induction therapy for inflammatory bowel disease (IBD), although immunosuppressive agents (azathioprine, mercaptopurine, and methotrexate; see also Chapter 41) are better for maintenance therapy
4. Anti-inflammatories exert their action by inhibiting prostaglandins and leukotrienes (mediators of inflammation)

B. Common medications are listed in Box 37–1

NCLEX® **C. Administration considerations**: give antispasmodics 30–60 minutes before meals and at bedtime; anti-inflammatories may be given with meals or after meals to slow intestinal transit time, but should be taken consistently in the same manner for best effect

D. Contraindications

1. Antispasmodics
   - **a.** Narrow-angle glaucoma, obstructive GI disease, paralytic ileus, obstructive uropathy
   - **b.** Excreted in breast milk; may cause infant toxicity and decreased milk production
   - **c.** Use with caution with renal dysfunction

Box 37–1

GI Antispasmodic and Anti-Inflammatory Medications

Antispasmodic	**Anti-inflammatory**
Dicyclomine (Bentyl)	Balsalizide (Colazal)
Hyoscyamine (Anaspaz)	Mesalamine (Asacol)
	Olsalazine (Dipentum)
	Sulfasalazine (Azulfidine)

2. Anti-inflammatories
   NCLEX® **a.** Hypersensitivity to salicylate (aspirin) for all in this class or sulfonamides for sulfasalazine
   b. Urinary obstruction
   c. Cautious use in hemotological disorders (risk of blood dyscrasias), liver disease (hepatotoxicity), dehydration (crystalluria), hyper- or hypoglycemia (increases insulin secretion)

E. Side/adverse effects

NCLEX® 1. Antispasmodics
   a. Common: dry mouth, blurred vision, drowsiness, constipation, urinary hesitancy, tachycardia
   b. Less common: confusion, paralytic ileus
2. Salicylate anti-inflammatories
   a. Common: headache, abdominal pain, nausea and vomiting (N/V), rash, allergic reactions
   b. Less common: hepatotoxicity, blood dyscrasias, salicylate hypersensitivity, crystalluria (sulfasalazine)

F. Nursing considerations

NCLEX® 1. Determine factors contributing to diarrhea to determine effective treatment
2. Clients who lose significant potassium with diarrhea are at risk for paralytic ileus and cardiac dysrhythmias
NCLEX® 3. Monitor for metabolic acidosis (loss of bicarbonate and impaired renal excretion of acids) and results of serum electrolytes
NCLEX® 4. Monitor vital signs (VS), intake and output (I&O), and visual changes

G. Client teaching

NCLEX® 1. Avoid exposure to high temperatures because of risk of hyperthermia if fluid losses occur
NCLEX® 2. Follow recommended dietary/fluid interventions to decrease constipation
3. Report any additional medications prescribed
4. Monitor own I&O for adequacy

II. ANTIDIARRHEALS

A. Overview

1. Slow and/or inhibit GI motility by acting on intestinal wall nerve endings to reduce stool volume, increase viscosity, and decrease fluid and electrolyte loss
2. Used for symptomatic relief of acute, nonspecific diarrhea and diarrhea of inflammatory disease

B. Common medications are listed in Box 37–2

C. Administration considerations

1. Shake suspensions well; chew tablets thoroughly
NCLEX® 2. Stool may appear gray-black (may mask GI bleeding)
3. Do not give concurrently with other medications
NCLEX® 4. Seek medical care if diarrhea persists for more than 2 days in an adult
5. Do not use to treat diarrhea in children; seek medical attention

D. Contraindications

NCLEX® 1. Bloody diarrhea, diarrhea associated with pathogens such as *E. coli*, salmonella, shigella or pseudomembranous colitis, or other bacterial toxins
2. Avoid use if obstructive bowel disease is suspected
NCLEX® 3. Avoid bismuth subsalicylate if allergic to aspirin or others salicylates; avoid concurrent use of aspirin with bismuth subsalicylate to prevent additive effects

Box 37–2

Antidiarrheals

Loperamide (Imodium)	Bismuth subsalicylate (Pepto-Bismol)
Diphenoxylate with atropine (Lomotil)	Octreotide (Sandostatin)
Difenoxin with atropine (Motofen)	

4. Difenoxin/atropine sulfate should not be used in children under age 2
5. Octreotide is used in severe diarrhea associated with cancer, ileostomy, and acquired immunodeficiency syndrome (AIDS)
6. Avoid concurrent use with monoamine oxidase inhibitors (MAOIs), which may increase risk of hypertensive crisis

E. Side/adverse effects

NCLEX® 1. Dry mouth, dizziness, drowsiness, constipation, N/V
2. Temporary darkening of stools and tongue may occur with bismuth salicylate
3. Central nervous system (CNS) depression, respiratory depression, hypotonic reflexes, angioedema, anaphylaxis, and paralytic ileus
4. Clinical signs and symptoms of overdose include drowsiness, decreased blood pressure (BP), seizures, apnea, blurred vision, dry mouth, and psychosis

F. Nursing considerations

1. Note allergies
2. Document onset, duration, and frequency of symptoms
3. Document previous therapies used and current medications
4. Identify any causative factors and presence of comorbid conditions; perform stool analysis as ordered
NCLEX® 5. Monitor for signs of dehydration or electrolyte imbalance
NCLEX® 6. Monitor vital signs and I&O
NCLEX® 7. Check abdomen for tenderness, distention, bowel sounds, or masses

G. Client teaching

1. Drink fluids to avoid dehydration and alleviate dry mouth
2. Follow BRAT diet—bananas, rice, applesauce, tea/toast—to reduce episodes of diarrhea if recommended by health care provider
3. Do not exceed prescribed dose
NCLEX® 4. Consult prescriber if diarrhea persists over 2 days
NCLEX® 5. Use caution in activities requiring alertness if dizziness/drowsiness is present (possible side effects)
6. Report occurrence of fever, N/V, abdominal pain or distention
NCLEX® 7. Avoid dairy products, which could aggravate diarrhea
8. Use hygiene measures to avoid skin irritation or breakdown due to diarrhea
9. Avoid alcohol ingestion while taking medication
10. Notify health care provider if pregnant or breastfeeding

III. LAXATIVES

A. Bulk-forming laxatives

1. Overview
   a. Include nonabsorbable polysaccharide and cellulose derivatives
   b. **Laxatives** swell in water, forming an emollient gel that increases bulk in intestines, which stimulates peristalsis and decreases bowel transit time
   c. Generally produce laxative effect within 12–14 hours but may require 2–3 days for full effect
2. Common medications are listed in Box 37–3

Box 37–3

Laxatives

Bulk-forming laxatives	Osmotic laxatives
Methylcellulose (Citrucel)	Lactulose (Constulose)
Calcium polycarbophil (Fibercon)	Polyethylene glycol (Miralax)
Psyllium (Metamucil)	Glycerin (Glycerol)
Stimulant laxatives	**Stool softener (surfactant)**
Senna (Senokot)	Docusate sodium (Colace)
Bisacodyl (Dulcolax)	**Saline laxatives**
Castor oil (Emulsoil)	Magnesium hydroxide (Milk of Magnesia)
Lubricant laxative	Sodium biphosphate (Fleets Phospho-Soda)
Mineral oil	

3. Administration considerations
   a. Since water is needed to increase bulk, give adequate fluids; may cause intestinal and esophageal obstruction if insufficient liquid is given with dose
   NCLEX® b. Give each dose with a full glass of liquid (240 mL)
   c. Use products that do not have phenylalanine in clients with phenylketonuria
4. Contraindications
   a. Not recommended for clients with intestinal stenosis, ulceration, or adhesions
   b. Use cautiously in clients with swallowing difficulties to prevent aspiration
   c. Do not use if fecal impaction is present
5. Side/adverse effects
   a. Abdominal discomfort and/or bloating, flatulence, N/V, diarrhea
   b. Rare reports of allergy to karaya (urticaria, rhinitis, dermatitis, bronchospasm)
   NCLEX® c. Esophageal obstruction, swelling, or blockage may occur if insufficient fluid used in mixing a bulk-forming laxative
6. Nursing considerations
   a. Check swallowing ability, adequately mix agents in liquid, and encourage additional fluid intake
   b. Monitor for aspiration
   NCLEX® c. If administered via feeding tube, use large bore tube; give rapidly with adequate flushing
   d. Add at least 8 oz (240 mL) of water or juice to drug
   e. Separate psyllium administration from digoxin, salicylates, and anticoagulants by 2 hours
   f. Use sugar-free preparations in diabetic clients
   NCLEX® g. Increase bulk or roughage (such as bran) in diet as ongoing therapy; provide 240–360 mL fluid with each tablespoon of bran to prevent fecal impaction
7. Client teaching
   a. Take in additional fluids, engage in exercise and increase dietary fiber
   NCLEX® b. Mix powder preparation with at least 8 oz fluid, drink immediately, and follow with another 8 oz of fluid
   c. Bulk-forming laxatives may decrease appetite if taken before meals
   d. Take medication 2 hours after meals and any oral medications
   e. Use sodium- and sugar-free preparations if appropriate for diet restrictions
   NCLEX® f. Full effect of medication may not occur for 2–3 days

B. Stimulant cathartics

1. Overview
   a. Stimulate peristalsis via mucosal irritation or intramural nerve plexus activity, which results in increased motility
   NCLEX® b. **Cathartics** are agents with purgative actions
   c. May modify permeability of colonic mucosal cells, which results in intraluminal fluid and electrolyte secretion
   d. Defecation occurs 6–12 hours after oral administration
   NCLEX® e. Rectal dose of bisacodyl and senna produces catharsis within 15 minutes to 2 hours
2. Common medications (see again Box 37–3)
3. Administration considerations
   NCLEX® a. Bedtime administration of dose promotes a morning bowel movement
   NCLEX® b. Swallow tablet whole; do not crush; do not take within 1 hour of antacids or milk
   c. Mix castor oil with 8 oz of water or juice; this drug is infrequently used
4. Contraindications
   NCLEX® a. Abdominal pain, N/V, symptoms of appendicitis, rectal bleeding, gastroenteritis, intestinal obstruction, fecal impaction
   b. Castor oil may induce premature labor
   c. Use senna cautiously during lactation; is excreted in breast milk
5. Side/adverse effects
   a. Abdominal cramps, diarrhea, N/V, laxative dependence
   b. Muscle weakness, hypokalemia, hypocalcemia, metabolic acidosis or alkalosis
   c. Rectal burning or irritation with suppository use
6. Nursing considerations
   a. Monitor for N/V, abdominal pain, diarrhea, fluid or electrolyte imbalances
   b. Administer dose either 1 hour before or after ingestion of milk or an antacid
   NCLEX® c. Encourage increased fluids and increased amounts of high-fiber foods in diet
   NCLEX® d. Monitor for laxative dependence and notify RN or health care provider

7. Client teaching
   NCLEX® a. Avoid chronic use of laxatives (beyond 1 week)
   NCLEX® b. These agents may produce a cathartic colon if used for several years; colon develops abnormal motor function, and resembles ulcerative colitis; usually discontinuation of laxative use restores normal bowel function
   c. Increase fluid intake and diet high in fiber; report side effects to prescriber
   d. Take dose 1 hour before or after ingestion of milk or an antacid

C. Hyperosmotic cathartics

1. Overview
   a. Increase osmotic pressure in intestinal lumen, resulting in retention of water, softening of stool
   b. Lactulose is an unabsorbed disaccharide metabolized by colon bacteria primarily to lactic, formic, and acetic acids, which may contribute to osmotic effect; it is used to treat occasional constipation or to reduce ammonia levels
2. Common medications (see again Box 37–3)
3. Administration considerations
   NCLEX® a. Glycerin is available only for rectal administration (suppository or enema) to treat acute constipation; laxative effect occurs within 15–30 minutes
   NCLEX® b. Lactulose may require 24–48 hours for effect; is more costly and should be used for acute constipation; dilute in water or juice to decrease sweet taste
   c. Dissolve Miralax in 8 oz of water and drink once daily for up to 2 weeks; results may take 2–4 days to occur
4. Contraindications: bowel obstruction; use lactulose cautiously in diabetic clients
5. Side/adverse effects
   a. Glycerin: rectal irritation and burning, hyperemia of rectal mucosa
   b. Lactulose and Miralax: flatulence, abdominal cramps/bloating, diarrhea
   NCLEX® c. Fluid and electrolyte imbalances
6. Nursing considerations: monitor frequency and consistency of stools and for electrolyte imbalances, especially in elderly
7. Client teaching
   a. Medication may take 2–4 days for effect
   b. Contact prescriber if unusual bloating, cramping, or diarrhea occurs
   c. Prolonged use may result in electrolyte imbalance and laxative dependence
   d. Take medication with juice to improve taste

D. Stool softeners (*surfactants*)

1. Overview
   a. Used on a scheduled basis for clients at risk for constipation, such as during hospitalization and bedrest, after surgery, or when receiving opioid analgesics
   b. Stool softeners are often called emollient laxatives; are anionic surfactants that lower fecal surface tension by allowing water and lipid penetration
   c. Some preparations combine a stool softener (docusate sodium) with a stimulant (casanthrol) to make a single combination product (e.g., Pericolace)
   NCLEX® d. Used for constipation associated with dry, hard stools and to decrease strain of defecation; fecal softening generally occurs in 1–3 days
2. Common medications (see again Box 37–3)
3. Administration considerations: do not give with mineral oil; offer fluids after each oral dose
4. Contraindications
   a. Hypersensitivity to drug
   NCLEX® b. Intestinal obstruction, undiagnosed abdominal pain, vomiting or other signs of appendicitis, fecal impaction, or acute abdomen
   c. Docusate sodium in congestive heart failure (CHF) because of sodium content
5. Side/adverse effects
   a. Bitter taste; mild abdominal cramping, diarrhea; dependence with long-term or excessive use
   b. Possible hepatotoxicity with docusate if used with oxyphenisatin or dantrolene
NCLEX® 6. Nursing considerations: monitor frequency and consistency of stools and electrolyte balance, especially in older adults
NCLEX® 7. Client teaching
   a. Take medication with milk or juice to decrease bitter taste

b. Increase high fiber foods in diet and fluid intake
c. May require 1–3 days to soften fecal matter; avoid prolonged use

E. Lubricant laxative

1. Overview
a. Lubricates feces and hinders water reabsorption into colon
b. Not commonly used today because of unintended effects
2. Common medication: mineral oil
3. Administration considerations
a. May take 24–48 hours to work
b. Do not give with food because it may delay gastric emptying; separate by 2 hours
c. May interfere with absorption of some drugs; alter administration times as needed

NCLEX® 4. Contraindications: abdominal pain, N/V; symptoms of appendicitis or acute abdomen; fecal impaction or bowel obstruction

5. Side/adverse effects
a. N/V, diarrhea, abdominal cramps
b. Laxative dependence may occur with excessive or long-term use
c. Nutritional deficiencies and impaired absorption of fat-soluble vitamins (A, D, E, K)
d. Aspiration may cause lipoid pneumonia
6. Nursing considerations

NCLEX® a. Because of possible aspiration and diminished vitamin absorption, do not give to children under 6, pregnant women, or debilitated clients

NCLEX® b. Use cautiously in older adults because of risk of aspiration; do not administer to client lying flat in bed

c. Do not administer medication at bedtime or within 2 hours of food because of possible decrease in gastric emptying
7. Client teaching

NCLEX® a. Avoid chronic use; mineral oil may leak through anal sphincter; report side effects to prescriber

b. Do not take medication when lying flat or at bedtime (risk of aspiration)

F. Saline laxatives

1. Overview
a. Magnesium, sulfate, phosphate, and citrate salts used for rapid bowel evacuation, such as in preparation for procedures or surgery
b. Mechanism of action is unclear, but may produce an osmotic effect that increases intraluminal volume and stimulates peristalsis
c. Magnesium may cause cholecystokinin release from duodenal mucosa, promoting increased fluid secretion and motility of small intestine and colon
d. Orally administered magnesium and sodium phosphate salts are effective within 30 minutes to 6 hours
e. Phosphate-containing rectal enemas evacuate bowel within 2–15 minutes
2. Common medications (see again Box 37–3)

NCLEX® 3. Administration considerations

a. Use magnesium salts cautiously in renal impairment because absorption may cause hypermagnesemia
b. Use sodium phosphate salts cautiously in clients with sodium restriction
c. Concurrent use with antacids may inactivate both
4. Contraindications
a. Not recommended for children under 2 because of risk for hypocalcemia
b. Contraindicated in presence of abdominal pain, N/V, signs of appendicitis or acute abdomen, intestinal obstruction, edema, CHF, megacolon, or impaired renal function
5. Side/adverse effects
a. Cramping and urgency to defecate

NCLEX® b. Safe when administered for short-term management; may cause significant fluid and electrolyte imbalances with prolonged use or in certain clients

6. Nursing considerations
a. Encourage increased fluid intake to avoid dehydration since these drugs are salts
b. Monitor drug effectiveness
7. Client teaching
a. Avoid frequent or prolonged use to avoid laxative dependence; report side effects or lack of effectiveness to prescriber
b. Increase fluid intake and dietary fiber as additional measures

IV. ANTIEMETICS

A. Overview

1. **Emesis** is a complex reflex brought about by activation of vomiting center in medulla oblongata
2. Certain stimuli activate vomiting center directly (e.g., GI irritation), while others (e.g., drugs, toxins, radiation) stimulate chemoreceptor trigger zone (CTZ) in medulla
3. Emetogenic compounds and antiemetic drugs produce their effects by affecting neuroreceptors (which are influenced by acetylcholine, histamine, serotonin, dopamine, benzodiazepines, and cannabinoids)
4. Phenothiazines suppress emesis by blocking dopamine receptors in CTZ
5. Cannabinoids are approved to treat N/V associated with cancer chemotherapy; mechanism of action is unknown; dronabinol also approved as appetite stimulant in AIDS

Memory Aid

Cannabinoids can be recognized on sight because they end with the suffix *-abinol.*

6. Benzodiazepines: primary effect is suppression of anxiety; most effective for management of N/V associated with cancer chemotherapy when combined with metoclopramide (Reglan) and dexamethasone (Decadron)
7. Glucocorticoids: mechanism for suppression of chemotherapy-associated emesis is unknown; are effective alone and in combination with other antiemetics
8. Antihistamines: anticholinergic effect reduces motion sickness and vomiting
9. Serotonin receptor antagonists: block serotonin receptors to reduce nausea

B. Common medications are listed in Box 37–4

Memory Aid

Serotonin antagonists can be recognized on sight because they end with the suffix *-setron.*

C. Administration considerations

1. Often antiemetic combinations work better than single-drug treatment, particularly for cancer chemotherapy induced emesis, suggesting more than one mechanism may trigger emesis

Box 37–4

Antiemetics

Anithistamine type

Cyclizine (Marezine)

Dimenhydrinate (Dramamine)

Diphenhydramine (Benadryl)

Hydroxyzine (Vistaril)

Meclizine (Antivert)

Scopolamine (Transderm Scop)

Benzodiazepines

Lorazepam (Ativan)

Cannabinoids

Dronabinol (Marinol)

Nabilone (Cesamet)

Glucocorticoids

Dexamethasone (Decadron)

Methylprednisolone (Solu-Medrol)

Phenothiazine and Phenothiazine-like

Metoclopramide (Reglan)

Perphenazine (Phenazine)

Prochlorperazine (Compazine)

Promethazine HCl (Phenergan)

Serotonin Receptor Antagonists

Dolasetron (Anzemet)

Granisetron (Kytril)

Ondansetron (Zofran)

Palonosetron (Aloxi)

Neurokinin Receptor Antagonist

Aprepitant (Emend)

2. Prophylactic drugs are often given by mouth; however, active emesis is usually managed with parenteral or rectal dosing
3. Anticipatory N/V should be treated 1 hour before meals or therapy
4. Parenteral doses should be given deep IM to avoid drug leakage into subcutaneous tissues

D. Contraindications
1. CNS depression and coma
2. Use cautiously in clients with glaucoma, seizures, intestinal obstruction, prostatic hyperplasia, asthma, cardiac, pulmonary, or hepatic disease

E. Side/adverse effects
1. Phenothiazines: extrapyramidal reactions, anticholinergic effects, hypotension, and sedation
2. Cannabinoids: temporal disintegration, dissociation, depersonalization, and dysphoria
3. Phenothiazines: agranulocytosis, thrombocytopenia

F. Nursing considerations
1. Dronabinol and nabilone have a high potential for abuse
2. Check VS regularly for hypotension or tachycardia
3. Observe for side effects and adverse reactions
4. Monitor I&O for urine retention
5. Observe for mood changes or involuntary movements
6. Monitor lab values: liver function tests, electrolytes, blood urea nitrogen (BUN) and creatinine
7. May mask response of skin testing; discontinue 4 days prior to testing
8. Monitor for anticholinergic effects: dry mouth, constipation, visual changes

G. Client teaching
1. Avoid activities that require alertness; avoid alcohol and CNS depressants
2. Monitor blood glucose if diabetic
3. Avoid excessive sunlight/ultraviolet light because of potential photosensitivity
4. Use sugarless hard candy or ice chips to avoid dry mouth
5. Increase fluids and dietary fiber to decrease risk of constipation
6. Take medication 30–60 minutes before any activity that causes nausea

V. HISTAMINE H_2 ANTAGONISTS

A. Overview
1. Reduce gastric acid secretion by blocking histamine$_2$ in gastric parietal cells
2. Histamine **H_2 antagonists** (agents that decrease gastric secretion) are used to treat duodenal ulcer, gastric ulcer, hypersecretory conditions such as Zollinger-Ellison syndrome, reflux esophagitis
3. Used to prevent stress ulcers in critically ill clients; used in combination therapy to treat ***Helicobacter pylori*** (bacteria found in gastric mucosa) infection
4. Prototype agent, cimetidine, has highest rate of side effects

B. Common medications are listed in Box 37–5

Memory Aid

Histamine 2 antagonists can be recognized on sight because they end with the suffix *-tidine.*

C. Administration considerations
1. Drugs administered intravenously (IV) should not be mixed with other medications
2. Avoid antacid use within 1 hour of administration

D. Contraindications: hypersensitivity to drug; use caution in clients with impaired renal or hepatic function

E. Side/adverse effects
1. Cimetidine: common unintended effects are constipation, diarrhea, nausea, headache, fatigue, gynecomastia; rarely hepatitis, blood dyscrasias, dysrhythmias, skin reactions, confusion, anaphylaxis, galactorrhea

Box 37–5
Histamine 2 (H_2) Antagonists

Cimetidine (Tagamet)	Famotidine (Pepcid)
Ranitidine (Zantac)	Nizatidine (Axid)

2. Other drugs: more common unintended effects are headache, nausea, and dry mouth; rarely musculoskeletal pain, tachycardia, blood dyscrasias, blurred vision

F. Nursing considerations

NCLEX® 1. Dosages are usually reduced with hepatic or renal impairment
2. Check medications for possible interactions
3. Monitor nutritional status and dietary interventions
4. Evaluate need for smoking cessation and alcohol abuse programs

G. Client teaching

1. Avoid smoking, which causes gastric stimulation
NCLEX® 2. Avoid **antacid** (agent reducing acidity) use within 1 hour of dose
3. Take once-a-day dose at bedtime; otherwise take before meals
4. Avoid gastric irritants such as alcohol, aspirin, and nonsteroidal anti-inflammatory drugs (NSAIDs)
5. Report side effects to prescriber

VI. PROTON PUMP INHIBITORS (PPIs)

A. Overview

1. Block acid secretion by inhibiting H^+–K^+ ATPase at secretory surface of gastric parietal cells
2. Used to treat gastroesophageal reflux disease (GERD) or duodenal ulcers, active benign gastric ulcers, and NSAID-associated gastric ulcers
3. Used to treat pathological hypersecretory conditions such as Zollinger-Ellison syndrome

B. Common medications are listed in Box 37–6

Memory Aid

Proton pump inhibitors can be recognized on sight because they end with the suffix *-prazole.*

C. Administration considerations

1. May give with antacids
2. If unable to swallow capsules, lansoprazole and esomeprazole capsules may be opened and sprinkled on applesauce before taking
3. Omeprazole, pantoprazole, and rabeprazole must be swallowed whole
4. Pantoprazole IV: administer over 15 minute period at rate not more than 3 mg/min (7 mL/min)
5. To give per nasogastric (NG) tube, dilute capsule contents in 40 mL juice

D. Contraindications: not recommended in children or nursing mothers

E. Side/adverse effects

1. More common are headache, diarrhea, nausea, rash, dizziness, and abdominal pain
2. Rarely agranuloxytosis or other blood disorder can occur

F. Nursing considerations

NCLEX® 1. Document reason for therapy, duration of symptoms, and drug efficacy
2. Monitor for side effects
3. Monitor liver function tests, CBC, BUN and creatinine; dose may be reduced in liver disease

G. Client teaching

1. Follow prescribed diet and activities to decrease symptoms
2. Medication is often for short-term therapy; keep health care appointments for continued signs and symptoms
3. Take early in morning 30–60 minutes before breakfast
NCLEX® 4. Notify prescriber of any difficulty swallowing because omeprazole, pantoprazole, and rabeprazole must be swallowed whole
5. Lansoprazole and esomeprazole capsules may be opened and sprinkled

Box 37–6

Proton Pump Inhibitors

Esomeprazole (Nexium)	Pantoprazole (Protonix)
Lansoprazole (Prevacid)	Rabeprazole sodium (Aciphex)
Omeprazole (Prilosec)	

VII. MUCOSAL PROTECTIVE AGENTS

A. Overview

1. Misoprostol (Cytotec) is a synthetic prostaglandin E2 that stimulates production of protective mucus and inhibits gastric secretion; is often used to prevent gastric ulcers with high-dose NSAID or corticosteroid therapy
2. Sucralfate (Carafate) enhances mucosal defenses and produces a thick protective coating over ulcer, which protects against further erosion and aids healing

B. Common medications: misoprostol (Cytotec), sucralfate (Carafate)

C. Administration considerations

NCLEX®
1. Sucralfate should be taken 1 hour before meals and bedtime, or 2 hours after meals or medications and not within 2 hours of antacids
2. Misoprostol should be taken with food

D. Contraindications

NCLEX®
1. Misoprostol is contraindicated in clients who are allergic to prostaglandins, or who are pregnant or lactating; misoprostol is labeled as a pregnancy category X drug; safety not established for those under age 18; use cautiously with clients with renal impairment and/or older than 64 years
2. Sucralfate has no known contraindications but safety in children and during lactation is not fully established

E. Side/adverse effects

1. Misoprostol: diarrhea, abdominal cramping, dysmenorrhea, menstrual disorders, and postmenopausal bleeding
2. Sucralfate: constipation; minimal adverse effects because little drug absorbed from GI tract

F. Nursing considerations

NCLEX®
1. Monitor effect of medication on GI symptoms and monitor side effects

NCLEX®
2. Screen for pregnancy
3. Monitor concurrent medications

G. Client teaching

NCLEX®
1. Avoid gastric irritants such as caffeine, alcohol, smoking, and spicy foods
2. Report side effects to prescriber for possible dosage change

NCLEX®
3. Follow contraceptive practices while on misoprostol
4. Do not take misoprostol if pregnant; discontinue use if pregnancy occurs or is suspected; report any abnormal vaginal bleeding; avoid pregnancy at least 1 month or 1 menstrual cycle after stopping medication
5. Increase fluids and fiber to decrease constipation
6. Follow instructions for antacid use to decrease interaction

VIII. ANTACIDS

A. Overview

1. Gastric acid–neutralizing agent used for relief of hyperacidity associated with GI disorders
2. Used as antiflatulent to alleviate symptoms of gas and bloating

B. Common medications are listed in Box 37–7

NCLEX®
C. Administration considerations: take at least 2 hours apart from other drugs where a drug interaction may occur

D. Contraindications

1. Safety has not been established for use of antacids by lactating women

Box 37–7

Antacids

- Aluminum hydroxide (AlternaGel, others)
- Calcium carbonate (Tums, Titralac)
- Calcium carbonate with magnesium hydroxide (Rolaids)
- Magaldrate (Riopan)
- Magnesium hydroxide (Milk of Magnesia)
- Magnesium trisilicate and aluminum hydroxide (Gaviscon)
- Magnesium hydroxide and aluminum hydroxide (Maalox)
- Magnesium hydroxide, aluminum hydroxide, and simethicone (Mylanta, others)
- Sodium bicarbonate (Alka-Seltzer, baking soda)

2. Magnesium hydroxide is contraindicated with abdominal pain, N/V, diarrhea, severe renal dysfunction, fecal impaction, rectal bleeding, colostomy, ileostomy
3. Aluminum carbonate antacids: prolonged use of high doses with low serum phosphate
4. Calcium carbonate antacids: hypercalcemia and hypercalciuria, severe renal disease, renal calculi, GI hemorrhage or obstruction, dehydration

E. Side/adverse effects

1. Antacids increase gastric pH, and may bind with other drugs, decreasing their absorption and effectiveness; separate their administration from other drugs by 1–2 hours or as recommended by drug literature
2. Prolonged use may alter aluminum, calcium, sodium, and phosphate levels
3. Belching, constipation, flatulence, diarrhea, and gastric distention
4. Hypophosphatemia (anorexia, malaise, tremors, muscle weakness)
5. Aluminum toxicity (dementia) may occur with repeated dosing of aluminum-based products
6. Hypercalcemia and metabolic alkalosis may occur with antacids containing calcium carbonate
7. Use of antacids containing sodium carbonate may worsen hypertension and risk for heart failure from increased sodium intake
8. NCLEX® Aluminum-containing antacids can cause constipation, while magnesium-containing antacids tend to cause diarrhea

NCLEX® **F. Nursing considerations**

1. Shake suspension well
2. Flush NG tube with water after administration
3. Observe for signs of altered phosphate levels: anorexia, muscle weakness, and malaise
4. Liquid preparations act more quickly than tablets; follow liquid dose with 4 ounces of water to speed effectiveness

NCLEX® **G. Client teaching**

1. Understand methods to avoid constipation; drink plenty of fluids
2. Take as directed; do not exceed maximum dose
3. Keep out of reach of children
4. May interact with certain medications; notify prescriber of other medications used
5. Do not use without medical advice if diagnosed with kidney disease

IX. TREATMENT REGIMENS FOR *HELICOBACTER PYLORI*

A. Overview

1. Antisecretory and antimicrobial action against most strains of *Helicobacter pylori (H. pylori)*
2. Used to eradicate *H. pylori* infection and to reduce risk of duodenal ulcer recurrence

B. Common medication combinations are listed in Box 37–8

C. Administration considerations

1. Swallow all pills whole except bismuth, which should be chewed
2. If dose is missed, continue with normal dosage regimen; do not double dose
3. NCLEX® Do not administer if client has allergy to any component of therapy
4. Pregnant women should not take regimens containing clarithromycin
5. Therapy usually continues for 7–14 days

D. Side/adverse effects

1. Rash, N/V, diarrhea, abnormal taste, abdominal pain, dyspepsia
2. Transient CNS reactions such as anxiety, behavior changes, tinnitus, and vertigo
3. Headache, photosensitivity, ventricular dysrhythmias

E. Nursing considerations

1. Note signs and symptoms, onset, and duration; document allergy status
2. NCLEX® Determine pregnancy status; do not adminster bismuth subsalicylate to children because of risk of Reye's syndrome
3. Document previous therapies used; document confirmation of infection

Box 37–8

Treatment Regimens for *Helicobacter pylori*

- Omeprazole, clarithromycin (Prilosec/Biaxin), and amoxicillin (Amoxil)
- Omeprazole (or other PPI), bismuth subsalicylate, metronidazole (Flagyl), and tetracycline
- Omeprazole (or other PPI), clarithromycin (Biaxin), and metronidazole (Flagyl)

F. Client teaching

1. Understand importance of compliance; review drug packaging (some combinations are prepackaged)
2. NCLEX® Avoid gastric irritants such as smoking, alcohol, and caffeine
3. Practice stress reduction techniques; avoid prolonged exposure to sun
4. Bismuth-containing preparations may cause darkening of tongue and stool
5. Report side effects or continued symptoms to prescriber
6. Do not double dose if dose is missed
7. Use additional contraceptive measures because antibiotics can decrease birth control pill effectiveness

X. GALLSTONE-DISSOLVING AGENT

A. Ursodiol (Actigall)

1. Natural occurring bile acid that inhibits hepatic synthesis and secretion of cholesterol; used to dissolve gallbladder stones smaller than 20 mm
2. Absorbed in small bowel, secreted into hepatic bile ducts, and expelled into duodenum in response to eating

B. Administration considerations: use beyond 24 months has not been established

C. Contraindications

1. Clients who have calcified cholesterol stones, radiopaque stones, or radiolucent bile pigment stones
2. Avoid in clients with acute cholecystitis, biliary obstruction, pancreatitis, allergy to bile acids, and chronic liver disease; excretion in breast milk is not known

D. Side/adverse effects

1. NCLEX® Abdominal pain, N/V, constipation, diarrhea, rash
2. Headache, fatigue, anxiety, sweating, thinning of hair, arthralgia

E. Nursing considerations

1. NCLEX® Document indications and length of therapy; if no dissolving of partial stone is noted in 12 months, drug will probably not be effective
2. Gallbladder ultrasound should be done every 6 months during first year of therapy
3. Determine pregnancy status

F. Client teaching

1. Avoid antacid use with drug unless prescribed
2. Therapy may take up to 24 months, and stones may recur; comply with follow-up visits and diagnostic tests
3. Report any side effects to prescriber
4. Be aware that birth control pills may decrease drug effect

XI. PANCREATIC ENZYME REPLACEMENT

A. Pancrelipase

1. Enzyme (lipase, amylase, and protease) replacement therapy for cystic fibrosis, chronic pancreatitis, ductal obstructions, or pancreatic insufficiency
2. Various formulations available with trade names of Cotazym, Pancrease, others

B. Administration considerations

1. Swallow tablets/capsules whole; do not crush or chew
2. If swallowing is difficult, open capsules and give contents in applesauce or pudding to swallow without chewing
3. Take medications with meals; do not give with antacids or iron

NCLEX® **C. Contraindications**: hypersensitivity to pork protein or enzymes, or with acute pancreatitis

NCLEX® **D. Side/adverse effects**: nausea, diarrhea, abdominal cramps, hyperuricemia

E. Nursing considerations

1. NCLEX® Determine swallowing ability or difficulty
2. Monitor for side effects and monitor steatorrhea (should diminish with appropriate drug dose)
3. Monitor to maintain good nutritional status; monitor uric acid levels
4. Document allergies

F. Client teaching

1. Follow dietary interventions; consult with dietitian for meal planning
2. Take before or with meals with plenty of water
3. Report side effects to prescriber

Check Your NCLEX–PN® Exam I.Q.

You are ready for testing on this content if you can

- Apply knowledge of expected actions and effects of gastrointestinal medications to client care.
- Correctly administer gastrointestinal medications to clients.
- Monitor for side effects and adverse effects of gastrointestinal medications.
- Take appropriate action if a client has an unexpected response to a gastrointestinal medication.
- Monitor a client for expected outcomes or effects of treatment with gastrointestinal medications.

PRACTICE TEST

1 A client who has been prescribed rabeprazole (Aciphex) for symptoms of gastroesophageal reflux disease (GERD) has trouble swallowing pills. What alternate medication should the nurse expect to be ordered for this client?

1. Omeprazole (Prilosec)
2. Pantoprazole (Protonix)
3. Lansoprazole (Prevacid)
4. IV esomeprazole (Nexium)

2 A nurse is reinforcing teaching to a female client newly diagnosed with *Helicobacter pylori* infection. The nurse expects that which medication will not be used after learning the client is pregnant?

1. Metronidazole (Flagyl)
2. Amoxicillin (Amoxil)
3. Clarithromycin (Biaxin)
4. Ciprofloxacin (Cipro)

3 A client is taking bismuth for diarrhea. For which side effect, unique to this medication, would a nurse monitor?

1. Darkening of the tongue
2. Dyspepsia
3. Abdominal pain
4. Diarrhea

4 A client's breath urease test is positive for *Helicobacter pylori* organisms. The nurse anticipates that which medications will be ordered to eradicate this infection most effectively?

1. Antacids and amoxicillin
2. Omeprazole, ranitidine, and amoxicillin
3. Combination of proton pump inhibitor, amoxicillin, and clarithromycin
4. Clarithromycin and bismuth salicylate

5 The nurse would consider that which medication is ordered at a safe and effective dosage range for an adult client who is experiencing nausea and vomiting?

1. Promethazine (Phenergan) 25 mg every 4–6 hours prn
2. Prochlorperazine (Compazine) 200 mg every 6 hours
3. Metoclopramide (Reglan) 30 mg ac and HS
4. Trimethobenzamide hydrochloride (Tigan) 20 mg t.i.d. prn

6 A client is receiving omeprazole (Prilosec) for esophageal reflux. The nurse should monitor the results of which laboratory studies? Select all that apply.

1. Urinalysis
2. Uric acid
3. Liver enzymes
4. Serum glucose
5. Complete blood count (CBC)

7 When caring for a client with onset of severe nausea, the nurse telephones the health care provider for an order for which emetic that has the fastest onset of action?

1. Oral promethazine (Phenergan)
2. Scopolamine transdermal (Transderm-Scop)
3. Oral metoclopramide (Reglan)
4. Haloperidol (Haldol)

PRACTICE TEST

8 A client has been diagnosed with severe erosive esophagitis. The nurse who is assisting in developing a medication teaching plan should recognize that which medication is most appropriate to treat the disorder?

1. Sucralfate (Carafate)
2. Omeprazole (Prilosec)
3. Nizatidine (Axid)
4. Amoxicillin (Amoxil)

9 A client has been advised to take an antacid to neutralize gastric acid in order to decrease gastric irritation pain. What administration issues related to antacids should be discussed with the client? Select all that apply.

1. Chew the tablets and follow with 4 ounces of water.
2. Take the antacid 2 hours after other prescribed oral medication.
3. Take prescribed antacids on a regular basis for up to 6 weeks.
4. Take antacids regularly after meals to prevent gastric irritation.
5. Breastfeeding mothers can safely be prescribed the use of antacids.

10 A client who has a history of glaucoma is diagnosed with a gastrointestinal disorder. The nurse should question the health care provider if which medication is prescribed?

1. Dicyclomine (Bentyl)
2. Omeprazole (Prilosec)
3. Metoclopramide (Reglan)
4. Magnesium hydroxide (Milk of Magnesia)

11 A client who needs to take a histamine (H_2) antagonist has a history of multiple health problems. The nurse would explain that which histamine antagonist should be avoided because it has the greatest number of drug interactions?

1. Famotidine (Pepcid)
2. Ranitidine (Zantac)
3. Nizatidine (Axid)
4. Cimetidine (Tagamet)

12 A client newly diagnosed with a gastric ulcer has been prescribed sucralfate (Carafate). Which beneficial effect related to this medication should the nurse reinforce with the client?

1. It will reduce GI spasms.
2. It will protect the eroded ulcer surface from stomach acid.
3. It will help relieve nausea and vomiting.
4. It will act as an anticholinergic.

13 A client with chronic pancreatitis has been prescribed pancrelipase (Pancrease). The nurse who is teaching the client about this medication would include that pancrelipase increases digestion of what foods?

1. Proteins and starches
2. Proteins and fats
3. Starches and fats
4. Vitamins and starches

14 A client, with diarrhea for the past 24 hours, reports taking loperamide (Imodium) the previous day per dosage instructions without relief. Currently, the client has a temperature of 102ºF, excessive thirst, and severe abdominal cramping. What is the highest-priority action for the nurse at this time?

1. Obtain a further history of digestive disorders.
2. Discuss dietary factors that might be causing the diarrhea.
3. Suggest acetaminophen (Tylenol) for fever and pain.
4. Notify the health care provider.

15 A parent of a 2-year-old child asks the nurse why bismuth subsalicylate (Pepto-Bismol) should not be used for diarrhea in children under 3 years. The nurse should include which rationale in response?

1. The taste is offensive to children.
2. It could lead to development of Reye's syndrome.
3. It has a higher-than-recommended lead content.
4. The side effect of a darkened tongue frightens children.

16 The nurse is giving follow-up instructions to a client with irritable bowel syndrome (IBS). The nurse provides information about which medication that would be beneficial to treat both the diarrhea and constipation associated with IBS?

1. Methylcellulose (Citrucel)
2. Docusate sodium (Colace)
3. Dicyclomine (Bentyl)
4. Bisacodyl (Dulcolax)

17 A 26-year-old female client comes to the clinic for an annual health examination. She has been taking misoprostol (Cytotec) for several years following diagnosis of a gastric ulcer. She is getting married next month. What is the priority nursing intervention for this client?

1. Discuss whether to continue taking her oral contraceptive.
2. Discuss family planning.
3. Provide sexually transmitted infection (STI) counseling.
4. Explain the risks of using misoprostol during pregnancy.

18 A client with compensated congestive heart failure comes to the ambulatory care center reporting increased fatigue, weakness, and dizziness. Laboratory results indicate a low sodium level. Current medications include daily doses of Lasix, K-Dur, Lanoxin, and a prn bisacodyl (Dulcolax) suppository. What information would help determine the cause of the client's hyponatremia?

1. How frequently a bisacodyl suppository is used.
2. Whether digoxin doses were skipped in the last week.
3. Validation of compliance with prescribed amount of K-Dur.
4. Frequency of dietary intake of salty foods in restaurants.

19 A client with constipation has history of coronary artery disease and congestive heart failure. Which type of laxative does the nurse expect to be prescribed for this client?

1. A bulk-forming laxative
2. A saline laxative
3. A stimulant laxative
4. PRN enemas

20 The client comes to the office to get a refill of a prescription for dicyclomine hydrochloride (Bentyl). She tells the nurse she is leaving the next day for a vacation to Florida. What information should the nurse provide this client?

1. "Don't be so concerned about taking the medication on vacation."
2. "This medication makes you more sensitive to high temperatures."
3. "If you anticipate drinking alcohol, discontinue themedication."
4. "Take antacids with this medication to decrease any symptoms of GERD."

ANSWERS & RATIONALES

1 **Answer: 3** **Rationale:** Lansoprazole capsules may be opened and sprinkled on applesauce or dissolved in 40 mL of juice; this is an appropriate substitution for the client who cannot swallow capsules or pills. Omeprazole and pantoprazole must be swallowed whole. Esomeprazole does not come in IV form; pantoprazole (when ordered IV) can be given over 15 minutes at a rate not more than 3 mg/min. **Cognitive Level:** Analyzing **Client Need:** Pharmacological and Parenteral Therapies **Integrated Process:** Nursing Process: Planning **Content Area:** Pharmacology **Strategy:** The core issue of the question is knowledge of the formulations of various proton pump inhibitors. Use medication knowledge and the process of elimination to make a selection. Eliminate the drug with the most invasive route of administration first.

2 **Answer: 4** **Rationale:** Ciprofloxacin is not recommended for *Helicobacter pylori* infection during pregnancy. Metronidazole, amoxicillin, and clarithromycin can be used by a pregnant client after consulting with the physician. **Cognitive Level:** Applying **Client Need:** Pharmacological and Parenteral Therapies **Integrated Process:** Nursing Process: Planning **Content Area:** Pharmacology **Strategy:** The core issue of the question is knowledge of what medications are safe for use in pregnancy for a client with *Helicobacter pylori* infection. Use medication knowledge and the process of elimination to make a selection.

3 **Answer: 1** **Rationale:** Bismuth-containing preparations, such as Pepto-Bismol, can cause all the listed side effects, but transient darkening of the tongue and stool is a side effect specific to bismuth. Dyspepsia, abdominal pain, and diarrhea are not unique to this medication. **Cognitive Level:** Applying **Client Need:** Pharmacological and Parenteral Therapies **Integrated Process:** Nursing Process: Data Collection **Content Area:** Pharmacology **Strategy:** The critical word in the stem of this question is *unique*. This means that the answer is a side effect that does not occur with other drugs that are antidiarrheals. Use specific medication knowledge and the process of elimination to make a selection.

4 **Answer: 3** **Rationale:** The highest rate of eradication of *Helicobacter pylori* infection is achieved by using a proton pump inhibitor and two antibiotics (usually clarithromycin and amoxicillin or metronidazole). The other options do not provide a level of effectiveness for eradication of *Helicobacter pylori*. **Cognitive Level:** Applying **Client Need:** Pharmacological and Parenteral Therapies **Integrated Process:** Nursing Process: Planning **Content Area:** Pharmacology **Strategy:** The core issue of the question is knowledge of what medications are commonly used in treating *Helicobacter pylori* infection. Use medication knowledge and the process of elimination to make a selection.

5 **Answer: 1** **Rationale:** Promethazine is usually given 25 mg every 4–6 hours prn. Dosing may start at 12.5 mg every 4–6 hours prn depending on client status; however, 25 mg is the usual dose. The normal dose of prochlorperazine is 5–10 mg t.i.d.–q.i.d; 200 mg is too high. The normal dose of metoclopramide is 10 mg, 30 minutes AC and HS; 30 mg is too high. The normal dose of trimethobenzamide hydrochloride is 250 mg t.i.d.–q.i.d. prn; 20 mg is too low. **Cognitive Level:** Applying **Client Need:** Pharmacological and Parenteral Therapies **Integrated Process:** Nursing Process: Planning **Content Area:** Pharmacology **Strategy:** The core issue of the question is knowledge of the dosage range for various antiemetics. Use medication knowledge and the process of elimination to make a selection.

6 **Answer: 1, 3, 5** **Rationale:** Urinalysis results should be monitored for hematuria and proteinuria. Omeprazole can cause an increase in liver enzyme levels (AST, ALT, alkaline phosphatase, and bilirubin), leading to adverse reactions of liver necrosis and hepatic failure. The nurse should monitor these lab values as they become available. It is rare, but agranulocytosis can occur; therefore, the CBC should be monitored to identify the development of any hematological disorders. Uric acid should be monitored only as indicated based on an individual client's identified health need; there is no health need that indicates a need for this test. Omeprazole does not affect the serum glucose levels; monitoring is not necessary in relation to this drug administration. **Cognitive Level:** Analyzing **Client Need:** Pharmacological and Parenteral Therapies **Integrated Process:** Nursing Process: Planning **Content Area:** Pharmacology **Strategy:** The core issue of the question is knowledge of the laboratory values that could be affected by administration of omeprazole. With this group of medications, it is necessary to remember the liver and kidneys. Use medication knowledge and the process of elimination to make a selection. When more than one answer is correct, consider each option as a true/false statement.

7 **Answer: 2** **Rationale:** All medications listed have antiemetic effects, but transdermal scopolamine has the fastest onset of action. For this reason, it is most effective in providing relief from nausea for a prolonged period of time. **Cognitive Level:** Applying **Client Need:** Pharmacological and Parenteral Therapies **Integrated Process:** Nursing Process: Implementation **Content Area:** Pharmacology **Strategy:** The core issue of the question is knowledge of onset of action of various antiemetics. Recall that transdermal systems begin to absorb into the skin immediately after application, while oral doses take various amounts of time to absorb through the GI tract. Use medication knowledge and the process of elimination to make a selection.

8 **Answer: 2** **Rationale:** Because of their antisecretory effect, proton pump inhibitors such as omeprazole are the drugs of choice for moderate-to-severe erosive esophagitis. The course of therapy is usually 4–8 weeks. The other options might be helpful for clients with *Heliobactor pylori*; however, proton pump inhibitors are the medication classification of choice for erosive esophagitis. **Cognitive Level:** Analyzing **Client Need:** Pharmacological and Parenteral Therapies **Integrated Process:** Nursing Process: Planning **Content Area:** Pharmacology **Strategy:** The core issue of the question is knowledge of the various GI medications that are useful in treating digestive system health problems. Recall that disorders that end in *-itis* involve inflammation, so the correct answer is one that reduces inflammation either by its own action or by inhibiting other irritants, such as gastric acid. Use medication knowledge of omeprazole as a proton pump inhibitor to make a selection.

9 **Answer: 1, 2, 4** **Rationale:** Antacids should be chewed well and followed with 4 ounces of water for optimal effect. The client should allow at least 2 hours between taking the antacid and any other oral medication to avoid any issues related to absorption. Antacids should be taken regularly after meals in order to prevent gastric upset and provide better symptom control. Antacids should not be taken for longer than 2 weeks without further evaluation. Safety has not been established for the use of antacids by lactating women. **Cognitive Level:** Analyzing **Client Need:** Pharmacological and Parenteral Therapies **Integrated Process:** Nursing Process: Planning **Content Area:** Pharmacology **Strategy:** The core issue of the question is knowledge of medication administration procedures for antacids. Recall that antacids are more effective when given with fluid to help disperse medication in the stomach. Use medication knowledge and the process of elimination to make a selection. When more than one answer is correct, consider each option as a true/false statement.

10 **Answer: 1** **Rationale:** Clients with glaucoma should not take anticholinergic agents such as dicyclomine, because the medication affects pupillary dilatation, and therefore indirectly affects the outflow of aqueous humor. Prescribing omeprazole should not pose a problem for a client with glaucoma. It is safe to prescribe metoclopramide for gastric issues in a client with glaucoma. There are no contraindications regarding a client with glaucoma taking magnesium hydroxide. **Cognitive Level:** Analyzing **Client Need:** Pharmacological and Parenteral Therapies **Integrated Process:** Nursing Process: Implementation **Content Area:** Pharmacology **Strategy:** The core issue of the question is knowledge of medications that are contraindicated with glaucoma. Specific medication knowledge is needed to answer the question. Use medication knowledge and the process of elimination to make a selection.

11 **Answer: 4** **Rationale:** Cimetidine decreases metabolism of beta-blockers, phenytoin, procainamide, quinidine, benzodiazepines, metronidazole, tricyclic antidepressants, and warfarin, leading to increased risk of drug toxicity. The other options are histamine blockers that are newer than cimetidine, and have fewer side effects. **Cognitive Level:** Applying **Client Need:** Pharmacological and Parenteral Therapies **Integrated Process:** Nursing Process: Implementation **Content Area:** Pharmacology **Strategy:** The core issue of the question is knowledge of histamine antagonists that are highest in side or adverse effects. Specific medication knowledge is needed to answer the question. Use medication knowledge and the process of elimination to make a selection.

12 **Answer: 2** **Rationale:** Sucralfate forms an adhesive barrier on the surface of the gastric mucosa, protecting it from gastric acid. Sucralfate does not reduce GI spasms, relieve nausea and vomiting, or have anticholinergic effects. **Cognitive Level:** Applying **Client Need:** Pharmacological and Parenteral Therapies **Integrated Process:** Nursing Process: Implementation **Content Area:** Pharmacology **Strategy:** The core issue of the question is knowledge of the mechanism of action of sucralfate (Carafate). Specific medication knowledge is needed to answer the question. Use this knowledge and the process of elimination to make a selection.

13 **Answer: 3 Rationale:** Pancrease, a pancreatic enzyme replacement, increases digestion of starches and fats, and thereby decreases the incidence of steatorrhea (fatty, frothy, foul-smelling stools). It does not increase the digestion of the other options. **Cognitive Level:** Applying **Client Need:** Pharmacological and Parenteral Therapies **Integrated Process:** Teaching and Learning **Content Area:** Pharmacology **Strategy:** The core issue of the question is knowledge of the mechanism of action of pancrease. Specific medication and physiology knowledge is needed to answer the question. Use this knowledge and the process of elimination to make a selection.

14 **Answer: 4 Rationale:** Associated symptoms of fever, abdominal pain, and dehydration might suggest pathological diarrhea. The health care provider should be contacted for further evaluation. Obtaining a history of digestive disorders is appropriate but it is not the highest nursing priority. Identifying dietary factors that might be the cause of the diarrhea is not the highest nursing priority. Suggesting Tylenol for fever and pain is an inappropriate nursing action. **Cognitive Level:** Analyzing **Client Need:** Pharmacological and Parenteral Therapies **Integrated Process:** Nursing Process: Implementation **Content Area:** Pharmacology **Strategy:** The stem of the question contains the critical words *highest-priority*. This tells you that more than one of the options could be partially or totally correct. Use general nursing knowledge about diarrhea associated with fever, and the process of elimination, to make a selection.

15 **Answer: 2 Rationale:** Reye's syndrome is a theorized complication of salicylate use in young children. Taste is not the primary or most important reason for not giving a child bismuth subsalicylate. Bismuth subsalicylate contains small amounts of naturally occurring lead, but it is not the most important reason for not giving the medication to a child. Darkening of the tongue may be frightening to a child, but it is not the primary issue for not giving a child bismuth subsalicylate. **Cognitive Level:** Analyzing **Client Need:** Pharmacological and Parenteral Therapies **Integrated Process:** Teaching and Learning **Content Area:** Pharmacology **Strategy:** Note the critical word *salicylate* in the stem of the question. Immediately associate this word with aspirin, which is contraindicated for use in children because of the risk of developing Reye's syndrome.

16 **Answer: 1 Rationale:** Methylcellulose is a bulk-forming cellulose that absorbs intestinal fluids. This action helps prevent constipation and reduce or eliminate diarrhea. Docusate sodium is a laxative, which would not be effective in eliminating diarrhea. Dicyclomine is an antispasmodic medication, and not prescribed for constipation or diarrhea. Bisacodyl is a laxative and would not be prescribed for diarrhea. **Cognitive Level:** Applying **Client Need:** Pharmacological and Parenteral Therapies **Integrated Process:** Nursing Process: Implementation **Content Area:** Pharmacology **Strategy:** The core issue of the question is knowledge of a medication that relieves both constipation and diarrhea. With this in mind, you need to select a medication that regulates the bowel. Use medication knowledge and the process of elimination to make a selection.

17 **Answer: 4 Rationale:** A serious adverse effect of misoprostol (Cytotec) is that a pregnant woman who takes the medication could experience a miscarriage. Misoprostol should be discontinued at least 1 month before pregnancy occurs. A discussion related to the client's use of oral contraceptives may be appropriate, but it has a lower priority than the discussion regarding adverse effects of misoprostol (Cytotec). A discussion related to family planning may be appropriate, but it has a lower priority than the discussion regarding adverse effects of misoprostol (Cytotec). Providing STI counseling is not supported by information in this question. **Cognitive Level:** Applying **Client Need:** Pharmacological and Parenteral Therapies **Integrated Process:** Nursing Process: Implementation **Content Area:** Pharmacology **Strategy:** The core issue of the question is associated risks of taking misoprostol during pregnancy. Eliminate the options that do not relate to misoprostol. Then choose the option that is more specific to the medication.

18 **Answer: 1 Rationale:** Bisacodyl is a stimulant laxative that can cause fluid and electrolyte imbalance. This can have additive effects, because the diuretic use would also contribute to this finding. For this reason, the nurse should assess the use of the laxative. The other options would not help determine the cause of the client's current symptoms. **Cognitive Level:** Analyzing **Client Need:** Pharmacological and Parenteral Therapies **Integrated Process:** Nursing Process: Data Collection **Content Area:** Pharmacology **Strategy:** Note that the question contains the critical word *hyponatremia*. With this in mind, evaluate each option in terms of its relevance to the low sodium value. Eliminate each of the incorrect options, because they would not cause the electrolyte imbalance stated in the question.

19 **Answer: 1 Rationale:** Bulk-forming laxatives, such as methylcellulose, absorb intestinal fluid which increases stool volume, stimulates peristalsis, and decreases straining on defecation. This type of laxative is the best choice for a client with a history of heart disease complicated by heart failure. A saline laxative is more likely to cause episodes of bearing down or straining at stool for the client, and is therefore less helpful for the client's overall status. A stimulant laxative is more likely to cause straining at stool for the client, and would increase cardiac workload. PRN enemas are more likely to cause sudden bearing down for the client, and therefore are less helpful for the client's overall status. **Cognitive Level:** Applying **Client Need:** Pharmacological and Parenteral Therapies **Integrated Process:** Nursing Process: Data Collection **Content Area:** Pharmacology **Strategy:** The critical words in the stem of the question are *best choice*. This tells you that more than one option might be partially or totally correct, but one option is best. Keeping in mind that the client has heart disease, use the process of elimination to choose the bulk-forming laxative as least likely to cause strain on the heart.

20 **Answer: 2 Rationale:** Dicyclomine HCl is an antispasmodic drug. Peripheral side effects include hot, flushed, dry skin; hyperthermia; and intolerance to high temperatures, manifested by dizziness. The client should not be advised to change the medication regimen because of vacation; this is an inappropriate comment by the nurse. The client should be reminded that any CNS effects of the medication will be enhanced by an intake of alcohol; the client should not be advised to change the medication regimen. There is nothing to indicate that the client has GERD. **Cognitive Level:** Analyzing **Client Need:** Pharmacological and Parenteral Therapies **Integrated Process:** Nursing Process: Planning **Content Area:** Pharmacology **Strategy:** The core issue of the question is adverse effects of dicyclomine. A clue in the question is the reference to Florida, which suggests that the effects of high temperature is the correct option.

Key Terms to Review

antacid p. 575
anticholinergic p. 567
antispasmodic p. 567
cathartic p. 570
emesis p. 573
H_2 antagonist p. 574
Helicobacter pylori p. 574
laxative p. 569
proton pump inhibitor p. 575
surfactant p. 571

References

Adams, M., Holland, L., & Urban, C. (2011). *Pharmacology for nurses: A pathophysiological approach* (3rd ed.). Upper Saddle River, NJ: Pearson Education, Inc.

Adams, M., & Koch, R. (2010). *Pharmacology: Connections to nursing practice.* Upper Saddle River, NJ: Pearson Education, Inc.

Deglin, J. H., & Vallerand, A. H. (2011). *Davis's drug guide for nurses* (12th ed.). Philadelphia: F. A. Davis.

Lehne, R. (2010). *Pharmacology for nursing care* (7th ed.). Philadelphia: W. B. Saunders.

Wilson, B., Shannon, M., & Shields, K. (2012). *Pearson nurse's drug guide 2012.* Upper Saddle River, NJ: Pearson Education.

Test Yourself

Are you ready for the NCLEX-PN® or course exams? Use the practice tests on the companion website to check.

Endocrine Medications

38

In this chapter

Cross Reference

Other chapters relevant to this content area are

Dosage Calculation and Medication Administration Chapter 28
Endocrine Disorders Chapter 56

I. MEDICATIONS AFFECTING PITUITARY GLAND

A. Growth hormone (GH)

1. Regulates growth of organs and tissues, specifically length of long bones; replacement therapy is approved for use in children to treat growth hormone deficiency; GH suppressants are used to treat GH excess in children (gigantism) and adults (acromegaly)
2. Common medications are listed in Table 38–1
3. Administration considerations
   a. Most are only given by subcutaneous (SubQ)route; oral dose is inactivated by digestive enzymes; exception is bromocriptine which is given orally
   b. Reconstitute per package directions; mixture must be clear, not cloudy, and be free of undissolved particles; label date of reconstitution and discard refrigerated drug according to manufacturer's directions
   c. *NCLEX®* Contraindicated to stimulate growth in children who are short unrelated to GH deficiency, during or after closure of epiphyseal plates in long bones, or with secondary intracranial tumors
   d. Use cautiously with diabetes or family history of same, hypothyroidism, or concurrent or previous use of thyroid or hormones in males before puberty
   e. Use of thyroid hormone, anabolic steroids, androgens, or estrogens may hasten closure of epiphyseal plates of long bones
4. Side/adverse effects of GH replacement
   a. Metabolic: glucose intolerance, adrenocorticotropic hormone (ACTH) deficiency, or hypothyroidism
   b. *NCLEX®* Renal: **hypercalciuria** (excess calcium excretion in urine) during first 2 to 3 months of treatment; risk of renal calculi with complaints of flank pain, colic, gastrointestinal (GI) upset, urinary frequency, chills, fever, and hematuria
   c. Other: recurrent intracranial tumor growth or presence of GH antibodies
   d. Local allergic reaction: pain and edema at injection site
   e. *NCLEX®* Systemic allergic reaction: peripheral edema, headache, myalgia, and weakness
   f. Excess dosage: diabetes mellitus, atherosclerosis, enlarged organs, hypertension, and features related to acromegaly
5. Side/adverse effects of GH suppressants
   a. Most common are nausea and vomiting (N/V), diarrhea, headache, flushing and injection site pain
   b. More serious ones are dysrhythmias (octreotide), elevated liver enzymes (pegvisomant), or hyper- or hypoglycemia (lanreotide)

Table 38–1 Drugs That Affect Growth Hormone (GH)

Generic (Trade) Name	Actions/Uses
Bromocriptine (Parlodel)	Suppresses GH level in children with GH excess in combination with octreotide
Lanreotide (Somatuline Depot)	Suppresses GH level in clients with acromegaly who have not responded to radiation therapy or are unable to tolerate surgery
Pegvisomant (Somavert)	GH receptor antagonist
Ocreotide (Sandostatin)	Suppresses intestinal peptide hormones, insulin, glucagons, and growth hormone
Somatropin (Humatrope, others)	Used as GH replacement therapy
Mecasermin (Increlex, Iplex)	Recombinant DNA insulinlike growth factor (IGF) with same actions as GH; used for growth failure in children only (before bone epiphyses close)

6. Nursing considerations
   a. Make sure there is documentation of growth rate for at least 6–12 months prior to initiating treatment
   b. Make sure annual bone age assessments are performed, especially for clients undergoing thyroid, androgen, or estrogen replacement therapy
7. Client teaching for GH replacement
   a. Advise parents or caregivers about need for regular bone age assessments
   NCLEX® b. A 3- to 5-inch growth rate is expected in first year and less in second year, with normal growth rate in subsequent years; sub fat diminishes during treatment but will return later
   c. Inform client/caregiver to document monthly height and weight measurements and to report any less-than-expected growth to prescriber
   NCLEX® d. Review signs and symptoms of slipped femoral epiphysis (hip or knee pain and limp) and to notify prescriber of same
8. Client teaching for GH suppressants
   a. Reconstitute gently (avoid shaking); allow solution to come to room temperature before injecting; rotate injection sites among abdomen, thighs, and buttocks
   b. Report jaundice, N/V, or right upper pain to prescriber (possible liver or gallbladder disease)
   c. Treatment is discontinued when adequate adult height is reached, epiphyseal plates fuse, or client fails to respond to GH

B. Antidiuretic hormone (ADH)

1. Promotes reabsorption of water; vasopressor effect due to constriction of smooth muscle; increases aggregation of platelets
2. NCLEX® Is pituitary hormone replacement therapy for clients with diabetes insipidus (DI); also for use in hemophilia A, von Willebrand's disease type 1
3. Common medications are listed in Box 38–1
4. Administration considerations

Memory Aid

Medications that are pituitary hormone replacements usually end with the suffix *-pressin.*

   a. Give by intranasal, SubQ, IV, IM, or intra-arterial route per order and preparation
   b. Infusion pump is needed for IV or intra-arterial routes
   NCLEX® c. Contraindicated with coronary artery or vascular disease; vasoconstriction causes blood pressure elevation
   d. Monitor serum and urine osmolality if given to treat diabetes insipidus
   e. Monitor Factor VIII coagulation level if given for hemostasis
5. Side/adverse effects
   a. Excess dosing can cause water intoxication; early signs are drowsiness, headache, and lethargy; later signs are seizures and coma
   b. Nasal congestion and irritation, rhinitis, abdominal cramps, nausea, heartburn, elevated BP, pain or swelling at injection site
   NCLEX® c. IV route may cause anaphylaxis

6. Nursing considerations
   a. Give initial dose in evening to aid in uninterrupted sleep
NCLEX® b. Check vital signs (VS), especially BP and pulse before giving by IV and SubQ routes
   c. Monitor for mental status changes such as disorientation, lethargy, and behavioral changes related to fluid overload
NCLEX® d. Measure daily intake and output (I&O) and daily weight to monitor water retention and sodium depletion; Check for edema in extremities
NCLEX® e. For nasal spray, inspect nares for intact nasal mucosa prior to dose
   f. Store nasal spray at room temperature; all other solutions need refrigeration
7. Client teaching
   a. Follow proper technique for nasal instillation (tube inserted into nostril to instill)
   b. Avoid over-the-counter (OTC) medicines containing epinephrine that can decrease drug's action
   c. Wear Medic-Alert identification
   d. May take missed dose up to 1 hour before next dose
NCLEX® e. Report nasal congestion or upper respiratory tract infection to prescriber; also report signs of water retention such as shortness of breath and increases in weight, pulse, and BP

II. MEDICATIONS AFFECTING ADRENAL GLANDS

A. Mineralocorticoids

1. A **mineralocorticoid** is a steroid hormone that acts on kidneys to retain sodium and water and release potassium; synthesis is regulated by renin-angiotensin system
NCLEX® 2. Replacement therapy is required with adrenal gland failure or hypofunction (hypoaldosteronism)
3. Common medication: fludrocortisone (Florinef)

Memory Aid

Medications that replace hormones from the adrenal cortex (either glucocorticoid or mineralocorticoid) often have the syllable *cort* somewhere in the name.

4. Administration considerations
   a. Use with caution in disorders where fluid accumulation could be harmful, such as heart failure, hypertension, renal and possibly liver disease
   b. Monitor serum electrolyte levels because drug's hypokalemic effect may potentiate action of other drugs and hypernatremia can result if given with high sodium drugs
5. Side/adverse effects
   a. Sodium and fluid retention, nausea, acne, thromboembolism
   b. Impaired wound healing, aggravation or masking of infection
   c. Anaphylactoid reactions are rare; may occur with hypersensitivity to glucocorticoids (fludrocortisone also has glucocorticoid properties)
6. Nursing considerations
NCLEX® a. Used with glucocorticoids for replacement therapy
   b. Monitor serum electrolyte levels, weight and I&O; report weight gain of 5 lb per week
   c. Monitor BP daily and more frequently during periods of dosage adjustment
NCLEX® d. Check for signs of overdosage related to hypercorticism (psychosis, excess weight gain, edema, congestive heart failure [CHF], increased appetite, severe insomnia, and elevated BP)
   e. Check for signs of underdosage: weight loss, poor appetite, N/V, diarrhea, muscular weakness, increased fatigue, and low BP
7. Client teaching
NCLEX® a. Report signs of low potassium associated with high sodium (muscle weakness, paresthesias, circumoral numbness, fatigue, anorexia, nausea, depression, delirium, diminished reflexes, polyuria, irregular heart rate, CHF, ileus)
NCLEX® b. Eat foods high in potassium if so advised
   c. Salt intake regulates drug's effect: report signs of edema

Box 38–1

Drugs to Treat Diabetes Insipidus

Desmopressin (DDAVP, Stimate)

Vasopressin (Pitressin)

NCLEX® d. Weigh daily and report weight gain of 5 pounds per week

NCLEX® e. Report any infections, trauma, or unexpected stress, which may require increased dosage

f. Wear/carry medical identification alert with drug use and prescriber's name

B. *Glucocorticoids*

1. A glucocorticoid is a steroid hormone with metabolic effects on carbohydrate, protein and fat metabolism, and anti-inflammatory and immunosuppressive activity
2. Synthesis is regulated by pituitary gland via negative feedback effect; may regulate metabolism of skeletal and connective tissues
3. Used in acute **adrenal insufficiency** (inability of adrenal glands to produce sufficient adrenocortical hormones) caused by trauma or thrombosis; chronic primary adrenal insufficiency (**Addison's disease**); and secondary adrenal insufficiency (diseased or destroyed adenohypophysis with inadequate production of ACTH)

NCLEX® 4. Many miscellaneous uses

a. Allergic conditions (asthma, angioedema, transfusion reactions, and serum sickness)
b. Dermatological conditions, such as dermatitis and pemphigus
c. Inflammatory GI disorders, such as Crohn's disease and ulcerative proctitis
d. Severe joint inflammation, bursitis, rheumatic disease (acute inflammatory states of arthritis and systemic lupus erythematosus)
e. With antineoplastic agents to treat leukemias and lymphomas
f. Transplant rejection prophylaxis

5. Common medications are listed in Table 38–2
6. Administration considerations

NCLEX® a. Routes of administration for systemic use to treat inflammatory conditions are IV, IM, and PO; routes for nonsystemic use are inhalation, nasal, ophthalmic, otic, and topical

b. Contraindicated with systemic fungal infections and known hypersensitivity

NCLEX® c. Monitor CBC and differential, serum electrolytes, and blood glucose (BG)

d. With long-term therapy, monitor hypothalamic-pituitary-adrenal (HPA) axis function to check adrenal function

NCLEX® 7. Side/adverse effects

a. Few side effects if high doses are given for only a few days
b. Higher doses and prolonged therapy may alter tissue and organ metabolism, leading to muscle wasting and increased fat tissue deposits in trunk and face; changes in behavior and personality may also occur
c. Prolonged therapy may suppress growth in children and lead to osteoporosis in adults; impaired glucose tolerance and diabetes mellitus may occur
d. Prolonged therapy can suppress the HPA axis; **adrenal crisis** (acute, life-threatening state of profound adrenocortical insufficiency) may result if drug is abruptly withdrawn; taper dose slowly as ordered
e. Toxicity may include anaphylactoid reactions, hypertriglyceridemia, peptic ulcers, acute pancreatitis, aseptic necrosis of bone, cataracts, glaucoma, hypertension, and opportunistic infections
f. **Osteoporosis** (abnormal loss of bone density), decreased muscle mass, **cushingoid state** (having the appearance and facies characteristic of Cushing's disease), activation of latent tuberculosis or diabetes mellitus, vertebral compression fractures

8. Nursing considerations

NCLEX® a. Check VS, BP, lung sounds, weight (including any history of gain or loss), N/V, and dependent edema

b. Conduct mental status exam and monitor for signs of depression, withdrawal, insomnia, and anorexia

Table 38–2 Drugs for Adrenal Replacement Therapy (Glucocorticoids)

Generic (Trade) Name	Notes
Betamethasone (Celestone, others)	Little or no mineralocorticoid action
Cortisone acetate (generic)	Both mineralocorticoid and glucocorticoid action
Dexamethasone (Decadron, others)	Little or no mineralocorticoid action
Hydrocortisone (Cortef, others)	Both mineralocorticoid and glucocorticoid action
Methylprednisolone (Medrol others)	Little mineralocorticoid action
Prednisolone (Delta-Cortef, others)	Both mineralocorticoid and glucocorticoid action
Prednisone (Meticorten, others)	Little mineralocorticoid action
Triamcinolone (Aristacort, others)	Little or no mineralocorticoid action

NCLEX® c. Check skin for striae, thinning, bruising, change in color, change in hair growth, and acne; with prolonged therapy, reposition immobilized clients carefully and limit use of adhesive tape on skin

d. In children on prolonged therapy, monitor height and growth pattern

e. Encourage regular ophthalmic examinations with long-term therapy

NCLEX® f. Check stool for occult blood periodically; GI bleeding could result

9. Client teaching

NCLEX® a. Take oral doses with meals

b. If ordered every other day, take any missed dose immediately if remembered on same day; if remembered next day, take dose and readjust schedule to be every other day; do not double up missed doses

NCLEX® c. It may be advisable to lose weight, limit sodium intake, and increase potassium intake if excessive weight gain occurs

NCLEX® d. If diabetic, carefully monitor for increased BG levels

NCLEX® e. Report any blood in stool or black tarry stools, mood changes or insomnia, vision changes or headache, weight gain of more than 5 lb per week, irregular menses or pregnancy, irregular heart rate, excessive fatigue, severe abdominal pain, serious injury, or infection

f. Avoid strenuous activities if skin is fragile and bruises easily

g. With long-term therapy, do not discontinue medication without notifying prescriber; do not increase or decrease dose on own; tapering of dose is necessary

h. Avoid immunizations during therapy and for 3 months after; avoid contact with anyone with measles or chicken pox or anyone receiving oral polio vaccine

i. Avoid skin testing during therapy

j. Wear specific medical identification during therapy

NCLEX® k. With long-term therapy, report any fever, cough, sore throat, malaise, and unhealed injuries; avoid contact with anyone with active infection

C. Adrenocorticotropic hormone (ACTH)

1. Directly stimulates adrenal cortex to synthesize adrenal steroids

NCLEX® 2. Used primarily to diagnose adrenal disorders such as Addison's disease and secondary adrenal insufficiency caused by pituitary dysfunction

3. Plasma cortisol levels are measured before and 1 hour after test dose; if no rise in cortisol then problem is at level of adrenal gland (Addison's disease; primary adrenocortical insufficiency); if cortisol level rises then problem is in hypothalamus or pituitary gland (secondary adrencortical insufficiency)

NCLEX® 4. Limited use in treatment of adrenal insufficiency; corticosteroids used instead

5. Common medications are listed in Box 38–2; corticotropin and cosyntropin are used to diagnose etiology of insufficiency (Addison's disease versus CNS); metapyrone has an inhibiting action and is used to diagnose excess (Cushing's disease versus CNS)

6. Administration considerations

a. Give according to manufacturer's instructions

b. Contraindicated with ocular herpes simplex, recent surgery, disorders such as CHF, scleroderma, osteoporosis, systemic fungoid infections, hypertension, sensitivity to porcine proteins, or conditions related to adrenocortical insufficiency or hyperfunction

7. Side/adverse effects

a. N/V, dizziness, drowsiness, or light headedness

NCLEX® b. Hypersensitivity including urticaria, pruritus, and anaphylactic shock

8. Nursing considerations

NCLEX® a. Shake bottle well before injecting into deep gluteal muscle; observe closely for 15 minutes after dose for hypersensitivity reactions

b. Monitor VS and BP, and check for dizziness, fever, flushing, rash, and urticaria

c. Monitor plasma or urinary cortisol levels and serum electrolytes

9. Client teaching: drug action and possible results

Box 38–2

Drugs Used to Diagnose Adrenal Gland Insufficiency

Corticotropin HP (Acthar Gel)

Cosyntropin (Cortrosyn)

Metyrapone (Metopirone)

III. MEDICATIONS AFFECTING THYROID GLAND

A. Thyroid hormones

1. Are replacement therapy for **hypothyroidism** (decreased activity of thyroid gland with a variety of specific causes); have same action as naturally produced thyroid hormones in body
2. Used to diagnose and treat thyroid deficiency and **myxedema** (most severe form of hypothyroidism characterized by swelling of face, feet, and periorbital tissues; may lead to coma and death), and to control goiter or thyroid carcinoma
3. Common medications are listed in Table 38–3
4. Administration considerations
   - NCLEX® **a.** Contraindicated in thyrotoxicosis, acute myocardial infarction (MI) and cardiovascular disease, morphologic hypogonadism, nephrosis, and uncorrected hypoadrenalism
   - **b.** Use cautiously with angina pectoris; hypertension; elderly with cardiac disease; renal insufficiency; pregnancy; concurrent use of **catecholamines** (drugs that mimic sympathetic nervous system effects); diabetes mellitus; **hyperthyroidism** (hyperfunction of thyroid gland), and malabsorption states
   - **c.** Note results of significant laboratory studies: serum T_4, free thyroxine, T_3 uptake, serum T_3, serum thyroid-stimulating hormone (TSH), protirelin test, thyroid uptake of radioiodine, TSH test, and thyroid suppression test
5. Side/adverse effects
   - NCLEX® **a.** Weight gain, vomiting, and tachycardia
   - NCLEX® **b.** Angina pectoris, coronary occlusion, or stroke in elderly or predisposed clients
   - **c.** Relative adrenal insufficiency in clients with inadequate pituitary function related to secondary hypothyroidism and secondary adrenal insufficiency; adrenal crisis
   - **d.** Overdosage causing signs of hyperthyroidism related to thyroid storm with shock and coma; thyrotoxicosis with CHF, angina, cardiac dysrhythmias, and shock
6. Nursing considerations
   - NCLEX® **a.** Monitor VS, BP, weight and history of weight change, normal diet, energy level, mood, subjective feeling, and response to temperature
   - **b.** In children, check height
   - NCLEX® **c.** Monitor thyroid function test results and BG levels
   - **d.** Start older adults on lower dose and increase dose by small increments; look for symptoms of stress that could lead to angina or stroke
7. Client teaching
   - **a.** Self-monitor pulse, weight, and height; wear medical alert identification
   - NCLEX® **b.** Adhere to dosage schedule and intervals; therapy is life-long; do not change brand of thyroid medication without prescriber approval because of differences in bioavailability
   - NCLEX® **c.** Immediately report chest pain or other signs of aggravated cardiovascular disease
   - **d.** With juvenile hypothyroidism therapy, dramatic weight loss and catch-up growth can occur
   - **e.** Understand side effects and related treatment if changes in insulin or anticoagulants are needed

B. Antithyroid medications

1. Used to treat hyperthyroidism and **Graves' disease** (pronounced hyperthyroidism often associated with enlarged thyroid gland and exophthalmos; also called thyrotoxicosis)
2. Common medications are listed in Table 38–4
3. Administration considerations
   - **a.** Give orally according to manufacturer's instructions
   - **b.** Contraindicated with previous allergic or other severe reactions to thioamides

Table 38–3 Drugs for Diagnosing and Treating Hypothyroid Disorders

Generic (Trade) Name	Notes
Levothyroxine (Levothroid, Synthroid, others)	Chemically pure form of T_4 and preferred therapy for hypothythroidism. Given IV for myxedema coma.
Liothyronine (Cytomel)	Chemically pure form of T_3; for adult hypothyroidism; not used for cretinism since T_3 does not cross blood–brain barrier as well as T_4 does.
Liotrix (Thyrolar, Euthroid)	Chemically pure T_4 and T_3 in 4:1 ratio; used for hypothyroidism.
Dessicated thyroid (Thyroid USP, others)	Older porcine formulation with less reliable concentrations than synthetic forms; used only by clients who have taken it for years.

Table 38–4 Drugs Used to Treat Hyperthyroidism and Graves' Disease

Generic (Trade) Name	Notes
Thioamides	
Methimazole (Tapazole)	Inhibits thyroid hormone synthesis but not release.
Propylthiouracil (generic)	Inhibits thyroid hormone synthesis but not release; in peripheral tissues inhibits conversion of T_4 to T_3.
Iodine	
Potassium iodide (Pima)	Has direct action on thyroid and used for short-term inhibition of thyroid hormone synthesis.
^{131}I as NaI (Iodotope)	Radioisotope concentrates in thyroid and destroys tissue.

c. Impaired hepatic function may require reduced doses

NCLEX® d. Monitor results of laboratory studies: serum T_4, serum T_3, free T_4, free T_3, T_3 resin uptake, serum thyroid uptake of radioiodine, and thyroid suppression test

4. Side/adverse effects
   a. Fever, itching, skin rash, blood dyscrasias and peripheral neuropathy
   b. Pain and swelling of joints or lupus like syndrome
   c. Dizziness and alteration in taste (NCLEX®)
   d. Overdosage results in hypothyroidism
   e. Rare instances of agranulocytosis
5. Nursing considerations
   a. Monitor for tingling of fingers and toes
   b. Monitor weight and check for hair loss and skin changes (NCLEX®)
   c. Check CBC, differential count, and thyroid and liver function tests
   d. Dilute oral iodine solutions well in milk, juice, or other beverage (NCLEX®)
   e. Monitor for metallic taste in mouth, sneezing, edematous thyroid, vomiting, and bloody diarrhea (NCLEX®)
6. Client teaching
   a. Wear/carry medical identification alert
   b. Side effects may not appear for days or weeks after treatment begins
   c. Report fever, chills, sore throat, and unusual bleeding/bruising (NCLEX®)
   d. Take dose at same time of day and with meals or snack; space additional daily doses throughout day (NCLEX®)
   e. With radioactive iodine, clients may become hypothyroid and require thyroid hormone replacement; periodic thyroid evaluation is needed

IV. MEDICATIONS AFFECTING PARATHYROID GLANDS

A. Medications to treat hypocalcemia

1. Calcium supplements replace calcium to supply body's metabolic needs, help maintain bone strength, and prevent calcium loss from bones (NCLEX®)
2. Used to treat mild hypocalcemia and to supplement dietary calcium; has additional use as antacid
3. Common medications are listed in Box 38–3
4. Administration considerations
   a. Given orally, dosage differs among different oral calcium salts
   b. Give with large glass of water and with meals or 1–1.5 hours after meals for better absorption (NCLEX®)

Memory Aid

Most drugs that directly or indirectly affect calcium levels will have *calci-* or *calc-* somewhere in the generic or trade name.

Box 38–3 Calcium Salts Used to Treat Mild Calcium Deficiency

- Calcium acetate (PhosLo)
- Calcium chloride (generic)
- Calcium carbonate (Tums, others)
- Calcium citrate (Citracal)
- Calcium gluconate (Kalcinate)
- Calcium lactate (Cal-Lac)
- Calcium phosphate tribasic (Posture)

NCLEX® c. When used as antacid, should be given 1 hour after meals and at bedtime
d. Contraindications: hypercalcemia, renal calculi, and hypophosphatemia
NCLEX® e. Foods such as spinach, Swiss chard, beets, bran, and whole grains may reduce calcium absorption
f. Monitor results of periodic calcium levels for effectiveness

5. Side/adverse effects
   a. Constipation and flatulence
   b. Hypercalcemia may occur if frequent or high doses are used, or in clients receiving calcium as part of renal dysfunction therapy
6. Nursing considerations
   NCLEX® a. Note number and consistency of stools; for constipation, a laxative or stool softener may be ordered
   b. With prolonged therapy, monitor weekly serum and urine calcium levels
   c. Observe for signs of hypercalcemia if client is receiving frequent or high doses
   d. Monitor for acid rebound if used as an antacid for more than 1–2 weeks
7. Client teaching
   NCLEX® a. Understand signs of hypercalcemia and report any N/V, constipation, frequent urination, lethargy, or depression
   NCLEX® b. Do not take with cereals or other foods high in oxalates that form insoluble, nonabsorbable compounds with calcium
   c. If used as antacid, understand risk of acid rebound if used for more than 2 weeks

B. Vitamin D

1. Is a fat-soluble vitamin (can accumulate in body) needed for proper calcium absorption
2. Used to control hypocalcemia or vitamin D deficiency
3. NCLEX® Used in treatment of rickets, **osteomalacia** (abnormal loss of calcification of lamellar bone matrix, resulting in bone softening and fracture), and **hypoparathyroidism** (insufficient secretion by parathyroid glands caused by primary parathyroid dysfunction or abnormal serum calcium level)
4. Common medications are listed in Box 38–4
5. Administration considerations
   a. Give PO or IV depending on formulation
   NCLEX® b. Adequate calcium is needed for optimal response to treatment
   c. Contraindications: hypercalcemia, vitamin D toxicity, malabsorption syndrome
6. Side/adverse effects
   a. Hypercalcemia from overuse (ataxia, fatigue, irritability, seizures, somnolence, tinnitus, hypertension, GI tract distress or constipation, and hypotonia in infants)
   NCLEX® b. Vitamin D hypercalcemia may lead to dysrhythmias in clients taking digoxin
   c. Hypervitaminosis D caused by large therapeutic doses may lead to hypercalcemia, hypercalciuria, bone pain, and calcium deposits in soft tissues
7. Nursing considerations
   NCLEX® a. Check for any CNS problems; monitor BP, pulse, and I&O
   NCLEX® b. Monitor BUN, serum creatinine levels, serum calcium and phosphorus levels, serum alkaline phosphatase and urinalysis
   c. If vitamin D toxicity occurs, make sure client stops drug immediately, drinks large amounts of fluid, and eats a low-calcium diet
8. Client teaching
   a. Make sure oral dose is swallowed intact without crushing or chewing tablet
   NCLEX® b. Consult prescriber before taking any OTC medications containing calcium, phosphorus, vitamin D, or substances high in vitamin D
   NCLEX® c. Do not drive or use heavy equipment if fatigue, vertigo, or weakness develop
   d. Avoid magnesium-containing antacids

C. Medications to treat hypercalcemia

1. Form complexes with free calcium in blood and promote urinary excretion of calcium
2. Decrease mobilization of calcium from bone

Box 38–4

Drugs Used to Treat Vitamin D Deficiency

Calcitriol (Rocaltrol)
Dihydrotachysterol (DHT)
Doxercalciferol (Hectoral)
Ergocalciferol (Calciferol, Drisdol)
Paricalcitol (Zemplar)

3. Decrease intestinal absorption of calcium
NCLEX® 4. Used in emergency treatment of hypercalcemia
5. Common medications are listed in Table 38–5
6. Administration considerations
   a. May be given IM, IV, PO, or SubQ
   b. Give injected doses at bedtime to minimize effects of flushing
   NCLEX® c. In emergency situations, dilute IV dose before administration to prevent extravasation; infuse over prescribed period of time
   NCLEX® d. Contraindicated with known hypersensitivity and impaired renal function
   e. Significant drug interactions occur with antacids, mineral supplements, calcium salts, and vitamin D
   f. Decreased effects of digoxin occur when serum calcium is reduced
7. Side/adverse effects
   a. N/V, diarrhea, and dyspepsia with oral route
   b. Facial flushing and occasional inflammatory reaction at injection site
   c. Transient influenza like symptoms with IV route
   d. Nasal dryness and irritation with intranasal spray
   NCLEX® e. Allergic reactions with calcitonin salmon
   NCLEX® f. IV dose may cause venous irritation, thrombophlebitis, and nephrotoxicity
   g. Varying effects of hypocalcemia
   h. Toxicity with higher doses causes more severe GI distress, such as esophagitis, severe nephrotoxicity, and severe hypocalcemia
8. Nursing considerations
   a. Monitor for hypercalcemia and hypocalcemia
   b. Monitor weight and I&O if vomiting and diarrhea occur
   c. Monitor serum electrolytes, serum alkaline phosphatase, serum creatinine, BUN, liver function tests, CBC with differential, and urinalysis
   NCLEX® d. Monitor vital signs and check for dysrhythmias with IV infusion
9. Client teaching
   a. Understand and demonstrate SubQ self-injection
   b. Do not discontinue therapy without notifying MD
   NCLEX® c. Taking dose in evening may lessen flushing
   d. Take PO doses on empty stomach
   e. Wear medical alert identification if on long-term therapy
   f. Eat a low-calcium and low–vitamin D diet (decrease in dairy products)
   NCLEX® g. Take sufficient fluid intake (at least 6–8 glasses of water daily and possibly more if not contraindicated by other health problems)

D. Medications to treat osteoporosis and *Paget's disease*

1. Reduce calcium release from bone, slow bone resorption and remodeling, and prevent high serum calcium concentrations
2. Used long-term for Paget's disease (a nonmetabolic disease of bone) and postmenopausal osteoporosis (abnormal loss of bone density)
3. Also used to treat heterotropic ossification after spinal cord injury and hip replacement
4. Common medications are listed in Box 38–5

Table 38–5 Drugs Used to Treat Hypercalcemia

Trade (Generic) Name	Notes
Calcitonin (Miacalcin)	Inhibits bone resorption.
Cinacalcet (Sensipar)	Decreases parathyroid hormone secretion by increasing parathyroid sensitivity to extracellular calcium.
Calcium disodium versenate (generic)	Strong chelating agent; used on short-term basis to remove excess calcium.
Etidronate (Didronel)	Inhibits bone resorption (bisphosphonate).
Gallium nitrate (Ganite)	Used for hypercalcemia caused by cancer.
Pamidronate (Aredia)	Acts directly on bone by slowing bone reabsorption and lowering release of calcium (bisphosphonate). Also used for Paget's disease.
Zolendronate (Zometa)	Inhibits bone resorption (bisphosphonate).

Box 38-5

Drugs to Treat Osteoporosis and Paget's Disease

Hormonal Agents
Calcitonin salmon (Fortical, Miacalcin)
Cinacalcet (Sensipar)
Raloxifene (Evista)
Teriparatide (Forteo)

Bisphosphonates
Alendronate (Fosamax)
Etidronate (Didronel)
Ibandronate (Boniva)
Pamidronate (Aredia)
Risedronate (Actonel)
Tiludronate (Skelid)
Zolendronate (Reclast, Zometa)

5. Administration considerations
   a. Is given PO, IV, SubQ or by intranasal spray (once daily in alternate nostrils)
   b. Contraindicated with known hypersensitivity or esophageal disorders
   c. Interacts with antacids, mineral supplements, calcium salts, vitamin D, and calcium-rich dairy products
6. Side/adverse effects
   a. N/V, diarrhea, and dyspepsia with oral route
   b. Facial flushing and occasional inflammatory reaction at injection site
   c. Transient influenza like symptoms with IV route
   d. Muscle spasms; leukopenia with chills, fever, or sore throat
   e. Nasal dryness and irritation with intranasal spray
   f. Allergic reactions with calcitonin salmon
   g. NCLEX® IV route may cause venous irritation, thrombophlebitis, nephrotoxicity
   h. Varying effects of hypocalcemia
   i. Toxicity with higher doses causes more severe hypocalcemia, GI distress such as severe esophagitis with ulceration, and severe nephrotoxicity
7. Nursing considerations
   a. Monitor for hypercalcemia and hypocalcemia
   b. Monitor weight and I&O if vomiting and diarrhea occur
   c. Monitor serum electrolytes, serum alkaline phosphatase, calcium and phosphorus, and 24-hour urinary hydroxyproline
   d. NCLEX® Monitor bone pain in clients with Paget's disease
   e. NCLEX® Check results of baseline values of bone mineral density (BMD) in hip, vertebrae, and forearm, and obtain periodic BMD values
8. Client teaching
   a. How to self-administer SubQ injection and to rotate sites
   b. Taking doses in evening may lessen flushing
   c. NCLEX® Take PO doses on empty stomach and remain upright for 30–60 minutes after taking
   d. NCLEX® Recognize signs of esophagitis; withhold drug and notify prescriber if difficulty swallowing or worsening heartburn occur
   e. Wear Medic-Alert identification if on long-term therapy
   f. NCLEX® Consume a diet sufficient in calcium and vitamin D; take in sufficient fluid
   g. Understand activation and use of metered dose pump for nasal spray use

V. MEDICATIONS USED TO TREAT DIABETES MELLITUS

A. Insulin

1. Restores cells' ability to use glucose for energy and corrects **hyperglycemia** (higher than normal BG levels; normal BG is 70–110 mg/dL)
2. Corrects many associated metabolic derangements
3. NCLEX® Treats both type 1 and type 2 diabetes mellitus (DM) and diabetic ketoacidosis (DKA)
4. Also lowers plasma potassium levels and regular insulin IV and dextrose IV are used as emergency treatment of severe hyperkalemia
5. NCLEX® Types of insulin are listed in Table 38–6; premixed insulin combinations are also available, see product literature (Humulin 70/30, Novolin 70/30, Humulin 50/50 Novolog Mix 70/30, and Humalog Mix 75/25)
6. Administration considerations
   a. Given only by injection (SubQ, IM, IV); only regular insulin may be given IV; inactivated by digestive enzymes if given orally
   b. NCLEX® Injection sites include upper arms, thighs, abdomen, and infrascapular area

Table 38-6 Types of Insulin Preparations

Action	Generic (Trade) Name	Timeframes	Notes
Rapid	Insulin lispro (Humalog)	Onset: 5–15 min Peak: 1–1.5 hr Duration: 3–4 hr	Give SubQ 5–10 min before meal; can give with NPH (draw lispro up first) and give immediately
	Insulin aspart (Novolog)	Onset: 10–20 min Peak: 1–3 hr Duration: 3–5 hr	Give SubQ 5–10 min before meal; can give with NPH (draw aspart up first) and give immediately
	Insulin glulisine (Apidra)	Onset: 15–30 min Peak: 1 hr Duration: 3–4 hr	Give SubQ 15 min before meal; can give with NPH (draw glulisine up first) and give immediately
Short	Insulin regular (Humulin R, Novolin R)	Onset: 30–60 min Peak: 1–5 hr Duration: 6–10 hr	Give SubQ 30–60 min before meal; can give with NPH (draw regular up first) but not glargine; can be given IV; can mix with sterile water or normal saline
Intermediate	Isophane susp (NPH, Humulin N)	Onset: 1–2 hr Peak: 6–14 hr Duration: 16–24 hr	Give SubQ; is cloudy in appearance; can mix with aspart, lispro, and regular; do not mix with glargine
Long	Insulin detemir (Levemir)	Onset: 3–8 hr Peak: None Duration: 24 hr	Give SubQ once or twice daily; do not mix with any other types of insulin
	Insulin glargine (Lantus)	Onset: 2–4 hr Peak: None Duration: 24 hr	Give SubQ once daily at same time of day; do not mix with any other types of insulin

NCLEX® **c.** One general location is used at one time to maintain consistent absorption rates although sites within each general location are used only once each month

NCLEX® **d.** Only mix insulins that are compatible with one another and use according to manufacturer's guidelines

NCLEX® **e.** Store unopened vials in refrigerator; opened vials can remain at room temperature for up to one month; label vial with date and time opened and/or due to expire according to agency policy

f. Alternate methods of delivery include jet injectors, pen injectors, and portable and implantable insulin pumps

g. Dosage must be monitored and linked with insulin needs

h. Insulin selection, doses and timing are individualized to achieve glucose regulation in each client

NCLEX® **i.** Concurrent use of beta-adrenergic blocking agents could mask signs of hypoglycemia normally triggered by sympathetic nervous system (tachycardia and palpitations)

NCLEX® **7.** Side/adverse effects

a. **Hypoglycemia** when BG level drops below 50 mg/dL (headache, confusion, drowsiness, fatigue, tachycardia, anxiety, sweating, and cool, clammy skin)

b. Coma related to inadequate insulin dosage as seen in uncontrolled diabetes with high BG levels and ketoacidosis or hyperosmolar coma

c. Coma related to insulin overdose caused by inadequate food intake, excessive exercise, or excessive insulin administration

8. Complications (fewer types of complications now with use of recombinant DNA technology)

NCLEX® **a.** **Lipodystrophy** (abnormal deposition of SubQ fat at injection sites)

b. Local allergic reaction related to a contaminant in insulin preparation

9. Nursing considerations

a. Monitor VS, weight, condition of skin and nails, and wound healing

b. Monitor for long-term complications related to acceleration of atherosclerosis (hypertension, heart disease, stroke); retinopathy leading to possible blindness; nephropathy leading to possible renal failure; neuropathy leading to lower limb ulcerations and amputation, impotence, and gastroparesis

c. Communicate with prescriber regarding insulin management when there is insufficient food intake or when client is NPO for surgery
d. Adhere to agency policy regarding insulin administration
NCLEX® e. Monitor results of random BG, fasting BG, glucose tolerance test, **glycosylated hemoglobin** A_{1c} (represents average BG over past several weeks), serum electrolytes
f. Increase frequency of BG monitoring with fever, N/V, diarrhea or other illness, to detect rises requiring adjustment of insulin dose
g. Check urine ketones if BG exceeds 250–300 mg/dL to detect early DKA
h. Be alert for signs of hypoglycemia and treat as indicated (15-gram carbohydrate snack or simple sugar if necessary)

10. Client teaching
a. Participate in individualized teaching plan about insulin management
NCLEX® b. Understand all aspects of insulin administration, including syringe use, mixing of insulins, stability of mixture, injection technique and sites
NCLEX® c. Do not switch type or source of insulin or brand of syringe and avoid taking any new drug before notifying prescriber
NCLEX® d. Understand (and ensure family understands) signs of hyper- and hypoglycemia and self-treatment measures
e. Learn how to test BG levels
f. Follow dietary restrictions and weight control measures; consult dietitian
g. Engage in regular aerobic exercise appropriate to health and abilities
h. Understand foot care and related aspects of personal hygiene
NCLEX® i. Learn sick-day management of DM and insulin administration (continue to eat and take liquids as able, check BG, maintain insulin schedule, and call prescriber if BG is higher than 250 mg/dL)
j. Obtain and wear a Medic-Alert tag or bracelet
k. Avoid smoking; avoid drinking alcoholic beverages unless approved by prescriber, since this can lead to hypoglycemia without proper food intake
l. Consult with prescriber before conceiving (if female)
m. Contact local home care agency and American Diabetes Association for additional follow-up and access to community-based resources

B. Oral antidiabetic (hypoglycemic) agents—sulfonylureas

1. Stimulate release of insulin from pancreatic islets
2. Used as an adjunct to nondrug therapy to reduce BG levels in type 2 DM
3. Common medications are listed in Box 38–6
4. Administration considerations
a. Dose is given orally 1–3 times a day
b. Different agents possess different durations of action
NCLEX® c. May be used alone or in combination with insulin
NCLEX® d. Contraindicated during pregnancy, in women who are nursing/lactating, or in clients allergic to sulfa or urea
NCLEX® e. Beta-adrenergic blocking agents can suppress insulin release and delay response to hypoglycemia

Memory Aid

The classification name *sulfonylurea* provides the clue as to what allergies to look for as contraindications for use. Break the word into component parts. The syllable *sulf* can trigger an assessment of sulfa allergy, while *urea* should trigger an assessment of allergy to urea.

Box 38–6

Oral Antidiabetics Agents (Sulfonylureas)

First-Generation Agents	Second-Generation Agents
Chlorpropamide (Diabinese)	Glimepiride (Amaryl)
Tolbutamide (Orinase)	Glipizide (Glucotrol)
Tolazamide (Tolinase)	Glyburide Nonmicronized (Diabeta)
	Glyburide Micronized (Glynase PresTab)

5. Side/adverse effects
   a. GI tract distress (nausea, heartburn)
   b. Neurologic symptoms such as dizziness, drowsiness, or headache
   NCLEX® c. Alcohol may cause a disulfiram-like reaction: flushing, palpitations, and nausea
   d. Allergy noted by skin reaction
   e. Blood dyscrasias and cholestatic jaundice
   f. Hypoglycemia related to drug overdosage, drug interactions, altered drug metabolism, or inadequate food intake, or because of renal or hepatic dysfunction
6. Nursing considerations
   NCLEX® a. Monitor VS, weight, condition of skin and nails, BG levels, glycosylated hemoglobin, and electrolyte and arterial blood gas levels as appropriate
   b. Monitor for long-term complications of diabetes as noted in previous section regarding nursing considerations with insulin
   NCLEX® c. Communicate with prescriber regarding management when client has insufficient food intake or is NPO for surgery
7. Client teaching
   NCLEX® a. Participate in individualized teaching plan based on previous knowledge, educational level, motivation to learn, and cultural considerations
   b. Understand all aspects of drug therapy; take with food if GI upset
   c. Take medication even if not feeling well
   d. Take dose with first daily meal and take any missed dose as soon as remembered unless time for next dose; do not double up doses
   NCLEX® e. Understand and be sure family understands signs and symptoms of hypoglycemia; notify prescriber if symptoms occur
   f. Learn how to test BG levels
   g. Follow dietary restrictions and weight control measures; consult dietitian (for help developing effective meal and weight management plans)
   h. Engage in regular aerobic exercise appropriate to health and abilities
   i. Understand foot care and related aspects of personal hygiene
   NCLEX® j. Understand sick-day management of diabetes and PRN insulin administration
   k. Obtain and wear Medic-Alert tag or bracelet
   l. Avoid drinking alcoholic beverages or smoking
   m. Consult with prescriber before conceiving (females); discontinue drug during pregnancy and lactation (may need insulin)
   n. Contact local home care agency and American Diabetes Association for additional follow-up and access to community-based resources

C. Oral antidiabetics (hypoglycemic) agents—nonsulfonylureas

1. Act in a variety of ways; combination drugs are also available
   a. Biguanides decrease production and release of glucose by liver, increase glucose uptake by cells, and lower lipid levels
   b. Alpha-glucosidase inhibitors interfere with carbohydrate breakdown and absorption; act locally in GI tract with little systemic absorption
   c. Thiazolidinediones or "glitazones" inhibit glucose production in liver and increase cellular sensitivity to insulin
   d. Metiglinides stimulate insulin release from pancreas
   e. Incretin enhancers increase synthesis and release of insulin, decrease glucagon production and glucose secretion, and increase satiety
2. NCLEX® All decrease BG levels after meals in clients with type 2 DM not controlled by diet and exercise
3. Common medications are listed in Box 38–7
4. Administration considerations
   a. Given orally 1 to 3 times a day
   b. Alpha-glucose inhibitors are contraindicated with GI disorders such as bowel inflammatory disease, bowel obstruction, and should be used cautiously in clients with GI distress or liver disease
   NCLEX® c. Thiazolidinediones should be used cautiously in clients with liver disease; may cause liver damage
   d. Biguanides and alpha-glucosidase inhibitors should not be taken together because of significant GI distress
   NCLEX® e. Alcohol may increase risk of hypoglycemia or lactic acidosis

Box 38-7

Oral Antidiabetics/ Hypoglycemics (Nonsulfonylureas)

Biguanide

Metformin (Glucophage)

Meglitinides

Nateglinide (Starlix)

Repaglinide (Prandin)

Alpha-glucosidase Inhibitors

Acarbose (Precose)

Miglitol (Glyset)

Incretin Enhancers

Exenatide (Byetta)

Sitagliptin (Januvia)

Thiazolidinediones

Pioglitazone (Actos)

Rosiglitazone (Advandia)

Combination Drugs

Glipizide/metformin (Metaglip)

Glyburide/metformin (Glucovance)

Rosiglitazone/metformin (Avandamet)

Pioglitazone/metformin (Actos plus met)

Pioglitazone/glimepiride (Duetact)

Repaglinide/metformin (Prandimet)

Sitagliptin/metformin (Janumet)

5. Side/adverse effects
    a. All groups except biguanides have risk of hypoglycemia (tremors, palpitations, sweating)
    b. Other common side effects include GI symptoms such as anorexia, N/V, diarrhea, abdominal discomfort or flatulence
    c. Decreased vitamin B_{12} levels can occur with biguanides and incretin enhancers
    d. Lactic acidosis can occur with biguanides
    e. Symptoms of upper respiratory infection can occur with metiglinides, thiazolidinediones, and incretin enhancers
    f. Miscellaneous adverse effects: anaphylaxis and pancreatitis (metiglinides); hepatotoxicity, bone fractures, heart failure and myocardial infarction (thiazolidinediones); and angioedema, Stevens-Johnson syndrome (sitagliptin)

NCLEX®

6. Nursing considerations
    a. Monitor VS, weight, condition of skin and nails, serum BG levels, glycosylated hemoglobin, and electrolyte and arterial blood gas levels as appropriate
    b. Review renal function and liver function studies (NCLEX®)
    c. Monitor for early signs of lactic acidosis (biguanides)
    d. Monitor for long-term complications of diabetes mellitus
    e. Communicate with prescriber regarding management when client has insufficient food intake or is NPO for surgery

NCLEX®

7. Client teaching
    a. Understand all aspects of diabetic management as outlined in previous client education section for sulfonylureas
    b. Understand early signs of hypoglycemia and lactic acidosis (hyperventilation, myalgia, malaise, unusual somnolence) and notify prescriber immediately if symptoms occur

D. Glucose-elevating medication—glucagon (Glucagen)

1. Promotes breakdown of glycogen in liver (glycogenolysis) and converts amino acids to glucose (gluconeogenesis)

NCLEX®

2. Used for emergency treatment of severe hypoglycemia in clients who are unconscious or unable to swallow
3. Administration considerations
    a. Reconstitute according to manufacturer's directions
    b. Give IM, SubQ or by direct IV push; flush IV line with 5% dextrose instead of sodium chloride (NaCl) solution; incompatible with NaCl solutions or additives (NCLEX®)
    c. Incompatible in syringe with any other medication
    d. Contraindicated with hypersensitivity to glucagon or protein compounds
    e. Use cautiously in insulinoma and pheochromocytoma

NCLEX®

4. Side/adverse effects: N/V, hypersensitivity, hyperglycemia, hypokalemia

5. Nursing considerations

NCLEX® a. Client usually responds/awakens within 5 to 20 minutes after administration, which is slower than response time to IV glucose

NCLEX® b. After client awakens and is able to swallow, give oral carbohydrate

c. After recovery, monitor for persistent headache, nausea, and weakness

NCLEX® 6. Client teaching

a. Proper testing of BG levels

b. Be sure responsible family member knows how to administer SubQ or IM dose to treat hypoglycemic reactions

c. Notify prescriber immediately after reaction to determine cause

Check Your NCLEX–PN® Exam I.Q.

You are ready for testing on this content if you can

- Apply knowledge of expected actions and effects of endocrine medications to client care.
- Correctly administer endocrine medications to clients.
- Monitor for side effects and adverse effects of endocrine medications.
- Take appropriate action if a client has an unexpected response to an endocrine medication.
- Monitor a client for expected outcomes or effects of treatment with endocrine medications.

PRACTICE TEST

1 A young child who has been taking growth hormone (Somatropin) for 1 month reports flank pain, colic, and GI symptoms. The nurse concludes that this client is at increased risk for which adverse effect that is more likely to occur during the first few months of treatment?

1. Acute glomerulonephritis
2. Renal calculi
3. Bowel obstruction
4. Duodenal ulcer

2 A client with coronary artery disease and hypertension was recently diagnosed with diabetes insipidus. For what reason should the nurse conclude that treatment with antidiuretic hormone (ADH) is contraindicated for this client?

1. Fluid overload and elevated BP could occur.
2. Volume depletion and decreased blood pressure could occur.
3. Overstimulation and agitation could occur.
4. Hypercalciuria and renal calculi could occur.

3 A client with cardiovascular disease has been recently diagnosed with hypothyroidism, and levothyroxine (Levoxyl) has been prescribed. Which manifestation related to this medication is most important for the client to report to the physician?

1. Increased urine output
2. Chest pain
3. Increase in appetite
4. Loose stools

4 A client with a history of cardiac disease is exhibiting severe symptoms of hypothyroidism, and is started on medication therapy with levothyroxine (Synthroid). The nurse anticipates that which principle will be followed for initiation of drug therapy?

1. Start with the highest dose, and titrate according to the client's response.
2. Start with the highest dose and give a beta blocker to prevent tachycardia.
3. Start with a low dose and gradually increase the dose over a period of weeks.
4. Administer a fixed dose calculated to client's weight; adjust as necessary.

5 A client with acute adrenal insufficiency (adrenal crisis) is admitted to the hospital. The nurse monitors for resolution of which manifestation to determine that drug therapy with cortisone (Cortone) has been effective? Select all that apply.

1. Hyperexcitability and restlessness
2. Decreased appetite and weight loss
3. Vitiligo and hyperpigmentation
4. Hypertension and hypernatremia
5. Episodes of angina and hypotension

PRACTICE TEST

6 The nurse is reviewing the laboratory data of a client diagnosed with Cushing's syndrome. The nurse would expect to note which laboratory values prior to initiation of drug therapy? Select all that apply.

1. Elevated plasma cortisol level
2. Decreased blood glucose level
3. Increased white blood cell count
4. Increased sodium level
5. Increased potassium level

7 The nurse is caring for a client who has just been diagnosed with Graves' disease. When reinforcing client education, the nurse should include what information?

1. Atropine-like medications are safe to use.
2. Thyroid hormone replacement therapy is necessary.
3. A low-calorie diet will be ordered.
4. Propylthiouracil (PTU) will be prescribed.

8 A client with Graves' disease has been taking medication therapy as prescribed. Which finding, noted on cardiac assessment indicates to the nurse that the client has not had a sufficient response to medication therapy?

1. Decreased systolic blood pressure
2. Narrowed pulse pressure
3. Bradycardia
4. Tachycardia

9 The nurse is caring for a client who recently was diagnosed with hypoparathyroidism. To note the effectiveness of medication therapy with calcitrol (Rocaltrol), the nurse should monitor laboratory findings to see if what change has occurred?

1. Hypercalcemia is resolving.
2. Hypocalcemia is resolving.
3. Hypermagnesemia is resolving.
4. Vitamin D levels are decreasing.

10 A client with type 2 diabetes mellitus has been prescribed pioglitazone (Actos). Which test does the nurse anticipate will be done before drug therapy is initiated with this medication?

1. Liver function tests
2. Thyroid function tests
3. Respiratory function tests
4. Pituitary function tests

11 A client newly diagnosed with adrenal insufficiency is to begin therapy with fludrocortisone (Florinef). What therapeutic effect of this medication should the nurse explain to the client?

1. Decreases resorption of sodium by decreasing hydrogen and potassium excretion in the distal tubule
2. Increases resorption of sodium by increasing hydrogen and potassium excretion in the distal tubule
3. Decreases inflammation by suppressing migration of leukocytes and eliminating the body's immune response to certain stimuli
4. Increases inflammation by stimulating the production of leukocytes and enhancing the body's immune response to many stimuli

12 A homebound client with type 2 diabetes mellitus calls the nurse to report nausea and flu-like symptoms for 2 days. What response should the nurse make to the client?

1. "Be sure to check your blood glucose level in the morning on a daily basis."
2. "Take half of your regular dose of insulin and oral hypoglycemic agent."
3. "Limit fluid intake, and eat only when you feel hungry."
4. "Test your urine for ketones if your blood glucose is higher than 240 mg/dL."

13 A client, just diagnosed with hypothyroidism, also takes sodium warfarin (Coumadin). Before giving any thyroid replacement hormone, the nurse should check the results of what laboratory value?

1. Complete blood count (CBC)
2. Prothrombin time (PT) or international normalized ratio (INR)
3. Activated partial thromboplastin time (APTT)
4. Warfarin (Coumadin) level

14 A client newly diagnosed with diabetes mellitus has begun taking insulin. The client asks the nurse about alcohol consumption. What information should the nurse provide to the client?

1. "Moderate-to-high alcohol consumption without food can cause your blood glucose level to go down too low."
2. "Moderate-to-high alcohol consumption without food can cause your blood glucose level to rise too high."
3. "Consumption of alcohol has no effect on your blood glucose, as long as you don't eat while drinking."
4. "As long as you only drink beer and wine, and not hard liquor, there should be no effect from the alcohol."

15 The nurse is instructing the newly diagnosed diabetic client how to mix regular insulin and NPH insulin. What should the nurse tell the client?

1. Shake the bottle of intermediate insulin before withdrawing the amount.
2. Withdraw the longer-acting insulin first.
3. Withdraw the shorter-acting insulin first.
4. Inject air into the bottle of shorter-acting insulin first.

16 Metformin (Glucophage) has been prescribed for a client newly diagnosed with type 2 diabetes mellitus. Which client statement about the action of this medication validates to the nurse that the client understood medication teaching?

1. Decreases sensitivity of peripheral tissue to insulin
2. Stimulates glucose production in the liver
3. Treats unstable type 2 diabetes mellitus
4. Decreases production of glucose by the liver

17 A client has been receiving high doses of glucocorticoids for several weeks. The client asks the nurse when he can stop taking the medication. The nurse's response incorporates which information in a response?

1. Even at high doses, adverse reactions are unlikely if the medication is abruptly withdrawn.
2. If steroid medication is withdrawn suddenly, a client could die of acute adrenal insufficiency.
3. The client could experience severe psychological symptoms when the medication is withdrawn.
4. Tapering of the medication requires daily assessment of serum chemistries.

18 A client newly diagnosed with hypothyroidism is placed on levothyroxine sodium (Synthroid). The client asks when his lack of energy will improve. What should the nurse include in a response?

1. Lack of energy is probably caused by depression, not hypothyroidism.
2. Dramatic improvement in energy levels can be experienced, usually in 1–2 days.
3. The drug works best when taken after a full meal.
4. Optimum effectiveness of the drug might not occur for several weeks.

19 A nurse is caring for a client who is receiving insulin. For which sign of hypoglycemic reaction should the nurse observe the client?

1. Fruity breath
2. Flushing of the face
3. Hunger
4. Dry, flaky skin

20 The nurse who is working in a women's health clinic has several clients to see during the day. Which client does the nurse anticipate will need medication teaching for calcium supplementation to treat primary osteoporosis?

1. A premenopausal client
2. An overweight client
3. An African-American client
4. A Caucasian client

ANSWERS & RATIONALES

1 **Answer: 2** **Rationale:** Adverse/side effects during the first 2–3 months of treatment with growth hormone include hypercalciuria, with resultant renal calculi. The client taking Somatropin is not at increased risk for the other options. **Cognitive Level:** Analyzing **Client Need:** Pharmacological and Parenteral Therapies **Integrated Process:** Nursing Process: Data Collection **Content Area:** Pharmacology **Strategy:** Note the critical words in the question are *first few months*. This tells you that the adverse effect occurs soon after the start of medication therapy. Use medication knowledge and the process of elimination to make a selection.

2 **Answer: 1** **Rationale:** Clients with coronary artery insufficiency and hypertensive cardiovascular disease who take ADH are at increased risk for developing fluid overload and edema. Volume depletion and decreased blood pressure are the opposite of what can occur with this client. Overstimulation and agitation are not related to the diagnosis. Hypercalciuria and renal calculi are not related to this client's situation. **Cognitive Level:** Analyzing **Client Need:** Pharmacological and Parenteral Therapies **Integrated Process:** Nursing Process: Planning **Content Area:** Pharmacology **Strategy:** Note that two of the options are opposite, which could be a clue that one of them is correct. Recall that ADH causes fluid retention to link this information with the associated risks for a client with cardiac disease.

3 **Answer: 2** **Rationale:** Clients with known cardiovascular disease who are prescribed thyroid hormone replacement therapy can develop chest pain that could lead to myocardial infarction. For this reason, it is the most important manifestation for the client to report. The other options should be reported, but are of lesser priority. **Cognitive Level:** Analyzing **Client Need:** Pharmacological and Parenteral Therapies **Integrated Process:** Nursing Process: Planning **Content Area:** Pharmacology **Strategy:** The critical words in the stem of the question are *most important*, which tell you that more than one answer might be correct, and that you must prioritize your answer. Use the ABCs (airway, breathing, and circulation) to select the answer most important to a client with cardiac disease (which affects circulation).

4 **Answer: 3** **Rationale:** Clients with severe symptoms of hypothyroidism and a history of cardiac disease must be started on the lowest dose possible of hormone therapy and have the dose gradually increased, in order to prevent onset of severe hypertension, heart failure, and myocardial infarction (MI). Weight would not be an appropriate calculation factor. The highest possible starting dose puts the client at risk for chest pain and subsequent MI. **Cognitive Level:** Analyzing **Client Need:** Pharmacological and Parenteral Therapies **Integrated Process:** Nursing Process: Planning **Content Area:** Pharmacology **Strategy:** The core issue of the question is knowledge of the principles of beginning a medication that stimulates metabolism in a client with heart disease. Use knowledge of pathophysiology to select the option that causes the least stress on the heart during initiation of therapy.

5 **Answer: 2, 3, 5** **Rationale:** Clients with acute adrenal insufficiency will complain of anorexia, nausea and vomiting, and weight loss. Clients with acute adrenal insufficiency will exhibit integumentary symptoms, such as of vitiligo and hyperpigmentation. Clients with acute adrenal insufficiency will exhibit cardiovascular symptoms related to anemia, such as angina; hypotension is also an expected manifestation. Hyperexcitability and restlessness are opposite manifestations from those seen with adrenal insufficiency. Hypertension and hypernatremia are opposite manifestations from those seen with adrenal insufficiency. **Cognitive Level:** Analyzing **Client Need:** Pharmacological and Parenteral Therapies **Integrated Process:** Nursing Process: Evaluation **Content Area:** Pharmacology **Strategy:** The wording of the question tells you that the core issue is knowledge of signs and symptoms of adrenal insufficiency that should respond to drug therapy. Use nursing knowledge and the process of elimination to make a selection. When more than one answer is correct, consider each option as a true/false statement.

6 **Answer: 1, 3, 4** **Rationale:** Clients with Cushing's syndrome, or hypercortisolism, have elevated levels of cortisol sodium and white blood cell counts; drug therapy will reduce serum cortisol levels when given as directed. A decreased blood glucose level and increased potassium level are opposite of what would be expected in Cushing's syndrome. **Cognitive Level:** Analyzing **Client Need:** Pharmacological and Parenteral Therapies **Integrated Process:** Nursing Process: Data Collection **Content Area:** Pharmacology **Strategy:** The core issue of the question is knowledge of laboratory values that are expected to change once drug therapy is initiated for Cushing's syndrome. Use nursing knowledge and the process of elimination to make a selection. When more than one answer is correct, consider each option as a true/false statement.

7 **Answer: 4** **Rationale:** Graves' disease is caused by elevated levels of thyroid hormone. Clients experience tachycardia, nervousness, insomnia, increased heat production, and weight loss. Medication therapy with an agent such as propylthiouracil will help control the disorder. Atropine-like drugs are contraindicated for clients with hyperthyroidism. Graves' disease is caused by elevated levels of thyroid hormone. Initiation of thyroid hormone replacement therapy is indicated for hypothyroidism. A client with Graves' disease needs a high-calorie diet, not a low-calorie one; behavioral and metabolic activity increases, which results in weight loss. **Cognitive Level:** Analyzing **Client Need:** Pharmacological and Parenteral Therapies **Integrated Process:** Nursing Process: Planning **Content Area:** Pharmacology **Strategy:** The core issue of the question is the type of medication therapy that will be effective in treating hyperthyroidism or Graves' disease. Use nursing knowledge and the process of elimination to make a selection.

8 **Answer: 4** **Rationale:** Cardiac problems related to Graves' disease and hyperthyroidism include increased systolic blood pressure, a widened pulse pressure, tachycardia, and other dysrhythmias. Appropriate control of the disorder with medication therapy would prevent these manifestations from occurring. **Cognitive Level:** Applying **Client Need:** Pharmacological and Parenteral Therapies **Integrated Process:** Nursing Process: Data Collection **Content Area:** Pharmacology **Strategy:** The core issue of the question is knowledge of which symptoms should resolve once medication therapy for Graves' disease has begun. Recall that Graves' disease represents a hypermetabolic state, and then eliminate each option that does not correlate with excessive metabolic activity.

9 **Answer: 2 Rationale:** Management of hypoparathyroidism is aimed at correcting hypocalcemia, vitamin D deficiency, and hypomagnesemia. **Cognitive Level:** Applying **Client Need:** Pharmacological and Parenteral Therapies **Integrated Process:** Nursing Process: Data Collection **Content Area:** Pharmacology **Strategy:** The core issue of the question is knowledge of abnormal laboratory values that should resolve with effective medication therapy for hypoparathyroidism. Use knowledge of medication actions to eliminate each of the incorrect options. Two options are opposite, which is a clue that one of them is likely to be the correct answer.

10 **Answer: 1 Rationale:** Actos is a thiazolidinedione type of oral antidiabetic agent; its action enhances insulin action and promotes glucose utilization in peripheral tissues. This drug improves sensitivity to insulin in muscle and fat tissue, and inhibits glucogenesis. Because of the potential for liver damage, clients taking drugs in this class must have liver function studies done before therapy is begun, and periodically thereafter. The other options are not necessary before beginning therapy with Actos. **Cognitive Level:** Applying **Client Need:** Pharmacological and Parenteral Therapies **Integrated Process:** Nursing Process: Planning **Content Area:** Pharmacology **Strategy:** The core issue of this question is knowledge of the adverse effects of thiazolidinedione antidiabetic agents. Recall as a general strategy that many drug classes have adverse effects on the liver. Use medication knowledge and the process of elimination to make a selection.

11 **Answer: 2 Rationale:** Adrenocortical replacement therapy medications are divided into mineralocorticoids and glucocorticoids. Mineralcorticoids such as fludrocortisone increase resorption of sodium by increasing hydrogen and potassium excretion in the distal tubule. Mineralcorticoids such as fludrocortisone increase resorption of sodium by increasing hydrogen and potassium excretion in the distal tubule. Glucocorticoids decrease inflammation by suppressing leukocyte migration, but they do not eliminate the body's immune response. Glucocorticoids decrease inflammation by suppressing leukocyte migration and modifying the body's immune response. **Cognitive Level:** Applying **Client Need:** Pharmacological and Parenteral Therapies **Integrated Process:** Teaching and Learning **Content Area:** Pharmacology **Strategy:** Specific medication knowledge about the effects of mineralocorticoid drug therapy is needed to answer this question. Use medication knowledge and the process of elimination to make a selection.

12 **Answer: 4 Rationale:** To prevent diabetic ketoacidosis, this client must regularly check urine ketone levels if the blood glucose level is higher than 240 mg/dL. If anorexia, nausea, or vomiting is present, sick-day diabetic management care requires clients to check their blood glucose level every 4–6 hours. Clients should not eliminate or adjust their doses of insulin or oral hypoglycemics. Meals should be eaten at regular times, and clients should consume foods and liquids that are more easily tolerated. **Cognitive Level:** Applying **Client Need:** Pharmacological and Parenteral Therapies **Integrated Process:** Teaching and Learning **Content Area:** Pharmacology **Strategy:** The core issue of the question is knowledge of how to manage medication therapy for a diabetic client during illness. With this in mind, choose the option that does not decrease the drug dose (since blood glucose rises during illness), and that provides for safe and effective treatment (calling the physician when the level is excessive).

13 **Answer: 2 Rationale:** Thyroid hormones increase the effects of anticoagulants. Assessment of PT or INR will determine if the anticoagulant dosage must be decreased. The nurse also assesses the client for evidence of bruising or bleeding. A CBC could detect anemia caused by bleeding as a complication of excessive warfarin therapy, which should be monitored on a regular basis; however, it is not an essential test prior to thyroid replacement hormone therapy. APTT measures the effectiveness of heparin, and would not be appropriate for a client on Coumadin therapy. Coumadin levels are not drawn. **Cognitive Level:** Analyzing **Client Need:** Pharmacological and Parenteral Therapies **Integrated Process:** Nursing Process: Data Collection **Content Area:** Pharmacology **Strategy:** The core issue of the question is an understanding of interactive effects of thyroid hormones and anticoagulants such as warfarin. Use knowledge of both medications and associated laboratory values to make a selection.

14 **Answer: 1 Rationale:** Because of the risk of alcohol-induced hypoglycemia, diabetic clients must ingest alcohol only with or shortly after meals. If diabetes is well controlled, blood glucose levels are not affected by mild consumption of alcohol; however, food should be ingested shortly before, after, or during alcohol intake. Because of the risk of alcohol-induced hypoglycemia, diabetic clients must ingest alcohol only with or shortly after meals. In all cases, the client should confer with the prescribing physician and dietitian to determine whether alcohol may be utilized as part of the overall caloric intake. The effects of alcohol on a diabetic client do not change in regard to the source of the alcohol. Male clients taking insulin may ingest two alcoholic beverages daily, and female clients may ingest one alcoholic beverage with, or in addition to, the regular meal plan. **Cognitive Level:** Applying **Client Need:** Pharmacological and Parenteral Therapies **Integrated Process:** Communication and Documentation **Content Area:** Pharmacology **Strategy:** The core issue of the question is knowledge of how alcohol can affect blood glucose levels in a client taking insulin. Use knowledge of interactive effects of medications and alcohol to make a selection.

15 **Answer: 3 Rationale:** The shorter-acting insulin should be withdrawn first to prevent the longer-acting insulin from mixing in the bottle with the shorter-acting insulin. Gently roll the bottle of intermediate insulin to mix, because vigorous shaking creates bubbles, leading to an inaccurate dose. Withdrawing the shorter-acting insulin first prevents the longer-acting insulin from mixing in the bottle with the shorter-acting insulin. Air must be injected into each bottle before withdrawing; first into the bottle of longer-acting insulin, and then into the bottle of shorter-acting insulin. **Cognitive Level:** Applying **Client Need:** Pharmacological and Parenteral Therapies **Integrated Process:** Teaching and Learning **Content Area:** Pharmacology **Strategy:** The core issue of the question is proper technique for drawing up mixed insulins. Choose the option that does not contaminate the shorter-acting insulin with the longer-acting one, which would necessitate discarding the contaminated vial.

16 **Answer: 4 Rationale:** Metformin is given to clients with stable type 2 diabetes mellitus to inhibit glucose production by the liver and increase sensitivity of peripheral tissue to insulin. **Cognitive Level:** Analyzing **Client Need:** Pharmacological and Parenteral Therapies **Integrated Process:** Nursing Process: Evaluation **Content Area:** Pharmacology **Strategy:** The core issue of the question is knowledge of the actions of metformin on reducing blood glucose. Use medication knowledge and the process of elimination to make a selection.

17 **Answer: 2 Rationale:** Abrupt cessation of long-term steroid therapy can cause acute adrenal insufficiency, which could

lead to death. Adverse reactions would be likely if the medication is abruptly withdrawn. Central nervous system symptoms such as confusion and psychosis are adverse effects of steroids such as prednisone. Daily chemistry measurements are not needed during drug dosage tapering. **Cognitive Level:** Applying **Client Need:** Pharmacological and Parenteral Therapies **Integrated Process:** Nursing Process: Implementation **Content Area:** Adult Health **Strategy:** Recall knowledge of the pathophysiological process of glucocorticoids to lead to the only correct selection. If this was difficult, review the action of glucocorticoids.

18 **Answer: 4** **Rationale:** After the start of therapy, peak levels of the drug should not be expected for many weeks to months. Lack of energy is a common symptom with hypothyroidism. After the start of therapy, peak levels of the drug should not be expected for many weeks to months. Thus, increased energy levels cannot be expected within a few days. The drug works best when taken before breakfast on an empty stomach. **Cognitive Level:** Analyzing **Client Need:** Physiological Adaptation **Integrated Process:** Nursing Process: Implementation **Content Area:** Pharmacology **Strategy:** Note the question being asked is when the energy level will increase. First eliminate two options that do not address the client's question. Since the medication is long-term therapy, immediate results cannot be expected, which would eliminate a third.

19 **Answer: 3** **Rationale:** Hunger; nausea; pale, cool skin; and sweating are signs of a hypoglycemic reaction. Fruity breath can accompany ketoacidosis. Flushing of the face can accompany hyperglycemia. Dry, flaky skin is unrelated to hypoglycemia. **Cognitive Level:** Applying **Client Need:** Physiological Adaptation **Integrated Process:** Nursing Process: Data Collection **Content Area:** Adult Health **Strategy:** Specific knowledge of the signs and symptoms of hypoglycemia is needed to answer the question. If this was difficult, learn to distinguish between hypoglycemia and hyperglycemia signs and symptoms.

20 **Answer: 4** **Rationale:** Primary osteoporosis is more prevalent in Caucasian and Asian women. Primary osteoporosis most often occurs in postmenopausal women. Primary osteoporosis most often occurs in women who are thin and lean. Primary osteoporosis is not as prevalent in African-American women. **Cognitive Level:** Analyzing **Client Need:** Pharmacological and Parenteral Therapies **Integrated Process:** Nursing Process: Planning **Content Area:** Pharmacology **Strategy:** The core issue of the question is knowledge of the clients at risk for osteoporosis and amenable to therapy with calcium supplementation. Use general nursing knowledge and the process of elimination to make a selection.

Key Terms to Review

Addison's disease p. 588
adrenal crisis p. 588
adrenal insufficiency p. 588
catecholamine p. 590
cushingoid state p. 588
glucocorticoid p. 588
glycosylated hemoglobin p. 596
Graves' disease p. 590
hypercalciuria p. 585
hyperglycemia p. 594
hyperthyroidism p. 590
hypoglycemia p. 095
hypoparathyroidism p. 592
hypothyroidism p. 590
lipodystrophy p. 595
mineralocorticoid p. 587
myxedema p. 590
osteomalacia p. 592
osteoporosis p. 588
Paget's disease p. 593

References

Adams, M., Holland, L., & Urban, C. (2011). *Pharmacology for nurses: A pathophysiological approach* (3rd ed.). Upper Saddle River, NJ: Pearson Education, Inc.

Adams, M., & Koch, R. (2010). *Pharmacology: Connections to nursing practice.* Upper Saddle River, NJ: Pearson Education, Inc.

Deglin, J. H., & Vallerand, A. H. (2011). *Davis's drug guide for nurses* (12th ed.). Philadelphia: F. A. Davis.

Lehne, R. (2010). *Pharmacology for nursing care* (7th ed.). Philadelphia: W. B. Saunders.

Wilson, B., Shannon, M., & Shields, K. (2012). *Pearson nurse's drug guide 2012.* Upper Saddle River, NJ: Pearson Education.

Test Yourself

Are you ready for the NCLEX-PN® or course exams? Use the practice tests on the companion website to check.

Integumentary Medications

39

In this chapter

Cross Reference

Other chapters relevant to this content area are

Dosage Calculation and Medication Administration	Chapter 28
Integumentary Disorders	Chapter 58

I. GENERAL AGENTS

A. Lotions

1. May be a liquid emulsion or a suspension of a powder in water; may have a drying effect on skin as water evaporates
2. Common preparations include calamine lotion (Calamox), zinc stearate, and others; may contain calamine, zinc oxide, glycerin, bentonite magma, calcium hydroxide, and other ingedients
3. *NCLEX®* Shake lotion before application
4. *NCLEX®* Some preparations of calamine lotion also contain diphenhydramine (Benadryl), which can cause drowsiness; use cautiously until effect is known

B. Emollients

1. Are occlusive agents that make skin soft by hydrating and filling gaps in stratum corneum created by dry, contracted skin cells
2. Include silicone oils, propylene glycol, isopropyl palmitate, and octyl stearate
3. *NCLEX®* Can also function as skin protectants if they soothe **pruritus** (intense itching) due to exposed, traumatized nerve endings
4. Moisturizers mimic function of sebum on skin, based on mechanisms of occlusion and humectancy
5. Occlusion function uses petrolatum, lanolin, cocoa butter, or mineral oil to prevent evaporation of water from skin
6. Humectancy function uses substances that attract moisture to skin, (e.g., glycerin, sorbitol, propylene glycol)
7. Common preparations are listed in Box 39–1
8. *NCLEX®* Nursing considerations; collect data about any skin symptom, beginning with a history; apply to skin after bathing while skin is slightly moist unless otherwise directed; teach client proper use of product

Box 39–1

Emollients

Aquaphor	Lac-Hydrin Lotion 12% (prescription only)
Cetaphil Lotion	Lubriderm Lotions and Oil
Curel Moisturizing Lotion	Moisturel Lotion
Dermasil Lotion	Neutrogena Emulsion
Eucerin Crème or Lotion	Penecare Lotion
Keri Lotion	White Petrolatum
Lac-Hydrin Cream or Lotion	

C. Protectants

1. Designed to protect skin from wetness or prevent and treat diaper rash, prickly heat, and/or chafing
2. Common preparations are listed in Box 39–2
3. Nursing considerations: collect data about any skin symptom, beginning with a history; monitor skin for desired effect

NCLEX®

4. Client teaching
   a. Keep powders away from face to avoid inhalation
   b. Some preparations should not be used on broken skin
   c. If diaper rash or skin irritation worsens or does not improve within 7 days of treatment, consult health care provider

D. Soaks and wet dressings

NCLEX®

1. Acute lesions that are oozing, weeping, and crusting tend to respond best to aqueous, drying preparations

NCLEX®

2. Scaling chronic lesions tend to respond best to moisturizing, lubricating preparations

NCLEX®

3. Open soaks are applied for 20 minutes, 3 times a day
4. Closed soaks use a water-impermeable substance (occlusion) over a wet soak, to cause heat retention, which is excellent for debridement but may lead to skin maceration; are applied for 1–2 hours 2 to 3 times a day
5. Continuous closed soaks are left in place for 24 hours to treat thick crusts; it is important to rewet dressing 4 to 5 times a day
6. Common preparations are listed in Table 39–1
7. Nursing considerations: collect data about any skin symptom, beginning with a history, and monitor for achievement of intended effects
8. Client teaching: proper procedure for type of soak recommended or prescribed

Box 39–2

Protectants

A & D Ointment (lanolin, petrolatum, others)

A & D Medicated Diaper Rash Ointment (white petrolatum, zinc oxide, cod liver oil, light mineral oil, others)

Balmex Ointment (zinc oxide, balsam Peru, beeswax, mineral oil, others)

Caldesene Medicated Powder or Ointment (powder: calcium undecylenate; ointment: white petrolatum, zinc oxide, others)

Clocream Skin Protectant Cream (each ounce contains vitamins A and D equivalent to 1 ounce of cod liver oil, many others)

Desitin Cornstarch Baby Powder (zinc oxide 10% with cornstarch, others)

Desitin Ointment (zinc oxide 40% with cod liver oil in a petrolatum-lanolin base, others)

Table 39–1 Soaks and Wet Dressings

Agent	Use
Burow's Solution (Bluboro Powder, Domeboro, others): yields 5% aluminum acetate solution or 1 tablet or packet added to 1 pint of tap water	Acts as astringent to decrease exudation by precipitation of protein
Acetic Acid 0.1–1% solution: ½-cup white vinegar to 1 quart water	May be helpful for wound infected with *Pseudomonas* organisms
Salt solution: 1 tbsp. of salt to 1 quart of water	Wetting action

E. Rubs and liniments

1. Are over-the-counter (OTC) preparations for temporary relief of minor aches and pains of muscles and joints associated with strains, bruises, sprains, sports injuries, simple backache, and arthritis
2. Contain various antiseptics, analgesics, local anesthetics; some contain salicylates that could lead to salicylate side effects (nausea and vomiting [N/V] or tinnitus) if used extensively
3. Common preparations: methyl salicylate (BenGay™, Icy Hot™), trolamine salicylate (Aspercreme™), capsaicin (Capsin™) with active ingredient from cayenne peppers; others
4. Nursing considerations: note causative symptom and monitor for achievement of intended effects

NCLEX®

5. Client teaching
   a. Remove other ointments (water in oil emulsions), creams, sprays, or liniments before applying product
   b. Apply to affected areas not more than 3 to 4 times daily
   c. Some products have specific directions (e.g., BenGay should not be used with heating pad or tight bandage because skin irritation or burning could occur)

II. PROTECTIVE AGENTS

A. Overview

1. This discussion is limited to sunscreen preparations and protective dressings
2. For other preparations that offer protection, see previous section on *protectants*

B. Sunscreen preparations

1. Can help to prevent sunburn and later skin cancer by absorbing rays of ultraviolet (UV) light
2. Chemical absorbers formulated against UVB rays include cinnamates, p-aminobenzoic acid (PABA) and PABA esters, or salicylates; those formulated against UVA rays include benzophenones
3. Physical sunscreens reflect or scatter light to prevent skin penetration and contain ingredients such as titanium dioxide, zinc oxide, talc

NCLEX®

4. Effectiveness is indicated by sun protection factor (SPF); a SPF of 15 means product offers 15 times greater protection than no sunscreen; SPFs range from 4 to 70+
5. Sunscreens should be applied 30–60 minutes before sun exposure and should be reapplied after swimming, sweating, and every 2–3 hours; a minimum SPF of 15 is recommended

C. Protective dressings

1. Includes occlusive biosynthetic dressings for certain wound therapies
2. Common dressings are listed in Table 39–2; other dressings are outlined in Chapter 26 in Table 26–6
3. Nursing considerations
   a. Collect data about any skin wound, beginning with a history
   b. *NCLEX®* Inspect dressing at least daily for leaks, dislodgment, wrinkling, or odor
   c. *NCLEX®* Change dressing when it becomes dislodged, leaks, or develops an odor
   d. *NCLEX®* If wound has substantial drainage, dressing might need changing every 24–48 hours but generally is left in place for 3–7 days
   e. When changing dressing, leave residue that is difficult to remove; it will wear off in time; attempts to remove can irritate surrounding skin
4. Client teaching: proper use of any prescribed occlusive biosynthetic dressing

Table 39–2 Common Protective Wound Dressings

Dressing	Transmits Oxygen	Transmits Water Vapor	Excludes Bacteria	Absorbs Fluids	Transparent	Adhesive
Bioclusive	+	+	–	–	+	+
DuoDERM	–	–	+	+	–	+
Geliperm	+	+	+	+	+	+
Intrasite	–	–	+	+	–	+
Op-site	+	+	+	–	+	+
Replicare	–	–	+	–	–	+
Tegasorb	–	–	+	+	–	+
Tegaderm	+	+	?	–	+	+
Vigilon	+	–	–	+	+	–
Zenoderm	+	+	+	+	+	+

+ has the stated action; – does not have the stated action; ? may or may not have the stated action

III. ANTIPRURITICS

A. Overview

1. Medications that stop intense itching of pruritis
2. Pruritus has a multitude of causes, and treatment must be tailored to specific cause
3. Types include winter pruritus, senior pruritus, lichen simplex chronicus, external otitis, pruritus ani (e.g., pinworm infestation in children), and genital pruritus
4. Antipruritic therapy for some types of pruritis might include topical corticosteroids to decrease inflammation and/or methods to promote skin hydration
5. Antipruritic therapy may also require use of a systemic antihistamine, such as hydroxyzine (Vistaril or Atarax), chlorpheniramine (Chlortrimetron), or cyproheptadine hydrochloride (generic)

B. Common topical preparations are listed in Box 39–3

C. Nursing considerations

1. Medications are often topical but oral medications may need to be added if relief is insufficient with topical products
2. Take a history of systemic symptoms and any associated skin symptoms
3. NCLEX® Monitor for local and systemic adverse effects of any topical preparation
4. NCLEX® Monitor for drowsiness or other anticholinergic side effects if systemic antihistamines are used

D. Client teaching (NCLEX®)

1. Bathe less frequently, use only mild soaps, and use soap sparingly
2. Understand need to interrupt itch-and-scratch cycle because of negative effect of scratching
3. Maintain cool environment, especially in bedroom for sleep
4. Try to eliminate environmental source of trigger if possible

IV. ANTI-INFECTIVES

A. Antibacterials

1. Certain topical antibiotics inhibit growth of *Propionibacterium acnes* and reduce inflammatory lesions of acne
2. Topical antibacterial therapy may be useful for prophylaxis of infections in wounds and injuries
3. Common medications are listed in Table 39–3
4. NCLEX® Nursing considerations
   a. Collect data about any skin symptom, beginning with a history
   b. Monitor for hypersensitivity to any ingredient in product to be used
   c. Monitor for skin irritation and superinfection
5. NCLEX® Client teaching
   a. Wash hands before using any topical antibacterial agent; may wear gloves
   b. Generally, apply products sparingly and gently to affected area
   c. With some, a dressing should be applied; with others, it should not: follow prescriber instructions
   d. Report worsening of condition or lack of healing

B. Antivirals

1. Used to treat cutaneous **herpes simplex** (an acute viral disease marked by groups of skin vesicles, often on borders of lips, nares, or genitals) or herpes zoster
2. With some infections an oral agent instead of a topical agent may be needed
3. Common medication: acyclovir 5% ointment (Zovirax)

Box 39–3

Local Antipruritic Agents

Lotion or Cream

Aveeno Anti-itch Lotion or Cream

Aveeno Moisturing Lotion or Cream

Eucerin Crème or Lotion

Sarna Topical Lotion (camphor, menthol, and phenol)

Zonalon Cream

Hydrating Baths

Aveeno (colloidal oatmeal)

Aveeno Oil (colloidal oatmeal, mineral oil, glyceryl stearate, etc.)

Table 39-3 Antibacterial Agents

Medication	Source	Mechanism of Action	Notes
Bacitracin (Baciguent Topical)	*Bacillus subtilis*	Cell wall inhibitor	Used with impetigo, furunculosis, pyodermas
Bacitracin, polymyxin B, neosporin (Triple Antibiotic Topical, others)	*Bacillus subtilis, Streptomyces fradiae*	Cell wall inhibitor, 30S ribosome inhibition	Available as ointment to treat secondarily infected skin problems
Clindamycin phosphate (Cleocin T, Clinda-Derm Topical Solution)	Semisynthetic	Binds to 50S ribosome; suppresses bacterial protein synthesis	Available in various forms; used primarily for treatment of acne
Erythromycin and benzoyl peroxide (Benzamycin)			Gel for acne vulgaris
Gentamicin sulfate (generic)	Fermentation product from *Micromonospora purpura*	Interferes with bacterial protein synthesis	Cream or ointment used prophylactically after ear surgery against otitis externa due to *Pseudomonas aeruginosa*
Metronidazole (MetroGel)		Possible antibiotic, antioxidant, and anti-inflammatory properties	Available as gel, topical treatment of rosacea
Mupirocin (Bactroban)	*Pseudomonas fluorescens*	tRNA synthetase inhibitor	Topical treatment of impetigo

Memory Aid

Antiviral agents often can be recognized on sight because they contain *vir* in the beginning, middle, or end of the name.

NCLEX®

4. Nursing considerations: collect data about skin symptoms (beginning with a history) and monitor for local adverse effects of topical product, such as mild pain, burning, stinging

NCLEX®

5. Client teaching
   a. Wash hands before use and apply gloves or finger cot when applying product to avoid autoinnoculation of other body sites
   b. Apply as soon as symptoms of herpes lesions begins
   c. Apply sparingly and gently to affected area
   d. Wear loose clothing and keep area clean and dry
   e. Avoid sexual activity when skin lesions are present

C. Antifungals

1. Topical agents can be used in clients with limited disease and if infection is limited to glabrous (smooth, hairless) skin; clients with extensive disease or infection of hair and nails are best treated with systemic therapy

NCLEX®

2. Advantages of topical use over systemic use: absence of serious adverse reactions or drug interactions, OTC availability of some preparations, ability to localize treatment to affected sites, no need to monitor laboratory tests
3. New drugs have decreased use of keratolytics and **antiseptics** (chemical agents that inhibit growth of microorganisms but may not kill them) used in past
4. Common medications
   a. Topical agents are listed in Box 39–4
   b. Oral agents include fluconazole (Diflucan), griseofulvin (Grifulvin V, Gris-peg), itraconazole (Sporanox), ketoconazole (Nizoral), and terbinafine (Lamisil); these are discussed in Chapter 41

Memory Aid

Antifungal agents are easy to recognize on sight because they generally end with the suffix *-azole*.

Box 39-4

Topical Antifungals

Allylamines

Naftifine hydrochloride (Naftin): cream gel

Terbinafine (Lamisal): cream

Imidazoles

Clotrimazole (Lotrimin AF, Mycelex): cream, solution, lotion, vaginal tablets, cream

Betamethasone dipropionate, clotrimazole (Lotrisone): cream, lotion

Econazole nitrate (generic): cream

Ketoconazole (Nizoral A-D): cream, shampoo

Miconazole (Monistat, others): cream, powder, spray, vaginal suppository or cream

Oxiconazole (Oxistat): cream, lotion

Sulconazole nitrate (Exelderm): cream, solution

Miscellaneous

Ciclopirox (Loprox): cream, lotion

Undecylenic acid (Trifungol): cream, powder

Nystatin (Mycostatin, others): cream, ointment, powder, vaginal tablet

Tolnaftate (Tinactin): cream, solution, spray, liquid, spray powder; (Aftate) gel, powder, spray liquid

5. Nursing considerations
   a. Collect data about any skin symptom, beginning with a history
   b. Monitor for predisposing factors, such as trauma, general health, suppressed immune status, hygiene practices, and exposure to infectious agent
   c. *NCLEX®* Monitor for local adverse effects (irritation, burning, or stinging)
   d. *NCLEX®* Monitor for skin sensitization, noted by increased redness, swelling, weeping, or any burning or itching not present before treatment began
   e. Systemic effects of topical products are negligible, since absorption rates generally are only 3–6%
6. *NCLEX®* Client teaching
   a. Use products as directed for full course of therapy (may be prolonged); apply liberally to clean and dry skin
   b. Leave exposed to air; do not apply protective dressing unless specifically ordered
   c. Wear shower shoes or foot thongs in public or communal showers and locker rooms (with **tinea pedis** or athlete's foot)
   d. Avoid going barefoot, and wear footwear of natural fibers (leather shoes, cotton or wool socks) to prevent tinea pedis; change socks daily
   e. To avoid other fungal infections, practice adequate hygiene by keeping affected areas clean, dry, and well ventilated (loose clothing), and use powders (with or without antifungal ingredients) to keep skin dry and prevent maceration

D. Antiparasitics

1. Used to treat infestations such as **scabies** (infestation caused by mites) or **pediculosis** (infestation caused by lice); may involve hair (tinea capitus), body (tinea corporis), or pubic area (tinea pubis)
2. Recurrence of scabies is generally related to reinfection from incomplete treatment rather than resistance of mite
3. Crotamiton can be used in clients with scabies and pediculosis capitis who are ragweed-sensitive
4. Common medications are listed in Table 39–4; oral ivermectin (Stromectol) may be used for hard to treat head lice
5. Nursing considerations
   a. Collect data about any skin symptom, beginning with a history
   b. Monitor for local adverse effects (irritation, pruritis, burning, stinging)
   c. *NCLEX®* Monitor for systemic effect of dizziness with lindane because it affects nervous system; avoid use in infants, children, and clients with known seizure disorders because of risk of seizures

Table 39-4 Antiparasitics

Agent	Uses
Crotamiton (Eurax)	Scabies
Malathion (Ovide)	Pediculosis capitis and their ova
Permethrin (Elimite, Nix)	Pediculosis capitis, scabies
Pyrethrin, piperonyl butoxide (Rid)	Pediculosis capitis, pediculosis corporis, pediculosis pubis
Lindane (generic)	Pediculosis capitis, pediculosis pubis, scabies

NCLEX® 6. Client teaching: scabies
   a. Apply thin layer to dry skin from neck down over body; rub in thoroughly
   b. Permethrin and lindane: leave on 8–12 hours, remove thoroughly with washing
   c. Crotamiton: apply again after 24 hours, remove with washing 48 hours after initial application

NCLEX® 7. Client teaching: pediculosis capitis
   a. Lindane lotion: apply lotion to dry hair, rub in thoroughly, leave on 12 hours, remove thoroughly
   b. Lindane shampoo: apply shampoo to dry hair, lather with small amount water, work into hair for 4 minutes, rinse thoroughly
   c. Second treatment in 7–10 days may be needed with malathion, Rid

V. CORTICOSTEROIDS

A. Overview

1. Topical or systemic corticosteroids may be used with skin disorders; clinical effectiveness relates to four properties
   a. Vasoconstriction: decreases erythema
   b. Antiproliferative effects: inhibits DNA synthesis and mitosis
   c. Immunosuppression: mechanism poorly understood
   d. Anti-inflammatory effects: inhibits formation of prostaglandins
2. Responsiveness to topical corticosteroids varies: highly responsive diseases include **psoriasis**, atopic dermatitis in children, seborrheic dermatitis, intertrigo
3. Penetration of preparation varies according to skin site
4. Increased incidence of adverse reactions can occur when used on thin skin, on older adult or pediatric clients, or under occlusive dressing
5. Adverse effects more common in higher potency preparations

NCLEX® 6. Local adverse reactions include atrophy, hypopigmentation, striae

NCLEX® 7. Topical corticosteroids can cause systemic adverse reactions, including suppression of adrenal function

8. Low-potency agents are best used for diffuse eruptions, those involving face or occluded areas such as axilla or groin, and chronic dermatoses
9. Medium-potency agents are appropriate for acute flare of chronic dermatoses and acute self-limited eruptions with treatment periods of 14–21 days
10. High-potency agents are best for acute localized eruptions for only 7–14 days
11. High-potency agents should be avoided on areas susceptible to increased penetration and adverse reactions, such as face, intertriginous areas, perineum
12. A twice-a-day application is usually sufficient; more frequent application does not appear to improve response

NCLEX® 13. Mid- or high-potency corticosteroids should not be discontinued abruptly; may result in rebound flare of disorder

Memory Aid

A corticosteroid drug often can be recognized because it ends in the suffix *-sone* or *-one*. As an alternative, it may contain *cort* in the beginning, middle, or end of the drug name.

B. Common medications are listed in Table 39–5

C. Nursing considerations

1. Collect data about any skin symptom, beginning with a history
2. Generally, corticosteroids are applied sparingly and gently in a thin film to affected area

NCLEX® 3. Monitor for local adverse effects (acneiform skin eruptions, dryness, itching, burning, allergic contact dermatitis, hypopigmentation, overgrowth of bacteria/fungi/viruses)

Table 39-5 Topical Corticosteroids

Potency Class	Generic Name	Sample Trade Name (if listed)
Lowest potency	Alclometasone 0.05%	Aclovate
	Desonide 0.05%	Desowen
	Dexamethasone 0.1%	Decaspray
	Hydrocortisone 1%	Ala-Cort
	Methylprednisolone 0.25–1% ointment	Medrol
Low potency	Clocortolone 0.1%	Cloderm
	Fluocinolone acetonide 0.01%	Derma-Smoothe/FS
	Flurandrenolide 0.025%	Cordran
	Hydrocortisone valerate 0.2%	Westcort
	Triamcinolone acetonide 0.025%	Kenalog
Intermediate potency	Betamethasone benzoate 0.025%	Uticort
	Betamethasone valerate 0.1%	Beta-Val
	Desoximetasone 0.05%	Topicort LP
	Fluocinolone acetonide 0.025%	Synalar
	Fluticasone propionate 0.05%	Cutivate
	Halcinonide 0.025%	Halog
	Mometasone furoate 0.1%	Elocon
	Triamcinolone acetonide 0.1%	Kenalog
High potency	Amcinonide 0.1%	Cyclocort
	Betamethasone dipropionate 0.05%	
	Desoximetasone 0.25% cream	Topicort
	Fluocinolone 0.25% cream	Synalar
	Halcinonide 0.1%	
	Triamcinolone acetonide 0.5%	
Very high potency	Augmented betamethasone dipropionate 0.05%	Diprolene AF
	Clobetasol propionate 0.05%	Temovate
	Diflorasone diacetate 0.05%	Maxiflor
	Halobetasol propionate 0.05%	Ultravate

NCLEX® 4. Monitor for systemic adverse effects, which are more likely to include hirsutism (usually of face), moon facies, alopecia (scalp area), and immunosuppression

NCLEX® **D. Client teaching**

1. Before using, wash and dry area gently; use exactly as directed; do not overuse
2. Do not apply to open wounds or weeping areas
3. Report worsening of condition, signs of infection, or lack of healing

VI. KERATOLYTICS

A. Overview

1. Reduce thickness of hyperkeratotic stratum corneum (remove or soften horny layer of skin)
2. Used to treat disorders such as ichthyosis, dermatitis, psoriasis, and eczema; some are used to treat certain warts
3. Concentration necessary for keratolytic action differs among available agents

B. Common medications are listed in Table 39–6

NCLEX® **C. Nursing considerations**

1. Collect data about any skin symptom, beginning with a history
2. Monitor for local adverse effects of topical preparations

NCLEX® **D. Client teaching**

1. Understand purpose, use, side effects, and anticipated length of treatment
2. Apply as directed; method will vary somewhat depending on use

VII. ANTI-ACNE MEDICATIONS

A. Overview

1. Generally, a staged approach is used
2. Mild **acne** (noninflammatory and inflammatory lesions often on face, chest, back) with some comedones or few inflammatory lesions) is treated with topical agents such as salicylic acid, azelaic acid, benzoyl peroxide, and topical antibiotics
3. Moderate acne consisting of *comedones* (blackheads) and **papules** (small, circumscribed, superficial, solid elevations of the skin) can be managed by gradually increasing strength of topical tretinoin
4. Severe acne consisting of inflammatory papules and nodulocystic disease requires systemic antibiotics and isotretinoin (Accutane)
5. Choice of vehicle for topical preparation depends on whether client has dry or oily skin
6. NCLEX® Local adverse reactions to some topical preparations include erythema, burning or stinging, excessive dryness, hypersensitivity and susceptibility to sunburn
7. Most clients develop tolerance to local side effects within 3–4 weeks

B. Common medications are listed in Table 39–7

C. Nursing considerations

1. Inspect skin lesions as baseline and periodically to evaluate effectiveness of therapy
2. Monitor for local adverse effects of topical preparations
3. NCLEX® Monitor for systemic adverse effects as particular to individual product

D. Client teaching

1. Understand purpose, use, side effects, and anticipated length of treatment
2. Treatment is designed to control, not cure; therefore, periodic breakouts (especially premenstrual flares) may still occur
3. NCLEX® With topical preparation, wash and dry skin; massage thin film gently into affected areas as ordered
4. NCLEX® Avoid getting product into eyes, mouth, and mucous membranes; wash hands after use
5. NCLEX® With certain preparations, minimize exposure to sun and UV light
6. NCLEX® Isotretinoin (Accutane) is a teratogen; females of child-bearing age must strictly avoid becoming pregnant; they should have negative pregnancy test within 2 weeks before starting therapy and monthly during therapy
7. NCLEX® Avoid excess vitamin A intake with isotretinoin (Accutane), which is a vitamin A metabolite, to prevent toxicity
8. Comply with monthly triglyceride levels with isotretinoin to detect elevation as adverse effect

Table 39–6 Keratolytics

Agent	Uses
Salicylic acid	Warts, psoriasis, lichen simplex or chronicus, calluses, seborrheic dermatitis
Resorcinol monoacetate (Resinol)	Acne vulgaris, rosacea, seborrheic dermatitis, psoriasis, eczema, corns, calluses, and warts
Imiquimod (Aldara)	Exfoliative for warts and to slough epidermal cells of skin cancer
Sulfur (sulfur, precipitated)	Tinea of any area of body, acne vulgaris, rosacea, seborrheic dermatitis, pyodermas, psoriasis
Alpha-hydroxy acids (lactic, glycolic, glucuronic, pyruvic acids)	Ichthyosis, hyperkeratotic eczema, photoaging, acne, hyperpigmentation
Podofilox (Condylox)	Exfoliative for warts (epidermal cells only)
Calcipotriene (Dovonex)	Psoriasis and related skin disorders

Table 39–7 Anti-Acne Medications

Medication	Action or Use	Preparation
Adapalene (Differin)	Retinoid	Alcohol-free gel, cream; solution with alcohol
Benzoyl peroxide (Benzac; Benzamycin)	Antibacterial, keratolytic	Gel, wash
Benzoyl peroxide, erythromycin (Benzamycin)	Antibacterial, keratolytic	Gel
Azelaic acid (Azelex)	Antibacterial, keratolytic	Cream
Clindamycin and tretinoin (Ziana)	Antibacterial, retinoid	Gel, capsules
Isotretinoin (Accutane)	Retinoid acid derivative	
Sulfacetamide sodium (Klaron)	Antibacterial	Lotion
Tazarotene (Tazorac)	Retinoid; also for plaque psoriasis	Aqueous gel
Tetracyclines (Monodox, Sumycin, Doryx, Vibramycin)	Antibacterial	Capsules, tablets
Tretinoin (Retin-A, Avita)	Retinoic acid derivative; loosens keratin debris	Gel, liquid, aqueous gel, cream

VIII. BURN MEDICATIONS

A. Overview

1. Goals of therapy are to decrease inflammation, prevent infection, relieve pain, and promote healing
2. Topical agents are used to prevent infection in burn wounds, which could rapidly lead to sepsis

B. Common medications are listed in Table 39–8

Table 39–8 Burn Medications

Medication	Use	Notes
Mafenide (Sulfamylon)	Bacteriostatic against *Pseudomonas aeruginosa* and *Clostridia*	Adverse reactions include pain, burning, or stinging at application site for first 20–30 minutes after application With impaired renal function, high blood levels of agent may lead to metabolic acidosis; watch for compensatory respiratory alkalosis
Silver sulfadiazine (Silvadene, others)	Silver is toxic to bacteria; prevents replication of several organisms	Application is generally painless Watch for adverse reactions, including leukopenia, skin necrosis, erythema multiforme, skin discoloration, rashes Up to 10% may be absorbed; hazardous to use in clients with G6PD deficiency
Nitrofurazone (Furacin)	Adjunctive therapy when bacterial resistance to other agents occurs	Use cautiously in clients with impaired renal function; polyethylene glycol in preparation can be absorbed through denuded skin and may not be excreted normally by compromised kidneys Watch for rash, itching, dermatitis, bacterial or fungal superinfection, and allergic reaction at site Drug darkens on exposure to light, but does not affect potency
Silver nitrate	Similar to silver sulfadiazine; is a solution effective against gram negative bacteria	Apply silver nitrate to dressings, not directly to burned or nonintact skin Ensure that dressings stay moist Note that silver nitrate discolors whatever it contacts, but this is not usually permanent

C. Nursing considerations

NCLEX® **1.** Apply agents under sterile conditions once or twice daily to a thickness of approximately $\frac{1}{16}$-inch to clean and debrided wound

2. If hospitalized, client may undergo hydrotherapy (bathing in whirlpool) to aid debridement prior to application

NCLEX® **3.** Premedicate client with analgesic whenever possible 30 minutes prior to burn wound cleansing

4. Wound may be covered or left open

NCLEX® **5.** Monitor for adverse effects as outlined in Table 39–8

NCLEX® **6.** Watch for signs of infection and monitor WBC count in clients receiving silver sulfadiazine because of leukopenic effect

D. Client teaching

1. Understand purpose, use, side effects, and anticipated length of treatment

2. Use as directed if using preparation as an outpatient

IX. DEBRIDING AGENTS

A. Overview

1. Debriding agents remove dirt, damaged tissue, and cellular debris from wound to prevent infection and promote healing

2. Effectiveness in removing necrotic tissue, clotted blood, purulent exudates, or fibrinous accumulations has been questioned

a. Appear most effective when wound base has collagen that must be removed before epithelialization can proceed

b. Specific indications may vary (e.g., collagenase is indicated for stage 3 and 4 pressure ulcers)

B. Common medications are listed in Table 39–9

Table 39–9 Debriding Agents

Agent	Action	Notes
Collagenase (Santyl)	Digests collagen; active at pH 6–8, takes 10–14 days	Inactivated by extremes of pH, hydrogen peroxide, heavy metals like silver, detergents, iodine, nitrofurazone, and hexachlorophene
Sutilains (Travase)	Digests necrotic soft tissues by proteolytic action	Same as for collagenase
Trypsin, Balsam Peru, castor oil (Granulex)	Source of trypsin is bovine pancreas	Balsam Peru is capillary bed stimulant used to improve circulation; castor oil used to reduce premature epithelial cornification

Memory Aid

Some enzymes that are used to debride wounds end in the suffix *-ase*. This may help you to choose an appropriate product at least some of the time.

C. Nursing considerations: observe skin problem before use and monitor progress in wound healing

D. Client teaching: understand purpose, use, and side effects of medications, and anticipated length of treatment

Check Your NCLEX-PN® Exam I.Q.

You are ready for testing on this content if you can

- Apply knowledge of expected actions and effects of integumentary medications to client care.
- Correctly administer integumentary medications to clients.
- Monitor for side effects and adverse effects of integumentary medications.
- Take appropriate action if a client has an unexpected response to an integumentary medication.
- Monitor a client for expected outcomes or effects of treatment with integumentary medications.

PRACTICE TEST

PRACTICE TEST

1. The nurse would include what information when explaining the skin emollient Dermasil to a client?
   1. It requires shaking before each use.
   2. It has a drying effect on the skin when the water evaporates.
   3. It includes a corticosteroid component.
   4. It fills the gaps in the stratum corneum.

2. What instructions should the nurse give the client who is receiving tretinoin (Retin-A)?
   1. Apply the preparation in the morning.
   2. Use gloves, and apply a thick layer four times a day.
   3. Avoid products containing vitamin C.
   4. Apply to dry skin 30 minutes after washing.

3. A client's burn is infected and mafenide (Sulfamylon) is prescribed. The nurse's knowledge about this medication would indicate that which organism is involved?
   1. *Pseudomonas aeruginosa*
   2. Tubercle bacillus
   3. Methicillin-resistant *Staphylococcus aureus* (MRSA)
   4. *Candida albicans*

4. A female client who is using salicylic acid to treat psoriasis asks how long she will have to use this drug. What would be the best response by the nurse?
   1. "The drug should not be needed after three months of therapy."
   2. "Prolonged remission is uncommon, and maintenance therapy is needed."
   3. "Each situation is so unique that the question cannot be answered accurately."
   4. "The dermatologist caring for you is the best resource for your question."

5. The nurse would recommend that a client with excessive dandruff use a medicated shampoo that contains which active ingredient?
   1. Silver sulfadiazine
   2. Selenium sulfide
   3. Corticosteroid
   4. Lindane

6. It is winter and the client has extremely dry skin. Which type of preparation should the nurse recommend first?
   1. Regular use of soap, such as Dial
   2. Shake lotion
   3. Emollient or emollient-containing lotion
   4. Antipruritic lotion

7. Which of the following client disorders might require the use of acyclovir (Zovirax)?
   1. Herpes simplex virus infection
   2. Chronic dermatitis
   3. Pseudofolliculitis
   4. Candidiasis

8. A child has scraped his finger on a sharp spot on a shower door edge. The mother would like to use a topical antibiotic to prevent infection. Which agent would the nurse recommend?
   1. Bacitracin (Baciguent Topical)
   2. Malathion (Ovide Lotion)
   3. Ketoconazole (Nizoral)
   4. Mafenide (Sulfamylon)

9. The older adult client is being treated for a pressure ulcer. The nurse would anticipate what type of agent being used to topically debride this ulcer?
   1. Hydrocolloid dressing
   2. Antibiotic-impregnated gauze packing
   3. Allylamine
   4. Enzyme

10. The nurse is preparing to do tracheostomy care, and notes that the client's tracheostomy has encrusted debris around the tube. If allowed by agency policy, the nurse should dilute which antiseptic solution to half strength to most effectively clean the skin around the tracheostomy?

1. Iodine
2. Hydrogen peroxide
3. Chlorhexidine
4. Isopropyl alcohol

11. The physician's order sheet calls for topical application of the proteolytic enzyme Elase. The nurse carries out this order by applying this product to which area on the client?

1. External ear canal
2. Rectal area
3. Dry skin on feet
4. Sacral pressure ulcer

12. A client is seeking treatment for a wart. The nurse should explain that which type of product would effectively remove this growth?

1. Astringent
2. Antiseptic
3. Keratinolytic
4. Proteolytic

13. The nurse would be most careful when using a topical drug for a client in which group, because of increased risk of toxicity?

1. Middle-aged adult
2. Older adult
3. Child
4. Adolescent

14. Which type of dermatological product would the nurse recommend as having the most benefit for a client with acne?

1. Drying agent
2. Steroid
3. Emollient
4. Lubricant

15. A client has been using hydrocortisone 1% cream (Ala-Cort) as a topical agent. For what medication actions should the nurse evaluate the client? Select all that apply.

1. Moisturizing
2. Drying
3. Antimicrobial
4. Anti-inflammatory
5. Vasoconstriction

16. A client with psoriasis needs to apply a lubricating lotion to a psoriatic plaque. The nurse plans to reinforce teaching with the client to use what type of substance?

1. Emollient
2. Antiseptic
3. Alcohol
4. Astringent

17. The nurse is choosing a protective wound dressing for a client. Which product should be used when selecting a dressing that is permeable to oxygen?

1. Tegaderm
2. DuoDERM
3. Replicare
4. Tegasorb

18. A child has been diagnosed as having impetigo. The nurse anticipates that which topical agent will be prescribed?

1. Ketoconazole (Nizoral)
2. Mupirocin (Bactroban)
3. Capsaicin (Capsin)
4. Acyclovir (Zovirax) ointment

19. The nurse explains to a client that sunscreen with an SPF of 6 means that the product has which characteristic?

1. Provides protection from sun's rays for 6 hours
2. Is water-resistant, but not waterproof
3. Is waterproof for six immersions in the water
4. Provides six times the sun exposure protection as use of no sunscreen

20 An 18-year-old female client has severe acne. There has been no improvement from the use of various preparations and isotretinoin (Accutane) is being prescribed. The nurse evaluates that the client understood medication instructions, if the client stated to do which of the following?

1. Apply a thick layer of isotretinoin twice a day.
2. Increase exposure to the sun for added benefit.
3. Have a pregnancy test prior to beginning therapy and use contraception.
4. Have blood drawn for hormonal studies monthly for the first 6 months.

ANSWERS & RATIONALES

1 **Answer: 4 Rationale:** Emollients contain petrolatum, oils, propylene glycol, or other substances, and make the skin soft and pliable by filling the gaps and increasing hydration of the dry stratum corneum. Shaking Dermasil prior to application is not always necessary. Emollients contain petrolatum, oils, propylene glycol, or other substances; they do not dry the skin. Dermasil does not contain corticosteroids. **Cognitive Level:** Applying **Client Need:** Pharmacological and Parenteral Therapies **Integrated Process:** Nursing Process: Implementation **Content Area:** Pharmacology **Strategy:** The core issue of the question is general knowledge of integumentary products that are emollients. Use knowledge regarding these ordinary products and the process of elimination to make a selection.

2 **Answer: 4 Rationale:** The area to be treated with tretinoin should be washed at least 30 minutes before applying. Tretinoin is a retinoic acid derivative that needs to be applied once daily in a thin layer before retiring. Tretinoin is to be applied once daily in a thin layer before retiring; gloves are not necessary when applying the medication. Increased intake of vitamin A, not vitamin C, needs to be avoided. **Cognitive Level:** Applying **Client Need:** Pharmacological and Parenteral Therapies **Integrated Process:** Nursing Process: Implementation **Content Area:** Pharmacology **Strategy:** The core issue of the question is knowledge of proper use of tretinoin. Use medication knowledge and the process of elimination to make a selection.

3 **Answer: 1 Rationale:** Mafenide is useful in treatment of partial- and full-thickness burns to prevent septicemia caused by organisms such as Pseudomonas aeruginosa. Mafenide does not have a defined use with infections caused by Tubercle bacillus. MRSA is not treated with mafenide. Mafenide is useful in treatment of partial- and full-thickness burns, not Candida albicans. **Cognitive Level:** Applying **Client Need:** Pharmacological and Parenteral Therapies **Integrated Process:** Nursing Process: Planning **Content Area:** Pharmacology **Strategy:** The core issue of the question is knowledge of the uses of mafenide in a client with a burn injury. Use medication knowledge and the process of elimination to make a selection.

4 **Answer: 2 Rationale:** There is no cure for psoriasis. Psoriasis is notoriously chronic and recurrent. The cause is unknown. For most clients the disease is recurrent, and therapy will need to be continued. **Cognitive Level:** Applying **Client Need:** Pharmacological and Parenteral Therapies **Integrated Process:** Teaching and Learning **Content Area:** Pharmacology **Strategy:** The core issue of the question is general knowledge about medications used to treat psoriasis. Use medication knowledge and the process of elimination to make a selection.

5 **Answer: 2 Rationale:** A 1% lotion of selenium sulfide is used to relieve the itching and flaking of the scalp associated with dandruff. Silver sulfadiazine is a cream used in the prevention and treatment of infection in partial- and full-thickness burns. Corticosteroids can be used for many things, but dandruff is not one of them. A shampoo with lindane 1% (Kwell) would be used for pediculosis capitis. **Cognitive Level:** Analyzing **Client Need:** Pharmacological and Parenteral Therapies **Integrated Process:** Teaching and Learning **Content Area:** Pharmacology **Strategy:** The core issue of the question is general knowledge about medications used to treat dandruff. Use medication knowledge and the process of elimination to make a selection.

6 **Answer: 3 Rationale:** Emollient lotions are dilute dispersions of emulsified lipids in water. These provide smooth application and the most rapid hydration if applied to dry skin. Emollients (e.g., petrolatum) are occlusive agents that make the skin soft and pliable by increasing hydration of the stratum corneum. Excessive washing with harsh soaps (such as Dial) strips stratum corneum of its natural lipids, and exacerbates dry skin. No shake lotion is made specifically for management of dry skin. Itching can occur with dry skin, but before an antipruritic lotion is used, an emollient lotion or emollient should be tried. **Cognitive Level:** Analyzing **Client Need:** Pharmacological and Parenteral Therapies **Integrated Process:** Nursing Process: Implementation **Content Area:** Pharmacology **Strategy:** The core issue of the question is general knowledge about products used to treat dry skin. Use product knowledge and the process of elimination to make a selection.

7 **Answer: 1 Rationale:** Acyclovir is an antiviral agent that is useful in the treatment of herpes simplex viruses. The other options would require therapy with an anti-infective, but not of the antiviral type. **Cognitive Level:** Applying **Client Need:** Pharmacological and Parenteral Therapies **Integrated Process:** Nursing Process: Implementation **Content Area:** Pharmacology **Strategy:** The core issue of the question is knowledge of the uses of acyclovir in a client with herpes infection. Use medication knowledge and the process of elimination to make a selection. Remember that an antiviral medication often contains *vir* somewhere in its name.

8 **Answer: 1 Rationale:** Bacitracin is a topical antibiotic that is bactericidal against Gram-positive cocci and bacilli, including staphylococci and streptococci. These organisms might cause infection in a skin wound. Malathion is an antiparasitic agent for pediculosis. Ketoconazole is an antifungal agent. Mafenide is an agent used for burns. **Cognitive Level:** Applying **Client Need:** Pharmacological and Parenteral Therapies **Integrated Process:** Nursing Process: Implementation **Content Area:** Pharmacology **Strategy:** The core issue of the question is knowledge of the types of medications used for various skin conditions. Use medication knowledge and the process of elimination to make a selection. Remember that cuts or open wounds often heal effectively when topical antibiotics are used to prevent infection at the site.

9 **Answer: 4** **Rationale:** Ulcers with necrotic material should be debrided, either by sharp debridement (e.g., using a scalpel) or chemical debridement (e.g., wound cleanser, such as an enzyme). An example of such a preparation is collagenase (Santyl), which is inactivated by metal salts, hexachlorophene, or acidic solutions. Hydrocolloid dressings can be helpful with uninfected wounds with fibrinous bases. Topical antibiotics will not help remove necrotic material. Allylamines are selected for fungal infections. **Cognitive Level:** Analyzing **Client Need:** Pharmacological and Parenteral Therapies **Integrated Process:** Nursing Process: Planning **Content Area:** Pharmacology **Strategy:** The core issue of the question is the type of topical agent to use when debridement is needed. Use medication knowledge and the process of elimination to make a selection. Enzymes often end in *-ase*, which makes them easy to recognize on sight.

10 **Answer: 2** **Rationale:** Hydrogen peroxide is an oxidizing antiseptic that can be used to clean wounds or tracheostomy tubes. Iodine, as a cleaning agent, does not have the bubbling action to remove debris. Chlorhexidine can be used as a cleaning agent, but it does not have the bubbling action to aid in cleansing. Isopropyl alcohol would be irritating or drying to the skin and should not be used. **Cognitive Level:** Applying **Client Need:** Pharmacological and Parenteral Therapies **Integrated Process:** Nursing Process: Implementation **Content Area:** Pharmacology **Strategy:** The core issue of the question is knowledge of the type of skin cleansing agent used for tracheostomy. Use knowledge of these agents and the process of elimination to make a selection.

11 **Answer: 4** **Rationale:** Proteolytic enzymes such as Elase ointment can be used to chemically debride tissue. These areas commonly include venous stasis ulcers, burn wounds, and pressure ulcers. Proteolytic enzymes would not be used on other areas. **Cognitive Level:** Applying **Client Need:** Pharmacological and Parenteral Therapies **Integrated Process:** Nursing Process: Implementation **Content Area:** Pharmacology **Strategy:** The core issue of the question is knowledge of the debriding agents appropriate for use at various skin sites. Use knowledge of these agents and the process of elimination to make a selection.

12 **Answer: 3** **Rationale:** A keratinolytic agent such as salicyclic acid is used to treat warts, as well as corns, calluses, and other keratin-containing skin lesions. Astringents cause topical vasoconstriction, and would not be effective to remove a wart. Antiseptics inhibit bacterial growth. Proteolytic enzymes are used to debride tissue, but not warts. **Cognitive Level:** Applying **Client Need:** Pharmacological and Parenteral Therapies **Integrated Process:** Teaching and Learning **Content Area:** Pharmacology **Strategy:** The core issue of the question is what type of medication is effective in treating warts. Begin to answer by reasoning that treatment of a wart includes breaking it down for removal. Next note the suffix *-lytic* in the correct option, which means "to break down."

13 **Answer: 3** **Rationale:** Children have an increased risk of systemic toxicity from topically applied drugs because of the greater ratio of surface area to weight. The other options have a smaller body surface area-to-weight ratio than a child; age is not a factor. **Cognitive Level:** Applying **Client Need:** Pharmacological and Parenteral Therapies **Integrated Process:** Nursing Process: Evaluation **Content Area:** Pharmacology **Strategy:** The core issue of this question is the age group that is at greatest risk because of its skin characteristics when topical drugs are used. Recall that the greater the area involved, the greater the risk of absorption and toxic effects. Finally, recall that infants and children have a greater body surface-to-weight ratio than an adult of any age.

14 **Answer: 1** **Rationale:** Acne can be successfully treated with drying agents. The other options would be of no benefit or might worsen the condition. **Cognitive Level:** Applying **Client Need:** Pharmacological and Parenteral Therapies **Integrated Process:** Nursing Process: Planning **Content Area:** Pharmacology **Strategy:** The core issue of the question is which type of medication is effective in treating acne. Since this condition is characterized by inflammation and drainage, consider that an agent that has a drying effect would be opposite to the characteristics of the condition and would help reduce symptoms.

15 **Answer: 4, 5** **Rationale:** Corticosteroids such as hydrocortisone are anti-inflammatory drugs. Corticosteroids such as hydrocortisone decrease erythema through vasoconstriction. Corticosteroids are not moisturizing agents. Corticosteroids do not act as drying agents. Corticosteroids do not exert antimicrobial action, and, in fact, they can increase risk of infection by suppressing the inflammatory response. **Cognitive Level:** Analyzing **Client Need:** Pharmacological and Parenteral Therapies **Integrated Process:** Nursing Process: Evaluation **Content Area:** Pharmacology **Strategy:** The core issue of the question is knowledge of the intended effects of corticosteroids as anti-inflammatory agents. Use this information and the process of elimination to make a selection. When there is more than one correct answer, consider each option as a true/false statement.

16 **Answer: 1** **Rationale:** Psoriatic plaques need to be lubricated so that they are easier to loosen and remove. Emollients and lubricants are fatty or oily substances that can be used for this purpose because they keep skin soft, and prevent water evaporation. The other options are harsher substances and might have a drying effect. **Cognitive Level:** Applying **Client Need:** Pharmacological and Parenteral Therapies **Integrated Process:** Teaching and Learning **Content Area:** Pharmacology **Strategy:** Note the word *lubricating* in the stem of the question. This tells you that regardless of the client's health problem, the agent is one that has a moisturizing effect on the skin. Use the process of elimination and knowledge of the categories of skin products to make a selection.

17 **Answer: 1** **Rationale:** Tegaderm is a protective dressing that is permeable to oxygen. The other products listed do not have this advantage. DuoDERM is an absorbent product that excludes bacteria and adheres to the site. Replicare excludes bacteria. Tegasorb is an absorbent product that excludes bacteria and adheres to the site. **Cognitive Level:** Applying **Client Need:** Pharmacological and Parenteral Therapies **Integrated Process:** Nursing Process: Planning **Content Area:** Pharmacology **Strategy:** The core issue of the question is the type of dressing that is permeable to oxygen. Use the process of elimination and knowledge of wound care products to make a selection.

18 **Answer: 2** **Rationale:** Mupirocin is a topical antimicrobial agent effective against impetigo caused by *Staphylococcus aureus*, beta-hemolytic streptococci, and *Streptococcus pyogenes*. Ketoconazole is an antifungal agent. Capsaicin is a topical agent that has been useful in certain painful syndromes. Acyclovir is an antiviral agent. **Cognitive Level:** Analyzing **Client Need:** Pharmacological and Parenteral Therapies **Integrated Process:** Nursing Process: Planning **Content Area:** Child Health **Strategy:** Knowing the causative agent for the diagnosis will assist in selecting the correct answer.

Recall the classification of the medications in determining which is the best option. If this was difficult, review the diagnosis and usual method of treatment.

19 **Answer: 4** **Rationale:** The effectiveness of a sunscreen when compared to no use of sunscreen is usually indicated by its sun protection factor (SPF) (e.g., 6, 15, 30). The number assigned to the sunscreen does not refer to the hours of effectiveness. Rather, it is the effectiveness of the sunscreen against sun exposure compared to not using a sunscreen. Sunscreens can be classified as either waterproof or water-resistant, but the SPF number does not indicate this information. **Cognitive Level:** Applying **Client Need:** Health Promotion and Maintenance **Integrated Process:** Nursing Process: Implementation **Content Area:** Adult Health **Strategy:** Recall knowledge that SPF is an abbreviation for "sun protection factor" to allow selection of the correct option.

20 **Answer: 3** **Rationale:** Accutane is an oral preparation that is a known teratogen; strict adherence to avoidance of pregnancy is mandatory. Accutane is contraindicated with pregnancy because of the occurrence of spontaneous abortions, as well as major abnormalities in the fetus at birth, such as hydrocephalus. The medication should be applied thinly. Sun exposure provides no added benefit. Elevated triglyceride levels might occur, but changes in hormone functioning are not anticipated. **Cognitive Level:** Analyzing **Client Need:** Pharmacological and Parenteral Therapies **Integrated Process:** Nursing Process: Evaluation **Content Area:** Pharmacology **Strategy:** Knowing that isotretinoin (Accutane) has terotogenic effects, as well as that the client is an 18-year-old female, should assist in selecting the correct option. The other options are incorrect, since they do not address the teratogenic effects of the medication.

Key Terms to Review

acne p. 613
antiseptics p. 609
herpes simplex p. 608
papules p. 613
pediculosis p. 610
pruritus p. 605
psoriasis p. 611
scabies p. 610
tinea pedis p. 610

References

Adams, M., Holland, L., & Urban, C. (2011). *Pharmacology for nurses: A pathophysiological approach* (3rd ed.). Upper Saddle River, NJ: Pearson Education, Inc.

Adams, M., & Koch, R. (2010). *Pharmacology: Connections to nursing practice.* Upper Saddle River, NJ: Pearson Education, Inc.

Deglin, J. H. & Vallerand, A. H. (2011). *Davis's drug guide for nurses* (12th ed.). Philadelphia: F. A. Davis.

Lehne, R. (2010). *Pharmacology for nursing care* (7th ed.). Philadelphia: W. B. Saunders.

Wilson, B., Shannon, M., & Shields, K. (2012). *Pearson nurse's drug guide 2012.* Upper Saddle River, NJ: Pearson Education, Inc.

Test Yourself

Are you ready for the NCLEX-PN® or course exams? Use the practice tests on the companion website to check.

Eye and Ear Medications

40

In this chapter

Cross Reference

Other chapters relevant to this content area are

Dosage Calculation and Medication Administration **Chapter 28**
Eye, Ear, Nose, and Throat Disorders **Chapter 59**

I. MEDICATIONS TO TREAT GLAUCOMA

A. Beta-adrenergic blockers (antagonists)

1. Decrease production of **aqueous humor** (fluid formed by ciliary body in eye)
2. Reduce **intraocular pressure** (IOP; pressure within eye) in **open-angle glaucoma** (a change in appearance of optic disk resulting in visual loss)
3. Are commonly used to manage chronic, primary open-angle glaucoma
4. Common medications are listed in Box 40–1

> ***Memory Aid*** Remember that a beta-blocking drug can be recognized easily because it ends with the suffix *-olol* or *-lol*.

5. Administration considerations
   a. Available in ophthalmic solutions and suspensions
   b. Drugs cross placenta, enter breast milk
   NCLEX® c. Use nasolacrimal occlusion (press on inner canthus of eye) to minimize **systemic absorption** (entry of drug into body and circulating fluids)
   NCLEX® d. Use cautiously in clients with renal failure, diabetes, asthma, and chronic obstructive pulmonary disease (COPD)
   NCLEX® e. Administer with caution to clients receiving cardiovascular agents such as antihypertensives and antiarrhythmics
   f. May mask symptoms of hyperthyroidism
   g. Drug may be $beta_1$ selective (cardiac), $beta_2$ selective (pulmonary), or both $beta_1$ and $beta_2$ selective
   h. Because it is $beta_1$ selective, betaxolol (Betoptic) is usually preferred for clients with pulmonary disease
6. Contraindicated in hypersensitivity, sinus bradycardia or second- or third-degree heart block, cardiogenic shock or congestive heart failure (CHF)
7. *NCLEX®* Adverse cardiovascular effects may occur when beta-adrenergic blockers are used in combination with other cardiovascular agents such as antihypertensives and antidysrhythmics

Box 40–1

Medications to Treat Glaucoma

Beta-Adrenergic Blockers (Antagonists)

Betaxolol (Betoptic)

Carteolol (Ocupress)

Levobunolol (Betagan)

Metipranolol (OptiPranolol)

Timolol (Timoptic)

Alpha$_2$-Adrenergic Agonists

Apraclonidine (Iopidine)

Brimonidine tartrate (Alphagan P)

Cholinergic Agonists

Carbachol (Isoptocarbachol)

Echothiophate iodide (Phospholine Iodide)

Pilocarpine (Isopto Carpine, others)

Carbonic Anhydrase Inhibitors

Acetazolamide (Diamox)

Brinzolamide (Azopt)

Dorzolamide (Trusopt)

Methazolamide (Neptazane)

Sympathomimetics

Dipivefrin (Propine)

Prostaglandin Agonists

Bimatoprost (Lumigan)

Latanoprost (Xalatan)

Travoprost (Travatan)

8. Side/adverse effects
   - NCLEX® **a.** Primarily local reactions: eye irritation, burning, stinging
   - NCLEX® **b.** Systemic adverse cardiovascular effects: bradycardia or tachycardia, CHF, dysrhythmias, hypotension, and edema of lower extremities
   - NCLEX® **c.** Systemic adverse respiratory effects: wheezing, cough, exacerbation of asthma, and bronchospasm
   - **d.** Systemic adverse central nervous system (CNS) effects: weakness, ataxia, confusion, and depression
   - **e.** Systemic adverse gastrointestinal (GI) effects: nausea and vomiting (N/V)
9. Nursing considerations
   - NCLEX® **a.** Obtain baseline vital signs (VS), neurologic status, vision and intraocular pressure data
   - **b.** Review history for cardiovascular disease, renal failure, diabetes, lactation, or thyrotoxicosis
   - **c.** Observe for signs of hypersensitivity such as burning, itching, redness, and swelling occurring after medication administration
   - NCLEX® **d.** Refer to Box 40–2 for administration of ophthalmic medications
10. Client teaching
    - NCLEX® **a.** Beta-blocking agents may mask symptoms of hypoglycemia
    - **b.** Inform prescriber if surgery is being considered; gradual withdrawal of beta-blocking agent 48 hours before surgery may be required (withdrawal is controversial)
    - **c.** Have routine eye examinations and measurement of IOP
    - **d.** Do not stop medication unless instructed to do so by prescriber
    - NCLEX® **e.** Report symptoms of breathing difficulty, swelling of extremities, slow heart rate
    - NCLEX® **f.** Wear dark glasses and avoid bright light if photophobia is present

B. Adrenergic medications (alpha$_2$-adrenergic agonists)

1. Decrease production of aqueous humor and decrease IOP
2. Used to manage open-angle glaucoma (often in combination with other drugs), glaucoma secondary to **uveitis** (intraocular inflammatory disorder), to produce **mydriasis** (pupil dilation) for ocular examination, and to produce local hemostasis during eye surgery to control bleeding
3. Common medications: see again Box 40–1
4. Administration considerations
   - **a.** Drugs cross placenta, enter breast milk
   - **b.** Do not administer ophthalmic solution that contains precipitates or has turned brown
5. NCLEX® Contraindicated in treatment of narrow-angle (angle-closure) glaucoma or abraded cornea, because pupil dilation further restricts ocular fluid outflow, precipitating an acute attack of glaucoma
6. Side/adverse effects
   - NCLEX® **a.** Local reactions include eye pain and stinging on initial instillation
   - **b.** CNS side effects include headache, blurred vision, brow ache, photophobia, and difficulty with night vision

Box 40–2

Administration of Ophthalmic Medications

Instillation of Eyedrops

- ➤ Wash hands.
- ➤ Cleanse exudates from eye(s) if necessary.
- ➤ Tilt client's head toward side of affected eye.
- ➤ Gently pull lower eyelid down and have client look up (this forms a "sac").
- ➤ Instill drops in conjunctival sac formed by lower lid, *not* onto eye.
- ➤ Unless specifically indicated otherwise, apply gentle pressure for 30 seconds to 1 minute over inner canthus next to nose. This prevents absorption through lacrimal (tear) duct and drainage of medication.
- ➤ Unless specifically indicated otherwise, client should close eye(s) gently. Avoid squeezing eye(s) tightly as this forces medication out.

Instillation of Eye Ointment

- ➤ Follow same procedure for instillation of eyedrops except that ointment is expressed directly into lower conjunctival sac from inner canthus to outer canthus.
- ➤ Unless specifically indicated otherwise, client should close eye(s) and gently massage eye(s) to distribute medication.

Note: To avoid contamination and risk of infection, do not touch dropper or tube to eye, eyelashes, or any other surface. Remove contact lenses before instilling ophthalmic medications.

c. Systemic adverse effects are unusual but may include hypertension in clients with cardiovascular disease

7. Nursing considerations
   a. Obtain history of allergies or hypersensitivity to specific agents
   b. Obtain baseline VS, vision and intraocular pressure data *(NCLEX®)*
   c. Monitor cardiac, respiratory, and renal function routinely
8. Client teaching *(NCLEX®)*
   a. Drugs may discolor contact lenses
   b. Do not blink for at least 30 seconds after instilling medication
   c. Report a decrease in visual acuity, floating spots, sensitivity to light, eye redness, or headache to health care provider

C. Cholinergic agonists (miotics, cholinesterase inhibitors)

1. Increase outflow of aqueous humor, decrease resistance to aqueous flow in open-angle and angle-closure glaucoma
2. Produce miosis before ophthalmic examination or after ophthalmic surgery
3. Generally used for clients who fail to respond to first-line agents (beta-blockers)
4. Common medications: see again Box 40–1
5. Administration considerations
   a. Drug crosses placenta, enters breast milk
   b. Do not administer ophthalmic solution that contains precipitates or has turned brown *(NCLEX®)*
   c. Pilocarpine can be stored at room temperature
   d. Contraindicated in acute iritis or conditions in which pupillary constriction is not desirable
   e. Concurrent use with beta-adrenergic blocking agents may increase risk of cardiovascular reactions *(NCLEX®)*
6. Side/adverse effects
   a. Visual blurring, myopia, irritation, reduced visual acuity in low light, and headache
   b. Systemic reactions include abdominal pain with diarrhea, bronchoconstriction, hypotension, N/V diuresis, diaphoresis, exacerbation of asthma
   c. Toxic effects produce ataxia, confusion, seizures, coma, respiratory failure, hypotension, and death *(NCLEX®)*
   d. Prolonged use of cholinergics may lead to retinal detachment, obstruction of tear drainage, and cataracts
   e. Acute toxicity is reversible by IV atropine, an anticholinergic agent that acts as antidote *(NCLEX®)*
7. Nursing considerations
   a. Obtain baseline VS, neurologic status, vision, and IOP data

b. Monitor for cardiovascular disease, renal failure, diabetes, lactation, or thyrotoxicosis
c. Monitor for signs of hypersensitivity such as burning, itching, redness, and swelling occurring after medication administration

8. Client teaching: miosis may cause difficulty adjusting quickly to changes in lighting; use proper administration technique

D. Carbonic anhydrase inhibitors (CAIs)

1. Are nonbacteriostatic sulfonamides that lower IOP by decreasing aqueous humor production
2. Oral CAIs are used to treat open-angle, secondary, and angle-closure glaucoma
3. Ophthalmic CAIs are used to treat open-angle glaucoma and ocular hypertension
4. NCLEX® Commonly used preoperatively in intraocular surgery
5. Common medications: see again Box 40–1

Memory Aid

Carbonic anhydrase inhibitors can often be recognized because many of them end with the suffix *-zolamide*.

6. Administration considerations
   a. NCLEX® Oral acetazolamide (Diamox) is administered for maintenance
   b. NCLEX® IV route is used preoperatively or to rapidly reduce increased IOP
   c. Give oral form with food or milk to decrease GI side effects
   d. May crush tablets and suspend in liquid
   e. Do not use alcohol or glycerin in administration of drug
   f. To minimize nocturia, schedule doses early in day
   g. Administer with caution to clients with adrenocortical insufficiency
   h. NCLEX® Contraindicated with hypersensitivity to antibacterial sulfonamides, chronic noncongestive angle-closure glaucoma, hyponatremia, hypokalemia, or other electrolyte imbalances, or hepatic or renal dysfunction
7. Side/adverse effects
   a. Oral agents: anorexia, diarrhea, diuresis, N/V, lethargy, weakness, weight loss, metallic bitter taste, and paresthesia of fingers, hands, and toes
   b. NCLEX® Topical agents: topical allergic reaction, photosensitivity, superficial **keratitis** (inflammation of cornea)
   c. NCLEX® Stevens-Johnson syndrome and bone marrow depression with acetazolamide (Diamox)
   d. Acidosis, blood dyscrasias, hypokalemia
8. Nursing considerations
   a. Potential exacerbation of renal stones; monitor renal function
   b. NCLEX® Monitor for fluid volume depletion related to diuresis; monitor intake and output (I&O), skin turgor, mucous membranes, and weight
   c. NCLEX® Monitor urinalysis, complete blood cell count (CBC), electrolytes
9. NCLEX® Client teaching
   a. Unless contraindicated, eat diet high in potassium and low in sodium
   b. Unless contraindicated, increase fluid intake to at least 2 liters per day to decrease risk of renal stones
   c. Report changes in urine color, rashes, fever

E. Sympathomimetic agents

1. Lower IOP by decreasing aqueous humor production and increasing its outflow; used to manage open-angle glaucoma
2. Common medications (ophthalmic): dipivefrin (Propine) and epinephrine
3. Administration considerations
   a. Administer with caution to clients with cardiovascular disease, hypertension, asthma, diabetes mellitus, hyperthyroidism, and parkinsonism
   b. Onset of action for epinephrine is 1 hour; peak effect occurs in 4–8 hours
   c. Onset of action for dipivefrin (Propine) is 30 minutes; peak effect in 1 hour
   d. NCLEX® Question client about sensitivity to sulfites
   e. NCLEX® Avoid concurrent use with monoamine oxidase inhibitors (MAOIs)
   f. NCLEX® Contraindicated with **narrow-angle glaucoma** (increased IOP from impaired rate of aqueous humor flow) or predisposition to narrow-angle glaucoma
4. Side/adverse effects
   a. Local: brow pain, burning, eye irritation, headache, watering eyes, stinging, **photophobia** (sensitivity to light)

NCLEX® b. Systemic: hypertension, diaphoresis, tachycardia, palpitation, tremors, light-headedness

5. Nursing considerations
   a. Monitor VS; obtain baseline IOP and vision data
   NCLEX® b. Maintain pressure on lacrimal sac for 1–2 minutes after instillation of drug to minimize systemic absorption
   NCLEX® c. Obtain heart rate and BP periodically to detect systemic effects
6. Client teaching
   a. Prolonged use of epinephrine may result in pigment deposits in the conjunctiva
   b. Discuss use of contact lenses with prescriber; use may or may not be permitted
   c. Report increased heart rate, heart palpitations, or elevated BP to prescriber

F. Prostaglandin agonists

1. Increases aqueous humor outflow
2. Used to manage open-angle glaucoma and ocular hypertension
3. Common medications: see again Box 40–1

> **Memory Aid**
>
> Prostaglandin agonists can often be recognized because many of them end with the suffix *-prost*.

4. Administration considerations
   NCLEX® a. Administer 5 minutes apart from other antiglaucoma ophthalmic medications
   b. If pilocarpine (Isopto Carpine) is included in drug regimen, it should be administered 1 hour after prostaglandin agonist
   c. May be used in conjunction with other agents to lower IOP
5. Contraindications: hypersensitivity to latanoprost or benzalkonium
6. NCLEX® Side/adverse effects
   a. Blurred vision, photophobia, burning, stinging, and itching
   b. Longer, thicker, darker eyelashes; increasing iris pigmentation
   c. Conjunctival hyperemia
7. Nursing considerations
   a. Monitor for hypersensitivity to latanoprost or benzalkonium chloride
   b. Check for burning, itching, stinging after initial administration of medication
8. NCLEX® Client teaching
   a. Drug may cause an increase in iris pigmentation
   b. Do not exceed once-a-day dose
   c. Remove contact lenses before dose and leave out for 15 minutes after
   d. Report burning, itching, stinging after administration to prescriber

II. MYDRIATICS AND CYCLOPLEGICS

A. Anticholinergic cycloplegics

1. Produce mydriasis (pupil dilation) and/or **cycloplegia** (paralysis of ciliary muscle)
2. Used to treat ocular pain secondary to inflammatory disorders such as uveitis and keratitis or for relaxation of ciliary muscle to improve measurement of refractive errors
3. NCLEX® Used preoperatively and postoperatively for intraocular surgery
4. Common medications: see Box 40–3
5. Administration considerations
   NCLEX® a. Use cautiously with primary glaucoma or predisposition to angle-closure glaucoma
   b. Apply ointment several hours before vision examination
   NCLEX® c. Compress lacrimal duct during administration and for 2–3 minutes after
   d. Contraindicated with severe systemic reactions to atropine or hypersensitivity to anticholinergic drugs
6. Side/adverse effects
   a. Local: blurred vision, photophobia, allergic lid reactions
   NCLEX® b. Systemic: confusion, delirium, drowsiness, dry mouth, flushing, and tachycardia
   NCLEX® c. Acute glaucoma can be precipitated by pupillary dilation; if not recognized and treated, acute glaucoma can result in blindness
   d. Dry mouth and tachycardia may be symptoms of scopolamine toxicity

Box 40–3

Mydriatic and Cycloplegic Ophthalmic Medications

Anticholinergics: Cycloplegics

Atropine sulfate (Isopto Atropine, others)

Cyclopentolate (Cyclogyl, Pentolair)

Cyclopentolate and phenylephrine (Cyclomydril)

Homatropine (Isopto Homatropine, others)

Scopolamine hydrobromide (Isopto Hyoscine)

Tropicamide (Midriacyl, Tropicacyl)

Tropicamide and hydroxyamphetamine (Paremyd)

Sympathomimetics: Mydriatics

Phenylephrine (Neo-synephrine)

7. Nursing considerations
   a. Obtain baseline IOP and vision status data
   b. Combination drugs produce greater mydriasis
   c. Systemic side effects are more pronounced in infants and children with blond hair and blue eyes
   d. (NCLEX®) Monitor for tachycardia, confusion, slurred speech, dry mouth, dry skin, weakness, drowsiness
8. Client teaching
   a. Mydriasis may last from 3 days (scopolamine) to 12 days (atropine)
   b. Blurred vision may occur
   c. (NCLEX®) Wear dark sunglasses and avoid bright light for photophobia
   d. (NCLEX®) IOP and vision should be monitored over course of therapy
   e. Withhold dose if experiencing tachycardia or dry mouth (symptoms of toxicity)
   f. (NCLEX®) Use sugarless hard candy to relieve dry mouth
   g. Report tachycardia and dry mouth to prescriber

B. Sympathomimetics

1. Usually used to treat minor eye injuries and before eye examination
2. Common medication: phenylephrine (Neo-Synephrine)
3. Administration and nursing considerations, and client teaching: same as in adrenergic section earlier in chapter
4. Side/adverse effects
   a. Rebound **miosis** (constriction of pupils) may occur with phenylephrine
   b. Older adults with cardiac disease may experience BP elevations with phenylephrine

III. ANTI-INFLAMMATORY AND ANTI-INFECTIVE EYE MEDICATIONS

A. Nonsteroidal anti-inflammatory drugs (NSAIDs)

1. Flurbiprofen (Ocufen) is used to inhibit intraoperative miosis
2. Diclofenac (Voltaren) is used to treat postoperative inflammation after cataract extraction
3. Ketorolac (Acular) is used to treat conjunctivitis and seasonal allergic ophthalmic pruritis
4. Common medications: see Box 40–4

Box 40–4

Anti-Inflammatory Drugs for Ophthalmic Use

Anti-Inflammatory Drugs (Nonsteroidal)

Diclofenac (Voltaren)

Flurbiprofen (Ocufen)

Ketorolac (Acular)

Corticosteroids: Steroidal Anti-Inflammatory Drugs

Dexamethasone (Maxidex)

Fluorometholone (FML Forte)

Hydrocortisone (generic)

Prednisolone (Pred-Forte)

5. Administration considerations
   a. Systemic effect may be produced if absorbed
   NCLEX® b. NSAIDs may cause increased bleeding; therefore, clients with increased bleeding tendencies should be monitored closely and have periodic CBC and coagulation studies done
   NCLEX® c. Contraindicated with sensitivity to aspirin or phenylacetic acid derivatives or to systemic NSAIDs
6. Side/adverse effects
   a. Local: transient burning or stinging on application, itching, allergic reaction, pain, and redness
   b. Systemic toxicity: bleeding
7. NCLEX® Nursing considerations: watch for bleeding and hypersensitivity symptoms (burning, itching, redness, and swelling occurring after administration of dose)
8. Client teaching: NSAIDs may potentiate bleeding in clients with known bleeding tendencies

B. Corticosteroids

1. Indicated for allergic and inflammatory ophthalmic disorders of conjunctiva, cornea, and anterior segment of eye
2. Common medications: see again Box 40–4
3. Administration considerations
   NCLEX® a. Corticosteroids should be used for short-term treatment only
   b. Use with caution in clients with cataracts and chronic open-angle glaucoma
4. NCLEX® Contraindicated with hypersensitivity and corneal abrasion; may mask hypersensitivity reactions to other drugs
5. Side/adverse effects
   a. Local: stinging after application
   NCLEX® b. Toxicity: visual disturbances, headache, and eye pain
6. NCLEX® Nursing considerations
   a. May mask symptoms of infection and hypersensitivity reactions
   b. May increase susceptibility to infection
7. NCLEX® Client teaching: avoid use of contact lenses during and for prescribed time after use of corticosteroid therapy; have eye(s) examined for progress

C. Antibacterial, antifungal, and antiviral agents

1. Antibacterial agents are used to manage bacterial infections such as conjunctivitis, blepharitis, keratitis, uveitis, and hordeolum (external stye) or chalazion (internal stye)
2. Antifungal agents are used to manage fungal blepharitis, conjunctivitis, and keratitis
3. Antiviral agents are used to manage herpes simplex virus keratitis and herpes simplex virus keratoconjunctivitis
4. Common medications are listed in Box 40–5
5. Administration considerations
   NCLEX® a. If indicated, obtain culture from eye(s) before administering first dose
   b. Remove exudates from eyes before administering medication
   NCLEX® c. Contraindicated with hypersensitivity to drug
   d. Do not administer ophthalmic anesthetics within 30 minutes of sulfonamides (sulfacetamide sodium); sulfonamides are incompatible with thimerosol and silver preparations

Box 40–5

Antibacterial, Antifungal, and Antiviral Agents for Ophthalmic Use

Antibacterial

Bacitracin

Ciprofloxacin (Ciloxan)

Erythromycin

Gentamicin sulfate (Genoptic)

Ofloxacin (Ocuflox)

Polymyxin B sulfate

Sulfacetamide sodium (Bleph-10)

Tobramycin (Tobrex)

Antiviral

Idoxuridine (Herplex)

Trifluridine (Viroptic)

Antifungal

Natamycin (Natacyn)

6. Side/adverse effects
   a. Local: dermatitis, itching, stinging, swelling
   b. Stevens-Johnson syndrome, systemic lupus erythematosus (SLE) with sulfacetamide sodium

NCLEX®
7. Nursing considerations
   a. Monitor infected eye(s) for pain, drainage, redness, swelling
   b. Store idoxuridine (Stoxil, Herplex) and trifluridine (Viroptic) in cool place or refrigerator

NCLEX®
8. Client teaching: inform prescriber of photosensitivity, redness, swelling, increased drainage, pain, or if no improvement seen within a few days

IV. ANESTHETIC EYE MEDICATIONS

A. Action and use
1. Prevent initiation and transmission of nerve impulses
2. Prevent pain during diagnostic procedures such as **tonometry** (measurement of IOP, used to detect glaucoma), subconjunctival injections, removal of foreign bodies, surgical procedures, and removal of sutures

B. Common medications
1. Proparacaine hydrochloride (Alcaine, Ophthaine)
2. Tetracaine hydrochloride (Altacaine, Pontocaine)

C. Administration considerations
1. Rapid onset within 20 seconds, and duration is 15–20 minutes
2. Tetracaine hydrochloride can cause systemic toxicity

D. Contraindications: hypersensitivity

E. Side/adverse effects
1. Proparacaine causes allergic contact dermatitis, cycloplegia, conjunctival congestion, delayed corneal healing
2. CNS excitation symptoms (rare, systemic effect) include blurred vision, dizziness, nervousness, restlessness, trembling, followed by CNS depression (dyspnea, drowsiness, dysrhythmias)

NCLEX®
F. Nursing considerations
1. Protect eye from injury while anesthetized to avoid corneal damage
2. To protect cornea, as follow-up, apply eye patch until blink reflex has returned
3. Observe for hypersensitivity symptoms such as burning, itching, stinging

NCLEX®
G. Client teaching: do not touch or rub the eye until anesthesia has worn off

V. AUDITORY MEDICATIONS

A. Antibiotics for ear
1. Used to manage infections of external ear (external auditory canal surface)
2. Common medications
   a. Gentamicin sulfate (Garamycin): 3 or 4 drops instilled in ear canal 3 times daily; note: otic preparation of gentamicin sulfate has not been approved by the Food and Drug Administration (FDA); prescribers in United States use *ophthalmic* preparation for otic infections
   b. A variety of standard antibiotics may be ordered orally to treat otitis media (middle ear infections)
3. Administration considerations
   a. Unless contraindicated, warm ear drops by running medication bottle under warm water, immersing bottle in a cup of warm water, or holding bottle in hand or pocket for 30 minutes prior to administration
   b. Determine client's baseline hearing status, and presence of ear drainage, earache, erythema, pain, and **vertigo** (dizziness)
   c. Inspect that ear canal is clear and not impacted with *cerumen* (earwax) before medication administration
   d. Inspect for intact tympanic membrane

   NCLEX®
   e. Contraindicated in hypersensitivity and perforation of tympanic membrane
4. Side/adverse effects
   a. Local: burning, rash, redness, swelling, blurred vision
   b. Systemic: hypersensitivity reaction
   c. Rare occurrence of systemic hematologic toxicity
5. Nursing considerations

   NCLEX®
   a. Monitor for local adverse effects
   b. Discontinue use if hypersensitivity reaction occurs

c. Monitor auditory canal for drainage and pain
d. Monitor for hearing disturbances
6. Client teaching
a. Inform prescriber of increased pain, drainage, or no improvement in symptoms within a few days of treatment
NCLEX® b. Refer to Box 40–6 for instillation of otic medications

B. Corticosteroids

1. Used for anti-inflammatory, antipruritic, or antiallergenic effects; may be given with antibacterial or antifungal agents
2. Common medications are listed in Box 40–7
3. Administration considerations
a. Monitor client's hearing status and presence of ear drainage, earache, erythema, pain, and vertigo
b. Inspect that ear canal is clear and not impacted with cerumen before medication administration
c. Inspect for intact tympanic membrane
d. May be given in combination with antibiotics to treat infections of external ear canal or mastoid cavity
e. Contraindicated in hypersensitivity to sulfites or perforation of tympanic membrane
NCLEX® 4. Side/adverse effects: corticosteroids may mask infection or exacerbate an existing infection
NCLEX® 5. Nursing considerations: monitor for hypersensitivity after administration of medication
6. Client teaching
a. Hearing should be monitored during duration of treatment
b. Inform prescriber of new onset of ear drainage, heat, fever, odor, or pain, or if no improvement is seen within a few days of treatment

C. Other medications (over-the-counter medications)

1. Acetic acid (alcohol, glycerin, or propylene glycol) is used after swimming or bathing to restore normal acid pH to the ear canal
2. Glycerin, mineral oil, and olive oil are emollients to relieve itching and burning in ear
3. Propylene glycol enhances antibacterial effects and acidity of acetic acid
4. Carbamide peroxide is an antibacterial agent used to help remove accumulated cerumen
5. Common medications are listed in Box 40–8
6. General considerations: generally considered safe and effective; contraindicated with hypersensitivity

Box 40–6

Administration of Otic Medications

For instillation of eardrops in older children and adults

- Inspect ear canal for cerumen or edema.
- Tilt client's head toward unaffected side.
- Gently pull pinna of ear up and back.
- Instill eardrops—*do not* insert dropper into ear canal.
- Gently massage area anterior to ear to facilitate entry of drops into ear canal.

For instillation of eardrops in children 3 years and younger

- Inspect ear canal for cerumen or edema.
- Tilt client's head toward unaffected side.
- Gently pull pinna of ear slightly down and back.
- Instill eardrops—*do not* insert dropper into ear canal.
- Gently massage area anterior to ear to facilitate entry of drops into ear canal.

Box 40–7

Corticosteroid Agents for Otic Use

Betamethasone (generic)
Hydrocortisone (generic)
Dexamethasone (Decadron)
Hydrocortisone with acetic acid (Acetasol HC)

Box 40-8

Common OTC Agents for Otic Use

Acetic acid; aluminum acetate (Otic Domeboro)

Boric acid and isopropyl alcohol (Auro-Dri Ear Drops)

Carbamide peroxide (Auro Ear Drops)

Carbamide peroxide and glycerin (Dent's Ear Wax Drops, E.R.O. Ear drops, Ear Wax Removal System)

Hydrocortisone, propylene glycol, alcohol, benzyl benzoate (Earsol-HC Drops)

Isopropyl alcohol (Aurocaine 2)

Isopropyl alcohol in glycerin (Swim-Ear Drops)

7. Client teaching
   a. Seek evaluation by prescriber if symptoms do not improve within several days
   b. Inform prescriber if adverse reactions occur or if symptoms worsen

D. Medications that cause ototoxicity

1. Analgesics: aspirin and other salicylates, NSAIDs
2. Antibiotics: aminoglycosides (clarithromycin, tobramycin), erythromycin, vancomycin, chloramphenicol
3. Antineoplastic agents: cisplatin, mechlorethamine, nitrogen mustard
4. Loop diuretics (bumetanide [Bumex], ethacrynic acid [Edecrin], furosemide [Lasix]) and carbonic anhydrase inhibitor diuretic acetazolamide (Diamox)
5. Miscellaneous: quinine, quinidine

Check Your NCLEX-PN® Exam I.Q.

You are ready for testing on this content if you can

- Apply knowledge of expected actions and effects of eye and ear medications to client care.
- Correctly administer eye and ear medications to clients.
- Monitor for side effects and adverse effects of eye and ear medications.
- Take appropriate action if a client has an unexpected response to an eye or ear medication.
- Monitor a client for expected outcomes or effects of treatment with eye and ear medications.

PRACTICE TEST

1 A client being treated for glaucoma with eye drops complains of photophobia. What instructions should the nurse include in the client teaching?

1. Discontinue use of the medication.
2. Wipe eyes with a tissue after instilling eye drops.
3. Wear dark glasses when outside, or when around bright lights.
4. Special glasses are necessary while being treated for glaucoma.

2 Which statement by the client indicates to the nurse that the client has an understanding regarding pilocarpine (Isopto Carpine)?

1. "I will see better at night."
2. "I may have trouble adjusting to darkness."
3. "I will adjust quickly to changes from light to dark."
4. "I will not use the medication if I plan to drive."

3 The nurse is providing care to a client taking methazolamide (Neptazane), a carbonic anhydrase inhibitor for glaucoma. The nurse should include monitoring for which electrolyte imbalances when implementing the plan of care? Select all that apply.

1. Hyperkalemia
2. Hypokalemia
3. Hypocalcemia
4. Hypercalcemia
5. Hypernatremia

4 A client has a prescription for otic chloramphenicol (Chloromycetin). Which statement by the client should indicate a need for further instruction by the nurse?

1. "I will inform my doctor of increased ear pain."
2. "I will inform my doctor if my ear has not improved in seven days."
3. "I will inform my doctor if I have an increase in drainage from my ear."
4. "I will inform my doctor if I experience any hearing disturbances."

5 A client is receiving pilocarpine (Isopto Carpine) for the treatment of glaucoma. Which symptom, if experienced by the client, does the nurse attribute to systemic absorption?

1. Diaphoresis
2. Constipation
3. Tachycardia
4. Hypertension

6 A client is receiving cyclopentolate and phenylephrine (Cyclomydril) before an ocular examination. How should the nurse explain the purpose of the medication?

1. To constrict the pupil
2. To dilate the pupil
3. To provide anesthesia
4. To provide a prophylactic antibiotic

7 Which symptoms, if described by a client, would lead the nurse to suspect a systemic side effect of atropine ophthalmic solution? Select all that apply.

1. Tachycardia
2. Slurred speech
3. Salivation
4. Diaphoresis
5. Confusion

8 Which statement demonstrates the client's understanding of proper administration of ophthalmic solutions?

1. "I will discard a medication if it has turned brown."
2. "I will discontinue medication that causes eye burning."
3. "I will use a cotton swab to apply my medication."
4. "I will replace medications that are more than 1 month old."

9 When describing side effects of over-the-counter medications, for which medications would the nurse discuss ototoxicity? Select all that apply.

1. Salicylates (aspirin)
2. Vitamin C
3. Diphenhydramine (Benadryl)
4. Vitamin A
5. Ibuprofen

10 During a follow-up visit at the clinician's office a client states, "I insert the ear dropper deep into my ear so the medication doesn't run back out." What should be the nurse's response and priority teaching to the client?

1. The client's ear canal is likely obstructed with cerumen.
2. The client is using the appropriate technique for administering an otic solution.
3. The client should lie on the affected side for 5 minutes to promote absorption.
4. The medication dropper should not be inserted into the ear canal.

11 Which action, if observed by the nurse, demonstrates appropriate client technique for self-administering an ophthalmic medication?

1. Administers two different ophthalmic solutions 5 minutes apart.
2. Administers ophthalmic solution 5 minutes after ophthalmic ointment.
3. Administers two different ophthalmic solutions 2 minutes apart.
4. Administers ophthalmic ointment 2 minutes after ophthalmic solution.

PRACTICE TEST

12 The nurse is observing a client give a return demonstration of the administration of eye drops. Which client actions indicate a need for further teaching? Select all that apply.

1. The client pulls the lower lid of the eye down, forming a sac.
2. The client instills the medication into the conjunctival sac.
3. The client cleanses the eyelid with cotton balls moistened with warm tap water.
4. The client cleanses the eye from inner canthus to outer canthus.
5. The client promotes drainage of the medication toward the inner canthus.

13 The nurse is monitoring a client with open-angle glaucoma who is receiving timolol (Timoptic) for treatment. The nurse should expect the timolol to exert which action that leads to the therapeutic response?

1. A decrease in the outflow of aqueous humor
2. An increase in the outflow of aqueous humor
3. A decrease in aqueous humor production
4. An increase in aqueous humor production

14 The nurse is providing information on safety measures to the family of an older adult client being treated with carbachol (Carboptic), an ophthalmic cholinesterase inhibitor, to counteract which drug side effect?

1. Difficulty in making quick changes in illumination due to miosis
2. Difficulty in making quick changes in illumination due to mydriasis
3. Medication side effect of constipation
4. Medication side effect of hypertension

15 A client who just self-administered the first dose of vidarabine (Vira-A) calls the clinic and reports eye redness and swelling not present before treatment began. The nurse should instruct the client to take which action?

1. No action is necessary, because these are normal manifestations of the medication.
2. Discontinue the medication, and return to clinic immediately for evaluation.
3. If redness continues after 3 days, return to the clinic for evaluation.
4. Discontinue the medication until the next scheduled clinic appointment.

16 Which statement, if made by a client being treated with ophthalmic trifluridine (Viroptic), indicates an understanding of the medication instructions?

1. "I will stop the medication once healing has occurred."
2. "I will administer the treatment for 7 days."
3. "I will keep the medication in my pocket to avoid missing a dose."
4. "I will continue the medication for 5–7 days after healing has occurred."

17 The parent of a 2-year-old child exhibits correct administration technique for otic solutions by which action in a return demonstration?

1. The child's pinna is pulled down and back before administering the medication.
2. The child's pinna is pulled up and back before administering the medication.
3. The dropper is placed into the child's ear canal for instilling the medication.
4. The child's head is tilted towards the affected side for medication instillation.

18 A client who takes acetazolamide (Diamox) reports frequent urination during the night. The nurse should collect data regarding which of the following, which is likely to be the cause of the nocturia?

1. The client takes oral acetazolamide (Diamox) every morning.
2. The client consumes 2000 mL of fluid per day.
3. The client takes oral acetazolamide before supper.
4. The client takes oral acetazolamide with juice.

19 Which of the following is the priority in nursing care of the client prior to administering the first dose of an ophthalmic medication?

1. Determining the client's understanding of the purpose of the medication
2. Observing the client's eye and vision status
3. Checking the client's history of hypersensitivity to medications
4. Questioning the client's understanding of the action of the medication

20 Which technique performed by the client demonstrates an understanding of appropriate administration of ophthalmic medications?

1. Pulls the lower lid down, and instills the medication directly onto the eye.
2. Pulls the lower lid down, and instills the medication into the conjunctival sac.
3. Pulls the lower lid up, and instills the medication directly onto the eye.
4. Pulls the lower lid up, and instills the medication into the conjunctival sac.

ANSWERS & RATIONALES

1 **Answer: 3 Rationale:** Clients experiencing photophobia are instructed to wear dark sunglasses and to avoid bright lights. Not enough information is provided to warrant discontinuing the medication. Eyes should not be wiped with tissue immediately after instillation of drops. No special glasses are required. **Cognitive Level:** Applying **Client Need:** Pharmacological and Parenteral Therapies **Integrated Process:** Teaching and Learning **Content Area:** Pharmacology **Strategy:** Focus on the word *photophobia* and use the process of elimination to choose the answer that shields the eyes from light.

2 **Answer: 2 Rationale:** Difficulty in adjusting quickly to changes in illumination occurs as a result of miosis, an effect of pilocarpine. The client will experience more difficulty seeing at night. Driving is not contraindicated; however, nighttime driving might not be possible because of the miosis. **Cognitive Level:** Analyzing **Client Need:** Pharmacological and Parenteral Therapies **Integrated Process:** Nursing Process: Evaluation **Content Area:** Pharmacology **Strategy:** Specific knowledge of the important teaching points related to pilocarpine is needed to answer the question. Use this knowledge and the process of elimination to make a selection.

3 **Answer: 2, 5 Rationale:** The diuretic effects of methazolamide could lead to electrolyte disturbances of hypokalemia and hypernatremia. The diuretic effects of methazolamide will not cause the other options. **Cognitive Level:** Analyzing **Client Need:** Pharmacological and Parenteral Therapies **Integrated Process:** Nursing Process: Data Collection **Content Area:** Pharmacology **Strategy:** The core issue of the question is knowledge of electrolyte disturbances for which the client is at risk during therapy with methozolamide. Recall that the medication has a diuretic effect, and reason that potassium might be lost while sodium is retained. Use this knowledge and the process of elimination to make a selection. When there is more than one correct answer, consider each option as a true/false statement.

4 **Answer: 2 Rationale:** Superinfections are known to occur with this medication; therefore, 7 days is too long to seek further evaluation and treatment; this statement indicates a need of additional instruction. The other options are correct actions by the client. **Cognitive Level:** Analyzing **Client Need:** Pharmacological and Parenteral Therapies **Integrated Process:** Nursing Process: Evaluation **Content Area:** Pharmacology **Strategy:** The wording of the question tells you that the correct answer is an inaccurate statement. Use the process of elimination, and select the option that represents incorrect information.

5 **Answer: 1 Rationale:** Symptoms of systemic absorption of pilocarpine include diaphoresis, diarrhea, bradycardia, and hypotension. The other options are not symptoms of systemic absorption of pilocarpine. **Cognitive Level:** Applying **Client Need:** Pharmacological and Parenteral Therapies **Integrated Process:** Nursing Process: Evaluation **Content Area:** Pharmacology **Strategy:** The core issue of the question is recognition of signs of systemic absorption of pilocarpine. Specific knowledge of systemic effects of this medication is needed to answer the question. Use this knowledge and the process of elimination to make a selection.

6 **Answer: 2 Rationale:** Cyclomydril and other mydriatics are applied topically to produce mydriasis (dilated pupil) to facilitate ocular examination. Cyclomydril and other mydriatics do not provide anesthesia, nor do they prevent infection. **Cognitive Level:** Applying **Client Need:** Pharmacological and Parenteral Therapies **Integrated Process:** Teaching and Learning **Content Area:** Pharmacology **Strategy:** The core issue of the question is knowledge of the intended effects of cyclomydril. Note that the name of the drug contains the letters *myd*, which is also the beginning of the word *mydriasis* (meaning to dilate the pupils). Using simple word association will sometimes assist in making the correct selection.

7 **Answer: 1, 2, 5 Rationale:** Systemic side effects of ophthalmic atropine include tachycardia, slurred speech, dry mouth, and confusion. Diaphoresis is unrelated to the use of ophthalmic atropine. **Cognitive Level:** Analyzing **Client Need:** Pharmacological and Parenteral Therapies **Integrated Process:** Nursing Process: Data Collection **Content Area:** Pharmacology **Strategy:** The core issue of the question is knowledge of side/adverse effects of atropine. Recall that when used for cardiac reasons and as a pre-op medication, the medication speeds up heart rate. A common side effect of many medications is confusion. When there is more than one correct answer, consider each option as a true/false statement.

8 **Answer: 1 Rationale:** Ophthalmic solution that has darkened or become cloudy should be discarded. Many eye medications can cause the sensation of eye burning; medications should not be discontinued without first consulting the physician. Swabs should not be used to apply ophthalmic medication. Ophthalmic medications generally have a shelf life of 3 months. **Cognitive Level:** Analyzing **Client Need:** Pharmacological and Parenteral Therapies **Integrated Process:** Nursing Process: Evaluation **Content Area:** Pharmacology **Strategy:** The core issue of the question is safe self-administration of ophthalmic medications. Use nursing knowledge and the process of elimination to answer the question.

9 **Answer: 1, 5 Rationale:** Salicylates can cause tinnitus, vertigo, and hearing loss, if ingested in high doses. Over-the-counter ibuprofen, if ingested in high doses, can cause ototoxicity. The other options do not present concerns regarding ototoxicity. **Cognitive Level:** Applying **Client Need:** Pharmacological and

Parenteral Therapies **Integrated Process:** Nursing Process: Implementation **Content Area:** Pharmacology **Strategy:** The core issue of the question is an understanding of the types of drugs that can cause ototoxicity. Use nursing knowledge and the process of elimination to make a selection. When there is more than one correct answer, consider each option as a true/false statement.

10 **Answer: 4 Rationale:** Inserting objects, including medication droppers, into the ear canal can perforate the tympanic membrane; this is the priority teaching need. The ear canal may or may not be obstructed with cerumen, the client needs teaching about the appropriate instillation technique; addressing the issue of cerumen is not the priority. The client is not demonstrating the proper technique for instilling ear medication. The client is instructed to lie on the unaffected side, not the affected side, to allow flow of medication into the ear. While important, this is not the priority teaching need. **Cognitive Level:** Analyzing **Client Need:** Pharmacological and Parenteral Therapies **Integrated Process:** Nursing Process: Planning **Content Area:** Pharmacology **Strategy:** The core issue of the question is an understanding of the procedure for safe self-administration of an otic medication. Use nursing knowledge and the process of elimination to make a selection.

11 **Answer: 1 Rationale:** The recommended wait time between administrations of two ophthalmic solutions is 5 minutes. If an ophthalmic ointment is instilled, the waiting time is 10 minutes between the ointment and the next medication. **Cognitive Level:** Applying **Client Need:** Pharmacological and Parenteral Therapies **Integrated Process:** Nursing Process: Evaluation **Content Area:** Pharmacology **Strategy:** The core issue of the question is an understanding of the procedure for safe self-administration of an ophthalmic medication. Use nursing knowledge and the process of elimination to make a selection.

12 **Answer: 3, 5 Rationale:** The eye is cleansed with sterile irrigating solution or sterile normal saline, to decrease risk of contamination; this action indicates a need for additional teaching. Drainage of the medication should be directed toward the outer canthus and gentle pressure applied to the inner canthus to prevent systemic absorption of the medication; this action requires additional teaching. The other options represent appropriate technique. **Cognitive Level:** Analyzing **Client Need:** Pharmacological and Parenteral Therapies **Integrated Process:** Nursing Process: Evaluation **Content Area:** Pharmacology **Strategy:** The wording of the question tells you that the correct options are inappropriate actions. Analyze each option to decide if it is a true or false statement, and make the selection that represents false information.

13 **Answer: 3 Rationale:** Timolol is a beta-adrenergic blocker that decreases the production of aqueous humor, thereby decreasing intraocular pressure. Sympathomimetics also decrease aqueous humor production. A decrease in the outflow of aqueous humor is contraindicated for a client with glaucoma. Prostaglandins increase the outflow of aqueous humor to decrease intraocular pressure. An increase in aqueous humor production would be harmful for a client with glaucoma. **Cognitive Level:** Analyzing **Client Need:** Pharmacological and Parenteral Therapies **Integrated Process:** Nursing Process: Evaluation **Content Area:** Pharmacology **Strategy:** Note that the drug name ends in *-olol*, and reason that the medication is a beta-blocking agent. With this in mind, recall the actions of beta-blocker medications in the eye. Use nursing knowledge and the process of elimination to make a selection.

14 **Answer: 1 Rationale:** Carbachol causes miosis (pupil constriction), making quick changes in illumination difficult. Nighttime is particularly hazardous for the elderly client. The client and family are instructed on methods such as lighting hallways and bathrooms at night, to reduce the potential for injury. Mydriasis, pupil dilation, is not a concern when taking carbachol. Systemic side effects of carbachol include diarrhea, not constipation. Systemic side effects of carbachol include hypotension, not hypertension. **Cognitive Level:** Applying **Client Need:** Pharmacological and Parenteral Therapies **Integrated Process:** Teaching and Learning **Content Area:** Pharmacology **Strategy:** Note that two options are opposites and when two options are opposite, consider the possibility that one of them is the correct answer. In this case, note that the client is elderly, and is not in a situation (such as an eye exam) when the pupils would be dilated. With this in mind, eliminate the option that represents pupil dilation.

15 **Answer: 2 Rationale:** Redness and swelling are signs of hypersensitivity to vidarabine. The medication should be discontinued, and the client should return to the clinic immediately for evaluation. The other responses fail to recognize the significance of the finding or delay of treatment. **Cognitive Level:** Analyzing **Client Need:** Pharmacological and Parenteral Therapies **Integrated Process:** Nursing Process: Implementation **Content Area:** Pharmacology **Strategy:** Note that the question contains key information about adverse effects that began after the first dose of the medication. When symptoms suddenly appear, as in this question, consider the possibility of a hypersensitivity reaction, and choose an option accordingly.

16 **Answer: 4 Rationale:** Viroptic, used in the treatment of viral infections such as herpes, is administered for an additional 5–7 days after healing has occurred. Immediately discontinuing the medication is contraindicated and stopping at 7 days is too limited of a time frame. Ophthalmic medications are stored in a cool, dry place, and some are recommended for refrigeration; a pocket is too warm. **Cognitive Level:** Analyzing **Client Need:** Pharmacological and Parenteral Therapies **Integrated Process:** Nursing Process: Evaluation **Content Area:** Pharmacology **Strategy:** The core issue of the question is knowledge of appropriate information about Viroptic as an ophthalmic medication. Use nursing knowledge and the process of elimination to make a selection.

17 **Answer: 1 Rationale:** The child's pinna is pulled down and back for administration of otic solutions. The pinna in the adult is pulled up and back. Droppers should never be inserted into the ear canal. The head is tilted toward the unaffected side so that medication will run into the ear canal. **Cognitive Level:** Analyzing **Client Need:** Pharmacological and Parenteral Therapies **Integrated Process:** Nursing Process: Evaluation **Content Area:** Pharmacology **Strategy:** One quick way to remember the direction for pulling the pinna is to associate the direction with the height of the person. Since an adult is taller, pull the pinna up and back, while for a child, who is shorter, pull the pinna down and back.

18 **Answer: 3 Rationale:** Acetazolamide may be taken with food to minimize gastrointestinal irritation. Acetazolamide, a carbonic anhydrase inhibitor, causes diuresis. The nurse should instruct the client to take the medication early in the day, to avoid nocturia. Clients receiving acetazolamide are encouraged to consume at least 2000 mL of fluid per day to avoid

fluid volume depletion. Acetazolamide may be taken with juice to minimize gastrointestinal irritation. **Cognitive Level:** Analyzing **Client Need:** Pharmacological and Parenteral Therapies **Integrated Process:** Nursing Process: Data Collection **Content Area:** Pharmacology **Strategy:** The core issue of the question is recognition of and client teaching to prevent nocturia, a side effect of carbonic anhydrase inhibitors. Use medication knowledge and general principles for timing the administration of diuretics to answer the question.

19 **Answer: 3 Rationale:** Data collection of allergies and reactions to medications is essential when administering a new medication. Hypersensitivity responses can occur with ophthalmic medications, and severe adverse reactions can occur with hypersensitivity to the medication because it is systemically absorbed. Collecting data regarding eye and vision status and client's understanding of the medication are important; however, avoiding reactions to the medication is the priority. **Cognitive Level:** Applying **Client Need:** Pharmacological and Parenteral Therapies **Integrated Process:** Nursing Process: Data Collection **Content Area:** Adult Health **Strategy:** Knowing that one of the safety factors prior to administering any medication is collecting data for any allergies or hypersensitivities will lead to the correct option. Recognize that while the other options are important, safe care is the priority action.

20 **Answer: 2 Rationale:** Correct technique for administration of ophthalmic medications includes pulling the lower eyelid down and instilling the medication into the conjunctival sac. Medication is not applied directly to the eye. The lower lid is pulled down rather than up, and medication is not applied directly to the eye. The lid is pulled down rather than up. **Cognitive Level:** Analyzing **Client Need:** Pharmacological and Parenteral Therapies **Integrated Process:** Nursing Process: Evaluation **Content Area:** Adult Health **Strategy:** Use the process of elimination and knowledge of basic care in the instillation of eye medications to choose the correct option.

Key Terms to Review

aqueous humor p. 621
cycloplegia p. 625
intraocular pressure p. 621
keratitis p. 624
miosis p. 626
mydriasis p. 622
narrow-angle glaucoma p. 624
open-angle glaucoma p. 621
photophobia p. 624
systemic absorption p. 621
tonometry p. 628
uveitis p. 622
vertigo p. 628

References

Adams, M., Holland, L., & Urban, C. (2011). *Pharmacology for nurses: A pathophysiological approach* (3rd ed.). Upper Saddle River, NJ: Pearson Education, Inc.

Adams, M., & Koch, R. (2010). *Pharmacology: Connections to nursing practice*. Upper Saddle River, NJ: Pearson Education, Inc.

Deglin, J. H., & Vallerand, A. H. (2011). *Davis's drug guide for nurses* (12th ed.). Philadelphia: F. A. Davis.

Lehne, R. (2010). *Pharmacology for nursing care* (7th ed.). Philadelphia: W. B. Saunders.

Wilson, B., Shannon, M., & Shields, K. (2012). *Pearson nurse's drug guide 2012*. Upper Saddle River, NJ: Pearson Education, Inc.

Test Yourself

Are you ready for the NCLEX-PN® or course exams? Use the practice tests on the companion website to check.

41 Immunological and Anti-Infective Medications

In this chapter

Cross Reference

Other chapters relevant to this content area are

Dosage Calculation and Medication Administration	Chapter 28
Immunological Disorders	Chapter 62
Communicable or Infectious Diseases	Chapter 63

I. IMMUNOMODULATORS

A. Description

1. Immunomodulators can either suppress or enhance immune response
2. Depending on intended immune response, client is administered either an immune stimulant or an **immunosuppressant**, which suppresses body's response to an **antigen** (a substance that stimulates production of antibodies)
3. Can be used to stimulate platelet production to prevent severe thrombocytopenia (abnormally low platelet count) caused by platelet destruction
4. Increase development of bone marrow, which is adversely affected by chemotherapy agents used after bone marrow transplantation (BMT) or to treat cancer

B. *Colony-stimulating factors*

1. Action and use
   a. Glycoproteins that increase white blood cell (WBC) production, which enhances cellular immunity (immunity of host affecting body cells)
   b. Are described as granulocyte colony-stimulating factors (G-CSF) or macrophage and granulocyte colony stimulating factors (GM-CSF)
   c. Reduce **neutropenia** (abnormally low neutrophil count) and decrease incidence of infection; they assist in mobilizing stem cells, allowing for stem cell collection
2. Common medications are listed and described in Table 41–1

Table 41-1 Common Immunostimulant Medications

Generic/Trade Names	Actions
Sargramostim (Leukine)	Increases production of granulocytes and macrophages before and after bone marrow transplantation, so labeled as a GM-CSF
Epoetin alfa (Epogen)	Increases RBC count in clients with chronic renal failure, cancer, or human immunodeficiency virus; is actually a hematological, not an immunological, colony stimulating factor, but is used in clients who have immunodeficiency
Filgrastim (Neupogen) Pegfilgrastim (Neulasta)	Increases neutrophil (granulocyte) production in clients with cancer to prevent infection, so labeled as a G-CSF

Memory Aid

Associate the *e* in epoetin alfa with the *e* in erythrocyte to recall that it stimulates red blood cell growth. Use the same strategy to associate *Neu*pogen with *neu*trophil count (WBC).

3. Administration considerations
   a. Sargramostim (Leukine): reconstitute with sterile water; avoid shaking vial; use for 21 days after BMT and, in clients with acute myelogenous leukemia, around either day 11 following chemotherapy dose or 4 days after chemotherapy induction
   NCLEX® b. Epoetin alfa (Epogen, Procrit): goal of administration is to raise hematocrit (Hct) to 30–33% (maximum 36%); usually given 3 times per week; do not shake during or after reconstitution
   NCLEX® c. Filgrastim (Neupogen): do not give during or 24 hrs after a dose of cytotoxic chemotherapy; dosage may be titrated depending on neutrophil count, stop drug if absolute neutrophil count (ANC) exceeds 20,000/mm^3 or 10,000/mm^3 after nadir of drug

NCLEX® 4. Contraindications
   a. Sargramostim: pregnancy, hypersensitivity to yeast or *E. coli* products; leukemic myeloblasts in bone marrow; use cautiously with hepatic or renal insufficiency and lactation
   b. Epoetin alfa: uncontrolled hypertension, pregnancy, hypersensitivity to albumin
   c. Filgrastim: pregnancy, hypersensitivity to *E. coli* products
5. Side/adverse effects
   a. Nausea and vomiting (N/V), anorexia, constipation, diarrhea
   b. Headache, stomatitis, edema, rash, mucositis, generalized pain, bone pain
   c. Supraventricular dysrhythmias, tachycardia
   d. Renal or hepatic dysfunction, dyspnea, seizures, porphyria
   e. Report ANC as noted above
   f. Adult respiratory distress syndrome (ARDS), pleural effusion
   g. Myocardial infarction (MI), gastrointestinal (GI) hemorrhage, thrombus formation
6. Nursing considerations for sargramostim (Leukine)
   a. Monitor baseline CBC and platelet count and 2 times per week during therapy
   b. Monitor renal and hepatic function
   c. Monitor for excessive myeloid blasts in bone marrow
   d. Do not administer during pregnancy; use cautiously during lactation
   e. Store in refrigerator; dilute with normal saline; administer only one dose per vial
7. Nursing considerations for epoetin alfa (Epogen)
   a. Measure blood pressure (BP) before administration and regularly during therapy; hypertension may occur if Hct level rises rapidly
   b. Use cautiously during lactation
   c. Provide diet rich in iron; client may need an iron supplement to increase effectiveness of therapy
   d. Monitor Homan's sign periodically to detect thrombus development with increased RBC counts
   e. Measure Hct; a rapid elevation of 4 points in 2 weeks may lead to hypertension and seizures

NCLEX® 8. Nursing considerations for filgrastim (Neupogen)
   a. Monitor CBC, differential, and platelet count at baseline and 2 times per week during therapy
   b. Do not administer 24 hours before or after chemotherapy
   c. Check for hypersensitivity to *E. coli* products
   d. Filgrastim is pregnancy category C; use cautiously with lactation
   e. Administer only one dose per vial, and discard after 24 hours; store medication in refrigerator

f. Reconstitute in dextrose 5%, and avoid shaking bottle to prevent damage to protein
g. Avoid exposure to infection because client's lowered WBC count increases risk of infection

9. Client education for sargramostim (Leukine)
   a. Avoid exposure to infection and be aware of signs and symptoms of infection
   b. Report difficulty breathing and fever
   c. CBC and platelet counts must be done periodically
   d. Address body image with client because of alopecia
10. Client education for epoetin alfa (Epogen)
   a. Administration of medication at home with home dialysis; action, side effects, and nursing implications associated with administration
   b. Signs and symptoms of clot formation
   c. Self-monitor BP
   d. Eat a diet high in iron and take iron supplement if ordered
11. Client education for filgrastim (Neupogen)
   a. Report pain in joints and bones
   b. Maintain good hygiene and avoid exposure to crowds to reduce risk of infection

C. Cell-stimulating medications

1. Action and use
   a. Interleukins are biologic response modifiers that prevent thrombocytopenia and stimulate platelet production
   b. In helper T cells, cellular immunity is increased along with number of lymphocytes
   c. Interleukins are a group of proteins, produced by lymphocytes, that have antitumor activity, causing cells to change to a nonproliferative type
   d. Aldesleukin (Proleukin) is used to treat renal carcinoma and prevents severe thrombocytopenia
   e. Levamisole (Ergamisol) increases immune response by increasing activity of B cells, T cells, and macrophages; it is used in combination with fluorouracil to treat Duke's stage C colon cancer
   f. Oprelvekin (Neumega) is used following chemotherapy that causes **myelosuppression** (suppressed bone marrow function in manufacture of blood cells); it increases thrombocyte and megakaryocyte production to prevent and treat thrombocytopenia in clients receiving chemotherapy
2. Common medications are listed in Table 41–2
3. Administration considerations
   a. Aldesleukin (Proleukin): because of serious side effects, this drug is given in a hospital that has an intensive care unit with medical specialists available; after 14 doses, a waiting period ensues, followed by another 14 doses
   b. Levamisole (Ergamisol): therapy should begin 7–30 days after bowel resection surgery; maintenance dose: 50 mg every 8 hours for 3 days with fluorouracil
   c. Oprelvekin (Neumega): can be given for 21 days or until platelet count is greater than 100,000 cells/mm^3; reconstitute in an isotonic solution; do not agitate; administer within 3 hours of reconstitution
4. Side/adverse effects
   a. Aldesleukin: cardiac dyshythmias, fluid retention, lethargy, myalgia
   b. Levamisole: flulike symptoms, bone marrow depression, GI upset
   c. Oprelvekin: cardiac dysrhythmias, fluid retention
5. Nursing considerations
   a. Monitor CBC, with WBC differential, and platelet count
   b. Monitor heart rate, BP, respirations, and lung sounds
   c. Maintain fluid and electrolyte balance, particularly during flu-like symptoms
   d. Provide good hygiene practices
6. Client and family education
   a. Home medication administration
   b. Measurement of fluid retention and irregular heart rate

Table 41–2 Common Cell-Stimulating Medications

Generic/Trade Names	Actions
Aldesleukin (Proleukin)	Increases lymphocytes, platelets, and tumor necrosis factor
Levamisole (Ergamisol)	Increases B cell activity and antibody formation by increasing monocyte and macrophage action
Oprelvekin (Neumega)	Increases thrombocyte and megakaryocyte production, thus preventing thrombocytopenia

Table 41–3 Common Immunosuppressant Medications

Generic/Trade Names	Actions
Azathioprine (Imuran)	Prevents renal transplant rejection; administered for life
Basiliximab (Simulect)	Prevents acute renal transplant rejection in combination with cyclosporine and a glucocorticoid
Daclizumab (Zenapax)	Prevents renal transplant rejection
Cyclosporine (Sandimmune)	Prevents rejection in solid organ transplant
Muromonab CD3 (Orthoclone OKT3)	Suppresses T cells to prevent renal transplant rejection
Mycophenolate (CellCept)	Prevents rejection in renal, liver, and cardiac transplants
Sirolimus (Rapamune)	Prevents renal transplant rejection in combination with cyclosporine and a glucocorticoid
Tacrolimus (Prograf)	Prevents rejection in solid organ transplant, primarily liver transplant

c. Measures to assist in preventing infection
d. Care and management of flulike symptoms

D. Immunosuppressants

1. Action and use
   a. Inhibit inflammatory response and block immune response to an antigen; inhibit T cells and block production of antibodies by B cells
   b. Prevent rejection of organs that have been transplanted

NCLEX®

2. Common medications are listed in Table 41–3
3. Administration considerations
   a. Azathioprine (Imuran): reaches peak level in 1–2 hours after dose; duration of action is 10 hours
   b. Cyclosporine (Sandimmune): reaches peak level in 4–5 hours after dose; duration of action is 20–54 hours
   c. Basiliximab (Simulect): given IV 24 hours post-transplant, then 4 days after transplant
   d. Daclizumab (Zenapax): given IV 24 hours post-transplant for total of 5 doses
   e. Muromonab CD3 (Orthoclone OKT 3): therapy should begin as soon as rejection is identified
   f. Mycophenolate (CellCept): renal transplant clients receive 1 gram 2 times per day; therapy should begin 72 hours after transplant
   g. Tacrolimus (Prograf): administered 6 hours after transplant
4. Side/adverse effects
   a. Increased risk for infection; hypertension; acne
   b. Hepatotoxicity and/or renal toxicity
   c. Flulike symptoms and/or headache, diarrhea, nausea and/or vomiting
   d. Contraindicated with allergy to drug, or during pregnancy or lactation
5. Nursing considerations
   a. Check for signs and symptoms of infection
   b. Provide supportive care for flulike symptoms
   c. Monitor results of CBC, platelet count, BUN, creatinine, and liver enzymes
   d. Monitor nutritional status; encourage nutritious meals with small, frequent feedings
6. Client education: need for lab studies, prevention of infection, and all aspects of medication administration, including action, side effects, and nursing implications

II. MEDICATIONS TO TREAT MULTIPLE SCLEROSIS (MS)

A. Action and use

1. Goal is to decrease inflammation, suppress immune system to prevent nerve tissue destruction, and decrease fatigue and ataxia
2. A wide variety of medications are used to treat multiple sclerosis; they include beta-adrenergic blockers, corticosteroids, anti-inflammatory agents, and interferon

NCLEX®

B. Common medications are listed in Table 41–4

C. Administration considerations

1. Interferon Beta 1b (Betaseron) is discontinued in 6 months if disease does not enter remission
2. Should be administered cautiously with hepatic or renal insufficiency and when client has been diagnosed with a neoplasm
3. Contraindicated in pregnancy, lactation, and hypersensitivity to drug

Table 41–4 Common Medications to Treat Multiple Sclerosis

Generic/Trade Names	Actions
Interferon Beta 1a (Avonex) Interferon Beta 1b (Betaseron)	Interferon that reduces severity of acute exacerbations; decreases demyelination in brain tissue; can be used for long-term treatment of relapsing forms
Glatiramer acetate (Copaxone)	Immunomodulator that prevents destruction of brain and nerve tissue; used for long-term treatment
Mitoxantrone (Novantron)	An antineoplastic that suppresses activity of T and B cells and macrophages to slow disease process; approved for use in MS
Natalizumab (Tysabri)	Monoclonal antibody that may inhibit movement of damaging immune cells across blood–brain barrier

D. Side/adverse effects

1. Azathioprine (Imuran): increased risk of infection, renal or hepatic insufficiency; leukopenia and thrombocytopenia
2. Interferons: muscle aches, flu-like symptoms, local reactions, headache, anemia, myelosuppression, hepatotoxicity
3. Glatiramer acetate (Copaxone): anxiety, arthralgia, back pain, malaise, flu-like symptoms, lymphadenopathy, pain at injection site
4. Mitoxantrone (Novantrone): myelosuppression, cardiotoxicity, stomatitis, N/V, pain at injection site; also potentially fatal opportunistic viral brain infection (progressive multifocal leukoencephalopathy)
5. Natalizumab (Tysabri): headache, depression, fatigue, menstrual dysfunction, infections, and rarely anaphylaxis

E. Nursing considerations

1. Monitor for signs of adverse effects
2. Monitor results of laboratory tests ordered by prescriber
3. Provide comfort measures when client experiences flu-like symptoms
4. Observe injection sites for inflammation and pain
5. Monitor for effects of treatment and exacerbations of disease

F. Client education

1. Side effects of medication and need for periodic laboratory studies
2. Report any side effects to prescriber
3. Supportive care of flu-like symptoms, including adequate fluid intake, rest, and use of acetaminophen for relief of pain and fever
4. Signs and symptoms of cardiotoxicity for mitoxantrone

III. MEDICATIONS TO TREAT MYASTHENIA GRAVIS

A. Action and use

1. Anticholinesterase drugs treat symptoms of myasthenia gravis (MG) by increasing concentration of acetylcholine at neuromuscular junction
2. Increase nerve impulse conduction and muscle strength

NCLEX® **B. Common medications are listed in Table 41–5**

Table 41–5 Common Medications to Treat Myasthenia Gravis

Generic/Trade Names	Actions
Ambenonium (Mytelase)	Long-acting medication to treat MG
Edrophonium (Tensilon)	Used for diagnostic purposes; clients who exhibit temporary improvement in muscle strength, posture, and respiratory function with injected dose have MG
Neostigmine (Prostigmin)	Has a duration of action of 2–4 hours; increases acetylcholine concentration, facilitating neuromuscular function
Pyridostigmine (Mestinon)	Increases acetylcholine concentration facilitating neuromuscular function; taken every 3–6 hours

NCLEX® **C. Administration considerations**

1. Edrophonium (Tensilon): single dose is for diagnostic purposes only; may be repeated once to aid in uncertain diagnosis
2. Neostigmine (Prostigmin): can be administered subcutaneously (SubQ) during an acute exacerbation
3. Pyridostigmine (Mestinon): a timed-release preparation can be administered at bedtime; can also be administered IM during acute exacerbation
4. Contraindicated in pregnancy and lactation, bradycardia, intestinal or urinary obstruction
5. Use cautiously in clients with asthma, heart disease, Parkinson's disease, and seizure disorders

D. Side/adverse effects

1. Bradycardia, hypotension, or cardiac arrest
2. Increased gastric secretions, N/V, diarrhea
3. Increased urinary urgency and involuntary incontinence of stool
4. NCLEX® Severe cholinergic reactions: excessive salivation, sphincter relaxation, diarrhea, and vomiting

E. Nursing considerations

1. NCLEX® Monitor respirations, heart rate, and general muscle strength, including swallowing, before dose
2. Administer with meals to enhance absorption and decrease GI irritation
3. NCLEX® Administer on time to prevent difficulty with respirations and swallowing caused by undermedication or late medication administration
4. Administer IV preparations slowly to prevent cholinergic reaction
5. NCLEX® Have atropine available as antidote to counteract cholinergic reaction
6. Monitor response to medication and ability to perform activities of daily living

F. Client education

1. All aspects of drug administration, side effects; take with food to decrease GI irritation
2. Coordination of medication administration with activities of daily living
3. Overmedication will result in cholinergic reaction
4. Measurement of apical pulse

IV. MEDICATIONS TO TREAT RHEUMATOID ARTHRITIS

A. Action and use

1. Early stage rheumatoid arthritis (RA) is managed with NSAIDs, which have antiinflammatory and analgesic action, along with selected disease-modifying antirheumatic drugs (DMARDs)
2. DMARDs are a diverse group of drugs that modify immune or inflammatory response
3. DMARDs used early in treatment of RA tend to include hydrochloroquine (Plaquenil), methotrexate (Rheumatrex), or sulfasalazine (Azulfidine)
4. Multiple drugs may be used at one time to adequately control symptoms and delay disease progression
5. Less frequently used drugs are gold salts, D-penicillamine (Cuprimine), and cyclophosphamide (Cytoxan) because they are more toxic than other DMARDs
6. Corticosteroids are used to relieve symptoms of flares in moderate to severe RA, but are used in smallest possible doses and are not used long-term because of their adverse effects

B. Common medications are listed in Table 41–6

Table 41–6 Common Medications to Treat Rheumatoid Arthritis

Generic/Trade Names	Actions
Abatacept (Orencia), etanercept (Enbrel), infliximab (Remicade), adalimumab (Humira)	Are tumor necrosis factor (TNF) inhibitors that block steps in TNF mediated cellular response, thus reducing inflammation and slowing progression of joint damage; are called biologic therapies
Anakinra (Kineret)	Inhibits interleukin-1 (IL-1), an important chemical mediator of inflammation
Azathioprine (Imuran), cyclosporine (Sandimmune)	Immunosuppressants that inhibit lymphocyte replication or disrupt T helper cells
Hydroxychloroquine (Plaquenil)	Not completely understood; reduces migration of eosinophils and neutrophils and probably inhibits synthesis of histamine and prostaglandins
Leflunomide (Arava)	Inhibits inflammatory process by blocking enzyme DHODH
Methotrexate (Rheumatrex)	Inhibits DNA synthesis and folic acid reductase to reduce inflammation; is a cytotoxic drug
Sulfasalazine (Azufidine)	An anti-inflammatory drug that is also a sulfonamide and a salicylate

C. Administration considerations
1. Check medications for RA with other ordered medications for interactions
2. Check CBC, uric acid levels, urinalysis, and liver and renal function tests as baseline and periodically during therapy
3. Check to see if specific drug is contraindicated with pregnancy, lactation, liver disease, renal disease
4. Inject etanercept into abdomen, thigh, or upper arm SubQ

NCLEX®
5. Penicillamine is contraindicated with a known hypersensitivity to penicillin; sulfasalazine is contraindicated with allergy to sulfonamides or salicylates

D. Side/adverse effects
1. Biologic therapies: local reactions at injection site, headache, nasopharyngitis, infections, lupus-like syndrome, heart failure exacerbations, Stevens-Johnson syndrome
2. Azathioprine (Imuran): chills, fever, malaise, myalgia, myelosuppression, hepatotoxicity
3. Hydroxychloroquine (Plaquenil): anorexia, N/V, headache, personality changes, retinopathy, agranulocytosis, aplastic anemia, seizures
4. Methotrexate (Rheumatrex): headache, glossitis, gingivitis, nausea, myelosuppression, hepatic cirrhosis, nephrotoxicity, pulmonary fibrosis, and teratogenicity
5. Sulfasalazine (Azulfidine): headache, anorexia, N/V, leukopenia, Stevens-Johnson syndrome, reversible oligospermia

E. Nursing considerations
1. Avoid antacid use for at least 2 hours following medication administration
2. Monitor for drug adverse effects

NCLEX®
3. Observe for signs of infection
4. Monitor effects of medication therapy on RA symptoms and joint function

F. Client education
1. Protect self from infection
2. Comply with periodic laboratory studies
3. If taking gold preparations, report signs of gold toxicity, including metallic taste and pruritus
4. All aspects of medication administration, including side effects, action, use, and contraindications

V. MEDICATIONS TO TREAT SYSTEMIC LUPUS ERYTHEMATOSUS

A. Action and use
1. Cytotoxic drugs or purine analogs are used along with NSAIDs, and corticosteroids to treat symptoms of systemic lupus erythematosus (SLE)
2. Provide immunosuppressive action to treat autoimmune diseases

NCLEX®
B. Common medications
1. NSAIDS (off-label use)
2. Methotrexate (off-label use)
3. Immunosuprressants such as cyclosporine (Sandimmune), mycophenolate (CellCept), azathioprine (Imuran)

C. See previous section on RA and immunosuppressants for discussion of these drugs

VI. ANTIBIOTICS

A. Aminoglycosides
1. Action and use
   a. **Bactericidal**: aminoglycosides kill bacteria cells
   b. Used in infections caused by *Acinetobacter, Citrobacter, E. coli, Klebsiella pneumoniae, proteus, pseudomonas, Providencia, Salmonella, Serratia,* and *staphylococcus* organisms; also active against protozoal infections
   c. Used to sterilize bowel prior to surgery
   d. Used to destroy urease-producing bacteria to prevent absorption of ammonia in hepatic encephalopathy
   e. Toxicity limits use to serious Gram-negative infections and specific conditions involving Gram-positive cocci

NCLEX®
2. Common medications are listed in Box 41–1

Memory Aid

Recognize an aminoglycoside by the suffix *-mycin*. Note that not all drugs that end in *-mycin* are aminoglycosides, but all aminoglycosides end in *-mycin* or *-micin*.

Box 41–1

Aminoglycosides

Amikacin (Amikin)	Paromomycin (Humatin)
Gentamicin (Garamycin, others)	Streptomycin (generic)
Kanamycin (Kantrex)	Tobramicin (Nebcin)
Neomycin (generic)	

3. Administration considerations
  a. IV route preferred for optimal distribution to tissues; used intramuscularly (IM)
  b. Oral route: poorly absorbed, so effective orally only to decrease bacteria in bowel before surgery or prevent absorption of ammonia in hepatic encephalopathy
  c. Intrathecal or intraventricular injection: can be used to counteract poor penetration of cerebral spinal fluid (CSF) by other routes
  d. Periocular instillations: because of poor penetration of eye fluids, direct instillations are used
  e. Contraindicated with allergy to aminoglycosides; preexisting renal disease; if receiving renal toxic agents such as amphotericin B (Fungizone), vancomycin (Vancocin), or loop diuretics such as furosemide (Lasix); in myasthenia gravis; and cautious use in pregnancy and lactation

4. Significant laboratory studies
  NCLEX® **a. Peak drug level**: blood specimen drawn 30 minutes after completion of IV infusion of aminoglycoside to determine that toxic levels do not occur; dose may need to be decreased if peak too high
  NCLEX® **b. Trough drug level**: blood specimen drawn immediately prior to starting next IV infusion of aminoglycoside to assure that therapeutic drug levels are maintained between administrations; if drug level is too low, an increase in dose and/or dosing frequency may be indicated
  c. WBC count to monitor effectiveness of drug therapy; counts decrease as infection resolves
  d. Serum creatinine and blood urea nitrogen (BUN) to monitor renal function; expected BUN to creatinine ratio is 20:1 or 15:1 depending on laboratory criteria; creatinine is most specific test for renal function; if creatinine level rises 3–4 days into treatment, renal damage has occurred

5. Side/adverse effects
  a. Headache, paresthesias, skin rash, fever
  b. Nephrotoxicity and ototoxicity (two common toxicities with aminoglycosides)
  c. Nephrotoxicity: increased with risk factors such as advancing age (with associated declining renal function), hypotension, dehydration, preexisting renal disease, coadministration of other nephrotoxic drugs
  d. Ototoxicity: may be irreversible; auditory impairment and vestibular damage; possible damage to 8th cranial nerve; risk is increased with nephrotoxic drugs, prolonged treatment with aminoglycosides, impaired renal function, and other ototoxic drugs, such as furosemide (Lasix), vancomycin (Vancocin), amphotericin B, and certain antineoplastic agents
  e. Neuromuscular blockade: by inhibiting acetylcholine release; may be seen in clients with myasthenia gravis or those receiving neuromuscular blockers such as pancuronium bromide (Pavulon) or succinylcholine (Anectine); use calcium salts to reverse blockade
  NCLEX® **f. Candidiasis** superinfection: secondary infection usually of skin and mucous membranes caused by *Candida albicans*; appears as discrete white plaques that are not easily removed
  NCLEX® **g. Pseudomembranous colitis** superinfection: secondary infection of bowel, usually caused by *Clostridium difficile*; manifested by 4–6 watery stools per day with blood and/or mucus, abdominal pain, and fever; antibiotic is discontinued and vancomycin (Vancocin) PO or Flagyl IV or PO is prescribed

6. Nursing considerations
  a. See Box 41–2 for general nursing considerations with antibiotic therapy
  b. Empiric therapy (based on probable offending organism) is usually begun before test results available because of seriousness of infection
  c. Monitor peak and trough aminoglycoside levels
  d. Monitor for nephrotoxicity: monitor serum creatinine, BUN, urine creatinine clearance and urinalysis (urinary casts and proteinuria)
  e. Make certain the client is not taking other nephrotoxic drugs
  f. Keep accurate record of intake and output (I&O)
  g. Monitor for ototoxicity: look for dizziness, lightheadedness, tinnitus, fullness in ears, and hearing loss; monitor vestibular integrity with Romberg's test

Box 41–2

General Nursing Considerations for Antibiotic Therapy and Other Anti-Infectives

- Collect appropriate specimen for culture and sensitivity (C&S), whenever possible, before starting antibiotic therapy to ensure proper drug selection; empiric therapy may be started so that infection can be treated promptly.
- Review client's medication profile (including OTC and herbal products) for agents that may cause drug interactions.
- Check for allergy before administration and withhold dose and notify prescriber for documented hypersensitivity reaction (such as hives, urticaria, stridor, dyspnea, and anaphylaxis).
- Administer doses on time to maintain therapeutic blood levels; when IV antibiotic is scheduled at same time as another IV medication (e.g. ranitidine [Zantac]); give IV antibiotic first to assist in maintaining standardized times and keep drug level within therapeutic range.
- Monitor for, document, and report adverse effects of prescribed antibiotic.
- Monitor for superinfection:
  - Candidiasis: vaginal yeast infection or oral thrush; is treated with appropriate anti-infective agent.
  - Pseudomembranous colitis: 4–6 or more watery stools per day, accompanied by blood and mucus in stools, abdominal cramps, and fever; usually caused by overgrowth of *clostridium difficile;* is treated with oral or IV metronidazole (Flagyl) or oral vancomycin; place client on contact precautions; original antibiotic is discontinued and another is selected.
- Maintain adequate fluid hydration and increase fluids if indicated (up to 3 liters daily) depending on antibiotic class.
- Ensure that client takes full course of therapy for full beneficial effects, even if signs of infection resolve; otherwise, microorganism regrowth and drug resistance can occur.
- Observe for evidence that infection is resolving with symptom improvement within 48–72 hours of beginning therapy (decreased temperature, WBC count, and local signs of infection); report to prescriber if infection is not resolving and prepare to do additional cultures as ordered.

NCLEX®
h. Maintain fluid hydration to protect kidneys; intake should be 2500 to 3000 mL/day unless contraindicated by other conditions
i. Provide small, frequent, nutritious meals with high-quality proteins; drugs may cause less GI upset if doses can be taken with food

7. Client education

NCLEX®
a. See general teaching points for antibiotic therapy (Box 41–3)
b. Keep liquid drug refrigerated if so recommended
c. Take oral drug with food if not contraindicated to reduce risk of GI upset
d. Eat small, frequent meals with at least 6 to 8 glasses of fluid a day

B. Cephalosporins

1. Action and use

a. Related to penicillins structurally and chemically, as well as in mechanism of action, drug actions, therapeutic effects, side and adverse effects, and drug interactions; **cross-sensitivity** may occur between penicillins and cephalosporins, meaning that allergy to one class may indicate hypersensitivity to the other in some clients
b. Four generations of cephalosporins exist with various uses but generally include Gram-negative organisms and anaerobes; fourth generation has increased activity against Gram-positive cocci and Gram-negative bacilli
c. Usually bactericidal
d. Used to treat sexually transmitted infections (STIs); respiratory infections such as bronchitis, pharyngitis, otitis media, sinusitis, and pneumonia; urinary tract infections (UTIs); skin and tissue infections; and Lyme disease

Box 41-3

General Client Teaching Points for Antibiotic Therapy

- Know drug, dose, purpose, route, and schedule of drug regimen.
- Take at evenly spaced intervals around the clock without disrupting sleep to maintain serum levels.
- Take with food, if not contraindicated, to minimize GI upset.
- If medication must be taken on empty stomach, take 1 hour before or 2 hours after a meal.
- Ensure adequate fluid intake of 2000–3000 mL fluid intake daily if not contraindicated by heart failure, kidney disease, or other condition.
- If using liquid preparation, use calibrated measuring device rather than household measurement (kitchen teaspoons can vary by 2 to 10 mL).
- Know side and adverse effects of drug and which ones require notification of prescriber.
- Report signs of possible superinfection: sore throat or white patches in mouth (candida), or watery stools more often than 4–6 times per day (pseudomembranous colitis).
- Before taking any over-the-counter (OTC) drugs, check efficacy and possible adverse reactions with prescriber.
- Take full course of therapy as ordered; do not discontinue drug on own even if feeling better and symptoms have resolved; do not "save" medication for future illnesses.
- Do not take drugs with expired date; discard any drug that is not used (full course of therapy should be taken).
- Report to prescriber if symptoms aren't resolving or not feeling better after 48–72 hours.

e. Used prophylactically and therapeutically in orthopedic disorders; cefazolin (Ancef) is drug of choice to prevent or treat bone infections associated with orthopedic surgery
f. Used for endocarditis prophylaxis before surgery in clients with history of rheumatic heart disease
g. Important to reserve use for appropriate clinical infections because bacterial resistance is increasing
h. Most cephalosporins are excreted through urine; exceptions are cefoperazone (Cefobid) and ceftriaxone (Rocephin), which are excreted in bile

2. Common medications are listed in Box 41–4

Memory Aid

Recognize a cephalosporin by the prefix or root *cef-* or *ceph-*.

3. Administration considerations
a. Well absorbed from GI tract; do not readily enter CSF except for cefuroxime; third-generation drugs readily enter CSF in presence of meningeal inflammation
b. Check renal function before and during therapy; renal impairment significantly extends drug half-life; use extreme caution if creatine clearance is less than 50 mL/min
c. Crosses placenta
d. Separate oral administration of antacids, H_2-receptor antagonists, iron supplements, and foods fortified with iron by 2 hours before and after oral doses
e. Intramuscular administration is painful and irritating; administer deep IM into large muscle; avoid repeated IM injections; IV is preferred parenteral route
f. Shake suspensions to disperse or dissolve particles of drug immediately before measurement
g. Continue therapy for at least 10 days to decrease risk of rheumatic fever in beta-hemolytic streptococcal bacterial infections such as strep throat; also, acute glomerulonephritis can become a sequela of this infection if treatment is inadequate

Box 41–4

Cephalosporins

First-generation cephalosporins

Cefadroxil (Duricef)

Cefazolin (Ancef, Kefzol)

Cephalexin (Keflex)

Cephradine (Velosef)

Second-generation cephalosporins

Cefaclor (Ceclor)

Cefotetan (Cefotan)

Cefoxitin (Mefoxin)

Cefprozil (Cefzil)

Cefuroxime (Ceftin, Zinacef)

Third-generation cephalosporins

Cefdinir (Omnicef)

Cefditoren (Spectracef)

Cefixime (Suprax)

Cefoperazone (Cefobid)

Cefotaxime (Claforan)

Cefpodoxime (Vantin)

Ceftazidime (Fortaz, Tazicef)

Ceftibuten (Cedax)

Ceftizoxime (Cefizox)

Ceftriaxone (Rocephin)

Fourth-generation cephalosporins

Cefepime (Maxipime)

h. Contraindications may include cross-sensitivity with penicillins; not recommended for those who have had a type I (anaphylactic) reaction to penicillin
i. Hepatotoxicity with cefoperazone and ceftriaxone
j. Caution in pregnancy and lactation

4. Side/adverse effects
   a. Central nervous system (CNS): lethargy, hallucinations, anxiety, depression, twitching, convulsions, coma
   b. GI: N/V, mild diarrhea, abdominal cramps or distress, elevated liver enzymes such as aspartate aminotransferase (AST) and alanine aminotransferase (ALT), abdominal pain, colitis; pseudomembranous colitis
   c. Hematologic: anemia, increased bleeding time, bone marrow depression, granulocytopenia
   d. Metabolic: hyperkalemia, hypokalemia, alkalosis
   e. Other: taste alteration, sore mouth; dark, discolored, or sore tongue; hives, pruritis, rash, edema
   NCLEX® **f.** Hypersensitivity occurs in 5–16% of clients; cross-sensitivity with penicillins occurs
   g. Serum sickness–like illness: usually follows second course of treatment and is noted by erythema multiforme and other skin rashes, arthralgia, and fever; treated with antihistamines and corticosteroids
   h. Seizure activity: especially in renal impairment; discontinue drug to resolve
   i. Increased risk for coagulation disturbances with coexisting renal impairment, cancer, malnutrition, impaired vitamin K synthesis or low vitamin K stores when given parenterally
   j. Use of alcohol with some cephalosporins such as cefoperazone and cefotetan can cause disulfiram-like reaction during therapy and up to 72 hours after drug is discontinued; can occur within 30 minutes of alcohol ingestion; manifestations include weakness, pulsating headache, and abdominal cramps
5. Nursing considerations as per Box 41–2
   a. Monitor injection site for induration and tenderness; provide warm compresses and gentle massage to site if painful or swollen; if phlebitis or redness at IV site develops, remove IV device and restart IV
   b. Monitor for renal toxicity: check serum creatinine, BUN, urine creatinine clearance; keep accurate I&O
   c. Monitor for unusual lethargy beginning after drug started; provide safety measures, including adequate lighting, use of side rails, and assistance with ambulation to protect client if CNS effects occur
   NCLEX® **d.** For client with diabetes mellitus, use blood glucose monitoring; false-positive urine glucose can occur with copper sulfate technique (Clinitest)
   e. Offer small, frequent meals with quality protein as tolerated
   f. Provide frequent oral care; offer ice chips or sugarless candy if stomatitis and sore mouth occur
   g. Monitor for increased bleeding if taking anticoagulants
   h. Monitor for hemolytic anemia (rare): check RBCs with indices, fatigue or weakness, jaundice (in dark-skinned clients, check hard palate)

6. Client education as per Box 41–3
   a. Take safety precautions, including changing position slowly and avoiding driving and hazardous tasks, if CNS effects occur
   NCLEX® b. Drink fluids and maintain nutrition, especially protein, to ensure adequate protein for drug binding and efficacy of action
   c. Shake suspensions well to dispense or dissolve particles of drug immediately before measurement; use a measuring device for liquid/suspension and not a kitchen teaspoon (may vary from 2 to 10 mL/teaspoon)
   NCLEX® d. Report manifestations of hypersensitivity to health care provider: difficulty breathing, severe rash, hives, severe headache, dizziness or weakness, aching joints
   e. Report side effects to prescriber: anorexia, epigastric pain, N/V indicating biliary sludge or pseudolithiasis if on ceftriaxone; discontinue drug and manifestations will resolve
   f. Do not drink alcohol during therapy and for 72 hours after drug is discontinued to avoid disulfiram-like reaction

C. Fluoroquinolones

1. Action and use
   a. Newer class of broad-spectrum bactericidal antibiotics
   b. Used against Gram-negative and selected Gram-positive organisms; used in various bacterial infections: lower respiratory tract infections, sinusitis, bone and joint infections, infectious diarrhea, UTIs, skin and soft tissue infections, intra-abdominal infections, and STIs
   c. Many oral formulations are as effective as parenteral forms
2. Common medications are listed in Box 41–5

Memory Aid Recognize a fluoroquinolone by the suffix *-oxacin*.

3. Administration considerations
   a. Administer around the clock, evenly spaced, to maintain therapeutic blood level; avoid interrupting sleep if possible
   b. Oral drug is tolerated better with food
   c. Use cautiously in clients with renal dysfunction, advanced age, children, pregnant or lactating women, and those with history of seizures
   d. Elimination of caffeine is decreased with ciprofloxacin (Cipro), enoxacin (Penetrex), and norfloxacin (Noroxin)
4. Side/adverse effects
   a. Headache, dizziness, fatigue, lethargy, insomnia, depression, restlessness, confusion, and seizure
   b. N/V, diarrhea, constipation, flatulence, epigastric distress, oral candidiasis, dysphagia, pseudomembranous colitis, and elevated liver enzymes (ALT, AST, bilirubin, alkaline phosphatase)
   c. Rash, pruritus, urticaria, photosensitivity, flushing
   d. Fever, chills, piloerection, blurred vision, tinnitus
   e. Hypersensitivity reaction
5. Nursing considerations as per Box 41–2
   a. Separate drug from oral antacids, iron and zinc salts, or sucralfate by 2 hours
   NCLEX® b. Monitor PT, INR, and increased bleeding or bruising if also on oral anticoagulants

Box 41–5 Fluoroquinolones

First Generation	Third Generation
Cinoxacin (Cinobac)	Gatifloxacin (Tequin)
Nalidixic acid (NegGram)	Levofloxacin (Levaquin)
Second Generation	**Fourth Generation**
Ciprofloxacin (Cipro)	Gemifloxacin (Factive)
Norfloxacin (Noroxin)	Moxifloxacin (Avelox)
Ofloxacin (Floxin)	

c. Monitor renal function
d. Provide more frequent meals with complete or complementary proteins to better ensure adequate albumin levels for drug efficacy
e. Monitor for increased CNS irritability if client has history of epilepsy, alcohol abuse, or is concurrently taking theophylline
f. Maintain hydration with 3 L fluid/day, if not contraindicated

6. Client education as per Box 41–3
a. Take safety precautions including changing position slowly and avoiding driving and hazardous tasks if CNS effects occur
b. Drink fluids and maintain nutrition, especially protein, to provide adequate protein for drug-binding and drug efficacy
c. Report difficulty breathing, severe headache, dizziness, weakness to prescriber
d. Baseline electrocardiogram may be necessary if client receives sparfloxacin or moxifloxacin
NCLEX® e. Wear sunglasses, long-sleeves and long-legged garments, and hat to protect from direct sunlight; sunscreen or sunblock may not prevent photosensitivity reaction; avoid ultraviolet lights, tanning beds, and direct sunlight

D. Macrolides and lincosamides

1. Action and use
a. **Bacteriostatic** (inhibiting bacterial growth) but can be bactericidal in high doses with some bacteria
b. Highly protein-bound
c. Action is similar to other antibiotics
d. Used in upper and lower respiratory tract infections, skin and soft tissue infections caused by *Streptococcus* or *Haemophilus* organisms
e. Used to treat syphilis, gonorrhea, chlamydia, Lyme disease, and *mycoplasma, listeria,* and *corynebacterium* infections
f. Clarithromycin (Biaxin) is used with omeprazole (Prilosec) to treat *Helicobacter pylori* associated with peptic ulcers
g. Lincosamides may be bactericidal and bacteriostatic; used to treat chronic bone infections, genitourinary (GU) infections, intra-abdominal infections, pneumonia, and streptococcal or staphylococcal septicemia

2. Common medications are listed in Box 41–6

3. Administration considerations
a. If erythromycin form has bitter taste, give with juice or applesauce; give with food to reduce GI irritating effects
b. Give clindamycin (Cleocin) and lincomycin (Lincocin) with at least 8 ounces of fluid or on an empty stomach
c. If clindamycin (Cleocin) is given IV, do not give by intravenous push (IVP) method; instead, give by IV infusion
d. Zithromax: longer half-life with less frequent dosing, shorter term of therapy, and fewer or less intense GI side effects (may enhance compliance)
e. Contraindicated with hypersensitivity, ulcerative colitis/enteritis (lincosamides), and children under 1 year (lincosamides)
f. Use caution with liver or renal dysfunction, GI disorders, older adults, and pregnant or lactating women

4. Side/adverse effects
a. Stimulation of smooth muscle and GI motility results in diarrhea (may be used therapeutically as a GI stimulant to facilitate passage of intestinal tube or to prevent gastroesophageal reflux)
b. Palpitations and chest pain
c. Headache, dizziness, vertigo, lethargy, somnolence, confusion, hearing loss usually preceded by tinnitus
d. Stomatitis, flatulence, epigastric distress, anorexia, N/V, abnormal taste (clarithromycin/Biaxin)

Box 41–6

Macrolides and Lincosamides

Azithromycin (Zithromax, Z-Pak)	Clindamycin (Cleocin)
Clarithromycin (Biaxin)	Lincomycin (Lincocin)
Dirithromycin (Dynabac)	Telithromycin (Ketek)
Erythromycin (E-Mycin, Erythrocin)	

e. Jaundice, rash, pruritis, urticaria
f. Thrombophlebitis at peripheral IV site
g. Toxicities: hepatotoxicity, nephrotoxicity, and ototoxicity (erythromycin)
h. Superinfections such as pseudomembranous colitis, candidiasis

5. Nursing considerations as per Box 41–2
   a. Collect data such as age, hypersensitivity to drugs, hepatic and renal function; also check cardiac status if appropriate for prescribed drug
   b. Monitor GI function and elimination pattern; monitor for superinfections
   c. Observe for bleeding if taking oral anticoagulants
   d. Monitor ALT, AST, bilirubin, and alkaline phosphatase as indicated for hepatic dysfunction before and during therapy
   e. Monitor serum creatinine, BUN, creatinine clearance, I&O as appropriate for development of renal dysfunction
   f. Determine baseline hearing and monitor for hearing loss; arrange for discontinuation of drug if hearing loss occurs
   g. Hydrate with at least 2000–2400 mL/day if not contraindicated
6. Client education as per Box 41–3; include protein in diet because these drugs are highly protein bound and require protein for therapeutic efficacy

E. Penicillins (beta-lactams) and penicillinase-resistants

1. Action and use
   a. Derived from fungus or mold evidenced on bread or fruit
   b. Similarities exist among penicillins, cephalosporins, monobactams, carbapenems, and beta-lactamase inhibitors; they share many actions and uses; cross-sensitivity is possible
   c. Most effective against Gram-positive organisms; less effective against Gram-negative ones
   d. Used to treat infections caused by meningococci, pneumococci, streptococci, treponema pallidum, staphylococci such as in upper respiratory infections, pneumonia, STIs such as syphilis but not gonorrhea, wound infections, and UTI
   e. Used prophylactically against endocarditis for oral, GI, pulmonary procedures when bacteria may enter circulation; usually amoxicillin (Amoxil) or ampicillin (Omnipen) are used
   f. Used in beta-hemolytic streptococci Group A infections associated with rheumatic fever or acute glomerulonephritis, such as pharyngitis; penicillin V often used with PO route preferred
   g. Increasing resistance developing, especially in facility-acquired or nosocomial infections
2. Common medications are listed in Box 41–7

Memory Aid

Recognize a penicillin by the suffix *-cillin*.

3. Administration considerations
   a. Oral dosing needs to be 3 to 4 times greater than parenteral dose because of hepatic first-pass effect and instability of penicillin in acid environment of stomach
   b. For serious systemic infections, parenteral route is recommended

Box 41–7

Penicillins (Beta-Lactams) and Penicillinase-Resistants

Amoxicillin (Amoxil)	Carbenicillin (Geocillin)
Amoxicillin/clavulanate (Augmentin)	Mezlocillin (Mezlin)
Ampicillin (Principen)	Cloxacillin (Cloxapen)
Ampicillin/sulbactam (Unasyn)	Dicloxacillin
Bacampicillin (Spectrobid)	Methicillin (Staphcillin)
Piperacillin	Nafcillin
Piperacillin/tazobactam (Zosyn)	Oxacillin
Ticarcillin (Ticar)	Penicillin G (Bicillin)
Ticarcillin/clavulanate (Timentin)	Penicillin V (V-Cillin)

c. Absorption erratic from IM route; limit due to irritability of tissue; IM injection should be slow and steady over 12–15 seconds to minimize discomfort and prevent needle obstruction, especially with thick preparations
d. Nafcillin (Unipen): IV extravasation can cause necrosis; avoid IM route or, if not possible, inject by Z-track method
e. Contraindicated with hypersensitivity reaction and anaphylaxis, serum sickness, exfoliative dermatitis, blood dyscrasias
f. Penicillin G procaine or benzathine not to be given IV: lethal
g. Most likely drug category to cause allergic reactions
h. Use caution in anemia, thrombocytopenia, bone marrow depression, and concurrently with anticoagulants because some penicillins cause increased bleeding

4. Side/adverse effects

NCLEX®
a. Most common allergic responses are skin rash, urticaria, pruritis, angioedema; a maculopapular, pruritic rash that is like measles with ampicillin or amoxocillin is not a true allergic reaction but develops after 7–10 days of therapy and may last several days after discontinuing penicillin; is not a contraindication to give drug in future

NCLEX®
b. Most common adverse effects are GI, such as N/V, diarrhea, epigastric distress, abdominal pain, colitis, elevated liver enzymes; also taste alteration, sore mouth, or dark, discolored, sore tongue
c. Anemia, bone marrow suppression, granulocytopenia, increased bleeding time
d. Lethargy, anxiety, depression, hallucinations, twitching, convulsions, coma
e. Hypokalemia or hyperkalemia, metabolic alkalosis

NCLEX®
f. Type I hypersensitivity often fatal immediately if untreated within 2 to 30 minutes; noted by urticaria, pruritis, severe dyspnea, stridor, tachycardia, hypotension, diaphoresis, vertigo, loss of consciousness and circulatory collapse
g. Serum sickness–like reaction: skin rash, arthralgia, fever
h. Exfoliative dermatitis: red, scaly skin

NCLEX®
5. Nursing considerations as per Box 41–2
a. Monitor renal studies, liver enzymes, and electrolytes; many of the penicillins contain sodium salts that can result in hypokalemia
b. Monitor for adverse effects; may not be necessary to discontinue penicillin if mild diarrhea develops; give yogurt or buttermilk to restore normal flora; use absorbent antidiarrheal agents (kaolin and pectin [Kao-Tin]); avoid antiperistaltic agents that delay or prevent elimination of intestinal toxins
c. Provide adequate nutrition and hydration
d. Some penicillins cause false-positive results on urine glucose testing; use blood glucose monitoring

6. Client education as per Box 41–3
a. Take oral drug on empty stomach, 1 hour before meals or 2 hours after meals, except amoxicillin (not affected by food)
b. Chewable tablets must be crushed or chewed for penicillin to be effectively absorbed

NCLEX®
c. Shake suspensions to disperse particles before measuring; use a calibrated device; most suspensions maintain potency for 14 days if refrigerated
d. Ensure antibiotic drops are used for correct route: oral, eye, ear
e. Take missed doses as soon as possible; do not double dose if one missed

NCLEX®
f. Report rash, urticaria, pruritis, difficulty breathing
g. Eat small, frequent meals with high-quality protein and drink 6–8 glasses or more of water per day if not contraindicated by other conditions

F. Sulfonamides

1. Action and use
a. First effective group of antibiotics; bacteriostatic
b. Used to treat UTIs (especially caused by *Escherichia coli,* most common cause of cystitis), *Chlamydia trachomatis* causing blindness, pneumonia, brain abscesses, mild to moderate ulcerative colitis, active Crohn's disease, and RA drugs of choice for treatment of nocardiosis
c. Silver sulfadiazine (Silvadene) and mafenide (Sulfamylon) prevent bacterial growth in burns and wounds
d. Cross-sensitivity possible with penicillins and cephalosporins

2. Common medications are listed in Box 41–8

Memory Aid

Recognize a sulfonamide by the root *sulf* in the drug name.

Box 41–8

Sulfonamides

Systemic	**Topicals**
Sulfisoxazole (Gantrisin)	Silver sulfadiazine (Silvadene)
Sulfadiazine	Sulfacetamide
Sulfamethoxazole–Trimethoprim (Bactrim)	Mafenide (Sulfamylon)
Sulfasalazine (Azulfidine)	

3. Administration considerations
   a. Provide fluid intake of 3000–4000 mL/day to promote urine output of at least 1500 mL/day to prevent crystalluria/stone formation; if not possible, antacids or sodium bicarbonate may alkalinize urine; alkaline ash diet may help, which includes fruit (except plums, prunes, and cranberries), vegetables, and milk
   b. Store in light-resistant, tightly closed container at room temperature
4. Contraindications
   a. History of hypersensitivity to sulfonamides, and possibly salicylates, penicillins, cephalosporins
   b. In lactation and children younger than 2 months unless used to treat congenital toxoplasmosis
   c. In porphyria, advanced or severe renal or hepatic dysfunction, or with intestinal and urinary blockage; use cautiosly in impaired renal or hepatic function, asthma, blood dyscrasias, or glucose-6-phosphate dehydrogenase (G6PD) deficiency
5. Side/adverse effects
   a. Rash common; most are urticaria and maculopapular
   NCLEX® b. N/V, diarrhea, abdominal pain, jaundice, stomatitis, crystalluria
   c. Headache, insomnia, drowsiness, depression, psychosis, photosensitivity
   d. Hepatitis, pancreatitis, blood dyscrasias
   NCLEX® e. Exfoliative dermatitis, Stevens-Johnson syndrome (an adverse reaction of skin that resembles appearance of partial thickness burns)
   f. Serum sickness, drug fever
6. Nursing considerations as per Box 41–2
   a. Check baseline laboratory tests for liver and renal function, and monitor during therapy
   NCLEX® b. Hydration to assure daily urine output of 1500 mL or more to prevent crystalluria; alkalinize urine as indicated; keep accurate I&O record
   c. Provide small, frequent, nutritious meals with high-quality proteins; drugs that may be taken with food may decrease GI upset
7. Client education as per Box 41–3
   a. Take with food, if not contraindicated, to minimize GI upset
   b. Eat small, frequent meals with at least 2500 to 3000 mL fluid intake a day
   c. Empty bladder frequently, such as every 2 hours while awake
   NCLEX® d. Report flank or suprapubic pain, increased dysuria, disruption of skin integrity to health care provider

G. Tetracyclines

1. Action and use
   a. Broad spectrum; bacteriostatic; can be bactericidal in high concentrations
   b. Effective against most chlamydia, mycoplasmas, rickettsiae, cholera, and certain protozoa
   c. Suppress *Proprionibacterium acnes* in treating acne; topical or oral forms may be used for severe acne
   d. Used prophylactically for traveler's diarrhea
   e. Used to treat Rocky Mountain Spotted Fever, **amebiasis** (a protozoan infection), brucellosis, shigellosis, cholera, tetanus, chronic bronchitis, Lyme disease
   f. Used to treat syphilis and gonorrhea in clients with penicillin allergy
   g. Used as a sclerosing agent for pleural and pericardial effusion, such as in cancer metastasis; causes inflammation resulting in fibrosis, leaving scar tissue that does not allow fluid to accumulate
   h. Used in *Helicobacter pylori* peptic ulcer disease, Q fever, Rickettsia pox, typhus, Mycoplasma pneumonia, epididymo-orchitis, pelvic inflammatory disease (PID)
   i. Used with quinine for treatment of malaria
   j. Treat syndrome of inappropriate antidiuretic hormone (SIADH) with demeclocyline (Declomycin) by inhibiting antidiuretic hormone (ADH)
2. Common medications (generic name ends in *-cycline*; see Box 41–9)

Box 41–9

Tetracyclines

Demeclocycline (Declomycin)	Tetracycline (Sumycin, others)
Doxycycline (Vibramycin, others)	Tigecycline (Tygacil)
Minocycline (Minocin, others)	

Memory Aid

Recognize a tetracycline by the suffix *-cycline* in the drug name.

3. Administration considerations
   - **a.** Avoid administering outdated drug: Fanconi-like syndrome with polyuria, polydipsia, N/V, glycosuria, proteinuria, acidosis can occur; renal tubular dysfunction and lupus erythematosus–like syndrome have occurred and are attributed to preparations used beyond expiration date
   - **b.** Oral: give with full glass of water on empty stomach at least 1 hour before or 2 hours after meals; food, and milk products decrease absorption by half
   - **c.** IM injection contains procaine; check for allergies to local anesthetics ending with *-caine*
   - **d.** Administer deep IM into large muscle such as the gluteus; alternate sites; do not administer IV
   - **e.** If topical, clean area with soap and water, rinse and dry well prior to application
   - NCLEX® **f.** Tetracyclines bind to calcium, preventing normal bone growth and causing tooth hypoplasia in developing fetus or child younger than 8 years old; contraindicated during last half of pregnancy when tooth development occurs, from birth to 8 years of age, and in lactating women
   - **g.** Use caution with renal or liver dysfunction, allergy, asthma, hay fever, urticaria, or in myasthenia gravis
4. Side/adverse effects
   - **a.** N/V, diarrhea, epigastric or abdominal discomfort, flatulence, dry mouth, bulky or loose stools
   - **b.** Headache, photosensitivity, dizziness
   - **c.** Maculopapular rash, urticaria, exfoliative dermatitis, angioedema
   - **d.** Stinging/burning with topical application
   - **e.** Discoloration of developing teeth
   - **f.** Drug fever, serum sickness, and anaphylaxis
   - NCLEX® **g.** Hepatotoxicity; nephrotoxicity in clients with preexisting renal disease
   - **h.** Topical application can cause stinging and burning; allergic reaction is possible
5. Nursing considerations as per Box 41–2
   - **a.** Monitor for history of renal or liver problems and related laboratory results
   - **b.** Monitor I&O
6. Client education as per Box 41–3
   - NCLEX® **a.** Unstable with age and light exposure; store in tightly covered container in dry area, protected from light at room temperature
   - **b.** Report side effects, particularly severe diarrhea
   - **c.** Practice good oral care and hygiene
   - NCLEX® **d.** Avoid exposure to direct sunlight or ultraviolet light or tanning beds; wear hat, long sleeves, long-legged pants, and sunglasses outside during and for a few days after treatment; sunscreen or sunblock may not prevent erythema
   - **e.** Take oral doses with full glass of water on empty stomach (1 hour before or 2 hours after meal or dairy product) to promote absorption and decrease risk of esophagitis; report sudden dysphagia to prescriber
   - **f.** Topical form may stain clothing or cause affected skin to reflect yellow or green fluorescence under an ultraviolet or "black" light

H. Urinary tract antiseptics

1. Action and use: drugs that act against bacteria in urine (UTIs) but have little or no systemic antibacterial effects
2. Common medications are listed in Box 41–10

Box 41–10

Urinary Tract Antiseptics

Fosfomycin (Monourol)	Nalidixic acid (NegGram)
Methenamine mandelate (Mandelamine)	Nitrofurantoin (Furadantin)
Methenamine hippurate (Hiprex)	

3. Administration considerations
   a. Use caution with impaired renal and/or hepatic function and during lactation and pregnancy
   b. Controversial if pH of urine has any effect on UTI
   c. Alkaline ash diet may interfere with the required acidity of urine for antiseptic action; alkaline ash foods include fruits (except cranberries, prunes, plums), milk, vegetables

   NCLEX® d. Acid ash foods that may or may not increase urine acidity include meat, cheese, eggs, whole grains, as well as cranberries, prunes, and plums

   NCLEX® e. Fluids that may acidify urine and potentially facilitate drug action include cranberry and prune juice
4. Side/adverse effects
   a. N/V, anorexia, diarrhea, epigastric distress
   b. Rash, pruritus, photosensitivity, photophobia, tinnitus, insomnia, headache, dizziness, drowsiness
   c. Low back pain, dysuria
   d. Nitrofurantoin: urine may become brown
5. Nursing considerations as per Box 41–2
   a. Monitor for previous renal or liver dysfunction
   b. Encourage at least 3000 mL/day fluids, including cranberry juice, if not contraindicated by fluid restriction or other conditions
   c. Monitor urine pH at bedside with test strip as indicated
   d. Give medication with or after food to limit GI adverse effects
6. Client education as per Box 41–3
   a. Take with or after food to minimize GI distress

   NCLEX® b. Drink at least 3 liters of fluid a day, including cranberry and prune juice, unless contraindicated by other conditions

   c. Include acid ash foods in diet (cranberries, prunes, plums, cheese, eggs, meat, whole grains); limit alkaline ash foods (citrus fruits and juices, vegetables)
   d. Do not take other medications unless approved by prescriber; avoid drugs that may alkalinize urine, such as antacids, Alka-Seltzer
   e. Nalidixic acid (NegGram) can cause photophobia; avoid bright sunlight, wear sunglasses, and report visual disturbances; photosensitivity can also occur several weeks after drug is discontinued so avoid direct sunlight or ultraviolet light
   f. Nitrofurantoin may cause urine to be brown; may stain clothing
   g. Do not drive or perform hazardous tasks if drowsiness or dizziness occurs
   h. If diabetic, urine glucose test with Clinitest can yield a false-positive result; test blood glucose

I. Miscellaneous antibiotics are listed in Box 41–11

1. Quinupristin/dalfopristin (Synercid): used to treat bacteremia and life-threatening infections caused by vancomycin-resistant *Enterococcus faecium* (VREF); also complicated skin and skin structure infections
   a. Administration considerations: IV use only, preferably via central line
   b. Side/adverse effects: arthralgias, myalgias (possibly severe); with peripheral IV administration, frequently pain, inflammation, edema, and thrombophlebitis
   c. Nursing considerations and client education: same as for other antibiotics
2. Vancomycin (Vancocin): bactericidal; parenteral antibiotic of choice for methicillin-resistant *Staphylococcus aureus* (MRSA) and other Gram-positive bacteria, yeast, and fungi; antibiotic-induced pseudomembranous colitis caused by *Clostridium difficile* and staphylococcal enterocolitis (oral drug form)

Box 41–11

Miscellaneous Antibiotics

Generic/Trade Names

Monobactam

Aztreonam (Azactam)

Carbapenems

Doripenem (Doribax)

Imipenem/Cilastatin (Primaxin)

Ertapenem (Invanz)

Meropenem (Merrem)

Ketolide

Telithromycin (Ketek)

Streptogramin

Quinupristin/dalfopristin (Synercid)

Other

Daptomycin (Cubicin)

Metronidazole (Flagyl)

Vancomycin (Vancocin)

NCLEX® a. Administration considerations: poorly absorbed from GI tract so indicated for local surface-infected areas of GI tract; IV dose should be through a central venous access device (CVAD) because of high risk for phlebitis; can cause necrosis if it extravasates

b. Side/adverse effects: nausea, hypotension, flushing; pain and thrombophlebitis at injection site; ototoxicity, nephrotoxicity, temporary leukopenia; "red neck (or man) syndrome": too rapid IV infusion results in profound hypotension, erythematous rash on face, neck, upper chest, and arms

NCLEX® c. Nursing considerations: as for other antibiotics; give IV dose over 60 to 90 minutes to avoid hypotension and red neck syndrome

d. Client education: as for other antibiotics; also, if client is receiving IV therapy in home, ensure appropriate knowledge and ability to perform procedures correctly, including monitoring BP and heart rate

3. Carbapenems
   a. May be used in serious infections of urinary tract, lower respiratory tract, bones, joints, skin and skin structures; intraabdominal, gynecologic, and mixed infections
   b. Meropenem (Merrem) is used in bacterial meningitis because of its ability to enter CSF, especially if inflammation is present
   c. Administration considerations: preparations are specific for IM or for IV use; do not interchange; give IM deep into gluteal muscle
   d. Contraindicated with known hypersensitivities to components of drugs or penicillins or cephalosporins; also allergy to amide local anesthetics
   e. Side/adverse effects: headache, dizziness, mental changes, somnolence, tremors, paresthesia, heartburn, N/V, diarrhea, glossitis, rash, urticaria, candidiasis, flushing, sweating, facial edema, fever, pain/phlebitis at injection site, hyperkalemia, hyponatremia, polyuria, oliguria, weakness, arthralgias
   f. Nursing considerations and client education: same as for other antibiotics; eat meals with high-quality protein; drink at least 6–8 glasses of fluids a day
4. Aztreonam: a cell wall inhibitor with a beta lactam ring but does not have cross-sensitivity to penicillins or cephalosporins; given by parenteral route; adverse effects include N/V, diarrhea, candidiasis, pain at injection site; anaphylaxis and pseudomemebranous colitis are rare
5. Telithromycin: a ketolide (new class) similar to macrolides; used primarily for respiratory infections, including those resistant to macrolides; most adverse effects are minor and GI-related, but can cause hepatotoxicity and visual disturbances
6. Metronidazole (Flagyl): active against bacteria and multicellular parasites; antibacterial uses include anaerobic infections and peptic ulcer disease; resistance is rare; adverse effects include nausea, dry mouth, headache; neurotoxicity can occur in high doses

VII. ANTIMYCOBACTERIALS

A. Antituberculins

1. Action and use
   a. Inhibit cell wall synthesis, protein synthesis, RNA synthesis; effects limited primarily to *Mycobacterium tuberculosis* and other mycobacterium strains
   b. Primary use is prophylaxis or treatment of pulmonary tuberculosis and extrapulmonary tuberculosis in adults and children
   c. Used to prevent or delay onset of *Mycobacterium avium* bacteremia in clients with acquired immunodeficiency syndrome (AIDS) in combination with another antituberculin antibiotic
   d. Rifampin also eradicates meningococci from nasopharynx of asymptomatic *Neisseria meningitides* carriers when there is increased risk for infection outbreaks in a community, and is used prophylactically with exposure to *Haemophilus influenzae* type B (HIB) infection
   e. Antituberculins are used in combination to treat leprosy, endocarditis with methicillin-resistant staphylococci, chronic prostatitis with staphylococcal organisms, and anti-infective-resistant pneumococci
2. Common medications are listed in Box 41–12
3. Administration considerations
   a. Effectiveness depends on correct drug, correct combination therapy, adequate dosing and duration of therapy, and compliance
   b. See Box 41–13 for typical treatment regimens; second-line agents are less effective and have greater toxicity, and are used when resistance develops to first-line agents
   c. Multicombination drug therapy decreases risk or rate of developing resistance to any single drug
   d. Give isoniazid 1 hour before meals on empty stomach
   e. Contraindications: hypersensitivity to drug, hepatic or renal damage, use caution in pregnancy unless risk is significant

Box 41–12

Antituberculin Drugs

First-Line Agents

Ethambutol (Myambutol)

Isoniazid (INH, Nydrazid)

Pyrazinamide (PZA)

Rifabutin (Mycobutin)

Rifampin (Rifadin)

Rifapentine (Priftin)

Second-Line Agents

Aminosalicylic acid (Paser)

Amikacin (Amikin)

Capreomycin (Capastat Sulfate)

Ciprofloxacin (Cipro)

Cycloserine (Seromycin)

Ethionamide (Trecator-SC)

Kanamycin (Kantrex)

Ofloxacin (Floxin)

Streptomycin

Box 41–13

Drug Treatment Regimens for Tuberculosis

Standard Regimen

- Initial Phase. Daily therapy for 2 months with first line agents: isoniazid, rifampin, pyrazinamide and ethambutol; ethambutol is later dropped if C&S shows strain is sensitive to first 3 drugs
- Continuation phase. Isoniazid and rifampin given 2–3 times per week for 4 months

Chemoprophylaxis Regimens

- Nine months of therapy with isoniazid (standard treatment); dosing is daily or twice weekly depending on anticipated adherence
- Two months of therapy with rifampin and pyrazinamide; improves adherence and eliminates most strains
- Four months of therapy with rifampin; used if unable to take isoniazid or pyrazinamide or for organisms resistant to these drugs

f. Caution in renal or liver dysfunction, history of seizures, ethanol abuse

g. Caution in older clients, children, diabetics, those with gout or blood dyscrasias, and optic neuritis or defects

4. Side/adverse effects

a. Fairly well tolerated; N/V, anorexia, constipation, diarrhea, dyspepsia

b. Headache, dizziness, malaise, fever, chills, arthralgia, flu-like symptoms, weakness

c. Skin rash, dry skin, photophobia, photosensitivity, vision changes

d. Dysrhythmias

e. Urinary retention (in males)

NCLEX® f. Change in color to orange-red of excretions/secretions such as urine, tears, feces, perspiration (with rifampin and rifabutin)

Memory Aid

Remember the *r* for rifampin can indicate a reddish-orange discoloration to body fluids.

g. Electrolyte imbalances

h. Metallic taste with ethionamide (Trecator-SC)

i. Disulfiram-like effect with alcohol ingestion

j. Nephrotoxicity or hepatotoxicity, or ototoxicity

Memory Aid

Remember the *H* in INH can stand for *H*epatotoxicity as an adverse drug effect.

k. Hematologic disorders: agranulocytosis, thrombocytopenia, eosinophilia, anemia
l. Seizures, depression, confusion, ataxia, paresis, paresthesias, drowsiness

5. Nursing considerations as per Box 41–2
   a. Monitor baseline and periodic liver and renal function, C&S results, CBC with WBC differential, RBC indices, and platelet count
   b. Screen for pregnancy
   c. Coadminister pyridoxine (vitamin B_6) and/or cyanocobalamin (vitamin B_{12})
   d. *NCLEX®* Encourage food high in B-complex vitamin (especially pyridoxine), such as meat (chicken, beef, and pork), liver, soybeans, baked potato with skin, raw avocado
   e. Evaluate compliance with therapy to lessen risk of reinfection, drug resistance
   f. Encourage adequate hydration and good nutrition with high-quality protein
6. Client education as per Box 41–3
   a. Take isoniazid (INH) 1 hour before meals
   b. Rifampin (Rifadin): may discolor urine, tears, saliva; may stain contact lens and undergarments
   c. Keep follow-up appointments with health care provider and for tests
   d. Use infection control measures to protect self and others
   e. Avoid alcohol because of increased risk for hepatitis or disulfiram-like effect
   f. Use alternative contraception during therapy and for at least 1 month after therapy is discontinued if using oral contraceptives
   g. For dry skin, use emollients or oils

B. Leprostatics

1. Action and use: treat leprosy and some AIDS-related opportunistic infections
2. Common medications dapsone (DDS) and clofazimine (Lamprene)
   a. Dapsone is bacteriostatic against *Mycobacterium leprae* and *tuberculosis, Pneumocystis carinii, Plasmodium*
   b. Clofazimine (Lamprene) is bactericidal against *Mycobacterium leprae* and *avium*
3. Administration considerations
   a. Give clofazimine with food
   b. Contraindicated with hypersensitivity to DDS and possible sulfonamides
   c. Use cautiously in clients with hepatic disease or G6PD deficiency (an inherited type of hemolytic anemia associated with stress or certain drug interactions)
   d. Not established for safe use in pregnant and lactating clients
4. Side/adverse effects
   a. Skin pigmentation changes (pink to brownish black); may resolve in weeks to months
   b. Dry skin, N/V, diarrhea, abdominal pain
   c. Headache, insomnia, malaise, paresthesias, nervousness, tinnitus, vertigo, vision changes
   d. Agranulocytosis, hepatotoxicity, phototoxicity
   e. Dose-related hemolysis (increased in G6PD deficiency)
   f. Methemoglobinemia (rhinitis, fatigue, difficulty breathing, cyanosis)
   g. Male infertility with DDS
5. Nursing considerations as per Box 41–2; monitor hemoglobin and reticulocyte count
6. Client education as per Box 41–3
   a. Take clofazimine with meals; skin discoloration may be pink to brownish-black; resolves in months to years after drug is discontinued
   b. Ensure infection control measures are used
   c. Encourage hydration and good nutrition with complete or complementary proteins for tissue healing

VIII. ANTIVIRALS

A. Medications to treat herpes and cytomegalovirus

1. Action and use
   a. Virustatic; drugs convert to compound that is a counterfeit nucleotide, which terminate developing viral DNA chain and results in cell death with help from host's immune system
   b. Drug has little effect on host cells; effective only during acute phase of infection, not latent phase; virus must be in living cell to survive and replicate
   c. Used to treat broad spectrum of diseases, including cold sores, viral encephalitis, shingles, and genital infection

d. Viruses include herpes simplex virus-1 (HSV-1) in oral herpes or herpes labialis, HSV-2 in genital herpes, herpes zoster in shingles, herpes varicella zoster virus (VZV) in chickenpox, and some Epstein-Barr viruses
e. Acyclovir (Zovirax) is drug of choice in herpes simplex encephalitis and frequently used for genital herpes; used prophylactically with immunosuppressed seropositive clients before bone marrow transplantation and after other organ transplants; not found to be beneficial in treating those who are not immunosuppressed, although it may help prevent shedding of virus
f. Ganciclovir (DHPG) is approved to treat only cytomegalovirus (CMV) retinitis in immunosuppressed clients; has good intraocular penetration; foscarnet (Foscavir) is used to treat ganciclovir-resistant CMV retinitis and shingles; cidofovir (Vistide) is also given IV for CMV retinitis
g. Trifluridine is used topically for herpes simplex keratoconjunctivitis
h. Valacyclovir (Valtrex), an improved oral form of acyclovir, is drug of choice for genital herpes
i. Penciclovir (Denavir) is used topically to treat herpes infections; is negligibly absorbed so is well tolerated and shortens pain and healing by one-half day
j. Cidofovir (Vistide) IV is used to treat CMV retinitis in clients with AIDS

2. Common medications are listed in Box 41–14

Memory Aid

Recognize an antiviral drug by the root *vir* in the drug name.

3. Administration considerations
   a. Hydrate client to decrease risk or extent of nephrotoxicity
   b. Administer as soon as possible to improve effectiveness
   c. Wear gloves for topical application to limit exposure to drug or lesions
   d. Preferred central venous access for IV administrations
   e. Foscarnet: precipitates with many drugs when used IV; use with D_5W or NaCl solutions
4. Contraindicated with hypersensitivity to drug; use caution in preexisting hepatic or renal dysfunction, concurrent use of nephrotoxic drugs, and in pregnant and lactating women
5. Side/adverse effects
   a. Anemia, neutropenia, headache, mood changes, seizures, N/V, diarrhea
   b. Local irritation including phlebitis at IV site
   c. Fever, hypocalcemia, hypomagnesemia, hypokalemia, metabolic acidosis, dysrhythmias
   d. Increased risk for CNS disturbances and fluid overload in clients with impaired hepatic or renal function
   e. Ocular hypotony
   f. Carcinogenic, embryotoxic
   g. Infertility in males and females: ganciclovir
   h. Nephrotoxicity, hepatoxicity; thrombocytopenic purpura; pancreatitis

NCLEX®

6. Nursing considerations
   a. Check allergies, including allergy to antiviral agents
   b. Determine baseline data to monitor effectiveness of drug and side effects
   c. Monitor for neutropenic infection if immunosuppressed

Box 41–14

Antivirals to Treat Herpes and Cytomegalovirus

Systemic Agents	Topical Agents
Acyclovir (Zovirax)	Docusanol (Abreva)
Cidofovir (Vistide)	Penciclovir (Denavir)
Famciclovir (Famvir)	Trifluridine (Viroptic)
Foscarnet (Foscavir)	
Ganciclovir (Cytovene)	
Valacyclovir (Valtrex)	
Valganciclovir (Valcyte)	

d. Monitor renal function: creatinine, BUN, creatinine clearance, I&O
e. Check hepatic function: ALT, AST, alkaline phosphatase, bilirubin
f. Collaborate with prescriber if reduced dosage needed for hepatic or renal disease
g. Monitor CBC with differential, CD4 count, platelet count for bone marrow activity and effectiveness of therapy
h. May exacerbate preexisting CNS disturbances; check orientation and reflexes; implement safety measures as indicated
i. Monitor skin and lesions regularly
j. Hydrate to decrease risk of nephrotoxicity (e.g., 2000–3000 mL/fluids per day) if not contraindicated by other conditions
k. Monitor relief of infection and of pain
l. Monitor nutritional status, especially if GI side effects occur; ensure adequate protein intake

7. Client education
a. Similar principles as in antibiotic therapy (Box 41–3); importance of completing full course of therapy with evenly distributed dosing that does not interrupt sleep (to improve effectiveness and prevent drug resistance)
b. Self-administration techniques if indicated
c. Clinical manifestations to report: severe side effects; increased bleeding, edema, fatigue; severe rash (especially if accompanied by blisters), fever, and other indications of infection
NCLEX® d. Avoid sexual intercourse if genital herpes being treated
NCLEX® e. Avoid touching lesions to avoid spreading infection to new sites
f. Avoid hazardous tasks and driving if drowsiness, dizziness, seizure activity occurs
g. Ensure client follows up with labs and appointments with prescriber
h. Offer frequent, small, high-protein meals; encourage 2000–3000 mL/day intake
NCLEX® i. Female clients should have annual Pap smear since there is increased risk of cervical cancer with genital herpes infection
j. Antiviral agents do not cure herpes and CMV infections
k. Notify prescriber if lesions do not heal or if they recur

B. Protease inhibitors

1. Most potent of antiviral agents; inhibit cell protein synthesis to interfere with viral replication
2. Not curative but slow progression of AIDS and prolong life
3. Used prophylactically because viral replication peaks before manifestations of infection emerge, which limits antiviral efficacy; increased risk for toxicity to host cell
4. Used in AIDS and AIDS-related complex (ARC) to decrease viral load and opportunistic infections
5. Used in combination to decrease viral load, increase CD4 counts, and decrease incidence or rate of development of drug resistance
6. Common medications are listed in Box 41–15
7. Administration considerations
a. Give saquinavir (Invirase) with high-fat meals or within 2 hours of full meal
b. Give ritonavir (Norvir) with chocolate milk, nutritional supplement, or food (ritonavir is unpalatable)
c. Indinavir (Crixivan) requires an acidic gastric environment for absorption, so give dose 1 hour before or 2 hours after a light, low-fat snack and client should drink 1.5 liters or more of fluid daily
d. Contraindicated in pregnant or lactating women, children, and hypersensitivity to drug
8. Side/adverse effects
a. Headache, fatigue, N/V, diarrhea, abdominal discomfort, anemia, taste perversion, asthenia, circumoral paresthesia with ritonavir
b. Reversible hyperbilirubinemia and nephrolithiasis with indinavir (Crixivan): 1.5 liters or more of fluid daily are needed to prevent nephrolithiasis
c. Hepatotoxicity; reduce dose in liver dysfunction

Box 41–15

Antivirals for HIV and AIDS: Protease Inhibitors

Atazanavir (Reyataz)	Nelfinavir (Viracept)
Darunavir (Prezista)	Ritonavir (Norvir)
Fosamprenavir (Lexiva)	Saquinavir (Invirase)
Indinavir (Crixivan)	Tipranavir (Aptivus)
Lopinavir/ritonavir (Kaletra)	

9. Nursing considerations
   a. Similar principles as for antibiotic therapy (Box 41–2)
   b. Monitor for hepatotoxicity: ALT, AST, alkaline phosphatase, bilirubin; observe for N/V, jaundice, enlarged or tender liver
   c. Monitor for nephrotoxicity: creatinine, BUN, creatinine clearance, urinalysis; keep accurate I&O
   d. Monitor CBC for blood dyscrasias such as neutropenia, thrombocytopenia, or anemia, and for improvement as evidenced by increased T-cell count
   e. Monitor for side effects; if neutropenic, observe for occult signs of infection (e.g., low back, flank, or suprapubic pain), normal temperature or low-grade fever related to UTI
   f. Saquinavir (Invirase): take with high-fat foods or within 2 hours of full meal
   g. Ritonavir (Norvir): take with chocolate milk, nutritional supplement, or food to counteract unpleasant taste
   h. Indinavir (Crixivan): take 1 hour before or 2 hours after light, low-fat snack; drink more than 1500 mL/day of fluids
   i. Provide neutropenic care as appropriate
10. Client education
   a. Similar principles as for antibiotic therapy (Box 41–3)
   b. Ensure fluid intake of at least 1500 mL/day
   c. Take with food: saquinavir (Invirase) (high-fat foods recommended) and ritonavir (unpalatable taste)
   d. Take 1 hour before or 2 hours after light, low-fat snack: indinavir
   e. Eat small, frequent meals with complete or complementary proteins
   f. Use neutropenic precautions

C. Reverse transcriptase inhibitors

1. Block viral reverse transcriptase; stops replication/growth; effectiveness diminishes over time
2. Used for all symptomatic HIV clients with a CD4 count less than 500/mm^3 and some with higher counts; possible prophylaxis for known occupational HIV exposure
3. Penetrates blood–brain barrier
4. AZT is used to prevent maternal transmission of HIV
5. A major advantage of nonnucleoside reverse transcriptase inhibitors (NNRTIs) is that they do not adversely affect development of blood cells
6. There is no cross-resistance between nucleoside reverse transcriptase inhibitors (NRTIs) and NNRTIs
7. Used in combination because resistant strains rapidly evolve if used alone
8. Common medications are listed in Box 41–16
9. Administration considerations
   a. Crush or chew buffered tablets that are chewable because drug has acid lability
   b. Food may slow absorption but does not affect total absorption
   c. May administer at bedtime for better tolerance of CNS adverse effects
   d. Contraindicated with concurrent use of drugs that cause peripheral neuropathy
10. Side/adverse effects
   a. Neurological side effects of insomnia, confusion, peripheral neuropathies (numbness and tingling of extremities), dizziness, anxiety, tremors, or seizures
   b. Diarrhea, pancreatitis, hypermagnesemia

Box 41–16

Antiviral Medications for HIV and AIDS: Reverse Transcriptase Inhibitors and Miscellaneous Drugs

Nucleoside Reverse Transcriptase Inhibitors

Abacavir sulfate (Ziagen)

Didanosine (DDI, Videx)

Emtricitabine (Emtriva)

Lamivudine (Epivir, 3TC)

Stavudine (Zerit, 4DT)

Zidovudine (AZT, Retrovir)

Nonnucleoside Reverse Transcriptase Inhibitors

Delavirdine (Rescriptor)

Efavirenz (Sustiva)

Etravirine (Intelence)

Nevirapine (Viramune)

Miscellaneous

Enfuvirtide (Fuzeon)

Raltegravir (Isentress)

Maraviroc (Selzentry)

c. Discolored fingernails, rash, myalgias, altered taste sensations, cough
d. Anemia, leukopenia, thrombocytopenia with nucleosides
e. Nevirapine (Viramune): severe hepatotoxicity and dermatologic effects such as Stevens-Johnson syndrome

11. Nursing considerations
   a. Similar principles as for other anti-infective drugs (Box 41–2)
   b. Monitor baseline and periodic renal and liver test results
   c. Ensure client takes complete course and all drugs included in the regimen to improve effectiveness and retard risk for resistant strains emerging
   d. Administer around the clock as needed to maintain therapeutic levels
   e. Stop administration if severe rash or other hypersensitivity reaction occurs
   f. Monitor client for complications of HIV infection (e.g., opportunistic infections, cancer, neurologic disease)
   g. Monitor level of consciousness (LOC), strength, appropriateness of activity, short-term memory, ability to follow complex commands, reasoning and calculation abilities, and peripheral sensation
   h. Provide safety measures to protect from injury if CNS adverse effects occur
   i. Observe for compromised respiratory or cardiovascular status
   j. Monitor nutritional intake and tolerance
   k. Monitor skin and mucous membranes frequently
   l. Monitor renal function with labs, I&O, daily weight; monitor for reduced symptoms of AIDS or ARC and for increase in CD4 count
12. Client education
   a. Similar principles as for other anti-infective therapy (Box 41–3)
   b. Caution about risks of dizziness or altered mentation; do not drive or perform hazardous tasks
   c. Avoid crowds and persons with infections
   d. Hair loss possible with zidovudine (AZT)
   e. Drug does not cure but helps manage infection; it reduces viral load, decreases risk for complications, and extends survival
   f. Practice good hygiene and safe sex practices

D. Miscellaneous drugs for HIV and AIDS (see again Box 41–16)

1. Enfuvirtide (Fuzeon)
   a. Interferes with fusion of viral and cell membranes, blocking entry of HIV into host cell
   b. Given by SubQ injection twice daily
   c. Injection site reaction is almost certain in first week, with severe pain, pruritus, erythema, cysts, abscesses and cellulitis at injection site
   d. Other common adverse effects are nausea, diarrhea and fatigue, and increased risk for pneumonia
2. Raltegravir (Isentress)
   a. An integrase inhibitor that inhibits viral integrase enzyme needed to insert viral DNA into human chromosome
   b. Given orally with headache and GI symptoms as most common adverse effects
3. Maraviroc (Selzentry)
   a. A CCR5 inhibitor that blocks CCR5 coreceptor needed for viral entry into human cell
   b. Significantly reduces viral load and increases T-cell production
   c. Given orally
   d. Common adverse effects are abdominal pain, cough, dizziness, fever, rash, respiratory infections, and musculoskeletal symptoms
   e. Risk for hepatotoxicity and in clients with cardiac disease, increased risk for myocardial ischemia or infarction

E. Medications for influenza and respiratory viruses

1. Have both treatment and prophyactic applications; see product literature
2. Are virustatic; most viral replication has occurred before symptoms appear; bacterial replication occurs as signs of infection emerge, so antibacterial agents are more effective against bacterial infections than antiviral agents are against viral infections, since drug therapy relies on viral replication for effectiveness
3. Administration considerations
   a. Initiate drug therapy as soon as possible to enhance effectiveness and prevent complications of infection
   b. Administer before flu season for prophylactic purpose

Box 41–17 Medications for Influenza and Respiratory Viruses
Amantadine (Symmetrel)
Rimantadine (Flumadine)
Oseltamivir (Tamiflu)
Zanamivir (Relenza)

4. Side/adverse effects
   a. Most are transient and resolve quickly after drug is discontinued
   b. Dizziness, lightheadedness, headache, palpitations, mood and mental changes, drowsiness, insomnia, irritability, nightmares
   c. Dyspnea, rash, peripheral edema, leukopenia, possibly digoxin toxicity
   d. Orthostatic hypotension, N/V, mouth dryness, urinary retention
   e. Slurred speech, ataxia, convulsions; possible teratogenic
5. Nursing considerations
   a. Similar principles as for other anti-infectives (Box 41–2)
   b. Monitor hepatic and renal dysfunction, and baseline neurological status (orientation, affect, coordination, reflexes)
   c. Initiate drug therapy as soon as possible after exposure
   d. Monitor for respiratory deterioration in infants
   e. Provide safety precautions if CNS adverse effects develop
   f. Keep accurate I&O; monitor for urinary retention
   g. Provide oral care with water or saline rinses
6. Client education
   a. As per other types of anti-infectives (Box 41–3)
   b. Change position slowly to minimize risk of orthostatic hypotension
   c. Report increased respiratory distress or severe adverse effects to prescriber
   d. If drowsiness, dizziness, lightheadedness, confusion, ataxia, or blurred vision occur, do not drive or perform hazardous tasks
   e. If dry mouth develops, rinse mouth with plain warm water or with one teaspoon of salt added; avoid commercial mouthrinses with alcohol or hydrogen peroxide that increase dry mouth; hard sugarless candy may stimulate salivation
   f. Drink at least 6–8 glasses of fluids a day

F. Locally active antiviral agents

1. Action and use: not absorbed systemically
2. Common medications are listed in Box 41–18
   a. Idoxuridine (Herplex): topical ophthalmic agent to treat herpes simplex keratitis
   b. Imiquimod (Aldara): genital and perianal warts
   c. Penciclovir (Denavir): herpes simplex 1 or herpes labialis; cold sores on face and lips; do not apply to mucous membranes
   d. Fomivirsen (Vitravene): ophthalmic solution injected into eye to treat CMV retinitis in clients with AIDS
   e. Trifluridine (Viroptic): ophthalmic agent to treat herpes simplex infection of the eye
   f. Docusanol (Abreva): a nonprescription agent used topically for cold sores and fever blisters; blocks fusion of HSV with target cells to shorten symptoms and healing time; is not absorbed so has few significant adverse effects
3. Administration considerations
   a. Wash hands well before applying medication
   b. *NCLEX®* Wear gloves or use cotton-tipped applicator to apply to skin lesions, being cautious not to contaminate drug or other sites on skin
   c. Stop drug if severe local adverse effect or open lesions develop

Box 41–18 Locally Active Antiviral Agents	
Docusanol (Abreva)	Penciclovir (Denavir)
Idoxuridine (Herplex)	Trifluridine (Viroptic)
Imiquimod (Aldara)	

4. Contraindications use: caution in known hypersensitivity, pregnancy, lactation
5. Side effects
   a. Local burning, stinging, discomfort on application; usually resolve without intervention
   b. Temporary visual impairment possible with optic application
6. Adverse effects/toxicity: skin eruptions and hypersensitivity
7. Nursing considerations: monitor for comfort, safety, and compliance
8. Client education
   a. Similar principles as for other anti-infectives (Box 41–3)
   b. Does not cure but alleviates pain and discomfort and prevents extended damage to uninvolved tissue; report severe local discomfort or reaction to prescriber

IX. ANTIFUNGALS

A. Systemic antifungals

1. Fungistatic or fungicidal depending on therapeutic serum levels and sensitivity to fungi
2. Treat candida infections, cryptococcus, blastomycosis, histoplasmosis, aspergillus fumigates, and **tinea** infections (a fungal infection caused by ringworm)
3. Increased cell membrane permeability allows other drugs to enter fungus cell
4. Common medications are listed in Box 41–19
5. Administration considerations
   a. Administer carefully as ordered, especially IV dosages
   b. Combination of antifungal agents may deter or retard drug resistance
   c. May premedicate amphotericin with an antipyretic such as acetaminophen (Tylenol), an antihistamine such as diphenhydramine (Benadryl), an antiemetic, and meperidine (Demerol) to reduce severity of fever/chills response; heparin or hydrocortisone (Cortaid) added to IV solution may reduce risk for thrombophlebitis at IV site
   d. Give amphotericin B with heparin or hydrocortisone and over 4 to 6 hours to avert clinical manifestations of hypersensitivity or drug toxicity
   NCLEX® e. Hydrate with IV fluids usually 2 hours before and 2 hours after amphotericin B administration to decrease risk for nephrotoxicity
   f. To test for hypersensitivity to amphotericin B before administration, deliver 1 mg/20 mL D_5W IV over 10 to 30 minutes; if test elicits response, a lipid preparation such as amphotericin B liposomal complex (Ambisome) may be given to minimize severe fever, shaking, and chills; premedicate as above
   g. Mix amphotericin B in D_5W only; sodium chloride solutions cause precipitation
   h. Contraindicated in hypersensitivity; use cautiously in pregnant and lactating clients, or those with renal impairment or severe bone marrow depression
6. Side/adverse effects
   a. Thrombophlebitis when given through peripheral vein; fever, chills, shaking, headache, anorexia, N/V, piloerection
   b. Anorexia, N/V during or after dose; heartburn, diarrhea, flatulence
   c. Myalgia, arthralgia, weakness, hypotension, insomnia, vertigo, confusion
   d. Taste acuity diminished or causes unpleasant taste
   e. Photosensitivity, rash, pruritus, dry skin, urticaria
   f. Hypokalemia or hypomagnesemia, especially with concurrent use of glucocorticosteroids or diuretics
   g. Ketoconazole (Nizoral): sexual impotency, hair loss, and gynecomastia
   h. Bone marrow depression resulting in neutropenia, thrombocytopenia, anemia
   i. Ototoxicity and nephrotoxicity with amphotericin B preparations
   j. Stevens-Johnson syndrome, **superinfections** (candidiasis, diarrhea)
   k. Cardiovascular collapse with too rapid infusion

Box 41–19

Systemic Antifungal Medications

Amphotericin B (Fungizone, Ambisone)	Itraconazole (Sporanox)
Anidulafungin (Eraxis)	Ketoconazole (Nizoral)
Caspofungin (Cancidas)	Micafungin (Mycamine)
Fluconazole (Diflucan)	Voriconazole (Vfend)
Flucytosine (Ancobon)	

7. Nursing considerations
   a. Similar principles as for other anti-infectives (Box 41–2); check for incompatibility of solutions as there are many
   b. Screen for pregnancy, lactation, liver or renal dysfunction; monitor liver and renal laboratory studies throughout therapy
   c. Monitor serum levels of antifungal agents
   d. Monitor WBC for improvement and for early detection of developing neutropenia, platelet count (thrombocytopenia), red blood cell count (anemia)
   e. Give potassium supplements if hypokalemia occurs
   f. Protect amphotericin B from light, and monitor client's I&O
8. Client education
   a. Similar principles as for other anti-infectives (Box 41–3); know length of therapy (e.g., Amphotericin B may be given over weeks or months)
   b. Report adverse effects such as burning at IV site, increased bleeding or bruising, evidence of superinfection
   c. Febrile reaction may decrease over time
   d. Fluid intake of 2000–3000 mL/day if not contraindicated by other conditions
   e. Eat small, frequent meals with high-quality protein
   f. Take oral agents with food to minimize GI distress

B. Topical antifungals

1. Action and use
   a. Local infections of skin and mucous membranes of oropharynx, vagina, or intestines caused by Candida species; infections of tinea pedis (athlete's foot), tinea cruris (in scrotal, crural, anal, and genital areas, called "jock itch"), tinea corporis (skin), tinea unguium or onychomycosis (nail fungus), tinea manus, tinea versicolor (infection of skin with yellow or beige brawny patches)
   b. Use vaginal tablets up to 6 weeks prior to delivery to prevent newborn thrush
2. Common medications are listed in Box 41–20
3. Administration considerations
   a. Oral tablets or lozenges/troches are not to be chewed or swallowed whole; swallow saliva as lozenge/troche dissolves slowly over 5–30 minutes; avoid food or drink during and for 30 minutes after dose
   b. For oral infections in client with dentures, remove dentures at bedtime; with oral suspension, remove dentures before each rinse or before each oral lozenge/troche
   c. NCLEX® For application to skin: wear latex gloves, cleanse area with tepid water (soap if prescribed), dry thoroughly (without application of heat), and apply antifungal to infected area sparingly; do not cover with an occlusive dressing or tight clothing; wash hands well after removing gloves
   d. For treatment of tinea pedis (athlete's foot), apply antifungal powder such as nystatin (Mycostatin) to inside of shoes and stockings
   e. For vulvovaginal use: insert one full applicator or one vaginal tablet at bedtime as instructed; continue therapy during menstruation
   f. Avoid contact of antifungal with eyes; with certain agents, avoid contact with mucous membranes
   g. NCLEX® Do not apply occlusive dressing unless prescribed; client should avoid restrictive clothing in areas of infection

Box 41–20

Topical Antifungal Medications

Butenafine (Mentax)	Econazole (Spectazole)
Ciclopirox (Loprox, Penlac)	Fluconazole (Diflucan)
Griseofulvin (Fulvicin)	Itraconazole (Sporanox)
Naftifine (Naftin)	Ketoconazole (Nizoral)
Nystatin (Mycostatin)	Miconazole (Micatin)
Terbinafine cream (Lamisil)	Oxiconazole (Oxistat)
Tolnaftate (Tinactin)	Sulconazole (Exelderm)
Undecylenic acid (Fungi-Nail, others)	Terconazole (Terazol)
Butoconazole (Femstat)	Tioconazole (Monistat-1, others)
Clotrimazole (Lotrimin, others)	

h. Store creams, vaginal application, and topical preparation at room temperature; if specified for vaginal tablets and troches, refrigerate but do not freeze
i. Contraindicated with drug hypersensitivity

4. Side/adverse effects
   a. Topical: stinging, burning, erythema, edema, dry skin, vesication, pruritis, urticaria, desquamation, skin fissures
   b. Vaginal: slight burning, lower abdominal discomfort, bloating, erythema, itching, vaginal soreness during intercourse
   c. Oral troches or swish and swallow: N/V
   d. Possible hepatotoxicity in client with liver impairment
5. Nursing considerations
   a. Ensure complete course of therapy taken
   b. Observe for clinical signs of improvement
   c. Observe for clinical evidence of liver dysfunction, such as upper right quadrant tenderness, abdominal discomfort or bloating, lethargy, mentation changes, icterus, enlarged liver, elevated liver enzymes
   d. Stop application if severe burning or exacerbation of lesions occur and collaborate with prescriber
6. Client education
   a. Know drug name, purpose, dose, strength, how to apply, schedule of administration, length of therapy
   b. Observe site for improvement within first week of therapy; some infections require 2–4 weeks of treatment; notify prescriber if condition worsens or no improvement is noted in 1–2 weeks
   c. Store in tightly covered container at room temperature; if vaginal tablet or suppository, store as recommended, usually in refrigerator or above 59° F; avoid freezing or excess heat with all products
   d. If taken vaginally, refrain from sexual intercourse or have partner wear condom to avoid burning or irritation of penis or urethra

   NCLEX®

   e. Clothing and linens in contact with infectious sites should be washed after each treatment with soap and water; ointments may be removed from fabric with commercial cleaning products
   f. If severe burning, stinging, or eruptions occur, discontinue use and notify prescriber

X. ANTIPROTOZOALS

A. Antimalarials

1. Action and use
   a. Treatment or prophylaxis of malarial infection
   b. Chloroquine treatment for **giardiasis** (a protozoan intestinal infection) and amebiasis outside GI tract
2. Common medications are listed in Box 41–21
3. Administration considerations
   a. Separate drug from antacid administration by 4 hours before or after antacids
   b. Take quinine with food to decrease GI distress and mask bitter taste; do not crush capsule

Box 41–21

Antiprotozoal Medications

Antimalarials

Atovaquone and proguanil (Malarone)
Chloroquine HCl (Aralen HCl)
Hydroxychloroquine (Plaquenil)
Mefloquine (Lariam)
Primaquine
Pyrimethamine (Daraprim)
Quinine (Quinamm)

Other Antiprotozoal Medications

Eflornithine (Ornidyl)
Iodoquinol (Yodoxin)
Melarsoprol (Arsobol)
Metronidazole (Flagyl)
Nifurtimox (Lampit)
Nitazoxanide (Alinia)
Paromomycin (Humatin)
Pentamidine (Pentam)
Pyrimethamine and sulfadiazine (Fansidar)
Sodium stibogluconate (Pentostam)
Suramin (Germanin)
Tinidazole (Tindamax)

c. Chloroquine HCL (Aralen HCL), hydroxychloroquine (Plaquenil), and pyrimethamine (Daraprim): take with food to minimize GI distress

NCLEX®

d. For prophylaxis, take as prescribed, such as same day every week when entering high-risk area and for 10 weeks after departing
e. Mefloquine (Lariam): take with at least 8 ounces water; separate by at least 8 hours from ingestion of quinine or quinidine, an antidysrhythmic

4. Side/adverse effects
   a. Dizziness, vertigo, headache, visual impairment, angina
   b. N/V, diarrhea, gastric distress, abdominal cramps
   c. Confusion, apprehension, insomnia, nightmares, syncope, delirium
   d. Cutaneous flushing, pruritus, rash, paresthesia, dyspnea, weight loss, fatigue
   e. Chloroquine HCL (Aralen HCL) and hydroxychloroquine (Plaquenil): alopecia, bleaching of scalp or hair (including eyebrows, body hair) and freckles; bluish-black hue of skin or mucous membranes, rash, pruritis, photophobia
   f. Tinnitus, hearing loss, visual halos, blurring, inability to focus
   g. Cardiotoxicity in clients with atrial fibrillation
   h. Hypotension, tachypnea, tachycardia, hypothermia, blood dyscrasias
   i. Seizures, coma, cardiovascular collapse, blackwater fever (extensive intravascular hemolysis with renal failure), death
5. Nursing considerations
   a. Similar principles as for other anti-infectives (Box 41–2)
   b. Monitor hepatic and cardiac function at intervals
   c. Monitor for electrolyte disturbances, blood disorders as anemia, thrombocytopenia
   d. If client is taking antiepileptics, monitor drug levels of these agents
   e. Ensure regular ophthalmic exams, electcardiograms, and lab tests as ordered
   f. Check for G6PD deficiency as indicated
   g. Monitor for muscle weakness and depressed deep tendon reflexes periodically; monitor for CNS side effects; collaborate with prescriber regarding discontinuation of agent
6. Client education
   a. Similar principles as for other anti-infectives (Box 41–3)
   b. If weekly, take on same day every week
   c. Do not drive or perform hazardous tasks if drowsiness, dizziness, vertigo, visual disturbances occur
   d. Report fever, sore throat, myalgias, visual disturbances, anxiety, mental changes, hallucinations

NCLEX®

e. Chloroquine HCl: sunglasses may decrease risk of photophobia or ocular changes; urine may become rusty yellow or brown

B. Other antiprotozoals

1. Action and use
   a. Amebic dysentery, hepatic amebiasis, or abscess
   b. Some are bacteriocidal as well as amebicidal, especially in GI tract
   c. Paromomycin (Humatin): bactericidal and amebicidal related to tape worms
   d. Destroy intestinal bacteria that form nitrogen to decrease ammonia in hepatic disease and coma
   e. Pentamidine (Pentam): treat *pneumocystis carinii* pneumonia, an opportunistic infection in client with AIDS
2. Common medications are listed in Box 41–21
3. Administration considerations
   a. Pentamidine: decreased doses in renal dysfunction
   b. Rotate IM injection sites
   c. Use caution in pregnancy and lactation; contraindicted with hypersensitivity to drug or to iodine or primaquin
4. Side/adverse effects
   a. Hypotension, tachycardia, dizziness, headache, syncope, dysrhythmias
   b. Flushing, pruritis, dyspnea, pain at injection site
   c. Abdominal cramps, diarrhea, N/V, epigastric distress, unpleasant taste
   d. Myalgia, precordial stiffness, tremors, restlessness
   e. Nephrotoxicity: mild, reversible
   f. Leukopenia, neutropenia, anemia, thrombocytopenia
   g. Large doses can cause abscess, cellulitis, or lesion in muscle in the GI tract, heart, liver, and kidneys

NCLEX® 5. Nursing considerations: ensure complete course of therapy is taken for full benefit

NCLEX® 6. Client education
   a. Know drug, dose, purpose, schedule, proper administration technique
   b. Take full course of therapy for best effect
   c. Report side or adverse effects to prescriber
   d. Know clinical manifestations of infections to recognize and report

XI. ANTIHELMINTHICS

A. Action and use
1. Intestinal worms: *Ascaris lumbricoides, Trichostrongylus*
2. Pinworm: *Enterobius vermicularis*
3. Hook worms: *Ancytostoma duodenale, Necator americanus*

B. Common medications are listed in Box 41–22

C. Administration considerations
1. Mebendazole: may be chewed, swallowed whole, crushed, mixed with food
2. Pyrantel: may take with food
3. Thiabendazole: take after meals

D. Contraindications
1. Known hypersensitivity
2. Paromomycin: in intestinal obstruction
3. Caution with other antihelminthics in clients with hepatic or renal dysfunction
4. Safety not established in pregnancy and lactation

E. Side/adverse effects
1. N/V, diarrhea, abdominal cramps, anorexia
2. Rash, urticaria, erythema multiforme, photosensitivity, muscle aches, nephrotoxicity, or elevated liver enzymes
3. Dizziness, headache, fever, dose-related agranulocytosis and leukopenia
4. Thiabendazole: urinary odor

F. Nursing considerations
1. Similar principles as for other anti-infectives (Box 41–2)
2. Monitor hepatic, renal, or hematological laboratory results
3. Collect stool specimen for ova and parasites (O&P) for baseline and follow-up to verify eradication of infectious agents

G. Client education
1. Similar principles as for other anti-infectives (Box 41–3)
2. Agents may be taken with or after food to minimize GI distress
3. Store drug at room temperature protected from light and heat
4. Do not repeat drug therapy for continued infection until 1 week after initial treatment
5. Practice personal hygiene to prevent transmission
6. Urine odor may occur with thiabendazole

Box 41–22

Antihelminthics

Albendazole (Albenza)	Praziquantel (Biltricide)
Ivermectin (Stromectol)	Pyrantel (Antiminth, others)
Mebendazole (Vermox)	Thiabendazole (Mintezol)

Check Your NCLEX–PN® Exam I.Q.

You are ready for testing on this content if you can

- Apply knowledge of expected actions and effects of anti-infective and immunological medications to client care.
- Correctly describe administration of anti-infective and immunological medications to clients.
- Monitor for side effects and adverse effects of anti-infective and immunological medications.
- Take appropriate action if a client has an unexpected response to an anti-infective or immunological medication.
- Monitor a client for expected outcomes or effects of treatment with anti-infective and immunological medications.

PRACTICE TEST

1 Gentamicin (Garamycin) therapy is to be initiated. Which laboratory test result would indicate to the nurse that the client is manifesting a common adverse effect?

1. Elevated urine creatinine clearance
2. Increased prothrombin time (PT)
3. Increased serum creatinine
4. Hypokalemia

2 A client who is taking isoniazid (INH) is experiencing paresthesia as a common side effect. The nurse should teach the client to include what foods in the diet? Select all that apply.

1. Liver
2. Peanuts
3. Raw avocados
4. Raw apples
5. Baked potato with skin

3 A client is receiving levofloxacin (Levaquin) in addition to an oral anticoagulant. What treatment should the nurse anticipate administering if the client experiences an adverse drug effect as a result of this combination?

1. Albumin
2. Platelets
3. Protamine sulfate
4. Phytonadione (vitamin K)

4 The nurse notes that a client taking doxycycline (Vibramycin) is jaundiced and lethargic. What laboratory test result would be most specific for the nurse to review?

1. Bilirubin
2. Alkaline phosphatase (ALP)
3. Alanine aminotransferase (ALT or SGPT)
4. Aspartate aminotransferase (AST or SGOT)

5 A client taking ampicillin (Omnipen) develops a macular rash on the chest. What conclusion should the nurse make about this finding?

1. This reaction is Stevens-Johnson syndrome.
2. A minor rash usually precipitates the development of more severe reactions.
3. A minor rash requires notification of the prescriber, but might be well tolerated, and might fade with continued treatment.
4. Hypersensitivity reactions requiring discontinuation of the antibiotic occur to some extent with all clients taking a penicillin agent.

6 A client is started on erythromycin (Erythrocin) as treatment for pneumonia. The nurse should teach the client to contact the health care provider for which reasons? Select all that apply.

1. Improvement of fever, cough, or respiratory effort is not observed in 48–72 hours.
2. Fluids can be taken orally, but the client still cannot eat after 24 hours.
3. Anorexia and nausea develop within 24 hours.
4. Fever fluctuates.
5. Changes in response to verbal stimuli are noted.

7 A child with otitis media is taking trimethoprim-sulfamethoxazole (TMP-SMZ) as a suspension. What instructions should the nurse provide to the mother?

1. Do not allow the child to drink water immediately after taking the medication.
2. The medication is to be taken on an empty stomach.
3. The medication must be kept refrigerated.
4. Use a calibrated measuring device.

8 A client receiving an anti-infective drug begins to wheeze. The nurse anticipates initial administration of what drug?

1. Epinephrine HCL (Adrenalin Chloride)
2. Methylprednisolone (Solu-Medrol)
3. Atropine sulfate (Atropine)
4. Dopamine HCL (Intropin)

PRACTICE TEST

9. An adult client is ordered to take one 250 mg tablet of metronidazole (Flagyl) three times a day for a confirmed diagnosis of trichomoniasis. After taking the medication for 24 hours, the client reports flushing, dizziness, pounding headache, sweating, abdominal cramps, nausea, and irritability. What important data should the nurse gather? Select all that apply.

1. History of alcohol use
2. Current over-the-counter medications
3. History of liver disease
4. Tablets were crushed before administration
5. Food was given with the medication

10. The nurse assesses the client receiving cefotazime (Claforan), and notes three diarrhea stools in the past 24 hours, rectal itching, glossitis, and fever. What adverse effects should the nurse conclude that the client is exhibiting?

1. Leukocytosis
2. Opportunistic infection
3. Bone marrow depression
4. Drug failure against original infective organism

11. What teaching or intervention is appropriate for a client taking an antibiotic that causes diarrhea secondary to elimination of normal intestinal flora?

1. Test stool for occult blood.
2. Include yogurt or buttermilk products in the diet.
3. Arrange for IV administration instead of oral route.
4. Take antacids with antibiotic to reduce diarrhea.

12. A disulfiram-like reaction occurs in a client taking cefoperazone sodium (Cefobid). The nurse suspects this reaction is a drug interaction resulting from the client's ingestion of which of the following substances within the last few hours?

1. Caffeine in tea or coffee
2. Sulfamethoxazole (Gantonol) for a chronic urinary tract infection
3. Over-the-counter cough suppressant
4. Ampicillin (Omnipen), which has a cross-sensitivity to cephalosporins

13. The nurse evaluates for an adverse reaction to tobramycin sulfate (Tobrex) by collecting which data?

1. Capillary refill
2. Romberg test
3. Chvostek sign
4. Babinski reflex

14. What instruction should the nurse reinforce with a premenopausal client receiving griseofulvin microsize (Grisfulvin V) for a systemic antifungal condition?

1. If taking oral contraceptives, use an alternative form of contraception during and for one month after use of griseofulvin.
2. Record number of absorbent products used daily to monitor for increased menstrual flow while taking griseofulvin.
3. Check blood pressure (BP) daily if taking oral contraceptive and griseofulvin, as both can increase BP.
4. Avoid taking calcium supplements concurrently with griseofulvin.

15. A client is receiving long-term oral anticoagulation therapy and is also taking a beta-lactam penicillin. What laboratory result should the nurse monitor during this therapy?

1. Decreased bleeding time
2. Increased thrombin time (TT)
3. Increased prothrombin time (PT)
4. Increased activated partial thromboplastin time (aPPT)

16. During a routine screening, a client has a positive response to intradermal injection of purified protein derivative (PPD or Mantoux test). The nurse draws which of the following conclusions about this result?

1. The client is currently infectious with tuberculosis.
2. The client tests positively for active tuberculosis.
3. The client has been exposed to the tubercle bacillus within the past 2 weeks.
4. The client has been infected with tuberculosis, and has developed a cellular (T cell) response to the tubercle bacillus.

17. Appropriate teaching for a young adult female related to a new prescription for ampicillin (Omnipen) orally would include which of the following? Select all that apply.

1. May notice the development of red, scaly skin.
2. Observe for clinical extrapyramidal tract manifestations.
3. Change positions slowly to avoid orthostatic hypotension.
4. Oral contraceptives may lose effectiveness.
5. Vaginal itching and discharge can occur.

18. The nurse should collect data frequently for clients receiving oprelvekin (Neumega) to detect which manifestations? Select all that apply.

1. Dehydration
2. Congestive heart failure (CHF)
3. Anxiety
4. Hyperuricemia
5. Irregular apical pulse

19. A client is admitted to the emergency department with a 3-inch laceration over the left eye. The nurse should observe for which priority factors related to the risk of infection before beginning drug therapy to prevent infection?

1. The client's temperature
2. The date of the client's last tetanus vaccine
3. If the client's blood pressure is decreased
4. Whether the client is taking corticosteroid medication

20. In reinforcing client teaching about Beta 1b (Betaseron), what should the nurse explain as the goal for administering this medication?

1. Cure the client of multiple sclerosis.
2. Prevent signs and symptoms of anaphylaxis.
3. Destroy nerve tissue that is laden with plaque.
4. Decrease the demyelination in the brain tissue.

21. What should the nurse instruct the client to do in order to decrease renal insufficiency side effects in clients receiving cyclophosphamide (Sandimmune)?

1. Consume a diet high in fiber.
2. Have creatinine level assessed weekly.
3. Drink 3000 mL of fluid per day.
4. Take hydrochlorothiazide (HCTZ).

22. To determine a client's baseline prior to the administration of azathioprine (Imuran), the nurse should put highest priority on evaluating which laboratory test result(s)?

1. Creatinine
2. Uric acid
3. PT and PTT
4. Red blood cell count

23. Azathioprine (Imuran) and allopurinol (Zyloprim) are administered to a client diagnosed with multiple sclerosis and gout. It is important for the nurse to monitor the results of which laboratory test in this client?

1. Creatinine
2. Uric acid
3. Blood glucose
4. Blood urea nitrogen (BUN)

24. A client is scheduled for diagnostic testing for myasthenia gravis. What medication is necessary for the nurse to have available for this testing?

1. Ambenonium (Mytelase)
2. Edrophonium (Tensilon)
3. Neostigmine (Prostigmine)
4. Physostigmine (Eserine)

25. What points should the nurse reinforce in a teaching plan for a client receiving medications to treat multiple sclerosis? Select all that apply.

1. Indication of pulmonary edema
2. Restriction of oral fluids
3. Requirement to avoid crowds
4. Enhancement of muscle strength
5. Chest pain

26 A client has been exposed to hepatitis A. Which client factor would be an indication to the nurse for withholding administration of immune serum globulin to the client?

1. The client has received a hepatitis B vaccine.
2. The client has recently fallen and suffered a hip fracture.
3. The client has a history of a coagulation disorder.
4. The client is scheduled for foreign travel.

27 A client with Parkinson's disease is admitted to the emergency department with lethargy, hypotension, and a weakened gait. The nurse should be prepared to administer what medication?

1. Carbidopa (Lodosyn)
2. Levodopa (Dopar)
3. Atropine (generic)
4. Physostigmine (Eserine)

28 The client taking isoniazid (INH) reports paresthesia of the extremities. The nurse initially monitors the client for which of the following?

1. Hyperactive motor reflex responses
2. Other clinical manifestations of hypercalcemia
3. Concurrent self-administration of aluminum antacids
4. Compliance with taking pyridoxine (vitamin B_6) supplement

29 Rifampin (Rifadin) is being initiated prophylactically for a client who lives with a family member who has *Haemophilus influenzae* meningitis. What client teaching would be most appropriate for the nurse to reinforce?

1. Explain that rifampin is being prescribed to treat meningitis.
2. Adverse effects might be severe such as convulsions and coma.
3. Protect undergarments, because with rifampin, urine will become orange-red and will stain.
4. The client will need to keep follow-up visits with her health care provider, but it will not be necessary to continue blood test monitoring.

30 A client with benign prostatic hyperplasia (BPH) is receiving amantadine (Symmetrel) for *influenza A*. The nurse monitors the client for which of the following side effects?

1. Increased risk for urinary retention
2. Hypermotility of bowel
3. Increased lacrimation
4. Nephrotoxicity

31 A client with *herpes zoster* infection (shingles) has started therapy with acyclovir (Zovirax). The nurse should perform which important intervention during the course of this treatment?

1. Monitor for jaundice and elevated liver enzymes.
2. Teach the client to avoid sexual intercourse during therapy.
3. Administer the dose early in the day, as it could cause insomnia.
4. Encourage fluid intake of 2500–3000 mL daily, if not contraindicated by other client conditions.

32 The nurse determines that the client understands an important principle of self-administration of an oral antibiotic when the client makes which of the following statements?

1. "I will continue to take the antibiotic as it is ordered, even though I no longer have a cough with yellow sputum."
2. "When I missed a dose of my antibiotic this morning, I made up for it by taking 2 doses when it was time to take the next dose."
3. "I am careful to take the antibiotic every day at breakfast, lunch, and dinner."
4. "Even though the doctor prescribed amoxicillin (Amoxil) chewable tablet, I have no problem swallowing it whole."

33 A client who has been on anti-infective therapy for 10 days has developed diarrhea, with 10 watery stools a day. The nurse should anticipate an order for which of the following?

1. Monitor for clinical manifestations of metabolic alkalosis.
2. Administer an antiperistaltic agent, such as dicyclomine HCl (Bentyl).
3. Administer an antidiarrheal agent, such as kaolin and pectin (Kaopectolin).
4. Collect a stool specimen for cytotoxin assay to detect *Clostridium difficile*.

34 The client with pneumonia is being treated with amoxicillin (Amoxil). The nurse monitors for therapeutic effectiveness by noting which of the following?

1. Normalization of fever beginning 96 hours after therapy starts
2. No clinical manifestations of hypersensitivity
3. Resolution of orthostatic hypotension
4. Pulse oximetry of 98%

35 A client receiving sodium penicillin G (PCN) for several days reports weakness, numbness, tingling in the extremities, and nausea. The nurse palpates a weak pulse, and auscultates an irregular heart rate and decreased bowel sounds. The nurse further monitors the client for specific signs of which electrolyte imbalance?

1. Hypokalemia
2. Hypochloremia
3. Hypercalcemia
4. Hypophosphatemia

ANSWERS & RATIONALES

1 **Answer: 3 Rationale:** Increased serum creatinine indicates renal dysfunction. Nephrotoxicity is a common adverse effect of aminoglycosides such as gentamicin. The urine creatinine clearance would be decreased in renal impairment. Coagulation disturbances are not attributed to this class of antibiotic as a direct adverse reaction. Hypokalemia is not attributed to this class of antibiotic as a direct adverse reaction. **Cognitive Level:** Analyzing **Client Need:** Pharmacological and Parenteral Therapies **Integrated Process:** Nursing Process: Data Collection **Content Area:** Pharmacology **Strategy:** Note the critical words *common adverse effect* in the stem. Recall that aminoglycosides often adversely affect the kidneys. Identify the option that indicates renal impairment as the correct answer.

2 **Answer: 1, 3, 5 Rationale:** Peripheral neuritis is the most common side effect of isoniazid (INH). Adding vitamin B_6 (pyridoxine) to the client's intake is the therapy to correct this side effect. The diet may be supplemented with vitamin B_6. Foods highest in vitamin B_6 include beef liver and chicken liver. A food other than meat that could be included is raw avocados, as well as baked potato with skin, raw banana, figs, and soybeans. Raw apples and peanuts are not high in pyridoxine. **Cognitive Level:** Applying **Client Need:** Pharmacological and Parenteral Therapies **Integrated Process:** Nursing Process: Implementation **Content Area:** Pharmacology **Strategy:** The core issue of the question is knowledge of what nutrient will reduce adverse drug effects of INH. Recall that vitamin B_6 will assist in this action, and then choose the food that is highest in this vitamin. When more than one answer is correct, consider each option as a true/false statement.

3 **Answer: 4 Rationale:** Absorption of vitamin K from the intestines can be interrupted, and prolonged bleeding can result due to inadequate serum level of prothrombin (hypothrombinemia). Appropriate therapy in this case is to administer phytonadione or menadiol sodium diphosphate (Synkayvite). Albumin, a plasma expander, is not indicated unless there is notable blood loss. The nurse must assess for and protect against increased bleeding exacerbated by eradication of intestinal flora with levofloxacin (Levaquin); however there is no indication that the client has notable blood loss. Protamine sulfate is an antidote to heparin and is not appropriate or effective if bleeding should occur from the administration of levofloxacin (Levaquin). **Cognitive Level:** Analyzing **Client Need:** Pharmacological and Parenteral Therapies **Integrated Process:** Nursing Process: Planning **Content Area:** Pharmacology **Strategy:** The core issue of the question is knowledge of drug interaction between levofloxacin and oral anticoagulants. Recall that vitamin K reverses bleeding to help identify the drug that reverses the effect of oral anticoagulant drugs.

4 **Answer: 3 Rationale:** ALT is specific for diagnosing and monitoring liver disease or impairment. Differential diagnosis of etiology of jaundice between hepatic dysfunction and hemolysis of red blood cells is indicated by the bilirubin. Alkaline phosphatase (ALP) is a protein found in all body tissues, and while liver tissue has a high amount of ALP, this test is not as liver-specific as the ALT or SGPT results. AST can help to diagnose or monitor heart disease or disease of the liver. **Cognitive Level:** Analyzing **Client Need:** Pharmacological and Parenteral Therapies **Integrated Process:** Nursing Process: Data Collection **Content Area:** Pharmacology **Strategy:** The core issue of the question is the laboratory test that will help evaluate the presence of jaundice as an adverse effect of doxycycline. Use specific nursing knowledge and the process of elimination to make a selection.

5 **Answer: 3 Rationale:** A minor rash might not signify an allergic reaction, and does not prohibit future administration of penicillin. However, the nurse reports this finding and closely monitors for further hypersensitivity reaction because other clinical manifestations could develop. Stevens-Johnson syndrome is a more serious aberration of the skin associated with antimicrobial adverse reactions; it resembles a second-degree burn in that necrolysis separates the epidermis from the dermis, causing blisters. A minor rash is the most common side effect of penicillins, and might be relatively insignificant. All available antimicrobials are capable of stimulating an exaggerated immune response, but not all clients experience allergy with antibiotic therapy. **Cognitive Level:** Analyzing **Client Need:** Pharmacological and Parenteral Therapies **Integrated Process:** Nursing Process: Data Collection **Content Area:** Pharmacology **Strategy:** The core issue of the question is the significance of a rash that develops in a client

taking ampicillin. Use specific nursing knowledge and the process of elimination to make a selection. Recall that not all drug rashes indicate hypersensitivity to aid in choosing the correct option.

6 **Answer: 1, 5** **Rationale:** Improvement in clinical manifestations of the infection should be noted within 48–72 hours. Otherwise, compliance with prescribed drug therapy should be monitored, and adjustment of drug, dose, and/or administration frequency might be needed. A side effect of erythromycin (Erythrocin) is ototoxicity, resulting in hearing loss preceded by tinnitus. A baseline hearing assessment should be made prior to administering the drug. The client's ability to take in fluids can temporarily sustain his nutritional status for a few days, particularly if dietary supplements are also included, which is appropriate for client education. Anorexia and nausea can be common sequelae in systemic infections, and would not warrant contacting the physician unless the manifestations became increasingly worse. A fluctuating febrile state can be common sequelae in systemic infection, and in itself, would not be considered a reason to contact the physician. **Cognitive Level:** Analyzing **Client Need:** Pharmacological and Parenteral Therapies **Integrated Process:** Teaching and Learning **Content Area:** Pharmacology **Strategy:** The core issues of the question are unsatisfactory progress or adverse side effects after beginning erythromycin and indicators that need to be reported to the prescriber. Use specific nursing knowledge and the process of elimination to make a selection. When there is more than one correct answer, consider each option as a true/false statement.

7 **Answer: 4** **Rationale:** The volume of a household teaspoon can vary by 2–10 mL, so a calibrated device is necessary for accurate dosing. The suspension is to be shaken to disperse the particles just prior to measurement. It is recommended that a glass of water be given with the medication, and that adequate urinary output be maintained. Food does not interfere with absorption of the medication, and could help to minimize gastrointestinal side effects. The medication is stable at room temperature, but the taste might be more palatable if cold. **Cognitive Level:** Applying **Client Need:** Pharmacological and Parenteral Therapies **Integrated Process:** Teaching and Learning **Content Area:** Pharmacology **Strategy:** The core issue of the question is the proper method of administration of trimethoprim-sulfamethoxazole to a child. Use specific nursing knowledge and the process of elimination to make a selection.

8 **Answer: 1** **Rationale:** Epinephrine is the primary drug used when bronchoconstriction causes inadequate respiratory exchange, as in anaphylactic shock. Marked improvement in respiration occurs within a few minutes after subcutaneous administration of 0.1–0.5 mL of 1:1000 strength epinephrine. Corticosteroids may be given to minimize the inflammation and edema, but are not the initial agent given. Atropine might minimize secretions, but would not be given unless vagal-induced bradycardia or asystole occurred; then atropine could be given as an IV bolus rapidly before, during, or after cardiopulmonary arrest. Dopamine HCL, a catecholamine (as is epinephrine), may be given to increase blood pressure if shock develops. **Cognitive Level:** Analyzing **Client Need:** Pharmacological and Parenteral Therapies **Integrated Process:** Nursing Process: Implementation **Content Area:** Pharmacology **Strategy:** The core issue of the question is knowledge of drugs that are used to treat hypersensitivity or anaphylactic reactions. Think of the necessity to preserve the airway first. Use specific nursing knowledge and the process of elimination to make a selection.

9 **Answer: 1, 2** **Rationale:** A disulfiram-like effect is associated with certain drugs, including metronidazole (Flagyl). Onset is usually within 15–30 minutes of ingestion of alcohol, but can occur up to 72 hours after Flagyl has been discontinued. The reaction lasts approximately 20–30 minutes but can remain up to 24 hours. Over-the-counter drugs, such as cold and cough preparations may contain alcohol, and could cause a disulfiram-like effect. Metronidazole (Flagyl), if prescribed for clients with liver disease, should be given in smaller doses; however, this information should be noted prior to this medication being prescribed. Metronidazole (Flagyl) tablets can be crushed for the client who cannot swallow the medication whole, except for the extended release form. There is no indication that the medication is the extended release form. Metronidazole (Flagyl) tablets can be taken safely before, with, or after meals or with food or milk to decrease GI distress. **Cognitive Level:** Analyzing **Client Need:** Pharmacological and Parenteral Therapies **Integrated Process:** Nursing Process: Implementation **Content Area:** Pharmacology **Strategy:** The core issue of the question is to determine the connection between Flagyl and the presenting manifestations. Use specific nursing knowledge and the process of elimination to make a selection. When more than one answer is correct, consider each option as a true/false statement.

10 **Answer: 2** **Rationale:** Opportunistic infections or superinfections are manifested commonly by vaginal and GI tract infections, including candidiasis and diarrhea. They often result from broad-spectrum antibiotic use that destroys bacteria in the normal flora, allowing the resistant pathogens to proliferate. Early recognition and intervention with administration of sensitive anti-infectives is important in controlling discomfort and the severity of the reaction. The manifestations exhibited by the client do not represent the other options. **Cognitive Level:** Analyzing **Client Need:** Pharmacological and Parenteral Therapies **Integrated Process:** Nursing Process: Data Collection **Content Area:** Pharmacology **Strategy:** The core issue of the question is knowledge of adverse drug effects of cefotazime and their significance. Use specific nursing knowledge and the process of elimination to make a selection.

11 **Answer: 2** **Rationale:** Yogurt and buttermilk products can decrease the diarrhea as well as add protein to the diet to provide albumin for drug binding. Clients are not usually taught to test their stool for occult blood. Blood or mucus in the stool with increased number of stools indicates the possibility of pseudomembranous colitis that should be reported to the health care provider. The route of administration of antibiotics is not the cause of destruction of normal flora. Antacids would interfere with the effectiveness of the antibiotic and should not be taken; yogurt or buttermilk products are a more beneficial treatment for the diarrhea. **Cognitive Level:** Applying **Client Need:** Pharmacological and Parenteral Therapies **Integrated Process:** Nursing Process: Implementation **Content Area:** Pharmacology **Strategy:** The core issue of the question is knowledge of client teaching points related to antibiotic therapy that has diarrhea as a side effect. Use specific nursing knowledge and the process of elimination to make a selection.

12 **Answer: 3** **Rationale:** Disulfiram- or antabuse-like reactions can occur when cephalosporins are taken with ingestion of alcohol during and up to 72 hours after discontinuation of the cephalosporin. Caffeine would not cause this reaction.

Sulfamethoxazole (Gantonol) prescribed for a chronic urinary tract infection would not cause this reaction. Cross-sensitivity is not responsible for this reaction. **Cognitive Level:** Analyzing **Client Need:** Pharmacological and Parenteral Therapies **Integrated Process:** Nursing Process: Data Collection **Content Area:** Pharmacology **Strategy:** The core issue of the question is knowledge of the causes of disulfiram-like drug reactions. Use specific nursing knowledge and the process of elimination to make a selection.

13 **Answer: 2 Rationale:** Vestibular ototoxicity as well as cochlear otoxicity can occur with administration of an aminoglycoside such as tobramycin. A positive Romberg test indicates vertigo or loss of balance, and can suggest a vestibular problem. Capillary refill is one method of monitoring peripheral circulation; it is not an appropriate method for detection of adverse reactions to tobramycin sulfate. Chvostek sign is seen in tetany and hypocalcemia. Babinski reflex, if present in the adult, reflects a possible lesion in the corticospinal tract. **Cognitive Level:** Analyzing **Client Need:** Pharmacological and Parenteral Therapies **Integrated Process:** Nursing Process: Data Collection **Content Area:** Pharmacology **Strategy:** The core issue of the question is knowledge of assessment techniques that will help determine whether ototoxicity is occurring in a client taking tobramycin. Use specific nursing knowledge and the process of elimination to make a selection.

14 **Answer: 1 Rationale:** Griseofulvin can interfere with the effectiveness of estrogen-containing oral contraceptives. Griseofulvin does not cause increased bleeding unless the client is also on anticoagulant therapy. Griseofulvin has no known effect on blood pressure. Griseofulvin has no known interaction with calcium supplement intake. **Cognitive Level:** Applying **Client Need:** Pharmacological and Parenteral Therapies **Integrated Process:** Teaching and Learning **Content Area:** Pharmacology **Strategy:** The core issue of the question is knowledge of key teaching points regarding systemic griseofulvin. Use specific nursing knowledge and the process of elimination to make a selection.

15 **Answer: 3 Rationale:** The prothrombin time (PT) and the international normalization ratio (INR) values are standard tests to monitor warfarin (Coumadin) levels. The beta-lactam antibiotics can cause increased PT and INR. The bleeding time evaluates the integrity of the vascular and platelet factors associated with stagnated blood. Thrombin time evaluates the fibrinogen-to-fibrin conversion factor that can be used to gauge heparin effectiveness; if the client is receiving oral anticoagulant therapy it is with warfarin. The APPT is currently used most often in regulating heparin therapy; the client is receiving oral anticoagulant therapy. **Cognitive Level:** Analyzing **Client Need:** Pharmacological and Parenteral Therapies **Integrated Process:** Nursing Process: Data Collection **Content Area:** Pharmacology **Strategy:** The core issue of the question is the expected change in laboratory results for a client taking a beta-lactam penicillin and an oral anticoagulant. Use specific nursing knowledge and the process of elimination to make a selection.

16 **Answer: 4 Rationale:** The PPD injection stimulates a local inflammatory response at the injection site in the client who has been exposed to the tubercle bacillus in the past. A positive PPD result does not indicate that the client is in an infectious state. Follow-up sputum tests for tubercle bacillus and/or chest films are done to clarify current status. A positive PPD result alone does not indicate that the client currently has active tuberculosis; follow-up testing needs to be done to clarify current status. The client develops a cellular response to tubercle bacillus at 3–10 weeks after infection. **Cognitive Level:** Analyzing **Client Need:** Pharmacological and Parenteral Therapies **Integrated Process:** Nursing Process: Data Collection **Content Area:** Pharmacology **Strategy:** The core issue of the question is the significance of PPD test results. Use specific nursing knowledge and the process of elimination to make a selection.

17 **Answer: 1, 4, 5 Rationale:** The development of exfoliative dermatitis, which presents as red, scaly skin, is possible with ampicillin therapy. All skin changes should be reported to the physician for evaluation; they may be nonallergenic and not an absolute contraindication to future therapy. Antibiotics, especially aminopenicillins such as ampicillin, can decrease the effectiveness of oral contraceptives; therefore, alternative contraceptive methods should be used during and for one month following ampicillin therapy. Ampicillin can cause superinfections, which may be manifested by the presence of vaginal itching and vaginal discharge. Extrapyramidal tract manifestations are not noted with ampicillin therapy. Orthostatic hypotension does not occur with ampicillin therapy. **Cognitive Level:** Analyzing **Client Need:** Pharmacological and Parenteral Therapies **Integrated Process:** Teaching and Learning **Content Area:** Pharmacology **Strategy:** The core issue of the question is client teaching that is needed for a client beginning drug therapy with ampicillin. Use specific nursing knowledge and the process of elimination to make a selection. When there is more than one correct answer, consider each option as a true/false statement.

18 **Answer: 2, 5 Rationale:** Oprelvekin (Neumega) can cause cardiopulmonary insufficiency with irregular heart rate and fluid retention. Thus, it is a nursing priority to monitor the client frequently for signs and symptoms of congestive heart failure. Dehydration is not a probable or priority concern with oprelvekin (Neumega) therapy. While anxiety can occur with the development of CHF, as a result of oprelvekin (Neumega) therapy, it is not the priority concern. Hyperuricemia is not a priority concern with oprelvekin (Neumega) therapy. **Cognitive Level:** Analyzing **Client Need:** Pharmacological and Parenteral Therapies **Integrated Process:** Nursing Process: Data Collection **Content Area:** Pharmacology **Strategy:** The core issue of the question is knowledge of adverse drug effects of oprelvekin. Use specific nursing knowledge and the process of elimination to make a selection. When there is more than one correct answer, consider each option as a true/false statement.

19 **Answer: 2 Rationale:** It is recommended that every client have a tetanus vaccine every 10 years to prevent infection caused by tetanus. The primary opportunity for this assessment is following a laceration. Temperature does not address the risk of infection caused by trauma while the client is in the emergency department. A decreased blood pressure measurement does not address the risk of infection caused by trauma while the client is in the emergency department. Delayed wound healing is a possibility with corticosteroid therapy, but assessment of tetanus immunization status takes priority. **Cognitive Level:** Understanding **Client Need:** Pharmacological and Parenteral Therapies **Integrated Process:** Nursing Process: Data Collection **Content Area:** Pharmacology **Strategy:** The critical words in the question are *laceration* and *emergency department*, which indicates that the injury is the result of trauma and is subject to contamination. Recall that the skin is the first line of defense

against infection, and the client will need to be assessed for the need for a tetanus vaccine.

20 **Answer: 4** **Rationale:** Interferon Beta 1b (Betaseron) reduces the severity of acute exacerbations of multiple sclerosis by decreasing demyelination in brain tissue. There is no cure for multiple sclerosis; the manifestations can only be managed through the use of medications. Preventing signs and symptoms of anaphylaxis does not accurately reflect the action of interferon Beta 1b. The destruction of nerve tissue that is laden with plaque is not a desirable or effective goal in treating multiple sclerosis. **Cognitive Level:** Applying **Client Need:** Pharmacological and Parenteral Therapies **Integrated Process:** Nursing Process: Implementation **Content Area:** Pharmacology **Strategy:** The core issue of the question is knowledge of goals of drug therapy with interferon Beta 1b (Betaseron). Use specific nursing knowledge and the process of elimination to make a selection.

21 **Answer: 3** **Rationale:** Adequate fluid intake greater than 2000–3000 mL per day allows for the kidneys to flush renal toxins, and prevents renal insufficiency. Consuming a diet high in fiber is a general measure to prevent constipation. Having a weekly assessment of creatinine level would be a monitoring function, but would not prevent renal insufficiency. The nurse would not instruct the client to take additional medication that is not specifically part of the plan of care. **Cognitive Level:** Applying **Client Need:** Pharmacological and Parenteral Therapies **Integrated Process:** Teaching and Learning **Content Area:** Pharmacology **Strategy:** The core issue of the question is knowledge of measures to prevent the development of renal side effects with use of cyclophosphamide. Use specific nursing knowledge and the process of elimination to make a selection.

22 **Answer: 1** **Rationale:** The most significant laboratory test to utilize prior to medication therapy with azathioprine is creatinine level, because renal and hepatic function should be assessed for baseline parameters. Monitoring uric acid levels is irrelevant for the administration of azathioprine. A decreased platelet count can occur with the administration of azathioprine, but laboratory values for PT and PTT provides information related to blood clotting. An RBC evaluates an important component of the blood; however, a risk related to the administration of azathioprine would be a change in white blood cell count (risk for infection). **Cognitive Level:** Applying **Client Need:** Pharmacological and Parenteral Therapies **Integrated Process:** Nursing Process: Data Collection **Content Area:** Pharmacology **Strategy:** The core issue of the question is knowledge of adverse drug effects of azathioprine and which laboratory test to use as a baseline measure. Use specific nursing knowledge and the process of elimination to make a selection.

23 **Answer: 2** **Rationale:** Azathioprine (Imuran) is administered to treat multiple sclerosis, and allopurinol (Zyloprim) is administered to treat symptoms of gout. When these two medications are administered together, the dose of azathioprine should be reduced. The uric acid level and client symptoms should be monitored to determine the control of gout. The creatinine indicates kidney function. Blood glucose levels are not important during the administration of Imuran and Zyloprim. BUN is a laboratory indicator related to renal function. **Cognitive Level:** Applying **Client Need:** Pharmacological and Parenteral Therapies **Integrated Process:** Nursing Process: Data Collection **Content Area:** Pharmacology **Strategy:** The core issue of the question is knowledge of drug interactive effects of azathioprine and allopurinol. Use specific nursing knowledge and the process of elimination to make a selection.

24 **Answer: 2** **Rationale:** Edrophonium (Tensilon) is used for diagnostic purposes. Clients who receive an injection of edrophonium and exhibit a temporary relief of symptoms are diagnosed with myasthenia gravis, which is characterized by a decrease in the concentration of acetylcholine in the neuromuscular junction. The other options are not used to diagnose myasthenia gravis. **Cognitive Level:** Applying **Client Need:** Pharmacological and Parenteral Therapies **Integrated Process:** Nursing Process: Planning **Content Area:** Pharmacology **Strategy:** The core issue of the question is knowledge of medications used for diagnosis of myasthenia gravis. Use specific nursing knowledge and the process of elimination to make a selection.

25 **Answer: 1, 5** **Rationale:** Medications used to treat symptoms of multiple sclerosis have been noted to increase pulmonary edema. Medications used to treat symptoms of multiple sclerosis have been noted to increase pulmonary edema, leading to chest pain, and shortness of breath. The restriction of oral fluids could increase risk of urinary tract infection. Avoiding crowds is useful to avoid infection, but does not specifically relate to medication teaching. Activities that could effectively enhance muscle strength could increase fatigue; if done to excess, it could lead to exacerbation of symptoms. **Cognitive Level:** Applying **Client Need:** Pharmacological and Parenteral Therapies **Integrated Process:** Teaching and Learning **Content Area:** Pharmacology **Strategy:** The core issue of the question is knowledge of essential teaching points for a client being treated with drug therapy for multiple sclerosis. Use specific nursing knowledge and the process of elimination to make a selection. When more than one answer is correct, consider each option as a true/false statement.

26 **Answer: 3** **Rationale:** Immune serum globulin should not be administered to clients with a history of coagulation disorders. Having received a hepatitis B vaccine does not represent contraindication to administration of immune serum globulin. Immune serum globulin is safe to administer to a client who recently experienced a traumatic hip fracture. Immune serum globulin is safe to administer to a client scheduled for foreign travel. **Cognitive Level:** Analyzing **Client Need:** Pharmacological and Parenteral Therapies **Integrated Process:** Nursing Process: Data Collection **Content Area:** Pharmacology **Strategy:** The core issue of the question is knowledge of safe administration of serum immune globulin. Use specific nursing knowledge and the process of elimination to make a selection.

27 **Answer: 4** **Rationale:** Physostigmine (Eserine) is an anticholinesterase agent that crosses the blood–brain barrier. It is used as an agent to correct anticholinergic poisoning. The other options do not have this effect. **Cognitive Level:** Applying **Client Need:** Pharmacological and Parenteral Therapies **Integrated Process:** Nursing Process: Planning **Content Area:** Pharmacology **Strategy:** The core issue of the question is knowledge of drug therapy to reverse excessive effects of medications used to treat Parkinson's disease. Use specific nursing knowledge and the process of elimination to make a selection.

28 **Answer: 4** **Rationale:** Administration of vitamin B_6 is recommended during therapy with isoniazid (INH), to reduce the incidence of peripheral neuritis, which could be associated

with isoniazid. Monitoring motor reflexes would not be indicated. Paresthesia is not usually a clinical manifestation of hypercalcemia, but rather of hypocalcemia. Antacids interfere with absorption of INH when taken within 1–2 hours of the INH, but would not cause the symptoms reported by the client. **Cognitive Level:** Applying **Client Need:** Pharmacological and Parenteral Therapies **Integrated Process:** Nursing Process: Data Collection **Content Area:** Adult Health **Strategy:** In order to answer this question, recall nursing interventions associated with the administration of this medication. If this was difficult, review the nursing interventions in the administration of the medication.

29 **Answer: 3 Rationale:** Rifampin causes an orange red discoloration of body fluids, including urine. The client needs to be aware of this. The drug is being ordered prophylactically to prevent the development of meningitis, not to treat it. Adverse effects are generally minor with rifampin. Because the drug is metabolized by the liver, regular liver function tests should be monitored. Rifampin should be used with caution in the presence of elevated liver enzymes or hepatic dysfunction. **Cognitive Level:** Applying **Client Need:** Physiological Adaptation **Integrated Process:** Nursing Process: Implementation **Content Area:** Pharmacology **Strategy:** Recall the side effects and client responses to listed medications. If this was difficult, review side effects and client responses to the medications.

30 **Answer: 1 Rationale:** Amantadine (Symmetrel) can cause anticholinergic effects, two of which are bladder relaxation and detrusor muscle contraction. Urinary retention could become more of a problem for a client with BPH on this medication. Hypermotility of the bowel is a cholinergic effect, not an anticholinergic effect. Increased lacrimation is a cholinergic effect, not an anticholinergic effect. Amantadine is not particularly nephrotoxic. **Cognitive Level:** Applying **Client Need:** Physiological Adaptation **Integrated Process:** Nursing Process: Planning **Content Area:** Pharmacology **Strategy:** In order to answer this question correctly, recall the side effects and client responses to listed medications. If this was difficult, review side effects and client responses to the medications.

31 **Answer: 4 Rationale:** Agents for herpes virus as herpes zoster can be nephritic. Important interventions include monitoring renal function and ensuring good hydration to decrease toxic effects. This drug is not reported to be particularly hepatotoxic. Sexual intercourse is to be avoided if the client is being treated with the acyclovir for genital herpes. Insomnia is not a side effect of acyclovir. **Cognitive Level:** Applying **Client Need:** Pharmacological and Parenteral Therapies **Integrated Process:** Nursing Process: Implementation **Content Area:** Fundamentals **Strategy:** In order to select the correct answer to this question, recall that the medication is toxic to the kidneys. The other answers do not apply to nephrotoxicity.

32 **Answer: 1 Rationale:** A full course of antibiotic therapy must be taken in order to decrease the risk of resistance to the antibiotic, or reoccurrence of the infection. Missed doses should be taken as soon as they are remembered, but the dose should not be doubled by taking 2 doses at the same time. Antibiotic doses are to be taken at regular intervals spaced throughout the 24 hours, without interrupting sleep when possible, in order to maintain effective therapeutic blood level of the antibiotic. Chewable tablets must be crushed or chewed, or the drug might not absorb adequately. **Cognitive Level:** Analyzing **Client Need:** Pharmacological and Parenteral Therapies **Integrated Process:** Nursing Process: Evaluation **Content Area:** Fundamentals **Strategy:** Note that the question stem asks for selection of the answer that indicates that the client understands correct administration of medication. Thus, the correct answer is also a true statement of fact. Use basic medication administration principles to choose correctly.

33 **Answer: 4 Rationale:** More than 4–6 watery stools per day and stools with blood are clinical manifestations of pseudomembranous colitis. C. *difficile* is the causative microorganism for this superinfection. The client is at risk for developing metabolic acidosis due to increased loss of bowel contents with loss of base. Antiperistaltic agents can promote retention of toxins, and should not be given. Antidiarrheal agents may be given for mild diarrhea, but not when toxins need to be eliminated. **Cognitive Level:** Applying **Client Need:** Pharmacological and Parenteral Therapies **Integrated Process:** Nursing Process: Planning **Content Area:** Fundamentals **Strategy:** The key information in the question stem is that the client has been on anti-infective therapy for 10 days, and has now developed diarrhea with watery stools. The length of time should direct selection of the first intervention before any treatment can begin, which would lead to first collecting the stool specimen.

34 **Answer: 4 Rationale:** Specific indicators of improvement, such as the resolution of pulmonary infiltrates, improved breath sounds, and normalization of pulse oximetry, are important outcomes to monitor in pneumonia. Systemic signs including fever, malaise, and leukocytosis are expected to demonstrate improvement within 48–72 hours of antibiotic therapy. Absence of hypersensitivity does not indicate therapeutic effectiveness. Orthostatic hypotension is unrelated to the question. **Cognitive Level:** Analyzing **Client Need:** Physiological Adaptation **Integrated Process:** Nursing Process: Evaluation **Content Area:** Fundamentals **Strategy:** Note that the respiratory system is addressed in the question to assist in selecting the correct answer. Look for an answer that addresses respiration.

35 **Answer: 1 Rationale:** The penicillins are structured with a sodium or potassium salt. When a high-sodium-content penicillin is administered, serum sodium can be elevated, which often results in hypokalemia. This client is demonstrating clinical manifestations of hypokalemia. With the elevated sodium, the accompanying anion would most likely be chloride, resulting in hyperchloremia, and not hypochloremia. Hypercalcemia is unrelated to this medication. Hypophosphatemia is unrelated to this medication. **Cognitive Level:** Analyzing **Client Need:** Pharmacological and Parenteral Therapies **Integrated Process:** Nursing Process: Data Collection **Content Area:** Fundamentals **Strategy:** In reviewing the question stem, the client is experiencing cardiovascular changes. Knowing that low potassium will result in cardiovascular changes will lead to the answer of hypokalemia.

Key Terms to Review

amebiasis p. 651
antigen p. 636
bactericidal p. 642
bacteriostatic p. 648
candidiasis p. 643
colony-stimulating factors p. 636
cross-sensitivity p. 644
empiric therapy p. 643
giardiasis p. 664
immunosuppressant p. 636
myelosuppression p. 638
neutropenia p. 636
peak drug level p. 643
pseudomembranous colitis p. 643
superinfection p. 662
tinea p. 662
trough drug level p. 643

References

Adams, M., Holland, L., & Urban, C. (2011). *Pharmacology for nurses: A pathophysiological approach* (3rd ed.). Upper Saddle River, NJ: Pearson Education, Inc.

Adams, M., & Koch, R. (2010). *Pharmacology: Connections to nursing practice.* Upper Saddle River, NJ: Pearson Education, Inc.

Deglin, J. H., & Vallerand, A. H. (2011). *Davis's drug guide for nurses* (12th ed.). Philadelphia: F. A. Davis.

Lehne, R. (2010). *Pharmacology for nursing care* (7th ed.). Philadelphia: W. B. Saunders.

Wilson, B., Shannon, M., & Shields, K. (2012). *Pearson nurse's drug guide 2012.* Upper Saddle River, NJ: Pearson Education.

Test Yourself

Are you ready for the NCLEX-PN® or course exams? Use the practice tests on the companion website to check.

Common Laboratory Tests 42

In this chapter

Cross Reference

Other chapters relevant to this content area are

Common Diagnostic Tests and Procedures	Chapter 43
Fluid and Electrolyte Imbalances	Chapter 49
Acid–Base Imbalances	Chapter 50

I. GENERAL PRINCIPLES OF SPECIMEN COLLECTION

A. Routine specimens

NCLEX® **1.** Usually collected in early morning before intake of food and fluids; if done in fasting state, withhold food and fluids for 8–12 hours prior to test

2. Collect using standard precautions for protection against exposure to blood or other body fluids; also use strict aseptic technique to protect client from infection

NCLEX® **3.** Label specimens with client name, date, exact time of collection, and type of specimen

NCLEX® **4.** On laboratory requisition slip, note client name, age, gender, room, physician, possible diagnosis, and test (or tests) being requested; record any factors that could interfere with results, such as foods or drugs

NCLEX® **5.** Avoid shaking blood specimens to avoid hemolysis and send promptly to lab

6. Values that fall within laboratory reference range are considered normal

NCLEX® **7.** Critical (panic) values are abnormal results that could increase risk of harm to client; these are telephoned to nursing unit and must be reported to charge nurse and/or health care provider

NCLEX® **B. Twenty-four-hour urine specimens**

1. Obtain a 24-hour specimen collection container from lab

2. Place container on ice, if indicated for test, and place 24-hour specimen collection sign above client bed, in bathroom, and on chart as a reminder not to discard urine

3. Have client void prior to test and discard this urine; save all urine for next 24 hours
4. Instruct client to void each time into container, such as a specimen hat, and avoid contaminating specimen with feces or bathroom tissue
5. Transfer voided specimen into collection device using standard precautions
6. At end of collection time, have client void and save this specimen
7. Label container with client's name, date, type of specimen, and exact time of collection (e.g., 12/29/11 07:00 to 12/30/11 07:00)

II. ARTERIAL BLOOD GASES (SEE ALSO CHAPTER 50)

A. Analysis of *serum* pH, partial pressure of arterial oxygen (PaO_2), partial pressure of carbon dioxide ($PaCO_2$), bicarbonate (HCO_3^-), and base excess
B. See Table 42–1 for normal reference ranges
C. See Chapter 50 for further discussion of arterial blood gases (ABGs)

Table 42–1 Normal Arterial Blood Gases

Test	Normal Reference Range
Serum pH	7.35–7.45
Oxygen (PaO_2)	80–100 mm Hg
Carbon dioxide ($PaCO_2$)	35–45 mm Hg
Bicarbonate (HCO_3^-)	22–26 mEq/L
Base excess	+3 to −3

III. SERUM ELECTROLYTES (SEE ALSO CHAPTER 49)

A. Consist of cations sodium, potassium, calcium, and magnesium; and anions chloride and phosphorus
B. Standard reported values include sodium, potassium, chloride, bicarbonate; others are ordered as needed; see Table 42–2 for normal reference ranges
C. See Chapter 49 for further discussion of full range of electrolytes

Table 42–2 Normal Serum Electrolytes

Test	Normal Reference Range
Sodium	135–145 mEq/L
Potassium	3.5–5.1 mEq/L
Chloride	98–107 mEq/L
Bicarbonate (venous)	23–29 mEq/L
Calcium	9–10.5 mg/dL total or 4.6–5.1 mg/dL ionized
Magnesium	1.8–3 mg/dL
Phosphorus	3–4.5 mg/dL

IV. GLUCOSE STUDIES

A. Fasting blood glucose (FBG)
1. Glucose is an end product of carbohydrate digestion, glycogenolysis, and gluconeogenesis
2. It is primary fuel source for cellular energy, especially for brain, which is only fueled by glucose and oxygen

NCLEX®
3. FBG is used to diagnose diabetes mellitus (DM) type 1 or 2 and hypoglycemia; see Table 42–3 for normal reference range

NCLEX®
4. Client must fast for 8 to 12 hours prior to drawing lab sample, with no ingestion of foods, beverages, or medications (oral antidiabetics or insulin)

B. Random blood glucose
1. Measures blood glucose as above but in nonfasting state
2. May be checked using capillary blood as in fingerstick blood glucose measurements

NCLEX®
3. See Table 42–3 for normal reference range

Table 42–3 Normal Adult Glucose Levels

Test	Normal Reference Range
Fasting blood glucose	70–110 mg/dL
Random (capillary) glucose	60–110 mg/dL
2-hour postprandial blood glucose	< 140 mg/dL
Oral glucose tolerance test (OGTT)	
Fasting baseline	70–110 mg/dL
30-minute sample	110–170 mg/dL
60-minute sample	120–170 mg/dL
90-minute sample	100–140 mg/dL
120-minute sample	70–120 mg/dL
Glycosylated hemoglobin A_{1c}	
Normal	3.5–6%
Good diabetic control	7.5% or lower
Fair diabetic control	7.6–8.9%
Poor diabetic control	9% or higher

C. Two-hour postprandial blood glucose: measures serum glucose 2 hours after eating

D. Glucose tolerance test (GTT)

1. Used as a screening test for clients at risk of DM and as diagnostic aid
2. Glucose levels should rise and fall in predictable amounts following ingestion of a specific glucose load (see Table 42–3); with DM, glucose levels peak at higher levels and fall more slowly than normal

NCLEX®

3. Client teaching
   a. Eat high-carbohydrate (CHO) diet (200–300 grams daily) for 3 days prior to test (give client list of high-CHO foods as needed)
   b. Do not drink alcohol or coffee or smoke for 36 hours before test (eliminates alcohol, caffeine, and nicotine as interfering factors with test results)
   c. Fast for 10 to 16 hours before test as instructed by health care provider
   d. Do not take any oral antidiabetic medications or insulin prior to test
   e. Do not exercise vigorously for 8 hours before or after test; sit quietly during test
   f. Test consists of baseline glucose level, ingestion of oral or IV glucose load, and series of blood glucose samples
   g. Two-hour GTT takes about 3 hours to complete; abnormal results may require a longer (3–5 hour) GTT

E. Glycosylated hemoglobin A_{1c}

1. Measures glucose that binds irreversibly to hemoglobin for life of red blood cell (RBC lifespan is 120 days)

NCLEX®

2. Indicates glycemic control over period of 3–5 weeks (takes into account continuous production and destruction of RBCs in body)
3. See Table 42–3 for interpretation of results
4. No fasting is required before test

V. COAGULATION STUDIES

A. Prothrombin time (PT) and international normalized ratio (INR)

1. Measures time needed for prothrombin (a vitamin K–dependent glycoprotein) to form a fibrin clot via extrinsic clotting pathway
2. Commonly used to evaluate effectiveness of oral anticoagulant such as sodium warfarin (Coumadin) or to diagnose disseminated intravascular coagulopathy (DIC), vitamin K deficiency, or liver dysfunction

NCLEX®

3. Normal reference ranges vary slightly by lab (9.6–11.8 seconds for adult males and 9.5–11.3 seconds for adult females); normal level is control value plus or minus 2 seconds; therapeutic range for warfarin is 1.5 to 2 times the control value

NCLEX®

4. INR is similar to PT but standardizes normal values across all lab systems; it measures effectiveness of oral anticoagulation

NCLEX®

5. Normal reference ranges are 2.0–3.0 for standard warfarin therapy and 3.0–4.5 for high-dose therapy
6. Draw baseline PT before beginning oral anticoagulation and repeat at specified intervals to monitor progress of therapy

7. Report abnormals or any values outside therapeutic ranges; low values indicate ineffective therapy and high values indicate risk for bleeding or hemorrhage

NCLEX® 8. Teach client to limit green leafy vegetables in diet because they are rich in vitamin K and will decrease PT/INR

B. Activated partial thromboplastin time (aPTT)

1. Measures time needed for recalcified, citrated plasma to clot after adding activated thromboplastin reagent
2. Commonly used to evaluate heparin therapy; can screen for all clotting factor deficiencies except VII and XIII
3. Elevated in liver disease and DIC

NCLEX® 4. Normal reference range is 20–35 seconds, and therapeutic range for heparin therapy is 1.5–2.5 times the control in seconds

5. Draw baseline aPTT before beginning heparin therapy and repeat at specified intervals to monitor progress of therapy

NCLEX® 6. Do not draw lab sample from vein in same arm in which heparin is infusing

NCLEX® 7. Report abnormals or any values outside therapeutic ranges; low values indicate ineffective therapy and high values indicate risk for bleeding or hemorrhage

C. Clotting time

1. Measures time required to complete all steps in clotting process
2. Normal reference range: 8–15 minutes
3. Results can be affected by anticoagulant therapy, high temperatures, and test tube agitation

VI. COMPLETE BLOOD COUNT

A. Hematocrit (Hct)

1. Measures proportion of RBCs in a volume of whole blood
2. Blood is centrifuged and proportions of **plasma** and solid components are measured and reported as a percentage
3. Can be falsely elevated when white blood cell (WBC) counts are markedly elevated (referred to as "buffy coat")
4. Can be falsely lowered with hemodilution (increased water component of blood)

NCLEX® 5. Normal reference range for males is 40–50% and for females is 38–47%

B. Hemoglobin (Hgb)

1. Heme consists of red pigment porphyrin and iron and is capable of combining loosely with oxygen (O_2) and carbon dioxide (CO_2)
2. Globin is a complex protein that can result in hemoglobinopathies when abnormal amino acid sequencing is present
3. Abnormal hemoglobinopathies include sickle cell disease and thallasemias; decreased Hgb commonly indicates anemia
4. Normally, Hgb and Hct levels parallel each other; Hct is usually 3 times higher than Hgb level

NCLEX® 5. Normal reference range for males is 13.5–18 grams/dL and for females is 12–16 grams/dL

C. RBC count

1. RBCs are formed in bone marrow and removed by liver, spleen, and bone marrow
2. Life span of RBC is approximately 120 days
3. Carry hemoglobin molecules responsible for O_2 transport to tissues
4. Normal reference range: 4.0–5.5 million cells/microliter for adult females and 4.5–6.2 million cells/microliter for adult males

NCLEX® 5. Abnormal values indicate anemia or blood dyscrasias

D. Platelet count

NCLEX® 1. Normal reference range: 150,000–450,000 per cubic mm (mm^3)

2. When microtrauma occurs and damages blood vessels, platelets aggregate and adhere to altered surface to form hemostatic plug to initiate clot formation
3. Platelets produce prostaglandins, which also promote platelet adherence and aggregation
   a. Aspirin is an antiplatelet drug that inhibits platelet aggregation
   b. Aspirin is given to prevent platelet aggregation along walls of atherosclerotic lesions (and initiating clot formation that could occlude vessel)
4. Decreased levels occur with cancer chemotherapy from bone marrow suppression, idiopathic thrombocytopenic purpura (ITP), most leukemias, uremia, and some infections such as infectious mononucleosis
5. Normal platelet life span is about 10 days

Table 42–4 White Blood Cell Differential Counts

Cells	Normal Adult Reference Range
Neutrophils (total)	50–70% or 2500–7000 cells/microliter
Segments (mature)	50–65% or 2500–6500 cells/microliter
Bands (immature)	0–5% or 0–500 cells/microliter
Eosinophils	1–3% or 100–300 cells/microliter
Basophils	0.4–1.0% or 40–100 cells/microliter
Lymphocytes	25–35% or 1700–3500 cells/microliter
Monocytes	4–6% or 200–600 cells/microliter

E. WBC

1. Consist of agranulocytes (monocytes and lymphocytes; no stainable granules in nucleus) and granulocytes (neutrophils, eosinophils, and basophils)

NCLEX®

2. Normal total WBC reference range: 5000–10,000 cells/mm^3
3. Normal WBC differential reference ranges: see Table 42–4
4. Neutrophils function as immune system defenses against inflammation, tissue injury, and infection

NCLEX®

   a. A "shift to the left" indicates a greater number of neutrophils are immature (bands) because of need for more rapid production to combat inflammation or infection
   b. A "shift to the right" indicates cells with excessive nuclear segments, seen with liver disease, megaloblastic and pernicious anemias, and Down syndrome
5. Eosinophils increase during allergic and parasitic conditions and decrease with higher levels of steroids
6. Basophils increase during healing process and decrease when steroid levels rise
7. Monocytes ("monos") are second line of defense against bacterial infection and foreign substances; they are macrophages that ingest larger particles and debris from cellular destruction; may also kill tumor cells—mechanism unclear
8. Lymphocytes ("lymphs") elevate during chronic and viral infections and lymphocytic leukemia; consist of B lymphocytes and T lymphocytes
   a. B lymphocytes lie dormant in lymph nodes until stimulated by antigenic substance and provide for humoral immunity by transforming into plasma cells that secrete immunoglobulins; IgG is immunoglobulin responsible for antiviral, antitoxin, and antibacterial work
   b. T lymphocytes mature in thymus, although they reside in lymph nodes, spleen, and other peripheral lymphoid tissue; are also stimulated when presented with an antigen that has been preprocessed by a macrophage; see immune studies section later in this chapter for additional information on T cells

VII. CARDIOVASCULAR FUNCTION STUDIES

A. Serum lipids

1. Primary measurements include total cholesterol, low-density lipoproteins (LDLs), high-density lipoproteins (HDLs), and triglycerides
2. Normal reference ranges: see Table 42–5

NCLEX®

3. Elevated levels (except for HDLs) increase risk of heart disease, stroke, and peripheral vascular disease; high HDL levels seem to have cardioprotective function; elevated triglycerides indicate hyperlipidemia (possibly familial)

Table 42–5 Serum Lipid Levels

Type of Lipid	Normal Reference Range
Cholesterol (total)	< 200 mg/dL
LDL	< 130 mg/dL
HDL	30–70 mg/dL
Triglycerides	< 200 mg/dL

Table 42-6 Cardiac Enzymes

Enzyme/Isoenzyme	Normal Reference Range	Pattern of Elevation and Decline
Creatine kinase (CK)	Males 55–170 units/L Females 30–135 units/L	Begins to rise 4–6 hours after myocardial or skeletal muscle damage
CK-MM	94–100%	Peaks at 18–24 hours
CK-MB	0–6%	Returns to normal within 3–4 days
CK-BB	0%	
Lactic dehydrogenase (LDH)	140–280 units/L	Begins to rise 24 hours after myocardial damage
LDH_1	14–26%	Peaks in 48–72 hours
LDH_2	29–39%	Returns to normal within 7–14 days
LDH_3	20–26%	
LDH_4	8–16%	
LDH_5	6–16%	
Cardiac Troponins		Rise within 3 hours of myocardial infarction
Troponin I	<0.1 to <1.0 ng/mL	
Troponin T	<0.2 to <1.0 ng/mL	Returns to normal in 5–9 days (I) or 10–14 days (T)

NCLEX® 4. Teach client to avoid alcohol intake for 24 hours before test and avoid high-cholesterol foods the evening before blood is drawn

5. Client must fast (except water) for 12 to 14 hours prior to test

B. Creatine kinase (CK) or creatinine phosphokinase (CPK)

NCLEX® 1. An enzyme found in large amounts in cardiac and skeletal muscle and in low amounts in brain tissue; enzyme is released from cells upon cell death

2. Enzyme can be fractionated into isoenzymes to identify tissue of origin; CK-MB is cardiac band; CK-MM is skeletal muscle band; CK-BB is brain tissue band

NCLEX® 3. Normal reference range and pattern of elevation: see Table 42–6

4. Avoid intake of alcohol 24 hours prior to test
5. Avoid injections, which could lead to falsely elevated value
6. Instruct client to avoid excessive physical exertion if monitoring skeletal muscle band; make note of soft tissue injury or falls that could cause false elevations

NCLEX® 7. Monitor results serially over 3 days if monitoring myocardial infarction (MI) and correlate with clinical picture

C. Lactic dehydrogenase (LDH)

1. An enzyme sometimes used to detect MI; elevates with myocardial cell death
2. Normal reference range and pattern of elevation: see Table 42–6

NCLEX® 3. Considered diagnostic for MI when level of LDH_2 rises or "flips" above LDH_1

4. Monitor results serially over 3 days and correlate with clinical picture

D. Troponins

1. Regulatory proteins found in skeletal and cardiac muscle (striated muscle cells)
2. Released into bloodstream with myocardial cell death; early indicator of cardiac damage; myoglobin also rises (12–90 mcg/L normal); peaks in 8–12 hrs

NCLEX® 3. Normal reference range and pattern of elevation: see Table 42–6

NCLEX® 4. Monitor results serially over 3 days and correlate with clinical picture

VIII. THYROID FUNCTION STUDIES

A. Thyroxine (T_4)

1. Major hormone secreted by thyroid gland
2. Aids in diagnosis of hypo- or hyperthyroidism with low or high levels respectively
3. Normal reference range: 4.5–11.5 mcg/mL T_4 or 1.0–2.3 ng/dL free T_4

B. Triiodothyronine (T_3)

1. A short-acting but potent thyroid hormone; present only in small amounts in blood
2. More useful for diagnosing hyperthyroidism than hypothyroidism
3. Normal reference range: 80–200 ng/dL

C. Thyroid-stimulating hormone (TSH)

1. A hormone secreted via negative feedback loop by anterior pituitary gland in response to decreased T_4
2. Used with results of T_4 level to differentiate between pituitary and thyroid dysfunction
   a. Decreased T_4 and normal or elevated TSH is consistent with thyroid disorder
   b. Decreased T_4 and decreased TSH is consistent with pituitary disorder
3. Normal reference range: 0.5–4 microinternational units/mL

D. No special preparation is needed for any thyroid test, but results can be affected by antithyroid drugs

IX. RENAL FUNCTION STUDIES

A. Blood urea nitrogen (BUN)

1. Formed in liver as end product of protein metabolism; consists of nitrogen portion of urea
2. Excreted via kidneys with only small amounts reabsorbed in renal tubules
3. *NCLEX®* Normal reference range: see Table 42–7
4. *NCLEX®* Rises with reduced glomerular filtration rate (GFR), increased dietary protein, increased catabolism (such as starvation), crush injuries, febrile illness, absorption of blood from intestines, and with hemoconcentration from dehydration
5. Decreases with overhydration, inadequate protein intake, or liver disease (liver is not adequately converting ammonia to urea)
6. *NCLEX®* Evaluate concurrently with serum creatinine for true indication of renal status; if BUN and creatinine rise together, indicates renal insufficiency or failure

B. Serum creatinine

1. End product of muscle creatine metabolism; is a specific indicator of GFR and renal status
2. *NCLEX®* Elevated levels commonly indicate renal insufficiency or failure
3. Teach client to avoid eating red meat for 24 hours prior to test and heavy exercise 8 hours prior in order to avoid falsely high values
4. Normal reference range: see Table 42–7

C. Creatinine clearance

1. Compares serum creatinine with creatinine excreted in a volume of urine over a period of hours (2, 12, 24)
2. Collection procedure is same as for a 24-hour urine; no preservative is needed in collection device
3. Normal reference range: see Table 42–7
4. Decreases progressively with renal insufficiency and failure as GFR declines

D. Serum osmolality

1. Reflects concentration of serum (number of osmotically active particles in solution)
2. Can be calculated using serum Na^+, BUN, and BG levels (see Box 42–1) but calculated value can be up to 9 mOsm less than drawn value
3. Normal reference range: see Table 42–7
4. Values rise with dehydration (more particles per volume of solution) and decrease with fluid overload (fewer particles per volume of solution)
5. Often used to detect risk of increased intracranial pressure

Table 42–7 Renal Function Tests

Renal Function Test	Normal Reference Range
Blood urea nitrogen (BUN)	8–22 mg/dL
Serum creatinine	0.6–1.3 mg/dL
Creatinine clearance	95–135 mL/min men, 85–125 mL/min women
Serum osmolality	280–296 mOsm/kg water
Urine osmolality	500–800 mOsm/kg water (average), 50–1,400 mOsm/kg water (extremes)

Box 42–1 Estimating Serum Osmolality Using Laboratory Values

Formula **2(Na+) + BUN/2.8 + Blood glucose/18**

Example: 2(137) + 10/2.8 + 110/18

276 + 3.57 + 6.11 = 286

Note: Na+ = serum sodium, BUN = blood urea nitrogen

E. Urine osmolality

1. Measures concentration of urine, as does specific gravity
2. Normal reference range: see Table 42–7
3. High values indicate kidneys are conserving water, while low values may reflect increased fluid intake, effect of diuretics, diabetes insipidus, or renal damage; clinical correlation is needed

X. URINALYSIS

A. Normal results: see Table 42–8

B. Possible causes of abnormal results: see Table 42–9

C. Nitrites

1. If present, nitrites suggest urinary tract infection (UTI)
2. Mechanism
   a. Dietary nitrates are excreted in urine
   b. When Gram-negative bacteria (such as common *E. coli*) are present in urine, these nitrates are converted to nitrites
   c. Test *suggests* a UTI with Gram-negative bacteria
   d. False-negatives can result if urine does not sit in bladder long enough (≥ 4 hours), for reaction to take place, if infection is not caused by Gram-negative organism, or if dietary nitrate is absent

D. Leukocyte esterase

NCLEX®
1. Simple test that may be done on a voided urine sample; positive result suggests UTI
2. Mechanism: WBCs contain esterases that react with substances in urine
3. More than 100,000 colonies of bacteria (per high-powered field) needed for UTI diagnosis

XI. LIVER FUNCTION STUDIES

A. Alanine aminotransferase (ALT) or serum glutamic pyruvic transaminase (SGPT)

1. An enzyme found primarily in liver cells but also found in small amounts in heart, kidney, and skeletal muscle
2. Normal reference range: see Table 42–10
3. Rises as high as 200–400 units with hepatitis or liver damage from drugs and chemicals

NCLEX®
4. Used to differentiate between jaundice caused by liver disease (often > 300 units/L) and causes outside liver (often < 300 units/L)
5. There is no food or fluid restriction before test

B. Aspartate aminotransferase (AST) or serum glutamic oxaloacetic transaminase (SGOT)

1. An enzyme found mainly in heart muscle and liver, with moderate amounts also found in skeletal muscle, kidneys, and pancreas
2. Normal reference range: see Table 42–10
3. Rises with cellular injury and release of enzyme into circulation
4. Rises following MI in 6–10 hours, peaks in 24–48 hours, and returns to normal in 4–6 days; rarely used because not specific to myocardial tissue

NCLEX®
5. With liver injury (hepatitis, necrosis), levels rise by 10 times or more and stay elevated longer; also rises with pancreatitis and musculoskeletal trauma, including injections
6. There is no food or fluid restriction before test

Table 42–8 Normal Urinalysis Findings

Component	Normal Finding
Color	Ranges from pale yellow to amber
Clarity	Clear when first excreted
Odor	Faintly aromatic
Specific gravity	1.005–1.030
pH	4.6–6.0
Protein	Trace to none
Glucose	None
Ketones	None
Sediment	0–3 RBCs, 0–4 WBCs; occasional cast; occasional renal epithelial cell

Table 42–9 Possible Causes of Abnormal Urinalysis Findings

Urinalysis	Significance of Abnormal Findings
Color	Pale: diabetes insipidus, drinking of excess free water Reddish: RBCs Burgundy: porphyria Orange: phenazopyridine HCl (Pyridium) or rifampin (Rifadin) Green: bile Black-brown: mercury poisoning Milky: pus, fat globules
Clarity	Cloudy: infection, phosphate precipitation from standing Turbid: spermatozoa, prostatic fluid
Odor	Sweet: acetonuria Strong: drugs, asparagus Ammonia: after standing for a time
Specific gravity	Decreased: diabetes insipidus, diuretics, excessive intake of free water Increased: diabetes mellitus, hypovolemia, liver disease, heart failure, SIADH, IV contrast medium
pH	Acid: acidosis, diabetes mellitus, fever, starvation, dehydration Alkaline: citrus, salicylate poisoning, sodium bicarbonate, urinary tract infection; urine becomes alkaline after standing because urea-splitting bacteria result in ammonia production
Protein	Transient: fever, stress 0.5 gram/day: chronic pyelonephritis 0.5–4 grams/day: multiple myeloma, diabetic nephropathy 5 grams/day: nephrotic syndrome, glomerulonephritis
Glucose	Present: diabetes mellitus
Ketones	Present: acidosis, diabetic ketoacidosis, starvation, or dieting (fat breakdown)
Sediments	Casts: clumps of material or cells that form in renal collecting tubule, assuming shape of tubule; are seen in various renal disease states Granular casts: acute tubular necrosis, glomerulonephritis, UTI, stress, renal transplant rejection Pus: glomerulonephritis RBC casts: glomerulonephritis WBCs: UTI RBCs: bleeding within glomeruli, transfusion reaction, malaria, hemolytic anemia

C. Bilirubin

1. A by-product of hemoglobin breakdown; produced also by liver, spleen, and bone marrow
2. Consists of total bilirubin, direct or conjugated bilirubin (excreted by GI tract), and indirect or unconjugated bilirubin (circulates protein-bound in blood)
3. Normal reference ranges: see Table 42–10

NCLEX®

4. Levels are elevated with jaundice and liver disease

Table 42–10 Liver Function Tests

Liver Function Test	Normal Reference Range
Alanine aminotransferase (ALT)	10–25 units/L
Aspartate aminotransferase (AST)	8–38 units/L
Bilirubin	Total: 0.1–1.2 mg/dL adults and 1–12 mg/dL newborn Direct: 0.1–0.3 mg/dL Indirect: calculate by subtracting direct from total
Ammonia	35–65 micrograms/dL

5. Draw infant blood sample from heel of foot
NCLEX® 6. Protect specimen from sunlight and artificial light and avoid hemolysis
7. Alcohol and many drugs will increase levels; write medications given on lab requisition
8. Teach client to reduce intake of yellow vegetables (beans, carrots, sweet potatoes, squash) for 3–4 days before test and to fast for 4 hours prior to test

D. Ammonia

1. End product of nitrogen breakdown during protein metabolism
2. Metabolized by liver and excreted via kidneys
3. Normal reference range: see Table 42–10
4. Elevated results indicate liver disease and possibly encephalopathy (and hepatic coma)
NCLEX® 5. Degree of elevation does not correlate directly with risk of developing hepatic coma
6. Teach client not to smoke for 24 hours prior to test and to fast (except for water) for 8–10 hours before test

XII. PANCREATIC ENZYMES

A. Amylase

1. Produced by pancreas and salivary glands for CHO digestion and excreted via kidneys
2. Normal reference range: 25–151 units/L
NCLEX® 3. Increased with pancreatitis; elevation begins 3 to 6 hours after pain begins, peaks in 24 hours and returns to normal in 2 to 3 days
4. Many drugs affect results, so list them on lab requisition; false results can occur if measured within 72 hours of cholecystography with radiopaque dyes

B. Lipase

1. Produced by pancreas to break down fats and triglycerides into fatty acids and glycerol
2. Normal reference range: 10–140 units/L
NCLEX® 3. Increased with pancreatic disorders; may rise as late as 24 to 36 hours after onset of disorder and return to normal as much as 14 days later

XIII. METABOLIC FUNCTION STUDIES

A. Albumin

1. A plasma protein that maintains oncotic pressure (to prevent edema) and transports water-insoluble substances (fatty acids, hormones, bilirubin, drugs)
NCLEX® 2. Normal reference range: see Table 42–11
NCLEX® 3. May be decreased in malnourished states and monitored as an indicator of nutritional status

B. Total protein

1. Consists of circulating albumin and globulins in serum; serve many functions, including tissue growth and repair, pH buffering, enzymes, hormones, and coagulation factors
NCLEX® 2. Normal reference range: see Table 42–11
NCLEX® 3. May be decreased with malnutrition, low-protein diet, GI disorders, severe liver disease, chronic renal failure, severe burns, or water intoxication
4. May be increased with dehydration (hemoconcentration), vomiting, diarrhea, and myeloma
5. Teach clients to avoid high-fat foods for 24 hours prior to test

C. Pre-albumin

1. Is also known as thyroxin-binding pre-albumin or transthyretin
2. Is a sensitive indicator of recent changes in catabolism because half-life is less than 2 days
3. Used to screen for nutritional problems and gauge effectiveness of nutrition therapy

Table 42-11 Tests Reflecting Metabolic Function

Test	Normal Reference Range
Prealbumin	12–50 mg/dL (adults)
Albumin	3.4–5.0 grams/dL
Total protein	6.0–8.0 grams/dL
Alkaline phosphatase	4.5–1.3 King-Armstrong units/dL
Uric acid	3.5–8.0 mg/dL adult males, 2.8–6.8 mg/dL females

4. Normal reference range: see Table 42–11
5. Low values indicate need for comprehensive nutritional evaluation (history, weight, anthropometric measurements, calorie count)
6. High values are found in renal failure because of poor renal excretion

D. Alkaline phosphatase

1. Enzyme present in intestines, liver, bone, and placenta
2. Normal reference range: see Table 42–11
3. NCLEX® Rises with periods of bone growth and with liver disease or bile duct obstruction
4. Results may be affected by hepatotoxic drugs administered during 12 hours prior to test
5. Fasting may be required for 12 hours prior to test

E. Uric acid

1. NCLEX® By-product of purine metabolism; is elevated in gout; is affected by diet and renal function
2. Normal reference range: see Table 42–11
3. Excessive uric acid can lead to kidney stone formation as renal clearance occurs
4. NCLEX® Teach client to avoid high-purine foods (liver, kidney, brain, heart, sweetbreads, scallops, sardines) for 24 hours prior to test; otherwise, no food or drink restriction
5. Write medications taken on lab requisition, since many drugs affect results

XIV. IMMUNE FUNCTION STUDIES

A. Human immunodeficiency virus (HIV) tests

1. Consist of enzyme-linked immunosorbent assay (ELISA) and Western blot
2. NCLEX® ELISA is tested first, and if positive, Western blot is done; if second test is negative, client should be retested in 3 to 6 months
3. NCLEX® Positive Western blot confirms diagnosis of HIV
4. Recent infections can be detected using standard ELISA test and a second detuned (weaker) version of this test
   a. Standard ELISA is positive 3–4 weeks after exposure, while detuned test is only positive 4 months later
   b. A positive ELISA and negative detuned test helps identify newer infections to help clients and at-risk partners get treatment sooner and also aid Public Health departments to track transmission patterns

B. CD4 T cell counts

1. Function of T helper cells is primarily to help B cells and increase immunoglobulin production
2. Normal reference range: 500–1600 cells/microliter (mcL)
3. NCLEX® CD4 counts decrease with HIV, causing increased risk of infection at levels of 200–499 cells/mcL and severe risk when count is less than 200 cells/mcL

C. CD4 to CD8 ratio

1. CD8 or T suppressor cells are responsible for down-regulation of immune response or once an infection has been eradicated
2. Normal ratio of CD4 to CD8 cells is 2:1
3. With decrease in CD4 counts as HIV progresses to acquired immunodeficiency syndrome (AIDS) and client condition worsens, this ratio decreases

D. Viral load testing

1. Measures amounts of HIV viral RNA or other viral protein in blood
2. NCLEX® Values increase or decrease according to current level of infection

XV. THERAPEUTIC DRUG LEVELS

A. Measure amount of drug circulating in bloodstream, usually before scheduled daily dose

B. NCLEX® If measurement is required before and after drug administration, referred to as peak and trough drug levels

1. Trough level is drawn when dose circulating in bloodstream is lowest (just prior to next dose)
2. Peak level is drawn when dose circulating in bloodstream is highest (approximately 30 minutes after drug has finished infusing and dose has equilibrated in bloodstream)

C. Drug levels need to remain within therapeutic range at all times

D. NCLEX® High drug levels could cause signs of toxicity; low levels could result in symptoms of original health problem (ineffective dose)

E. NCLEX® Teach client not to take daily dose before routine drug level is drawn

F. Alert prescriber immediately of abnormal levels so dosage adjustment can be made

G. NCLEX® See Table 42–12 for common therapeutic drug levels

Table 42–12 Common Therapeutic Drug Levels

Drug	Therapeutic Range
Acetaminophen (Tylenol)	10–20 mcg/mL
Amitriptyline (Elavil)	120–150 ng/mL
Carbamazepine (Tegretol)	5–12 mcg/mL
Digoxin (Lanoxin)	0.5–2.0 ngmL
Ethosuximide (Zarontin)	40–100 mcg/mL
Lidocaine (Xylocaine)	1.5–5.0 mcg/mL
Lithium (Lithobid)	0.5–1.3 mEq/L
Magnesium sulfate	4.0–7.0 mg/dL
Phenytoin (Dilantin)	10–20 mcg/mL
Procainamide (Pronestyl)	4–10 mcg/mL
Quinidine (Cardioquin)	2–5 mcg/mL
Salicylate	100–250 mcg/mL
Theophylline (Theo-Dur)	10–20 mcg/mL
Valproic acid (Depakene)	50–100 mcg/mL

Check Your NCLEX-PN® Exam I.Q.

You are ready for testing on this content if you can

- Collect blood and body fluid specimens correctly for laboratory analysis.
- Perform client teaching about specimen collection for laboratory analysis.
- Identify normal and abnormal values for common laboratory tests.
- Correlate pathophysiology with results of laboratory tests.
- Make appropriate clinical decisions after reviewing laboratory test results, including notification of primary care provider.

PRACTICE TEST

1 Eighteen hours after surgery, the urine output of a client who underwent removal of a pituitary tumor is markedly increased, and the urine specific gravity is 1.002. The nurse expects to note which corresponding findings when reviewing results of laboratory tests? Select all that apply.

1. Serum sodium 148 mEq/L
2. Serum potassium 3.4 mEq/L
3. Serum osmolality 263 mOsm/L
4. Blood urea nitrogen 7 mg/dL
5. Hematocrit 51%

2 The nurse would be most concerned about which laboratory value obtained for a client receiving furosemide (Lasix) therapy?

1. Blood urea nitrogen 20 mg/dL
2. Hematocrit 46%
3. Creatinine 1.1 mg/dL
4. Potassium 3.2 mEq/L

3 A client has just undergone insertion of a nasogastric tube, and it immediately drains 1000 mL of fluid. Which electrolyte monitoring becomes the nurse's greatest concern at this time?

1. Sodium
2. Potassium
3. Chloride
4. CO_2 content

4 A client who was just admitted to the nursing unit has a uric acid level of 9.5 mg/dL. Which question would the nurse ask initially?

1. "Do you have a history of gallbladder disease?"
2. "Do you drink large amounts of green tea?"
3. "Do you have a history of gout?"
4. "Do you have any pains in the flank area?"

5 The nurse is caring for a client who received a renal transplant 24 hours previously. Which trend in laboratory studies indicates to the nurse that the new kidney is functioning? Select all that apply.

1. Hemoglobin 12%, increased from 11.8%
2. Serum creatinine 1.6 mg/dL, decreased from 1.9 mg/dL
3. Serum sodium 140 mEq/L, increased from 136 mEq/L
4. Serum phosphate 4.4 mg/dL, decreased from 4.8 mg/dL
5. Blood urea nitrogen level 29 mg/dL, decreased from 35 mg/dL

6 The nurse is caring for a client who has just returned from the operating room. Blood loss was minimal, but the client was given large volumes of crystalloid fluid during the procedure. Which laboratory test results suggest overhydration? Select all that apply.

1. Sodium 147 mEq/L
2. Hemoglobin 14%
3. Hematocrit 33%
4. Calcium level 8.8 mg/dL
5. Blood urea nitrogen 8 mg/dL

7 A client is being evaluated for possible appendicitis. An elevation of which laboratory test result suggests most strongly to the nurse the presence an acute bacterial infection?

1. Neutrophils
2. Erythrocytes
3. Lymphocytes
4. Platelets

8 The nurse is assigned to care for a client admitted with meningitis who has had a spinal tap performed. Which cells in the cerebrospinal fluid (CSF) suggest that the client has a viral meningitis infection?

1. Platelets
2. Neutrophils
3. Red blood cells
4. Lymphocytes

9 In caring for a female client who has a urinary tract infection (UTI) with more than 100,000 colonies of *Escherichia coli* bacteria, what corresponding findings would the nurse expect to see on the client's urinalysis report? Select all that apply.

1. Positive nitrites
2. Positive leukocyte esterase
3. Negative red blood cells (RBCs)
4. Negative white blood cells (WBCs)
5. Positive glucose

10 The nurse is reviewing the results of follow-up laboratory studies on a client diagnosed with hyperlipidemia. The nurse concludes that the client has been compliant with diet and medication therapy if the total cholesterol level is less than how many mg/dL? Provide a numeric answer.

Fill in your answer below:

_____mg/dL

11 A nurse notes the client's albumin level is 2.4 grams/dL. The nurse should plan to monitor the client for which of the following at this time? Select all that apply.

1. Peripheral edema
2. Inelastic skin turgor
3. Hypoactive bowel sounds
4. Dry mucous membranes
5. Lung crackles

12 A client is admitted with complaints of severe nausea and vomiting for several days. The nurse expects arterial blood gases to reveal which acid–base imbalance?

1. Metabolic acidosis
2. Metabolic alkalosis
3. Respiratory acidosis
4. Respiratory alkalosis

13 Troponin levels are ordered on a client to confirm a myocardial infarction. When should the nurse expect to have blood drawn for this test?

1. Within 1–2 hours of onset of chest pain
2. Within the first 24 hours of onset of chest pain
3. Between 6 and 24 hours of onset of chest pain
4. Between 24 and 48 hours of onset of chest pain

14 The nurse would anticipate that a client with cirrhosis of the liver would have increased levels of which laboratory values? Select all that apply.

1. Albumin
2. Bilirubin
3. Ammonia
4. Prothrombin time
5. Calcium

15 The nurse notes that the international normalized ratio (INR) of a client with aortic valve replacement taking sodium warfarin (Coumadin) is 2.6. What action should the nurse take at this time?

1. Encourage the client to eat foods high in vitamin K.
2. Administer the daily dose of Coumadin as ordered.
3. Monitor the client closely for signs of a deep vein thrombosis.
4. Withhold the next scheduled dose of Coumadin, and notify the prescriber.

16 A client is being evaluated for primary hypothyroidism, and has had blood drawn to determine thyroid stimulating hormone (TSH) and T_4 levels. The nurse observes that which test results pattern would support this diagnosis?

1. Elevated TSH and elevated T_4 levels
2. Elevated TSH and decreased T_4 level
3. Decreased TSH and elevated T_4 level
4. Decreased TSH and decreased T_4 level

17 A client is admitted with dehydration secondary to prolonged nausea and vomiting. Which serum laboratory test results would the nurse expect to note as a result of the dehydration? Select all that apply.

1. Sodium 138 mEq/dL
2. Potassium 4.2 mEq/dL
3. Blood urea nitrogen (BUN) 30 mg/dL
4. Hematocrit 49%
5. Total protein 6.8 mg/dL

18 The nurse should observe for Trousseau's sign in a client after noting which electrolyte abnormality?

1. Potassium 3.3 mEq/L
2. Sodium 131 mEq/L
3. Chloride 94 mEq/L
4. Calcium 7.7 mEq/L

19 The white blood cell (WBC) count of a client is 18,000 cells/microliter. The nurse recognizes that this value is associated with what health problem of this client?

1. Rheumatoid arthritis
2. History of alcoholism
3. Viral infection
4. Wound dehiscence

20 The nurse would monitor the client for fever and other signs of infection if the client's white blood cell (WBC) count was noted to be greater than _____ cells/mm^3 on the laboratory report. Provide a numerical response that is a whole number.

Fill in your answer below:

_____ cells/mm^3

ANSWERS & RATIONALES

1 **Answer: 1, 5 Rationale:** Diabetes insipidus is a potential complication following surgery on the pituitary gland. Edema of the remaining pituitary gland can inhibit release of antidiuretic hormone (ADH), resulting in loss of water from glomeruli into collecting tubules of the nephrons. The client excretes large volumes of urine with a low urine specific gravity. As water is removed from the vascular compartment, the serum sodium and hematocrit become concentrated. The blood urea

nitrogen and serum osmolality would be expected to be elevated rather than low as the client loses body water. The serum potassium would not be low. **Cognitive Level:** Analyzing **Client Need:** Reduction of Risk Potential **Integrated Process:** Nursing Process: Data Collection **Content Area:** Adult Health **Strategy:** This question calls for specific knowledge of altered ADH secretion that can occur after pituitary surgery. Remember that ADH results in movement of free water (that is, water without sodium) into collecting tubules of the nephron, which results in large volumes of water being removed from the blood. The specific gravity (concentration) of the urine decreases. In addition, removal of water from the serum concentrates (and thereby elevates) the serum sodium and hematocrit. Recall also that hemoconcentration could also raise, not lower, other lab values.

2 **Answer: 4** **Rationale:** Furosemide inhibits reabsorption of sodium, water, and potassium from the distal renal tubules and the loop of Henle, leading to a diuresis. The most common electrolyte disturbance associated with furosemide administration is hypokalemia. The creatinine value is within normal limits. The BUN and hematocrit could rise or fall, depending on the amount of fluid retained in the vascular compartment. **Cognitive Level:** Analyzing **Client Need:** Reduction of Risk Potential **Integrated Process:** Nursing Process: Data Collection **Content Area:** Adult Health **Strategy:** This question calls for specific knowledge of the action of furosemide, and knowledge that hypokalemia is a common side effect. Use nursing knowledge and the process of elimination to make a selection.

3 **Answer: 2** **Rationale:** Hypokalemia is an almost universal complication of loss of gastric hydrochloric acid. In this scenario, loss of the hydrogen ions results in a metabolic alkalosis. In turn, compensation for this loss takes place in the nephron, where hydrogen ions are retained. The nephron is obligated to excrete potassium, which could result in profound hypokalemia and require vigilant IV replacement. Other electrolytes might be affected, but not to the degree that potassium homeostasis is altered. The CO_2 content might be affected, but is of less concern than potassium depletion, which could lead to cardiac dysrhythmias. **Cognitive Level:** Applying **Client Need:** Reduction of Risk Potential **Integrated Process:** Nursing Process: Data Collection **Content Area:** Adult Health **Strategy:** This question calls for specific knowledge that loss of hydrochloric acid triggers the mechanism whereby the kidneys lose potassium. Use nursing knowledge and the process of elimination to make a selection.

4 **Answer: 3** **Rationale:** Elevated uric acid levels are commonly seen with gout, which is a disorder of purine metabolism, and this is the initial question to ask the client. Uric acid does not rise with gallbladder disease, and is not affected by green tea. Although the client could experience renal stones from precipitation of uric acid crystals (causing flank pain), this is not the initial question to ask, since renal stones are a complication of gout. **Cognitive Level:** Analyzing **Client Need:** Reduction of Risk Potential **Integrated Process:** Nursing Process: Data Collection **Content Area:** Adult Health **Strategy:** Note the stem of the question has the critical word *initially*, which indicates more than one option might be technically correct but one is best. Use nursing knowledge related to uric acid level and gout, and the process of elimination, to make a selection.

5 **Answer: 2, 5** **Rationale:** Serum creatinine and blood urea nitrogen (BUN) are often associated with renal function, although serum creatinine is the most reliable indicator of kidney function. Decreases in serum creatinine and BUN often are dramatic following renal transplantation. Regular monitoring of these levels is imperative in assessing the function of the transplanted kidney. Hemoglobin levels can increase postoperatively due to blood transfusions. Serum phosphate might decrease long-term as the kidney increases excretion of phosphates; however, this is not a reliable indicator of renal function. Serum sodium levels might fluctuate according to an individual client's sodium–water balance. **Cognitive Level:** Analyzing **Client Need:** Reduction of Risk Potential **Integrated Process:** Nursing Process: Data Collection **Content Area:** Adult Health **Strategy:** This question calls for the specific knowledge that creatinine is the best indicator of renal function and that BUN is another key indicator. Note the wording of the question indicates that more than one option may be correct.

6 **Answer: 3, 5** **Rationale:** The hematocrit is an indicator of the proportion of red blood cells in a given volume of blood. The hematocrit might decrease when cell volume of the blood is decreased because of blood loss or when the liquid portion of the blood volume increases, such as when large volumes of intravenous (IV) fluid are administered. The blood urea nitrogen varies according to hydration status; it rises with dehydration and falls with fluid overload, such as when large volumes of IV fluid are administered. Hemoglobin, sodium and calcium levels would not be altered. **Cognitive Level:** Analyzing **Client Need:** Reduction of Risk Potential **Integrated Process:** Nursing Process: Data Collection **Content Area:** Adult Health **Strategy:** This question requires understanding of how fluid overload affects laboratory values. Specifically, it requires knowledge that the BUN can decrease and that hematocrit can be reduced even if there is no blood loss. Note that the wording of the question suggests that more than one option is likely to be correct.

7 **Answer: 1** **Rationale:** Neutrophils are responsible for destruction of bacterial invaders. In acute bacterial infections, such as appendicitis, the percentage of neutrophils (especially immature bands) in the complete blood count will increase. This presence of an increased number of bands is known as a "shift to the left." Lymphocytes are responsible for destruction of viruses. Erythrocytes and platelets are not affected by infections. **Cognitive Level:** Analyzing **Client Need:** Reduction of Risk Potential **Integrated Process:** Nursing Process: Data Collection **Content Area:** Adult Health **Strategy:** This question calls for specific knowledge that neutrophils are responsible for destroying bacteria, and will be elevated in acute bacterial infections. Use nursing knowledge and the process of elimination to make a selection.

8 **Answer: 4** **Rationale:** Lymphocytes are responsible for the destruction of viruses. Thus, the presence of lymphocytes in the CSF suggests that the meningitis is viral in etiology. This is significant because the infection is most commonly self-limiting, and will not respond to antibiotic therapy (as would bacterial meningitis). The presence of neutrophils would suggest bacterial meningitis. Normally, CSF is free of all cell types. **Cognitive Level:** Applying **Client Need:** Reduction of Risk Potential **Integrated Process:** Nursing Process: Data Collection **Content Area:** Adult Health **Strategy:** This question calls for the specific knowledge that lymphocytes are responsible for destruction of viruses. Use nursing knowledge and the process of elimination to make a selection.

9 **Answer: 1, 2** **Rationale:** Nitrites are likely to be positive with UTI. A positive leukocyte esterase suggests a UTI. Leukocytes (white blood cells) contain esterases that react

with substances contained in urine. More than 100,000 colonies of bacteria (per high-powered field) are needed before the client can be diagnosed with a UTI. RBCs are also usually positive because of the effect of infection on tissue. WBCs are present in the urine to fight infection. Glucose in the urine should be negative and a positive finding would indicate glucose intolerance rather than UTI. **Cognitive Level:** Applying **Client Need:** Reduction of Risk Potential **Integrated Process:** Nursing Process: Data Collection **Content Area:** Adult Health **Strategy:** This question calls for specific knowledge that leukocyte esterase will be positive in urine infected with bacteria. Use nursing knowledge and the process of elimination to make a selection.

10 **Answer: 200 Rationale:** To maintain health, the recommended total cholesterol level should be less than 200 mg/dL. **Cognitive Level:** Analyzing **Client Need:** Reduction of Risk Potential **Integrated Process:** Nursing Process: Data Collection **Content Area:** Adult Health **Strategy:** The core issue of the question is knowledge of normal serum cholesterol levels. Use nursing knowledge and the process of elimination to make a selection.

11 **Answer: 1, 5 Rationale:** Albumin is a protein responsible for increasing osmotic pressure and maintaining intravascular fluid volume. Low albumin levels reduce intravascular colloid osmotic pressure, which allows fluid to move out of blood vessels and into interstitial tissues. This fluid retention will be assessed as peripheral edema, lung crackles, and fluid weight gain. Skin turgor will be elastic when fluid shifts into the interstitial spaces. Bowel sounds and mucous membranes would not be affected. **Cognitive Level:** Analyzing **Client Need:** Reduction of Risk Potential **Integrated Process:** Nursing Process: Planning **Content Area:** Adult Health **Strategy:** Determine that this test result is an abnormally low albumin level. Recall that albumin is necessary for maintenance of fluid balance between body compartments and then select all options that indicate fluid retention.

12 **Answer: 2 Rationale:** The loss of stomach acids creates an imbalance, leading to an excess of alkaline fluids in the body. The source of the loss is metabolic, not respiratory. **Cognitive Level:** Applying **Client Need:** Reduction of Risk Potential **Integrated Process:** Nursing Process: Data Collection **Content Area:** Adult Health **Strategy:** First, determine if the imbalance is metabolic or respiratory. Loss of GI fluids is a metabolic function, so options indicating a respiratory problem can be eliminated. Next, determine if the imbalance is acid or base. Loss of body acids will lead to an excess of bicarbonate in the body and an alkaline state.

13 **Answer: 3 Rationale:** Troponin is a specific marker for cardiac injury. Elevations in serum levels usually begin 4–6 hours after onset of symptoms, and peak in 12–24 hours. Drawing the blood in the first 2 hours would be too soon, and waiting longer than 24 hours would miss the times for peak levels. **Cognitive Level:** Applying **Client Need:** Reduction of Risk Potential **Integrated Process:** Nursing Process: Planning **Content Area:** Adult Health **Strategy:** The question calls for specific knowledge of troponin release times following myocardial infarction. Recall the times for elevation and return to normal and choose the option that is closest and most specific to this pattern.

14 **Answer: 2, 3, 4 Rationale:** The cirrhotic liver is unable to completely break down bilirubin, and serum levels are elevated. Ammonia is normally converted to urea in the liver; serum levels are increased with liver damage. Prothrombin times are increased when the liver is unable to synthesize clotting factors. In cirrhosis, the damaged liver is unable to properly metabolize amino acids and synthesize albumin, resulting in decreased serum concentrations. Calcium levels should be unaffected by cirrhosis. **Cognitive Level:** Applying **Client Need:** Reduction of Risk Potential **Integrated Process:** Nursing Process: Data Collection **Content Area:** Adult Health **Strategy:** This question tests knowledge of liver functions and cirrhosis. Recall the liver's function as related to each of the laboratory values, and systematically eliminate incorrect options.

15 **Answer: 2 Rationale:** The usual therapeutic INR level during medication therapy with sodium warfarin (Coumadin) is 2–3. The next dose should be given as scheduled, not withheld. Encouraging the client to eat foods high in vitamin K would reduce effectiveness of the drug. The client would be at risk for deep vein thrombosis when blood clotting is accelerated, not slowed. **Cognitive Level:** Analyzing **Client Need:** Reduction of Risk Potential **Integrated Process:** Nursing Process: Implementation **Content Area:** Adult Health **Strategy:** First, determine if the level is expected. Recall that in order to be therapeutic, the INR usually needs to fall within the 2–3 range. With this in mind, select the option that is consistent with routine nursing care.

16 **Answer: 2 Rationale:** In primary hypothyroidism, the thyroid gland does not produce thyroxine (T_4), despite being stimulated by the pituitary gland (with elevated TSH) to do so. Elevated TSH and T_4 levels are seen with secondary hyperthyroidism caused by excessive TSH production by the pituitary. A decreased TSH and elevated T_4 are seen with primary hyperthyroidism, not hypothyroidism. Decreased TSH and T_4 levels are seen in secondary hypothyroidism due to insufficient pituitary secretions. **Cognitive Level:** Applying **Client Need:** Reduction of Risk Potential **Integrated Process:** Nursing Process: Data Collection **Content Area:** Adult Health **Strategy:** The question requires knowledge of pituitary and thyroid hormone functions. First eliminate options with an increased T_4 level, which would not be seen with hypothyroidism. Next recall the negative endocrine feedback loop to differentiate between test results expected with primary and secondary hypothyroidism.

17 **Answer: 3, 4 Rationale:** Dehydration results in loss of fluids, causing a hemoconcentration of BUN, which is elevated. The hematocrit would be elevated secondary to hemoconcentration from dehydration. The sodium is normal and would be more likely to be elevated from hemoconcentration with dehydration. The potassium level is normal, and would most likely be lower because of losses from the vomiting. The total protein level is normal, and would not likely be influenced by dehydration. **Cognitive Level:** Analyzing **Client Need:** Reduction of Risk Potential **Integrated Process:** Nursing Process: Data Collection **Content Area:** Adult Health **Strategy:** The question requires analysis of fluid losses on common lab values. Recall that vomiting leads to a loss of sodium, potassium, and water. Eliminate values that are normal; look for abnormal values.

18 **Answer: 4 Rationale:** Hypocalcemia causes excitability of skeletal, cardiac, and smooth muscle tissues. Evidence of this is seen in Trousseau's sign, a carpopedal spasm. Hypokalemia, hyponatremia, and hypochloremia would not cause this sign. **Cognitive Level:** Applying **Client Need:** Reduction of Risk Potential **Integrated Process:** Nursing Process: Data Collection **Content Area:** Adult Health **Strategy:** Specific knowledge of Trousseau's sign is needed to answer this question. Recall this carpopedal spasm is seen with low calcium and

magnesium levels. Eliminate the other options because low levels of the other electrolytes would lead to muscle weakness, not neuromuscular excitability.

19 **Answer: 4** **Rationale:** Tissue injury, such as with wound dehiscence, can cause a significant increase in WBCs. The WBC count may not increase with rheumatoid arthritis. The WBC count does not increase with alcoholism. Viral infection could lead to an increase in lymphocytes, but the overall WBC count does not rise to such high levels overall with viral infections. **Cognitive Level:** Analyzing **Client Need:** Reduction of Risk Potential **Integrated Process:** Nursing Process: Data Collection **Content Area:** Adult Health **Strategy:** First, determine that the WBC is abnormally high. Recall conditions that elevate the WBC, such as bacterial infections, stress, and tissue injury. Evaluate each option to eliminate conditions in which the WBC is decreased or unaffected.

20 **Answer: 10,000|10000** **Rationale:** The normal range for the WBC count is 5000–10,000/mm^3. For this reason, the nurse would be concerned about the risk of infection if the WBC exceeded 10,000. **Cognitive Level:** Analyzing **Client Need:** Reduction of Risk Potential **Integrated Process:** Nursing Process: Data Collection **Content Area:** Adult Health **Strategy:** The core issue of the question is knowledge of normal laboratory values. Use this knowledge to choose an answer. Since specific knowledge is needed to answer correctly, memorize this value if you found the question difficult.

Key Terms to Review

plasma p. 680

serum p. 678

References

Corbett, J. (2008). *Laboratory tests and diagnostic procedures with nursing diagnoses* (7th ed.). Upper Saddle River, NJ: Pearson Education.

Fischbach, F., & Dunning, M. (2009). *A manual of laboratory and diagnostic tests* (8th ed.). Philadelphia: Lippincott Williams & Wilkins.

Kee, J. (2010). *Laboratory and diagnostic tests with nursing implications* (8th ed.). Upper Saddle River, NJ: Pearson Education.

Leeuwen, A., & Poelhuis-Leth, D. (2009). *Davis's comprehensive handbook of laboratory and diagnostic tests with nursing implications* (3rd ed.). Philadelphia: F.A. Davis.

Smith, S., Duell, D., & Martin, B. (2012). *Clinical nursing skills: Basic to advanced skills* (8th ed.). Upper Saddle River, NJ: Pearson Education, Inc.

Test Yourself

Are you ready for the NCLEX-PN® or course exams? Use the practice tests on the companion website to check.

ANSWERS & RATIONALES

43 Common Diagnostic Tests and Procedures

In this chapter

Cross Reference

Another chapter relevant to this content area is

Common Laboratory Tests **Chapter 42**

I. GENERAL DIAGNOSTIC TESTS

A. Client safety in diagnostic testing

1. Ensuring client safety is required by The Joint Commission (formerly known as JCAHO)
2. Client safety for any diagnostic test implies knowledge of procedure, risks and benefits, and pre- and postcare
3. *NCLEX®* Ensure that informed consent form is signed and witnessed, especially for invasive diagnostic tests involving penetration of tissues or blood vessels (contrast dye, radioisotopes)
4. *NCLEX®* Before beginning a diagnostic test, a *time out* or pause is called to double-check that right procedure is being carried out on right client at right site

B. Biopsy

1. Overview
   a. Removes and examines body tissue to detect malignancy or other disease process
   b. Methods include aspiration by suction, brush method (scrapes cells using stiff bristles), excision by surgical cutting, needle aspiration, or punch biopsy (using punch-type instrument)
   c. Common sites are bone marrow, breast, endometrium of uterus, kidney, colon, and liver
2. Preprocedure care
   a. Take baseline vital signs (VS)
   b. Explain that biopsy site will be anesthetized just prior to procedure
   c. Explain that with needle biopsy client may be asked to take a breath and hold it
   d. Keep client NPO for 6 hours prior to liver biopsy to decrease liver congestion
3. Postprocedure care
   a. Monitor VS as prescribed
   b. *NCLEX®* Apply pressure to site for 20 minutes (kidney) or place client on right side (liver) to reduce risk of bleeding; apply pressure dressing
   c. Observe for bleeding at site and instruct client to report bleeding
   d. *NCLEX®* Instruct client to rest and avoid heavy lifting for 24 hours or longer if indicated (liver, kidney)

e. Increase fluid intake and teach client to report decreased urine output or burning on urination (kidney)
f. Do not administer aspirin, anticoagulants (heparin or warfarin), or nonsteroidal anti-inflammatory drugs (NSAIDs) from immediately after biopsy until 2 weeks postbiopsy to prevent bleeding

C. *Computed tomography (CT) scan*

1. Overview
   a. Screens commonly for abscesses, infection, vascular disease, stroke, bone destruction, tumors, edema, lesions in head, liver, and kidney and soft tissue foreign bodies
   b. Common areas for scanning are head and brain, chest (thoracic), abdominal, spine, long bones, joints, and pelvis; may be done with or without contrast dye (most are without contrast)
   c. Produces narrow x-ray beam that examines body sections from many angles
   d. Protective shields must be worn by personnel and over client's reproductive area to prevent adverse effects of x-ray exposures
   e. Clients of child-bearing age should have urine pregnancy testing done before CT scan
2. Preprocedure care
   a. Ensure informed consent when contrast is used
   NCLEX® b. See Box 43–1 for general nursing care of clients having diagnostic tests using contrast dye
   c. No food or fluid restriction if contrast dye is not used
   d. Ensure client has patent IV access
   e. Remove metal objects prior to scanning
   f. Explain that machine is circular and makes series of "clicking" sounds, test is not painful, and takes usually about 15 minutes
3. Postprocedure care
   NCLEX® a. See Box 43–1 for postprocedure care of clients receiving contrast dye
   b. Explain that client can resume usual diet and activity unless otherwise ordered

D. Fluoroscopy

1. Overview
   a. Views functions of organs in motion on fluorescent screen
   b. Often used with many diagnostic tests for visualization and guidance
   c. Common areas include thorax, abdomen, heart, and brain
   d. Room is darkened for visualization and those remaining in room should wear protective aprons to prevent exposure

Box 43–1

General Nursing Care with Diagnostic Tests Using Contrast Dye

Preprocedure

1. Ask client about allergies to shellfish, iodine, or contrast media.
2. If client is allergic to contrast medium, hypoallergenic contrast may be used or client may be premedicated with prednisone (corticosteroid) or diphenhydramine (antihistamine).
3. Obtain informed consent because injection of contrast is an invasive procedure.
4. Client may be ordered to be NPO for 4–8 hours preprocedure, depending on study.
5. Obtain baseline VS and note adequacy of preprocedure urine output (contrast is cleared by kidneys).
6. Ensure client has patent IV access.
7. Explain contrast media may cause a warm, flushed feeling or salty, fishy, or metallic taste in mouth, and possibly nausea for 1–2 minutes after injection.

Postprocedure

1. Monitor urine output to ensure clearance of contrast via kidneys.
2. Increase fluid intake to aid contrast dye excretion unless contraindicated by heart failure or renal disease.
3. Monitor for and report delayed reaction to contrast dye (dyspnea, rash, flushing, urticaria, tachycardia, decreased urine output, and others); prepare to treat with ordered antihistamines or corticosteroids.

2. Preprocede care
   a. Explain that there is no discomfort with procedure
   b. Ask if client is pregnant or suspects pregnancy (procedure contraindicated during pregnancy); complete a pregnancy test if indicated
   c. Barium sulfate is given to clients undergoing abdominal procedures
   d. Advise that x-ray personnel may give specific instructions during test
3. Postprocedure care
   a. Food and fluids permitted after abdominal and thorax fluoroscopy, but cardiac catheterization aftercare is performed following fluoroscopy of heart (see section later in chapter)
   b. Laxative is usually ordered postfluoroscopy of abdomen

E. *Magnetic resonance imaging (MRI)*

1. Overview
   a. Produces images similar to CT scanning but does not use ionizing radiation, so client is free of hazards caused by exposure to x-rays
   b. Consists of magnet enclosed in large, doughnut-shaped cylinder; client is guided into cylinder until area being diagnosed is within magnetic field
   NCLEX® c. Implanted metal devices (pacemakers or wires, aneurysm or surgical clips, metal rods or screws in bones, some hearing aids, nerve stimulators) are contraindications to MRI
   d. Detects central nervous system (CNS) lesions, vascular problems with blood flow or hemorrhage, cardiac perfusion problems, injury, edema, or tumors
2. Preprocedure care
   a. Screen for implanted metal objects, which are contraindications for test
   NCLEX® b. Remove all jewelry and other metal objects (eyeglasses, hearing aids, hair pins, cosmetics that may have metallic fragments)
   c. Food and fluids are not restricted for adults; children may be NPO for 4 hours
   NCLEX® d. IV access may be inserted for contrast (usually gadolinium is used—nonallergenic, but may affect calcium absorption for next 24 hours)
   e. Explain that procedure involves lying on narrow table that will slide into machine; clients with claustrophobia may need sedation or use of open machine if available; test is painless
   NCLEX® f. Advise that machine makes series of loud noises (clicks and thumps) but earplugs are available and client can communicate with personnel via intercom; family member or friend may remain in room with client (no radiation)
   g. MRI machines have weight limits; obese and claustrophobic clients may need to use newer open scanner if available
3. Postprocedure care: none specific

F. *Nuclear scan* (also called radionuclide imaging or radioisotope scan)

1. Overview
   a. Scintillation camera records distribution of radioisotope in specific organ(s) after inhalation, oral, or IV administration
   b. Common radioisotopes: technetium 99m, iodine 123 or 125, thallium 201, xenon, indium 111 (to label white blood cells), and gallium citrate
2. Preprocedure care
   a. Keep NPO for scan of heart, GI tract and gallbladder, and thyroid; no restriction for lung, bone, brain, kidney (keep well hydrated), liver, and spleen
   NCLEX® b. Administer ordered blocking agent (Lugol's solution, potassium perchlorate) prior to radioiodine study except for thyroid scan
   c. Adhere to specific preparation protocols for administering radioisotopes and waiting periods before scanning; ensure client arrives for appointment on time
   d. Instruct to avoid high-iodine foods and iodized salt for 3 days prior to thyroid scan
   NCLEX® e. Explain that radionuclide leaves body in 6–24 hours and should not affect other people
   f. Explain that scans cause no discomfort, to lie still during procedure unless asked to change position, and more than one imaging session may be needed (client may need to return at specified times)
   NCLEX® g. Remove jewelry and other metal objects in area under study
3. Postprocedure care: none specific

G. Positron emission tomography (PET) scan

1. Overview
   a. Most common purpose is to detect blood flow to brain and heart

b. Other uses include to differentiate between types of dementia, identify stages of cranial tumors, differentiate between benign and malignant lesions, and stage malignant lesions and disease
c. Measures concentrations of positron-emitting isotope after receiving a substance tagged with a radionuclide (radioactive glucose, rubidium 82, oxygen 15, nitrogen 13)
2. Preprocedure care
a. Ensure that client has patent IV access and measure VS
b. Request client follow instructions given during test, Velcro straps may be used to limit movement during test, and radiation from test is short-lived
3. Postprocedure care
a. Monitor VS; avoid postural hypotension by moving client slowly to upright position
b. Increase fluid intake to aid in clearing radioisotope via kidneys

H. *Ultrasonography* (sonogram)

1. Overview
a. Uses a probe (transducer) over skin surface or in body cavity to produce ultrasound beam that is reflected or echoed from tissues and can be captured by computer into scans, graphs, or audible sounds (Doppler)
b. Detects tissue abnormalities such as masses, cysts, edema, fluid, and stones; evaluates blood flow in arteries and veins
c. Can be used for many body tissues, including abdominal aorta, brain, breast, arteries and veins, gallbladder, heart, kidney, liver, pelvis including pregnant or nonpregnant uterus, pancreas, prostate, scrotum, spleen, thorax, and thyroid
2. Preprocedure care
a. Restrict food and fluids for 4–8 hours prior to tests of abdomen, abdominal aorta, gallbladder, liver, spleen, and pancreas
NCLEX® b. Have client eat fat-free meal on evening prior to abdominal, gallbladder, liver, pancreas, kidney, or liver sonogram
NCLEX® c. For pelvic and renal ultrasound (including obstetrics), client should drink 24 ounces water 1 hour prior to exam or three to four 8-ounce glasses of clear fluid 90 minutes prior to exam; teach client not to void until after test is completed
d. Explain that ultrasound gel is applied to skin surface of site being examined; probe is moved smoothly with light pressure over area
e. Tell client that test is usually painless and no radiation is involved
3. Postprocedure care: none specific

I. *X-rays*

1. Overview
a. Detect abnormal size, structure, and shape of bone or tissues; may be done as initial screening test
b. Common tests include chest, heart, abdominal (flat plate), KUB (kidneys, ureter, bladder), skull, and skeletal
NCLEX® c. Because of risk of radiation, protective garb is provided to personnel and client to wear over reproductive organs; pregnant clients should avoid x-rays, especially during first trimester (perform urine pregnancy test prior to x-rays)
2. Preprocedure care
a. Food and fluids are generally not restricted unless it is anticipated that client may go to surgery following tests (such as to repair bone fractures)
NCLEX® b. Remove hairpins, glasses, jewelry, and other metallic objects prior to test
c. Explain that more than one x-ray film may be needed and that client may need to wait while staff ensures that films are of good quality
3. Postprocedure care: none specific

II. RESPIRATORY DIAGNOSTIC TESTS

A. Bronchoscopy

1. Overview
a. Allows for direct inspection or visualization of larynx, trachea, and bronchi using a metal or flexible fiberoptic bronchoscope
b. Indicated to diagnose tracheobronchial tumor or bleeding site, remove foreign body or mucus plugs, or obtain secretions for cytologic examination or culture
c. Client generally receives premedication and local anesthetic sprayed in throat and sometimes nose (if fiberoptic instrument used) before insertion of bronchoscope

2. Preprocedure care
   a. Ensure that informed consent form and complete preprocedure or preoperative checklist are completed
   NCLEX® b. Ask client about allergies to drugs (especially analgesics, anesthetics, and antibiotics), food, and latex
   NCLEX® c. Have client void before giving premedication
   d. Remove dentures, contact lenses, and jewelry
   e. Obtain baseline VS; ensure admission VS also available for comparison
   f. Instruct client to relax during test if using local anesthesia (general anesthesia could be used); throat may be sore after procedure but will resolve
3. Postprocedure care
   a. Monitor VS every 15 minutes for first hour, every 30 minutes for second hour, and then hourly until stable
   NCLEX® b. Keep head of bed (HOB) elevated in semi-Fowler's position; if unconscious, position client on side with head slightly elevated to prevent aspiration
   c. Observe for and notify physician of respiratory distress (dyspnea, wheezing, apprehension, decreased breath sounds)
   NCLEX® d. Explain that coughing with minimal blood-tinged mucus may be expected; monitor for and immediately report hemoptysis (coughing up of excessively bloody secretions)
   NCLEX® e. Do not give food or fluids until gag and swallow reflexes have returned (usually 2–8 hours postprocedure); offer ice chips and sips of water before giving food
   f. Offer throat lozenges to relieve sore throat once client is taking food and fluids
   g. Monitor for and report complications, including laryngeal edema, bronchospasm, pneumothorax, cardiac dysrhythmias, and bleeding from biopsy site

B. Pulmonary function tests

1. Overview
   a. Detect pulmonary dysfunction, differentiate obstructive and restrictive lung disease, evaluate response to drug therapy (e.g., bronchodilators or steroids), and obtain baseline parameters for pulmonary rehabilitation
   b. Common pulmonary tests include vital capacity tests, lung volume studies, flow volume loop, diffusion capacity test, bronchial provocation studies, exercise studies, pulse oximetry, nutritional studies (indirect calorimetry), and body plethysmography
2. Preprocedure care
   a. Contact laboratory for specific restrictions, which can vary among labs
   NCLEX® b. Instruct client to avoid eating heavy meal prior to test and to avoid smoking for 4–6 hours before test
   c. Record age, height, and weight for predicting normal range of results
   d. Tell client to wear nonrestrictive clothing
   e. Cancel test if client has active cold, fever, or is under influence of alcohol
   NCLEX® f. Withhold medications that affect results, including sedatives and narcotics; check whether bronchodilators are allowed (may be withheld prior and given during test)
   g. Help client practice breathing patterns for test, such as normal breathing, rapid breathing, forced deep inspiration, and forced deep expiration
3. Postprocedure care: none specific

C. Ventilation scan (pulmonary ventilation scan)

1. Overview
   a. A nuclear lung scan after inhaling a mixture of air, oxygen, and radioactive gas
   b. Often performed with pulmonary perfusion scan to differentiate between ventilatory problem and vascular abnormality in lungs
   c. Also done to detect lung cancer, sarcoidosis, or tuberculosis, and to determine hypoventilation caused by excessive smoking or chronic obstructive pulmonary disease (COPD)
2. Preprocedure care
   a. There is no food or fluid restriction
   b. Remove all jewelry and other metal objects from neck and chest area
   NCLEX® c. Explain that client will inhale radioactive gas and will be asked to take deep breath and hold it while single image of lung is taken; other images will be recorded during three phases of test: wash-in (gas builds up in lungs), equilibrium (steady state), and wash-out (gas is expelled while breathing room air)
3. Postprocedure care
   NCLEX® a. Monitor respiratory status and breath sounds; report changes in rate and difficulty breathing
   b. Monitor for and report chest pain, especially if pulmonary embolism is suspected as underlying problem being diagnosed

III. CARDIOVASCULAR DIAGNOSTIC TESTS

A. Angiography (angiogram)

1. Overview
    a. Injection of contrast dye via catheter into femoral, brachial, subclavian, or carotid arteries to visualize blood vessels; also called arteriography
    b. Used to detect aneurysms, thrombosis, emboli, space-occupying lesions, stenosis, and plaques, and to evaluate cerebral, pulmonary, and renal blood flow
    c. Type is generally specified by prefacing *angiography* or *angiogram* with name of area being studied, such as cerebral angiography or pulmonary angiogram; may also be used to evaluate extent of peripheral arterial disease
2. Preprocedure care
    NCLEX® a. Keep client NPO for 8–12 hours prior to test
    NCLEX® b. Shave access site per agency policy
    c. Discontinue anticoagulants, such as heparin, for specified time prior to test (e.g., 6 hours)
    d. See again Box 43–1 for preprocedure care of clients receiving contrast dye
    e. Have client void before procedure
    NCLEX® f. Ensure that client has patent IV access before procedure and begin any ordered IV fluids at time specified; administer any ordered premedication
    g. Give cleansing enema as ordered prior to renal angiography to enhance visualization; perform vascular studies before any barium studies are done
    h. Explain that client will receive local anesthetic and must remain still during procedure
3. Postprocedure care
    NCLEX® a. Apply pressure for up to 30 minutes or longer until bleeding has stopped; check site for bleeding, swelling, or hematoma with each set of VS
    NCLEX® b. Monitor VS every 15 minutes for first hour, every 30 minutes for 2 hours, every hour for next 4 hours, or longer until stable, then routine
    NCLEX® c. Palpate peripheral pulses in affected area (femoral and dorsalis pedis or radial) with VS and document and report diminished or absent pulses
    NCLEX® d. Note neurovascular status of affected extremity (color, temperature, motion, sensitivity) when taking pulses and report abnormal findings (pale, cool, numbness, weakness)
    e. Monitor body temperature every 4 hours for 24–48 hours as ordered
    f. Maintain bedrest for 6–8 hours; restrict activities until following day
    NCLEX® g. Apply sandbag, pressure device, cold compress, or ice bag to site as ordered to relieve edema or discomfort
    NCLEX® h. See Box 43–1 for postprocedure care of clients receiving contrast dye
    i. Explain that coughing may be expected following pulmonary angiography
    NCLEX® j. Monitor for and report dysphagia and respiratory distress after cerebral angiography, and also for weakness or numbness in an extremity, confusion, slurred speech, visual changes (possible transient ischemic attack)

B. Cardiac catheterization

1. Overview
    a. Also known as cardiac angiography, angiocardiography, and coronary arteriography
    b. Right-heart catheterization uses femoral vein access to diagnose tricuspid or pulmonic valve stenosis or regurgitation, pulmonary hypertension, and septal defects
    c. Left-heart catheterization uses brachial or femoral artery access up through aorta to diagnose mitral or aortic valve stenosis or regurgitation, coronary artery disease, left ventricular hypertrophy, and ventricular aneurysm
    d. Left-sided catheterization is more commonly performed and uses principles of angiography outlined in previous section
2. NCLEX® Preprocedure care
    a. Ensure that informed consent is signed and witnessed and that provider has discussed possible risks with client and family
    b. Restrict food and fluids for 8 hours before test or as per agency policy
    c. Provide preprocedure care to clients receiving contrast dye (see again Box 43–1); administer any ordered antihistamines and steroids on evening before or on day of test
    d. Withhold medications, including anticoagulants such as heparin, for 6–8 hours as ordered by provider
    e. Cleanse and shave/prep insertion site on morning of procedure

f. Measure and record client's height and weight to calculate dye needed (1mL/kg body weight), and record baseline VS and peripheral pulses
g. Ensure client voids before administering any premedication (given 30 minutes to 1 hour prior)
NCLEX® h. Explain that client will be in cardiac cath room on a padded table; IV fluids will be given; cardiac rhythm will be monitored; skin anesthetic will be applied to injection site; client may feel flushed or warm with dye injection and this will pass; client may be asked to cough or deep breathe during procedure; coughing can reduce nausea from dye and possible cardiac dysrhythmias

NCLEX® 3. Postprocedure care
a. Monitor VS (BP, pulse, respirations) every 15 minutes for an hour, every 30 minutes until stable, then every hour as ordered, and then every 4 hours; monitor temperature every 4 hours
b. Observe catheter insertion site for bleeding or hematoma; change dressing as needed
c. Monitor peripheral pulses, neurovascular status of affected extremity, pain or discomfort
d. Observe cardiac rhythm and report rate or rhythm abnormalities
e. Report chest pain, chest heaviness, shortness of breath, and abdominal or groin pain
f. Administer prescribed analgesics for comfort and antibiotics if ordered
g. Maintain client on bedrest for 8–12 hours or per agency policy
h. Client may turn from side to side and HOB may be elevated to no more than 30 degrees (some agencies have head flat or only 15 degrees elevation); affected leg must be kept straight for 8–12 hours; if arm used for access, it must be immobilized for 3 hours (smaller blood vessel)
i. Provide postprocedure care to clients receiving contrast dye (see again Box 43–1)
j. Monitor for and report complications, including myocardial infarction, dysrhythmias, cardiac tamponade, and pulmonary or cerebral embolism

C. Echocardiography

1. Overview
a. A noninvasive ultrasound test to identify abnormalities in heart size, structure, and function, and to diagnose valvular disease
b. Handheld transducer is moved over chest in area of heart and other identified areas; sound waves are emitted and reflected back to produce images that appear on a video screen and are recorded on videotape and paper
c. Several specific types of studies are available, including M-mode, two-dimensional, spectral Doppler, color Doppler, transesophageal, contrast, and stress echocardiography

2. Preprocedure care
a. Measure and record baseline VS
b. There is no food or fluid restriction and no medications need to be withheld unless ordered by provider; exceptions are transesophageal and stress echocardiography, which require NPO status 4 hours prior to test
NCLEX® c. For transesophageal test, client will be given IV sedation
NCLEX® d. For contrast test, an IV access line must be inserted
e. Have client undress from waist up and wear hospital gown
f. Explain procedure to client (outlined earlier in general ultrasound section)
g. Explain that client will lie supine or on left side

3. Postprocedure care: none for most tests; client is monitored during recovery for 1–2 hours after transesophageal test

D. Electrocardiography (electrocardiogram or ECG, EKG)

1. Overview
a. Measures electrical activity of heart
NCLEX® b. Detects cardiac dysrhythmias and electrolyte imbalance (hyperkalemia—tall peaked T wave)
NCLEX® c. Electrodes are placed on extremities and chest (excess hair may be shaved in small spots) and electrical activity is recorded with each heartbeat
d. Records cardiac waveforms or complexes in 12 leads: six limb leads (three bipolar: leads I, II, and III; three unipolar: leads aVR, aVL, and aVF), and six chest or precordial leads (V1 through V6)

NCLEX® 2. Preprocedure care
a. No food or fluid restriction is needed; no consent form is required
b. Position client supine and expose arms and legs for lead placement
c. Clothing should be removed to waist, with females given a gown to wear
d. Note medications client is receiving, since some drugs (e.g., antidysrhythmics and beta-blockers) may alter readings

e. Ask client to relax muscles and breathe normally during ECG; explain that procedure does not cause pain or electric shock
f. Ask client to state if chest pain is experienced during ECG
3. Postprocedure care: remove electrode paste or jelly if used and assist client to dress if needed

E. Holter monitoring

1. Overview
a. Evaluates heart rate and rhythm during normal activities over a 24-hour period; identifies cardiac dysrhythmias
b. Consists of a recording device and clock inside a 1-pound monitor that is worn by client
NCLEX® c. Client keeps a diary to record timing of symptoms such as palpitations, chest pain, shortness of breath, syncope, vertigo, and usual daily activities (eating, exercise, sleep) for correlation with ECG readings
2. Preprocedure care
a. No food or fluid restriction is necessary
b. Clean and shave as necessary skin areas needed for electrode placement
c. Place five to seven electrodes on chest as per particular monitor
NCLEX® d. Tell client to avoid vigorous exercise or sweating, and not to shower, take a bath, or swim until electrodes are removed
3. Postprocedure care: none specific except to review items in diary with client for clarification if necessary

F. Stress/exercise tests

1. Overview
a. Include a variety of specific tests, such as treadmill exercise electrocardiography, exercise myocardial perfusion imaging test (thallium or technetium stress test), nuclear dipyridamole (Persantine) or dobutamine stress test
b. Used to screen for coronary artery disease, evaluate myocardial perfusion, differentiate between cardiac ischemia and infarct, develop cardiac rehabilitation program, evaluate cardiac status for work capability, and evaluate effectiveness of cardiac drug therapy
c. Electrodes are applied to chest; baseline VS are recorded and monitored periodically during test, and client exercises per age-based protocol on treadmill or bicycle (except persantine test, prescribed for those who cannot tolerate exercise)
2. Preprocedure care
a. Maintain NPO status after midnight (dipyridamole, dobutamine) or for 2–3 hours prior to test (others)
NCLEX® b. Avoid alcohol, caffeine, and nicotine during NPO status
NCLEX® c. Have client wear comfortable clothes (shorts or slacks with belt, sneakers or tennis shoes with socks, shirt with buttons in front for ECG electrodes)
NCLEX® d. Tell client to inform staff so that test can be stopped if client has dyspnea, severe fatigue, chest pain, rapid increase in pulse rate or BP, life-threatening dysrhythmias, or palpitations
e. Make note of any medications, such as beta-blockers, that could interfere with test results
3. Postprocedure care
a. Return client to department for any follow-up testing
b. Record VS and ECG tracings at end of test and 5–10 minutes later
NCLEX® c. Explain client can resume usual activity but may need to avoid strenuous activity or taking hot baths or showers posttest, depending on procedure

G. Venography (venogram), also called phlebography

1. Overview
a. A fluoroscopic or x-ray exam of deep leg veins after contrast dye injection
b. Detects deep vein thrombosis (DVT) and congenital venous abnormalities, and aids in selecting vein for arterial bypass grafting
2. Preprocedure care
a. NPO for 4 hours before test (some hospitals permit clear liquids)
b. Provide preprocedure care to clients receiving contrast dye (see again Box 43–1)
c. Record baseline VS and have client void prior to procedure
d. Explain that client will lie on x-ray table tilted at 40- to 60-degree angle, tourniquet is applied above ankle, and dye is injected into vein over 2–4 minutes
3. Postprocedure care
a. Monitor VS until stable, then as per routine
b. Palpate peripheral pulses (femoral, popliteal, dorsalis pedis)

NCLEX® c. Observe injection site for bleeding, hematoma, or infection (redness, edema, pain); document and report if any of these are found

NCLEX® d. Elevate extremity as ordered; if DVT is found, expect client to have orders for bedrest, heparin, leg elevation, and warm moist compresses

IV. RENAL OR URINARY DIAGNOSTIC TESTS

A. Cystoscopy and cystography (cystogram)

1. Overview
   a. *Cystoscopy* is direct visualization of bladder wall and urethra using a cystoscope (tubular lighted telescopic lens), usually by urologist
   b. *Cystography* is instillation of contrast dye into bladder using a catheter
   c. Purposes are to detect and remove urinary calculi, determine cause of hematuria or urinary tract infection (UTI), and detect tumors or prostatic hyperplasia
2. Preprocedure care
   NCLEX® a. Ensure informed consent is signed and witnessed before giving any ordered premedication (usually 1 hour before test)
   NCLEX® b. Record baseline VS and urine characteristics (amount, color, odor, specific gravity)
   c. Question regarding allergy to medications, food, and latex
   NCLEX® d. Explain that procedure will be done under local or general anesthesia; local anesthesia will be injected into urethra several minutes before cystoscope is inserted
   e. Complete preoperative or preprocedure checklist as per agency policy
3. Postprocedure care
   NCLEX® a. Monitor VS every 15 minutes for an hour, then possibly every half-hour until stable
   NCLEX® b. Monitor urine output for 48 hours after cystoscopy; increase fluid intake if less than 240 mL in 8 hours; report low urine output to provider
   c. Apply heat to lower abdomen to relieve pain and muscle spasm as ordered; explain that some pressure or burning may be present after test
   NCLEX® d. Monitor for and report gross hematuria; blood-tinged urine may be expected
   e. Monitor for complications of cystoscopy, such as hemorrhage, bladder perforation, urinary retention, and infection
   NCLEX® f. Explain that slight burning on urination is expected for 1 to 2 days after procedure; use analgesic if prescribed and avoid alcoholic beverages for 2 days after test (bladder irritant)

B. Intravenous pyelography (IVP)

1. Overview
   a. Also called excretory urography, because test visualizes entire urinary tract rather than just pelvis of kidney
   b. Consists of injecting IV radiopaque contrast and taking series of x-rays at specified times (3, 5, 10, 15, and 20 minutes postinjection), and a final x-ray after client voids to visualize residual dye in bladder
   c. Used to identify abnormal size, shape, and function of kidneys and detect renal calculi, tumors, and cysts
2. Preprocedure care
   a. Keep client NPO for 8–12 hours prior to test
   NCLEX® b. Administer laxative on evening before test and enema on morning of test as ordered
   c. Provide preprocedure care to clients receiving contrast dye (see again Box 43–1)
   NCLEX® d. Check blood urea nitrogen (BUN) lab result (test might be canceled if greater than 40 mg/dL [normal 8–22 mg/dL])
NCLEX® 3. Postprocedure care
   a. Monitor VS and urine output
   b. Provide postprocedure care to clients receiving contrast dye (see again Box 43–1)

C. Retrograde pyelography (retrograde pyelogram)

1. Overview
   a. May be performed after or in place of IVP and is usually done in conjunction with cystoscopy
   b. Consists of injecting contrast dye via catheter into ureters and renal pelvis to diagnose suspected nonfunctioning kidney, unlocated calculus, tumor, or renal stricture
   c. Not as frequently performed today
2. Preprocedure care
   NCLEX® a. NPO for 8 hours prior to test; some clients may be allowed water to avoid dehydration unless undergoing general anesthesia

b. Administer laxative and/or cleansing enema as ordered

NCLEX® c. Provide preprocedure care to clients receiving contrast dye (see again Box 43–1)

d. Explain that legs are placed in stirrups; there should be little to no pain or discomfort although pressure and urge to void may occur with insertion of cystoscope

3. Postprocedure care

a. Monitor vitals signs as per protocol

b. Provide postprocedure care to clients receiving contrast dye (see again Box 43–1)

NCLEX® c. Monitor urine output and report if less than 240 mL in 8 hours or if client does not void in 8 hours

d. Observe for and report hematuria; explain to client that blood-tinged urine is common

e. Provide ordered analgesics for pain or discomfort and report severe pain

NCLEX® f. Observe for and report signs of infection (fever, chills, abdominal pain, tachycardia, and later hypotension)

V. NEUROLOGICAL DIAGNOSTIC TESTS

A. Electroencephalography (EEG)

1. Overview

a. Measures electrical impulses produced by brain cells to detect seizure disorder, brain tumor, abscess, intracranial hemorrhage, and to assist in determinating brain death

b. Consists of applying electrodes to scalp and in specific positions, and recording brain activity on moving paper

c. Procedure may be performed while client is awake, drowsy, asleep, undergoing stimuli (hyperventilation, flashes of bright light), or combinations of these

2. Preprocedure care

NCLEX® a. Shampoo hair night before test and instruct client not to use oil or hair spray on hair

NCLEX® b. Food and fluids are permitted and encouraged (hypoglycemia could affect results) but client may not have alcohol (CNS depressant) or coffee, tea, cola (CNS stimulants) before test

c. Do not administer sleep aids or other sedatives on night before test because they affect readings; check with provider whether other medications should be given or withheld (such as antiepileptic drugs)

d. Explain that procedure is painless and may be done with client lying down or seated in reclining chair

e. Explain electrode placement and that electric shock will not occur; alleviate any client fears including that machine cannot determine intelligence and cannot read client's mind

NCLEX® f. Observe for and report seizure activity; note whether client is extremely anxious, restless, or upset

3. Postprocedure care

NCLEX® a. Shampoo client's hair to remove paste or collodion; acetone may be used to remove paste

b. Allow client to resume normal activity unless client was sedated

B. Myelography (myelogram)

1. Overview

a. A fluoroscopic and radiologic exam of spinal subarachnoid space (spinal canal) using contrast agent (oil- or water-based)

b. Detects spinal lesions (herniated intervertebral disks, cysts or tumor in spinal column, or spinal nerve root injury)

2. Preprocedure care

NCLEX® a. NPO for 4 to 8 hours prior to test; client may have light breakfast or clear liquids in morning if test is scheduled for afternoon

b. Administer cleansing enema if ordered to remove feces and gas to improve visualization

c. Administer ordered premedications such as sedative or narcotic analgesic and atropine

d. Provide preprocedure care to clients receiving contrast dye (see again Box 43–1)

NCLEX® e. Explain that spinal puncture will be performed and dye will be injected; table may be tilted as dye enters spinal column to enhance visualization of structures

f. Inform client to tell physician of any discomfort (such as pain going down legs)

3. Postprocedure care

a. Monitor vital signs until stable, then per protocol

NCLEX® b. Monitor urine output and notify physician if client does not void in 8 hours

NCLEX® c. Position client properly: keep head of bed flat if oil-based contrast used and elevated to 60 degrees for 8 hours or longer if water-based contrast was used (to prevent irritation from residual dye; oil-based dye is aspirated out but some microdroplets could remain)

NCLEX® d. Increase fluid intake to excrete dye via kidneys and to replace lost spinal fluid

e. Provide postprocedure care to clients receiving contrast dye (see again Box 43–1)
f. Monitor for signs of chemical or bacterial meningitis (severe headache, fever, chills, stiff neck, irritability, photophobia, and seizures)
g. Encourage use of good body mechanics

VI. MUSCULOSKELETAL DIAGNOSTIC TESTS

A. Arthroscopy

1. Overview
   a. An endoscopic examination of interior joint (usually knee) using fiberoptic endoscope; usually preceded by arthrography (x-ray exam of joint using air, contrast media, or both)
   b. Performed to diagnose meniscal, patellar, extrasynovial, and synovial problems
   c. Also used to perform joint surgery
2. Preprocedure care
   a. No food or fluid restriction if done using local anesthetic; NPO after midnight for spinal and general anesthesia
   b. Observe involved skin area for lesion or infection; document and report if found
3. Postprocedure care
   a. Monitor vital signs and local bleeding or swelling; report abnormal findings
   b. Apply covered ice bag to area if ordered
   c. Administer ordered analgesics for pain or discomfort
   d. Instruct client to rest joint for specified amount of time and avoid excessive use of joint for 2 to 3 days after procedure; minimize walking

B. Bone densitometry

1. Overview
   a. Detects early osteoporosis by determining density of bone mineral content
   b. Normal result is determined according to client age, gender, and height
   c. Most frequent population is postmenopausal women, who are at risk for greatest annual bone loss
2. Preprocedure care
   a. Food and fluids do not need to be restricted
   NCLEX® b. Have client remove all metal objects in area to be scanned; inform that test takes 30 to 60 minutes and is not painful
3. Postprocedure care: none

VII. GASTROINTESTINAL DIAGNOSTIC TESTS

A. Barium enema

1. Overview
   a. An x-ray examination of large intestine (colon) to detect polyps, tumor, diverticuli, intestinal stricture or obstruction, intussusception, or ulceration
   b. Consists of administering barium sulfate (alone as single contrast or with air as double contrast) via rectal tube into large intestine
   c. Filling process is monitored by fluoroscopy, and then x-rays are taken
   d. Indicated for clients who have lower abdominal pain or cramps; stool that contains blood, mucus, or pus; changes in bowel habits or stool characteristics

NCLEX® 2. Preprocedure care
   a. Some institutions ask that clients eat low-residue diet for 2 to 3 days before test (tender meats, eggs, bread, clear soup, pureed bland fruits and vegetables, boiled milk, potatoes)
   b. Ensure that ordered abdominal x-rays, ultrasound studies, radionuclide studies and proctosigmoidoscopy are done prior to this test
   c. Withhold oral medications for 24 hours prior to test unless ordered by provider
   d. Provide, or instruct client to take, clear liquid diet for 18–24 hours before test and maintain water and clear liquid intake 24 hours prior to maintain hydration
   e. Administer laxatives (such as magnesium citrate) in late afternoon or early evening (4–8 p.m.) of day before test
   f. Administer cleansing enema or laxative suppository such as bisacodyl (Dulcolax) on evening before test as ordered
   g. Administer saline enemas in early morning of day of procedure until clear (maximum of three) if ordered
   h. Black coffee or tea is permitted up to 1 hour prior to test

3. Postprocedure care
   a. Have client try to expel barium in bathroom or on bedpan immediately after test
   NCLEX® b. Increase fluid intake for hydration and prevent constipation from retained barium
   NCLEX® c. Administer ordered laxative or oil retention enema to expel barium; laxative may need to be repeated on day following test

B. Cholangiography

1. Overview
   a. May be done as IV, percutaneous, or T-tube cholangiography
   b. IV test examines biliary ducts to detect strictures, stones, or tumor, but gallbladder may not be well visualized
   c. Percutaneous test is indicated when biliary obstruction is indicated because contrast is injected directly into biliary tree
   d. T-tube test may be done 7 to 8 hours after cholecystectomy to explore common bile duct for patency and determine if any gallstones are blocking duct after gallbladder removal; dye is injected into T-shaped tube, which is placed into common bile duct during surgery to promote drainage
2. Preprocedure care
   a. NPO for 8 hours prior to test
   b. Take usual precautions regarding allergy to contrast media
   c. Provide laxative (evening before test) and cleansing enema (morning of test) as ordered; for T-tube test, only cleansing enema may be ordered
3. Postprocedure care
   a. Check vital signs as ordered and instruct client to remain in bed for 6 hours after percutaneous test
   b. T-tube may or may not be taken out after procedure
   c. Provide postprocedure care to clients receiving contrast dye (see again Box 43–1); otherwise, no specific aftercare is indicated

C. Cholecystography (oral)

1. Overview
   a. An x-ray test to visualize stones in gallbladder or determine obstruction in cystic duct
   b. Oral contrast media is administered, which concentrates in gallbladder in 12–14 hours
   c. Specific sequence of dietary instructions must be followed for best results
   d. Liver disease, inadequate client preparation, obstruction of cystic duct, and diarrhea (eliminates contrast agent) can interfere with results
2. Preprocedure care
   NCLEX® a. Obtain allergy history; observe for signs of jaundice (yellow sclera, skin or serum bilirubin greater than 3 mg/dl); notify provider if found
   b. Provide fat-free diet for 24 hours before test (some agencies suggest high-fat meal at noon to empty gallbladder and low-fat meal in evening)
   NCLEX® c. Begin NPO status with sips of water after dinner the evening before test
   d. Administer radiopaque tablets 2 hours after dinner meal according to package directions with total of 240 mL (8 ounces) of water
   e. Saline enema may be ordered on morning of test in some agencies to clear GI tract
   f. Explain to client that fasting x-rays will be taken and then high-fat meal or fat-containing substances (Bilevac) will be given in x-ray department; follow-up x-rays will be done over next 1–2 hours to monitor gallbladder emptying
   g. Explain that test does not cause discomfort
   h. Explain that client should not become alarmed if test needs to be repeated but should remain on low-fat diet until repeat test is completed
3. Postprocedure care: none specific

D. Colonoscopy

1. Overview
   a. An endoscopic procedure that inspects large intestine (colon) using long, flexible fiberoptic tube (colonoscope)
   b. Tube is inserted anally and advanced through rectum, sigmoid colon, and large intestine to cecum, and air is used to insufflate area for better visualization
   c. Detects lower GI bleeding, polyps, diverticulitis, and benign or malignant lesions in colon
2. Preprocedure care
   a. Withhold medications that interfere with coagulation (aspirin, NSAIDs) and alcohol 1 week prior to test

b. Explain that another person must be available to drive client home if performed on outpatient basis
c. Follow preprocedure preparation to clear bowel of feces: usually GoLytely or Colyte solution or Fleet PhosphoSoda beginning on day prior to test
d. Avoid soap solution enemas, which could irritate wall of colon
e. Record baseline VS
NCLEX® f. Client will lie in Sims or left lateral position, will receive IV moderate sedation immediately before test, and will be asked to breathe deeply during insertion of colonoscope
3. Postprocedure care
a. Monitor VS and report abnormal changes
b. Do not administer anything by mouth following IV moderate sedation until gag and swallow reflexes have returned
c. Observe for and report anal bleeding, abdominal distention, severe pain or abdominal cramps, or fever
NCLEX® d. Maintain client safety postsedation

E. Endoscopic retrograde cholangiopancreatography (ERCP)
1. Overview
a. Examines biliary and pancreatic ducts endoscopically after injection of contrast medium into duodenal papilla
b. Identifies causes of biliary obstruction (usually accompanied by jaundice), such as stricture, cyst, stones, or tumor
c. May be done as follow-up to ultrasound, CT scan, liver scan, or biliary tract x-rays
2. Preprocedure care
a. Inquire about allergies to contrast media
b. Maintain NPO status for 8 hours prior to test
c. Obtain baseline VS
d. Ensure that informed consent is obtained and that client voids before premedication (mild sedative or narcotic and atropine, usually)
NCLEX® e. Explain that local anesthetic is sprayed in throat to decrease gag reflex prior to insertion of endoscope
3. Postprocedure care
a. Monitor vital signs including temperature (fever could indicate infection) and respiratory rate (respiratory status could be compromised from anesthetic spray in throat and/or endoscope)
NCLEX® b. Ensure gag and swallow reflexes are present before offering food and fluids
c. Provide warm saline gargles or lozenges to reduce sore throat caused by endoscope; may be needed for a few days
NCLEX® d. Note and report presence of persistent abdominal pain, discomfort, or fullness

F. Esophagogastroduodenoscopy
1. Overview
a. Also includes or is known as gastroscopy, esophagoscopy, esophagogastroscopy, duodenoscopy, endoscopy
b. Directly visualizes esophagus, stomach, and duodenum with flexible fiberoptic endoscope
c. Used to diagnose esophageal, gastric, or duodenal disease; diverticulosis or *H. pylori* infection; to obtain cytologic specimens; or to remove foreign bodies
2. Preprocedure care
NCLEX® a. NPO status for 8–12 hours before test; if done as emergency and NPO status not possible, perform stomach lavage/suction to prevent aspiration
b. Record baseline VS and have client void
c. Administer any prescribed premedication; client's usual prescribed medications may often be taken at 6 a.m. on day of test; check with provider
NCLEX® d. Give client hospital gown to wear and remove dentures, eyeglasses, and jewelry; note any loose teeth
e. Explain that client may feel some pressure with insertion of scope, but that IV sedation and local anesthetic to throat will be used
3. Postprocedure care
NCLEX® a. NPO for 2–4 hours after test as ordered; ensure that gag and swallow reflexes have returned before offering fluids or food
b. Monitor VS
c. Explain that "burping up air" or passing gas is expected because air is instilled during procedure to visualize area

d. Provide gargles, lozenges, or analgesics for throat discomfort, which is expected and caused by endoscope
e. Observe for possible complications, such as perforated GI tract; monitor for and report epigastric, abdominal, or back pain; dyspnea; fever; tachycardia; and subcutaneous emphysema in neck

G. Gastric analysis

1. Overview
   a. Examines acidity of gastric secretions via nasogastric (NG) tube during basal state (without stimulation) and at peak secretion (with drug stimulation)
   b. Decreased levels indicate pernicious anemia, gastric malignancy, and atrophic gastritis
   c. Increased levels indicate peptic ulcer (duodenal) or Zollinger-Ellison syndrome
2. Basal gastric analysis
   NCLEX® a. NPO for 8 to 12 hours prior to test and restrict smoking for 8 hours
   b. Restrict selected drugs (antacids, steroids, cholinergics, and anticholinergics) and coffee and alcohol for at least 24 hours prior; note on test request form if not complied with
   c. Record baseline VS and remove loose dentures
   d. Insert NG tube and obtain residual gastric specimen as well as four additional specimens 15 minutes apart
   e. Properly label first set of specimens as basal specimens with client name, date, time, and specimen number
3. Stimulation test (a continuation of basal gastric analysis test)
   a. Administer gastric stimulant such as Histalog, histamine, or pentagastrin
   b. Obtain four to eight specimens 15 minutes apart depending on agent used
   c. Label peak specimens obtained after stimulation with client name, date, time, and specimen number
   d. Monitor VS postprocedure; remove NG tube if inserted only for test

H. Gastrointestinal (GI) series

1. Overview
   a. Also known as upper GI series, barium swallow, or small bowel series
   b. Consists of fluoroscopic and x-ray exams of esophagus, stomach, and small intestine after ingestion of oral barium sulfate or water-soluble contrast such as Gastrografin
   c. Used to detect esophageal, gastric, or duodenal ulcer, polyps, tumors, hiatal hernia, foreign bodies, esophageal varices, or esophageal or small bowel strictures
2. Preprocedure care
   NCLEX® a. Low-residue diet may be ordered for 2–3 days prior to test
   NCLEX® b. Maintain NPO status with no smoking for 8–12 hours before test
   c. Withhold medications for 8 hours before test unless otherwise ordered; withhold narcotics and anticholinergics for 24 hours because they reduce gastric motility
   d. Administer laxatives as ordered on evening before test
   e. Explain that client swallows a chalk-flavored (chocolate or strawberry) barium meal or Gastrografin and x-rays are taken periodically over 1–2 or 4–6 hours depending on length of area to be visualized; follow-up film (post–GI series) at 24 hours may be ordered as well
3. Postprocedure care
   a. Check with radiology department that studies are completed before giving late breakfast or late lunch
   NCLEX® b. Administer ordered laxative following test to excrete barium
   NCLEX® c. Explain to client that stool will be light in color for some days after test and to notify physician if no bowel movement in 2 to 3 days

VIII. REPRODUCTIVE DIAGNOSTIC TESTS

A. Fetal nonstress test (NST)

1. Overview
   a. Evaluates fetal functioning and well-being in response to fetal movement
   b. Is inexpensive, rapidly accomplished, lacks side effects, and helps identify at-risk fetuses for mothers with high-risk pregnancy conditions (such as diabetes and gestational hypertension)
   c. Monitors fetal heart rate (FHR) with fetal movement, which should accelerate 15 beats per minute for 15 seconds
   d. If FHR does not increase within 20 minutes, can rub mother's abdomen or make loud noise nearby to stimulate fetal movement
   e. If no increase in FHR after 40 minutes, test indicates a nonreactive fetus; normal is a reactive fetus
2. Preprocedure care
   a. Obtain informed consent and measure baseline VS and FHR

b. Position mother in semi-Fowler or lateral position with roll or wedge under right hip to displace uterus to left slightly

NCLEX® c. Instruct client to press pressure transducer when she feels fetus move so FHR acceleration can be monitored

3. Postprocedure care
   a. Encourage client to rest
   b. Provide general teaching that instructs client to report bleeding, continuous contractions, or lack of fetal movement
4. Nonreactive test may be followed up with contraction stress test
   a. Evaluates fetal functioning during spontaneous or induced uterine contractions
   b. May also be performed as routine test for selected high-risk mothers
   c. Uses nipple stimulation or oxytocin to stimulate uterine contraction

NCLEX® d. Normal result is absence of late decelerations in FHR during three contractions; presence of late decelerations indicates condition that leads to placental dysfunction or insufficient blood supply

B. Hysteroscopy

1. Overview
   a. Visualizes uterine cavity; allows for endometrial biopsy or polyp removal
   b. Contraindicated with cervical or vaginal infection, pelvic inflammatory disease, purulent vaginal discharge, or if cervical surgery performed previously
   c. Risks to procedure include perforation of uterus and infection
2. Preprocedure care
   a. Obtain menstrual history because test should be done after menses but before ovulation
   b. Restrict food and fluids for 8 hours before test
   c. Have client void before test
   d. Explain that client will be in lithotomy position; hysteroscope will be inserted and carbon dioxide will be instilled to distend uterus for visualization
3. Postprocedure care
   a. Monitor VS and check for excessive bleeding or discharge
   b. Explain that cramping may occur following test and mild analgesic will reduce discomfort; report severe discomfort or shortness of breath immediately
   c. Advise to avoid sexual intercourse or douching for 2 weeks or as instructed by provider

C. Mammography

1. Overview
   a. X-ray examination of breasts to detect cysts or tumors
   b. Detects approximately 90% of breast malignancies

NCLEX® c. Recommended annually for women over 40 years and every 2 years for women ages 35 to 40

2. Preprocedure care
   a. Food and fluids are not restricted prior to test

NCLEX® b. Instruct client not to use ointment, powder, or deodorant on breasts or under arms on day of test; client will need to remove clothes to waist and wear a paper gown that opens in front

   c. Explain that procedure will not cause pain but some discomfort may occur during breast compression during test
   d. Explain that client will need to wait while films are developed, and reassure client that additional films are sometimes needed and not to be alarmed
3. Postprocedure care: none specific

D. Papanicolaou (Pap) smear

1. Overview
   a. A cytological test to detect precancerous lesions or cancerous cells of cervix
   b. Also identifies viral, fungal, and parasitic conditions and evaluates response to chemotherapy or radiation therapy
2. Preprocedure care
   a. Food and fluids are not restricted

NCLEX® b. Client should not douche, insert vaginal medications, or have sexual intercourse for 24 hours before test

   c. Obtain menstrual history, including any problems, and document whether or not client is taking any hormones or oral contraceptives

d. Ask client to remove all clothes; provide paper gown; breast examination is done after Pap smear is taken
e. Explain that client will lie on examining table in lithotomy position and speculum will be inserted into vagina to aid in specimen collection

3. Postprocedure care: none specific; provide tissues so client can remove lubricant before dressing

IX. INTEGUMENTARY DIAGNOSTIC TESTS

A. Tuberculin skin test

1. Overview
   a. Screens for tuberculosis
   b. Tine test or Mono-Vacc test is multipuncture test that uses tines impregnated with purified protein derivative (PPD); used for mass screening and is read in 48–72 hours
   NCLEX® c. Mantoux test involves injection of PPD intradermally using a tuberculin (1 mL) syringe with a 25- to 27-gauge needle, and is read in 48–72 hours
2. Preprocedure care
   a. Food and fluids are not restricted
   NCLEX® b. Determine whether client has tested positive to test before; test should only be performed if previous results were negative
   c. Cleanse inner aspect of forearm with alcohol and let dry before injecting 0.1 mL of antigen intradermally
3. Postprocedure care
   NCLEX® a. Explain that client needs to return to have results read in 48–72 hours; a 72-hour reading is more accurate; client may be asked to return for reading at 72 hours if 48-hour result is questionable
   NCLEX® b. Explain that positive test does not always indicate active infectious disease but that organism is present in body in either an active or dormant state; follow-up x-ray and sputum cultures are indicated

B. Other skin tests

1. Include tests for blastomycosis, coccidioidomycosis, histoplasmosis, trichinosis, and toxoplasmosis
2. Procedures are similar to that described above for tuberculosis
3. NCLEX® For allergy skin tests, injected area may be outlined with a marker and a diagram made of injection sites, especially if more than one antigen is planted concurrently; antihistamines are withheld 3–4 days prior to avoid false negatives

Check Your NCLEX–PN® Exam I.Q. *You are ready for testing on this content if you can*

- Apply knowledge from foundational sciences to the care of clients undergoing diagnostic testing.
- Carry out specific nursing interventions needed before and after diagnostic testing.
- Monitor a client appropriately before and after diagnostic testing.
- Compare the results of client assessments before and after diagnostic testing.
- Monitor the results of serial or periodic diagnostic tests.
- Reinforce client teaching about diagnostic tests.

PRACTICE TEST

1 A client is about to undergo skin biopsy to determine if a skin lesion is malignant. The client asks how much the biopsy will hurt. Which response by the nurse is best?

1. "We will give you a pain pill in just a moment that will minimize any pain during the biopsy."
2. "Luckily, this type of procedure does not cause any pain for most people."
3. "You may feel some discomfort while the local anesthetic is injected, but this will numb the area for the actual biopsy."
4. "The procedure is fairly painful, but you can manage it afterward with acetaminophen (Tylenol)."

PRACTICE TEST

2 The client is about to undergo a computerized tomography (CT) scan of the head with contrast. Which question by the nurse is most important to ask while preparing the client for the test?

1. "Have you ever had a procedure like this before?"
2. "Do you have an allergy to iodine or shellfish?"
3. "Would you like something to drink before you go to the radiology department?"
4. "Have you voided in the bathroom in the last few hours?"

3 The client is scheduled for a magnetic resonance imaging (MRI) study of the spine. The outpatient nurse gives the client which instructions as part of preprocedure care? Select all that apply.

1. "Do not eat anything after midnight the day before the test."
2. "You will be able to drive yourself home after the test."
3. "Expect to stay in the MRI department for an hour afterward for observation."
4. "Do not wear any metal, such as jewelry or hairclips."
5. "Do not drink any liquids for 6 hours before the test."

4 A client will undergo a radionuclide scan of the thyroid. A nursing assistant asks what needs to be done to protect staff from any residual radiation after the scan. What is an appropriate response by the nurse? Select all that apply.

1. "Everyone must stand 6 feet away from the client for 24 hours. I should put a sign above the bed."
2. "Using standard precautions for handling body fluids will be sufficient to protect staff."
3. "I have arranged for the client to be moved to a private room for 48 hours after the test."
4. "The client will need to be on contact precautions. Can you call the central processing department for a cart with gowns and gloves?"
5. "The amount of residual radiation is quite small."

5 A 17-year-old girl is brought to the emergency department for x-rays after twisting her ankle. Which question is most important for the nurse to ask the client before sending her to the radiology department?

1. "Do you experience claustrophobia when in small spaces?"
2. "Are you wearing any necklaces or other metal objects?"
3. "When was your last monthly period?"
4. "Have you ever had an x-ray before?"

6 A female client is returning to the nursing unit following a pelvic ultrasound. What should the nurse plan to do for the client at this time? Select all that apply.

1. Make the client comfortable.
2. Instruct the client to drink at least one quart of water over the next hour.
3. Explain that analgesic medication is available to relieve the expected cramping pain.
4. Tell the client that she will be able to eat in one hour.
5. Ask the client if she needs anything.

7 A client who underwent bronchoscopy 4 hours ago is asking for something to drink to ease his sore throat. The nurse obtains some juice for the client after noting which data?

1. Respiratory rate has ranged from 16 to 18.
2. Breath sounds are clear bilaterally.
3. The client has had no hemoptysis.
4. Gag and swallow reflexes have returned.

8 A client underwent angiography of the left leg. Which of the following findings obtained during current data collection is of concern to the nurse? Select all that apply.

1. Skin paler on left foot than right.
2. Skin temperature cooler on left foot than right.
3. Left dorsalis pedis pulse audible by Doppler, previously 2.
4. Dressing at femoral access site has trace amount of dark red blood.
5. Client reports slight numbness and tingling in the left leg.

9 The client who will undergo a cardiac catheterization says to the nurse: "I am nervous about having a cardiac catheterization. Can you tell me what to expect during this test?" Which response by the nurse is appropriate? Select all that apply.

1. "The procedure will be done in the operating room to help ensure sterile conditions."
2. "The room will be brightly lit at all times."
3. "The insertion of the catheter in the femoral area will be one of the few painful moments of the procedure."
4. "The physician will ask you to lie still except to do specific things, such as cough or take a deep breath."
5. "There will be a fluoroscopy screen in the room, which may looked at by the staff during the procedure."

10 A client on the medical unit scheduled for a cardiac echocardiogram at 9 a.m. the next day asks the nurse if eating breakfast before the test is possible. What response by the nurse is appropriate?

1. "Yes, we can arrange for your breakfast tray to arrive a half hour early so that you have time to eat before the test."
2. "Yes, but you will need to get up at 5 a.m. so that you will be without food or fluids for four hours before the test."
3. "Yes, but you can only drink clear liquids, such as apple juice, and you cannot eat solid food until after the test."
4. "No, you cannot eat or drink before the test, but you can have a full breakfast after the test."

11 A client has just received a Holter cardiac monitor to wear for the next 24 hours. The nurse determines that the client understands its use when the client makes which statement?

1. "I should write in the diary what I am doing every half-hour."
2. "I should only take a bath, not a shower, for the next 24 hours."
3. "I can continue with my usual activity and exercise pattern while wearing the monitor."
4. "I need to try to walk a total of 3 miles over the next 24 hours while wearing the monitor."

12 A client who underwent cystography 16 hours ago has a urinary output of 180 mL in the previous 8 hours. Which of the following actions should the nurse take at this time? Select all that apply.

1. Measure the specific gravity of the urine.
2. Document the volume on the client's flowsheet.
3. Encourage the client to drink more fluids.
4. Notify the physician.
5. Compare the output to the client's intake during the previous shift.

13 The nurse has assigned a nursing assistant (NA) to work with a client who just returned to the nursing unit at 0945 after electroencephalography. What direction should the nurse give the NA regarding care to the client?

1. "Do not give any food or fluids until lunchtime."
2. "Wash the client's hair at your earliest opportunity."
3. "Keep the client on bedrest for the remainder of the shift."
4. "Encourage the client to drink fluids to flush dye through the kidneys."

14 A client has just returned to the nursing unit after a myelogram using water-based contrast to diagnose a herniated intervertebral disk. The nurse should assist the client to which position in bed after transferring from the stretcher?

1. Supine, with the head of the bed elevated 60 degrees
2. Supine, with the head of the bed elevated 15 degrees
3. Left side-lying, with the head of the bed flat
4. Any position of the client's choice, with the head of the bed elevated 30 degrees

15 A client has received discharge instructions after undergoing arthroscopy of the knee earlier in the day. The nurse concludes that the client understands self-care after discharge when the client makes which statement?

1. "I should not expect to need pain medication following this procedure."
2. "I should apply warm, moist heat to my knee to maintain comfort."
3. "I should limit my activities, including walking, for 2–3 days."
4. "I should expect increased swelling and perhaps some bleeding in the knee area after going home."

PRACTICE TEST

16 A client with gastroesophageal reflux disease has just undergone esophagogastroscopy. The nurse places highest priority on continuing to monitor which client data?

1. Inability to swallow saliva
2. Temperature of 99.4°F oral
3. Client report of heartburn
4. Client report of sore throat

17 The nurse has reinforced instructions to a client who will have a barium swallow in 3 days. The nurse determines that the client understands how to properly prepare for the test after the client makes which statement?

1. "I should eat a low-fat meal for 2 days, and then have clear liquids the day before the test."
2. "I should stop taking all medication except antacids the day before the test."
3. "I should not eat or drink anything after midnight just prior to the test."
4. "I should eat a high-carbohydrate diet for 3 days before the test."

18 The nurse is providing instructions to a client who is returning home following colonoscopy. Which statement would be appropriate for the nurse to include? Select all that apply.

1. "You may drive in about 6 hours, after the medication given during the procedure has fully worn off."
2. "It is alright to eat and drink, but it is helpful to resume the diet gradually."
3. "You should call the doctor if you feel distended, or begin passing gas."
4. "Bleeding from the rectum is expected after this procedure, but call the physician if it gets severe."
5. "Avoid activities requiring mental alertness for 24 hours after the test."

19 The nurse would give which instruction regarding preprocedure care to a woman who is scheduled for a mammogram?

1. "Drink liquids, but don't eat breakfast on the morning of the mammogram."
2. "Do not use any lotions or deodorant on the chest or underarms before the mammogram."
3. "Take a mild analgesic such as acetaminophen (Tylenol) before coming in for the mammogram."
4. "Plan a light schedule for the day of the mammogram, so you can rest after the procedure."

20 The nurse has given an intradermal injection of purified protein derivative (PPD) to a client to screen for tuberculosis. After noting that the current day is Monday, when should the nurse instruct the client to return to have the result read?

1. Tuesday or Wednesday
2. Wednesday or Thursday
3. Thursday or Friday
4. Friday or the following Monday

21 A client will undergo basal gastric acid secretion analysis. The client is taking several medications. Which types of drugs should the nurse withhold prior to the test? Select all that apply.

1. Anticholinergic
2. Cardiac glycoside
3. Antacid
4. Diuretic
5. Corticosteroid

ANSWERS & RATIONALES

1 **Answer: 3** **Rationale:** The area is anesthetized using a local anesthetic before skin biopsy, so the client should only feel discomfort while the anesthetic is administered. Analgesics are not given before the procedure. The procedure is not pain free. The client may take medication such as acetaminophen following the procedure, but this does not address the client's question about pain during the procedure. **Cognitive Level:** Analyzing **Client Need:** Reduction of Risk Potential **Integrated Process:** Communication and Documentation **Content Area:** Adult Health **Strategy:** The core issue of the question is pain during skin biopsy. Use knowledge that local anesthesia is used during the procedure to make your selection.

2 **Answer: 2 Rationale:** Because a contrast agent will be used for the test, it is most important for the nurse to ask about an allergy to iodine or shellfish. While it is good to know if the client has had a similar test to determine possible anxiety, it is not the priority. The client should not have anything to eat or drink for 4 hours prior to the test. It is generally helpful for the client to void before leaving the unit to avoid having to do so during the test, but this is a lower-priority item than assessing for allergy. **Cognitive Level:** Analyzing **Client Need:** Reduction of Risk Potential **Integrated Process:** Nursing Process: Data Collection **Content Area:** Adult Health **Strategy:** The core issue of the question is knowledge that a client who is allergic to iodine or shellfish is likely to have an allergic reaction to iodinated contrast media. Memorize this important point if this question was difficult.

3 **Answer: 2, 4 Rationale:** The client can drive home after the test. Because the MRI scanner uses magnets, the client cannot wear any metal, and clients who have implanted metal might be ineligible for this study. The client does not need to withhold food after midnight on the evening before the test. The client does not need to remain in the department for additional observation after the test. The client does not need to withhold fluids before the test. **Cognitive Level:** Applying **Client Need:** Reduction of Risk Potential **Integrated Process:** Communication and Documentation **Content Area:** Adult Health **Strategy:** The core issues of the question are that the client does not need to withhold food or fluids before the test, and also that metal cannot be worn in the vicinity of an MRI scanner because of the magnetic field. Note the wording of the question suggests more than one option is likely to be correct.

4 **Answer: 2, 5 Rationale:** The amount of residual radioactivity following radionuclide scanning is very small, and poses no risk to visitors or staff. Using standard precautions in handling blood or body fluids is sufficient for protection. It is unnecessary to stand six feet away from the client, use a private room, or place the client on contact precautions. **Cognitive Level:** Applying **Client Need:** Reduction of Risk Potential **Integrated Process:** Communication and Documentation **Content Area:** Adult Health **Strategy:** The core issue of the question is knowledge that the amount of radioactivity following radionuclide imaging is very small. With this in mind, eliminate each of the incorrect options, which contain excessive and unnecessary steps for protection of staff.

5 **Answer: 3 Rationale:** The most important question is to determine whether the client could be pregnant, since x-rays are contraindicated during pregnancy, especially during the first trimester. Asking about fear of small or enclosed spaces would be important for MRI machines and possibly for CT scanning machines. The question second in importance would be whether the client is wearing any metal, but possible pregnancy is a priority. It is helpful, but not of highest priority, to know if the client has had an x-ray before, to alleviate concerns. **Cognitive Level:** Analyzing **Client Need:** Reduction of Risk Potential **Integrated Process:** Nursing Process: Data Collection **Content Area:** Adult Health **Strategy:** The core issue of the question is knowledge that x-rays are contraindicated during pregnancy. Note the critical words *most important* in the question, which indicates more than one option could be correct, and you must prioritize your answer. Use knowledge of x-rays and the process of elimination to make a selection.

6 **Answer: 1, 5 Rationale:** There is no special aftercare following pelvic ultrasound. For this reason, the nurse should make the client comfortable and ask if she needs anything before leaving the room. The client does not need to drink fluids, should not have cramping pains, and does not need to wait an hour before eating. **Cognitive Level:** Applying **Client Need:** Reduction of Risk Potential **Integrated Process:** Nursing Process: Planning **Content Area:** Adult Health **Strategy:** The core issue of the question is knowledge that there is no special aftercare following ultrasound. Use nursing knowledge and the process of elimination to answer. Note the wording of the question suggests that more than one option is likely to be correct.

7 **Answer: 4 Rationale:** Before offering food or fluids to a client following bronchoscopy, it is essential to ensure that gag and swallow reflexes have returned. A local anesthetic is used to numb the throat to ease passage of the bronchoscope, and if protective reflexes have not returned, the client could aspirate. The other client data are also normal, but would not indicate whether the client can safely swallow. **Cognitive Level:** Analyzing **Client Need:** Reduction of Risk Potential **Integrated Process:** Nursing Process: Data Collection **Content Area:** Adult Health **Strategy:** The core issue of the question is knowledge that gag and swallow reflexes need to be present before offering clients food or beverages to prevent aspiration. Think of gag and swallow reflexes as a possible priority concern whenever a client has had a procedure ending in *-oscopy*.

8 **Answer: 1, 2, 3, 5 Rationale:** The findings that should be of concern to the nurse are those that indicate adverse circulatory changes in the leg where the femoral artery was used as an access site for the angiography. These would include skin that is paler and cooler than the other leg, decreased pulse, and numbness and tingling in the affected limb. A bandage that has a small amount of old blood is expected, and is not of concern at this time. **Cognitive Level:** Analyzing **Client Need:** Reduction of Risk Potential **Integrated Process:** Nursing Process: Data Collection **Content Area:** Adult Health **Strategy:** The core issue of the question is adverse change in the neurovascular status of a client who underwent angiography. The critical words in the stem of the question are *of concern*, which guides you to look for data that is abnormal. Note that the wording of the question indicates that more than one option is likely to be correct.

9 **Answer: 4, 5 Rationale:** The client is asked to lie still except for specific requests, such as to cough or deep-breathe to aid in catheter movement, or to terminate cardiac dysrhythmias caused by irritation of the catheter. The fluoroscopy screen may be used to view catheter movement, and also the flow of dye after injection. The procedure is done in a special cardiac catheterization room in the radiology department, not in the operating room. The lights in the room may be dimmed at times so catheter movement can be visualized on a fluoroscopy screen. The catheter insertion site is anesthetized with a local anesthetic, so the client should feel pressure but not pain. **Cognitive Level:** Applying **Client Need:** Reduction of Risk Potential **Integrated Process:** Teaching and Learning **Content Area:** Adult Health **Strategy:** The core issue of the question is knowledge of typical events during a cardiac catheterization. Knowledge of these factors helps alleviate client fears. Use nursing knowledge and the process of elimination to make a selection.

10 **Answer: 1 Rationale:** There is no restriction of food or fluids prior to a cardiac (or any) echocardiogram. This test uses sound waves emitted from and reflected back to a transducer, and it is noninvasive. Each of the other options are variations of an incorrect response. **Cognitive Level:** Analyzing

Client Need: Reduction of Risk Potential **Integrated Process:** Teaching and Learning **Content Area:** Adult Health **Strategy:** The core issue of the question is knowledge of client preparation for echocardiography. Recall that this is a noninvasive test and uses only ultrasound waves (and thus has no special restrictions) to eliminate each of the incorrect options.

11 **Answer: 3 Rationale:** The client should go about his usual daily activities and exercise pattern while wearing the monitor, and should record activities and any symptoms experienced in the diary. The client does not need to make diary entries every 30 minutes, but as needed to provide an overview of activity so that it can be correlated with any cardiac abnormalities on the time-stamped electrocardiogram being recorded. The client should not take a bath or a shower while wearing the device, which has electrical circuitry. The client does not need to walk a total of 3 miles during the 24-hour period. **Cognitive Level:** Analyzing **Client Need:** Reduction of Risk Potential **Integrated Process:** Nursing Process: Evaluation **Content Area:** Adult Health **Strategy:** The core issue of the question is knowledge of proper use of a Holter monitor. The wording of the question indicates only one option is a correct statement. Use nursing knowledge and the process of elimination to make a selection.

12 **Answer: 2, 3, 4, 5 Rationale:** The client has 60 mL less than the expected minimum urine output of 240 mL in 8 hours. It is appropriate to assess the client's fluid intake and encourage the client to drink increased fluids. Documenting the value would also be done as part of routine care. The nurse should notify the physician because the urine output is only 75% of the minimum volume (240 mL) that is acceptable in an 8-hour period. Measuring the urine specific gravity is not a routine nursing action at this time. **Cognitive Level:** Analyzing **Client Need:** Reduction of Risk Potential **Integrated Process:** Nursing Process: Implementation **Content Area:** Adult Health **Strategy:** The critical words in the question are *at this time*. The wording of the question also suggests that more than one answer is likely to be correct. Use this nursing knowledge of routine actions for decreased urine output to make a selection.

13 **Answer: 2 Rationale:** The NA should wash the client's hair to remove the paste or collodion that was used to secure the electrodes to the head for the diagnostic test. The client should be able to eat and drink and can resume usual activity unless otherwise ordered. There is no dye used in this diagnostic test. **Cognitive Level:** Applying **Client Need:** Reduction of Risk Potential **Integrated Process:** Nursing Process: Implementation **Content Area:** Adult Health **Strategy:** Recall that electroencephalography requires no special aftercare except to cleanse the client's scalp because of the electrode paste. Use this knowledge and the process of elimination to make a selection.

14 **Answer: 1 Rationale:** Following myelogram with water-based contrast, the head of the bed needs to be elevated to 60 degrees to reduce the risk of meningeal irritation from any residual contrast in the spinal fluid. The head of the bed at 15 or 30 degrees is too low to prevent headache from meningeal irritation as a complication of the procedure. If an oil-based contrast was used, the head of the bed would need to remain flat. **Cognitive Level:** Applying **Client Need:** Reduction of Risk Potential **Integrated Process:** Nursing Process: Implementation **Content Area:** Adult Health **Strategy:** The core issue of the question is knowledge of correct head position following myelogram using water-based contrast. Use nursing knowledge and the process of elimination to make a selection.

15 **Answer: 3 Rationale:** The client should limit joint movement, including walking, for 2–3 days after arthroscopy. Analgesics are often needed to manage pain, and the client should be instructed about what to use and how often to take it. The physician may order ice to control swelling, but not heat, which would aggravate swelling. Increased swelling and bleeding after discharge should be reported, because these are abnormal findings, and could indicate a complication of the procedure. **Cognitive Level:** Analyzing **Client Need:** Reduction of Risk Potential **Integrated Process:** Nursing Process: Evaluation **Content Area:** Adult Health **Strategy:** The core issue of the question is knowledge of measures to prevent complications and aid healing after arthroscopy. Use nursing knowledge about arthroscopy care and the process of elimination to make a selection.

16 **Answer: 1 Rationale:** Because the throat is anesthetized so the client can tolerate the endoscope, the client's gag and swallow reflexes are temporarily lost during any upper endoscopy procedure, such as esophagogastroscopy. The nurse's priority is to monitor for return of these protective airway reflexes. While mildly elevated temperature and reports of heartburn also warrant continued monitoring, they are of lesser priority than concerns related to the client's airway. A temporary sore throat is expected and warrants routine follow-up. **Cognitive Level:** Analyzing **Client Need:** Reduction of Risk Potential **Integrated Process:** Nursing Process: Data Collection **Content Area:** Adult Health **Strategy:** Use the ABCs (airway, breathing, and circulation) to answer the question. Options that involve the airway are frequently the highest priority items. Use nursing knowledge and the process of elimination to make a selection.

17 **Answer: 3 Rationale:** The client should not eat or drink anything for 8–12 hours before the test, so the client should not eat or drink anything after midnight. Oral medications including antacids are usually withheld before the procedure. A low-fat diet or a high-carbohydrate diet is unnecessary before this test. **Cognitive Level:** Analyzing **Client Need:** Reduction of Risk Potential **Integrated Process:** Nursing Process: Evaluation **Content Area:** Adult Health **Strategy:** The core issue of the question is knowledge of dietary preparation before a barium swallow or upper GI series. Use ordinary logic to determine that the GI organs would be difficult to visualize if they contained food or fluid. Use nursing knowledge and the process of elimination to make a selection.

18 **Answer: 2, 5 Rationale:** The diet may be resumed after colonoscopy, but the client usually tolerates it better if it is resumed gradually. The client should not drive or perform other activities requiring mental alertness for about 24 hours, until all medications have fully worn off. It is normal to pass gas and feel bloated because of the carbon dioxide used to insufflate the colon to visualize the area. It is abnormal for bleeding to be present, and the client should notify the physician if it occurs. **Cognitive Level:** Analyzing **Client Need:** Reduction of Risk Potential **Integrated Process:** Teaching and Learning **Content Area:** Adult Health **Strategy:** The core issue of the question is knowledge of self-care following colonoscopy. Use nursing knowledge and the process of elimination to make a selection.

19 **Answer: 2 Rationale:** The client should avoid using any skin products, such as lotions or deodorant, on the skin of the breast or underarm prior to mammogram. The client may

eat and drink as usual. Although the procedure might cause some women discomfort with compression of the breast, it is not necessary to premedicate with analgesics. There is no activity restriction following the test. **Cognitive Level:** Applying **Client Need:** Reduction of Risk Potential **Integrated Process:** Teaching and Learning **Content Area:** Adult Health **Strategy:** The core issue of the question is knowing to avoid skin products to prevent possible skin damage before a radiographic procedure such as a mammogram. The wording of the question tells you that only one option is correct. Use nursing knowledge and the process of elimination to make a selection.

20 **Answer: 2** **Rationale:** A Mantoux test (or PPD test) to screen for tuberculosis should be read in 48–72 hours. If the test was planted on Monday, the result must be read in 2–3 days, which is Wednesday or Thursday. The other options are either partially or completely incorrect. **Cognitive Level:** Applying **Client Need:** Reduction of Risk Potential **Integrated Process:** Nursing Process: Implementation **Content Area:** Adult Health **Strategy:** The core issue of the question is knowledge of specific time frames for reading a PPD test. Remember when there is more than one part to an option, the entire option must be correct for that option to be the correct answer. Use nursing knowledge and the process of elimination to make a selection.

21 **Answer: 1, 3, 5** **Rationale:** Selected drugs (antacids, corticosteroids, cholinergics, and anticholinergics) and coffee and alcohol should be restricted for at least 24 hours prior to test; note on the test request form if the client has not complied with the restrictions. There is no reason to withhold a cardiac glycoside or a diuretic, because these medications would not affect the test results. **Cognitive Level:** Applying **Client Need:** Reduction of Risk Potential **Integrated Process:** Nursing Process: Implementation **Content Area:** Adult Health **Strategy:** The core issue of the question is knowledge of drugs that could interfere with basal gastric acid testing and analysis. The wording of the question tells you that more than one option might be correct. Use nursing knowledge and the process of elimination.

Key Terms to Review

computed tomography (CT) scan p. 695
magnetic resonance imaging (MRI) p. 696
nuclear scan p. 696
ultrasonography p. 697
x-ray p. 697

References

Corbett, J. (2008). *Laboratory tests and diagnostic procedures with nursing diagnoses* (7th ed.). Upper Saddle River, NJ: Pearson Education.

Kee, J. (2010). *Laboratory and diagnostic tests with nursing implications* (8th ed.). Upper Saddle River, NJ: Pearson Education.

Fischbach, F. & Dunning, M. (2009). *A manual of laboratory and diagnostic tests* (8th ed.). Philadelphia: Lippincott Williams & Wilkins.

Leeuwen, A. & Poelhuis-Leth, D. (2009). *Davis's comprehensive handbook of laboratory and diagnostic tests with nursing implications* (3rd ed.). Philadelphia: F.A. Davis.

Smith, S., Duell, D., & Martin, B. (2012). *Clinical nursing skills: Basic to advanced skills* (8th ed.). Upper Saddle River, NJ: Pearson Education, Inc.

Test Yourself

Are you ready for the NCLEX-PN® or course exams? Use the practice tests on the companion website to check.

44 Perioperative Care

In this chapter

Cross Reference

Other chapters relevant to this content area are
Preventing and Controlling Infection **Chapter 7**
Maintaining Function of Tubes and Drains **Chapter 27**

I. OVERVIEW OF PERIOPERATIVE NURSING

NCLEX®

A. Perioperative phases

1. **Preoperative phase** begins with decision to have surgery and ends with transport of client to operating room (OR); general nursing activities include client identification, client assessment, identifying potential or actual health problems, and beginning teaching about postoperative self-care
2. **Intraoperative phase** (surgical period) begins when client is transferred to operating table and ends with admission to postanesthesia care unit (PACU); general nursing activities include
   a. Preparing client for induction of anesthesia
   b. Maintaining homeostasis and asepsis throughout procedure
   c. Assisting surgeon and team as needed by providing an aseptic, hazard-free environment and necessary supplies in a timely manner
3. **Postoperative phase** begins with client's admission to PACU and ends with a follow-up evaluation in either a clinical setting or home; general nursing activities include
   a. Evaluating for physical adaptation following anesthesia and surgical intervention
   b. Assisting in orienting client back to consciousness
   c. Providing continuity of information between nursing units about client progress and adaptation following procedure

B. Summary of nursing responsibilities during preoperative period

1. Interview: current health status, allergies, medication currently taking, previous surgical experiences, mental status, understanding of surgical procedure and anesthesia, smoking habit, alcohol and drug use, coping strategies, social resources, and cultural considerations
2. Arranging for preadmission testing, consultations, and education about recovering from surgery and anesthesia
   a. Scheduling appropriate ordered laboratory tests, electrocardiogram, x-rays
   b. Ensuring reports are available on chart

c. Reporting to surgeon or anesthesiologist any pertinent abnormalities
d. Asking client if arrangements for autologous or directed blood donation (family/friends) have been made; if so, attach pertinent lab requisitions

NCLEX®
3. Day of surgery: after appropriate identification of client, verify completion of paperwork and secure valuables; if procedure is being performed on an outpatient basis, verify transportation home; then complete these activities:
   a. Determine client's cognitive understanding of procedure and obtain signed **informed consent** form; ensure consent is obtained before administering premedication with sedative effects; some agencies have client mark limb that will be operated on, if appropriate
   b. Perform a physical examination and record vital signs (VS)
   c. Implement preoperative teaching for postoperative care
   d. Physical preparation: may include skin preparation, antiembolism stockings, catheterization, and starting an intravenous (IV) infusion
   e. Complete preoperative checklist; note client status and pertinent recent lab results; assist client to remove clothing, jewelry, and other articles, and to don hospital gown
   f. If client refuses to remove wedding band, tape in place and notify operating room personnel; leave eyeglasses in place if consistent with hospital policy; keep hearing aid(s) in place; remove dentures

C. Summary of nursing responsibilities during intraoperative period

1. Administer IV infusions and medications as needed

NCLEX®
2. Provide safe, effective care
   a. Position client to ensure functional alignment and exposure of surgical site
   b. Apply grounding device
   c. Provide emotional and physical support if awake
   d. Account for all equipment and supplies
   e. Maintain aseptic environment
   f. Perform physiologic monitoring
   g. Monitor fluid loss or gain
   h. Monitor cardiac, respiratory, and neurological status
   i. Monitor client response to preoperative medications
3. Nursing roles during surgery
   a. Circulating nurse assists scrub nurses and surgeons; sterile scrubbing and gloving not necessary
   b. Scrub nurses assist surgeons; maintain sterile gowns, gloves, shoe covers; wear eye protection and caps
   c. Circulating nurse and scrub nurse account for used sponges, needles, and instruments during case

D. Summary of nursing responsibilities during postoperative period

1. Immediate care
   a. Monitor effects of anesthetic agents and surgical procedure
   b. Monitor vital functions
   c. Provide comfort and pain relief

NCLEX®
2. Ongoing care
   a. Monitor for client adaptation to effects of surgery
   b. Provide pain management
   c. Position client appropriately
   d. Promote use of incentive spirometry
   e. Assist with postoperative exercises
   f. Maintain hydration
   g. Promote urinary elimination
   h. Maintain suction to devices as needed
   i. Provide wound care
   j. Continue to reinforce client teaching and discharge planning

II. PURPOSES AND TYPES OF SURGERY AND ANESTHESIA

NCLEX®
A. Purposes

1. Diagnostic or exploratory: establishes a diagnosis, such as a breast biopsy
2. Curative: removes pathological cause, such as removal of cancer
3. Ablative: removes a diseased body part, such as tonsils for tonsillitis
4. Reconstructive: restores function or appearance, such as cleft lip repair
5. **Palliative**: relieves or reduces pain or symptoms of a disease, such as removal of sensory nerves for intractable pain

Table 44–1 Urgency Classification of Surgery

Classification	Description	Example
Emergent	Performed immediately to save client's life, limb, or organ	Testicular torsion
Urgent	Requires prompt attention, usually within 24 hrs	Fracture reduction
Required	Needed for client's well-being, often within weeks to months	Cholecystectomy, if not acute
Elective	Needed but condition is not imminently life threatening; surgery will improve client's life	Plastic surgery
Optional	Based on client preference	Gastric stapling

B. General classification of surgery

1. Major (higher risk) versus minor (lower risk)
   a. Major: may include prolonged intraoperative period, a large loss of blood, involvement of a vital organ, or postoperative complications; examples are lung surgery, colectomy
   b. Minor: usually associated with few complications, may be described as "one-day surgery" or outpatient surgery; examples are cyst removal, ingrown toenails

NCLEX® 2. Urgency classification (see Table 44–1)

C. Administration of *anesthesia* (partial or complete loss of sensation)

1. Anesthetic agents are drugs used to effect a partial or complete loss of pain sensation; client may be conscious or unconscious

NCLEX® 2. **Moderate sedation** (or conscious sedation)
   a. An anesthesia state involving minimal depression of level of consciousness (LOC), allowing client to respond to verbal and physical stimuli; client maintains a patent airway while pain threshold is raised; examples are with burn dressings, balloon angioplasty
   b. Uses IV narcotics and anti-anxiety agents

NCLEX® 3. **Regional anesthesia**: loss of sensation in one part of body; see Table 44–2

NCLEX® 4. General anesthesia
   a. Anesthesia that involves loss of all sensation and consciousness
   b. It is usually administered by IV infusion or by inhalation of gases
   c. Examples of use: major surgery, exploratory laparotomy

D. Stages of general anesthesia (see Table 44–3)

E. Preanesthesia classification of client's physical condition

1. Anesthesiologist reviews client's medical history as well as current data related to diagnosis, medication use, allergies, and drug reactions
2. Client is then assigned a risk category for surgery, from I (healthiest) to VI (brain dead; organs being donated) or E for emergency surgery

NCLEX® 3. General health problems that increase overall surgical risk are malnutrition (delayed wound healing and infection), obesity (impaired respiratory and cardiac function, impaired wound healing), cardiac conditions, blood coagulation disorders (bleeding), lung disease (reduced pulmonary function), renal disease (impaired regulation of fluids, electrolytes, and drug excretion), diabetes mellitus (delayed healing, wound infection), and liver disease (impaired drug detoxification, prothrombin production for clotting, and nutrient metabolism for healing)

Table 44–2 Types of Regional Anesthesia

Type	Description
Local	Injected in a specific area for minor surgical procedures, such as lidocaine for suturing a small wound.
Nerve block	Anesthetic agent is injected into and around a nerve or group of nerves, such as a pudendal block used to numb perineum for an episiotomy.
Epidural block	Anesthetic agent injected into epidural space to anesthetize larger areas, such as in vaginal childbirth; client is awake and aware of surroundings but feels no pain.
Spinal anesthesia	Anesthesia is injected through a lumbar puncture into subarachnoid space, such as for hernia repairs or cesarean section deliveries; client is conscious but has no sensation or movement of lower extremities up to a specific area.

Table 44–3 Stages of Anesthesia

Stage	Characteristics
Stage I	Beginning of anesthesia; client is drowsy and dizzy; pain sensation is depressed
Stage II	Excitement stage; client has irregular breathing, involuntary motor movements; avoid stimulating client, which can trigger vomiting, holding the breath, and increased activity; ensure client safety by proper use of safety straps
Stage III	Stage of anesthesia appropriate for surgical procedures; client has skeletal muscle relaxation, constricted pupils, absence of eyelid reflex
Stage IV	Medullary depression; client is near death; pupils are fixed and dilated, respirations are weak, pulse is rapid and thready

F. Anesthetic agents may be administered by either inhalation or IV routes

1. Inhalation anesthetic agents are inhaled in gaseous forms
   - **a.** Administered by mask or by endotracheal tube
   - **b.** Induction is usually rapid
   - **c.** Drugs are eliminated by respiratory system
   - **d.** With normal lung function, recovery rate is predictable
2. IV anesthesia
   - **a.** Administered alone or in combination with inhalation anesthesia
   - **b.** Rapid onset of unconsciousness
   - **c.** Metabolized primarily by liver and excreted by kidneys
   - **d.** Reversal agents may be required to stop drug effects

III. COMPONENTS OF PREOPERATIVE DATA COLLECTION

A. Client's history

1. Medical history: current and past
   - NCLEX® **a.** Family history of malignant hyperthermia
   - **b.** Current health status including any chronic disease that might affect response to surgery and anesthesia
   - **c.** Past medical illnesses and treatments; previous surgical experiences including complications that occurred with previous surgical or anesthesia experience (such as malignant hyperthermia)
   - **d.** Report of severe anxiety associated with surgery
2. NCLEX® Medication use: all current medications, including prescription, over-the-counter, and herbal or other agents
3. NCLEX® Allergies
   - **a.** Food or medication
   - **b.** Environmental: latex allergies, tape, soap, and antiseptic agents
4. Tobacco use: may indicate potential problems of respiratory tract; identify type of product and amount and frequency of use; when possible, urge client to stop smoking 6–8 weeks before major surgery
5. Alcohol and controlled substance use: determine type of product, amount and frequency, and potential for problems with withdrawal
6. Psychosocial and economic factors
   - **a.** Occupation and financial concerns
   - **b.** Support systems
   - **c.** Spiritual needs and cultural beliefs
   - **d.** Coping mechanisms used in the past
   - **e.** Fear and anxiety about procedure (e.g., changes in body image, pain, grieving loss of a body part)

B. Physical examination

1. Determine factors that will affect response to surgery or anesthesia
2. NCLEX® See Table 44–4 for summary of important preoperative data

C. Diagnostic screening

1. Laboratory tests are done before surgery to screen for existing abnormalities and to use as a baseline for future assessments
2. Additional tests may be ordered related to specific condition
3. NCLEX® Verify that ordered test results are available because abnormal findings may need to be corrected prior to surgery
4. See Table 44–5 for routine preoperative screening tests

Table 44-4 Components of Preoperative Physical Examination

Focus	Specific Data Collection Items
General	Overall appearance, gestures, facial expression Height and weight (obesity increases risk) Vital signs (hypertension increases risk)
Head and neck	Oral mucous membranes (hydration status) Loose teeth, dentures, and orthodontia work Soft palate, nasal sinuses, cervical lymph nodes Presence of jugular venous distention
Integumentary	Skin over entire body noting areas where skin is thin, dry, has poor turgor or breakdown
Chest and lungs	Adventitious breath sounds Degree of chest expansion, presence of cough, upper airway congestion, and/or obstructed nasal passages
Cardiovascular	Apical rate and rhythm Color and temperature of extremities Presence of pacemaker, A-V fistula or graft
Gastrointestinal	Distinguish between obesity and distention of abdomen Monitor baseline bowel sounds and elimination patterns Note gag reflex and history of nausea/vomiting postoperatively Validate NPO (nothing by mouth) status when applicable; anesthetics are known to depress GI functioning; clients are usually NPO for 6–8 hours before surgery to reduce risk of vomiting and aspiration
Genitourinary and reproductive	Determine alterations in urinary elimination, color, appearance, and usual amount of urine output Note presence of abnormal vaginal discharge, uterine bleeding in women Pregnancy status
Neurological and mobility status	Determine baseline LOC Note presence of sensory or perceptual deficits Evaluate range of motion and ability to perform activities of daily living

Table 44-5 Routine Preoperative Screening Tests

Test	Purpose for Assessment
Urinalysis	Urine composition and possible abnormal components
Chest x-ray	Respiratory status and heart size
Electrocardiogram	Preexisting cardiac disease or rhythm abnormalities
Complete blood count (CBC)	RBCs, hemoglobin, and hematocrit for O_2-carrying capacity; WBCs as indicator of immune function (infection)
Blood typing and cross-matching	Blood transfusion, ABO and Rh matching
Serum electrolytes	Electrolyte balance (Na^+, K^+, Ca^{++}, Mg^{++}, Cl^-, HCO_3^-)
Fasting blood glucose	Detection or control of diabetes mellitus
BUN and creatinine	Renal function
ALT, AST, LDH, bilirubin	Liver function
Serum albumin and total protein	Nutritional status

IV. INFORMED CONSENT

A. Description

1. Written permission obtained from client prior to any invasive procedure or one that has potentially serious side effects or complications
2. Client has right to accept or reject procedure after receiving explanation

NCLEX® 3. Informed consent includes providing client with information about the following:
 a. Nature and purpose of a treatment or procedure
 b. Expected outcomes and probabilities of success, material risks, benefits and consequences of treatment
 c. Alternatives to procedure and supporting information
 d. Effect of not having procedure or treatment, including effect on prognosis

B. Three elements of informed consent

1. It is given voluntarily
2. It is given by an individual with capacity and competence to understand what procedure involves (NCLEX®)
 a. Adults have legal authority to make decisions for themselves
 b. If client is a minor, parent or legal guardian has right to provide consent
 c. Many states recognize emancipated minors who can provide consent for themselves
 d. Many states allow minors to provide consent for treatment in cases related to sexually transmitted infections, pregnancy, abortion, and contraception
 e. Legal power of attorney for health care allows another person to make decisions should client become incapacitated
3. Sufficient information must be provided to client to allow for an informed decision
 a. Health care workers must communicate in a way client can understand
 b. An interpreter may be needed to ensure adequate communication
4. In emergencies, when informed consent cannot be obtained from client or next of kin, consent is implied by law; specific information about emergency situation and reason informed consent was not obtained must be documented in medical record

C. Nurse's role with informed consent

1. Informed consent is part of physician–client relationship
2. Physician has obligation to obtain consent (NCLEX®)
3. Because nurse does not perform surgery or procedures, obtaining informed consent is not a nursing responsibility; nurses can reinforce physician explanations
4. Nurse can serve as witness to the following: (NCLEX®)
 a. Authority on consent form is authentic
 b. Client has capacity to make informed consent
 c. Client has authority to consent
 d. Consent is being given voluntarily

V. DEVELOPMENTAL CONSIDERATIONS OF CLIENTS HAVING SURGERY

A. Children and adolescents (NCLEX®)

1. Take care with all children and adolescents while explaining procedures because they may misinterpret meaning
2. Infancy: surgery and separation from parents may interfere with bonding; infants have no understanding of events but are aware of adult emotions; no explanations about procedures are required for infant, but parents will need complete preparation
3. Toddlers: may experience separation anxiety; their security lies in presence of their caregivers; when caregivers are not present, child may suffer; immediately prior to a procedure, give toddler a brief, simple explanation
4. Preschoolers: often view illness as punishment for bad behavior; have an inadequate understanding of cause–effect and thus misinterpret relationships; continue to give simple explanations in close proximity to time of procedure; play therapy may help preschooler to express feelings
5. School-age children: are better able to withstand separation from parents and are accustomed to dealing with adults other than family; they fear pain and mutilation and require more complete, yet age-appropriate instructions; they may benefit from pictures, dolls, and videos as teaching aids
6. Adolescents: concerns are separation from peers and body image/physical attractiveness; protect child's privacy

B. Adults

1. Fear of unknown and separation from support systems
2. Dependence and loss of control
3. Disruption in career goals, family living patterns, and financial worries
4. Concern over disability and/or death

VI. PHYSICAL PREPARATION OF CLIENTS HAVING SURGERY

A. Preparing for anesthesia

1. Anesthetic needs and risks are assessed by anesthesiologist
2. Type of anesthetic along with method of administration, risks, and recovery is explained

B. Preparing skin

1. Purpose: cleansing and removing transient microbes from skin
2. Components
   a. Cleansing: begins with morning shower or bath; surgical site is then cleansed with an antimicrobial agent immediately prior to surgical procedure
   b. Hair removal from surgical site: may be ordered to further reduce microbial growth; take care to maintain intact skin (clip but do not shave)

C. Preparing GI tract

NCLEX®

1. Client is placed on NPO status prior to OR to reduce risk of vomiting or aspiration, prevent contamination of operative site from fecal material, and reduce postoperative nausea, vomiting, gastric distention, or bowel obstruction
2. Colon cleansing may be ordered for surgical procedures involving GI tract to reduce contamination of surgical field; postoperative constipation may be prevented; cleansing may occur using enemas, laxatives, and oral antibiotics (such as neomycin)

D. Preparation on day of surgery

NCLEX®

1. Routine care for most outpatient as well as hospitalized clients
   a. Consent form is signed
   b. Preoperative medications are given
   c. Emotional support to client and family is provided
   d. Preoperative teaching is completed, including postoperative routine

NCLEX®

2. General care
   a. Record VS for baseline information
   b. Remove dentures, bridgework (or both); note on chart presence of loose teeth
   c. Have client put on hospital gown without undergarments in many cases (for children and minor procedures, there may be exceptions)
   d. Have client void to empty bladder
   e. Remove cosmetics and nail polish
   f. Remove jewelry per agency policy and place in secure area for safekeeping; if client does not want to remove wedding band, it can be taped in place; in certain situations, removal of wedding band may be required because of risk of postoperative edema
   g. Leave hearing aids in place and note on preoperative checklist
   h. Remove eyeglasses, contact lenses, and other prostheses
   i. Antiembolism stockings may be ordered to promote venous return from legs

E. Preoperative medications

1. May be ordered at a scheduled time or "on call" to OR
2. Purposes
   a. Sedate or tranquilize
   b. Decrease respiratory tract secretions
   c. Provide analgesia

Table 44–6 Classifications of Possible Preoperative Medications

Drug Class	Preoperative Use	Major Side Effects
Anti-infectives	Reduce risk of infection prophylactically	Antibiotic resistance; first dose hypersensitivity
Anticholinergics	Reduce body fluid secretion (ex: saliva)	GI system depression
Antiemetics	Reduce risk of emesis and aspiration	Respiratory depression
H_2-receptor blockers	Reduce gastric acidity and reflux	Rebound acidity
Opioid analgesics	Reduce dosages needed of anesthetics	CNS depression
Benzodiazepines	Reduce anxiety and as a medication enhancer	CNS depression
Barbiturates	Sedation and as narcotic enhancer; not often used	CNS, respiratory depression

   d. Reduce nausea and prevent vomiting
   e. Reduce gastric acid
3. Classifications of preoperative medication: see Table 44–6

VII. INTRAOPERATIVE FACTORS AFFECTING POSTOPERATIVE PHASE

A. Principles of perioperative asepsis

1. General
   a. Keep sterile supplies dry and unopened
   b. Check package sterilization expiration date to verify sterility
   c. Maintain general cleanliness in surgical suite
   NCLEX® d. Maintain **surgical asepsis** (techniques to keep sites free of micro organisms) throughout procedure (see Box 44–1)
2. Personnel with signs of illness should not report to work
3. **Surgical scrub**, a specific handwashing technique used by OR personnel to reduce microorganisms on hands and arms; is done for length of time designated by hospital policy
   a. A sensor-controlled or knee- or foot-operated faucet allows water to be turned on and off without use of hands
   b. Remove all rings and watches
   c. Use liquid soaps to prevent spread of microorganisms
   d. Keep fingernails short and well-trimmed; clean fingernails with a nail stick under running water; artificial nails pose risk of infection and are prohibited
   e. Hold hands higher than elbows throughout procedure so run-off goes to elbows; this allows hands to be cleanest area
   f. A scrub brush facilitates removal of microorganisms; clean all areas of skin on hands and arms in sequence, starting at hands and ending at elbows
   g. After rinsing, dry hands with sterile towels, drying first one arm from hand to elbow, then using a second towel to dry second hand
4. NCLEX® Maintaining a **sterile field** (a microoganism-free area)
   a. Create a sterile field using sterile drapes
   b. Use sterile field to place sterile supplies to be available during procedure
   c. Drape equipment prior to use
   d. Keep drapes dry and out of contact with nonsterile objects
   e. Utilize sterile technique while adding or removing supplies from sterile fields
5. NCLEX® Sterile supplies and solutions
   a. Check expiration dates for sterility
   b. Don't use solutions that were opened prior to current use
   c. "Lip" solutions after initial use by pouring a small amount of liquid out of bottle into a waste container to cleanse bottle lip

Box 44–1

Principles of Surgical Asepsis

All objects used in a sterile field must be sterile.

Sterile objects become unsterile when touched by unsterile objects.

Objects that are below waist or table level or out of vision are considered unsterile.

Sterile objects become unsterile with prolonged exposure to airborne microorganisms.

Fluids flow in the direction of gravity.

Moisture that passes through a sterile object draws microorganisms from unsterile surfaces above or below to the sterile surface by capillary action (also called *strikethrough*).

A 1-inch (2.5 cm) margin at each edge of a sterile field is considered unsterile because it is in contact with an unsterile surface.

The skin cannot be sterilized and is unsterile.

Maintaining surgical asepsis requires conscientiousness, alertness, and honesty.

Adapted from Berman, A. & Snyder, S. *Kozier & Erb's fundamentals of nursing: Concepts, process, and practice* (9th ed.), p. 701. (c) 2012. Reprinted by permission of Pearson Education, Inc., Upper Saddle River, NJ 07458.

B. Potential environmental health hazards during intraoperative period

1. Injuries caused by equipment
   a. Laser tools used for a surgical procedure can cause burns
   b. Improperly grounded cautery devices can cause burns
   c. Ensure proper grounding for electrical equipment and check equipment prior to beginning surgical procedure

NCLEX®

2. Latex allergy affects many people, both clients and hospital personnel
   a. Clients with spina bifida and those who have had multiple surgical procedures are at greatest risk
   b. Exposure can occur percutaneously, mucosally, parenterally, and via inhalation
   c. Symptoms can vary from contact dermatitis to anaphylaxis
   d. Symptoms in an anesthetized client would include flushing, facial swelling, urticaria, bronchospasm, hypotension, and cardiac arrest
   e. Be aware of equipment that contains latex, including tourniquets, manual resuscitation (Ambu) bags, balloon catheters, surgical gowns, boots, and drapes

NCLEX®

3. Exposure to blood and body fluids
   a. Is a concern for client and staff alike
   b. Use goggles and fluid-protectant shields; gloves worn for extended period can leak and should be changed periodically
   c. Use caution with sharps

C. Potential intraoperative complications

1. Nausea and vomiting: ensure that client is NPO for prescribed time period
2. Hypoxia and respiratory complications
   a. Loss of pharyngeal and cough reflexes may lead to aspiration of secretions or vomitus
   b. Respiratory depression can occur from anesthetic agents
   c. Respiratory muscles become weakened or paralyzed by neuromuscular agents
   d. Positioning can negatively affect lung expansion
   e. Tissue perfusion is monitored by anesthesiologist
   f. Use of a pulse oximeter assists with monitoring oxygenation
3. Hypothermia
   a. Related to OR temperature and exposure of internal organs
   b. Minimized by preventing exposure of nonsurgical body parts, use of head covering and blankets, warmed IV fluids and anesthetic agents

NCLEX®

4. Malignant hyperthermia
   a. Excessive heat production related to stress, trauma, infection; may be attributed to anesthetic agent; seen more commonly in males; there is a tendency toward development if inherited as an autosomal-dominant trait
   b. Symptoms include rapid rise in body temperature, tachycardia, tachypnea, and respiratory and metabolic acidosis
   c. Skin initially appears flushed, then becomes mottled and cyanotic
   d. Treatment includes use of 100% oxygen, cooling blankets and ice packs, cool IV fluids, and stomach irrigation
   e. Can be fatal
5. Paresthesia and impaired skin integrity related to positioning
6. Excessive fluid and blood loss

VIII. POSTOPERATIVE NURSING CARE

A. Data collection in immediate period following surgery in PACU (see Box 44–2)

1. Confirm client's identity
2. Receive report from surgical nurse: surgical procedure, anesthesia, drugs and IV fluids administered, and estimated blood loss
3. Note location, types, and conditions of catheters, **drains**, or packs; drains are tubes inserted into wounds to allow removal of excessive **serosanguineous** (fluid composed of serum and blood) or **purulent** (containing pus) material from wound

B. Nursing management in PACU

NCLEX®

1. Maintain a patent airway: priority nursing concern
   a. May be impaired by continued effects of anesthesic drugs, relaxation of tongue, oropharyngeal secretions, or vomitus
   b. Position client on side unless contraindicated

Box 44-2

Clinical Assessment in the Postanesthetic Phase

- Adequacy of airway
- Oxygen saturation
- Adequacy of ventilation: respiratory rate, rhythm, and depth; use of accessory muscles; breath sounds
- Cardiovascular status: heart rate and rhythm; peripheral pulse amplitude and equality, BP, capillary filling
- Level of consciousness: not responding; arousable with verbal simuli, fully awake, oriented to time, person, and place
- Presence of protective reflexes (e.g., gag, cough, swallow)
- Activity, ability to move extremities
- Skin color (pink, pale, dusky, blotchy, cyanotic, jaundiced)
- Fluid status: intake and output, status of IV infusions (type of fluid, rate, amount in container, patency of tubing), signs of dehydration or fluid overload
- Condition of operative site: status of dressing, drainage (amount, type, and color)
- Patency, character, and amount of drainage from catheters, tubes, and drains
- Discomfort (i.e., pain: type, location, and severity), nausea, vomiting
- Safety (e.g., necessity for side rails, call bell within reach)

Source: Berman, A. & Snyder, S. (2012). *Kozier & Erb's fundamentals of nursing: Concepts, Process, and Practice* (9th ed.). Upper Saddle River, NJ: Pearson Education, 976.

  c. Monitor respiratory rate (should be 10–30 breaths/minute)
  d. Auscultate breath sounds for crackles (fluid) or rhonchi (secretions) and suction as necessary
  e. Wheezing or stridor may signal broncho- or laryngospasm; monitor carefully and maintain airway; notify surgeon or anesthesiologist immediately
  f. Monitor for return of cough, gag, and swallow reflexes

NCLEX®

2. Maintain cardiovascular stability
  a. Client is typically on a cardiac and respiratory monitor
  b. Monitor vital signs (VS) according to hospital policy (often every 15 minutes) until stable and then every 30 minutes until PACU discharge
  c. Report changes in VS immediately; small but persistent trends are early signs that client's condition is deteriorating
  d. Apply pneumatic boots or antiembolism stockings as ordered to promote circulation in lower extremities

3. Monitor for hypotension or shock
  a. May be related to fluid or blood loss or as a reaction to drugs
  b. Symptoms: restlessness, decreased urine output (UO), cool moist skin, pallor followed by cyanosis, and dropping BP with increasing pulse
  c. Monitor and maintain IV infusion flow rates to prevent hypovolemia as a cause of shock

NCLEX®

4. Monitor for hemorrhage
  a. Monitor dressings and drains for amount of discharge; observe appearance and amount of urine (concentrated and decreased volume with hypovolemia); observe for distention of body tissues
  b. A client with excessive blood loss may require a transfusion; ensure blood product and type are correct

5. Monitor for hypertension and dysrhythmias

6. Relieve pain and anxiety
  a. Pain can negatively affect VS and recovery
  b. Determine location and cause of pain
  c. Administer analgesics (often opioids by IV) as ordered
  d. Observe effectiveness of analgesics

7. Neurological status
  a. Monitor LOC with vital signs and prn
  b. Frequently attempt to arouse client until fully awake
  c. Orient to environment when awake
  d. Maintain quiet environment during recovery period from anesthesia

8. Temperature
   a. Measure temperature
   b. Apply warm blankets or Bear hugger to keep client warm if hypothermic from cool operating room and exposure during surgery

NCLEX®
9. Integumentary
   a. Monitor status of incision if visible; otherwise, monitor status of incisional dressing
   b. Observe for skin redness or breakdown because of surgical positioning or burns from cautery or grounding pad; report and complete incident report if found

NCLEX®
C. Discharge criteria from PACU
1. VS are stable and spontaneous respirations have returned
2. Gag reflex is present
3. Client is easily arousable
4. Additional client discharge criteria from ambulatory surgical unit:
   a. Is alert and oriented
   b. Has no respiratory distress
   c. Is able to cough, swallow, and walk
   d. Is free of vomiting
   e. Has voided (may not be required in minor procedures per some agency policies)
   f. Has mild or minimal pain
   g. Has minimal, if any, bleeding from incisional area
   h. Has responsible adult to drive client home

D. Nursing management on clinical unit

NCLEX®
1. Immediate nursing interventions
   a. Monitor breathing and apply oxygen if prescribed
   b. Check VS and skin warmth, moisture, color
   c. Observe surgical site and wound drains; partial or total rupture of a sutured wound is termed **dehiscence**; dehiscence may be preceded by sudden straining as occurs during coughing (see also section on complications that follows)
   d. Note and document wound **exudate** (fluid and cells that accumulate in a wound); exudate varies in appearance: **serous** (like serum—watery and clear), purulent (thick and contains pus; may be blue, green, or yellow tinged), **sanguineous** (bloody and may be dark red or bright red depending on freshness of blood)
   e. Connect tubes to drain devices or suction
   f. Perform pain assessment and utilize appropriate pain relief interventions
   g. Position client properly using support devices as necessary
   h. Monitor IV fluids and infusion pumps
   i. Monitor UO hourly or less frequently as ordered; hourly UO should be 30 mL or more
   j. Bladder distention is possible for up to 24 hours following spinal anesthesia; client should void spontaneously within 6–8 hours postoperatively; if unable to void, catheterization may be ordered and repeated as necessary
2. Ongoing nursing interventions

NCLEX®
   a. Encourage incentive spirometer, deep breathing and coughing exercises every 2 hours while awake to prevent atelectasis and pneumonia; encourage client to sit up in bed and place hands one on top of the other directly on wound (splint incision) to reduce discomfort of coughing; monitor oxygen saturation with VS
   b. Reinforce and encourage leg exercises (such as foot circles, ankle pumps), use of support stockings or sequential compression devices; check for Homan's sign or calf pain with dorsiflexion during routine assessments
   c. Keep call light, emesis basin, ice chips, bedpan, urinal within reach
   d. Communicate with family and significant others

NCLEX®
   e. Monitor for infection by noting wound characteristics, temperature, and WBC test results; administer prophylactic or other antibiotics on time to maintain therapeutic blood levels
   f. Reinforce self-care measures according to surgical procedure and client and family needs
   g. Encourage activity as tolerated

NCLEX®
   h. Promote GI status: perform abdominal examination including bowel sounds each shift; provide diet and fluids once bowel sounds return; begin with clear liquids and advance to full liquids, soft and regular as ordered and tolerated (no N/V, abdominal distention); encourage early ambulation to promote bowel function

Box 44–3

Common Postsurgical Discharge Instructions

Diet

- Drink at least 6 to 8 glasses of fluid daily unless otherwise ordered (water is beneficial)
- Adhere to any diet restrictions (provide individualized instruction according to diet)
- Eat well-balanced meals that are high in vitamin C and protein to aid wound healing

Activity

- Maintain activity restriction if ordered by surgeon
- Resume activities gradually (all clients)
- Avoid heavy lifting for 6 weeks after major surgery
- Avoid lifting more than 10 pounds or performing activities involving pushing or pulling with an abdominal incision
- Often may return to work in 6 to 8 weeks (depending on surgery and client status preoperatively)

Medications

- Continue to take pain medication as needed; follow directions on prescription bottle
- Take other medications as ordered (teach specifics about medication action, dose, how to take, and side/adverse effects to watch for and report)

Wound Care

- Take care of incision and/or change dressing as taught (specific information is individualized to client and surgery; provide 1 to 2 days of dressing materials or according to hospital policy)
- Cover incision with plastic wrap before showering (if allowed)
- Sutures or staples are often removed in surgeon's office 7 to 14 days postoperatively
- Steri-Strips will fall off by themselves (if used instead of sutures or if applied for support when sutures are removed before discharge)

Follow-up Care

- Contact surgeon if signs of complications occur (fever, signs of wound infection, increased pain, other signs specific to surgery)
- Keep follow-up appointments to aid in continued recovery from surgery

NCLEX® **i.** Continue to monitor UO and compare to intake; diuresis from mobilization of fluids given during surgery can occur by second postoperative day

j. Provide wound care as ordered (monitor incision, change dressing as ordered); document findings

NCLEX® **k.** Provide for adequate pain management using patient-controlled analgesia or other opioids; monitor for pain at least every 4 hours; document pain rating, location, quality and other characteristics; evaluate effectiveness of pharmacological and nonpharmacological (e.g., music, distraction, massage) measures

NCLEX® **l.** Participate in discharge planning according to client needs: include in discharge teaching diet, activity, medications, and when to call surgeon for complications; schedule follow-up care; ensure that home care or other support services are in place (see Box 44–3)

IX. POSTOPERATIVE COMPLICATIONS (SEE TABLE 44–7)

Table 44–7 Potential Postoperative Problems

Problem	Description	Cause	Clinical Signs	Preventive Interventions
Respiratory				
Pneumonia	Inflammation of alveoli	Infection, toxins, or irritants causing inflammatory process Immobility and impaired ventilation result in atelectasis and promote growth of pathogens	Elevated temperature, cough, expectoration of blood-tinged or purulent sputum, dyspnea, chest pain	Deep-breathing exercises and coughing, moving in bed, early ambulation

(continued)

Table 44–7 Potential Postoperative Problems *(continued)*

Problem	Description	Cause	Clinical Signs	Preventive Interventions
Atelectasis	A condition in which alveoli collapse and are not ventilated	Mucous plugs blocking bronchial passageways, inadequate lung expansion, analgesics, immobility	Dyspnea, tachypnea, tachycardia; diaphoresis, anxiety; pleural pain, decreased chest wall movement; dull or absent breath sounds; decreased oxygen saturation (SpO_2)	Deep-breathing exercises and coughing, moving in bed, early ambulation
Pulmonary embolism	Blood clot that has moved to lungs and blocks a pulmonary artery, thus obstructing blood flow to a portion of lung	Stasis of venous blood from immobility, venous injury from fractures or during surgery, use of oral contraceptives high in estrogen, preexisting coagulation or circulatory disorder	Sudden chest pain, shortness of breath, cyanosis, shock (tachycardia, low blood pressure)	Turning, ambulation, antiemboli stockings, sequential compression devices
Circulatory				
Hypovolemia	Inadequate circulating blood volume	Fluid deficit, hemorrhage	Tachycardia, decreased urine output, decreased BP	Early detection of signs; fluid and/or blood replacement
Hemorrhage	Internal or external bleeding	Disruption of sutures, insecure ligation of blood vessels	Overt bleeding (dressings saturated with bright blood; bright, free-flowing blood in drains or chest tubes), increased pain, increasing abdominal girth, swelling or bruising around incision	Early detection of signs
Hypovolemic shock	Inadequate tissue perfusion resulting from markedly reduced circulating blood volume	Severe hypovolemia from fluid deficit or hemorrhage	Rapid weak pulse, dyspnea, tachypnea; restlessness and anxiety; urine output less than 30 mL/hr; decreased BP; cool, clammy skin, thirst, pallor	Maintain blood volume through adequate fluid replacement, prevent hemorrhage; early detection of signs
Thrombophlebitis	Inflammation of veins, usually of legs and associated with a blood clot	Slowed venous blood flow due to immobility or prolonged sitting; trauma to vein, resulting in inflammation and increased blood coagulability	Aching, cramping pain; affected area is swollen, red, and hot to touch; vein feels hard; discomfort in calf when foot is dorsiflexed or when client walks (Homans' sign)	Early ambulation, leg exercises, antiemboli stockings, SCDs, adequate fluid intake
Thrombus	Blood clot attached to wall of vein or artery (most commonly leg veins)	As for thrombophlebitis for venous thrombi; disruption or inflammation of arterial wall for arterial thrombi	*Venous:* same as thrombophlebitis *Arterial:* pain and pallor of affected extremity; decreased or absent peripheral pulses	*Venous:* same as thrombophlebitis *Arterial:* maintain prescribed position; early detection of signs
Embolus	Foreign body or clot that has moved from its site of formation to another area of body (e.g., lungs, heart, or brain)	Venous or arterial thrombus; broken intravenous catheter, fat, or amniotic fluid	In venous system, usually becomes a pulmonary embolus (see pulmonary embolism); signs of arterial emboli may depend on location	Turning, ambulation, leg exercises, sequential compression devices; careful maintenance of IV catheters
Urinary				
Urinary retention	Inability to empty bladder, with excessive accumulation of urine in bladder	Depressed bladder muscle tone from narcotics and anesthetics; handling of tissues during surgery on adjacent organs (rectum, vagina)	Fluid intake larger than output; inability to void or frequent voiding of small amounts, bladder distention, suprapubic discomfort, restlessness	Monitoring of fluid intake and output, interventions to facilitate voiding, urinary catheterization as needed
Urinary tract infection	Inflammation of bladder, ureters, or urethra	Immobilization and limited fluid intake, instrumentation of urinary tract	Burning sensation when voiding, urgency, cloudy urine, lower abdominal pain	Adequate fluid intake, early ambulation, aseptic straight catheterization only as necessary, good perineal hygiene

Table 44-7 Potential Postoperative Problems *(continued)*

Problem	Description	Cause	Clinical Signs	Preventive Interventions
Gastrointestinal				
Nausea and vomiting		Pain, abdominal distention, ingesting food or fluids before return of peristalsis, certain medications, anxiety	Complaints of feeling sick to stomach, retching or gagging	IV fluids until peristalsis returns; then clear fluids, full fluids, and regular diet; antiemetic drugs if ordered; analgesics for pain
Constipation	Infrequent or no stool passage for abnormal length of time (e.g., within 48 hours after solid diet started)	Lack of dietary roughage, analgesics (decreased intestinal motility), immobility	Absence of stool elimination, abdominal distention, and discomfort	Adequate fluid intake, high-fiber diet, early ambulation
Tympanites	Retention of gases within intestines	Slowed motility of intestines due to handling of bowel during surgery and effects of anesthesia	Obvious abdominal distention, abdominal discomfort (gas pains), absence of bowel sounds	Early ambulation; avoid using a straw, provide ice chips or water at room temperature
Postoperative ileus	Intestinal obstruction characterized by lack of peristaltic activity	Handling bowel during surgery, anesthesia, electrolyte imbalance, wound infection	Abdominal pain and distention; constipation; absent bowel sounds; vomiting	
Wound				
Wound infection	Inflammation and infection of incision or drain site	Poor aseptic technique; laboratory analysis of wound swab identifies causative microorganism	Purulent exudate, redness, tenderness, elevated body temperature, wound odor	Keep wound clean and dry, use surgical aseptic technique when changing dressings
Wound dehiscence	Separation of a suture line before incision heals	Malnutrition (emaciation, obesity), poor circulation, excessive strain on suture line	Increased incision drainage, tissues underlying skin become visible along parts of incision	Adequate nutrition, appropriate incisional support and avoidance of strain
Wound evisceration	Extrusion of internal organs and tissues through incision	Same as for wound dehiscence	Opening of incision and visible protrusion of organs	Same as for wound dehiscence
Psychological				
Postoperative depression	Mental disorder characterized by altered mood	Weakness, surprise nature of emergency surgery, news of malignancy, severely altered body image, other personal matter; may be a physiologic response to some surgeries	Anorexia, tearfulness, loss of ambition, withdrawal, rejection of others, feelings of dejection, sleep disturbances (insomnia or excessive sleeping)	Adequate rest, physical activity, opportunity to express anger and other negative feelings

Source: Berman, A. & Snyder, S. *Kozier & Erb's fundamentals of nursing: Concepts, Process, and Practice* (9th ed.), p. 976. (c) 2012. Reprinted by permission of Pearson Education, Inc., Upper Saddle River, NJ 07458.

Check Your NCLEX-PN® Exam I.Q.

You are ready for testing on this content if you can

- Determine a client's readiness for surgery.
- Prepare a client for surgery.
- Monitor a client before, during, and after surgery.
- Provide preoperative, intraoperative, and postoperative care to a client.
- Monitor a client's response to recovery from various types of anesthesia.
- Provide client education about preoperative and postoperative care.
- Monitor a client's response to a surgical procedure.
- Evaluate effectiveness of interventions designed to prevent postoperative complications.

PRACTICE TEST

PRACTICE TEST

1 The nurse has taught the postoperative client to perform deep-breathing and coughing exercises. The nurse determines that the client needs more teaching when the client is observed doing which activity? Select all that apply.

1. Sitting upright before deep breathing and coughing
2. Taking deep breaths before attempting to cough
3. Placing both hands vertically and lightly on either side of the incision
4. Using a pillow for splinting during coughing
5. Use gentle coughing efforts that sound like clearing the throat

2 A toddler who has not had surgery before is being prepared for a surgical procedure. The child's mother expresses concern about the child's psychological adaptation to surgery. While planning for postoperative care, the nurse recognizes that the child is likely to have which greatest concern based on age?

1. Anticipated pain
2. Body image changes
3. Communication difficulties
4. Separation from parents

3 A female client is being prepared for surgery. When the nurse asks the client to remove her wedding ring, the client refuses. What would be an appropriate response by the nurse? Select all that apply.

1. Encourage the client to use soapy water to remove the ring, if it is tight.
2. Explain that the hospital cannot be responsible for jewelry worn during surgery.
3. Notify the surgeon's office that the surgeon must see the client in the preoperative holding area.
4. Tape the ring in place before the client is transported to the preoperative holding area.
5. Make a notation on the preoperative checklist that the ring is in place.

4 The nurse is caring for clients in the preanesthesia room. The nurse notes that one client, who is an older adult, has an increased surgical risk based on which factor?

1. Decreased kidney function leading to potential fluid and electrolyte imbalances
2. Increased hunger sensations leading to postoperative complications from hyperacidity
3. Inability to comprehend the seriousness of surgical interventions, leading to noncompliance
4. Poor cardiovascular status leading to decreased pain sensation

5 The nurse is preparing a client for surgery. Prior to completing the skin preparation, the nurse observes the surgical site for which finding?

1. Presence of pustules or abrasions
2. Absence of hair growth
3. Presence of lanugo
4. Absence of pulsation

6 A male client who arrives for an outpatient surgical procedure has the odor of alcohol on his breath. Before completing preoperative data collection, the nurse reports this finding to the surgeon, after drawing which conclusion about the significance of this finding?

1. Alcohol can affect the client's response to anesthesia and surgery.
2. Alcohol can increase the risk for respiratory complications.
3. Alcohol can decrease the effectiveness of preoperative sedatives or hypnotics.
4. Physiological and psychological responses are slowed down by recent alcohol intake.

7 When the nurse asks questions about the preoperative client's vision and hearing, a family member asks the nurse why the questions are important. What information should the nurse provide as the primary reason for seeking this information?

1. "This will help us determine the need for additional resources after discharge."
2. "This will help determine the risk of accidents in the home after surgery, which could affect the surgical outcome."
3. "This helps identify any unanticipated needs prior to beginning the surgery."
4. "This will help us to individualize how we provide preoperative and postoperative teaching."

8 A client is admitted for surgery. During preoperative data collection, the nurse learns the client was taking warfarin sodium (Coumadin) but stopped it a few days ago per surgeon instructions. The nurse would plan to monitor for which specific problem when implementing postoperative care?

1. Delirium tremens
2. Respiratory depression
3. Bleeding or oozing at the surgical wound site
4. Hypovolemia

9 The postsurgical unit nurse is implementing measures to prevent thrombophlebitis. Which measure would be the priority action by the nurse?

1. Apply ordered pneumatic compression boots.
2. Reinforce importance of smoking cessation.
3. Observe the legs with each set of vital signs.
4. Teach the client to report calf pain.

10 A client has been admitted for surgery for resection of nerve roots. The client, observing the written comment that the surgery is palliative, asks what this means. The nurse would offer which explanation?

1. The surgery schedule is overbooked, so the client's surgery could be delayed.
2. The surgeon is against performing the surgery.
3. The exact surgical procedure has not been decided.
4. The procedure will be done to relieve pain, but will not cure the problem.

11 The physician progress note indicated a plan to let a client's wound heal by tertiary intention. The nurse concludes that healing has occurred after making which observation of the wound?

1. The wound is smaller but irregular.
2. Very little scarring has occurred.
3. Tissue loss prevents the edges from approximating.
4. A wide scar is present over the area of wound closure.

12 The nurse observes that the wound of a postoperative client has moderate drainage with a greenish tinge. The nurse should take which priority action next?

1. Document the expected findings.
2. Check for bleeding at the base of the wound.
3. Take the pulse and blood pressure, and compare with previous readings.
4. Note the latest temperature and white blood cell (WBC) count.

13 A client experiences wound dehiscence when coughing. After assisting the client to a low Fowler's position with legs slightly elevated, what is the next best action?

1. Push the internal organs back into the abdominal opening.
2. Cover the wound with a moist hydrocolloid dressing.
3. Cover the wound with a sterile, saline-moistened dressing.
4. Use Steri-Strips to hold the wound together.

14 A client is scheduled for surgery, and has been placed on NPO status. The client reports thirst and hunger, and asks for breakfast. The nurse explains that NPO status has which purpose?

1. To make anesthesia induction easier
2. To avoid the risk of aspiration
3. To prevent excessive bleeding
4. To allow for more rapid wound healing

15 A client has just entered the postanesthesia care unit (PACU) from surgery. The postoperative client's immediate needs include initial monitoring of which set of items?

1. Vital signs, level of consciousness, and presence of pain
2. Skin coloring, surgical incision, and limb movements
3. Skin temperature, blood pressure, and mental status
4. Temperature, emotional status, and social support

16 The postoperative client questions why the nurse encourages repositioning from side to side at least once every two hours. The nurse explains this intervention is to achieve which of the following?

1. Aids return of peristalsis at a faster rate
2. Lessens muscle weakness
3. Increases the client's ability to sleep
4. Lets the lungs alternately achieve maximum expansion

17 The nurse is observing the client's surgical wound in the postoperative period. Which finding indicates the first stage of healing?

1. Inflammation in the wound edges
2. Bleeding around the incision
3. Clot binding the wound edges
4. Collagen synthesis

18 The client arrives in the post-anesthesia care unit (PACU) in an unconscious state. In what position would the nurse place this client in this immediate postanesthetic stage?

1. Side-lying, with the face slightly down
2. Side-lying, with a pillow under the client's head
3. Semi-prone, with the head tilted to the side
4. Dorsal recumbent, with the head turned to the side

ANSWERS & RATIONALES

1 **Answer: 3, 5 Rationale:** Placing the hands directly on the incision during coughing (instead of lightly to each side) will diminish the discomfort associated with coughing. The client should cough forcefully (instead of weakly as in clearing the throat) to eliminate secretions effectively. The other actions listed (sitting up before coughing, taking deep breaths before coughing, and using a pillow to splint incision) are correct and do not require further teaching by the nurse. **Cognitive Level:** Applying **Client Need:** Reduction of Risk Potential **Integrated Process:** Nursing Process: Evaluation **Content Area:** Fundamentals **Strategy:** The words *needs more teaching* in the stem of the question indicates the incorrect client statement is the correct option. Note the wording of the question indicates more than one option is likely to be correct. Use knowledge of nursing fundamentals to answer the question.

2 **Answer: 4 Rationale:** The child fears separation from her parents during the toddler years. The child has no previous experiences to compare to this experience, so she will not anticipate pain before the surgery. A toddler cannot anticipate any changes in her body. Communication may be difficult, but it would not be the greatest concern. **Cognitive Level:** Applying **Client Need:** Reduction of Risk Potential **Integrated Process:** Nursing Process: Planning **Content Area:** Fundamentals **Strategy:** The critical word *greatest* in the stem of the question provides a clue that more than one option could be partially true. Use knowledge of growth and development to make a selection, recalling that toddlers fear separation from their parents.

3 **Answer: 4, 5 Rationale:** Taping a wedding band in place is acceptable for the client who does not wish to remove it, unless there is danger the finger might swell during or after surgery. Documenting the presence of the ring on the preoperative checklist alerts staff in the surgical suite of its presence. Encouraging the client to use soapy water assumes the ring is tight, and that the client wishes to remove it. Explaining that the hospital cannot be liable creates unnecessary anxiety at a time when it already is likely to be increased. The surgeon does not need to see the client in the preoperative holding area. **Cognitive Level:** Applying **Client Need:** Reduction of Risk Potential **Integrated Process:** Nursing Process: Implementation **Content Area:** Fundamentals **Strategy:** Identify the core issue of the question, which is the method of safeguarding client property during surgery. Choose options that meet the needs of the client and protect both the hospital and the client's property.

4 **Answer: 1 Rationale:** With increased age, there is a greater likelihood that the kidneys start to degenerate. This can lead to reduced glomerular filtration rate and makes the client generally more at risk for fluid and electrolyte imbalances. Hunger does not necessarily lead to complications from hyperacidity. Other factors (when diet is resumed, whether a nasogastric tube is in place, and whether drugs are ordered to decrease stomach acidity) will all affect stomach acidity. Comprehension is not altered in older adults unless the client has a form of dementia, which is a clinical diagnosis and not an age-related change. Cardiovascular problems do not necessarily diminish pain sensations. **Cognitive Level:** Analyzing **Client Need:** Reduction of Risk Potential **Integrated Process:** Nursing Process: Data Collection **Content Area:** Fundamentals **Strategy:** For questions that ask you to choose one client over others, determine which client description indicates the worst client status or greatest risk for complications. In this case, note that fluid and electrolyte balance poses the greatest risk in the intraoperative period, which is the core issue of the question.

5 **Answer: 1 Rationale:** Abrasions, pustules, or other skin conditions have to be inspected and documented because they can interfere with wound healing, or increase the risk of infection. Lack of hair growth or presence of lanugo or fine hair will not interfere with the skin preparation. Pulsation is not always visible or available to inspect, depending upon the part of the body being operated on. **Cognitive Level:** Applying **Client Need:** Reduction of Risk Potential **Integrated Process:** Nursing Process: Data Collection **Content Area:** Fundamentals **Strategy:** The core issue of the question is knowledge of integumentary risks to a surgical procedure. Use the process of elimination, focusing on skin breaks or alterations as the option that interferes with the protective function of the skin.

6 **Answer: 1 Rationale:** Alcohol affects the central nervous system, and therefore the client's response to surgery and the anesthetic itself. Smoking, not alcohol (in small amounts), poses respiratory risks. Alcohol could have an addictive or synergistic effect with any preoperative sedatives or hypnotics, because both depress the central nervous system. Past and recent intake of alcohol can impact responses, which can be either slowed down or escalated. **Cognitive Level:** Analyzing **Client Need:** Reduction of Risk Potential **Integrated Process:** Nursing Process: Data Collection **Content Area:** Fundamentals **Strategy:** The core issue of the question is knowledge that alcohol has an interactive effect with anesthesia and possibly other medications used during surgery. Focus on the option that safeguards the client's physical status as the reason for notifying the surgeon.

7 **Answer: 4 Rationale:** The ability of the client to see and hear could affect the preoperative and postoperative teaching methods used. The need for referrals for post-discharge resources depends not only on the client's vision and hearing, but also on family supports and the client's physical and mental status. Vision and hearing impairments could interfere with safety post-discharge, but this is not a primary reason for the assessment at this time. *Unanticipated needs* is a very general term that can be applied not just to vision and hearing but also to any area of client functioning. **Cognitive Level:** Applying **Client Need:** Reduction of Risk Potential **Integrated Process:** Teaching and Learning **Content Area:** Fundamentals **Strategy:** Focus on the critical word *preoperative*, which should help you select an option that is linked in time with the reason for the assessment.

8 **Answer: 3** **Rationale:** Anticoagulants inhibit clotting of the blood, putting the client at increased risk for bleeding postoperatively. If the client was abusing alcohol, the nurse would need to assess for onset of delirium tremens caused by alcohol withdrawal. Respiratory compromise might occur if the client takes sedatives or hypnotics. Hypovolemia is a general risk in the intraoperative and postoperative period, but this risk would be heightened if the client is taking diuretics. **Cognitive Level:** Applying **Client Need:** Reduction of Risk Potential **Integrated Process:** Nursing Process: Planning **Content Area:** Fundamentals **Strategy:** The core issue of the question is knowledge that warfarin sodium is an anticoagulant, and that this medication increases risk of bleeding unless stopped for a sufficient amount of time before surgery (approximately 7 days, depending on client and surgery). Of the two options that relate to bleeding, choose *bleeding or oozing at the surgical wound site* over *hypovolemia* because of the critical word *specific* in the stem of the question.

9 **Answer: 1** **Rationale:** Pneumatic compression boots facilitate venous return from the lower extremities by alternately inflating and deflating. Smoking can contribute to cardiovascular events, but cessation will not necessarily lessen the chance of thrombophlebitis in the immediate postsurgical period. Observation of the leg will help with detection but not prevention of thrombophlebitis. Calf pain can occur with dorsiflexion of the leg in a client with thrombophlebitis and is a means of detection, but not prevention. **Cognitive Level:** Applying **Client Need:** Reduction of Risk Potential **Integrated Process:** Teaching and Learning **Content Area:** Fundamentals **Strategy:** Focus on the critical word in the stem, *prevent*. Discriminate between those options that address data collection and those that address prevention.

10 **Answer: 4** **Rationale:** A surgical procedure that relieves symptoms of disease or pain but does not cure is described as palliative. The scheduling of the surgery would not have anything to do with the name or category of surgery. There is no term to describe a surgery that the surgeon does not want to perform. A surgical procedure that has not been decided would not be named or documented. **Cognitive Level:** Applying **Client Need:** Reduction of Risk Potential **Integrated Process:** Teaching and Learning **Content Area:** Fundamentals **Strategy:** Use the process of elimination, selecting the answer that is an accurate description of the meaning of the term *palliative*. Recall that the word *palliate* means to lessen or reduce, which may help in selecting the correct option.

11 **Answer: 4** **Rationale:** A wide scar occurs in tertiary intention because the edges are not approximated, and they regenerate via granulation. A wound that is smaller but irregular is consistent with a wound that has healed by secondary intention. Very little scarring is expected in a wound that heals by primary intention. Tissue loss that prevents edges from approximating is consistent with a wound that is healing by secondary intention. **Cognitive Level:** Analyzing **Client Need:** Reduction of Risk Potential **Integrated Process:** Nursing Process: Evaluation **Content Area:** Fundamentals **Strategy:** First, recall the definition of *tertiary intention*. Then, visualize the appearance of the wound to make your selection.

12 **Answer: 4** **Rationale:** Purulent drainage, which often indicates wound infection, is made up of tissue debris, WBCs, and bacteria, and can have different colors, depending upon the type of bacteria. The next action by the nurse would be to gather additional data that could indicate infection, such as elevated temperature and WBC count. The nurse would document the findings at some point, but this is not the priority action because green drainage is not an expected finding. It is not a priority to assess for bleeding within the wound at this time. There is no specific reason to measure pulse and BP at this time, since these vital signs are not precise indicators of infection. **Cognitive Level:** Analyzing **Client Need:** Reduction of Risk Potential **Integrated Process:** Nursing Process: Data Collection **Content Area:** Fundamentals **Strategy:** The critical words in the stem of the question are *priority action*. This means that the correct option is one that contains a critical-thinking sequence based on the information presented. Correlate the word *greenish* with infection, and then choose the option that assesses for signs of infection.

13 **Answer: 3** **Rationale:** Covering the wound with sterile, saline-moistened gauze keeps the wound moist, and protects it from infection. In wound dehiscence, the layers of the wound are disrupted, but there is no protrusion of vital organs. In addition, pushing back organs such as the intestines is extremely dangerous because it could cause strangulation. A hydrocolloid dressing is not indicated because its absorptive properties are not needed. The use of Steri-Strips would be ineffective, and does not protect underlying tissue. **Cognitive Level:** Applying **Client Need:** Reduction of Risk Potential **Integrated Process:** Nursing Process: Implementation **Content Area:** Fundamentals **Strategy:** The core issue of the question is nursing management of wound dehiscence. Recall that the priority sequence of actions is to remove the effects of gravity on the wound, and then to protect the wound. Choose the saline dressing because it is moist and saline is isotonic.

14 **Answer: 2** **Rationale:** By keeping the stomach empty during surgery, the risk of vomiting and aspiration is decreased. NPO status does not make anesthesia induction easier, prevent excessive bleeding, or allow for more rapid wound healing. **Cognitive Level:** Applying **Client Need:** Reduction of Risk Potential **Integrated Process:** Nursing Process: Implementation **Content Area:** Fundamentals **Strategy:** Use knowledge of basic principles of preoperative care to make a selection. The wording of the question tells you that there is only one correct choice.

15 **Answer: 1** **Rationale:** Although all the options contain aspects that need ongoing monitoring, vital signs, level of consciousness and pain are the most important for data collection initially because they relate to physiological needs and are more global indicators of overall functioning. The other observations would be part of routine postoperative care. **Cognitive Level:** Applying **Client Need:** Reduction of Risk Potential **Integrated Process:** Nursing Process: Data Collection **Content Area:** Fundamentals **Strategy:** When an option contains more than one part, all parts need to be correct for the option itself to be correct.

16 **Answer: 4** **Rationale:** Turning side-to-side allows the lungs alternately to expand properly. Peristalsis increases with movement even without the turning. Muscle weakness can be lessened with any type of movement. Turning does not necessarily induce sleep. **Cognitive Level:** Applying **Client Need:** Reduction of Risk Potential **Integrated Process:** Nursing Process: Implementation **Content Area:** Fundamentals **Strategy:** Select the option that is of greatest concern in the postoperative client, which is respiratory function.

17 **Answer: 3** **Rationale:** The first signs of healing are absence of bleeding and wound edges bound by fibrin in the clot.

Inflammation at the wound edges follows the first sign, and then, when the clot diminishes, inflammation decreases, and collagen forms a scar. **Cognitive Level:** Analyzing **Client Need:** Physiological Adaptation **Integrated Process:** Nursing Process: Data Collection **Content Area:** Fundamentals **Strategy:** The critical word in the question is *first*. Use specific knowledge of wound healing to select an answer.

18 **Answer: 1 Rationale:** In a side-lying and slightly face-down position, gravity keeps the tongue forward, which helps to prevents aspiration. A side-lying position is good but a pillow elevates the head which could increase the risk of aspiration on own secretions. Semi-prone position is unsafe in most cases, as it can interfere with breathing. Dorsal recumbent position could increase the risk of aspiration by interfering with drainage of oral secretions, and head turned to the side could interfere with arterial circulation and venous drainage from the brain. **Cognitive Level:** Applying **Client Need:** Reduction of Risk Potential **Integrated Process:** Nursing Process: Implementation **Content Area:** Fundamentals **Strategy:** Select the option that provides the highest level of airway protection.

Key Terms to Review

anesthesia p. 718
dehiscence p. 726
drain p. 726
exudate p. 726
informed consent p. 717
intraoperative phase p. 716
moderate sedation p. 718
palliative p. 717
postoperative phase p. 716
preoperative phase p. 716
purulent p. 724
regional anesthesia p. 718
sanguineous p. 726
serosanguineous p. 724
serous p. 726
sterile field p. 723
surgical asepsis p. 723
surgical scrub p. 723

References

Ball, J., Bindler, R, & Cowen, K. (2010). *Pediatric nursing: Partnering with children and families* (2nd ed.). Upper Saddle River, NJ: Pearson Education.

Berman, A. & Snyder, S. (2012). *Kozier & Erb's fundamentals of nursing: Concepts, process, and practice* (9th ed.). Upper Saddle River, NJ: Pearson Education.

LeMone P., Burke, K., & Bauldoff, G. (2012). *Medical surgical nursing: Critical thinking in patient care* (5th ed.). Upper Saddle River, NJ: Pearson Education.

Perry, A., & Potter, P. (2010). *Clinical nursing skills and techniques* (7th ed.). St. Louis, MO: Elsevier.

Smith, S. Duell, D., & Martin, B. (2012). *Clinical nursing skills: Basic to advanced skills* (8th ed.). Upper Saddle River, NJ: Pearson Education, Inc.

Test Yourself

Are you ready for the NCLEX-PN® or course exams? Use the practice tests on the companion website to check.

Complicated Antenatal Care 45

In this chapter

Cross Reference

Other chapters relevant to this content area are

Reproduction, Family Planning, and Infertility	**Chapter 8**
Uncomplicated Antenatal Care	**Chapter 9**
Uncomplicated Labor and Delivery Care	**Chapter 10**
Uncomplicated Postpartum Care	**Chapter 11**
Uncomplicated Newborn Care	**Chapter 12**
Complicated Labor and Delivery Care	**Chapter 46**
Complicated Postpartum Care	**Chapter 47**
Complicated Newborn Care	**Chapter 48**

I. DATA COLLECTION AND DIAGNOSTIC TESTING FOR HIGH-RISK PRENATAL CLIENT

A. Introduction

1. Identifying clients at risk begins with first prenatal visit and continues through puerperium
2. Risk factors (physiological, psychological, sociodemographic, or environmental) may be associated with a negative pregnancy outcome
3. *NCLEX®* More frequent monitoring of high-risk clients is important during pregnancy, labor, birth, and puerperium to identify potential complications, ensure early treatment, and improve maternal–fetal outcomes
4. Ongoing care consists of routine antenatal care plus special considerations as noted in following text

B. Diagnostic tests

1. **Biophysical profile (BPP)**
   - **a.** Overview: a method of determining fetal well-being by determining scores on five criteria: fetal breathing movements, body movements, muscle tone, fetal heart rate (FHR), and amniotic fluid volume
   - **b.** Total score ranges from 0 to 10; criterion scores are 2 (normal) or 0 (abnormal)
   - **c.** A total score of 8 to 10 is normal, 4 to 6 is possibly abnormal, and less than 4 may indicate a need for delivery
2. **Doppler blood flow analysis**
   - **a.** Overview: a noninvasive assessment of fetal blood flow across placenta
   - **b.** Provides data about blood flow and resistance in placental circulation; helps detect intrauterine growth restriction (IUGR)
   - **c.** Can be done as early as 15 weeks
   - **d.** Velocity waveforms from umbilical and uterine arteries are reported as systolic/diastolic (S/D) ratios
   - **e.** Persistently elevated ratios of greater than 3 after 30 weeks' gestation are considered abnormal and have been associated with IUGR

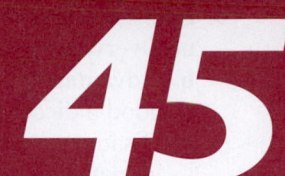

3. **Nonstress test (NST)**
   a. Overview: a screening test that assesses fetal well-being; analyzes response of FHR to fetal movement
   b. Advantages: noninvasive, easily interpreted, and can be done in outpatient setting at low cost; is a good indicator of fetal well-being
   c. Disadvantages: high number of false-positive results caused by fetal sleep cycles, medications, fetal immaturity; is not a good predictor of poor fetal outcomes
   NCLEX® d. Test procedure: semi-Fowler's position used; an ultrasound transducer and tocodynamometer record contractions and FHR; client may be asked to press a handheld button that graphs FHR when fetal movement is felt
   e. Episodes of fetal movement can then be compared to changes in FHR; acoustical stimulation can be done if absence of fetal movement
   NCLEX® f. Findings: normal (reactive) if there are two or more accelerations of 15 beats per minute lasting for 15 seconds over a 20-minute period, normal baseline, and long-term variability of 10 or more beats per minute
   NCLEX® g. If these criteria are not met within 40 minutes, test is considered nonreassuring (nonreactive) and further testing is indicated
4. **Contraction stress test (CST)**
   a. Overview: assesses fetal ability to withstand stress of uterine contractions and evaluates placental capacity for O_2/CO_2 exchange; since contractions reduce blood flow to fetus, can predict a fetus that may not tolerate stress of labor
   b. Indications: factors that place fetus at risk for asphyxia such as IUGR, diabetes, postdates, nonreactive NST, and BPP score less than 6
   c. Contraindications: third-trimester bleeding and previous cesarean birth with classical uterine incision; advantages of CST should be weighed against danger of preterm labor if this is a risk, such as with premature rupture of membranes or incompetent cervix
   NCLEX® d. Test procedure: explain procedure and obtain signed consent; electronic monitoring of contractions and FHR are begun; after obtaining baseline fetal heart tracing, contractions (if not spontaneous) are initiated with IV oxytocin or breast self-stimulation
   NCLEX® e. Findings: when at least three contractions of 40- to 60-second duration occur in a 10-minute time period, the FHR pattern is assessed; result is reassuring (negative) if no late decelerations occur; is not reassuring (positive) if late decelerations occur with at least two of three contractions; is suspicious (equivocal) if there is late deceleration with one of three contractions or contractions every 2 minutes for 10 minutes (hyperstimulation pattern)
5. **Amniocentesis**
   a. Overview: used to assess fetal well-being and maturity; a needle is inserted through abdominal wall (see Figure 45–1) to collect sample of amniotic fluid; can be done after 14 to 16 weeks' gestation

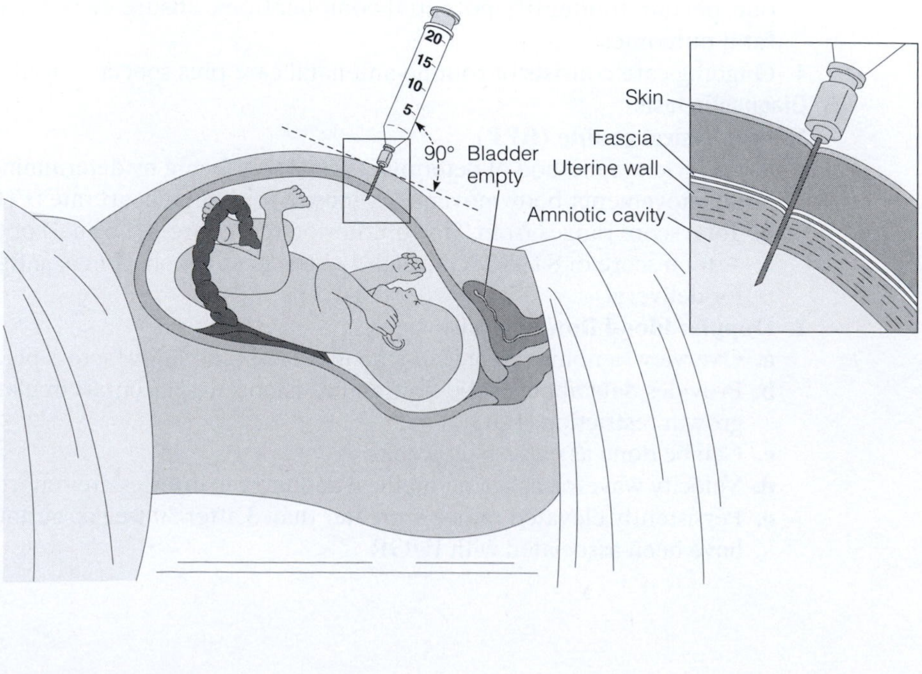

Figure 45–1

Amniocentesis.

b. Purpose: prenatal diagnosis of genetic disorders or congenital anomalies, assessment of pulmonary maturity, and diagnosis of fetal hemolytic disease

NCLEX® c. Complications: occur in fewer than 1% of cases; possible maternal complications include hemorrhage, infection, labor, **abruptio placentae**, damage to intestines or bladder, and amniotic fluid leakage or embolism; possible fetal complications include death, hemorrhage, infection, and direct needle injury

d. Test procedure: explain procedure is done on an ouptatient basis and obtain signed consent; if client is more than 20 weeks' gestation, she should empty bladder and assume supine position with possibly a wedge under left hip to avoid pressure of uterus on vena cava; using sterile technique, physician inserts a needle through abdomen into uterus; ultrasound assists in guiding needle; 15 to 20 mL of fluid are withdrawn

NCLEX® e. Monitor FHR and maternal vital signs during procedure and for 30 minutes after

NCLEX® f. Rh-negative clients should receive RhoGAM after procedure because of risk of isoimmunization from fetal blood

g. Follow-up: inform client to contact physician for fluid loss, bleeding, fever, abdominal pain, increased or decreased fetal activity

h. Inform client that test results will be available in about 2 weeks

6. **Lecithin to sphingomyelin (L/S) ratio**
   a. Obtained via amniocentesis to assess fetal lung maturity
   b. Ratio of 2:1 or greater indicates probable lung maturity; contamination with meconium or blood may alter results
7. **Phosphatidylglycerol (PG)**
   a. Obtained via amniocentesis; is a phospholipid found in pulmonary surfactant
   NCLEX® b. Presence in amniotic fluid indicates fetal lung maturity
8. **Karyotype**
   NCLEX® a. Obtained via amniocentesis; analyzes chromosomes to determine gender and chromosomal aberrations
   b. Gender identification is important in assessment of sex-linked diseases
   c. Bilirubin pigment level in amniotic fluid assesses Rh isoimmunization status and severity of hemolytic anemia
   d. Alpha-fetoprotein (AFP) levels, either increased or decreased, can indicate anatomic abnormalities; fetal blood contamination of amniotic fluid can alter AFP results
9. **Chorionic villus sampling (CVS)**
   a. Involves collecting small specimen of tissue from fetal portion of placenta for fetal genetic studies
   b. Specimen can be obtained either transcervically or transabdominally
   c. Indications: over 35 years old (increased risk for Down syndrome), frequent spontaneous **abortions**, fetuses with chromosomal anomalies or other defects, or a client with a genetic defect
   d. Advantages: earlier diagnosis and rapid return of results compared to amniocentesis; can be performed at 10 to 12 weeks' gestation with results returned in 1 to 2 weeks
   e. Test preparation: instruct client to come for procedure with full bladder; explain procedure and obtain signed consent; use lithotomy position
   f. Test procedure: using sterile technique, physician visualizes cervix using ultrasound guidance, a suction cannula is used to collect specimen transvaginally or transabdominally (if necessary)
   g. Rh-negative clients should receive RhoGAM postprocedure
   h. Complications (rare): vaginal spotting or bleeding, miscarriage, rupture of membranes, and chorioamnionitis; limb anomalies if procedure done before 10 weeks' gestation
   i. Follow-up includes reinforcing client signs of complications to report, stating when results will be available, and arranging genetic counseling as needed

II. PREGESTATIONAL CONDITIONS

A. Cardiac disease

1. Pregnancy increases workload on heart; cardiac output increases 30–50% by midpregnancy (cardiac workload greatest at 28 to 30 weeks' gestation when blood volume peaks)
2. A compromised heart with inadequate cardiac capacity and decreased reserves may be unable to adapt to added requirements of pregnancy
3. Treatment options and outcome depend on degree of cardiac compromise
4. Clients with class I and II cardiac disease have potential for good pregnancy outcome, while class III or IV clients may have serious maternal or fetal compromise (Table 45–1)

Table 45–1 Classification of Functional Capacity for Clients with Cardiac Disease (NYHA 1979)

Classification	Functional Capacity
I	Uncompromised: No limitation on physical activity due to angina or symptoms of cardiac insufficiency
II	Slightly compromised: Normal activity causes fatigue, palpitation, dyspnea, or angina
III	Markedly compromised: May be comfortable at rest but less than usual activity causes fatigue, dyspnea, palpitations, or angina
IV	Severely compromised: Cannot perform any activity without increasing discomfort; may experience angina and cardiac insufficiency while at rest.

NCLEX® **5.** Nursing data collection: most common complication of heart disease during pregnancy is congestive heart failure (CHF)
   a. Edema of varying degree from pedal edema, pitting edema, generalized edema (anasarca), and pulmonary edema
   b. Dyspnea on exertion, increasing fatigue, dyspnea at rest, moist cough, basilar crackles, pallor then cyanosis of nail beds, circumoral cyanosis
   c. Tachycardia, irregular pulse, murmurs, chest pain

6. Collaborative management
   a. Monitor client and fetal well-being more frequently during pregnancy; changes in maternal vital signs or signs of fetal compromise may indicate inability to handle increasing demands on heart
   NCLEX® **b.** Encourage adequate nutrition for pregnancy and provide prenatal vitamins and iron to prevent anemia; monitor for signs of infection
   NCLEX® **c.** Reinforcing instructions to avoid excessive weight gain and emotional stress, which place added stress on cardiac reserves
   d. Inform client to report signs of infection so treatment may begin early
   e. Diagnostic procedures may include auscultation, electrocardiogram, echocardiogram, and possible cardiac catheterization
   NCLEX® **f.** Prophylactic antibiotics are used for invasive procedures, including dental work and at time of birth, to prevent bacterial endocarditis; penicillin (PCN) is usually prescribed unless client is allergic
   g. Cardiac glycosides (digoxin [Lanoxin]) may increase myocardial contractility and slow heart rate for effective filling
   h. Antidysrhythmia agents may reduce incidence of cardiac dysrhythmias
   i. The diuretic furosemide (Lasix) may decrease fluid excess; take care to ensure adequate circulating volume to maintain uteroplacental perfusion
   NCLEX® **j.** Heparin is considered safe for use in pregnancy if an anticoagulant is indicated (pregnancy category C); warfarin (Coumadin) is a pregnancy category X drug (Table 45–2) and must be avoided
   NCLEX® **k.** Reinforce client teaching to avoid exertion and to plan frequent rest periods

Table 45–2 FDA Pregnancy Categories for Prescription Drugs

Category	Risk to the Fetus	Examples of Drugs
A	Controlled studies in women do not demonstrate risk to fetus in first trimester, and possibility of fetal harm appears remote.	RDA dose of Vitamin C
B	Animal studies have not demonstrated fetal risk but there are no controlled studies in women, or animal studies show an adverse effect not confirmed in controlled studies in women in first trimester.	Acetaminophen (Tylenol) Penicillins
C	Animal studies show adverse effects and there are no controlled studies in women, or studies in women and animals are not available. Drug should be given only if potential benefit justifies potential risk to fetus.	Zidovudine (Retrovir) Heparin
D	Positive evidence of fetal risk in humans, but benefits to mother may be acceptable despite risk in certain situations.	Phenobarbitol (Luminol)
X	Risks to fetus clearly outweigh any possible benefit to mother. Drug is contraindicated in women who may become pregnant.	Warfarin (Coumadin) Diethylstilbestrol (DES)

l. Provide adequate pain relief during labor to avoid excessive maternal stress
m. Vaginal delivery is preferred with epidural anesthesia, continuous maternal oxygen administration, and low-forceps delivery to decrease maternal straining
NCLEX® n. Observe client carefully for complications from hemodynamic changes immediately after delivery

B. Diabetes mellitus

1. Description
   a. A pancreatic endocrine disorder affecting carbohydrate (CHO) metabolism
   b. Results from insufficient insulin production in beta cells of islets of Langerhans
   c. Insulin facilitates transport of glucose from blood into cells for storage or energy
   d. **Gestational diabetes** results when pancreas is unable to meet increased demands for insulin production during pregnancy
2. Effect of pregnancy on glucose metabolism
   a. During first half of pregnancy, maternal hormones increase demand for insulin production to facilitate increased storage of glycogen in maternal tissue
   NCLEX® b. During last half of pregnancy, human placental lactogen (hPL) from placenta causes resistance to action of maternal insulin, increasing circulating glucose for fetal use and demand on maternal pancreas to produce more insulin
   c. Fetus produces own insulin but obtains glucose from mother across placenta; amount of glucose available in maternal circulation stimulates fetal pancreas to produce insulin
3. Effects of diabetes on pregnancy and fetus relate to degree of blood glucose (BG) control within 70 to 110 mg/dL range and degree of vascular involvement
4. Complications are more common with type 1 diabetes mellitus and include
   a. Polyhydraminos, preeclampsia, eclampsia, ketoacidosis and worsening retinopathy
   b. Dystocia and stillbirth (usually after 36 weeks)
   NCLEX® c. Neonatal **macrosomia** (excessively large body), hypoglycemia, hyperbilirubinemia, delayed fetal lung maturity resulting in respiratory distress syndrome (RDS), and increased incidence of congenital anomalies including neural tube defects (NTD)
5. Nursing data collection
   a. Risk factors: family history of diabetes, maternal obesity, previous large-for-gestational-age (LGA) infants, previous unexplained stillbirth
   b. Classic symptoms of diabetes mellitus: polyuria, polydipsia, polyphagia
   NCLEX® c. Possible increasing frequency of urinary tract infections and vaginal candidiasis (yeast) infections caused by altered pH in reproductive tract
   d. Urine testing for ketones as part of routine prenatal care
   NCLEX® e. Diabetes screening at about 28 weeks' gestation with a 50-gram oral glucose tolerance test (GTT); if BG is greater than 140 mg/dL at 1 hour, a 3-hour 100-gram oral GTT is performed
   NCLEX® f. Long-term BG control is estimated with glycosylated hemoglobin (HbA_{1c}), which measures percent of hemoglobin with glucose bound to it (glycohemoglobin); levels depend on amount of circulating glucose in previous weeks (see Chapter 42)
6. Collaborative management
   a. Reinforce teaching about prescribed ADA diet regulation with no concentrated sweets
   b. Dietary regulation is usually adequate; excessive weight gain should be avoided; caloric needs will increase as pregnancy progresses
   NCLEX® c. Medications: oral hypoglycemic medications are contraindicated during pregnancy, although glyburide (Micronase) is now an alternative to insulin in women whose BG is not controlled by diet and exercise; insulin (human) of the intermediate, regular, and/or analog (lispro and aspart) types should be carefully regulated and adjusted as pregnancy progresses with up to a fourfold dose increase needed at term
   NCLEX® d. Instruct client in frequent BG and urine ketone testing and to keep a diary of test results and activity levels
   NCLEX® e. Encourage regular nonstrenuous exercise such as walking for weight and BG control
   f. Monitor fetal well-being: quadruple screening at 15–20 weeks, ultrasound for anomalies, amniotic fluid volume, and fetal size; fetal movement counts, weekly NST from 28–32 weeks, possible oxytocin challenge test (OCT), BPP, and amniocentesis for lung maturity; L/S ratio needs to be 1:3 (normal is 1:2); PG should be present
   g. Monitor client for development of complications: infection, preeclampsia, and diabetic ketoacidosis

h. Prepare for possible induction of labor at 38–39 weeks for clients with type 1 diabetes mellitus to reduce risk for stillbirth caused by premature placental aging

NCLEX® i. Insulin requirements drop dramatically after delivery of placenta and removal of hormonal influences; client may need no insulin or a very decreased dose; those with gestational diabetes generally eat a regular diet

C. Substance abuse

1. Description and etiology
   a. As many as 10% of pregnant women use tobacco, alcohol, or other drugs, often in combination; clients using illegal drugs may delay seeking care for fear of prosecution; all pregnant women should be screened for substance abuse
   b. Substances frequently used are tobacco, alcohol, marijuana, cocaine, crack cocaine, MOMA (Ecstasy), and heroin; effects on pregnancy include spontaneous abortion, IUGR, preterm labor, placental abruption, stillbirth, neonatal addiction, and fetal alcohol syndrome (FAS)
2. Nursing data collection
   NCLEX® a. Establish trusting relationship with client by remaining open, matter-of-fact, and nonjudgmental; women seeking prenatal care are interested in improving and safeguarding their health and that of fetus
   b. Encourage client to describe all substances used, amounts, times, and triggers to use, and any previous attempts to discontinue use
   c. Determine client's motivation, support systems, and personal strengths that may be elicited to change behaviors
3. Collaborative management
   NCLEX® a. Monitor client for complications: anemia, inadequate nutrition and weight gain, hypertension, preterm labor; random urine toxicology screens may be ordered
   NCLEX® b. Monitor fetal growth and well-being: fundal height, ultrasound, NST, BPP
   c. Describe potential negative effects of substances used on pregnancy and fetus/neonate
   NCLEX® d. Assist with referrals for client as indicated: smoking cessation classes, Alcoholics Anonymous, addiction counseling, psychological counseling, and possible hospitalization
   e. Reinforce teaching about nutrition and effects on fetal development; teach client danger signs of pregnancy including signs of preterm labor and abruption of placenta
   NCLEX® f. Support client's efforts to change negative behaviors
   g. Client may need to be followed by a perinatologist during pregnancy; an addicted neonate will require intensive care at birth
   h. Client should not go through "cold turkey" drug withdrawal during pregnancy; clients with heroin addiction may receive methadone hydrochloride (Dolophine)—a narcotic agonist analgesic that blocks more severe symptoms of heroin withdrawal

D. HIV/AIDS

1. Overview
   a. Human immunodeficiency virus (HIV) leads to acquired immunodeficiency syndrome (AIDS) over years of time
   b. HIV is transmitted through contact with infected blood and body secretions, usually during sexual contact or use of contaminated needles
   c. AIDS is characterized by decreased immunity and increased susceptibility to opportunistic infections
   NCLEX® d. Pregnancy does not appear to change course of illness for mother; fetus may contract HIV transplacentally or through breast milk, but generally fetal infection is considered to occur during vaginal birth
   NCLEX® e. Current maternal treatment with highly active antiretroviral therapy (HAART) consists of at least three drugs; these include zidovudine (ZDV), a nucleoside reverse transcriptase inhibitor or NRTI, and a second NRTI combined with a non-nucleoside reverse transcriptase inhibitor (NNRTI), with an overall aim to reduce perinatal transmission; see Chapter 41 for specific drug information
   NCLEX® f. Maternal HIV antibodies cross placenta so all infants of HIV-positive mothers will test positive at birth and until maternal antibodies are depleted at between 15 to 18 months of age
2. Nursing data collection
   a. Antibodies to HIV are detected with ELISA test and results confirmed by Western blot test; alternative rapid testing for women in active labor who do not know HIV status or for those who did not receive prenatal care include Ora-Quick HIV-1 Antibody test and SUDS HIV-1 test; a small blood sample is required and results are sensitive, specific, and can be read in about 20 minutes
   b. All pregnant women should be offered HIV testing because most clients are asymptomatic for 5 to 10 years before signs of opportunistic infection appear

3. Collaborative management
   a. Provide emotional support and reproductive counseling to client and family
   b. Evaluate client for other sexually transmitted infections and hepatitis B
   c. Review lab results for signs of anemia, thrombocytopenia, leukopenia, and decreased CD-4 T-lymphocyte counts
   NCLEX® d. Monitor client for signs of opportunistic infection: fever, weight loss, fatigue, candidiasis, cough, skin lesions
   e. Administer prophylactic antiretroviral drugs as ordered during pregnancy and labor and delivery
   f. Monitor fetal growth and well-being
   NCLEX® g. Be meticulous in use of standard blood and body fluid precautions with all clients
   h. Protect fetus from maternal secretions by not using fetal scalp electrode or invasive devices during labor
   NCLEX® i. Wash infant's eyes and face at birth before administering prophylactic eye drops or ointment
   NCLEX® j. Bathe entire newborn as soon as possible after delivery to remove all maternal secretions; delay any newborn injections or heel-sticks until after bath
   NCLEX® k. Encourage mother to formula-feed infant to avoid transmission by breast milk

E. Rh-sensitization

1. Overview
   a. Rh-negative women who have Rh-positive embryo/fetus (from an Rh-positive father) may become sensitized to Rh antigen with contact between maternal and fetal blood
   b. Other causes of Rh-sensitization might be blood transfusion of Rh-positive blood to an Rh-negative woman or fetomaternal blood contact during amniocentesis or other invasive procedure
   c. Sensitized Rh-negative women develop anti-Rh antibodies, which may cross placenta in subsequent Rh-positive pregnancies and attack and destroy fetal RBCs
   d. Sensitized effects of Rh incompatibility and sensitization are progressively severe

NCLEX® 2. Hemolysis of fetal erythrocytes leads to greatly increased immature RBC production, termed **erythroblastosis fetalis**

NCLEX® 3. Breakdown of RBCs releases bilirubin, causing jaundice; high levels of circulating bilirubin can cause **kernicterus**, a yellow staining of basal ganglia and brain, and may result in permanent neurological damage

NCLEX® 4. Continued RBC destruction and anemia results in jaundice and marked fetal edema known as **hydrops fetalis**; may lead to fetal CHF

5. Nursing data collection
   a. All pregnant women should be tested for blood group, Rh factor, and have routine antibody screening; note history of previous miscarriage, blood transfusions, or infants experiencing jaundice
   NCLEX® b. If client is Rh-negative, infant's father is tested for Rh status; an Rh-negative father and mother will only produce Rh-negative offspring who will not be affected by Rh-incompatibility
   NCLEX® c. An indirect **Coombs' test** on maternal blood determines whether Rh-negative client has developed antibodies to Rh antigen; serial antibody screening should continue throughout pregnancy; a direct Coombs' test on infant's blood after birth identifies maternal antibodies attached to fetal RBCs

6. Collaborative management
   a. Provide support and education to client and family; client should carry Rh-negative identification card and recognize that she may need medication (RhoGAM) with future pregnancies
   b. Unsensitized Rh-negative clients should receive 300 mcg of Rh-immune globulin (RhoGAM) IM at 28 weeks and also within 72 hours of delivery
   c. Antibodies in immune globulin bind with Rh antigens in maternal circulation to provide passive immunity (mother will not become sensitized to Rh antigens and will not produce antibodies)
   NCLEX® d. RhoGAM is not given to mothers who are already sensitized and have antibodies (positive indirect Coombs' test)
   NCLEX® e. Rh-immune globulin is also given after abortion, **ectopic** pregnancy, amniocentesis, and any other situation that might result in maternal exposure to fetal Rh antigen
   f. Kleihauer-Betke test estimates amount of fetal blood in maternal circulation; used to determine dose of Rh-immune globulin when a larger fetal–maternal bleed is suspected
   NCLEX® g. Evaluate fetus for onset of complications by serial ultrasound for amniotic fluid volume, fetal size, and development of edema or enlarged heart
   h. A sinusoidal electronic fetal monitoring pattern indicates severe fetal anemia; BPP may be used to identify a compromised fetus

i. Amniocentesis or percutaneous umbilical cord blood sampling (PUBS) may be used to determine fetal Rh; both procedures carry risk of causing maternal exposure and sensitization, so RhoGAM should be given

NCLEX® j. An early delivery with phototherapy and exchange transfusions may be planned if fetus is developing anemia close to term

k. Intrauterine exchange transfusion may be performed for severely affected fetus until viability is reached

III. GESTATIONAL CONDITIONS

A. Hyperemesis gravidarum (pernicious vomiting of pregnancy)

1. Overview
   a. Extreme nausea and vomiting (N/V) during first half of pregnancy associated with dehydration, weight loss, and electrolyte imbalances
   b. Emesis is much more severe than in common "morning sickness" of early pregnancy, although it is more rare
   c. Theories about etiology include psychological and physiological factors but actual cause remains unknown; condition is rare in developing countries
   d. High levels of hCG, as are found in **gestational trophoblastic disease** (hydatidiform mole, molar pregnancy), are associated with severe N/V
   e. Fetus is at risk for abnormal development, IUGR, or death from lack of nutrition, hypoxia, and maternal ketoacidosis
2. Nursing data collection
   a. Intractable vomiting during first 20 weeks of pregnancy
   NCLEX® b. Dehydration with weight loss of greater than 5% of prepregnancy weight, poor skin turgor, dry mucous membranes, possible hypotension, tachycardia, and increased hematocrit and urine specific gravity
   c. Manifestations of electrolyte or acid–base imbalance (acidosis): ketosis, confusion, drowsiness, muscle weakness, cramps, clumsiness, tremors, irregular heartbeat, decreased level of consciousness (LOC)
   d. Manifestations of starvation: muscle wasting, ketonuria, jaundice, bleeding gums (vitamin deficiency)
3. Collaborative management
   NCLEX® a. Client may need hospitalization with IV fluid therapy with glucose, electrolytes, and vitamins to begin treatment and then continue at home once stabilized
   NCLEX® b. Monitor daily weight and measure intake and output (I&O); observe vital signs as appropriate, hydration, and nutritional status
   c. Administer ordered antiemetic medications such as phenothiazines or antihistamines as prescribed to control N/V
   NCLEX® d. Encourage 6 small feedings/day after acute N/V pass; salty foods and clear liquids such as lemonade and herbal teas are sometimes better tolerated at first
   e. Total parenteral nutrition (TPN) may be required in severe cases when client cannot tolerate oral feedings
   f. Monitor fetal growth with serial ultrasounds
   g. Provide emotional support; help client to identify healthy coping mechanisms and support systems to rely on during pregnancy
   h. Refer for additional counseling and support as indicated

B. Ectopic pregnancy

1. Overview
   a. Implantation of fertilized ovum outside uterus; most common site is a fallopian tube narrowed by scarring or adhesions; other sites may include ovary or elsewhere in abdominal cavity
   b. Risk factors for tubal damage that can lead to ectopic pregnancy include ascending infections, pelvic inflammatory disease (PID), use of IUD contraception, or tubal surgery
2. Nursing data collection
   a. Last normal menstrual period (LNMP) is consistent with possible pregnancy; possible subjective symptoms of pregnancy, such as breast tenderness and nausea, are present
   NCLEX® b. Unilateral lower abdominal pain: may be slowly increasing or sudden and severe with abdominal rigidity and referred right shoulder pain
   NCLEX® c. Possible irregular vaginal bleeding or signs of hypovolemic shock if fallopian tube has ruptured; prioritize care accordingly
   d. Laboratory tests: β-hCG confirms pregnancy
   e. Ultrasound confirms an extrauterine pregnancy

3. Implementation and collaborative care

NCLEX® **a.** Monitor BP, pulse, and respirations every 15 minutes or more often if indicated by client condition

b. Start an IV of ordered fluid with at least an 18-gauge needle in case blood products need to be given

NCLEX® **c.** Provide oxygen as indicated for shock

d. Medicate for pain as ordered

e. Obtain laboratory tests: β-hCG, CBC, and blood group and type; type and cross-match if hemorrhage is suspected

f. Medical treatment is methotrexate as a single or two-dose approach (second dose 4 days later); this is an option for stable healthy client with unruptured ectopic pregnancy of 4 cm or less and no fetal heart movement

g. Surgical treatment is salpingostomy via laparoscope if future pregnancy is desired

NCLEX® **h.** Provide standard preoperative and postoperative care and teaching; offer emotional support to client and family; facilitate grieving; provide RhoGAM for Rh-negative mothers with an Rh-positive partner

C. *Gestational trophoblastic disease (GTD)*

1. Overview

a. An abnormal growth of trophoblastic tissue with three types: hydatiform mole (molar pregnancy), invasive mole (chorioadenoma destruens), and choriocarcinoma (a form of cancer)

b. **Hydatiform mole** is characterized by abnormal development of placenta (with either complete or partial hydatiform mole); chorionic villi grow rapidly into fluid-filled, grapelike clusters; a complete mole develops from an empty ovum that contains no maternal genetic material; a partial mole may have an abnormal embryo that usually spontaneously aborts in first trimester

c. A complete mole may lead to development of choriocarcinoma, a rapidly growing malignant neoplasm

d. An invasive mole (chorioadenoma destruens) is similar to a complete mole but involves uterine myometrium

2. Nursing data collection

a. Variable vaginal bleeding usually occurs during first trimester; may be brown, like prune juice, and may contain some grapelike vesicles

NCLEX® **b.** Unusual uterine growth measured by fundal height; no fetal parts can be palpated and no FHR heard; "snowstorm" pattern seen on ultrasound

c. Abnormal labs include very high hCG levels and very low maternal AFP levels

NCLEX® **d.** Complications include hyperemesis gravidarum (probably associated with high hCG levels) and severe hypertension that occurs during first half of pregnancy; others include hyperthyroidism and possible trophoblastic pulmonary embolism

3. Collaborative management

NCLEX® **a.** Monitor client for signs of hemorrhage, hypertension, or other complications, including disseminated intravascular coagulopathy (DIC)

b. Prepare client and assist with suction uterine evacuation of molar pregnancy; hysterectomy may be chosen for clients who do not want to preserve fertility

c. Provide RhoGAM to appropriate clients (Rh-negative with Rh-positive partners) postprocedure

NCLEX® **d.** Reinforce need for frequent follow-up care during next year to rule out development of cancer (choriocarcinoma)

e. Weekly hCG levels are done initially with other testing to rule out cancer; reinforce need for diligent follow-up care because 1 in 5 women develop cancer

NCLEX® **f.** Client should not become pregnant for 1 year following molar pregnancy in case chemotherapy is indicated; provide contraceptive counseling

g. Provide emotional support for client and family who are grieving pregnancy loss and living with fear of developing a malignancy

D. Incompetent cervix

1. Overview

NCLEX® **a.** A painless cervical effacement and dilatation not associated with contractions (usually occurs in second trimester and results in spontaneous abortion or very preterm birth)

b. Maternal DES (diethylstilbestrol) exposure or congenital uterine anomalies may be associated with incompetent cervix

c. Other possible contributing factors: cervical inflammation, previous cervical trauma

2. Nursing data collection

a. Previous unexplained second-trimester pregnancy losses may indicate undiagnosed incompetent cervix

NCLEX® **b.** Cervical effacement and dilatation without contractions or pain; client may present for care completely dilated with bulging membranes

3. Collaborative management
   a. Provide emotional support and grief support group referral for client with pregnancy loss from an incompetent cervix
   NCLEX® b. Provide client teaching if client is managed on bedrest at home for a cervix just beginning to efface (shorten)
   NCLEX® c. Provide teaching about cervical **cerclage** if this is treatment method chosen; cerclage is a technique of reinforcing closure of cervix with sutures during pregnancy
   d. Monitor for signs of preterm labor or infection; client may be placed in Trendelenburg position and receive tocolytics; provide appropriate nursing assessments and care related to medication
   NCLEX® e. Instruct client to return if contractions begin because cesarean section is performed or suture must be removed before vaginal birth can be accomplished

E. Spontaneous abortion

1. Overview
   a. An unintended pregnancy loss before 20 weeks' gestation or weight of 500 grams; lay term is *miscarriage*
   b. Most common cause of bleeding in first trimester; usually results from chromosomal abnormalities in embryo
   c. Other causes may be teratogen exposure, inadequate implantation, and maternal endocrine disorders or chronic illness
   d. Late spontaneous abortion may be caused by incompetent cervix; classification of spontaneous abortion is presented in Box 45–1
2. Nursing data collection
   NCLEX® a. Vaginal spotting or bleeding is common; client may pass clots and tissue
   b. Pelvic cramping or dull backache is usually present
   c. Falling hCG levels indicate death of embryo; ultrasound is used to identify gestational sac and note whether there is current cardiac movement
3. Collaborative management
   NCLEX® a. Instruct client with threatened abortion about bedrest at home and when to return if bleeding or cramping worsens
   NCLEX® b. Monitor amount of bleeding; instruct client to save all clots and tissue that may be passed for further examination
   c. Monitor BP, pulse, and respirations frequently if bleeding is heavy; evaluate client for signs of impending shock
   d. Initiate IV therapy with at least an 18-gauge needle as ordered
   e. Assist with dilatation and curettage (D&C) as indicated for an incomplete abortion
   NCLEX® f. Provide emotional support, without false hope, to client and family; never discount importance of even a very early pregnancy

Box 45–1

Classification of Spontaneous Abortion

Terminology associated with spontaneous abortion helps to classify the clinical condition.

- Threatened abortion: Client has vaginal bleeding, but cervix remains closed; there may be some mild cramping or backache.
- Imminent/inevitable abortion: Client experiences cramping and bleeding; cervix dilates, and membranes may rupture.
- Incomplete abortion: Client experiences bleeding, cramping, and expulsion of some products of conception; tissue remains in uterus, and cervix is dilated; hemorrhage is possible.
- Complete abortion: Client experiences bleeding, cramping, and expulsion of all products of conception; cervix is closed, and uterus contracts.
- Missed abortion: Client experiences decreasing signs of pregnancy because fetus has died in utero but is not expelled; client may be at risk for DIC if products of conception are not removed with 6 weeks of fetal death.
- Recurrent abortion: Abortion occurs in three or more consecutive pregnancies.
- Septic abortion: Infection is present; can occur with unknown rupture of membranes, pregnancy with IUD in place, or attempt to end pregnancy by unqualified person.

g. Refer to pregnancy loss or grief support groups

NCLEX® h. Give RhoGAM to Rh-negative clients with Rh-positive partners within 72 hours of abortion

F. *Placenta previa*

1. Overview
   a. Placenta is abnormally implanted near to or over internal cervical os; as cervix softens and begins to efface and dilate, placental sinuses are opened causing progressive hemorrhages
   b. May be a low implantation near cervix, a partial previa covering part of os, or a complete placenta previa that covers entire internal cervical os
   c. Incidence of placenta previa is higher with multiple gestation and multiparity
   d. Delivery of client with complete previa is by cesarean section, usually with a classical uterine incision to avoid placenta
   e. Vaginal birth may be possible with a low-lying placenta if fetal head is down to press against placenta and occlude sinuses
2. Nursing data collection
   NCLEX® a. Episodic painless vaginal bleeding after 20th week of pregnancy (usually first episode is around 29th week) without contractions; each successive bleeding episode is usually heavier than previous one; profuse hemorrhage can occur as cervix dilates under placenta
   b. Ultrasound identification of placental location
3. Collaborative management
   NCLEX® a. Never perform vaginal exam on pregnant client presenting with painless vaginal bleeding to avoid profuse hemorrhage
   NCLEX® b. Maintain preterm clients on bedrest with bathroom privileges as long as there is no active bleeding until fetal maturity is reached or until hemorrhage warrants immediate cesarean delivery
   NCLEX® c. Monitor maternal vital signs to rule out ascending infection or shock
   NCLEX® d. Measure blood loss by weighing peripads and bed pads that are bloody (1 gram = 1 mL)

Memory Aid

Remember when weighing small amounts of blood or other fluids that one gram equals one milliliter (1 gram = 1 mL); weigh the dry object (such as peripad) and subtract weight from that of wet object to obtain weight of blood or other fluids.

   e. Monitor serial hemoglobin and hematocrit levels; obtain blood group and type, have two units of cross-matched blood available
   f. Assist with external fetal monitoring and other testing as indicated
   g. Maintain IV access with at least an 18-gauge needle and provide replacement fluids (Lactated Ringers) as ordered
   NCLEX® h. Provide emotional support to client on bedrest; facilitate family visits
   NCLEX® i. Promote adequate nutrition with prenatal vitamins and iron to prevent maternal anemia
   j. Assist with double setup procedure if indicated: physician performs a careful vaginal exam in OR with equipment and staff ready to perform either cesarean or vaginal delivery depending on whether bleeding is caused by placenta previa or is increased bloody show of advanced labor
   k. Provide routine preoperative and postoperative cesarean care if indicated; instruct client about location of uterine incision as it relates to future desire for a vaginal birth after cesarean (VBAC)

G. Abruptio placentae

1. Overview
   a. Premature separation of placenta from uterine wall during pregnancy
   b. Placenta may separate only at margins (marginal abruption), causing vaginal bleeding but perhaps little pain
   c. A central (concealed) abruption may not result in vaginal bleeding but does cause increasing uterine irritability and tenderness
   d. A complete (total) separation from uterine wall leads to profuse hemorrhage
   e. Most common identified precipitating factors are maternal hypertension, cocaine abuse, and abdominal trauma
   f. Client is at increased risk of depleting clotting factors and developing DIC

2. Nursing data collection
   - NCLEX® **a.** A painful, rigid, boardlike abdomen with vaginal bleeding is classic sign; abdomen may increase in size as bleeding continues; ultrasound confirms diagnosis
   - **b.** A central abruption causes severe pain from bleeding behind placenta that distends uterine muscle but there may be little or no vaginal bleeding; uterus is very irritable and fetus shows consistent late decelerations
   - NCLEX® **c.** Bleeding behind placenta is forced into myometrium and may result in a Couvelaire uterus, which becomes bluish-purple, extremely irritable, distended, and rigid; uterus does not contract efficiently after delivery, leading to postpartum hemorrhage
   - **d.** Marginal placental abruption may present with more vaginal bleeding but less pain than a concealed abruption
   - **e.** Fetal outcome depends on degree of placental separation and fetal maturity at delivery
3. Collaborative management
   - **a.** Monitor maternal BP, pulse, and respiration for signs of impending shock
   - NCLEX® **b.** Monitor fetus continuously for signs of distress: increased fetal movement, decreased FHR variability, changes in baseline FHR, late decelerations
   - NCLEX® **c.** Monitor client for bleeding, uterine activity, and abdominal pain; place on external fetal monitor to evaluate uterine irritability and fetal well-being; palpate uterine tone
   - **d.** Measure client's abdominal girth at umbilicus for baseline size and repeat periodically to evaluate occult bleeding
   - **e.** Review lab values to estimate blood loss (hemoglobin and hematocrit) and monitor for potential development of DIC (decreased platelets and fibrinogen; increased fibrin degradation products, PT, and PTT)
   - **f.** Monitor client for signs of developing coagulation defects: unusual bleeding from injection sites, gums, development of petechiae
   - **g.** Start and maintain IV fluids with at least an 18-gauge needle; monitor I&O; a urinary catheter may be inserted with expected urine output of 30 mL/hour or greater
   - NCLEX® **h.** Provide oxygen as indicated at 8 to 12 L/min via snug-fitting face mask
   - **i.** Carefully monitor client and fetus if vaginal delivery is attempted; prepare for emergency cesarean delivery if fetus develops distress
   - **j.** Provide ongoing information and emotional support for client and family

H. Premature rupture of membranes

1. Overview
   - **a.** Premature rupture of membranes (PROM) refers to amniotic membrane rupture before labor begins; labor usually begins spontaneously within 24 hours of rupture
   - **b.** Preterm PROM (PPROM) refers to membrane rupture prior to term gestation or before 37 weeks; risk factors include infection, incompetent cervix, and trauma
   - **c.** Prolonged rupture of membranes refers to membranes ruptured more than 12 hours before birth; many caregivers will induce labor rather than risk prolonged rupture with possible ascending infection
2. Nursing data collection
   - **a.** Gush of watery, clear, or meconium-stained fluid from vagina with continued leakage
   - NCLEX® **b.** Amniotic fluid turns nitrazine paper blue, indicating an alkaline pH; urine is almost always acidic and does not change the yellow color of nitrazine paper
   - NCLEX® **c.** Amniotic fluid shows characteristic ferning pattern on microscopic examination of a slide containing dried fluid; urine and vaginal secretions do not display ferning
   - **d.** An unengaged fetus is at risk for prolapsed cord when membranes rupture
3. Collaborative management
   - NCLEX® **a.** Monitor FHR when membranes rupture to rule out prolapsed cord; note time, color, and amount of fluid; obtain a baseline maternal temperature
   - **b.** Measure client's temperature every 2 hours; other vital signs may be routine; if temperature elevates, monitor hydration status
   - NCLEX® **c.** Avoid vaginal exams to avoid introducing microorganisms that may cause an ascending infection
   - NCLEX® **d.** Monitor for onset of uterine contractions and evaluate fetal well-being; decreased amniotic fluid may cause variable decelerations of FHR
   - **e.** Monitor client for signs of **chorioamnionitis** (inflammation and infection of fetal membranes and amniotic fluid): elevated temperature, abdominal tenderness, increased WBCs and erythrocyte sedimentation rate

f. Obtain vaginal culture for group B streptococcus as ordered
g. Provide client teaching and reassurance that amniotic fluid is continuously produced and that there is no such thing as a "dry birth"
h. Administer antibiotics if ordered; some caregivers prefer to wait and treat newborn

I. Preeclampsia and eclampsia

1. Overview

NCLEX® a. Hypertension during pregnancy may be classified as gestational (transient) hypertension, chronic hypertension, hypertension with superimposed preeclampsia or eclampsia, and preeclampsia/eclampsia
b. Gestational hypertension is a high BP during pregnancy that resolves after delivery; it is not associated with proteinuria
c. *Preeclampsia* is associated with vasospasm and vascular endothelial damage; it is more common in young primigravidas, women over 35, multiple gestation and diabetes mellitus, GTD, and large placental mass; client is at risk for CVA, DIC, renal failure, hepatic rupture, and hemorrhage

NCLEX® d. Mild preeclampsia is characterized by BP higher than 140/90 after 20 weeks' gestation and proteinuria of 1–2+ by dipstick
e. Severe preeclampsia is characterized by a BP of 180/110 or higher or an increase of 30/15 from previous visit and proteinuria 3^+ or greater
f. Sudden onset of severe edema indicates a need for evaluation for preeclampsia or renal disease

NCLEX® g. Eclampsia is the term for preeclampsia that has progressed to include maternal generalized seizures or coma

NCLEX® h. HELLP (hemolysis, elevated liver enzymes, and low platelet count) syndrome may be associated with severe preeclampsia; the client is at risk for hemorrhage, pulmonary edema, and hepatic rupture
i. Fetal complications include IUGR, fetal distress from hypoxia, and death

Memory Aid

Remember HELLP to recall a syndrome that is a complication of pregnancy-induced hypertension:
Hemolysis, **E**levated **L**iver enzymes and **L**ow **P**latelet count

2. Nursing data collection

NCLEX® a. Symptoms usually develop during third trimester (most frequently in last 10 weeks of gestation) except in cases of GTD; client is at risk for seizures and other complications up to 48 hours after delivery; see Table 45–3
b. Systemic responses: CNS irritability causes severe or continuous headache, hyperreflexia (greater than +2, baseline, or clonus), or visual disturbance (blurred vision, seeing spots or flashing lights); renal damage is indicated by oliguria (less than 30 mL/hr); portal hypertension may result in epigastric pain and may precede hepatic rupture

NCLEX® c. Lab values: increased hematocrit (as fluid moves out of intravascular space), serum uric acid and BUN; increased liver enzymes (alanine aminotransferase [ALT] and aspartate aminotransferase [AST]); decreased RBCs and platelets as condition worsens

Table 45–3 Comparison of Mild and Severe Preeclampsia

	Mild Preeclampsia	Severe Preeclampsia
Blood pressure	140/90 or increase of 30/15 from baseline	160/110 or higher on 2 occasions
Proteinuria	Trace to +1	3+ to 4+ or more than 5 grams in a 24-hour urine specimen
Edema	Possible mild to moderate pretibial edema	Facial edema and pitting pretibial edema
Weight gain	2 to 2.5 pounds/week	Sudden large weight gain
Other	——	Possible signs of CNS irritation

3. Collaborative management: the only cure for preeclampsia is delivery; goal is to deliver healthy, viable infant while safeguarding mother's health
   - NCLEX® **a.** Bedrest at home is indicated if preeclampsia is mild; hospitalization if severe until fetus is mature enough for delivery; bedrest on left side to facilitate uteroplacental perfusion
   - **b.** Maintain quiet, calm environment to decrease CNS stimulation; keep siderails up and padded for clients with severe preeclampsia who are at risk of progressing to seizures
   - NCLEX® **c.** A high-protein diet without salt restriction is indicated; restricting salt intake may result in hypovolemia and fetal distress
   - NCLEX® **d.** Implement frequent assessments (every 15 minutes to 1 to 4 hours as indicated by client condition) to include BP, pulse and respirations, edema, deep tendon reflexes, and clonus checks; check client for headache, visual disturbances, and epigastric pain
   - **e.** Urinary catheter is inserted to monitor renal function, record strict I&O; evaluate urine for protein; measure daily weight
   - **f.** Monitor fetal well-being by continuous electronic fetal monitoring, serial NSTs, BPP, or amniocentesis as indicated
   - NCLEX® **g.** Administer magnesium sulfate as ordered for seizure prevention; monitor client for signs of magnesium toxicity (see also Chapter 31)
   - **h.** Prepare for induction or cesarean birth when fetus is mature or if maternal condition worsens
   - **i.** Reinforce teaching and provide support to client and family about condition and interventions; clients with mild preeclampsia frequently do not feel ill and may have difficulty maintaining bedrest
   - **j.** Observe newborn for signs of depression related to magnesium sulfate
   - **k.** Continue to monitor client for complications; seizures may occur for 48 hours after delivery

Check Your NCLEX–PN® Exam I.Q.

You are ready for testing on this content if you can

- Implement nursing care for pregnant clients undergoing diagnostic testing.
- Determine whether the condition of a pregnant client undergoing diagnostic testing has changed from preprocedure to postprocedure.
- Position clients appropriately for diagnostic testing.
- Take action to prevent complications of diagnostic procedures.
- Implement nursing care for clients experiencing complications of pregnancy.
- Reinforce client teaching about ongoing care for clients who have a complication of pregnancy.

PRACTICE TEST

1 A 37-year-old gravida 1 at 38 weeks' gestation is scheduled for an amniocentesis. After learning the client was diagnosed with diabetes at age 17, the nurse concludes that the procedure is most likely being done to assess for what potential problem?

1. Neural tube defects
2. Down syndrome
3. Effects of TORCH syndrome
4. Lung maturity

2 A client at 24 weeks' gestation has been scheduled for an amniocentesis. Which actions should the nurse plan to take in the care of this client? Select all that apply.

1. Monitor maternal vital signs and fetal heart rate (FHR) during procedure.
2. Explain that an ultrasound machine will be used during the procedure.
3. Assist the woman in assuming a supine position with a wedge under left hip.
4. Have a consent signed for epidural analgesia.
5. Explain that 60 mL of amniotic fluid will be withdrawn.

3 The client is scheduled to have an amniocentesis for assessment of lung maturity. She seems upset, and says that she doesn't understand how this test could tell if a baby's lungs are mature. What is the best response by the nurse?

1. "Please try not to worry about that. Your doctor knows the procedure well."
2. "The fluid changes color as the fetal lungs mature. We look at the color to determine lung maturity."
3. "A chemical called lecithin is made by the fetal lungs and increases as pregnancy continues. It flows into amniotic fluid, where we can measure it."
4. "The amount of bilirubin in amniotic fluid increases as the lungs mature. We check for yellow colored fluid to assess lung maturity."

4 The nurse recognizes that which maternal condition in the third trimester would be a contraindication for conducting a contraction stress test? Select all that apply.

1. Intrauterine growth restriction
2. Diabetes mellitus
3. Pregnancy at 42 weeks' gestation
4. Marginal abruptio placentae
5. Third trimester bleeding

5 A primigravida is hospitalized at 32 weeks' gestation after a second hemorrhage from a complete placenta previa. The client appears subdued and sad after learning she will remain hospitalized until delivery. She says she is worried about her husband, who will be at home alone much of the time. The nurse interprets the client's response as indicating which psychological state?

1. Anxiety
2. Denial
3. Immaturity
4. Ineffective coping

6 The nurse reviews the client's chart for results of which diagnostic test that will best indicate a diagnosis of erythroblastosis fetalis?

1. Amniocentesis
2. Biophysical profile
3. Indirect Coombs' test
4. Percutaneous umbilical blood sampling

7 The nurse caring for a client with a concealed abruptio placentae prepares to monitor the client for which complication as a priority after delivery?

1. Retained placental fragments
2. Urinary tract infection
3. Uterine atony
4. Vaginal hematoma

8 A pregnant client with class II heart disease progressed through pregnancy without complications and is admitted to the hospital in active labor. Soon after admission, the client reports shortness of breath and the nurse auscultates lung crackles. The nurse anticipates administering which medication based on the client's history? Select all that apply.

1. Penicillin (generic)
2. Metoprolol (Lopressor)
3. Furosemide (Lasix)
4. Digoxin (Lanoxin)
5. Procainamide (Pronestyl)

9 The nurse reinforces client teaching with a pregnant client who has placenta previa and who states her religious beliefs prohibit receiving blood or blood products. The nurse recognizes that the teaching has been effective if the client makes which statement?

1. "A judge will force me to accept a transfusion if I really need it."
2. "I might have to sign out of the hospital against medical advice (AMA)."
3. "I will meet with the dietician to increase the amount of iron in my diet."
4. "There is little chance that I will bleed heavily during this pregnancy."

10 The nurse would monitor the pregnant client with a history of multiple sexual partners for which complication of pregnancy of greatest concern in this situation?

1. Ectopic pregnancy
2. Premature rupture of membranes
3. Preeclampsia
4. Rh incompatibility

PRACTICE TEST

11 The nurse anticipates that a pregnant client with a history of which health problem might benefit from a scheduled cesarean birth to have an improved outcome for the infant? Select all that apply.

1. Diabetes mellitus
2. Active genital herpes lesions
3. Human immunodeficiency virus
4. Systemic lupus erythematosus
5. Class I heart disease

12 A prenatal client with type 1 diabetes mellitus asks the clinic nurse whether she will be able to breastfeed her baby. Which response by the nurse is most accurate?

1. "Breastfeeding is contraindicated for insulin-dependent moms."
2. "Certainly, breastfeeding will be beneficial for both of you."
3. "I think this is a good idea because it also prevents pregnancy."
4. "You will have a lot of difficulty maintaining a stable blood sugar."

13 A client is admitted with membranes that ruptured 4 hours ago and occasional mild contractions. The term fetus looks healthy on external monitoring. What is the priority intervention in the nursing plan of care for this client?

1. Encourage ambulation
2. Monitor vital signs
3. Promote rest
4. Provide clear liquids

14 A prenatal client at 14 weeks' gestation reports continuous nausea and vomiting, and a severe headache. The blood pressure is elevated and fundal height is 21 centimeters. Which diagnostic test does the nurse anticipate will be ordered to confirm a hydatidiform mole?

1. Biophysical profile
2. Human chorionic gonadotropin
3. Maternal serum alpha-fetoprotein
4. Sonography

15 A human immunodeficiency virus (HIV)-positive client in active labor with newly ruptured membranes is being transported to the hospital via ambulance. The nurse assisting in the labor and delivery unit anticipates priority administration of which medication to this client?

1. Antibiotics
2. Immune globulin
3. Oxytocin (Pitocin)
4. Zidovudine (Retrovir)

16 A client who admits to crack cocaine use during her pregnancy asks the nurse not to inform the baby's father about the substance abuse. Which response by the nurse is appropriate? Select all that apply.

1. "You must be worried about how he will react to that information."
2. "This is your pregnancy and your body, so I'll keep your information private."
3. "Your baby will probably not survive, so there is no need for him to know."
4. "Have you considered that he deserves to know that the baby may be at risk?"
5. What reaction do you think the baby's father will have?

17 A client experiencing profuse hemorrhage from placenta previa is being prepared for an emergency cesarean birth. The client exhibits signs of hypovolemia. The nurse makes it a priority to place the client in which position?

1. Knee–chest
2. Left lateral
3. Semi-Fowler's
4. Trendelenburg

18 A client with premature rupture of membranes (PROM) at 33 weeks' gestation is to be given betamethasone (Celestone) to increase fetal lung maturity. The nurse checks the client's record to ensure that the client does not have what disorder that could be affected by this drug?

1. Diabetes mellitus
2. History of alcohol abuse
3. Incompetent cervix
4. Intrauterine growth restriction (IUGR)

19 The nurse concludes that a client is at risk for preeclampsia when the vital signs taken today show that the blood pressure has shown which pattern of elevation since the previous prenatal visit?

1. 90/56 to 110/70
2. 100/60 to 130/76
3. 122/80 to 138/86
4. 134/80 to 140/88

20 A client who has experienced a spontaneous abortion at 8 weeks asks the nurse why this happened. What would the nurse include in a response to address the most common cause of "miscarriage?"

1. Chromosome abnormalities
2. Environmental teratogens
3. Excessive activity
4. Substance abuse

21 A client who received no prenatal care delivers a 9-pound, 4-ounce baby boy who exhibits signs of respiratory distress. The nurse obtains a blood sample from the infant per protocol to screen for which potential problem?

1. Hemolysis
2. Hyperbilirubinemia
3. Hypoglycemia
4. Sepsis

22 The nurse reinforces to a client who had a cervical cone biopsy several years ago that she is now at increased risk for which complication of pregnancy?

1. Ectopic pregnancy
2. Incompetent cervix
3. Gestational trophoblastic disease
4. Placenta previa

23 A 20-year-old gravida 2, para 0 at 37 weeks' gestation calls the nurse because she is experiencing contractions every 7–8 minutes. Her first pregnancy ended with a spontaneous abortion at 18 weeks, and the client had a MacDonald cerclage placed early in the current pregnancy. Which instruction by the nurse is most appropriate?

1. "Try a warm bath and relaxation techniques to see if the contractions will go away."
2. "You must wait until your contractions are every 5 minutes before going to the hospital."
3. "You need to go to the hospital, so we can stop your premature labor this time."
4. "You should go to the hospital to be evaluated and have the cerclage removed."

24 A pregnant client comes to the hospital at 36 weeks reporting that her "water broke," but denies any contractions. Which data collected by the nurse provides the most reliable indication of premature rupture of membranes?

1. A dried specimen shows a microscopic fern pattern.
2. Fluid from the perineum turns nitrazine paper dark blue.
3. No membranes are felt on a sterile vaginal exam.
4. The client has a visible watery vaginal discharge.

25 During which procedure should the nurse wear protective goggles in addition to gloves?

1. Changing a soaked disposable bed pad
2. Performing an amniotomy
3. Starting an intravenous line
4. Washing dirty instruments

ANSWERS & RATIONALES

1 **Answer: 4 Rationale:** Amniocentesis for a client with diabetes mellitus at 38 weeks' gestation is probably being done to assess lung maturity in anticipation of delivery. Neural tube defects can be initially screened using a blood test. Amniocentesis for genetic testing is usually done early in the second trimester. Amniocentesis for effects of TORCH syndrome would not be conducted so late in the pregnancy. **Cognitive Level:** Analyzing **Client Need:** Physiological Adaptation **Integrated Process:** Nursing Process: Implementation **Content Area:** Maternal-Newborn **Strategy:** The critical words in the question are *38 weeks' gestation.* Use knowledge of the timing of tests used to diagnose genetic defects to systematically eliminate the incorrect options. As an alternative, consider that lung maturity is a key concern as a pregnant client approaches the due date.

2 **Answer: 1, 2, 3 Rationale:** Maternal vital signs and FHR are monitored during procedure. The test is completed on an outpatient basis under guidance of ultrasound visualization. The client is positioned on her back with a wedge under her left hip to avoid hypotension from pressure of the uterus on the vena cava. Epidural analgesia is not used for the procedure. Approximately 15–20 mL of amniotic fluid is aspirated for the procedure. **Cognitive Level:** Applying **Client Need:** Reduction of Risk Potential **Integrated Process:** Nursing Process: Planning **Content Area:** Maternal-Newborn **Strategy:** The wording of the questions indicates that more than one option is likely to be correct. Visualize the procedure and choose standard safe actions for a pregnant client (positioning, monitoring vital signs). Recall that the procedure uses ultrasound to choose that option. Recall that a local skin

anesthetic may be used, but not epidural analgesia, to eliminate that option. Finally, realize that 60 mL is a large amount of fluid to consider that option incorrect.

3 **Answer: 3 Rationale:** The amount of lecithin increases as the fetal lungs mature. The ratio of lecithin to sphingomyelin is used to assess lung maturity. To ask a client not to worry or state the doctor knows the procedure well does not provide information to the client. The color of the amniotic fluid is not useful in determining lung maturity. Bilirubin levels in amniotic fluid do not determine lung maturity. **Cognitive Level:** Applying **Client Need:** Reduction of Risk Potential **Integrated Process:** Communication and Documentation **Content Area:** Maternal-Newborn **Strategy:** Recall that amniotic fluid is clear to eliminate options referring to color change of amniotic fluid. Next, eliminate the response that is not therapeutic.

4 **Answer: 5 Rationale:** Intrauterine growth restriction, diabetes mellitus, and postterm (42 weeks) pregnancy are all indications for completing a contraction stress test. Contractions elicited during the test could cause increased bleeding if an abruption is present or if there is already bleeding in the third trimester. **Cognitive Level:** Analyzing **Client Need:** Reduction of Risk Potential **Integrated Process:** Nursing Process: Data Collection **Content Area:** Maternal-Newborn **Strategy:** Note the critical word *contraindication* in the stem of the question. This tells you that the correct answer is likely an item that could pose risk of harm to the fetus. From there, recall that abruptio placentae can lead to bleeding to help you choose correctly.

5 **Answer: 1 Rationale:** The client has stated that she is worried, which creates anxiety. The information presented does not represent denial or immaturity. There is not enough data to determine whether the client's coping is effective at this time. **Cognitive Level:** Analyzing **Client Need:** Physiological Adaptation **Integrated Process:** Communication and Documentation **Content Area:** Maternal-Newborn **Strategy:** Note that the client exhibits appropriate nonverbal behavior (*subdued* and *sad*), and is able to articulate a concern (*worried about her husband*). Consider that all of these are expected reactions to choose Anxiety over the other options.

6 **Answer: 4 Rationale:** Percutaneous umbilical blood sampling (PUBS) obtains an actual sample of fetal blood for analysis. Amniocentesis, biophysical profile, and indirect Coombs' test provide information about fetal well-being, but do not directly sample the fetal erythrocytes. **Cognitive Level:** Analyzing **Client Need:** Reduction of Risk Potential **Integrated Process:** Nursing Process: Data Collection **Content Area:** Maternal-Newborn **Strategy:** Note the word *erythroblastosis* in the question, and correlate that with erythrocytes or red blood cells. Eliminate amniocentesis and biophysical profile first because they are not related to red blood cells. Then choose option PUBS over indirect Coombs' test because it allows access to fetal cells, not to maternal cells.

7 **Answer: 3 Rationale:** A concealed abruption could result in a Couvelaire uterus, which does not contract effectively after delivery, leading to uterine atony. Retained placental fragments, vaginal hematoma, or urinary tract infection could occur in any client. **Cognitive Level:** Analyzing **Client Need:** Physiological Adaptation **Integrated Process:** Nursing Process: Data Collection **Content Area:** Maternal-Newborn **Strategy:** Specific knowledge of the risks of concealed abruptio placentae is needed to answer the question. Use nursing knowledge and the process of elimination to make your selection.

8 **Answer: 1, 3, 4 Rationale:** Prophylactic antibiotics such as penicillin are given during labor to prevent bacterial endocarditis. A cardiac glycoside such as digoxin and a diuretic such as furosemide may help counteract the new signs of decreased cardiac output (crackles and shortness of breath). An antihypertensive such as metoprolol or antidysrhythmic such as procainamide would be used only as needed. **Cognitive Level:** Analyzing **Client Need:** Physiological Adaptation **Integrated Process:** Nursing Process: Planning **Content Area:** Maternal-Newborn **Strategy:** The core issue of the question is the significance of adverse cardiopulmonary assessment findings with class II heart disease during labor. Use nursing knowledge and the process of elimination to make your selection. Consider that an antibiotic is the only drug listed that could prevent a new problem (infection), while a cardiac glycoside and diuretic will manage symptoms of decreased cardiac output because of increased cardiac demand during labor.

9 **Answer: 3 Rationale:** The client is likely to lose some blood with a placenta previa. Increasing iron in her diet is a positive response that does not interfere with her religious beliefs. A judge will not force a transfusion. The client will not need to sign out AMA to avoid receiving a transfusion, even if one is indicated. It is not possible to predict that amount of bleeding that could be experienced by a specific client with placenta previa. **Cognitive Level:** Analyzing **Client Need:** Physiological Adaptation **Integrated Process:** Nursing Process: Evaluation **Content Area:** Maternal-Newborn **Strategy:** The core issue of this question is culturally competent care to reduce risk of complications. First, eliminate options that fail to provide care or go against the client's wishes. Next, choose the option about iron because it is a positive behavior and avoids having to guess about the unknown (amount of bleeding to expect during pregnancy).

10 **Answer: 1 Rationale:** The client with multiple partners is at high risk for sexually transmitted diseases and ascending infection that can lead to blockage in the fallopian tubes. Ultimately, this process could lead to ectopic pregnancy. The other options do not address this particular pathophysiological concern. **Cognitive Level:** Analyzing **Client Need:** Physiological Adaptation **Integrated Process:** Nursing Process: Data Collection **Content Area:** Maternal-Newborn **Strategy:** Note the critical words *multiple sexual partners* and *greatest concern* in the question. This tells you that the correct answer has a connection to risks associated with multiple sex partners. Use knowledge of complications of sexually transmitted infections to choose correctly.

11 **Answer: 2, 3 Rationale:** A client with active herpes lesions should be delivered by cesarean to prevent transmission of the virus during vaginal birth. The chance of transmission of HIV is less than 1% if the infant is delivered by cesarean prior to membrane rupture. A client with diabetes mellitus does not require cesarean delivery based on this diagnosis alone. A client with systemic lupus erythematosis does not require cesarean delivery based on this diagnosis alone. A client with Class I heart disease may be successful with a vaginal delivery. **Cognitive Level:** Applying **Client Need:** Physiological Adaptation **Integrated Process:** Nursing Process: Planning **Content Area:** Maternal-Newborn **Strategy:** The core issue of the question is knowledge of methods of transmitting infection from mother to newborn during the delivery process. Choose the options that represent risk of neonatal infection and eliminate all of the remaining options.

12 **Answer: 2 Rationale:** Breastfeeding should be encouraged because it benefits both the mother and her infant. Breastfeeding is not contraindicated for diabetic mothers.

Breastfeeding might or might not help prevent future pregnancy during lactation. Breastfeeding does not necessarily lead to loss of blood glucose control with careful management. **Cognitive Level:** Applying **Client Need:** Physiological Adaptation **Integrated Process:** Nursing Process: Implementation **Content Area:** Maternal-Newborn **Strategy:** Note the critical words *most accurate*, which indicates the correct answer is one that is a true statement, while the others are false to a greater or lesser degree. First eliminate the options that contain the words *contraindicated* and *a lot of difficulty*. Then choose the option that is most true.

13 **Answer: 2** **Rationale:** The client with premature ruptured membranes is at risk for developing an infection and should have vital signs, specifically temperature, monitored every 2 hours. The client may be on bedrest, not ambulating, following rupture of the membranes. Promoting rest and providing clear liquids are slightly lower priorities for this client. **Cognitive Level:** Analyzing **Client Need:** Physiological Adaptation **Integrated Process:** Nursing Process: Planning **Content Area:** Maternal-Newborn **Strategy:** The core issue of the question is knowledge of infection as the key risk following rupture of the membranes. Eliminate options that do not address this risk.

14 **Answer: 4** **Rationale:** Ultrasound confirms the diagnosis of molar pregnancy that is indicated by the client's symptoms. The client will have high hCG levels and low maternal serum alpha-fetoprotein levels, but these are not conclusive for hydatidiform mole. Biophysical profile is inappropriate before the third trimester because that test evaluates the fetus. **Cognitive Level:** Applying **Client Need:** Reduction of Risk Potential **Integrated Process:** Nursing Process: Data Collection **Content Area:** Maternal-Newborn **Strategy:** The core issue of the question is the best method to determine hydatidiform mole. Choose sonography over the others because it is the only one that allows direct visualization of the reproductive structures and differentiates true pregnancy from hydatidiform mole.

15 **Answer: 4** **Rationale:** The rate of transmission of HIV to the newborn decreases sharply if the mother is given prophylactic zidovudine (Retrovir) orally during pregnancy and by IV during labor. An antibiotic could be administered if the membranes were ruptured for an extended time before delivery. There is no indication in the question for immune globulin, which would provide passive immunity against a specific type of infection. There is no indication in the question for pitocin, which would induce labor. **Cognitive Level:** Analyzing **Client Need:** Physiological Adaptation **Integrated Process:** Nursing Process: Planning **Content Area:** Maternal-Newborn **Strategy:** The core issue of the question is management of the HIV client in active labor to prevent HIV transmission to the newborn. Eliminate oxytocin first because it stimulates labor. Choose zidovudine over the others listed that related to infection because it is an antiviral rather than antibacterial and the immunity is needed by the neonate rather than the mother.

16 **Answer: 1, 5** **Rationale:** Addressing the client's worry is a therapeutic response to the client's concerns. Asking about the father's reaction gathers more data and also provides an opportunity to assess possible client safety concerns. Stating to keep the information private is nontherapeutic because it does not explore the client's concern. Stating the baby is not likely to survive is inaccurate. Asking whether the father deserves to know is judgmental. **Cognitive Level:** Applying **Client Need:** Psychosocial Integrity **Integrated Process:** Communication and Documentation **Content Area:** Maternal-Newborn **Strategy:** The core issue of the question is a therapeutic response to a concern shared by the client. Eliminate each of the incorrect options systematically because they do not invite further sharing of information between client and nurse.

17 **Answer: 2** **Rationale:** The left lateral position facilitates uteroplacental perfusion. Knee–chest position will not aid circulation and is unlikely to be maintained by a client in shock. Semi-Fowler's position would decrease maternal cerebral perfusion. Trendelenburg puts the weight of the gravid uterus against the maternal lungs. **Cognitive Level:** Analyzing **Client Need:** Physiological Adaptation **Integrated Process:** Nursing Process: Implementation **Content Area:** Maternal-Newborn **Strategy:** The core issue of the question is how to maintain uteroplacental perfusion for the client in shock. Choose the position that turns the client to the left side and takes pressure of the gravid uterus off the great vessels in the abdomen.

18 **Answer: 1** **Rationale:** Glucocorticoids raise the blood glucose and this has implications for diabetic control in a client with diabetes mellitus. A history of alcohol abuse, incompetent cervix, and IUGR are not contraindications for giving betamethasone. **Cognitive Level:** Applying **Client Need:** Physiological Adaptation **Integrated Process:** Nursing Process: Data Collection **Content Area:** Maternal-Newborn **Strategy:** The core issue of the question is knowledge of key side effects of betamethasone, which helps to select the client for whom it has implications. Recall that the glucocorticoids often end in *-sone* to help you recognize the drug as a glucocorticoid. Recall next the risk of elevating blood glucose levels to choose diabetes mellitus over the others.

19 **Answer: 2** **Rationale:** An increase of 30 mm Hg systolic and 15 mm Hg diastolic is diagnostic for preeclampsia. The blood pressures in each of the other options do not meet the criteria for increase in either the systolic or the diastolic blood pressure reading. **Cognitive Level:** Analyzing **Client Need:** Physiological Adaptation **Integrated Process:** Nursing Process: Data Collection **Content Area:** Maternal-Newborn **Strategy:** Specific knowledge of the criteria for preeclampsia is needed to answer this question. Choose the option that has the greatest degree of change in both systolic and diastolic measurements.

20 **Answer: 1** **Rationale:** The majority of early abortions are related to abnormal chromosomes. The client might fear that she has caused the loss, and should be provided with accurate information. The majority of early abortions are not related to environmental teratogens, excessive activity, or substance abuse. **Cognitive Level:** Applying **Client Need:** Physiological Adaptation **Integrated Process:** Communication and Documentation **Content Area:** Maternal-Newborn **Strategy:** Specific knowledge of the etiologies of spontaneous abortion is needed to answer the question. Use nursing knowledge and the process of elimination to make your selection.

21 **Answer: 3** **Rationale:** A 9-pound, 4-ounce infant is large for gestational age (LGA). An LGA infant who demonstrates respiratory distress could have a diabetic mother. The infant produces his own insulin during pregnancy, and stores the excess glucose as fat to compensate for high maternal glucose loads. After delivery the infant is at high risk for hypoglycemia because excess maternal glucose is now absent from the infant's circulation. The blood sample is not being drawn to assess for hemolysis, sepsis, or hyperbilirubinemia. **Cognitive Level:** Analyzing **Client Need:** Physiological Adaptation **Integrated Process:** Nursing Process: Data Collection **Content Area:** Maternal-Newborn **Strategy:** The core issues of the question

are prenatal risks for LGA infants and the consequences after delivery. Use nursing knowledge and the process of elimination to make your selection.

22 **Answer: 2 Rationale:** Cervical trauma and scarring, such as from cervical cone biopsy, can result in cervical incompetence during pregnancy. The client who had a cervical cone biopsy is not at greater risk for ectopic pregnancy, gestational trophoblastic disease, or placenta previa. **Cognitive Level:** Analyzing **Client Need:** Physiological Adaptation **Integrated Process:** Teaching and Learning **Content Area:** Maternal-Newborn **Strategy:** Note the critical word *cervical* in the stem of the question, and choose the option that also refers to the cervix.

23 **Answer: 4 Rationale:** The MacDonald cerclage is a purse-string suture that ties the cervix closed. The suture needs to be removed before vaginal delivery is possible. The cerclage is usually removed at 37 weeks to allow natural labor to begin. A warm bath and relaxation delays care and could place the client at risk for cervical injury. The cerclage needs to be removed. Waiting for contractions to occur every 5 minutes places the client at risk of cervical injury. Labor at 37 weeks may not be considered to be premature. **Cognitive Level:** Applying **Client Need:** Physiological Adaptation **Integrated Process:** Nursing Process: Implementation **Content Area:** Maternal-Newborn **Strategy:** Knowledge of the need to remove the cerclage at 37 weeks' gestation, prior to labor and delivery, will help to identify the correct response and the correct answer.

24 **Answer: 1 Rationale:** During pregnancy, only amniotic fluid will dry to a ferning pattern. Urine occasionally might be alkaline, and turn nitrazine paper blue, or old nitrazine paper might be unreliable. Performing a vaginal exam places the client at unnecessary risk for an ascending infection, and feeling for membranes is unreliable. A watery vaginal discharge is not necessarily amniotic fluid. **Cognitive Level:** Applying **Client Need:** Physiological Adaptation **Integrated Process:** Nursing Process: Data Collection **Content Area:** Maternal-Newborn **Strategy:** The core issue of the question is the most objective data to document rupture of membranes. Eliminate one option because it jeopardizes the safety of the client, and can result in inaccurate data. Eliminate two others that are not conclusive for amniotic fluid.

25 **Answer: 2 Rationale:** Consider routes of disease transmission and associate the use of goggles with an item that can result in splash of fluids. **Cognitive Level:** Analyzing **Client Need:** Safety and Infection Control **Integrated Process:** Nursing Process: Planning **Content Area:** Maternal-Newborn **Strategy:** Recall that goggles are indicated to prevent contamination of the eyes. Eliminate incorrect options because they place the nurse at risk for contamination from skin contact, necessitating the use of gloves, not goggles.

Key Terms to Review

abortion p. 737
abruptio placentae p. 737
amniocentesis p. 736
biophysical profile (BPP) p. 735
cerclage p. 744
chorioamnionitis p. 746
chorionic villus sampling (CVS) p. 737
contraction stress test (CST) p. 736
Coombs' test p. 741
Doppler blood flow analysis p. 735
ectopic p. 741
erythroblastosis fetalis p. 741
gestational diabetes p. 739
gestational trophoblastic disease (GTD) p. 743
Hydatiform mole p. 743
hydrops fetalis p. 741
karyotype p. 737
kernicterus p. 741
lecithin to sphyngomyelin (L/S) ratio p. 737
macrosomia p. 739
nonstress test (NST) p. 736
placenta previa p. 745
phosphatidylglycerol (PG) p. 737

References

Davidson, M., London, M., & Ladewig, P. (2012). *Olds' maternal newborn nursing and women's health across the lifespan* (9th ed.). Upper Saddle River, NJ: Pearson Education, Inc.

Ladewig, P., London, M., & Davidson, M. (2010). *Contemporary maternal-newborn nursing care* (7th ed.). Upper Saddle River, NJ: Pearson Education, Inc.

London, M., Ladewig, P., Ball, J., Bindler, R., & Cowen, K. (2011). *Maternal & child nursing care* (3rd ed.). Upper Saddle River, NJ: Pearson Education, Inc.

Perry, S., Hockenberry, M., Lowdermilk, D., & Wilson, D. (2010). *Maternal child nursing care* (4th ed.). St. Louis, MO: Elsevier.

Smith, S., Duell, D., & Martin, B. (2012). *Clinical nursing skills: Basic to advanced skills* (8th ed.). Upper Saddle River, NJ: Pearson Education.

Test Yourself

Are you ready for the NCLEX-PN® or course exams? Use the practice tests on the companion website to check.

Complicated Labor and Delivery Care

46

In this chapter

Cross Reference

Other chapters relevant to this content area are

Reproduction, Family Planning, and Infertility	Chapter 8
Uncomplicated Antenatal Care	Chapter 9
Uncomplicated Labor and Delivery Care	Chapter 10
Uncomplicated Postpartum Care	Chapter 11
Uncomplicated Newborn Care	Chapter 12
Complicated Antenatal Care	Chapter 45
Complicated Postpartum Care	Chapter 47
Complicated Newborn Care	Chapter 48

I. GENERAL NURSING CARE OF CLIENT

A. High-risk factors

1. May develop at any time during labor in client who was healthy throughout pregnancy
2. Etiology may be related to fetus, birth passage, relationship between birth passage and fetus, and psychosocial considerations

B. Client response to onset of high-risk factors in labor

1. Stress, fear, and anxiety brought about by unexpected complications during labor may have profound effects on maternal and fetal outcomes
2. Maternal anxiety can increase tension, produce higher pain perception, and may make labor contractions less effective
3. Catecholamines released during stress produce vasoconstriction that may negatively affect uterine blood flow

C. Family members

1. May be overwhelmed with concern
2. May become less capable of providing needed emotional support for client

D. Nursing care

1. Basic intrapartal care is still important
2. Nursing care during complicated labor requires additional special knowledge and skill in assessment and care of mother and fetus

II. PROBLEMS WITH THE FETUS

A. Fetal *malpositions*

1. Ideal fetal position is flexed with occiput in right or left anterior quadrant of maternal pelvis
2. Various types of malpositions are possible
3. Occiput posterior (OP) position
   a. Right or left OP position occurs in about 25% of all term pregnancies but usually rotates to occiput anterior (OA) as labor progresses
   b. Failure to rotate is termed persistent occiput posterior; may be related to small maternal pelvis, poor contractions, inadequate pushing effort (often from epidural anesthesia), abnormal flexion of head, or large fetus
   NCLEX® c. Maternal risks include prolonged labor, potential for operative delivery, extension of midline episiotomy, or 3rd- or 4th-degree perineal laceration
   NCLEX® d. Maternal symptoms include intense back pain in labor, dysfunctional labor pattern, prolonged active phase, hypotonic labor (not enough pressure of head on cervix), arrest of dilatation and/or descent
4. Occiput transverse (OT) position
   a. Incomplete rotation of OP position to OA results in fetal head being in horizontal or transverse position
   b. Persistent OT position occurs because of ineffective contractions or flattened bony pelvis
   c. If pelvic structure is adequate, vaginal delivery can be accomplished by stimulating contractions with oxytocin (Pitocin) and use of forceps
5. Collaborative management of fetal malpositions
   a. Key maternal assessments are pain and coping skills
   NCLEX® b. Knee-chest position may provide a downward slant to vaginal canal and pelvic rocking may facilitate rotation
   NCLEX® c. Apply sacral counterpressure with heel of hand to reduce back pain
   d. If rotation accomplished, encourage client to lie in Sims position on side opposite from fetal back
   e. Provide support and encouragement by keeping client and family informed of progress, praising efforts to maintain control, and encouraging relaxation with contractions
   f. Anticipate forceps rotation and forceps-assisted birth or vacuum extraction if rotation not accomplished
   g. Forceps: metal instruments applied to fetal head to provide traction or a means to rotate fetal head
   NCLEX® h. Risks of forceps use are fetal ecchymosis or edema of face, transient facial paralysis, maternal lacerations, or episiotomy extensions
   i. Vacuum extraction: a suction cup applied to fetal head to provide traction to shorten second stage of labor
   NCLEX® j. Risks of vacuum extraction are newborn cephalohematoma, retinal hemorrhage, and intracranial hemorrhage

B. Fetal *malpresentations*

1. Normal presentation is occipital; fetal malpresentations include brow, face, shoulder (transverse lie), breech, and compound presentation
2. With brow presentation, fetal forehead is presenting part; includes military presentation (fetal head is between flexion and extension) and occipitomental presentation (fetal head enters birth canal at widest diameter of head)
   a. Occurs more often in multiparas than nulliparas
   b. May be due to weakened or lax pelvic or abdominal musculature
   c. Many convert spontaneously to occipital or face presentations
   d. Maternal risks include longer labor and possible cesarean birth
   e. Neonatal risks include facial edema, bruising, exaggerated molding of head, and increased mortality from cerebral and neck compression, and damage to trachea and larynx
3. With face presentation, fetal head is hyperextended more than in brow presentation; occurs more often in multiparas, there is increased risk of prolonged labor and operative (cesarean) delivery
   a. Anticipate vaginal delivery if mother's pelvis is adequate and infant's chin (mentum) is in anterior position
   NCLEX® b. Anticipate cesarean delivery if mentum is posterior and does not rotate to anterior in late stages of labor, or if signs of fetal distress occur
   NCLEX® c. Do not place fetal monitor electrode on presenting part (infant's face); requires external fetal heart rate (FHR) monitoring
   NCLEX® d. Edema and bruising of face, eyes, and lips are common; prepare clients for this before seeing infant for first time

4. Breech presentations
   a. Three types (see Figure 46–1)
   b. Is frequently associated with preterm birth, placenta previa, hydramnios, multiple gestation, uterine anomalies, and fetal anomalies such as anencephaly and hydrocephaly

   NCLEX®
   c. Maternal concern is increased likelihood of cesarean delivery, while fetal risks include compressed or prolapsed umbilical cord, entrapment of fetal head in incompletely dilated cervix, risk of cervical cord injury from hyperextension of fetal head during birth, aspiration and asphyxia at birth, and birth trauma from manipulation and use of forceps to free fetal head

   NCLEX®
   d. Current therapy includes using **external cephalic version** (ECV) at 36–38 weeks, which involves manipulating fetus through abdominal wall to convert from breech (or shoulder) to cephalic presentation prior to onset of labor
   e. Collaborative management during ECV includes applying external fetal monitor, starting IV fluids, administering terbutaline (Brethine) via a piggybacked IV line to relax uterine muscle, closely monitoring FHR during version attempt, and discontinuing version if undue maternal or fetal distress occurs
   f. **Cesarean section**: most breech presentations are delivered by planned cesarean section (abdominal delivery) to reduce risk of complications
5. Shoulder presentation (transverse lie): acromium process is presenting part
   a. Occurs more often with grand multiparity with relaxed uterine muscles, preterm fetus, abnormal uterus, placenta previa, excess amniotic fluid, and contracted pelvis
   b. ECV is attempted at 36–37 weeks, because of significant risk of prolapsed cord; is followed by induction of labor if successful

   NCLEX®
   c. Vaginal delivery is not considered possible in term infant; cesarean birth is preferred method of delivery
6. Compound presentations: more than one part of fetus presents
   a. Most common type is a hand or arm prolapsing beside head

   NCLEX®
   b. Risk of cord compression and prolapse is increased
   c. Vaginal versus cesarean delivery depends on size of fetus, presence of fetal distress, and progress in labor

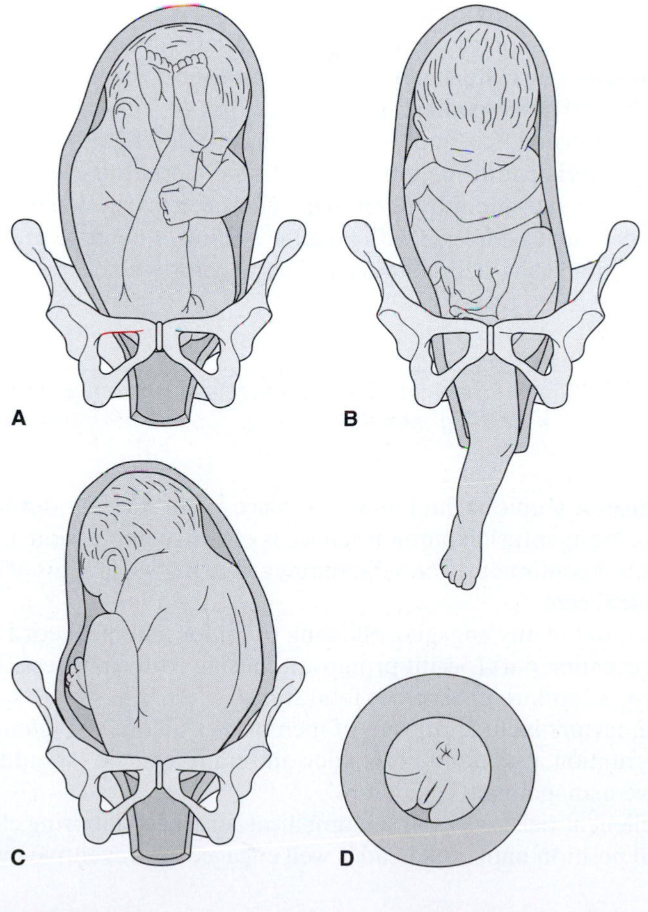

Figure 46–1

Breech presentation. *A.* Frank breech: sacrum is presenting part, knees extended. *B.* Incomplete (footling) breech: one or both feet presenting, increasing risk of umbilical cord prolapse. *C.* Complete breech: sacrum is presenting part, knees flexed, left sacral anterior position shown. *D.* On vaginal exam, nurse may feel anal sphincter; tissue of fetal buttocks feels soft.

7. Collaborative management of clients with fetal malpresentations
   NCLEX® a. Leopold's maneuvers may help detect abnormal presentation
   NCLEX® b. Observe closely for abnormal labor patterns; monitor FHR and contractions continuously
   c. Provide client and family teaching, client support and encouragement
   d. Anticipate forceps-assisted birth
   e. Anticipate cesarean birth for incomplete breech, shoulder, or posterior chin presentations
   f. Be prepared for childbirth emergencies such as neonatal resuscitation

C. Nonreassuring fetal status (fetal distress): transient or chronic insufficient oxygen supply to meet demands of fetus

1. Causes include compression of umbilical cord and uteroplacental insufficiency (from placental abnormalities or maternal condition)
2. Most common initial signs are variations from normal FHR pattern and decreased fetal movement; other signs are meconium-stained (green-tinged) amniotic fluid (excluding breech presentation)
3. Changes in FHR baseline
   NCLEX® a. Tachycardia (above 160): early sign of distress
   b. Bradycardia (below 110): late sign of distress
4. Decreased or absence of variability of heart rate
   a. Heart rate varies less than 2 to 5 beats per minute (bpm), causing a flattened appearance to heart rate
   b. Indicates depression of the autonomic nervous system that controls heart rate
   c. Fetal sleep, sedation, and hypoxia may affect variability
5. Late deceleration pattern
   NCLEX® a. FHR slows following peak of contraction and slowly returns to baseline rate during resting phase
   b. Indicates fetal response to hypoxia from uteroplacental insufficiency
   c. Considered an omnious pattern regardless of depth of deceleration of FHR and requires immediate intervention
6. Severe variable deceleration pattern
   NCLEX® a. FHR repeatedly decelerates below 90 bpm for more than 60 seconds before returning to baseline
   b. Indicates interference of fetal blood flow from cord compression
   c. Leads to fetal hypoxia and low APGAR scores unless corrective steps taken
7. Collaborative management
   a. Monitor FHR baseline, variability, and pattern of periodic changes; evaluate results of fetal acoustic stimulation test (FAST) or scalp stimulation test (SST) for acceleration with sound or manual stimulation (a reassuring result)
   b. Monitor contraction pattern and maternal response to labor
   NCLEX® c. Institute **intrauterine resuscitation** (corrective measures to improve oxygen exchange within maternal-fetal circulation) based on FHR pattern (see Box 46–1); for late deceleration, take steps to improve uteroplacental blood flow and for severe variable deceleration, take steps to relieve cord compression
   d. Provide appropriate information and emotional support to client and family
   e. Maintain continuous monitoring of FHR, uterine activity, and labor progress
   NCLEX® f. Prevent meconium aspiration with possible suction of neonate's nasopharynx prior to delivery of chest and abdomen; visualize larynx and vocal cords with deep suction immediately after delivery and before first breath is taken

Memory Aid

To correctly perform nasotracheal suction on an infant, slightly hyperextend head to a "sniffing" position with chin up and head tilted back slightly.

   g. **Amnioinfusion**: amniotic fluid may be replaced with warmed sterile saline through an intrauterine catheter using an infusion pump when signs of cord compression are present during labor; monitor FHR monitor continuously and discontinue infusion when signs of cord compression disappear

D. Prolapsed umbilical cord

1. Cause: fetus is not firmly engaged, allowing room for umbilical cord to move beyond (prolapse) or alongside presenting part (occult prolapse), causing cord compression that can lead to decreased oxygen transport and nonreassuring fetal status
2. Contributing factors include rupture of membranes before engagement of presenting part, small fetus, breech presentation, multifetal pregnancy, and transverse lie (shoulder presentation)
3. Collaborative management
   a. Identify client at risk for prolapsed umbilical cord; keep laboring client with ruptured membranes in horizontal position until fetal head is well engaged as preventive measure

Box 46-1

Nursing Management of Nonreassuring Fetal Status

Late decelerations (uteroplacental insufficiency)
Goal is to improve maternal blood flow to placenta

- Reposition mother on her left side
- Administer O_2 by face mask at 8–10 L/min
- Maintain continuous electronic fetal monitoring
- Increase IV fluids
- Discontinue oxytocin infusion if labor is being induced
- Notify health care provider immediately

Severe variable decelerations or prolonged bradycardia (cord compression)
Goal is to relieve pressure on umbilical cord

- Reposition mother on either side; if no improvement, reposition to opposite side
- Administer O_2 by face mask at 8–10 L/min
- Trendelenburg or knee-chest position if not corrected
- Perform vaginal examination and apply upward digital pressure on presenting part to relieve pressure on umbilical cord

NCLEX® b. Place mother's hips higher than head: either knee-chest or Trendelenburg position
c. Administer O_2 by face mask at 8–10 L/min
d. Maintain continuous electronic fetal monitoring
NCLEX® e. Perform sterile vaginal exam, pushing fetal presenting part upward with fingers to relieve pressure on cord until physician or midwife arrives
NCLEX® f. If cord protrudes through vagina, determine that pulsation is present and wrap cord loosely with warm sterile saline soaked towel or dressing to prevent drying; do not allow dressing or towel to cool, which could cause spasms of umbilical cord vessels and decrease fetal oxygenation
g. Prepare for rapid delivery vaginally or by cesarean section

E. Macrosomia

1. A fetal weight of more than 4500 grams at birth (some sources indicate 4000 grams)
2. More common with prepregnancy maternal obesity, excessive maternal weight gain, grand multiparity, prolonged gestation and maternal diabetes mellitus
3. Maternal risks include cephalopelvic disproportion (CPD), dysfunctional or prolonged labor, soft-tissue lacerations during vaginal birth, and postpartum hemorrhage
4. Fetal risks include asphyxia, meconium aspiration, shoulder dystocia, upper brachial plexus injury and fractured clavicles, hypoglycemia, polycythemia, and hyperbilirubinemia
5. Cesarean delivery is planned for fetus weighing 4500 grams or more, with mixed views about vaginal versus cesarean birth if weight is 4000–4500 grams

III. PROBLEMS WITH PELVIC STRUCTURES

A. *Cephalopelvic disproportion (CPD)*

1. Occurs when fetal head is larger than bony maternal pelvis (at inlet, outlet or between these) and cannot pass through birth canal
2. Android and platypelloid pelvic types predispose to CPD
3. Contracted pelvic inlet: anterior–posterior diameter less than 10 centimeters (cm); transverse diameter less than 12 cm
   a. Makes engagement difficult
   b. Influences fetal position and presentation
4. Contracted midpelvic plane: interspinous diameter less than 9.5 cm
   a. Hampers internal rotation of fetal head
   b. Secondary arrest of dilatation or arrest of descent of fetal head occurs
5. Contracted pelvic outlet: interischial tuberous diameter less than 8 cm

NCLEX® 6. Signs and symptoms: fetal head does not descend despite strong contractions
7. Maternal risks include prolonged labor, exhaustion, hemorrhage, and infection
8. Fetal risks include hypoxia and birth trauma

9. **Trial of labor (TOL)**: physician may allow labor to continue or may even stimulate labor with oxytocin when pelvic measurements are borderline to see if fetal head will descend, making vaginal delivery possible; if progressive changes in dilatation and station do not occur, or if obvious CPD is present, a cesarean delivery is performed

B. Shoulder dystocia: an obstetric emergency resulting from difficulty or inability to deliver shoulders

1. Inability to deliver shoulders leads to fetal hypoxia and death; fetal macrosomia increases risk
NCLEX® 2. Maternal risks: lacerations and tears of birth canal and postpartum hemorrhage
NCLEX® 3. Neonatal risks: hypoxia, fractures of clavicle, and injury to neck and head
4. Collaborative management
   a. Identify client at risk for shoulder dystocia: obesity, increased fundal height, history of macrosomia, maternal diabetes or gestational diabetes, prolonged second-stage labor
   NCLEX® b. Assist with positioning during delivery: use McRoberts maneuver, flexing thighs up onto abdomen to change angle of pelvis, increase pelvic diameters, and facilitate delivery of shoulders
   c. Monitor for maternal and newborn injury following delivery

IV. PROBLEMS WITH UTERINE CONTRACTIONS

A. *Induction of labor*

1. Methods consist of pharmacologic (see also Chapter 31) and nonpharmacologic measures to initiate contractions and cervical change
2. Cervical ripening with prostaglandins gel (Cervidil), misoprostol (Cytotec) or with laminaria (hydrophilic agent): when inserted into cervix, absorbs water from cervical mucus, expands, and dilates cervix
3. **Amniotomy** or artificial rupture of membranes (AROM)
   NCLEX® a. Auscultate FHR prior to and immediately after AROM to detect prolapse of umbilical cord or fetal distress
   NCLEX® b. Take maternal temperature every 1–2 hours after AROM to detect infection

Memory Aid

Remember that *-otomy* means "cutting into"; amniotomy is thus artificial rupture of amniotic membranes.

4. Misoprostol (Cytotec)
   a. A synthetic prostaglandin agent administered intravaginally and/or orally to stimulate onset of contractions
   b. Continuous monitoring of FHR, uterine activity, and maternal vital signs (VS) is essential
5. Oxytocin (Pitocin) administration (see also Chapter 31)
   a. Use **Bishop score** to determine maternal readiness for induction by determining dilatation, effacement, station, cervical consistency, and position of cervix
   NCLEX® b. Begin external fetal monitoring and monitor FHR closely throughout induction
   NCLEX® c. Monitor and record maternal VS, intake and output (I&O), and contraction frequency and intensity
   NCLEX® d. Always administer using IV infusion pump for safety; stop infusion immediately if contractions are closer than 2 minutes, last longer than 90 seconds, or for any indication of fetal distress
6. Absolute contraindications to induction of labor
   a. Placenta previa
   b. Transverse lie and other fetal malpresentations
   c. Prior classic uterine incision
   d. Pelvic structure abnormality
   e. Prolapsed umbilical cord
   f. Active genital herpes
   g. Invasive cervical cancer

B. *Dystocia* or difficult labor

1. **Hypertonic labor pattern**: poor quality, ineffective uterine contractions occur in latent phase of labor, with increased uterine resting tone; contractions often become more frequent but have decreased intensity and are ineffective in dilating and effacing cervix
   a. Maternal risks are prolonged or nonprogressive labor, pain, fatigue and stress

b. Fetal risks include hypoxia caused by decreased uteroplacental blood flow and possible prolonged pressure on fetal head (leading to cephalhematoma, caput succedaneum, excessive molding)
c. Medical treatment includes bed rest and sedation to stop contractions, reduce pain, and allow a normal labor pattern to develop; if unsuccessful, oxytocin infusion or amniotomy may be considered after CPD and fetal malpresentation are ruled out

NCLEX®
d. Provide hydration, monitor I&O, and promote relaxation

2. **Hypotonic labor pattern**: infrequent contractions with decreased intensity
   a. More commonly occurs in active phase of labor
   b. Maternal risks are maternal exhaustion, stress on coping ability, intrauterine infection if prolonged labor, and postpartum hemorrhage from insufficient uterine contractions after birth
   c. Fetal risks are nonreassuring fetal status from prolonged labor and fetal sepsis from pathogens ascending birth canal

NCLEX®
   d. Medical treatment includes ruling out CPD and initiating active management of labor (AMOL), which includes amniotomy, timed cervical exams and **augmentation of labor**, or stimulation of contractions, with oxytocin

3. Abnormal progress in labor: a **labor graph**, or **Friedman curve**, identifies deviations from normal progress in labor by plotting cervical dilatation and descent of fetal head over time
   a. Prolonged latent phase: more than 20 hours for nulliparous client or more than 14 hours for multiparous client; may indicate CPD; may be caused by false labor; medical treatment is sedation and rest
   b. Protracted active phase: dilatation less than 1.2 cm per hour in nulliparous client or less than 1.5 cm per hour in multiparous client; may be caused by malposition; check for CPD and fetal presentation and position
   c. Protracted descent: less than 1 cm per hour change in station in nulliparous client or less than 2 cm per hour in multiparous client; rule out CPD; monitor contraction intensity and duration; labor may be augmented with oxytocin
   d. Secondary arrest of dilatation: cessation of dilatation for more than 2 hours in nulliparous client or more than 1 hour in multiparous client; rule out CPD and, if absent, augment labor with oxytocin
   e. Arrest of descent: no progress in fetal station for more than 1 hour; check for CPD and, if absent, augment labor

4. Retraction rings
   a. Physiologic retraction ring is a boundary between upper and lower uterine segments that normally forms during labor; upper segment contracts and becomes thicker as muscle fibers shorten; lower segment distends and becomes thinner

NCLEX®
   b. Bandl's ring: a pathological retraction ring that forms when labor is obstructed due to CPD or other complications; upper segment continues to thicken while lower segment continues to distend; risk of uterine rupture increases if contractions continue, so cesarean delivery is indicated
   c. Constriction ring: retraction ring forms and impedes fetal descent; relaxation of constriction ring with analgesics, anesthetics, or both allows vaginal delivery

C. Premature labor: contractions occurring between 20 to 37 weeks' gestation

1. Reinforce client teaching to prevent preterm labor
   a. Rest 2–3 times daily lying on left side
   b. Drink 2–3 quarts of liquid each day; avoid caffeine
   c. Void every 2 hours or more during waking hours
   d. Avoid lifting heavy objects; pace activities to avoid overexertion
   e. Avoid prenatal breast preparation (nipple-rolling or rubbing with towel) or nipple stimulation during sexual activity to reduce uterine irritability

NCLEX®
2. Reinforce client teaching about signs and symptoms of premature labor
   a. Contractions occurring every 10 minutes or less with or without pain
   b. Low abdominal cramping with or without diarrhea
   c. Intermittent sensation of pelvic pressure, urinary frequency
   d. Low backache (constant or intermittent)
   e. Increased vaginal discharge, may be pink-tinged
   f. Leaking amniotic fluid

NCLEX®
3. Immediate actions to be taken by clients experiencing suspected premature labor
   a. Empty bladder
   b. Assume a side-lying position, left preferred
   c. Drink 3 to 4 cups of water
   d. Palpate abdomen for uterine contractions; if 10 minutes apart or closer, contact health care provider

e. Rest for 30 minutes and slowly resume activity if symptoms disappear
f. If symptoms do not subside within 1 hour, contact health care provider

4. Medical management
   a. Bedrest
   b. Continued monitoring of uterine activity and FHR
   NCLEX® c. Administer ordered **tocolytic agents**, drugs to stop contractions, if labor continues (see also Chapter 31), including ritodrine (Yutopar), terbutaline (Brethine), and magnesium sulfate
   NCLEX® d. Administration of betamethasone (Celestone) or dexamethasone to stimulate fetal lung maturity
5. Collaborative management
   a. Identify clients at risk for premature labor
   b. Provide client and family teaching regarding signs and management of premature labor
   NCLEX® c. Promote bedrest encouraging left lateral position
   NCLEX® d. Monitor uterine activity and FHR
   e. Administer tocolytics and monitor for adverse reactions
   f. Provide emotional support encouraging client and family to express feelings and concerns

D. ***Premature labor***: labor lasting less than 3 hours and resulting in rapid birth

1. Contributing factors include multiparity, large pelvis, previous **precipitous labor**, small fetus in favorable position, and recent maternal cocaine use
2. *NCLEX®* Maternal risks: cervical, vaginal, or rectal lacerations and postpartum hemorrhage from undetected lacerations or inadequate uterine contractions after birth
3. *NCLEX®* Fetal risks: hypoxia (decreased perfusion to intervillous spaces), cerebral trauma and brachial plexus injuries from rapid descent through birth canal
4. Collaborative management
   a. Identify client at risk for precipitous labor and birth
   NCLEX® b. Do not leave client; send someone or call for help
   c. Don sterile gloves if time allows
   d. Instruct client to pant or blow to decrease urge to push
   NCLEX® e. Support perineum with a sterile towel as crowning occurs
   NCLEX® f. Apply gentle pressure on fetal head to prevent rapid delivery; lacerations of perineum can occur and subdural or dural tears may occur with sudden expulsion of infant's head

Memory Aid

Remember to "protect the head" during a precipitous birth. Apply enough pressure to guide the descent and prevent rapid intracranial pressure changes within the infant's molded skull.

   NCLEX® g. After delivery of head, suction infant's mouth then nose with bulb syringe
   NCLEX® h. Check around infant's neck for possible tight umbilical cord; if present, cord must be clamped and cut before delivery

Memory Aid

Remember that an umbilical cord could choke the fetus and is dangerous. If, during delivery, it can't be loosened and slipped away from infant's neck, two clamps should be applied to cord and cord should be cut between these clamps.

   i. Place hands on each side of infant's head and instruct client to push
   j. Gentle downward pressure facilitates birth of anterior shoulder
   k. Gentle upward traction facilitates birth of posterior shoulder
   l. Support infant's body with a towel during expulsion from birth canal
   m. Suction and dry infant thoroughly
   n. Place infant on mother's abdomen as soon as stable
   o. Clamp and cut umbilical cord
   p. Observe for signs of placental separation: gush of bright blood; lengthening of the cord
   q. Gently pull cord while massaging fundus to deliver placenta
   NCLEX® r. Continue to massage fundus to prevent hemorrhage or put infant to breast
   s. Inspect perineum for lacerations or tears

E. Prolonged (postterm) pregnancy

1. Extends more than 294 days or 42 weeks past first day of last menstrual period (2 weeks past estimated date of birth at 40 weeks)
2. Maternal risks include probable labor induction, increased risk for large-for-gestational-age (LGA) infant and subsequent perineal trauma, increased risk of infection, and increased risk of forceps-assisted, vacuum-assisted, or cesarean delivery
3. Fetal risks include decreased placental perfusion, oligohydramnios (less amniotic fluid), meconium aspiration, and low 5-minute Apgar score
4. Treatment includes nonstress test (NST) and biophysical profile (BPP) 2–3 times weekly to evaluate fetal well-being, and induction of labor (some prefer this at 41 weeks) or cesarean delivery

F. Uterine prolapse

1. Vigorous massage of fundus and pulling on umbilical cord to speed placental separation may cause prolapse of cervix and lower uterine segment through introitus
2. **Uterine inversion**: turning inside out of uterus; may be complete (visible outside introitus) or incomplete (partially inverted and not visible): either can result in hemorrhage and shock and requires correction manually by physician

G. *Uterine rupture:* tearing open or separation of uterine wall

NCLEX® 1. Rare but serious complication, caused by separation of scar from previous classical cesarean, uterine trauma, intense uterine contractions, overstimulation of labor with oxytocin, difficult forceps-assisted birth, and external cephalic or internal version
2. Risk factors: multiparity, overdistension of uterus with multifetal pregnancy, malpresentation, or previous uterine surgery
3. Types
   a. Complete: extends through uterine wall into peritoneal cavity
   b. Incomplete: extends into peritoneum but not into peritoneal cavity; often due to partial separation of cesarean scar; may go unnoticed until repeat cesarean is performed
4. Collaborative management
   a. Attempt to prevent by identifying clients at risk and avoiding hyperstimulation of uterus during induction
   NCLEX® b. May be silent or have dramatic signs and symptoms: sudden, sharp, lower abdominal pain, tearing sensation, signs of shock, cessation of contractions, cessation of FHR
   c. Note that blood loss is often concealed and that fetal parts may be easily palpated through abdominal wall

NCLEX® 5. Specific medical management: complete rupture requires management of shock, blood transfusion, and hysterectomy, while incomplete rupture may require laparotomy, repair, and blood transfusion

V. PROBLEMS WITH MATERNAL PSYCHOLOGICAL STATUS

A. Factors influencing psyche of client in labor

1. Fear, anxiety, and perception of situation
2. Self-image
3. Preparation for childbirth
4. Support systems and coping ability
5. Underlying psychological disorder such as depression or anxiety

B. Effects of fear and anxiety on labor progress

1. Epinephrine secreted in response to stress
2. Vascular changes divert blood from uterus to skeletal muscles
3. Oxygen and glucose supplies decrease with accumulation of lactic acid in uterine muscle
4. Higher perception of pain
5. Decrease in available energy supply to support effective contractions
6. Labor progress is slowed

C. Collaborative management

1. Review client's past experiences with, preparation for, and expectations of labor and birth

NCLEX® 2. Observe client's current coping behaviors and their effectiveness with current situation; expect client with a psychological disorder to exhibit behaviors characteristic of disorder, although they may be exaggerated
3. Establish trusting relationship with client and family

NCLEX® 4. Remain at bedside with client and family as able during labor
5. Encourage relaxation
6. Keep client and family informed about progress and procedures

NCLEX®

7. Encourage positive coping behaviors and discourage negative ones
8. Promote self-image by praising efforts

VI. CESAREAN DELIVERY

A. Overview

1. Is delivery of infant by an abdominal incision
2. Purpose is to facilitate delivery to preserve health of mother and fetus
3. Major indications for cesarean delivery include dystocia or CPD, fetal distress, fetal malpresentation, and previous cesarean birth

NCLEX®

B. Maternal risks

1. Aspiration or pulmonary embolism
2. Hemorrhage or infection
3. Injury to bowel or bladder
4. Thrombophlebitis

NCLEX®

C. Fetal/neonatal risks

1. Prematurity
2. Injury at birth
3. Respiratory problems caused by delayed absorption of fetal lung fluid

D. Surgical techniques

1. Skin incisions: vertical or transverse (Pfannenstiel)
2. Uterine incisions
   a. Classical: through upper uterine segment
   b. Low transverse cervical: in lower uterine segment (Kerr incision)
   c. Lower uterine segment vertical (Selheim incision)

E. Collaborative management

1. Determine reason for cesarean delivery
2. Determine client's understanding of indication, procedure, and implications for recovery from abdominal delivery
3. Determine whether cesarean birth was discussed in childbirth preparation classes
   a. Clients and families cope better if they have time to learn about cesarean birth
   b. Emergency cesarean birth increases anxiety and alters couple's expectations about childbirth

NCLEX®

4. Preoperative care
   a. Institute NPO status (being NPO decreases risk of aspiration)
   b. Explain procedure so that client and family know what to expect
   c. Obtain client signature on consent form
   d. Perform abdominal prep
   e. Insert urinary catheter to prevent bladder trauma during surgery
   f. Start IV fluids using a large bore catheter
   g. Administer an antacid PO or agent to lower gastric acidity IV to decrease risk of lung damage from aspirating acidic gastric contents during surgery
   h. Administer antibiotics as ordered
   i. Assist with positioning and administration of regional anesthesia if used
5. Intraoperative care

   NCLEX®

   a. Provide heated crib and supplies to receive newborn
   b. Provide immediate care to newborn or assist nursery personnel as needed
   c. Provide assistance to surgical team and immediate care for mother

NCLEX®

6. Postoperative care
   a. Begin postanesthesia (recovery room) monitoring of VS, pulse oximetry, and cardiac monitoring; monitor VS every 15 minutes for first hour and until stable
   b. Monitor fundus for firmness and location (if boggy, massage until firm); monitor vaginal bleeding
   c. Observe abdominal dressing
   d. Observe urinary catheter and urine output
   e. Apply and maintain sequential compression devices (SCDs) to prevent deep vein thrombosis
   f. Turn, cough, and deep breathe hourly
   g. Monitor for return of sensation post-anesthesia
   h. Administer medications for pain as needed
   i. Administer maternal–infant contact and bonding

F. *Trial of labor after cesarean (TOLAC)*

1. Labor and vaginal birth after a previous cesarean is considered a safe option if indication for cesarean delivery is not likely to be repeated
2. Contraindications
   a. Previous classical incision into uterus
   b. Large infant (over 4000 grams)
   c. Malpresentation
   d. Pelvic measurements inadequate
   e. Any fetal or placental problem that may require cesarean section
   f. Delivery in an alternative birth setting: access to a facility where emergency cesarean may be performed is necessary

NCLEX®

3. Risks of TOLAC
   a. Possible uterine rupture and hemorrhage: less likely to occur if previous uterine incision was in the lower uterine segment
   b. Failure of trial of labor, requiring a repeat cesarean
4. Benefits of TOLAC
   a. Ability to experience labor and vaginal delivery (desired by some clients)
   b. Vaginal delivery is less costly than cesarean delivery with faster, easier recovery period and less risk of complications
   c. Does not preclude induction or augmentation of labor
5. Collaborative management
   a. (NCLEX®) Monitor uterine activity and progress in labor; identify deviations from normal progress in labor and report to physician (essential)
   b. (NCLEX®) Monitor FHR and response to contractions, identify and report indications of fetal distress quickly
   c. Provide teaching before onset of labor that early period of labor carries greatest risk of uterine rupture for TOLAC clients
   d. (NCLEX®) Observe for indications of uterine rupture, including signs of shock or hemorrhage, report of "ripping or tearing" sensation or sharp uterine pain, abrupt cessation of contractions, abrupt onset of fetal distress, and more easily palpable fetus (lying outside uterus)
   e. Be alert and prepared for possible emergency cesarean delivery
   f. Provide support and encouragement for client attempting TOLAC

Check Your NCLEX–PN® Exam I.Q. *You are ready for testing on this content if you can*

- Monitor the client experiencing complications of labor and delivery.
- Provide care to the client experiencing complications of labor and delivery.
- Take action to prevent fetal distress during complications of labor and delivery.
- Evaluate client's response to interventions to treat complications of labor and delivery.
- Communicate effectively to increase client and family understanding of complications of labor and delivery.

PRACTICE TEST

1 The nurse caring for a high-risk client in labor observes the presence of variability of the fetal heart rate (FHR) of 10–12 beats per minute as recorded by the internal fetal monitor. What interpretation should the nurse make about the fetal condition or state?

1. Fetal hypoxia
2. Fetal well-being
3. Umbilical cord compression
4. Uteroplacental insufficiency

2 The nurse locates fetal heart tones in the right upper quadrant of the abdomen. This finding should cause suspicion that the fetus is in what presentation?

1. Occiput posterior
2. Occiput transverse
3. Breech
4. Shoulder

3 A client's contractions have become less frequent and less intense in the past hour. Vaginal examination reveals 6 cm dilatation and 0 station, which is unchanged since the last examination over 2 hours ago. The nurse understands that which action needs to be taken at this time?

1. Notify the physician of the last exam.
2. Continue to observe for one hour for further progress.
3. Encourage the client to turn on her side and rest.
4. Prepare for cesarean delivery.

4 The nurse is assisting in the delivery of a client whose infant has shoulder dystocia. How should the nurse have the client move to perform McRoberts maneuver to assist with delivery?

1. Flex the thighs against the abdomen
2. Place her legs in stirrups
3. Assume a side-lying position for delivery
4. Sit upright for delivery

5 The nurse reinforces an explanation to a client with premature labor that betamethasone (Celestone) will be administered for which purpose?

1. Stop uterine contractions
2. Prevent infection
3. Hasten fetal lung maturity
4. Prevent cervical dilatation

6 After reinforcing teaching with the pregnant client and her husband about premature labor, the nurse recognizes the instruction was effective when the client makes which statement? Select all that apply.

1. "I will call the office if I notice excessive fetal movement."
2. "I will call the office if I have back pain that does not go away."
3. "I will lie down and rest awhile if I notice watery vaginal discharge."
4. "I will call the office for abdominal cramps or pressure that don't stop after I drink 3–4 cups of liquid and rest for an hour."
5. "I don't need to worry about occasional irregular contractions."

7 The client is admitted in active labor with a breech presentation. Which sign would indicate to the nurse that there is fetal distress?

1. Meconium-stained amniotic fluid
2. Fetal heart rate (FHR) of 180 beats/minute
3. Mild variable decelerations
4. Increased FHR variability

8 The labor graph (Friedman curve) shows that a nulliparous client has not made any progress in cervical dilatation or station since she was 7 cm and 0 station over 2 hours ago. What would this information represent to the nurse?

1. A prolonged deceleration phase
2. Protracted active phase
3. Arrest of descent
4. Secondary arrest of dilatation

9 A client asks the nurse about the significance of the presence of a Bandl's ring, which the client overheard from the physician. What description would the nurse use when explaining this to the client?

1. A serious complication requiring cesarean section.
2. A constriction ring that could prolong labor.
3. The normal physiologic division between the upper and lower uterine segments.
4. An abnormal depression in the lower uterine segment.

10 The client in labor says she was told she is having hypertonic uterine contractions but does not understand how these could harm the baby. How would the nurse explain the relationship between hypertonic contractions and risk of fetal distress?

1. Maternal exhaustion occurs, producing a build-up of lactic acid.
2. Umbilical cord compression occurs, decreasing oxygen supply to the fetus.
3. Increased uterine tone and frequent contractions interfere with blood flow to fetus through the uterine arteries.
4. Placental separation can occur, which can be harmful to both mother and fetus.

11 After the initial care following amniotomy, the nurse should monitor which of the following data every 2 hours?

1. Maternal blood pressure and pulse
2. Fetal movement
3. Color and consistency of amniotic fluid
4. Oral temperature

12 Which condition of the pregnant client places her at increased risk for uterine inversion during the current labor and delivery?

1. Forceps delivery of a previous infant
2. Fundal pressure during delivery of the head and body
3. Precipitous birth of less than 3 hours' duration
4. Traction on the umbilical cord and vigorous fundal massage in the third stage

13 What is the priority goal of the nurse in helping a client during a complicated labor?

1. Establish a trusting relationship.
2. Ensure that the client knows what to expect.
3. Prevent invasion of privacy.
4. Prevent fear and anxiety.

14 A client asks what *trial of labor* means. What is the best response by the nurse?

1. "The doctor is giving you more time to make progress in labor before considering cesarean delivery."
2. "You will need to make progress in the next hour, or a cesarean delivery will be done."
3. "Even though your pelvis is small, sometimes it is possible to deliver your baby vaginally."
4. "A cesarean delivery will be done because you already went into labor and have not made much progress."

15 The nurse should suspect cephalopelvic disproportion (CPD) after noting documentation of which data for a laboring client?

1. Pelvic outlet is less than 9 cm.
2. Midpelvis is contracted.
3. Fetal shoulders are too large to pass through the bony pelvis.
4. Fetal head is too large to pass through the bony pelvis.

16 The nurse explains to a pregnant client at 37 weeks' gestation that a Bishop score is being completed to determine which of the following?

1. The client's readiness for labor
2. The fetus's readiness for labor
3. Progress during induction
4. Cervical changes in labor

17 Which of the following priority items should the nurse monitor due to the potential impact on the laboring client's psychological status?

1. Attitude about parenting
2. Relationship with the client's own mother
3. Self-image
4. Beliefs about health

18 A pregnant client in the active phase of labor has contractions that occur every 3–4 minutes, are 35-seconds' duration and have mild intensity. What conclusion about the client's status does the nurse draw from this data?

1. Hypertonic uterine dysfunction
2. Hypotonic uterine dysfunction
3. Normal uterine activity
4. Progressive labor pattern

19 In preparing the client in labor for vacuum extraction, it is important to reinforce that the infant might initially have which appearance after delivery? Select all that apply.

1. Edema of the caput
2. Red marks on the face
3. Edema of the face
4. Swelling of the eyes
5. Bruising of the scalp

20 The nurse should encourage the pregnant client not to push during vaginal delivery of a breech infant to avoid which of the following?

1. Prolapsed cord
2. Fetal distress
3. Fetal head entrapment
4. Cervical lacerations

ANSWERS & RATIONALES

1 **Answer: 2** **Rationale:** Variability of FHR indicates fetal well-being. The presence of variability is assessed by internal fetal monitoring, since there is less artifact that could be mistaken for variability of heart rate. Hypoxia can cause loss of variability of the FHR. Umbilical cord compression can cause severe variable decelerations or prolonged bradycardia of FHR. Uteroplacental insufficiency can cause late decelerations of FHR. **Cognitive Level:** Analyzing **Client Need:** Physiological Adaptation **Integrated Process:** Nursing Process: Data Collection **Content Area:** Maternal-Newborn **Strategy:** The core issue of the question is knowledge of the significance of variability in FHR. Recall that less or loss of variability may be a cause for concern, depending on the circumstances leading to it. Use nursing knowledge and the process of elimination to make a selection.

2 **Answer: 3** **Rationale:** Fetal heart tones are heard loudest over the fetal back. In breech presentation, this tends to be above the umbilicus. Fetal heart tones are heard just below the midline of the umbilicus in shoulder presentation or transverse lie. The terms occiput posterior and occiput transverse refer to head positions (fetal malpositions) rather than fetal malpresentations. **Cognitive Level:** Analyzing **Client Need:** Physiological Adaptation **Integrated Process:** Nursing Process: Data Collection **Content Area:** Maternal-Newborn **Strategy:** Specific knowledge related to fetal position and associated location of fetal heart sounds is needed to answer the question. Use nursing knowledge and the process of elimination to make your selection.

3 **Answer: 1** **Rationale:** The nurse should suspect cephalopelvic disproportion CPD because of the lack of progress since the last exam. The physician might assess the maternal pelvis by CT, MRI, or other means, or could stimulate contractions with oxytocin (Pitocin), opting for a trial of labor (TOL). Lack of progress could be caused by inadequate contractions, and a vaginal delivery could be possible, so it is too early to anticipate cesarean delivery. Encouraging rest and continued observation will do nothing to resolve the problem. **Cognitive Level:** Analyzing **Client Need:** Physiological Adaptation **Integrated Process:** Nursing Process: Implementation **Content Area:** Maternal-Newborn **Strategy:** The core issues of the question are recognition of lack of progress in labor and the nurse's decision-making ability once this is detected. Eliminate options that do nothing to help labor progress again, and choose notifying the physician over preparing for cesarean delivery because there is not enough information yet to indicate that cesarean delivery is needed.

4 **Answer: 1** **Rationale:** Flexing the thighs against the abdomen (McRoberts maneuver) increases the pelvic angle from symphysis pubis to sacrum, and facilitates delivery by making the bony pelvis less restrictive. Placing the legs in stirrups is not sufficient to make the bony pelvis less restrictive. Assuming a side-lying position or sitting upright for delivery will not make the bony pelvis less restrictive. **Cognitive Level:** Applying **Client Need:** Physiological Adaptation **Integrated Process:** Nursing Process: Implementation **Content Area:** Maternal-Newborn **Strategy:** Specific knowledge of the McRoberts maneuver is needed to answer this question. Use nursing knowledge and the process of elimination to make your selection.

5 **Answer: 3** **Rationale:** Corticosteroids such as betamethasone have been shown to enhance fetal lung maturity and prevent respiratory distress. Betamethasone does not stop labor or cervical changes. A side effect of betamethasone is increased risk of infection. **Cognitive Level:** Applying **Client Need:** Pharmacological and Parenteral Therapies **Integrated Process:** Nursing Process: Implementation **Content Area:** Maternal-Newborn **Strategy:** Specific knowledge of the purpose of betamethasone late in pregnancy is needed to answer this question. Use nursing knowledge and the process of elimination to make your selection.

6 **Answer: 2, 4, 5** **Rationale:** Signs of premature labor can include persistent back pain. The client should be instructed to empty her bladder, lie down on her side, and drink 3–4 cups of water. If symptoms do not disappear within an hour, the health care provider should be notified. Excessive fetal movement can sometimes indicate fetal distress, but is not a sign of premature labor. Watery vaginal discharge should be reported sooner rather than later after lying down and resting because the fluid could be amniotic fluid. Occasional irregular contractions are called Braxton Hicks contractions and are normal during pregnancy. **Cognitive Level:** Analyzing **Client Need:** Physiological Adaptation **Integrated Process:** Teaching and Learning **Content Area:** Maternal-Newborn **Strategy:** The wording of the question indicates that correct answers are options that contain a true statement. Eliminate the option with watery discharge, because this symptom should not be ignored and would not be relieved by rest. Eliminate the option about excessive movement because this is not of concern.

7 **Answer: 2** **Rationale:** An FHR greater than 160 beats per minutes is considered fetal tachycardia, an early sign of distress. Meconium passage often occurs in breech presentation because of pressure on the presenting part, and is not an indication of fetal distress in this situation. Mild variable decelerations and increased variability are not indications of fetal distress, and occur more frequently in breech presentations. **Cognitive Level:** Analyzing **Client Need:** Physiological Adaptation **Integrated Process:** Nursing Process: Data Collection **Content Area:** Maternal-Newborn **Strategy:** The core issue of this question is the ability to correlate knowledge of breech presentation with knowledge of fetal distress. Choose correctly by recalling that the normal FHR is 120–160 beats per minute. An FHR outside this range is generally a cause for concern regardless of the specific situation.

8 **Answer: 4** **Rationale:** Dilatation has stopped (arrested) after considerable progress. The cause could be hypotonic uterine contractions, malposition, or cephalopelvic disproportion. The terms *prolonged* and *protracted* when describing labor indicates that progress occurs at a very slow rate. Arrest of descent occurs when the station, rather than cervical dilatation, does not change. **Cognitive Level:** Analyzing **Client Need:** Physiological Adaptation **Integrated Process:** Nursing Process: Data Collection **Content Area:** Maternal-Newborn **Strategy:** Note the critical phrases *not made any progress* and *over 2 hours ago*. Correlate these phrases with the word *arrest* to eliminate options using the term *prolonged* or *protracted*. Choose *secondary arrest of dilation* because dilatation has not changed and because the word *secondary* implies that labor was active at one time, which is true in this case.

9 **Answer: 1 Rationale:** Bandl's ring forms when labor is obstructed. The upper uterine segment continues to thicken while the lower segment thins and retracts. If left untreated, uterine rupture can occur and thus it requires cesarean delivery. **Cognitive Level:** Understanding **Client Need:** Physiological Adaptation **Integrated Process:** Nursing Process: Implementation **Content Area:** Maternal-Newborn **Strategy:** Specific knowledge of Bandl's ring is needed to answer this question. Use nursing knowledge and the process of elimination to make your selection.

10 **Answer: 3 Rationale:** Frequent contractions and increased uterine muscle tone impede the blood flow through uterine arteries to the placenta. While maternal exhaustion and lactic acid accumulation can occur over time, they do not immediately threaten fetal well-being. The incidence of umbilical cord compression is not increased. Hypertonic contractions are not necessarily associated with placental separation. **Cognitive Level:** Applying **Client Need:** Physiological Adaptation **Integrated Process:** Communication and Documentation **Content Area:** Maternal-Newborn **Strategy:** The core issue of the question is how hypertonic uterine contractions affect fetal well-being. Eliminate maternal exhaustion and placental separation as least likely to happen, and then eliminate umbilical cord compression because this may or may not occur, depending on the position of the fetus.

11 **Answer: 4 Rationale:** The risk of infection is increased after amniotomy (rupture of membranes). The nurse should assess temperature every 2 hours. Blood pressure, pulse, and fetal movement are checked more often during active labor. Color and consistency of amniotic fluid are noted immediately after rupture, and each time the underpad is changed. **Cognitive Level:** Applying **Client Need:** Physiological Adaptation **Integrated Process:** Nursing Process: Data Collection **Content Area:** Maternal-Newborn **Strategy:** Recognize that the term *amniotomy* (*-otomy* means "cutting into") refers to artificial rupture of the membranes. Correlate this with increased risk for infection as a complication to choose temperature as the answer.

12 **Answer: 4 Rationale:** Although not always preventable, uterine inversion can occur because of excessive traction on the umbilical cord during the third stage of labor with or without vigorous fundal massage to remove the placenta, especially if the placenta is implanted in the fundus. Previous forceps delivery, fundal pressure during delivery of head and body, and precipitous birth are not associated with inversion. **Cognitive Level:** Analyzing **Client Need:** Physiological Adaptation **Integrated Process:** Nursing Process: Planning **Content Area:** Maternal-Newborn **Strategy:** Specific knowledge of the etiology and risks of uterine inversion is needed to answer this question. Use nursing knowledge and the process of elimination to make your selection.

13 **Answer: 1 Rationale:** Establishing a trusting relationship with the client and her family is a priority. A trusting relationship increases the likelihood of cooperation and compliance during a crisis. In an emergency situation such as a complicated labor, the nurse might have little time to ensure that the client knows what to expect, or to protect her privacy. It is not always possible to prevent fear and anxiety. **Cognitive Level:** Applying **Client Need:** Psychosocial Integrity **Integrated Process:** Nursing Process: Planning **Content Area:** Maternal-Newborn **Strategy:** Note the critical word *priority* in the question, which tells you all options might be partially or totally correct, and you must choose the most important one. A client experiencing a complicated labor is likely to experience both fear and lack of knowledge. Choose a trusting relationship over the others as it is the foundation for assisting the client through the labor process and reducing fear and lack of knowledge.

14 **Answer: 1 Rationale:** A trial of labor means that the client will be followed closely and given more time to show progress before considering a cesarean delivery. Placing a time limit of 1 hour or stating that vaginal delivery is sometimes possible makes cesarean delivery seem inevitable, and can increase the client's anxiety. Cesarean delivery is incorrect because the client will be allowed to continue laboring as long as some progress is made. **Cognitive Level:** Applying **Client Need:** Physiological Adaptation **Integrated Process:** Communication and Documentation **Content Area:** Maternal-Newborn **Strategy:** Recall the definition of the term *trial of labor*. Eliminate systematically those options that are not consistent with its meaning. The wording of the question indicates only one option is correct.

15 **Answer: 4 Rationale:** CPD means that the fetal head is too large to pass through the bony pelvis. A pelvic outlet of less than 9 cm and a contracted midpelvis refer to a smaller-than-normal pelvis, but do not take into account the fetal head size. Fetal shoulders that are too large to pass through the bony pelvis refers to shoulder dystocia. **Cognitive Level:** Analyzing **Client Need:** Physiological Adaptation **Integrated Process:** Nursing Process: Evaluation **Content Area:** Maternal-Newborn **Strategy:** Specific knowledge of CPD is needed to answer this question. Consider the word *disproportion* in the question to determine the correct answer must have two elements that are compared. Use nursing knowledge and the process of elimination to make your selection.

16 **Answer: 1 Rationale:** The Bishop score, an assessment of the mother's physical readiness for labor, takes into account cervical dilatation, effacement, consistency, cervical position, and station before contractions begin. The higher the score, the more likely a client can be successfully induced. The Bishop score does not evaluate the condition of the fetus, progress during labor, or cervical changes during labor. **Cognitive Level:** Analyzing **Client Need:** Physiological Adaptation **Integrated Process:** Nursing Process: Implementation **Content Area:** Maternal-Newborn **Strategy:** Recall that a Bishop score focuses primarily on the mother rather than the fetus, and on readiness for labor (rather than progress during labor) to choose correctly. Note also that the client in the question is at 37 weeks' gestation, which suggests that the client is not in labor.

17 **Answer: 3 Rationale:** Self-image refers to how a client feels about herself. A positive self-image enables a client to deal with labor and delivery realistically, even in the event of complications. Research has shown that self-image impacts the laboring client's psyche. Attitude about parenting, relationship with own mother, and health beliefs have not been identified as having a significant impact during labor. **Cognitive Level:** Analyzing **Client Need:** Psychosocial Integrity **Integrated Process:** Nursing Process: Data Collection **Content Area:** Maternal-Newborn **Strategy:** Note that the focus of the question is on the client in active labor. With this in mind,

choose the self-image option because it is the only one that specifically relates to the client's current status.

18 Answer: 2 Rationale: Hypotonic uterine dysfunction occurs most often during the active phase. It is characterized by contractions that have become further apart, less intense, and of shorter duration. Normal uterine contractions are typically 2–3 minutes apart, strong, and last 45–60 seconds in the active phase of labor. Hypertonic uterine dysfunction would be characterized by long, strong contractions with little resting time between contractions. A progressive labor pattern would show contractions that get longer, stronger, and closer together. **Cognitive Level:** Analyzing **Client Need:** Physiological Adaptation **Integrated Process:** Nursing Process: Data Collection **Content Area:** Maternal-Newborn **Strategy:** Note that the question contains the critical words *mild intensity* and *active phase*. Reasoning that active labor should be characterized by strong contractions, you would select hypotonic uterine contractions because it contains the word *hypotonic*. Alternatively, eliminate normal uterine activity and progressive labor pattern because they are similar, and eliminate hypertonic uterine dysfunction because the word *hypertonic* conveys the opposite of what the client in the question is experiencing.

19 Answer: 1, 5 Rationale: Suction applied over the occiput commonly causes edema and bruising of the scalp. Although it might appear to be a deformity of the fetal head, the edema disappears in 2–3 days and the bruising resolves more gradually. Suction is not applied to the face and thus would not cause facial red marks, facial edema, or swelling of the eyes. **Cognitive Level:** Applying **Client Need:** Physiological Adaptation **Integrated Process:** Nursing Process: Planning **Content Area:** Maternal-Newborn **Strategy:** Note the critical word *vacuum* in the stem of the question, and eliminate as incorrect any options that refer to a part of the face, rather than to the head itself.

20 Answer: 3 Rationale: Molding of the fetal head does not occur during labor in the breech presentation. The fetal body can pass through an incompletely dilated cervix, leaving the larger, firmer fetal head entrapped. The woman might feel a strong urge to push before complete dilatation due to pressure from the fetal body, increasing the risk of head entrapment. Prolapsed cord is a risk inherent with breech delivery whether the woman pushes or not. Fetal distress is a risk inherent with breech delivery whether the woman pushes or not. Cervical lacerations most often occur at the time of delivery from the application of forceps or manipulation of the fetus to deliver the after-coming head. **Cognitive Level:** Applying **Client Need:** Physiological Adaptation **Integrated Process:** Nursing Process: Planning **Content Area:** Maternal-Newborn **Strategy:** The core issue of the question is the risk from pushing during vaginal breech delivery. Eliminate two options because prolapsed cord and fetal distress are risks inherent with breech delivery whether the woman pushes or not. Eliminate a third because cervical lacerations most often occur at the time of delivery from the application of forceps or manipulation of the fetus to deliver the after-coming head, rather than from pushing.

Key Terms to Review

amnioinfusion p. 758
amniotomy p. 760
augmentation of labor p. 761
Bishop score p. 760
cephalopelvic disproportion (CPD) p. 759
cesarean section p. 757
dystocia p. 760
external cephalic version p. 757
hypertonic labor pattern p. 760
hypotonic labor pattern p. 761
induction of labor p. 760
intrauterine resuscitation p. 758
labor graph (Friedman's curve) p. 761
malpresentation p. 756
malposition p. 756
precipitous labor p. 762
premature labor p. 761
tocolytic agents p. 762
trial of labor after cesarean (TOLAC) p. 765
trial of labor (TOL) p. 760
uterine inversion p. 763
uterine rupture p. 763

References

Davidson, M., London, M., & Ladewig, P. (2012). *Olds' maternal newborn nursing and women's health across the lifespan* (9th ed.). Upper Saddle River, NJ: Pearson Education, Inc.

Ladewig, P., London, M., & Davidson, M. (2010). *Contemporary maternal-newborn nursing care* (7th ed.). Upper Saddle River, NJ: Pearson Education, Inc.

London, M., Ladewig, P., Ball, J., Bindler, R., & Cowen, K. (2011). *Maternal & child nursing care* (3rd ed.). Upper Saddle River, NJ: Pearson Education, Inc.

Perry, S., Hockenberry, M., Lowdermilk, D., & Wilson, D. (2010). *Maternal child nursing care* (4th ed.). St. Louis, MO: Elsevier.

Test Yourself

Are you ready for the NCLEX-PN® or course exams? Use the practice tests on the companion website to check.

Complicated Postpartum Care

47

In this chapter

Cross Reference

Other chapters relevant to this content area are

I. NURSING CARE OF HIGH-RISK POSTPARTUM CLIENT

NCLEX®

A. Data collection

1. Degree of homeostasis, amount of intrapartum blood loss, hematocrit, hemoglobin, and complete blood cell (CBC) count results
2. Vital signs: elevated temperature, blood pressure (BP), heart rate; low BP, symptoms of shock
3. Fundus: height, tone, and position
4. Lochia: amount, color, consistency, odor, and presence/size of clots (larger than quarter-size is of concern)
5. Perineum: edema, ecchymosis, pain, hemorrhoids
6. Bladder: distension and displacement, ability to void
7. Bowel: constipation, distended abdomen, decreased or absent bowel sounds (risk of ileus)
8. Breasts: cracked, bleeding, or blistered nipples; engorgement, red streaks, lumps, clogged milk ducts
9. Homan's sign (nonspecific), redness, tenderness, areas of heat in calves, severe abdominal or flank pain
10. Rest, activity tolerance
11. Bonding or attachment behaviors, maternal–infant interaction

B. Planning

1. Participate in developing a nursing care plan that reflects etiology, pathophysiology, and current clinical management for client experiencing a postpartum complication
2. Goals/expected outcomes of care: client will be free from undetected problems and will maintain physiological and psychosocial integrity

C. Implementation

1. Reinforce teaching to client about normal adaptation
2. Observe for actual or potential problems in immediate postpartum period (first 2 hours after delivery) and continue into later postpartum period
3. Administer treatment or medication as ordered
4. Reinforce client teaching about signs of complications prior to discharge
5. Reinforce importance of keeping appointment for postpartum check-up
6. Provide client with telephone numbers to call if questions arise

II. POSTPARTUM HEMORRHAGE

A. *Early-postpartum hemorrhage*

NCLEX® 1. Traditional definition: a blood loss greater than 500 mL in first 24 hours after vaginal delivery; may be greater with cesarean delivery; is currently being questioned because clinical estimates of blood loss may be underestimated by 50%; alternative criterion is decrease in hematocrit of 10% from admission to postbirth period

2. Predisposing factors: early postpartum hemorrhage occurs within first 24 hours of birth; at term, 600 mL/minute of blood perfuse pregnant uterus; most common causes are uterine atony (75%) and lacerations
3. Other causes include genital tract lacerations, episiotomy, retained placental fragments, hematomas (vulvar, vaginal, or subperitoneal), uterine inversion, uterine rupture, problems of placental implantation, and coagulation disorders
4. ***Uterine atony***
   - NCLEX® **a.** Description: lack of uterine muscle tone; after birth, contraction of interlacing uterine muscles occludes open areas at site of placental attachment; absent or ineffective uterine contractions can cause significant blood loss
   - NCLEX® **b.** Predisposing factors that overdistend uterus: delivery of a large infant (macrosomia), multiple gestation, hydramnios/polyhydramnios
   - NCLEX® **c.** Predisposing factors that affect uterine contractility: multiparity, precipitous labor, dysfunctional or prolonged labor, prolonged third stage of labor, retained placental fragments
   - **d.** Predisposing medications: general anesthesia, magnesium sulfate, oxytocin induction or augmentation of labor, tocolytics
   - **e.** Predisposing maternal condition: preeclampsia or placenta previa, coagulation disorders
5. Lacerations
   - **a.** Description: more common after operative obstetrics, a firm uterus with bright red blood or a steady stream or trickle of unclotted blood
   - **b.** Types/locations: perineal, vaginal, cervical
   - NCLEX® **c.** Predisposing factors: nulliparity, epidural anesthesia, precipitous childbirth (less than 3 hrs), macrosomia, forceps or vacuum-assisted birth, use of oxytocin
6. ***Hematoma***
   - **a.** Overview: a collection of blood, often vulvar or vaginal, that results from injury to a blood vessel during spontaneous delivery; in an assisted vaginal delivery, most common site is lateral wall in area of ischial spine; can rarely occur as subperitoneal (involves uterine artery branches or broad ligament blood vessels) but this is most dangerous because significant blood loss can occur without signs until client becomes hemodynamically unstable
   - NCLEX® **b.** Predisposing factors: preeclampsia, first full-term birth, prolonged pressure of fetal head on vaginal mucosa, forceps or vacuum-assisted births, prolonged second stage of labor, precipitous labor, macrosomia, pudendal anesthesia
7. Retained placental fragments
   - **a.** May be a cause of either early or late postpartum hemorrhage
   - **b.** Predisposing factor: partial separation of placenta during fundal massage before fundus spontaneously separates
8. ***Disseminated intravascular coagulopathy (DIC)***
   - **a.** Overview: complex disorder of clotting mechanisms in blood; consumption of clotting factors because of widespread clotting, leads to widespread and diffuse hemorrhage; oozing from puncture sites or development of petechiae may be initial clues of coagulopathy
   - NCLEX® **b.** Predisposing factors: preeclampsia, amniotic fluid embolism, sepsis, abruptio placentae, prolonged intrauterine fetal demise, excessive blood loss
9. Other causes of early postpartum hemorrhage: uterine rupture or uterine inversion

B. ***Late-postpartum hemorrhage***
1. **Subinvolution**: failure of uterus to return to normal size after pregnancy
NCLEX® 2. Late-postpartum hemorrhage occurs most often within 1–2 weeks after childbirth because of retained placental tissue; blood loss may be excessive but usually poses less risk than immediate postpartum hemorrhage
3. Lochia often fails to progress from rubra to serosa to alba normally; lochia rubra that exists longer than 2 weeks is suggestive of subinvolution
4. Subinvolution is most commonly diagnosed at 4- to 6-weeks postpartum exam

C. **Data collection**
NCLEX® 1. Review client's history and labor and delivery record for predisposing factors to postpartum hemorrhage
NCLEX® 2. Monitor vaginal bleeding after delivery every 10–15 minutes for 1 hour, then every 30 minutes for 1 hour until stable; more frequent assessments may be needed depending on condition
   a. Bleeding may be slow and continuous or rapid and profuse
   b. Blood may escape from vagina or pool in uterus and vagina, becoming evident as clots
NCLEX® c. Bleeding from a laceration occurs in presence of a firm uterus and may be noted as a slow, steady trickle
   d. Large and numerous clots may occur
NCLEX® e. Assist client to a side-lying position and check pad underneath frequently; blood may accumulate under client
   f. Weigh peri-pads to estimate blood loss if careful measurement is needed
NCLEX® 3. Palpate fundus for firmness, assess for height in relation to umbilicus and position
4. Monitor for signs of shock
5. Examine bladder for fullness and distension
6. Monitor for pelvic pain or backache

D. **Implementation**
1. Remain with client
NCLEX® 2. Massage boggy uterus gently but firmly, cupping uterus between two hands and avoiding overmassage
NCLEX® 3. Administer uterine stimulants as prescribed to prevent or manage uterine atony and hemorrhage; these often include oxytocin (Pitocin) IV or IM, methylergonovine maleate (Methergine) or ergonovine maleate (Ergotrate) IM or PO (commonly used for subinvolution); or prostaglandin (Hemabate) IM; hypertension is a common adverse effect; see Chapter 31 for additional information
4. If bleeding is excessive, health care provider may perform bimanual massage
NCLEX® 5. Monitor vital signs up to every 15 minutes as indicated, intake and output (I&O), level of consciousness (LOC), fundal tone and placement, and amount of bleeding during episode of acute hemorrhage; elevate legs 15 to 30 degrees (modified Trendelenburg position)
6. Initiate perineal pad counts if steady free flow of blood and possible pad weighing (1 mL=1 gram); also have client turn to side in bed to assess for pooling of blood underneath client
NCLEX® 7. Encourage frequent voiding to prevent bladder distension that contributes to uterine atony; a client may be catheterized during postpartum hemorrhage if unable to void
8. Monitor hematocrit values if available and notify provider if a decrease of 10% or more occurs
9. Replace fluids by IV and administer blood products as ordered
10. Provide adequate rest and assistance with self-care because of fatigue associated with anemia from blood loss; assist also with infant care or encourage partner to assist in client and infant care as appropriate
11. Assist with any preoperative preparation as necessary for surgical removal of placental fragments, ligation of bleeding vessel, suturing of laceration, or to correct more serious causes of bleeding, such as uterine rupture (see also Chapter 46)
12. Maintain asepsis
13. Ensure that surgical consent form is signed if necessary
14. Support significant other

III. POSTPARTUM INFECTIONS

A. **Reproductive tract infections (see Table 47–1)**
1. Overview: any infection in reproductive system within 6 weeks of delivery
2. Predisposing factors: prolonged rupture of amniotic membranes, obstetric trauma (episiotomy and lacerations of perineum, vagina, or cervix), invasive procedures including internal fetal monitoring, multiple vaginal examinations, retained placental fragments, chorioamnionitis, pre-existing bacterial

vaginosis, manual removal of placenta, use of forceps or vacuum-extraction, compromised health status (nutrition, anemia, obesity, smoking, alcohol or drug use), lapses in aseptic technique by staff

NCLEX® **3.** Cesarean delivery is single most significant risk (10 times greater than vaginal births)

4. Localized infections of perineum, vulva, and vagina

   a. Local infection may extend through venous circulation, resulting in infectious thrombophlebitis or septicemia

   b. Local infection may extend through lymphatic vessels, resulting in **pelvic cellulitis/parametritis**, an infection involving connective tissue of broad ligament or connective tissue of all pelvic structures

   c. Can lead to **peritonitis**, an infection involving peritoneal cavity

5. **Endometritis or endomyometritis**: localized infection of uterine lining, usually beginning at placental site; is more common after cesarean delivery; antibiotic prophylaxis at time of cord-clamping reduces incidence of postpartum endometritis in both elective and emergent cesarean sections

6. Bacterial causative agents are many and include *Escherichia coli*, *staphylococcus aureus*, *chlamydia trachomatis*, *beta-hemolytic streptococcus*, and others

7. Nursing data collection

NCLEX® **a.** Temperature higher than 100.4°F on any 2 of first 10 days postpartum excluding first 24 hours

NCLEX® **b.** Abnormal lochia: prolonged rubra phase, foul odor, scant or profuse in amount

   c. Tachycardia

   d. Delayed involution: fundal height does not descend as expected; uterus may feel larger and softer; pain or tenderness over uterus

   e. Pain, tenderness, or inflammation of perineum

   f. Backache, chills, malaise, and fatigue

NCLEX® **g.** Abnormal laboratory results: increased erythrocyte sedimentation rate (nonspecific indicator of inflammation); postpartum leukocytosis—white blood cell (WBC) level of 14,000 to 16,000/mm^3 is not unusual; an increase in WBC level greater than 30% in 6 hours indicates infection

8. Implementation

   a. Administer antibiotics, analgesics, and antipyretics as ordered

   b. Promote comfort; change linen frequently

NCLEX® **c.** Promote adequate nutrition and hydration (3000–4000 mL/day); monitor and record I&O

NCLEX® **d.** Use aseptic technique and good hand hygiene; provide frequent perineal care and educate client in correct technique

Table 47–1 Summary of Specific Reproductive System Infections and Associated Findings

Type of Infection	Findings
Metritis	Fever initially 101–102°F, (38.3–38.9°C); then sawtooth temperature elevations between 101 and 104°F (38.3 and 40°C) Uterine tenderness on palpation of fundus or on bimanual exam Grimacing, guarding, reports of pain; prolonged or bothersome afterpains Subinvolution of uterus Positive bacteria culture of lochia
Parametrial cellulitis (parametritis)	Prolonged elevation of temperature to 102–104°F (38.9–40°C) with fluctuations Abdominal pain extending laterally; possible rebound tenderness Hypotension, subinvolution, chills, decreased bowel sounds, nausea, and vomiting
Peritonitis	Elevated temperature up to 105°F (40.5°C) and severe pain Paralytic ileus and abdominal rigidity; frequent vomiting with dehydration Possibly weak and thready pulse; rapid, shallow respirations Excessive thirst and marked anxiety
Septic pelvic thrombophlebitis	Elevation of temperature to 105°F (40.5°C); dramatic fluctuations possible Pain in flank or lower abdomen
Bacteremia and septic shock	Rapid elevation of temperature to 103–104°F (39.4–40°C) Profuse, foul-smelling lochia Symptoms of shock, including urine output less than 30 mL/hr, tachycardia, hypotension

NCLEX®
e. Monitor vital signs; monitor laboratory results
f. Monitor fundus for involution and lochia; encourage semi-Fowler's position to facilitate drainage
g. Promote adequate rest and sleep; allow family and friends to visit per client's wishes
h. Encourage client to care for self first before caring for infant; allow client to care for and feed infant per client's condition; provide positive reinforcement

B. Wound infections

1. Description: infection of abdominal incision for cesarean delivery or episiotomy; infection rate following cesarean births is 3% to 5%, with highest rate occurring after emergency cesarean because of greater tissue trauma; culture of wound drainage commonly reveals mixed pathogens

NCLEX®
2. Predisposing factors: obesity, diabetes mellitus, prolonged postpartum hospitalization, premature rupture of membranes (PROM), metritis, prolonged labor, anemia, steroid therapy, immunosuppression
3. Nursing data collection

NCLEX®
a. REEDA assessment; see Box 47–1

Memory Aid

Use the mnemonic **REEDA!** See Box 47–1 to remember to inspect episiotomies and wounds for **r**edness, **e**dema, **e**cchymosis, **d**ischarge, and **a**pproximation of wound edges.

b. Generalized fever and/or induration (hardening) of site, localized tissue warmth
c. Tenderness

4. Implementation

NCLEX®
a. Monitor incision or episiotomy site every 8 to 12 hours for signs of infection; document and report adverse REEDA signs and induration
b. Assess vital signs; monitor laboratory results

NCLEX®
c. Use aseptic technique and good handwashing; provide frequent wound or perineal care; educate client in correct technique
d. Administer antibiotics, analgesics, and antipyretics as ordered

NCLEX®
e. Promote adequate nutrition and hydration (3000–4000 mL/day); monitor and record I&O
f. Promote comfort, change linen frequently
g. Promote adequate rest and sleep; allow family and friends to visit per client's wishes
h. Encourage client to care for self first before taking care of baby; allow client to care for and feed infant per client's condition; provide client positive reinforcement

C. Breast infection (*mastitis*)

1. Overview: an infection of breast connective tissue, primarily in women who are lactating; usual causative organisms are *Staphylococcus aureus*, *Escherichia coli*, *Haemophilus parainfluenzae*, *H. influenzae*, *Streptococcus* species, and occasionally *Candida albicans*
2. Predisposing factors
a. Traumatized tissue, fissured or cracked nipples
b. Engorgement, milk stasis or failure to empty breasts, missed feedings
c. Lowered maternal defenses caused by fatigue or stress
d. Poor hand hygiene practices or breasts not air-dried after feeding
e. Restrictive clothing or constricting or underwire bra

NCLEX®
3. Nursing data collection
a. Breast consistency, nipple condition
b. Warm, reddened, painful area on breast, often wedge-shaped

Box 47–1

REEDA Assessment

Redness: erythema around wound
Edema: swelling of tissues
Ecchymosis: skin discoloration
Discharge: purulent drainage from incision site
Approximation of skin edges: gaping of the wound edges

c. Axillary lymph nodes enlarged or tender
d. Flu-like symptoms (fever, chills, headache, muscle aches, and malaise)

4. Implementation
a. Culture and sensitivity of breast milk may be ordered (first 3 mL expressed and discarded before mid-stream sample obtained); note that infection usually is not transmitted to breast milk
b. Administer antibiotics (or antifungal if candida is responsible), analgesics compatible with breastfeeding, such as nonsteroidal anti-inflammatory drugs (NSAIDs), and antipyretics as ordered
NCLEX® c. Promote comfort: a well-fitting, supportive bra is needed 24 hours a day
d. Promote adequate nutrition, hydration, rest, and sleep; bedrest is ordered for at least 24 hours; increase fluid intake to 2–2.5 L/daily
e. Provide local application of warm moist-heat compresses for comfort
NCLEX® f. Remind mother and staff to use meticulous handwashing technique before handling breasts or assisting with breastfeeding; continue and increase breastfeeding as advised by health care provider
NCLEX® g. Reinforce teaching regarding breast care, proper positioning of infant on breast and latch on, let-down reflex, necessity for frequent breastfeeding, signs of complications, and telephone numbers client can call with questions, provide client positive reinforcement
NCLEX® h. Change position of infant for feeding to relieve pressure on same area of nipple; breastfeed frequently to prevent stasis of milk

D. *Urinary tract infections* (UTI)

1. Overview: can occur as **cystitis** (lower urinary tract infection) and often appears 2 to 3 days after birth, or as **pyelonephritis** (upper urinary tract infection); postdelivery urinary tract infections are usually caused by *E. coli* bacteria and generally occur soon after vaginal delivery

NCLEX® 2. Predisposing factors
a. Increased bladder capacity
b. Decreased bladder sensitivity from stretching or trauma
c. Possible inhibited neural control of bladder following use of general or regional anesthesia
d. Contamination from catheterization
e. Obesity

NCLEX® 3. Nursing data collection
a. Overdistension of bladder in early postpartum period
b. Frequent urination of small amounts, burning, dysuria
c. Hematuria
d. Elevated temperature; low-grade temperature occurs with cystitis, higher fever occurs with pyelonephritis
e. Flank pain, costovertebral angle tenderness, chills, nausea and vomiting (N/V) with pyelonephritis

4. Implementation
NCLEX® a. Monitor bladder frequently during recovery period to institute preventative measures
b. Culture and sensitivity of urine may be ordered prior to giving antibiotics
c. Administer antibiotics as ordered; commonly sulfamethoxazole/trimethoprim (Bactrim), nitrofurantoin (Macrobid) or amoxicillin-clavunate (Augmentin) if allergic to sulfa
d. Promote comfort; administer analgesic, antispasmodic, antipyretic medications
NCLEX® e. Promote nutrition and hydration; increase oral fluids to at least 8 to 10 8-ounce glasses daily, especially water, avoid carbonated beverages which increase alkalinity of urine, and increase acidity of urine with cranberry juice/tablets or vitamin C
f. Encourage voiding every 2–4 hours while awake; wear underwear with a cotton panel to facilitate air circulation
g. Measure vital signs, especially temperature and assess for resolution of symptoms

IV. THROMBOEMBOLIC DISORDERS

A. Overview

1. Usually occur antepartally but are often considered a postpartum complication
2. When thrombus forms in response to inflammation in vein wall, it is called **thrombophlebitis**; in this type of thrombosis, the clot is more firmly attached and is less likely to result in an embolism
3. Thromboembolic disorders are more likely to occur after a cesarean birth

B. Contributing factors

1. Increased amounts of blood clotting factors in postpartum period
2. Postpartum thrombocytosis (increased number and adhesiveness of circulating platelets)

3. Release of thromboplastin substances from placental tissue and fetal membranes
4. Increased amounts of fibrinolysis inhibitors

NCLEX® **C. Predisposing factors**

1. Maternal factors such as obesity, cigarette smoking, increased maternal age, multiparity, anemia, or hypothermia
2. Anesthesia or surgery (such as cesarean birth) resulting in injury to leg (incorrect positioning or prolonged time in stirrups), venous stasis, immobility
3. Disorders such as diabetes mellitus, heart disease, endometritis, varicosities or injury to leg, and history of deep vein thrombosis (DVT)

D. Types of thromboembolic disorders

1. Superficial thrombophlebitis (more common in postpartum period)
2. DVT
   - **a.** More frequently seen in women with a history of thrombosis
   - NCLEX® **b.** Increased incidence in women with obstetric complications such as hydramnios, preeclampsia, and operative birth
3. Septic pelvic thrombophlebitis
   - **a.** Develops in conjunction with infections of reproductive tract
   - **b.** More common in women with a cesarean birth
   - **c.** DVT and septic pelvic thromboemboli predispose clients to pulmonary embolization

E. Nursing data collection

1. Superficial thrombophlebitis
   - **a.** Symptoms become apparent about third or fourth postpartum day
   - **b.** Tenderness in portion of vein, cord-like vein
   - **c.** Local heat and redness is present; may have low-grade fever
   - **d.** Pulmonary embolism is extremely rare
2. Deep vein thrombosis
   - **a.** Frequently occurs in women with history of thrombosis
   - NCLEX® **b.** Characterized by edema of ankle and leg; increased calf circumference by more than 2 cm (0.8 inch)
   - NCLEX® **c.** Initial low-grade fever followed by chills and high fever
   - **d.** Pain located in lower leg, popliteal or inguinal area, or lower abdomen depending on which vein is involved
   - NCLEX® **e.** Homan's sign may or may not be positive, but pain results from calf pressure
   - **f.** Peripheral pulses may or may not be decreased
   - NCLEX® **g.** May result in pulmonary embolism; signs include dyspnea and chest pain, diagnosis may be verified by VQ (ventilation quotient) scan, blood gas studies, or x-ray
3. Septic pelvic thrombophlebitis
   - **a.** Infection ascends upward along the venous system, and thrombophlebitis develops in uterine, ovarian, or hypogastric veins
   - **b.** Usually unresponsive to antibiotics
   - **c.** Characterized by abdominal or flank pain present with guarding
   - **d.** Occurs on second to third postpartum day with fever and tachycardia
   - **e.** Intermittent fever and chills may persist
   - **f.** Pulmonary embolism may result; signs include dyspnea and chest pain, diagnosis may be verified by VQ scan, blood gas studies, or x-ray

F. Implementation

1. Evaluate regarding need for support hose during labor and postpartum period
2. NCLEX® Encourage early ambulation following birth; women who have had a cesarean birth should perform regular leg exercises to promote venous return
3. NCLEX® If diagnosis of DVT is made, monitor for signs of pulmonary embolism
4. NCLEX® Monitor for signs of bleeding related to heparin or sodium warfarin (Coumadin) therapy, and keep protamine sulfate (antagonist for heparin) available; keep vitamin K available if receiving warfarin
5. Keep legs elevated and use warm, moist soaks if ordered
6. Obtain clotting times as ordered in client who is on anticoagulant therapy
7. Maintain bedrest as ordered; if client can get up, educate client to avoid standing or sitting for long periods of time; advise client against crossing legs
8. Review need for client to wear support stockings, if ordered, and to plan for rest periods with legs elevated
9. Promote increased fluid intake

10. Promote comfort
    a. Administer nonaspirin analgesic for pain
    b. Elevate extremities on pillow to decrease venous aching
    c. Promote adequate rest and sleep

NCLEX® 11. Take serial bilateral calf measurements daily to compare for any increase in swelling

NCLEX® 12. Report to physician any heavy vaginal bleeding, generalized petechiae, bleeding from mucous membranes, hematuria, or oozing from venipuncture sites as adverse effects of anticoagulant therapy

V. POSTPARTUM PSYCHIATRIC DISORDERS

A. Overview

1. Various psychiatric problems may occur during postpartum period
2. *Adjustment reaction* with depressed mood is also known as postpartum, maternal, or baby blues; may be associated with rapid alteration in estrogen, progesterone, and prolactin levels after birth
    a. Is characterized by mild depression interspersed with happier feelings
    NCLEX® b. Typically occurs within a few days after baby's birth and is self-limiting, lasting from 1 to 10 days, more severe in primiparas
    NCLEX® c. New mothers feel overwhelmed, unable to cope, fatigued, anxious, irritable, and oversensitive; episodic tearfulness occurs without any reason
3. *Postpartum major mood disorder*, also known as postpartum depression
    a. Develops in about 4.5–28% of postpartum women across studies
    b. May occur anytime in first postpartum year, most often occurs around the fourth week, just before start of menses, or upon weaning
    NCLEX® c. Symptoms: sadness, frequent crying, insomnia, appetite change, difficulty concentrating and making decisions, feelings of worthlessness, obsessive thoughts of inadequacy as a person/parent, lack of interest in usual activities, lack of concern about personal appearance; possible irritability and hostility toward new baby
    d. Risk factors: primiparity, ambivalence about pregnancy, history of postpartum depression or bipolar illness, lack of social support or stable relationship with parents or partner, body image and eating disorders
    NCLEX® e. Treatment: medication, primarily selective serotonin reuptake inhibitors such as sertraline (Zoloft) as first-line treatment and paroxetine (Paxil) as alternative first-line treatment; only small amounts of these drugs found in breast milk; fluoxetine (Prozac) not recommended during breastfeeding because of long drug half-life; individual or group psychotherapy, and practical assistance with child care and other demands of daily life
4. Postpartum psychosis
    a. Evident within the first 3 months postpartum
    NCLEX® b. Symptoms: agitation, hyperactivity, insomnia, mood lability, confusion, irrationality, difficulty remembering or concentrating, poor judgment, delusions, and hallucinations
    c. Risk factors: previous postpartum psychosis, history of bipolar disorder, prenatal stressors such as lack of support, obsessive personality, and a family history of mood disorder
    d. Up to 20–30% recurrence rate in subsequent pregnancies
    NCLEX® e. Treatment: hospitalization, antipsychotic medications, sedatives, electroconvulsive therapy, removal of the infant, social support, and psychotherapy
5. *Postpartum onset panic disorder:* characterized by frightening panic attacks that include acute onset of anxiety, fear, rapid breathing, palpitations, and sense of doom

B. Nursing data collection

1. History of previous psychological problems; assessment using Edinburgh Postnatal Depression Scale (score above 12 likely to occur with postpartum depression) or Beck's Revised Postnatal Depression Predictors Inventory
2. NCLEX® Adequacy of coping skills
3. Degree of self-esteem
4. NCLEX® Presence of mood swings, emotional distress, restlessness, irritability, guilt, extreme anxiety about the baby, anorexia, inability to complete activities of daily living, or trouble concentrating or expressing self

C. Implementation

1. NCLEX® Observe client with baby, by herself, and with family and friends; arrange home visits especially for early-discharge families
2. Telephone follow-up at 2–3 weeks postpartum to see if mother is having difficulties; recognize early signs of problems

3. Seek client referral to psychiatrist for evaluation of psychological status
NCLEX® 4. Support positive parenting behaviors
5. Discuss client's plans for her baby and herself
NCLEX® 6. Refer client to social services if indicated

Check Your NCLEX-PN® Exam I.Q.

You are ready for testing on this content if you can

- Identify signs and symptoms of complications in the postpartum period.
- Implement nursing interventions to prevent postpartum complications or assist the client to recover from them.
- Reinforce client teaching about postpartum complications and their management.
- Monitor the client and family responses to therapy for postpartum complications.

PRACTICE TEST

1 The nurse determines that the client who is at greatest risk for postpartum hemorrhage is the one who delivered which infant?

1. A 5-pound, 12-ounce infant
2. A 6-pound infant after a 2-hour labor
3. A 7-pound, 3-ounce infant after a 9-hour labor
4. A 7-pound, 14-ounce infant after a 12-hour labor

2 The nurse is preparing for beginning-of-shift rounds on assigned postpartum clients. After reviewing the assignment, the nurse plans to observe for hematoma formation in which client, who is at greatest risk for this complication?

1. A 17-year-old client who gave birth to a small-for-gestational-age infant
2. A 26-year-old client with gestational diabetes and forceps delivery of a large-for-gestational-age infant
3. A 35-year-old client having twins
4. A 40-year-old client having her first infant

3 The clinic nurse receives a telephone call from a 7-day postpartum client who states she is having increased vaginal bleeding and asks if it is serious and what could be the cause. The nurse suspects which most common etiology of late-postpartum hemorrhage?

1. Uterine atony
2. Disseminated intravascular coagulopathy (DIC)
3. Retained placental fragments
4. Laceration

4 The postpartum nurse would use which therapeutic measure to help prevent a urinary tract infection (UTI) in an assigned client who has just delivered an infant?

1. Promote bedrest for 12 hours postdelivery.
2. Discourage voiding until the bladder regains the sensation of being full.
3. Encourage fluids to 3000 mL per day.
4. Encourage the intake of orange, grapefruit, or apple juice.

5 A newly postpartum client is going into hypovolemic shock as a result of uterine inversion. Which initial order should the nurse expect to implement to restore fluid volume?

1. Administer oxygen at 3–4 L/min via nasal cannula.
2. Administer an oxytocic drug via IV.
3. Monitor heart rate every 5 minutes.
4. Increase the IV infusion rate.

6 A client who previously had an infant by cesarean delivery has successfully delivered an infant by vaginal birth. During postpartum recovery, she suddenly reports severe pain in the abdomen and between her scapulae. There is minimal amount of vaginal bleeding. What is the nurse's priority action?

1. Put the client in Trendelenburg position.
2. Continue to monitor for uterine atony.
3. Maintain the rate of IV fluids.
4. Notify the physician promptly.

7 The nurse interprets that a postpartum client has early postpartum hemorrhage if the amount of vaginal bleeding in the first 24 hours post-delivery exceeds _____ mL. Provide a numeric answer.

Fill in your answer below:

_____ mL

8 A client has been taking methylergonovine maleate (Methergine) for uterine subinvolution but it has not been effective. Which procedure does the clinic nurse anticipate will be ordered to correct the cause of this late-postpartum hemorrhage?

1. Dilatation and curettage
2. Laparotomy
3. Hysterotomy
4. Hysterectomy

9 The husband of a 4-day postpartum client calls the nursing unit saying that his wife is happy one minute and cries the next. He states, "She never was like this before the baby was born." What is the best initial response by the nurse?

1. Tell him to ignore the mood swings, as they will go away.
2. Reassure him that this is normal in the postpartum period because of hormonal changes.
3. Advise him to contact a psychiatrist immediately; this is the first step in postpartum psychosis.
4. Instruct the husband in signs and symptoms of postpartum psychiatric disorders.

10 The postpartum nurse who is reviewing the client assignment realizes that which client is at greatest risk for early postpartum hemorrhage?

1. A client with an infant weighing 5 pounds, 7 ounces
2. A client who is 17 years old
3. A client with endometritis
4. A client with uterine atony

11 While performing postpartum data collection, the nurse notices the client's lochia is very heavy. What should be the nurse's first response?

1. Palpate and massage the uterus.
2. Elevate the head of the bed to Fowler's position.
3. Reevaluate in 10 minutes to see if the problem has corrected itself.
4. Place the client in modified Trendelenburg position.

12 The postpartum nurse would use which measure that would be most effective in detecting development of thrombophlebitis?

1. Monitoring the client's temperature
2. Asking if the client has calf pain when getting out of bed
3. Asking if the client has pain during leg massage
4. Checking for petechiae on the lower extremities

13 What would the postpartum nurse expect to document about the client's lochia and location of uterine fundus on the second day after delivery?

1. Yellowish-white lochia with no clots, fundus three fingerbreadths below the umbilicus
2. Dark red lochia with small clots, fundus midline and two fingerbreadths below the umbilicus
3. Pinkish-brown lochia with no clots, fundus midline and four fingerbreadths below the umbilicus
4. A large amount of bright red lochia with large clots, fundus midline and at the umbilicus

14 The clinic nurse working with women during the postpartum period would recognize that which of the following behaviors exhibited by a client is typical during this time? Select all that apply.

1. The mother experiences feelings of depression as she assumes responsibility for her new baby.
2. The mother does not take care of herself, but attends well to her infant.
3. The mother is receptive to learning about her baby.
4. The mother does not sleep or eat well, but tries to take care of herself.
5. The mother talks to the newborn and looks often at the newborn's face.

15 The nurse is assigned to a postpartum client diagnosed with a right labial hematoma. What instruction should the nurse reinforce at this time?

1. A hot pack will be used to increase comfort and to decrease blood loss.
2. Witch hazel pads will be applied to reduce discomfort.
3. She needs to give informed consent for surgery to incise and drain the hematoma.
4. A cold pack will help to decrease bleeding and reduce the swelling.

16 A postpartum client receiving heparin asks whether she can continue to breastfeed. What is the best response for the nurse to give?

1. She should stop breastfeeding immediately.
2. She can continue to breastfeed, but must assess the baby daily for ecchymotic spots.
3. Heparin will not affect the breastfeeding, and requires no special precautions for the infant.
4. She should alternate breastfeeding and bottle-feeding.

17 During a clinic visit, a 10-day postpartum client reports development of a reddened, swollen, and tender breast. What should the nurse include in a response to the client?

1. These symptoms suggest an inflammatory or infectious process, and require immediate physician notification.
2. She should mention it to her physician at her 2-week check-up, because it will be abnormal if it continues after two weeks.
3. This is normal breast engorgement, and should subside within another week.
4. She has to stop breastfeeding immediately until the swelling and redness resolve on their own.

18 A client has developed disseminated intravascular coagulopathy (DIC) following a placenta previa. Which nursing action is important at this time? Select all that apply.

1. Monitor for Homans' sign hourly.
2. Frequently monitor her vaginal bleeding.
3. Administer antibiotics.
4. Monitor reflexes hourly.
5. Monitor results of D-dimer blood tests.

19 The postpartum nurse is caring for a client with thrombophlebitis. The nurse monitors the client for which symptoms of complications? Select all that apply.

1. Confusion
2. Sudden high fever
3. Dyspnea
4. Diaphoresis
5. Sudden onset of chills

20 The nurse observes that a postpartal client who delivered 3 hours ago has saturated four peripads with bright red blood during the past hour. Her vital signs are stable. The nurse interprets her bleeding to be which of the following?

1. A normal indication of subinvolution
2. Abnormal, requiring inspection for a hematoma
3. Abnormal, indicating the need to palpate the uterine fundus
4. Normal, requiring no further action by the nurse

ANSWERS & RATIONALES

1 **Answer: 2** **Rationale:** A rapid (precipitous) labor and delivery can cause exhaustion of the uterine muscle and prevent contraction of the uterus after delivery, which controls the amount of bleeding. A 5-pound, 12-ounce infant is of normal size while delivery of a large infant is a predisposing factor for postpartum hemorrhage. A labor of 9 hours and 12 hours with birth of infants of normal size does not increase risk of postpartum hemorrhage. **Cognitive Level:** Analyzing **Client Need:** Physiological Adaptation **Integrated Process:** Nursing Process: Data Collection **Content Area:** Maternal-Newborn **Strategy:** First, eliminate options that are similar (normal size infants and 9- and 12-hour labors), because they identify infants of similar size who were delivered within reasonably similar time frames. Choose the 6-pound infant because of the very short duration of labor (2 hours).

2 **Answer: 2** **Rationale:** A hematoma is a collection of blood in the pelvic tissue caused by damage to a blood vessel wall without tissue laceration. A client with gestational diabetes is more prone to have a large infant that could cause tissue trauma during delivery. This client was also delivered with forceps, which is another high-risk factor for developing a postpartum hematoma. Increasing maternal age and delivery of an SGA infant do not increase risk of hematoma formation. A large newborn, rather than the number of newborns, determines risk for hematoma formation. **Cognitive Level:** Analyzing **Client Need:** Physiological Adaptation **Integrated Process:** Nursing Process: Data Collection **Content Area:** Maternal-Newborn **Strategy:** The core issue of the question is knowledge that large fetal size at delivery is a risk factor for hematoma formation. Evaluate each option carefully, considering the client with diabetes mellitus is more likely to have a large for gestational age (LGA) infant.

3 **Answer: 3** **Rationale:** Retained placental fragments are a cause of late-postpartum hemorrhage (which occurs any time after the first 24 hours postdelivery). The retained fragments undergo necrosis, forming fibrin deposits. These deposits form polyps, which eventually detach from the myometrium, causing hemorrhage. Uterine atony, DIC, and lacerations are causes of early postpartum hemorrhage. **Cognitive Level:** Analyzing **Client Need:** Physiological Adaptation **Integrated Process:** Nursing Process: Evaluation **Content Area:** Maternal-Newborn **Strategy:** Specific knowledge of how to discriminate etiology of early- and late-postpartum hemorrhage is needed to answer this question. Use nursing knowledge and the process of elimination to make your selection.

4 **Answer: 3** **Rationale:** Adequate fluid intake (up to 3000 mL/day) prevents urinary stasis, dilutes urine, and flushes out waste products, all of which help to prevent UTI. Bedrest is of no value in preventing UTI, although urinary stasis can actually increase risk. The client should attempt to void every few hours, rather than waiting to regain a sense of a full bladder. While intake of juices is healthy, it is the large volume of fluid consumed that aids in flushing out wastes. **Cognitive Level:** Applying **Client Need:** Physiological Adaptation **Integrated Process:** Nursing Process: Implementation **Content Area:** Maternal-Newborn **Strategy:** The core issue of the question is knowing how to decrease risk for UTIs. Recall that the risk can be diminished by decreasing risk of urinary stasis, and increasing fluid intake as well as foods and beverages that yield acidic urine (cranberry juice, ascorbic acid in high doses).

5 **Answer: 4** **Rationale:** Increasing the rate of IV fluids is an effective initial measure necessary to replace lost fluid volume that occurs in uterine inversion caused by hemorrhage. Blood products might also be necessary, but generally take some time to obtain from the blood bank. Oxygen would be given to increase perfusion to tissues, but does not restore circulating volume. An oxytocic drug will help to limit further bleeding, but will not restore circulating volume. Monitoring heart rate will not limit the condition because it is an assessment rather than an intervention. **Cognitive Level:** Applying **Client Need:** Physiological Adaptation **Integrated Process:** Nursing Process: Planning **Content Area:** Maternal-Newborn **Strategy:** The core issue of the question is fluid volume replacement. Eliminate each of the incorrect options because they do not replace fluids, although they might be helpful in a specific way.

6 **Answer: 4** **Rationale:** A common risk associated with vaginal delivery after cesarean is uterine rupture. Pain in the abdomen and between the scapulae can occur when the uterus ruptures. The hemorrhage is concealed and blood accumulates under the diaphragm, leading to scapular pain. This is an emergency, and requires immediate medical intervention, which is initiated by calling the physician. The client may be put in modified Trendelenburg position to manage shock, not Trendelenburg. Uterine atony is not the problem and an action rather than monitoring is required. IV fluids would be increased rather than maintained. **Cognitive Level:** Applying **Client Need:** Physiological Adaptation **Integrated Process:** Nursing Process: Implementation **Content Area:** Maternal-Newborn **Strategy:** Note the core issue of the question is recognition of internal hemorrhage due to uterine rupture. Eliminate each of the incorrect options because they fail to initiate or provide effective treatment for this medical emergency.

7 **Answer: 500** **Rationale:** The traditional definition of early postpartum hemorrhage after a vaginal birth is greater than 500 mL in 24 hours. **Cognitive Level:** Analyzing **Client Need:** Physiological Adaptation **Integrated Process:** Nursing Process: Data Collection **Content Area:** Maternal-Newborn **Strategy:** The core issue of the question is an understanding of criteria for postpartum hemorrhage. Use nursing knowledge to make your selection.

8 **Answer: 1** **Rationale:** Late-postpartum hemorrhage most frequently occurs due to retained placental tissue. Dilatation and curettage is the vaginal procedure of choice to remove retained tissue from the uterus. Laparotomy, hysterotomy, and hysterectomy are abdominal surgeries but they are not used to treat this condition. **Cognitive Level:** Analyzing **Client Need:** Physiological Adaptation **Integrated Process:** Nursing Process: Planning **Content Area:** Maternal-Newborn **Strategy:** Consider first that the client is bleeding, and determine the most likely cause, retained placental fragments. Then visualize each of the surgeries described, and use the process of elimination and nursing knowledge to choose the one that will effectively treat the condition.

9 **Answer: 2** **Rationale:** Before providing further instructions, the nurse should explain that these are signs of postpartum blues, which is a normal process related to hormonal changes. Telling the husband to ignore the mood swings fails to address the client's concern. In this case, the husband is the client. Advising the husband to consult a psychiatrist immediately is an excessive response. Teaching the client about various postpartum psychiatric disorders is unnecessary and excessive. **Cognitive Level:** Applying **Client Need:** Psychosocial Integrity **Integrated Process:** Communication and Documentation **Content Area:** Maternal-Newborn **Strategy:** The core issue of the question is recognition and appropriate instruction regarding mood changes in the postpartum period. Use nursing knowledge and the process of elimination to make your selection.

10 **Answer: 4** **Rationale:** Uterine atony accounts for 80–90% of all early (within first 24 hours) hemorrhage. Infants weighing between 5 and 7 pounds would not overdistend the uterus and thus not cause increased risk of postpartum hemorrhage. The client's age does not increase the incidence of postpartum hemorrhage. Endometritis could cause late postpartum hemorrhage, not early postpartum hemorrhage. **Cognitive Level:** Analyzing **Client Need:** Physiological Adaptation **Integrated Process:** Nursing Process: Evaluation **Content Area:** Maternal-Newborn **Strategy:** First, recall the causes of early postpartum hemorrhage, which might help you to easily select the correct option. Alternatively, eliminate endometritis first because it

is a different postpartum complication, then the 5-pound, 7-ounce infant because of small size, and finally the age of 17 years because it is irrelevant.

11 **Answer: 1** **Rationale:** Excessive bleeding must be evaluated and managed immediately to prevent excessive loss of blood and shock. The nurse should palpate the uterus to determine whether it is boggy, and massage the uterus. Elevating the head of the bed will not address the possible complication of early postpartum hemorrhage. Waiting represents a failure to act and will only cause the client harm. Bleeding should be addressed immediately. A modified Trendelenburg position is the classic shock position, but the nurse should first try measures to reduce bleeding and thus prevent onset of shock. **Cognitive Level:** Applying **Client Need:** Physiological Adaptation **Integrated Process:** Nursing Process: Implementation **Content Area:** Maternal-Newborn **Strategy:** The core issue of the question is knowledge of measures to reduce postpartum bleeding. With this in mind, eliminate options that delay action or focus on positioning, since these will not correct a boggy uterus.

12 **Answer: 2** **Rationale:** Calf pain upon dorsiflexion of the foot (such as when getting out of bed) indicates a positive Homans' sign, a sign of thrombophlebitis. Thrombophlebitis may cause a mild temperature elevation, but monitoring temperature is not the most direct or effective measure to assess thrombophlebitis. The legs (especially the calves) should not be massaged with risk of thrombophlebitis, because doing so could dislodge a potential clot. Petechiae are not a clinical sign of thrombophlebitis. **Cognitive Level:** Analyzing **Client Need:** Physiological Adaptation **Integrated Process:** Nursing Process: Data Collection **Content Area:** Maternal-Newborn **Strategy:** Specific knowledge of assessment of thrombophlebitis is needed to answer this question. First eliminate the option with leg massage, which is contraindicated. Next eliminate petechiae because the problem is not evidenced by bleeding into skin tissue. Finally choose calf pain over monitoring for temperature because it is a more specific sign than mild fever.

13 **Answer: 2** **Rationale:** The fundus should be midline, two fingerbreadths below the umbilicus, with dark red lochia, which might contain small clots (lochia rubra). Yellowish-white color with no clots explains lochia alba, which does not occur until about 10 days postpartum. Pinkish-brown lochia with no clots describes lochia serosa, which usually occurs between days 4 and 9 of postpartum. A large amount of bright red lochia with large clots describes findings that occur with subinvolution. **Cognitive Level:** Analyzing **Client Need:** Physiological Adaptation **Integrated Process:** Nursing Process: Data Collection **Content Area:** Maternal-Newborn **Strategy:** Specific knowledge of changes in lochia during the postpartum period is needed to answer this question. Use nursing knowledge and the process of elimination to make your selection.

14 **Answer: 3, 5** **Rationale:** Typical behavior during the postpartum period includes accepting responsibility for infant care. Typical behavior during the postpartum period includes activities that demonstrate maternal-newborn bonding. The presence of feelings of depression indicates potential psychiatric problems and requires additional investigation. Lack of self care indicates potential psychiatric problems and requires additional investigation. An inability to eat or sleep well requires investigation as to the cause, as both are especially important during the postpartum period. **Cognitive Level:** Analyzing **Client Need:** Psychosocial Integrity **Integrated Process:** Nursing Process: Data Collection **Content Area:** Maternal-Newborn **Strategy:** The core issue of the question is healthy adaptation to life with a new infant. Choose the options that indicate the greatest resemblance to healthy behavior and adaptive coping.

15 **Answer: 4** **Rationale:** Applying a cold pack will minimize swelling, bleeding, and discomfort. A hot pack is incorrect because it will increase engorgement at the site via vasodilation. Witch hazel will not decrease the swelling in the area. Labial hematomas do not necessarily need to be drained; they usually resolve on their own. **Cognitive Level:** Applying **Client Need:** Physiological Adaptation **Integrated Process:** Nursing Process: Implementation **Content Area:** Maternal-Newborn **Strategy:** The core issue of the question is knowledge of hot and cold applications to aid in reabsorption of hematoma. Use basic nursing knowledge and the process of elimination to make your selection.

16 **Answer: 3** **Rationale:** Heparin does not pass to the breast milk. Thus, heparin will not affect breastfeeding and requires no special infant precautions. A woman can continue to breastfeed while on heparin. The infant does not need to be assessed for ecchymoses. It is unnecessary to alternate with bottle-feeding. **Cognitive Level:** Applying **Client Need:** Physiological Adaptation **Integrated Process:** Nursing Process: Implementation **Content Area:** Maternal-Newborn **Strategy:** Specific knowledge of acceptable medication to use while breastfeeding is needed to answer this question. Use nursing knowledge and the process of elimination to make your selection.

17 **Answer: 1** **Rationale:** These symptoms are suggestive of mastitis, and require prompt attention by the client's physician. It is not therapeutic to wait for the symptoms to resolve on their own. These symptoms are not characteristic of normal breast engorgement. Breastfeeding does not have to be stopped if mastitis is present. **Cognitive Level:** Analyzing **Client Need:** Physiological Adaptation **Integrated Process:** Nursing Process: Data Collection **Content Area:** Maternal-Newborn **Strategy:** The core issues of the question are recognition of mastitis and applying knowledge of appropriate intervention. Use nursing knowledge and the process of elimination to make your selection.

18 **Answer: 2, 5** **Rationale:** DIC is a disorder of widespread microvascular clotting that can result in bleeding once clotting factors are consumed. Vaginal bleeding can be excessive if a coagulation disorder is present. A D-dimer test monitors fibrinogen level, platelet count, fibrin degradation products, and various coagulation times, all of which are altered during DIC. Homans' sign is associated with thrombophlebitis, not with DIC. Antibiotics will not affect a clotting disorder. DIC does not affect a client's reflexes. **Cognitive Level:** Analyzing **Client Need:** Physiological Adaptation **Integrated Process:** Nursing Process: Data Collection **Content Area:** Maternal-Newborn **Strategy:** The core issue of the question is knowledge that DIC can be evidenced by bleeding once clotting factors have been consumed. When answering questions about DIC, look for options that address bleeding in some way.

19 **Answer: 1, 3, 4** **Rationale:** Classic symptoms of pulmonary embolus include sudden onset of dyspnea, chest pain, anxiety, diaphoresis, elevated pulse, and hypotension. Confusion can occur because of decreased oxygenation to the brain resulting from loss of adequate gas exchange in the affected area of the lung. The client would not experience chills or fever; these are more indicative of infection. **Cognitive Level:** Analyzing **Client Need:** Physiological

Adaptation **Integrated Process:** Nursing Process: Data Collection **Content Area:** Maternal-Newborn **Strategy:** Specific knowledge of manifestations of pulmonary embolism is needed to answer this question. Use nursing knowledge and the process of elimination to make your selection.

20 **Answer: 3** **Rationale:** Heavy bleeding is an abnormal postpartal finding. Early hemorrhage can be caused by uterine atony or by a lacerated cervix. Palpation of the uterine fundus can determine uterine atony. Subinvolution causes the majority of late-postpartal hemorrhages occurring after the first 24 hours following delivery. The client did not report excessive perineal pain or pressure, which would be caused by a hematoma. Blood is retained in the tissue with a hematoma, and is not usually visible on the perineal pad. Heavy bleeding is an abnormal postpartal finding. **Cognitive Level:** Analyzing **Client Need:** Physiological Adaptation **Integrated Process:** Nursing Process: Data Collection **Content Area:** Maternal-Newborn **Strategy:** Recognize the data in the question as abnormal; the time period indicates early-postpartal hemorrhage.

Key Words to Review

cystitis p. 776
disseminated intravascular coagulopathy (DIC) p. 772
early-postpartum hemorrhage p. 772
endometritis/endomyometritis p. 774
hematoma p. 772
late-postpartum hemorrhage p. 773
mastitis p. 775
pelvic cellulitis/parametritis p. 772
peritonitis p. 774
postpartum psychiatric disorders p. 778
pyelonephritis p. 776
subinvolution p. 773
thrombophlebitis p. 776
urinary tract infection p. 776
uterine atony p. 772

References

Davidson, M., London, M., & Ladewig, P. (2012). *Olds' maternal newborn nursing and women's health across the lifespan* (9th ed.). Upper Saddle River, NJ: Pearson Education, Inc.

Ladewig, P., London, M., & Davidson, M. (2010). *Contemporary maternal-newborn nursing care* (7th ed.). Upper Saddle River, NJ: Pearson Education, Inc.

London, M., Ladewig, P., Ball, J., Bindler, R., & Cowen, K. (2011). *Maternal & child nursing care* (3rd ed.). Upper Saddle River, NJ: Pearson Education, Inc.

Perry, S., Hockenberry, M., Lowdermilk, D., & Wilson, D. (2010). *Maternal child nursing care* (4th ed.). St. Louis, MO: Elsevier.

Test Yourself

Are you ready for the NCLEX-PN® or course exams? Use the practice tests on the companion website to check.

Complicated Newborn Care

48

In this chapter

Cross Reference

Other chapters relevant to this content area are

Reproduction, Family Planning, and Infertility	Chapter 8
Uncomplicated Antenatal Care	Chapter 9
Uncomplicated Labor and Delivery Care	Chapter 10
Uncomplicated Postpartum Care	Chapter 11
Uncomplicated Newborn Care	Chapter 12
Maternal and Newborn Medications	Chapter 31
Complicated Antenatal Care	Chapter 45
Complicated Labor and Delivery Care	Chapter 46
Complicated Postpartum Care	Chapter 47

I. GENERAL NURSING CARE OF HIGH-RISK NEWBORN

A. Identification of high-risk newborns

1. Certain prenatal and intrapartal risk factors increase risk of neonatal complications after delivery
   a. Maternal preexisting diabetes or development of gestational diabetes during the pregnancy can lead to hypoglycemia after delivery for infants of diabetic mothers (IDMs)
   b. Opioid analgesics/anesthetics administered during labor, especially systemically and immediately before delivery, cross placenta and cause respiratory depression in neonate after delivery
   c. Fetal asphyxia causes fetus to pass meconium into amniotic fluid, which could be aspirated during delivery; common causes include placental insufficiency, prolapsed cord, placental abruption, and placenta previa
   d. Difficult or prolonged labor, which increases risk of birth trauma
   e. Multiple gestation pregnancy
   f. Preterm or postterm delivery

g. Life-threatening congenital anomalies
h. Maternal or neonatal infection
i. Small for gestational age (SGA) or large for gestational age (LGA)

NCLEX® 2. Apgar scores: an Apgar score of less than 6 at 1 minute or 7 at 5 minutes indicates unsatisfactory transition to extrauterine life and requires careful monitoring

NCLEX® 3. Changes in physical signs are often vague, so thorough examination is essential (see Box 48–1)

4. Gestational age

NCLEX® a. Gestational age less than 37 weeks based on due date
b. Perform a quick examination if due date unknown; follow up with a thorough gestational age estimate as soon as possible
c. Eyelids fused until 26 weeks' gestation
d. Creases cover a third of soles of feet at 36 weeks' gestation
e. Breast buds are absent until 37 weeks' gestation
f. Ear cartilage has little recoil until 30 weeks' gestation
g. Vernix covers body by 31 to 33 weeks' gestation
h. Lanugo covers shoulders by 33 to 36 weeks' gestation

B. General planning and implementation for all high-risk newborns

1. Constantly monitor infant for subtle changes in condition and intervene promptly when necessary

NCLEX® 2. Decrease risk of hospital-acquired infections; provide each neonate with own supplies; handwashing is most important method of preventing infection

NCLEX® 3. Conserve infant's energy and decrease physiologic stress by organizing care and minimizing interruptions; monitor each neonate for signs of stress

4. Provide appropriate stimulation for infant growth and development; high-risk neonates have same developmental needs as healthy neonate

5. Pulse oximeter; estimates arterial oxygen saturation through sensor placed on skin
a. Place sensor on palm of hand, sole of foot, or wrap around finger

NCLEX® b. Monitor skin integrity at sensor site every 4 hours and rotate site every 12 hours

NCLEX® c. Pulse oximeter reading of 88–92% reflects safe clinical range

6. Arterial blood gas (ABG)
a. Direct measurement of amount of oxygen (O_2), carbon dioxide (CO_2), and select electrolytes in a sample of arterial blood by arterial puncture or from **umbilical arterial line (UAL)**
b. Compare oximeter reading at time of blood sample to correlate values

NCLEX® c. Apply pressure to arterial puncture site for 3 to 5 minutes

7. Blood glucose monitoring (Dextrostick, Accucheck)
a. Warm foot prior to obtaining blood sample to increase circulation
b. Lance heel to obtain blood sample; heel is preferred site

8. Umbilical lines
a. An umbilical arterial line (UAL) is inserted into an umbilical artery primarily to obtain ABG
b. An **umbilical venous line (UVL)** is inserted into umbilical vein to give IV fluids and medications and to obtain blood for lab tests

NCLEX® c. Monitor all neonates with umbilical lines closely for blue discoloration or blanching on lower extremities or buttocks, which could indicate an embolus or vasospasm and may necessitate removal of line

NCLEX® d. Monitor closely for line placement, bleeding from umbilicus, or disconnected tubing; position infant in a side-lying or prone position for close monitoring

Box 48–1

Critical Neonatal Data Collection Indicators

The appearance of any of these signs in a neonate could indicate the presence of a serious complication:

- Respiratory: bradypnea or tachypnea, respiratory distress, weak or absent respiratory effort
- Cardiovascular: bradycardia or tachycardia, murmur
- Neuromuscular: lethargy, temperature instability, tremors, unusual behaviors such as lip-smacking
- Gastrointestinal: poor feeding tolerance, poor suck/swallow reflex
- Skin color: cyanosis (acrocyanosis is normal for first 24 to 48 hours after delivery), jaundice (especially within first 24 hours)
- Obvious major anomalies

9. Oxygen administration
   a. Administered by **oxygen hood** (hood placed over infant's head), nasal cannula, **continuous positive airway pressure (CPAP)** (pressurized air), or endotracheal tube (ET)

NCLEX®
   b. Warm and humidify O_2 prior to administration to decrease insensible fluid loss and heat loss

NCLEX®
   c. Monitor amount of O_2 being administered and O_2 saturation and/or ABGs; administer minimum amount of O_2 to meet infant's O_2 needs to prevent complications

10. Gavage tubes
    a. Used to decompress stomach or administer formula, breast milk, or oral medications
    b. It is preferred to insert tube orally instead of nasally because infants are obligate nose-breathers

NCLEX®
    c. A 5 Fr. or 8 Fr. tube is commonly used; measure tube from earlobe to nose and then to tip of xyphoid process; insert tube and secure placement

NCLEX®
    d. Check placement of tube prior to administering any feeding or medication; administer feedings over 3 to 5 minutes to avoid dumping syndrome; offer a pacifier during feeding

11. Parenting the high-risk newborn
    a. Parents are initially in a state of shock and disbelief and may grieve loss of "perfect baby"
    b. Observe bonding
    c. Explain equipment and infant's condition
    d. Present positive, realistic attitude and establish trust

NCLEX®
    e. Encourage parents to touch infant and perform care-taking activities as infant's condition allows
    f. Encourage parents to verbalize feelings
    g. Give Polaroid pictures of infant to parents prior to transfer to neonatal intensive care unit (NICU)
    h. Reinforce teaching about infant care in preparation for discharge

II. PROBLEMS RELATED TO MATURITY

A. Prematurity

1. Description: infant born before completion of 37th week of pregnancy
   a. Prognosis and severity of complications related to level of maturity: the earlier infant is born, the greater chance of complications
   b. Earliest age of viability is 23 to 24 weeks' gestation

NCLEX®
   c. Major complications are related to **respiratory distress syndrome (RDS)** (disorder caused by lack of surfactant), difficulty regulating body temperature, infection, and hemorrhage
   d. Generally ready for discharge near their due date

2. Etiology

NCLEX®
   a. Maternal risk factors: age, smoking, poor nutrition, placental problems (placenta previa, placental abruption, preeclampsia/eclampsia), previous preterm delivery, incompetent cervix
   b. Fetal risk factors: multiple gestation pregnancy, infection
   c. Other risk factors: low socioeconomic status, environmental exposure to harmful substance

3. Respiratory data
   a. Insufficient surfactant allows alveoli to collapse with each expiration
   b. Inadequate number and maturity of alveoli makes adequate alveolar gas exchange difficult
   c. Skeletal muscles weak so may not be able to reposition head and body to maintain patent airway

NCLEX®
   d. Signs of respiratory distress typically develop within 1 to 2 hours after delivery (see Box 48–2)
   e. Respiratory failure is most common cause of death in preterm infants in first 72 hours of life

Memory Aid

Remember respiratory distress in a premature infant by the mnemonic SIN:

S	Substernal retractions
I	Inspiratory grunting
N	Nasal flaring

NCLEX®

4. Respiratory interventions
   a. Maintain respirations at 30 to 60/min, check every 1 to 2 hours and as needed
   b. Monitor oxygenation and administer O_2 as ordered
   c. Auscultate breath sounds
   d. Monitor for signs of respiratory distress
   e. Suction prn
   f. Monitor O_2 saturation and/or ABGs

Box 48-2

Signs of Neonatal Respiratory Distress

- Tachypnea
- Intercostal and/or subcostal retractions
- Nasal flaring
- Expiratory grunting
- Seesaw respiratory movements
- Diminished breath sounds
- PaO_2 less than 50 mm Hg
- PCO_2 above 60 mm Hg
- Increasing exhaustion
- Cyanosis (late finding)

5. Monitor thermoregulation
   a. Lack of subcutaneous fat to insulate body and small muscle mass
   b. Large body surface area in proportion to body weight, so more likely to lose heat quickly
   c. Absent sweat or shiver mechanisms
   d. Increased insensible fluid loss
   e. Increased risk of hypothermia
6. Interventions to assist thermoregulation
   a. Maintain **neutral thermal environment** (temperature that prevents heat loss) and prevent cold stress
   b. Place infant under radiant warmer or in double-wall isolette (NCLEX®)
   c. Warm equipment and linen before contact with infant (NCLEX®)
   d. Generally, infant can be weaned to an open bassinet when temperature is stable and infant is gaining weight
   e. Measure infant's temperature every 2 to 3 hours and as needed
7. Low resistance to infection
   a. Lack of immunoglobulins from mother (usually cross placenta in third trimester)
   b. Difficulty localizing infection and poor white blood cell (WBC) response
   c. Increased risk of infection, so monitor carefully for signs of infection
8. Hepatic data
   a. Liver is immature at birth
   b. Increased risk of hyperbilirubinemia caused by difficulty in eliminating bilirubin released by normal breakdown of red blood cells (RBCs); monitor for jaundice
   c. Immature production of clotting factors resulting in increased risk of bleeding disorders
   d. Increased risk of hypoglycemia related to inadequate glucose stores
   e. Prolonged drug metabolism related to immature liver
9. Hematopoetic data: bruises easily related to fragile capillaries and prolonged prothrombin time
10. Gastrointestinal (GI) data
    a. Weak suck/swallow reflex until 33 to 34 weeks' gestation and poor gag/cough reflexes increase risk of aspiration (NCLEX®)
    b. Increased risk of **necrotizing enterocolitis (NEC)**, a neonatal disorder related to immature GI system and hypoxia
11. Feeding
    a. Feed according to abilities
    b. Monitor tolerance of feedings
    c. Monitor suck/swallow reflex to determine risk of aspiration; if poor, gavage feed as indicated (NCLEX®)
    d. Use "preemie" nipple if bottle-feeding; burp frequently (NCLEX®)
    e. Observe for abdominal distention and emesis, as signs that neonate is not tolerating feedings
    f. Monitor intake and output (I&O), daily weight; check for dehydration
    g. Monitor for hypoglycemia
12. Renal data
    a. Unable to concentrate urine effectively, increasing risk of dehydration
    b. Prolonged drug excretion time related to immature kidneys
13. Neuromuscular data
    a. Immature control of vital functions
    b. Increased risk of **intraventricular hemorrhage (IVH)**, which is bleeding into ventricles of brain
    c. Increased risk of apnea
    d. Poor muscle tone and weak or absent reflexes
    e. Weak, feeble cry

14. Organize care to minimize stress
15. Provide skin care with special attention to cleanliness and careful positioning to prevent skin breakdown
16. Measure apical heart rate for 1 min every 1 to 2 hours
17. Monitor potential bleeding sites (umbilicus, injection sites)
18. Monitor overall growth and development; check daily weight, measure length and occipital frontal circumference (OFC) weekly
19. NCLEX® Monitor closely for medication side effects caused by decreased ability to metabolize and excrete medications

B. Potential complications related to prematurity

1. RDS, also known as hyaline membrane disease
   a. Usually appears during first 24 to 48 hours after birth and peaks around 72 hours
   b. Other predisposing factors include fetal hypoxia and postnatal hypothermia
   c. Protection against RDS can be achieved with prenatal betamethasone to mother to accelerate fetal lung maturity and artificial surfactant (Exosurf, Survanta) in infant's airway after delivery to keep alveoli from collapsing and causing atelectasis
2. **Bronchopulmonary dysplasia (BPD)**, a chronic pulmonary disease requiring mechanical ventilation and high oxygen levels in first weeks of life
3. **Retinopathy of prematurity (ROP)**
   a. Etiology: prolonged exposure to high concentrations of O_2 causes hemorrhage within retina and leads to retinal detachment and loss of vision
   b. NCLEX® Preventable with cautious administration of O_2; it is critical to administer minimum amount of O_2 needed to maintain a PaO_2 of 50 to 70 mm Hg
   c. All premature infants who receive O_2 should be screened prior to discharge by an ophthalmologist
4. Intraventricular hemorrhage (IVH)
   a. Etiology: rupture of thin, fragile capillaries within ventricles of brain leading to increased intracranial pressure
   b. Prematurity and hypoxia are primary risk factors
   c. Data collection: neurological changes such as hypotonia and lethargy, bulging fontanels, increasing OFC, bradycardia, apnea
5. Necrotizing enterocolitis (NEC)
   a. Etiology: intestinal ischemia related to shunting of blood to brain and heart in response to fetal or neonatal distress
   b. Data collection: abdominal distention, poor feeding, vomiting, blood in stool
   c. Treatment involves nothing by mouth (NPO), IV fluids and antibiotics until intestines healed
6. Apnea and bradycardia
   a. Preterm neonates are at risk for apnea related to immature regulation of vital functions; if apnea is prolonged, eventually bradycardia occurs
   b. Infants almost always experience respiratory arrest before cardiac arrest; by supporting respiratory function, heart rate should return to normal range
   c. NCLEX® If apnea occurs, first stimulate respirations with gentle tactile stimulation; if unsuccessful, reposition neonate, and finally, support respirations with a manual resuscitation bag if necessary

C. Postmaturity

1. Overview
   a. Born after completion of 42 weeks of pregnancy
   b. Problems caused by progressively less efficient actions of placenta
   c. At risk for birth injury related to dystocia
   d. Placental insufficiency may occur with an aging placenta that can no longer meet fetal needs; increases risk of fetal asphyxia that results in passage of meconium in utero and increased risk of **meconium aspiration syndrome (MAS)**, inhalation of meconium into lungs
2. Nursing data collection
   a. Absence of vernix and minimal lanugo
   b. Dry, cracked skin related to metabolism of fat to meet energy needs in utero
   c. Hypoglycemia related to metabolism of glycogen to meet energy needs in utero
   d. Minimal subcutaneous fat
   e. Skin and cord yellow/green caused by meconium staining
   f. Long fingernails and often has scratches on face and trunk
3. NCLEX® Interventions: check for presence of meconium at delivery, birth injuries, and hypoglycemia

III. PROBLEMS RELATED TO SIZE

A. Small for gestational age

1. Overview
   a. Defined as birth weight below 10th percentile (under 2500 grams or 5 pounds, 8 ounces)
   NCLEX® b. Etiology: placental insufficiency, infections, smoking, hypertension, malnutrition

Memory Aid

Remember that a low-birth-weight infant weighs 2500 grams (5 pounds, 8 ounces) at birth or less.

2. Nursing data collection
   a. Skin: loose and dry, little fat or muscle mass
   b. Little scalp hair
   c. Hypoglycemia
   d. Weak cry
3. Interventions
   NCLEX® a. Observe for presence of meconium during labor and delivery; thoroughly suction airway immediately after delivery if present
   b. Measure temperature and provide neutral thermal environment
   c. Monitor for signs of hypoglycemia
   NCLEX® d. Weigh daily and note changes in weight
4. Outcomes: infant maintains stable temperature and blood glucose level and gains weight

B. Large for gestational age

1. Overview
   a. Defined as birthweight above 90th percentile (over 4000 grams or 8 pounds 13 ounces)
   b. Primary etiology: infant of diabetic mother (IDM)
2. Risks
   a. Hyperbilirubinemia related to increased bilirubin released from damaged RBCs secondary to traumatic delivery
   b. Birth injury: fractured clavicle, Erb-Duchenne paralysis secondary to shoulder dystocia
   c. If preterm, risk for RDS
   d. If postterm, risk for meconium aspiration
3. Nursing data collection
   a. Macrosomia (large body size and high birthweight)
   b. Signs of birth trauma related to cephalopelvic disproportion (CPD)
   NCLEX® c. Hypoglycemia, especially in an IDM
NCLEX® 4. Interventions: monitor for signs of birth injury, and/or hypoglycemia

IV. PROBLEMS RELATED TO BIRTH TRAUMA

A. Facial paralysis

1. Etiology: temporary problem caused by pressure on facial nerve during delivery
NCLEX® 2. Nursing data collection: face on affected side is unresponsive when neonate cries, eye remains open, forehead does not wrinkle
3. Self-resolves within hours or days of delivery; permanent paralysis is rare
NCLEX® 4. Monitor and support ability to feed orally

B. Erb-Duchenne paralysis

1. Definition: brachial paralysis of upper portion of arm
2. Etiology
   a. Most common type of paralysis associated with difficult delivery
   b. Related to stretching or pulling head away from shoulder during difficult delivery
NCLEX® 3. Nursing data collection
   a. Flaccid arm with elbow extended and hand rotated inward
   b. Moro reflex absent on affected side
   c. Grasp reflex intact
4. Interventions
   NCLEX® a. Intermittent immobilization using a brace or splint, or pinning sleeve to mattress

b. Position arm for 2–3 hours at a time with arm abducted 90 degrees, shoulder externally rotated, elbow flexed 90 degrees, and wrist supinated with palm angled slightly toward face ("Statue of Liberty" pose)
c. Reposition every 2 to 3 hours but avoid positioning on affected side
NCLEX® d. Delay range of motion until 10th day to prevent further damage

C. Fractures

1. Etiology
   a. Clavicle is bone most frequently fractured during delivery
   b. Other bones fractured during delivery are skull, humerus, and femur
   c. CPD is often a predisposing factor
2. NCLEX® Nursing data collection (fractured clavicle): limited range of motion, crepitus over affected bone and absence of Moro reflex on affected side
3. Interventions (fractured clavicle)
   a. NCLEX® Instruct parents to handle affected arm gently
   b. Usually self-resolves

D. Asphyxia

1. Definition: inadequate tissue perfusion that fails to meet metabolic needs of tissues
2. Etiology
   a. Nonreassuring fetal heart rate (FHR) pattern during labor (late or variable decelerations, loss of variability, bradycardia), difficult delivery, prematurity, passage of meconium in utero
   b. Initial goal is to identify neonates at risk so resuscitation can begin immediately if necessary
3. Nursing data collection
   a. Fetal scalp pH during labor; 7.20 or less is considered ominous sign of fetal asphyxia
   b. NCLEX® Apgar score of 4 to 7 indicates need for stimulation; score less than 4 indicates need for resuscitation; resuscitative efforts should begin immediately if needed
   c. Passage of meconium prior to or during delivery
4. Interventions
   a. At delivery, hold neonate in head-down position and thoroughly suction mouth and nares
   b. Place neonate under prewarmed radiant warmer
   c. NCLEX® Stimulate respiratory effort by rubbing back and feet
   d. NCLEX® If respirations inadequate, place neonate in "sniffing" position; inflate neonate's lungs with positive pressure using bag and mask with 100% O_2 at rate of 40 to 60 breaths/min
   e. NCLEX® Once breathing established, check heart rate; if less than 60, or if 60 to 80 and not increasing, begin cardiac compressions; compress lower third of sternum with two fingertips or both thumbs at rate of 90 beats/min; use a 3:1 ratio of compressions to assisted ventilation; see also Chapter 64
   f. Administer as ordered resuscitative medications, primarily epinephrine, after 30 seconds of assisted ventilation and compressions if neonate's heart rate is not more than 80 beats/min
   g. NCLEX® Administer naloxone (Narcan) as ordered if mother received narcotics near time of delivery

V. GENERAL CARE OF NEONATE WITH RESPIRATORY DISTRESS

A. Common causes of neonatal respiratory distress

1. RDS, typically in preterm infants
2. Meconium aspiration syndrome (MAS), typically in term and postterm infants
3. **Transient tachypnea of the newborn (TTN)** from delayed absorption of fluid in lungs from delivery; typically in term and postterm infants

NCLEX® **B. Nursing data collection (see Box 48–1 again)**

C. Interventions

1. Maintain neutral thermal environment due to increased O_2 demand if neonate is hypothermic
2. Administer warmed, humidified O_2 as ordered, generally attempting to keep O_2 saturation higher than 90% and PaO_2 between 50 and 70 mm Hg
3. NCLEX® Withhold oral feedings if respiratory rate is higher than 60 breaths/min because of increased risk of aspiration; notify health care provider
4. NCLEX® Position neonate side-lying or supine with neck slightly extended (sniffing position); arms at sides
5. Suction prn to maintain a patent airway
6. Monitor O_2 saturation and/or ABGs as ordered

D. Meconium aspiration syndrome

1. Definition: aspiration of meconium into tracheobronchial tree during first few breaths after delivery in a term neonate

2. Etiology
   a. Prenatal asphyxia causes increased fetal intestinal peristalsis, relaxed anal sphincter, and passage of meconium into amniotic fluid, which may be aspirated into lungs during first few breaths after delivery
   b. Meconium in lungs produces a ball-valve action (air is allowed in but cannot be exhaled) and is irritating to airway; as lungs become hyperinflated, pulmonary perfusion decreases, leading to increasing hypoxia
   c. Can lead to persistent pulmonary hypertension of the newborn (PPHN)
3. Nursing data collection
   a. May demonstrate signs of fetal distress during labor and delivery
   b. Apgar score less than 6 at 1 and 5 minutes
   NCLEX® c. Immediate signs of respiratory distress at delivery (cyanosis, tachypnea, retractions)
   d. Overdistended, barrel-shaped chest
   e. Diminished breath sounds
   f. Yellow staining of skin, nails, and umbilical cord
4. Interventions
   NCLEX® a. Suction oropharynx then nasopharynx after neonate's head is born, and while shoulders and chest are still in birth canal, to remove as much meconium as possible before baby's first breath
   NCLEX® b. If meconium is thick in amniotic fluid, place neonate under radiant warmer, visualize glottis, and suction any meconium from trachea before stimulating respirations
   c. Administer O_2 to maintain adequate PO_2 and O_2 saturation
   d. Anticipate need for mechanical ventilation, high-frequency ventilation, or **extracorporeal membrane oxygenation (ECMO)**, which is used for prolonged heart–lung bypass to allow lungs to heal
   e. Perform chest physiotherapy routinely

E. Transient tachypnea of the newborn

1. Etiology
   a. Failure to clear airway of excess lung fluid at delivery
   b. Primarily occurs in term infants, especially if delivered by cesarean because they have not experienced mechanical squeezing that occurs during vaginal delivery
2. Nursing data collection
   a. Expiratory grunting, nasal flaring, mild cyanosis
   NCLEX® b. Tachypnea by 6 hours of age, respiratory rate may climb to 100 to 140 breaths/min
3. Interventions
   a. Administer O_2 as needed to maintain PO_2 and O_2 saturation within normal limits
   b. Usually self-resolves within 72 hours

VI. CONGENITAL INFECTIONS

A. TORCH (see also Chapter 9)

1. Toxoplasmosis
   a. Overview: protozoan *Toxoplasma gondii*; contracted by mother's ingestion of raw or undercooked meat or contact with feces of infected cats; maternal–fetal transmission occurs during pregnancy
   b. Often results in spontaneous abortion if contracted during first trimester
   c. Severe neonatal disorders associated with congenital infection include seizures, coma, microcephaly, and hydrocephalus
   NCLEX® d. Advise pregnant client to practice good hand hygiene, avoid eating raw meat, avoid exposure to cat litter during pregnancy, and have toxoplasma titer checked prenatally if cats live in household
2. Other infections, usually hepatitis B (HBV)
   a. Transmitted from mother to neonate in about 90% of cases
   b. Transmitted transplacentally and by contact with blood and body fluids
   c. Associated with 32% increase in risk of preterm labor
   d. Infected neonates may be symptom-free or have acute hepatitis, with a 75% mortality rate
   NCLEX® e. Infants of mothers with positive HbsAg should receive hepatitis B immune globulin (HBIG) 0.5 mL IM within first 12 hours of life
   NCLEX® f. Infants of mothers with positive HbsAg should also receive hepatitis B vaccine, with first dose within first 12 hours of life, second dose at 1 month, and third dose at 6 months
   g. Centers for Disease Control (CDC) recommends all women be screened prenatally for HbsAg to determine newborns at risk

3. Rubella
   a. Overview: also called German measles; up to 20% of women of childbearing age are not rubella immune; a rubella titer of 1:8 or greater indicates immunity
   b. Of fetuses exposed during first trimester, 80–90% will be affected by either spontaneous abortion or congenital anomalies
   c. Nursing data collection: clinical signs of congenital infections are congenital heart disease, **intrauterine growth restriction (IUGR)** or fetal undergrowth, and hearing loss
   NCLEX® d. Intervention: infants born with congenital rubella syndrome are infectious and should be isolated
4. Cytomegalovirus (CMV)
   a. Respiratory or sexual transmission; neonate can contract during delivery through an infected birth canal
   b. Most common cause of congenital viral infection (1% of all newborns); most (90–95%) are asymptomatic at birth; remaining 5–10% may experience hemolytic anemia and jaundice, hydrocephaly or microcephaly, pneumonitis, deafness, and fetal or neonatal death
   c. Disease is usually progressive through infancy and childhood
5. Herpes simplex virus (HSV)
   a. Overview: HSV type 1 or type 2
   b. Nursing data collection: maternal symptoms include vesicles on genitalia that are usually painful; fetal symptoms include fever or hypothermia, jaundice, seizures, poor feeding; 50% develop vesicular skin lesions
   c. There is no known cure
   NCLEX® d. Virus can be lethal to fetus and is transmitted during birth; cesarean delivery is indicated if mother has active lesions at time of delivery

B. Sexually transmitted infections, or STIs (see also Chapter 9)

1. Syphilis
   a. Overview: caused by *treponema palladium,* a spirochete that crosses placenta after 16 weeks' gestation and infects fetus; Langhans' layer in chorion prevents fetal infection early in pregnancy until this layer begins to atrophy between 16 and 18 weeks' gestation
   b. There is no increased risk of anomalies, but spirochete may cause inflammatory and destructive changes in liver, spleen, kidneys, and bone marrow
   NCLEX® c. If syphilis is untreated during pregnancy, 25% will end in stillbirth and 40–50% of neonates will have symptomatic congenital syphilis
   NCLEX® d. Data collection: clients with syphilis have a positive rapid plasma reagin (RPR) test
2. Gonorrhea
   a. Causative organism is *Neisseria gonorrhea*
   b. Neonate can be exposed to organism during birth, which can result in sepsis or ophthalmia neonatorum, possibly leading to permanent blindness
   c. Penicillin is treatment of choice
   NCLEX® d. Eye prophylaxis with erythromycin (Ilotycin) ointment within 4 hours after birth decreases risk of ophthalmia neonatorum
3. Chlamydia
   a. Overview: most common STI; caused by *Chlamydia trachomatis*
   b. Can be transmitted to neonate during delivery and cause neonatal conjunctivitis and pneumonia
   NCLEX® c. Eye prophylaxis with erythromycin ointment shortly after birth can prevent neonatal conjunctivitis
4. Candidiasis
   a. Overview: a neonatal oral yeast infection commonly called thrush; most commonly caused by vaginal *Candida albicans*
   b. Excessive yeast growth occurs more commonly in sick newborns and those receiving antibiotics or steroids
   c. Neonate may contract thrush during birth process or from contaminated hands or feeding equipment
   NCLEX® d. Nursing data collection: white patches on oral mucosa, gums, and tongue, which cannot be manually removed and may bleed when touched; occasional difficulty in swallowing
   NCLEX® e. Interventions: antifungal medications to affected area (feed sterile water prior to administration to rinse out milk); nystatin (Mycostatin) using medicine dropper or swab to mucosa, gums, and tongue after a feeding; Gentian violet swabbed over mucosa, gums, and tongue (avoid staining skin, clothes, and equipment)

5. HIV/AIDS
   a. Overview: transmission can occur across placenta during childbirth or through breastmilk or contaminated blood; transmission rate 20–30%; decreases by two thirds when zidovudine (AZT) given prenatally and intrapartally to mother, and to newborn after delivery
   b. It may take up to 15 months for infants to form their own antibodies against HIV
   c. For infants, average survival time between testing positive for HIV infection and death is 9 months, with a 70–80% mortality rate by 2 years of age

NCLEX®
   d. HIV testing should be done at birth and 3 to 6 months of age
   e. Nursing data collection: typically asymptomatic at birth, failure to thrive with developmental delays, hepatomegaly and/or splenomegaly, lymphoid interstitial pneumonitis, recurrent infections, persistent thrush, chronic diarrhea

NCLEX®
   f. Interventions: standard precautions; specific isolation not required; promote comfort; keep well nourished (bottle-feeding to prevent HIV transmission in breast milk); thorough cord care to prevent infection, prevent exposure to infections; provide all routine vaccines; (no live virus vaccines) give skin and mouth care; administer AZT as ordered

C. Sepsis

1. Overview: generalized infection that spreads rapidly through bloodstream; aided by immature neonatal immune system, inability to localize infection, and lack of IgM immunoglobulin (necessary to protect against bacteria and does not cross placenta)
2. Etiology
   a. Prolonged rupture of membranes
   b. Long, difficult labor
   c. Resuscitation and other invasive procedures
   d. Maternal infection

NCLEX®
   e. Beta-hemolytic streptococcal vaginosis is most common cause of neonatal sepsis and meningitis; obtain cervical culture prior to delivery; if positive, antibiotics given during intrapartum period decrease risk of transmission
   f. Aspiration of amniotic fluid, formula, or mucus
   g. Nosocomial: caused by infected health care workers or equipment
3. Data collection
   a. Symptoms often vague initially
   b. Temperature instability, especially hypothermia
   c. Feeding intolerance as evidenced by decreased intake, abdominal distention, vomiting, poor sucking
   d. Subtle behavior changes, "infant just doesn't look right," lethargy, seizure activity, pallor
   e. Progressive respiratory distress
   f. Hyperbilirubinemia
   g. Tachycardia initially, followed by periods of apnea and bradycardia
4. Interventions

NCLEX®
   a. Obtain cultures (blood, urine, cerebral spinal fluid) before antibiotics are initiated
   b. Administer antibiotics as ordered
   c. After 72 hours of treatment, antibiotics may be discontinued if final culture reports are negative and symptoms have subsided; antibiotics are generally continued for 10 to 14 days if final culture reports are positive
   d. Observe for changes in vital signs and physical assessment

VII. COLD STRESS

A. Overview

1. Neonates produce body heat by nonshivering thermogenesis; this process requires increased O_2 and glucose consumption to burn brown fat
2. Subcutaneous fat acts as an insulator and helps conserve body heat
3. A flexed position decreases exposed surface area and conserves body heat
4. Can cause infant to develop hypoglycemia, hypoxemia, and acidosis

B. Etiology

1. Hypothermia because of large surface-area-to-mass ratio

NCLEX®
2. Large amount of heat lost from head
3. All newborns are at risk for hypothermia, especially preterm and SGA infants

C. Interventions

1. Maintain neutral thermal environment

   a. Reduce or eliminate heat lost through drafts and contact with cold objects
   b. Postpone initial bath until temperature has stabilized
   c. Dry infant immediately after delivery and when bathing
2. Place newborn under servo-controlled warmer or on mother's abdomen immediately after delivery
3. Monitor body temperature; keep axillary temperature 97.6° to 99.2°F
4. If axillary temperature is less than 97.6°F
   a. Put hat on infant's head
   b. Wrap newborn with warm blankets
   c. Monitor oxygenation status and evaluate for hypoglycemia
   NCLEX® d. Rewarm infant slowly to prevent hypotension and apnea
5. Chronic hypothermia could be an early sign of sepsis

VIII. HYPERBILIRUBINEMIA

A. Etiology

1. Bilirubin is formed by breakdown of hemoglobin from RBCs; direct (conjugated) is water-soluble and easier to eliminate, and indirect (unconjugated) is fat-soluble so it can more easily cross blood–brain barrier and is harder to eliminate
2. Before birth, unconjugated bilirubin is eliminated via placenta; after delivery, bilirubin converts from unconjugated to conjugated form in liver and is excreted via bile ducts into intestines; it can be reabsorbed from intestines if peristalsis slows
3. **Kernicterus** is a potential complication; bilirubin is deposited in basal ganglia of brain and causes permanent impaired neurological function; bilirubin level, gestational age, condition, and poor fluid–caloric balance increase risk of kernicterus at low serum bilirubin levels

B. Physiologic jaundice

1. Healthy newborn has twice as much bilirubin as an adult related to higher concentration of circulating RBCs; immature liver has impaired ability to conjugate bilirubin during transition from fetal to neonatal circulation; a shorter life span of fetal RBCs is also a factor
2. Factors that increase risk of physiologic jaundice
   a. Resolution of enclosed hemorrhage (cephalhematoma, large amount of bruising from difficult delivery)
   b. Infection or sepsis
   c. Dehydration
3. *NCLEX®* Physiologic jaundice usually begins after first 24 hours of life

C. Pathologic jaundice

1. Rh incompatibility (hemolytic anemia)
   a. RBCs from Rh-positive fetus enter Rh-negative maternal bloodstream late in pregnancy and after separation of placenta at delivery, causing maternal antibody formation, and destruction of fetal RBCs (erythroblastosis fetalis)
   b. In subsequent pregnancy with fetus of same blood type, maternal antibodies attack fetal RBCs, causing hemolysis and anemia
   c. RhoGAM prevents development of antibodies, but cannot reverse reaction once it occurs
   d. Hydrops fetalis is most severe hemolytic reaction, causing severe anemia, cardiac decompensation, edema, ascites, hypoxia, and possible fetal death
2. ABO blood type incompatibility (hemolytic anemia)
   a. Type O mother carries type A, B, or AB fetus
   b. Maternal antibodies cross placenta, enter and attack fetal RBCs, causing hemolysis and fetal anemia
   c. Reaction tends to be less severe than with Rh incompatibility
3. *NCLEX®* Pathologic jaundice begins within first 24 hours of life

D. Nursing data collection

1. Determine mother's blood type and Rh factor; if mother is Rh-negative or type O blood, determine infant's blood type and Rh factor
2. *NCLEX®* Evaluate results of Coombs' tests
   a. Indirect Coombs' determines presence of antibodies (sensitization) in maternal blood; a positive test indicates presence of antibodies
   b. Direct Coombs' determines presence of maternal Rh antibodies in fetal blood; cord blood is generally used; a positive test indicates presence of antibodies
3. Golden-colored amniotic fluid indicates severe hemolytic disease
4. *NCLEX®* Monitor for jaundice by gently pressing on sternum or forehead; in dark-skinned infants, observe sclera, palms of hands, soles of feet, nose, or palate

Memory Aid Remember that natural light is best for identifying jaundice; apply slight pressure to blanche the forehead (preferred), tip of nose or gum line and watch for yellow discoloration when pressure is released.

5. Evaluate results of bilirubin levels
   a. Bilirubin can be monitored noninvasively with a bilimeter
   NCLEX® b. Total serum bilirubin levels higher than 13 to 15 mg/dL indicate hyperbilirubinemia
6. Enlarged liver and spleen
7. Anemia
8. Concentrated, dark urine

E. Interventions

1. Early and frequent feedings to stimulate peristalsis
2. **Phototherapy** (exposure of infant to bright light)
   NCLEX® a. Cover infant's closed eyes when under phototherapy light; remove eye covers every 2 hours during light therapy to monitor for conjunctivitis and when not under phototherapy to promote bonding
   b. Undress infant to maximize amount of circulating blood exposed to phototherapy light; genitalia can be covered to prevent soiling
   NCLEX® c. Change infant's position every 2 hours and monitor for skin breakdown
   d. Observe for loose green stools as bilirubin is excreted through intestines
   e. Increase fluid intake to prevent dehydration
   NCLEX® f. Measure temperature every 2 hours and monitor for hypothermia or hyperthermia
   g. Monitor bilirubin levels
3. **Exchange transfusion**
   a. Used to quickly decrease high bilirubin level by exchanging infant's circulating blood volume with donor blood; also removes anti-Rh antibodies and fetal cells coated with antibodies from infant's blood and corrects anemia
   NCLEX® b. Only use Type O Rh-negative blood to decrease risk of transfusion reaction
   NCLEX® c. Warm blood to room temperature to prevent cardiac arrest
   d. Give calcium gluconate, as ordered, after each 100 mL
   NCLEX® e. Measure vital signs before procedure, every 15 minutes during procedure and postprocedure
   f. Record time, and amount of blood withdrawn, time and amount injected, medications given
   g. Monitor for dyspnea, listlessness, bleeding, cyanosis, bradycardia or arrythmias, hypoglycemia

IX. HYPOGLYCEMIA

A. Etiology

1. Definition: blood glucose (BG) lower than 30 to 35 mg/dL in a term newborn
2. BG levels are measured with a heel-stick
3. Newborns at risk: IDM, SGA, premature, and infants experiencing cold stress, hypothermia, or delayed feedings
4. Poor prognosis if hypoglycemia is not treated
5. BG usually stabilizes within 48 to 72 hours

B. Nursing data collection

NCLEX® 1. Tremors, jitteriness
2. Lethargy, apathy, limpness, decreased muscle tone
3. High-pitched or weak cry
4. Apnea, irregular respirations, possible respiratory distress
5. Poor feeding, poor sucking, vomiting

C. Interventions

NCLEX® 1. Check BG on all infants at risk by 1 hour of age (30 minutes if IDM) and any symptomatic newborn
NCLEX® 2. Treat hypoglycemia by breastfeeding immediately or giving formula (avoid glucose water to prevent rebound hyperglycemia followed again by hypoglycemia); do not feed a lethargic infant orally because of increased risk of aspiration; give lethargic infant or any infant with BG less than 25 mg/dL dextrose 10% via IV
3. If treated for hypoglycemia, measure BG level again before next feeding

X. INFANT OF A DIABETIC MOTHER

A. Etiology

1. Hormones secreted during pregnancy (human placental lactogen, or HPL) increase maternal resistance to insulin, increasing insulin requirements; in diabetic clients, pancreas cannot secrete additional insulin and BG levels increase
2. Maternal insulin cannot cross placenta but glucose can; fetal glucose levels rise; fetal pancreas secretes more insulin, which metabolizes additional glucose and acts as a growth hormone; increased insulin needs decrease surfactant production

B. Nursing data collection

NCLEX®
1. LGA; birth trauma more likely
2. Maternal dystocia related to CPD
3. Enlarged internal organs: cardiomegaly, hepatomegaly, splenomegaly

NCLEX®
4. Hypoglycemia
5. Hypocalcemia
6. Hyperbilirubinemia
7. RDS

NCLEX®
8. False positive lecithin to sphingomyelin (L/S) ratio
9. Increased risk for congenital anomalies, particularly cardiac and spinal defects

C. Interventions

1. Observe for birth trauma

NCLEX®
2. Measure BG at 30 minutes and at 1, 2, 4, 6, 9, 12, and 24 hours after birth
3. Treat hypoglycemia per orders

XI. SUBSTANCE ABUSE

A. Fetal alcohol syndrome (FAS)

1. Etiology
   a. Alcohol crosses placenta and interferes with protein synthesis
   b. Increased risk of congenital anomalies, mental deficiency, IUGR
2. Nursing data collection
   a. Small for gestational age
   b. Facial features: epicanthal folds, maxillary hypoplasia, long and thin upper lip
   NCLEX® c. Irritable, hyperactive
   NCLEX® d. High-pitched cry
3. Interventions
   NCLEX® a. Reduce environmental stimuli
   NCLEX® b. Swaddle to increase feeling of security
   c. Administer sedatives as ordered to decrease side effects of withdrawal
   d. Maintain nutrition and hydration

B. Neonatal abstinence syndrome (NAS)

1. Etiology
   a. Repeated intrauterine absorption of drugs from maternal bloodstream causes fetal drug dependency
   b. Increased risk of spontaneous abortion, preterm labor, stillbirth
   c. Degree of drug withdrawal depends on type and duration of addiction and maternal drug levels at delivery
2. Nursing data collection
   NCLEX® a. Hyperactivity, jitteriness
   b. Absence of "step" reflex and "head-righting" reflex
   c. Shrill, persistent crying
   d. Frequent yawning and sneezing; nasal stuffiness
   e. Respiratory distress
   f. Sweating
   NCLEX® g. Feeding difficulties (regurgitation, vomiting, and diarrhea), increased need for nonnutritive sucking
   h. Developmental delays

NCLEX®
3. Interventions
   a. Position infant on side to facilitate drainage of mucus
   b. Suction as needed to maintain patent airway
   c. Decrease environmental stimuli, swaddle for comfort
   d. Monitor I&O; measure daily weight

Memory Aid

Remember that infants are jittery during withdrawal. Create a soothing environment by keeping the room dark and quiet.

e. Obtain meconium and/or urine for drug screening as ordered
f. Administer medications as ordered: paregoric elixir to wean infant; chlorpromazine (Thorazine) and diazepam (Valium) to decrease hyperirritability (diazepam predisposes to hyperbilirubinemia and is contraindicated in jaundiced newborns); methadone; phenobarbital to decrease hyperirritability and hyperbilirubinemia
g. Provide pacifier for nonnutritive sucking

Check Your NCLEX–PN® Exam I.Q.

You are ready for testing on this content if you can

- Identify signs and symptoms of neonatal complications after delivery.
- Implement nursing interventions to prevent neonatal complications or assist the client to recover from them.
- Reinforce teaching about neonatal complications and their management.
- Evaluate the client and family response to therapy for neonatal complications.

PRACTICE TEST

1 The following neonates are admitted to the nursery. The nurse should withhold the scheduled initial feeding on which newborn?

1. A neonate with a sustained heart rate of 118 beats/min
2. A neonate with an axillary temperature of 97.5°F
3. A neonate with a sustained respiratory rate of 68 breaths/min
4. A neonate who is small for gestational age (SGA)

2 The nurse hears the parents of a 26-week gestation newborn tell family members, "We'll be ready to bring the baby home in a few weeks." What is the most therapeutic response by the nurse?

1. "I'm glad he's doing so well."
2. "He probably won't be ready to come home for a few months."
3. "A therapist could help you resolve your feelings of denial."
4. "Do you have the nursery ready yet?"

3 While observing parents whose newborn is in the neonatal intensive care unit, the nurse interprets that reinforcement of instructions has been effective when the parents perform which activity?

1. Wear gloves every time they touch their baby.
2. Attach family pictures to the side of the isolette.
3. Bring a 2-year-old sibling to visit.
4. Turn off the cardiac monitor when at the newborn's bedside.

4 The nurse is assisting in developing a plan of care for an infant born at 28 weeks' gestation. What would be a realistic goal for this infant to be achieved within one week?

1. Drinking from a bottle
2. Recognizing the parents
3. Maintaining respiratory rate at 30–60 breaths/minute
4. Maintaining her body temperature in a bassinet

5 A newborn is receiving phototherapy for the treatment of hyperbilirubinemia. The nurse recognizes that teaching has been effective when the parents do which of the following? Select all that apply.

1. Cover the infant with a loose blanket while under the bililights.
2. Continue breastfeeding during the jaundice.
3. Limit the infant's intake due to loose green stools.
4. Cover the infant's eyes before placing him under the bililight.
5. Keep the genitalia covered to prevent soiling.

6 Which data would be most important for the nurse to note as part of an initial review of a newborn's history?

1. Mother received morphine sulfate 4 mg IV 20 minutes before delivery.
2. Mother reports drinking a glass of wine with dinner each night.
3. Mother's age is 14.
4. Mother's blood type is O negative.

7 The parents of a preterm neonate ask why their baby gets cold so easily. The nurse responds with which explanation about preterm neonates?

1. Preterm neonates are able to shiver to produce body heat.
2. Preterm neonates have minimal body fat to retain body heat.
3. Preterm neonates have blood vessels that are deep under the skin surface.
4. Preterm neonates lose heat faster because they lie in a fetal position.

8 While feeding an infant, the nurse notices white, adherent patches on the infant's gums and buccal cavity. Which action should the nurse should take at this time?

1. Document this normal finding.
2. Further evaluate for yeast infection.
3. Verify that vitamin K (AquaMEPHYTON) was given at delivery.
4. Review for maternal history of herpes simplex.

9 Which data would alert the nurse that a newborn infant is experiencing dehydration? Select all that apply.

1. Urine-specific gravity 1.006
2. Urine volume 2 mL/kg/hr
3. Low serum sodium
4. Sunken anterior fontanel
5. Poor skin turgor

10 A newborn male is admitted to the nursery 15 minutes after delivery. His skin is mottled, and mucous membranes are blue; he is active, and is wrapped in a blanket. The nurse should monitor which of the following as a priority?

1. Umbilical cord for bleeding
2. Infant's temperature
3. Visible deformities
4. Patent airway

11 Which nursing intervention is appropriate in the care of an infant with respiratory distress syndrome (RDS)?

1. Maintain a neutral thermal environment.
2. Perform a complete gestational age assessment.
3. Perform chest physiotherapy twice a day.
4. Suction meconium from airway as needed.

12 A 26-week-gestation neonate has received 80–100% oxygen via mechanical ventilation for 2 weeks, and has received several blood transfusions for anemia. The nurse should plan for which intervention needed by the infant?

1. Begin phototherapy.
2. Arrange for eye exam by ophthalmologist prior to discharge.
3. Wean supplemental oxygen rapidly.
4. Administer surfactant via endotracheal tube.

13 The nurse is caring for a neonate born to a mother who is human immunodeficiency virus (HIV)-positive. Which sign in the newborn should be evaluated further?

1. Absence of tears
2. White bumps on nose
3. Enlarged liver
4. Fine, red rash over trunk

14 An infant of a diabetic mother (IDM) is admitted to the newborn nursery. Which nursing intervention has highest priority at this time?

1. Clean the umbilical cord.
2. Administer vitamin K (AquaMEPHYTON) intramuscularly.
3. Complete a gestational age assessment.
4. Monitor the infant's blood glucose level.

15 A father asks how the bilirubin lights make the newborn's bilirubin level go down. What is the best reply by the nurse?

1. "The lights prevent more bilirubin from being released into your baby's body."
2. "Exposing the skin to the air helps get rid of the jaundice. The bililights really just keep the baby warm while this occurs."
3. "The bililights help convert the bilirubin to a form the baby can get rid of."
4. "The bililights release a substance in the body that attacks the bilirubin and destroys it."

16 The nurse examines a newborn and obtains the following information: Left arm limp and extended; left hand internally rotated; positive grasp reflex bilaterally; no response on left side to Moro reflex. What is the most appropriate nursing intervention for this infant? Select all that apply.

1. Examine for congenital hip dysplasia.
2. Avoid positioning infant on left side.
3. Provide passive range of motion exercises after 24 hours
4. Prepare supplies for a cast application.
5. Immobilize the arm by securing the infant's sleeve to the shirt

17 An infant with fetal alcohol syndrome is about to be discharged home with foster parents. Place in order the priority of the nurse in reinforcing teaching about the following topics to the foster parents.

1. Toy safety
2. Infection prevention
3. Feeding methods
4. Immunizations

18 A baby's mother is hepatitis B–positive. Which nursing intervention is most important when planning care for this newborn?

1. Administer hepatitis B vaccine within 12 hours after delivery.
2. Monitor for HIV risk factors.
3. Prepare for exchange transfusion.
4. Isolate the newborn.

19 The nurse realizes that a neonate born at 34 weeks' gestation might not have enough surfactant, so the nurse should observe closely for which of the following? Select all that apply.

1. Abdominal distention
2. Jaundice
3. Jitteriness
4. Sternal retractions
5. Tachypnea

20 The maternal newborn nurse considers that which infant is at greatest risk for infection?

1. 38 weeks' gestation, small for gestational age (SGA)
2. 39 weeks' gestation, diagnosed with caput succedaneum
3. 38 weeks' gestation, cesarean delivery for breech presentation
4. 41 weeks' gestation, infant of a diabetic mother (IDM)

ANSWERS & RATIONALES

1 **Answer: 3** **Rationale:** Feeding a baby with a respiratory rate greater than 60 breaths/min orally increases the risk of aspiration. A heart rate of 118 is slightly below the normal range of 120–160 beats/min, but it is not a contraindication to feeding the infant. A hypothermic or SGA infant is at risk for hypoglycemia, and requires a consistent source of glucose. **Cognitive Level:** Analyzing **Client Need:** Physiological Adaptation **Integrated Process:** Nursing Process: Implementation **Content Area:** Maternal-Newborn **Strategy:** Simply recall that breathing and swallowing cannot be done at the same time. This will help you to select the infant with an elevated respiratory rate as the one who is at risk if given feedings orally.

2 **Answer: 2** **Rationale:** Families are often in a state of denial with the birth of a sick newborn. It is important for nurses to gently encourage the parents to be realistic by sharing truthful information. Agreeing with the parent's statement (by being glad the infant is doing well) prolongs the state of denial and makes it more difficult for the parents to see the situation realistically. Some parents do benefit from professional counseling, but nurses still need to provide support when working with families. It is not important if the nursery is ready yet, and this question distracts from the real issues this family is facing at this time. **Cognitive Level:** Applying **Client Need:** Psychosocial Integrity **Integrated Process:** Communication and Documentation **Content Area:** Maternal-Newborn **Strategy:** Use knowledge of therapeutic communication techniques to answer the question. The correct response is one that provides factual information about the infant's status while respecting the parent's potentially vulnerable status.

3 **Answer: 2** **Rationale:** The act of taping family pictures to the sides of the isolette promotes bonding and infant stimulation. Parents should wash their hands when they enter the unit, but do not need to wear gloves when in contact with their infant. Young children often harbor organisms that could be transmitted to vulnerable newborns, and should not have contact until the infant is moved out of the neonatal intensive care unit. The cardiac monitor should not be turned off unless specifically allowed by staff. **Cognitive Level:** Analyzing **Client Need:** Physiological Adaptation **Integrated Process:** Nursing Process: Evaluation **Content Area:** Maternal-Newborn **Strategy:** The wording of the question tells you that the correct answer is an option that contains an appropriate action on the part of the parents. Use nursing knowledge and the process of elimination to make a selection.

4 **Answer: 3** **Rationale:** A healthy respiratory rate for all newborns is 30–60 breaths/min. Drinking from a bottle, recognizing parents, and maintaining body temperature in a bassinet are not timely goals for a 28-week-gestation infant at 1 week of age. **Cognitive Level:** Applying **Client Need:** Physiological Adaptation **Integrated Process:** Nursing Process: Planning **Content Area:** Maternal-Newborn **Strategy:** Specific knowledge of expected fetal development by gestational age is needed to answer this question. Use nursing knowledge and the process of elimination to make your selection.

5 **Answer: 2, 4, 5** **Rationale:** Breastfeeding is not contraindicated with hyperbilirubinemia. It is important to protect the infant's eyes from the bililight to prevent permanent damage. It is acceptable practice to keep the genitalia covered to prevent soiling from urine or feces. The infant should be unclothed to allow as much skin exposure to the bililight as possible. Increased fluid intake will aid excretion of bilirubin and loose green stools are an indication that bilirubin is being excreted. **Cognitive Level:** Applying **Client Need:** Physiological Adaptation **Integrated Process:** Nursing Process: Evaluation **Content Area:** Maternal-Newborn **Strategy:** The core issue of the question is knowledge of hyperbilirubinemia and its treatment with phototherapy. Use specific nursing knowledge about hyperbilirubinemia and the process of elimination to make your selection.

6 **Answer: 1** **Rationale:** Opioid analgesics cross the placenta and, if given close to delivery, can cause respiratory depression in the newborn, making this the priority item. Maternal drinking, young maternal age, and maternal Rh-negative status might warrant further investigation and follow up, but the priority at delivery is to establish and maintain an airway. **Cognitive Level:** Analyzing **Client Need:** Physiological Adaptation **Integrated Process:** Nursing Process: Data Collection **Content Area:** Maternal-Newborn **Strategy:** Note that critical words in the stem of the question are *most important*. This tells you that some or all of the options are correct, but you must select the priority option. Use nursing knowledge and the process of elimination to make your selection.

7 **Answer: 2** **Rationale:** Preterm infants have minimal adipose tissue, so they lose heat more quickly through their skin. In general, infants are not able to shiver to produce body heat when they are cold. The skin of a neonate is thin, with blood vessels near the surface, which increases heat loss through the skin. Because they are weak and neurologically immature, they aren't able to lie in a tight fetal position, allowing greater exposure of the body to the air, which results in heat loss. **Cognitive Level:** Applying **Client Need:** Physiological Adaptation **Integrated Process:** Communication and Documentation **Content Area:** Maternal-Newborn **Strategy:** The wording of the question tells you that the correct option must be a true statement. Use knowledge about the physical characteristics of premature infants and the process of elimination to make your selection.

8 **Answer: 2** **Rationale:** The primary sign of an oral yeast infection, or thrush, is the presence of white patches in the mouth that tend to bleed if they are touched. The presence of white adherent patches in the mouth is not a normal finding. This finding is unrelated to whether vitamin K was given at delivery. Maternal history of herpes simplex is not relevant. **Cognitive Level:** Applying **Client Need:** Physiological Adaptation **Integrated Process:** Nursing Process: Implementation **Content Area:** Maternal-Newborn **Strategy:** The core issue of the question is the significance of white patches in the infant's mouth. First recall this is not a normal finding. Then recall that vitamin K aids in blood clotting to determine it is unrelated. Finally, recall that herpes simplex (cold sores) would present as vesicles, not white patches.

9 **Answer: 4, 5** **Rationale:** Signs of dehydration in a newborn infant include dry mucous membranes, sunken fontanels, and poor skin turgor. A urine specific gravity of 1.006, urine volume of 2 mL/kg/hr, and low serum sodium are expected findings in a newborn infant. **Cognitive Level:** Analyzing **Client Need:** Physiological Adaptation **Integrated Process:** Nursing Process: Data Collection **Content Area:** Maternal-Newborn **Strategy:** Specific knowledge of manifestations of dehydration is needed to answer this question. Use nursing knowledge and the process of elimination to make your selection.

10 **Answer: 4** **Rationale:** The highest priority after delivery is to maintain and support respiratory function. This infant is demonstrating initial signs of respiratory deficiency. Once airway and breathing are noted, the nurse may check the umbilical cord for bleeding, measure temperature, and, finally, check for visible deformities. **Cognitive Level:** Analyzing **Client Need:** Physiological Adaptation **Integrated Process:** Nursing Process: Data Collection **Content Area:** Maternal-Newborn **Strategy:** Follow the ABCs of resuscitation (airway, breathing, and circulation) to select the correct answer to this question. Airway and breathing are assessed before circulation (bleeding).

11 **Answer: 1** **Rationale:** Infants use additional oxygen and glucose when faced with cold stress. Infants with RDS are already compromised, so it is important to keep environmental temperatures stable to minimize their oxygen and glucose requirements. A complete assessment could increase oxygenation requirements even further. Chest physiotherapy might or might not be needed. There is no specific evidence in the question that meconium is present. **Cognitive Level:** Analyzing **Client Need:** Physiological Adaptation **Integrated Process:** Nursing Process: Implementation **Content Area:** Maternal-Newborn **Strategy:** Note that the core issue of the question is care of an infant with respiratory distress. First, eliminate complete gestational assessment because of the word *complete*. Choose temperature control over chest physiotherapy or suctioning the airway because there is no evidence in the question that these are needed.

12 **Answer: 2** **Rationale:** This infant has been receiving high levels of oxygen for two weeks, and is at risk for retinopathy of prematurity (ROP). All preterm infants who receive oxygen should have a thorough eye exam done by an ophthalmologist prior to discharge. It is important to administer the minimum amount of oxygen to infants to decrease the risk that this condition will develop. Phototherapy is indicated for treatment of high bilirubin levels. Oxygen should be weaned as tolerated but this may or may not be rapidly. Artificial surfactant may be administered within the first several days of life to decrease the risk of respiratory distress syndrome (RDS). **Cognitive Level:** Applying **Client Need:** Physiological Adaptation **Integrated Process:** Nursing Process: Planning **Content Area:** Maternal-Newborn **Strategy:** The core issue of the question is knowledge of the effects of long-term oxygen

therapy for a neonate. Use nursing knowledge and the process of elimination to make your selection.

13 **Answer: 3 Rationale:** Hepatosplenomegaly (enlarged liver and spleen) can be an early sign of HIV infection in an infant. The absence of tears, the presence of milia on the nose, and a fine red rash over the trunk are data that are within normal limits for a neonate. **Cognitive Level:** Applying **Client Need:** Physiological Adaptation **Integrated Process:** Nursing Process: Data Collection **Content Area:** Maternal-Newborn **Strategy:** The core issue of the question is discriminating normal findings from abnormal findings in a newborn whose mother is HIV-positive. Use nursing knowledge and the process of elimination to make your selection.

14 **Answer: 4 Rationale:** An infant of a diabetic mother is at risk for hypoglycemia, and blood glucose should be monitored closely after delivery and treated if necessary. All other interventions are important, but are not the highest priority. **Cognitive Level:** Applying **Client Need:** Physiological Adaptation **Integrated Process:** Nursing Process: Implementation **Content Area:** Maternal-Newborn **Strategy:** Note the critical word *priority* in the stem of the question. This tells you that multiple options are technically correct, but you must decide which has the greatest importance at this time. Note the connection between the word *diabetic* in the stem and the word *glucose* in the correct option to help you make a selection.

15 **Answer: 3 Rationale:** Phototherapy assists the body in converting unconjugated bilirubin to conjugated bilirubin, which is water-soluble and easier for the body to eliminate. The other statements are not accurate explanations. **Cognitive Level:** Applying **Client Need:** Physiological Adaptation **Integrated Process:** Communication and Documentation **Content Area:** Maternal-Newborn **Strategy:** The core issue of the question is knowledge of how phototherapy assists in lowering the bilirubin levels of a jaundiced newborn. Use nursing knowledge and the process of elimination to make your selection.

16 **Answer: 2, 5 Rationale:** The infant should not be positioned on the affected side. The arm may be secured by securing the infant's sleeve to the shirt or using a brace or splint. Congenital hip dysplasia is characterized by a clicking sound with hip rotation, while this infant has Erb-Duchenne's paralysis (Erb's palsy) of the left arm. Passive range of motion is delayed until the 10th day to prevent further damage. Occasionally a splint may be applied, but a cast is not indicated. **Cognitive Level:** Analyzing **Client Need:** Physiological Adaptation **Integrated Process:** Nursing Process: Implementation **Content Area:** Maternal-Newborn **Strategy:** The core issue of this question is recognition of and appropriate intervention for an infant with Erb's paralysis. Note the wording of the question indicates more than one option may be correct. Use nursing knowledge and the process of elimination to make your selections.

17 **Answer: 3, 2, 4, 1 Rationale:** Infants with fetal alcohol syndrome have an increased risk of feeding difficulties related to hyperactivity. Nutrition is a key concern for this infant for proper growth and development. Infection prevention is the second priority concern, since this will help to maintain healthy physiological condition. The immunization schedule has third priority because it is also related to prevention of communicable diseases and infection. Although toy safety is important, it is the fourth priority because newborns are not developed sufficiently to play with toys. **Cognitive Level:** Analyzing **Client Need:** Physiological Adaptation **Integrated Process:** Nursing Process: Planning **Content Area:** Maternal-Newborn **Strategy:** Use Maslow's hierarchy of needs to guide priority setting. Physiological needs come first, followed by safety needs, then psychosocial needs.

18 **Answer: 1 Rationale:** Infants born to mothers who are hepatitis B–positive should receive a hepatitis B vaccine within 12 hours of birth to decrease their risk of acquiring the infection from maternal exposure. It is appropriate to monitor for HIV risk factors in all infants, not just those at risk for hepatitis B. An exchange transfusion is not appropriate in this situation. Isolating the infant is not appropriate in this situation. **Cognitive Level:** Applying **Client Need:** Physiological Adaptation **Integrated Process:** Nursing Process: Implementation **Content Area:** Maternal-Newborn **Strategy:** The key focus of the question is the risk of transmission of hepatitis B from mother to infant. The correct answer would be the option that contains a nursing action to reduce the risk of disease transmission for this infant.

19 **Answer: 4, 5 Rationale:** Preterm infants lack adequate surfactant to keep their alveoli open during expiration. This can lead to development of respiratory distress syndrome (RDS), which would be evidenced by signs of respiratory distress, including tachypnea. Abdominal distention, jaundice, and jitteriness are not directly related to RDS. **Cognitive Level:** Applying **Client Need:** Physiological Adaptation **Integrated Process:** Nursing Process: Data Collection **Content Area:** Maternal-Newborn **Strategy:** The focus of the question is assessment findings in a premature infant with the potential for developing respiratory distress. Eliminate incorrect options because abdominal distention, jaundice, and jitteriness are not directly related to RDS.

20 **Answer: 1 Rationale:** SGA infants often experience intrauterine growth restriction related to decreased blood flow to the placenta, which increases their risk for infection. In comparison, the infants in the other options are at less risk for infection. **Cognitive Level:** Analyzing **Client Need:** Physiological Adaptation **Integrated Process:** Nursing Process: Evaluation **Content Area:** Maternal-Newborn **Strategy:** The wording of the question tells you the correct answer is the infant who is at greatest risk for infection. Recall the relative risk for infection in each neonate listed to answer this question. Use nursing knowledge and the process of elimination to make your selection.

Key Terms to Review

bronchopulmonary dysplasia (BPD) p. 789
continuous positive airway pressure (CPAP) p. 787
exchange transfusion p. 796
extracorporeal membrane oxygenation (ECMO) p. 792
intrauterine growth restriction (IUGR) p. 793
intraventricular hemorrhage (IVH) p. 788
kernicterus p. 795
meconium aspiration syndrome (MAS) p. 789
necrotizing enterocolitis (NEC) p. 788
neutral thermal environment p. 788
oxygen hood p. 787
phototherapy p. 796
retinopathy of prematurity (ROP) p. 789
respiratory distress syndrome (RDS) p. 787
transient tachypnea of the newborn (TTN) p. 791
umbilical arterial line (UAL) p. 786
umbilical venous line (UVL) p. 786

References

Davidson, M., London, M., & Ladewig, P. (2012). *Olds' maternal newborn nursing and women's health across the lifespan* (9th ed.). Upper Saddle River, NJ: Pearson Education, Inc.

Ladewig, P., London, M., & Davidson, M. (2010). *Contemporary maternal-newborn nursing care* (7th ed.). Upper Saddle River, NJ: Pearson Education, Inc.

London, M., Ladewig, P., Ball, J., Bindler, R., & Cowen, K. (2011). *Maternal & child nursing care* (3rd ed.). Upper Saddle River, NJ: Pearson Education, Inc.

Perry, S., Hockenberry, M., Lowdermilk, D., & Wilson, D. (2010). *Maternal child nursing care* (4th ed.). St. Louis, MO: Elsevier.

Test Yourself

Are you ready for the NCLEX-PN® or course exams? Use the practice tests on the companion website to check.

49 Fluid and Electrolyte Imbalances

In this chapter

Cross Reference

Other chapters relevant to this content area are

Meeting Nutritional Needs	**Chapter 25**
Common Laboratory Tests	**Chapter 42**

I. CONCEPTS OF FLUID AND ELECTROLYTE BALANCE

A. Fluid transport

1. Body fluid compartments
   a. Intracellular fluid (ICF): fluid within cells; two thirds of body fluid is ICF
   b. Extracellular fluid (ECF): fluid outside of cells; made up of two components, interstitial fluid (surrounding cells) and fluid within vascular space (blood vessels)
   c. Fluid constantly moves among intracellular, interstitial, and vascular spaces to maintain body fluid balance
   d. ICF is most stable and is fairly resistant to major fluid shifts
   e. Vascular fluid is least stable; it is quickly lost or gained in response to fluid intake or losses
   f. Interstitial fluid is reserve fluid, replacing fluid either in blood vessels or cells, depending on need
2. Osmosis
   a. Water moves through a semipermeable membrane (allows water and small particles, but not large particles, to easily pass through) from an area of lower concentration (fewer particles, more water) to an area of higher concentration (more particles, less water) until concentrations are equalized
   b. Osmosis is a major force in body fluid movement and intravenous (IV) fluid therapy; cell membranes and capillary membranes are semipermeable; water moves into and out of cells and capillaries by osmosis

3. Osmolality and osmotic pressure
   a. Osmolality and osmalarity refer to concentration of a solution, which creates its osmotic pressure (pulling power of a solution for water)
   b. Osmolality is concentration of solute (particles) measured per *kilogram* of water, while osmolarity is concentration of solute (particles) measured per *liter* of solution (solvent does not have to be water)
   c. Because body fluid solvent is water and one liter of water weighs one kilogram, the terms can be used interchangeably in discussing human fluids
   d. The higher the osmolality of a solution, the greater its pulling power for water
   e. Serum osmolality is concentration of particles (major particles are sodium and protein) in plasma: normal is 275 to 295 mOsm/L
   f. Isotonic: having same osmolality as normal plasma (see Table 49–1 for examples of IV solutions that are isotonic; also see Chapter 30)
   g. **Hypotonic**: having a lower osmolality than normal plasma; water is pulled out of blood vessels into cells, resulting in decreased vascular volume and increased cell water (see Table 49–1 for examples of hypotonic IV solutions; also see Chapter 30)
   h. **Hypertonic**: having a higher osmolality than normal plasma; water is pulled from cells into blood vessels, resulting in increased vascular volume and decreased cell water (see Table 49–1 for examples of hypertonic IV solutions; also see Chapter 30)
4. Diffusion
   a. Particles move from an area of higher concentration (more particles, less water) to lower concentration (fewer particles, more water) until equalized
   b. Electrolytes (e.g., sodium, potassium, chloride, calcium, magnesium, and phosphate) are small particles that move easily through semipermeable membranes
   c. Urea, glucose, and albumin are large particles that do not pass easily through semipermeable membranes

B. Capillary fluid movement

1. Hydrostatic pressure: pushing force of a fluid against walls of space it occupies; generated in blood vessels by heart's pumping action and varies within vascular system
2. Oncotic pressure (also called colloid osmotic pressure, or COP): pulling force exerted by colloids (such as albumin, other plasma proteins) that normally remain in bloodstream
3. Starling's Law of the capillaries
   a. Filtration (net fluid movement into or out of capillary) is determined by difference between forces favoring filtration and those opposing it (like a tug of war—pushing and pulling)
   b. Interstitial hydrostatic pressure (pushing water into capillary) and interstitial oncotic pressure (pulling water out of capillary) are very low and essentially equal, thus normally exerting little influence on fluid movement into or out of capillaries
   c. Capillary hydrostatic pressure (pushing water out of capillary) and capillary oncotic pressure (pulling water into capillary) are not equal, and fluid movement is seen in capillary bed

Table 49–1 Tonicity of Typical IV Solutions

Tonicity	Examples of IV Solutions	Comments
Isotonic	0.9% sodium chloride (normal saline, NS, 0.9% NaCl) Ringer's solution Lactated Ringer's solution (LR) 5% dextrose in water (D_5W)	Same osmolality as normal plasma; no osmotic pressure difference is created, so fluids remain primarily in ECF; isotonic IV fluids replace ECF losses and expand vascular volume quickly D_5W is isotonic in bag but has hypotonic effect in body after dextrose is metabolized; two thirds of water goes to body cells
Hypotonic	0.45% sodium chloride (½ NS) 0.225% sodium chloride (¼ NS)	Provides free water and small amounts of sodium and chloride to cells
Hypertonic	5% dextrose in 0.45% sodium chloride (D_5 ½ NS) 5% dextrose in 0.225% sodium chloride (D_5 ¼ NS) 5% dextrose in 0.9% sodium chloride (D_5 NS) 3% sodium chloride (3% NaCl) 5% sodium chloride (5% NaCl) 10% dextrose 50% dextrose	D_5 ½ NS and D_5 ¼ NS are hypertonic in IV bag and provide dextrose and some water to cells D_5NS is isotonic after dextrose is metabolized 3% and 5% NaCl: used to treat specific problems; administered in carefully controlled, limited doses to avoid vascular volume overload and cell dehydration; also used to pull excess fluid from cells and promote osmotic diuresis

C. Chemical regulation of fluid and electrolyte balance

1. Antidiuretic hormone (ADH): a hormone synthesized by hypothalamus and secreted by posterior pituitary that regulates water (see also Chapter 56); is released and inhibited in a feedback loop
2. Aldosterone: hormone produced by adrenal gland that conserves sodium by causing renal retention of sodium and excretion of potassium; water follows sodium because of osmosis, thus aldosterone has an indirect effect on water; is released and inhibited in a feedback loop as part of the renin-angiotensin-aldosterone (RAA) system
3. Glucocorticoid (cortisol): hormone produced and released by adrenal gland and increased when body is stressed; promotes renal retention of sodium and water
4. Atrial natriuretic peptide (ANP): a cardiac hormone found in atria of heart and released when atria are stretched by high blood volume or high BP; ANP causes vasodilation by direct effects on blood vessels, suppresses RAA system, decreases ADH release, and increases glomerular filtration rate (GFR) in kidneys; these actions all promote fluid excretion
5. Thirst mechanism: occurs with fluid losses or increases in serum osmolality; stimulated by receptors in hypothalamus that can detect as little as 1 mOsm/L change in plasma concentration; stimulates ADH and aldosterone release, which promotes reabsorption of water; thirst is depressed in people over 60 years as an age-related change, including healthy people and those with debilitating illnesses
6. Fluid losses occur mainly via kidneys (approx. 1500 mL/day), but also via skin through diffusion (400 mL/day) and perspiration (100 mL), lungs via moisture in exhaled air (350 mL/day), and feces (150 mL/day); fluid losses that are not measureable are called insensible losses

II. DEFICIENT FLUID VOLUME (DEHYDRATION)

A. Overview

1. Occurs when fluid intake is inadequate for bodily needs; goal is to replace fluid and any necessary electrolytes and eliminate cause of deficit
2. Types of fluid loss: isotonic, hypotonic, hypertonic (see Table 49–2)
   - **a.** Isotonic dehydration involves equal losses of all fluid components and is most common type of fluid volume deficit
   - **b.** Hypertonic dehydration involves greater losses of ECF volume than electrolytes, leading to an increased plasma osmolality; fluid shifting occurs as body tries to compensate to restore balance

Table 49–2 Comparison of Isotonic, Hypertonic, and Hypotonic Dehydration

Type of Dehydration	Description	Causes
Isotonic	Fluid and solutes are lost in proportional or equal amounts; serum osmolality remains normal, and no osmotic force is created Intracellular water is not disturbed, and fluid losses are primarily ECF (especially vascular), which can quickly lead to shock Is primarily an ECF loss that requires ECF replacement, with emphasis on vascular volume	Hemorrhage Gastrointestinal losses (mild nausea and vomiting, gastric suction, etc.) Fever, environmental heat, and diaphoresis Burns (especially large burns) Diuretics Third space fluid shifts (when fluid moves from blood vessels into physiologically useless extracellular spaces (becoming unavailable as reserve fluid or to transport nutrients)
Hypertonic	More water than solute (primarily sodium) is lost, creating a fluid volume deficit and a relative solute excess Solute (sodium or glucose more commonly) can also be gained in excess of water, creating a similar imbalance Serum osmolality is elevated, resulting in hypertonic ECF that pulls fluid into blood vessels from cells by osmosis and causes cells to shrink and become dehydrated	Inadequate fluid intake (those unable to respond to thirst, nausea, anorexia, dysphagia) Severe or prolonged isotonic fluid losses (vomiting, watery diarrhea, diabetes insipidus) Increased solute intake (salt, sugar, protein) without proportional fluid increase, such as concentrated enteral feedings, hyperglycemia, excess salt or sugar ingestion, excess osmotic diuretic use
Hypotonic	More solute than water is lost Fluid moves into cells, causing cellular swelling	Chronic illness Malnutrition Excess hypotonic fluid replacement

c. Hypotonic dehydration involves greater losses of electrolytes, leading to a decreased plasma osmolality; fluid shifting occurs as ECF volume decreases

3. Third spacing
   a. Occurs when fluid is deposited into extracellular body spaces that do not normally hold large amounts of fluid but in which fluids can accumulate; fluid is useless because it is not available as reserve fluid or to transport nutrients
   b. Common locations for third space fluid to accumulate include tissue spaces (edema), abdomen (ascites), pleural spaces (pleural effusion), and pericardial space (pericardial effusion); see Box 49–1 for causes of third spacing

NCLEX®

B. Nursing data collection (see Table 49-3 to compare signs of Deficient Fluid Volume and Excess Fluid Volume)

1. Presence of risk factors: age (very young or old), acute or chronic illness, vigorous exercise or heat injuries, dysphagia, malnutrition, and medications (diuretics, chemotherapy agents that cause vomiting)
2. Thirst (an early sign), unreliable as an indicator in older adults and in children who cannot express needs
3. Low urine volume: less than 1 to 2 mL/kg/hour in children; less than 30 mL/hour (240 mL/8 hours) or 0.5 mL/kg/hour for adults
4. Concentrated, dark urine with specific gravity higher than 1.035 (normal 1.010 to 1.030); note that if diabetes insipidus is causing fluid loss, urine will be pale, dilute, and high in volume

Box 49–1

Causes of Third Spacing

Injury or inflammation (increases capillary permeability, allowing fluid, electrolytes, and proteins to leak from blood vessels)

Massive trauma

Crush injuries

Burns

Sepsis

Cancer

Intestinal obstruction

Abdominal surgery

Malnutrition or liver dysfunction (prevents liver from producing albumin, thus lowering capillary oncotic pressure)

Starvation

Cirrhosis

Chronic alcoholism

High vascular hydrostatic pressure (pushes abnormal volumes of fluid from vessels)

Heart failure

Renal failure

Other forms of vascular fluid overload

Table 49-3 Fluid Volume Imbalances: Quick Summary of Findings

Deficient Fluid Volume (Dehydration)	Fluid Volume Excess (Fluid Overload)
Thirst	Peripheral edema
Low urine output, concentrated, dark urine	Increased urine output that is dilute (if normal kidney function)
Acute weight loss	Acute, rapid weight gain
Dry mucous membranes, tongue	Tense or bulging fontanels in infants
Dry skin and decreased turgor	Distended neck veins (high central venous pressure (CVP), delayed peripheral vein emptying,
Decreased tearing and dry conjunctiva, sunken eyeballs	S_3 heart sound in adults
Sunken or depressed fontanels in infants	Possible hepatomegaly and splenomegaly from venous congestion
Flat neck veins (low central venous pressure), poor peripheral vein filling	Tachypnea, dyspnea, crackles and other signs of pulmonary edema
Hypotension (late sign); postural or frank	Full or bounding peripheral pulses, warm extremities, brisk capillary refill
Tachycardia	Mental status changes (headache, confusion, lethargy; seizures possible)
Delayed capillary refill	
Tachypnea (usually without dyspnea)	
Weakness, dizziness, lightheadedness, syncope	
Mental status changes (irritability, restlessness, lethargy, confusion, drowsiness, seizures or coma)	

5. Dry mucous membranes, dry tongue with longitudinal furrows in all ages, dry skin and decreased skin turgor (tenting, which occurs when skin is pinched gently and it takes time to return to normal—forming a "tent")
    a. Skin of older clients loses elasticity with aging, so tenting is not a reliable sign in older adults; test skin on sternum, forehead, inner thigh, or top of hip bone rather than arms or legs
    b. Decreased tearing and dry conjunctiva
6. Sunken eyeballs; sunken or depressed anterior and possibly posterior fontanels in infants under 18 months old
7. Flat neck veins (with head of bed 30 to 45 degrees) and poor peripheral vein filling when hand is placed lower than heart (normally fill within 3 to 5 seconds)
8. Hypotension (late sign in infants and young children); may be postural or frank
    a. Reports of weakness, dizziness, lightheadedness
    b. Syncope when rising from lying position
9. Tachycardia (early sign, especially in infants and young children); weak, thready pulse; cool extremities with delayed capillary refill
10. Tachypnea (usually without dyspnea)
11. Low-grade fever (higher fever can occur in severe dehydration)
12. Mental status changes (e.g., irritability, restlessness, lethargy, confusion, drowsiness)
    a. Often first signs noticed in older adults and also often cause alarm in parents of infants and small children
    b. Are a serious sign of significant fluid loss; if fluid loss is severe, client can progress to seizures and coma
13. Acute weight loss (an important sign in infants and young children)
    a. 1 liter (L) water = 1 kg (2.2 pounds)

    NCLEX®

    b. Monitoring weight is considered more accurate than monitoring intake and output (I&O) because of difficulty in keeping accurate records
14. Laboratory findings: normal or high hematocrit (Hct) and blood urea nitrogen (BUN), high urine specific gravity (>1.030) except in diabetes insipidus (<1.010); possible elevated serum osmolality (>300 mOsm/kg), hypernatremia over 150 mEq/L

NCLEX®

C. Therapeutic management

1. Oral replacement therapies if deficit is mild, thirst is intact, and client can drink; during initial rehydration, avoid fluids with sugar or salts, which can worsen fluid loss, and caffeinated beverages, which have diuretic effect
2. Parenteral replacement therapies: IV fluid replacement depending on type of fluid loss (isotonic, hypertonic, hypotonic)
3. Monitor specific parameters (vital signs, urine output, mental status, IV site, I&O, and daily weight)
4. Provide comfort measures such as mouth care and lip moisturizer; avoid giving client hard candy or chewing gum with sugar, which have drying effect
5. Provide measures to prevent fluid volume deficit and dehydration
    a. Provide additional plain water boluses periodically during enteral feedings
    b. Implement measures to control nausea, vomiting, diarrhea, and high fever, which may cause further complications
    c. Recognize acutely ill clients who are at risk for dehydration and initiate measures to provide adequate fluids by oral, enteral, or parenteral routes
6. Medication therapy as needed: antiemetics, antidiarrheals, ADH (vasopressin), antipyretics for fever

D. Client teaching

1. Awareness of predisposing or risk factors; contact physician if illness lasts more than 24 hours, if client is an older adult or very young, or if client has a chronic illness (such as diabetes, heart disease, kidney or liver disease)
2. Measures to help prevent fluid deficit and dehydration (frequent fluid intake during day in hot weather even if not thirsty; avoid highly salty fluids and excess table salt; avoid caffeine)
3. Specific measures that treat underlying cause

III. EXCESS FLUID VOLUME (FLUID OVERLOAD)

A. Overview

1. A state in which rate of fluid intake or retention exceeds rate of fluid loss in body; goal is to restore fluid balance
2. Types of fluid volume excess (FVE)

a. Isotonic fluid excess is caused by renal failure, heart failure, excess fluid intake, high corticosteroid levels, or high aldosterone levels
b. Hypotonic fluid excess (water intoxication) is caused by repeated plain water enemas or repeated plain water NG tube or bladder irrigations, overuse or excessive speed of hypotonic IV fluid infusions, excessive plain water intake (such as in extreme dieting), syndrome of inappropriate ADH (SIADH) secretion (SIADH), or psychogenic polydipsia
c. Hypertonic: caused by excessive salt intake

NCLEX®
B. Nursing data collection (see again Table 49–3)

1. Predisposing risk factors: age (very old or young), surgery, chronic illess (especially cardiac or renal failure), medications such as long-term glucocorticoids
2. Peripheral edema
3. Tense or bulging fontanels in children under 18 months old
4. High central venous pressure (CVP) with venous engorgement (distended neck veins with head of bed at 45 degrees or higher), delayed peripheral vein emptying, S_3 heart sound in adults, hepatomegaly and splenomegaly are signs of venous congestion
5. Signs of pulmonary edema because of increasing extravascular fluid retention
   a. Tachypnea and dyspnea, irritated cough (often early sign of fluid in alveoli)
   b. Hacking cough that eventually becomes moist and productive (clear to white sputum); a late sign of fluid in alveoli and larger airways
   c. Labored breathing (seen as intercostal and substernal retractions, nasal flaring, and expiratory grunting in infants)
   d. Wet lung sounds (moist crackles) on auscultation (first appear in bases bilaterally and progress upward as FVE worsens)
   e. Decreased O_2 saturation due to inadequate or mismatched ventilation and perfusion as a result of FVE
   f. Cyanosis (a late sign of hypoxemia)
6. Vital signs (reflect normal or increased cardiac output): normal heart rate, full or bounding peripheral pulses, warm extremities, brisk capillary refill
7. Third space fluid accumulations may be present (ascites, pleural effusion, pericardial effusion)
8. Acute, rapid weight gain
9. Increased urine output that is dilute
10. A weight gain of 3 pounds or more can occur over 2 to 5 days
11. Hct and BUN are decreased because of hemodilution (plasma has more water than normal, thus is more dilute), possible significant decreases in serum osmolality (<275 mOsm/kg) or serum sodium (<125 mEq/L); chest x-ray may show pleural effusions
12. Mental status changes such as headache, confusion, and lethargy, can also progress to seizures

NCLEX®
C. Therapeutic management

1. Restrict fluid intake (sometimes as low as 1000–1500 mL per 24-hour period) and restrict sodium (helps decrease water retention); keep IV access with saline lock instead of infusing IV fluids
2. Involve client in dividing fluid allowances over 24-hour period; plan for more fluids during meals and with oral medications
3. Promote excretion (diuretics, cardiac glycosides in heart failure to increase cardiac output and renal perfusion)
4. Increase protein intake in clients who are malnourished and have low serum proteins to increase capillary oncotic pressure (and pull fluid into blood vessels for excretion)
5. Monitor cardiac, and respiratory status
6. Monitor fluid I&O carefully, ice chips count as fluid intake (1 cup ice chips equals ½ cup water); improved urine output indicates response to therapy
7. Monitor daily weights (same time, same clothing, same scale); a change of 2.2 lbs (1 kg) equals a 1 liter water loss or gain
8. Observe for peripheral edema (differentiate dependent, or stasis, edema from more generalized edema related to heart, kidney, or liver problems)
9. Observe for developing or worsening water intoxication (hypotonic fluid volume excess), often associated with neurological changes
10. Monitor for overcorrection, in which signs of fluid volume deficit begin to appear
11. Review follow-up electrolytes, BUN, serum osmolarity for return to normal values
12. Use an infusion pump to help prevent inadvertent administration of excess fluid
13. Institute measures to prevent fluid volume excess: irrigate NG tube and bladder with normal saline rather than plain water; avoid repeated plain tap water enemas; mix infant formula according to package directions; do not use a water bottle as a pacifier for infants

D. **Client teaching**
1. Risk factors for excess fluid volume
2. Weigh self (adult) daily and report a gain of more than 2 pounds per week
3. Elevate extremities and change position frequently if peripheral edema present
4. Dietary education: sodium-restricted diet and use of alternative seasonings (natural, sodium-free herbs and spices); clients taking potassium-sparing diuretics and/or ACE inhibitors (which cause potassium retention) should not use salt substitutes because most contain potassium; avoid adding salt while cooking or at table; monitor sodium content by reading food/OTC drug labels

IV. HYPONATREMIA

A. **Overview**
1. **Hyponatremia**: a serum sodium (Na^+) level below 135 mEq/L (normal range 135–145 mEq/L)
2. Usually associated with **hypervolemia** (increased fluid volume), which can then be referred to as dilutional hyponatremia or **water intoxication** (excess fluid that dilutes serum Na^+); can also occur in euvolemia (normal volume) and **hypovolemia** (low volume) states (see Table 49–4)
3. Predisposing conditions (see Box 49–2)

NCLEX® B. **Nursing data collection**
1. Common signs relate to shift of water into cells and role of Na^+ in nerve impulse transmission and muscle contraction (see Table 49–5)
2. Decreased BUN and Hct
3. Dietary: prolonged NPO status; excess infusion of nonelectrolyte solutions, causing free water accumulation

C. **Therapeutic management**
1. Focuses on restoring normal levels, preventing complications, and treating underlying problems
2. NCLEX® Encourage inclusion of high Na^+ foods in diet (refer to Box 49–3 for Na^+ food sources)
3. For hyponatremia with normal fluid volume (euvolemic) or hypertonic dehydration, use water restriction and treat underlying cause
4. Use isotonic saline NS for wound or other irrigations
5. Salt and fluid restrictions and even dialysis may have to be used if clinical picture indicates
6. Continue to monitor laboratory results; aim is to raise Na^+ level no more than 25 mEq/L in the first 48 hours with a rate not to exceed 1 to 2 mEq/L/hr
7. Keep accurate I&O records
8. NCLEX® Obtain daily weights; a weight loss of more than 0.5 pound in 24 hours is considered to be caused by fluid loss
9. NCLEX® Monitor for resolution of signs of hyponatremia, including CNS changes such as confusion, lethargy, and seizures

Table 49–4 Hyponatremia in Various Fluid Volume States

Euvolemic State	Hypervolemic State	Hypovolemic State
Description		
Decrease in fluids in both intravascular and interstitial spaces Results in a normal serum osmolality Use of sodium-free solutions that dilute the ECF	High-glucose states that pull water from cells, leading to cellular dehydration as seen in diabetic ketoacidosis (DKA) Fluid loss from ECF is greater than solute loss, leading to increased serum osmolality	Glucose in isotonic solutions is oxidized, leading to cellular swelling Loss of solute from ECF is greater than excess of water, resulting in a decreased serum osmolality
Clinical presentations		
SIADH, medications, hypothyroidism, psychiatric disorders	CHF, cirrhosis, nephrotic syndrome, and renal failure	GI fluid loss, diuretic therapy, osmotic diuresis, adrenal insufficiency, burns, sweating, hypotonic dehydration
Treatment		
Water restriction, correct underlying cause, treat SIADH with demeclocycline (unlabeled use), and increase dietary salt intake	Water restriction, treat existing disease states, loop diuretics such as furosemide (Lasix), and restrict dietary salt intake	NS to correct ECF deficits, increase dietary salt intake; hypertonic saline to raise Na^+ level

Box 49–2

Causes of Hyponatremia

- Loss of sodium
- Renal losses through excretion, diuretics, renal disease (salt-wasting nephropathy)
- GI losses through vomiting, diarrhea, suctioning, tap water enemas (TWE), GI surgery, bulimia
- Skin losses through perspiration, environmental heat and humidity, burns, tissue destruction
- Conditions that increase extracellular water
- Hormone regulation of ADH and aldosterone, leading to fluid shifts and water gain
- Disorders that add to increased volume, such as CHF, cirrhosis, and nephrotic syndrome
- Conditions such as psychiatric disorders that involve compulsive water drinking
- Disorders such as tumors, SIADH, and adrenal insufficiency that affect hormonal response, leading to increased secretion
- Hyperglycemic states such as diabetic ketoacidosis (DKA) that cause cellular dehydration
- Prolonged or excessive use of hypotonic fluid administration
- Conditions that lead to inadequate dietary intake of sodium
- Prolonged use of fluids without sodium replacement
- Anorexia and other eating disorders

Table 49–5 Sodium Imbalances: Quick Summary of Findings

	Hyponatremia (Na^+ < 135 mEq/L)	Hypernatremia (Na^+ > 145 mEq/L)
Cardiovascular	Bounding pulse, tachycardia, hypotension (↓ ECV), hypertension (↑ ECV)	Tachycardia, hypertension, ↓ cardiac contractility
Integument	Pale, dry skin and mucous membranes (↓ ECV), edema and weight gain (↑ ECV)	Dry and sticky mucous membranes; rough, dry tongue; flushed skin
Renal	↑ urine output with low specific gravity (<1.010)	Thirst, ↑ urine output as kidneys try to eliminate Na^+
Neuromuscular	Lethargy, agitation, dizziness, weakness, headache, confusion, seizures	Twitching, tremor and hyperreflexia, agitation and CNS irritability, hallucinations, seizures, coma
Gastrointestinal (GI)	Anorexia, vomiting, diarrhea, hyperactive bowel sounds, abdominal cramping	Watery diarrhea, nausea, thirst

Box 49–3

Sodium Food Sources

The following foods are considered adequate sources of sodium:

- Processed food products (highest sources of sodium in the diet)
- Lunch meats
- Ham, bacon, and pork products (high sodium levels)
- Dill pickles, corned beef, and products that are "pickled" in brine solutions
- Potato chips and other salted snack foods
- Butter, cheese, and milk
- Condiments such as ketchup, mustard, soy sauce, relishes
- Anchovies, mackerel, and other saltwater fish products

NCLEX®

10. Protect client from injury and maintain a safe environment if client experiences neurological changes due to hyponatremia
11. Medication therapy: salt tablets, loop diuretics, LR or NS (isotonic dehydration) or 3% or 5% hypertonic saline (severe deficits)

D. Client teaching

1. Predisposing factors: age (older adults and very young), environmental conditions (heat and humidity)
2. Dietary education: high-sodium foods
3. Preventing a recurrence: observe for and report early signs and symptoms of hyponatremia such as abdominal cramps, muscle weakness, and nausea
4. Observe for changes in mental status, especially if client already has cardiac, renal, or endocrine problems that might exacerbate hyponatremia

V. HYPERNATREMIA

A. Overview

1. **Hypernatremia**: a serum Na^+ level greater than 145 mEq/L (normal range 135–145 mEq/L)
2. Sodium excess always exists in a **hyperosmolar** (osmotic pressure greater than normal plasma pressure) state
3. Sodium excess can exist in hypovolemic, euvolemic, and hypervolemic states (see Table 49–6 for summary of this disorder)
4. Predisposing clinical conditions
   a. Disturbances in water regulation such as decreased intake, increased insensible loss, or watery diarrhea
   b. Water loss due to fever, hyperventilation, diuretic therapy, and burns
   c. Increased Na^+ intake either from food or sodium-containing fluids
   d. Renal water losses or disease, or hormonal states such as Cushing's syndrome (increased cortisol production) or diabetes insipidus
   e. Clients who experience near-drowning in salt water are at risk for developing hypernatremia

NCLEX®

B. Nursing data collection

1. Common signs relate to water shifting from cells into vascular space (cellular dehydration) and sodium's role in nerve impulse transmission and muscle contraction (see again Table 49–5)
2. Risk factors: age (very young or old), OTC or prescribed medications, high Na^+ diet or excessive use of salt as flavoring

NCLEX®

C. Therapeutic management

1. Focuses on restoring normal levels, preventing complications, and treating underlying problems
2. Decrease Na^+ intake depending on severity to 3 grams, 2 grams, 1 gram, or 500 mg/day
3. Refer client to a dietitian to evaluate dietary intake for hidden sources of Na^+
4. Maintain safe environment because of CNS irritability and risk of seizure activity; initiate seizure precautions
5. Monitor I&O and daily weight
6. Medication therapy: loop diuretics (sodium excess), IV fluids as needed

Table 49–6 Hypernatremia in Various Fluid Volume States

Euvolemic State	Hypervolemic State	Hypovolemic State
Description		
Decrease in water that leads to elevated serum sodium; does not present with contracted volume unless severe water loss occurs	Greater gain of sodium in relation to fluids, leading to elevated serum sodium	Greater loss of water than sodium, leading to elevated serum sodium
Clinical conditions		
Increased fluid loss via skin or lungs (hyperventilation)	Administration of hypertonic saline solutions or $NaHCO_3$, hyperaldosteronism or hypertonic dehydration	Renal losses (osmotic diuresis), insensible loss (sweating and/or fever), GI losses (diarrhea) Young and older adult clients are most at risk
Treatment		
Free water replacement either orally or by fluid-hydrating IV solutions	Remove sodium source, administer diuretics, and replace water	NS to correct intravascular volume deficit, then hypotonic fluids can be used to restore Na^+ level

D. Client teaching

1. Awareness of predisposing factors in older adults: limited mobility, multiple medication profile, and restricted access to fluids
2. Report recurrence of early signs of hypernatremia to health care provider

NCLEX®

3. Dietary education
   a. Na^+ content of foods and sources of hidden Na^+
   b. Follow a low-sodium diet after discharge
   c. Read all labels for Na^+ content prior to ingestion
   d. Use herbs, lemon juice, spices, and vinegar instead of salt or salt substitutes
   e. Do not routinely salt food prior to tasting

VI. HYPOKALEMIA

A. Overview

1. **Hypokalemia**: a serum potassium (K^+) level below 3.5 mEq/L (normal range 3.5–5.1 mEq/L)
2. Has widespread effects on body, and if severe or not corrected quickly, death can result from cardiac and respiratory arrest
3. Predisposing factors
   a. Increased secretion of aldosterone leading to excretion of K^+ from renal tubules (adrenal adenomas, cirrhosis, nephrosis, heart failure and hypertensive crisis, Cushing's syndrome, diabetes insipidus)
   b. Excessive loss of K^+ by loop diuretics, thiazide diuretics, corticosteroids, cardiac glycosides, penicillins, amphotericin B, gentamicin, theophylline, cisplatin, and tocolytic agents
   c. GI loss by vomiting, diarrhea, prolonged nasogastric suctioning, newly created ileostomy, villous adenoma on intestinal tract, laxative abuse, or enema administration
   d. Heat induced diaphoresis
   e. Renal disease affecting reabsorption of K^+ seen in diuretic phase of renal failure
   f. Hemodialysis and peritoneal dialysis
   g. Reduced intake (K^+ restricted diets), NPO status without sufficient IV replacement therapy, starvation, malnutrition, alcoholism, anorexia, high glucose levels (leading to diuresis), large ingestion of black licorice (causes aldosterone effects)

NCLEX®

B. Nursing data collection (see Table 49–7)

NCLEX®

C. Therapeutic management

1. Focuses on restoring normal levels, preventing complications, and treating underlying problems
2. If client also has hypocalcemia and/or hypomagnesemia, all electrolyte levels must be corrected together
3. Check for signs of metabolic alkalosis (including irritability and paresthesias) because hypokalemia is present in alkalotic states
4. Monitor pertinent client data for potential effects related to hypokalemia and for response to therapeutic treatment
   a. Vital signs, especially BP (hypokalemia can lead to orthostatic hypotension) and respiratory rate, depth, and pattern

Table 49–7 Potassium Imbalances: Quick Summary of Findings

	Hypokalemia (K^+ < 3.5 mEq/L)	Hypernatremia (K^+ > 5.1 mEq/L)
Cardiovascular	Weak, thready pulse with variable rate; pedal pulses difficult to palpate; ECG changes (ST segment depression, flattened T wave, onset of U wave, ventricular dysrhythmias, heart block); digitalis toxicity is potentiated	Irregular, slow heart rate, ↓ BP, ECG changes (narrow, peaked T waves, widened QRS complexes, prolonged PR intervals, flattened P waves, frequent ectopy, ventricular fibrillation and standstill)
Respiratory	↓ breath sounds; weak, shallow respirations; dyspnea	Unaffected until level is very high, leading to muscle weakness and paralysis and causing respiratory failure
Neuromuscular	Anxiety, lethargy, depression, confusion, paresthesias, weakness, leg cramps	Muscle twitching (early) and cramps, irritability, anxiety; a late sign is ascending flaccid paralysis involving arms and legs
Gastrointestinal (GI)	Nausea, diarrhea or constipation (from ↓ peristalsis), polydipsia	Hyperactive bowel sounds, diarrhea, nausea
Other	Renal: polyuria and nocturia, ↓ urine specific gravity	Not applicable

Box 49–4

Potassium Food Sources

The following foods are considered adequate sources of potassium:

- Vegetables such as spinach, broccoli, carrots, green beans, tomato juice, acorn squash, and potatoes
- Fruits such as bananas, cantaloupe, apricots, oranges, and raisins
- Milk, milk products, yogurt, and meat
- Legumes, nuts, and seeds
- Whole grains

b. Serum electrolyte levels
c. ECG changes and heart rate and rhythm pattern
d. I&O and possibly daily weight

5. Monitor therapeutic serum drug levels for clients taking cardiac glycosides (digoxin) and serum K^+ levels for clients taking loop and thiazide diuretics
6. Protect client from injury and maintain a safe environment because client may experience weakness due to hypokalemia
7. Dietary interventions to promote normal K^+ levels
   a. Encourage high-fiber diet and increased fluid intake, if not on fluid restriction, to prevent constipation
   b. Provide adequate dietary sources of K^+; see Box 49–4 for good food sources of K^+
   c. Avoid foods such as black licorice that, when eaten in large quantities, can cause hypokalemia
8. Oral replacement therapy (note: K^+ supplements should never be given unless client has a urine output of at least 0.5 mL/kg/hour)
   a. Usual dose is 20 mEq; higher doses (up to 100 mEq in divided doses) may be given depending on client's baseline
   b. Medication can be given in either liquid or pill form
9. Administer parenteral K^+ carefully
   a. Verify additive K^+ in solution prior to hanging infusion
   NCLEX® b. Always use an infusion pump, paying attention to rate, intake and output
   c. Do not exceed an infusion rate of 5 to 10 mEq/hr unless there is moderate hypokalemia
   d. Dilute K^+ in a solution that provides no more than 1 mEq/10 mL
   e. If more than 20 mEq/hr is given, use continuous ECG monitoring and check serum level every 4 to 6 hours until normal
   f. Monitor IV site closely because potassium chloride (KCl) is irritating to blood vessels and can lead to infiltration, phlebitis, and tissue necrosis; this could cause sloughs that may require skin grafts
   NCLEX® g. Never administer K^+ by IV push or intramuscular routes because these methods can lead to fatal dysrhythmias

D. Client teaching

1. Report signs and symptoms of hypokalemia to physician
2. Take K^+ supplements with at least 4 ounces fluid or with food
3. Never crush or break K^+ tablets or capsules
4. Dissolve powder form of K^+ in at least 4 ounces of water or other fluids (no carbonated beverages)
5. Take K^+ after meals to prevent GI upset
6. Do not use salt substitutes when taking K^+ supplements
7. NCLEX® Know and report signs and symptoms of hyperkalemia to health care provider
8. Get regular serum K^+ levels drawn per health care provider's recommendations

VII. HYPERKALEMIA

A. Overview

1. **Hyperkalemia**: a serum K^+ level greater than 5.1 mEq/L (normal range 3.5–5.1 mEq/L)
2. Actual hyperkalemia (K^+ level in the ECF is elevated)
   a. Excessive K^+ intake from K^+-rich food or medications, use of salt substitutes, or rapid infusion of K^+-containing IV solutions
   b. Decreased K^+ excretion due to adrenal insufficiency (Addison's disease), renal failure, K^+-sparing diuretics, or use of ACE inhibitors
3. Relative hyperkalemia (movement of K^+ from ICF to ECF leading to elevated serum K^+ levels without a true body increase of K^+)

a. Excessive cellular release: massive cell damage, burns, hyperuricemia in tumor lysis syndrome, major surgeries, and hypercatabolism
b. Pseudohyperkalemia: hemolysis of blood sample
c. Excessive transcellular shifting: metabolic acidosis, insulin deficiency, rapid increase in blood osmolality
d. Medication therapy: digoxin use, overdose of replacement therapy, administration of stored blood (hemolysis of RBCs in solution increases serum K^+), use of K^+-sparing diuretics
e. Addison's disease is associated with decreased aldosterone that leads to Na^+ depletion and K^+ retention

NCLEX® **B. Nursing data collection (see again Table 49–7)**

NCLEX® **C. Therapeutic management**

1. Decrease K^+ intake: implement prescribed K^+ restrictions; do not administer K^+ supplements; refer client to dietitian to evaluate hidden dietary intake of K^+
2. Promote K^+ excretion: increase urinary output and monitor adequate renal function
3. Continued monitoring of client: serum K^+ levels; report abnormals; monitor cardiac status, and signs and symptoms of hyperkalemia and metabolic acidosis
4. Whenever possible, determine and treat underlying cause to restore balance
5. Dialysis may be performed for intractable conditions to prevent development of potentially lethal problems
6. Monitor for response to therapeutic treatment
7. Sodium polystyrene sulfonate (Kayexalate), to reduce K^+ levels, can be given either orally or as an enema with an osmotic agent (sorbitol) to decrease possible constipation
8. Intravenous medications
   a. Calcium gluconate
   b. Regular insulin and dextrose (usually 50%) solution (shifts K^+ from ECF to ICF)
   c. Sodium bicarbonate
9. K^+ wasting diuretics (loop diuretics and thiazide and thiazide-like diuretics)

D. Client teaching

1. Recognize predisposing factors
2. Avoid foods that are high in K^+
3. Examine food labels and medication packages to determine K^+ content
4. Avoid salt substitutes

VIII. HYPOCALCEMIA

A. Overview

1. **Hypocalcemia**: a serum calcium (Ca^{++}) level less than 8.5 mg/dL (normal range 8.5–10.5 mg/dL) or decreased availability of ionized Ca^{++}
2. Predisposing clinical conditions result from decreased physiologic availability of Ca^{++}, decreased Ca^{++} intake or absorption, or increased Ca^{++} excretion (see Box 49–5)
3. Other risk factors
   a. Postmenopausal women not taking estrogen
   b. Family history of hereditary hypoparathyroidism
   c. History of Crohn's or small bowel dysfunction
   d. Increased incidence of fractures; osteoporosis and/or osteopenia

Box 49–5

Clinical Conditions That Lead to Hypocalcemia

- Hypoparathyroidism or post-thyroidectomy
- Hypomagnesemia
- Alkalotic states
- Multiple blood transfusions
- Hypoalbuminemia
- Acute pancreatitis
- Hyperphosphatemia
- Vitamin D deficiency
- Malabsorptive states
- Renal disease
- Alcoholism
- Neonatal hypocalcemia
- Gram-negative sepsis
- Medullary thyroid carcinoma
- Burns

e. Immobility
f. Dietary patterns that lack adequate Ca^{++} and vitamin D sources
g. Excessive use of dietary phosphorus supplements
h. Eating disorders with laxative use as part of dietary pattern
i. Lactose-intolerance unless alternative products are used
j. Dietary factors that limit absorption of Ca^{++} (oxalates such as spinach and rhubarb, phytates such as bran and whole grains, and tannins as in tea)
k. Medications (loop diuretics, antiepileptics, citrate-buffered blood products, phosphates, antineoplastic agents, radiographic contrast media, corticosteroids, bisphosphonates, antacids, and heparin)

NCLEX®

B. Nursing data collection

1. See Table 49–8
2. Other systems: laryngospasm can occur, leading to respiratory compromise, airway failure and respiratory arrest; development of cataracts; dry, brittle nails and dry hair; increased bleeding or bruising

C. Therapeutic management

1. Treatment focuses on restoring normal levels, preventing complications, and treating underlying problems

NCLEX®

2. Replacement therapies
   a. Calcium gluconate (more common) or calcium chloride (less common; irritating to vein) by slow IV push in an emergency; may give slow IV infusion of calcium gluconate until tetany has been controlled or until calcium reaches 8 to 9 mg/dL
   b. Daily oral doses of elemental Ca^{++}, usually 1.0 to 3.0 grams/day
   c. Calcitriol, vitamin D supplements, or phosphorus-binding antacids based on need
   d. Thiazide diuretics may be used to decrease urinary excretion of calcium
3. Continue monitoring client (laboratory values and clinical condition) for treatment effectivesss
   a. Continuous ECG monitoring, especially during calcium gluconate or calcium chloride administration
   b. Continually monitor neurologic, respiratory, and cardiac status
   c. Monitor clients receiving Ca^{++} replacement who are also on digitalis for enhanced digitalis effect—check pulse

NCLEX®

4. Protect client from injury and maintain a safe environment
   a. Be prepared for emergencies that may result from hypocalcemia, such as tetany, seizures, laryngospasm, and respiratory and cardiac arrest
   b. Initiate seizure precautions and maintain a quiet environment

Table 49–8 Calcium Imbalances: Quick Summary of Findings

	Hypocalcemia (Ca^{++} < 8.5 mEq/L)	Hypercalcemia (Ca^{++} > 10.5 mEq/L)
Cardiovascular	↓ BP; ECG changes include prolonged QT interval and lengthened ST segment; cardiac arrest	Hypertension, shortened ST segments and QT interval on ECG, cardiac dysrhythmias such as heart block; cardiac arrest
Neuromuscular	Paresthesias in hands and feet; muscle cramps, positive Chvostek sign (twitching of cheek) and Trousseau sign (spasm of arm when BP cuff inflated); ↑ deep tendon reflexes (DTRs), ↑ irritability and apprehension; mental status changes ranging from depression, memory impairment, delusions and hallucinations to seizures	Headache and confusion, subtle changes in personality to acute psychosis, fatigue, ↓ DTRs; impaired memory and bizarre behavior, lethargy, or coma (seizures are rare)
Renal	↓ serum Ca^{++} levels are associated with renal failure, along with other electrolyte disturbances	Polyuria and polydipsia due to altered renal function; ↓ ability of kidneys to concentrate urine; renal colic from development of kidney stones due to high Ca^{++} levels; renal failure may occur
Gastrointestinal (GI)	Possible hyperactive bowel sounds and diarrhea, intestinal cramps	Anorexia, nausea and vomiting; abdominal pain; constipation, hypoactive bowel sounds
Musculoskeletal	Possible bone fractures from bone demineralization; bone pain; chronic hypocalcemia may retard growth and cause rickets in children; can lead to osteomalacia and osteoporosis in adults	Pathologic bone fractures; bone thinning, deep bone pain

c. Closely observe respiratory and airway status; have emergency tracheostomy kit available and IV calcium gluconate at bedside for postoperative thyroidectomy clients (may have inadvertent removal of parathyroid gland)
d. Observe for signs of tetany in clients receiving multiple blood transfusions
e. Observe for signs of bleeding or increased bruising

5. Monitor for possible hypercalcemia resulting from replacement therapy
6. Encourage foods high in Ca^{++}, such as dairy products

D. Client teaching

1. Predisposing factors
2. Paresthesias, tingling and numbness in extremities are early warning signs of tetany
3. Report onset of signs of tetany or seizures immediately to health care provider
4. Take oral replacements as prescribed
5. Avoid overuse of antacids and/or laxatives containing phosphorus
6. Increase intake of foods rich in Ca^{++} (dairy products) and protein
7. Vitamin D and protein are important to keep Ca^{++} within normal limits
8. Use appropriate substitutes for milk and dairy products if lactose intolerant
9. Avoid foods high in phosphorus
10. Limit foods that decrease absorption of Ca^{++} in diet

IX. HYPERCALCEMIA

A. Overview

1. **Hypercalcemia**: a serum Ca^{++} level greater than 10.5 mg/dL (normal range 8.5–10.5 mg/dL); symptoms may not appear until serum Ca^{++} level is higher than 12 mg/dL
2. Predisposing clinical conditions (see Box 49–6)
3. Other risk factors
   a. Excessive dietary intake of Ca^{++} rich foods
   b. Excessive intake of antacids for gastric distress

NCLEX® **B. Nursing data collection (see again Table 49–8)**

NCLEX® **C. Therapeutic management**

1. Decrease Ca^{++} intake
   a. Limit milk and dairy products
   b. Eliminate use of calcium carbonate antacids until Ca^{++} levels return to normal
2. Promote calcium excretion
   a. Use loop diuretics, such as furosemide (Lasix) or bumetanide (Bumex) to promote increased urine output so that more Ca^{++} will be excreted
   b. Maintain hydration of 3000 to 4000 mL (3–4 L) of fluid/day; oral fluids should be high in acid ash, such cranberry or prune juice
   c. Give 0.9% NaCl IV at 300 to 500 mL/hr up to 6 liters as ordered until volume status restored, then 0.45% NaCl may be used; watch for fluid overload as a complication, especially with preexisting cardiac or respiratory disease
   d. Corticosteroids to decrease GI absorption of Ca^{++}: prednisone 20 to 50 mg po BID is usual dose or 40 to 100 mg daily in four divided doses; may take 5 to 10 days for Ca^{++} levels to fall
   e. Chronic management of hypercalcemia is effective only with parathroidectomy for primary hyperparathyroidism
3. Continued monitoring of client: strict I&O, daily weight, serum Ca^{++} and phosphorus levels, possible ECG monitoring

Box 49–6

Clinical Conditions That Lead to Hypercalcemia

- Hyperparathyroidism
- Metastatic cancer
- Use of thiazide diuretics
- Sarcoidosis
- Immobility
- Hypophosphatemia
- Hyperthyroidism (thyrotoxicosis)
- Renal tubular acidosis
- Milk-alkali syndrome
- Familial hypocalciuric hypercalcemia
- Lithium therapy
- Vitamin D intoxication

4. Treatment of hypercalcemic crisis
   a. 0.9% NaCl at 300 to 500 mL/hr initially and up to 6 liters until intravascular volume restored or calcium level is 8 to 9 mg/dL
   b. Bisphosphonates, such as pamidronate (Aredia) IV to inhibit bone resorption; returns Ca^{++} to normal within 24 to 48 hours with effects lasting for weeks in most clients
   c. Salmon calcitonin may temporarily lower Ca^{++} level by 1 to 3 mg/dL in clients with severe hypercalcemia
   d. Phosphorus IV to decrease Ca^{++} because of inverse relationship in emergency situations only
5. Dialysis: during oliguric/anuric stage, severe renal dysfunction can lead to life-threatening fluid and electrolyte imbalances
6. Prevent injuries and maintain safe environment
   a. Monitor for pathologic fractures in clients with long-term hypercalcemia
   b. Assist client with mobility to prevent injury and maintain safety

D. Client teaching

1. Predisposing factors
2. Take phosphorus agents or other medications as prescribed
3. Notify health care provider if flank pain develops (risk of kidney stones)
4. How to strain urine (check for kidney stones) if indicated
5. Notify health care professional if symptoms worsen
6. Avoid foods and OTC antacids that are high in Ca^{++}
7. NCLEX® Increase fluid intake to 2 to 3 L in 24 hours, especially fluids high in acid-ash such as prune or cranberry juice
8. Increase dietary fiber and fluid to prevent constipation
9. Do not take large doses of vitamin D supplements

X. HYPOMAGNESEMIA

A. Overview

1. **Hypomagnesemia**: a serum magnesium (Mg^{++}) level less than 1.4 mEq/L (normal range 1.4–2.1 mEq/L)
2. Usually occurs with nutritional or metabolic abnormalities, decreased absorption, increased renal loss, or redistribution of body magnesium
3. Predisposing clinical conditions
   a. Chronic alcoholism is most common cause
   b. Decreased dietary intake or prolonged IV therapy without Mg^{++} supplementation; in parenteral nutrition therapy, Mg^{++} moves into cells from bloodstream, leading to low serum Mg^{++} levels
   c. Decreased absorption: inflammatory bowel disease, small bowel resection (less surface available to absorb), GI cancer, chronic pancreatitis, or medications such as gentamicin (Garamycin, an aminoglycoside antibiotic) or cisplatin (Platinol, an antineoplastic agent)
   d. Increased intestinal (lower GI) losses: prolonged diarrhea, draining intestinal fistulas, and ileostomy
   e. Increased renal excretion: loop diuretics, hyperaldosteronism that leads to volume expansion, diabetes that leads to osmotic diuresis
   f. Losses can also occur because of burns and debridement therapy

NCLEX® **B. Nursing data collection**

1. Clinical manifestations usually appear when serum Mg^{++} level drops below 1 mEq/L
2. Respiratory: laryngeal stridor
3. Cardiovascular: supraventricular tachycardia, premature ventricular contractions and ventricular fibrillation, and increased susceptibility to digitalis toxicity (possibly enhanced by concurrent hypokalemia)
4. ECG changes: diminished voltage of P wave; broad, flat, or inverted T waves; depressed ST segments; prolonged QT interval; possible prominent U wave
5. Neuromuscular: mood changes, such as apathy, depression, and confusion; muscle twitching, tremors, hyperreactive reflexes
6. GI: nausea and vomiting, diarrhea, and anorexia (from concurrent hypokalemia)
7. Growth failure in children can occur
8. Severe deficiency can lead to convulsions, hallucinations, or tetany
9. Signs and symptoms are similar to hypokalemia or hypocalcemia (all are cations and may occur together); positive Chvostek's sign (twitching of cheek when stimulated) can occur

Memory Aid

Rember the *Ch* in *Ch*vostek and in *ch*eek to help remember how Chvostek's sign is manifested.

NCLEX®

C. Therapeutic management

1. Identify risk factors: malabsorption and/or GI dysfunction, renal disease, diabetes, alcohol intake, and medications such as diuretics
2. Monitor client with continuous IV fluid therapy without Mg^{++} replacement
3. Monitor client with hyperaldosteronism because volume expansion may result in decreased Mg^{++}
4. Monitor client taking a diuretic for increased renal excretion of Mg^{++}
5. Institute ECG monitoring and seizure precautions
6. Monitor for stridor and/or difficulty swallowing
7. Keep bed rails raised if client is confused; take other safety precautions as needed
8. Maintain accurate intake and output records
9. Monitor DTRs in clients receiving IV solutions containing Mg^{++}; depressed DTRs indicate a rebound elevated Mg^{++} level
10. Medication therapy
    a. Oral replacement therapy: Mg^{++}-containing antacids; magnesium oxide; use caution because they may cause diarrhea, leading to decreased absorption
    b. Parenteral magnesium sulfate or magnesium chloride
    c. Ensure urine output of at least 30 mL/hr or 120 mL every 4 hours during therapy to avoid rebound hypermagnesemia if renal insufficiency is present
    d. Monitor DTRs (such as patellar reflex) before each dose of parenteral Mg^{++}; if reflex is present, hypermagnesemia from previous doses has not occurred
11. Dietary therapy: for mild hypomagnesemia, encourage foods high in Mg^{++}, such as legumes, whole grain cereals, nuts, dark green vegetables, seafood, bananas, oranges, and chocolate

D. Client teaching

1. Predisposing factors
2. Increase intake of foods high in Mg^{++}
3. Increase intake of hard water or mineral water, which are high in Mg^{++}
4. Take 300 to 350 mg magnesium daily with an extra 150 mg for pregnant or lactating women

XI. HYPERMAGNESEMIA

A. Overview

1. **Hypermagnesemia**: serum Mg^{++} level greater than 2.1 mEq/L (normal range 1.4–2.1 mEq/L)
2. Predisposing factors
    a. Decreased renal excretion of Mg^{++}, such as with decreased urine output or renal failure
    b. Increased Mg^{++} intake, such as with overuse of Mg^{++}-containing antacids, cathartics, or enemas; total parenteral nutrition; or hemodialysis using hard water dialysate
3. Predisposing clinical conditions
    a. Untreated diabetic ketoacidosis (glucose carries cations across cell membranes)
    b. Adrenal insufficiency (Addison's disease): causes fluid and electrolyte shifts
    c. Mg^{++} treatment in preeclampsia of pregnancy
    d. Lithium ingestion
    e. Volume depletion

NCLEX®

B. Nursing data collection

1. Neuromuscular symptoms (most common): decreased DTRs and depressed neuromuscular activity; symptoms are similar to those seen in hyperkalemia
2. Cardiovascular: hypotension, bradycardia, bradyarrhythmias, flushing and sensation of warmth, possible cardiac arrest
3. ECG may show prolonged PR interval, widened QRS complex, and elevated T wave
4. CNS: somnolence, weakness and lethargy, respiratory depression, and coma

NCLEX®

C. Therapeutic management

1. Decrease Mg^{++} intake; withhold Mg^{++}-containing drugs (antacids) and enemas
2. Promote Mg^{++} excretion using diuretics (in stable renal function)
3. Provide rehydration to promote increased urine output and Mg^{++} excretion

4. Emergency treatment includes IV calcium gluconate to antagonize effect of Mg^{++} and counteract cardiac and respiratory symptoms
5. Dialysis: in clients with renal failure, dialysis may be necessary for Mg^{++} removal; if hemodialysis is not feasible, peritoneal dialysis is an option
6. Monitor I&O
7. Identify risk factors such as antacid use, laxative use, diabetic instability, and renal failure
8. Promote client safety

D. Client teaching

1. Predisposing factors
2. Signs and symptoms of hypermagnesemia to report
3. Avoid foods high in Mg^{++} such as legumes, whole-grain cereals, nuts, dark green vegetables, and cocoa

XII. HYPOCHLOREMIA

A. Overview

1. **Hypochloremia**: a serum chloride (Cl^-) level less than 95 mEq/L (normal range 95–108 mEq/L)
   - a. Decreases in Cl^- usually are accompanied by decreases in Na^+ and K^+
   - b. A reduction in hydrochloric acid decreases Cl^-
   - c. Chloride is excreted with cations during massive diuresis and when HCO_3^- is elevated
2. Predisposing clinical conditions
   - a. Hyponatremia, metabolic alkalosis, hypokalemia, prolonged D_5W IV therapy
   - b. Chronic respiratory acidosis
   - c. Chronic lung disease accompanied by high pCO_2 and HCO_3^- levels that result in decreased serum Cl^-
   - d. Diabetic ketoacidosis because of increased anion gap
   - e. Acute infections, although how they lower serum Cl^- is unclear
   - f. Vomiting (loss of HCl), GI suctioning, perspiration, diarrhea, and fistulas
   - g. Metabolic stress conditions, such as severe burns, fever, heat and exhaustion states
   - h. Disease states such as Addison's disease, anorexia, salt-wasting renal nephropathy, SIADH, and hypervolemic states such as congestive heart failure (CHF) and cirrhosis
   - i. Medications that promote electrolyte loss, are diuretics, or promote alkalosis

B. Nursing data collection

1. Neuromuscular: tremors and twitching
2. Respiratory: slow and shallow breathing
3. Cardiac: hypotension if severe Cl^- and ECF losses
4. Seldom a primary problem; usually associated with hyponatremia, hypokalemia, metabolic alkalosis or hypokalemic alkalosis

C. Therapeutic management

1. Administer oral salt tablets
2. Provide IV infusion of Cl^- (as NaCl or KCl) if levels are critical or client is unable to tolerate oral dose
3. Monitor I&O because excess water administration can cause dilutional hypochloremia and hyponatremia
4. Monitor BP (a drop can occur if hypochloremia is caused by ECF volume loss)
5. Monitor ABG results if clinical presentation or underlying medical history suggests accompanying acid–base imbalance
6. Maintain safety precautions: keep bed rails up and assist with ambulation if client has muscle tremors and/or decreased BP
7. Dietary therapy: foods high in Cl^-, such as salt, processed foods, canned vegetables, dates, bananas, cheese, spinach, milk, eggs, celery, crabs, fish, olives, and rye

D. Client teaching

1. Predisposing factors
2. Include in diet Na^+ and processed foods that are also high in Cl^-
3. Electrolyte replacement as well as fluid replacement is important if activity level is increased and client perspires excessively

XIII. HYPERCHLOREMIA

A. Overview

1. **Hyperchloremia**: a serum Cl^- level greater than 108 mEq/L (normal range 95–108 mEq/L)
2. Predisposing clinical conditions
   - a. Fluid and electrolyte imbalances such as hypernatremia and metabolic acidosis

b. Drugs that promote Cl^- retention, such as IV saline, certain diuretics, salicylate intoxication, corticosteroids, guanethidine, and phenylbutazone
c. Dehydration
d. Endocrine disturbances that result in diabetes insipidus and certain cases of hyperparathyroidism (seen in association with hypercalcemia)
e. Hyperaldosteronism (increased sodium and chloride reabsorption)
f. Renal changes that manifest as renal tubular acidosis or acute renal failure

B. Nursing data collection

1. Neuromuscular: weakness and lethargy; can progress to significant CNS damage
2. Respiratory: deep, rapid, vigorous breathing that can lead to unconsciousness (results from attempt to compensate for acidotic state due to loss of bicarbonate)
3. Cardiac: dysrhythmias due to retained Cl^- and result acid–base imbalance
4. Increased aldosterone leads to greater reabsorption of both Na^+ and Cl^-
5. Fluid volume disturbances: dehydration, retention of salt and water due to drug administration, and a greater Na^+ loss than Cl^- loss
6. Increased Cl^- sweat levels are seen in diabetes insipidus, hypothyroidism, malnutrition, acute renal failure, and certain genetic disorders such as cystic fibrosis and glucose-6-phosphate-dehydrogenase (G6PD) deficiency
7. Associated electrolyte imbalances that usually occur with elevated Cl^- levels are elevated K^+ and Na^+ levels and decreased HCO_3^- levels

C. Therapeutic manageme

1. Decrease Cl^- intake; stop all chloride-containing agents used as treatment measures
2. Promote Cl^- excretion by administering diuretics
3. Continue monitoring client, including acid–base, respiratory, and cardiac status
4. Monitor vital signs and I&O parameters
5. Promote client safety
6. Hypotonic IV solutions such as 0.45% NaCl or D_5W to correct dehydration or IV diuretics to promote Cl^- loss

D. Client teaching

1. Predisposing factors
2. Avoid foods high in Cl^- and restrict processed foods (high in both Na^+ and Cl^-)
3. Maintain adequate hydration status

XIV. HYPOPHOSPHATEMIA

A. Overview

1. **Hypophosphatemia**: serum phosphorus level of less than 2.5 mg/dL (normal range 2.5–4.5 mg/dL)
2. May be associated with increased Ca^{++} levels (hypercalcemia)
3. Predisposing factors
   a. A complication of refeeding after severe malnourishment (has high mortality rate) or administering total parenteral nutrition without adequate phosphorus
   b. Poor dietary intake or decreased absorption from vitamin D deficiency, malabsorption disorders, and starvation
   c. Prolonged use of aluminum- and Mg^{++}-based antacids (bind to phosphorus)
   d. Severe vomiting and diarrhea; prolonged gastric suction
   e. Increased renal excretion from hyperparathyroidism, hypomagnesemia, hypokalemia, thiazide diuretic therapy, the diuretic phase of acute tubular necrosis, renal tubular disorders, polyuria, and glycosuria from uncontrolled diabetic ketoacidosis
   f. Respiratory alkalosis (may stimulate glycolysis, which enhances movement of phosphorus into cells)

B. Nursing data collection

1. Hematologic effects (anemia from increased RBC fragility from low ATP levels), impaired granulocyte functioning (immunosuppression), bruising and bleeding from platelet dysfunction and destruction
2. Neuromuscular: slurred speech, confusion, apprehension, seizures, coma
3. Cardiac: chest pain, dysrhythmias related to decreased oxygenation, heart failure and shock from decreased myocardial contractility
4. Respiratory: alkalosis from an increased rate/depth of breathing in response to hypoxemia; respiratory muscle fatigue leading to respiratory failure

5. GI: hypoactive bowel sounds, anorexia, dysphagia, vomiting, gastric atony and ileus related to reduced gastric motility

C. **Therapeutic management**

1. Administer phosphorus via oral supplements; dissolve dose in a full glass of water and give after meals to minimize gastric irritation and laxative effect
2. Provide IV replacement and monitor infusion site for infiltration, which may lead to tissue necrosis or sloughing
3. Avoid use of phosphorus-binding antacids
4. Monitor clients for difficulty speaking; note weakening respiratory efforts; have appropriate size airway available
5. Check serial hand grasps for increasing weakness
6. Investigate episodes of bleeding and/or bruising
7. Monitor for other associated fluid and electrolyte imbalances, especially in clients with nausea, vomiting, and/or diarrhea
8. Monitor orientation and neurologic status with each set of vital signs; incorporate seizure precautions into care
9. Carefully monitor fluid I&O
10. Increase intake of foods high in phosphorus, such as red and organ (brain, liver, kidney) meats, fish, poultry, eggs, milk and milk products, legumes, whole grains, and nuts
11. Reduce dietary sources of oxalates (spinach and rhubarb) and phytates (bran and whole grains), which bind phosphates in GI tract and reduce absorption

D. **Client teaching**

1. Predisposing factors and signs and symptoms of hypophosphatemia
2. Avoiding phosphorus-binding antacids
3. Increase intake of foods high in phosphorus

XV. HYPERPHOSPHATEMIA

A. **Overview**

1. **Hyperphosphatemia**: serum phosphorus level of greater than 4.5 mg/dL (normal range 2.5–4.5 mg/dL)
2. Predisposing factors
   a. Acute and chronic renal failure
   b. Hypocalcemia from antacids, diuretic agents, steroids
   c. Chemotherapy for malignant tumors
   d. Hypoparathyroidism (primary or secondary), which causes a decrease in Ca^{++} and increased renal absorption of phosphorus
   e. Excessive intake of phosphorus or its supplements
   f. Vitamin D excess or increased GI absorption
   g. Massive transfusions (phosphorus can leak from cells during blood storage)
   h. Hyperthyroidism, hyperparathyroidism
   i. Large milk intake
   j. Overzealous administration of oral or IV phosphorus supplements
   k. Rhabdomyolysis (breakdown of striated muscle), which releases cellular phosphorus

NCLEX® B. **Nursing data collection**

1. Most signs relate to development of hypocalcemia or soft tissue calcification (calcium phosphate deposits in nonosseous sites such as kidney and heart)
2. Metastatic calcification includes oliguria, corneal haziness, conjunctivitis, irregular heart rate
3. ECG changes and conduction disturbance, tachycardia
4. Paresthesias (especially lips and fingertips), muscle spasms, and tetany (positive Chvostek and Trousseau signs) from decreased Ca^{++} that accompanies increased phosphorus)
5. Anorexia, nausea, vomiting

NCLEX® C. **Therapeutic management**

1. Restrict dietary phosphorus; avoid medications or enemas with phosphorus
2. Administer phosphate binding agents
3. Perform renal dialysis in clients with renal failure
4. Treat concurrent hypocalcemia
5. Monitor renal function carefully, particularly urine output, BUN, creatinine
6. Monitor I&O; keep clients well hydrated; pay particular attention to types of fluids being ingested (avoid carbonated beverages, which are high in phosphates)

D. Client teaching

1. Purpose of phosphate binders; take them with or after meals to maximize effectiveness
2. Avoid OTC phosphorus in laxatives, enemas, and vitamin-mineral supplements
3. Use bulk-building supplements or stool softeners to combat constipating effects of some phosphate-binders, especially those with an aluminum base
4. Avoid or limit foods high in phosphorus, as previously described, and avoid carbonated beverages, which have low nutrient value and are also high in phosphates

Check your NCLEX–PN® Exam I.Q.

You are ready for testing on this content if you can

- Describe the pathophysiology and etiology of fluid and electrolyte imbalances.
- Discuss expected data and diagnostic test findings for fluid or electrolyte imbalance.
- Discuss therapeutic management of a client experiencing a fluid or electrolyte imbalance.
- Discuss nursing management of a client experiencing a fluid or electrolyte imbalance.
- Identify expected outcomes for the client experiencing a fluid or electrolyte imbalance.

PRACTICE TEST

1 A 10-month-old infant is admitted to the emergency department with a 102°F rectal temperature and a history of vomiting and diarrhea for 48 hours. For what signs should the nurse look related to this client's likely fluid imbalance?

1. Bulging fontanels, tearless cry, and low urine output
2. Sunken eyes, lethargy, and dry, furrowed tongue
3. Weight loss, dilute urine, and peripheral edema
4. Dry skin, thready pulse, and neck vein distention

2 Which observation of an adult client is a reliable indicator that therapy for fluid volume excess is achieving the desired outcome? Select all that apply.

1. Full, bounding peripheral pulses
2. Flat neck veins with the head of the bed elevated
3. Hand vein emptying longer than 20 seconds
4. S_3 heart sound clearly audible on auscultation
5. Lung sounds are clear.

3 The nurse concludes that which sign reliably indicates that ascites fluid is being effectively mobilized in response to therapy? Select all that apply.

1. Weight gain of 1 pound in 24 hours
2. Increase in urine output
3. Drop in blood pressure
4. Hand veins fill slowly.
5. Abdominal girth has decreased by 1 inch in 24 hours.

4 What instruction should the nurse anticipate will be included in an education program to prevent dehydration for a high school hiking club that is planning a 12-mile hike in early summer?

1. Take water and commercial sports drinks to sip often along the way.
2. Drink large amounts of water, at least 16 ounces every hour, while hiking.
3. Take salt tablets every 3–4 hours, and drink plenty of water while in the heat.
4. Stop every 4 hours along the way, and drink a few ounces of water while resting.

5 The nurse considers that which postoperative client could be at risk for developing a sodium imbalance?

1. A client who has just had a tonsillectomy
2. A client who has a primary cesarean section for failure to progress in labor
3. A client who has a transurethral resection of the prostate (TURP)
4. A client who has a right knee arthroscopy

6 The nurse is caring for a client who has a sodium level of 128 mEq/L. As part of the care, the nurse will restrict which item for this client?

1. Sports drinks, such as Gatorade
2. Eggs and cheese products
3. Salt on the diet tray
4. Water

7 The nurse is caring for a client who has a sodium level of 149 mEq/L. The nurse concludes that it is important to administer which of the following to this client?

1. Cough suppressant to treat symptomatic cough
2. 3% saline solution
3. Water
4. Lactulose (Chronulac)

8 The nurse is assisting in the care of a client who has sustained partial and full thickness burns over 30% of his body 18 hours ago. The nurse monitors for which fluid and electrolyte imbalances at this time? Select all that apply.

1. Hyperkalemia
2. Hypokalemia
3. Hypervolemia
4. Hypercalcemia
5. Hypovolemia

9 The nurse concludes that a history of which condition places a client at risk for possible hypokalemia?

1. Chronic obstructive pulmonary disease (COPD)
2. Cirrhosis
3. Addison's disease
4. Chronic renal failure (CRF)

10 Which health care provider order for potassium chloride (KCl) should the nurse question regarding a client with severe hypokalemia?

1. Infuse 1000 mL normal saline with 20 mEq KCl IV over 8 hours.
2. Give KCl 20 mEq PO daily after meals.
3. Infuse 1000 mL normal saline with 40 mEq KCl IV at 200 mL/hour.
4. Give 20 mEq KCl IV over 10 minutes.

11 Which treatment option does the nurse anticipate will be most appropriate for a client with a potassium level of 3.5 mEq/L?

1. Give sodium polystyrene sulfate (Kayexalate) per rectum.
2. Use salt substitutes in the diet.
3. Administer oral potassium chloride (KCl).
4. Continue to monitor and offer foods high in potassium.

12 The nurse who is assisting to develop a plan of care includes periodically monitoring which items for a client who is at risk for developing hypocalcemia? Select all that apply.

1. Blood urea nitrogen (BUN) and creatinine levels
2. Constipation
3. Serum albumin level
4. Fluid overload related to intravenous saline therapy
5. Serum magnesium level

13 A client with hypocalcemia is taking supplemental vitamin D. When the client asks the purpose of this therapy, what explanation should the nurse reinforce?

1. It directly opposes calcitonin.
2. It prevents renal disease in clients with hypocalcemia.
3. Calcium is absorbed in the intestines only under the influence of activated vitamin D.
4. The only way to obtain vitamin D is with oral supplementation.

14 Which medication reported by a client during a nursing history could be associated with the development of hypocalcemia?

1. Phenytoin (Dilantin)
2. Calcium carbonate (TUMS)
3. Calcitriol
4. Hydrochlorothiazide (HydroDIURIL)

15 The family of a client with hypercalcemia states that the client is "not acting like himself." The nurse focuses data collection on which manifestation?

1. Personality change
2. Anxiety
3. Seizure activity
4. Carpal spasms

16 The nurse monitoring a client for signs of hypocalcemia would conclude that this electrolyte imbalance exists after noting which finding?

1. Negative Chvostek's sign
2. Positive Trousseau's sign
3. Positive Kernig's sign
4. Hypoactive bowel sounds

17 The nurse would review a client's electrolyte levels to detect a possible increase in magnesium if the client had which condition? Select all that apply.

1. Cushing's syndrome
2. Diabetes
3. Addison's disease
4. Splenomegaly
5. Dehydration

18 The nurse concludes that a client does not have an increased magnesium level based on which finding?

1. Hypotension
2. Bradycardia
3. Supraventricular tachycardia (SVT)
4. Flushing and sweating

19 A client with end stage renal disease is experiencing hypermagnesemia. The nurse explains that which treatment will decrease the magnesium level most effectively?

1. Dialysis
2. Diuretics
3. Fluid restriction
4. High-volume IV fluids

20 The nurse reviews the laboratory test results for a client with preeclampsia, expecting to find which value?

1. Sodium 148 mEq/L
2. Sodium 125 mEq/L
3. Magnesium 3.1 mEq/L
4. Magnesium 1.2 mEq/L

21 A client admitted to the hospital with a 30-pound weight gain over the past month has a fat pad at the back of the neck and moon facies. Admission laboratory results indicate decreased serum potassium and magnesium, and elevated serum chloride and sodium levels. The nurse interprets that which disorder is most consistent with these electrolyte abnormalities?

1. Addison's disease
2. Cushing's syndrome
3. Burns
4. Syndrome of inappropriate ADH (SIADH)

22 An older adult client with a history of heart failure (HF) was prescribed diuretics twice a day and a low-sodium diet. The nurse should be most concerned about which current laboratory result?

1. Sodium 145 mEq/L
2. Chloride 90 mEq/L
3. K^+ 4.2 mEq/L
4. HCO_3^- 27 mEq/L

23 Which finding in a client's history would alert the nurse to look for signs of hypophosphatemia?

1. Alcohol abuse
2. The oliguric phase of acute tubular necrosis
3. Short-term gastric suction
4. Occasional use of aluminum-containing antacids

24 The nurse would report to the charge nurse that an assigned client has hyperkalemia after noting that the serum potassium level drawn that morning was greater than how many mEq/L? Provide a numerical answer.

Fill in your answer below:

____ mEq/L

25 Which intervention should the nurse perform when caring for a client on a fluid restriction? Select all that apply.

1. Involve the client in dividing fluid allowances over the 24-hour period.
2. Use an infusion pump to control the infusion of any required intravenous fluids.
3. Include ice chips in the client's oral intake measurement.
4. Provide unlimited ice chips to help keep the client's mouth and lips moist.
5. Do not include fluid taken with medications.

ANSWERS & RATIONALES

1 **Answer: 2 Rationale:** The client's history suggests fluid volume deficit and dehydration. Sunken eyes, altered mental status and behavior, and dry, furrowed tongue are reliable signs of fluid volume deficit in infants. Bulging fontanels, peripheral edema, and neck vein distention are seen with fluid volume excess. **Cognitive Level:** Applying **Client Need:** Physiological Adaptation **Integrated Process:** Nursing Process: Data Collection **Content Area:** Adult Health **Strategy:** The core issue of the question is the ability to correlate a clinical picture with risk for hypovolemia. Use nursing knowledge of signs of dehydration and the process of elimination to make a selection.

2 **Answer: 2, 5 Rationale:** Venous congestion results from fluid volume excess, and causes full, bounding pulses, delayed hand vein emptying, and S_3 heart sounds. Flat neck veins with the head of the bed elevated are an indicator of the absence of venous congestion. With fluid overload, crackles can often be auscultated in lung fields. Absence of crackles is consistent with normal fluid balance. **Cognitive Level:** Applying **Client Need:** Physiological Adaptation **Integrated Process:** Nursing Process: Evaluation **Content Area:** Adult Health **Strategy:** The core issue of the question is knowledge of signs of fluid overload and normal findings. Use nursing knowledge and the process of elimination to make a selection.

3 **Answer: 2, 5 Rationale:** Ascites is a form of third space fluid in the abdomen. Therapy is aimed at moving third space fluid back into the circulation, where it can be eliminated by the kidneys. When this fluid is drawn back into the vascular space (leading to a rise in BP and venous pressure), the kidneys increase the urine output to eliminate the excess fluid. Loss of fluid results in loss of weight and abdominal girth decreases. **Cognitive Level:** Analyzing **Client Need:** Physiological Adaptation **Integrated Process:** Nursing Process: Evaluation **Content Area:** Adult Health **Strategy:** The core issues of the question are recognition of ascites as a third space fluid and knowledge of effective mobilization of that fluid. Recall that mobilized fluid must be eliminated via the kidneys to assist in making a selection.

4 **Answer: 1 Rationale:** Drinking a combination of water and sports drinks is helpful. Sports drinks provide carbohydrates, water, and electrolytes. Drinking large amounts of only water fails to replace electrolytes, which can lead to water intoxication. Salt tablets are no longer recommended, because too much salt has a hypertonic effect, causes diuresis, and can actually worsen fluid loss. Those who exercise in hot climates need to continuously replace both fluid and electrolyte losses. A few ounces of fluid every 4 hours is insufficient. **Cognitive Level:** Analyzing **Client Need:** Physiological Adaptation **Integrated Process:** Nursing Process: Planning **Content Area:** Adult Health **Strategy:** The core issue of the question is knowledge of measures to prevent fluid and electrolyte imbalance during exercise. Use nursing knowledge and the process of elimination to make a selection.

5 **Answer: 3 Rationale:** A TURP procedure can place a client at risk for developing hyponatremia in the postoperative period due to increased fluid irrigation used during and after surgery. Clients with a TURP procedure have a CBI (continuous bladder irrigation) as a routine part of their postoperative care. The other options do not place a client at risk for development of sodium imbalances, because they do not require lengthy fluid and dietary restrictions, or excessive fluid irrigation. **Cognitive Level:** Applying **Client Need:** Physiological Adaptation **Integrated Process:** Nursing Process: Data Collection **Content Area:** Adult Health **Strategy:** The core issue of the question is knowledge that procedures and surgeries requiring use of water for irrigation can lead to dilutional hyponatremia. Use nursing knowledge and the process of elimination to make a selection.

6 **Answer: 4 Rationale:** Hyponatremia can also be referred to as dilutional hyponatremia or water intoxication. Water restriction would be an important part of the treatment plan when caring for a client who has hyponatremia. Restrictions of Gatorade (electrolyte-rich solution), eggs, cheese products, and salt on the diet tray are not indicated, because the client is experiencing a sodium deficit. **Cognitive Level:** Analyzing **Client Need:** Physiological Adaptation **Integrated Process:** Nursing Process: Implementation **Content Area:** Adult Health **Strategy:** The core issue of the question is effective treatment measures for hyponatremia. Use nursing knowledge and the process of elimination to make a selection.

7 **Answer: 3 Rationale:** Clients with hypernatremia are thirsty, and need water replacement to balance their increased sodium levels. Cough medication and lactulose can further increase sodium levels, and should not be administered

unless there is sufficient clinical information to warrant their use. Three-percent saline is a hypertonic solution that would also increase serum sodium levels, and should not be given to this client. **Cognitive Level:** Analyzing **Client Need:** Physiological Adaptation **Integrated Process:** Nursing Process: Implementation **Content Area:** Adult Health **Strategy:** The core issue of the question is knowledge of measures that effectively treat hypernatremia. Use nursing knowledge and the process of elimination to make a selection.

8 **Answer: 1, 5 Rationale:** During major burn injury, potassium shifts from the intracellular fluid to the extracellular fluid because of cell death, leading to high serum levels of potassium. Hypokalemia is not seen in burn clients during the time of fluid shifting secondary to trauma. The client with burns is more likely to be hypovolemic rather than hypervolemic and hypocalcemic rather than hypercalcemic at this time because of fluid and electrolyte loss caused by altered capillary integrity. **Cognitive Level:** Applying **Client Need:** Physiological Adaptation **Integrated Process:** Nursing Process: Data Collection **Content Area:** Adult Health **Strategy:** The core issue of the question is knowledge that burn injury causes fluid loss and increases the risk of hyperkalemia. Use nursing knowledge and the process of elimination to make selections.

9 **Answer: 2 Rationale:** In clients with cirrhosis, increased amounts of aldosterone are secreted, which leads to sodium retention and potassium excretion from the kidneys; these clients are likely to become hypokalemic. Clients with COPD are likely to develop hyperkalemia due to retention of acids, which lead to loss of hydrogen ions and retention of potassium as an alternate cation. Clients with Addison's disease (hypofunction of adrenal gland) are likely to develop hyperkalemia because of high sodium loss. Clients with CRF are likely to develop hyperkalemia because of inadequate potassium excretion. **Cognitive Level:** Analyzing **Client Need:** Physiological Adaptation **Integrated Process:** Nursing Process: Data Collection **Content Area:** Adult Health **Strategy:** The core issue of the question is the ability to discriminate predisposing factors for hypokalemia from factors for hyperkalemia. Use nursing knowledge and the process of elimination to make a selection.

10 **Answer: 4 Rationale:** Potassium is never given as a bolus when it is administered intravenously. KCl should never be given rapidly or by IV push, because serious arrhythmias or cardiac arrest can occur. All of the other orders are within a safe and therapeutic range. **Cognitive Level:** Analyzing **Client Need:** Pharmacological and Parenteral Therapies **Integrated Process:** Nursing Process: Planning **Content Area:** Adult Health **Strategy:** The core issue of the question is knowledge of safe and unsafe methods of administering potassium as replacement therapy in hypokalemia. Use nursing knowledge and the process of elimination to make a selection.

11 **Answer: 4 Rationale:** A serum potassium level of 3.5 mEq/L is at the low end of the normal range. With a low normal level, it is better to continue to monitor the client and offer foods that are good sources of potassium. In the absence of additional medical history, it is not advisable to use oral KCL or salt substitutes as sources of additional potassium. Kayexelate reduces the potassium level and is contraindicated in this client. **Cognitive Level:** Applying **Client Need:** Physiological Adaptation **Integrated Process:** Nursing Process: Planning **Content Area:** Adult Health **Strategy:** The core issue of the question is knowledge of treatment measures depending on the severity of hypokalemia. First, recognize that this is a value at the low end of normal, and then select the mildest intervention of the choices provided. Note the critical word *most*, which indicates that some options may be plausible, but one is better than the others.

12 **Answer: 3, 5 Rationale:** A client who is at risk for developing hypocalcemia requires monitoring of serum albumin (provides information relative to physiologically available calcium) level. Decreased magnesium levels are usually seen concurrently with low serum calcium levels. Assessing BUN and creatinine, constipation would be included for a client at risk for hypercalcemia, and assessing for fluid overload would be important for a client being treated with fluid therapy for hypercalcemia. **Cognitive Level:** Applying **Client Need:** Physiological Adaptation **Integrated Process:** Nursing Process: Planning **Content Area:** Adult Health **Strategy:** The core issue of the question is the ability to choose assessments to detect hypocalcemia. Use nursing knowledge and the process of elimination to make a selection.

13 **Answer: 3 Rationale:** Calcium is absorbed in the intestines only under the influence of vitamin D, which is activated in the kidneys. Parathyroid hormone, not activated vitamin D, directly opposes calcitonin. Vitamin D does not prevent renal disease in hypocalcemia, but renal disease prevents activation of vitamin D, thereby reducing the body's ability to absorb calcium. There are other ways besides supplementation to obtain vitamin D in the body, such as exposure to sunlight. **Cognitive Level:** Applying **Client Need:** Pharmacological and Parenteral Therapies **Integrated Process:** Nursing Process: Implementation **Content Area:** Adult Health **Strategy:** The core issue of the question is knowledge of the purpose and effects of vitamin D in a client with hypocalcemia. Use nursing knowledge and the process of elimination to make a selection.

14 **Answer: 1 Rationale:** Antiepileptics such as phenytoin (Dilantin) alter vitamin D metabolism and lead to hypocalcemia. Calcium carbonate and calcitriol represent calcium sources, and the inclusion of these in a treatment plan would lead to increased serum calcium levels. Hydrochlorothiazide is incorrect because thiazide diuretics can lead to calcium retention. **Cognitive Level:** Applying **Client Need:** Physiological Adaptation **Integrated Process:** Nursing Process: Data Collection **Content Area:** Adult Health **Strategy:** The core issue of the question is knowledge of medications that increase the risk of hypocalcemia. Use nursing knowledge and the process of elimination to make a selection.

15 **Answer: 1 Rationale:** Clinical manifestations of hypercalcemia include personality changes. Anxiety, seizures, and carpal spasms are manifestations of hypocalcemia. **Cognitive Level:** Applying **Client Need:** Physiological Adaptation **Integrated Process:** Nursing Process: Data Collection **Content Area:** Adult Health **Strategy:** The core issue of the question is knowledge of manifestations of hypercalcemia. Use nursing knowledge and the process of elimination to make a selection.

16 **Answer: 2 Rationale:** Clinical manifestations of hypocalcemia include a positive Trousseau's sign, which is presence of carpopedal spasm. A positive Chvostek's sign (twitching of muscles of cheek) is associated with hypocalcemia. Kernig's sign is an indication of meningeal irritation. Hypoactive bowel sounds are a sign of hypercalcemia. **Cognitive Level:** Applying **Client Need:** Physiological Adaptation **Integrated Process:** Nursing Process: Data Collection **Content Area:** Adult Health **Strategy:** The core issue of the question is knowledge

of manifestations of hypocalcemia. Use nursing knowledge and the process of elimination to make a selection.

17 **Answer: 3, 5** **Rationale:** Addison's disease, known also as adrenal insufficiency, can cause increased magnesium levels resulting from volume depletion. Dehydration, or Deficient Fluid Volume, can lead to an elevated magnesium level because of hemoconcentration. Cushing's syndrome is hyperfunction of the adrenal gland and could lead to low magnesium levels from fluid overload. Diabetes mellitus could lead to low magnesium levels if osmotic diuresis is present from hyperglycemia. Splenomegaly is an unrelated finding. **Cognitive Level:** Applying **Client Need:** Physiological Adaptation **Integrated Process:** Nursing Process: Data Collection **Content Area:** Adult Health **Strategy:** The core issue of the question is knowledge of risk factors for hypermagnesemia. Use nursing knowledge and the process of elimination to make a selection.

18 **Answer: 3** **Rationale:** SVT is seen with decreased magnesium levels, as are premature ventricular contractions and ventricular fibrillation. Hypotension, bradycardia, and flushing and sweating are associated with hypermagnesemia. **Cognitive Level:** Analyzing **Client Need:** Physiological Adaptation **Integrated Process:** Nursing Process: Data Collection **Content Area:** Adult Health **Strategy:** The core issue of the question is the ability to discriminate signs of hyper- and hypomagnesemia. Use nursing knowledge and the process of elimination to make a selection.

19 **Answer: 1** **Rationale:** Either hemodialysis or peritoneal dialysis is used to remove excess magnesium in the client with renal failure. Diuretics will not be effective if the kidneys are not functional. Fluid restriction will be part of the treatment for end stage renal disease but will be ineffective alone in decreasing magnesium level. High-volume IV fluid replacement is contraindicated in renal failure. **Cognitive Level:** Applying **Client Need:** Physiological Adaptation **Integrated Process:** Nursing Process: Implementation **Content Area:** Adult Health **Strategy:** The core issue of the question is knowledge of effective therapies for increased magnesium levels. Note the critical words *end stage renal disease*, which lead you to look for a treatment that does not involve functional kidneys. Use nursing knowledge and the process of elimination to make a selection.

20 **Answer: 4** **Rationale:** A decreased magnesium level can occur in toxemia of pregnancy, preeclampsia, and eclampsia, causing seizures. A magnesium level of 3.1 mEq/L is an increased level, the opposite of the concern for this client. Sodium is not the electrolyte of concern in a client with preeclampsia. **Cognitive Level:** Applying **Client Need:** Physiological Adaptation **Integrated Process:** Nursing Process: Data Collection **Content Area:** Adult Health **Strategy:** The core issue of the question is knowledge of conditions that are consistent with decreased magnesium levels, and the ability to determine a reduced level. Use nursing knowledge and the process of elimination to make a selection.

21 **Answer: 2** **Rationale:** Cushing's syndrome causes low potassium and magnesium levels and an increase in sodium and chloride levels. The moon facies and fat pad at the back of the neck are also symptoms of excess corticosteroids. Addison's disease causes low sodium and increased magnesium and potassium levels. Burn states cause significant fluid and electrolyte disturbances (loss of sodium, chloride, and magnesium, with alterations in potassium depending on the stage of burn), but the presence of a moon facies and fat pad at the back of the neck is characteristic of Cushing's syndrome. SIADH is associated with hyponatremia. **Cognitive Level:** Analyzing **Client Need:** Physiological Adaptation **Integrated Process:** Nursing Process: Data Collection **Content Area:** Adult Health **Strategy:** The core issue of the question is the ability to synthesize electrolyte results with a clinical picture in a client with Cushing's syndrome. Use nursing knowledge and the process of elimination to make a selection.

22 **Answer: 2** **Rationale:** The decreased chloride level is of greatest concern because it can be associated with dilutional hypochloremia from fluid overload. The client's history of HF places the client in a higher risk category for fluid retention. The sodium, potassium, and bicarbonate levels are within normal range and are reassuring. **Cognitive Level:** Analyzing **Client Need:** Physiological Adaptation **Integrated Process:** Nursing Process: Data Collection **Content Area:** Adult Health **Strategy:** The core issue of the question is the ability to determine abnormal electrolyte levels. Use nursing knowledge and the process of elimination to make a selection.

23 **Answer: 1** **Rationale:** Poor nutritional intake, such as occurs in clients with alcoholism, can lead to hypophosphatemia. During oliguria, the kidneys are unable to excrete phosphorus, leading to hyperphosphatemia. Clients with prolonged (not short-term) gastric suction are more likely to experience hypophosphatemia. Prolonged or continuous use of aluminum-containing antacids (not occasional use) leads to hypophosphatemia. **Cognitive Level:** Analyzing **Client Need:** Physiological Adaptation **Integrated Process:** Nursing Process: Data Collection **Content Area:** Adult Health **Strategy:** The core issue of the question is knowledge of risk factors for hypophosphatemia. Use nursing knowledge and the process of elimination to make a selection.

24 **Answer: 5.1** **Rationale:** Hyperkalemia exists when the serum potassium level rises above the upper limit of normal, which is 5.1 mEq/L. **Cognitive Level:** Analyzing **Client Need:** Physiological Adaptation **Integrated Process:** Nursing Process: Data Collection **Content Area:** Adult Health **Strategy:** The core issue of the question is knowledge that hypocalcemia accompanies hypermagnesemia. To answer correctly, you must also be able to recognize abnormal laboratory values. Use nursing knowledge to make a selection.

25 **Answer: 1, 2, 3** **Rationale:** Actions that are helpful to maintain a fluid restriction are involving the client in dividing fluid allowances, using an infusion pump, and including oral ice chips and fluids with medications in the intake record. Unlimited ice chips could contribute to excess fluid intake. **Cognitive Level:** Applying **Client Need:** Basic Care and Comfort **Integrated Process:** Nursing Process: Implementation **Content Area:** Adult Health **Strategy:** The critical term is *fluid restriction*. Note the word *unlimited* is opposite of restriction and recognize that all fluid intake must be measured to eliminate the proper options.

Key Terms to Review

hypercalcemia p. 817
hyperchloremia p. 820
hyperkalemia p. 814
hypermagnesemia p. 819
hypernatremia p. 812
hyperosmolar p. 812
hyperphosphatemia p. 822
hypertonic p. 805
hypervolemia p. 810
hypocalcemia p. 815
hypochloremia p. 820
hypokalemia p. 813
hypomagnesemia p. 818
hyponatremia p. 810
hypophosphatemia p. 821
hypotonic p. 805
hypovolemia p. 810
water intoxication p. 810

References

Berman, A., & Snyder, S. (2012). *Kozier & Erb's fundamentals of nursing: Concepts, process, and practice* (9th ed.). Upper Saddle River, NJ: Pearson Education, Inc.

Ignatavicius, D., & Workman, L. (2010). *Medical-surgical nursing: Patient-centered collaborative care* (6th ed.). Philadelphia: Saunders.

Kee, J. (2010). *Laboratory and diagnostic tests* (8th ed.). Upper Saddle River, NJ: Pearson Education, Inc.

LeMone, P., Burke, K., & Bauldoff, G. (2012). *Medical surgical nursing: Critical thinking in patient care* (5th ed.). Upper Saddle River, NJ: Pearson Education.

Lewis, S., Dirksen, S., Heitkemper, M., & Bucher, L. (2011). *Medical surgical nursing: Assessment and management of clinical problems* (8th ed.). St. Louis, MO: Elsevier.

Smeltzer, S., Bare, B., Hinkle, J., & Cheever, K. (2010). *Textbook of medical-surgical nursing* (12th ed.). Philadelphia: Lippincott Williams & Wilkins.

Test Yourself

Are you ready for the NCLEX-PN® or course exams? Use the practice tests on the companion website to check.

50 Acid–Base Imbalances

In this chapter

Cross Reference

Other chapters relevant to this content area are

Common Laboratory Tests Chapter 42
Fluid and Electrolyte Imbalances Chapter 49

I. NORMAL ACID–BASE BALANCE

A. Nature of acids and bases

1. An **acid** is a substance that releases a hydrogen (H^+) ion when dissolved in water
2. A **base** is a substance that will bind to an H^+ ion when dissolved in water
3. Weak acids do not completely separate in water; they only release some of H^+ ions
4. A weak base accepts H^+ ions less easily, but it is extremely valuable in preventing major alterations in **pH** of extracellular fluid (ECF)

B. Chemical buffer systems in body

1. A **buffer** prevents major changes in ECF by releasing or accepting H^+ ions
2. The major chemical buffers (found in blood) include bicarbonate–carbonic acid buffer system, phosphate buffer system, and protein buffer system
3. Chemical buffers are present in both intracellular fluid (ICF) and ECF
4. Buffers are found in all body tissues, including bone
5. Chemical buffers act within seconds to neutralize acids and bases, and keep pH within narrow normal range of 7.35 to 7.45
6. Bicarbonate buffer system
   a. Consists of a water solution that contains a weak acid, carbonic acid (H_2CO_3), and a bicarbonate salt, usually sodium bicarbonate ($NaHCO_3$)
   b. Normally, body maintains pH by keeping ratio of bicarbonate (**HCO_3^-**) to H_2CO_3 at a proportion of 20:1; this ratio is changed if pH goes up or down
   c. Once compensation occurs, ratio becomes stable again
   d. The bicarbonate–carbonic acid buffer system is linked to both respiratory and renal systems
   e. H_2CO_3 is respiratory compensatory component; it can dissociate into carbon dioxide (CO_2) and water, with CO_2 being exhaled by lungs
   f. HCO_3^- is the primary renal compensatory component; it can be excreted by kidneys or retained with excretion of H^+ ions
   g. This function is illustrated by the following equation:
      $CO_2 + H_2O \leftrightarrow H_2CO_3 \leftrightarrow HCO_3^- + H^+$
7. The phosphate buffer system buffers both ICF and ECF to maintain a normal pH

8. The protein buffer system acts similarly to bicarbonate–carbonic acid buffer system because it releases or accepts H^+ readily and can exist as either an acid or a base; it is a major intracellular buffer
9. The hemoglobin-oxyhemoglobin buffer system helps to maintain pH within normal range in both arterial and venous blood, which have different amounts of CO_2

C. Physiologic buffers in body

1. Pulmonary regulation
   a. Lungs control the respiratory carbonic acid buffer system and compensate for acid–base disturbances that are primarily metabolic in nature (e.g., lactic acidosis that occurs with exercise)
   b. Under control of medulla oblongata, lungs increase or decrease respiratory rate and depth in response to amount of CO_2 in ECF
   c. Respiratory system is extremely sensitive to changes in pH and begins compensatory efforts within seconds to minutes but can become quickly exhausted and is not as efficient as renal compensation
   d. Older adults have reduced gas exchange during breathing and less alveolar membrane so CO_2 retention and increased H^+ ion concentrations may be a problem
2. Renal regulation
   a. Kidneys control the metabolic buffer $NaHCO_3^-$ by excreting an acidic urine or an alkaline urine
   b. This system works within several hours to days but is powerfully effective by eliminating either acids or bases as needed
   c. Kidneys control HCO_3^- in ECF by either reabsorbing or excreting H^+ ions; they also combine ammonia (NaH_3) with hydrochloric acid (HCl) to form ammonium (NH_4Cl), which is excreted by kidneys; approximately 50% of excess H^+ can be excreted by this mechanism
   d. Kidneys can also excrete weak acids into urine
   e. Body depends on kidneys to excrete acids from cellular metabolism; thus urine is normally acidic (average pH 6)
   f. Renal function decreases with age, so older adults do not excrete H^+ ions or synthesize HCO_3^- as efficiently, making their acid–base imbalances more difficult to correct

NCLEX®

3. **Compensation** occurs when body uses regulatory mechanisms to return pH to normal by transforming acids and bases within body; pH becomes normal, but there are abnormal amounts of CO_2 and/or HCO_3^-
   a. A primary metabolic disturbance will cause respiratory compensation
   b. A primary respiratory disturbance will activate blood buffers and cause metabolic compensation by kidneys
   c. Complete compensation means that buffers have achieved homeostasis and pH is fully corrected
   d. Partial compensation means that buffers are working to restore homeostasis
   e. Decompensation refers to a worsening state of acid–base imbalance
4. Correction of acid–base imbalance occurs when lungs and/or kidneys eliminate offending substance(s) from body, and both CO_2 and HCO_3^- levels (not just pH) are returned to normal

D. Indicator measures of acid–base status

1. pH: the negative logarithm of H^+ ion concentration in mEq per liter

NCLEX®

   a. Normal pH in arterial blood is 7.35 to 7.45; in venous blood, it is 7.32 to 7.42
   b. A pH less than 7.35 is labeled acidotic; acidosis has depressant effect on central nervous system (CNS)
   c. A pH greater than 7.45 is labeled alkalotic; alkalosis has excitatory effect on CNS

Memory Aid

The pH is like the center of a seesaw; it wants to stay balanced.

2. **$PaCO_2$** (partial pressure of carbon dioxide): measurement of CO_2 pressure being exerted on plasma; is directly related to amount of CO_2 being produced
   a. $PaCO_2$ is regulated by lungs and indicates amount of H_2CO_3 that is available to act as a buffer
   b. $PaCO_2$ indicates whether condition is a respiratory disturbance

NCLEX®

   c. Normal value of $PaCO_2$ is 35 to 45 mm Hg
   d. Values less than 35 mm Hg indicate alkalosis
   e. Values greater than 45 mm Hg indicate acidosis

Memory Aid

Carbon dioxide (CO_2) acts as an acid in the body. It is also the indicator of how the respiratory system is functioning.

3. HCO_3^- (bicarbonate): measurement of HCO_3^- in plasma and is directly related to attraction and release of H^+ ions from H_2CO_3
   a. HCO_3^- is regulated by kidneys and indicates body's ability to buffer H^+ ions (acid) by combining to form H_2CO_3
   b. HCO_3^- is the value that indicates whether there is a metabolic disturbance
   NCLEX® c. Normal value of HCO_3^- is 22 to 26 mEq/L in arterial blood gas
   d. Values less than 22 mEq/L indicate acidosis
   e. Value greater than 26 mEq/L indicate alkalosis

Memory Aid

Bicarbonate (HCO_3^-) acts as a base in the body. It is also the indicator of how the metabolic system is functioning.

4. **PaO_2** (partial pressure of oxygen): measurement of amount of pressure exerted by oxygen on plasma
   a. Range of normal values for PaO_2 is 80 to 100 mm Hg for adults under 60 years of age; for every year above 60, there is an expected decrease in PaO_2 of 1 mmHg
   b. If PaO_2 drops dramatically, then O_2 saturation also decreases greatly
5. **SaO_2**: percentage of hemoglobin saturated with O_2; since most O_2 is carried on hemoglobin, total O_2 concentration is measured using hemoglobin saturation (SaO_2)
   a. A relationship between PaO_2 and SaO_2 influences binding affinity and dissociation of oxygen and hemoglobin (called oxygen–hemoglobin dissociation curve)
   b. Acidosis causes a shift toward right on oxygen–hemoglobin dissociation curve that results in a decreased affinity; oxygen is more easily released to tissues
   c. Alkalosis causes a shift toward left on oxygen–hemoglobin dissociation curve that results in an increased affinity; oxygen is held more tightly and is less available to tissues
   d. Other factors that affect oxygen affinity include body temperature and transfusion of banked blood
6. Electrolyte interactions
   NCLEX® a. HCO_3^- is a direct reflection of renal system's ability to compensate for pH changes; a decreased HCO_3^- level is consistent with acidosis, and an increased HCO_3^- level is consistent with alkalosis
   b. Base excess (BE) indicates amount of HCO_3^- available in ECF, and normal values range from –3.0 to +3.0 in adults; values above +3.0 indicate metabolic alkalosis, while values below –3.0 indicate metabolic acidosis
   c. Serum anion gap (AG) (normal range 10 to 12 mEq/L) calculates concentrations of anions (HCO_3^-, chloride [Cl^-], proteins, phosphates, and sulfates) and cations (sodium [Na^+], potassium [K^+], magnesium [Mg^{++}], calcium [Ca^{++}]) by using the following equation:
   $Na^+ - [Cl^- + HCO_3^-]$
   d. Increased AG of more than 12 mEq/L indicates metabolic acidosis (AG acidosis); however, a normal AG can exist with a metabolic acidosis (non-AG acidosis) when there is a decrease in HCO_3^- balanced by an increase in Cl^-
   e. Decreased AG of less than 10 mEq/L can be seen with low albumin levels or in conditions in which there is an increase in unmeasured cations (multiple myeloma, lithium toxicity, or nephrotic syndrome)
   f. Potassium (K^+) helps to maintain acid–base balance by exchanging for H^+ ions across cell membranes; in acidosis, K^+ comes out of cell and allows H^+ in to reduce circulating acids; in alkalosis, K^+ goes into cell and allows H^+ to come out to increase circulating acids
   g. Chloride levels are used to evaluate clients who are at risk for metabolic alkalosis to determine cause of alkalosis and thus corrective treatment

E. Arterial blood gas (ABG) analysis (see Table 50–1 for normal values)

NCLEX® 1. Follow a systematic approach (see Figure 50–1)
2. Interpret pH: a pH less than 7.35 indicates acidosis, while a pH greater than 7.45 indicates alkalosis
3. Identify primary cause—respiratory or metabolic
   a. Examine first $PaCO_2$ value and then HCO_3^- value
   b. If $PaCO_2$ is abnormal and direction of change in value is inversely related to direction of change in pH, then primary problem is respiratory
   c. If HCO_3^- is abnormal and direction of change in value is same as direction of change in pH, then problem is metabolic

Table 50–1 Normal Arterial Blood Gas Values

	Normal Reference Ranges		
Serum Laboratory Value	**Adult**	**Child**	**Infant**
pH (arterial)	7.35–7.45	7.37–7.43 (c) 7.35–7.41 (a)	7.36–7.42
PCO_2 (mm Hg)	35–45	35–41 (c) 38–44 (a)	30–34
HCO_3^- (mEq/L)	22–26	18–25 (c) 23–25 (a)	17.2–23.6
PO_2 (mm Hg)	80–100	80–100	80–100
SaO_2 (%)	95–100	95–100	95–100
Anion Gap Base Excess	10–12 mEq/L +3 to – 3 (+/– 2 mEq/L)	10–12 mEq/L +3 to –3 (+/–2 mEq/L)	10–12 mEq/L +3 to –3 (+/–2 mEq/L)

c, children; a, adolescents

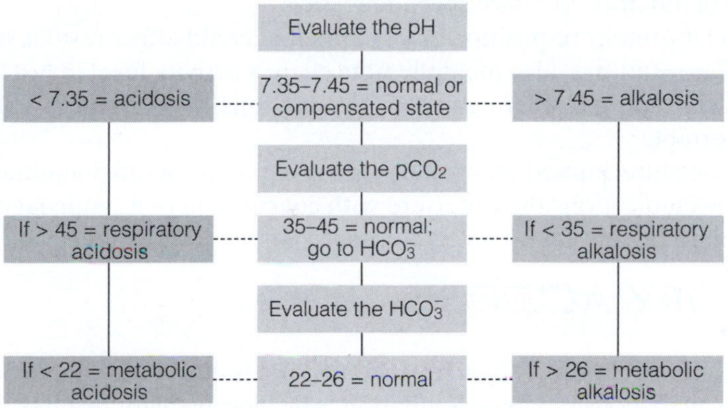

Figure 50–1

Interpreting ABGs: If CO_2 and HCO_3^- are both abnormal, look to see which one has a change that *matches* the change in the pH (CO_2 acts as an acid; HCO_3^- acts as a base). This match will be the primary imbalance, while the other system is compensating.

Memory Aid

Interpret ABGs by looking first at the pH, then at the CO_2, then at the HCO_3^-. Determine first whether there is acidosis or alkalosis, then evaluate whether the imbalance is respiratory (CO_2) or metabolic (HCO_3^-) in origin. The cause will be the value that *matches* or correlates with the change in the direction of the pH.

4. Determine presence of compensation

a. Determine if $PaCO_2$ and HCO_3^- are decreased or increased as body attempts to maintain ratio of HCO_3^- to H_2CO_3 at 20:1

b. Partial compensation exists when pH remains abnormal but parameter that did not originally alter pH now changes (e.g., pH indicates an acidotic state and CO_2 is high, indicating respiratory origin, but HCO_3^- is also increased, indicating that body is utilizing buffer systems to bring pH back into line)

Memory Aid

The pH is like a seesaw. The CO_2 and the HCO_3 are like riders on the ends of the see-saw. When one side goes up, the other tries to go up to compensate. When one side goes down, the other side also tries to go down to compensate and bring the pH back toward normal.

c. Full or complete compensation occurs when buffer system is working effectively and brings pH back to a value of 7.35 to 7.45 (e.g., respiratory acidosis exists as indicated by an elevated $PaCO_2$; however, pH is normal and HCO_3^- is increased)

Memory Aid

If CO_2 and HCO_3^- are both abnormal, again look to see which one has a change that *matches* the direction of the change in the pH (e.g., CO_2 acts as an acid; HCO_3^- acts as a base). This match will be the primary imbalance, while the other system is compensating. If the pH is back in normal range, the value will be a number that is nearer to the side of the primary imbalance (e.g., 7.43 is nearer to alkalosis than acidosis, while 7.36 is nearer to acidosis than alkalosis). Remember that the body does not overcompensate!

F. Assisting with obtaining an ABG specimen

1. Determine site of specimen collection (radial or femoral artery, intra-arterial line) and obtain baseline vital signs
2. *NCLEX®* Perform Allen test prior to radial artery puncture
   - **a.** Apply simultaneous pressure to radial and ulnar arteries of affected hand
   - **b.** Ask client to repeatedly make a fist and open it; note that hand should blanch
   - **c.** Maintain pressure on radial artery and release pressure on ulnar artery; note color of hand
   - **d.** A return of normal pink color within 6 seconds indicates adequate collateral circulation from ulnar artery, making it safe to use radial artery for puncture; otherwise, site should not be used
3. Assist with specimen preparation by preparing heparinized syringe and placing ice in collection bag prior to blood draw; prepare specimen labels
4. Note on laboratory requisition any factors that could affect results, such as body temperature and O_2 or ventilator settings; also mentally note client's activity level in last 20 minutes
5. Explain procedure to client and provide emotional support during blood draw, which may be uncomfortable
6. *NCLEX®* After procedure, immediately apply firm pressure for a full 5 minutes by the clock, and longer if client takes any medications that interfere with coagulation (e.g., anticoagulants, aspirin); arrange for specimen to be sent immediately for analysis

II. RESPIRATORY ACIDOSIS

A. Overview

1. In **respiratory acidosis**, CO_2 is retained and pH is decreased (Table 50–2)
2. *NCLEX®* It occurs in response to hypoventilation, which occurs with respiratory depression, inadequate chest expansion, airway obstruction, or interference with alveolar-capillary exchange

B. Nursing data collection

1. See Table 50–2 for clinical manifestations
2. *NCLEX®* Diagnostic findings
   - **a.** pH decreased below 7.35
   - **b.** $PaCO_2$ elevated above 45 mm Hg
   - **c.** Hyperkalemia
3. Compensation
   - **a.** *NCLEX®* Increased rate and depth of respirations to blow off CO_2
   - **b.** Kidneys eliminate H^+ ions and retain HCO_3^- (urine pH less than 6)
   - **c.** HCO_3^- levels rise when body is compensating for acidosis

C. Collaborative management

1. Treatment is aimed at correcting underlying cause and improving ventilation
2. Use pulmonary hygiene measures to clear respiratory tract of mucus and purulent drainage
3. *NCLEX®* Provide adequate fluid intake to liquefy secretions
4. *NCLEX®* If indicated, administer supplemental O_2 cautiously to a client with chronic respiratory acidosis
   - **a.** Note that clients with chronic acidosis have compensated and are adjusted to living with higher $PaCO_2$ levels
   - **b.** Remember CO_2 level is the mechanism that stimulates respiratory drive
   - **c.** O_2 administration at higher levels can lead to a decreased ventilatory drive and can cause further hypoxia
   - **d.** Low-flow oxygen is expected treatment
   - **e.** Collaborate with physician and respiratory therapist to manage chronic respiratory disease
5. Mechanical ventilation may be required to improve respiratory status; CO_2 is decreased gradually to prevent alkalosis and seizures from occurring
6. *NCLEX®* Monitor respiratory rate and depth
7. *NCLEX®* Position to facilitate maximum lung expansion (upright as tolerated)

Table 50–2 Overview of Acid–Base Imbalances

Primary Abnormality	Compensation	Common Etiologies	Clinical Manifestations
Respiratory acidosis pH ↓ < 7.35 CO_2 ↑ > 45	HCO_3^- ↑ to raise pH	COPD, sedative or barbiturate overdose, chest wall abnormalities, pneumonia, atelectasis, respiratory muscle weakness, hypoventilation	Respiratory rate ↑ and shallow to attempt to blow off CO_2, hypotension, heart block, peaked T waves, prolonged PR interval, weak and thready pulse, tachycardia, warm and flushed skin, headache, papilledema, decreased level of consciousness, drowsiness, coma
Respiratory alkalosis pH ↑ > 7.45 CO_2 ↓ < 35	HCO_3^- ↓ to lower pH	Hyperventilation caused by hypoxia, fever, fear, pain, exercise, anxiety, or pulmonary embolus; mechanical ventilation, septicemia (respiratory center stimulation), brain injury, encephalitis, salicylate poisoning	↑ myocardial irritability, ↑ heart rate, ↑ sensitivity to digitalis preparations, dyspnea, chest tightness, dizziness, anxiety, panic, tetany, seizures, blurred vision
Metabolic acidosis pH ↓ < 7.35 HCO_3^- ↓ < 22	CO_2 ↓ to raise pH	DKA, lactic acidosis, starvation, severe diarrhea, renal tubule acidosis, renal failure, GI fistulas, shock	Hypotension, dysrhythmias, peripheral vasodilation, cold, clammy skin, deep rapid respiratory pattern (Kussmaul respirations), drowsiness, headache, confusion, lethargy, weakness, coma, nausea and vomiting, diarrhea, abdominal pain
Metabolic alkalosis pH ↑ > 7.45 HCO_3^- ↑ < 26	CO_2 ↑ to lower pH	Severe vomiting, excessive nasogastric suctioning, diuretic therapy, hypokalemia, excess licorice intake, excessive $NaHCO_3$ use, excessive mineralocorticoids	↑ heart rate, dysrhythmias secondary to hypokalemia, hypotension, premature ventricular contractions, atrial tachycardia, hypoventilation, respiratory failure, dizziness, irritability, nervousness, confusion, tremors, muscle cramps, tetany, hyper-reflexia, parasthesias in fingers and toes, seizures

NCLEX®
8. Take apical pulse and check for tachycardia and irregularities; note color of skin, nail beds, and mucous membranes

NCLEX®
9. Monitor LOC
10. Monitor ECG for dysrhythmias
11. Monitor results of ABGs and serum electrolytes, especially potassium
12. Administer medications as ordered
    a. Bronchodilators to decrease bronchospasm; inhalation medications may be administered by respiratory therapists per agency policy
    b. Antibiotics to treat infections in respiratory tract
    c. Respiratory agents to decrease viscosity of pulmonary secretions, such as acetylcystine (Mucomyst)
    d. Anticoagulants and thrombolytics to prevent or treat pulmonary emboli
    e. Medications are usually administered IV in acute situations and then changed to oral route as client's condition stabilizes
13. Provide good oral hygiene frequently and provide adequate fluid intake
14. Keep side rails up, bed at lowest level, and call bell within client's reach
15. Maintain a calm, quiet environment; if client is confused, orient frequently to person, place, and time
16. Satisfactory outcomes include ABGs improved to client's baseline, decreased anxiety, improved breathing with less effort, freedom from injury, absence of cardiac dysrhythmias, improved LOC, and decreased rate but increased depth of respirations

D. Client education
1. Teach preventive measures to clients at risk
2. Teach deep breathing techniques
3. Report signs of infections, shortness of breath, fatigue, and increased pulse rate to health care provider

III. RESPIRATORY ALKALOSIS

A. Overview
1. In **respiratory alkalosis**, the pH is elevated and $PaCO_2$ is decreased (Table 50–2)

NCLEX®
2. Occurs with hyperventilation and leads to a decreased level of CO_2; sometimes called an H_2CO_3 deficit
3. Other causes can include infection, excessive mechanical ventilation, and respiratory center stimulation from fever, salicylate intoxication, and trauma to CNS

B. Nursing data collection

NCLEX® 1. See Table 50–2 for clinical manifestations

NCLEX® 2. Diagnostic findings

a. High pH (over 7.45)

b. Low $PaCO_2$ (under 35 mm Hg)

c. Hypokalemia

d. Hypocalcemia (as pH increases, calcium binding occurs in plasma and calcium levels decrease)

3. Compensation

a. Kidneys conserve H^+ and excrete HCO_3^- (urine pH greater than 6)

b. Low HCO_3^- indicates body is attempting to compensate

C. Collaborative management

1. Treat underlying cause
2. Assist client to breathe more slowly; if needed, have client rebreathe CO_2 by using a rebreather mask or a paper bag

NCLEX® 3. Give oxygen therapy if client is hypoxic

4. Medicate as needed with anti-anxiety drugs to control anxiety or sedatives to control hyperventilation associated with anxiety
5. Provide support and reassurance

NCLEX® 6. Monitor vital signs and ABGs

NCLEX® 7. Protect from injury

8. Satisfactory outcomes include decreased respiratory rate, absence of numbness and tingling in extremities, return of ABGs to normal or client's baseline, and diminished anxiety; additionally, client remains free from injury

D. Client education

1. Teach client relaxation techniques
2. Encourage client to attend stress management classes as indicated

NCLEX® 3. Teach parents to keep aspirin and other salicylates out of reach of children and to follow current poison control guidelines if exposure occurs

IV. METABOLIC ACIDOSIS

A. Overview

1. In **metabolic acidosis**, the pH decreases and HCO_3^- decreases (Table 50–2)

NCLEX® 2. Occurs when there is a loss of HCO_3^- or when acids other than carbonic acid (H_2CO_3) accumulate in ECF

3. This condition rarely occurs spontaneously but rather is accompanied by other problems, such as gastrointestinal (GI) conditions (starvation, malnutrition, and chronic diarrhea), renal (kidney failure), diabetic ketoacidosis (DKA), hyperthyroidism, trauma, shock, increased exercise, severe infection, and fever

B. Nursing data collection

NCLEX® 1. See Table 50–2 for clinical manifestations

Memory Aid Acidosis of any origin tends to be a CNS depressant.

NCLEX® 2. Diagnostic findings

a. pH less than 7.35

b. HCO_3^- less than 22 mEq/L

c. Hyperkalemia frequently seen

d. ECG may show changes related to K^+ levels

e. AG calculation increases

f. BE decreases

3. Compensation

a. Lungs eliminate CO_2; kidneys conserve HCO_3^-

b. Urine pH less than 6

c. $PaCO_2$ decreases when compensation is occurring

C. Collaborative management

1. Treatment is aimed at correcting underlying problem
2. Provide hydration to restore water, nutrients, and electrolytes
3. An alkalotic IV solution (sodium bicarbonate or sodium lactate) may be indicated to correct acidosis
4. Mechanical ventilation is used only if other treatment modalities are ineffective
5. Monitor ABGs
6. *NCLEX®* Monitor I&O and measure daily weights; monitor serum electrolytes
7. *NCLEX®* Check vital signs, especially respiration for rate and depth
8. Monitor LOC
9. Observe GI function
10. Monitor ECG for conduction problems
11. *NCLEX®* Protect from injury
12. *NCLEX®* Administer IV fluids and medications as ordered, based on underlying cause
    a. If cause is secondary to DKA, implement hydration with normal saline, regular insulin, and possibly potassium
    b. If diarrhea is cause, treat with hydration and antidiarrheal agents
    c. Administer $NaHCO_3$ cautiously and only when HCO_3^- levels are very low (below 16 to 18 mEq/L); can cause metabolic alkalosis and hypokalemia; titrate closely to avoid further acid–base imbalances
13. Satisfactory outcomes include that client is free from injury and has no dysrhythmias, ABGs return to normal, fluid volume deficits are corrected, LOC returns to normal, and GI upset is relieved

D. Client education

1. Teach clients to seek health care for prolonged diarrhea
2. Teach diabetic clients importance of preventing occurrences of DKA and how to manage DKA should it occur

V. METABOLIC ALKALOSIS

A. Overview

1. In **metabolic alkalosis**, there is an increased pH and increased HCO_3^- (see Table 50–2)
2. *NCLEX®* Occurs when there is a loss of H^+ ions (e.g., because of vomiting or nasogastric suctioning) or an increase in HCO_3^- level (such as with ingestion of bicarbonate-based antacids)

B. Nursing data collection

1. See Table 50–2 for clinical manifestations

Memory Aid

Alkalosis of any origin tends to have an excitatory effect on the CNS.

2. *NCLEX®* Diagnostic findings
    a. pH greater than 7.45
    b. HCO_3^- above 26 mEq/L
    c. Hypokalemia
    d. Hypocalcemia (as pH increases, Ca^{++} binding occurs and serum Ca^{++} levels decrease)
    e. Hyponatremia and hypochloremia
    f. Urine chloride levels reveal whether client is chloride responsive (under 10 mEq/L) or chloride resistant (over 10 mEq/L)
    g. BE increases
3. Compensation
    a. Lungs retain CO_2; kidneys conserve H^+ and excrete HCO_3^-
    b. $PaCO_2$ increases with compensation
    c. Urine pH greater than 6

C. Collaborative management

1. Treatment aimed at correcting underlying problem
2. Provide sufficient Cl^- to enhance renal absorption of Na^+ and excretion of HCO_3^-
3. Restore normal fluid balance
4. *NCLEX®* Monitor LOC
5. *NCLEX®* Note vital signs, especially respiratory rate and depth

6. Administer medication and IV fluids as ordered
   a. Normal saline-based IV fluid replacement
   b. Potassium supplementation if hypokalemic
   c. Histamine-2 receptor antagonists such as ranitidine (Zantac) or famotidine (Pepcid) to reduce secretion of H^+ ions and loss of H^+ ions from GI drainage
   d. If client is chloride responsive, then administer acetazolamide (Diamox) to increase renal bicarbonate excretion
   e. If client is chloride resistant, then correct K^+ and Mg^{++} deficits with appropriate supplementation
7. Monitor I&O
8. NCLEX® Protect from injury
9. Monitor ECG for conduction abnormalities
10. Monitor results of ABGs and serum electrolytes
11. Satisfactory outcomes include that client is free from injury, ABGs return to normal, hypertension is corrected, electrolytes are restored to normal, cardiac conduction is normal, and client states ways to prevent reoccurrance

D. Client education

1. Teach clients to take antacids correctly to prevent excessive dosing
2. Teach signs and symptoms to report to health care provider for those at risk, especially older adults
3. Teach signs and symptoms of hypokalemia to report to health care provider

VI. MIXED ACID–BASE DISORDERS

A. Identification and treatment of primary disorder

1. A **mixed acid–base disorder** occurs when two or more independent acid–base disorders occur at same time
2. pH depends on type and severity of each simple disorder
3. Respiratory acidosis and alkalosis cannot occur concurrently; it is impossible to have hyperventilation and hypoventilation at same time
4. Treatment is aimed at correcting underlying cause of each disorder
5. When identifying acid–base imbalances, mathematical formulas can be used to determine degree of expected compensation
6. AG and urine pH values will also help determine which imbalance is occurring

B. Chronic and superimposed acid–base disturbances

1. Mixed metabolic acidosis and respiratory acidosis
   a. Clients with acute pulmonary edema
   b. Clients with cardiac arrest as a result of buildup of lactic acidosis and CO_2 retention due to inadequate ventilation
   c. NCLEX® pH values decrease and are more pronounced because of decreasing HCO_3^- level coupled with increasing CO_2 level
2. Mixed metabolic alkalosis and respiratory acidosis
   a. NCLEX® Clients with chronic obstructive pulmonary disease (COPD) and who have treatment with potassium-wasting diuretics, severe vomiting, or development of diarrhea
   b. Clients with COPD who have a quick improvement in ventilation
   c. pH values tend to become balanced because of an increase in both HCO_3^- and $PaCO_2$ values
3. Mixed metabolic acidosis with respiratory alkalosis
   a. Clients with a rapid correction of metabolic acidosis
   b. NCLEX® Clients with salicylate intoxication
   c. Clients with Gram-negative septicemia
   d. pH values tend to become balanced because of decreases in both HCO_3^- and $PaCO_2$
4. Mixed metabolic alkalosis and respiratory alkalosis
   a. Postoperative clients with severe hemorrhage
   b. Clients who have massive transfusions
   c. Clients with excessive nasogastric (NG) drainage
   d. pH values increase and are more pronounced because of increasing HCO_3^- coupled with decreasing CO_2 levels
5. Mixed metabolic acidosis and metabolic alkalosis
   a. NCLEX® Seen in clients with gastroenteritis, vomiting, and diarrhea
   b. If imbalance is present in same proportion, there is usually no change in values (pH, HCO_3^-, and $PaCO_2$) even though there is volume depletion

6. Chronic and acute respiratory acidosis

NCLEX®
   a. Chronic respiratory conditions with an acute condition superimposed can lead to increased $PaCO_2$ levels, causing further pulmonary dysfunction and leading to serious consequences that can compromise both treatment and expected response to treatment
   b. Clients with both a chronic and a superimposed acute respiratory acid–base imbalance should be closely monitored by a pulmonologist
   c. Respiratory therapist should be part of collaborative health care team plan during client's treatment

C. Diagnostic and laboratory findings

1. Increased $PaCO_2$ with decreased pH
   a. Respiratory acidosis
   b. Respiratory acidosis with incompletely compensating metabolic alkalosis
   c. Respiratory acidosis with coexisting metabolic acidosis
2. Increased $PaCO_2$ with increased pH
   a. Metabolic alkalosis with incomplete compensating respiratory acidosis
   b. Metabolic alkalosis with coexisting respiratory acidosis
3. Decreased $PaCO_2$ with decreased pH
   a. Metabolic acidosis with incomplete respiratory alkalosis
   b. Metabolic acidosis with coexisting respiratory alkalosis
4. Decreased $PaCO_2$ with increased pH
   a. Respiratory alkalosis
   b. Respiratory alkalosis with incomplete compensating metabolic acidosis
   c. Respiratory alkalosis with coexisting metabolic alkalosis
5. Normal pH values
   a. Increased $PaCO_2$ leads to respiratory acidosis with compensated metabolic alkalosis
   b. Decreased $PaCO_2$ leads to respiratory alkalosis with compensated metabolic acidosis
6. Changes in AG levels and $NaHCO_3^-$ levels
7. Abnormal serum electrolyte levels can reflect changes in acid–base balance
8. ECG results may show electrolyte disturbances
9. Chest x-ray (CXR) may show underlying cardiac or pulmonary disease
10. Hemoglobin and hematocrit levels can indicate O_2-carrying potential

D. Collaborative management

1. Treatment focuses on correcting underlying causes of disorder
2. Mixed disorders must be treated before acid–base balance can be restored
3. A collaborative team approach (including a pulmonologist, respiratory therapist, nurses, and dietitian) is needed to assist client in restoring acid–base balance, increasing activity tolerance, and improving physiological function
4. Monitor vital signs and LOC (NCLEX®)
5. Monitor ABGs, pulmonary function tests, pulse oximetry, and CXR
6. Protect from injury (NCLEX®)
7. Monitor ECG, hemoglobin and hematocrit levels, and serum electrolytes
8. Ensure adequate fluid intake
9. Implement therapeutic measures such as O_2 therapy and medications to resolve underlying causes of imbalances (NCLEX®)
10. Satisfactory outcomes include that client remains free from injury, ABGs return to normal or baseline, cardiac conduction is normal; fluid balance and electrolyte levels are restored, LOC is improved, and client is able to report ways to prevent problem from reoccurring

E. Client education

1. Clients with chronic respiratory conditions should report exacerbations to health care provider
2. Clients who experience fluid losses through emesis or diarrhea are at increased risk for acid–base imbalance and should notify health care provider if condition is not self-limiting (lasts more than 2 or 3 days)
3. Clients with diabetes are at risk for acid–base imbalance due to alterations in glucose levels and should closely monitor serum glucose levels and use appropriate interventions to maintain normal levels
4. Clients who have renal problems are prone to develop acid–base imbalance due to alterations in electrolyte levels; closely monitor renal status to identify potential disturbances and allow for intervention

PRACTICE TEST

Check your NCLEX-PN® Exam I.Q.

You are ready for testing on this content if you can

- Use knowledge from the biological and physical sciences to determine acid–base status.
- Apply concepts of pathophysiology to acid–base imbalances.
- Identify signs and symptoms of acid–base imbalances.
- Describe interventions to treat acid–base imbalances.
- Monitor the client's response to treatments for acid–base imbalances.

PRACTICE TEST

1 A client has been admitted for dehydration after fasting for five days. For which acid–base imbalance would the nurse monitor this client?

1. Metabolic acidosis
2. Metabolic alkalosis
3. Respiratory acidosis
4. Respiratory alkalosis

2 A client is admitted to the hospital after vomiting for three days. Which arterial blood gas (ABG) result would the nurse expect?

1. pH 7.30; $PaCO_2$ 50; HCO_3^- 27
2. pH 7.47; $PaCO_2$ 43; HCO_3^- 28
3. pH 7.34; $PaCO_2$ 50; HCO_3^- 28
4. pH 7.48; $PaCO_2$ 30; HCO_3^- 23

3 A client is admitted to the hospital with a diagnosis of respiratory acidosis secondary to overdose of barbiturates. Which finding would the nurse expect upon chart review and data collection? Select all that apply.

1. Slow, shallow respirations
2. Tetany symptoms
3. Increased deep tendon reflexes
4. Palpitations
5. Headache

4 A client is admitted with a diagnosis of renal failure. Which arterial blood gas (ABG) result would the nurse expect to see with this client?

1. pH 7.49; $PaCO_2$ 36; HCO_3^- 30
2. pH 7.30; $PaCO_2$ 35; HCO_3^- 18
3. pH 7.31; $PaCO_2$ 50; HCO_3^- 23
4. pH 7.43; $PaCO_2$ 48; HCO_3^- 30

5 A client is admitted to the hospital with atelectasis and reports of chest pain. For which acid–base imbalance would the nurse monitor this client?

1. Respiratory alkalosis
2. Metabolic acidosis
3. Metabolic alkalosis
4. Respiratory acidosis

6 A client is admitted to the hospital with respiratory acidosis. The nurse considers that which condition most likely led to development of this state? Select all that apply.

1. Severe diarrhea for several days
2. Diabetic ketoacidosis
3. Obesity
4. Diuretics
5. Sedative overdose

7 The nurse would monitor for which signs and symptoms in a client who has metabolic acidosis? Select all that apply.

1. Weight gain
2. Rapid, deep respirations
3. Drowsiness
4. Decreased respiratory rate and depth
5. Melena

8 Which client medication should the nurse review first for its potential interaction in a client admitted to the hospital in a state of alkalosis?

1. Warfarin (Coumadin)
2. Metformin (Glucophage)
3. Digoxin (Lanoxin)
4. Ibuprofen (Motrin)

9 A client is admitted to the hospital with sudden onset of severe abdominal pain. Which arterial blood gas (ABG) value would the nurse expect to see with this client?

1. $PaCO_2$ 48
2. HCO_3^- 18
3. pH 7.32
4. SaO_2 90

10 A client is admitted to the hospital with an acid–base imbalance. Arterial blood gas (ABG) results are pH 7.33; $PaCO_2$ 49; HCO_3^- 28. The nurse recognizes these results indicate which of the following?

1. Uncompensated respiratory acidosis
2. Metabolic alkalosis, uncompensated
3. Partially compensated respiratory acidosis
4. Partially compensated metabolic acidosis

11 A client is admitted to the hospital with numerous episodes of muscle weakness and twitching. Arterial blood gas (ABG) results are pH 7.44; $PaCO_2$ 49; HCO_3^- 30. How would the nurse interpret these findings?

1. Uncompensated metabolic acidosis
2. Compensated respiratory alkalosis
3. Uncompensated respiratory alkalosis
4. Compensated metabolic alkalosis

12 The nurse would suspect that a client who frequently uses which medication is at risk for developing metabolic alkalosis?

1. Calcium carbonate (Tums)
2. Ibuprofen (Motrin)
3. Acetylsalicylic acid (aspirin)
4. Acetaminophen (Tylenol)

13 The nurse is assisting in the admission of a client who has metabolic alkalosis. The nurse plans to monitor for manifestations of which electrolyte imbalance? Select all that apply.

1. Hypernatremia
2. Hypochloremia
3. Hypermagnesemia
4. Hypocalcemia
5. Hypokalemia

14 A client's arterial blood gas (ABG) results are pH 7.48; $PaCO_2$ 30; HCO_3^- 23. How will the nurse interpret these results?

1. Compensated respiratory alkalosis
2. Uncompensated metabolic alkalosis
3. Uncompensated respiratory alkalosis
4. Compensated metabolic alkalosis

15 The nurse monitors a client with a nasogastric tube that has been on low suction for five days because this client is at risk for developing which acid–base imbalance?

1. Respiratory acidosis
2. Metabolic alkalosis
3. Metabolic acidosis
4. Respiratory alkalosis

16 The following arterial blood gas (ABG) results are on the client's chart: pH 7.50; $PaCO_2$ 36; HCO_3^- 30. How will the nurse interpret this report?

1. Partially compensated metabolic alkalosis
2. Compensated respiratory alkalosis
3. Uncompensated metabolic alkalosis
4. Uncompensated respiratory alkalosis

17 A client is admitted to the hospital. Arterial blood gas (ABG) results are pH 7.50; $PaCO_2$ 40; HCO_3^- 29. Which question should the nurse ask the client to help determine an etiology for these results?

1. "Have you had diarrhea lately?"
2. "Do you have a history of COPD?"
3. "How long have you had nausea and vomiting?"
4. "Do you smoke?"

PRACTICE TEST

18 A client's arterial blood gas (ABG) results are pH 7.36; $PaCO_2$ 50; HCO_3^- 28. What do these results indicate to the nurse?

1. Compensated respiratory acidosis
2. Compensated metabolic acidosis
3. Uncompensated metabolic acidosis
4. Uncompensated respiratory acidosis

19 Which statement by the client indicates that discharge teaching for respiratory alkalosis is understood? Select all that apply.

1. "I will not take so many antacids anymore."
2. "I will take a stress management class."
3. "I will not take my furosemide (Lasix) without taking my potassium supplement."
4. "I will tell the doctor the next time I have diarrhea for so long."
5. "I am more aware of how my breathing changes when I get nervous."

20 A client is admitted with severe diarrhea. Arterial blood gas (ABG) results are pH 7.33; $PaCO_2$ 42; HCO_3^- 20. The nurse recognizes this client has which acid–base imbalance?

1. Uncompensated metabolic acidosis
2. Compensated respiratory acidosis
3. Compensated metabolic acidosis
4. Uncompensated respiratory acidosis

ANSWERS & RATIONALES

1 **Answer: 1 Rationale:** A prolonged fasting state can lead to dehydration. During fasting, the body reverts to cellular breakdown to maintain energy, and lactic and pyruvic acids build up in the body. This accumulation of acids leads to the development of metabolic acidosis. Metabolic and respiratory alkalosis are incorrect because alkalosis would not occur. Respiratory acidosis is incorrect because the primary disturbance is not respiratory. **Cognitive Level:** Applying **Client Need:** Physiological Adaptation **Integrated Process:** Nursing Process: Data Collection **Content Area:** Adult Health **Strategy:** Note the critical word *fasting* that indicates this is a metabolic rather than respiratory problem, which eliminates respiratory acidosis and alkalosis. Choose metabolic acidosis because metabolic by-products are acidic in nature, not alkaline.

2 **Answer: 2 Rationale:** Vomiting leads to the loss of hydrochloric acid from gastric acids. Hydrogen ions must leave the blood to replace this acidity in the stomach. Metabolic alkalosis occurs and is reflected by elevated pH and HCO_3^-, and normal $PaCO_2$. The ABG with the pH of 7.30 is incorrect because it reflects respiratory acidosis with partial compensation (decreased pH, and elevated $PaCO_2$ and HCO_3^-). The ABG with the pH of 7.34 is incorrect because it reflects a mixed acid–base imbalance (metabolic alkalosis with respiratory acidosis) with a normal pH, and elevated $PaCO_2$ and HCO_3^-. The ABG with the pH of 7.48 is incorrect because it reflects respiratory alkalosis (increased pH, decreased $PaCO_2$, and normal HCO_3^-). **Cognitive Level:** Applying **Client Need:** Physiological Adaptation **Integrated Process:** Nursing Process: Data Collection **Content Area:** Adult Health **Strategy:** Note the critical word *vomiting*, and recall that stomach contents are rich in acid. Loss of acid would raise the pH (eliminating options with pH of 7.30 and 7.34) and lead to increased free circulating HCO_3^-, eliminating the ABG with the pH of 7.48.

3 **Answer: 1, 5 Rationale:** Clients with respiratory acidosis from ingestion of barbiturates would have slow and shallow respirations, leading to hypoventilation. Tetany symptoms, increased deep tendon reflexes, and palpitations are associated with respiratory alkalosis. Headache is associated with respiratory acidosis because the increased CO_2 level causes cerebral vasodilation, which leads to headache. **Cognitive Level:** Applying **Client Need:** Physiological Adaptation **Integrated Process:** Nursing Process: Data Collection **Content Area:** Adult Health **Strategy:** Recall that barbiturates are central nervous system (CNS) depressants, while palpitations, tetany and increased deep tendon reflexes indicate CNS excitation. Choose slow shallow respirations as consistent with CNS depression, and choose headache because of the dilating effect of retained CO_2 on cerebral blood vessels.

4 **Answer: 2 Rationale:** Clients with renal failure have difficulty synthesizing HCO_3^- in the renal tubules secondary to the renal failure. These clients also retain K^+, and subsequently develop metabolic acidosis. The ABG with the pH of 7.30 reflects uncompensated metabolic acidosis. The ABG with the pH of 7.49 is incorrect because it reflects metabolic alkalosis (increased pH and HCO_3^-) and normal $PaCO_2$. The ABG with the pH of 7.31 is incorrect because it reflects respiratory acidosis (decreased pH, increased $PaCO_2$) and normal HCO_3^-. The ABG with the pH of 7.43 is incorrect because it reflects a mixed acid–base imbalance metabolic alkalosis with a respiratory acidosis (normal pH, and increased $PaCO_2$ and HCO_3^-). **Cognitive Level:** Applying **Client Need:** Physiological Adaptation **Integrated Process:** Nursing Process: Data Collection **Content Area:** Adult Health **Strategy:** First, recognize renal failure as a metabolic condition in which there is an impaired ability to eliminate metabolic acids and wastes, leading to acidosis. With this in mind, eliminate options that have elevated or normal pH. Then choose the option with the HCO_3^- of 18 rather than 23 because 18 is low while 23 is normal.

5 **Answer: 4 Rationale:** A client with atelectasis has collapsed alveoli that retain CO_2, which can lead to respiratory acidosis.

The client most likely would have hypoventilation as a respiratory pattern, which would further contribute to the development of respiratory acidosis. Respiratory and metabolic alkalosis are incorrect because the client would not be in an alkalotic state. Metabolic acidosis is incorrect because the primary disturbance is respiratory. **Cognitive Level:** Applying **Client Need:** Physiological Adaptation **Integrated Process:** Nursing Process: Data Collection **Content Area:** Adult Health **Strategy:** The critical word in the stem of the question is *atelectasis*. Recall that this term is associated with respiratory problems to eliminate options referring to metabolic disorders. Choose respiratory acidosis over alkalosis recalling that CO_2 retention characterizes many respiratory conditions, leading to acidosis (since CO_2 acts as an acid in the body).

6 **Answer: 3, 5 Rationale:** Obesity can lead to chest wall abnormalities and hypoventilation, which can lead to respiratory acidosis. Sedative overdose depresses the central nervous system, which leads to hypoventilation and respiratory acidosis. Prolonged diarrhea can lead to the development of metabolic acidosis. DKA leads to the development of metabolic acidosis. Diuretic administration leads to the development of metabolic alkalosis. **Cognitive Level:** Analyzing **Client Need:** Physiological Adaptation **Integrated Process:** Nursing Process: Data Collection **Content Area:** Adult Health **Strategy:** Note the term *respiratory acidosis* in the stem of the question. First evaluate each option to determine whether it would lead to acidosis and alkalosis. Then differentiate between respiratory and metabolic acidosis to choose correctly. Note the wording of the question suggests that more than one option is correct.

7 **Answer: 2, 3 Rationale:** Clients who have metabolic acidosis develop Kussmaul's breathing (rapid and deep respirations). Drowsiness occurs because of the CNS depressant effect of acidosis. Weight gain is not an associated finding with metabolic acidosis. Shallow breathing is associated with the development of metabolic alkalosis. Melena (blood in stool) is not associated with metabolic acidosis. **Cognitive Level:** Applying **Client Need:** Physiological Adaptation **Integrated Process:** Nursing Process: Implementation **Content Area:** Adult Health **Strategy:** The critical words in the stem of the question are *metabolic acidosis*. Recall that in metabolic abnormalities, the respiratory system helps to compensate; this will help to eliminate weight gain and melena. Choose rapid breathing over slower shallower breathing because this option assists the body to "blow off" acid in the form of CO_2. Finally, choose drowsiness recalling that acidosis causes CNS depression, while alkalosis causes CNS excitation.

8 **Answer: 3 Rationale:** Alkalosis, especially respiratory alkalosis, makes the client more sensitive to the effects of digoxin; toxicity can develop even at therapeutic levels. A serum digoxin level should be obtained, and the client evaluated for potential digoxin toxicity. Warfarin affects clotting factors. Metformin can cause the development of lactic acidosis. Ibuprofen can cause gastric irritation. **Cognitive Level:** Applying **Client Need:** Physiological Adaptation **Integrated Process:** Nursing Process: Planning **Content Area:** Adult Health **Strategy:** Specific knowledge of medications that are affected by alkalosis is needed to answer this question. Use nursing knowledge and the process of elimination to make your selection.

9 **Answer: 2 Rationale:** Acute pain usually leads to hyperventilation, which causes CO_2 to be blown off, leading to an increased pH and decreased CO_2 level. If the client has not compensated, the bicarbonate level will be normal. If the client is compensating, then the bicarbonate level will decrease in an attempt to restore the pH. A $PaCO_2$ of 48 is incorrect because it reflects a slight elevation; if the client were in severe pain, the level would likely be lower as the client would have increased respirations. A pH of 7.32 is incorrect because the pH is slightly acidotic. An SaO_2 of 90 is incorrect because the oxygen saturation should be within normal limits. **Cognitive Level:** Analyzing **Client Need:** Physiological Adaptation **Integrated Process:** Nursing Process: Data Collection **Content Area:** Adult Health **Strategy:** Visualize a picture of the client in pain. This person is most likely to have an increased respiratory rate, which blows off CO_2 and decreases the bicarbonate level as a compensatory mechanism. This will help you to easily choose the correct option.

10 **Answer: 3 Rationale:** The pH is low, indicating acidosis; the $PaCO_2$ is elevated, indicating a respiratory basis; and the HCO_3^- is elevated, indicating that compensatory mechanisms are partially working. Uncompensated respiratory acidosis is incorrect because compensation is taking place due to increased HCO_3^- level. Uncompensated metabolic alkalosis is incorrect because the client is not alkalotic. Partially compensated metabolic acidosis is incorrect because the primary disturbance is respiratory. The change in the $PaCO_2$ level is greater than the change in the HCO_3^- level, which indicates a respiratory disturbance. **Cognitive Level:** Analyzing **Client Need:** Physiological Adaptation **Integrated Process:** Nursing Process: Data Collection **Content Area:** Adult Health **Strategy:** First, eliminate the option with alkalosis because the pH of 7.33 indicates acidosis. Next, note that both the CO_2 and HCO_3^- levels are abnormal, indicating that the body is attempting to compensate (eliminating uncompensated). Choose correctly from the remaining options noting the elevated CO_2 "matches" a respiratory acidosis, and the HCO_3^- (an alkaline substance) is rising to try to compensate.

11 **Answer: 4 Rationale:** The pH is just below the high limit, and the HCO_3^- is elevated, indicating a metabolic problem. The $PaCO_2$ is elevated, indicating compensation, so the correct interpretation is compensated respiratory alkalosis. Uncompensated metabolic acidosis is incorrect because the client is not acidotic. Compensated respiratory alkalosis is incorrect because the CO_2 would be decreased rather than elevated. Uncompensated respiratory alkalosis is incorrect because the primary disturbance is metabolic, and the CO_2 is elevated rather than decreased. **Cognitive Level:** Analyzing **Client Need:** Physiological Adaptation **Integrated Process:** Nursing Process: Data Collection **Content Area:** Adult Health **Strategy:** Note that the pH is within normal range, which indicates that the condition is compensated, thus eliminating acidosis options. Note the high HCO_3^- is a metabolic indicator (not respiratory), and is consistent with a pH near the high end of normal, to help you choose the compensated respiratory alkalosis option.

12 **Answer: 1 Rationale:** Excessive use of oral antacids can lead to metabolic alkalosis. Use of ibuprofen and Tylenol is not associated with the development of metabolic alkalosis. Overdoses of aspirin can be associated with the development of respiratory alkalosis, and eventually can lead to metabolic acidosis. **Cognitive Level:** Applying **Client Need:** Physiological Adaptation **Integrated Process:** Nursing Process: Data Collection **Content Area:** Adult Health **Strategy:** Knowledge of medication side effects is needed to answer this question. First, eliminate ibuprofen and Tylenol because they are similar (non-opioid analgesics). Then, eliminate aspirin because acid would not lead to alkalosis.

Alternatively, recall that calcium carbonate is an antacid, which in excess could lead to metabolic alkalosis.

13 **Answer: 2, 4, 5 Rationale:** Clinical manifestations of metabolic alkalosis are associated with the presence of tetany-like symptoms. Clients should be monitored for the presence of these symptoms because they usually correlate with low levels of calcium. Hypomagnesemia (not hypermagnesmia) can occur with hypocalcemia. Hyponatremia, hypochloremia, and hypokalemia can occur with metabolic alkalosis. **Cognitive Level:** Applying **Client Need:** Physiological Adaptation **Integrated Process:** Nursing Process: Data Collection **Content Area:** Adult Health **Strategy:** Specific knowledge of the association between metabolic alkalosis and various electrolytes is needed to answer this question. Use nursing knowledge and the process of elimination to make your selection.

14 **Answer: 3 Rationale:** The client's pH is high, indicating alkalosis. The $PaCO_2$ is abnormal, indicating a respiratory basis. The HCO_3^- is normal, indicating that compensation has not started. Compensated respiratory alkalosis is incorrect because the HCO_3^- level would decrease with compensation. Uncompensated metabolic alkalosis is incorrect because the primary disturbance is respiratory, as indicated by the decrease in the CO_2 parameter. Compensated metabolic alkalosis is incorrect because the primary disturbance is respiratory, as indicated by the decrease in the CO_2 parameter. **Cognitive Level:** Analyzing **Client Need:** Physiological Adaptation **Integrated Process:** Nursing Process: Data Collection **Content Area:** Adult Health **Strategy:** Note that the pH is high, so the condition is not compensated, eliminating compensated states. Choose respiratory because a low CO_2 correlates with a high pH, whereas HCO_3^- at the lower end of the normal range does not correlate with a high pH.

15 **Answer: 2 Rationale:** A client who has prolonged nasogastric suction is apt to have higher levels of bicarbonate because of hydrogen ion loss. Bicarbonate excess leads to a metabolic disturbance and the development of metabolic alkalosis. Respiratory and metabolic acidosis are incorrect because the client will not experience acidosis. Respiratory alkalosis is incorrect because the primary disturbance is caused by retained levels of bicarbonate (not elimination of carbon dioxide) in the body. **Cognitive Level:** Applying **Client Need:** Physiological Adaptation **Integrated Process:** Nursing Process: Data Collection **Content Area:** Adult Health **Strategy:** Eliminate respiratory imbalances first because nasogastric suction is a metabolic problem. Choose alkalosis recalling that pancreatic juices are rich in bicarbonate and are not neutralized because the nasogastric suction eliminates hydrochloric acid that would neutralize the alkaline pancreatic secretions.

16 **Answer: 3 Rationale:** The pH indicates alkalosis; HCO_3^- is high, indicating a metabolic origin, and the $PaCO_2$ is normal, which indicates that compensation has not taken place. Partially compensated metabolic acidosis is incorrect because with compensation, the $PaCO_2$ level would be increased. Compensated and uncompensated respiratory alkalosis options are incorrect because the primary disturbance is metabolic, as reflected by the increased bicarbonate level. **Cognitive Level:** Analyzing **Client Need:** Physiological Adaptation **Integrated Process:** Nursing Process: Data Collection **Content Area:** Adult Health **Strategy:** First, note that the pH is high, and so the imbalance cannot be compensated. Then note that HCO_3^- is the abnormally high value (not CO_2), so the imbalance must be metabolic rather than respiratory. Choose uncompensated over compensated metabolic alkalosis because the CO_2 (normally 35–45) has made no attempt to rise to compensate for the high HCO_3^-.

17 **Answer: 3 Rationale:** ABG results reflect elevated pH, indicating alkalosis, and normal $PaCO_2$ and an increased HCO_3^-, indicating metabolic alkalosis. Vomiting is a common cause of this condition. The presence of diarrhea is associated with metabolic acidosis. COPD is associated with respiratory acidosis. Smoking can be associated with respiratory acidosis if it leads to respiratory disease. **Cognitive Level:** Analyzing **Client Need:** Physiological Adaptation **Integrated Process:** Nursing Process: Data Collection **Content Area:** Adult Health **Strategy:** An ability to interpret ABGs and specific knowledge of manifestations of metabolic alkalosis are needed to answer this question. Use nursing knowledge and the process of elimination to make your selection.

18 **Answer: 1 Rationale:** The pH is just within normal range, so the blood gas results are either normal or compensated. However, the $PaCO_2$ is high, indicating a respiratory problem, and thus the ABGs cannot be normal. The HCO_3^- is also high, which along with a normal pH indicates complete compensation. The metabolic acidosis options are incorrect because the primary disturbance is respiratory, as reflected by the correlation between an elevated $PaCO_2$ and a pH toward the low end of normal. Uncompensated respiratory acidosis is incorrect because the HCO_3^- level would be normal if no compensation is taking place. **Cognitive Level:** Analyzing **Client Need:** Physiological Adaptation **Integrated Process:** Nursing Process: Data Collection **Content Area:** Adult Health **Strategy:** Because the pH is within normal range, eliminate the uncompensated options. Choose respiratory over metabolic acidosis because the pH is near the acidic end of the range and the high CO_2 correlates with acidosis, whereas a high HCO_3^- would correlate with an alkalotic state.

19 **Answer: 2, 5 Rationale:** Respiratory alkalosis is caused by hyperventilation, which can be caused by stress and anxiety, as examples. It is important that clients who are prone to develop respiratory alkalosis be aware of how to manage causative factors. Antacids and diuretics are associated with metabolic alkalosis. Diarrhea is associated with metabolic acidosis. **Cognitive Level:** Analyzing **Client Need:** Physiological Adaptation **Integrated Process:** Teaching and Learning **Content Area:** Adult Health **Strategy:** The critical word in the question is *respiratory*. Eliminate each of the incorrect options that would correlate better with a metabolic condition than with a respiratory one. Alternatively, consider that a common cause of respiratory alkalosis is hyperventilation, which is often caused by anxiety, and managed with stress management.

20 **Answer: 1 Rationale:** The pH and HCO_3^- are decreased, indicating metabolic acidosis. The $PaCO_2$ is normal, indicating that compensatory mechanisms have not started working. Compensated or uncompensated respiratory acidosis is incorrect because the primary disturbance is metabolic, as indicated by the low bicarbonate level. Compensated metabolic acidosis is incorrect because with compensation, a decrease in $PaCO_2$ to restore balance would be expected. **Cognitive Level:** Analyzing **Client Need:** Physiological Adaptation **Integrated Process:** Nursing Process: Data Collection **Content Area:** Adult Health **Strategy:** First, correlate diarrhea with a metabolic problem to eliminate compensated respiratory acidosis and uncompensated respiratory acidosis. Then, note that the pH is not within normal limits to choose uncompensated metabolic acidosis over compensated metabolic acidosis.

Key Terms to Review

acid p. 830
base p. 830
buffer p. 830
compensation p. 831
HCO_3^- p. 830
metabolic acidosis p. 836
metabolic alkalosis p. 837
mixed acid–base disorder p. 838
$PaCO_2$ p. 831
PaO_2 p. 832
pH p. 830
respiratory acidosis p. 834
respiratory alkalosis p. 835
SaO_2 p. 832

References

Berman, A., & Snyder, S. (2012). *Kozier & Erb's fundamentals of nursing: Concepts, process, and practice* (9th ed.). Upper Saddle River, NJ: Pearson Education, Inc.

Ignatavicius, D., & Workman, L. (2010). *Medical-surgical nursing: Patient-centered collaborative care* (6th ed.). Philadelphia: Saunders.

Kee, J. (2010). *Laboratory and diagnostic tests with nursing implications* (8th ed.). Upper Saddle River, NJ: Pearson Education.

LeMone, P., Burke, K., & Bauldoff, G. (2012). *Medical-surgical nursing: Critical thinking in patient care* (5th ed.). Upper Saddle River, NJ: Pearson Education.

Lewis, S., Dirksen, S. Heitkemper, M. & Bucher, L. (2011). *Medical surgical nursing: Assessment and management of clinical problem* (8th ed.). St. Louis, MO: Elsevier.

Smeltzer, S., Bare, B., Hinkle, J., & Cheever, K. (2010). *Textbook of medical-surgical nursing* (12th ed.). Philadelphia: Lippincott Williams & Wilkins.

Test Yourself

Are you ready for the NCLEX-PN® or course exams? Use the practice tests on the companion website to check.

51 Respiratory Disorders

In this chapter

Cross Reference

Other chapters relevant to this content area are

I. OVERVIEW OF ANATOMY AND PHYSIOLOGY

A. Respiratory system structures

1. Upper respiratory tract (conducting airways)
   a. Nose: filters, humidifies, and heats inspired air; nasal hairs trap airborne particles in mucus; olfactory nerve receptors allow for sense of smell
   b. Paranasal sinuses: air-filled cavities in frontal, maxillary, ethmoid, and sphenoid bones that contribute to mucus production and voice resonance
   c. Pharynx: nasopharynx, laryngopharynx, and oropharynx; lymphatic tissue in adenoids (nasopharynx) and tonsils (oropharynx) contribute to immune function
   d. Larynx: contains vocal cords that vibrate to produce voice; epiglottis closes during swallowing to prevent passage of food into trachea
   e. Trachea: connects upper and lower respiratory tract; divides into right and left mainstem bronchi
2. Lower respiratory tract (conducting airways and gas exchange airways)
   a. Bronchi: right and left mainstem bronchi (conducting airways) lead into smaller bronchioles that eventually terminate in alveoli; right mainstem bronchus curves less sharply than left, making it a more common passage for aspirated gastric contents and dislocated endotracheal tubes
   b. **Alveoli**: air-filled sacs in lungs; oxygen (O_2) diffuses from alveoli (gas exchange airways) into blood across alveolar-capillary membrane (primary site of gas exchange); carbon dioxide (CO_2) diffuses back into alveoli; surfactant decreases surface tension
   c. Lungs: right lung has three lobes (upper, middle, and lower); left lung has two lobes (upper and lower); upper area is called apex; lower area is called base
   d. Pleura: two-layer membrane covering lungs (visceral pleura) and thoracic cavity (parietal pleura); pleural fluid lubricates pleural layers and holds them together during inspiration and expiration
   e. Pleural cavity: air-filled space of thoracic cavity housing structures of lower respiratory tract
3. Accessory structures: contribute to mechanics of breathing and/or provide support and protection
   a. Rib cage: 12 pairs of ribs and sternum
   b. Intercostal muscles: located between ribs
   c. Diaphragm: separates thoracic cavity from abdominal cavity; flattens (contracts) during inspiration via phrenic nerve to allow greater chest expansion

B. Respiratory system functions

1. Primary function is gas exchange; **respiration** (process of O_2 and CO_2 exchange) involves ventilation, perfusion, diffusion, and nervous system control
2. Ventilation: passage of gases between atmosphere and lungs during inspiration and expiration; adequacy is influenced by tissue properties, airway resistance, lung volumes and capacities, body position, and disease processes
   a. **Pulmonary ventilation**: total volume of gas exchange between atmosphere and lungs
   b. **Alveolar ventilation**: volume of air that undergoes gas exchange
   c. **Inspiration**: stimulation of phrenic nerve causes diaphragm to contract and increase diameter of thoracic cavity; intrapleural pressure becomes more negative; air moves from atmosphere to alveoli and pulmonary capillaries where gas exchange occurs
   d. **Expiration**: diaphragm relaxes and pushes upward; intrapulmonic pressure becomes higher than atmospheric pressure, allowing passive air flow from lung into atmosphere; smaller airways may collapse during expiration, particularly in supine position
   e. Intrapulmonary (intra-alveolar) pressure: equals atmospheric pressure (760 mm Hg) when glottis is open and there is no air movement
   f. Intrapleural pressure: negative pressure produced by opposite forces of elastic recoil between lungs and chest wall; normally negative intrapleural pressure prevents lung collapse
   g. Intrathoracic pressure: generally has negative pressure that equals intrapleural pressure; with forced expiration against a closed glottis (Valsalva maneuver), it becomes positive
   h. **Compliance**: elastic property of lung because of elastic and collagen fibers; higher compliance allows for easier lung distention; lower compliance (lung stiffness) makes distention more difficult
   i. Elastic recoil: ability of lungs to return to original shape after air is expelled
   j. Airway resistance: obstruction to airflow caused by conditions of respiratory system tissues (elastic recoil, compliance), changes in airway diameter (bronchoconstriction, mucus obstruction), and/or pressure differences between atmospheric air and intrapulmonary air
   k. Lung volumes and capacities: volumes are normal individual quantities of air exchanged during specific period of breathing cycle; capacities are combined quantities of lung volumes during specific periods of breathing cycle (see Box 51–1)

Box 51–1

Lung Volumes and Capacities

- Tidal volume (V_T): total air volume inspired and expired during one breathing cycle.
- Inspiratory reserve volume (IRV): maximum air volume inspired with forced inspiration (i.e., movement of air from atmosphere into respiratory system) following normal inspiration.
- Expiratory reserve volume (ERV): air volume that can be expired with force following normal expiration.
- Residual volume (RV): air volume remaining in lungs following forced expiration.
- Total lung capacity (TLC): maximum capacity of air volume of lungs. TLC = IRV + V_T + ERV + RV
- Inspiratory capacity (IC): maximum air volume that can be inhaled following a normal exhalation. IC = V_T + IRV
- Vital capacity (VC): maximum air volume that can be exhaled after a maximum inhalation. VC = IRV + V_T + ERV
- Functional residual capacity (FRC): residual air volume in lungs after a normal exhalation. FRC = ERV + RV

l. Body position: gravity accounts for greater ventilation in dependent areas of lung; with upright body (sitting, standing) during inspiration, airflow has less resistance in reaching lung bases

3. **Perfusion**: blood flow through pulmonary capillary bed in pulmonary and bronchial circulation to respiratory system structures
   a. Pulmonary circulation: pulmonary artery carries deoxygenated (venous) blood from right ventricle, branches into pulmonary capillaries, and connects to alveoli; CO_2 is exchanged for O_2 at pulmonary capillary membranes; capillary membranes merge into pulmonary venules and pulmonary veins that carry oxygenated blood back to left atrium of heart
   b. Bronchial circulation: bronchial arteries branch from thoracic aorta to circulate blood to conducting airways and other respiratory tract tissues; bronchial blood does not circulate to alveoli and is not included in gas exchange
   c. Characteristics of respiratory system circulation: blood pressure (BP) and resistance to blood flow are lower in pulmonary blood vessels than systemic blood vessels
4. **Diffusion**: movement of air and O_2 from atmosphere into alveoli; O_2 crosses into pulmonary capillaries; CO_2 diffuses out of pulmonary capillaries into alveoli;
   a. Variables that influence gas exchange (see Table 51–1)
   b. Ventilation–perfusion relationship: adequate gas exchange requires alveolar ventilation of about 4 L/min balanced with alveolar capillary perfusion of about 5 L/min (see Figure 51–1); normal ventilation-perfusion (V/Q) ratio: 4:5
5. Nervous system control of breathing: initiates within medulla oblongata (inspiration, expiration, breathing pattern) and pons (rate, depth) of brainstem
   a. Sensory inputs to brainstem that influence respiration: chemoreceptors (increased PCO_2 and/or decreased blood pH), stretch receptors (alveolar septa, bronchi, bronchioles), proprioceptors (muscles and tendons of moveable joints), baroreceptors (aortic arch, carotid sinus), and external environment factors (cold, physical stress, air pollution, smoking, pain, infection, fever)
   b. Motor nerve impulses travel from brain stem via phrenic nerve to diaphragm and stimulate muscle contraction for breathing

Table 51–1 Variables That Influence Gas Exchange

Variable	Example
Partial pressure of gas	Supplemental oxygen increases partial pressure of inspired air
Surface area	Loss of lung tissue by surgery or disease decreases surface area available for gas exchange
Molecular weight and gas solubility	CO_2 is more soluble in membranes and diffuses more quickly than oxygen
Thickness of membrane	Membrane is thickened by some disease processes, such as pneumonia, pulmonary edema; a thicker membrane impedes effective air exchange

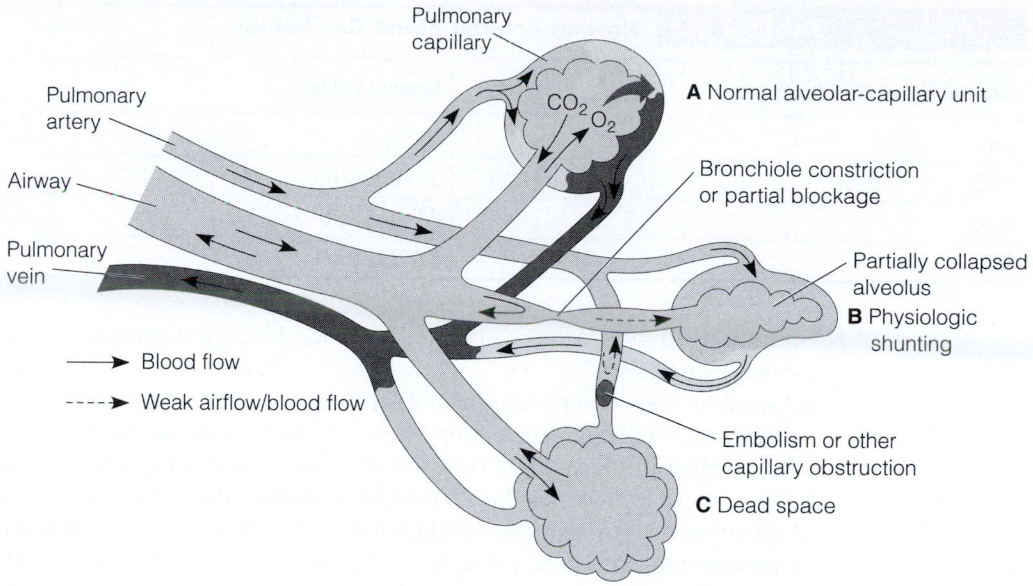

Figure 51–1

Ventilation perfusion relationships. *A.* Normal alveolar-capillary unit with an ideal match of ventilation and blood flow. Maximum gas exchange occurs between alveolar wall and blood. *B.* Physiologic shunting: a unit with adequate perfusion but inadequate ventilation. *C.* Dead space: a unit with adequate ventilation but inadequate perfusion. In the latter two cases, gas exchange is impaired.

II. DIAGNOSTIC TESTS AND DATA COLLECTION

A. Radiological studies

1. Chest x-ray: visualizes structures, fluid, and air in thoracic cavity; anterior–posterior and lateral views are most common; appropriate use of lead shielding reduces overall exposure to x-rays
2. Computed tomography (CT): provides a cross-sectional view of tissue; detects lesions not identified by x-ray; performed with or without contrast media (check allergies to iodine or seafood if contrast used)
3. Magnetic resonance imaging (MRI): computerized images similar to CT identify subtle changes in tissue structure; check client to ensure metal sources are removed; clients with metal implants may be ineligible for MRI
4. Pulmonary angiogram: outlines pulmonary vasculature; radioactive contrast medium is injected through a central venous catheter into right side of heart and pulmonary artery; identifies tumors and circulation abnormalities (congenital, thromboembolism); inquire about iodine and/or seafood allergies
5. Ventilation–perfusion scan: radioactive isotope injected to identify areas of ventilation and perfusion within lungs; also called VQ (ventilation quotient) scan

B. Pulse oximetry

NCLEX® 1. Monitors arterial **oxygen saturation** (SpO_2 or percentage of O_2 bound to hemoglobin [Hgb] compared to volume that Hgb is capable of binding); normal is usually 95% or greater if no lung disease; in clients with lung disease, target SpO_2 is 90% or greater; may be measured intermittently (such as with vital signs or ambulation) or continuously

2. Uses a light spectroscopy probe attached to a finger, earlobe, or nose

NCLEX® 3. Accuracy is lower with diminished peripheral perfusion, brightly lit environment, acrylic fingernails, and dark skin color

C. Pulmonary function test

1. Uses a spirometer to measure lung volumes and capacities during forced breathing techniques; identifies normal or abnormal pulmonary functions
2. Differentiates restrictive versus obstructive lung disease, and measures effects of bronchodilator therapy; see also Chapter 43

D. Bronchoscopy (see Chapter 43)

E. Thoracentesis

1. Introduction of a needle into thoracic cavity for diagnostic and/or therapeutic reasons
2. Allows withdrawal of pleural fluid for laboratory analysis (microbiology, cytology), such as to determine if cancerous cells are present
3. Permits drainage of pleural effusion to relieve dyspnea

F. Laboratory

1. Arterial blood gases (ABGs): blood specimen obtained by arterial puncture or drawn from arterial line; identifies oxygenation status, acid–base balance and compensatory mechanisms
   a. Results can indicate acidosis (pH <7.35) or alkalosis (pH >7.45) and may be of respiratory (CO_2) or metabolic (HCO_3^-) origin

NCLEX® b. See Table 51–2 for normal values and refer to Chapter 50 for additional information

Table 51-2 Normal Arterial Blood Gas Values

Arterial Blood Gas Parameter	Normal Value
pH	7.35–7.45
PCO_2	35–45 mm Hg
HCO_3^-	22–26 mEq/L
PO_2	80–100 mm Hg

2. Sputum analysis: specimen obtained for microbiology (Gram stain, culture and sensitivity) or cytology analysis
   - a. Sputum collection procedure: obtained by expectoration, suctioning, saline-induced from airways, thoracentesis, lung needle biopsy, or transtracheal aspiration; for sputum collection from clients who can cooperate, have them rinse mouth prior to obtaining expectorated specimen
   - NCLEX® b. Specimens for acid-fast bacilli (mycobacterium tuberculosis or TB) may be collected on three different days; specimen collection following a long sleep period (early morning) is best because of greater concentration; if unable to obtain a sputum specimen for acid-fast bacilli, gastric specimen may be obtained because mycobacterium tuberculosis is not altered by acidic gastric contents
   - NCLEX® c. Specimen processing: collect specimens in appropriate container and send to laboratory promptly
3. Skin testing: detects allergic reactions to specified antigens (type I hypersensitivity), exposure to tuberculosis-causing organisms (type IV hypersensitivity), or fungi
   - a. Administer by intradermal route; circle injection site with a long-lasting marker; diagram forearm injection site on chart
   - NCLEX® b. Measure area of induration (if present), *not* reddened area; read result 48 to 72 hrs after placement; an uncertain reading at 48 hrs may be reread at 72 hrs
   - NCLEX® c. Positive result: indicates exposure to antigen; does not indicate client currently has active disease, only that there has been exposure/infection
   - d. Induration of 5 mm or greater: indicates recent exposure to TB or possible HIV infection; chest x-ray findings with characteristic Ghon tubercles are likely healed and not active sites of TB infection
   - e. Induration of 10 mm or greater: indicates typical finding of active TB infection in populations with chronic, complicating diseases such as diabetes, end-stage renal disease, gastrointestinal (GI) cancer; finding is compatible in high-risk populations such as intravenous (IV) drug users, homeless, and residents of high infection incidence areas
   - f. Negative result: indicates no exposure; false-negative findings occur with suppression of cell-mediated immunity such as occurs with HIV infection
   - NCLEX® g. When performing skin tests to check for type I allergies, ensure that antihistamines, which could interfere with test results, are discontinued 72 hours prior to testing

III. COMMON NURSING TECHNIQUES AND PROCEDURES

A. Airway management: goal is to maintain patent airway

1. Head and jaw position
   - a. Upper airway obstruction is often caused by foreign object or loss of local muscle tone
   - NCLEX® b. Open airway by head tilt and anterior chin lift maneuver
   - NCLEX® c. In clients with suspected neck injury, open airway by anterior chin displacement and/or jaw thrust; do *not* perform head tilt
   - d. Perform Heimlich maneuver in conscious clients with suspected foreign body obstruction of airway
2. Oropharyngeal airway: maintains airway patency by preventing posterior tongue displacement
   - a. Is intended only for use in unconscious clients because of possible vomiting or laryngeal spasms
   - b. Airway must be sized for each client
   - c. Examine oral cavity for possible foreign body or vomitus
   - d. Tongue blade may be needed to temporarily displace tongue during insertion
   - e. Head and jaw position must be maintained independent of airway placement
3. Nasopharyngeal airway: maintains airway patency via nasal route in semiconscious client or when placement of oropharyngeal airway is not feasible
   - a. Airway must be sized for client; an excessively long tube may pass into esophagus, causing stomach distention and inadequate ventilation
   - b. Maintain head and jaw position even when an airway is in place

4. Endotracheal (ET) intubation: a long, cuffed ET tube is inserted with a laryngoscope by specially trained personnel for long-term airway management or connection to a mechanical ventilator; see Chapter 27
5. Tracheostomy: surgical placement of cuffed airway into trachea by specially trained personnel to assist in maintaining an effective airway in clients who cannot maintain an airway or require prolonged mechanical ventilation; see Chapter 27
6. Cricothyrotomy: emergency surgical opening of cricothyroid membrane to maintain patent airway when other methods fail or are not feasible
7. Techniques for airway clearance
   a. Oropharyngeal suctioning: nonsterile procedure to remove secretions from upper airway; alert clients may be taught to do self-suctioning
   b. Nasotracheal suctioning: sterile procedure to remove secretions from tracheal area; may be performed to obtain a sterile sputum specimen
   c. Tracheobronchial suctioning: sterile procedure using individual suction catheters or in-line suction catheter for clearing secretions via ET tube
   d. Ensure that catheter diameter is no more than two thirds of airway lumen
   NCLEX® e. Limit suctioning to 10 seconds per catheter pass (5 in children) to reduce risk of inadequate oxygenation and cardiac dysrhythmias from hypoxia

B. Body positioning

1. Physiology: fluid shift theory
   a. Lung ventilation and perfusion are gravity-dependent
   b. Changes in body position from supine (0 degrees) to varying degrees of head elevation or lateral positioning activates reflexive cardiovascular changes that produce fluid shifts in lungs and chest blood vessels
2. Acute respiratory failure
   NCLEX® a. Elevate head at least 45 degrees to increase chest expansion
   b. Elevation also mobilizes fluid from chest to more dependent areas
3. Unilateral lung disease
   NCLEX® a. Position with unaffected lung in dependent position ("good lung down")
   b. Position by using gravity to promote ventilation–perfusion matching
4. Adult respiratory distress syndrome (ARDS)
   a. Prone positioning may be used for clients on maximal mechanical ventilation with unresponsive hypoxemia
   b. Prone position allows previously nondependent air-filled alveoli to become dependent, increasing perfusion to air-filled alveoli and possibly improving ventilation–perfusion matching
   c. Use caution to avoid unintentional dislodgment of ET tube during position changes

C. Oxygen (O_2) administration

1. Nasal cannula
   NCLEX® a. Typical O_2 flow of 1 to 6 L/min will provide O_2 concentrations of 24–44%
   b. For each 1 L of O_2 flow, O_2 concentration increases by about 4% (room air is about 21% O_2)
   NCLEX® c. Clients with chronic obstructive pulmonary disease (COPD) should receive low flow oxygen, about 1 to 2 L/min, to prevent respiratory depression; these clients are used to high CO_2 levels and low O_2 levels, so increased O_2 (greater than 2 L/min) can cause a loss of respiratory drive
2. Face mask
   a. Provides O_2 concentration of 40–60%
   b. Exhaled CO_2 trapped by mask can be rebreathed
   c. Oxygen flow should be greater than 5 L/min to minimize rebreathing CO_2
3. Face mask with O_2 reservoir (partial rebreather)
   a. Constant flow of O_2 into attached reservoir bag attached to mask allows rebreathing of ⅓ of exhaled air along with O_2
   b. Typical O_2 flow of 6 to 10 L/min provides 60–90% O_2 concentration
4. A nonrebreather mask is used for clients who require higher O_2 concentrations; provides 95–100% O_2 with flow rate of 10 to 15 L/min
5. Venturi mask
   a. Delivers O_2 in precise concentrations of 24%, 28%, 35%, and 40%
   b. Used in clients with COPD and chronic CO_2 retention

D. Pulmonary hygiene

1. Pursed lip breathing: client exhales through pursed lips, which slows exhalation and reduces airway collapse, thus enhancing respiration

2. Coughing
   a. Coughing adequate for airway clearance requires higher airway pressures
   b. Augmented coughing: caregiver places hand below xiphoid process and thrusts downward on abdomen as client ends inspiration

   NCLEX®

   c. Huff coughing: client attempts sequential coughing while saying "huff"; maneuver keeps glottis open during coughing; beneficial in clients with COPD
3. Chest physiotherapy (CPT)
   a. Mobilizes bronchial secretions into larger airways for removal by coughing or suctioning; useful for clients with more than 30 mL secretions per day, secretions with artificial airway, and/or atelectasis
   b. Percussion: client is positioned for maximal drainage from affected area; involves use of cupped hands alternately percussing indicated area; contraindicated with lung cancer, hemoptysis, and bronchospasm
   c. Vibration: pressure is applied with palm of hand or electrical vibrator over affected area of chest; may be used in some clients when percussion is contraindicated
   d. Postural drainage: uses gravity to mobilize bronchial secretions; nebulized bronchodilators may be used prior to postural drainage; contraindicated about 1 hour before and within 3 hours after a meal to reduce risk of vomiting and/or aspiration (see Box 51–2)

E. Mechanical ventilation

1. Purpose: to assist with breathing and provide for adequate gas exchange using a ventilator attached to ET or tracheostomy tube
2. Types of ventilators
   a. Positive-pressure volume-cycled, which exerts a positive pressure on airway to deliver a predetemined volume of gas; this type of ventilator allows for pressure and time limits to be set and is the most common ventilator used
   b. Positive-pressure time-cycled ventilator, which exerts a positive pressure on airway, delivering a set volume of gas over a preset time
   c. Positive-pressure pressure-cycled ventilator, which exerts positive pressure on airway within pressure limits set to stop inspiration if that pressure is exceeded
   d. Positive-pressure jet ventilator, which exerts a positive pressure on airway and delivers small volumes of gas at a very high rate
   e. Negative-pressure ventilator, which exerts a negative pressure on external chest and does not require intubation; rarely used; an iron lung previously used for clients with polio is an example
3. Modes of ventilation
   a. Intermittent mandatory ventilation (IMV): delivers a preset tidal volume (V_T) at a preset rate despite client breathing spontaneously at his or her own rate and V_T
   b. Assist control ventilation (ACV): delivers a preset volume for every breath set on machine as well as those initiated by client; allows for hyperventilation which may or may not be beneficial to a specific client
   c. Controlled mandatory ventilation (CMV): delivers a preset volume at a preset rate and is most frequently utilized for those clients with no ventilatory effort; sometimes requires neuromuscular blockade in clients not tolerating ventilation
   d. Synchronized intermittent mandatory ventilation (SIMV): delivers a preset, mandatory volume synchronized to client's inspiratory effort; most common ventilation currently used

Box 51–2

Chest Physiotherapy (CPT)

- Client is dressed in a lightweight shirt.
- Percussion is performed with a cupped hand striking chest over a portion of lung; if done properly, a popping sound will be heard.
- Postural drainage facilitates removal of secretions that are loosened during percussion; for drainage, various head-down positions drain all lung segments.
- Positioning for bronchial drainage can be achieved by child standing on his head, hanging upside down on monkey bars, and other playground activities that are fun for child.
- Avoid performing CPT immediately after eating.

NCLEX®

4. Key ventilator settings
   a. Rate: number of breaths per minute delivered by ventilator; is a number that is combined with mode often in clinical practice (e.g., SIMV of 6/min)
   b. FiO_2: fraction of inspired O_2 or O_2%; amount of O_2 in air inhaled via ventilator; is expressed as a decimal instead of a percentage (e.g., FiO_2 of .40 versus 40%)
   c. Tidal volume (V_T): amount of air delivered with each breath; often expressed in milliliters or liters (e.g., 700 mL or 0.7 L)
   d. PEEP: abbreviation for positive end-expiratory pressure; is amount of positive pressure set in system at end of exhalation; keeps alveoli open during exhalation to increase gas exchange; is expressed in terms of centimeters of pressure (e.g., 5 cm)
5. Indications: ineffective breathing pattern or hypoxia (e.g., dyspnea, cyanosis, altered mental status, absent breath sounds, tachycardia with no underlying cardiac disease); O_2 saturation levels under 80%, pH less than 7.35, $PaCO_2$ greater than 50 mm Hg, V_T less than 5 mL/kg, or minute volumes less than 10 L/min

NCLEX®

6. Nursing management
   a. Position client for maximum alveolar ventilation and comfort; maintain soft restraints to avoid accidental extubation
   b. Monitor for any changes in respiratory status or effort
   c. Maintain ventilator settings as ordered and know how to troubleshoot ventilator alarms (high pressure frequently indicates need for suctioning or kinking/compression of ET tube; low pressure indicates leak or disconnection); manually ventilate client if alarms sound without apparent cause
   d. Monitor ABGs and maintain continuous SpO_2 monitoring
   e. Complete a thorough physical examination with emphasis on cardiac, neurological, and respiratory areas
   f. Administer antibiotics, neuromuscular blocking agents, and sedatives as ordered
   g. Maintain nasogastric suction to prevent aspiration
   h. Supply nutritional support as ordered
   i. Perform frequent oral care and suctioning to maintain airway patency
   j. Provide emotional support to client and family as well as alternative communication method
7. Potential complications: pneumothorax, GI stress ulcers, hypotension caused by decreased venous return from increased intrathoracic pressure, increased intracranial pressure, infection

F. Laryngectomy

1. Purpose: excision of larynx as treatment for cancer; may be partial or total
2. Preoperative teaching: educate client and family about long-term implications, including loss of voice, swallowing difficulties, altered route for nutrition, and permanent tracheostomy

NCLEX®

3. Postoperative care
   a. Maintain patent airway
   b. Provide pain management
   c. Provide appropriate nutritional support
   d. Teach client and family how to care for tracheostomy and feeding tube (if applicable)
   e. Communicate using devices such as writing supplies, picture or word board, speaking tracheostomy valve; teach client about esophageal speech, transesophageal puncture, or use of electrolarynx as indicated
   f. Provide emotional support to client and family; make appropriate referrals

G. Respiratory isolation

1. Employers must provide protective materials to caregivers at risk for exposure to infectious substances per Occupational Safety and Health Administration (OSHA)
2. Standard precautions include hand hygiene, gloves, and protective face gear used with all clients regardless of actual or potential risk for infection; use these precautions whenever there is possible contact with blood, mucous membranes, nonintact skin, or parenteral devices

NCLEX®

3. Droplet precautions (transmission-based precautions)
   a. In addition to standard precautions, mask should be worn when near client who has known or suspected pathogen transmitted by droplet route
   b. Limit client transport within facility; when transport is necessary, place mask on client
   c. Limit contamination of equipment and/or environment
   d. Place client in private room or with a cohort (client with same diagnosis)
4. Airborne precautions: use same principles as droplet precautions but use fit-tested N95 respirator and place client in private room with negative air pressure; keep door closed (see also Chapter 7)

IV. NURSING MANAGEMENT OF CLIENT HAVING LUNG SURGERY

NCLEX®

A. Preoperative period

1. Reduce anxiety with preoperative teaching about procedure and postoperative course and care
2. Determine client's support systems and ability to care for self after surgery
3. Administer preoperative medications, such as antibiotics, opioid analgesics, and anti-anxiety agents, as ordered
4. Obtain baseline vital signs (VS), oxygen saturation (SpO_2), and cognitive status for comparison postoperatively

B. Postoperative period

1. Perform baseline data collection for VS, SpO_2, and cognitive status as for all postoperative clients
2. NCLEX® Maintain patent airway
3. NCLEX® Position client for optimal ventilation and perfusion; note any specific surgeon's orders for positioning; be prepared to initiate respiratory support (intubation, emergency tracheostomy, mechanical ventilation) as needed
4. Provide standard care to client with a chest tube, if present; see also Chapter 27
5. Maintain sterility of operative dressing
6. NCLEX® Maintain client safety
7. Administer antibiotics, bronchodilators, corticosteroids, inhalation agents, or other medications as ordered
8. Administer analgesics as ordered; adequate pain management facilitates chest expansion and optimal ventilation
9. NCLEX® Monitor for and report possible surgical complications to maintain oxygenation
   - a. Change in level of consciousness (LOC) ranging from restlessness and agitation to lethargy or unresponsiveness
   - b. Increase in respiratory rate, unequal chest expansion, decreased breath sounds, and/or use of accessory muscles for breathing
   - c. Loss of water seal drainage in closed chest drainage system
   - d. Greater than desired volume of chest drainage (75–100 mL drainage over 1 hour is an average acceptable upper limit); orders should specify volume of acceptable chest tube drainage; should decrease over first 24 hours
10. Reinforce teaching to client and family about postdischarge home care and follow-up
11. Refer to community health resources for help with postdischarge care if needed

C. Positioning client after lung surgery: orders should specify turning parameters for individual client

1. NCLEX® Lobectomy: positioning includes lying on back or turned to either side
2. NCLEX® Segmental resection: positioning includes lying on back and tilted to nonoperative side; positioning on operative side may place tension on sutures and promote bleeding
3. NCLEX® Pneumonectomy
   - a. Positioning includes lying on back and tilted toward operative side but not full lateral positioning
   - b. Client may be turned temporarily and slightly toward nonoperative side but should not remain in this position
   - c. Positioning client with operative side tilted slightly down promotes desired consolidation of fluid in pleural space previously occupied by removed lung, prevents remaining lung from shifting into operative side, and aids ventilation and perfusion
   - d. NCLEX® Avoid complete lateral turning to either side, which changes pressure dynamics within chest and could lead to mediastinal shift

V. OBSTRUCTIVE PULMONARY DISEASES

A. Emphysema

1. Overview
   - a. Progressive destruction of alveoli related to chronic inflammation
   - b. Decreased surface area of alveoli and alveolar ducts available for gas exchange
   - c. Airway collapse due to loss of elasticity in respiratory system tissues
   - d. A chronic form of obstructive pulmonary disease (COPD)
   - e. Common symptom is difficulty with exhalation caused by airways obstructed by edema or excessive mucus production
   - f. Lung hyperinflation causes alveolar air trapping and leads to frequent pulmonary infections
   - g. Cigarette smoking is primary etiology associated with emphysema

h. Contributing factors include chronic respiratory inflammation from air pollution or occupational substances such as coal, glass, and asbestos
i. Diagnosis may be associated with hereditary deficiency of alpha-1-antitrypsin, an enzyme that prevents breakdown of lung tissue protein, especially when combined with exposure to cigarette smoke
j. Air trapping in respiratory bronchioles, alveoli, and alveolar ducts leads to repeated infections and characteristic **barrel chest** appearance
k. Work of breathing requires more energy and greater use of accessory muscles

NCLEX®
2. Data collection
a. "Pink puffer" is a classic clinical description characterized by barrel chest, pursed-lip breathing (caused by forced exhalation), obvious use of accessory muscles when breathing, and underweight appearance
b. Exertional dyspnea progresses with advancing disease
c. Persistent tachycardia is related to inadequate oxygenation
d. Overall diminished breath sounds, and possible wheezes or crackles
e. ABGs: slightly decreased PO_2; PCO_2 is not elevated until later stages
f. Chest x-ray: hyperinflated lungs and flattened diaphragm; normal or small heart size
g. Pulmonary function tests: low VC and forced expiratory volume (FEV_1)

NCLEX®
3. Therapeutic management
a. Goals are to improve ventilation and promote patent airway by removing secretions
b. Remove environmental pollutants and encourage smoking cessation
c. Prescribed treatments include bronchodilator therapy, beta-adrenergic agonists, corticosteroid therapy, low-flow oxygen and nebulizer therapy, chest physiotherapy, intermittent positive-pressure breathing (IPPB), possibly mechanical ventilation, and possible surgical procedures such as bullectomy, lung volume reduction surgery, or lung transplantation
d. Provide education and referrals for clients with behaviors (such as smoking) that increase risk for COPD
e. Refer clients to a structured pulmonary conditioning program and provide reinforcement as appropriate
f. Reinforce teaching for clients to avoid pulmonary irritants
g. Assist clients to eat a nutrient dense diet and smaller, more frequent meals to provide adequate calories if dyspnea and fatigue interfere with eating
h. Ensure adequate but not excessive nutritional intake
i. Administer supplemental low-flow O_2 as necessary; be prepared to initiate mechanical ventilatory support
j. Administer and teach clients about antibiotic therapy, bronchodilator therapy, and use of measured-dose (metered dose) inhalants
k. Position clients to optimize and maintain airway and effective breathing patterns, usually with head elevated according to comfort
l. Provide immunization against pneumonia (one-time or every 5 years) and influenza (yearly)

4. Reinforce client teaching: smoking cessation, avoid occupational/environmental pollutants, maintain adequate nutrition (emphasis on higher calorie intake), energy conservation techniques

B. Chronic bronchitis

1. Overview
a. A disorder of chronic airway inflammation with a chronic productive cough lasting at least 3 months during 2 years; is a form of COPD
b. Cigarette smoking is primary etiology of chronic bronchitis
c. Contributing factors include chronic respiratory inflammation from air pollution or occupational substances such as coal, glass, and asbestos
d. Chronic inflammation of airways produces hyperplasia of mucous glands, resulting in excessive sputum production
e. Cilia disappear, and their airway clearance function is lost
f. Goblet cells develop in abnormal sites of terminal bronchioles, also increasing sputum production
g. Mucosal edema and increased production of thick mucus progressively obstructs airflow
h. Work of breathing increases with progressive airway obstruction
i. Repeated pulmonary infections result from increased sputum production with ineffective airway clearance
j. Polycythemia develops as a compensatory response to chronic hypoxemia

NCLEX®

2. Data collection
   a. Frequent cough, occurring during winter season, with foul-smelling sputum
   b. Frequent pulmonary infections
   c. Classic appearance of "blue bloater" includes tendency for obesity and bluish-red skin discoloration from cyanosis and polycythemia
   d. Dyspnea and activity intolerance occurs as disease progresses
   e. Increased anterior–posterior chest diameter
   f. Elevated red blood cell count; hemoglobin and hematocrit elevated in later stages
   g. Chest x-ray reveals enlarged heart, congested lung fields, and normal or flattened diaphragm
   h. Pulmonary function indicates increased residual volume, decreased VC, FEV_1, and FEV_1/FVC ratio

NCLEX®

3. Therapeutic management
   a. Includes measures previously described in section on emphysema
   b. Provide education or referrals to clients with behaviors that increase risk of developing COPD
   c. Refer clients to a structured pulmonary conditioning program and provide reinforcement as appropriate
   d. Reinforce client teaching about how to avoid pulmonary irritants
   e. Assist clients to develop nutritional plans that provide adequate calories but maintain ideal weight
   f. Administer supplemental low-flow O_2 as necessary; be prepared to initiate mechanical ventilation
   g. Surgical interventions include bullectomy, lung volume reduction surgery, and lung transplantation
   h. Medication therapy includes immunization against pneumonia (one-time or every 5 years) and influenza (yearly), antibiotics, possible bronchodilators (beta-adrenergic agonists, anticholinergics such as ipratropium (Atrovent), long-acting theophylline (strengthens diaphragmatic contractions and respiratory drive), corticosteroids (if asthma is a component of COPD)
4. Reinforce client teaching: smoking cessation, avoiding occupational or environmental pollutants, nutritional therapies for adequate energy needs and weight management

C. Asthma

1. Overview
   a. Chronic inflammation of airways leads to intermittent obstruction
   b. Severity and duration of symptoms are unpredictable
   c. Progressive airway obstruction that is unresponsive to treatment can lead to status asthmaticus, an emergency condition
   d. Intrinsic etiologies: uncertain causes; physical or psychological stress; exercise-induced
   e. Extrinsic etiologies: antigen–antibody (allergic) reaction to specific irritants; common **triggers** (initiators) include air pollutants, sinusitis, cold and dry air, medications, food additives, hormonal influences, and gastroesophageal reflux
   f. Episodes of widespread spasms of bronchial smooth muscle with airway edema
   g. Excessive secretion of thick mucus contributes to airway obstruction, and lungs become hyperinflated and alveolar air trapping occurs
   h. Gas exchange becomes impaired as **ventilation–perfusion mismatching** occurs

NCLEX®

2. Data collection
   a. Severe **dyspnea** (difficulty breathing)
   b. Wheezing with expiration; intensity of wheezing is not related to severity of airway obstruction; clients with severe airway obstruction may not be able to move enough air to produce wheezing sound
   c. Cough
   d. Feelings of chest tightness
   e. Prolonged expiration
   f. Mild to greatly diminished breath sounds; may be related to **atelectasis** or narrowed airway lumens
   g. Hyperresonant sound on percussion
   h. Increased heart rate and blood pressure (BP)
   i. Extreme restlessness, anxiety, agitation
   j. **Tachypnea** (rapid respirations) with use of accessory muscles
   k. Decreased PaO_2, mild respiratory alkalosis during "attack"
   l. Elevated eosinophil count
   m. Increased residual volume, decreased VC, FEV_1 and peak expiratory flow rate (PEFR)

NCLEX®

3. Therapeutic management
   a. Acute episodes are managed with inhaled beta agonists, bronchodilators, anti-inflammatory agents, corticosteroids, and oxygen therapy; in severe cases, mechanical ventilation may be instituted
   b. Chronic management: depends on disease severity and whether in a state of exacerbation; may include a short-acting or long-acting beta-agonist inhaler, anti-inflammatory inhaler, corticosteroid inhaler, or systemic corticosteroids (for severe exacerbations)

c. Monitor respiratory and oxygenation status; administer supplemental O_2 as needed
d. Observe characteristics of sputum
e. Identify, avoid, and remove precipitating factors
f. Reinforce client relaxation techniques during nonacute periods
g. Allergy desensitization therapy if appropriate
h. Be prepared to establish IV access
i. Be prepared to initiate mechanical ventilation if indicated
j. Diagnostic testing during nonacute period includes chest x-ray, pulmonary function studies, allergy skin testing, serum eosinophils, and IgE
k. Provide emotional support to client and family

4. Reinforce client teaching
   a. Asthma triggers
   b. Proper use of metered-dose inhaler
   c. Use of peak-flow meter for self-assessment of asthma status; goal is to remain in green zone (80–100% of personal best); use action plan for medications when PEFR is in yellow zone (50–80%); use action plan and seek health care when in red zone (less than 50%)
   d. How to recognize asthma symptoms requiring emergency intervention

VI. PLEURAL EFFUSION

A. Overview

1. Accumulation of fluid in pleural space that indicates underlying pulmonary disease or abnormality; pressure exerted by fluid compresses normal lung tissue; a form of restrictive lung disease
2. Transudative pleural effusion: contains small amounts of protein and may be associated with increased hydrostatic pressure (heart failure) or decreased oncotic pressure from low albumin level (chronic renal or liver disease); fluid moves from capillaries into pleural space
3. Exudative pleural effusion: contains larger quantity of protein; results from increased capillary permeability and fluid shift out of capillaries associated with inflammatory processes such as pulmonary tumors, infection, or emboli
4. Empyema: pleural fluid containing pus associated with infections such as pneumonia, lung abscess, and tuberculosis
5. Chylothorax: pulmonary lymph vessels disrupted by surgery or trauma can lead to abnormal accumulation of lymph fluid in pleural space; produces fat malabsorption from GI tract

NCLEX®

B. Data collection

1. Worsening dyspnea with diminished or absent breath sounds on affected side from lung compression
2. Dullness to percussion on affected side
3. Chest wall pain
4. Fever, persistent cough, night sweats, and weight loss with empyema
5. Visible on chest x-ray if greater than 250 mL fluid accumulates
6. Diagnostic thoracentesis: differentiates source of pleural fluid

NCLEX®

C. Therapeutic management

1. Goal is to treat underlying cause
2. Thoracentesis to drain pleural cavity
3. Surgery may include decortication, or the separation of pleural membranes
4. Monitor respiratory and oxygenation status; provide supplemental O_2 if indicated
5. Provide adequate nutrition with focus on adequate protein intake
6. Medication therapy: analgesics, antipyretics, antibiotics if indicated; IV lipids if chylothorax present

D. Reinforce client teaching

1. Underlying cause of pleural effusion
2. How to monitor for changes in respiratory and oxygenation status
3. Purpose of thoracentesis/thoracostomy

VII. PNEUMOTHORAX AND HEMOTHORAX

A. Overview

1. Pneumothorax: air accumulation in pleural space
   a. Spontaneous: rupture of air-filled bleb allows air to move between respiratory system and pleural space; collapse of involved tissue may seal leak with minimal client symptoms; air leak may progress until pressure between thoracic cavity and atmosphere equalizes and client is symptomatic
   b. Primary: spontaneous rupture of bleb in otherwise healthy individual; occurs more often in tall, slender males aged 20 to 40

c. Secondary: rupture of overly distended alveolus/alveoli; occurs in those with known COPD; severity of symptoms varies with size of pneumothorax

NCLEX® d. Tension: disruption of chest wall or lungs causes air accumulation in pleural space; pressure on mediastinum causes pressure on other lung and interrupts venous return to heart; is a medical emergency that requires emergency placement of chest tube to relieve increasing pressure in thoracic cavity and restore adequate cardiac output

e. Traumatic: disruption of pleura, bronchi, or lung tissue caused by blunt or penetrating trauma with air accumulation in pleural space

f. Iatrogenic: disruption of pleura, bronchi, or lung tissue during central venous line placement, lung biopsy, or thoracentesis produces unintentional air leak within respiratory system; clinical manifestations and treatment are same as for spontaneous pneumothorax

2. Hemothorax: blood accumulation in pleural space; clinical manifestations and treatment are same as for pneumothorax

NCLEX® **B. Data collection**

1. Dyspnea
2. Tracheal deviation toward unaffected side
3. Diminished breath sounds on affected side
4. Percussion dullness on affected side
5. Unequal chest expansion (reduced on affected side)
6. Crepitus over chest
7. Chest x-ray reveals pneumothorax
8. ABG shows decreased PO_2

NCLEX® **C. Therapeutic management**

1. In mild cases, no chest tube is required; if pneumothorax is significant, a chest tube is inserted and attached to water seal drainage
2. Spontaneous pneumothorax: in otherwise healthy client, may resolve without invasive treatment
3. If spontaneous pneumothorax occurs repeatedly, may require pleurodesis, an instillation of an agent (such as talc or tetracycline) in pleural spaces to allow pleura to adhere together; other procedures include partial pleurectomy, stapling, or laser pleurodesis for pleural sealing
4. Care of client with a chest tube: previously discussed in Chapter 27
5. Monitor respiratory and oxygenation status
6. Provide supplemental O_2 as indicated
7. Maintain infection control practices
8. Medication therapy: analgesics and antibiotics

D. Reinforce client teaching: purpose of chest tube, activity limitations, and pain management

VIII. ATELECTASIS

A. Overview

1. Incomplete expansion or collapse of lung tissue resulting from obstruction of air passages by secretions or a foreign body
2. Common complication among postoperative or immobilized clients
3. Pulmonary secretions and/or exudates contribute to airway obstruction
4. Airway obstruction increases intra-alveolar pressure, causing alveolar collapse
5. Surface area available for gas exchange is decreased

NCLEX® **B. Data collection**

1. Low-grade fever
2. Breath sounds diminished or absent in affected area
3. Diminished rate and depth of respiration
4. Physical inactivity caused by immobility or pain
5. Diagnostic and laboratory test findings: chest x-ray reveals area of collapse

NCLEX® **C. Therapeutic management**

1. Primary goal is prevention of atelectasis
2. Chest physical therapy and general pulmonary hygiene measures
3. Possible IPPB treatments
4. Supplemental oxygen as indicated
5. Monitor respiratory and oxygenation status
6. Deep breathing and coughing exercises; incentive spirometry hourly while awake
7. Frequent position change

8. Ambulation as soon as feasible with client condition
9. Maintain adequate hydration and nutrition
10. Medication therapy: analgesics and antipyretics

D. Reinforce client teaching: diaphragmatic and abdominal breathing, nonpharmacologic pain control measures

IX. PNEUMONIA

A. Overview

1. Acute inflammation of lung parenchyma (alveoli and respiratory bronchioles)
2. Classified as viral versus bacterial, community-acquired versus hospital-acquired, atypical, aspiration or pneumocystis
3. Causative agent can be infectious (bacteria, viruses, fungi, and other microbes) or noninfectious (aspirated or inhaled substances)
4. Most common organism for both community-acquired and hospital-acquired pneumonia is the Gram-positive bacteria *Streptococcus pneumoniae*
5. Other common organisms associated with community-acquired pneumonia include *Klebsiella pneumoniae, Pseudomonas aeruginosa, Escherichia coli, haemophilus influenzae,* and other influenzae viruses
6. Spread of microbes in alveoli activates inflammatory and immune response
7. Antigen–antibody response damages mucous membranes of bronchioles and alveoli resulting in edema
8. Microbe cellular debris and exudate fill alveoli and can impair gas exchange

B. Data collection

NCLEX®

1. Viral
   a. Fever: low-grade
   b. Cough: nonproductive
   c. White blood cell count: normal to low elevation
   d. Chest x-ray: minimal changes evident
   e. Clinical course: less severe than pneumonia of bacterial origin

NCLEX®

2. Bacterial
   a. Fever: high
   b. Cough: productive
   c. White blood cell count: high elevation
   d. Chest x-ray: obvious infiltrates
   e. Clinical course: more severe than pneumonia of viral origin

NCLEX®

C. Therapeutic management

1. Antibiotic therapy, analgesics, antipyretics
2. Supplemental oxygen therapy to treat hypoxemia
3. Maintain patent airway; monitor respiratory and oxygenation status
4. Be prepared to initiate mechanical ventilatory support
5. Provide nutritional support and fluids (2 liters per 24 hours or greater if no contraindications) via appropriate route
6. Provide adequate opportunities for physical rest
7. For all hospitalized clients, take measures to prevent pneumonia
   a. Identify clients at high risk for pneumonia
   b. Maintain appropriate infection control measures
   c. Maintain adequate nutrition
   d. Initiate aspiration precautions for clients at risk (ex: stroke)
   e. Encourage activity and mobility as soon as feasible
8. Medication therapy: antibiotics or other indicated anti-infectives, analgesics, antipyretics

D. Reinforce client teaching

1. Immunization against influenza and pneumococcal pneumonia
2. Activity limitations and importance of rest
3. Effects and dosages of medications
4. Need to avoid pollutants and irritants such as smoke
5. Symptoms to report: return of fever, worsening respiratory status

X. PULMONARY TUBERCULOSIS

A. Overview

1. Lung infection caused by *Mycobacterium tuberculosis* (although any tissue can be infected)
2. *M. tuberculosis* is an acid-fast, Gram-positive bacillus with transmission via airborne droplets

3. Infection usually results from frequent close contact with an infected individual
4. Inhaled bacilli inhabit respiratory bronchioles and alveoli
5. Bacilli travel through lymph circulation and may spread throughout body before cell-mediated immunity can contain its movement
6. Eventual activation of cell-mediated immunity produces a granuloma lesion
7. Liquified necrotic material from Ghon tubercle portion of granuloma lesion allows passage of infectious particles into major airways for exhalation into air

NCLEX®

B. Data collection

1. Nonproductive cough develops first as an early symptom (especially in early morning), followed by frequent cough with copious purulent or blood-tinged sputum
2. Late afternoon low grade fever and night sweats
3. Anorexia and weight loss
4. Fatigue
5. History may indicate recent exposure to infected individual
6. Positive tuberculin skin test (indicates exposure)
7. Appearance of characteristic Ghon tubercle on chest x-ray
8. Positive acid-fast bacillus sputum cultures (provides definitive diagnosis of infection)

NCLEX®

C. Therapeutic management

1. Monitor respiratory and oxygenation status
2. Provide adequate nutrition and hydration
3. Institute standard precautions (Centers for Disease Control [CDC] Tier 1) and airborne precautions (Tier 2, transmission-based precautions); see also Chapter 7
   a. Use a private room with negative air pressure that has 6 to 12 full air exchanges per hour and is vented to the outside or has its own air filtration system
   b. Wear specially fitted mask (N95 respirator) whenever entering client's room; fit-test mask with each use
   c. Provide visitors with appropriate masks
   d. Wear gown as well as mask if client does not reliably cover mouth during coughing or sneezing to reduce risk of transmission to others
   e. Provide client with a surgical mask if client must be transported to another department; choose shortest and least busy route and alert department ahead of time about client's status; schedule tests for least busy times of day
   f. Administer antimicrobial therapy as prescribed
   g. Provide supplemental O_2 as indicated
   h. Obtain periodic sputum cultures following onset of antimicrobial therapy
4. Medication therapy (see also Chapter 41)
   a. Antibiotic prophylaxis: for individuals exposed to clients with active disease; isoniazid (INH) is drug of choice for 6 months if no clinical evidence of disease
   b. INH drug of choice for 12 months if abnormal chest x-ray or high-risk population such as with HIV or drug-induced immunosuppression
   c. Active disease option 1 (CDC): INH, rifampin (Rifadin), pyrazinamide (Tebrazid), and ethambutol (Myambutol) or streptomycin given daily or two to three times weekly (if therapy verified); if cultures report sensitivity to rifampin or INH, ethambutol or streptomycin can be stopped; minimal 6 months of drug therapy; drug therapy continues for at least 3 months after first negative sputum culture obtained
   d. Active disease option 2 (CDC): INH, rifampin, pyrazinamide, and ethambutol or streptomycin given daily for 2 weeks, then twice weekly for 6 weeks, then twice weekly INH and rifampin for 16 weeks
   e. Active disease option 3 (CDC): INH, rifampin, pyrazinamide, and ethambutol or streptomycin three times weekly for 6 months
   f. Active disease option 4 (CDC): active TB with HIV; option 1, 2, or 3 for minimum of 9 months and to continue for at least 6 months after first negative sputum culture

D. Reinforce client teaching

NCLEX®

1. Infection control measures, including hand hygiene, coughing into tissues and disposing of them in a closed bag
2. No special precautions need to be taken with clothing, books, personal objects, or eating utensils because inanimate objects do not easily spread these bacteria

NCLEX®

3. Mechanisms of transmission and antimicrobial therapy, including need to take medication for full course of therapy to prevent recurrence and/or development of drug-resistant organisms

4. Adverse effects of medications; see also Chapter 41
5. Need for adequate nutrition for healing and rest periods to reduce fatigue

XI. PULMONARY EMBOLISM

A. Overview

1. Emboli lodge in pulmonary vasculature and impede blood flow through pulmonary capillaries
2. Ventilation–perfusion mismatch: a clinically significant imbalance between volume of air and volume of blood circulating to gas exchange area of lungs; leads to impaired gas exchange
3. Pulmonary embolism (PE) more commonly occurs in immobilized clients who develop deep vein thrombosis
4. Other sites of origin of emboli include veins in pelvis, or thrombi in right side of heart
5. Risk factors for PE include immobility, hypercoagulability, trauma to endothelial layer of blood vessels, and long bone fractures
6. Venous thrombus dislodges and circulates to pulmonary vasculature; fat emboli travel from site of long bone fractures and traumatized vessels
7. Emboli obstruct small to large areas of pulmonary vasculature, preventing adequate perfusion and gas exchange
8. A massive area of obstructed tissue leads to pulmonary infarction
9. Severe impairment of gas exchange can be rapidly fatal

NCLEX®

B. Data collection

1. Restlessness, anxiety, agitation, apprehension
2. Vital signs: tachycardia, tachypnea, hypotension, low-grade fever
3. Dyspnea, shortness of breath and chest pain
4. Cough and possible hemoptysis
5. Mental status changes with possible decreasing level of consciousness (LOC)
6. Possible diaphoresis and cyanosis
7. Recent history of thromboembolism and/or long bone fractures
8. Lung crackles upon auscultation
9. S_3 and/or S_4 gallop; atrial fibrillation may result in mural thrombi that may be cause of PE
10. Chest x-ray may be normal or show pulmonary infiltration
11. Pulmonary angiogram reveals site of PE
12. Ventilation–perfusion scan indicates areas of mismatch
13. Abnormal ABGs (significantly low PaO_2)

NCLEX®

C. Therapeutic management

1. Supplemental O_2 therapy; maintain patent airway
2. Be prepared to initiate mechanical ventilation
3. Maintain IV access and provide circulatory support as needed
4. Anticoagulant and/or thrombolytic therapy
5. Opioid analgesics and anti-anxiety agents as needed
6. Embolectomy
7. To prevent future pulmonary emboli, a vena cava filter may be inserted to trap emboli from a recurrent known source

D. Reinforce client teaching

1. Prevention of thromboembolism
2. Avoid immobility as much as feasible
3. Signs/symptoms of venous occlusion
4. Anticoagulant therapy if indicated

XII. BRONCHOGENIC CARCINOMA

A. Overview

1. Lung cancer is leading cause of death from malignancy, with a 5-year survival rate less than 15%
2. Greater than 90% of lung cancers originate in bronchus epithelium
3. Cigarette smoking is leading cause; cancer risk increases with length of smoking exposure
4. Contributing factors: inhaled environmental substances such as air pollution, arsenic, asbestos, iron, radon, and aromatic hydrocarbons
5. Some individuals have a genetic predisposition to bronchogenic carcinoma
6. Tumor growth commonly begins in bronchus then migrates to upper lobes of lungs
7. Nonspecific inflammatory cellular changes lead to excessive mucus production, desquamation, metaplasia of epithelium, and slow-growing bronchogenic carcinoma

8. Tumor types include small cell and non-small cell
9. Metastasis occurs by direct contact and transport in blood and lymph

NCLEX® **B. Data collection**

1. Symptom onset is often late in course of disease
2. Persistent cough with or without hemoptysis
3. Localized chest pain
4. Dyspnea
5. Unilateral wheeze upon auscultation
6. Swallowing difficulty
7. Anorexia and weight loss
8. Enlarged neck lymph nodes
9. Mass visible on chest x-ray, CT scan or MRI
10. Sputum for cytology reveals tumor cells
11. Bronchoscopy for direct biopsy or washings for cytology reveal tumor cells

NCLEX® **C. Therapeutic management**

1. Surgical resection
   - **a.** Pneumonectomy: removal of entire lung
   - **b.** Lobectomy: removal of a lobe of lung
   - **c.** Segmentectomy (segmental resection): removal of a segment or segments of a lung
   - **d.** Wedge resection: dissection and removal of a defined area in lung
2. Non-surgical therapies (see also Chapter 61): chemotherapy, radiation therapy, laser therapy, immunotherapy
3. Provide psychological support for client and family
4. Provide preoperative and postoperative care for client having surgery
5. Administer O_2 therapy as prescribed
6. Assist client with pain management
7. Position to optimize oxygenation (see previous discussion)
8. Provide care of chest tubes (see also Chapter 27)
9. Medication therapy: opioid analgesics and antiemetics

D. Reinforce client teaching: treatment plan, pain management, and assistance with coping skills

XIII. CANCER OF LARYNX

A. Description

1. Most laryngeal tumors are benign
2. Most common form of malignant laryngeal cancer is squamous cell carcinoma
3. Primary etiologies include long-term cigarette smoking and alcohol ingestion
4. Contributing factors: chronic laryngeal irritation caused by singing, air pollution, and environmental hazards
5. Tumor growth occurs in glottis, supraglottis, and subglottis; symptoms are specific to site of tumor
6. Chronic laryngeal irritation leads to precancerous lesions, leukoplakia, and erythroplakia
7. Carcinoma may develop at site of precancerous lesions
8. Most common site for laryngeal metastasis is lungs; larynx is, however, a rare site for metastasis of other tumors

NCLEX® **B. Data collection**

1. Hoarseness and/or change in voice characteristics
2. Palpable jugular nodes
3. Pain when swallowing
4. Unexplained earache
5. Diagnostic test results: laryngeal biopsy findings, x-ray visualization, MRI or CT findings, barium swallow visualization

NCLEX® **C. Therapeutic management**

1. Depends on stage of disease and general condition of client
   - **a.** Radiation therapy or brachytherapy (placement of a radioactive source next to tumor)
   - **b.** Chemotherapy
   - **c.** Surgery: laryngectomy or radical neck dissection
2. Maintain patent airway (tracheostomy performed with laryngectomy)

3. Pain management
4. Provide adequate hydration and nutrition (temporary or permanent altered route for nutrition)
5. Provide alternate means for communication (word or picture board, paper and pencil) and plan for permanent means of communication (electrolarynx, esophageal speech, or transesophageal puncture [TEP])
6. Monitor respiratory and oxygenation status
7. Provide supplemental O_2 as indicated
8. Medication therapy: opioid analgesics and antipyretics

D. Reinforce client teaching
1. Smoking cessation
2. Changes in body image
3. Care of tracheostomy
4. Use of artificial larynx
5. Supraglottic swallowing for voice production (esophageal speech)
6. Nutritional access device if indicated
7. Pain management
8. Signs of tumor spread

XIV. THORACIC TRAUMA

A. Overview
1. Alteration of breathing mechanics and/or gas exchange caused by respiratory system trauma
2. Blunt trauma: injury to chest wall without disruption of pleura
   a. Rib fractures
   b. Flail chest
   c. Soft tissue rupture: diaphragm, trachea, bronchi, and major blood vessels
   d. Tension pneumothorax
   e. Contusion: lungs, heart
   f. Mechanism of injury commonly involves motor vehicle collisions, falls, and assaults
3. Penetrating trauma: injury involves disruption of pleura
   a. Internal wounds communicate with external atmosphere
   b. Open air-sucking wounds
   c. Pneumothorax and hemothorax
   d. Tissue wounds: heart, lungs, major blood vessels
   e. Mechanism of injury commonly involves firearms, knives, motor vehicle collisions, falls, or assaults
4. Flail chest
   a. Multiple rib fractures in two or more places (separated from bony skeleton)
   b. Chest wall unstable with paradoxical chest expansion (flail segment moves inward with inhalation and outward with exhalation)
   c. Ventilation–perfusion mismatch
   d. Possible underlying lung injury
5. Rupture of diaphragm
   a. Abdominal contents dislocate upward into thoracic cavity
   b. Decrease in diaphragmatic control of breathing

NCLEX® **B. Data collection**
1. Varies with cause
2. Chest pain, may be severe such as with flail chest, or worse on inspiration (such as with fractured ribs)
3. Shallow breathing with splinting
4. Possible unequal chest expansion
5. Tachycardia, tachypnea, hypotension
6. Crepitus over chest
7. Chest x-ray findings show white opacifications (pulmonary contusion), site of fracture, or accompanying pneumothorax or hemothorax
8. ABGs reveal hypoxemia

NCLEX® **C. Therapeutic management:** same as pneumothorax and hemothorax
1. Ventilation support with O_2 therapy; be prepared to initiate mechanical ventilation
2. Maintain IV access
3. Possible placement of chest tube with water seal drainage
4. Medication therapy: opioid analgesics, patient-controlled or epidural analgesia may be appropriate

D. Reinforce client teaching

1. Techniques for pulmonary hygiene
2. Pain management: patient-controlled analgesia or oral analgesics
3. Prevention of thromboembolism
4. Measures to decrease anxiety

XV. CYSTIC FIBROSIS (CF)

A. Overview

1. Multisystem disorder of exocrine glands, leading to increased production of thick mucus in bronchioles, small intestines, and pancreatic and bile ducts
2. Increased viscosity of secretions obstructs small passageways of these organs and interferes with normal pulmonary and digestive functioning
3. Respiratory problems are most serious threat to life; thick, sticky secretions pool in bronchioles, cause atelectasis, and serve as a medium for bacterial growth
4. Pancreatic ducts become clogged with thick secretions and prevent pancreatic enzymes from reaching duodenum, impairing digestion and absorption
5. Small intestines, without aid of pancreatic enzymes, are unable to absorb fats and protein; thus, growth and puberty are retarded
6. Inherited as an autosomal-recessive trait; gene on chromosome 7 responsible for functioning of cystic fibrosis transmembrane regulator (CFTR) is defective; absence of CTFR as a chloride channel interferes with sodium-chloride (Na^+–Cl^-) transport, prohibiting movement of water across cell membranes
7. Usually diagnosed in infancy and early childhood; affects white children primarily; rarely seen in children of Asian of African descent; males and females are affected equally
8. Life expectancy has increased to median age of 30 years, but disease is terminal; death usually results from resistant pulmonary organisms and fibrosis and destruction of lung tissues

NCLEX® **B. Data collection**

1. **Sweat test** (pilocarpine iontophoresis) analyzes Na^+ and Cl^- content in sweat; a chloride concentration greater than 60 meq/L is diagnostic of cystic fibrosis; parents often report that infants taste salty when kissed
2. 72-hour fecal fat analysis
3. Chest x-ray
4. Prior to delivery, prenatal DNA analysis of amniotic fluid shows intestinal alkaline phosphatase is reduced in a fetus with cystic fibrosis
5. History usually reveals frequent bouts of respiratory infections
6. Observe for respiratory impairment (i.e., cough, presence and color of sputum, dyspnea, retractions) color of nailbeds and mucous membranes, O_2 saturation; auscultate breath sounds for equality, crackles, wheezes, or any increased effort during breathing; observe for clubbing of fingers and toes; **digital clubbing**, an indication of hypoxia, produces nails with increased rounding and a loss of normal angle at base of nail
7. Monitor nutritional status by obtaining height and weight and plot on growth charts; monitor skin turgor and mucous membranes for hydration status; record diet history and activity tolerance; signs of malabsorption include bulky, frothy, foul-smelling stools called steatorrhea and unusually protruberant abdomen and thin extremities; often first sign of CF is meconium ileus, where intestine is blocked with thick, tenacous secretions in newborn period and neonate is unable to pass first meconium stool

NCLEX® **C. Therapeutic management**

1. Respiratory: ensure pulmonary hygiene is performed; auscultate breath sounds before and after treatments; encourage coughing and deep breathing exercises and physical activity as tolerated; administer prescribed antibiotics and bronchodilator(s)
2. Digestive: provide high-calorie (150% above normal recommendations), high-protein diet and snacks; give infants a predigested formula such as pregestimil or nutramigen; administer pancreatic enzymes with all meals and snacks; individualize to achieve stools as near normal as possible; administer fat-soluble vitamins; determine food preferences to encourage acceptance of diet; weigh daily; avoid pulmonary treatments immediately after meals to decrease risk of vomiting
3. Medications: antibiotics for pulmonary infection and purulent secretions, pancreatic enzymes for fat absorption, vitamin supplementation, mucolytics to decrease viscosity of sputum, bronchodilators to improve lung function; see Chapter 33 for overview of commonly ordered respiratory medications

D. Reinforce child and family teaching

1. Avoid exposure to respiratory infections; report immediately any fever, increase in cough, or change in sputum

2. Chest percussion and postural drainage must be performed 3 to 4 times daily; noncompliance will result in increased infections and hospitalizations; see Box 51–2 for instructions on CPT and postural drainage (p. 852)

NCLEX®

3. High-calorie, high-protein diet is essential; give pancreatic enzymes with all meals and snacks; may need extra salt in hot weather
4. Physical activity and exercise loosen secretions and promote lung expansion
5. Reinforce information on community resources, such as Cystic Fibrosis Foundation, American Lung Association; provide social service consults, home-health referrals with visiting nurses and respiratory therapists
6. Genetic counseling
7. Provide written information on medications, breathing exercises, CPT, and postural drainage
8. Suggest clergy, mental health services, respite care, and families of other children with CF to assist with psychologic and emotional coping with chronic, progressive illness

XVI. *BRONCHOPULMONARY DYSPLASIA (BPD)*

A. Overview

1. A chronic obstructive pulmonary disorder occurring in infants as a sequela to prolonged O_2 therapy and mechanical ventilation
2. Premature infants with BPD have usually survived respiratory distress syndrome (RDS) at birth; term infants who develop BPD also generally had serious respiratory problems that required ventilatory assistance
3. High O_2 concentrations and mechanical ventilation damage bronchial epithelium and alveoli; thickened alveolar walls, scarring, and fibrosis lead to atelectasis, poor airway clearance of mucus, and poor gas exchange; chronic low oxygenation results in decreased lung compliance and altered function
4. Lung immaturity is a major contributor to BPD, and improved survival rates of premature infants have increased incidence of BPD; as little as 3 days of positive pressure ventilation can increase an infant's risk of developing BPD
5. There may be a genetic predisposition; males have increased morbidity

NCLEX® **B. Data collection**

1. Diagnosed by chest x-ray, which reveals lung changes and air trapping with or without hyperinflation
2. ABGs reveal hypercapnia (increased CO_2) and respiratory acidosis
3. Respiratory signs include tachypnea, tachycardia, increased work of breathing, retractions, wheezing, and barrel chest
4. Pallor, activity intolerance, and poor feeding result from chronic hypoxia

NCLEX® **C. Therapeutic management**

1. Infants with BPD are cared for in intensive care units and require an artificial airway; avoid pressure or trauma to ET tube and infant's airway
2. Suctioning, turning, and weighing is done carefully to ensure adequate O_2 saturation levels are maintained
3. Monitor respiratory status continuously; infant's condition can worsen in a short period of time
4. Monitor for fluid overload because of increased risk for pulmonary edema; weigh daily; maintain strict intake and output (I&O)
5. Strict hand hygiene; avoid exposure to respiratory infections
6. Cluster nursing care to minimize O_2 requirements and caloric expenditure
7. Plan quiet stimulation and activities to foster normal infant development and parental bonding with extended and often repeated hospitalizations of infants with BPD
8. Medications
   a. Bronchodilators open airways and increase lung compliance
   b. Corticosteroids reduce airway edema and inflammation
   c. Diuretics remove excess fluid from lungs and help prevent pulmonary edema
   d. Antibiotics may be given prophylactically

D. Reinforce client and family teaching

1. Infants are discharged with multiple needs; review family's understanding and ability to follow treatment regimen
2. Importance of knowing cardiopulmonary resuscitation (CPR), use of home monitoring equipment and O_2 therapy; infants are usually discharged with a tracheostomy when O_2 concentration requirements are low

Box 51–3

Tracheostomy Home Care and Oxygen Therapy

Discharge instructions for child with tracheostomy (trach):

- Keep small toys, talcum powder, plastic bibs and bedding, and any small particles away from child to decrease risk for aspiration or occlusion of trachea.
- Be sure child wears cloth bib loosely over trach when eating to prevent food particles from entering tube.
- Be careful when bathing to keep water from entering trachea; showers are not recommended.
- Cover trach loosely when outside in strong wind or cold to prevent tracheal spasms.
- Observe skin around trach daily for redness, breakdown, or signs of infection.
- Change trach ties weekly; be sure to use nonfraying material; always have assistance to change ties.
- Clean area around trach daily with half-strength saline and cotton applicators.
- Suction trach tube when needed to remove secretions from airway; use sterile gloves and limit suctioning to 5 seconds; insert suction catheter only to length of trach tube and apply intermittent suction while withdrawing catheter.
- Allow child to rest between suctioning if catheter is passed more than once.
- Notify physician if tracheal secretions are increased or become purulent or fever develops.
- Keep written instructions available at all times.
- Keep emergency bag with extra suction catheters and trach tubes available.
- Notify utility companies and emergency medical services that child in the home requires emergency equipment.
- Do not allow smoking in the home of child with oxygen therapy.
- Keep oxygen tanks away from any heat source; keep a fire extinguisher nearby.

3. Infection control practices such as hand hygiene and avoiding family members with respiratory infections; review warning signs of illness
4. Safety precautions regarding O_2 therapy and tracheostomy care; see Box 51–3 for instructions on home tracheostomy care; before discharge, notify utility companies, emergency services, and telephone companies of a technology-dependent infant or child
5. Basic care—feeding, bathing, playing, holding; provide parents with opportunities to care for child in hospital before discharge; after basic care is mastered, medical treatment plan is developed with assistance of parents
6. Community agencies that can assist with supplies, medications, nutrition, parental support, and stimulation programs to foster growth and development

XVII. *LARYNGOTRACHEOBRONCHITIS (LTB)*

A. Overview

1. Viral infection that causes inflammation, edema, and narrowing of larynx, trachea, and bronchi; usually LTB is preceded by a recent upper respiratory infection (URI)
2. LTB is most common in infants and toddlers and affects boys more often than girls; is most common croup syndrome
3. LTB is usually caused by parainfluenzae virus, influenzae A and B, respiratory syncytial virus (RSV), and mycoplasma pneumoniae
4. Inflammation and narrowing of airways cause inspiratory stridor and suprasternal retractions as child struggles to inhale air; increased production of thick secretions and edema further obstruct airway and cause hypoxia and CO_2 accumulation, and lead to respiratory acidosis and failure

NCLEX®

B. Data collection

1. Onset is gradual after URI
2. Child awakens with low-grade fever, barking cough, and acute stridor; noisy breathing and use of accessory muscles increase

3. Child is agitated, restless, has a frightened appearance, sore throat, and rhinorrhea
4. Pulse oximetry is used to detect hypoxemia (via SpO_2 or O_2 saturation); anteroposterior (AP) and lateral upper airway x-rays are ordered

NCLEX® **C. Therapeutic management**

1. Monitor child's respiratory effort continuously to ensure a patent airway; observe for diminished breath sounds, circumoral cyanosis, diminishing noisy breathing, and drooling
2. Quiet respiratory effort is a sign of physical exhaustion and impending respiratory failure
3. Provide humidity and supplemental O_2; IV fluids prevent dehydration and help liquefy secretions
4. Assist child to assume upright position or any position of comfort; promote a calm, quiet environment; keep parents nearby to reduce child's stress/crying
5. Keep emergency intubation equipment available at bedside; readily respond to call bell or requests for assistance
6. Monitor parental and child's anxiety level; provide emotional support
7. Medications
   a. Bronchodilators decrease mucosal constriction and laryngeal edema; nebulized racemic epinephrine has a rapid onset with improvement of symptoms, although relapse may occur within 2 hours
   b. Corticosteroids decrease inflammation and edema

D. Reinforce child and family teaching

1. Symptoms are usually worse at night and may recur for several nights; instruct parents that child can be cared for at home if able to take fluids by mouth and has no stridor at rest
2. NCLEX® Cool mist humidifier and parental presence can be initial treatment of crisis; comforting measures include cuddling, rocking, singing, and any calming measures until breathing becomes easier
3. NCLEX® Seek medical attention immediately if breathing becomes labored, child seems exhausted or very agitated, or if symptoms do not improve after cool air humidity treatment
4. LTB is a viral illness; avoid contact with large groups of people and practice infection control measures

XVIII. *EPIGLOTTITIS*

A. Overview

1. Inflammation and swelling of epiglottis, primarily affecting children ages 2 to 8
2. Epiglottis covers larynx during swallowing to prevent food from entering trachea
3. Bacteria, usually *Haemophilus influenzae,* cause epiglottis to become cherry red, swollen, and so edematous that it obstructs airway; secretions pool in pharynx and larynx above epiglottis; child has a sore throat and is unable to swallow; complete airway obstruction can occur within 2 to 6 hours
4. Onset is sudden in a previously healthy child; Hib vaccine has reduced incidence of epiglottitis, although causative organisms may also be streptococcus and staphylococcus

NCLEX® **B. Data collection**

1. Child awakens with sudden onset of high fever (102°F), extremely sore throat, and pain on swallowing
2. Child is very anxious, restless, looks ill, and insists on sitting upright leaning on arms, with chin thrust out and mouth open (tripod position)
3. Dysphonia (muffled voice), dysphagia (difficulty swallowing), drooling of saliva, and distressed respiratory effort are classic signs
4. Edematous, cherry-red epiglottis is most reliable diagnostic sign
5. Examination of throat is contraindicated, however, unless emergency intubation equipment and trained personnel are available; physical manipulation of hypersensitive and irritated airway muscles may result in spasm and complete obstruction
6. Lateral neck x-ray confirms an enlarged epiglottis; portable x-rays are completed in exam room with child on parent's lap to minimize stress and maximize comfort and calm behavior
7. Complete blood count (CBC) and blood cultures are taken once child is intubated and stabilized

NCLEX® **C. Therapeutic management**

1. Monitor continuously for respiratory distress and decrease in respiratory effort; report changes in status
2. Never leave child unattended; support child in position of comfort; encourage parents to hug and cuddle child
3. Keep ET and tracheotomy tubes and suction equipment at bedside; assist with emergency ventilation if needed before child is taken to operating room (OR) for airway insertion
4. Child is usually intubated for 24 hours; restraints may be needed to prevent tube dislodgment, because swelling of epiglottis may prohibit reintubation

5. Provide support for child and family and alleviate anxiety; explain all procedures clearly and calmly
6. All invasive procedures, including starting an IV infusion, ABGs, and blood cultures are performed in OR
7. Keep child NPO; IV fluids provide hydration; administer antipyretics and antibiotics as prescribed
8. After extubation, monitor child closely in intensive care unit to ensure immediate observation if respiratory effort is compromised
9. Medications
   a. Antibiotics treat bacterial infection (usually given for 7 to 10 days); child is discharged in about 3 days with oral antibiotics
   b. Antipyretics treat fever and manage pain of sore throat
   c. Corticosteroids may be given for 24 hours before extubation to decrease edema

D. Reinforce client and family teaching

1. Need for airway insertion in OR
2. Importance of completing antibiotic regimen after discharge; explain medications, how to administer, and side effects to expect
3. Importance of Hib vaccine
4. Recurrence of epiglottitis is uncommon

XIX. BRONCHIOLITIS

A. Overview

1. Inflammation of bronchioles with edema and excess accumulation of mucus; air trapping and atelectasis result from increased airway resistance because of small obstructed bronchioles
2. A major cause of hospitalization of high-risk infants
3. RSV is primary causative organism; virus is spread by contact with contaminated objects; RSV is not airborne but can live for several hours on nonporous surfaces
4. RSV bronchiolitis is most prevalent during first 2 years of life, with most occurrences in spring and winter; bronchiolitis usually begins with a mild URI; as disease progresses, gas exchange is compromised, hypoxemia results, and metabolic acidosis develops

NCLEX® **B. Data collection**

1. Clinical manifestations include worsening of URI with tachypnea, retractions, low-grade fever, anorexia, thick nasal secretions, and increasingly labored breathing; older infants may have a frequent, dry cough
2. Auscultation of lungs reveal wheezing or crackles
3. Nasopharyngeal washing to obtain respiratory secretions identifies causative virus; chest x-ray may be normal or indicate hyperinflation or nonspecific inflammation

NCLEX® **C. Therapeutic management**

1. Monitor respiratory status hourly; provide humidified O_2 to ease respiratory effort; use pulse oximetry to measure O_2 saturation
2. Clear nasal passages with bulb syringe; elevate head of bed
3. Cluster nursing care to allow for rest; monitor anxiety level of parents and provide support; maintain a calm environment
4. IV fluids may be needed if oral intake is compromised; monitor strict I&O; weigh daily to measure fluid loss
5. Maintain strict hand hygiene and contact precautions; caregivers should not care for other high-risk children
6. Medications: bronchodilators and steroids are sometimes used; prevention of bronchiolitis in high-risk children under age 2 may be achieved with use of palivizumab (Synagis) or IV RSV immunoglobulin

D. Reinforce child and family teaching

1. Disease process and provide support to lessen anxiety
2. How to assist in care of infant; explain all procedures and treatments
3. How to use bulb syringe as needed to keep nasal passages clear
4. Need to provide frequent oral fluids; notify physician if child demonstrates symptoms of dehydration, including crying without tears, sunken eyes, lethargy, or "acts sick"
5. Notify physician if child refuses to eat or breathing becomes worse
6. How and why to use humidifier in child's bedroom
7. Need to avoid smoking in child's vicinity
8. Importance of strict hand hygiene and keeping child away from those with upper respiratory infections; RSV can reoccur

XX. *FOREIGN BODY ASPIRATION*

A. Overview

1. Inhalation of an object into respiratory tract, intentional or otherwise
2. Peak age for foreign body aspiration is children under 3 years; is a leading cause of death in children under 1 year
3. Foreign bodies usually lodge in right main bronchus (which is shorter and wider than left); obstruction may be partial or complete and causes atelectasis, air trapping, and hyperinflation distal to site of obstruction
4. *NCLEX®* The type and shape of object, as well as small diameter of an infant's airway, determine severity of problem; round objects such as hot dogs, round candy, nuts, and grapes do not break apart and are more likely to occlude airway; latex balloons are particularly hazardous; objects with irregular shapes may irritate airway and partially obstruct airflow
5. Failure to remove a foreign object is usually fatal; a delay in removal may cause aspiration pneumonia

NCLEX® **B. Data collection**

1. Sudden coughing and gagging is first sign, and objects in upper airway may be expelled by coughing
2. Partial obstruction may cause symptoms of respiratory infection for days or even weeks; child may have hoarseness, croupy cough, wheezing, and dyspnea
3. If obstruction is complete, child will demonstrate stridor, cyanosis, difficulty swallowing and speaking
4. A child who cannot speak, is cyanotic, and collapses requires immediate attention for complete airway obstruction
5. Fluoroscopy and chest x-ray reveal foreign body in respiratory tract

NCLEX® **C. Therapeutic management**

1. Monitor respiratory status to determine severity of problem and degree of obstruction; continuously monitor and provide assistance if obstruction worsens
2. If total airway obstruction occurs, perform back blows and chest thrusts for infants and Heimlich maneuver in children older than 1 year
3. Keep NPO; foreign body is usually removed in surgery
4. Position for comfort and to optimize airway; provide emotional support to parents and child and alleviate anxiety
5. After removal of object, examine for additional obstruction that may result from laryngeal edema and tissue swelling
6. Medications: antibiotics may be administered if secondary infection is suspected, or if purulent secretions are present in airway, with or without signs of pneumonia

D. Reinforce child and family teaching

1. Hazards leading to aspiration and importance of child-proofing home
2. Age-appropriate foods and most frequently aspirated objects: coins, hot dogs, balloons, nuts, popcorn, grapes, round candy, peanut butter
3. Toy safety and avoiding toys with small, removable parts; caution against allowing child to run and play with objects in mouth
4. Importance of knowing CPR and techniques of chest thrusts, back blows, abdominal thrusts

Check Your NCLEX-PN® Exam I.Q.

You are ready for testing on this content if you can

- Identify basic structures and functions of the respiratory system.
- Describe the pathophysiology and etiology of common respiratory disorders.
- Discuss expected data and diagnostic test findings for selected respiratory disorders.
- Discuss therapeutic management of a client experiencing a respiratory disorder.
- Discuss nursing management of a client experiencing a respiratory disorder.
- Identify expected outcomes for the client experiencing a respiratory disorder.

PRACTICE TEST

PRACTICE TEST

1 What should the nurse reinforce regarding health maintenance strategies to the client with chronic obstructive pulmonary disease (COPD)? Select all that apply.

1. Yearly influenza immunization
2. Immunization against pneumonia
3. Limitation of physical activity
4. Oral fluid restriction
5. Adequate caloric intake

2 The nurse who is explaining the pathophysiology of chronic obstructive pulmonary disease (COPD) to a client includes the fact that alveolar destruction results in which manifestations? Select all that apply.

1. Decreased surface area for gas exchange
2. Increased dead space air
3. Development of pulmonary emboli
4. Chronic dilation of bronchioles
5. Airway collapse related to loss of elasticity

3 A client who develops acute respiratory distress syndrome (ARDS) is exhibiting hypoxemia unresponsive to oxygen therapy. What concept should the nurse reinforce when working with the family regarding the client's condition?

1. Blood is shunted past alveoli with no ventilation.
2. The individual has difficulty expelling air trapped in the alveoli.
3. There is excess surfactant production by the alveoli.
4. Thick secretions block the airways.

4 What intervention should the nurse identify as the priority for the client with a nursing diagnosis of Ineffective Airway Clearance related to tumor mass?

1. Provision of supplemental oxygen.
2. Keep the head of the bed elevated.
3. Coughing, deep breathing, and hydration maintenance.
4. Preparation for insertion of a tracheostomy tube.

5 When assisting with psychological issues for the client with lung cancer, which epidemiological factor should the nurse keep in mind?

1. The 5-year survival rate for lung cancer is less than 15 percent.
2. Symptoms usually occur early during lung cancer progression.
3. Tumor growth usually begins in a bronchus, and then migrates upward in the tissue.
4. Risk of lung cancer is associated with length of exposure to cigarette smoking.

6 A client is hospitalized with a diagnosis of pneumonia. Which findings, based on the nurse's knowledge, are indicative of a deteriorating clinical state? Select all that apply.

1. Increased respiratory rate
2. Tachycardia
3. Agitation
4. Cyanosis
5. Increased urinary output

7 For the hospitalized client, which manifestation would the nurse recognize as a symptom of pulmonary embolism?

1. Slow increase in heart rate and respiratory rate
2. Cyanosis of the upper torso
3. Abrupt onset of dyspnea and apprehension
4. Significant bilateral wheezing

8 A client underwent a thoracentesis a few hours earlier. What finding should the nurse report immediately to the registered nurse?

1. Oozing of blood from the puncture site
2. Onset of crepitus
3. Diminished sounds in the affected lung base would occur with atelectasis.
4. Fever that is gradually elevating

9 The nurse assisting the client with obstructive pulmonary disease would use which of the following statements to explain why dyspnea occurs?

1. "Decreased surfactant causes many of your alveoli to collapse."
2. "You have difficulty breathing in enough air."
3. "Your airways open wider on inspiration, and trap air on expiration."
4. "Your lung compliance is decreased."

10 A client is admitted to the hospital with a medical diagnosis of viral pneumonia. The nurse needs to monitor for which of the following most frequent manifestations? Select all that apply.

1. Presence of Ghon's tubercle on chest x-ray
2. Nonproductive cough
3. Normal or near normal white blood cell count
4. High fever that is intermittent
5. Profuse pleural diffusion on chest x-ray

11 The nurse would question an order for ipratropium bromide (Atrovent) to be administered to a client with asthma if the client had which concurrent medical history?

1. Glaucoma
2. Cushing's syndrome
3. Warfarin therapy
4. Fluid retention

12 A client newly diagnosed with asthma has infrequent acute episodes. The nurse should reinforce which teaching concept regarding the medication that is most effective for providing quick relief in acute episodes?

1. Corticosteroid via metered-dose inhaler as needed
2. Beta-agonist via metered-dose inhaler
3. Anti-inflammatory via metered-dose inhaler
4. Daily use of a bronchodilator inhaler

13 The nurse caring for a client diagnosed with acute respiratory distress syndrome (ARDS) should consider that, in this client, impaired gas exchange is mostly likely related to which factor?

1. Air trapping in the alveoli
2. Accumulation of exudative fluid into the alveoli
3. Shunting of blood around nonventilated alveoli
4. Excessive alpha-1-antitrypsin

14 A child with laryngotracheobronchitis (LTB) is being treated in the emergency department. What action should the nurse do to ease respiratory distress? Select all that apply.

1. Place the child in a high-Fowler's position.
2. Administer racemic epinephrine.
3. Administer corticosteroids.
4. Administer intravenous antibiotics.
5. Ask parent to help keep child calm.

15 The parents of an infant with bronchiolitis ask the nurse why their baby's room has a sign on the door that says "Contact Precautions," and why the nurses all wear gowns and gloves when they hold him. What is the nurse's best response?

1. "Extra precautions prevent the virus from spreading to other babies."
2. "Your baby is very ill, we don't want to have another baby catch what he has."
3. "It's because we need to protect your baby from other illnesses."
4. "We always wear gowns when babies are coughing."

16 What would be a priority nursing intervention for a child with bronchiolitis?

1. Keep the child well stimulated.
2. Maintain strict intake and output.
3. Encourage visitors.
4. Encourage oral fluids, if tachypneic.

17 When taking the nursing history of a child with cystic fibrosis, what piece of information about the child's newborn period would the nurse expect the mother to report?

1. That the child required resuscitation in the delivery room
2. That labor was longer than 24 hours
3. That the child had a meconium ileus
4. That labor was less than 4 hours

PRACTICE TEST

18 The parents of a child with asthma are about to perform postural drainage exercises. The nurse should observe to see if the parents perform which action first before continuing with the exercises?

1. Administer the child's bronchodilator.
2. Change the child's clothes.
3. Administer the child's antibiotic.
4. Suction the child's throat.

19 What symptom should the nurse monitor for to indicate that the treatment of acute epiglottitis in a child was effective?

1. Pale lips and mucous membranes
2. Maintains tripod position
3. Tachypneic and dysphonic
4. Clear, bilateral breath sounds

20 The parents of a child with bronchopulmonary dysplasia (BPD) are performing tracheostomy care. With regard to suctioning, the nurse should monitor that the parents are taking no longer than _____ seconds with each suction pass. Provide a numerical answer.

Fill in your answer below:

_____ seconds

21 A young toddler is being discharged after an emergency admission for foreign body aspiration. The parents ask what they can do to prevent another accident. What advice is appropriate for the nurse to give the parents?

1. Watch the child very carefully.
2. Reinforce to the child not to eat nonfood items.
3. Keep small objects and toys out of the child's reach.
4. Keep the child under continuous observation while awake.

22 The nurse wears gloves when working with a child with respiratory syncytial virus (RSV). After removing the gloves, what should be the nurse's next action?

1. Discard the gloves in the laundry basket.
2. Inspect the gloves for holes or fraying.
3. Remind the parents to wear gloves.
4. Perform careful hand hygiene.

23 A 6-year-old child is hospitalized following an acute asthmatic episode. Which statement by the parents indicates the need for the nurse to further reinforce teaching?

1. "Next time, we'll be sure he takes his cromolyn before soccer."
2. "After this episode, he will need to quit the swim team."
3. "We think this was an exercise-induced asthma episode."
4. "We need to make sure he has his inhaler at all times."

24 The nurse is preparing to administer respiratory medications to a child hospitalized with asthma. By which most frequently used route will the medication be administered?

1. Aerosol
2. Intravenous
3. Subcutaneous
4. Oral

25 The nurse anticipates using postural drainage as a treatment modality for which of the following conditions?

1. Epiglottitis
2. Foreign body aspiration
3. Cystic fibrosis
4. Bronchopulmonary dysplasia

26 The nurse attaches a spacer to the metered-dose inhaler for a young child. What is the purpose of the spacer?

1. Makes the device look less intimidating to a small child
2. Makes it unnecessary to shake the inhaler before administering the drug
3. Concentrates the medication in the upper respiratory tract
4. Reduces the risk for oral yeast by depositing medication more deeply into the airways

27 The nurse documents which expected finding after auscultating the lungs of a child with bacterial pneumonia?

1. Wheezes
2. Crackles
3. Apnea
4. Retractions

28. An infant with respiratory syncytial virus (RSV) is receiving ribavirin. While caring for this infant, what actions should the nurse avoid? Select all that apply.

1. Maintaining contact precautions
2. Clearing nasal passages with a bulb syringe
3. Wearing contact lenses
4. Staying in the room with the door closed
5. Caring for other high-risk children

29. The mother of an infant who has had recurrent respiratory infections asks the nurse why infants are at increased risk for complications from respiratory infections. The best response by the nurse provides which explanation about infants?

1. The airway structures are larger, allowing for entry of a greater number of organisms.
2. The respiratory rate is slower than in adults.
3. Parents are unable to monitor respiratory problems accurately.
4. The airways are narrower and more easily obstructed.

30. One day postoperative, the client reports dyspnea, respiratory rate (RR) is 35, slightly labored, and there are no breath sounds in the lower-right base. The nurse would suspect which of the following?

1. Cor pulmonale
2. Atelectasis
3. Pulmonary embolus
4. Cardiac tamponade

ANSWERS & RATIONALES

1. **Answer: 1, 2, 5 Rationale:** Clients with COPD are highly susceptible to respiratory infections such as influenza, so they should be immunized yearly. Clients with COPD are highly susceptible to respiratory infections such as pneumonia so they should be immunized as prescribed by their physician. Clients with COPD use a large amount of calories because of labored respiratory function; increased caloric intake is necessary to maintain a healthy weight. Clients with COPD should undergo a progressive rehabilitation program to increase their activity tolerance. Fluid restriction is not needed with COPD unless there is fluid retention from another etiology. **Cognitive Level:** Applying **Client Need:** Health Promotion and Maintenance **Integrated Process:** Teaching and Learning **Content Area:** Adult Health **Strategy:** The critical words in the stem of the question are *health maintenance*. This phrase indicates that you should focus on the option that prevents a health problem rather than diagnoses or treats it. When there is more than one correct answer, consider each option as a true/false statement.

2. **Answer: 1, 5 Rationale:** The loss of elasticity in the airway of a client with COPD can be attributed to repeated infections and inflammation, which leads to airway collapse. Airway collapse can cause alveolar destruction because of either over- or under-inflation of alveolar sacs. The impaired gas exchange occurring with COPD is caused by the loss of alveolar surface area available for gas exchange. Destruction of alveoli is not related to increased dead space air, pulmonary emboli, or chronic dilation of bronchioles. With COPD, there is progressive narrowing of bronchioles. **Cognitive Level:** Analyzing **Client Need:** Physiological Adaptation **Integrated Process:** Communication and Documentation **Content Area:** Adult Health **Strategy:** The core issue of the question is the nature of the pathophysiology of COPD. Use general nursing knowledge and the process of elimination to make a selection. When more than one answer is correct, consider each option as a true/false statement.

3. **Answer: 1 Rationale:** One of the primary alterations occurring with ARDS is the collapse of alveoli and therefore loss of ventilation in those areas. Air does not become trapped in hyperinflated alveoli in ARDS; instead, alveoli collapse. Surfactant production decreases with ARDS, a factor that impairs adequate gas exchange. One of the primary alterations occurring with ARDS is the collapse of alveoli and therefore loss of ventilation in those areas; thick secretions blocking the airways are not a consideration. **Cognitive Level:** Applying **Client Need:** Physiological Adaptation **Integrated Process:** Teaching and Learning **Content Area:** Adult Health **Strategy:** The core issues of the question are an understanding of disease process and how to select appropriate concepts for family education. Use nursing knowledge and the process of elimination to make a selection.

4. **Answer: 3 Rationale:** Coughing, deep breathing, and adequate hydration are essential for achieving effective airway clearance. The provision of supplemental oxygen is important, but it is not related to the nursing diagnosis of Ineffective Airway Clearance. Elevating the head of the bed might help the client to cough more forcefully, but head elevation alone is not an effective maneuver related to Ineffective Airway Clearance. Insertion of a tracheostomy is not a primary treatment to maintain airway clearance. **Cognitive Level:** Analyzing **Client Need:** Physiological Adaptation **Integrated Process:** Nursing Process: Implementation **Content Area:** Adult Health **Strategy:** The critical word in the stem of the question is *priority*, which tells you that more than one option could be correct, and you must choose the most important one. Use nursing knowledge and the process of elimination to make a selection.

5. **Answer: 1 Rationale:** The nurse should help the client and family to approach the diagnosis of lung cancer from a realistic perspective. Symptoms of lung cancer usually appear late in the course of the disease. Tumor growth does typically begin in a bronchus and progress upward, but this

information has no relation to the client's psychological adaptation to the disease. The risk of lung cancer is associated with multiple causes, with exposure to cigarette smoking being just one factor. **Cognitive Level:** Applying **Client Need:** Psychosocial Integrity **Integrated Process:** Communication and Documentation **Content Area:** Adult Health **Strategy:** The core issue of the question is the knowledge of the interrelationship between prognosis and the communication approaches used by the nurse. Use nursing knowledge and the process of elimination to make a selection.

6 **Answer: 1, 2, 3, 4 Rationale:** Increased respiratory rate, tachycardia, and agitation are early signs of respiratory distress, and can be interpreted by the nurse as deteriorating clinical state. Cyanosis develops later in the progression of respiratory distress, but is still an indication of client deterioration. Increased urinary output is the opposite of what the nurse would expect in a client with respiratory distress whose condition is deteriorating. **Cognitive Level:** Analyzing **Client Need:** Physiological Adaptation **Integrated Process:** Nursing Process: Data Collection **Content Area:** Adult Health **Strategy:** The critical word in the stem of the question is *deteriorating*, which indicates that the nurse should be collecting data for both early and late manifestations of respiratory distress. In an adult, cyanosis is always a late sign; but is occurs early in children. Use nursing knowledge and the process of elimination to make a selection. When there is more than one correct answer, consider each option as a true/false statement.

7 **Answer: 3 Rationale:** Symptoms associated with pulmonary embolism typically have a sudden onset. The client often feels panic because of the sudden dyspnea. Increase in heart rate and respiratory rate is abrupt, not slow, with a pulmonary embolism. Cyanosis of the upper torso is associated with embolism of a central vein other than the pulmonary vasculature. Bilateral wheezing is more often associated with asthma than with pulmonary embolism. **Cognitive Level:** Applying **Client Need:** Physiological Adaptation **Integrated Process:** Nursing Process: Data Collection **Content Area:** Adult Health **Strategy:** The critical words in the stem of the question are *symptom* and *pulmonary embolism*. They tell you that the question is seeking an answer that is a correct data collection. Use nursing knowledge and the process of elimination to make a selection.

8 **Answer: 2 Rationale:** The finding of crepitus at any time is associated with pneumothorax, and should be reported immediately to the physician. Oozing of blood from the thoracentesis puncture site is not uncommon, and does not require emergency intervention, as would crepitus. Diminished sounds in the affected side might or might not be related to the thoracentesis. Fever might or might not be related to the thoracentesis. **Cognitive Level:** Analyzing **Client Need:** Physiological Adaptation **Integrated Process:** Nursing Process: Data Collection **Content Area:** Adult Health **Strategy:** The core issue of the question is the ability to recognize and prioritize complications that need to be reported to the health care provider. Use nursing knowledge and the process of elimination to make a selection.

9 **Answer: 3 Rationale:** The primary physiological alterations occurring with COPD are alveolar air trapping and alveolar hyperinflation, which lead to alveolar rupture and loss of area available for gas exchange. Decreased surfactant production is associated with ARDS, and is not a primary alteration of COPD. The difficulty that a COPD client has with breathing in is related to alveolar air trapping and hyperinflation; newly inhaled air has no place to enter. Lung compliance is decreased, but this is due to the alveolar air trapping and hyperinflation. **Cognitive Level:** Applying **Client Need:** Physiological Adaptation **Integrated Process:** Teaching and Learning **Content Area:** Adult Health **Strategy:** The core issues of the question are knowledge of the underlying changes associated with COPD and how to communicate that information effectively to a client or family. Use nursing knowledge and the process of elimination to make a selection.

10 **Answer: 2, 3 Rationale:** Viral pneumonia is considered less serious for the client because symptoms are not as apparent compared with bacterial pneumonia. Viral pneumonia is associated with a nonproductive cough and normal or near normal white blood cell count. Ghon's tubercles are seen on x-ray in clients with tuberculosis. Viral pneumonia is associated with low-grade fever. The client with viral pneumonia will display normal or minimal chest x-ray findings. **Cognitive Level:** Analyzing **Client Need:** Physiological Adaptation **Integrated Process:** Nursing Process: Data Collection **Content Area:** Adult Health **Strategy:** The critical words in the stem are *most frequent*. With this in mind, you must compare options in terms of their frequency. Use nursing knowledge and the process of elimination to make a selection. When there is more than one correct answer, consider each option as a true/false statement.

11 **Answer: 1 Rationale:** Anticholinergics such as ipratropium are contraindicated in clients with angle-closure glaucoma because they can inhibit flow of aqueous humor and raise intraocular pressure. The other medical conditions would not cause the nurse to question an order for Atrovent. **Cognitive Level:** Applying **Client Need:** Pharmacological and Parenteral Therapies **Integrated Process:** Nursing Process: Implementation **Content Area:** Adult Health **Strategy:** The core issue of the question is knowledge of contraindications to medication therapy. Use nursing knowledge and the process of elimination to make a selection.

12 **Answer: 2 Rationale:** Clients with mild and infrequent asthma symptoms are treated with a short-acting beta-agonist inhaler for quick relief in acute episodes. Corticosteroids as oral or inhaled medication are used for clients with more severe and frequent episodes of asthma. Clients with mild and infrequent asthma symptoms are treated with regular *daily* administration of an anti-inflammatory inhaler. Bronchodilators as oral or inhaled medication are used for clients with more severe and frequent episodes of asthma. **Cognitive Level:** Applying **Client Need:** Physiological Adaptation **Integrated Process:** Nursing Process: Planning **Content Area:** Adult Health **Strategy:** The core issue of the question is knowledge of the rapid management of symptoms in a client with asthma. Use nursing knowledge and the process of elimination to make a selection.

13 **Answer: 3 Rationale:** A primary physiological alteration occurring with ARDS is shunting of blood around nonventilated alveoli. Alveoli collapse in ARDS, preventing air from entering the alveoli, and ventilation decreases. The development of ARDS is not associated with the accumulation of exudative fluid in the alveoli or excessive alpha-1-antitrypsin. A primary physiological alteration occurring with ARDS is shunting of blood around nonventilated alveoli. Blood perfusing to these areas cannot undergo adequate gas exchange. **Cognitive Level:** Applying **Client Need:** Physiological

Adaptation **Integrated Process:** Nursing Process: Implementation **Content Area:** Adult Health **Strategy:** The core issue of the question is knowledge of pathophysiology in the development of ARDS. Use nursing knowledge and the process of elimination to make a selection.

14 **Answer: 1, 2, 5** **Rationale:** The best position is semi- to high-Fowler's position. Epinephrine is a bronchodilator used to increase the diameter of the airways. Calming the child will ease respiratory function; crying and anxiety will cause an escalation in respiratory distress. Corticosteroids may be used, but will not ease respiratory distress immediately. Antibiotics may be used, but will not ease respiratory distress immediately. **Cognitive Level:** Analyzing **Client Need:** Physiological Adaptation **Integrated Process:** Nursing Process: Implementation **Content Area:** Child Health **Strategy:** The core issue of the question is the expected plan of care for a client with laryngotracheobronchitis. Use nursing knowledge and the process of elimination to make a selection. When there is more than one correct answer, consider each option as a true/false statement.

15 **Answer: 1** **Rationale:** RSV is the cause of bronchiolitis in most cases; RSV can live for several hours on nonporous surfaces, and can be transferred by the hands; gowns and gloves will prevent the nurses from spreading the RSV to other clients. The infant with RSV does not need to be protected from other illnesses; the objective is to protect the virus from spreading to other children. The nurse's statement should be therapeutic and not cause the parents additional stress. **Cognitive Level:** Analyzing **Client Need:** Physiological Adaptation **Integrated Process:** Nursing Process: Implementation **Content Area:** Child Health **Strategy:** The core issue of the question is the ability of the nurse to explain the rationale and use of isolation techniques. Use nursing knowledge and the process of elimination to make a selection.

16 **Answer: 2** **Rationale:** Maintaining strict I&O will provide immediate notification of signs of dehydration; children with bronchiolitis could already have a history of poor fluid intake when initially seen by medical personnel. The child with bronchiolitis should be kept quiet, with limited stimulation and visitors. Limited visitors will prevent over stimulation and promote a quiet environment. If the child is tachypneic, oral fluids present a risk of aspiration; fluids would be provided intravenously. **Cognitive Level:** Analyzing **Client Need:** Physiological Adaptation **Integrated Process:** Nursing Process: Implementation **Content Area:** Child Health **Strategy:** The core issue of the question is knowledge that a client with bronchiolitis has a priority need for hydration. Use nursing knowledge and the process of elimination to make a selection.

17 **Answer: 3** **Rationale:** Meconium ileus in the newborn period is often the first indication of cystic fibrosis. The other options are not indications that a child has cystic fibrosis. **Cognitive Level:** Applying **Client Need:** Physiological Adaptation **Integrated Process:** Nursing Process: Data Collection **Content Area:** Child Health **Strategy:** The core issue of the question is knowledge of the association between meconium ileus and cystic fibrosis in the neonate. Use nursing knowledge and the process of elimination to make a selection.

18 **Answer: 1** **Rationale:** Bronchodilators open the airways and afford easier removal of secretions. Changing the child's clothes prior to the postural drainage exercises is unnecessary. Administering the child's antibiotic before the postural drainage is not necessary. Suctioning of the child's throat could be done after the procedure, if necessary. **Cognitive Level:** Analyzing **Client Need:** Physiological Adaptation **Integrated Process:** Nursing Process: Implementation **Content Area:** Child Health **Strategy:** The core issue of the question is knowledge of the proper sequence of actions when a client undergoes chest physiotherapy. Use nursing knowledge and the process of elimination to make a selection.

19 **Answer: 4** **Rationale:** Clear breath sounds indicate effective airway clearance and decreased mucosal swelling and obstruction. Pale lips and mucous membranes could indicate hypoxia. Tripod position is a clinical manifestation of a child in distress due to epiglottitis. Tachypneic and dysphonic are symptoms of the disease. **Cognitive Level:** Analyzing **Client Need:** Physiological Adaptation **Integrated Process:** Nursing Process: Data Collection **Content Area:** Child Health **Strategy:** The core issue of this question is correctly identifying when an appropriate outcome measure has been achieved. Use nursing knowledge and the process of elimination to make a selection.

20 **Answer: 5** **Rationale:** Tracheostomy suctioning can be stressful to the child, and increases risk for hypoxia, infection, and mucosal damage. Each pass of the suction catheter should be limited to no more than 5 seconds, and the child should be allowed to rest between passes with supplemental oxygen, if needed. **Cognitive Level:** Applying **Client Need:** Physiological Adaptation **Integrated Process:** Nursing Process: Implementation **Content Area:** Child Health **Strategy:** The critical issue of this question is the appropriate length of time for suctioning without impairing the respiratory status of a child. Use nursing knowledge to make a selection.

21 **Answer: 3** **Rationale:** Toddlers should be supervised but this may not be sufficient to prevent aspiration of another object if the environment has not been cleared of unsafe objects. This advice is judgmental, implying that the parents did not watch the child carefully enough to prevent the accident. It is developmentally inappropriate to attempt to reinforce teaching to a toddler to stop normal hand-to-mouth activity. While toddlers need to be observed and supervised, it may not be possible to monitor them continually. **Cognitive Level:** Applying **Client Need:** Safety and Infection Control **Integrated Process:** Nursing Process: Implementation **Content Area:** Child Health **Strategy:** The core issue of the question is the best method to provide a safe environment for a toddler, while understanding the normal patterns of growth and development. Use nursing knowledge and the process of elimination to make a selection.

22 **Answer: 4** **Rationale:** Hand hygiene is the most important infection control practice, and decreases the spread of RSV and other organisms. Gloves worn when working with a child with RSV should be discarded in the trash basket. Defects in gloves should be noted before they are worn to work with a client. An activity is not as timely immediately after glove removal because the nurse is still engaged in infection control activities. **Cognitive Level:** Applying **Client Need:** Safety and Infection Control **Integrated Process:** Nursing Process: Implementation **Content Area:** Child Health **Strategy:** The core issue of the question is basic principles of infection control using medical asepsis. Use nursing knowledge and the process of elimination to make a selection.

23 **Answer: 2** **Rationale:** Swimming is recommended for children with asthma because prolonged expiration under water is

ANSWERS & RATIONALES

beneficial. Cromolyn sodium is used prophylactically to prevent exercise-induced asthma. When an asthma episode occurs in conjunction with high-level physical activity, it is considered to be an exercise-induced episode. Immediate access to a rescue inhaler is recommended. **Cognitive Level:** Analyzing **Client Need:** Physiological Adaptation **Integrated Process:** Teaching and Learning **Content Area:** Child Health **Strategy:** The core issue of the question is an understanding of the relationship of exercise to episodes of asthma. Use nursing knowledge and the process of elimination to make a selection. When the stem of a question is negative, look for the option that is wrong.

24 **Answer: 1** **Rationale:** Aerosol therapy such as a nebulizer is frequently used during hospitalization to administer medications. An advantage is that this route delivers medication directly to the airways. Intravenous is not a frequently used route to administer respiratory medications to a child hospitalized with asthma. Some respiratory drugs can be administered subcutaneously but aerosol is most direct. Oral respiratory medications take time to be effective. **Cognitive Level:** Applying **Client Need:** Pharmacological and Parenteral Therapies **Integrated Process:** Nursing Process: Implementation **Content Area:** Child Health **Strategy:** The core issue of the question is an understanding of medication routes used in children, specifically those with respiratory problems. Use nursing knowledge and the process of elimination to make a selection.

25 **Answer: 3** **Rationale:** Chest physiotherapy and postural drainage for children with cystic fibrosis help loosen pulmonary secretions and facilitate removal from airways. This treatment would not be helpful with the other conditions listed. **Cognitive Level:** Applying **Client Need:** Physiological Adaptation **Integrated Process:** Nursing Process: Planning **Content Area:** Child Health **Strategy:** The core issue of the question is the purpose of doing chest physiotherapy in a child with cystic fibrosis. Use nursing knowledge and the process of elimination to make a selection.

26 **Answer: 4** **Rationale:** Steroids given via metered-dose inhaler on oral mucosa increase the risk for yeast infection. A spacer avoids the mucous membranes and works directly on the airways. The purpose of the spacer is not related to the appearance of the inhaler. Use of a spacer on a metered-dose inhaler does not change the need to shake the medication before administration. It is desirable for the medication to penetrate into the lower respiratory tract to be most effective. **Cognitive Level:** Applying **Client Need:** Safety and Infection Control **Integrated Process:** Nursing Process: Implementation **Content Area:** Child Health **Strategy:** The core issue of the question is the rationale for using a spacer. Use nursing knowledge and the process of elimination to make a selection.

27 **Answer: 2** **Rationale:** Excess fluid in the alveoli is a manifestation of bacterial pneumonia. The sound produced by fluid in the airways is crackles. Wheezes are often typical of pneumonia caused by RSV, or conditions where the air passages are narrowed, such as asthma. Apnea is a pause in respirations, which is under the control of the central nervous system. Retractions are asymmetrical chest wall movements that are seen in any client having respiratory difficulty. **Cognitive Level:** Analyzing **Client Need:** Physiological Adaptation **Integrated Process:** Communication and Documentation **Content Area:** Child Health **Strategy:** The core issue of the question is the type of adventitious breath sound that is expected in bacterial pneumonia. Eliminate apnea because the focus is respiratory, not the central nervous system. Eliminate retractions next because they are seen rather than heard. Choose crackles over wheezes, recalling that the infection process leads to fluid accumulation, not to bronchoconstriction.

28 **Answer: 3, 5** **Rationale:** Ribavirin is an antiviral drug used to treat RSV, which causes crystallization of soft contact lenses, and is associated with conjunctivitis. Because RSV is easily transferred, it is advisable that the nurse caring for the child with the virus not care for other high-risk children. Strict hand hygiene and contact precautions will help prevent transfer of the virus. Clearing the nasal passages with a bulb syringe will promote breathing; infants are nose breathers and are not able to blow their noses. Staying in the room with the door closed will help prevent the transfer of RSV. **Cognitive Level:** Applying **Client Need:** Safety and Infection Control **Integrated Process:** Nursing Process: Planning **Content Area:** Child Health **Strategy:** The core issue of the question is providing care for a client with RSV. Because the stem of the question is negative, the correct answers address actions that should not be taken by the nurse. When more than one answer is correct, consider each option as a true/false statement.

29 **Answer: 4** **Rationale:** Infants and young children have narrower airways, and shorter distance between structures; accessory muscles generally used for breathing are immature. The respiratory rate of infants is faster than that of adults, and parents can be taught to monitor the child for respiratory problems. **Cognitive Level:** Analyzing **Client Need:** Physiological Adaptation **Integrated Process:** Nursing Process: Implementation **Content Area:** Child Health **Strategy:** Critical words are *why infants are at increased risk for complications from respiratory infections*. The core knowledge is the physiological differences between infants and older children. After eliminating two options as inaccurate; recall infant anatomy to choose correctly.

30 **Answer: 2** **Rationale:** The first three symptoms could be indicative of any of the conditions. The distinguishing symptom is the lack of breath sounds in the lower right base when a portion of the lung has collapsed. Three symptoms could be indicative of any of the conditions. The distinguishing symptom is the lack of breath sounds in the lower right base when a portion of the lung has collapsed. **Cognitive Level:** Analyzing **Client Need:** Physiological Adaptation **Integrated Process:** Nursing Process: Planning **Content Area:** Adult Health **Strategy:** Select the option that is common in the postoperative period, atelectasis.

ANSWERS & RATIONALES

Key Terms to Review

alveolar ventilation p. 847
alveoli p. 847
atelectasis p. 856
barrel chest p. 855
bronchopulmonary dysplasia (BPD) p. 865
compliance p. 847
diffusion p. 848
digital clubbing p. 864
dyspnea p. 856
epiglottitis p. 867
expiration p. 847
foreign body aspiration p. 869
inspiration p. 847
laryngotracheobronchitis p. 866
oxygen saturation p. 849
perfusion p. 848
pulmonary ventilation p. 847
respiration p. 847
sweat test p. 864
tachypnea p. 856
trigger p. 856
ventilation–perfusion mismatch p. 856

References

Ball, J., Bindler, R., & Cowen, K. (2010). *Child health nursing: Partnering with children and families* (2nd ed.). Upper Saddle River, NJ: Pearson Education.

Berman, A., & Snyder, S. (2012). *Kozier & Erb's fundamentals of nursing: Concepts, process, and practice* (9th ed.). Upper Saddle River, NJ: Pearson Education.

Black, J., & Hawks, J. (2009). *Medical surgical nursing: Clinical management for positive outcomes* (8th ed.). Philadelphia: Saunders.

Ignatavicius, D., & Workman, L. (2010). *Medical-surgical nursing: Patient-centered collaborative care* (6th ed.). Philadelphia: Saunders.

LeMone, P., Burke, K., & Bauldoff, G. (2011). *Medical surgical nursing: Critical thinking in patient care* (5th ed.). Upper Saddle River, NJ: Pearson Education.

Lewis, S., Heitkemper, M., & Bucher, L. (2011). *Medical surgical nursing: Assessment and management of clinical problems* (8th ed.). St. Louis, MO: Elsevier.

Smeltzer, S., Bare, B., Hinkle, J., & Cheever, K. (2010). *Brunner & Suddarth's textbook of medical surgical nursing:* (12th ed.). Philadelphia: Lippincott Williams & Wilkins.

Smith, S., Duell, D., & Martin, B. (2012). *Clinical nursing skills: Basic to advanced skills* (8th ed.). Upper Saddle River, NJ: Pearson Education.

Test Yourself

Are you ready for the NCLEX-PN® or course exams? Use the practice tests on the companion website to check.

52 Cardiovascular Disorders

In this chapter

Cross Reference

Other chapters relevant to this content area are

Cardiovascular Medications **Chapter 34**
Common Laboratory Tests **Chapter 42**
Common Diagnostic Tests and Procedures **Chapter 43**

I. OVERVIEW OF ANATOMY AND PHYSIOLOGY OF CARDIOVASCULAR SYSTEM

A. Structures of heart

1. Hollow muscular organ enclosed in a protective sac, divided into four chambers—two atria and two ventricles—divided by septum into right and left sides
2. Heart wall has three layers: *epicardium*, fibrous outside protective layer; *myocardium*, middle layer of specialized cardiac muscle; *endocardium*, endothelial lining of chambers
3. *Pericardium*: protective sac encasing heart
4. Valves of heart
   - **a.** Atrioventricular (AV) valves (tricuspid on right and mitral on left) separate and control blood flow between atria and ventricles
   - **b.** Semilunar valves (pulmonic on right and aortic on left) separate ventricles from pulmonary artery and aorta, respectively, and control blood flow from heart
   - **c.** S_1, first heart sound ("lub"), is heard when AV valves close during systole
   - **d.** S_2, second heart sound ("dub"), is heard when semilunar valves close during diastole
5. Coronary circulation
   - **a.** Left anterior descending (LAD) artery supplies anterior left ventricle, anterior ventricular septum, and left ventricle apex; circumflex artery supplies left atrium and lateral and posterior left ventricle
   - **b.** Right coronary artery (RCA): supplies right atrium and ventricle, inferior left ventricle, posterior septal wall, and sinoatrial (SA) and atrioventricular (AV) nodes

B. Functions of heart

1. Circulation: right side circulates deoxygenated blood to lungs; left side pumps oxygenated blood throughout body to perfuse tissues
2. Coronary arteries branch off aorta to supply oxygenated blood to heart
3. Cardiac conduction system transmits electrical impulses, stimulates depolarization and cardiac muscle contraction; cells have electrophysiologic properties: *automaticity* (ability to initiate an electrical impulse), *excitability* (ability of a cell to respond to a stimulus), and *conductivity* (ability to transmit impulses from one cell to another); see Table 52–1
4. Cardiac cycle: one complete heartbeat; includes two parts—systole (ventricular contraction) and diastole (relaxation and ventricular refilling)
5. **Cardiac output (CO)**: volume of blood in liters ejected by heart each minute; indicator of pumping function of heart; normal adult CO is 4–8 L/min

   $$CO = HR \times SV$$

   - **a.** Heart rate (HR): number of complete cardiac cycles per minute
   - **b.** **Stroke volume (SV)**: volume of blood ejected from left ventricle with each cardiac cycle; SV and ultimately CO are influenced by preload, afterload, and contractility
   - **c.** **Preload**: degree of myocardial fiber stretch at end of ventricular diastole; influenced by ventricular filling volume and myocardial compliance
   - **d.** **Afterload**: resistance that ventricles must overcome to eject blood into systemic circulation; directly related to arterial blood pressure (BP)
   - **e.** **Contractility**: strength of contraction regardless of preload; decreased by hypoxia and some drugs (e.g., beta-blockers and calcium channel blockers); increased by drugs (e.g., digoxin and dopamine)

Table 52–1 Functions within Cardiac Conduction System

Area	Function
Sinoatrial (SA) node	Natural pacemaker; generates heart rate normally at 60 to 100 beats per minute (bpm)
Internodal pathways	Carry impulse from SA node to AV node; depolarization results in myocardial contraction of both atria
AV node	Slows electrical impulse; allows atria to fully empty before transmitting impulse to depolarize ventricles; when SA node is not functioning, AV node can initiate an impulse at rate of 40 to 60 bpm
Bundle of His	Short branch of conductive cells connecting AV node to bundle branches at intraventricular septum
Bundle branches	Right (RBB) and left (LBB) split off on either side of intraventricular septum; carry impulses to Purkinje fibers
Purkinje fibers	Terminal branches of conduction system; initiate rapid depolarization wave causing ventricular contraction; when SA and AV nodes fail, can initiate impulses at rate of 20 to 40 bpm

6. Autonomic nervous system: responds to chemoreceptors, baroreceptors, and stretch receptors
   a. Sympathetic: produces norepinephrine; results in increased HR, myocardial contractility, peripheral vasoconstriction, and arterial BP
   b. Parasympathetic: produces acetylcholine, results in decreased HR and contractility

C. Fetal circulation

1. Ductus venosus
   a. Umbilical vein carries oxygenated blood from placenta to fetus; blood bypasses liver through ductus venosus
   b. At birth when umbilical cord is clamped and cut, blood flow from maternal circulation ceases and ductus venosus closes; blood flows into liver
2. Foramen ovale
   a. Oxygenated systemic blood enters right atrium; flows from right to left atria through foramen ovale
   b. Blood bypasses lungs, which are nonfunctional
   c. Blood flows from left atria to left ventricle and out to aorta
   d. Foramen ovale closes after birth with change in pressure in cardiac chambers
3. Ductus arteriosus
   a. A fistula that allows blood flowing through pulmonary artery to enter aorta; this is normal and desired in fetus
   b. Closes after birth with first few breaths so neonate's heart can circulate oxygenated blood to body

D. Structure and function of blood vessels

1. Distribute blood to body tissues
2. Walls of an artery or vein consist of three layers: tunica intima, tunica media, and tunica adventitia; amount of pressure in vessel determines thickness of walls and amount of connective tissue and smooth muscle
3. Arterial system consists of high-pressure vessels, beginning with aorta, then arteries, arterioles, and ending with capillaries; delivers blood to various tissues for nourishment and contributes to tissue temperature regulation
4. Venous system begins after capillaries and consists of venules and veins (large-diameter, thin-walled vessels) under much less pressure; some veins, most commonly in legs, contain valves to regulate one-way flow; returns blood from capillaries to right atrium and acts as a reservoir for blood volume

E. Regulation of BP

1. Autonomic nervous system
2. Baroreceptors in aortic arch and carotid sinus; chemoreceptors
3. Antidiuretic hormone (ADH)
4. Renin-angiotensin-aldosterone system; angiotensin I is converted to angiotensin II, a powerful vasoconstrictor
5. Others: temperature (cold results in vasoconstriction, heat results in **vasodilation**), substances such as nicotine (vasoconstrict) and alcohol (vasodilate), diet (sodium and fat intake), and factors such as age, gender, ethnicity, weight, physical health, and emotional state

II. DIAGNOSTIC TESTS AND DATA COLLECTION

A. Laboratory tests (see also Chapter 42)

NCLEX®
1. Serum cardiac enzymes: myoglobin, troponins, creatinine kinase (CK), and lactic dehydrogenase (LDH); increase with heart damage, such as myocardial **infarction** (MI); serial testing over days detects trend and determines peak time and extent of injury
2. Serum drug levels:

NCLEX®
   a. Digoxin: therapeutic range is 0.5 to 2.0 ng/mL; early signs of toxicity include nausea, vomiting, anorexia; abdominal pain, bradycardia, other dysrhythmias, and visual disturbances (yellow to green halos) may occur
   b. Quinidine: therapeutic range is 2 to 6 mcg/mL; signs of toxicity include tinnitus, hearing loss, visual disturbances, nausea, dizziness, widened QRS, ventricular dysrhythmias
3. Electrolytes: normal levels of sodium (135–145 mEg/L), potassium (3.5–5.1 mEg/L), calcium (8.6–10.2 mg/dL), and magnesium (1.8–2.6 mg/dL) are essential for proper cardiac function; cardiac disorders and medications can alter electrolyte balance; see Chapter 49 for detailed information

NCLEX®
   a. Potassium (K^+): hypokalemia such as with diuretic therapy increases risk of digitalis toxicity, ventricular dysrhythmias; hyperkalemia from renal disease or excess potassium supplements can lead to ventricular dysrhythmias and asystole;

NCLEX®
   b. Sodium (Na^+): hyponatremia with long-term diuretic therapy; hypernatremia could occur with excess saline IV infusion

c. Calcium: cardiac effects of hypocalcemia include ventricular dysrhythmias, prolonged QT interval and cardiac arrest; hypercalcemia shortens QT interval and causes AV block, digitalis hypersensitivity, and cardiac arrest

d. Magnesium: cardiac effects of decreased magnesium include ventricular tachycardia and fibrillation, while increased magnesium causes bradycardia, hypotension, prolonged PR and QRS intervals

4. Serum lipid profile: a measurement used to determine risk of developing atherosclerosis (see also Chapter 42)

a. Includes total serum cholesterol (< 200 mg/dL) triglycerides (10–190 mg/dL) and lipoproteins

NCLEX® b. High-density lipoproteins (HDL): transport cholesterol to liver for excretion ("good" cholesterol); normal is 30 to 70 mg/dL

NCLEX® c. Low-density lipoproteins (LDL): transport cholesterol to peripheral tissues ("bad" cholesterol) and increases risk of heart disease; normal is under 130 mg/dL

B. Electrocardiography (see also Chapter 43)

1. A graphic recording of electrical activity of heart; diagnoses myocardial ischemia, injury, and necrosis areas of cell death (MI); hypertrophy, electrolyte imbalance and effects of antidysrhythmic drugs
2. Resting electrocardiogram (ECG): represents a single recorded picture of electrical activity of heart
3. Holter monitoring: continuous ambulatory ECG monitoring over time (usually 24 hours) with small, timed, portable ECG recording device
4. Stress test: continuous multilead ECG monitoring during controlled and supervised exercise, usually on treadmill

C. Echocardiography: ultrasound that evaluates structure and function of heart chambers and valves

D. Phonocardiography: a graphic recording of heart sounds with simultaneous ECG; is not painful

E. Coronary angiography and arteriography (see also Chapter 43): an invasive procedure during which dye is injected into coronary arteries and flow of dye is recorded to determine structure of arteries

F. Cardiac catheterization:

1. Insertion of a catheter into heart and surrounding vessels to obtain diagnostic information about heart structure and function (see also Chapter 43)

NCLEX® 2. Client preparation, nursing care during procedure, and postprocedure nursing care are summarized in Box 52–1

G. Radionuclide tests

1. Safe, nonpainful methods of evaluating left ventricular muscle function and coronary artery blood distribution; radionuclide contrast is injected via venipuncture; encourage client to drink fluids postprocedure to facilitate excretion of contrast; examine venipuncture site for bleeding or hematoma; may be used in conjunction with stress testing
2. Allows visualization of ventricles through several cardiac cycles; calculate **ejection fraction (EF)**, portion of blood ejected during systole compared to total ventricular filling volume, (normal EF = 55 to 65%)
3. MUGA (gated pool imaging or multigated acquisition) scan
4. Thallium imaging: used to assess myocardial **ischemia** (decreased supply of oxygenated blood) during stress testing
5. PET (positron emission tomography) scan: evaluates cardiac metabolism and assesses tissue perfusion

H. Electron beam computed tomtography (EBCT): easily detects calcium deposits, which correlate with heart disease but also occur in greater frequency with advancing age; is a controversial "screening" tool that may or may not be useful for a specific client

I. Doppler ultrasound: a noninvasive test that measures speed of blood flow through a vessel and emits an audible signal; can determine blood flow when arterial palpation is difficult or impossible because of occlusive disease; a palpable pulse and a Doppler pulse are not equivalent, so document clearly

J. Plethysmography: records volume changes in an extremity associated with cardiac contractions or in response to pneumatic venous occlusion; can detect and quantify vascular disease by changes in pulse contour, BP, or arterial and venous blood flow

K. Digital intravenous angiography: utilizing computer technology, visualizes blood vessels after IV injection of contrast medium; allows for small peripheral venous injections of contrast medium instead of large doses used with arterial cannulation

L. Venography: injection of radiopaque dye into veins with serial x-rays taken to detect deep-vein thrombosis and incompetent valves

Box 52–1

Care of the Client Undergoing Cardiac Catheterization

Client Preparation

- Obtain written consent.
- Determine client history of allergies to iodine, dye, or shellfish.
- Explain that client will be awake and may experience various sensations during procedure, including flushing sensation as dye is injected or fluttering feeling as catheter passes through heart.
- Explain postprocedure routine (see Postprocedure Nursing Care).
- Prepare insertion site by shaving and cleansing with antiseptic.
- Nothing by mouth (NPO) except sips of water with cardiac medications as indicated for 6 to 8 hours.
- Initiate IV site with fluids as ordered.
- Administer preprocedure medications as ordered.

Nursing Care During Procedure

- Procedure is performed in catheterization laboratory by cardiologist; nurse monitors ECG and vital signs continuously, administers conscious sedation as ordered, and provides emotional support.

Postprocedure Nursing Care

- Maintain client on bedrest, often for 4 to 6 hours.
- Keep affected extremity straight; after 1 to 2 hours, head may be elevated up to 30 degrees for those who had femoral artery used as insertion site.
- Maintain pressure dressing at insertion site.
- Monitor BP, heart rate, distal pulses, color and temperature of extremity, and look for signs of bleeding at the site (with leg site, check under client for bleeding) according to agency schedule (routinely q 15 minutes for 1 hour, q 30 minutes for 2 hours, q hour for 4 hours, or q 8 hours for associated procedure of percutaneous transluminal coronary angioplasty [PTCA]).
- Report signs of chest pain, dysrhythmias, bleeding, hematoma formation, or other changes; report significant changes in vital signs, pulses, color or temperature of extremity immediately to physician; bleeding may be reported by client as a feeling of warmth in insertion area.
- If bleeding occurs, restore manual pressure to site (manual pressure also applied immediately post-procedure to achieve hemostasis, often for up to 20 minutes because of heparin use during procedure).
- Maintain IV and encourage oral fluids as ordered to eliminate contrast dye, which can be nephrotoxic.
- Monitor I&O to determine whether client is becoming dehydrated from increased urine output because of dye excretion.

M. **Angiography**: injection of radiopaque dye into arteries to detect plaques, occlusions, injury, and so on; similar to care for postcardiac catheterization

N. **Ankle-brachial index**: most commonly used parameter for overall evaluation of extremity status; ankle pressure normally is same or higher than brachial systolic pressure

O. **Computed tomography**: allows for visualization of arterial wall and its structures; used to diagnose abdominal aortic aneurysm (AAA) and postoperative vascular complications such as graft occlusion and hemorrhage

P. **Magnetic resonance imaging (MRI)**: uses magnetic fields rather than radiation; used with angiography to detect abnormalities, especially in clients who cannot have dye injected

III. COMMON NURSING TECHNIQUES AND PROCEDURES

A. Dysrhythmia monitoring

1. Continuous ECG monitoring in one lead with portable telemetry unit; indicated for high-risk clients with cardiac disease, taking medications affecting heart, and undergoing surgery or diagnostic or therapeutic procedures

2. Lead placements (ECG continuous monitors have 3 leads or 5 leads)
   a. Placement of leads with 3-lead monitor are below right clavicle (right arm—white lead), below left clavicle (left arm—black lead), and at lowest rib, left midclavicular line (left leg—red lead)
   b. Placement of leads with 5-lead monitor are same as 3-lead with fourth lead placed at lowest rib, right midclavicular line (right leg—green lead) and fifth lead on site of one of six chest leads (V leads—brown lead)

NCLEX®
3. Preparation of client: explain procedure and reassure that client will not receive electrical impulses or shocks; identify proper placement, cleanse skin with soap and water, shave hairy areas, use alcohol or skin prep according to agency policy, dry with cloth or gauze, and apply fresh electrodes

NCLEX®
4. Interpretations of ECG patterns originating in sinus node
   a. See Table 52–2 for descriptions of sinus rhythm (normal), sinus tachycardia, sinus bradycardia, and sinus arrhythmia

   NCLEX®
   b. Nursing and therapeutic interventions: with sinus arrest, tachycardia, or bradycardia, monitor for signs of inadequate cardiac output and tissue perfusion, including changes in blood pressure, activity tolerance, and level of consciousness (LOC); identify and treat cause of sinus tachycardia; atropine and possible pacemaker indicated for symptomatic or extreme low rates (<50)
5. ECG patterns originating in the atria

   NCLEX®
   a. See again Table 52–2 for descriptions of premature atrial contractions (PAC), paroxysmal supraventricular tachycardia (SVT), atrial flutter, and atrial fibrillation

   NCLEX®
   b. Nursing and therapeutic interventions: carotid massage, synchronized cardioversion, antidysrhythmia medications including beta-blockers, calcium channel blockers, and digoxin; anticoagulant therapy to reduce the risk of thrombus
6. ECG patterns originating from the AV node
   a. See again Table 52–2 for descriptions of first-degree heart block, second-degree heart block, Mobitz type I (Wenckebach) and Mobitz type II, third-degree (complete) heart block and junctional escape rhythm

   NCLEX®
   b. Nursing and therapeutic interventions include monitoring and observation; atropine, isoproterenol or pacemakers for symptomatic heart block (external or transthoracic, temporary, or permanent)
7. ECG patterns originating from ventricles

   NCLEX®
   a. See again Table 52–2 for descriptions of premature ventricular contractions (PVC), ventricular tachycardia (VT), and ventricular fibrillation (VF)

   NCLEX®
   b. Nursing and therapeutic interventions: for PVCs monitor for signs of decreased CO; instruct client to avoid caffeine and nicotine; with VT, examine immediately to determine LOC and if client has stable BP and pulse; if stable, treat with lidocaine, procainamide, and cardioversion; if client becomes unconscious or unstable or has pulseless VT or VF, immediate defibrillation is required

B. Percutaneous transluminal coronary angioplasty (PTCA)

1. Increases blood flow to coronary arteries by inserting a catheter with a balloon tip into narrowed segment of affected artery, inflating balloon to expand vessel lumen and removing catheter; may also include insertion of an expandable intracoronary stent, which is inserted over balloon and remains in place after balloon is removed
2. Client preparation, nursing care during procedure, and postprocedure nursing care are as outlined previously in Box 52–1
3. Administer anticoagulants as ordered to prevent thrombus formation, and monitor coagulation studies as indicated

NCLEX®
4. Because of anticoagulants used during procedure, site may have a vice-type pressure device requiring a longer period of hourly site checks; monitor closely for any changes in ECG or signs of chest pain (even minor changes may indicate ischemia); obtain a 12-lead ECG and notify physician of any complications

C. Coronary artery bypass grafting (CABG)

1. Surgery is indicated for more than 50% occlusion in left main coronary artery or severe blockage in several vessels; diseased arteries are "bypassed" with saphenous veins, mammary arteries, or less frequently, artificial grafts; indicated for myocardial ischemia not managed by medical treatment; client is typically maintained on cardiopulmonary bypass machine during surgery
2. Client preparation
   a. Ensure that all consents are signed
   b. Perform routine preoperative teaching, including turning, coughing, and deep breathing (vigorous coughing is discouraged because increased intrathoracic pressure may cause instability in sternal area), use of incentive spirometer (IS) to prevent respiratory complications, and leg exercises and sequential leg compression devices to prevent thrombus formation

Table 52–2 Selected Cardiac Rhythms and Dysrhythmias

Rhythm/ECG Appearance	ECG Characteristics	Management
Supraventricular Rhythms		
Normal sinus rhythm (NSR) 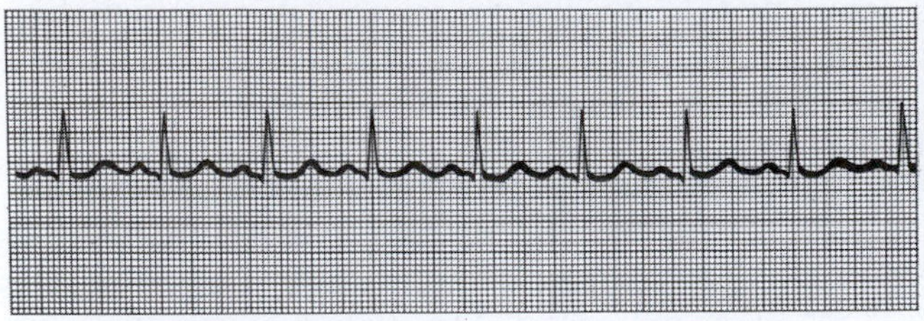	Rate: 60–100 bpm Rhythm: regular P:QRS ratio is 1:1 PR interval: 0.12–0.20 sec QRS complex: 0.06–0.10 sec	None; normal heart rhythm
Sinus arrhythmia 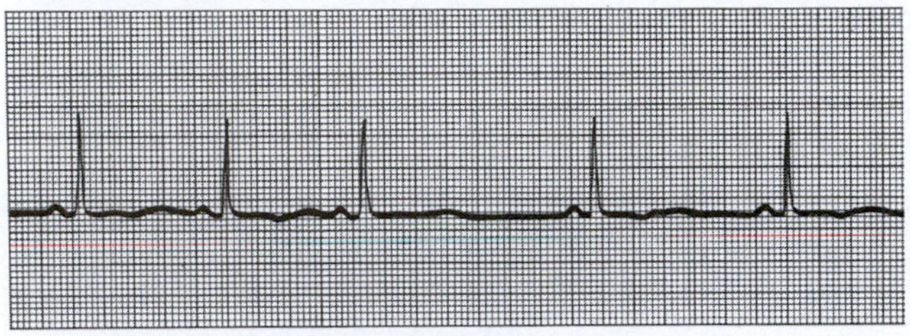	Rate: 60–100 bpm Rhythm: irregular, varying with respirations P:QRS ratio is 1:1 PR interval: 0.12–0.20 sec QRS complex: 0.06–0.10 sec	Generally none; considered a normal rhythm in the very young and very old
Sinus tachycardia 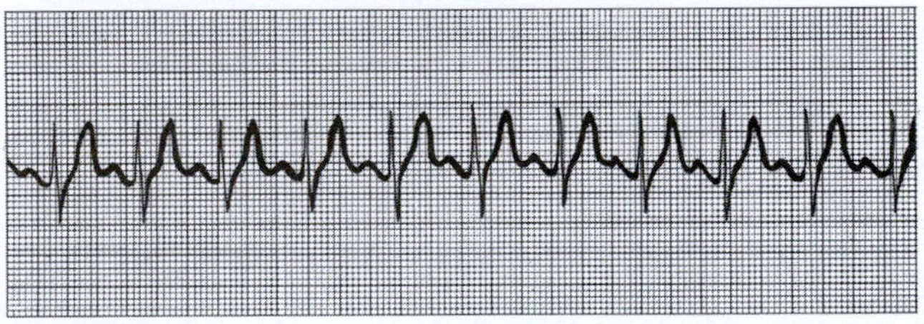	Rate: 101 to 150 bpm Rhythm: regular P:QRS ratio is 1:1 (with very fast rates, P wave may be hidden in preceding T wave) PR interval: 0.12–0.20 sec QRS complex: 0.06–0.10 sec	Treat only if client is experiencing symptoms or is at risk for myocardial damage; treat underlying cause (e.g., hypovolemia, fever, pain); beta-blockers or verapamil may be used
Sinus bradycardia 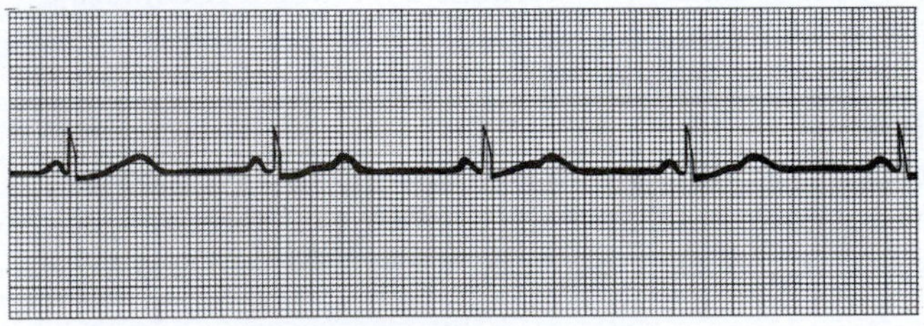	Rate: less than 60 bpm Rhythm: regular P:QRS ratio is 1:1 PR interval: 0.12–0.20 sec QRS complex: 0.06–0.10 sec	Treat only if client is experiencing symptoms; intravenous atropine, isoproterenol, and/or pacemaker therapy may be used
Premature atrial contractions (PAC) 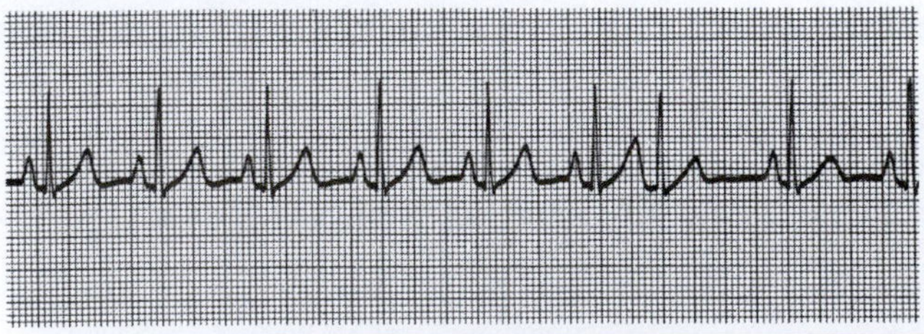	Rate: variable Rhythm: irregular, with normal rhythm interrupted by early beats arising in the atria P:QRS ratio is 1:1 PR interval: 0.12–0.20 sec but may be prolonged QRS complex: 0.6–0.10 sec	Usually requires no treatment; advise client to reduce alcohol and caffeine intake, to reduce stress, and to stop smoking
Paroxysmal supraventricular tachycardia (PSVT) 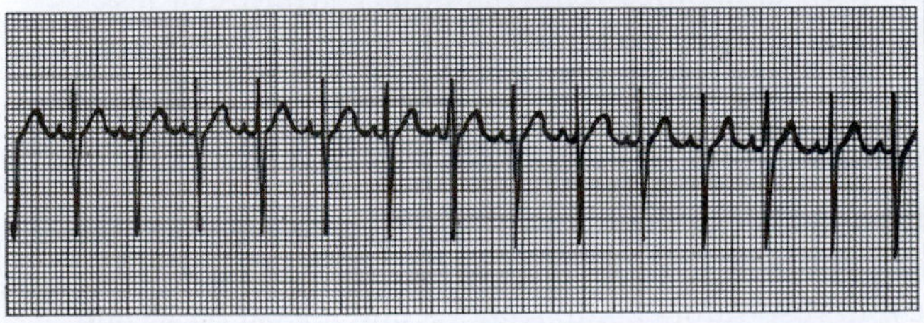	Rate: 100–280 bpm (usually 150–200 bpm) Rhythm: regular P:QRS ratio: P waves often not identifiable PR interval: not measured QRS complex: 0.06–0.10 sec	Treat if client is experiencing symptoms; treatment may include vagal maneuvers (Valsalva, carotid sinus massage); oxygen therapy; adenosine or a beta-blocker; temporary pacing or synchronized cardioversion

Table 52–2 ***(continued)***

Rhythm/ECG Appearance	ECG Characteristics	Management
Atrial flutter 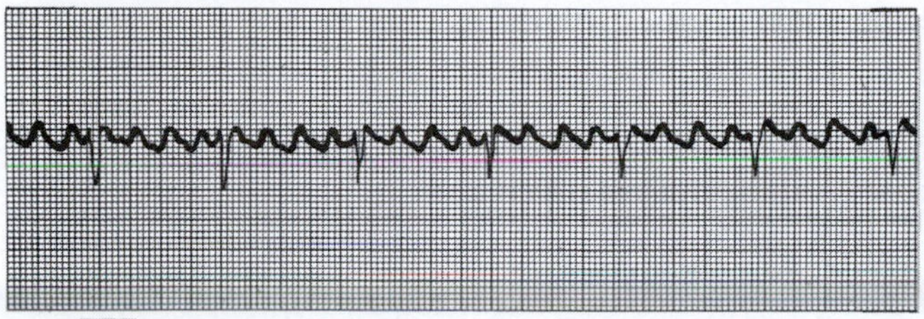	Rate: atrial 240–360 bpm; ventricular rate depends on degree of AV block; usually is less than 150 bpm Rhythm: atrial regular, ventricular usually regular P:QRS ratio may be 2:1, 4:1, 6:1 or may be variable PR interval: not measured QRS complex: 0.06–0.10 sec	Synchronized cardioversion; medications to slow ventricular response, such as beta-blocker or calcium channel blocker (verapamil), followed by class I antidysrhythmic or amiodarone
Atrial fibrillation 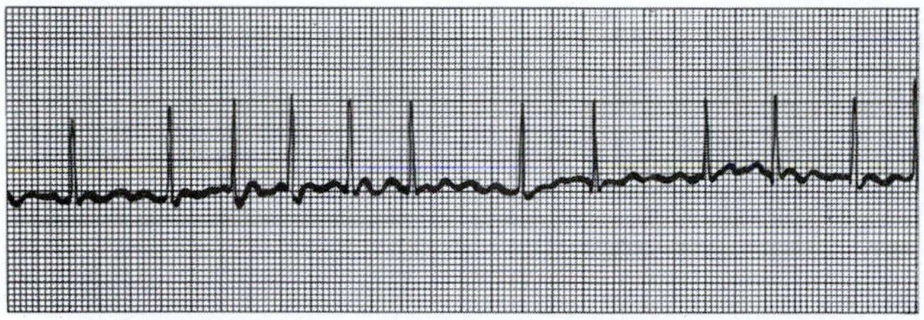	Rate: atrial 300–600 bpm (too rapid to count); ventricular 100–180 bpm in untreated clients Rhythm: irregularly irregular P:QRS ratio is variable PR interval: not measured QRS complex: 0.06–0.10 sec	Synchronized cardioversion; medications to reduce ventricular response rate: metoprolol, diltiazem, digoxin; anticoagulant therapy to reduce risk of clot formation and stroke
Junctional escape rhythm 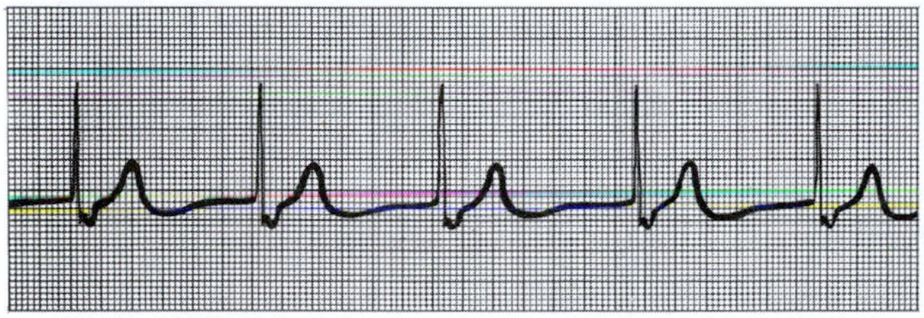	Rate: 40–60 bpm; junctional tachycardia 60–140 bpm Rhythm: regular P:QRS ratio: P waves may be absent, inverted, and immediately before, after, or hidden in QRS complex PR interval: less than 0.10 sec if P wave is prior to QRS complex QRS complex: 0.06–0.10 sec	Treat cause if client is experiencing symptoms
Ventricular Rhythms *Premature ventricular contractions (PVC)* 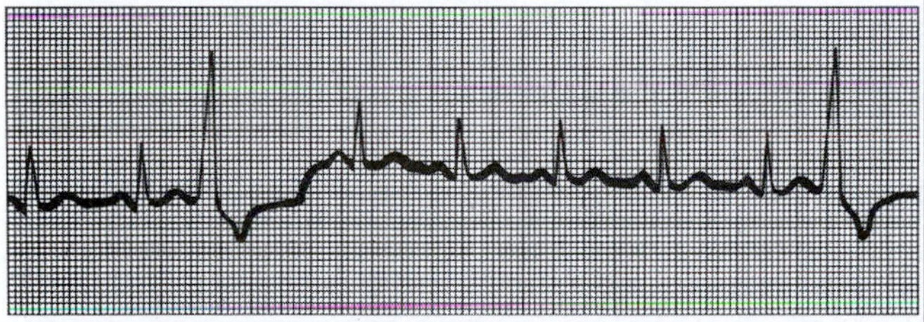	Rate: variable Rhythm: irregular; PVC interrupts underlying rhythm and followed by compensatory pause P:QRS ratio: no P wave noted before PVC PR interval: absent with PVC QRS complex: wide (greater than 0.12 sec), bizarre in appearance; differs from normal QRS complex	Treat if client is experiencing symptoms; advise against stimulant use (caffeine, nicotine); drug therapy includes class I and III antidysrhythmics and possibly addition of beta-blocker
Ventricular tachycardia (VT or V tach) 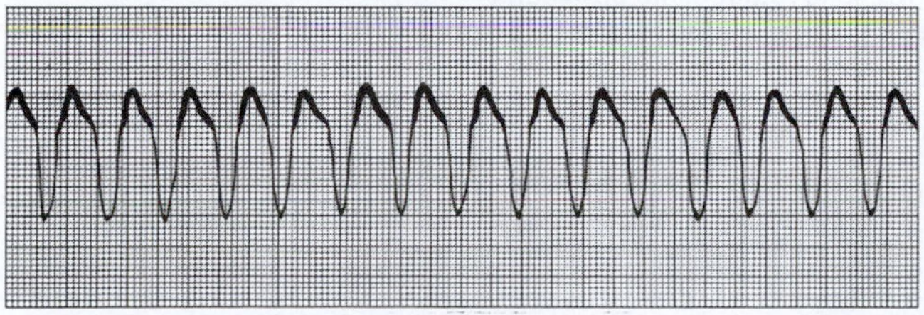	Rate: 100–250 bpm Rhythm: regular P:QRS ratio: P waves usually not identifiable PR interval: not measured QRS complex: 0.12 sec or greater; bizarre shape	Treat if VT is sustained or if client is experiencing symptoms; treatment includes intravenous procainamide, lidocaine or if unstable, a class III antidysrhythmic, and immediate DC cardioversion; ablation surgery or implanted cardioverter/defibrillator (IACD) for repeated episodes

(continued)

Table 52–2 ***(continued)***

Rhythm/ECG Appearance	ECG Characteristics	Management
Ventricular fibrillation (VF or V fib) 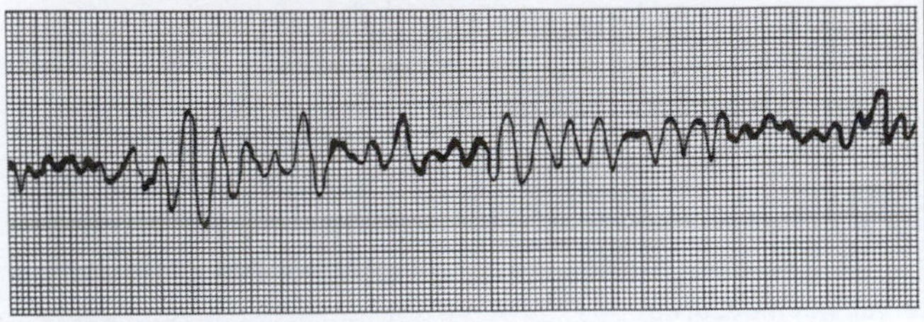	Rate: too rapid to count Rhythm: grossly irregular P:QRS ratio: no identifiable P waves PR interval: none QRS: bizarre, varying in shape and direction	Immediate defibrillation
Atrioventricular Conduction Blocks		
First-degree AV block 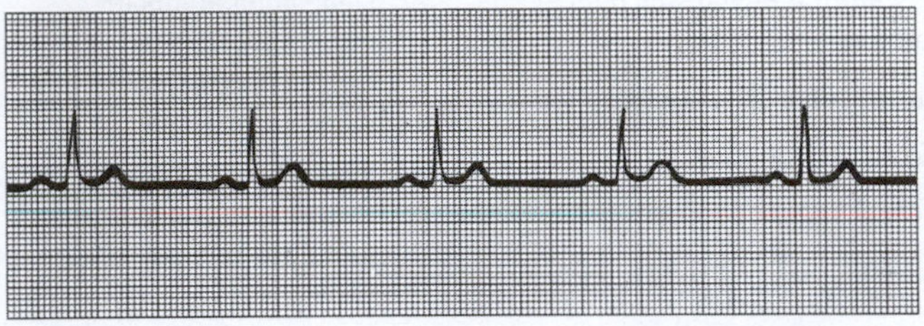	Rate: usually 60–100 bpm Rhythm: regular P:QRS ratio is: 1:1 PR interval: greater than 0.20 sec QRS complex: 0.06–0.10 sec	None required
Second-degree AV block, type I (Mobitz I, Wenckebach) 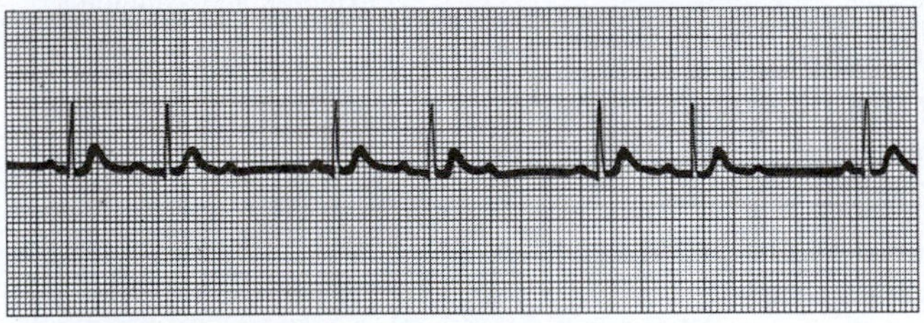	Rate: 60–100 bpm Rhythm: atrial regular; ventricular irregular P:QRS ratio is: 1:1 until P wave blocked with no QRS following PR interval: progressively lengthens in a regular pattern QRS complex: 0.06–0.10 sec; sudden absence of QRS complex	Monitoring and observation; atropine or isoproterenol if client is experiencing symptoms but this rarely occurs and client rarely progresses to higher level of block
Second-degree AV block, type II (Mobitz II) 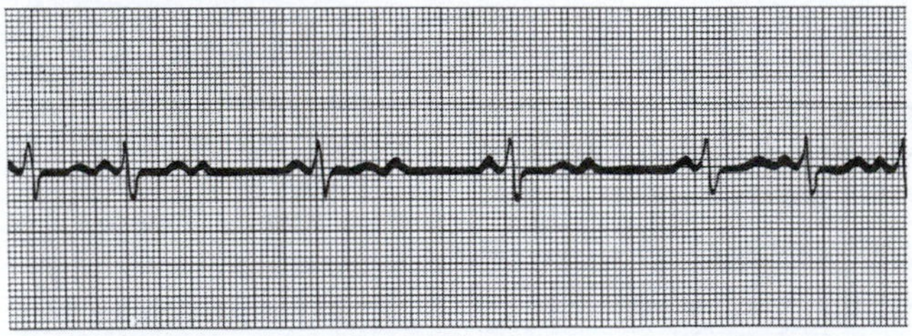	Rate: atrial 60–100 bpm; ventricular less than 60 bpm Rhythm: atrial regular; ventricular irregular P:QRS ratio is: typically 2:1, may vary PR interval: constant PR interval for each conducted QRS complex QRS complex: 0.06–0.10 sec	Atropine or isoproterenol; pacemaker therapy
Third-degree AV block (complete heart block) 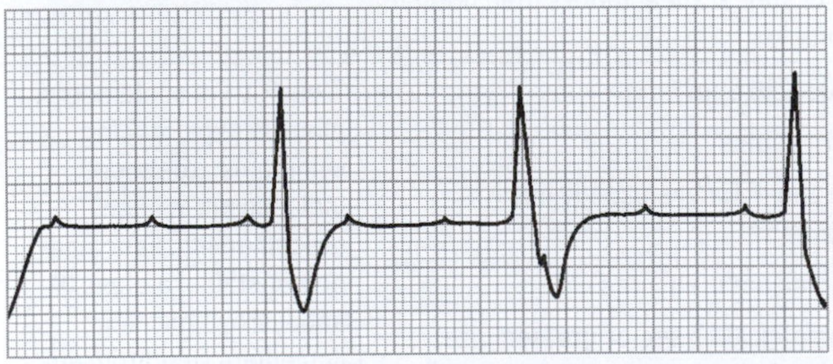	Rate: atrial 60–100 bpm; ventricular 15–60 bpm Rhythm: atrial regular; ventricular regular P:QRS ratio: no relationship between P waves and QRS complexes; independent rhythms PR interval: not measured QRS complex: 0.06–0.10 sec if junctional escape rhythm; 0.12 sec if ventricular escape rhythm	Immediate pacemaker therapy

Source: LeMone P., Burke, K. & Bauldoff, G. *Medical surgical nursing: Critical thinking for collaborative care* (5th ed.), © 2011, pp. 947–949, Table 30–7. Reprinted by permission of Pearson Education, Inc., Upper Saddle River, NJ 07458.

c. Explain postoperative course, including respiratory support on ventilator with an endotracheal tube; suctioning; surgical incisions, chest tubes, multiple IV lines, tubes, drains, and monitors with alarms and noises; pain management, communication techniques, visiting policies, and expected length of hospitalization and recovery period

NCLEX®

3. Postprocedure nursing care: immediate postoperative care given in cardiac critical care units; within 1 to 2 days client is transferred to a step-down/telemetry unit where care includes the following:
   a. Monitor client for signs of decreased CO; evaluate ECG via continuous monitoring; I&O; full data collection with lung sounds and heart sounds every 4 hours initially, then at least every 8 hours
   b. Monitor for and treat postoperative pain
   c. Monitor indicators of CO with client's increasing activity
   d. Monitor respiratory status and encouraging deep breathing and IS
   e. Monitor surgical wounds and treat as needed
   f. Reinforce teaching about new medication regime, activity plan for home, cardiac rehabilitation, resuming sexual activity (usually allowed by surgeon when client can walk up two full flights of stairs without shortness of breath [SOB] or chest pain; client should be rested, not after a heavy meal or alcohol consumption)
   g. Instruct client about symptoms to report to physician after discharge including chest pain, SOB, decrease in activity tolerance, fever, redness, swelling or drainage from surgical incisions
   h. Instruct client that clinical depression occurs in about 20% of clients up to 6 months after cardiac surgery, and client should notify physician because antidepressants have been shown to be effective; include family in teaching and planning for discharge

D. Valvular surgery repair or replacement of dysfunctional valve

1. Repair
   a. *Valvuloplasty*: reconstruction including repair or removal of calcification or vegetation
   b. *Annuloplasty*: narrowing a dilated valve with a prosthetic ring or purse-string sutures, or enlarging a stenosed valve with a balloon
   c. Repair is the preferred option because of lower incidence of postsurgical complications and mortality than occur in valve replacement
2. Replacement: valve is completely replaced
   a. Mechanical valves: more durable and longer lasting; subject to mechanical failure; require lifetime anticoagulation with warfarin (Coumadin), and infections are harder to treat; an example is the St. Jude medical valve
   b. Tissue valves: may deteriorate; frequent replacement is required; not associated with thrombus formation, no long-term anticoagulation; infections are easier to treat

NCLEX®

3. Client preparation and postprocedure nursing care: (same as for cardiac surgery, discussed previously); provide instructions for preventing infection, including precautions such as prophylactic antibiotic therapy prior to invasive procedures (e.g., dental care), gentle oral care to prevent bacteria from entering the bloodstream through the gums; provide instruction on management of anticoagulation therapy if applicable

E. Pacemakers

1. Permanent pacemakers are inserted to treat permanent cardiac conduction defects; generator box is implanted under chest wall and wires are threaded into blood vessel through right atrium for implantation in right ventricle (commonly)
2. Client preparation: obtain informed written consent; bedrest is required for 24 hours and activity is gradually increased to prevent dislodging leads; daily 1-minute pulse count will be required (should be equal to or higher than preset rate)

NCLEX®

3. Postprocedure nursing care
   a. Monitor ECG continuously to ensure that pacing impulses are being captured (e.g., pacer spike is followed by QRS with ventricular pacing) and that client rhythm is sensed (pacemaker does not fire when client rhythm is present)
   b. Monitor pacemaker site for signs of bleeding or infection
   c. Dressing should remain clean and dry with no temperature elevation or swelling, redness, or tenderness of incision
   d. Minimize right arm and shoulder movements immediately postprocedure to ensure that pacemaker wire remains in contact with ventricular wall

4. Temporary pacemakers are utilized for heart block that occurs suddenly or as temporary reponse to cardiac surgery or myocardial infarction as examples
   a. May be placed transvenously with external pacemaker box used to set milliamps of energy and rate
   b. Monitor cardiac rhythm for lack of capture and watch for site infection as risks
   c. May also utilize external pacemaker as initial measure, which is noninvasive and easy to use but may be uncomfortable to client

F. Blood pressure (BP) measurement

1. Is primarily a function of CO and systemic vascular resistance (SVR); arterial BP equals CO multiplied by SVR
2. Have client sit with arm bared, supported, and at heart level; ensure no smoking or caffeine intake 30 minutes prior
3. Take BP in both arms initially using appropriate-sized cuff (rubber bladder should at least encircle arm by 80%)
4. If averaging two or more readings, separate measurements by at least 2 minutes
5. If both client's arms are inaccessible (from combination of IV lines, dialysis shunt, mastectomy, burns, etc.), obtain readings from thigh or calf, auscultating popliteal or posterior tibial arteries, respectively

IV. MYOCARDIAL INFARCTION (MI)

A. Overview

1. Myocardial injury from sudden restriction of blood supply to a portion of heart; is a life-threatening condition
2. Main cause is **coronary artery disease** (CAD), build up of atherosclerotic plaque in coronary arteries that restricts blood flow to heart
   a. Nonmodifiable risk factors include age, gender, family history, and ethnic background
   NCLEX® b. Modifiable risk factors include smoking, obesity, stress, elevated cholesterol, diabetes mellitus, and hypertension
3. Coronary artery blood flow is blocked by atherosclerotic narrowing, thrombus formation, or (less frequently) persistent vasospasm; myocardium supplied by arteries is deprived of O_2; persistent ischemia may rapidly lead to tissue death
4. *NCLEX®* **Angina pectoris** is chest pain resulting from this restricted blood flow; may occur in three forms:
   a. *Stable angina,* a predictable response to increased activity
   b. *Unstable angina* with unpredictability (at rest) and increasing severity
   c. *Prinzmetal angina* caused by arterial spasm often awaking client from sleep
5. Angina pectoris may change in character and may progress to MI

NCLEX® B. Nursing data collection

1. Chest pain unrelieved by nitroglycerine or rest often indicates MI; may be a crushing substernal pain; may radiate to jaw, neck, back, or left arm (some clients, especially diabetic clients and women, report no pain)
2. Other symptoms may include diaphoresis, cool mottled skin, nausea and vomiting, fear, anxiety and sense of impending doom, dyspnea and shortness of breath, palpitations and dysrhythmias, hypertension or hypotension
3. ECG (12-lead): ST elevation, accompanied by T-wave inversion in leads that monitor affected area of heart; these changes resolve as treatment progresses; new pathologic Q wave in affected leads develops as a permanent change if ischemia not reversed before cell death occurs
4. Lab findings: elevated troponins (early or late diagnosis); elevated CK-MB isoenzymes over 5% (early diagnosis); or elevated LDH with "flipped" isoenzymes (late diagnosis)

NCLEX® C. Therapeutic management

1. Monitor pain status frequently with pain scale or other appropriate tool to estimate changes in pain level; pain is usually first presenting sign of new or extended MI
2. Monitor hemodynamic status including BP, HR, LOC, skin color, and temperature frequently (every 5 minutes during pain; every 15 minutes postpain) during acute phase to evaluate CO; continue to monitor frequently (every 1 to 2 hours) for first 24 hours post-MI
3. *NCLEX®* Emergency treatment usually includes MONA: morphine, oxygen, nitrates, and aspirin (see Memory Aid)

4. Monitor continuous ECG to detect dysrhythmias (PVCs and tachycardia common); perform 12-lead ECG immediately with new pain or changes in level or character of pain to identify ischemia and injury
5. Monitor respirations, breath sounds, and I&O to detect early signs of heart failure as a complication
6. Monitor O_2 saturation and administer O_2 (usually via nasal cannula at 2 to 4 L/min) as prescribed to increase oxygenation to heart

Memory Aid

Remember MONA as a key treatment approach to MI:
***M**orphine* to relieve chest pain
***O**xygen* to increase oxygenation
***N**itrates* to vasodilate coronary blood vessels and increase blood supply
***A**spirin* as an antiplatelet agent to interfere with thrombus formation in affected artery

7. Provide for physiological rest to decrease O_2 demands on heart
8. Keep client NPO or progress to liquid diet as ordered; maintain IV access for medications as needed
9. Provide care in specialized cardiac critical care unit; provide a calm environment and reassure client and family to decrease stress, fear, and anxiety
10. Report significant changes immediately to physician to ensure rapid treatment of complications
11. Interventions in recovery phase: maintain bedrest (with bedside commode) for 24–36 hours and gradually increase activity as ordered while closely monitoring CO, ECG, and pain status; reinforce to client importance of reporting any new pain immediately; progress diet from NPO or liquids to soft, low fat, and low sodium diet as ordered
12. Administer nitroglycerine as prescribed to dilate coronary vessels and increase blood flow
13. Administer morphine sulfate as ordered to relieve chest pain
14. Administer anticoagulants (IV heparin) and aspirin (antiplatelet) as ordered to prevent additional clot formation; monitor PTT to maintain heparin at therapeutic level (often 60–80 seconds)
15. Administer thrombolytic therapy if no contraindications (recent hemorrhagic stroke, surgery, childbirth, trauma); common drugs include alteplase recombinant (Activase), tissue plasminogen activator (TPA), or streptokinase (Streptase); they dissolve clot, stop progress of MI, and decrease myocardial damage; monitor frequently for signs of bleeding
16. Monitor neurological status frequently for changes; alteplase recombinant and streptokinase are not clot-specific and will dissolve other clots—can cause thrombolytic (hemorrhagic) CVA, a life-threatening complication
17. Administer beta-blockers post-MI as ordered to decrease cardiac work and decrease O_2 demands on heart
18. Administer antidysrhythmic drugs as prescribed or by emergency protocol
19. Surgical interventions: PTCA, CABG (see previous discussion)

D. Reinforce client teaching

1. Include appropriate family members whenever possible
2. Cardiac rehabilitation program if ordered
3. Modifiable risk factors and a plan to change lifestyle to decrease these factors (including supportive services)
4. Medication regime as prescribed; side effects to report (with written instructions for later reference)
5. Importance of reporting chest pain or signs of decreased CO
6. *NCLEX®* Bleeding precautions if client is on anticoagulant therapy: use soft toothbrush, electric razor, avoid trauma or injury; wear or carry Medic-Alert identification

V. HEART FAILURE

A. Overview

1. Inability of heart to pump adequate blood to meet metabolic needs of body
2. May be called congestive heart failure
3. Multiple causes include myocardial damage from MI, incompetent valves, inflammatory conditions of heart, cardiomyopathy, hypertension, and pulmonary hypertension (right-sided failure, called **cor pulmonale**)

4. Compensatory phase (early): CO falls → sensed by baroreceptors → stimulate sympathetic nervous system → release norepinephrine → increase in HR and vasoconstriction → increas in filling pressures → increase in SV and CO (because CO = HR × SV, CO is increased); compensatory mechanisms increase cardiac metabolic demands and over time decrease cardiac function and ability to compensate
5. Depending upon cause, heart failure (HF) presents initially as right-sided failure or left-sided failure; other side becomes affected as it progresses
   a. Left HF: left ventricle has reduced capacity to pump blood into systemic circulation, causing decreased CO and stasis or "backup" of fluid into pulmonary circulation
   b. Right HF: right ventricle has reduced capacity to pump blood into pulmonary circulation, causing stasis or "backup" of fluid in venous circulation
6. Onset of HF
   a. Acute, with significant overload in lungs (**pulmonary edema**, characterized by acute restlessness, anxiety, increased crackles, tachypnea, tachycardia, pink, frothy sputum, decreased SO_2 and PO_2)
   b. Chronic, with fatigue and activity intolerance as main features; clients with advanced chronic HF require careful management to prevent acute exacerbations

NCLEX®

B. Nursing data collection

1. Presenting symptoms
   a. Left HF: dyspnea on exertion (often first clinical sign), orthopnea, paroxysmal nocturnal dyspnea, crackles, new S_3 (ventricular gallop) as early sign; pulmonary edema is acute life-threatening left heart failure
   b. Right HF: lower extremity edema; **jugular venous distention (JVD)** is visible more than a few millimeters above clavicle with client supine with 45-degree head elevation; abdominal discomfort and nausea occur from fluid congestion in abdominal organs
   c. Both sides: unexplained fatigue or altered mental status, decreased exercise tolerance
2. Diagnostic findings
   a. Elevated atrial natriuretic factor or hormone (ANF or ANH) and B-type natriuretic peptide (BNP) elevate in HF but are not singly diagnostic since they can elevate also in women and those over age 60 years
   b. Chest x-ray may show cardiomegaly or vascular congestion
   c. Echocardiogram shows decreased ventricular function and decreased ejection fraction
   d. CVP elevated in right HF
   e. PA pressure monitoring may guide treatment in serious cases of pulmonary edema

C. Therapeutic management

1. Acute phase
   a. Monitor and record BP, pulse, respirations, ECG, and CVP or PCWP (if appropriate) to detect changes in CO
   NCLEX®
   b. Raise head of bed to decrease pulmonary congestion and improve gas exchange
   c. Auscultate heart and lung sounds frequently: increasing crackles, increasing dyspnea, decreasing lungs sounds, or new S_3 heart sound indicate worsening HF
   d. Administer O_2 as ordered to improve gas exchange and increase oxygenation of blood; monitor SO_2 and arterial blood gases (ABG) to determine effectiveness
   e. Administer prescribed medications on time
   f. Monitor serum electrolytes to detect hypokalemia secondary to diuretic therapy
   g. Monitor accurate I&O to evaluate fluid status (may require urinary catheter for accurate measurement of urine output)
   h. If fluid restriction is prescribed, spread fluid throughout day to reduce thirst
   NCLEX®
   i. Encourage physical rest and organize activities with frequent rest periods to reduce cardiac work
   j. Provide a calm, reassuring environment to reduce anxiety, thus decreasing O_2 consumption and demands on heart
2. Chronic HF
   a. Reinforce rationale for therapeutic regime to client and family
   b. Establish baseline data for fluid status and functional abilities: it is baseline "normal" for some clients with HF to have bilateral crackles in bases, some amount of peripheral edema, or to be unable to walk more than a specific number of feet before tiring
   NCLEX®
   c. Monitor daily weights to evaluate changes in fluid status
   d. Monitor at regular intervals for changes in fluid status or functional activity level

3. Angiotensin-converting enzyme (ACE) inhibitors such as lisinopril (Prinivil) and angiotensin II receptor blockers (ARBs) are used to reduce afterload and thus increase CO (primarily used in ongoing management); monitor for hypotension, especially orthostatic hypotension

NCLEX®

4. Diuretics (often loop diuretics such as furosemide/Lasix) to decrease preload and pulmonary congestion, which decreases cardiac work and increases CO; carefully monitor potassium levels for hypokalemia or hyperkalemia, depending on whether potassium-losing or potassium-sparing diuretics are used
5. Vasodilators including nitroglycerine to reduce preload; monitor for hypotension
6. Beta-blockers to inhibit sympathetic nervous system activity and improve CO; must be used cautiously because their effect could also decrease CO; typically used in conjunction with ACE inhibitors for best effect
7. Morphine to sedate and vasodilate during acute pulmonary edema; decreases cardiac work; monitor for hypotension or respiratory depression

NCLEX®

8. Digoxin (Lanoxin) to improve contractility and correspondingly increase stroke volume and CO; take apical pulse for 1 full minute and withhold if heart rate is less than 60 and notify prescribing physician
9. Other: inotropic agents such as dopamine (Intropin) and dobutamine (Dobutrex) are used in critical care settings to increase force of cardiac contraction when decompensation of CO includes hypotension; monitor BP and IV site frequently

D. Reinforce client teaching

1. Include family members or others in teaching as appropriate

NCLEX®

2. Weight monitoring: measure and record daily weights (with same amount of clothing before breakfast but after voiding) and report unexplained increase of 3 to 5 pounds—most sensitive indicator of increased fluid overload

NCLEX®

3. Diet: sodium restriction to decrease fluid overload; increase intake of potassium-rich foods if taking potassium-losing diuretics; restriction of high-potassium foods and salt substitutes if taking potassium-sparing diuretics; do not restrict water intake unless directed (this will not decrease fluid retention)
4. Medication regime: follow all medication instructions; although frequent urination is bothersome, regular diuretic therapy prevents fluid overload and acute exacerbation; take radial pulse for one full minute before taking digoxin; withhold dose and call prescriber if pulse is lower than 50 or 60 as instructed (variability exists) or is higher than 120
5. Activity: plan paced activity to maximize available CO
6. Symptoms: report promptly any chest pain, new onset of dyspnea on exertion, paroxysmal nocturnal dyspnea
7. Other: report even minor changes to physician or home care nurse because they may be early signs of decompensation

VI. ENDOCARDITIS (INFECTIVE, SUBACUTE BACTERIAL)

A. Overview

1. Inflammation of inner layer of heart; usually involves cardiac valves
2. Caused by microorganisms in blood: risk factors include IV drug use, structural defects in heart or valves (which increase number of platelet and fibrin strands in endothelium)
   a. Acute endocarditis: sudden onset with *Staphylococcus aureus* being most common organism
   b. Subacute endocarditis: gradual onset with *Streptococcus viridans* or other less virulent bacteria
3. Microorganisms in bloodstream colonize on fibrin and platelet strands in endothelium, multiply and develop new strands; seen as "vegetation" attached to endothelium, particularly valves, causing damage; segments of vegetation may break off and travel to extremities manifested as petechiae

NCLEX®

B. Nursing data collection

1. Acute: spiking fever and chills; signs of HF (see previous section); WBC elevation
2. Subacute: fever of unknown origin; cough; dyspnea; anorexia; malaise; normal WBC; anemia; and elevated erythrocyte sedimentation rate (ESR)
3. Both: positive blood cultures; new cardiac **murmurs** (abnormal heart sounds heard during systole or diastole) or change in existing murmur; petechiae (small hemorrhagic spots) on trunk, conjunctiva, or mucous membranes as embolic complications from segments of vegetation circulating in body; splinter hemorrhages (streaks) in nail beds; Janeway lesions (purple-red macular lesions on palms and soles); Roth's spots (small, whitish "cotton wool" spots on retina)

NCLEX®

C. Therapeutic management

1. Manage IV therapy; observe for any signs of infection
2. Determine appropriateness of home infusion therapy; client may require inpatient treatment in a subacute care facility if home infusion therapy is contraindicated (such as IV drug abuse)

3. Provide periods of rest and moderate periods of exercise to prevent venous stasis
4. Use antiembolism stockings to prevent thrombus formation
5. Provide for diversional activity; client is restricted from resuming normal activity for 4–6 weeks
6. Antibiotics given by IV route are needed for 6 weeks

D. Reinforce client teaching

1. Role in home infusion therapy
2. After one episode of endocarditis, client is susceptible to repeated infections because of lesions on endocardium; tell future caregivers about infection
3. Symptoms to report to physician, such as fever, anorexia, malaise
4. Gentle, thorough, oral care because infectious organisms can easily enter bloodstream through gums with vigorous brushing or oral treatments
5. Need for prophylactic antibiotics before invasive procedures and routine dental care

VII. VALVULAR DISORDERS

A. Overview

1. Defects in cardiac valve structure or function that interfere with proper cardiac circulation
2. **Stenosis**: heart valve leaflets are fused together; opening is narrow, stiff, and unable to open or close properly
3. **Regurgitation**: there is improper or incomplete closure of heart valves, resulting in back flow of blood
4. Multiple causes including rheumatic heart disease (most common), congenital, MI, endocarditis
5. Calcium deposits or scar tissue from endocarditis or MI may cause valve stiffening in stenosis

NCLEX® **B. Nursing data collection**

1. Heart sounds: valve dysfunctions have distinctive characteristic changes in heart sounds (see Table 52–3)
2. Symptoms and severity depend on extent of valve dysfunction, from asymptomatic to severe HF, and on type of valve dysfunction (stenosis or regurgitation); see Table 52–3

NCLEX® **C. Therapeutic management**

1. Refer again to Table 52–3
2. Monitor heart sounds to note changes
3. With signs of decreased CO, restrict activity to decrease demands on heart
4. Monitor for signs of endocarditis
5. Report changes to health care provider
6. Medication therapy is determined by symptoms; may include antidysrhythmics, anticoagulants (atrial fibrillation), antibiotics (endocarditis), and drugs to treat HF as needed
7. Surgery: valve repair or replacement (see discussion earlier in chapter)

D. Reinforce client teaching

1. Management of anticoagulants (warfarin, Coumadin) to prevent thrombus formation, including monitoring PT/INR and regulation of vitamin K in diet (green leafy vegetables)
2. Relationships among valve disorders, surgical valves, and increased risk for bacterial endocarditis
3. Methods to prevent endocarditis

VIII. CARDIOMYOPATHY

A. Overview

1. An abnormality of heart muscle that leads to functional changes in heart
2. Cause is unknown if primary; secondary cardiomyopathy may occur because of ischemia, infectious disease, exposure to toxins, connective tissue or metabolic disorders, or nutritional deficiencies
3. Three types: dilated, hypertrophic, and restrictive
   a. Dilated cardiomyopathy (most common): enlargement of all four chambers, starting with enlarged ventricles, followed by decreased contractility; CO progressively decreases
   b. Hypertrophic cardiomyopathy: unexplained progressive thickening of ventricular muscle mass causing increased pulmonary and venous pressures; CO progressively decreases
   c. Restrictive cardiomyopathy (least common): excessively rigid ventricular walls do not stretch during diastolic filling, creating back pressure and right HF as well as reduced SV and consequently, lowered CO

B. Nursing data collection

1. Fatigue with all types
2. Dilated: weakness, signs of left HF, S_3 (ventricular gallop heard immediately after S_2 with left ventricular failure or mitral regurgitation) and S_4 (atrial gallop heard immediately before S_1 with coronary heart disease, left ventricular hypertrophy, or aortic stenosis)

Table 52-3 Heart Valve Disorders

Valve Disorder	Specific Data Items	Planning and Implementation
Mitral stenosis	Murmur: low-pitched rumbling diastolic Common in young women Atrial dysrhythmias, especially atrial fibrillation (A-fib)	Monitor closely during pregnancy Administer diuretics and digoxin as prescribed Maintain sodium-restricted diet Anticoagulant therapy if A-fib present Prepare for surgery
Mitral regurgitation (insufficiency)	Murmur: high-pitched blowing systolic Clients generally asymptomatic A-fib common with low incidence of embolization	Administer diuretics, nitrates and ACE inhibitors as prescribed Maintain sodium-restricted diet
Mitral prolapse	Murmur: systolic click Most clients asymptomatic May have PVCs and palpitations, syncope, weakness, and anxiety	Administer beta-blockers as prescribed for syncopy and palpitations Monitor for signs of infective endocarditis Administer prophylactic antibiotics with invasive procedures
Aortic stenosis	Murmur: harsh systolic Late course symptoms: angina; S_3 and S_4; syncope	In symptomatic client, restrict activity to decrease myocardial oxygen consumption Monitor for signs of infective endocarditis Administer prophylactic antibiotics with invasive procedures Prepare for surgery: symptomatic aortic stenosis has poor prognosis without surgical intervention
Aortic regurgitation (insufficiency)	Murmur: blowing diastolic Widened pulse pressure Palpitations; tachycardia and PVCs	Medical management same as aortic stenosis Prepare for surgery, which is the only effective long-term therapy for aortic regurgitation

3. Hypertrophic: exertional dyspnea, syncope, angina, signs of HF, S_4, sudden death often first sign in asymptomatic individuals
4. Restrictive: dyspnea, right-sided HF, S_3, and S_4, emboli formation

C. Therapeutic management

1. Monitor indicators of level of HF (VS, lung sounds, edema, dyspnea, activity tolerance) *NCLEX®*
2. Encourage rest and minimize stressful situations to reduce cardiac workload *NCLEX®*
3. Provide counseling and psychological support because of poor prognosis
4. Medications such as digoxin are used to treat signs of HF
5. Anticoagulation therapy is used with restrictive cardiomyopathy to prevent emboli
6. Beta-blockers, calcium channel blockers, antidysrhythmics or implanted dual chamber pacemaker or IACD may be needed with hypertrophic type; surgical excision of part of ventricular septum may also be done

D. Reinforce client teaching

1. Avoid alcohol because of its cardiac-depressant effects
2. How to pace activities to reduce cardiac workload
3. Medication and dietary management of HF
4. Anticoagulation therapy and monitoring if appropriate to prevent emboli formation
5. Usual post-surgical teaching after pacemaker or IACD insertion or surgery on septum

IX. PERICARDITIS

A. Overview

1. Inflammation of pericardium
2. Acute pericarditis: may have multiple causes, including infection (viral most common), post-MI status (Dressler's syndrome), neoplasms, trauma, uremia, connective tissue diseases, or endocrine diseases

3. Chronic pericarditis: leads to fibrous thickening of pericardium, constricting movement of myocardium and restricting diastolic filling

NCLEX® **B. Nursing data collection**

1. Acute: substernal pain, radiating to neck, aggravated by breathing (particularly during inspiration) or coughing; friction rub (scratchy, high-pitched sound on auscultation); elevated WBC; fever; malaise; ECG changes including ST and T wave elevations followed by inverted T waves when ST returns to baseline
2. Chronic restrictive pericarditis: increasing dyspnea, fatigue leading to progressive signs of heart failure

NCLEX® **C. Therapeutic management**

1. Monitor for and relieve chest pain
2. Administer O_2 as ordered and monitor SO_2
3. NCLEX® Monitor for complications, especially cardiac **tamponade** (medical emergency; excess fluid collection in pericardial sac that interferes with heart filling and function); signs include the following:
   a. JVD with clear lungs
   b. Elevated CVP
   c. Narrowing pulse pressure
   d. Decreased CO
   e. Muffled heart sounds
4. Report significant changes immediately
5. Position client for comfort: high Fowler's, sitting, or side-lying
6. Provide for periods of rest and limit activity to decrease cardiac workload
7. Medication therapy: analgesics for pain, nonsteroidal anti-inflammatory drugs (NSAIDs) followed by corticosteroids if needed, antibiotics if caused by infection; avoid anticoagulants because of risk of tamponade
8. Pericardiocentesis: aspiration of fluid from pericardial sac to determine cause or as emergency treatment for tamponade
9. Dialysis for inflammation caused by uremia
10. Radiation to treat neoplasms

D. Reinforce client teaching

1. Disease process and medication management
2. Take anti-inflammatory drugs with food, milk, or antacids to reduce gastric distress
3. Risk for repeat episodes of pericarditis; report similar pain or dyspnea promptly

X. PRIMARY HYPERTENSION

A. Overview

1. BP of 140 mm Hg or higher systolic, or 90 or greater diastolic, based on average of 3 or more readings done on separate occasions
2. Hypertension can be primary (essential) or secondary; risk factors for primary hypertension include family history, age, race (more common in Blacks), high sodium intake, obesity, inactivity, excessive alcohol intake, and insulin resistance (with resulting hyperinsulinemia and effects on vascular smooth muscle and sympathetic nervous system)
3. Is classified by stage: prehypertension (120–139 systolic or 80–89 diastolic), stage 1 (140–159 systolic or 90–99 diastolic), or stage 2 (160 or higher systolic or 100 or higher diastolic)
4. A hypertensive crisis or emergency occurs when BP is 180/120 or higher; treatment is required within 1 hour to prevent cardiac, vascular, and renal damage

NCLEX® **B. Nursing data collection**

1. Past history of cardiovascular, cerebrovascular, renal, or thyroid diseases, diabetes, smoking, or alcohol use
2. Family history of hypertension or cardiovascular disease
3. Often silent with absence of symptoms if no target organ damage
4. Possible fatigue, nocturia, dyspnea on exertion (DOE), palpitations, angina, headaches, weight gain, edema, muscle cramps, or blurred vision may be caused by target organ damage
5. Possible retinal vessel changes, diminished or absent peripheral pulses, bruits, murmurs, and S_3 and S_4 heart sounds
6. Possible cardiomegaly on x-ray or left ventricular hypertrophy on ECG
7. Signs of hypertensive crisis include blurred vision, papilledema (swelling of optic nerve), headache, confusion, motor and sensory deficits

NCLEX® **C. Therapeutic management**

1. Tell client numeric BP readings for ongoing record-keeping

2. Accurately record I&O and daily weights of hospitalized clients
3. Medication therapy
   a. A stepped care approach is often used to guide treatment; this begins with lifestyle changes and adds medications based on response to previous therapy
   b. Medications follow a treatment algorithm for hypertensive stage and include thiazide-type diuretics, ACE inhibitors, angiotensin receptor blockers (ARBs), beta-blockers, calcium channel blockers, and, if needed, vasodilators
4. Hypertensive crisis is treated using parenteral vasodilators; goal is to reduce BP by no more than 25% in minutes to one hour, and then toward 160/100 within 2–6 hours to prevent organ ischemia caused by rapid reduction in BP; monitor BP every 5–30 minutes during this time

D. Reinforce client teaching

1. Hypertension is usually asymptomatic, and symptoms will not reliably indicate BP levels
2. *NCLEX®* Lifestyle modification
   a. Sodium restriction
   b. Weight reduction and exercise
   c. DASH (dietary approaches to stop hypertension) diet: includes prescribed number of servings of following foods: grains and grain products; vegetables; fruits; low-fat or nonfat dairy foods; meats, poultry, and fish; nuts, seeds, and legumes; fats and oils; and sweets
   d. Moderation of alcohol intake
   e. Relaxation techniques and stress management
   f. No smoking
3. *NCLEX®* Prevent **orthostatic hypotension** (a drop in blood pressure of 10–20 mm Hg with upright posture) by rising out of bed or chair slowly
4. Avoid hot baths and strenuous exercise within 3 hours of taking vasodilators
5. Adhere to treatment plan, even if asymptomatic, to reduce risk of target organ damage

XI. PERIPHERAL ARTERIAL DISEASE

A. Overview

1. Disorders that impede arterial peripheral blood flow; primarily caused by **atherosclerosis** (local accumulation of lipid and fibrous tissue along intimal layer of artery), but also by trauma, embolism, thrombosis, vasospasm, inflammation, or autoimmunity
2. By the time symptoms appear, vessel is about 75% narrowed
3. Femoral-popliteal area is most common site in nondiabetics; clients with diabetes most often develop disease in arteries below knees
4. Chronic arterial obstruction leads to inadequate tissue oxygenation, causing **intermittent claudication**, ischemic muscle pain precipitated by a predictable amount of exercise and relieved by rest

NCLEX® **B. Nursing data collection**

1. Intermittent claudication, an early sign of disease
2. **Rest pain**, which may awaken client at night; pain is usually in distal extremity (toes, arch, forefoot, heel) and is relieved when foot is placed below heart level; indicates more advanced disease
3. Extremities may be cool, pale, and numb with a cyanotic color on elevation
4. Bruits may be auscultated
5. Diminished or absent peripheral pulses
6. Thickened and opaque nails (trophic change)
7. Skin on legs may be shiny with sparse hair growth (trophic change)
8. Ulcers may be present on lower extremities in areas affected by reduced circulation
9. Diagnostic testing: digital subtraction angiography (DSA), angiography, Doppler ultrasound, plethysmography
10. See Table 52–4 for a comparison of arterial and venous vascular disease

NCLEX® **C. Therapeutic management**

1. Palpate and record strength of pulses
2. Encourage smoking cessation
3. Change position at least hourly and avoid crossing legs
4. Encourage client to exercise and walk to point of pain; stop walking when pain occurs and resume when pain stops to build exercise tolerance and stimulate growth of collateral circulation
5. Collect data about pain on a 1-to-10 scale and provide analgesics as ordered
6. If an ulcer develops, healing will be slow unless arterial blood flow is improved through surgery
7. If surgery is indicated, provide appropriate postoperative care

Table 52–4 Comparison of Arterial and Venous Vascular Disease

Data Item	Arterial Disease	Venous Disease
Color	Pale	Ruddy; cyanotic if dependent
Edema	None or minimal	Usually present
Nails	Thick and brittle	Normal
Pain	Worse with elevation and exercise; may be sudden or severe; rest pain; claudication	Better with elevation; possible Homan's sign, dullness or heaviness
Pulses	Decreased, weak, or absent	Normal
Temperature of extremity	Cool	Warm
Ulcers	Dry and necrotic	Moist; malleolar

8. Angioplasty
   NCLEX®
   a. Monitor **neurovascular status** (color, motion, sensitivity, temperature, and presence of distal peripheral pulses) to affected extremity every 15 minutes for 4 hours, every 30 minutes for 4 hours, then every 1 to 4 hours after sheath removal
   b. Notify physician if client experiences weak or thready pulses, coolness, numbness, or tingling in extremity
   c. Monitor sheath site for external and subcutaneous bleeding
   d. Explain to notify nurse and apply manual pressure to site if warm or wet sensation is felt at site
   e. Keep affected extremity immobilized for at least 6 hours by reminding client to keep extremity still, or lightly immobilize ankle with sheet tucked under both sides of mattress
   f. Maintain a pressure dressing and sand bag at site
9. Bypass grafting
   a. Provide standard postoperative care
   b. Monitor for signs of graft occlusion: severe ischemic pain, loss of pulses, decreasing ankle-brachial index, numbness, tingling or coolness of extremity
10. **Endarterectomy** (opening artery and removing obstructing plaque) or amputation in severe cases; use same principles of care as for other procedures
11. Medication therapy: aspirin inhibits platelet aggregation; pentoxifylline (Trental) decreases blood viscosity and increases blood flow; cilostazol (Pletal) inhibits platelet aggregation and enhances vasodilation; clopidogrel (Plavix) and ticlopidine (Ticlid) prevent thrombi formation with recent MI or stroke

D. Reinforce client teaching

NCLEX®

1. See Box 52–2
2. Relaxation techniques (stress increases vasoconstriction)

Box 52–2

Client and Family Education for Peripheral Arterial Disease

- Stop smoking
- Lose weight and eat a low-fat diet
- Do not cross legs while sitting
- Elevate feet at rest, but not above heart level
- Do not stand or sit for long periods of time
- Do not wear restrictive clothing
- Keep affected extremity warm but never apply direct heat
- Inspect feet daily and keep them clean and dry
- Avoid walking barefoot; wear proper-fitting shoes
- Avoid mechanical or thermal injury to the legs and feet; have nail care performed by podiatrist
- Begin and maintain an exercise and walking program
- Notify health care provider of any changes in color, sensation, temperature, or pulses in extremities

XII. ARTERIAL EMBOLISM

A. Overview

1. Arterial emboli usually develop in heart from atrial fibrillation, MI, HF, or prosthetic valves
2. Thrombi become detached and are carried from left heart into arterial system where they may lodge and cause obstruction
3. Symptoms may be abrupt and depend on size and location of embolus
4. Ischemia will progress to necrosis and gangrene within hours if untreated

NCLEX®

B. Nursing data collection: the "six Ps"

1. Pain
2. Pallor (pale color)
3. Pulselessness (diminished or absent pulses)
4. Parasthesias (altered local sensation)
5. Paralysis (weakness or inability to move extremity)
6. **Poikilothermia** (body temperature that varies with environment, usually is decreased)

NCLEX®

C. Therapeutic management

1. Monitor peripheral pulses and neurovascular status every 2 to 4 hours
2. Place affected extremity in a neutral position with no restrictive bedding or clothing
3. Determine level of pain using a 1-to-10 scale
4. Change position every 2 hours to improve collateral circulation
5. Monitor for and report unusual bleeding from anticoagulant therapy
6. Monitor lab values, including aPTT, PT, and INR levels
7. An emergency embolectomy should be performed within 4–5 hours to prevent permanent damage
8. If necrosis or infection is present, surgery is required for definitive treatment
9. Medication therapy (if no necrosis present): thrombolytic therapy with streptokinase, TPA or anticoagulant therapy with heparin; warfarin therapy at home

D. Reinforce client teaching

1. Pre- and postoperative teaching if embolectomy is performed
2. Measures to promote peripheral circulation and maintain tissue integrity (refer back to Box 52–2)

XIII. BUERGER'S DISEASE (THROMBOANGIITIS OBLITERANS)

A. Overview

1. Inflammatory disease of small- and medium-sized veins and arteries accompanied by thrombi and sometimes vasospasm; may occur in upper or lower extremities but is most common in leg or foot
2. Etiology is uncertain but is currently thought to involve an autoimmune reaction (occurs mostly in young men who are heavy smokers); higher incidence of HLA-B5 and 2A9 antigens suggest a genetic link
3. Inflammation occurs; microthrombi form; both can lead to vasospasm, and this process ultimately obstructs blood flow

NCLEX®

B. Nursing data collection

1. Initially, a bluish cast to a toe or finger and a feeling of coldness in affected limb is common
2. Rest pain, possibly severe
3. Excessive sweating in feet is possible from overactive sympathetic nerves, even though feet feel cold
4. Intermittent claudication and other symptoms similar to those of chronic obstructive arterial disease often appear gradually after occlusion
5. Ischemic ulcers and gangrene are common complications of progressive Buerger's disease

NCLEX®

C. Therapeutic management

1. Arrest progress of disease by smoking cessation
2. Take measures to promote vasodilation (similar to other arterial disorders)
3. Provide for pain relief
4. Provide emotional support
5. Medication therapy: analgesic pain medications, calcium channel blockers to ease vasospasm, pentoxifylline (Trental) to reduce blood viscosity
6. Surgical treatment includes sympathectomy (to vasodilate or eliminate vessel spasm) or arterial bypass grafting when larger arteries are involved

D. Reinforce client teaching

1. Stop smoking
2. Take measures to promote peripheral circulation and maintain tissue integrity (refer back to Box 52–2)

XIV. RAYNAUD'S DISEASE

A. Overview

1. Localized, intermittent episodes of vasoconstriction of small arteries of hands and, less commonly, feet, causing pallor, coolness, and cyanosis; primarily affects young women
2. Vasospastic attacks tend to be bilateral and symmetrical and usually begin at tips of digits, causing pallor, numbness, and sensation of cold
3. Attacks are triggered by exposure to cold, emotional stress, caffeine ingestion, and tobacco use

B. Nursing data collection

1. Classic triphasic color changes (pallor, cyanosis, and rubor) in hands with accompanying reduction in skin temperature
2. Intensity of pain increases as disease progresses
3. Skin of fingertips may thicken, and nails may become brittle

C. Therapeutic management

1. Keep hands warm and free from injury
2. Avoid stressful situations
3. In severe cases, a **sympathectomy** (surgical dissection of nerve fibers to relieve symptoms) may be performed
4. Medication therapy: analgesics for pain and possibly vasodilators and calcium channel blockers (vasospasm)

D. Reinforce client teaching

1. Keep hands warm: wear gloves when outdoors, in air-conditioned area, or handling cold food
2. Avoid injury to hands
3. Lifestyle changes: stop smoking; employ stress relief such as biofeedback

XV. AORTIC ANEURYSM

A. Overview

1. Localized dilation or outpouching of weakened area in aorta, classified by region as thoracic or abdominal, or as dissecting (layers of blood vessels separated by a layer of blood)
2. More common in abdominal aorta below level of renal arteries but can occur in thoracic area
3. Growth rate is unpredictable, and large aneurysms tend to rupture, a life-threatening emergency
4. Major risk factor is atherosclerosis

B. Nursing data collection

1. Thoracic aneurysms are often asymptomatic, with first sign being rupture
   - a. Symptoms may include pain in back, neck, and substernal area that may occur only when lying supine
   - b. Possible dysphagia and dyspnea, stridor, or cough when pressing on esophagus or laryngeal nerve
2. Abdominal aneurysms may also be asymptomatic until rupture
   - a. Client may report a "heartbeat" in abdomen when lying down
   - b. Possible pulsating abdominal mass; do not palpate (risk of rupture)
   - c. Moderate to severe abdominal or lumbar back pain may be present (severe pain may be a sign of impending rupture)
   - d. Client may experience claudication
   - e. Cool or cyanotic extremities may be noted
   - f. Systolic bruit may be heard
3. Dissecting aneurysms present with sudden, severe, and persistent pain described as "tearing" or "ripping" in anterior chest or back
   - a. Pain may extend to shoulder, epigastric area, or abdomen
   - b. Pallor, sweating, and tachycardia are evidenced
   - c. Initially, client may have an elevated BP that may be different in one arm than other
   - d. Possible syncope and paralysis of lower extremities

C. Therapeutic management

1. Diagnosed by chest x-ray, transesophageal echocardiography, aortography, ultrasound, and CT scan or MRI
2. Hematomas into scrotum, perineum, flank, or penis indicate retroperitoneal rupture
3. Surgery may be performed on an emergency or elective basis (not usually performed if less than 4 to 5 cm); involves excision of aneurysm with insertion of synthetic graft
4. Preoperatively mark and measure all peripheral pulses for comparison postoperatively

5. Postoperatively monitor neurovascular status and monitor for complications, such as graft occlusion, hypovolemia (renal failure), respiratory distress, cardiac dysrhythmias, paralytic ileus, and paraplegia (paralysis); use overbed cradle
6. Medication therapy
   a. Antihypertensives and diuretics to control blood pressure
   b. Postoperative anticoagulant therapy: heparin during hospitalization and warfarin (Coumadin) after discharge

D. Reinforce client teaching

1. If under medical care, get routine physical exams to monitor status of aneurysm
2. Signs and symptoms of impending rupture (see data collection of dissecting aneurysms above)
3. Monitor BP and report increases immediately; take medications as ordered
4. Postoperative teaching
   a. Do limited lifting for 4–6 weeks after surgery (no heavy lifting at all)
   b. Monitor incision site for bleeding and infection
   c. Self-assessment of neurovascular status of and pulses in extremities
5. Clients with a synthetic graft may require prophylactic antibiotics before invasive procedures

XVI. THROMBOPHLEBITIS

A. Overview

1. Formation of a thrombus (clot) associated with vein inflammation; classified as superficial or deep
2. Etiology: Virchow's triad (at least two of three conditions must be present for thrombosis to occur)
   a. Stasis of venous flow
   b. Damage to inner lining of vein (endothelial layer)
   c. Hypercoagulability of blood
3. If detachment occurs, emboli travel through veins to heart and into pulmonary circulation

NCLEX® **B. Nursing data collection**

1. History of thrombophlebitis, pelvic or abdominal surgery, obesity, neoplasm (hepatic and pancreatic), HF, atrial fibrillation, prolonged immobility, MI, pregnancy and/or postpartum period, IV therapy, hypercoagulable states (polycythemia, dehydration, or malnutrition)
2. Superficial
   a. Palpable, firm, subcutaneous, cordlike vein
   b. Surrounding area warm, red, tender to touch
   c. Edema may or may not be present
   d. Most common cause in arms is IV therapy; in legs it is often related to varicose veins
3. Deep
   NCLEX® a. Unilateral edema, pain, warm skin, and elevated temperature
   b. If inferior vena cava is involved, both legs will be edematous
   c. If superior vena cava is involved, both upper extremities, neck, back, and face may become edematous or cyanotic
   NCLEX® d. If calf is involved, **Homan's sign** may be present (pain on dorsiflexion of foot, especially when leg is raised, nonspecific sign)
4. Diagnostic studies: venous duplex scanning; Doppler ultrasonic flowmeter, MRI, and lung scan

NCLEX® **C. Therapeutic management**

1. Provide analgesics for pain relief
2. Elevate affected leg higher than heart to promote venous drainage
3. Apply warm, moist compresses, intermittent or continuous, to affected extremity; never massage affected extremity to reduce risk of embolism
4. Measure and monitor limb circumference when edema is present
5. Monitor status of peripheral pulses
6. Keep bed covers from touching affected limb by using an overbed cradle to avoid pressure and subsequent skin breakdown
7. Maintain strict bedrest
8. Instruct client to report any pink-tinged sputum and monitor for tachypnea, tachycardia, shortness of breath, chest pain, and apprehension, which may indicate a pulmonary embolism
9. Medication therapy: anticoagulants, thrombolytics, analgesics (NSAIDs to reduce pain and relieve inflammation)

D. Reinforce client teaching

1. Prevention
   a. Early ambulation postoperatively
   b. Use of compression stockings or pneumatic compression boots
   c. Low-dose anticoagulant therapy
   d. Avoid prolonged standing or sitting and sitting with crossed legs
   e. Avoid restrictive clothing
   f. Stop smoking
2. Anticoagulant therapy

XVII. VENOUS INSUFFICIENCY

A. Overview

1. Inadequate venous return over time causes venous hypertension, which stretches veins and damages valves, reducing blood return
2. Risk factors include thrombus formation, prolonged standing or sitting (teachers, waitresses, nurses, office workers), pregnancy, and obesity

NCLEX® **B. Nursing data collection**

1. Past history of thrombophlebitis, hypertension, varicosities
2. Past history of long periods of sitting and/or standing
3. Edema of lower legs, may extend to knee
4. Thick, coarse, brownish skin around ankles and feet
5. Stasis ulcers, usually in malleolar area
6. Refer back to Table 52–4 for a general comparison of signs of arterial and venous disorders

NCLEX® **C. Therapeutic management**

1. Bedrest with legs elevated above heart level
2. Avoid long periods of standing
3. Wear elastic support or compression hose (apply *before* getting out of bed and placing leg in a dependent position); remove at night
4. Never push hosiery down around leg—will further impair circulation
5. Treat venous stasis ulcer(s)
   a. Open lesions: hydrocolloid dressing and compression wraps; possible topical ointment, such as low-dose hydrocortisone, zinc oxide, or an antifungal
   b. Unna Boot or other compression wrap that is changed every 1–2 weeks and usually applied over a base dressing
   c. Severe ulcers may need surgical debridement
6. Medication therapy
   a. Topical agents to skin ulcers, such as hydrocortisone, antifungals, or zinc oxide
   b. Oral or IV antibiotics may be prescribed (infected ulcer or cellulitis)

D. Reinforce client teaching

1. Elevate legs for at least 20 minutes four times a day
2. Keep legs above level of heart when in bed
3. Avoid prolonged sitting or standing and do not cross legs when sitting
4. Do not wear tight, restrictive pants, socks, or boots; avoid girdles and garters that restrict circulation in upper leg
5. Wear support stockings as instructed

XVIII. VARICOSE VEINS

A. Overview

1. A vein or veins in which blood has pooled, producing distended, tortuous, and palpable vessels; valve leaflets become defective
2. Risk factors: women over 35, obesity, positive family history, prolonged standing
3. As vein swells, increased hydrostatic pressure pushes plasma through stretched vessel walls and edema may occur

NCLEX® **B. Nursing data collection**

1. Reports of aching, heaviness, itching, swelling, and unsightly appearance to leg(s)
2. Dilated, tortuous, superficial veins along upper and lower leg
3. Superficial inflammation may develop along path of varicose vein

4. Positive Trendelenburg test (evaluates valve competence; veins fill from proximal rather than distal end after sitting up from supine position with legs raised)

NCLEX®

C. Therapeutic management

1. Analgesics as needed
2. Improve venous circulation as described for venous insufficiency
3. Monitor pulses and neurovascular status of lower extremities
4. Apply support stockings
5. Elevate feet above heart level when lying down
6. Prevent skin breakdown; teach proper skin care and importance of avoiding trauma to legs
7. Sclerotherapy: injection of sclerosing agent into varicosed vein, usually in physician's office (palliative but not curative; elastic bandages often worn for several weeks)
8. Vein ligation surgery involves ligation (tying off) of entire vein (usually saphenous) and dissection and removal of incompetent tributaries
   a. Perform hourly circulation checks postoperatively in postanesthesia area
   b. Elevate extremity to a 15-degree angle to prevent stasis and edema
   c. Apply compression-gradient stockings from foot to groin
9. Medication therapy: no specific medications are used

D. Reinforce client teaching: prevention as for venous insufficiency; lose weight if necessary

XIX. *ACYANOTIC HEART DEFECTS*

A. Heart conditions that do not cause deoxygenation or low O_2 levels; blood flows from left to right side of heart, increasing pulmonary blood flow; skin and mucous membrane color is usually normal pink

B. Atrial septal defect (see Figure 52–1A)

1. Defect in atrial septal wall allowing blood to flow from left atrium to right atrium, called a left-to-right shunt; caused by failure of foramen ovale to close

NCLEX®

2. Data collection: often asymptomatic if defect is small; dyspnea, fatigue, poor growth, and soft systolic murmur in pulmonic area, splitting S_2
3. Diagnosed by echocardiogram (right ventricular overload and shunt size), cardiac catheterization (visualization of defect)
4. Therapeutic intervention includes surgical closure or patch of defect, transcatheter device closure during cardiac catheterization

NCLEX®

5. Nursing management of child with acyanotic heart disease (see Table 52–5)
6. Reinforce child and family education
   a. Purpose of tests and procedures
   b. Ways to support nutrition, reduce stress on heart, promote rest, and support growth and development during preoperative period
   c. Signs of HF and infection
   d. Prepare parents and child for surgery by visiting intensive care unit, explaining equipment and sounds
   e. Prepare older child for postoperative experience, including coughing and deep breathing and need for movement
   f. Need for antibiotic prophylaxis to prevent subacute bacterial endocarditis

C. Ventricular septal defect (VSD) (see Figure 52–1B)

1. Defect in ventricle septal wall allowing blood to flow from left ventricle to right ventricle (**left-to-right shunt**) because of higher pressue in left ventricle
2. Shunting of blood causes an increased load on right ventricle and increases pulmonary blood flow

NCLEX®

3. Data collection: tachypnea, dyspnea, poor growth, reduced fluid intake, palpable thrill, systolic murmur at left lower sternal border; ECG and radiology detect larger septal defects; signs of HF

NCLEX®

4. Therapeutic management (see Table 52–5)
   a. Occasionally spontaneous closure occurs
   b. Surgical patching if failure to thrive occurs
   c. Prophylactic antibiotics treatment to prevent endocarditis
   d. Preoperative nursing care involves promoting oxygenation and growth and development (see Table 52–5)
   e. Postoperative nursing care continues with activities of preoperative care, providing analgesics for pain relief, and maintaining sterile dressing on incision
5. Reinforce child and family education (same as for atrial septal defect)

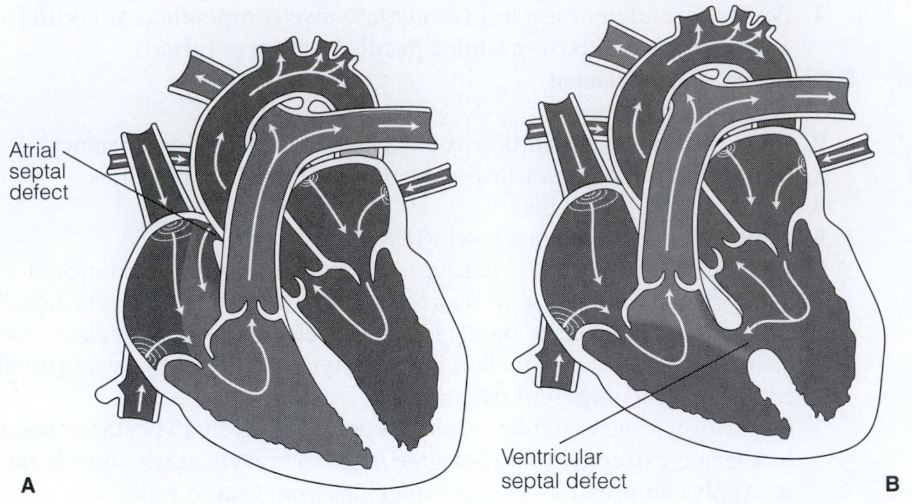

Figure 52–1

Heart defects with increased pulmonary blood flow. *A.* Atrial septal defect. *B.* Ventricular septal defect.

Table 52–5 Nursing Management of Child with an Acyanotic Heart Defect

Problem	Nursing Management
Anxiety and inadequate coping	1. Monitor coping mechanisms of family. 2. Provide family with information about condition. 3. Refer family to American Heart Association.
Possible delayed growth and development	1. Treat child as normally as possible. Teach parents that children are more comfortable when they know what to expect. 2. Promote mental development activities as appropriate for age and condition.
Risk for infection	1. Limit exposure to individuals with infections. 2. Promote good pulmonary hygiene—change position, use percussion and postural drainage. 3. Use prophylactic antibiotics when undergoing surgical or dental treatments to prevent subacute bacterial endocarditis.
Inadequate nutrition	1. Offer small, frequent meals. 2. Use soft nipple for infant to ease stress of sucking. 3. Organize nursing care to allow for rest.
Impaired gas exchange	1. Promote good pulmonary hygiene. 2. Monitor intake and output. Limit fluids as ordered. 3. Administer diuretics as ordered. 4. Change position every 2 hours.

D. Coarctation of aorta (see Figure 52–2)

1. Narrowing of descending aorta that restricts blood flow leaving heart
2. Often near ductus arteriosus
3. Progressive disorder that leads to HF

NCLEX®

4. Data collection: may be asymptomatic; BP difference of 20 mm between upper and lower extremities, brachial and radial pulses full, femoral pulses weak, headache, vertigo, epistaxis, exercise intolerance, left ventricular hypertrophy, dyspnea, cerebrovascular accident (CVA) secondary to hypertension in upper circulation

NCLEX®

5. Therapeutic management
   a. Balloon cardiac catheterization
   b. Surgical resection and patch of coarctation
   c. Prophylaxis for endocarditis when undergoing surgical or dental procedures
   d. Prior to correction, monitor BP in upper and lower extremities
   e. Rebound hypertension occurs in immediate postoperative period

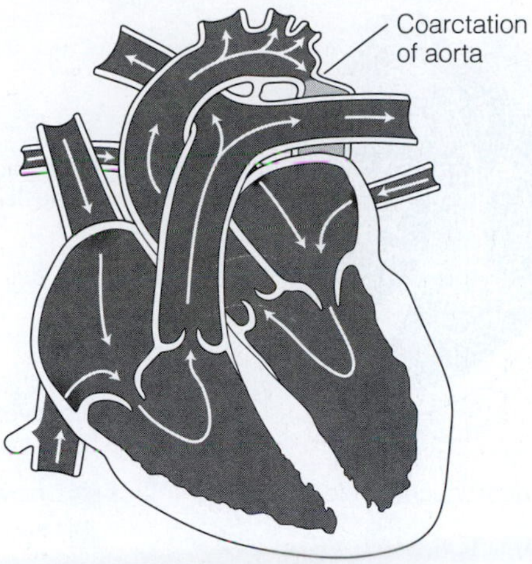

Figure 52–2

Coarctation of aorta.

6. Reinforce child and family education
   a. Tests and procedures child will undergo
   b. Signs and symptoms of worsening condition
   c. Administration of cardiac and vasoactive drugs
   d. Need for prophylactic antibiotics for all surgical and dental procedures

XX. *CYANOTIC HEART DEFECTS*

A. **Heart conditions that cause blood to contain inadequate O_2 by decreasing pulmonary blood flow**; skin and mucous membrane color is usually pale to blue; include pulmonic stenosis, tetralogy of Fallot, and pulmonary atresia (see Figure 52–3)

B. **Tetralogy of Fallot**

1. Four defects that combine to allow blood flow to bypass lungs and enter left side of heart, called a **right-to-left shunt**
   a. Four defects: pulmonic stenosis, right ventricular hypertrophy, ventricular septal defect, and overriding aorta
   b. Atrial septal defect occurs at times as a fifth defect
   c. Deficient O_2 in tissues leads to acidosis
   d. Hypercyanosis (TET) spells occur, which are transient periods when there is an increase in right-to-left shunting of blood
2. Deoxygenated blood enters systemic circulation, accounting for cyanosis

NCLEX®

3. Data collection
   a. TET spells: hypoxia, pallor, and tachypnea; precipitated by crying, defecation, and feeding; older children assume a squatting position to decrease blood return from lower extremities; treatment involves placing child in knee-chest position and administering morphine or propranolol and oxygen
   b. Clubbing of digits
   c. **Polycythemia** (excess number of RBCs), metabolic acidosis
   d. Poor growth, exercise intolerance
   e. Systolic murmur in pulmonic area
   f. Right ventricular hypertrophy
   g. Cardiac catheterization visualizes anomalous structures
4. Therapeutic management
   a. **Prostaglandin E1**: to maintain open ductus arteriosus
   b. Palliative surgery to improve oxygenation includes modified Blalock-Tassig shunt
   c. Corrective surgery includes patching VSD and relieving pulmonary stenosis

NCLEX®

   d. See Table 52-6 (p. 906) for associated nursing care
5. Reinforce child and family education
   a. Promote nutrition in light of weak suck
   b. Discuss activities to promote oxygenation
   c. Symptoms of respiratory infections
   d. Treatments and procedures child will undergo

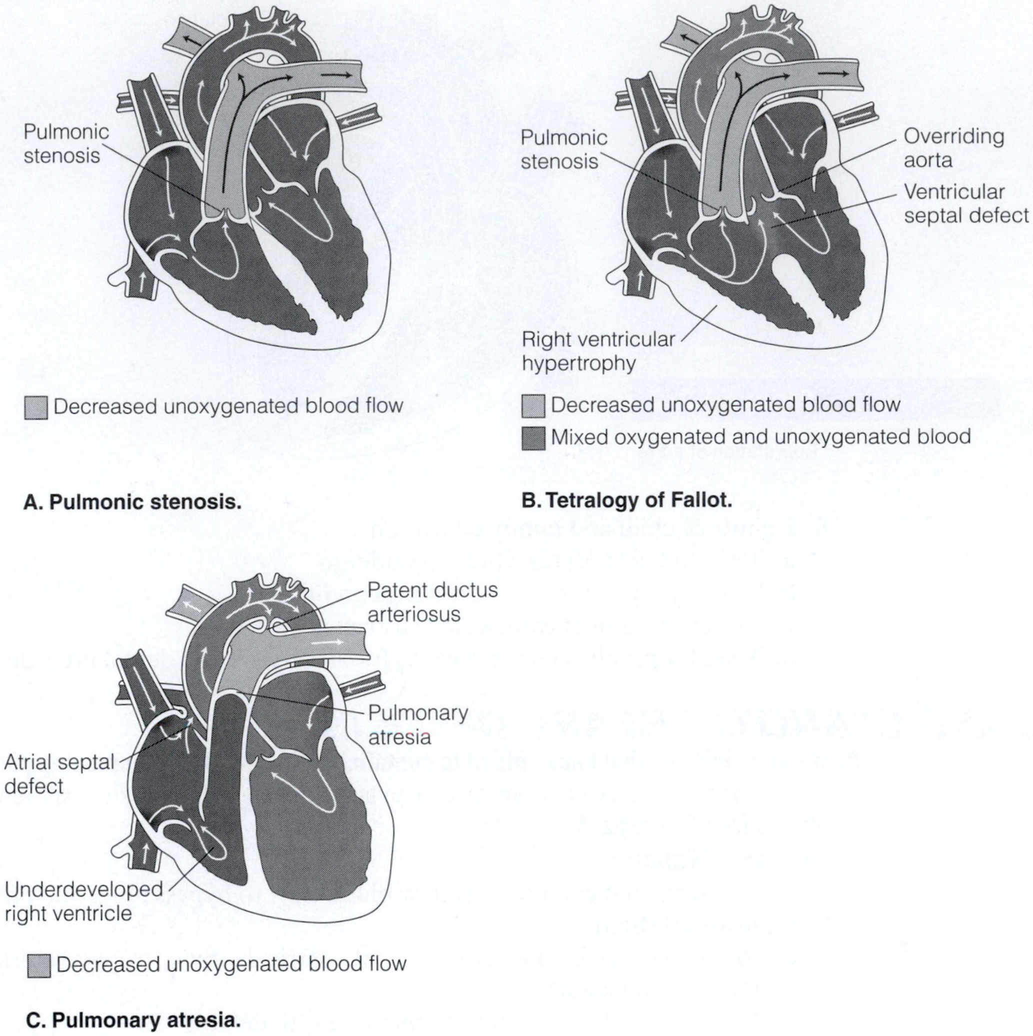

Figure 52–3

Heart Defects with Decreased Pulmonary Blood Flow.

C. Mixed heart defect: transposition of great vessels (see Figure 52–4)

1. Pulmonary artery originates from left ventricle; blood travels from left ventricle to pulmonary artery, then to lungs, and then back into left atrium
2. Aorta originates from right ventricle; blood leaves right ventricle by aorta, travels to body cells, and returns to right atrium by way of vena cava
3. There are two closed circulation pathways
4. Survival depends on foramen ovale remaining open to mix oxygenated and deoxygenated blood
5. *NCLEX®* Data collection: progressive cyanosis leads to hypoxia and then acidosis; signs of heart failure, tachypnea, poor feeding, failure to grow; echocardiogram identifies misplacement of arteries
6. *NCLEX®* Therapeutic management
   - a. Prostaglandin E1 to maintain open ductus arteriosus
   - b. Palliative surgical interventions
   - c. Corrective surgery
   - d. Prophylactic antibiotic therapy to prevent endocarditis
   - e. Nursing activities to promote nutrition and reduce respiratory congestion (see Table 52–6)
7. Reinforce child and family education
   - a. Home care requirements related to nutrition, rest, and oxygenation
   - b. Preparation for procedures and treatments
   - c. Safe administration of cardiac drugs and diuretics

D. Hypoplastic left heart syndrome (see Figure 52–5, p. 906)

1. Abnormally small left ventricle noted at birth, causing inadequate oxygen supply
2. Absent or stenotic mitral and aortic valves
3. Abnormally small left ventricle and aortic arch with major resistance to aortic blood flow
4. Hypertrophy of right ventricle
5. Prognosis poor

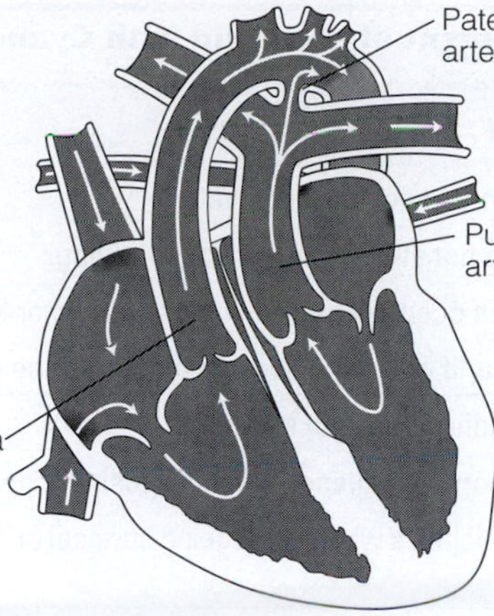

Figure 52–4

Mixed heart defect: Transposition of great arteries.

6. Data collection
   a. Tachypnea, chest retractions, dyspnea
   b. Cyanosis
   c. Decreased pulses, poor peripheral perfusion
   d. Increased right ventricular impulse
   e. Echocardiogram indicates small and weak left ventricle
   f. HF
7. Therapeutic management
   a. Prostaglandin E1 given to prevent closure of patent ductus arteriosus
   b. Palliative surgery
   c. Transplant may be performed
   d. Survival rate is low

XXI. RHEUMATIC FEVER

A. Overview

1. Systemic inflammatory disease involving heart, joints, and possibly CNS and connective tissue
2. Follows 2–6 weeks after a group A beta-hemolytic streptococcal infection
3. May be an autoimmune reaction against microorganisms; strep organisms cannot be cultured out of lesions of rheumatic fever
4. Acute phase lasts 2 to 3 weeks and is characterized by inflammation of connective tissue in heart, joints, and skin
5. Proliferative phase primarily affects heart, with Aschoff bodies developing on heart valves; cardiac valve leaflets scar and lead to valvular stenosis and regurgitation
6. Episode of rheumatic fever lasts up to 3 months and is self-limiting
7. *NCLEX®* Long-term consequence is rheumatic heart disease, which is often manifested in valvular damage
8. Difficult to diagnose because it mimics other diseases; diagnosis is usually based on **Jones criteria**, which lists major and minor manifestations according to likelihood of rheumatic fever infection; diagnosis is based on presence of two major or one major and two minor criteria

B. Data collection using Jones criteria *NCLEX®*

1. Major criteria
   a. Inflammation of multiple joints; most frequently large joints—knees, elbows, and wrists
   b. Carditis (most severe criteria): a new murmur, pericardial friction rub, changes on ECG; tachycardia in form of a sleeping pulse greater than 100
   c. CNS: chorea, which involves involuntary movement of limbs; emotional lability and slurred speech; tends to have a latent period of 2 months or more from strep infection
   d. Erythema marginatum is a erythematous, macular rash that occurs primarily on trunk and proximal limbs; frequently associated with carditis
   e. Subcutaneous nodules (nontender) on skin over flexor surfaces of joints and vertebrae
2. Minor criteria: fever (spiking temperature), arthralgia; elevated ESR, C-reactive protein, and decreased RBC count; prolonged PR and/or QT interval on ECG
3. Supporting evidence (of recent streptococcal infection): history of same, history of scarlet fever, positive throat culture for streptococcus, elevated antistreptolysin O (ASO) titer

Table 52-6 Nursing Management of the Child with Cyanotic Heart Disease

Problem	Nursing Management
Inadequate tissue perfusion	1. Monitor hemoglobin and hematocrit levels. 2. Keep child calm. Do not allow long periods of crying. 3. When hypercyanosis occurs, assist child to squatting or knee-chest position. 4. Administer oxygen and morphine as ordered during these spells.
Risk for infection	1. Limit exposure to individuals with infections. 2. Promote good pulmonary hygiene—change position, percussion, and postural drainage. 3. Use prophylactic antibiotics when undergoing surgical or dental treatments to prevent subacute bacterial endocarditis.
Inadequate nutrition	1. Offer small, frequent meals. 2. Use soft nipple for infant to ease stress of sucking. 3. Organize nursing care to allow for rest.
Possible impaired gas exchange	1. Limit activity. 2. Maintain clear airways. 3. Monitor electrolytes.
Possible decreased cardiac output	1. Note vital signs. 2. Monitor for signs of congestive heart failure. 3. Note peripheral edema. 4. Weigh child daily. 5. Maintain strict I&O measurement. 6. Administer diuretics as ordered. 7. Administer oxygen as ordered. 8. Palpate liver every 4–12 hours (indicates right-sided failure). 9. Administer digoxin as ordered: a. Check for apical pulse—monitor for bradycardia or arrhythmias. b. Be consistent in measurement of medication and time of administration. c. Do not repeat dose if child vomits.
Risk for injury	1. Monitor hemoglobin and hematocrit. 2. Observe for signs of thrombus formation.

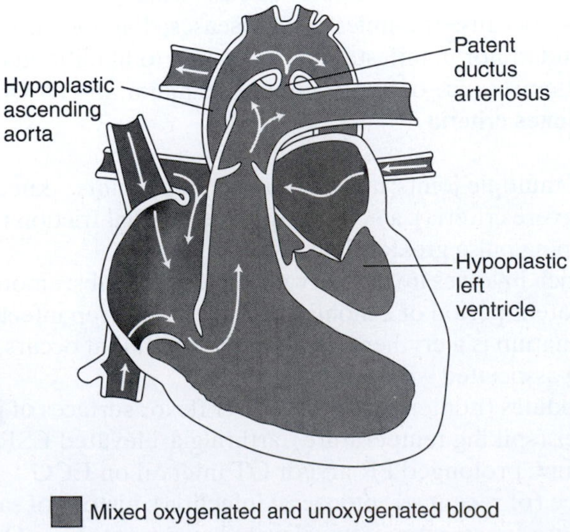

Figure 52-5

Hypoplastic left heart syndrome.

C. Therapeutic management

1. Bedrest until ESR returns to normal
2. Aspirin and prednisone as ordered; anti-inflammatory agents to reduce inflammation; aspirin will also promote relief from painful joints
3. Monitor client for cardiac function
4. Give penicillin as ordered in either an oral daily dose or monthly long-acting injection after recovery from rheumatic heart disease to reduce risk of recurrence of strep infection; erythromycin given if client is allergic to penicillin

NCLEX®

5. Design nursing activities to promote rest and to encourage diversional activities that do not stress heart; maintain bedrest with bathroom privileges
6. Reinforce child and family education
   a. Pathology of disease and rationale for bedrest
   b. Diversional activities that allow for mental stimulation without physical activity
   c. Planning for home care of child

XXII. KAWASAKI'S DISEASE

A. Overview

1. A multisystem disorder involving **vasculitis** (inflammation of tunica intima lining of arteries and veins)
2. Also called mucocutaneous lymph node syndrome
3. Unknown cause but generally affects young children; most frequently affected are boys under 2 years of age
4. Three phases of disease
   a. Acute phase characterized by fever, conjunctival hyperemia, swollen hands and feet, rash, and enlarged cervical lymph nodes
   b. Subacute phase is characterized by cracking lips, desquamation of skin on tips of fingers and toes, cardiac disease, and thrombocytosis
   c. Convalescent phase has lingering signs of inflammation
5. Significantly increased platelet count
6. Possible cardiac pathology, including dysrhythmias, HF, and MI

NCLEX®

B. Nursing data collection

1. Phase one (days 1 to 10): fever lasting longer than 5 days and unresponsive to antipyretics, conjunctivitis, crusted and fissured lips, swelling of hands and feet, erythema, **lymphadenopathy** (a condition that causes swollen glands and can be caused by infection or cancer)
2. Phase two (days 10 to 25): fever diminishes, irritability, anorexia, desquamation of hands and feet, arthritis and arthralgia, cardiovascular manifestations
3. Phase three (days 26 to 40): drop in ESR and diminishing signs of illness

C. Therapeutic management

1. Administer aspirin 80 to 100 mg/kg/day as ordered while temperature is elevated
2. Administer intravenous immune globulin (IVIG) as ordered to reduce risk of coronary artery lesions and aneurysms

NCLEX®

3. Nursing management
   a. Promote comfort
   b. Small, frequent feedings; encourage fluids
   c. Passive range of motion to extremities
   d. Cool baths and gentle oral care
   e. Monitor for complications: aneurysms; side effects of aspirin therapy (bleeding, GI upset); side effects of IVIG therapy (elevated BP, facial flushing, tightness in chest)
   f. Monitor temperature
   g. Monitor eyes for conjunctivitis

D. Reinforce child and family education

1. Safe administration of aspirin therapy
2. Keep skin clean and avoid soaps and lotions
3. Offer liquids high in calories, low in acids
4. Low-cholesterol diet
5. Call physician if child refuses to walk
6. Monitor temperature in morning and at night prior to giving aspirin

PRACTICE TEST

Check Your NCLEX-PN® Exam I.Q.

You are ready for testing on this content if you can

- Identify basic structures and functions of the cardiovascular system.
- Describe the pathophysiology and etiology of common cardiovascular disorders.
- Discuss expected data and diagnostic test findings for selected cardiovascular disorders.
- Discuss therapeutic management of a client experiencing a cardiovascular disorder.
- Discuss nursing management of a client experiencing a cardiovascular disorder.
- Identify expected outcomes for the client experiencing a cardiovascular disorder.

PRACTICE TEST

1 A client has been admitted to the emergency room with reports of chest pain for the past 2 hours. There are no clear changes on the 12-lead electrocardiogram (ECG). The nurse would expect which laboratory test to provide confirmation of a myocardial infarction (MI)? Select all that apply.

1. Potassium of 5.2 mEq/L
2. Creatinine kinase (CK) of 545
3. CK of 460 with MB of 11%
4. WBC of 11,400/mm^3
5. CK-MB isoenzyme of 6%

2 A client scheduled for discharge after coronary artery bypass grafting (CABG) reports new onset of anorexia and nausea. The client's new medications include digoxin (Lanoxin), metoprolol (Lopressor), and furosemide (Lasix). The nurse plans to report this finding to the registered nurse after checking the result of which laboratory test drawn earlier in the morning?

1. Potassium level
2. Sodium level
3. Creatinine kinase level
4. Digoxin level

3 A client with hypertension is being treated with metoprolol (Lopressor), hydrochlorothiazide (HydroDiuril), and captopril (Capoten). Other scheduled medications include docusate (Colace) and a multivitamin. The client's current blood pressure is 124/86 mm Hg and the pulse rate is 48. Which scheduled medication doses should the nurse administer? Select all that apply.

1. Metoprolol
2. Captopril
3. Hydrochlorothiazide
4. Docusate
5. Multivitamin

4 The nurse has finished reviewing the shift report on a cardiac unit. The nurse should plan to see which assigned client first?

1. A client with hypertrophic cardiomyopathy who is reporting dyspnea
2. A client who had a cardiac catheterization and will be ambulating for the first time
3. A client taking antibiotics for endocarditis who has sudden dyspnea and anxiety
4. A client who is recovering from coronary artery bypass grafting (CABG) surgery with a temperature of 101°F

5 The nurse is caring for a client with a history of renal failure and a new myocardial infarction. The nurse who is reviewing laboratory findings would notify the registered nurse to report which result?

1. Potassium level of 5.0 mEq/L
2. Sodium level of 145 mEq/L
3. Calcium level of 7.0 mg/dL
4. Digoxin level of 0.8 ng/mL

6 The nurse is caring for a client with a diagnosis of aortic stenosis who has surgery scheduled in 2 weeks. The client reports episodes of angina and passing out recently at home. What would be the nurse's best explanation about recommended activity at this time?

1. "It is best to avoid strenuous exercise, stairs, and lifting before your surgery."
2. "Take short walks three times daily to prepare for postoperative rehabilitation."
3. "There are no activity restrictions unless the angina reoccurs; then please call the office."
4. "Gradually increase activity before surgery to build stamina for the postoperative period."

7 A client who has just undergone cardiac angiography has a catheter insertion site that has no bleeding or hematoma. Vital signs and distal pulses remain in the client's normal range. Intravenous fluids have been discontinued. The client refuses any food or fluids, and asks the nurse to be left alone to rest. What is the nurse's best response?

1. "You are recovering well from the procedure and resting is a good idea."
2. "It is important for you to walk, so I will be back in 1 hour to walk with you."
3. "It is important to drink fluids after this procedure. I will bring you some water, and I encourage you to drink."
4. "You should do leg exercises to keep good circulation to your legs. After your exercises, you can rest."

8 A client's angiogram demonstrates the final stage of atherosclerosis. The nurse concludes that this client's pathophysiology includes which late developing element?

1. The presence of atheromas
2. Fatty deposits in the intima
3. Lipoprotein accumulation in the intima
4. Inflammation of the arterial wall

9 When caring for a client with peripheral arterial disease (PAD), the nurse monitors the client for which signs and symptoms that would be consistent with tissue ischemia? Select all that apply.

1. Peripheral edema
2. Thickened toenails
3. Leg pain while walking
4. Brownish discoloration to the skin on the leg
5. Cooler skin temperature on affected extremity

10 In assisting with community education on prevention of peripheral arterial disease (PAD), the nurse is careful to include which of the following as a major risk factor? Select all that apply.

1. Dysrhythmias
2. Low-protein intake
3. Exposure to cool weather
4. Cigarette smoking
5. Hypertension

11 When reinforcing teaching to a client with an aneurysm about signs and symptoms that may indicate impending rupture, the nurse first considers which of the following?

1. Medication therapy the client is receiving
2. Client's usual blood pressure
3. Age and gender of the client
4. Size and location of the aneurysm

12 The nurse concludes that an important outcome of care for a female client with hypertension has been met when the client is able to do which of the following?

1. Return to usual activities of daily living (ADLs)
2. Identify actions to counteract two modifiable risk factors
3. Lower blood pressure by 10%
4. Discontinue lifestyle modifications

13 A client with endocarditis develops sudden leg pain with pallor, tingling, and a loss of peripheral pulses. What should be the nurse's initial action?

1. Elevate the leg above the level of the heart.
2. Wrap the leg in a loose blanket.
3. Notify the registered nurse about the findings.
4. Perform passive ROM exercise to stimulate circulation.

PRACTICE TEST

14 Which client assigned to the nurse is most at risk for developing a deep vein thrombosis (DVT)?

1. A 30-year old client who is 1-week postpartum
2. A 63-year old client post-CVA on anticoagulant therapy
3. A 40-year old woman who smokes and uses oral contraceptives
4. A 41-year old female who underwent laparoscopic cholecystectomy

15 The nurse is caring for a 2-month old child with transposition of the great vessels. Which nursing intervention has highest priority?

1. Providing comfort for parents
2. Maintaining proper caloric intake
3. Reducing stressors for infant
4. Documenting vital signs

16 During the acute phase of rheumatic fever, what is a priority action of the nurse?

1. Encourage ambulation at least four times per day.
2. Monitor for early signs of endocarditis.
3. Maintain hydration by encouraging sips of water.
4. Manage pain with routine opioid analgesics.

17 A 6-year-old boy has been diagnosed with coarctation of the aorta. Lately, he has been complaining when he comes in from recess. The school health nurse should question the child about which of the following?

1. Weakness and pain in legs
2. Blurred vision
3. Increased respiratory rate
4. A bruise on the shin

18 A toddler with Kawasaki disease is going home on salicylate (aspirin) therapy. What is the priority element in parent teaching that needs to be reinforced at the time of discharge?

1. Monitor child for gastrointestinal bleeding
2. Avoid contact with other children
3. Report complaints of tingling extremities
4. Maintain a low-calorie diet

19 A toddler requires supplemental oxygen therapy for a cyanotic heart defect. The nurse would reinforce which information with the parents prior to discharge?

1. Need to maintain child on bedrest
2. Promoting mobility while providing supplemental oxygen
3. Symptoms of oxygen toxicity
4. How to draw blood for arterial blood gases

20 The nurse would monitor for which manifestations in a client with suspected arterial embolism to the left hand? Select all that apply.

1. Pain
2. Pale skin
3. Bounding radial pulse
4. Paresthesias
5. Pitting edema

21 The pediatric nurse is caring for two children with heart disease. The nurse concludes that which laboratory finding would be seen in the client with cyanotic heart disease but not in the client with acyanotic heart disease?

1. Elevated pO_2
2. Elevated hemoglobin
3. Decreased hematocrit
4. Decreased pCO_2

22 The parents of a toddler who has undergone a successful repair of a ventricular septal defect (VSD) question why the child is being sent home on antibiotics when no infection is present. The nurse explains that this will help prevent which complication?

1. Infective endocarditis
2. Pulmonary embolism
3. Cerebrovascular accident (CVA)
4. Gastritis

23 In caring for children with congenital heart defects, the pediatric nurse would expect to see clubbing of the fingers and toes in the child diagnosed with which of the following? Select all that apply.

1. Transposition of the great vessels
2. Atrial septal defect
3. Tetralogy of Fallot
4. Patent ductus arteriosus
5. Coarctation of the aorta

24 A child has been diagnosed with tetralogy of Fallot and is taking prostaglandin E1 (Alprostadil). The child is very cyanotic, weak, and has moist respirations. Which data would indicate a therapeutic response to this drug?

1. Cyanosis does not increase
2. Blood pressure lowers
3. Respirations increase
4. Temperature drops

25 After a pediatric client has a cardiac catheterization, which intervention would the nurse consider to be of highest priority during the immediate post-procedure period?

1. Encourage intake of small amounts of food.
2. Discuss with the parents signs of congestive heart failure.
3. Monitor the site for signs of infection.
4. Apply direct pressure to entry site for 15 minutes.

26 The nurse is caring for an infant with a cyanotic heart defect. Symptoms that would indicate risk for congestive heart failure include which of the following? Select all that apply.

1. Respiratory crackles and frothy secretions
2. Increased blood pressure
3. Oxygen saturation increase
4. Hepatomegaly
5. Rapid weight gain

ANSWERS & RATIONALES

1 **Answer: 3, 5 Rationale:** A CK level above 150 with over 5% MB isoenzyme indicates myocardial damage from acute MI. Elevated potassium is not indicative of MI. Elevated WBC is an indicator of many conditions, including MI. **Cognitive Level:** Analyzing **Client Need:** Physiological Adaptation **Integrated Process:** Nursing Process: Data Collection **Content Area:** Adult Health **Strategy:** The core issue of the question is the ability to correlate indicators of myocardial damage with a client situation. Evaluate each option carefully, and use nursing knowledge of appropriate laboratory tests and the process of elimination to select answer choices. Note the wording of the question suggests more than one option is likely to be correct.

2 **Answer: 4 Rationale:** Nausea and anorexia are signs of digitalis toxicity, making the digoxin level high priority for monitoring. The potassium, sodium, and creatinine kinase levels would not explain the client's symptoms and therefore are not priorities to monitor before notifying the registered nurse. **Cognitive Level:** Applying **Client Need:** Physiological Adaptation **Integrated Process:** Nursing Process: Data Collection **Content Area:** Adult Health **Strategy:** The core issue of the question is the ability to correlate early signs of digoxin toxicity with a need to check digoxin level in a client with cardiac disease. Evaluate each option carefully, and use nursing knowledge and the process of elimination to make a selection.

3 **Answer: 2, 3, 4, 5 Rationale:** The captopril does not lower the heart rate and may be safely administered to maintain control of the hypertension. The hydrochlorothiazide does not lower the heart rate and may be safely administered to maintain control of the hypertension. Docusate is a stool softener and may be safely administered to the client. Straining at stool could cause the client to use the Valsalva maneuver, which could temporarily lower the heart rate further. A multivitamin would not adversely affect the client's pulse rate and may be safely administered. The client's heart rate is bradycardic, and metoprolol, a beta-blocker, decreases the heart rate. The dose of this medication should be withheld. **Cognitive Level:** Analyzing **Client Need:** Physiological Adaptation **Integrated Process:** Nursing Process: Planning **Content Area:** Adult Health **Strategy:** The core issue of the question is which medication(s) could be responsible for the client's bradycardia and act accordingly. Evaluate each option carefully, and use nursing knowledge and the process of elimination to make selections. The wording of the question suggests more than one option may be correct.

4 **Answer: 3 Rationale:** A client with endocarditis is at risk for thrombus formation, and chest pain and anxiety are signs of pulmonary embolism (PE), which is a life-threatening complication requiring immediate attention. Dyspnea is a chronic symptom with hypertrophic cardiomyopathy, which requires monitoring; a temperature of 101°F requires additional monitoring, and a client who is ambulating for the first time will be monitored by the nurse. However, the client who needs to be monitored for PE is the most emergent. **Cognitive Level:** Analyzing **Client Need:** Coordinated Care **Integrated Process:** Nursing Process: Planning **Content Area:** Adult Health **Strategy:** The key to determining the answer to priority-setting questions is to evaluate which client is most unstable or has the greatest risk for developing a complication. Evaluate each option carefully using these methods, and use nursing knowledge and the process of elimination to make a selection.

5 **Answer: 3 Rationale:** Renal failure is a common cause of hypocalcemia, and a value of 7.0 mg/dL is below the normal range of 8.5–10.5 mg/dL. The potassium level is within the upper limit of its normal range of 3.5–5.1 mEq/L. The sodium level is within the upper limit of its normal range of 135–145 mEq/L. Digoxin is within the therapeutic range of 0.5–2.0 ng/mL. **Cognitive Level:** Applying **Client Need:** Physiological Adaptation **Integrated Process:** Nursing Process: Implementation **Content Area:** Adult Health **Strategy:** The core issue of the question is knowledge of normal and abnormal values that are important to report in a client with an acute cardiac problem and a history of renal failure. The best strategy in questions such as these is to pick the value with the most abnormal number and/or one that relates to the underlying disorder(s).

6 **Answer: 1 Rationale:** Symptomatic aortic stenosis has a poor prognosis without surgery. Restricting activity limits myocardial

oxygen consumption. Since the incidence of sudden death is high in this population, it is prudent to decrease the strain on the heart while awaiting surgery. **Cognitive Level:** Analyzing **Client Need:** Physiological Adaptation **Integrated Process:** Nursing Process: Implementation **Content Area:** Adult Health **Strategy:** The core issue of the question is the level of activity that will minimize the client's risk of complications or sudden death until surgery. Evaluate each option carefully, and use nursing knowledge and the process of elimination to make a selection.

7 **Answer: 3 Rationale:** The dye used in angiography is nephrotoxic, and a client should have adequate fluids after the procedure to eliminate the dye. Stating the client is recovering well gives false reassurance to a client who could be at risk if fluids are not taken in. The client should lie with the affected leg extended for 6 to 8 hours. Leg exercises are not recommended because exercise could disrupt the clot that formed at the insertion site. **Cognitive Level:** Analyzing **Client Need:** Physiological Adaptation **Integrated Process:** Communication and Documentation **Content Area:** Adult Health **Strategy:** The core issue of the question is knowledge of the correlation between lack of fluid intake and risk of kidney complications following angiography. Evaluate each option carefully, and use nursing knowledge and the process of elimination to make a selection.

8 **Answer: 1 Rationale:** The final stage of the atherosclerotic process is the development of atheromas, which are complex lesions consisting of lipids, fibrous tissue, collagen, calcium, cellular waste, and capillaries. The calcified lesions may rupture or ulcerate, stimulating thrombosis. Earlier changes in development of atherosclerosis include fatty deposits and lipoprotein accumulation along the intima and inflammation of the arterial wall. **Cognitive Level:** Applying **Client Need:** Physiological Adaptation **Integrated Process:** Nursing Process: Evaluation **Content Area:** Adult Health **Strategy:** Note the critical words *final stage*. Evaluate each option carefully, and use knowledge of pathophysiology and the process of elimination to make a selection.

9 **Answer: 2, 3, 5 Rationale:** Trophic changes from hypoxia and tissue malnutrition in PAD consist of thickened toenails, hair loss on the extremity, and thin shiny skin. Leg pain (also called intermittent claudication) is a primary manifestation of peripheral arterial disease. Intermittent claudication is muscle pain caused by interruption in arterial flow, resulting in tissue hypoxia. Because of insufficient blood supply, expected temperature of the skin of the affected extremity would be cooler than normal. Peripheral edema on the affected leg would be consistent with venous disease. Brownish discoloration to the skin on the leg would be consistent with venous disease, while pale colored skin is consistent with arterial disease. **Cognitive Level:** Applying **Client Need:** Physiological Adaptation **Integrated Process:** Nursing Process: Data Collection **Content Area:** Adult Health **Strategy:** The critical words in the question are *peripheral arterial disease*, which direct you to look for manifestations that are abnormal and that are consistent with arterial but not venous disease. Evaluate each option carefully, and use nursing knowledge and the process of elimination to make a selection.

10 **Answer: 4, 5 Rationale:** Nicotine in cigarettes promotes vasoconstriction. The three most significant risk factors for development of PAD are smoking, hyperlipidemia, and hypertension. The presence of dysrhythmias, low-protein intake, and exposure to cool weather are not risk factors for the disease, although cool weather could worsen the symptoms when disease is already present. **Cognitive Level:** Applying **Client Need:** Physiological Adaptation **Integrated Process:** Teaching and Learning **Content Area:** Adult Health **Strategy:** Note the critical word *prevention* to focus on the option that contains information that will affect the likelihood of developing peripheral arterial disease. Evaluate each option carefully, using nursing knowledge and the process of elimination to make a selection.

11 **Answer: 4 Rationale:** Aneurysms vary by size and location. Signs of rupture depend on the location of the aneurysm. Dissection can occur anywhere but most often occurs in the ascending aorta where pressure is the highest. The medication the client is receiving is vague and is not directly related to risk of aneurysm rupture. The blood pressure relates to whether the aneurysm may rupture, not to the associated signs and symptoms. The age and gender of the client are unrelated to the signs and symptoms of aneurysm rupture. **Cognitive Level:** Analyzing **Client Need:** Physiological Adaptation **Integrated Process:** Nursing Process: Planning **Content Area:** Adult Health **Strategy:** With the critical words *signs and symptoms* in mind, choose the option that most directly relates to the core issue of the question. Evaluate each option carefully, and choose size and location as the only option that could affect the specific list of signs and symptoms that would relate to aneurysm rupture.

12 **Answer: 2 Rationale:** An important outcome in care of the hypertensive client is the ability to identify and counteract personal risk factors that the client has the ability to change. Modifiable risk factors for hypertension include smoking, hypercholesterolemia, diabetes mellitus, sedentary lifestyle, obesity, stress, and alcohol use. Returning to ADLs is not likely to be an issue. Lowering blood pressure by 10% may or may not be sufficient. Discontinuing lifestyle modifications is contraindicated because the blood pressure could rise again. **Cognitive Level:** Applying **Client Need:** Physiological Adaptation **Integrated Process:** Nursing Process: Data Collection **Content Area:** Adult Health **Strategy:** The core issue of the question is the ability to identify an indicator that is a positive effect of care for the hypertensive client. Evaluate each option carefully, and use nursing knowledge and the process of elimination to make a selection.

13 **Answer: 2 Rationale:** The client is exhibiting symptoms of acute arterial occlusion. Without immediate intervention, ischemia and necrosis will result within hours. The nurse should first wrap the leg to maintain warmth and protect it from further injury. The leg should not be elevated above heart level because doing so would worsen the tissue ischemia. The nurse should quickly notify the registered nurse after taking an action that will benefit the client's status. Passive range of motion will increase ischemia by increasing tissue demand for oxygen. **Cognitive Level:** Analyzing **Client Need:** Physiological Adaptation **Integrated Process:** Nursing Process: Implementation **Content Area:** Adult Health **Strategy:** The core issue of the question is recognizing the complication of acute arterial occlusion and then determining which action should be taken first. Choose an option that is client-focused rather than physician-notification focused, if one is available. In this case, the nurse can protect the client from further injury by wrapping the leg loosely in a blanket.

14 **Answer: 3 Rationale:** A major risk factor for DVT is oral contraceptive use in women who smoke. Being 1-week postpartum does not place a client at risk since mobility is usually restored. Anticoagulant therapy is used to prevent development of

thrombi. Laparoscopic surgical procedures are associated with more rapid recovery times with reduced immobility, keeping this client at lower risk for DVT. **Cognitive Level:** Applying **Client Need:** Physiological Adaptation **Integrated Process:** Nursing Process: Data Collection **Content Area:** Adult Health **Strategy:** The critical words in the question are *most at risk*, indicating the correct option is the one that contains the most severe or greatest number of risk factors for DVT. With this in mind, evaluate each option and use the process of elimination to make a selection.

15 **Answer: 3 Rationale:** The open ductus arteriosus will allow a small amount of mixing of oxygenated and unoxygenated blood. Stress will increase the cardiac workload (and thus decrease cardiac output) and therefore avoiding stress is a priority for the nurse. Providing comfort to parents meets a secondary need rather than a primary need using Maslow's hierarchy. Maintaining caloric intake is a physiological priority that can be considered after ensuring airway, breathing, and circulation. Documenting vital signs is a routine activity and not a priority when compared to actual care activities. **Cognitive Level:** Analyzing **Client Need:** Physiological Adaptation **Integrated Process:** Nursing Process: Implementation **Content Area:** Child Health **Strategy:** Use Maslow's hierarchy of needs to review each option and choose the one that most closely relates to the ABCs and thus, cardiac workload. Use this knowledge and the process of elimination to make a selection.

16 **Answer: 2 Rationale:** The main complication of rheumatic fever is carditis. The nurse must monitor for early signs of bacterial endocarditis. The client should be encouraged to rest during the acute phase. Hydration needs may not be sufficiently met with sips of water. Opioid analgesics may not be necessary, although nonsteroidal anti-inflammatory drugs (NSAIDs) are likely to be ordered. **Cognitive Level:** Applying **Client Need:** Physiological Adaptation **Integrated Process:** Nursing Process: Implementation **Content Area:** Child Health **Strategy:** The core issue of the question is the ability to set priorities for a client with rheumatic fever. Omit ambulation because of the words *at least*, knowing that rest is encouraged. Likewise, eliminate hydration because of the word *sips*. Choose monitoring for endocarditis over opioid analgesics knowing that NSAIDs are likely to be effective in managing pain and inflammation from rheumatic fever.

17 **Answer: 1 Rationale:** Decreased circulation to lower extremities would contribute to muscle fatigue and pain in the legs. Blurred vision is not related to coarctation. Many children returning from recess may have increased respiratory rate secondary to play activities. A bruise on the shin is not of special concern if it is related to a play-related fall, since risk of bleeding is not a concern in coarctation. **Cognitive Level:** Applying **Client Need:** Physiological Adaptation **Integrated Process:** Nursing Process: Data Collection **Content Area:** Child Health **Strategy:** The core issue of the question is knowledge of signs of exercise intolerance in a 6-year-old client with a cyanotic heart defect. Use principles of gas exchange and knowledge of normal and abnormal findings after exercise to make a selection.

18 **Answer: 1 Rationale:** Salicylates prevent platelet agglutination. Gastrointestinal bleeding is often a side effect of aspirin therapy. It is not necessary to avoid contact with other children. Tingling of extremities is not a related concern in Kawasaki disease, although ringing in the ears could be a sign of salicylate toxicity. A low-calorie diet is not indicated. **Cognitive Level:** Applying **Client Need:** Pharmacological and Parenteral Therapies **Integrated Process:** Teaching and Learning **Content Area:** Child Health **Strategy:** The core issue of the question is knowledge of adverse drug effects of salicylate therapy for the child with Kawasaki disease. Use this knowledge and the process of elimination to make a selection.

19 **Answer: 2 Rationale:** Allowing mobility is helpful to promote growth and development in the toddler. Strategies should be discussed to promote mobility while maintaining the supplemental oxygen. Bed rest is unnecessary. Signs of oxygen toxicity are not the priority based on the information in the question. Drawing arterial blood gases is unnecessary. **Cognitive Level:** Applying **Client Need:** Physiological Adaptation **Integrated Process:** Teaching and Learning **Content Area:** Child Health **Strategy:** The core issue of the question is home care needs of a toddler receiving oxygen therapy. Use principles of needs related to normal growth and development to help select the correct option.

20 **Answer: 1, 2, 4 Rationale:** The client would exhibit pain, pallor of the affected skin, diminished or absent radial pulse, paresthesias (altered local sensation), paralysis (weakness or inability to move extremity), and poikilothermia (cooler temperature) because of reduced circulation to the area. The client would not have a bounding radial pulse (opposite finding is true) or pitting edema, indicating a fluid volume excess or heart failure. **Cognitive Level:** Analyzing **Client Need:** Physiological Adaptation **Integrated Process:** Nursing Process: Data Collection **Content Area:** Adult Health **Strategy:** The core issue of the question is knowledge of findings in arterial embolism. Visualize a clot in the local circulation and use that image to determine the effect of the blockage on circulation to the affected area.

21 **Answer: 2 Rationale:** Chronic hypoxemia in cyanotic heart disease leads to polycythemia, an above-normal increase in the number of red cells in the blood. This change increases the amount of hemoglobin available to carry oxygen. The other answers do not differentiate between the cyanotic and acyanotic forms of heart disease in the child. **Cognitive Level:** Analyzing **Client Need:** Physiological Adaptation **Integrated Process:** Nursing Process: Planning **Content Area:** Child Health **Strategy:** The difference between acyanotic and cyanotic heart disease is that in cyanotic heart disease, the blood is partially unoxygenated. Consider how this will affect each of the lab values over time.

22 **Answer: 1 Rationale:** Infective endocarditis is the most common complication of the cardiac surgery. Children may need prophylactic antibiotic therapy for specific conditions as recommended by the American Heart Association. Antibiotics prevent infection; they do not prevent pulmonary embolism. Antibiotics prevent infection; they do not prevent CVA. Antibiotics prevent infection; they do not prevent gastritis. **Cognitive Level:** Applying **Client Need:** Pharmacological and Parenteral Therapies **Integrated Process:** Teaching and Learning **Content Area:** Child Health **Strategy:** The core concept is prophylactic antibiotic use. Of the options listed, infective endocarditis is the primary bacterial condition.

23 **Answer: 1, 3 Rationale:** Clubbing of the fingers and toes occurs in cyanotic heart defects, such as transposition of the great vessels. **Cognitive Level:** Analyzing **Client Need:** Physiological Adaptation **Integrated Process:** Nursing Process: Data Collection **Content Area:** Child Health **Strategy:** Any defect that

bypasses the lungs will lead to these symptoms. Those defects which recycle through the lungs will not.

24 **Answer: 1** **Rationale:** Prostaglandin E1 helps maintain a patent ductus arteriosus open and thereby allows for mixing of blood. If the ductus arteriosus closes, cyanosis will increase. Prostaglandin E1 helps maintain a patent ductus arteriosus open and thereby allows for mixing of blood. It does not lower blood pressure. Prostaglandin E1 helps maintain a patent ductus arteriosus open and thereby allows for mixing of blood. It does not increase respirations. Prostaglandin E1 helps maintain a patent ductus arteriosus open and thereby allows for mixing of blood. It does not lower temperature. **Cognitive Level:** Analyzing **Client Need:** Pharmacological and Parenteral Therapies **Integrated Process:** Nursing Process: Data Collection **Content Area:** Child Health **Strategy:** Consider the therapeutic effects of the drug to determine the correct answer.

25 **Answer: 4** **Rationale:** Direct pressure on the wound site helps to form a clot and reduce bleeding. Hemorrhage can be life threatening in the immediate postprocedure period. Food intake is a lesser concern than maintaining hemostasis. Signs of congestive heart failure could relate to the original disease process but are not a priority at this time. Infection would not be apparent immediately following the procedure. **Cognitive Level:** Applying **Client Need:** Reduction of Risk Potential **Integrated Process:** Nursing Process: Implementation **Content Area:** Child Health **Strategy:** Note that only two options identify interventions in the immediate post-catheterization period. Of those two, consider the highest priority would be preventing bleeding.

26 **Answer: 1, 4, 5** **Rationale:** Pulmonary overload occurs prior to congestive heart failure. Crackles and frothy secretions are signs of moist respirations, a symptom of pulmonary overload. Fluid volume excess, secondary to ineffective cardiac function, leads to hepatomegaly and rapid weight gain. **Cognitive Level:** Applying **Client Need:** Physiological Adaptation **Integrated Process:** Nursing Process: Data Collection **Content Area:** Child Health **Strategy:** The learner needs to remember that symptoms of congestive heart failure arise from impaired cardiac output, pulmonary venous congestion, and systemic venous congestion.

ANSWERS & RATIONALES

Key Terms to Review

References

Ball, J., Bindler, R., & Cowen, K. (2010). *Child health nursing: Partnering with children and families* (2nd ed.). Upper Saddle River, NJ: Pearson Education.

Berman, A., & Snyder, S. (2012). *Kozier & Erb's fundamentals of nursing: Concepts, process, and practice* (9th ed.). Upper Saddle River, NJ: Pearson Education, Inc.

Ignatavicius, D., & Workman, L. (2010). *Medical-surgical nursing: Critical thinking for collaborative care* (6th ed.). Philadelphia: Saunders.

Kee, J. (2010). *Laboratory and diagnostic tests with nursing implications* (8th ed.). Upper Saddle River, NJ: Pearson Education.

LeMone, P., Burke, K., & Bauldoff, G. (2011). *Medical surgical nursing: Critical thinking in patient care* (5th ed.). Upper Saddle River, NJ: Pearson Education.

Smith, S., Duell, D., & Martin, B. (2012). *Clinical nursing skills: Basic to advanced skills* (8th ed.). Upper Saddle River, NJ: Pearson Education.

Test Yourself

Are you ready for the NCLEX-PN® or course exams? Use the practice tests on the companion website to check.

Neurological Disorders

53

In this chapter

Cross Reference

Other chapters relevant to this content area are

Neurological and Musculoskeletal Medications	Chapter 35
Common Laboratory Tests	Chapter 42
Common Diagnostic Tests and Procedures	Chapter 43

I. OVERVIEW OF ANATOMY AND PHYSIOLOGY OF NERVOUS SYSTEM

A. Cells in nervous system (NS)

1. Neurons: basic anatomical and functional units in NS; have 3 parts: cell body, axon, and dendrites; nerve cells are separated by a synaptic cleft; neurotransmitters are secreted into cleft by one neuron to stimulate dendrites of another neuron and conduct nerve impulses
2. Glial cells: structures of NS that nourish, support, and protect brain neurons; 4 main types of glial cells in brain are astrocytes, oligodendrocytes, ependymal cells, and microglia; Schwann cells are in peripheral nervous system (PNS)

B. Central nervous system (CNS)

1. Consists of cerebrum, cerebellum, brain stem, and spinal cord
2. Cerebrum, largest division of brain, enables individuals to reason, function intellectually, express personality and mood, and interact with environment
   a. Includes two hemispheres, each divided into a frontal lobe, temporal lobe, parietal lobe, and occipital lobe; each lobe has specific functions
   b. Right hemisphere generally controls left side of body and left controls right side of body; usually one hemisphere is considered dominant
   c. Frontal lobe performs high-level cognitive function, has memory storage, influences somatic motor control, controls voluntary eye movements, and controls motor aspect of speech in **Broca's area**, located in dominant hemisphere (usually left)
   d. Temporal lobe has primary auditory receptive areas and auditory association area (**Wernicke's area**), which is usually found on dominant side and is responsible for interpreting speech; interpretive area integrates somatic, auditory, and visual data (this impacts perception, learning, memory, emotions, and intellectual abilities)
   e. Parietal lobe holds primary sensory cortex and sensory association areas that define and localize sensations such as size, shape, weight, texture, and consistency; also processes visual–spatial information and controls spatial orientation
   f. Occipital lobe is visual center for eyes; controls eye reflexes and interpretation of sight
3. Diencephalons and hypophysis of brain have many functions, including temperature control, water metabolism, pituitary secretion, visceral and somatic activities, visible physical expressions in response to emotions, sleep–wake cycle, and hunger
4. Cerebellum is a double-lobed area posterior to pons responsible for muscle synergy and coordination and maintains balance through feedback loops
5. Brainstem is an integration system that also controls basic functions; has 3 major divisions: the midbrain, pons, and medulla; reticular activating system (RAS) is responsible for alertness; substantia nigra is affected in Parkinson's disease; most cranial nerves originate in brainstem
6. The spinal cord is an elongated mass of nerve tissue that runs most of length of vertebral column
   a. Divided into four areas: cervical area (C1 to C7) near neck; thoracic area (T1 to T12) near chest; lumbar area (L1 to L5) near lower back; sacral area (S1 to S4) is in sacrum
   b. Sensory tracts (dorsal roots) carry afferent impulses from periphery to dorsal root ganglia where they are sent to brain; general somatic afferent fibers carry pain, temperature, touch, and proprioception from body wall, tendons, and joints; general visceral fibers carry sensory input from body organs
   c. Motor tracts (ventral roots) convey efferent impulses from spinal cord to somatic fibers that innervate voluntary striated muscle, smooth muscle, cardiac muscle, and that regulate glandular secretions

C. The PNS

1. Consists of 31 pairs of spinal nerves, 12 pairs of cranial nerves, and autonomic NS divided into sympathetic and parasympathetic NS
2. Each pair of spinal nerves has dorsal and ganglion roots that exit spinal cord via an intervertebral foramina; they carry input between specific areas called dermatomes and spine
3. Cranial nerves (CN): 12 pairs arise from brain; there are three pure sensory nerves, five pure motor nerves, and four mixed (sensory and motor) nerves; olfactory nerve (CN I) and optic nerve (CN II) arise from cerebrum; CN III and IV arise in midbrain; CN V through VIII arise in pons; CN IX to XII arise in medulla (see Table 53–1 for an overview of cranial nerves)
4. Autonomic NS: a collection of motor nerves that regulate activities of viscera, smooth muscles, and glands to maintain a stable internal environment; two parts of system (sympathetic and parasympathetic) work antagonistically
   a. Sympathetic nervous system (SNS) is active during times of stress, such as flight-or-fight response; it increases heart rate (HR) and blood pressure (BP) and vasoconstricts the peripheral blood vessels (BVs)
   b. Parasympathetic nervous system is a conservation, restoration, and maintenance system; it decreases HR and increases gastrointestinal (GI) activity

D. Blood supply

1. Brain is unique in that it can only use glucose for energy; a lack of glucose for 5 minutes results in irreversible brain damage; brain receives 750 mL/min of blood or 15–20% of resting cardiac output
2. Cerebral arteries are thinner, have more internal elasticity and less smooth muscle than arteries elsewhere in body; brain is supplied with blood by two sets of arteries: anterior and posterior circulation

Table 53–1 Overview of Cranial Nerves

Cranial Nerve Name	Type of Nerve	Physiological Functions
Olfactory (I)	Sensory	Ability to smell
Optic (II)	Sensory	Visual fields, visual acuity
Oculomotor (III)	Motor	Extraocular movements (EOM)
Trochlear (IV)	Motor	EOM
Trigeminal (V)	Mixed	Movement of eyelids, ability to clench jaw
Abducens (VI)	Motor	EOM
Facial (VII)	Mixed	Movement of eyelids, facial symmetry
Acoustic (VIII)	Sensory	Hearing ability
Glossopharyngeal (IX)	Mixed	Gag, swallow, and cough reflexes; voice quality
Vagus (X)	Mixed	Gag, swallow, and cough reflexes; voice quality
Spinal Accessory (XI)	Motor	Neck strength and shoulder shrug
Hypoglossal (XII)	Motor	Tongue movement

a. Anterior circulation, fed by internal and external carotids, delivers blood to a central area at base of cerebrum called circle of Willis; from there it feeds anterior cerebrum via anterior cerebral artery, middle of cerebrum via middle cerebral artery, and posterior cerebrum via posterior cerebral artery
b. Posterior circulation, fed by vertebral arteries, delivers blood to posterior fossa; at bottom of posterior fossa, blood flows together into one basilar artery and delivers it to cerebellum, midbrain, pons, and medulla
c. Meninges are supplied with blood from branches of external carotid arteries that ascend into brain at base of skull

3. Venous system of brain is unique
   a. Vessel walls are thinner than other veins of body; do not follow path of arteries but instead follow their own course
   b. There are no valves in brain's venous system and therefore drainage depends on venous pressure and gravity
   c. Dural sinuses collect blood from brain and empty it into jugular veins

E. Blood–brain barrier

1. A network of endothelial cells in wall of capillaries and astrocyte projections in close proximity that do not have pores between them
2. This tight junction does not allow normal nonspecific filtering process that occurs in rest of body; therefore, molecules must enter brain by active transport, endocytosis and exocytosis, which creates a highly selective barrier that guards entrance to neurons
3. Movement of substances across this barrier depends on particle size, lipid solubility, chemical dissociation, and protein-binding potential
4. Barrier is very permeable to water, oxygen (O_2), carbon dioxide (CO_2), other gases, glucose, and lipid soluble compounds

F. Protective structures

1. **Meninges**: covers brain and spinal cord to protect and support; divided into 3 layers from outer to inner (dura mater, arachnoid, and pia mater)
   a. Dura is a tough, membranous tissue that surrounds and extends into the brain tissue
   b. Arachnoid membrane lies below dura and is a network of delicate, elastic tissue that contains BVs of varying sizes
   c. Pia mater is a vascular membrane that covers entire brain with tiny BVs that extend into gray matter of brain
   d. Within meninges, there are important potential spaces (epidural, subdural, subarachnoid) where bleeding can occur
2. Skull: bony structure of head that includes 8 fused cranial bones and 14 facial bones; encloses brain in a protective vault
3. Spine: flexible column that encloses spinal cord, formed from stacking of 7 cervical, 12 thoracic, 5 lumbar, and 4 sacral vertebrae

4. Cerebrospinal fluid (CSF) and ventricular system
   a. CSF is a clear, colorless, odorless solution that fills ventricular system and subarachnoid space of brain and spinal cord; acts as a shock absorber; also has electrolytes, glucose, protein, O_2, and CO_2 dissolved in solution
   b. Ventricular system is composed of two lateral ventricles (one in each hemisphere of cerebrum), a third that lies midline in thalamic area, and a fourth that lies below third, anterior to cerebellum and subarachnoid space

II. DIAGNOSTIC TESTS AND DATA COLLECTION

A. Data collection for NS

1. Determine circumstances of injury and admission, pertinent family and social history

NCLEX®

2. Inquire about chief complaint: use mnemonic APQRST

Memory Aid

Remember the mnemonic APQRST to recall all important points to determine whenever a client has an acute onset symptom:
A—any associated symptoms with chief complaint
P—what provokes (makes worse) or palliates (makes better) symptoms
Q—quality of pain
R—region and radiation
S—severity of pain on a scale of 1 to 10
T—timing: when it stops and starts, whether it is intermittent or constant, its duration

3. Health information: including past medical history, current medications, recent surgeries or other treatments, alcohol or illegal drug use
4. Mental status exam

NCLEX®

   a. A screening mental status exam includes orientation to person, place, and time; appearance and behavior; mood; speech pattern; and thought and perception including insight, thought, content, and judgment
   b. To conduct this exam, client must be awake, alert, and able to understand and respond to questions
   c. A client with an altered **level of consciousness (LOC)** may have a range of behaviors; see Table 53–2 for terms used to describe LOC
   d. Acute confusion or delirium should be recognized and treated by eliminating the cause; try to avoid confusing delirium with dementia (a chronic problem)

Table 53–2 Terms Used to Describe Level of Consciousness

Term	Description
Full consciousness	Alert; oriented to person, place, and time; and comprehends written and spoken words
Confusion	Unable to think clearly and rapidly; easily bewildered, with poor memory and short attention span; misinterprets stimuli and judgment is impaired
Disorientation	Not aware of or oriented to time, place, or person
Obtundation	Lethargic, somnolent, responds to verbal or tactile stimuli but quickly drifts back to sleep
Stupor	Generally unresponsive; may be briefly aroused with vigorous, repeated, or painful stimuli; may grab at or shrink away from source of stimuli
Semicomatose	No spontaneous movement; unresponsive to stimuli; may moan or withdraw from vigorous or painful stimuli without actual arousal
Coma	Unarousable; does not stir or moan in response to stimuli; may have slight nonpurposeful movement in an area stimulated but no attempt to withdraw
Deep coma	Unarousable; unresponsive to any stimuli, including pain; absence of brainstem reflexes; corneal, pupillary, and pharyngeal reflexes; and deep tendon and plantar reflexes

Source: LeMone, P., Burke, M., & Bauldoff, G., *Medical surgical nursing: Critical thinking in patient care* (5th ed.), © 2011, p. 1432. Reprinted by permission of Pearson Education, Inc., Upper Saddle River, NJ 07458.

Table 53–3 Cranial Nerve Testing

Cranial Nerve (CN)	Data Collection
CN I (olfactory)	Observe ability to identify common odors
CN II (optic)	Use Snellen chart to test vision
CN III, IV, and VI (oculomotor, trochlear and abducens)	EOM: have client follow finger through cardinal fields of gaze Ptosis (III): a droopy eyelid PEARLA: assess pupils equal and reactive to light and accommodation Nystagmus: pupil movement is choppy Doll's eyes: in comatose client, doll's eyes is present when eyes stay center while head moves left and right; absent when eyes move with head
CN V (trigeminal)	Jaw clench: palpate masseter and temporal muscles when client's jaw is clenched; note differences on left or right Compare light, dull, and sharp sensations on both sides of face Corneal reflex: on an unconscious client, a wisp of cotton is touched to cornea; normal response is to blink Lids (V, VII): stroke each lid to elicit a blink response
CN VII (facial)	Facial symmetry: note droopiness of nasal labia fold, lower eyelid or corner of mouth when asking client to grin, raise eyebrows, and sniff; note accuracy of tasting sweet, sour, and salty items on anterior two thirds of tongue
CN VIII (acoustic)	Test hearing of each ear with a ticking watch or whispering; cold caloric testing: irrigating ear in ice cold water causes a slow movement of eyes toward irrigated side with a rapid return to midline; this is called oculovestibular reflex and indicates an intact brainstem
CN IX and X (glossopharyngeal and vagus)	Swallow reflex: determine whether client can swallow water or has dysphagia (difficulty swallowing) Gag reflex: test gag by touching back of both sides of throat; a unilateral loss may be noted Hoarseness: note client's voice for hoarseness Cough reflex: determine whether client's cough is strong, weak or absent Check sweet, salty, and sour taste on posterior third of tongue
CN XI (spinal accessory)	Neck strength: have client turn head against resistance Shoulder shrug: have client shrug shoulders against resistance
CN XII (hypoglossal)	Tongue deviation: have client stick out tongue and move it side to side against resistance; if there is a weakness, tongue will go to stronger side

5. Cranial nerves (CN): can be tested as described in Table 53–3; some methods test more than one cranial nerve at a time
6. Motor function
   a. Inspect all body muscles for size, tone, movement, and strength
   b. Compare left and right side for symmetry and equality
   c. Observe for tremors (rhythmic movements) and fasciculations (twitching)
   d. Criteria for grading muscle strength (see Box 53–1)

NCLEX®

7. Cerebellar examination: balance and coordination are under cerebellar control
   a. Gait: have client walk normally and then on heels and toes to observe coordination; perform a Romberg's test by having client stand with feet together and eyes closed while you stand close by to prevent falling; there should be minimal swaying for 20 seconds
   b. To note coordination, observe client's ability to touch own nose and then touch one of your fingers, then own nose again; next observe client's ability to touch each finger to thumb of same hand; finally, observe client's ability to run heel down shin on each side while lying in supine position
8. Sensory function
   a. Have client close eyes while you touch client on all dermatomes with objects that are sharp, dull, light to touch, and that vibrate (over bony prominence); client should be able to discriminate location and type of touch
   b. To test a client's sense of position (kinesthesia), have client close eyes and move client's finger or toe up or down and ask client to describe movement
   c. To test for stereognosis, have client identify with eyes closed an object placed in hand

Box 53–1

Criteria for Grading Muscle Strength

0 = No contraction

1 = Trace of contraction

2 = Active movement with gravity

3 = Active movement against gravity

4 = Active movement against gravity and resistance

5 = Normal power

Note: Findings are recorded as a fraction with 5 (highest possible score) as the denominator; for example, normal finding is 5/5.

Box 53–2

Standard Criteria for Grading Reflexes

0 = absent or no response

1 = hypoactive; weaker than normal (+)

2 = normal (++)

3 = stronger than normal (+++)

4 = hyperactive (++++)

d. To test for graphesthesia, have client identify a number or letter traced on palm of hand
e. Test two-point discrimination by touching a client with two simultaneous pinpricks and asking how many pinpricks there were; use dull points on a caliper and begin on finger pads

9. Reflexes
   a. Deep tendon reflexes (patellar, biceps, brachioradialis, triceps, and Achilles) are tested with a reflex hammer; see Box 53–2 for scoring criteria
   b. Test superficial abdominal reflex by lightly stroking abdomen from side to midline; normally, side stroked will contract
   c. Test cremasteric reflex by lightly stroking inside of thigh on a male client to raise testicle on that side
   d. Test Babinski reflex by stroking lateral aspect of sole of foot from heel to ball, curving medially in ball; its presence is noted with dorsiflexion of big toe and fanning of other toes; is considered normal in infants but abnormal in adults (normal adult response is curling of toes, called a negative Babinski)
10. Speech is usually described from interview
    a. Clear: normal, fluent speech
    b. **Dysarthria**: ineffective articulation of speech; may be a motor deficit of tongue and speech muscles
    c. **Aphasia**: a language disorder classified by type
    d. Expressive, motor, or nonfluent aphasia: sometimes called Broca's aphasia; it is an inability to express one's self using motor aspects of speech
    e. Receptive, fluent, or sensory aphasia: sometimes called Wernicke's aphasia; it is an inability to comprehend spoken words
    f. Global aphasia: a client can neither express nor comprehend language (mixed receptive and expressive)

NCLEX®

11. Specialized tests for meningeal irritation
    a. **Kernig's sign**: positive or present when client feels resistance or pain when leg is raised with knee flexed; indicates meningeal irritation, such as in meningitis
    b. **Brudzinski's sign**: positive or present when there is involuntary flexion of knees or hips when head is flexed while in supine position; commonly found also in meningitis

Memory Aid

Recall that the words *Kernig's* and *knee* both begin with *K*, while *Brudzinski's* and *brain* both begin with *B*. This will aid in recalling how to conduct each test.

B. Diagnostic studies of NS

NCLEX®

1. Lumbar puncture (LP): collects CSF for analysis via needle aspiration; CSF is studied; normal CSF is colorless, clear, and without blood or bacteria (white cells 0 to 5 cells/mm^3), glucose 40 to 80 mg/dL, and protein 16 to 45 mg/dL; following LP, position head elevated with water-based contrast and flat with oil-based contrast; examine site for leakage of CSF and for signs of infection
2. Cerebral angiography: outlines vascular structure of brain; detects arteriovenous (AV) malformations and/or aneurysms; use standard measures associated with use of contrast media (ask client about allergies to iodine or shellfish; encourage fluids following procedure to aid in excretion)
3. Computed tomography (CT): helps detect bleeding, hydrocephalus, and ischemic strokes older than 48 hours; may be done with or without contrast; see precautions noted above
4. Magnetic resonance imaging (MRI): detects soft tissue changes including necrotic tissue, tumors, edema, congenital disorders, and degenerative diseases; ask client about implanted sources of metal that would contradict use of this procedure

NCLEX®

5. Electroencephalography (EEG): diagnostic procedure that measures brain waves with multiple scalp electrodes; is helpful in diagnosing epilepsy, herpes simplex, encephalitis, and dementia disorders; EEG is also an important criterion in determining brain death
   a. Explain that test will not deliver electric shock
   b. Shampoo hair before procedure for cleanliness and after procedure to remove residual electrode gel or paste
   c. Withhold antiepileptics and other medications as ordered for 12–24 hours prior
   d. Have client eat regular meals to avoid hypoglycemia that could affect results
6. Electromyography (EMG) and nerve conduction studies: differentiate between peripheral nerve and muscle disorders; measures conduction velocity of muscles between two points and measurements are recorded at rest, with movement, and with electrical stimulation
7. Ultrasound
   a. Carotid Doppler scan: a noninvasive ultrasound of carotids that detects occlusions and stenosis; does not cause discomfort
   b. Transcranial Doppler ultrasonography (TCD): a portable, noninvasive technique that assesses intracranial circulation by measuring blood flow velocity; assesses vasospasm, transient ischemic attack (TIA), headache, subarachnoid hemorrhage (SAH), head injury, and AV malformations

III. ALTERED LEVEL OF CONSCIOUSNESS (LOC)

A. Overview

1. A change in arousal or alertness and/or a change in cognition or ability to solve complex problems (thought processes, memory, perception, problem solving, and emotion); often first sign of a change in neurologic status
2. Causes for unconsciousness vary from primary CNS disorders (such as damage to RAS or cerebrum) to dysfunction of other organ systems
3. In addition, metabolic disorders may alter cellular environment enough to inhibit neuronal activity
4. The term **coma** is reserved for those who have long periods of unconsciousness, lasting from hours to months; neurological origin of coma results from damage to both hemispheres of brain, damage to brainstem, or both

NCLEX®

B. Nursing data collection

1. Except for cases of damage to brainstem, brain function deterioration and changes in LOC follow a predictable pattern from higher functions to primitive functions
2. Confusion; forgetfulness; disorientation to time, then person, then place; agitation; poor problem-solving abilities; or any change in behavior may be an early change in cerebral function
3. Changes of lethargy and obtundation result from greater cerebral deterioration
4. A change from purposeful movements to decorticate posturing (see Figure 53–1A), small reactive pupils, and positive doll's eyes (positive oculocephalic reflex; eyes do not turn when head is moved and stay fixed in original direction) are manifestations of midbrain deterioration; decorticate posturing is characterized by elbows, wrists and fingers flexed while arms are close to sides, and leg extension with internal rotation and plantar flexion
5. Decerebrate posturing (see Figure 53–1B), fixed pupils, and positive cold calorics test (positive vestibuloocular reflex; sustained deviation of both eyes toward ear being stimulated with ice water) show deterioration at level of pons; decerebrate posturing is characterized by neck extension, clenched jaws, pronated and extended arms that are close to sides, and legs extended with plantar flexion
6. Fixed pupils, flaccidity, and negative cold calorics test indicate involvement at level of medulla

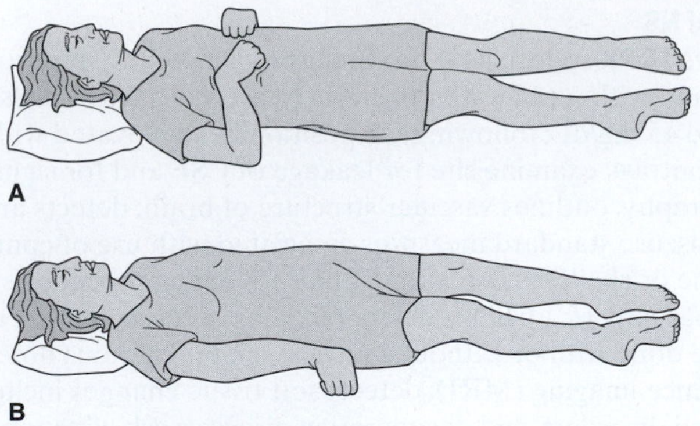

Figure 53–1

Abnormal posturing. *A.* Decorticate rigidity. *B.* Decerebrate rigidity.

7. Glasgow Coma Scale assessment includes components of eye opening (scored 1 to 4), best verbal response (scored 1 to 5), and best motor response (scored 1 to 6); total score ranges from 3 to 15; a score of 8 or lower usually indicates coma; see Table 53–4
8. Diagnostic and laboratory test findings
   a. CT and MRI may detect hemorrhage, tumor, cysts, edema, or brain atrophy
   b. EEGs evaluate unrecognized seizures as a cause for an altered LOC
   c. Cerebral angiography evaluates cerebral circulation for aneurysm and AV malformations
   d. Transcranial Doppler study is a less invasive method to study blood flow
   e. LP with CSF analysis determines presence or status of infection
   f. Laboratory tests such as glucose, serum electrolytes, osmolarity, creatinine, liver function, complete blood count (CBC), arterial blood gases (ABGs), and toxicology screens rule out metabolic, toxic, or drug-induced disorders

C. Therapeutic management

1. Depends on cause of altered mental status; in addition to treating cause, ongoing care focuses on maintaining airway, skin integrity and nutrition, and preventing contractures
2. *NCLEX®* Monitor for ability to clear secretions; observe breath sounds; maintain patent airway in unconscious client; maintain client with ineffective airway in side-lying position; provide tracheostomy care every 4 hours if client has tracheostomy
3. *NCLEX®* Monitor swallowing and gag reflex; provide interventions to prevent aspiration (such as elevated head of bed [HOB]); monitor for and report possible aspiration

Table 53–4 Glasgow Coma Scale

Data Item	Response	Score*
Eyes open (record C if eyes are closed by swelling)	Spontaneously	4
	To speech	3
	To pain	2
	No response	1
Best motor response (record best upper arm response)	Obeys commands	6
	Localized pain	5
	Flexion-withdrawal	4
	Abnormal flexion	3
	Abnormal extension	2
	No response	1
Best verbal response (record T if an endotracheal or tracheostomy tube is in place)	Oriented	5
	Confused	4
	Inappropriate words	3
	Incomprehensible sounds	2
	No response	1
Total Score:		—

*A higher score indicates a higher level of functioning.

Source: LeMone, P., Burke, K. M., & Bauldoff, G. *Medical surgical nursing: Critical thinking in patient care* (5th ed.), © 2011, p. 1421. Reprinted by permission of Pearson Education, Inc., Upper Saddle River, NJ 07458.

4. Monitor skin integrity every shift; reposition client every 2 hours; provide interventions to prevent skin breakdown; keep linens clean, dry, and wrinkle-free
5. Provide proper support devices to maintain extremities in functional condition; perform passive range of motion (ROM) regularly
6. Monitor nutritional status and daily weight; determine need for alternative methods of nutritional support
7. Provide emotional support to client and family
8. *NCLEX®* Provide for alternate means of communication as needed (such as questions with yes and no or other single-word answers)

D. Reinforce family teaching

1. Family anxiety is common when clients have altered mental status, especially if prognosis is uncertain
2. Reinforce information provided by physician
3. Encourage family to talk to client
4. Evaluate and provide information about client's care when family is ready
5. Offer support services as needed

IV. INCREASED INTRACRANIAL PRESSURE

A. Overview

1. Increased ICP is defined as a prolonged pressure greater than 15 mm Hg measured in lateral ventricles; exerted by brain tissue, CSF, and blood within cranial vault
2. Coughing, sneezing, straining, and bending forward cause a transient increase in ICP that does not cause significant tissue ischemia
3. *NCLEX®* **Cushing's triad**/response: involves three classic signs or responses to increased ICP: increased systolic BP with unchanged diastolic BP, widening pulse pressure, and reflex bradycardia from stimulation of carotid bodies
4. A prolonged increase in ICP causes tissue ischemia because cerebral blood flow and perfusion are compromised
5. Autoregulation, a compensatory mechanism to maintain cerebral blood flow, is disrupted and can lead to cellular hypoxia and ischemia
6. Untreated increased ICP leads to herniation and ultimately death
7. Because brain is encased in a closed cavity, expansion of brain can cause increased ICP
8. Cerebral edema is an increase in volume of brain tissue due to changes in capillary permeability (vasogenic edema) or functional or structural integrity of cell membrane (cytotoxic edema), or an increase in interstitial fluids (interstitial cerebral edema); edema is usually proportional to size of injury and may be localized or generalized
9. Hydrocephalus is an increase in CSF volume within ventricular system; it may be noncommunicating hydrocephalus in which drainage from ventricular system is impaired (such as tumor or mass) or communicating hydrocephalus, in which blood blocks CSF absorption, such as with subarachnoid hemorrhage

NCLEX® **B. Nursing data collection**

1. Earliest signs of increased ICP may be blurred vision, decreased visual acuity, and diplopia because of pressure on visual pathways; headache, papilledema, or swelling of optic disk and vomiting are next signs; most significant sign of increased ICP is a change in LOC; as pressure increases from front to back of brain, the LOC deteriorates
2. Diagnostic and laboratory test findings identify and treat underlying cause of increased ICP
   a. CT or MRI scanning is generally initial test
   b. LP is not usually performed because of possibility of brain herniation caused by sudden release of pressure
   c. Laboratory tests augment and monitor treatment approaches; serum osmolarity monitors hydration status; ABGs measure pH, O_2, and CO_2 (hydrogen ions and CO_2 are vasodilators that increase ICP)

C. Therapeutic management

1. Increased ICP is a medical emergency with little time for lengthy diagnostic studies; it centers on restoring normal pressure and can be accomplished through medications, surgery, and drainage of CSF from ventricles
2. A drainage catheter, inserted via ventriculostomy into lateral ventricle, can monitor ICP and drain CSF to maintain normal pressure; system is calibrated with transducer leveled 1 inch above ear (height of foramen of Munro); sterile technique is of utmost importance

NCLEX® 3. Monitor neurological status every 1 to 2 hours and report any deterioration; areas include LOC, behavior, motor/sensory function, pupil size and response, vital signs with temperature

NCLEX® 4. Maintain airway; elevate HOB 30 degrees or keep flat as prescribed; maintain head and neck in neutral position to promote venous drainage

NCLEX® 5. Monitor for bladder distention and bowel constipation; assist client when necessary to prevent Valsalva maneuver

NCLEX® 6. Plan nursing care so it is not too clustered because prolonged activity may increase ICP; provide for a quiet environment (lights kept low also) and limit noxious stimuli; limit stimulation such as radio, TV, and newspaper; avoid ingesting stimulants such as coffee, tea, cola drinks, and cigarette smoke

NCLEX® 7. Maintain fluid restriction as prescribed

8. Keep dressings over catheter dry and change dressings as prescribed; monitor insertion site for CSF leakage or infection; monitor client for signs and symptoms of infection; use aseptic technique when in contact with ICP monitor

NCLEX® 9. Medication therapy
   a. Osmotic diuretics such as mannitol (Osmitrol) and loop diuretics such as furosemide (Lasix) are mainstays used to decrease ICP; they draw water from edematous tissues into vascular system, but can also disturb glucose and electrolytes, so monitor their effect
   b. Corticosteroids may be effective in decreasing ICP, especially with tumors, although mechanism of action is unclear

NCLEX® 10. Reinforce client and family teaching
   a. Avoid coughing, blowing nose, straining for bowel movements, pushing against bed side-rails, or performing isometric exercises to reduce risk of increased ICP
   b. Maintain neutral head and neck alignment to enhance arterial and venous circulation
   c. Maintain a quiet environment and minimize stimuli
   d. Explain to family that upsetting client may increase ICP

V. HEAD INJURY

A. Skull fracture

1. Overview
   a. A break in skull that occurs with or without intracranial trauma; force of impact significantly increases risk of hematoma formation; disruption of skull can lead to infection and cranial nerve injury
   b. Occurs from trauma; may be labeled as open or closed, depending on whether or not skin is broken
   c. *Linear* fractures are most common of four types; risk of infection and CSF leakage is minimal because dura remains intact; hematoma formation is possible
   d. *Comminuted* and *depressed* skull fractures have a higher risk of brain tissue damage and infection, especially if overlying skin and dura is torn or damaged; risk of secondary brain injury is reduced because energy of impact caused bone fracture instead of being transferred to brain tissue
   e. *Basilar* skull fractures involve base of skull and are usually secondary injuries; most are uncomplicated, but those that disrupt sinuses and middle ear bones can lead to CSF leakage and infection
2. Nursing data collection

   NCLEX® a. Clinical manifestations may give clues to area of fracture; basilar skull fracture may produce manifestations listed in Box 53–3

   b. Diagnostic and laboratory tests: plain x-ray films and CT or MRI scans; basilar skull fractures may be difficult to identify on plain x-ray
3. Therapeutic management: treatment depends on type and location of injury
   a. Linear skull fractures generally require bedrest and observation for underlying brain injury; no specific treatment is necessary

Box 53–3

Signs of Basilar Skull Fracture

- Battle's sign: ecchymosis over mastoid process
- Hemotympanum: blood visible behind tympanic membrane
- Raccoon eyes: bilateral periorbital ecchymosis
- Rhinorrhea: CSF leakage through nose
- Otorrhea: CSF leakage through ear

b. Comminuted and depressed skull fractures require surgical intervention within 24 hours
c. Basilar skull fractures do not require surgery unless there is persistent CSF leakage, but do require regular neurological tests for meningitis
d. Observe client for otorrhea or rhinorrhea

NCLEX® e. Test clear ear drainage and sinus drainage for glucose; only CSF has glucose; mucous secretions do not

NCLEX® f. Observe blood-tinged drainage for halo sign; glucose-containing CSF dries in concentric rings on gauze or tissues

g. Keep nasopharynx and external ear clean; use sterile technique and supplies when cleaning drainage from nose and/or ears

NCLEX® h. Instruct client not to blow nose, cough, or inhibit sneeze and to sneeze through an open mouth

i. Use aseptic technique when changing head dressings
j. Medication therapy: dexamethasone to decrease cerebral edema and antibiotics when there is a risk of infection

NCLEX® 4. Reinforce client teaching: go to emergency department if client develops drowsiness or confusion, difficulty waking, vomiting, blurred vision, slurred speech, prolonged headache, blood or clear fluid leaking from ears or nose, weakness in an arm or leg, stiff neck, or seizures

B. Intracranial hemorrhage

1. Overview
   a. An escape of blood into cranium (often because of blunt trauma); hemorrhage may cause a very slow to very rapid neurological deterioration
   b. Results directly from trauma or from shearing forces on cerebral arteries and veins from acceleration-deceleration injuries; they are classified by location
   c. Bleeding can be epidural, subdural, or intracranial (see Box 53–4)
2. Data collection
   a. **Epidural hematoma**: client may initially lose consciousness then have a short period of lucidness, followed by rapid deterioration from drowsiness to coma; other manifestations include headache, fixed dilated pupil on affected side, hemiparesis, hemiplegia, and possible seizures; this condition is a surgical emergency
   b. **Subdural hematoma**: manifestations may develop slowly and may be mistaken for dementia in an older adult; slow thinking, confusion, drowsiness, or lethargy are common; headaches, ipsilateral pupil dilation and sluggishness, and possible seizures are other signs

Box 53–4

Types of Intracranial Bleeding

Epidural Hematoma

- Develops between dura and skull
- As hematoma forms, it strips dura away from skull
- Usually develops from a tear in meningeal artery
- Because this is an arterial bleed, it rapidly expands, leading to a rapid deterioration in neurological status

Subdural Hematoma

- Forms between dura mater and arachnoid–pia mater layers of meninges
- Usually involves veins but may involve small arteries as well
- As blood collects, pressure is applied to underlying brain tissue
- May be acute (develops within 48 hours after an acute injury), subacute (2 days to 3 weeks after lesser injury), or chronic (3 weeks to months after a minor injury), or may develop spontaneously

Intracerebral Hemorrhage

- Bleeding into brain tissue
- Can occur anywhere in brain but most commonly in frontal or temporal lobes
- May result from closed head trauma, where shearing forces are applied deep in brain; this type of hemorrhage occurs, for example, in a motor vehicle accident in which client hits head on windshield, resulting in coup and contrecoup injury

c. Intracerebral hematomas vary in initial presentation depending on location; headache is common; as hematoma progresses, a decreased LOC, hemiplegia, and ipsilateral pupil dilation occurs; an expanding clot may lead to herniation
d. Diagnostic and laboratory tests: CT and MRI; laboratory values do not establish diagnosis but provide baseline data for client's overall health status

3. Therapeutic management
a. Small hematomas reabsorb spontaneously and may be treated conservatively
b. Surgical intervention is needed to drain epidural hematomas and larger subdural hematomas; surgery is less successful with intracerebral hematomas because of widespread tissue damage; supportive care and preventing complications are goals of therapy
c. Monitor neurological signs on a regular schedule; clear client's nose and mouth of secretions; suction airway as needed
d. Monitor respiratory pattern for rate, depth, and rhythm if client is not mechanically ventilated; prepare for O_2 administration and endotracheal (ET) intubation for respiratory distress
e. Prepare for cranial surgery for deteriorating neurological condition
f. Provide appropriate preoperative and postoperative care
g. Provide previously discussed measures to manage increased ICP
NCLEX® h. Medication therapy: none specific to hematomas; osmotic diuretics and steroids reduce increased ICP; antiepileptics treat seizures if they occur as complications

4. Reinforce client and family teaching: possible surgery to evacuate hematoma

C. Contusion

1. Overview
a. Bruising of brain tissue from blunt trauma or coup/contrecoup injuries
b. Usually involves damage to parenchyma with tears in vessels or tissue, pulling, and subsequent areas of necrosis or infarction

2. Nursing data collection: symptoms vary depending on site of injury; may have decreasing LOC

3. Therapeutic management
a. Monitor neurological status
b. Monitor for signs of complications; can have sequelae specific to area of injury

4. Reinforce client and family teaching
a. Symptoms of complications that may occur after discharge
NCLEX® b. Provide written instructions as well as clear information about when to seek medical care (worsening neurological status, increasing headache)

D. Concussion

1. Overview
a. Concussion or "mild traumatic brain injury" involves some transient loss of consciousness, usually from blunt head trauma
b. Is usually related to stretching, compression, or shearing of nerve fibers
c. Postconcussion syndrome occurs after initial head injury; poor concentration and problems with memory may be noted; client may report headache, dizziness, and photophobia; subtle change in personality may be noted

NCLEX® 2. Nursing data collection: symptoms include amnesia of event, headache, and nausea; clients are neurologically intact with a Glasgow Coma Score of 13 to 15; there are 3 levels of concussion severity
a. Grade 1: transient confusion with no loss of consciousness and a duration of abnormal mental status for less than 15 minutes
b. Grade 2: transient confusion with no loss of consciousness and a duration of abnormal mental status for more than 15 minutes
c. Grade 3: loss of consciousness for a few seconds or several minutes or longer

3. Therapeutic management
a. Treatment is supportive with close observation for 24 hours in an emergency room or at home under certain circumstances
b. Clients who had loss of consciousness for more than 5 minutes or amnesia of event are usually admitted for observation to rule out other potential injuries

4. Reinforce client and family teaching: client may be discharged home with caregivers who have received instructions for continued monitoring and what steps to take if complications arise; share information about postconcussion syndrome (headaches, dizziness, fatigue, irritability, anxiety, insomnia, impaired concentration and memory, noise and light sensitivity)

VI. SPINAL CORD INJURY (SCI)

A. Overview

1. Usually caused by trauma; young adults and adolescents are most at risk
2. Affects motor and sensory function at level of injury and below
3. Classified by complete versus incomplete cord injury, cause of injury, and level of injury; in clinical practice, these overlap
4. Perception, sexual function, and elimination are also affected
5. Usually results from excessive force applied to spinal cord and vertebral column; four types of injuries occur:
   a. Hyperflexion compresses vertebral bodies and disrupts ligaments and discs
   b. Hyperextension disrupts ligaments and causes vertebral fractures
   c. Axial loading is an application of excessive vertical force and may cause compression fractures
   d. Excessive rotation tears ligaments and fractures articular surfaces and causes compression fractures (see Figure 53–2)
6. Risk factors include age, gender, and alcohol and drug abuse

B. Nursing data collection

NCLEX®

1. Spinal shock, a temporary loss of reflex function, may occur after SCI: symptoms include bradycardia; hypotension; flaccid paralysis of skeletal muscles; loss of pain, touch, temperature, pressure, visceral, and somatic sensations; bowel and bladder dysfunction; and loss of ability to perspire; spinal shock has resolved once spinal reflexes return
2. **Paraplegia** is paralysis of lower body; occurs when injury level is in thoracic spine or lower
3. **Tetraplegia**, formally quadriplegia, is paralysis of arms, trunk, legs, and pelvic portions of body; occurs when level of injury is in cervical spine

NCLEX®

4. **Autonomic hyperreflexia** (also called dysreflexia) is an exaggerated sympathetic response that occurs with injuries at T6 or higher; response is seen only after recovery from spinal shock; it occurs when stimuli cannot ascend cord; a stimulus such as urge to void or abdominal discomfort triggers massive vasoconstriction below injury, vasodilation above injury, and bradycardia and rapidly occurring systolic hypertension with widening pulse pressure

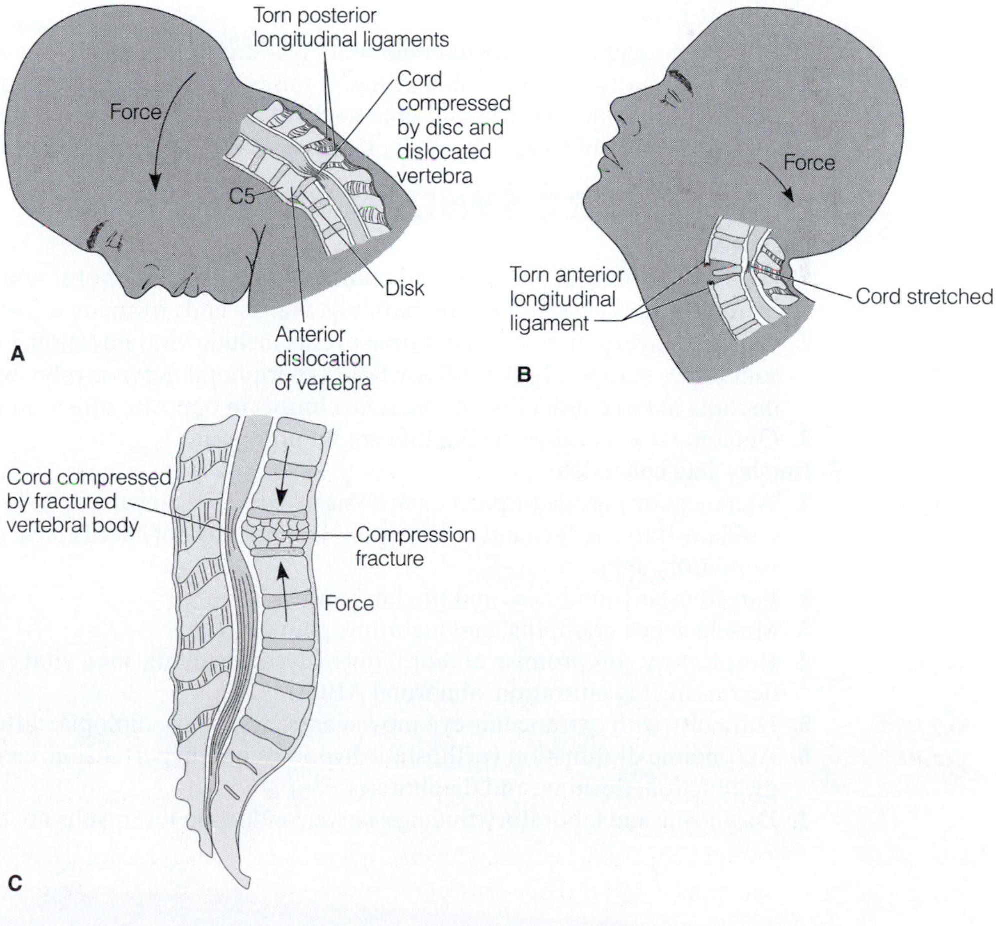

Figure 53–2

Spinal cord injury mechanisms. *A.* Hyperflexion. *B.* Hyperextension. *C.* Axial loading, a form of compression.

5. Diagnostic and laboratory test findings: x-ray films are done to visualize fractures; CT and MRI scans show changes in vertebrae, spinal cord, and tissues surrounding cord; an EMG is done after acute injury to locate level of injury

C. Therapeutic management

1. Acute management involves immobilizing injury and assessing and stabilizing client
2. Treat complications of respiratory distress, atonic bladder, paralytic ileus, and cardiovascular alterations
3. Stabilization of injury with devices such as halo traction and Gardner-Wells tongs or surgery as indicated
4. *NCLEX®* Monitor vital capacity and respiratory effectiveness; high cervical cord injuries (C4 or above or lower if edema ascends cord) may inhibit respirations requiring mechanical ventilation
5. Monitor for signs of ascending edema; may cause respiratory compromise
6. Assist client with quad coughing by pushing in and up at xiphoid process when client is coughing
7. *NCLEX®* Treat autonomic hyperreflexia immediately
   a. Elevate HOB and remove antiembolism stockings
   b. Measure BP every 2 to 3 minutes while determining stimuli that initiated response; remove stimulus immediately when found
   c. With severe hypertension unresolved by removing offending stimulus, notify physician and administer antihypertensives per protocol
8. Encourage client to verbalize feelings about loss of function and care
9. *NCLEX®* Institute bowel and bladder training programs to restore a regular schedule for elimination
10. Encourage self-care and independent decision making
11. Include family and important others in discussions
12. Clients with SCI because of fracture or dislocated cervical vertebrae may benefit from a Halo brace; it is an external fixation device that allows earlier mobility by eliminating need for skeletal cervical traction with Gardner-Wells tongs or other apparatus
13. *NCLEX®* Medication therapy: corticosteroids (such as methylprednisolone, [Solu-Medrol]) may decrease or control edema of cord; vasoactive drugs treat hypotension or hypertension due to spinal shock or autonomic hyperreflexia; antispasmodics (baclofen [Lioresal] and diazepam [Valium]) treat spasticity in clients; analgesics and tricyclic antidepressants treat pain

D. Reinforce client teaching

1. Promote independence in self-care, such as self-catheterization technique, bowel evacuation, activities of daily living
2. Information about variety of community resources available as needed
3. *NCLEX®* If client has a Halo vest, reinforce that it raises center of gravity; avoid bending over to reduce risk of falls; neck is immobilized in midline so client must learn to turn entire body to scan environment; eat soft foods and cut food into small pieces and use straw for liquids; driving is prohibited

VII. GUILLAIN-BARRÉ SYNDROME

A. Overview

1. An acute, rapidly progressive inflammation of peripheral motor and sensory nerves characterized by motor weakness and flaccid paralysis that ascends from lower extremities in most cases
2. Cause is uncertain, but precipitating events include viral infection, immunizations, fever, injury, and sometimes surgery; IgM antibody targets peripheral nerve **myelin**, which damages myelin sheath and disrupts nerve conduction; nerve remyelinizes in opposite direction of demyelination
3. Outcome is generally excellent if care is appropriate

B. Nursing data collection

1. *NCLEX®* Weakness or paresis or partial paralysis progressing upward from lower extremities (paralysis in Guillain-Barré is "ground to the brain"); about 20% of clients have respiratory paralysis requiring ventilatory support
2. Paresthesias (numbness and tingling) and pain
3. Muscle aches, cramping, and nighttime pain
4. *NCLEX®* Respiratory compromise and/or failure (dyspnea, diminished vital capacity and breath sounds), decreasing O_2 saturation, abnormal ABGs
5. *NCLEX®* Difficulty with extraocular eye movements, dysphagia, diplopia, difficulty speaking
6. *NCLEX®* Autonomic dysfunction (orthostatic hypotension), hypertension, change in HR, bowel and bladder dysfunction, flushing, and diaphoresis
7. Diagnostic and laboratory findings: nerve conduction test results are diminished, elevated protein in CSF

C. Therapeutic management

1. Supportive care to maintain function of all systems, including respiratory, cardiac, GI, renal, and skin; medications as ordered
2. Plasmapheresis: plasma is removed and separated from whole blood; blood cells are then returned without plasma to remove antibodies that cause disorder; monitor for complications of this therapy, which include bleeding from loss of clotting factors, and fluid and electrolyte imbalance

NCLEX®
3. Monitor respiratory status: rate, depth, breath sounds; vital capacity; note secretions; check gag, cough, and swallowing

NCLEX®
4. Monitor cardiac status: HR, BP, dysrhythmias
5. Administer chest physiotherapy and pulmonary hygiene measures
6. Maintain adequate nutrition as appropriate: administer enteral or parenteral nutrition as needed; if client can swallow, assist with small, frequent feedings of soft foods; weigh client weekly; check electrolyte status; provide mouth care every 2 hours
7. Monitor bowel and bladder function: note bowel sounds and frequency, amount, color of bowel movements; offer bedpan; check for distention and residuals in client who cannot void spontaneously; perform intermittent catheterization as needed; encourage fluid intake to 3500 mL/day
8. Prevent complications of immobility: encourage use of weak extremities as able; provide assistance with ROM and exercises prescribed by physical therapist; protect immobile extremities with use of air mattress or special bed and elbow and heel protectors; turn and reposition every 2 hours; elevate extremities to prevent dependent edema; use antiembolism compression devices/stockings
9. Provide eye care for client with inability to close eyelids completely; instill artificial tears, cleanse eyes as needed, use eye shields, and tape eyes closed if needed
10. Provide comfort and analgesics as needed
11. Promote communication with client and family; use alternative means of communication if client is on ventilator or cannot speak because of weak muscles
12. Initiate discharge planning at time of admission
13. Medication therapy: IV immunoglobulins (may result in low-grade fever, muscle aches, headache, or [rarely] acute renal failure or retinal necrosis); adrenocorticotropic hormone (ACTH) and corticosteroids or anti-inflammatory drugs; supportive medications include stool softeners, antacids or H_2-receptor antagonists, and analgesics

D. Reinforce client teaching: provide rationales for all care and information about disease progression; encourage client and family to express feelings and participate in care as able

VIII. CEREBROVASCULAR ACCIDENT (CVA, BRAIN ATTACK, STROKE)

A. Overview

1. A condition in which neurological deficits result from decreased blood flow to a localized area of brain; onset may be rapid or gradual

NCLEX®
2. Risk factors include hypertension, diabetes mellitus, sickle cell disease, substance abuse, cardiac dysrhythmias, and atherosclerosis
3. Severe and prolonged cerebral blood flow obstruction leads to ischemia and cell death; resulting deficits predict location of stroke; there are four types of brain attacks; CVAs can be further classified as ischemic or hemorrhagic

NCLEX®
   a. Transient ischemic attack (TIA) is a brief period of neurological deficits that resolve within 24 hours; is often a precursor to a CVA; causes of TIAs may be inflammatory arterial disorders, sickle cell anemia, or atherosclerotic changes in cerebral, jugular and/or carotid blood vessels, thrombosis, and emboli
   b. Thrombotic CVA (an ischemic CVA) is caused by a thrombus (blood clot) occluding a cerebral vessel; thrombi tend to form on atherosclerotic plaque in larger arteries while blood pressure is low (such as during sleep or rest); thrombosis occurs quickly but deficits progress slowly
   c. Embolic CVA (also an ischemic CVA) is caused by a traveling blood clot; source of clot is elsewhere in body; CVA has a sudden onset with immediate symptoms; if embolus is not absorbed, deficits will be persistent
   d. Hemorrhagic CVA or intracranial hemorrhage occurs when a blood vessel ruptures; most often occurs in presence of long-term, poorly controlled hypertension; other factors leading to hemorrhagic CVA include a ruptured intracranial aneurysm, embolic CVA, tumors, AV malformations, anticoagulant therapy, liver disease, and blood disorders; this type of CVA is often fatal because of rapidly increasing ICP; onset of symptoms is rapid; loss of consciousness occurs in about half of cases

B. Nursing data collection

1. Clinical manifestations: vary according to cerebral blood vessel involved
2. NCLEX® Internal carotid: contralateral motor and sensory deficits of arm, leg and face; in dominant hemispheric CVA, aphasia (loss of ability to use language); in nondominant hemispheric CVA, **apraxia** (inability to perform known tasks), **agnosia** (inability to recognize), and unilateral neglect and homonymous **hemianopsia** (loss of one half of visual field in each eye)
3. NCLEX® Middle cerebral artery: drowsiness; stupor; coma; contralateral hemiplegia and sensory deficits of arm and face; aphasia; and homonymous hemianopsia
4. Anterior cerebral artery: contralateral weakness or paralysis and sensory loss of foot and leg, loss of decision-making and voluntary action abilities, and urinary incontinence
5. Vertebral artery: pain in face, nose, or eye; numbness or weakness of face on ipsilateral side; problems with gait; **dysphagia** (difficulty swallowing); and dysarthria (difficulty speaking)
6. Diagnostic and laboratory test findings: CT and MRI demonstrate hemorrhage, tumors, ischemia, edema, and tissue necrosis; cerebral angiography detects abnormal vessel structure, vasospasm, carotid artery stenosis, and loss of vessel wall integrity; ultrasound evaluates blood flow

C. Therapeutic management

1. Drug therapy is most common treatment for CVAs; if it is an ischemic stroke, medications could include thrombolytics and/or heparin
2. NCLEX® It is imperative not to disrupt a clot that has formed following hemorrhagic CVA to avoid rebleed which is often fatal
3. Surgery is not usually indicated as a treatment modality
4. Rehabilitation is crucial to improve deficits
5. Encourage active ROM on unaffected side and passive ROM on affected side
6. Turn and reposition client every 2 hours
7. Monitor lower extremities for thrombophlebitis
8. Encourage use of unaffected arm for ADLs
9. Have client put clothing on affected side first
10. NCLEX® Resume diet orally only after successfully completing a swallowing evaluation; clients may need thickened liquids, foods with consistency of oatmeal, and to chew on unaffected side of mouth; this diet is sometimes called a dysphagia diet
11. Communicate with occupational and physical therapy about rehabilitation
12. Try alternate methods of communication for clients with aphasia and consult with speech pathologist as needed
13. Accept client's frustration and anger as normal to loss of function
14. NCLEX® Reinforce to client with homonymous hemianopsia to overcome deficit by turning head side to side to fully scan visual field
15. Medication therapy
    a. Antiplatelet agents are used to treat TIAs and clients with previous CVAs (except hemorrhagic CVAs)
    b. During acute phase of ischemic stroke, thrombolytic therapy may be administered within 3 hours to dissolve clot
    c. Anticoagulant therapy is provided with heparin initially and then continued with an oral anticoagulant after acute phase
    d. In clients with cerebral edema, hyperosmolar solutions (mannitol [Osmitrol]) or diuretics (furosemide [Lasix]) may be given
    e. In clients with seizures, antiepileptics such as phenytoin (Dilantin), barbiturates, diazepam (Valium), and lorazepam (Ativan) may be given

D. Reinforce client teaching: CVA and CVA prevention, community resources, physical care, and need for psychosocial support, medications

IX. SEIZURE DISORDER

A. Overview

1. A seizure is an episode of excessive and abnormal electrical activity in brain that is manifested by disturbances in skeletal motor activity, sensation, autonomic dysfunction of viscera, behavior, or consciousness
2. Seizures are classified as partial or generalized; partial seizures begin in one area of cortex; generalized seizures involve both hemispheres and deeper brain structures
3. Risk factors in adults include acute febrile state, head injury, infection, metabolic or endocrine disorders, and exposure to toxins

4. Risk factors during infancy include perinatal hypoxia, congenital diseases, infections, metabolic or degenerative diseases, drug withdrawal, and neoplasms
5. Risk factors during childhood include febrile infections, head injury, lead toxicity, drugs, genetic disorders, and neoplasms
6. If seizure activity is chronic (reoccurs within minutes, days, or even years), a diagnosis of epilepsy is made
7. Metabolic needs, O_2 requirements, metabolic by-products, and cerebral blood flow increase dramatically during seizure
8. As long as cerebral blood flow can meet demands of seizure, brain is protected from cellular exhaustion and destruction

B. Nursing data collection

NCLEX®
1. *Simple partial seizures* are limited to one hemisphere; manifestations include altered motor function, sensory signs, or autonomic or psychic symptoms

NCLEX®
2. *Complex partial seizures* originate in temporal lobe and may be preceded by an aura; an impaired LOC and repetitive nonpurposeful movements such as lip-smacking, picking, or aimless walking are noted; amnesia is common
3. *Generalized partial seizure* is a partial seizure that has spread to both hemispheres and deeper structures of brain
4. *Absence seizure* is a generalized seizure that lasts 5 to 30 seconds; there is a sudden, brief cessation of motor activity and a blank stare; they may occur occasionally or up to 100 per day; they may be accompanied by eyelid fluttering or automatisms such as lip-smacking; more common in children than adults

NCLEX®
5. **Tonic-clonic** seizures (grand mal) are most common type of seizure
   a. May be preceded by an aura but often occur without warning
   b. Typically start with a loss of consciousness and sharp muscle contractions
   c. Client falls to floor and may have urinary and/or bowel incontinence
   d. Breathing ceases and cyanosis develops during tonic phase (about 15 to 60 sec); see Figure 53–3A
   e. Clonic phase (60 to 90 sec) follows with alternating muscle contraction and relaxation in all extremities, hyperventilation, and eyes rolled back in head; see Figure 53–3B
   f. In next phase (postictal period), client is relaxed with quiet breathing and is unconscious and unresponsive; client gradually regains consciousness and may have transient confusion and disorientation; clients often report headache, muscle aches, and fatigue and may sleep several hours
   g. Clients will have amnesia of seizure and events just prior to seizure

NCLEX®
6. *Status epilepticus* is a life-threatening emergency that can occur during seizure activity; it is characterized by continuous cycles of tonic-clonic activity with short periods of calm between them; this cumulative effect can interfere with respiration; client is in great danger of developing hypoxia, hyperthermia, hypoglycemia, and exhaustion if seizure activity is not stopped
7. During actual seizure activity, observe order of events and duration of seizure; for tonic-clonic seizures, be certain to time length of seizure until jerking stops; tonic indicates continuous muscle contraction; clonic indicates alternating contraction and relaxation of muscles; for all other types of seizures, note duration from start of seizure to time that consciousness is regained; describe any precipitating events or unusual behavior; note parts of body involved and whether it begins in a specific body part

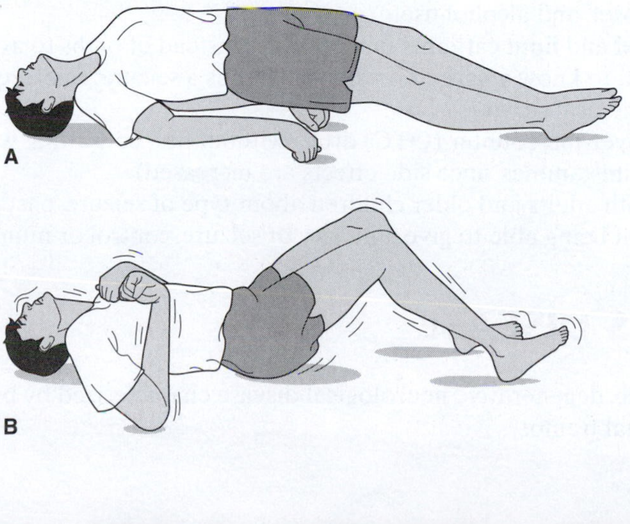

Figure 53–3

Tonic-clonic contractions in grand mal seizures. *A.* Tonic phase. *B.* Clonic phase.

8. Observe face for any color change, perspiration, and lack of expression; observe mouth for deviation to one side or other, clenched teeth, tongue biting, frothing, and/or flecks of blood or bleeding; if able to observe pupils, note any change in size, equality, reaction to light, and accommodation
9. Observe for presence or length of apnea; other general observations may be involuntary urination or defecation
10. Postictally, it is important to note duration of postictal period and LOC; orientation to time, person, place; and any alterations in motor ability or speech
11. Diagnostic and laboratory tests: complete neurological examination, EEG, skull x-ray series, CT scan, LP with CSF analysis, blood studies, and electrocardiogram

C. Therapeutic management

1. Provide interventions during seizure to maintain airway patency
   - NCLEX® a. Turn client to side if necessary to maintain airway and promote drainage of secretions without aspiration
   - b. Have O_2 and suction equipment at bedside for use following a seizure if needed
   - NCLEX® c. Do not try to force an object, such as a bite stick, into mouth of client who is seizing, as this may break teeth or cause other injury
2. NCLEX® Provide interventions during a seizure to reduce the risk of injury; do not restrain client but provide an environment that will not create further injury; teach family members how to protect client during seizures
3. Document seizure activity promptly and report it as appropriate
4. Provide support to client that concerns are normal; help client identify leisure activities that are safe; provide information about resources and support groups; provide accurate information about hiring practices and legalities of driving or operating heavy/dangerous equipment
5. Medication therapy
   - a. Antiepileptics that raise seizure threshold or limit spread of abnormal electrical activity are mainstay of epilepsy treatment
   - NCLEX® b. Some commonly used antiepileptics are phenytoin (Dilantin), divalproex sodium (Depakote), valproic acid (Depakene), carbamazepine (Tegretol), gabapentin (Neurontin), and lamotrigine (Lamictal)
   - c. Diazepam (Valium), lorazepam (Ativan), and phenobarbital are also used intermittently to stop seizure activity during acute episodes
6. If drug therapy fails to control seizures, surgery to excise tissue involved in seizure activity may be an alternative
7. Promote client's development of a positive self-image, especially if a child; talk with client about his or her feelings; plan strategies to promote acceptance and decrease fear among peers
8. Encourage client and family to express feelings

D. Reinforce client teaching

1. Correct misconceptions, fears, and myths about epilepsy
2. Provide information about community and national resources for epilepsy
3. Stress importance of follow-up care
4. Review laws (i.e., driving a motor vehicle) that apply to those with epilepsy
5. Refer for employment or vocational counseling as needed
6. Stress importance of wearing a medical alert band
7. Emphasize aura alert so client is aware of impending seizure
8. NCLEX® Stress importance of medication compliance
9. Stress importance of avoiding physical and emotional stress as triggers, including inadequate sleep, emotional upset, and alcohol use
10. NCLEX® Avoid alcohol and limit caffeine; take showers instead of baths to avoid drowning
11. Families need to know what to do when client has a seizure; reinforce safety measures and when to call emergency medical services
12. Do not use over-the-counter (OTC) drugs without first consulting with health care provider (for example, antihistamines since side effects are increased)
13. Reinforce with adults and older children about type of seizure, past and present medication, and importance of being able to give a history of seizure, control or number of seizures experienced and their timing

X. PARKINSON'S DISEASE

A. Overview

1. A progressive, degenerative neurological disease characterized by **bradykinesia**, muscle rigidity, and nonintentional tremor

2. Commonly affects older adults and is usually diagnosed between age 50 to 60; as disease progresses, burden of care increases
3. Atrophy occurs in substantia nigra, which produces dopamine; as dopamine decreases, acetylcholine is no longer inhibited; this neurotransmitter imbalance leads to symptoms

B. Nursing data collection

1. Clinical manifestations begin subtly with fatigue and a slight resting tremor as initial symptoms; in a small population of clients, dementia may be presenting symptom
2. *NCLEX®* Bradykinesia is slow movements caused by muscle rigidity; may also affect eyes, mouth, and voice; some clients exhibit a staring gaze
3. Uncoordinated movements and postural disturbance, trunk tilted forward
4. Short-stepped, shuffling and propulsive gait, leading to increased risk of falls
5. Seborrhea
6. Heat intolerance; excessive sweating of face and neck; absence of sweating on trunk and extremities
7. Constipation
8. Anxiety and depression, possible sleep disturbances
9. Dysphagia

C. Therapeutic management

1. Includes medications, surgery, and rehabilitation to optimize functional level; a team approach is essential to quality care
2. Client should perform active ROM twice a day; provide passive ROM when client is unable to do active ROM
3. Ambulate at least four times a day
4. *NCLEX®* Use assistive devices when recommended; consider velcro instead of buttons and slip-on shoes instead of those with ties
5. Monitor communication skills, speech, hearing, and writing
6. Consult with a speech pathologist if necessary
7. Monitor nutritional status and self-feeding abilities
8. *NCLEX®* Monitor diet to ensure foods high in bulk and fluids
9. *NCLEX®* Medication therapy: monoamine oxidase (MAO) inhibitors, dopaminergics, dopamine agonists, and anticholinergics; eventually all drugs lose effectiveness; a fluctuating response to drugs is called an on-off response; antidepressants, especially amitriptyline, treat depression; propranolol may be used to treat tremors

D. Reinforce client teaching

1. Preventive measures for malnutrition, falls, and other environmental hazards, constipation, skin breakdown from incontinence, and joint contractures
2. Gait training and exercises to improve ambulation, swallowing, speech, and self-care

XI. MULTIPLE SCLEROSIS

A. Overview

1. Chronic CNS disorder in which myelin and nerve axons in brain and spinal cord are destroyed
2. There are four forms based on rate of progression: benign, relapsing-remitting, primary progressive, and secondary progressive
3. Unknown etiology, possibly an autoimmune or genetic basis or may be associated with childhood viral infections
4. *NCLEX®* Destruction of myelin and nerve axons causes a temporary, repetitive, or sustained interruption in nerve impulse conduction, which causes symptoms of multiple sclerosis (MS)
5. Plaque formation occurs throughout white matter of CNS, which also affects nerve impulses of optic nerves, cervical spinal cord, thoracic and lumbar spine
6. Inflammation occurs around plaques as well as around normal tissue
7. Astrocytes appear in lesions, and scar tissue forms, replacing axons and leading to permanent disability

NCLEX® **B. Nursing data collection**

1. Visual disturbances or blindness (retrobulbar neuritis)
2. Sudden, progressive weakness of one or more limbs
3. **Spasticity** of muscles, nystagmus, tremors, and gait instability
4. Fatigue
5. Bladder dysfunction (UTIs, incontinence)

6. Depression
7. LP for CSF reveals clonal IgG bands
8. MRI, CT scans, muscle testing show characteristic changes

C. Therapeutic management

1. No cure is available; supportive care is indicated
2. Overall goal of care is to maintain as much independent function as possible
3. NCLEX® Include rest periods to prevent fatigue, which is an exacerbating factor
4. Help client to recognize choices in care and set priorities on a day-to-day basis whenever possible to maintain sense of control and independence
5. Assist client with ADLs on an as-needed basis; provide adaptive utensils or other assistive devices as needed
6. NCLEX® Maintain fluid intake of at least 2000 mL/day to promote bowel and bladder function and prevent impaction and/or urinary tract infection (UTI)
7. Communicate with client about issues of concern, such as coping skills, sexuality, changing body image, or others identified by client
8. NCLEX® Avoid sources of infection; illness can act as a stressor and trigger an exacerbation, as well as fatigue and rapid changes in temperature
9. Medication therapy: immunosuppressants, antivirals, corticosteroids, antibiotics for UTI, interferon-alpha, glatiramer (Copaxone), anticholinergics, and antispasmodics

D. Reinforce client teaching: medications, symptoms, bladder training, intermittent self-catheterization, sexual functioning, avoiding complications, and possible triggers (fatigue, temperature extremes, illness)

XII. MYASTHENIA GRAVIS

A. Overview

1. A chronic progressive disorder of peripheral NS affecting transmission of nerve impulses to voluntary muscles
2. Causes muscle weakness and fatigue that increases with exertion and improves with rest; eventually leads to fatigue without relief from rest
3. Causes include unknown etiology and family history of autoimmune disorders; has been associated with production of autoantibodies by thymus gland
4. An autoimmune process triggers autoantibody formation that decreases numbers of acetylcholine receptors and widens gap between neuronal axon and muscle fiber in neuromuscular (myoneural) junction
5. Muscle contraction is hindered because IgG autoantibodies prevent acetylcholine from binding with receptors; destruction of receptors at neuromuscular junction occurs
6. NCLEX® Onset is usually slow but can be precipitated by emotional stress, hormonal disturbance (pregnancy, menses, thyroid disorders), infections and vaccinations, trauma and surgery, temperature extremes, excessive exercise, drugs that interfere with neuromuscular transmission (opioids, sedatives, barbiturates, alcohol, quinidine, anesthetics), and thymus tumor

B. Nursing data collection

1. NCLEX® Mild diplopia (double vision) and unilateral ptosis (eyelid drooping) caused by weakness in extraocular muscles; weakness may also involve face, jaw, neck, and hip
2. NCLEX® Complications arise when severe weakness affects muscles of swallowing, chewing and respiration; respiratory distress is manifested by tachypnea, decreased depth, abnormal ABGs, O_2 saturation under 92%, and decreased breath sounds
3. Bowel and bladder incontinence, paresthesias, and pain in weak muscles
4. Myasthenic crisis: sudden motor weakness; risk of respiratory failure and aspiration; most often caused by insufficient dose of medication or an infection
5. Cholinergic crisis: severe muscle weakness caused by overmedication; also cramps, diarrhea, bradycardia, and bronchial spasm with increased pulmonary secretions and risk of respiratory compromise
6. ABGs and pulmonary function tests may show respiratory insufficiency
7. Electromyography (EMG) shows decreased amplitude when motor neurons are stimulated
8. NCLEX® Tensilon test: diagnosis is confirmed with IV edrophonium chloride (Tensilon), which allows acetylcholine to bind with receptors and temporarily improves symptoms; weakness returns after effects of Tensilon wear off

C. Therapeutic management

1. Focuses on medication management with anticholinesterases (see also Chapter 35): neostigmine (Prostigmin), pyridostigmine (Mestinon); immunosuppressants: corticosteroids, azathiopirine

(Imuran), and cyclosporine (Cytoxan); anti-inflammatory drugs; thymectomy (removal of thymus gland); plasmapheresis—removes IgG antibodies, atropine sulfate (Atropine) for cholinergic crisis

NCLEX® 2. Maintain effective breathing pattern and airway clearance; thoroughly monitor for respiratory distress

NCLEX® 3. Monitor meals and teach client to bend head slightly forward while eating and drinking to improve swallowing

4. Reinforce need for client to avoid exposure to infections, especially respiratory

5. Reinforce effective coughing, need for chest physiotherapy and incentive spirometry; have oral suction available, reinforce with client and family how to use it; be prepared to intubate if needed

NCLEX® 6. Provide adequate nutrition: schedule medications 30–45 minutes before eating for peak muscle strength while eating; frequently offer small amounts of foods that are easy to chew and swallow—soft or semisolid as needed; administer IV fluids and nasogastric tube feedings if client is unable to swallow

7. Promote improved function with referrals to physical and occupational therapy

NCLEX® 8. Provide eye care: instill artificial tears; use a patch over one eye for double vision (diplopia); wear sunglasses to protect eyes from bright lights

9. Promote positive body image and coping skills: encourage participation in treatment plan; actively listen to client and encourage expression of feelings; reinforce progress and explain all care

10. Medication therapy: as discussed in section above; see also Chapter 35

D. Reinforce client teaching

1. Plan rest periods and conserve energy; plan major activities early in day; schedule activities during peak medication effect

NCLEX® 2. Avoid extremes of hot and cold, exposure to infections, emotional stress and drugs that may worsen or precipitate an exacerbation (alcohol, sedatives, local anesthetics)

NCLEX® 3. Signs of myasthenic crisis (symptoms of disorder caused by inadequate medication related to need) and cholinergic crisis (over medication)

4. Encourage client to wear a Medic-Alert bracelet

5. Instruct in alternative methods of communication if necessary: eye blink, finger wiggle for yes or no; flash cards or communication board; teach to support lower jaw with hands to assist with speech

XIII. CRANIAL NERVE DISORDERS

A. Trigeminal neuralgia

1. Overview

a. A chronic disease of trigeminal nerve (CN V) that causes severe facial pain

b. Has an unknown cause; affects one or more of 3 divisions of trigeminal nerve (ophthalmic, maxillary, and mandibular); maxillary and mandibular divisions are affected most often

2. Nursing data collection

a. Brief, intense, skin surface pain is characteristic symptom; episodes may occur as frequently as 100 times a day or as infrequently as a few times each year

b. Pain typically starts peripherally and advances centrally

NCLEX® **c.** Motor or sensory deficits do not occur; some clients may have trigger zones that initiate onset of pain; in others, pain is triggered by light touch, eating, swallowing, talking, shaving, sneezing, brushing teeth, or washing the face

3. Therapeutic management

NCLEX® **a.** Centered on controlling pain with antiepileptic medications such as carbamazepine (Tegretol)

b. Surgery includes microvascular decompression (removal of blood vessel from posterior trigeminal root) or rhizotomy (surgical severing of nerve root)

NCLEX® **c.** Encourage client to chew on unaffected side

d. Monitor dietary intake, encouraging soft foods

NCLEX® **e.** Avoid triggers for pain, which include firm toothbrush, very hot or cold foods or liquids, or mechanical pressure on cheeks

f. Medication therapy: most useful drug for controlling pain is carbamazepine (Tegretol); when this is not effective, phenytoin (Dilantin) is tried

4. Reinforce client teaching: avoidance of triggers

B. Bell's palsy

1. Overview

a. A unilateral paralysis of facial muscles

b. Has an unknown cause, with inflammation of nerve and a viral cause suggested; 80% of clients recover completely within a few weeks to months; 15% recover some function but have permanent facial paralysis

NCLEX® 2. Nursing data collection

a. One-sided paralysis of facial muscles
b. Paralysis of upper eyelid with loss of corneal reflex on affected side
c. Loss or impairment of taste over anterior portion of tongue on affected side
d. Increased tearing from lacrimal gland on affected side

3. Therapeutic management

NCLEX® a. Assist with physiotherapy, including moist heat, gentle massage, and facial nerve stimulation with faradic current

NCLEX® b. Protect cornea with artificial tears, sunglasses, eye patch at night, and gentle intermittent closure of eye

NCLEX® c. Medication therapy: a corticosteroid such as prednisone (Deltasone) decreases edema of nerve tissue; antivirals may also be used

d. Assist with body image disturbance, which is often temporary

NCLEX® 4. Reinforce client teaching

a. Wear an eye patch at night and protective glasses when outside
b. Inspect inside of mouth on affected side for food that may collect between mouth and teeth

XIV. CEREBRAL PALSY

A. Overview

1. A nonprogressive motor CNS disorder resulting in altered movement and posture
2. Classified as spastic, athetoid, ataxic, or mixed
3. Topographic descriptions explain part(s) of body affected and include hemiplegia, diplegia, and quadriplegia (tetraplegia)
4. Causes include trauma, hemorrhage, anoxia, or infection before, during, or after birth
5. One third of children with cerebral palsy (CP) also have some degree of mental retardation

B. Nursing data collection

NCLEX® 1. Abnormal muscle tone and coordination: child with spastic cerebral palsy presents with spasticity (hypertonicity of muscle groups); child with athetoid cerebral palsy presents with wormlike movements of extremities; ataxic form of cerebral palsy involves disturbed coordination

2. May display hypertonia or hypotonia and may have varying degrees of tonicity on different extremities
3. Absence of expected reflexes or presence of reflexes that extend beyond expected age suggests cerebral palsy
4. Failure to meet developmental norms may be first suggestion that "something is wrong"

NCLEX® 5. Physical symptoms include altered speech and difficulty with swallowing and scissoring of legs when walking; visual and hearing defects may be present

6. Seizures may accompany CP and may be another indication of brain injury

C. Therapeutic management

1. Many individuals with CP require increased calorie intake because of spasticity or increased motor functioning

NCLEX® 2. If motor involvement causes child to have poor coordination or if child has seizure activity, a safe environment and precautions such as protective headgear and a padded bed are needed

NCLEX® 3. Communication can be a problem if there is oral involvement; child may need to use a communication board or computer-assisted communication; touch is an excellent means to communicate caring to a child

4. Self-care is a goal for all children; extensive collaboration with occupational therapists for strategies and devices to assist in this area may be necessary

NCLEX® 5. Risk for aspiration is present if oral muscles are involved; use of adaptive feeding devices and positioning during feedings can decrease risk; for some clients with severe spasticity, a gastrostomy tube might be surgically placed for enteral feedings

6. Collaborate with multidisciplinary team for speech, nutrition, occupation, and physical therapies
7. Regional early-intervention consortiums conduct community-based developmental screenings to identify children at risk or who have developmental delays from disorders such as CP; referrals for further examination help ensure that early intervention is initiated; Denver II is most widely used developmental screening test
8. Provide adequate nutrition and rest

NCLEX® 9. Maintain a safe environment

10. To control spasticity, traditional treatments have included surgery to release tendons to promote mobility, rehabilitation therapies, oral medications, and intramuscular injections of phenol and botulinum toxin
11. Newer treatment is use of a surgically implanted **intrathecal** pump, which administers a continuous infusion of baclofen (Lioresal); potential pump-related problems include infection and overdose; benefits include improved function, gait, and motor control and generally improved health

D. Reinforce client and family teaching

1. Physical therapy strategies such as ROM exercises to use at home
2. Special feeding techniques and use of adaptive devices such as special silverware and dishes, or how to do gastrostomy tube feedings if indicated
3. Child will need to learn self-care skills such as feeding and dressing self and performing hygiene activities

XV. NEURAL TUBE DEFECTS

A. Overview

1. Are also known as spina bifida or myelodysplasia, develop during first trimester of pregnancy; can occur at any place along spinal canal (see Figure 53–4)
2. *NCLEX®* Etiology is uncertain but incidence is decreasing with maternal folic acid supplementation; genetics, alcohol use, some medications, and maternal health problems (folic acid deficiency, diabetes mellitus, gestational diabetes, obesity) are possible causes
3. Degree of disability is determined by location of defect and number of spinal nerves encased in sac; higher defects are associated with greater neurologic dysfunction
4. There are several types of spina bifida or neural tube defects
   a. Spina bifida occulta: posterior vertebral arches fail to fuse, but there is no herniation of spinal cord or meninges (fibrous membrane that covers brain and lines vertebral canal); no loss of function
   b. Meningocele: posterior vertebral arches fail to fuse, and there is a saclike protrusion at some point along posterior vertebrae; sac contain meninges and CSF
   c. Myelomeningocele: posterior vertebral arches fail to fuse; saclike herniation contains meninges, CSF, and part of spinal cord or nerve roots; sometimes CSF leakage occurs
   d. Encephalocele: brain and meninges herniate through defect in skull into a sac

B. Nursing data collection

1. *NCLEX®* Prenatal diagnosis can be made by elevations in alpha-fetoprotein (AFP) in fluid obtained by amniocentesis; can also be determined on prenatal ultrasound
2. *NCLEX®* During postnatal period, monitor for leakage of CSF from sac and monitor skin integrity of sac; check for infection around sac and possible systemic or CNS infection
3. *NCLEX®* Determine degree of sensation at or below level of lesion; this can be evidenced by lack of movement or sensation in legs, and a **neurogenic** (lacking innervation) bladder or bowel
4. Measure head circumference because there is a high risk of hydrocephalus

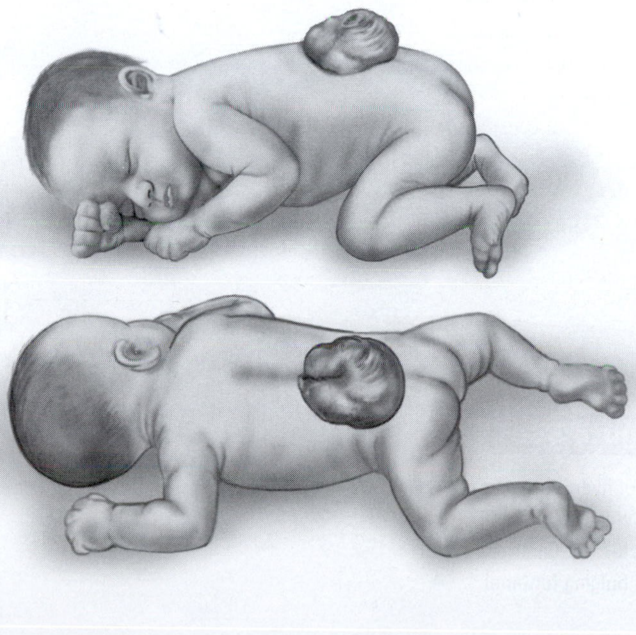

Figure 53–4

Infant with lumbarsacral myelomeningocele.

C. Therapeutic management

1. Collaborative management: defect/sac is surgically repaired during first 48 hours after birth
2. NCLEX® Focus preoperative care on maintaining skin integrity of sac and keeping it free of infection; position infant on side or abdomen to achieve this goal; keep sac moist with sterile, saline-soaked dressings; avoid contamination of sac area by urine or feces
3. NCLEX® Individuals with myelodysplasia have an increased incidence of latex allergies; monitor for this
4. NCLEX® Neurogenic bladder: frequent, clean, straight catheterization is preferred method of management; maintain home schedule as much as possible
5. NCLEX® Neurogenic bowel: work with family to develop a bowel management plan using control of high-fiber diet, adequate fluid intake, and pattern for evacuation of bowels; in some cases, laxatives and enemas are used as prescribed by physician
6. Work with physical therapy to develop modes of transport, such as using braces with crutches or wheelchair
7. Since areas with altered sensation are prone to skin breakdown, teach child and family to reposition frequently and inspect affected areas on a regular basis
8. Medication therapy: low-dose anti-infectives may be prescribed to prevent UTI

D. Reinforce client and family teaching

1. Possibility of child developing hydrocephalus, signs of increased ICP, and what to do if changes develop
2. Since most children with neural tube defects (except spina bifida occulta) have some neurogenic bladder, teaching about clean, intermittent, straight catheterization is important; work with family to develop bowel management program also

XVI. HYDROCEPHALUS

A. Overview

1. A condition characterized by imbalance between CSF production and absorption, resulting in enlarged ventricles and an increase in ICP; if untreated, this condition can cause permanent brain damage
2. Etiology: congenital causes include Arnold Chiari malformation associated with myelomeningocele; can be acquired from meningitis, trauma, or intraventricular hemorrhage in premature infants; etiology is idiopathic in up to 50% of cases

B. Nursing data collection

1. NCLEX® For infants, increased head circumference, split cranial sutures, high-pitched cry, bulging fontanel, irritability when awake, and seizures (see Figure 53–5)
2. NCLEX® Toddlers and older children may also present with sunset eyes, seizures, irritability, papilledema, decreased LOC, and change in vital signs (increased systolic BP and widening pulse pressure)
3. Older children and adults may report headaches and have difficulty with balance and coordination
4. All clients can present with vomiting, lethargy, and Cheyne-Stokes respiratory pattern
5. Diagnosis confirmed using CT and MRI to reveal location of CSF obstruction

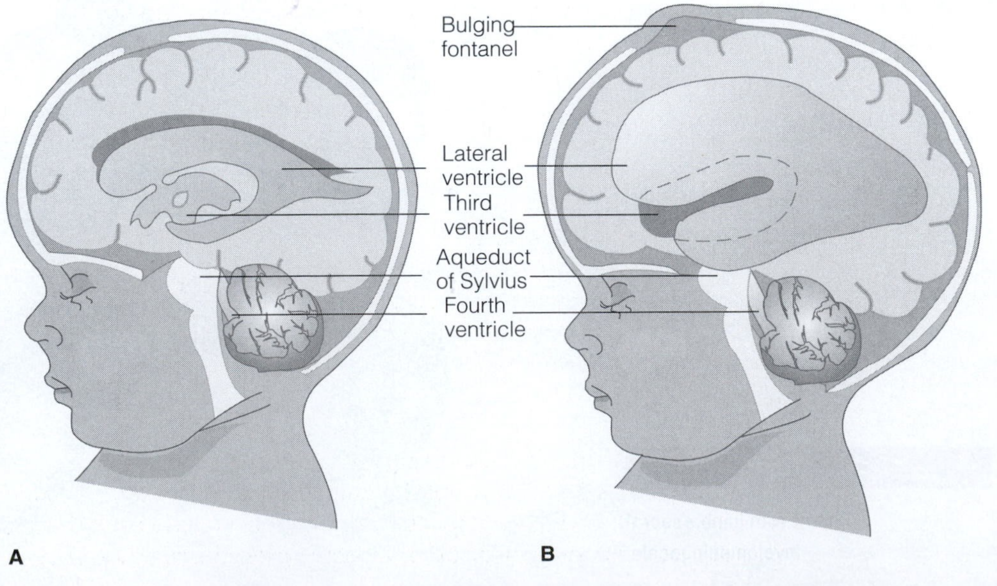

Figure 53–5

Development of hydrocephalus in a young child. *A.* Normal ventricles. *B.* Enlarged ventricles and bulging fontanel.

C. Therapeutic management

1. Surgical insertion of a tube (consistency of piece of cooked spaghetti) into ventricles with distal end in either the peritoneum or atrium
   a. Most common version of this shunt is ventriculoperitoneal
   b. Preoperatively monitor client for symptoms of increased ICP
   NCLEX® c. Postoperatively place client flat and on unoperative side; if an infant or child client is held by a caregiver, it is important not to allow head to be elevated
   NCLEX® d. Postoperatively, monitor client for symptoms of infection; notify physician if symptoms are present: fever, change in LOC, excessive redness at incision site or along shunt tract, elevated WBC count with leukocytosis or shift to left
2. Medication therapy: prophylactic antibiotics before and/or after surgery

D. Reinforce client and family teaching

1. Symptoms of shunt infection and malfunction and what actions to take
2. NCLEX® Signs of shunt malfunction
   a. Infant whose cranial suture lines have not fused; signs include increased head circumference, high-pitched cry, bulging fontanel, irritability when awake, and seizures
   b. Toddlers and older children display vomiting, irritability, and headache; as condition persists, sunset eyes, seizures, papilledema, decreased LOC, and change in vital signs (increased systolic BP and widening pulse pressure) occur
   c. Older clients have difficulty with balance and coordination
   d. All clients may have lethargy and Cheyne-Stokes respirations
3. Some children with hydrocephalus have brain damage that results in motor, language, perceptual, and intellectual disabilities; parents may need referrals to early-intervention professionals to provide long-term rehabilitation services
4. NCLEX® Children with hydrocephalus and myelomeningocele have an increased risk of latex allergies; avoid use of nipples, pacifiers, and toys made of latex products

XVII. CRANIOSYNOSTOSIS

A. Overview

1. Premature closure of cranial sutures in young children
2. There is some relationship between craniosynostosis and several inherited syndromes
3. Etiology is unknown; can be diagnosed by clinical exam, and is confirmed with skull films, CT scan, and MRI
4. Premature closure of skull bones may lead to increased ICP and resulting brain damage

B. Nursing data collection

1. A bony ridge is palpated along a suture line
2. Compensatory growth of skull in directions parallel to closed suture line creates skull deformities; monitor fontanels in all infants for premature closure of fontanels; head circumference also provides data related to this diagnosis

C. Therapeutic management

1. Medical treatment is surgical correction of skeletal defect
2. NCLEX® Follow all principles of postoperative care: keep incision dry and intact; monitor for signs of increased ICP, changing LOC, and infection postoperatively
3. Prepare parents and child for child's postoperative appearance; in addition to large, turbanlike bandage, child will have orbital edema and bruising; long-term results of surgery should be discussed, and "before and after" pictures may assist family in mentally preparing for surgery
4. NCLEX® Fluid restrictions may be ordered in postoperative period; child may be maintained with head of the bed elevated 30 degrees

D. Reinforce client and family teaching

1. Reassurance that surgery will improve child's appearance and that most children postoperatively are healthy and have normal brain development
2. Instructions about how to change dressing at home

XVIII. MENINGITIS

A. Overview

1. Inflammation of meninges of brain and spinal cord
2. Frequently caused by infection of meninges and CSF (rarely, chemicals are a cause)
3. Besides infectious disease exposure, risk factors include basilar skull fracture, otitis media, sinusitis, mastoiditis, neurosurgery or other invasive procedures, systemic sepsis, and impaired immune function

4. Bacterial causative organisms include *haemophilus influenzae* (type B), *streptococcus pneumoniae,* and *neisseria meningitides* (meningococcal)
5. Bacterial meningitis may be complicated by hydrocephalus, cerebral edema, arthritis, and cranial nerve damage
6. Viral meningitis is usually less severe; course of disease is often shorter and more benign

B. Nursing data collection

NCLEX®

1. Clinical manifestations in adults
   a. Restlessness, agitation, and irritability
   b. Abdominal and back pain
   c. Nausea and vomiting
   d. Severe headaches
   e. Signs of meningeal irritation: **nuchal rigidity** (stiff neck), positive Brudzinski's sign (pain, resistance, and hip and knee flexion occur when neck is flexed to chest while lying supine), positive Kernig's sign (pain and/or resistance occurs with flexion of knee and hip and straightening of knee in supine position), and **photophobia** (sensitivity of eyes to light)
   f. Chills and high fever
   g. Confusion, altered LOC
   h. Seizures
   i. Signs and symptoms of increasing ICP
   j. Diagnostic and laboratory test findings: LP with CSF analysis, including Gram stain and cultures, is definitive diagnostic measure for meningitis; cultures of blood, urine, throat, and nose identify possible source of infection

NCLEX®

2. Bacterial meningitis in infants and toddlers: poor feeding, vomiting, high-pitched cry, bulging fontanel, fever or hypothermia depending on maturity of infant's neurological system, and poor muscle tone; children and adolescents present similarly to adults; **opisthotonus** posture (hyperextending head and neck) may relieve some discomfort from meningeal irritation; petechial or purpuric rash will be seen if it is a meningococcal infection
3. Viral meningitis in infants and toddlers: irritability, lethargy, vomiting, and change in appetite; for older child and adult, usually preceded by a nonspecific febrile illness; presents with headache, malaise, muscle aches, nausea and vomiting, photophobia, and nuchal rigidity or spinal rigidity
4. Diagnosed by analysis of CSF obtained by LP; see Table 53–5

C. Therapeutic management

1. Bacterial meningitis is a medical emergency that, if not treated, can be fatal within days

NCLEX®

2. Treatment of bacterial meningitis focuses on eradicating bacterial infection with antibiotics
3. Surgical treatment may include placement of an Ommaya reservoir to allow intrathecal (into subarachnoid space) administration of antibiotics

NCLEX®

4. Monitor respiratory status, administer O_2, and maintain artificial airway
5. Monitor neurological status and vital signs (with temperature) regularly; report changes in neurological status or presence of cranial nerve dysfunction
6. Observe, prepare for, and report any seizure activity

NCLEX®

7. Provide an environment that will minimize ICP elevation; this can include elevating HOB 15 to 30 degrees, avoiding neck extension or flexion, and maintaining head in a neutral position; keep environment quiet and subdued, and handle client in a gentle manner; check for signs of increased ICP
8. Administer prescribed medications and maintain fluid restrictions
9. Monitor for fluid volume deficits; monitor I&O, daily weights, skin turgor, laboratory values, and urine concentration

Table 53–5 Comparison of Cerebrospinal Fluid in Meningitis

	Normal	Viral Meningitis	Bacterial Meningitis
Pressure	5–15 mm Hg	Normal or slightly elevated	Elevated
Appearance	Clear	Clear	Cloudy
Leukocytes (mm^3)	0–5	Slightly elevated	Elevated
Protein (mg/dL)	10–30	Slightly elevated	Elevated
Glucose (mg/dL)	40–80	Normal or decreased	Decreased

10. Medication therapy
    a. Bacterial meningitis is treated for 7 to 14 days with IV antibiotics sensitive to causative organism
    NCLEX® b. Preventive care includes Hib vaccine to protect all young children from haemophilus influenzae infection; medications for client also include ciprofloxacin (Cipro) or ceftriaxone (Rocephin); those who have close contact with clients diagnosed with meningococcal and *H. influenzae* meningitis may receive rifampin (Rifadin) prophylactically
    c. Antiepileptics (usually phenytoin [Dilantin]) to prevent or control seizures
    d. Antipyretic, antiemetic, and analgesic medications for symptom relief
    e. IV fluid replacement until client can resume oral intake
11. Monitor for evidence of pain with all routine assessments; administer nonopioid pain medication as prescribed; however, narcotics (opioids) should be avoided because they mask neuro signs and increasing ICP; pain relief should promote rest and reduce risk of increased ICP
12. NCLEX® Clients with bacterial meningitis must be isolated on droplet precautions until at least 24 hours of antibiotic therapy have been completed
13. NCLEX® Monitor for complications of meningitis (seizures, hearing loss, visual alterations); neurologic sequelae such as mental retardation, CP, and hydrocephalus may occur in children; a complication of meningococcal meningitis is meningococcemia, an overwhelming septic infection that can lead to circulatory collapse and tissue necrosis
14. Viral meningitis is treated symptomatically; usually only infants are hospitalized for viral meningitis

D. Reinforce client and family teaching

1. Importance of taking prescribed antibiotics until finished and other medications as ordered
2. Signs and symptoms of ear, throat, and upper respiratory infections to report so client can be tested for meningitis
3. Information about disease and its transmission, need for possible droplet precautions and antibiotic therapy, and need for prophylactic treatment for those in contact with client
4. Information about possible development of sequelae from disease and possible side effects of medications
5. Information about follow-up as well as rehabilitation services

XIX. ENCEPHALITIS

A. Overview

1. An inflammation of brain tissue
2. Presenting symptoms vary depending on causative organism and location of infection in brain; classic symptoms include an acute febrile illness accompanied by neurologic signs
3. Etiology is usually a viral organism; herpes simplex type 1 is most common cause during neonatal period; enteroviruses are frequently identified as causative agents; nonviral agents include bacteria, parasites, fungi, and rickettsiae
4. Infectious process usually begins elsewhere in body
5. Prognosis depends on degree of CNS involvement; permanent neurologic sequelae may result

NCLEX® **B. Nursing data collection**

1. Check for fever, severe headache, nausea, vomiting, and signs of an upper respiratory infection
2. Neurologic symptoms include those of nuchal rigidity, photophobia, and positive Kernig's and Brudzinski's signs
3. Other signs include disorientation, confusion with personality or behavior changes, speech disturbances, motor dysfunction, cranial nerve deficits, and focal or generalized seizures that alternate with periods of screaming, hallucinating, and bizarre movement; LOC can change from stupor to coma

C. Therapeutic management

1. Monitor client's vital signs, respiratory status, oxygenation, and urine output
2. NCLEX® Provide seizure precautions and have resuscitation materials close to bed; clients with encephalitis are best managed in an intensive care unit (ICU) during acute phase
3. Maintain skin integrity and prevent other complications of immobility through proper positioning, frequent turning, and chest physiotherapy
4. Work with family in planning for discharge; since many clients have neurologic sequelae, family will need support in giving physical and emotional care at home; parents will play an active role in child rehabilitation process; follow-up visits must be coordinated; families may need referral to home care, counseling, social services, and community support groups
5. Medication therapy: if suspected organism is bacterial, appropriate antibiotics will be ordered; acyclovir or other antiviral agents are administered for herpes virus infection

D. Reinforce client and family teaching

1. Information about causative agent and plan of treatment
2. Discharge plans must be started early; because of neurologic sequelae, plans for rehabilitation must be discussed

XX. REYE'S SYNDROME

A. Overview

1. An acute metabolic encephalopathy of childhood; fatty degeneration of liver leads to liver dysfunction
2. *NCLEX®* Characterized by five stages
   a. Vomiting and lethargy
   b. Combativeness and confusion
   c. Coma, decorticate posturing
   d. Decerebrate posturing
   e. Seizures, loss of deep tendon reflexes, respiratory arrest
3. While exact etiology is unclear, Reye's syndrome usually develops after a mild viral illness such as chickenpox
4. *NCLEX®* Research has linked development of Reye's syndrome to use of aspirin; incidence of Reye's syndrome has significantly decreased now that parents are taught to give children acetaminophen (Tylenol) or an NSAID such as naproxen (Naprosyn) or ibuprofen (Motrin)

B. Nursing data collection

1. *NCLEX®* Child presents with an abrupt change in LOC; history reveals child is recovering from a viral disease with sudden onset of vomiting and mental confusion
2. Liver enzymes and ammonia levels are elevated; blood glucose levels are below normal and prothrombin time is prolonged; bilirubin levels remain normal; liver biopsy shows small fat deposits

NCLEX® **C. Therapeutic management**

1. Most children are monitored in an ICU; care is focused on support and on child's physical status, such as monitoring for cerebral edema; enforce fluid restrictions (usually instituted); frequently measure vital signs and neurological status, which may include Glasgow Coma Scale
2. Monitor lab values for elevated ammonia, acidosis, or hypoglycemia; measure I&O
3. Provide all standard nursing measures to prevent complications of immobility
4. Provide emotional support to family; sudden onset and rapid deterioration in child's condition often overwhelm parents' ability to cope
5. Medication therapy
   a. Controlling cerebral edema is a primary concern; drug management may include corticosteroids to reduce swelling and barbiturates to induce a coma for severe cerebral edema; mannitol (Osmitrol; an osmotic diuretic) may be given
   b. Phenytoin may be used to control seizures
   c. Vitamin K may be given to aid in coagulation

D. Reinforce child and family teaching

1. Explanations of disease and its cause, treatment plan and prognosis, ICU environment and medical equipment in use; information helps parents to cope
2. Discharge planning includes rehabilitative needs of child and plans for follow-up
3. The public must be educated about Reye's syndrome and its connection with viral illnesses and administration of salicylates, and that if a child displays symptoms, early medical intervention is associated with a better prognosis

Check Your NCLEX-PN® Exam I.Q.

You are ready for testing on this content if you can

- Identify basic structures and functions of the neurological system.
- Describe the pathophysiology and etiology of common neurological disorders.
- Discuss expected data and diagnostic test findings for selected neurological disorders.
- Discuss therapeutic management of a client experiencing a neurological disorder.
- Discuss nursing management of a client experiencing a neurological disorder.
- Identify expected outcomes for the client experiencing a neurological disorder.

PRACTICE TEST

1 Which finding in a 35-year-old client with an intracranial hematoma should concern the nurse?

1. Hamstring pain when the hip and knee are flexed and then extended
2. Curling of the toes when the bottom of the foot is stroked in upward motion
3. Muscle aches and cramping, especially at night
4. Cogwheel and lead pipe rigidity

2 The nurse would prevent corneal abrasion in a client with myasthenia gravis by performing which nursing intervention?

1. Doing a saline eye irrigation every shift
2. Instilling artificial tears in the eyes every 1 to 2 hours
3. Ensuring the client's contact lenses are on while awake
4. Providing sunglasses when client is outside

3 The client with newly diagnosed Parkinson's disease states, "I just don't think I can handle having Parkinson's disease." What is the nurse's best first response?

1. "You sound overwhelmed. Can you tell me more?"
2. "I am sure you can. A lot of other people do!"
3. "What do you think will be the hardest thing to handle?"
4. "The entire health care team will help you manage the disease."

4 When monitoring the client with meningitis, the nurse looks for which manifestation as a frequent first sign of increased intracranial pressure?

1. A rising systolic blood pressure
2. Change in mood or attention level
3. Irregular respiratory rate and depth
4. A bounding radial pulse

5 The nurse is reinforcing teaching to a client who has been in the hospital with bacterial meningitis and will be going home soon. Which of the following will be of the highest priority?

1. Take all of the antibiotics as directed until completely gone.
2. Eat a high-protein, high-calorie diet.
3. Exercise daily, beginning with active ROM.
4. Get at least 8 hours of sleep per night with frequent rest periods.

6 What strategy would the nurse suggest to the family of the client with Parkinson's disease as the best approach to helping the client maintain as much functional independence as possible?

1. Assist the client to take a warm bath every morning.
2. Perform passive range of motion (ROM) three times a day.
3. Display an unhurried manner that allows the client sufficient time to respond or act.
4. Obtain assistive devices that will make activities of daily living (ADLs) easier.

7 The office nurse should direct a client on the phone to seek care at the hospital emergency department based on which statement?

1. "My legs are weak and now I'm having trouble getting a good breath."
2. "My shaky hand is no better than last visit. In fact, I think it's getting worse."
3. "The double vision went away when I put my eye patch on."
4. "My headache doesn't seem any better even though I gave up coffee."

8 A client seen in the neighborhood clinic reports "eye problems" and generalized weakness that became markedly worse after using a friend's hot tub. The client gives considerably long, detailed responses to initial demographic questions. What is the best question for the nurse to ask at this time?

1. "Was the weather the same each time you used the hot tub?"
2. "How do you feel the hot tub is responsible for your worsening condition?"
3. "Could you try to be a little briefer in your answers so I can best help you?"
4. "Can you tell me more about the eye problems?"

9 An abnormal electroencephalogram (EEG) indicates that a 2-year-old client has epilepsy, but the parents say they have never observed a seizure. The pediatric nurse concludes that the child may be experiencing which type of seizure?

1. Absence
2. Myoclonic
3. Jacksonian
4. Grand mal

10 The nurse is providing care for a 13-year-old who was placed in a halo brace within the last 24 hours because of a spinal cord injury. What action is the first priority?

1. Loosen the connections on the vest to monitor the skin.
2. Monitor the pin sites.
3. Ask how the client is able to reposition self in bed.
4. Ask about the client's ability to perform range of motion to legs.

11 In providing for the safety of the client during a grand mal seizure, the nurse performs which of the following interventions? Select all that apply.

1. Position the client on his back.
2. Gently place a padded tongue blade between the teeth.
3. Remove nearby objects that could lead to client injury.
4. Apply oxygen immediately via mask.
5. Note the length and progression of the seizure.

12 The client recently diagnosed with Guillain-Barré syndrome is drooling and having difficulty swallowing secretions. When the family asks why this occurs, the nurse indicates that which of the following is the cause?

1. Obstructed blood flow to the midbrain
2. Demyelination of cranial nerves responsible for swallow and gag reflex
3. Enlargement of the parotid and salivary glands
4. Deficiency in thiamine and pyridoxine in the central nervous system

13 A 1-year-old child has been diagnosed with cerebral palsy. The child has the spastic form that affects all extremities. Which nursing diagnosis would be appropriate for a child at this age? Select all that apply.

1. Risk for Injury
2. Feeding Self-care Deficit
3. Impaired Thought Processes
4. Impaired Verbal Communication
5. Disturbed Body Image

14 The nurse is reinforcing teaching to the parents of a 6-year-old child with a ventriculoperitoneal (VP) shunt to monitor for shunt malfunction. The nurse determines the parents understand the instructions if they state to notify the physician if the child develops which manifestation?

1. Bulging soft spot
2. Expanding head size
3. Sunset eyes
4. Altered level of consciousness

15 A child is admitted with a head injury after being in a motor vehicle accident. After noting the presence of clear drainage from the left ear, the nurse would suspect which underlying problem commonly associated with this finding?

1. Linear skull fracture
2. Basilar skull fracture
3. Subdural hematoma
4. Epidural hematoma

16 The nursing diagnosis of Ineffective Family Processes related to hospitalization of a child with a potentially fatal condition is being used for the family of a child who sustained a brain injury during an automobile accident. Which nursing interventions would have the highest priority for the LPN/VN?

1. Inform the family of the importance of using seatbelts.
2. Refer the family to support services in the community.
3. Encourage family to ask questions and express feelings.
4. Explain rules for visiting

17 A client arrives at the emergency department following a head injury and is diagnosed with a concussion. The client exhibits transient confusion with no loss of consciousness and a duration of abnormal mental status for less than 15 minutes. The nurse concludes that this client's symptoms are compatible with a concussion of what grade? Provide a numerical response that is a whole number.

Fill in your answer below:

Grade_____

18 The family who has a child with the chronic health problem of spina bifida experiences "chronic sorrow" throughout the child's life. The nurse can anticipate that this will be more prevalent at which time?

1. The child is admitted to the hospital for a planned procedure.
2. The child reaches the age of a "developmental milestone" that the child cannot attain.
3. The child attains independence by attending school.
4. A sibling is born without any health problems.

19 A newborn has been admitted to the unit with a myelomeningocele. The nurse would include which of the following as priority elements of care during the preoperative period? Select all that apply.

1. Measuring the head circumference on a daily basis
2. Preventing increased intracranial pressure by laying the baby in semi-Fowler's position
3. Positioning the infant on his abdomen to protect the spinal defect
4. Monitoring the child for signs of irritability and vomiting
5. Covering the sac with a sterile saline dressing to protect its integrity.

20 Which action has been shown to be effective in reducing the incidence of spina bifida in women of childbearing age?

1. Taking folic acid supplements or using fortified enriched grain products during pregnancy
2. Being immunized for rubella and rubeola
3. Avoiding pregnancy after the age of 45
4. Not having children with a man who also carries the spina bifida genetic trait

21 A 7-year-old child has just been diagnosed with a seizure disorder and the physician has prescribed carbamazepine (Tegretol) 500 mg/day. The nurse should reinforce teaching with the parents about which common side effects of this medication? Select all that apply.

1. Dizziness and headache
2. Hives and aching joints
3. Diaphoresis and vomiting
4. Blurred vision and papular skin rash
5. Drowsiness and vertigo

22 During a well-child visit for an 8-month-old girl, her parents express concern that their older child was already sitting alone at this age. The child was born six weeks premature but had no major difficulties during the neonatal period. What is the best response of the nurse to the parents?

1. "Your observations are good. Your child is demonstrating a developmental delay and probably has cerebral palsy."
2. "You shouldn't jump to conclusions. All children are individuals, and it is not fair to compare one child to another."
3. "You have nothing to worry about. Your child's development is completely normal."
4. "Can you tell me more about your child? Is she turning over?"

23 The nurse places a young child scheduled for a lumbar puncture in a side-lying position with the head flexed and knees drawn up to the chest. The mother asks why the child has to be positioned this way. The nurse uses which statement to explain the rationale?

1. Pain is decreased through this comfort measure.
2. Injury to the spinal cord is prevented.
3. Access to the spinal fluid is facilitated.
4. Restraint is needed to prevent unnecessary movement.

24 A 3-year-old child is admitted to the hospital unit with a diagnosis of viral meningitis. The nurse should take which actions in the care of this child? Select all that apply.

1. Allow the child to assume a position of comfort.
2. Keep the lights bright to monitor skin color.
3. Administer acetaminophen for pain.
4. Monitor the child for seizures.
5. Administer antibiotics.

25 A 2-year-old child is admitted to the neurosurgical unit following a head injury. The nurse is using the Glasgow Coma Scale to measure neurological functioning. Which finding indicates the lowest level of functioning for this child?

1. Confusion
2. Irritable and cries
3. Eyes open only to pain
4. No response to painful stimuli

26 A child with a history of a seizure was admitted 2 hours ago. The history reports fever, chills, and vomiting for the past 24 hours. In report, the nurse is told that the child has a positive Brudzinski's sign. The nurse concludes that this is most likely caused by which of the following?

1. Increased intracranial pressure
2. Meningeal irritation
3. Encephalitis
4. Intraventricular hemorrhage

ANSWERS & RATIONALES

1 **Answer: 1 Rationale:** Hamstring pain with hip and knee flexion and then extension is called positive Kernig's sign. This is common in intracranial hematomas. Curling of the toes with upward stroking on the bottom of the foot is called a negative Babinski; with a hematoma, the nurse should expect a positive Babinski (dorsiflexion of the toes in an adult). Muscle cramps and aching are common in many illnesses. Cogwheel and lead pipe rigidity is specific to Parkinson's disease. **Cognitive Level:** Applying **Client Need:** Physiological Adaptation **Integrated Process:** Nursing Process: Data Collection **Content Area:** Adult Health **Strategy:** The core issue of the question is knowledge of associated findings with intracranial hematoma. Use nursing knowledge and the process of elimination to make a selection.

2 **Answer: 2 Rationale:** Corneal abrasion in the client with myasthenia gravis is caused by dryness of the cornea from inability to close the eyelids and blink. It can be prevented by application of artificial tears every 1 to 2 hours. Saline eye irrigations, wearing contact lenses while awake, and wearing sunglasses when outside do not protect against corneal abrasion. **Cognitive Level:** Applying **Client Need:** Physiological Adaptation **Integrated Process:** Nursing Process: Implementation **Content Area:** Adult Health **Strategy:** Consider the effect of each intervention on preventing injury to the eye and use nursing knowledge and the process of elimination to make a selection.

3 **Answer: 1 Rationale:** The nurse should first encourage the client experiencing a loss to express his feelings. This answer acknowledges the client's feelings, is open-ended, and promotes further discussion. Stating "I am sure you can." provides false reassurance and saying "a lot of other people do!" draws attention away from the client's concern. Focusing on what will be most difficult to handle does not address the client's feelings. Stating the entire health team will help interrupts the opportunity for the client to share concerns by moving directly to attempted solutions. **Cognitive Level:** Analyzing **Client Need:** Psychosocial Integrity **Integrated Process:** Communication and Documentation **Content Area:** Adult Health **Strategy:** The core issue of the question is a therapeutic communication. For communication questions, look first for the option that addresses the client's feelings or concerns.

4 **Answer: 2 Rationale:** The first signs of increased intracranial pressure are often subtle changes in level of consciousness. Rising systolic BP, irregular respiratory rate, and bounding pulse are later signs of increased intracranial pressure. **Cognitive Level:** Analyzing **Client Need:** Physiological Adaptation **Integrated Process:** Nursing Process: Data Collection **Content Area:** Adult Health **Strategy:** The core issue of the question is the ability to discriminate early signs of rising intracranial pressure from later ones. Use nursing knowledge and the process of elimination to make a selection.

5 **Answer: 1 Rationale:** It is essential that the client recovering from bacterial meningitis take all of the prescribed antibiotics as directed. Failure to do so puts the client at risk for a relapse of symptoms and contributes to development of bacterial resistance to antibiotics. A high-protein and high-calorie diet, adequate exercise, and adequate rest and sleep are important aspects of self-care during recuperation but are not as essential as the completion of antimicrobial therapy. **Cognitive Level:** Applying **Client Need:** Physiological Adaptation **Integrated Process:** Teaching and Learning **Content Area:** Adult Health **Strategy:** The core issue of the question is the ability to prioritize the completion of antibiotic therapy with bacterial meningitis as essential. Use nursing knowledge and the process of elimination to make a selection.

6 **Answer: 3 Rationale:** While passive ROM, warm bath, and assistive devices are all useful and appropriate for the client with Parkinson's disease, the essential approach to enhance and encourage self-care abilities will be an unhurried one that allows sufficient time for self-expression and for the client to do as much as possible. **Cognitive Level:** Applying **Client Need:** Physiological Adaptation **Integrated Process:** Nursing Process: Implementation **Content Area:** Adult Health **Strategy:** The critical word in the question is *approach*, which implies a manner of behaving rather than a specific or single action. Use nursing knowledge and the process of elimination to make a selection.

7 **Answer: 1 Rationale:** What the client describes is a classic ascending progression of Guillain-Barré syndrome. The muscular weakness may ascend to include the diaphragm. Total respiratory paralysis can occur, requiring ventilatory support. The incorrect responses refer to chronic problems, not an acute one. **Cognitive Level:** Analyzing **Client Need:** Physiological Adaptation **Integrated Process:** Nursing Process: Implementation **Content Area:** Adult Health **Strategy:** Remember the ABCs and prioritize an answer that refers to a possible impaired airway. Use nursing knowledge and the process of elimination to make a selection.

8 **Answer: 4 Rationale:** A more detailed data collection, such as following up on the eye problems, is important in collecting data to meet client needs. A picture of multiple sclerosis may be unfolding. Focusing on the weather is not relevant to the client's situation. The client may not have an understanding of how the hot tub relates to the current condition. Asking the client to be briefer has a slightly judgmental tone. **Cognitive Level:** Analyzing **Client Need:** Physiological Adaptation **Integrated Process:** Communication and Documentation **Content Area:** Adult Health **Strategy:** The core issue of the question is the selection of an appropriate communication that focuses on data collection. Use nursing knowledge and the process of elimination to make a selection.

9 **Answer: 1** **Rationale:** Also known as petit mal seizures, absence seizures may be no more observable than brief staring instances. The parents should be instructed to note and report any change in the child's behavior, no matter how small. Myoclonic movements and Jacksonian or grand mal seizure activity would be very evident to the client's family. **Cognitive Level:** Analyzing **Client Need:** Physiological Adaptation **Integrated Process:** Nursing Process: Data Collection **Content Area:** Child Health **Strategy:** The core issue of the question is the ability to discriminate different types of seizures based on presentation (or lack of manifestations). Use nursing knowledge and the process of elimination to make a selection.

10 **Answer: 2** **Rationale:** The nurse would want to monitor the pin sites for redness, edema, and drainage as a first priority to detect infection as a complication. The nurse would want to ensure that the vest fits snugly to maintain traction. Asking about bed mobility is an important part of routine care to the client to prevent skin breakdown but is not as high a priority at this time as monitoring for signs of pin site infection. Monitoring the ability to perform range of motion is a routine part of care that can be completed once considerations related to the Halo traction are addressed. **Cognitive Level:** Applying **Client Need:** Physiological Adaptation **Integrated Process:** Nursing Process: Implementation **Content Area:** Child Health **Strategy:** The core issue of the question is knowledge of the importance of monitoring pin sites for a client who is in a halo vest. Use nursing knowledge and the process of elimination to make a selection.

11 **Answer: 3, 5** **Rationale:** The nurse's priority is to protect the client from injury. The nurse would note and then document when the seizure began, how it progressed, when it ended, and associated client findings. To promote drainage, it is more effective to secure an airway by turning the client onto the side rather than the back. Inserting a tongue blade can cause trauma. Oxygen should be available but does not have to be applied. **Cognitive Level:** Applying **Client Need:** Safety and Infection Control **Integrated Process:** Nursing Process: Implementation **Content Area:** Adult Health **Strategy:** The core issue of the question is priority concerns for a client experiencing a seizure. Use Maslow's hierarchy of needs, nursing knowledge, and the process of elimination to make a selection.

12 **Answer: 2** **Rationale:** Guillain-Barré syndrome is an acute demyelinating disorder that less commonly may present with initial weakness in the cranial nerves that progresses downward. Impairment of cranial nerves IX and X will affect swallowing. Guillain-Barré syndrome is not caused by obstructed blood flow to the brain. Parotitis could cause enlargement of parotid and salivary glands. Vitamin deficiencies could occur with any condition leading to malabsorption but are not an etiology for Guillain-Barré syndrome. **Cognitive Level:** Applying **Client Need:** Physiological Adaptation **Integrated Process:** Nursing Process: Implementation **Content Area:** Adult Health **Strategy:** The core issue of the question is the ability to explain the pathophysiology, underlying signs, and symptoms of Guillain-Barré syndrome. Use nursing knowledge and the process of elimination to make a selection.

13 **Answer: 1, 2, 4** **Rationale:** The client could be at risk for injury secondary to spasticity. Spasticity as well as age-related factors could lead to a feeding self-care deficit. At this age, a 1-year-old is beginning speech. This child will have trouble developing language because of the spasticity. Thought processes are difficult to evaluate in a 1-year-old. A 1-year-old client does not have the cognitive development to have acquired a self-image of the body. **Cognitive Level:** Analyzing **Client Need:** Physiological Adaptation **Integrated Process:** Nursing Process: Implementation **Content Area:** Child Health **Strategy:** The core issue of the question is the ability to determine appropriate nursing diagnoses for a client with cerebral palsy while taking into consideration growth and development. Use nursing knowledge and the process of elimination to make a selection.

14 **Answer: 4** **Rationale:** In most children, by age 6, the cranial suture lines have fused and the fontanelles are closed, so a bulging soft spot, expanding head size, and sunset eyes would not be common. An altered level of consciousness would be a symptom of shunt malfunction for the older child. **Cognitive Level:** Applying **Client Need:** Physiological Adaptation **Integrated Process:** Nursing Process: Evaluation **Content Area:** Child Health **Strategy:** The core issue of the question is knowledge of early signs of rising intracranial pressure, which is a sign of shunt malfunction. Use nursing knowledge and the process of elimination to make a selection.

15 **Answer: 2** **Rationale:** Drainage of cerebrospinal fluid (a clear fluid) from the ear is a symptom of basilar skull fracture. Children with linear skull fractures are often asymptomatic. Subdural and epidural hematomas present with signs of increasing intracranial pressure. **Cognitive Level:** Analyzing **Client Need:** Physiological Adaptation **Integrated Process:** Nursing Process: Data Collection **Content Area:** Child Health **Strategy:** The core issue of the question is the ability to correctly interpret signs of head injury. Use nursing knowledge and the process of elimination to make a selection.

16 **Answer: 3** **Rationale:** It is important for the nurse to learn about family members' perceptions of what is going on and their current needs. The best way to determine this is to encourage them to ask questions and express their feelings. While families may need education about seatbelts, this can occur at a later time. While families may benefit from community support services, this can occur after the child's likely outcome is better known. Timelines for visitation are appropriate but of less priority than open communication with the family. **Cognitive Level:** Analyzing **Client Need:** Psychosocial Integrity **Integrated Process:** Nursing Process: Planning **Content Area:** Child Health **Strategy:** The core issue of the question is the ability to determine priorities for the family of a critically ill child. Select the option that will most closely address the family's current issues and concerns.

17 **Answer: 1 or Grade 1** **Rationale:** In a grade 1 concussion, the client exhibits transient confusion with no loss of consciousness and a duration of abnormal mental status for less than 15 minutes. Grades 2 and 3 concussion consist of more severe neurological symptoms, with increasing levels of loss of consciousness and more significant abnormalities of mental status. **Cognitive Level:** Analyzing **Client Need:** Physiological Adaptation **Integrated Process:** Nursing Process: Evaluation **Content Area:** Adult Health **Strategy:** The core issue of the question is the ability to correctly interpret signs of head injury related to concussion. Use knowledge of the pathophysiology of concussions to determine an answer.

18 **Answer: 2** **Rationale:** All families deal with stressors, and the family of a child with a chronic health problem is no exception. Chronic sorrow is the emotional experience many families have in grieving the loss of the perfect child. This grief is intensified at times of developmental crisis

and traditional developmental milestones such as "first steps," when the parent is reminded of what the child will not be able to do. Planned hospitalizations are part of the treatment plan and are not as likely to evoke more prevalent feelings of chronic sorrow. Attaining a developmental milestone is not as likely to intensify chronic sorrow as it is a positive event for the child and family. The birth of an infant that is healthy is not likely to evoke more prevalent feelings of chronic sorrow. **Cognitive Level:** Applying **Client Need:** Psychosocial Integrity **Integrated Process:** Nursing Process: Planning **Content Area:** Child Health **Strategy:** Knowledge of the response of the parents to developmental crisis from inability of the child to achieve traditional milestones will aid in determining the correct answers.

19 **Answer: 3, 5 Rationale:** A priority concern preoperatively is maintaining the meningocele sac. A priority concern preoperatively is preventing infection. It is not a priority to measure head circumference daily. It is not a priority to use semi-Fowler's position. Prior to surgical repair of the meningocele, leaking cerebrospinal fluid usually reduces intracranial pressure. It is not a priority to monitor for irritability and vomiting (signs of increased intracranial pressure). **Cognitive Level:** Applying **Client Need:** Reduction of Risk Potential **Integrated Process:** Nursing Process: Implementation **Content Area:** Child Health **Strategy:** Note that three options related to increased intracranial pressure. Consider that the correct options deal with the spinal defect.

20 **Answer: 1 Rationale:** Research studies have shown a significant decrease in incidence of spina bifida in infants born to mothers who took folic acid supplements prior to pregnancy and during the first trimester. Spina bifida is not related to rubella or rubeola. No relationship has been seen between maternal age and the development of spina bifida, nor is there a genetic trait that can be linked to spina bifida. **Cognitive Level:** Applying **Client Need:** Physiological Adaptation **Integrated Process:** Teaching and Learning **Content Area:** Child Health **Strategy:** Each of the options describes known causative factors associated with a variety of conditions. Recall that folic acid has been associated with neural tubes defects to make the correct selection.

21 **Answer: 1, 5 Rationale:** Common side effects with antiepileptic medications include ataxia and rashes, which disappear when dosage is adjusted. Some drugs such as phenobarbital can adversely affect cognitive function, school performance, and behavior. Carbamazepine is considered relatively free of the sedative-like side effects but does have the side effects of blurred vision, diplopia, drowsiness, vertigo, headache, and, in rare cases, a rash (Stevens-Johnson syndrome). **Cognitive Level:** Applying **Client Need:** Pharmacological and Parenteral Therapies **Integrated Process:** Teaching and Learning **Content Area:** Pharmacology **Strategy:** This question requires specific knowledge about carbamazepine. Recall that many antiepileptic drugs have a side effect of drowsiness and dizziness. Eliminate hives because it would be an indication of an allergic reaction.

22 **Answer: 4 Rationale:** The best answer is to do further data collection of the child's abilities. At eight months, most infants can sit without support; however a remarkable piece of history for this child is her prematurity. Up until 2 years of age, it is important to remember to adjust for the weeks premature to have more realistic milestones for this individual child. Additional monitoring of motor skills is important to determine developmental progress while accounting for prematurity. Motor impairments associated with voluntary control are not usually apparent until after 2 to 4 months at the earliest so that motor dysfunction (and subsequent diagnosis of cerebral palsy) may not be confirmed until the second half of the first year. However, it is not the role of the nurse to make this statement. By using words such as "jump to conclusions" and "not fair," the nurse is engaging in communication that is not therapeutic and does not address the parents' concerns. The statement that there is "nothing to worry about" provides false reassurance and is not therapeutic. It is not unusual for the disorder to be overlooked in mildly affected infants until they exhibit a delay in some advanced motor skill such as walking. **Cognitive Level:** Applying **Client Need:** Health Promotion and Maintenance **Integrated Process:** Nursing Process: Data Collection **Content Area:** Child Health **Strategy:** Responses that deny the parents' concerns or tell them not to worry are usually not correct. In addition, for an option to be correct, every part of that option must be correct.

23 **Answer: 3 Rationale:** This position opens the intervertebral spaces and allows easier access to the spinal canal. This position does not decrease pain. All lumbar punctures are done below L4 (the level of the spinal nerves), so injury to the spinal cord is always avoided. The position does not help to restrain the child. **Cognitive Level:** Analyzing **Client Need:** Reduction of Risk Potential **Integrated Process:** Nursing Process: Implementation **Content Area:** Child Health **Strategy:** Visualize the procedure and positioning. Compare each option to the information in the stem looking for an option that fits with the question. To choose correctly, recall that the spinal vertebrae need to be separated to allow easier access by the spinal needle.

24 **Answer: 1, 3, 4 Rationale:** Viral meningitis does not require antibiotics. Treatment is aimed at reducing the symptoms. The child should be allowed to assume a position of comfort; the room should be kept dim and stimulation reduced. Seizures can occur, although the disease is usually self-limiting. Measuring the head circumference is of no benefit because the sutures are fused. **Cognitive Level:** Applying **Client Need:** Physiological Adaptation **Integrated Process:** Nursing Process: Implementation **Content Area:** Child Health **Strategy:** Viral infections do not require antibiotics. Consider the age of the child to determine if head measurement will provide any important data. Eliminate any options that would increase stimulation.

25 **Answer: 4 Rationale:** No eye opening, no verbal response, and no motor response are the lowest criteria on the scale. Confusion is a criterion applicable only for the older child and adult but is comparable to "irritable and cries" for the infant (which is a 4 out of 5 on the verbal response subscale). "Eyes open only to pain" is the next to the lowest level on the eye-opening category. **Cognitive Level:** Analyzing **Client Need:** Physiological Adaptation **Integrated Process:** Nursing Process: Data Collection **Content Area:** Child Health **Strategy:** Two options can be eliminated as these are normal findings. Consider the remaining two and determine which response shows the least brain functioning.

26 **Answer: 2 Rationale:** Brudzinski's sign indicates meningeal irritation. As the head and neck are flexed toward the chest, the legs flex at both the hips and the knees in response. Brudzinski's sign may be seen in the other options because of the meningeal irritation. **Cognitive Level:** Applying **Client Need:** Physiological Adaptation **Integrated Process:** Nursing Process: Implementation **Content Area:** Child Health **Strategy:** Consider how Brudzinski's sign is tested.

Key Terms to Review

agnosia p. 930
aphasia p. 920
apraxia p. 930
autonomic hyperreflexia p. 927
bradykinesia p. 932
Broca's area p. 916
Brudzinski's sign p. 920
coma p. 921
Cushing's triad p. 923
dysarthria p. 920
dysphagia p. 930
epidural hematoma p. 925
hemianopsia p. 930
intracranial pressure (ICP) p. 923
intrathecal p. 937
Kernig's sign p. 920
level of consciousness (LOC) p. 918
meninges p. 917
myelin p. 928
neurogenic p. 937
nuchal rigidity p. 940
opisthotonus p. 940
paraplegia p. 927
photophobia p. 940
spasticity p. 933
subdural hematoma p. 925
tetraplegia p. 927
tonic-clonic p. 931
Wernicke's area p. 916

References

Ball, J., Bindler, R., & Cowen, K. (2010). *Child health nursing: Partnering with children and families* (2nd ed.). Upper Saddle River, NJ: Pearson Education.

Berman, A., & Snyder, S. (2012). *Kozier & Erb's fundamentals of nursing: Concepts, process, and practice* (9th ed.). Upper Saddle River, NJ: Pearson Education, Inc.

Ignatavicius, D., & Workman, L. (2010). *Medical-surgical nursing: Critical thinking for collaborative care* (6th ed.). Philadelphia: Saunders.

Kee, J. (2010). *Laboratory and diagnostic tests with nursing implications* (8th ed.). Upper Saddle River, NJ: Pearson Education.

LeMone, P., Burke, K., & Bauldoff, G. (2011). *Medical surgical nursing: Critical thinking in patient care* (5th ed.). Upper Saddle River, NJ: Pearson Education.

Smith, S., Duell, D., & Martin, B. (2012). *Clinical nursing skills: Basic to advanced skills* (8th ed.). Upper Saddle River, NJ: Pearson Education.

Test Yourself

Are you ready for the NCLEX-PN® or course exams? Use the practice tests on the companion website to check.

54 Renal or Genitourinary Disorders

In this chapter

Cross Reference

Other chapters relevant to this content area are

Meeting Nutritional Needs	Chapter 25
Renal Medications	Chapter 36
Common Laboratory Tests	Chapter 42
Common Diagnostic Tests and Procedures	Chapter 43

I. OVERVIEW OF ANATOMY AND PHYSIOLOGY OF RENAL AND URINARY SYSTEMS

A. Renal structures

1. Kidneys: bean-shaped organs located on either side of spinal column behind peritoneal cavity; regulate fluid and acid–base balance
2. Adrenal glands: located atop each kidney; influence blood pressure (BP) and sodium (Na^+) and water retention
3. Renal cortex: outer region of kidneys; contains blood-filtering mechanisms
4. Renal medulla: middle region of kidneys; contains renal pyramids

5. Renal pyramids: triangular wedges containing tubular structures
   a. Apex: tapered section of each pyramid; empties into calyx (calyces)
   b. Calyces: channel urine from renal pyramids to renal pelvis
6. Renal pelvis: expansion of upper end of ureters, formed as calyces join together
7. **Nephron**: basic functional unit of kidneys; selectively secretes and reabsorbs ions; perform mechanical filtration of fluid, wastes, electrolytes, acids, and bases; contains a **glomerulus** surrounded by Bowman's capsule

B. Function of kidneys

1. Nephrons filter waste products as well as needed materials, such as electrolytes, from blood; necessary substances are returned to blood through reabsorption
2. Filtration: first step in blood processing; water and solutes move from plasma in glomerulus into Bowman's capsule; depends on pressure gradient between blood in glomeruli and filtrate in Bowman's capsule
3. Reabsorption: second step in urine formation; molecules move from tubules into blood through tubule cells; active and passive transport mechanisms are used in all parts of renal tubules
   a. Proximal tubules: reabsorb sodium (Na^+) and other major ions
   b. Loop of Henle: reabsorbs through countercurrent mechanism (passive); contents flow in opposite directions
   c. Distal tubules: reabsorb Na^+ in smaller amounts than proximal tubules
   d. Collecting ducts: prevent water from leaving filtrate
4. Tubular secretion: movement of substances out of blood into tubular fluid; tubules secrete certain substances in addition to performing reabsorption
5. Regulation of urine volume: hormones play a central part in urine regulation
6. Osmolality: osmotic pressure of a solution expressed as a number of osmols of pressure per kg of water; active transport and reabsorption mechanisms are based on osmolality of solutions

C. Renal hormones and enzymes (see Table 54–1)

D. Urinary excretion

1. Ureters: extend from renal pelvis of kidney to urinary bladder; conduct urine
2. Bladder: elastic sac located behind symphysis pubis; stores and excretes urine
3. Urethra: tube that carries urine from bladder to exterior of body
4. Urinary meatus: exterior opening of urethra

Table 54–1 Functions of Renal Hormones and Enzymes

Hormone or Enzyme	Function
Antidiuretic hormone (ADH)	Regulates urine volume by acting in distal tubule and collecting ducts to increase water reabsorption and urine concentration
Atrial natriuretic hormone (ANH)	Secreted by muscle fibers in atria of heart; promotes sodium (Na^+) loss via urine
Aldosterone	Secreted by adrenal cortex; increases Na^+ absorption in distal and collecting tubules and controls potassium (K^+) secretion, leading to osmotic imbalance that causes reabsorption of water; works in conjunction with ADH Increased serum K^+ levels lead to increased aldosterone secretion Increased aldosterone secretion increases Na^+ and water retention and depresses formation of renin
Renin	Enzyme secreted by kidneys; helps regulate Na^+ retention and therefore BP and fluid volume Renin-angiotensin system converts angiotensinogen to angiotensin I in liver Angiotensin I forms angiotensin II in lungs, which is a vasoconstrictor that stimulates adrenal cortex to produce aldosterone
Erythropoietin	Hormone produced by kidneys in response to low oxygen (O_2) levels in arterial blood; travels to bone marrow and stimulates increased red blood cell (RBC) production

5. Urination: an involuntary or voluntary reflex allowing urine to leave body
   a. Micturition reflex: parasympathetic response that stimulates relaxation and contraction of external sphincter, allowing urine to pass
   b. Internal sphincter muscle: helps control urine passage into urethra; relaxes in response to parasympathetic nerve fibers in bladder wall
   c. External sphincter muscle: voluntary muscle that allows urine to pass into urethra; controlled by micturition reflex

NCLEX®

6. Characteristics of normal urine
   a. Color: clear, pale amber
   b. Consistency: 95% water with many dissolved substances
   c. Output: 1000–2000 mL per 24-hour period; kidneys produce a minimum of 30 mL/hour (0.5 mg/kg/hr) under normal circumstances
   d. Specific gravity: commonly 1.015–1.025 (range 1.010–1.030)
   e. Odor: faint ammonia

E. Renal system differences between child and adult

1. Fluid is more important to body chemistry of infants and small children because it constitutes a larger fraction of total body weight
2. During first 2 years of life, kidneys are less efficient at regulating electrolyte and acid–base balance; infants are more prone to fluid volume excess and dehydration
3. Bladder capacity increases from 20–50 mL at birth to 700 mL in adulthood
4. Innervation of "stretch" receptors in bladder wall, which initiates urination and control of bladder sphincters (does not occur before age 2); children under 2 cannot maintain bladder control
5. Urethra is shorter in children than in adults and may contribute to frequency of urinary tract infections (UTIs) in children
6. Kidneys are more susceptible to trauma in children because they do not have as much fat padding

II. DIAGNOSTIC TESTS AND DATA COLLECTION

A. Physical examination

1. Appearance of meatus: normal position and lack of redness, swelling
2. Voiding pattern: frequency, amount, hesitancy, urgency, dysuria

B. Urine studies

1. Urinalysis: obtained for dipstick results, microscopic examination, or culture; refer to Chapter 42 for normal results and Table 54–2 for significance of color changes
2. Clean-catch specimen: urine specimen collected in a clean specimen container after cleaning urinary meatus and surrounding tissue; in infants and toddlers, catheterization may be performed; parental assistance is needed for school-age, toilet-trained children, and adolescents obtain own specimens after careful instruction
3. Sterile urine specimen: obtained by urinary catheterization only
4. Urine culture: checks urine for bacteria; urine is normally sterile

Table 54–2 Interpreting Changes in Urine Color

Color	Possible Meaning
Pale yellow	Normal
Yellow	Concentrated urine
Amber	Bile in urine
Orange	Alkaline or concentrated urine
Red-orange	Acidic urine, medication effect
Red	Blood, menses
Pink	Dilute blood
Burgundy	Laxatives
Tea	Melanin, hematuria
Dark gray	Medications, dyes
Blue	Dyes, medications

5. Twenty-four-hour urine specimen: urine is collected over 24 hours for these substances:
   a. **Creatinine**: nitrogenous waste product excreted by muscle tissue; normally found in urine (normal = 15–25 mg/kg in 24 hours)
   b. Creatinine clearance: test to measure how well the kidneys remove creatinine from blood (male = 95–135 mL/min; female = 85–125 mL/min)
   c. Protein: less than 150 mg/24 hours
   d. Urea nitrogen: end product of protein metabolism (normal 6–17 grams/24 hours)
6. Urine osmolality: osmotic pressure (concentration) of urine; average is 500–800 mOsm/kg water, with an extreme range of 50–1400 mOsm/kg water

C. **Renal scan**: intravenous (IV) radioactive substance (radionuclide) is injected, and then observed passing through kidneys; evaluates renal structures and blood flow, and nephron and collecting system function

D. **Radiographic studies (see also Chapter 43)**
1. Kidney-ureter-bladder (KUB) radiography: shows kidney size, position, and structure as well as ureters and bladder; provides limited diagnostic information
2. Renal angiography: detects abnormalities such as cysts, renal artery stenosis, and renal infarction
3. Renal venography: detects renal vein thrombosis
4. Retrograde cystography: contrast medium instilled into bladder via a catheter, followed by x-ray examination; several films are taken and dye is then drained via catheter; a final picture is taken when bladder is emptied; helps diagnose ruptured or neurogenic bladder and other conditions
5. Voiding cystourethrography: same process as a cystogram except when bladder is filled with contrast dye, urethral catheter is removed; client is allowed to void when urge is felt; films are taken during bladder filling, during **micturition** (voiding) and after voiding

E. **Computerized tomography (CT) scan**: identifies masses and other lesions; contrast medium may be injected

F. **Magnetic resonance imaging (MRI)**: produces three-dimensional images of renal tissue

G. **Ultrasonography**: evaluates kidney size, shape, and position

H. **Blood studies**
1. *Blood urea nitrogen (BUN)*: measures nitrogenous urea in blood from protein metabolism; insufficient excretion causes levels to rise and may indicate renal disorders; also rises with dehydration and intake of high-protein diet or other conditions in which excess protein is metabolized
   a. Normal: 8–25 mg/dL
   b. BUN levels best evaluated in conjunction with serum creatinine levels
2. Serum creatinine: a nitrogenous waste in blood resulting from muscle metabolism of creatine; creatinine levels reflect glomerular filtration rate
   a. Measures renal damage more reliably than BUN, because severe renal damage is single cause of significant elevation
   b. Normal: 0.6–1.5 mg/dL for adult males; 0.6–1.1 mg/dL for adult females

I. ***Intravenous pyelography (IVP)***: one or more x-rays of renal pelvis and ureters after injection of a contrast medium; special pre-procedure care may be necessary

J. **Cystoscopy or cystourethroscopy**: insertion of a cystoscope with a fiberoptic light source and telescopic lens into urethra for biopsy of bladder and prostate, lesion resection, calculi collection, or passage of catheter to renal pelvis

K. **Percutaneous renal biopsy**: client is positioned on abdomen while needle is inserted into kidney to remove tissue; x-ray may be used to guide needle; reveals renal disease, malignant tumors, and other conditions; risks include bleeding, hematoma, arteriovenous fistula, and infection

III. COMMON NURSING TECHNIQUES AND PROCEDURES

A. **Urinary catheterization: introduction of a catheter into urinary bladder**
1. Indwelling urinary catheter: a retention (Foley) catheter with balloon is inserted and remains in place; see Box 54–1
2. Intermittent catheterization: used for clients with neurogenic bladder dysfunction; may be done by nurse or at home by client after instruction on procedure (Box 54–2)

B. **Urine collection**
1. Twenty-four-hour urine collection
   a. Obtain specimen container with preservative from laboratory
   b. Provide clean receptacle to collect urine (bedpan, urinal, commode, or collection device on toilet) unless client already has an indwelling urinary catheter
   c. Post signs in client's room, chart, and bathroom alerting staff to save urine
   d. *NCLEX®* Have client void and discard first urine at beginning of collection period; if indwelling catheter used, empty collection bag at start time and discard

Box 54–1

Insertion of an Indwelling Urinary Catheter

- Explain procedure to client and ensure privacy.
- *Female*: assist client to supine position with knees flexed and thighs externally rotated; drape client.
- Wearing disposable gloves, cleanse perineal area; remove gloves.
- Prepare equipment and sterile field; don sterile gloves; drape client with sterile drape.
- Lubricate sterile cotton balls with antiseptic solution (specific to agency policy) and lubricate insertion tip of catheter with water-soluble jelly.
- Clean meatus with antiseptic (check agency policy).
- Use nondominant hand to separate labia minor and expose urinary meatus; check meatus for swelling, discharge, or redness.
- Grasp catheter near insertion end with sterile, gloved hand; gently insert catheter into meatus and advance catheter until urine flows; do not use forceful pressure; ask client to take deep breaths to relax external sphincter.
- Advance catheter farther into bladder (1–2 inches) and inflate balloon by injecting contents of prefilled syringe.
- Apply slight tension by pulling back on catheter until resistance is felt to confirm balloon placement in bladder.
- Anchor catheter to client's thigh with nonallergic tape and secure drainage bag to bed frame below level of bladder.
- *Male*: use same positioning except knees do not need to be flexed
- Wearing disposable gloves, wash penis and dry it well.
- Follow catheter preparatory steps as described above.
- Grasp insertion end of catheter with sterile, gloved hand; lift penis to 90-degree angle with body and exert slight traction.
- Insert catheter steadily about 20 cm (8 inches) until urine begins to flow; ask client to take deep breaths to relax external sphincter; rotate catheter during insertion if slight resistance is met because of curvature of urethra.
- Advance catheter farther into bladder (1 to 2 inches) and inflate balloon by injecting contents of prefilled syringe; secure as described above.

e. During collection period, save all urine in container; place container on ice or refrigerate as indicated; don't contaminate urine with bathroom tissue or feces

NCLEX®

f. Instruct client to empty bladder at end of collection period and save this urine

g. Send collected urine to laboratory with completed requisition

h. Document collection of specimen, time started and completed, and any observations

2. Clean catch (midstream)

a. Ask client to wash genital and perineal area with soap and water from front to back

b. Instruct to clean meatus with antiseptic towelettes

c. Female clients: use three towelettes, clean perineal area from front to back; use each towelette only once

d. Male clients: clean meatus with circular motion and distal portion of penis; use each towelette only once

e. For client who needs assistance: nurse may don gloves, clean perineal area, assist client to a comfortable position, and open clean-catch kit

f. Instruct client to begin voiding, then place specimen container in stream of urine; collect 30 to 60 mL of urine

g. Cap container, touching only outside

h. Label container, place in biohazard bag with requisition, and immediately send to laboratory

i. Document pertinent data, such as difficulty voiding, strong odor to urine, or sediment

C. ***Peritoneal dialysis***: removes toxins from blood of client with acute or chronic renal failure; uses peritoneal membrane as semipermeable dialyzing membrane (see Figure 54–1)

Box 54–2

Client Instructions for Intermittent Urinary Self-Catheterization

- Catheterize as often as needed; may be every 2–3 hours at first, then every 4–6 hours.
- Encourage client to void before procedure if appropriate; use catheter to obtain residual urine if amount voided is less than 100 mL.
- Assemble all supplies and use good lighting.
- Wash hands.
- Clean urinary meatus with towelette or soapy washcloth, then rinse and dry; female clients should clean perineum from front to back.
- Assume comfortable position, such as standing with one foot elevated, semireclining in bed, or sitting on chair or toilet.
- Apply lubricant to catheter tip.
- *Female*: locate meatus using a mirror or touch; separate labia with dominant hand; direct catheter through meatus, then forward and upward.
- *Male*: hold penis with slight upward tension to 90-degree angle and insert catheter.
- Hold catheter in place until all urine is drained, then withdraw slowly.
- Wash catheter with soap and water; store in clean container.
- Notify care provider of cloudy urine, sediment, bleeding, fever, or difficulty passing catheter.
- Drink at least 2000–2500 mL of fluid daily; cranberry and prune juices help to acidify urine to possibly reduce bacterial growth in bladder.

1. Hypertonic dialyzing solution (dialysate) is instilled through a catheter in peritoneal cavity
2. Excess electrolytes and uremic toxins move by diffusion across peritoneal membrane into dialysate; excess water also moves into solution by osmosis
3. Dialysate is drained after appropriate dwelling time
4. Procedure is performed manually or using a cycler machine; client may also perform continuous ambulatory peritoneal dialysis (CAPD)
5. NCLEX® Possible complications
    a. Peritonitis from bacteria entering peritoneal cavity (use surgical aseptic technique when handling catheter or tubing); is critical to prevent peritonitis because it could result in client having to change therapy to **hemodialysis** (removal of wastes in blood)
    b. Catheter obstruction from clots or kinking (keep all lines unobstructed; add heparin to dialysate per protocol)
    c. Insufficient outflow (reposition client as needed to bring fluid into contact with catheter; allow to ambulate if condition allows)
    d. Hypotension and hypovolemia from excess fluid removal (carefully monitor I&O records; report accordingly)
    e. Hyperglycemia (from glucose in dialysate; monitor diabetic clients closely; do not allow fluid to dwell longer than ordered)
6. NCLEX® Peritoneal dialysis procedure (see Box 54–3, p. 957)

D. Urinary diversion stoma care

1. NCLEX® Collection device should fit snugly around stoma; allow no more than ⅛-inch margin of skin between stoma and faceplate
2. Stoma should appear light or bright red; suspect a problem if it is deep red or bluish in color
3. NCLEX® Check peristomal skin for breakdown; main cause of irritation is urine leakage; change device and cleanse skin if leakage occurs
    a. Cleanse area with warm water and pat dry; apply light coating of karaya powder and thin layer of protective dressing
    b. Notify physician if severe skin excoriation occurs
4. Monitor I&O; note changes in urine color, odor, or clarity

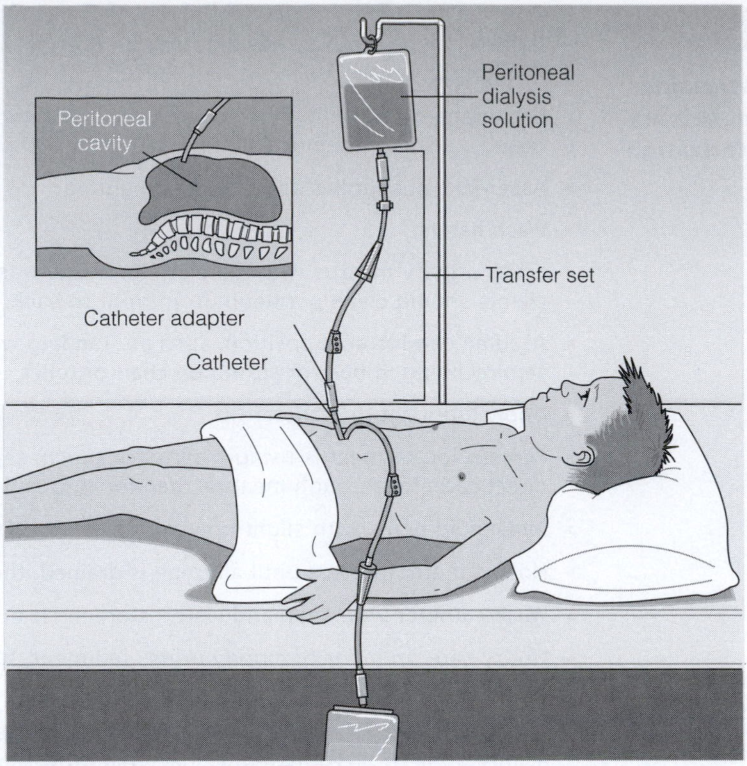

Figure 54–1
Peritoneal dialysis.

NCLEX® 5. Home care by client
   a. Expect stoma shrinkage within 8 weeks after surgery; may require smaller pouch opening
   b. Encourage client to change appliance as needed in early morning when urine production is less because of no fluid intake during sleep
   c. Appliance is often a one-piece unit (faceplate and collection bag) and must be emptied regularly and changed according to product directions
   d. Instruct client to report fever, chills, flank pain, abdominal pain, and pus in urine (**pyuria**) or blood in urine (**hematuria**)
   e. Refer client to support group, such as United Ostomy Association

E. **Care of an arteriovenous (AV) fistula**
1. An AV fistula provides vascular access to a vein and an artery for hemodialysis; most common sites are radial or brachial artery and cephalic vein
NCLEX® 2. Monitor circulation at access site by auscultating for bruits and palpating for thrills; lack of bruit may indicate blood clot and requires immediate surgical intervention
NCLEX® 3. Avoid using accessed arm for other procedures, such as IV insertion, BP monitoring, or venipuncture
4. Monitor site for bleeding after completion of hemodialysis
5. Home care instructions for client
   a. Keep fistula area clean and dry
   b. Notify health care provider of pain, swelling, redness, or drainage in accessed arm
   c. Exercise is beneficial and helps stimulate vein enlargement
   NCLEX® d. Don't allow any treatments or procedures on accessed arm
   NCLEX® e. Avoid excessive pressure to arm; don't sleep on it, wear constrictive clothing or jewelry, or lift heavy objects
   f. Avoid showering, bathing, or swimming for several hours after dialysis

F. **Hemodialysis**: removes wastes from body by filtering client's blood using a machine
1. Nurses who have undergone specialized instruction and training perform hemodialysis
NCLEX® 2. Before procedure, weigh client and take vital signs (VS); check BP in lying and standing positions (orthostatic blood pressures); check for routine medications that should be withheld until dialysis is completed (i.e., antihypertensives that could lower BP, medications that would be dialyzed out of client's system, or once-daily medications that can be given post-dialysis)
NCLEX® 3. Wear protective eyewear, gown, and gloves for protection during hemodialysis procedure

Box 54-3

Peritoneal Dialysis Procedure

- Explain procedure and check vital signs and weight.
- Have client urinate, if able, to avoid bladder puncture or discomfort; perform catheterization if client is unable to void.
- Warm dialysate to body temperature in a warmer.
- Use 1.5%, 2.5%, or 4.25% dextrose solution, usually with heparin added to prevent catheter clotting; dialysate should be clear and colorless; add prescribed medication as ordered.
- Put on surgical mask and prepare dialysis administration set, maintaining strict sterile technique at all times.
- Place drainage bag below client and connect outflow tubing.
- Connect dialysis infusion line to dialysate bags and hang on IV pole.
- Place client in supine position, prime tubing with solution, close clamps, and connect infusion line to abdominal catheter.
- Test catheter by instilling 500 mL of dialysate into peritoneal cavity; clamp tubing; unclamp outflow line and drain fluid into collection bag; if outflow is brisk, then catheter is patent.
- Unclamp infusion lines and infuse prescribed amount of dialysate; close clamps when bag is empty.
- Allow solution to dwell for prescribed time (usually up to 4 hours).
- Open outflow clamps and allow solution to drain.
- Wear protective eyewear when draining or handling outflow solution.
- Repeat cycle for prescribed number of times; when completed, clamp peritoneal catheter and disconnect inflow line while wearing sterile gloves.
- Apply sterile dressing to catheter site.
- During procedure, monitor vital signs every 10 minutes until stable, then every 2 to 4 hours.
- Observe for signs of peritonitis: fever; persistent abdominal pain and cramping; slow or cloudy dialysate drainage; swelling, redness, or tenderness around catheter; increased WBC count.
- Check outflow tubing periodically for clots or kinks; have client change position to increase flow.
- Clients lose protein during peritoneal dialysis and require fewer or no dietary restrictions of protein.
- Calculate fluid balance at end of each exchange (with manual dialysis), or at end of each session, or every 8 hours, depending on protocol; include oral and IV intake, urine output, and wound drainage in calculations.

4. Dialysis is continued usually for 3 to 4 hours, depending on client's status; monitor partial thromboplastin time (PTT) or other standard laboratory studies as ordered according to protocol (heparin is used as an anticoagulant during procedure)
5. At end of treatment, obtain blood samples as ordered, return blood remaining in dialyzer to client, and remove needles from vascular access device
6. Monitor access device for bleeding and maintain pressure on site as needed
7. *NCLEX®* Early in course of hemodialysis, monitor for and report disequilibrium syndrome, a condition in which cerebral edema forms from less rapid excretion of wastes behind blood–brain barrier, and subsequent uptake of fluid by brain cells
    a. Monitor client for headache, mental confusion, decreasing LOC, nausea, vomiting, twitching, and possible seizure activity
    b. Obtain necessary orders for antiepileptic medication
    c. Prevent occurrence by dialyzing for shorter times or at reduced blood flow rates early in therapy

IV. NURSING MANAGEMENT OF CLIENT HAVING RENAL OR BLADDER SURGERY

A. ***Lithotripsy***: also called extracorporeal shock-wave lithotripsy (ESWL); uses high-energy shock waves to break up calculi, restoring normal passage of urine

1. Perform preoperative teaching about procedure and postoperative course and care
   - **a.** Treatment takes 30 minutes to 1 hour
   - **b.** Client will receive a general or epidural anesthetic
2. Postprocedure care
   - **a.** Perform baseline data collection and check VS following agency policy
   - **b.** Maintain patency of indwelling urinary catheter and monitor I&O
   - NCLEX® **c.** Strain urine for calculi fragments and send these to laboratory for analysis
   - **d.** Slight hematuria is common, but report persistent bleeding
   - **e.** Encourage ambulation to aid passage of calculi fragments
   - NCLEX® **f.** Increase fluid intake as ordered to aid passage of calculi fragments
   - **g.** Give analgesics as needed; severe pain may indicate presence of new calculi—report such findings immediately
3. NCLEX® Home care instructions for client
   - **a.** Drink 3–4 L of fluid daily up to 1 month after treatment
   - **b.** Strain urine during first week and save any calculi fragments; bring these to first follow-up visit with physician
   - **c.** Expect blood-tinged urine, mild GI upset, and pain in treated side as calculi fragments pass; bruising on affected side will disappear
   - **d.** Report severe pain, persistent blood in urine, inability to void, fever and chills, or nausea and vomiting
   - **e.** Review prescribed medications or dietary regimen

B. **Ureterolithotomy, pyelolithotomy, nephrolithotomy**: involve making an incision into ureter, renal pelvis, or renal calyx to remove urinary calculi

1. Preoperative period
   - **a.** Explain procedure to client and postoperative care, including presence of a urinary catheter
   - **b.** Administer pre-anesthetic medications as ordered
2. NCLEX® Postoperative period
   - **a.** Perform baseline and ongoing postoperative data collection (VS, LOC, status of dressing)
   - **b.** Monitor urine output (UO) for amount, color, and clarity; urine may be bright red initially, but bleeding should diminish; cloudy urine may indicate infection
   - **c.** Maintain placement and patency of urinary catheters; irrigate gently as ordered
   - **d.** Monitor for pain and administer analgesics as needed
   - **e.** Increase client's fluid intake, as ordered, to aid passage of calculi fragments
   - **f.** Strain urine for calculi fragments and send them to laboratory for analysis
3. Home care for client
   - **a.** Follow agency policy for home incision care
   - NCLEX® **b.** Drink 3–4 liters of fluid daily up to a month after treatment
   - **c.** Report bloody, cloudy, or foul-smelling urine
   - **d.** Report inability to void, fever, chills, redness, swelling, or purulent drainage from incision
   - **e.** Strain urine during first week and save any calculi fragments; bring them to first follow-up visit with surgeon
   - **f.** Avoid strenuous exercise, sexual activity, heavy lifting, or straining until advised otherwise by surgeon
   - **g.** Mild activity aids passage of any retained calculi fragments
   - **h.** Review prescribed medications, dietary regimen, and explain catheter care if client is discharged with indwelling catheter

C. **Cystectomy with urinary diversion**

1. Complete radical **cystectomy** involves removal of bladder and adjacent muscles and tissues
   - **a.** In men, prostate gland and seminal vesicles are removed, which results in impotence
   - **b.** In women, uterus, Fallopian tubes, and ovaries are removed, resulting in sterility
   - **c.** A urinary diversion is created to provide for urine collection and drainage
2. **Urinary diversion**: a procedure that provides an alternative route for urine excretion when normal channels are damaged or defective
   - **a.** Ileal conduit: also called ileal loop; reroutes urine from kidneys to pouch in abdominal wall created from a segment of the ileum; urine drains continuously from the ileal pouch

b. Nephrostomy: drains urine through a catheter placed directly into kidney; used when a ureter is blocked or damaged; may be temporary

3. Preoperative period
   a. Reduce anxiety through preoperative teaching about procedure and postoperative course and care; client may awaken with nasogastric tube, IV, indwelling urinary catheter, Penrose drain, or other drains
   b. Note client's support systems and ability to care for self after surgery
   c. Address concerns about body image changes and loss of sexual or reproductive function
   NCLEX® d. Begin bowel preparations about 4 days prior to surgery
   e. Administer enema on night before surgery to clear fecal matter from bowel as prescribed or per protocol
   NCLEX® f. Administer antibiotics (usually erythromycin and neomycin) for 24 hours before surgery, as prescribed
   g. Administer preanesthetic medications as prescribed
4. Postoperative period
   a. Perform baseline and ongoing postoperative data collection (VS, LOC, status of dressing, patency of urinary catheter)
   NCLEX® b. Monitor amount and character of UO every hour; report output less than 30 mL/hour; irrigate catheter as ordered
   c. Observe for signs of hypovolemic shock, such as pallor, hypotension, and tachycardia
   NCLEX® d. Inspect stoma and incision for bleeding and observe urine for frank bleeding and clots; expect slight hematuria for several days
   e. Observe incision for signs of infection (redness and purulent drainage); change dressing per agency policy or surgeon's order
   f. Encourage frequent position changes, coughing and deep breathing, and early ambulation if appropriate
   g. Monitor respiratory status frequently
   h. Administer prescribed analgesic and antispasmodic medications as needed
5. Home care instructions for clients
   a. Report signs of infection, including fever, chills, cloudy urine, purulent drainage, or redness of incision
   b. Report persistent blood in urine, inability to void, or painful urination
   c. Reinforce stoma care and provide supplies as needed; refer client to support organization such as the United Ostomy Association
   d. Weakness, incisional pain, and fatigue may persist for several weeks

D. **Ureteral stent**: catheter used to maintain patency and promote healing of ureters; may be temporary after surgery or used for long periods in clients with a damaged ureter
1. Stent is positioned during surgery or cystoscopy
2. Nursing care
   a. If stent has been brought to surface, secure it and maintain its position
   b. Monitor UO, including color, consistency, and odor
   c. Observe for signs of infection, obstruction, or bleeding, including fever, tachycardia, cloudy urine, pain, hematuria
   d. Maintain fluid intake
   e. If stent is semipermanent, instruct client and family in its care

E. ***Nephrectomy***: removal of kidney
1. Preoperative period
   a. Reduce anxiety through preoperative teaching about procedure and postoperative course and care; client may awaken with nasogastric tube, IV, indwelling urinary catheter, Penrose drain, or other drains
   b. Note client's support systems and ability to care for self after surgery
   c. Administer preanesthetic medications as ordered
   d. Measure baseline urinary status
2. Postoperative period
   a. Perform baseline and ongoing postoperative data collection (VS, LOC, status of dressing, patency of urinary catheter)
   NCLEX® b. Monitor client's fluid and electrolyte status, and urine specific gravity; monitor hemoglobin and hematocrit because significant amount of blood is lost during nephrectomy
   NCLEX® c. Monitor amount and character of UO hourly; report UO less than 30 mL/hour; irrigate catheter as ordered

d. Observe for signs of urinary infection: fever, redness at surgical site, cloudy urine, or discharge
e. Determine patency of urinary or wound drainage tubes; reinforce or change dressing as needed

NCLEX® f. Monitor respiratory status frequently; encourage frequent position changes, coughing and deep breathing, and early ambulation if appropriate to reduce the risk of respiratory complications caused by pain from high abdominal/flank incision
g. Administer analgesic medications as needed

F. Renal transplantation

1. Preoperative period
   a. Reduce anxiety by teaching about procedure and postoperative course and care; encourage client to express feelings and ask questions
   b. Note support systems and ability to care for self after surgery and follow medical regime
   NCLEX® c. Reinforce that rejection of donated organ is major obstacle in transplantation (see Table 54–3); reassure client that rejection usually isn't life-threatening and client can resume dialysis if needed
   d. Begin administering immunosuppressant drugs; discuss purpose and possible adverse effects with client; monitor for increased BP and signs of anaphylaxis
   e. Plan for client to undergo dialysis on day before surgery, a cleansing enema, and many laboratory tests
2. Postoperative period
   a. Perform baseline and ongoing postoperative data collection (VS, LOC, status of dressing)
   b. Encourage frequent position changes, coughing and deep breathing, and early ambulation if appropriate
   NCLEX® c. Use special infection control measures: strict aseptic technique when changing dressings or performing catheter care; limit client's contact with staff and visitors; wear a surgical mask when in client's room; monitor WBC count and notify physician of significant drop
   NCLEX® d. Observe for signs of tissue rejection: fever; redness, tenderness, and swelling at surgical site; elevated WBC count; decreased UO with increased **proteinuria** (protein in urine); sudden weight gain; hypertension; elevated BUN and creatinine
   e. Provide analgesic medications as needed; pain should decrease after 24 hours
   f. Monitor UO closely; report output less than 100 mL/hour; decreased urine may indicate thrombus formation at renal artery anastomosis site
   g. Expect blood-tinged urine for several days; irrigate catheter as ordered, using strict aseptic technique
   NCLEX® h. With a living donor transplant, urine flow should begin immediately after revascularization and connection of ureter to client's bladder; with a cadaver transplant, expect **anuria** (urine output less than 100 mL in 24 hrs) for 2 days to 2 weeks, client will need dialysis during this period
   i. Monitor daily renal function tests: creatinine clearance, and BUN; urine creatinine, electrolytes, urine pH, and specific gravity

Table 54–3 Renal Transplant Rejection

Description	Manifestations	Management
Hyperacute		
Occurs within hours of surgery; results from antibody reaction to donor antigens; occurs rarely now because of better histocompatibility assessments	Urine output stops; examination of kidney shows a blue, flaccid appearance	Transplanted kidney must be removed; client must resume hemodialysis until (possibly) another kidney is available
Acute		
Occurs within days to months after surgery; body mounts an immune system defense against tissue in donor organ	Urine output drops sharply and BUN and creatinine rise; possible fever, graft tenderness, swelling	Increased dosage of immunosuppressant drugs, including steroids and monoclonal antibodies
Chronic		
Occurs from months to years after surgery; etiology is unclear but may involve immune response to donor tissue	More gradual decline in kidney function, including urine output, BUN, and creatinine; proteinuria may occur	No specific treatment; client must resume hemodialysis caused by loss of graft until or unless another donor kidney is transplanted

j. Observe for signs of hyperkalemia (weakness, irregular pulse, tall peaked T-waves on cardiac rhythm strip)
k. Weigh client daily; rapid weight gain may indicate fluid retention

3. Home care for client
   a. Carefully measure and record I&O; notify physician if UO falls below 600 mL for any 24-hour period
   b. Instruct client how to collect 24-hour urine samples
   NCLEX® c. Advise client to weigh self at least twice weekly
   d. Drink at least 1–2 liters of fluid daily unless advised otherwise
   NCLEX® e. Report signs of rejection: redness, warmth, tenderness, or swelling over kidney; fever; decreased UO; elevated BP (obtain and use home BP measuring device)
   NCLEX® f. Avoid crowds and persons with known infections for 3 months after surgery
   g. Practice regular, moderate exercise, but avoid heavy lifting or contact sports for at least 3 months; use shoulder but not lap-style seat belts
   h. Wait at least 6 weeks before engaging in sexual activity

V. URINARY CALCULI

A. Overview

1. Presence of stones in urinary tract
2. Stones form when chemicals and other elements in urine become concentrated and form crystals; usually related to metabolic or dietary causes
3. Types of stones: calcium phosphate and/or oxalate (most common type), struvite, uric acid, and cystine (least common type)
4. Most stones form in kidneys, but bladder stones are common in clients with indwelling urinary catheters or those unable to empty bladder completely (see Figure 54–2)
5. Stones may be single or multiple and vary in size; large calculi cause pressure necrosis and can also lead to obstruction
6. NCLEX® Risk factors
   a. Dehydration: concentrates calculus-forming substances
   b. Infection: damaged tissue and changing pH provide an environment for calculi to develop; bacteria may form nucleus of calculi
   c. Obstruction: urine stasis allows solid materials to collect; also promotes infection, which worsens obstruction
   d. Metabolic factors: hypoparathyroidism, renal tubular acidosis, elevated uric acid levels, defective oxalate metabolism, and excessive vitamin D or calcium intake

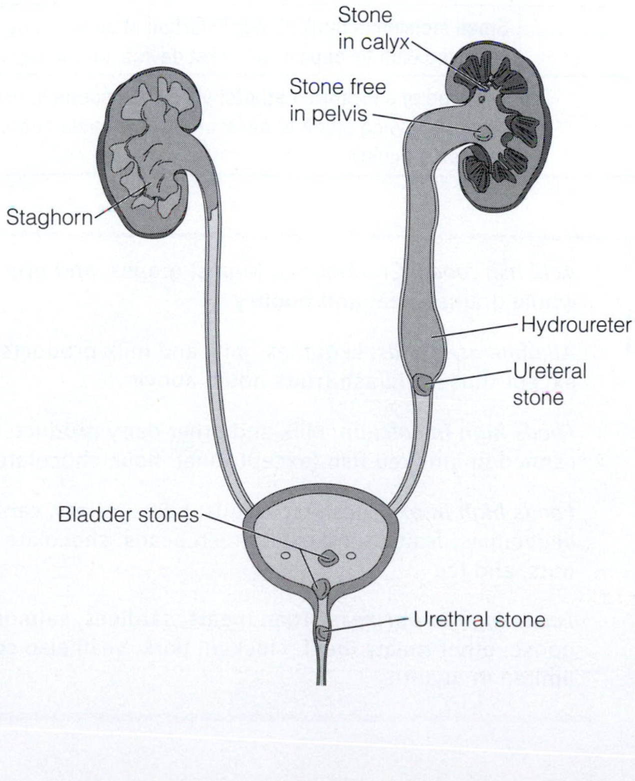

Figure 54–2

Development and location of calculi within kidneys and urinary tract.

B. Nursing data collection

1. Severe pain is most common symptom
2. NCLEX® Renal calculi cause flank pain on side of affected kidney; may radiate to groin, called renal colic
3. NCLEX® Fluctuates in intensity and may be severe; nausea and vomiting sometimes accompany severe pain
4. Other symptoms: abdominal distention, fever, and chills
5. Urinalysis (may reveal hematuria, pyuria, and crystal fragments)
6. Twenty-four-hour urine levels for calcium, uric acid, and oxalate
7. Serum levels for calcium, phosphorus, and uric acid
8. Chemical analysis of stones passed for content and type
9. KUB, IVP, retrograde pyelography, renal ultrasound, CT scan, cystoscopy, and MRI

C. Therapeutic management

1. Stones that are too large to pass spontaneously (diameter > 5 mm), multiple stones, and those that obstruct urinary tract usually require surgery (see Table 54–4)
2. NCLEX® Treatment for calcium phosphate and/or oxalate stones
   a. Acid-ash diet with limitations of foods high in calcium and oxalates (see Box 54–4)
   b. Increase hydration and exercise
3. NCLEX® Treatment for struvite stones: acid-ash diet
4. NCLEX® Treatment for uric acid stones: alkaline-ash and low-purine diet; increase hydration
5. NCLEX® Treatment for cystine stones: alkaline-ash diet; increase hydration
6. Goal of treatment is to relieve symptoms, remove or destroy calculi, and prevent future stone formation
7. Most calculi (90%) pass out of urinary system without invasive treatment
8. Provide pain relief measures and treat other symptoms as they occur
9. Monitor urinary function and monitor I&O
10. NCLEX® Strain all urine and save solid material for analysis
11. NCLEX® Encourage ambulation and large fluid intake to help client pass calculi

Table 54–4 Surgical Procedures to Treat Urinary Stones

Surgical Procedure	Description
Extracorporeal shock-wave lithotripsy (ESWL)	A procedure that uses externally generated waves to pulverize or shatter urinary stones and calculi, which are then excreted in urine
Ureterolithotomy, pyelolithotomy, or nephrolithotomy	Surgical removal of calculi from affected areas; requires a large flank incision and an extended recovery time
Percutaneous nephrostomy	Small incision in flank allows insertion of an endoscope to visualize renal pelvis; stones are removed with forceps or a basket device, or lithotripsy is used to crush stones
Transurethral uroscopy	Passage of a ureteral catheter via a cystoscope to drain urine proximal to a stone and dilate ureter, allowing stone to pass; or use of a basket catheter passed through cystoscope to remove calculus

Box 54–4

Dietary Considerations with Urinary Calculi

Acid-ash foods: Cranberries, plums, grapes, and prunes; tomatoes; eggs and cheese; whole grains; meat and poultry

Alkaline-ash foods: Legumes, milk and milk products, green vegetables, rhubarb, fruits except those acid-ash fruits noted above

Foods high in calcium: Milk and other dairy products, beans and lentils, dried fruits, canned or smoked fish (except tuna), flour, chocolate, and cocoa

Foods high in oxalates: Asparagus, beets, celery, cabbage, dark green leafy vegetables, fruits, tomatoes, green beans, chocolate and cocoa, beer, cola beverages, nuts, and tea

Foods high in purines: Organ meats, sardines, salmon, and herring, venison, and goose; other meats (beef, chicken, pork, veal) also contain purines and should be limited in quantity

12. Record daily weight to determine fluid status and renal function
13. Medication therapy: antimicrobial therapy for infection, analgesics for pain, and diuretics to prevent urine stasis

NCLEX® **D. Reinforce client teaching**

1. Proper diet is essential to prevent recurrence of stones; teach dietary needs related to type of calculus (refer again to Box 54–4)
2. Increase fluid intake to 2500–3500 mL/day
3. Maintain activity at level that will prevent urinary stasis and resorption of calcium from bone
4. If discharged prior to stone passage, collect and strain all urine and bring stones to follow-up visit; observe amount and character of urine and report to health care provider at follow-up visit also
5. Report increased pain, persistent blood in urine, inability to void, significant decrease in UO
6. Report signs of infection: burning with urination, cloudy urine, or fever
7. Review specific drug information and procedures for self-administration

VI. URINARY RETENTION

A. Overview

1. Inability to empty bladder leading to bladder distention, poor contractility of detrussor muscle, and further inability to urinate
2. Mechanical obstruction of bladder outlet is most often caused by benign prostatic hyperplasia (BPH) or acute inflammation
3. Functional problems
   a. Surgery may disrupt function of detrussor muscle, leading to retention of urine
   b. Many medications can interfere with detrussor muscle function, including anticholinergics, antidepressant and antipsychotic agents, anti-Parkinson drugs, antihistamines, and some antihypertensives

B. Nursing data collection

NCLEX® 1. Firm, distended bladder that may be displaced to one side of midline

NCLEX® 2. Overflow voiding or incontinence may occur, with 25–50 mL of urine eliminated at frequent intervals

NCLEX® 3. Residual urine (postvoiding catheterization) in amounts over 50 mL obtained from bladder catheterization

4. Positive urine culture indicates presence of urinary tract infection (UTI)
5. Elevated serum creatinine and BUN levels indicate disturbances in renal function
6. Elevated blood glucose may indicate diabetes mellitus
7. Cystometrography evaluates muscle function

C. Therapeutic management

1. Surgical correction of any condition causing mechanical obstruction to urine flow, including BPH and calculi
2. Palpate bladder for distention at regular intervals
3. Monitor I&O and observe urine characteristics
4. Attempt to stimulate relaxation of urethral sphincter by running water, providing warm water in which client can place fingers, pouring warm water over perineum, or providing warm sitz bath
5. Perform intermittent straight catheterization as ordered

NCLEX® 6. Review client's medication regime for drugs that cause urinary retention

NCLEX® 7. Medication therapy: cholinergic medications to promote detrussor muscle contraction and bladder emptying; anticholinesterase drugs to increase detrussor muscle tone

D. Reinforce client teaching

1. How to perform straight catheterization at home if necessary
2. Recognize and report signs of UTI: burning with urination, cloudy urine, pelvic pain, fever, and strong urine odor

NCLEX® 3. Moderate to high fluid intake and a diet that acidifies the urine; cranberry juice and ascorbic acid (vitamin C) help maintain acidity

4. Specific drug information and procedures for self-administration

VII. URINARY INCONTINENCE

A. Overview

1. Involuntary urination; five types according to North American Nursing Diagnosis Association International (NANDA-I)
   a. Stress incontinence: loss of urine with increased abdominal pressure

b. Reflex incontinence: involuntary loss of urine at somewhat predictable intervals when a specific bladder volume is reached
c. Urge incontinence: involuntary passage of urine soon after a strong urge to void
d. Functional incontinence: involuntary, unpredictable passage of urine
e. Total incontinence: continuous and unpredictable loss of urine

2. Incontinence is a symptom of other problems, not a disease in itself, although it has a significant impact on client's life
3. May be acute or chronic, and cause may be congenital or acquired
4. Occurs with any condition causing higher than normal bladder pressure or reduced urethral resistance
5. Common causes: relaxation of pelvic musculature, disruption of cerebral and nervous system control, and disturbances of bladder musculature
6. Risk factors in older clients: decreased bladder capacity, lax pelvic muscles in females, immobility, chronic degenerative diseases, low fluid intake, diabetes mellitus, and stroke

B. Nursing data collection

NCLEX® 1. Clinical manifestations: involuntary passage of urine
2. Weak abdominal and pelvic muscle tone in women
3. Enlarged prostate in men
4. Postvoiding residual urine greater than 50 mL
5. Cystometrography: reduced muscle function and tone
6. Ultrasonography and cystoscopy identify possible causes of the incontinence

C. Therapeutic management

1. Surgical suspension of bladder neck to treat stress incontinence associated with urethrocele
2. Prostatectomy to treat overflow incontinence due to enlarged prostate
3. Implantation of an artificial sphincter to treat clients with neurogenic bladder
4. Goal is to identify and correct cause of incontinence; if unable to correct underlying problem, client may learn techniques to manage UO
5. Monitor diagnostic tests to evaluate cause of incontinence
6. NCLEX® Employ behavioral techniques, such as bladder training, for clients who are cognitively and functionally intact
7. Insert urinary catheter as ordered and monitor client's UO
8. NCLEX® Medication therapy: anticholinergics for stress incontinence to increase bladder capacity and inhibit detrussor muscle contractions; antihistamines to enhance contraction of smooth muscles of bladder neck; estrogen therapy for incontinence associated with postmenopausal atrophic vaginitis

D. Reinforce client teaching

1. Care of indwelling urinary catheter at home
2. Recognize and report signs of UTI: burning with urination, cloudy urine, pelvic pain, fever; and strong urine odor
3. Moderate to high fluid intake and a diet that acidifies urine
4. Specific drug information and procedures for self-administration
5. Possible need to keep a voiding diary to help diagnose cause(s) of incontinence
6. NCLEX® Teach Kegel exercises to strengthen pelvic floor muscles (see Box 54–5)
7. Dietary and fluid intake modifications to reduce stress and urge incontinence; consume most fluids during times of day client is most able to remain continent
8. Wear clothing that is easily removed for ease in toileting
9. Use assistive devices, such as raised toilet seats, bedside commode, and urinal or bedpan as needed

Box 54–5

Teaching Kegel Exercises

- First, sit or stand with legs apart.
- Tense your muscles to pull your rectum, urethra, and vagina up inside, and hold for a count of 3 to 5 seconds; a pull should be felt at the cleft of your buttocks.
- Try to stop and start your stream of urine.
- Develop a schedule that will help remind you to do these exercises.
- To control episodes of stress incontinence, brace the muscles and use the Kegel maneuver when doing any activity that increases intra-abdominal pressure, such as coughing, laughing, sneezing, or lifting.

VIII. URINARY TRACT INFECTIONS (UTI)

A. Overview

1. Presence of microorganisms in urinary tract leading to inflammation
2. Infections are classified by region and primary site affected; infection in bladder is called **cystitis**
3. Urinary tract is sterile above urethra; pathogens enter by ascending from perineal area or are introduced from bloodstream; ascending route is most common
4. *Escherichia coli* is most frequent infective organism, causing about 80% of all cases; 5–15% are caused by *staphylococcus*
5. Free urine flow, large UO, and pH are antibacterial defenses
6. Females are prone to UTIs because female urethra is shorter than male urethra
7. Males are more likely to develop UTI with aging because of prostatic hyperplasia, which impedes urine flow and leads to incomplete bladder emptying and urinary stasis
8. Noninfectious cystitis results from exposure to radiation, chemical agents, or a metabolic disorder

B. Nursing data collection

NCLEX® 1. Burning, frequency, fever, cloudy urine, strong odor to urine, and pain in pelvic area

NCLEX® 2. Older clients may have nonspecific symptoms, such as nocturia, incontinence, confusion, lethargy, or anorexia

3. Urine cultures and Gram stain determine presence and number of bacteria
4. WBCs are elevated with an increase in neutrophils
5. Blood or urine tests are also done to rule out sexually transmitted infections, which produce similar symptoms

C. Therapeutic management

1. Surgery may be necessary if recurrent UTI is caused by structural abnormalities, including ureteroplasty (surgical repair of ureter) for stricture or placement of ureteral stent (catheter in ureter to provide free flow of urine)

NCLEX® 2. Increase fluid intake to 3000 mL per day

NCLEX® 3. Administer urinary antimicrobials as ordered

4. Administer analgesic and antispasmodic medications as needed
5. Encourage client to void every 2–3 hours and completely empty bladder to reduce urinary stasis
6. Monitor I&O and observe urine characteristics
7. Medication therapy: antimicrobials to eradicate bacteria; antispasmodics and analgesics to relieve pain, frequency, and burning

NCLEX® D. Reinforce client teaching

1. Avoid beverages that irritate bladder: carbonated or caffeinated drinks and alcohol
2. Hygiene measures for women to prevent reoccurrence: wipe from front to back, keep perineum clean and dry, do not douche, avoid tight-fitting pants; void after sexual intercourse
3. Finish complete course of antibiotics, even if symptoms subside
4. Correct use, purpose, and effects of medication
5. Phenazopyridine (Pyridium), a urinary analgesic, turns urine reddish orange; protect clothing and do not mistake color for bleeding (hematuria)
6. Signs of infection: frequency, burning, cloudy urine, fever, and malodorous urine
7. Maintain acidic urine with acid-ash diet, which may include cranberry juice or ascorbic acid daily (helps prevent bacteria from clinging to bladder wall)
8. Maintain fluid intake of at least 8–10 glasses per day
9. Practice frequent voiding (every 2–4 hours) to flush bacteria from urethra
10. Avoid harsh soaps, bubble bath, powder, or sprays in perineal area
11. Take showers rather than baths if recurrent infection is a problem

IX. *PYELONEPHRITIS*

A. Overview

1. Acute or chronic infection of one or both kidneys; usually begins in renal pelvis
2. Affects renal pelvis and parenchyma (functional portion of kidney)
3. Infection develops in scattered areas and spreads from renal pelvis to cortex; kidney becomes edematous and abscesses may develop; tissue destruction primarily affects tubules; with healing, scar tissue replaces normal tissue and affected tubules atrophy
4. *E. coli* causes 85% of cases; *Proteus* and *Klebsiella* bacteria are examples of less common causes
5. Acute form is a bacterial infection, which usually ascends from lower urinary tract

6. Risk factors: pregnancy, urinary tract obstruction, congenital malformation, urinary tract trauma, calculi, and diabetes
7. Asymptomatic bacteriuria or cystitis may lead to acute pyelonephritis
8. Chronic form is associated with nonbacterial infections and noninfectious processes caused by metabolic, chemical, or immunologic disorders
   a. Often results from an autoimmune process leading to inflammation
   b. Acute episodes may contribute to inflammation and scarring associated with chronic form
   c. Fibrosis and scarring lead to dilation of renal pelvis and gradual destruction of tubules
   d. May lead to chronic renal failure (CRF) and end-stage renal disease (ESRD)
9. **Vesicoureteral reflux** (urine moves from bladder back toward kidneys) is a common risk factor in children who develop pyelonephritis; is seen also in adults when bladder outflow is obstructed

NCLEX® **B. Nursing data collection**

1. Clinical manifestations: urinary frequency, dysuria, flank pain, costovertebral tenderness, tachypnea, GI symptoms, muscle tenderness, fever, chills, malaise
2. Urine culture: hematuria, pyuria, bacteriuria, leukocyte casts, leukocytosis

NCLEX® **C. Therapeutic management**

1. Maintain bedrest until symptoms subside
2. Encourage large fluid intake to maintain UO of 1500 mL/day
3. Continue monitoring for presence of bacteria
4. Monitor urinalysis: concentration and electrolytes
5. If **oliguria** (urine output less than 400 mL/day) is present, maintain diet low in protein and high in calories and vitamins
6. Observe for edema and signs of renal failure
7. Medication therapy: antimicrobials, urinary antiseptics, and analgesics for pain

D. Reinforce client teaching

1. Monitor UO and notify care provider if less than 1500 mL/day
2. Methods to prevent chronic renal insufficiency
3. Take high-calorie, low-protein diet if oliguria is present
4. Hygiene to prevent further infections (see previous section on UTI)
5. NCLEX® Encourage bedrest during acute stage
6. NCLEX® Finish complete course of antibiotics, even if symptoms resolve

X. NEOPLASTIC DISEASE

A. Overview

1. Excessive and pathologic tissue growth that may be benign or malignant
2. Other classifications: solid, cystic, superficial, invasive, primary, or metastatic
3. Most urinary tract tumors arise from epithelial tissue that lines entire urinary tract
4. Even nonmalignant tumors may lead to obstruction, renal failure, hemorrhage, and invasion and inflammation of surrounding tissues
5. Tissue destruction may cause fistulas, which can allow urine to leak into pelvis, vagina, or bowel
6. NCLEX® Major risk factors in bladder cancer are carcinogens in urine, chronic inflammation or infection of bladder mucosa, and cigarette smoking
7. NCLEX® Other risk factors: exposure to chemicals and dyes used in certain industries, chronic use of phenacetin-containing analgesic; carcinogen from these materials are excreted in urine and stored in bladder between voidings, leading to abnormal cell development

B. Nursing data collection

1. NCLEX® Painless hematuria is presenting symptom in 75% of cases; hematuria may be gross or microscopic and is often intermittent
2. Inflammation surrounding tumor may cause signs of UTI, such as frequency, urgency, and dysuria
3. With ureteral tumors, observe for colicky pain from obstruction
4. Neoplasms cause few outward symptoms and may not be discovered until urinary obstruction occurs or a fistula develops
5. Urinalysis shows gross or microscopic hematuria
6. Urine cytology shows abnormal tumor or pretumor cells
7. IVP, ultrasound, CT scan, cystoscopy, or ureteroscopy may show tumors

C. Therapeutic management

1. Radiation therapy
2. Surgical intervention for bladder tumors

a. Transurethral tumor resection
b. Partial cystectomy: resection of tumor
c. Complete or radical cystectomy: removal of bladder and adjacent structures

3. Urinary diversion may also be created
   a. Cutaneous ureterostomy: one or both ureters excised from bladder and brought to a stoma
   b. Ileal conduit: portion of ileum is isolated from small intestine and formed into a pouch; ureters are attached to pouch; pouch has open stoma
   c. Colon conduit: same as ileal conduit but a portion of sigmoid colon is used
   d. Kock pouch: same as ileal conduit but nipple valves are formed preventing leakage and reflux (see Figure 54–3)
   e. Indiana continent urinary reservoir: is formed from colon and cecum and portion of ileum is brought to surface
   f. Ileocystoplasty: section of ileum is used; is ideal for men because it allows client to void
4. *NCLEX®* Monitor urinary status, including I&O, signs of infection, hematuria, and BUN and creatinine levels
5. Monitor UO from all catheters, stents, and tubes for amount, color, and clarity
6. Prepare client for invasive tests to confirm location and size of neoplasm
7. *NCLEX®* Follow guidelines for care before and after surgery, chemotherapy, and radiation treatments
8. Encourage increased fluid intake unless contraindicated
9. Provide analgesics as needed for pain
10. Encourage client to express feelings about potentially life-threatening illness and to ask questions
11. Medication therapy: chemotherapeutic agents may be given IV or by intravesical instillation (into bladder)

D. Reinforce client teaching

1. Benefits and possible adverse effects of medical and nursing interventions
2. Explanations from health care provider about diagnosis
3. Importance of compliance with long-term treatment plan and follow-up care
4. *NCLEX®* Methods to prevent infection
5. For clients with a stoma or indwelling catheter, home care procedures and when to consult health care provider
6. *NCLEX®* For clients with a continent ileostomy, how to catheterize pouch (approximately every 4 hours) and wear a small dressing to protect the stoma and clothing
7. Relaxation techniques and other coping mechanisms

XI. *GLOMERULONEPHRITIS*

A. Overview

1. A group of kidney diseases caused by inflammation of capillary loops in glomeruli of kidney
2. Caused by an immunologic reaction to an antigen
   a. Endogenous antigens are already present in glomerulus or other body tissues
   b. Exogenous antigens come from infections occurring in body

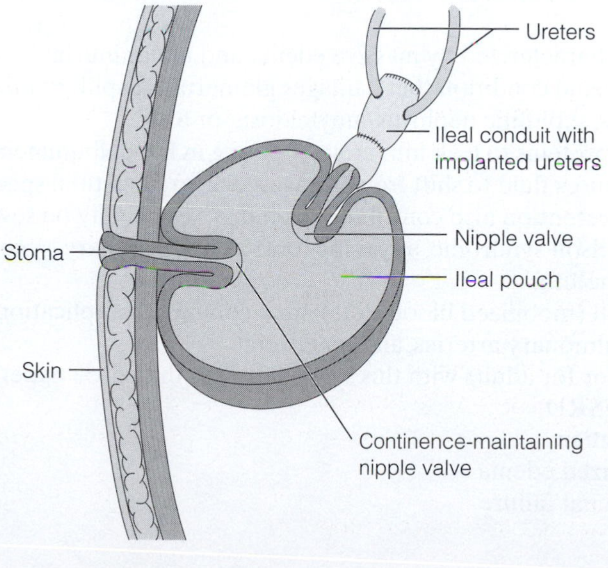

Figure 54–3

A continent urinary diversion. A segment of ileum is separated from the small intestine and formed into a pouch. Nipple valves are formed at each end of the pouch by intussuscepting tissue backward into a reservoir to prevent leakage.

3. Antigen–antibody complexes trapped within glomeruli produce an inflammatory response that damages glomeruli

NCLEX® 4. Most often follows infections with group A-beta-hemolytic streptococcus

NCLEX® 5. Upper respiratory infection, skin infection, and autoimmune processes (systemic lupus erythematosus [SLE]) predispose to glomerulonephritis

NCLEX® 6. Symptoms appear 2–3 weeks after original infection

7. Has higher incidence in men than in women; may occur at any age

NCLEX® **B. Nursing data collection**

1. Early symptoms may be mild: pharyngitis, fever, and malaise; weakness and fatigue
2. Recent upper respiratory or skin infections, pericarditis, or lower UTI
3. Anorexia, nausea, and vomiting
4. Coffee or cola-colored urine; hematuria, proteinuria (most important indicator of glomerular injury)
5. Peripheral edema
6. Hypertension
7. Hypoalbuminemia
8. Pulmonary infiltrates
9. Positive antibody response test for streptococcal exoenzymes: elevated antistreptinolysin O (ASO) titer
10. Elevated erythrocyte sedimentation rate (ESR)
11. Elevated BUN and creatinine; decreased creatinine clearance
12. Decreased serum sodium, elevated potassium, and decreased phosphate
13. Delayed uptake and excretion of radioactive dye in renal scan
14. Positive renal biopsy findings

C. Therapeutic management

NCLEX® 1. Plasmapheresis: removal of harmful components in plasma

2. Dialysis if disease progresses to renal failure

NCLEX® 3. Provide appropriate diet: protein restriction if oliguria is severe; high CHO to provide energy; K^+ usually restricted; Na^+ restriction for hypertension and edema

4. Maintain fluid restriction as needed

NCLEX® 5. Encourage complete bedrest during acute stage

6. Monitor VS frequently; observe for hypertension

NCLEX® 7. Monitor I&O and daily weight

8. Monitor for signs of renal failure: oliguria, azotemia, and acidosis
9. Medication therapy: antimicrobials (such as penicillin) for infection; analgesics for pain relief; and vitamin and electrolyte replacement as needed

D. Client teaching

1. Maintain strict bedrest during acute phase
2. Dietary changes and importance of maintaining diet
3. Importance of fluid restriction if oliguria present
4. Purpose of laboratory tests and other procedures

XII. NEPHROTIC SYNDROME

A. Overview

1. Renal disease characterized by massive edema and albuminuria
2. Seen with any renal condition that damages glomerular capillary membrane: glomerulonephritis, lipoid nephrosis, syphilitic nephritis, amyloidosis, or SLE

NCLEX® 3. Allows plasma proteins to leak into urine, resulting in hypoalbuminemia, with decreased plasma oncotic pressure that causes fluid to shift from intravascular to interstitial spaces and subsequent edema

4. Salt and water retention also contribute to edema, which may be severe
5. Kimmelstiel-Wilson syndrome, a specific form of intercapillary glomerulosclerosis, is associated with diabetes mellitus
6. Thromboemboli (mobilized blood clots) are a common complication and may occlude peripheral veins and arteries, pulmonary arteries, and renal veins
7. Prognosis is poor for adults with this syndrome; less than 50% experience complete remission; at least 30% develop ESRD

NCLEX® **B. Nursing data collection**

1. Severe generalized edema
2. Symptoms of renal failure

3. Loss of appetite and fatigue
4. Amenorrhea
5. Pronounced proteinuria, hypoalbuminemia, and hyperlipidemia
6. Positive renal biopsy finding

C. Therapeutic management

1. No specific treatment
2. Since 30% of adults with nephrotic syndrome progress to ESRD, care may involve management of renal failure

NCLEX®
3. Provide nursing care to control edema
   a. Na^+-restricted diet and avoiding Na^+ containing drugs (such as several OTC products)
   b. Administer diuretics that block aldosterone formation (such as furosemide [Lasix])
   c. Administer salt-poor albumin to reduce fluid retention

NCLEX®
4. Provide high-protein diet to restore body proteins, high-calorie diet, and a restricted Na^+ diet if edema is present
5. Administer drug therapy as prescribed

NCLEX®
6. Maintain bedrest until edema begins to subside
7. Monitor laboratory results, including BUN, creatinine, serum electrolytes, urinalysis, hemoglobin, and hematocrit
8. Observe for signs of pulmonary edema: tachypnea, dyspnea, crackles in lungs
9. Record total I&O every 4 to 8 hours and weigh client daily
10. Maintain fluid restriction; offer ice chips and provide frequent mouth care
11. Provide for adequate rest and energy conservation

NCLEX®
12. Be aware that immune system depression increases risk of infection
    a. Monitor for signs of infection, such as purulent wound drainage and signs of UTI
    b. Monitor CBC, with close attention to WBC and differential
    c. Use good hand hygiene and infection control techniques
    d. Avoid or minimize invasive procedures

NCLEX®
13. Medication therapy: immunosuppressives for autoimmune disorders; angiotensin converting enzyme (ACE) inhibitors to reduce protein loss; NSAIDs to reduce proteinuria; penicillin or other broad-spectrum antibiotics to kill bacteria; and antihypertensives as needed to lower BP

D. Reinforce client teaching

1. Take measures to maintain general health, as disorder may persist for months or years
2. Avoid sources of infection such as people with upper respiratory infections
3. Nutritious diet (low-sodium, high-protein)
4. Activity as tolerated
5. Use and potential effects of medications
6. Signs, symptoms, and implications of improving or declining renal function

XIII. *POLYCYSTIC KIDNEY DISEASE*

A. Overview

1. Hereditary disease characterized by cyst formation and massive kidney enlargement, affecting both children and adults
2. Autosomal-dominant form affects adults, while autosomal-recessive form is usually diagnosed in childhood
3. Renal cysts (fluid-filled sacs) develop in tubular epithelium of nephron and fill with glomerular filtrate or secreted solutes and fluid
4. Cysts range in size from microscopic to several centimeters

NCLEX®
5. As cysts enlarge and multiply, kidneys also enlarge; renal blood vessels and nephrons are compressed and obstructed, and functional tissue is destroyed
6. Disorder is slow and progressive; adult symptoms usually manifest by age 30 to 40

NCLEX®
7. Clients with this disorder often develop cysts elsewhere in body, including liver, spleen, pancreas, brain, and other organs

NCLEX®
B. Nursing data collection

1. Flank pain
2. Polyuria and nocturia
3. Gross hematuria, proteinuria
4. Signs of UTI and renal calculi
5. Hypertension
6. Palpable, enlarged, and knobby kidney

7. Signs of chronic renal failure as the client approaches age 50 to 60
8. Positive findings in renal ultrasonography, IVP, and CT scan

C. Therapeutic management

1. Provide supportive care to help client cope with symptoms; no effective treatment is available
2. NCLEX® Encourage fluid intake of 2000–2500 mL/day to help prevent UTI and calculi
3. Administer antihypertensive agents as prescribed
4. Discuss that hemodialysis and possibly renal transplant will be indicated as disease progresses
5. NCLEX® Provide nursing care directed toward edema control: Na^+ restricted diet and diuretics that block aldosterone formation
6. NCLEX® Medication therapy: ACE inhibitors to control hypertension; diuretics to control edema; and antibiotics if infection develops

D. Reinforce client teaching

1. Maintenance of general health because disorder is chronic and progressive
2. How to avoid UTI and to recognize early signs of infection
3. NCLEX® Avoid medications that are potentially toxic to kidneys and check with health care provider before taking any new drug
4. Need for genetic counseling and screening of family members for disease
5. NCLEX® Maintain fluid intake of at least 2500 mL/day

XIV. *ACUTE RENAL FAILURE*

A. Overview

1. Sudden loss of kidney function caused by failure of renal circulation or damage to the tubules or glomeruli
   a. Usually reversible, with spontaneous recovery in a few days to weeks
   b. Ischemia is primary cause; it produces irreversible damage to tubules if continues for more than 2 hours
2. Etiologic categories
   a. Prerenal: accounts for 55% of renal failure; caused by decreased blood flow to kidneys; readily reversible when recognized and treated early; may be caused by severe dehydration, diuretic therapy, circulatory collapse, hypovolemia, or shock
   b. Intrarenal: caused by a disease process, ischemia, or toxic conditions such as acute glomerulonephritis, vascular disorders, toxic agents, or severe infection
   c. Postrenal: caused by any condition that obstructs urine flow such as in benign prostatic hyperplasia (BPH), renal or urinary tract calculi, or tumors

NCLEX® **B. Nursing data collection (see also Table 54–5)**

1. Clinical manifestations follow three phases: initiation, maintenance, and recovery; initiation stage has very few manifestations; maintenance phase is characterized by oliguria; signs of improving UO and renal function characterize recovery stage
2. Muscle weakness, nausea, vomiting, and diarrhea may occur
3. Neurologic symptoms such as confusion, agitation, disorientation, seizures, and coma may also be present
4. Hyperkalemia, hyperphosphatemia, and hypocalcemia
5. Metabolic acidosis
6. **Azotemia** (retention of excess nitrogenous waste in blood)
7. Anemia
8. Elevated creatinine and BUN levels
9. Proteinuria
10. Urinalysis show specific gravity (SG) equal to SG of plasma; presence of casts, RBC, WBC, and renal tubular epithelial cells
11. Positive renal biopsy findings

C. Therapeutic management

1. Provide fluid and electrolyte management
2. Supportive therapy with dialysis
3. Monitor I&O
4. Observe for oliguria followed by **polyuria** (excess UO from diuresis)
5. NCLEX® Weigh daily and observe for edema
6. NCLEX® Monitor for complications of electrolyte imbalances, such as acidosis and hyperkalemia
7. Allow client to verbalize concerns regarding disorder
8. NCLEX® Encourage prescribed diet: moderate protein restriction, high in carbohydrates (CHO), restricted potassium (K^+) and sodium (Na^+)

Table 54–5 Clinical Manifestations of Renal Failure

Body System	Clinical Manifestations	Cause of Manifestations
Cardiovascular	Hypervolemia, hypertension, tachycardia, arrhythmias, congestive heart failure, pericarditis	Increased fluid volume, build up of metabolic wastes, chronic hypertension, change in renin-angiotension mechanism
Hematologic	Anemia, leukocytosis, decreased platelet function, thrombocytopenia	Decreased production of erythropoietin and RBCs, decreased survival of RBCs, decreased platelet activity; blood loss through dialysis and bleeding
Gastrointestinal	Anorexia, nausea, vomiting, abdominal distention, diarrhea, constipation, bleeding	Build up of uremic toxins, electrolyte imbalances, changes in platelet activity, conversion of urea to ammonia by saliva
Neurologic	Lethargy, confusion, convulsions, stupor, coma, sleep disturbances, behavioral changes, muscle irritability	Uremic toxins, electrolyte imbalances, cerebral swelling caused by fluid shifts
Dermatologic	Pallor, pigmentation, pruritus, ecchymosis, excoriation, uremic frost	Anemia, decreased activity of sweat glands, dry skin, phosphate deposits on skin
Urinary	Decreased urine output, decreased specific gravity, proteinuria, casts and cells in urine	Damage to nephron
Skeletal	Osteoporosis, renal rickets, joint pain	Decreased calcium absorption, decreased phosphate excretion

9. Once diuresis phase begins, evaluate slow return of BUN, creatinine, phosphorus, and K^+ to normal
10. Medication therapy
    - NCLEX® a. Avoid nephrotoxic drugs
    - b. Use volume expanders as prescribed to restore renal perfusion in hypotensive clients and dopamine (Intropin) IV to increase renal blood flow
    - c. Use loop diuretic to reduce toxic concentration in nephrons and establish urine flow
    - d. Use ACE inhibitors to control hypertension
    - e. Use antacids or histamine H_2-receptor antagonists to prevent gastric ulcers
    - f. Use sodium polystyrene sulfate (Kayexalate) to reduce serum K^+ levels and sodium bicarbonate to treat acidosis

D. Client teaching

NCLEX® 1. Dietary and fluid restrictions, including those that may be continued after discharge
2. Signs of complications, such as fluid volume excess, CHF, and hyperkalemia
NCLEX® 3. Monitor weight, BP, pulse, and UO
NCLEX® 4. Avoid nephrotoxic drugs and substances: NSAIDs, some antibiotics, radiologic contrast media, and heavy metals; consult health care provider before taking OTC drugs
5. Recovery of renal function requires up to 1 year; during this period, nephrons are vulnerable to damage from nephrotoxins

XV. END-STAGE RENAL DISEASE (ESRD)

A. Overview

1. Loss of renal function characterized by a glomerular filtration rate (GFR) less than 20% of normal
2. Final stage of **chronic renal failure** (CRF; slow, progressive loss of kidney function and glomerular filtration); ends fatally with **uremia** (excess urea and other nitrogenous waste products in blood)
NCLEX® 3. Most common causes of CRF are diabetes mellitus, hypertension, glomerulonephritis, SLE and polycystic kidney disease
4. Progressive loss of renal function occurs in four stages; fourth stage ends with ESRD (uremia)
5. As 90% or more of nephrons are destroyed, BUN and creatinine clearance rise, and urine specific gravity is fixed at 1.010 (normal up to 1.025)
6. Uremia: means "urine in blood"; term used for symptoms associated with ESRD
7. Loss of erythropoietin leads to chronic anemia and subsequent fatigue

NCLEX® 8. There is inadequate clearance of fluid and electrolytes, leading to fluid and Na^+ retention, as well as hyperkalemia, hypermagnesemia, hyperphosphatemia, and hypocalcemia; metabolic acidosis occurs because of impaired hydrogen ion excretion

NCLEX® **B. Nursing data collection**

1. Early: nausea, apathy, weakness, and fatigue; declining urine output
2. Late: possibly frequent vomiting, increasing weakness, lethargy, and confusion
3. Client may report "restless leg syndrome," paresthesia, and sensory loss
4. Personality changes, such as anxiety, irritability, and hallucinations; seizures and coma posible in late stages
5. Respirations may change to Kussmaul pattern, with deep coma following
6. Skin becomes pale and dry, with yellowish hue; metabolic wastes cause itching and uremic frost (crystallized deposits of urea on skin)
7. Urinalysis shows fixed specific gravity approximately 1.010, equivalent to plasma; abnormal proteins, blood cells, and casts are present.
8. Elevated creatinine and BUN and decreased creatinine clearance
9. Abnormal electrolyte values as noted above
10. Moderate anemia
11. Decreased platelets
12. Decreased renal size by ultrasonography
13. Positive renal biopsy if damage caused by cancer

C. Therapeutic management

NCLEX® 1. Provide diet low in protein (such as 60 grams protein) with supplemented amino acids; restrict fluids as ordered

NCLEX® 2. Provide electrolyte replacement or restriction
   a. Na^+ restriction (such as 2 grams daily)
   b. K^+ restriction (such as 2 grams daily)
   c. Replacement of bicarbonate stores to treat acidosis
3. Monitor and plan nursing care for hypertension and heart failure

NCLEX® 4. Prepare client for dialysis or kidney transplant
5. Monitor I&O and VS
6. Monitor laboratory results: BUN and serum creatinine, pH, electrolytes, and CBC
7. Provide symptomatic relief for nausea and vomiting
8. Observe for signs of infection

NCLEX® 9. Provide rest periods to combat fatigue, which is chronic in nature
10. Help client learn about and adjust to diagnosis; support coping strategies and work with client to develop realistic goals

NCLEX® 11. Medication therapy: limited by kidneys' inability to excrete
   a. Diuretics to reduce volume of extracellular fluid
   b. ACE inhibitors to maintain normal BP
   c. Electrolyte replacement
   d. Phosphate binding agents, such as calcium carbonate
   e. Kayexalate to reduce serum K^+ levels
   f. Folic acid, iron supplements, and possibly epoietin (Epogen) to combat anemia; multivitamins
   g. Medications for other health problems may require reduced dosage if excreted via kidneys

D. Reinforce client teaching

1. Monitor weight, VS, and UO at home

NCLEX® 2. Fluid and dietary restrictions (low-Na^+, low-K^+, low-protein) need to be followed carefully
3. Monitor symptoms of uremia

NCLEX® 4. Avoid nephrotoxic drugs and substances: NSAIDs, some antibiotics, radiologic contrast media, and heavy metals

NCLEX® 5. Share strategies to avoid thirst, yet continue fluid restrictions, such as frequent mouth care, sugarless hard candy, using ice chips instead of liquids, or using a spray bottle instead of a cup to limit fluids ingested
6. Discuss hemodialysis or renal transplant therapies as indicated
7. Suggest ways to combat nausea: antiemetics; mouth care; small, frequent meals
8. Provide referral to mental health counseling or support group

XVI. HYPOSPADIAS AND EPISPADIAS

A. Overview

1. **Hypospadias**: congenital defect in which urinary meatus is not at end of penis but is located on lower or underside of shaft
   a. Meatus can be anywhere on underside of penis to base of penis; most frequent anomalies are minor with openings off-center but still on glans
   b. Hypospadias is more common anomaly, and is often accompanied by **chordee**, a downward curvature of penis
2. **Epispadias**: congenital defect in which urinary meatus is not at end of penis but on upper side of penile shaft; less common than hypospadias
   a. Epispadias is often associated with **exstrophy** of bladder
   b. Both males and females can be affected by hypospadias or epispadias; in most instances, female anomaly does not require surgical correction

B. Nursing data collection: noted on admission to the newborn nursery

C. Therapeutic management

1. Does not interfere with voiding but could interfere with reproduction if not repaired before adulthood
2. Document findings carefully and report to physician
3. **Circumcision** (operation to remove part or all of prepuce) is delayed because prepuce may be used in reconstruction
4. If chordee is present, curvature of penis may be released before hypospadias repair

NCLEX® 5. Surgical correction is usually begun before age of 18 months

NCLEX® 6. Postoperative care
   a. Penis may have a urethral stent in place and be wrapped with a pressure dressing
   b. Arm and leg restraints may be needed to prevent accidental removal of stent
   c. Encourage increased fluid intake to maintain UO and stent patency
   d. Call physician if no UO occurs for 1 hour because there could be kinks in system or occlusion by sediment
   e. Medication therapy includes antibiotics until stent falls out, acetaminophen (Tylenol) for pain, and anticholinergics such as oxybutynin (Ditropan) for bladder spasms

D. Reinforce client and family teaching

1. Parents need explanation of disorder and surgical repair

NCLEX® 2. Postsurgical discharge teaching
   a. Double-diapering technique to protect stent (inner diaper collects stool and outer diaper collects urine)
   b. Limit activity for approximately 2 weeks; restrict activities that put pressure on site (riding toys, sitting on lap, or straddling child on hip); no tub baths while stent in place
   c. Medication administration, including full course of antibiotic therapy, anticholinergic for bladder spasm; acetaminophen (Tylenol) or ibuprofen (Motrin) for pain
   d. Maintain adequate fluid intake
   e. Monitor for signs of infection (strong smelling urine, redness, fever, pain, change in flow of urine stream)
   f. Call physician if urine leaks from anywhere but penis (urine will also be blood-tinged for several days)

XVII. EXSTROPHY OF BLADDER

A. Overview

1. Lower portion of abdominal wall and anterior bladder wall are missing, resulting in bladder being open and exposed on abdomen
2. Occurs more often in boys than girls and is most frequently associated with epispadias
3. Bladder appears as reddish mass glistening with urine
4. Continuous drainage of urine from ureters may lead to skin excoriation around bladder
5. Exstrophy of bladder can be life threatening and must be corrected as soon after birth as possible

B. Nursing data collection: immediately obvious at birth; evaluate for other anomalies

C. Therapeutic management

NCLEX® 1. Bladder closure is corrected during first 48–72 hours of life

NCLEX® 2. Correction of exstrophy of bladder is usually a staged surgical correction, with epispadias repair at about 9 months of age (if present) and bladder neck reconstruction with ureteral reimplantation at 2 to 3 years

NCLEX® 3. Preoperative nursing care involves covering bladder with sterile plastic wrap and maintaining integrity of surrounding skin using skin sealant to protect from excoriating effects of urine

NCLEX® 4. Postoperative nursing care may involve Bryant's traction to facilitate healing, and avoiding abduction of legs (puts stress on surgical area); change dressings as ordered by surgeon; monitor UO and characteristics, and watch for signs of obstruction, bladder spasms, and urine or blood draining from meatus

5. Emotional support of infant and parents is important; activities to support bonding and help parents accept deformity are a major component of care

D. Reinforce client and family teaching

1. Explanation of anomaly as well as instructions for care
2. As soon as possible, parents should participate in care of their infant

XVIII. *CRYPTORCHIDISM*

A. Overview

1. Failure of one or both testes to descend from inguinal canal into scrotum; normal descent of testes occurs late in gestation
2. More frequently seen in premature infants than in full-term infants

NCLEX® 3. Failure to descend exposes testes to body heat, leading to low sperm counts at sexual maturity

4. Undescended testicles are also at greater risk for torsion (twisting of a testis on its blood supply) and trauma; undescended testes have a higher incidence of cancer
5. Frequently associated with an inguinal hernia

B. Nursing data collection: absence of one or both testes in scrotal sac at birth

C. Therapeutic management

1. Often testes descend on own during first year of life; monitor periodically
2. If testes remain undescended, an orchiopexy is performed at one year of age before further damage occurs; if testes are damaged or absent, a prosthesis is placed in scrotum
3. Nursing care preoperatively is directed at preparing child and family for surgery

NCLEX® 4. Postoperatively, nursing care includes putting ice on surgical area, giving analgesics for pain, and monitoring child for infection; bedrest is maintained

D. Reinforce client and family teaching

1. Explanations of surgical repair
2. How to care for child at home postoperatively, since child will likely go home after recovering from anesthesia; instructions are similar to those after repair of hypospadias or epispadias, except there is no need for double diapering technique
3. Symptoms of infection to report

Check Your NCLEX–PN® Exam I.Q.

You are ready for testing on this content if you can

- Identify basic structures and functions of the renal system.
- Describe the pathophysiology and etiology of common renal disorders.
- Discuss expected data and diagnostic test findings for selected renal disorders.
- Discuss therapeutic management of a client experiencing a renal disorder.
- Discuss nursing management of a client experiencing a renal disorder.
- Identify expected outcomes for the client experiencing a renal disorder.

PRACTICE TEST

1 Which statement made by a client who has chronic renal failure and is on hemodialysis indicates the need to reinforce teaching?

1. "I will report any increase in my weight of 5 pounds in a 2-day period."
2. "I take my prescribed antihypertensive drugs daily."
3. "I am careful to take precautions in the arm with the AV fistula."
4. "I comply with salt restrictions in my diet by using salt substitutes."

2 What type of renal failure would the nurse expect to see in a client who overdosed accidentally on tobramycin (Nebcin)?

1. Prerenal failure
2. Postrenal failure
3. Extrarenal failure
4. Intrarenal failure

3 A client with urinary tract infection (UTI) is prescribed phenazopyridine (Pyridium). Which instruction would the nurse reinforce with the client?

1. "This drug will take care of the infection causing your symptoms."
2. "Your urine may turn reddish orange and may cause staining of your clothes."
3. "Take the drug before meals to minimize GI symptoms."
4. "Always keep this drug and use it at the first symptom of a UTI."

4 A client with a urinary diversion device has the nursing diagnosis Risk for Impaired Skin Integrity. Which interventions will the nurse use with this client? Select all that apply.

1. Change urine collection device every other day.
2. Reinforce teaching of self-catheterization technique.
3. Empty the bag reservoir every 2 hours.
4. Monitor for foul-smelling urine.
5. Ensure appliance wafer is not more than 1/8 inch larger than stoma.

5 A client with renal calculi is advised to restrict calcium in the diet. The nurse determines that the client understands the restriction when the client states to avoid which types of foods?

1. Chicken, beef, and salmon
2. Green vegetables, fruit, and legumes
3. Chocolate, smoked fish, and low-fat milk
4. Eggs, meat, and poultry

6 In assisting with teaching for a client who will undergo peritoneal dialysis at home, the nurse includes discussion of what common and significant complication of peritoneal dialysis?

1. Pulmonary embolism
2. Hypotension
3. Dyspnea
4. Peritonitis

7 The nurse is preparing to admit a client with urge incontinence. In reviewing the care plan, the nurse identifies interventions that target which manifestation?

1. Involuntary loss of urine without warning or stimulus
2. Loss of urine when coughing or sneezing
3. Inability to empty bladder
4. Inability to inhibit urine flow long enough to reach the toilet

8 A male client who presents to the emergency department with coffee-colored urine and edema states he had a bad sore throat a few weeks ago. His blood pressure is elevated, and urinalysis shows blood and protein in the urine. The nurse interprets that this clinical picture is consistent with which developing health problem?

1. Urinary tract infection
2. Urinary calculi
3. Acute glomerulonephritis
4. Acute prostatitis

9 Which discharge instructions would the nurse reinforce to a client who will receive an aminoglycoside antibiotic at home to address the risk of nephrotoxicity? Select all that apply.

1. Increase fluid intake to 2000–2500 mL fluid daily.
2. Report sudden weight gain or puffy eyes.
3. Don't be concerned with edema as a normal drug side effect.
4. Elevated blood pressure is an expected drug effect.
5. Eat a low protein diet while taking this antibiotic.

10 The nurse caring for a client undergoing a hemodialysis procedure places high priority on monitoring the client frequently for what common complication during the treatment?

1. Hyperglycemia
2. Infection and fever
3. Dialysis dementia
4. Hypotension

PRACTICE TEST

11 The nurse is explaining the process of peritoneal dialysis to a client who recently developed renal failure. Which statement would the nurse include in a discussion with the client?

1. "The solutes in the dialysate will enter the bloodstream through the peritoneum."
2. "The peritoneum is more permeable because of the presence of excess metabolites."
3. "The peritoneum acts as a semipermeable membrane through which wastes move by diffusion and osmosis."
4. "The metabolites will move from the interstitial space to the bloodstream mainly through diffusion and ultrafiltration."

12 Which statement made by a client who has received a renal transplant indicates that the desired outcome of discharge teaching has been met? Select all that apply.

1. "I will double my prednisone dose if my urine output is less than 300 mL/day."
2. "I will need to avoid crowds and prevent infection."
3. "Now I can eat whatever I want as long as I watch how much salt I use."
4. "Since I have not yet rejected the transplant, I never have to worry about rejection anymore."
5. "I should check my temperature and report increases to the physician."

13 Which statement by a female client indicates that instruction in ways to prevent urinary tract infection (UTI) was understood? Select all that apply.

1. "I should avoid tub baths and take showers instead."
2. "I should drink 8 to 10 glasses of fluid per day."
3. "I should only wear nylon underpants."
4. "I should void every 6 hours while I am awake."
5. "I should use powder or talc to aid in keeping the perineal skin dry."

14 A client with chronic renal failure asks the nurse why he is anemic. What response by the nurse is best?

1. "The increased metabolic waste products in your body depress the bone marrow."
2. "We will need to review your dietary intake of iron-rich foods."
3. "There is a decreased production by the kidneys of the hormone erythropoietin."
4. "It is most likely that you have hereditary traits for the development of anemia."

15 A child has been admitted to the unit with nephrotic syndrome. In talking with the mother, she reports that a cousin had acute glomerulonephritis (AGN) last year. The mother asks how these two diseases compare, as they both affect the kidneys. The nurse's response would include which piece of information?

1. Both disorders produce smoky colored urine.
2. Both disorders cause greatly reduced urine output.
3. Both disorders have a genetic basis.
4. Both disorders require treatment with antibiotic therapy.

16 In a child with acute renal failure, the nurse would help to prevent hyperkalemia by limiting which foods in the child's diet?

1. Grains, cheese, and citrus fruits
2. Potatoes, tomatoes, and oranges
3. Cereals, processed sugars, and wheat
4. Rice, leafy green vegetables, and carbonated beverages

17 A child has been admitted with acute glomerulonephritis (AGN). All of the following tests are positive for AGN. The nurse concludes that which laboratory test is most indicative of this disease?

1. Elevated antistreptinolysin O (ASO) titers
2. Elevated erythrocyte sedimentation rate (ESR)
3. Presence of hematuria according to urinalysis
4. Elevated creatinine concentrations

18 The mother of a child at the renal clinic asks why a radiological evaluation is performed on all children who have had one documented urinary tract infection (UTI). What information would the nurse include as the best explanation for use of x-ray?

1. It rules out structural abnormalities.
2. It confirms the absence of bacterial colonies after antimicrobial therapy.
3. It determines which kidney was infected.
4. It determines the probability of the infection recurring.

19 The nurse is caring for an adult client with poor urine output. The nurse would report to the registered nurse if the client had a urine output less than how many milliliters (mL) per hour for two consecutive hours? Provide a numeric answer.

Fill in your answer below:

_______mL

20 A 4-year-old child has been diagnosed with renal failure. The nurse would ensure that the diet for this child would contain which of the following?

1. Foods high in potassium and sodium
2. Adequate calories to optimize growth
3. Foods high in calcium content to promote bone growth
4. Increased fluid intake to flush the urinary system

21 The priority concern for the nurse in monitoring a child with acute renal failure (ARF) should be to look for which electrolyte imbalance?

1. Hyperkalemia
2. Hypernatremia
3. Hypercalcemia
4. Hypophosphatemia

22 The nurse would use which appropriate nursing diagnosis for a child receiving peritoneal dialysis? Select all that apply.

1. Deficient Fluid Volume related to sodium and water retention
2. Imbalanced Nutrition: Greater Than Body Requirements related to increased hunger
3. Risk for Infection related to invasive procedures and diminished immune functioning
4. Impaired Renal Tissue Perfusion related to hypervolemia
5. Ineffective Health Maintenance related to chronic condition

23 A child is admitted with acute renal failure (ARF). When reviewing the nursing history, the nurse notes a history of all of the following diseases. The nurse concludes that which most likely precipitated the onset of ARF?

1. Chickenpox
2. Influenza
3. Dehydration
4. Hypervolemia

24 A child has been admitted in renal failure. The nurse would expect to note which values in laboratory test results? Select all that apply.

1. Blood urea nitrogen (BUN) 5 mg/dL
2. Creatinine 2.9 mg/dL
3. Oliguria in 24-hour urine
4. Potassium 2.8 mEq/L
5. Phosphorus 6.5 mg/dL

25 A baby is born 6 weeks prematurely. On admission to the nursery, the nurse is unable to locate any testicles in the scrotum. What action should the nurse take?

1. Immediately notify the registered nurse as the child is at risk for renal failure.
2. Note the findings in the child's record and take no further action at this time.
3. Discuss with the parents the need for surgical correction of cryptorchidism.
4. Catheterize the child to determine if urine is present in the bladder.

26 A child returning to the unit after an intravenous pyelogram (IVP) has an order to drink extra fluids. How will the nurse explain the primary purpose of the extra fluids to the mother?

1. Overhydrate the child.
2. Increase serum creatinine levels.
3. Make up for fluid losses from NPO status before tests.
4. Flush any remaining dye from the urinary tract.

ANSWERS & RATIONALES

1 **Answer: 4** **Rationale:** Many salt substitutes use potassium chloride. Potassium intake is carefully regulated in clients with renal failure, and the use of salt substitutes will worsen hyperkalemia. Increases in weight do need to be reported to the health care provider as a possible indication of fluid volume excess. The control of hypertension is essential in the management of a client with renal failure. An AV fistula does need to be protected from injury that could be caused by constricting clothing, venipunctures, and other items. **Cognitive Level:** Analyzing **Client Need:** Physiological Adaptation **Integrated Process:** Nursing Process: Data Collection **Content Area:** Adult Health **Strategy:** The core issue of the question is the ability to determine accurate statements about self-care of clients with renal failure. Specifically, clients need to restrict both sodium and potassium, and salt substitutes are high in potassium. Use nursing knowledge and the process of elimination to make a selection.

2 **Answer: 4** **Rationale:** Nephrotoxic drugs, such as aminoglycoside antibiotics (tobramycin), can damage the nephrons and cause intrarenal (within the kidneys) failure. Prerenal causes of renal failure include any condition that reduces the blood flow to the kidney, such as heart failure, shock, and other conditions. Postrenal failure can be caused by conditions that obstruct urine outflow in the lower urinary system. There is no condition called extrarenal failure. **Cognitive Level:** Applying **Client Need:** Physiological Adaptation **Integrated Process:** Nursing Process: Planning **Content Area:** Adult Health **Strategy:** The core issue of the question is the ability to associate causes of renal failure with their categories in specific client situations. Use nursing knowledge and the process of elimination to make a selection.

3 **Answer: 2** **Rationale:** The drug makes the urine reddish orange in color, and the client should be advised that this might stain the underwear and other clothing. The client should also be reassured that it should not be confused with blood in the urine. Phenazopyridine does not target the cause of the infection. Taking the drug after meals minimizes GI symptoms associated with the use of this drug. Indiscriminate use of a urinary analgesic can mask symptoms and delay initiation of treatment. **Cognitive Level:** Analyzing **Client Need:** Pharmacological and Parenteral Therapies **Integrated Process:** Communication and Documentation **Content Area:** Adult Health **Strategy:** The core issue of the question is knowledge of expected adverse effects of phenazopyridine. Use nursing knowledge and the process of elimination to make a selection.

4 **Answer: 3, 5** **Rationale:** Emptying the reservoir bag every 2 hours prevents overfilling and possible leakage of urine into the skin surface. Ensuring that opening is not more than 1/8 inch larger than stoma reduces the risk of skin irritation and breakdown from urine on the skin. The urine collection device should be changed as needed to maintain integrity of the system. Self-catheterization is not appropriate for this nursing diagnosis. Monitoring for foul-smelling urine and monitoring for signs of infection are more appropriate interventions for the diagnosis risk for infection. **Cognitive Level:** Applying **Client Need:** Physiological Adaptation **Integrated Process:** Nursing Process: Implementation **Content Area:** Adult Health **Strategy:** The core issue of the question is knowledge of appropriate care for a client with a urinary diversion. Use nursing knowledge and the process of elimination to make a selection.

5 **Answer: 3** **Rationale:** Chocolate, smoked fish, milk products, beans, lentils, and dried fruits are high in calcium. In calcium phosphate and calcium oxalate calculi, dietary management includes an acid-ash diet and limiting foods high in calcium and oxalate. The other foods listed may be consumed as desired. **Cognitive Level:** Analyzing **Client Need:** Physiological Adaptation **Integrated Process:** Teaching and Learning **Content Area:** Adult Health **Strategy:** The core issue of the question is knowledge of high-calcium foods to avoid with renal calculi. Use nursing knowledge and the process of elimination to make a selection.

6 **Answer: 4** **Rationale:** Peritonitis is a grave complication of peritoneal dialysis, caused by bacteria that may enter through the catheter or dialysate solution. Hypotension is a common complication of hemodialysis but not peritoneal dialysis. Pulmonary embolism and dyspnea are not common complications of peritoneal dialysis. **Cognitive Level:** Applying **Client Need:** Physiological Adaptation **Integrated Process:** Nursing Process: Implementation **Content Area:** Adult Health **Strategy:** The core issue of the question is knowledge of complications of peritoneal dialysis and their relative frequency. Use nursing knowledge and the process of elimination to make a selection.

7 **Answer: 4** **Rationale:** Urge incontinence is the unpredictable passage of urine soon after a strong urge to void is felt. Total incontinence is involuntary loss of urine without warning or stimulus. Stress incontinence is loss of urine when intraabdominal pressure rises, such as with coughing or sneezing. Urinary retention is an inability to empty the bladder. **Cognitive Level:** Applying **Client Need:** Physiological Adaptation **Integrated Process:** Nursing Process: Implementation **Content Area:** Adult Health **Strategy:** Use nursing knowledge and the process of elimination to make a selection.

8 **Answer: 3** **Rationale:** The symptoms are typical of acute glomerulonephritis. Hematuria and proteinuria are caused by a damaged glomerular capillary membrane, which allows blood cells and proteins to escape into the renal filtrate. A urinary tract infection usually manifests with signs of infection including fever, malodorous urine, frequency, and urgency. Clients with urinary calculi usually present with renal colic. Prostatitis, or inflammation of the prostate gland, has presenting symptoms similar to a urinary tract infection. **Cognitive Level:** Analyzing **Client Need:** Physiological Adaptation **Integrated Process:** Nursing Process: Data Collection **Content Area:** Adult Health **Strategy:** The core issue of the question is the ability to identify signs and symptoms of glomerulonephritis and associate it with a common etiology. Use nursing knowledge and the process of elimination to make a selection.

9 **Answer: 1, 2** **Rationale:** The client should maintain a fluid intake of 2000 to 2500 mL per day to reduce the risk of nephrotoxicity. To detect nephrotoxicity early, the client should report signs of edema. Edema is not a normal side effect of the medication. To reduce the risk of nephrotoxicity, the client should report hypertension. It is unnecessary to eat a low protein diet while taking an aminoglycoside antibiotic.

Cognitive Level: Analyzing **Client Need:** Pharmacological and Parenteral Therapies **Integrated Process:** Nursing Process: Implementation **Content Area:** Adult Health **Strategy:** The core issue of the question is the ability to correctly institute client education about nephrotoxicity as an adverse effect of aminoglycoside medications. Use nursing knowledge and the process of elimination to make a selection.

10 **Answer: 4 Rationale:** Hypotension is the most common complication during hemodialysis and is related to several factors, including changes in serum osmolality and rapid removal of fluid from the intravascular compartment. Hyperglycemia could occur in peritoneal dialysis because of the glucose composition of the dialysate. Monitoring for infection and fever should be ongoing, not just when the client is undergoing hemodialysis. Dialysis dementia is a progressive, long-term complication. **Cognitive Level:** Applying **Client Need:** Physiological Adaptation **Integrated Process:** Nursing Process: Data Collection **Content Area:** Adult Health **Strategy:** The core issue of the question is the ability to identify important complications associated with hemodialysis. Use nursing knowledge and the process of elimination to make a selection.

11 **Answer: 3 Rationale:** The peritoneum acts as a semipermeable membrane, allowing substances to move from an area of high concentration (the blood) to an area of lower concentration (the dialysate). Metabolic waste products and excess water can be eliminated through osmosis and diffusion utilizing the peritoneum as a semipermeable membrane. **Cognitive Level:** Applying **Client Need:** Physiological Adaptation **Integrated Process:** Communication and Documentation **Content Area:** Adult Health **Strategy:** The core issue of the question is the ability to accurately relate the key elements of peritoneal dialysis. Use nursing knowledge and the process of elimination to make a selection.

12 **Answer: 2, 5 Rationale:** Clients with renal transplant need to be on long-term immunosuppressive drugs that predispose them to infection. The client must verbalize factors that potentially expose them to infection. Self-monitoring of temperature helps the client detect signs of early rejection that can be reported to the physician. The client must adhere to medication doses prescribed by the physician. Dietary restrictions for sodium must be discussed with the physician and the dietician. The success of transplantation is not guaranteed and the client could experience signs of rejection after discharge. **Cognitive Level:** Analyzing **Client Need:** Physiological Adaptation **Integrated Process:** Teaching and Learning **Content Area:** Adult Health **Strategy:** The core issue of the question is the knowledge that clients who have had organ transplant are greatly at risk for infection because of drug therapy needed to prevent organ rejection. Use nursing knowledge and the process of elimination to make a selection.

13 **Answer: 1, 2 Rationale:** Tub baths can promote migration of bacteria in the lower urinary tract; the client should shower instead. Maintaining an intake of 8 to 10 glasses of fluid daily will help prevent UTI. Cotton underpants are best, and nylon should be avoided because synthetic fibers retain body moisture and irritate the perineal area, which can promote the growth of bacteria. Emptying the bladder every 2 to 4 hours while awake is recommended to prevent urinary stasis. Powder or talc can be irritating to perineal skin and should be avoided. **Cognitive Level:** Analyzing **Client Need:** Physiological Adaptation **Integrated Process:** Teaching and Learning **Content Area:** Adult Health **Strategy:** The core issue of the question is knowledge of risk factors for UTIs that must be avoided by clients at risk. Use nursing knowledge and the process of elimination to make a selection.

14 **Answer: 3 Rationale:** Anemia is common in clients with renal failure because of decreased production of erythropoietin by the kidneys and shortened RBC life. Erythropoietin is involved in the stimulation of the bone marrow to produce RBCs. Metabolic wastes do not depress the bone marrow. Anemia is common in clients with renal failure but is not caused by iron deficiency. Heredity does not play a role in anemia associated with renal failure. **Cognitive Level:** Applying **Client Need:** Physiological Adaptation **Integrated Process:** Communication and Documentation **Content Area:** Adult Health **Strategy:** The core issue of the question is the pathophysiology of renal failure and associated changes. Use nursing knowledge and the process of elimination to make a selection.

15 **Answer: 2 Rationale:** Both AGN and nephrotic syndrome are characterized by a reduction in urine output. AGN presents with smoky urine while the urine in nephrotic syndrome is clear and frothy. AGN is a postinfectious disease with no genetic basis. Antibiotics are not used in nephrotic syndrome. **Cognitive Level:** Analyzing **Client Need:** Physiological Adaptation **Integrated Process:** Nursing Process: Planning **Content Area:** Child Health **Strategy:** The core issue of the question is knowledge of the similarities and differences between nephrotic syndrome and glomerulonephritis. Use nursing knowledge and the process of elimination to make a selection.

16 **Answer: 2 Rationale:** Potatoes, tomatoes, and oranges have a high level of potassium content. The other food options have less potassium in them. **Cognitive Level:** Applying **Client Need:** Physiological Adaptation **Integrated Process:** Nursing Process: Implementation **Content Area:** Child Health **Strategy:** The core issue of the question is knowledge of foods that are high in potassium to avoid in the client with renal failure. Use nursing knowledge and the process of elimination to make a selection.

17 **Answer: 1 Rationale:** An elevated ASO titer indicates a recent streptococcal infection, which is a precursor to AGN. An elevated ESR indicates inflammation in the body and is associated with many diseases. Hematuria is simply blood in the urine, which has many possible causes. Creatinine concentrations reflect the functioning of the kidney. **Cognitive Level:** Analyzing **Client Need:** Physiological Adaptation **Integrated Process:** Nursing Process: Data Collection **Content Area:** Child Health **Strategy:** The critical words in the question are *most indicative*. This tells you that all options are correct, and you must select the response that uniquely identifies glomerulonephritis as the disorder. Use nursing knowledge and the process of elimination to make a selection.

18 **Answer: 1 Rationale:** Radiological evaluations done after a documented UTI in children reveal structural abnormalities in 1% to 2% of girls and 10% of boys. Radiological tests cannot confirm bacterial colonies, determine the site of an old infection, or help predict whether infection will reoccur. **Cognitive Level:** Applying **Client Need:** Physiological Adaptation **Integrated Process:** Nursing Process: Implementation **Content Area:** Child Health **Strategy:** The core issue of the question is knowledge that UTIs are uncommon in children and could result from structural abnormalities that are yet undiagnosed. With this in mind, use the process of elimination to make a selection from the available options.

19 **Answer: 30** **Rationale:** The minimal urine output by the kidneys per hour is 30 mL. It is prudent for the nurse to report a drop below this amount if it persists for 2 hours or longer so that corrective treatment can be undertaken. **Cognitive Level:** Applying **Client Need:** Physiological Adaptation **Integrated Process:** Nursing Process: Implementation **Content Area:** Adult Health **Strategy:** The core issue of the question is knowledge of minimal hourly urine output based on normal kidney function. Use nursing knowledge to formulate an answer.

20 **Answer: 2** **Rationale:** Dietary intake is often inadequate in children with renal failure related to anorexia and dietary restrictions. Calories and nutrition are needed to optimize growth and to prevent growth retardation. Depending on the degree of renal failure, sodium, potassium and phosphorus may be restricted. Fluids are monitored closely for balance and may be restricted if oliguria is present. **Cognitive Level:** Applying **Client Need:** Physiological Adaptation **Integrated Process:** Nursing Process: Implementation **Content Area:** Child Health **Strategy:** Recognize that a child in renal failure will have problems excreting wastes. The only option that does not provide excessive volume or ingredients is the correct one.

21 **Answer: 1** **Rationale:** The kidney normally excretes potassium. Hyperkalemia occurs with decreased kidney function resulting in cardiac arrhythmias, which can be life-threatening. Hypernatremia can occur because of reduced excretion but fluid is also retained to hemodilute it. Renal failure is associated with hypocalcemia because of the inverse relationship between calcium and phosphorus (which is retained in renal failure). Renal failure is associated with hyperphosphatemia, not hypophosphatemia. **Cognitive Level:** Analyzing **Client Need:** Reduction of Risk Potential **Integrated Process:** Nursing Process: Data Collection **Content Area:** Child Health **Strategy:** Consider which of the electrolyte imbalances occur with renal failure. In renal failure, the normal imbalances are hyperkalemia, hyponatremia (due to excessive fluid retention), hypocalcemia, and hyperphosphatemia.

22 **Answer: 3, 5** **Rationale:** Peritoneal dialysis is an invasive procedure that places the child at risk for infection. Hypervolemia is secondary to poor kidney function and does not cause altered renal tissue perfusion. The child is anorexic and the child is not at risk for fluid volume deficit. The child's condition is chronic and routine health maintenance will need to be integrated with chronic disease management. **Cognitive Level:** Analyzing **Client Need:** Physiological Adaptation **Integrated Process:** Nursing Process: Implementation **Content Area:** Child Health **Strategy:** Consider typical symptoms of renal failure. There would not be fluid volume deficit and renal tissue perfusion would not be related to hypervolemia. That leaves two choices to choose between. Use knowledge of the disease to make a final selection.

23 **Answer: 3** **Rationale:** Dehydration results in hypovolemia, which can precipitate acute renal failure in infants and children. The other responses are incorrect because they don't directly impact renal perfusion. **Cognitive Level:** Analyzing **Client Need:** Physiological Adaptation **Integrated Process:** Nursing Process: Data Collection **Content Area:** Child Health **Strategy:** Consider which diseases directly relate to the kidneys. Also note that the options contain opposites, which usually indicate that one is the right answer.

24 **Answer: 2, 3, 5** **Rationale:** Creatinine is elevated in renal failure. Oliguria is associated with renal failure. Hyperphosphatemia is associated with renal failure. The BUN would be elevated, not reduced. Hyperkalemia, not hypokalemia, would be expected in renal failure. **Cognitive Level:** Applying **Client Need:** Reduction of Risk Potential **Integrated Process:** Nursing Process: Data Collection **Content Area:** Child Health **Strategy:** Recall that renal failure prevents the elimination of waste products from the body, so the nurse would expect excesses in most lab values.

25 **Answer: 2** **Rationale:** Premature males are often born with undescended testicles. The testes normally descend during the last few weeks of gestation or shortly after birth. This would not be a concern at this time. If surgery should be needed, it will be done prior to age two. Undescended testicles do not affect urine formation. **Cognitive Level:** Applying **Client Need:** Physiological Adaptation **Integrated Process:** Nursing Process: Implementation **Content Area:** Child Health **Strategy:** Be aware that the testicles have nothing to do with urination, so two options can be eliminated. Knowledge of cryptorchidism and the usual management will aid in choosing the correct answer.

26 **Answer: 4** **Rationale:** The additional fluids will increase urinary output, thereby flushing the nephrotoxic dye from the urinary system. Extra fluids are not intended to overhydrate the child. Extra fluids are not intended to increase creatinine levels, which directly reflect kidney function. Extra fluids are not intended to compensate for earlier NPO status, although this is a benefit. **Cognitive Level:** Analyzing **Client Need:** Reduction of Risk Potential **Integrated Process:** Teaching and Learning **Content Area:** Child Health **Strategy:** Consider the testing methods to determine the correct response. Knowledge that the test uses a dye to visualize the kidney's collection system and that the dye needs to be excreted will help to choose the correct answer.

Key Terms to Review

acute renal failure p. 970
anuria p. 960
azotemia p. 970
chordee p. 973
chronic renal failure p. 971
circumcision p. 973
creatinine p. 953
cryptorchidism p. 974
cystectomy p. 958
cystitis p. 965
epispadias p. 973
exstrophy p. 973
glomerulonephritis p. 967
glomerulus p. 951
hematuria p. 956
hemodialysis p. 955
hypospadias p. 973
intravenous pyelography (IVP) p. 953
lithotripsy p. 958
micturition p. 953
nephrectomy p. 959
nephron p. 951
nephrotic syndrome p. 968
oliguria p. 966
peritoneal dialysis p. 954
polycystic kidney disease p. 969
polyuria p. 970
proteinuria p. 960
pyelonephritis p. 965
pyuria p. 956
uremia p. 971
urinary diversion p. 958
vesicoureteral reflux p. 966

References

Ball, J., Bindler, R., & Cowen, K.(2010). *Child health nursing: Partnering with children and families* (2nd ed.). Upper Saddle River, NJ: Pearson Education.

Berman, A., & Snyder, S. (2012). *Kozier & Erb's fundamentals of nursing: Concepts, process, and practice* (9th ed.). Upper Saddle River, NJ: Pearson Education, Inc.

Ignatavicius, D., & Workman, L. (2010). *Medical-surgical nursing: Critical thinking for collaborative care* (6th ed.). Philadelphia: Saunders.

Kee, J. (2010). *Laboratory and diagnostic tests with nursing implications* (8th ed.). Upper Saddle River, NJ: Pearson Education.

LeMone, P., Burke, K., & Bauldoff, G. (2011). *Medical surgical nursing: Critical thinking in patient care* (5th ed.). Upper Saddle River, NJ: Pearson Education.

Smith, S., Duell, D., & Martin, B. (2012). *Clinical nursing skills: Basic to advanced skills* (8th ed.). Upper Saddle River, NJ: Pearson Education.

Test Yourself

Are you ready for the NCLEX-PN® or course exams? Use the practice tests on the companion website to check.

55 Gastrointestinal Disorders

In this chapter

Cross Reference

Other chapters relevant to this content area are

Meeting Nutritional Needs	**Chapter 25**
Maintaining Function of Tubes and Drains	**Chapter 27**

Gastrointestinal Medications **Chapter 37**
Common Laboratory Tests **Chapter 42**
Common Diagnostic Tests and Procedures **Chapter 43**

I. OVERVIEW OF ANATOMY AND PHYSIOLOGY OF GI SYSTEM

A. **Oral cavity and pharynx**: consists of mouth, oropharynx and laryngopharynx; passageway for food, fluids, and air
B. **Esophagus**: extends from pharynx to stomach; enters stomach at gastroesophageal sphincter (also called lower esophageal sphincter, or LES), which prevents reflux
C. **Stomach**: distensible organ located high on left side of abdomen; continues mechanical breakdown of food and mixes food with gastric secretions forming a mixture called chyme; divided into four regions (cardiac, fundus, body, and pyloric; digests food with assistance of pepsin and hydrochloric acid; produces intrinsic factor for vitamin B_{12} absorption in small intestine; churns gastric contents via peristalsis
D. **Small intestine**: begins at pyloric sphincter and ends at ileocecal valve; contains three regions: duodenum, jejunum, and ileum; pancreatic enzymes (trypsin, chymotrypsin, lipase, and amylase) and bile enter duodenum near pyloric sphincter to further digest chyme; most absorption occurs in villae of small intestine
E. **Large intestine**: also called colon; extends from ileocecal valve to anus; divided into five areas: cecum, appendix, colon (ascending, transverse, and descending), rectum, and anus; major function is to absorb water, salts, and vitamins formed by bacteria in large intestine and eliminate undigestible food and residue
F. **Hepatobiliary system**
1. Liver
   a. Located in right upper quadrant (RUQ) of abdomen, beneath diaphragm; produces bile, an alkaline, yellow-green fluid containing bile salts (conjugated bile acids), cholesterol, bilirubin (byproduct of red blood cell [RBC] destruction), electrolytes, and water
   b. Stores vitamin B_{12} and fat-soluble vitamins (A, D, E, and K)
   c. Stores and releases blood during hemorrhage
   d. Synthesizes plasma proteins to maintain plasma oncotic pressure
   e. Synthesizes prothrombin, fibrinogen, and clotting factors I, II, VII, IX, X
   f. Converts amino acids to carbohydrates through deamination
   g. Stores and releases glucose and copper; stores iron as ferritin
   h. Detoxifies alcohol and certain drugs
2. Biliary tract: composed of gallbladder and associated ducts (cystic, hepatic, and common bile ducts); transports bile formed in liver to bile ducts, gallbladder, and eventually duodenum
3. Gallbladder: saclike organ located on inferior surface of liver; stores and concentrates bile; releases bile into cystic duct and common bile duct in response to presence of fat in duodenum, which leads to hormone secretion and relaxation of sphincter of Oddi
4. Pancreas: has exocrine and endocrine functions; head is located within curve of duodenum, tail touches spleen, and body lies behind stomach
   a. Pancreatic secretions flow into duodenum
   b. Endocrine pancreas secretes insulin and glucagon hormones from islets of Langerhans; insulin is a protein hormone that promotes storage and utilization of food, primarily glucose and fats; glucagon stimulates glycogenolysis in liver
   c. Exocrine pancreas secretes enzymes in response to hormonal and vagal stimuli; produces about 1 to 1.5 L of alkaline pancreatic juice/day, which neutralizes acidic chyme as it empties into duodenum; produces lipase (fat breakdown); amylase (carbohydrate breakdown); and trypsin, chymotrypsin, and carboxypeptidase (protein breakdown)

II. DIAGNOSTIC TESTS AND DATA COLLECTION

A. **Laboratory tests**: serum chemistry study, liver profile, lipid profile, gastrin levels, Schilling test, erythrocyte sedimentation rate (ESR), C-reactive protein (CRP), thyroid function (see Chapter 42)
B. **Upper GI series**: series of x-rays using contrast medium (barium sulfate or Gastrografin) to diagnose hiatal hernia, tumors, ulcerations, inflammation, varices, or obstruction
1. After client drinks barium, a series of x-rays document progression of contrast as client is placed in different positions
2. Gastroesophageal reflux (from stomach into esophagus) can be determined with client in a flat or head-down position

3. Contraindications: complete bowel obstruction, esophageal or gastric perforation (may use Gastrografin instead of barium), pregnancy, or unstable vital signs (VS)

NCLEX® 4. Possible complications: aspiration of contrast medium, constipation (if barium used), partial bowel obstruction, or significant diarrhea (Gastrografin)

C. Lower GI series: series of x-rays utilizing contrast medium (barium enema)

1. Visualizes colon, including appendix, for anatomic abnormalities, polyps, ulcers, tumors, inflammatory bowel disease, fistulas, and diverticula

NCLEX® 2. Scheduling considerations: perform before an upper GI study to prevent residual barium remaining in colon, and colon should also be empty
   - **a.** Clear liquid diet day before test
   - **b.** Magnesium citrate or other bowel prep night before test
   - **c.** NPO after midnight and continue until test is complete
   - **d.** Cleansing enemas may be ordered before test
   - **e.** Contraindications: perforated colon, uncooperative client
   - **f.** Possible complications: colonic perforation or barium impaction

D. Upper GI endoscopy: *esophagogastroduodenoscopy (EGD)*, gastroscopy

1. Allows direct visualization of esophagus, stomach, and duodenum through lighted endoscope; detects mucosal inflammations (gastroesophageal reflux, gastritis), tumors, varices, hiatal hernias, polyps, ulcers, and obstruction
2. Used also to directly sample tissues and fluids, to stop areas of active GI bleeding with injection of sclerosing agents or cautery, and to perform GI surgery using laser beams
3. Contraindications: perforated colon, fulminant ulcerative colitis, toxic megacolon, pregnancy, uncooperative clients

NCLEX® 4. Possible complications: pulmonary aspiration of GI contents; perforation of esophagus, stomach, or duodenum; bleeding from biopsy site; and reactions to sedative medication given during test

NCLEX® 5. Special nursing considerations postprocedure: NPO until client is completely alert and swallowing/gag reflexes have returned (2–4 hours); general safety precautions because of sedation; monitor for signs of bleeding, dyspnea, or dysphagia

E. Colonoscopy: fiberoptic direct visualization of colon from anus to cecum to detect tumors (benign or malignant), polyps, inflammation, ulcerations, and bleeding; suspicious tissue may be biopsied

1. Contraindications: suspected colon perforation, acute diverticulitis, peritonitis, or fulminant ulcerative colitis

NCLEX® 2. Possible complications: perforation of colon, bleeding from biopsy sites, oversedation

NCLEX® 3. Special nursing considerations: requires complete bowel prep; monitor VS postprocedure for signs of bleeding and colon perforation

F. Sigmoidoscopy: direct visualization of anus, rectum, and sigmoid colon with either a rigid or flexible sigmoidoscope; similar to colonoscopy in procedure, contraindications, complications, and nursing considerations, but is a less extensive study

G. Ultrasonography: non-invasive visualization of abdominal organs using high-frequency sound waves that penetrate organ and bounce back to a transducer where they are converted to an electronic pictorial image

1. Can detect organ size, cyst formation, tumors, and filling defects
2. No contrast medium or radiation is involved, so there are no contraindications and no complications

H. Computed tomography (CT) scan: radiologic procedure (with or without contrast) used to diagnose conditions such as tumors, cysts, abscesses, perforation, bleeding inflammation, aneurysms, and obstruction (see also Chapter 43)

1. Take usual precautions with use of iodinated contrast medium; contraindicated with pregnancy, unstable VS, morbid obesity, and claustrophobia

NCLEX® 2. Special nursing considerations: encourage clients to drink fluids to promote contrast elimination and monitor client for delayed reaction to contrast medium

I. Gastric analysis: stomach contents are aspirated via NG tube; pH is measured at a basal rate (BAO—basal acid output) and also during a stimulated state (MAO—maximal acid output); may be done via tubeless gastric analysis whereby a resin dye (Diagnex Blue) is ingested, gastric acid displaces dye from resin, and dye is absorbed by bowel and excreted by kidneys

1. Differentiates causes of hypergastrinemia, including **Zollinger-Ellison syndrome** (elevated gastrin levels from pancreatic tumor), chronic antacid ingestion, and atrophic gastritis
2. Frequently used to determine effect of medical or surgical antiulcer therapy

NCLEX® 3. Precautions: clients with heart failure, carcinoid syndrome, or hypertension may have symptoms exacerbated with this test because histamine is used to stimulate gastric acid

Box 55–1

Common Substances Affecting Results for Occult Blood in Stool

Causes False-Positive Results	Causes False-Negative Results
➤ Red meat	➤ Vitamin C
➤ Fish	➤ Turnips
➤ Oral iron supplements	➤ Horseradish
➤ Iodine	➤ Beets
➤ Boric acid	➤ Melons
➤ Colchicine	
➤ Drugs irritating to gastric mucosa: aspirin, NSAIDs, corticosteroids	

J. Stool examination: examines fecal specimen for obvious and occult blood and fat, assays it for clostridial toxin and cultures it for bacterial, viral, and parasitic pathogens

1. Stool culture, ova, and parasites: detects bacterial pathogens and parasitic pathogens such as (hookworm), *Strongyloides* (tape worm), and *Giardia* (protozoans)
2. Stool for occult blood: stool is tested with a reagent to detect blood that is not visible; caused by benign and malignant GI tumors, ulcers, inflammatory bowel disease, diverticulosis, and hemorrhoids; see Box 55–1 for substances that cause a false-positive or false-negative result for blood
3. *NCLEX®* Fecal fat: measures fat content of stool over 24 hours from conditions such as cystic fibrosis, celiac disease, sprue, Crohn's disease (regional enteritis), Whipple's disease, and maldigestion from pancreato-biliary tree obstruction; instruct client to abstain from alcohol and eat a diet that contains 100 grams of fat per day for 3 days before and during stool collection
4. *NCLEX®* Stool for clostridial toxin: *Clostridium difficile* bacteria release a toxin that causes necrosis of bowel epithelium; infection occurs in people who are immunocompromised or after taking broad-spectrum antibiotics

III. NURSING MANAGEMENT OF CLIENT HAVING GI SURGERY

A. ***Colostomy***: fecal diversion to an external collection device; named for portion of colon from which it is formed: ascending, transverse, descending, or sigmoid

1. Preoperative period
   - **a.** Reinforce client and family teaching about procedure and postoperative course, including pain relief, breathing exercises, and appearance of stoma (reduces client anxiety and promotes postoperative participation in care); encourage client to verbalize concerns about lifestyle changes; participate in appropriate referrals for support (such as United Ostomy Assoc.)
   - **b.** Communicate with enterostomal therapist, who will advise surgeon about optimal ostomy placement
   - *NCLEX®* **c.** Carry out bowel preparation orders, which usually include low-residue diet for 1 to 2 days before surgery; bowel cleansing with cathartics and enemas as well as oral or parenteral antibiotics (to reduce bacteria count)
   - **d.** Complete usual preoperative activities and checklist
2. Postoperative period
   - **a.** Routine care for surgical client: monitor VS and bowel sounds; monitor I&O including wound drainage and drainage from tubes (NG, urinary drainage, etc.); evaluate incision(s) and perianal area; monitor LOC and encourage deep breathing, use of incentive spirometer (IS), and splinting of incision
   - *NCLEX®* **b.** Monitor appearance and drainage from stoma, identify any changes, and notify surgeon if stoma becomes pale, darkened, cyanotic, sunken, stenosed (narrowed opening) or if bleeding increases
   - *NCLEX®* **c.** Inspect pouch system for proper fit (only ⅛ inch space between stoma and appliance) and any signs of leakage; empty when one third full; inspect skin surrounding stoma to be sure it is intact when changing ostomy appliance
   - **d.** Monitor pain control and take appropriate actions if pain is not controlled (check patency of IV access, notify physician, provide comfort measures)
   - **e.** Encourage ambulation as ordered to stimulate peristalsis
   - **f.** Resume oral intake as ordered and monitor for nausea, abdominal distension, and adequacy of bowel sounds

NCLEX® g. Begin reinforcing discharge teaching: possible postoperative complications and preventative measures (infection, bowel obstruction, abdominal abscess); colostomy care (irrigation depending on stoma location, pouch management, skin care)

B. ***Ileostomy***: large intestine is removed and fecal diversion is created at level of ileum

1. Preoperative period: same care as before colostomy surgery
2. Postoperative period
   a. Provide routine postoperative care as per colostomy surgery
   b. Apply ostomy appliance (pouch) over stoma and reinforce teaching to client and family about procedure and nature of effluent (initially dark green, more liquid than colostomy, but will thicken slightly over time and become yellow-brown)
   NCLEX® c. Protect skin around stoma with a skin barrier from irritating effects of liquid effluent, which contains digestive enzymes and bile salts
   d. Begin showing client and family early about how to manage stoma, appliance, and skin care, and when to report abnormalities in stoma, effluent, or abdomen
   NCLEX® e. Emphasize importance of good nutrition and need for adequate fluid and electrolyte intake and symptoms of an imbalance; because of liquid effluent, clients are at high risk for dehydration and electrolyte imbalance, especially during hot weather, sustained exercise, or fever

C. **Gastrectomy**: removal of stomach with anastomosis of esophagus to jejunum (esophagojejunostomy); rarely performed, usually only for extensive gastric cancer or Zollinger-Ellison syndrome unresponsive to medical treatment

1. Preoperative period
   a. Reinforce physician teaching and obtain signature on surgical consent form
   b. Reinforce what to expect postoperatively, including pain relief, breathing exercises, expected tubes (nasogastric [NG], drains, jejunostomy feeding tube), and ambulation
2. Postoperative period
   a. Monitor VS, lung and bowel sounds, I&O including drainage from NG tube, wound drainage (amount and character), effectiveness of pain-control measures
   NCLEX® b. Do not reposition, irrigate, or check placement of NG tube because of risk of disrupting esophagojejunostomy sutures (check agency policy and surgeon's orders)
   c. Implement standard postoperative care (pain management, progressive activity to ambulation)
   d. Discuss limitations in oral intake and alternate methods to maintain nutrition; may require jejunostomy tube with an elemental (requires no digestion) enteral feeding
   NCLEX® e. Reinforce information about postoperative complications, including pernicious anemia (requiring vitamin B_{12} injections monthly), abdominal abscess or infection, and decreased nutrition

D. **Gastric resection**: portion of stomach removed for diseases such as cancer and peptic ulcer disease refractory to medical management (removing antrum eliminates most gastrin-producing cells)

1. Preoperative period
   a. Insert NG tube if ordered and connect to suction (may be inserted in operating room)
   b. Provide standard preoperative care for client having abdominal surgery
2. Postoperative period
   a. Monitor VS, lung and bowel sounds, I&O including drainage from NG tube, wound drainage (amount and character), effectiveness of pain-control measures
   NCLEX® b. Do *not* reposition, irrigate, or check placement of NG tube (unless there is a specific physician order) because of risk of disrupting stomach sutures
   c. Encourage ambulation to promote peristalsis and prevent postoperative complications such as paralytic ileus and obstruction
   d. Implement standard postoperative care for clients with abdominal surgery
   NCLEX® e. Monitor for acute gastric dilation as a postoperative complication; signs and symptoms include epigastric pain, fullness, hiccups, tachycardia, and hypotension; this complication results from a malfunctioning NG tube and rapidly improves after tube is flushed (physician order) or replaced (by surgeon or designee)
3. NCLEX® **Dumping syndrome** is a common complication of gastric resection when pylorus is bypassed; after eating there is rapid emptying of food into jejunum without proper mixing and duodenal digestion
   a. Early manifestations: occur 15 to 30 minutes postprandial (after eating) and include vertigo, tachycardia, syncope, sweating, pallor, and palpitations; believed to be caused by a rapid shift of extracellular fluid into bowel to dilute hypertonic chyme, thereby decreasing blood volume
   b. Late manifestations occur 2 to 3 hours postprandial and include epigastric fullness, distension, diarrhea, abdominal cramping, nausea and high-pitched bowel sounds; caused by excessive release

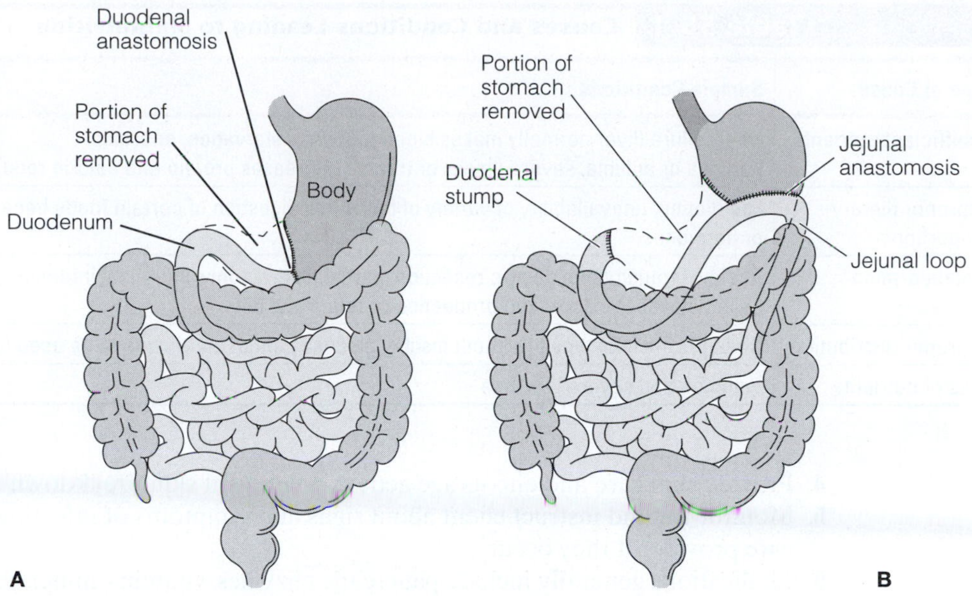

Figure 55–1

Partial gastrectomy.
A. Gastroduodenostomy or Billroth I.
B. Gastrojejunostomy or Billroth II.

of insulin in response to a rapid rise in blood glucose due to high-carbohydrate (CHO) bolus entering jejunum

c. Can be minimized by a low-CHO, high-protein, high-fat diet; suggest also that client avoid drinking fluids with meals and lie down after eating; prescribed antispasmodics or sedatives may delay gastric emptying

E. **Billroth I (gastroduodenostomy)**: a partial gastrectomy in which distal portion of stomach (including antrum) is removed and remainder is anastomosed to duodenum (see Figure 55–1A); gastrin-producing cells in antrum, as well as some parietal cells (acid-pepsinogen secreting cells), are removed

1. Preoperative and postoperative care is same as for any client having gastric surgery
2. Dumping syndrome is a common complication of this procedure

F. **Billroth II (gastrojejunostomy)**: a partial gastrectomy in which lower portion of stomach is removed and proximal remnant is anastomosed to jejunum (see Figure 55–1B); used to treat gastric and duodenal ulcers refractory to medical treatment

1. Preoperative and postoperative care is same as for any client having gastric surgery
2. *NCLEX®* Dumping syndrome is a common complication of this procedure

IV. MALNUTRITION

A. **Overview**

1. Insufficient amounts, improper proportions, malabsorption, or improper distribution of foods needed to provide body with energy for normal functions
2. Can also result from loss of nutrients as in vomiting
3. When more energy is expended than is consumed, body uses stored forms of energy in a certain order: first CHOs stored as glycogen, then fat stores, and finally protein stores in form of muscle tissue
4. *NCLEX®* Malnutrition can result from a variety of conditions (see Table 55–1)

B. **Nursing data collection**

1. Body mass index (BMI) estimates total body fat stores in relation to height and weight (weight in kg divided by body surface area)
2. *NCLEX®* Clinical manifestations include cheilosis, glossitis, stomatitis, muscle wasting, anemia, edema, alopecia, spongy bleeding gums, dry scaling skin, subcutaneous fat loss, bone pain, confusion, disorientation, paresthesia, heart failure, and decreased hair pigmentation
3. Diagnosed by history, physical exam, and laboratory results (protein, iron stores, vitamin levels, serum cholesterol, and electrolytes)

NCLEX® C. **Therapeutic management**

1. Ensure that client receives proper diet ordered (high-calorie, high-protein), and provide a pleasant dining environment, removing sources of unpleasant odors (bedpans, urinals, soiled dressings)
2. Encourage client to eat in a slow, relaxed manner
3. Provide enteral nutrition if ordered (see also Chapter 25)

Table 55–1 Causes and Conditions Leading to Malnutrition

Type of Cause	Sample Conditions
Insufficient nutrients	Liver failure (liver normally makes blood proteins), starvation, anorexia nervosa or bulimia, severe illness or trauma (increases protein and calorie requirements)
Improper dietary proportions	Fad dieting, unavailability of variety of foods, maldigestion of certain foods because of a loss of enzymes, acid, or hormones
Malabsorption	Rapid GI transit time, gastric resection, partial gastrectomy, intestinal infections, absence of some enzymes (as in celiac disease), decreased production or release of bile
Improper distribution	Diabetes mellitus type I (without insulin, glucose cannot enter cells to be used for energy)
Loss of nutrients	Vomiting and severe diarrhea

4. Provide skin care and encourage activity to prevent skin breakdown
5. Monitor for and instruct client about signs and symptoms of infection and to report them to health care provider if they occur
6. Medications generally include pancreatic enzymes, vitamins, minerals, antiemetics, antidiarrheals, antibiotics (for infectious diarrhea), insulin, and possibly total parenteral nutrition (TPN)

D. Reinforce client teaching

NCLEX® 1. Importance of adhering to diet prescription from dietitian; safe weight gain is 1–2 lbs/wk

NCLEX® 2. How to choose high-calorie, high-protein foods

3. Use of any prescribed medications for digestion, vomiting, diarrhea, or intestinal infections
4. Proper administration of enteral or parenteral feedings if prescribed

V. GASTROESOPHAGEAL REFLUX DISEASE (GERD)

A. Overview

1. Backward movement of stomach contents into esophagus without vomiting
2. Caused by relaxation of lower esophageal sphincter (LES), decreased LES tone, increased intra-abdominal pressure, increased gastric volume, or a combination (see Box 55–2 for factors influencing LES tone)
3. Reflux of gastric contents is irritating to esophagus and causes breakdown of mucosal barrier, leading to inflammation and erosion
4. Healing of esophageal erosion involves substitution of columnar epithelium (Barrett's epithelium) for normal squamous epithelium in lower esophagus
5. Barrett's epithelium resists acid (and thus supports healing) but is a premalignant tissue associated with an increased incidence of esophageal cancer
6. Occurs at any age but incidence increases over age 50; availability of over-the-counter (OTC) H_2 receptor antagonists have decreased reporting of mild cases

NCLEX® **B. Nursing data collection**

1. Heartburn or substernal burning pain is most common symptom and is exacerbated by bending over, recumbent position, or straining
2. Other symptoms include regurgitation not associated with vomiting or nausea; bad or sour taste upon awakening; coughing, hoarseness, or wheezing at night; belching, and flatulence

Box 55–2

Factors Decreasing Lower Esophageal Sphincter (LES) Tone

- Nicotine
- Caffeine (coffee, tea, cola)
- Chocolate
- Fatty foods
- Alcohol
- Peppermint, spearmint
- High levels of estrogen and progesterone
- Tight, restrictive clothing
- Bending, straining
- Hiatal hernia
- Medications: anticholinergics, beta-adrenergic blockers, calcium channel blockers, nitrates, theophylline, diazepam

3. Adult onset asthma is most often caused by GERD
4. Chronic GERD may cause dysphagia, indicating possible stricture or cancer
5. Diagnosis is most accurate through 24-hour pH monitoring
6. Esophagoscopy may be necessary in long-standing GERD to rule out malignancy

C. Therapeutic management

NCLEX® 1. Avoid foods and medication that reduce LES tone (see Box 55–2)
NCLEX® 2. Do not eat within 2 hours of bedtime or lie down after eating
3. Avoid restrictive clothing that increases intra-abdominal pressure
NCLEX® 4. Avoid large meals; eat smaller meals more often (such as six small meals/day)
NCLEX® 5. Elevate head of bed for sleeping
6. Stop smoking
7. Prescription and OTC medications
   a. Antacids neutralize stomach acid; treat mild to moderate symptoms
   b. H_2 receptor antagonists: ranitidine (Zantac), famotidine (Pepcid), nizatidine (Axid), and cimetidine (Tagamet)
   c. Proton pump inhibitors: omeprazole (Prilosec), lansoprazole (Prevacid), esomeprazole (Nexium), pantoprazole (Protonix), and rabeprazole (AcipHex)

D. Reinforce client teaching

1. Importance of smoking cessation and avoidance of caffeine
2. Avoid bending over and other activities that increase intra-abdominal pressure, especially after eating
3. Take medications as prescribed
4. Lose weight if overweight to decrease intra-abdominal pressure
5. Raise head of bed using wedge under mattress to reduce nighttime reflux

VI. HERNIAS

A. Diaphragmatic hernia in children

1. Overview
   a. A **hernia** is a protrusion of bowel through an abnormal opening in abdominal wall
   b. Congenital diaphragmatic hernia (CDH) is rare and results when abdominal contents protrude into thoracic cavity through an opening in diaphragm
   c. CDH occurs when there is failure of transverse septum and pleuroperitoneal folds to completely develop and form diaphragm
   d. Intestines and other abdominal structures enter thoracic cavity
   e. Lung growth may cease; after birth, respiration becomes further compromised by pulmonary hypoplasia and lung compression, including airways and blood vessels
2. Nursing data collection
   a. Clinical findings depend on severity of defect
   b. Fetal ultrasound shows abdominal organs in chest
   c. Postnatal diagnosis is confirmed by chest x-ray
   NCLEX® d. Diminished or absent breath sounds on affected side
   NCLEX® e. Bowel sounds may be heard over chest
   f. Cardiac sounds may be heard on right side of chest
   NCLEX® g. Dyspnea, cyanosis, nasal flaring, tachypnea, retractions
   h. Sunken abdomen, barrel-shaped chest

NCLEX® 3. Preoperative therapeutic management
   a. Monitor VS frequently with ongoing respiratory observation
   b. Elevate head of bed and position on affected side
   c. Maintain patency of NG tube to decompress stomach
   d. Monitor IV fluids
   e. Maintain mechanical ventilation, extracorporeal membrane oxygenator (ECMO), chest tubes
   f. Provide minimal stimulation

NCLEX® 4. Postoperative therapeutic management
   a. Focuses on promoting lung function
   b. Monitor for signs of infection and respiratory distress
   c. Continue to support respirations by positioning in semi-Fowler's position on affected side; organize care to decrease exertion
   d. Promote nutrition when feeding is resumed
   e. Support family through crisis

5. Reinforce client and family teaching
   a. Information for parents on wound care, prevention of infection, and feeding techniques
   b. Written and verbal information on growth and developmental needs
   c. Information regarding long-term problems and necessity of regular follow-up visits

B. Hiatal hernia in adults

1. Overview
   a. Diaphragmatic weakness through which a portion of stomach protrudes into thoracic cavity
   b. Caused by congenital weakness of diaphragm, trauma, obesity, aging, increased intra-abdominal pressure, or a combination of these factors
   c. Two major types: sliding hernia (90% of hernias), in which esophagogastric junction and portion of fundus move into thorax through esophageal hiatus; and rolling hernia (paraesophageal), in which only fundus and (less frequently) part of greater curvature roll into thorax
2. Nursing data collection
   a. Many cases are asymptomatic
   NCLEX® b. Symptoms include heartburn (pyrosis), substernal burning or pain, feeling of fullness, dysphagia, belching; these are usually worse when reclining
   c. Diagnosed by upper GI series and symptom history
3. Therapeutic management
   NCLEX® a. Conservative treatment: diet therapy and lifestyle modifications (same as discussed for GERD)
   NCLEX® b. Avoid straining
   c. Avoid excessive vigorous exercise
   NCLEX® d. Sleep with head of bed elevated 8 to 12 inches
   e. Assist client in decision making about surgical procedure (used only when conservative treatment has failed)
   f. Nissen fundoplication (used for GERD as well) most common; fundus of stomach is wrapped 360 degrees around lower portion of esophagus
   g. Hill repair: similar to Nissen repair but fundus is wrapped around esophagus only 180 degrees
   h. Provide preoperative and postoperative care as discussed previously for client undergoing gastric surgery
   NCLEX® i. Medication therapy: antacids and H_2 receptor antagonists (see treatment for GERD)
4. Client teaching
   a. Report any increase in symptoms
   b. Do not take antacids within 2 hours of other medications
   NCLEX® c. Avoid alcohol, caffeine, NSAIDs, and any medication containing aspirin (such as Alka-Seltzer)
   d. Reinforce diet and lifestyle modifications

C. Umbilical hernia

1. Overview
   a. A soft, skin-covered protrusion of intestine and omentum (double fold of peritoneum) through a weakness in abdominal wall around umbilicus
   b. In an umbilical hernia, incomplete closure of umbilical ring results in protrusion of portions of omentum and intestine through opening
   c. Defect usually closes spontaneously by age 3 or 4 years; surgical correction is needed if closure does not occur or if incarceration of herniated bowel occurs
   d. Most common in low-birthweight infants or black infants and commonly occurs in children with Down syndrome, hypothyroidism, and Hurler syndrome
NCLEX® 2. Nursing data collection
   a. Soft swelling or protrusion around umbilicus, usually reducible using a finger
   b. An incarcerated hernia is one that cannot be reduced and increases risk of bowel ischemia; it produces symptoms such as irritability, tenderness at site, anorexia, abdominal distention, and difficult defecation
3. Therapeutic management
   a. Most umbilical hernias disappear spontaneously by 1 year of age
   NCLEX® b. No surgical repair is needed unless it causes symptoms, persists past 5 years of age, becomes strangulated, or continues to grow
   c. Binding is not effective in reducing or minimizing the protrusion
   d. Monitor for changes in size of hernia
   NCLEX® e. Monitor for increased bowel sounds and irreducible mass, which may indicate strangulation
   NCLEX® f. Postoperatively, inspect for wound infection, maintain hydration, monitor and manage pain, allow for self-expression

4. Reinforce client and family education
   a. Signs of strangulation, such as vomiting, pain, and an irreducible mass at umbilicus; signs and symptoms of wound infection
   NCLEX® b. Avoid ineffective and potentially harmful home remedies such as "belly binders"
   c. Any precautions and restrictions, such as tub bathing or strenuous activity if surgery was performed

VII. PEPTIC ULCER DISEASE (PUD)

A. Overview

1. A generic term for ulcers or breaks in mucosal lining of GI tract that come in contact with gastric secretions; can occur in stomach (gastric ulcers, less common), duodenum (duodenal ulcers, more common), or lower esophagus (esophageal ulcers, rare)
2. Gastric ulcer
   a. Occurs most often on lesser curvature near pylorus
   b. Results from a disruption in normal protective mechanism that keeps gastric epithelial pH normal
   c. Prostaglandins in gastric mucosa increase resistance to acid; therefore, medications that reduce prostaglandins (such as aspirin, NSAIDs, alcohol), will decrease gastric mucosal resistance
   d. Gastric ulcers are associated with *H. pylori*, gastritis, alcohol, smoking, use of NSAIDs, stress, and an increased incidence of gastric cancer
3. Duodenal ulcer
   a. A chronic break in duodenal mucosa to muscularis mucosae layer; is most common type of ulcer
   b. Results from increased gastric acid from increased number of parietal cells, vagal activity, or secretion of gastrin
   c. Rarely associated with an increase in gastric cancer
   d. Associated with chronic *H. pylori* infection, alcohol, smoking, cirrhosis, and stress
4. Etiology and pathophysiology of PUD
   a. *H. pylori* is associated with a majority of duodenal ulcers
   b. Chronic NSAID use (aspirin is worst) is associated with increased risk for gastric ulcers
   c. Other factors that increase risk for PUD include cigarette smoking, family history, blood group O (duodenal ulcer), alcohol use
   d. Incidence of ulcers increases steadily with age and peaks in sixth decade
   e. Men and women are affected equally

NCLEX® B. Nursing data collection

1. Pain: gnawing, burning, aching, hungerlike, in epigastrium
2. Duodenal ulcers: pain relieved by eating
3. Gastric ulcers: pain not relieved by food and may be exacerbated by food
4. Upper GI series often done initially; diagnosis is made most conclusively by EGD
5. Tests for *H. pylori* usually positive
6. Observe for complications: perforation (pain, signs of peritonitis, shock), hemorrhage (hematemesis, tarry stool, stool positive for occult blood), or pyloric obstruction (vomiting, feeling of fullness)

C. Therapeutic management

1. Reinforce importance of following treatment plan to reduce symptoms
2. NCLEX® No foods are known to be ulcerogenic but some foods aggravate active PUD (coffee, cola, tea, chocolate, foods high in sodium, and spicy foods) and should be avoided during acute phase; even decaffeinated coffee stimulates gastrin release
3. Provide smoking cessation information and refer to smoking cessation program
4. NCLEX® Medication therapy
   a. Antacids are used to neutralize acid
   b. H_2 receptor antagonists block histamine-stimulated gastric secretions; proton pump inhibitors suppress the production of hydrochloric acid
   c. Prostaglandin analogs: misoprostol (Cytotec) contributes to mucosal barrier preventing NSAID-induced ulcers
   d. Mucosal barrier fortifier: sucralfate (Carafate) forms protective barrier over ulcer crater and prevents further erosion by acid and pepsin
   e. Treatment for *H. pylori* changes frequently but generally includes antimicrobials such as metronidazole (Flagyl) or erythromycin, proton pump inhibitors, and bismuth subsalicylate (Pepto-Bismol)

D. Reinforce client teaching

1. Take medications as prescribed
2. Learn signs of complications: blood in stool, vomiting, increased pain
3. Follow diet recommendations restricting caffeine, alcohol, and nicotine

VIII. IRRITABLE BOWEL SYNDROME (IBS)

A. Overview

1. Common noninflammatory functional bowel disorder also known as spastic bowel, functional colitis, and mucous colitis; is a motility disorder of lower GI tract
2. Cause is unknown, but aggravating factors are stress, anxiety, depression, certain foods and food additives in some clients, drugs, toxins, and hormones
3. There is no change in physical characteristics of intestinal mucosa
4. Usually manifests in three patterns: predominantly diarrhea, predominantly constipation, or combination of diarrhea and constipation; each pattern may or may not include abdominal pain

B. Nursing data collection

NCLEX® 1. Abdominal pain: relieved by defecation, intermittent and colicky, or continuous and dull

NCLEX® 2. Change in bowel motility and character
   a. Diarrhea or constipation
   b. Presence of mucus
   c. Feeling of incomplete evacuation
   d. Possible bloating, flatulence, urgency

3. Diagnosis is made by excluding organic causes of symptoms
4. Sigmoidoscopy may show spastic contractions that may be painful; mucosa is normal in appearance

C. Therapeutic management

1. Possibly tegaserod maleate (Zelnorm)

NCLEX® 2. Dietary fiber 30–40 grams/daily may help in predominantly constipation type

3. Assist client to identify and eliminate foods that exacerbate problem

NCLEX® 4. Common offenders: fruit, berries, lettuce, lactose, caffeinated drinks, preservatives (sodium sulfite), alcohol

5. Encourage relaxation and stress reduction; regular exercise may help control symptoms
6. Medication therapy
   a. No standard pharmacologic treatment

NCLEX® b. Bulk-forming agents (Metamucil, Fibercon) may help predominantly constipation-type IBS

NCLEX® c. Antidiarrheal agents (Imodium, Lomotil) may be used for predominantly diarrhea-type IBS

   d. Antidepressants, anxiolytics, antispasmodics, or anticholinergics may be used

D. Reinforce client teaching

1. Information about fiber content of various foods
2. Importance of following prescribed regimen
3. Encourage bathroom privacy and a regular time for defecation
4. Information about programs of relaxation or support groups

IX. CHRONIC INFLAMMATORY BOWEL DISEASE (IBD)

A. Ulcerative colitis

1. Overview
   a. Area of chronic inflammation of mucosa and submucosa in colon and rectum
   b. Peak incidence is between 15 and 35 years of age with a second peak between age 50 and 70
   c. Characterized by periods of exacerbation and remission
   d. Cause is unknown but may be related to stress, genetics, infection, dietary factors (low fiber intake), or antibody formation
   e. Inflammation (at base of crypts of Lieberkuhn, usually in rectum) develops into abscesses that penetrate mucosa and spread laterally
   f. Begins in rectum and can progress proximally, but is usually limited to sigmoid colon and rectum
   g. Can range in severity from mild to severe

NCLEX® 2. Nursing data collection
   a. Diarrhea; 10 to 20 liquid stools per day often containing blood and sometimes mucus; nocturnal diarrhea is common
   b. May report fatigue resulting from blood loss, lack of sleep, and/or fluid imbalance
   c. May affect quality of life; client may be afraid to leave house because of severe diarrhea
   d. Complications include hemorrhage, abscess formation, toxic megacolon, malabsorption, bowel obstruction, bowel perforation, increased risk of colon cancer, and extraintestinal symptoms (arthritis, uveitis)
   e. Diagnosed by sigmoidoscopy: characteristic edematous, friable mucosa with a granular appearance with evident crypt abscesses; lesions are contiguous

3. Therapeutic management
   a. Provide standard pre- and post-sigmoidoscopy or colonoscopy care
NCLEX® b. Rest is required to decrease intestinal activity
NCLEX® c. Diet therapy may include a low-residue, high-protein, high-calorie diet with vitamins and iron; in severe cases, nothing by mouth (NPO) to rest bowel; TPN will be ordered in severe cases
   d. Surgery (proctocolectomy with colostomy or ileostomy) may be needed if IBD not controlled medically
   e. Encourage client to talk about concerns related to disease and effect on lifestyle
NCLEX® f. Medications: corticosteroids during exacerbations to decrease bowel inflammation; salicylate compounds (sulfasalazine [Azulfidine], mesalamine [Asocol]) to decrease prostaglandin formation and bowel inflammation; immunomodulators such as azathioprine (Imuran) to alter immune response; antidiarrheals for symptom management
4. Reinforce client teaching
   a. Take medications as ordered
NCLEX® b. Avoid foods that exacerbate symptoms: raw vegetables and fruits, whole-grain breads and cereals, seeds, nuts, popcorn, and any highly spiced or flavorful food
   c. Notify health care provider if symptoms increase or there is blood in stool
   d. Information about ulcerative colitis support groups
   e. Importance of good perianal skin care to prevent complications
   f. Exacerbation and remission nature of disease and symptom management
   g. Postoperative stoma and incision care if applicable as described in earlier section

B. Crohn's disease (regional enteritis)

1. Overview
   a. Chronic inflammation of GI mucosa occurring anywhere from mouth to anus but most often in terminal ileum
   b. Characterized by exacerbations and remissions
   c. Cause is unknown, but possible factors are autoimmune, genetics, infectious agents, and environmental (stress)
   d. Lesions extend to all thicknesses of bowel wall and are prone to fistula formation
   e. Lesions have a "cobblestone appearance" with sections of normal mucosa between lesions called "skip" lesions
   f. Over time, chronic inflammation causes fibrotic changes in bowel wall, leading to obstruction
   g. Depending on severity and location of lesions, malabsorption may occur as well as losses of protein from lesions themselves
2. Nursing data collection
NCLEX® a. Diarrhea (5–6 liquid to semiformed stools/day) is most common symptom (usually without blood); depending on location, steatorrhea (fatty stool) may occur
NCLEX® b. Abdominal pain in RLQ that is unrelieved by defecation
NCLEX® c. Systemic signs include fever, fatigue, malaise, weight loss
   d. Complications include abscess and fistula formation, intestinal obstruction, malnutrition, and bowel perforation; hemorrhage is uncommon
   e. Barium enema and upper GI series often show areas of ulceration, narrowing, strictures, and fistulas; upper GI tract shows classic "string sign" of terminal ileum
   f. Diagnosed by colonoscopy; characteristic aphthoid ulcers, strictures, and segmental involvement is visualized; lesion is biopsied
   g. Laboratory tests (serum albumin, folic acid, hemoglobin, and hematocrit) monitor for complications and rule out other causes of diarrhea
3. Therapeutic management
NCLEX® a. Provide prescribed diet: usually high-calorie, high-protein; involve client in making appropriate menu choices
   b. Encourage intake of prescribed nutritional supplements
NCLEX® c. Weigh daily, maintain calorie count, and monitor I&O
   d. Allow client to express fears and anxiety about course of illness and possible surgery (not as common as for ulcerative colitis because is not necessarily curative)
NCLEX® e. Medications are same as for ulcerative colitis (antidiarrheals, salicylate-containing compounds, corticosteroids, immunomodulators)
   f. Metronidazole (Flagyl), a broad-spectrum antimicrobial, may also be given
   g. Antispasmodics decrease abdominal cramping after eating
   h. TPN may be ordered during periods of severe exacerbation to provide total bowel rest

4. Reinforce client teaching
   a. Information about disease, medications and diet
   b. Signs of complications: increased pain, rectal bleeding, fever, chills, lethargy
   c. If TPN is ordered, information about proper catheter care and administration techniques
   d. Nutritional supplements, such as Ensure, may enhance optimum nutrition

X. DIVERTICULITIS

A. Overview

1. Inflammation of diverticula, which are outpouchings in intestinal wall (diverticulosis is presence of multiple diverticula)
2. Most diverticula occur in sigmoid colon; incidence increases with age
3. Caused by increased pressure in intestinal lumen and herniation of mucosa through defects in bowel wall; decreased fecal bulk (low-fiber diet) contribute to bowel wall hypertrophy and result in increased intraluminal pressure
4. Diverticula become inflamed when undigested food or bacteria are trapped; abscess formation contributes to disease and diverticulum may rupture

B. Nursing data collection

NCLEX® 1. Pain, usually in LLQ, ranging in severity from mild to severe and can be constant or cramping; if perforation occurs, abdominal pain is generalized
NCLEX® 2. Most cases of diverticular disease are asymptomatic
NCLEX® 3. May note pattern of constipation alternating with increased bowel movements
NCLEX® 4. Fever, chills, and tachycardia along with generalized abdominal pain may indicate perforation of diverticulum and onset of peritonitis
5. Diverticular disease is diagnosed with barium enema, but is contraindicated when diverticulitis is present because of risk of rupturing diverticulum when barium is instilled
6. CT scan or ultrasonography can diagnose acute diverticulitis

C. Therapeutic management

NCLEX® 1. Reinforce dietary modifications to reduce complications of diverticulosis
   a. Bowel rest: NPO or low-residue diet during initial acute phase
   b. High-fiber diet after acute phase
   c. Addition of bran to everyday foods
   d. Common advice is to avoid intake of nuts, seeds, and foods with small seeds such as berries and figs
2. Monitor for signs of bleeding: check stool for occult blood
3. Prepare for possible surgery; colon resection is done in 25% of cases of diverticulitis
NCLEX® 4. Medication therapy includes antibiotics to decrease bowel flora and reduce infection, opioid analgesics to relieve pain, and stool softeners, although laxatives and enemas are contraindicated

D. Reinforce client teaching: fiber content of various foods, self-administration and side effects of medications, signs and symptoms of complications of diverticulitis

XI. INTESTINAL OBSTRUCTION

A. Overview

1. Failure of bowel contents to move forward; can be partial or complete
2. Mechanical obstruction results from forces outside of intestines, (adhesions, hernia, fibrosis); or blockage in lumen (fecal impaction, edema, tumor, stricture, volvulus, intussusception)
3. Nonmechanical obstruction or paralytic ileus results from impairment of muscle tone or nervous system innervation preventing forward movement of intestinal contents (anesthesia, abdominal surgery, spinal injuries, peritonitis, vascular insufficiency)
4. Obstructions occur most often in ileum where intestinal diameter is smallest
5. Peristalsis increases in intestine above blockage, leading to increased secretions, edema, and increased capillary permeability and resulting in fluid and electrolyte imbalances and hypovolemia

B. Nursing data collection

NCLEX® 1. Early in bowel obstruction, bowel sounds may be high-pitched and tinkling proximal to obstruction and hypoactive or silent distal to obstruction
NCLEX® 2. Late in bowel obstruction bowel sounds become absent
3. Abdominal pain can be colicky and more intense as obstruction progresses
NCLEX® 4. Vomiting is common and may have a fecal odor
NCLEX® 5. Abdominal distension is common, and peristalsis may be visible in early stages of obstruction

NCLEX® 6. Vital signs may be normal in early obstruction but client can demonstrate signs of shock as obstruction progresses (tachycardia, fever, tachypnea, hypotension)
7. Diagnosed by history, physical findings, and abdominal x-ray; dilated loops of bowel can be seen (barium studies are contraindicated)

C. Therapeutic management

1. Prepare client for possibility of surgery: exploratory laparotomy, colon resection, colostomy
2. Prepare client for insertion of nasogastric or nasointestinal tube
3. Provide mouth care to minimize effect of fecal-type secretions
4. NCLEX® Provide IV therapy as prescribed
5. NCLEX® Maintain NPO status until peristalsis returns
6. Provide comfort measures such as frequent position changes
7. NCLEX® Monitor VS including I&O; early detection of hypovolemic shock can prevent complications (bowel ischemia and necrosis)
8. NCLEX® Monitor level of pain; sudden change in nature of pain may indicate complications (ischemia and necrosis)
9. Monitor progression and drainage from intestinal tube
10. NCLEX® Medication therapy
    a. Analgesics are generally limited because opioids decrease GI motility, which further compromises bowel
    b. IV fluid with appropriate electrolyte replacement prevents hypovolemia and shock

D. Reinforce client teaching

a. Information about insertion and maintenance of NG tube or intestinal tube
b. Postoperative use of incentive spirometer, coughing and deep breathing exercises, ambulation, activity, and wound care
c. Importance of maintaining a healthy lifestyle on discharge
d. Provide support to client and family in coping with possibility of a colostomy

XII. JAUNDICE

A. Overview

1. Yellow-orange discoloration of skin and mucous membranes; caused by a disturbance of bilirubin metabolism causing ***hyperbilirubinemia*** (serum bilirubin greater than 2.5 mg/dL); also known as icterus
2. Associated with diffuse hepatocellular disorders or present in newborns because of impaired bilirubin uptake and conjugation
3. Hyperbilirubinemia and jaundice can result from hemolysis or from disorders of bile ducts (obstruction) or liver cells
4. Caused by accumulation of bilirubin pigments in skin and can be classified as obstructive or hemolytic
5. Obstructive jaundice is classified as extrahepatic (gallstones or tumor, with increased direct bilirubin) or intrahepatic (drug reactions or hepatitis, with increased indirect bilirubin)
6. Hemolytic jaundice is caused by excessive breakdown of red blood cells (RBCs)
    a. Amount of bilirubin produced exceeds liver's ability to conjugate it, so level of unconjugated or indirect bilirubin in serum increases
    b. Unconjugated bilirubin is insoluble in water and is not found in urine; causes include blood transfusion reactions, membrane defects of RBCs, severe infection, or toxic substances

NCLEX® **B. Nursing data collection**

1. Recent appetite and color of urine and stool
2. Abdominal swelling, RUQ pain, and hepatomegaly
3. Yellowish discoloration of skin and mucous membranes
4. Scleral icterus (yellowish discoloration of sclera)
5. Pruritus (severe itching) because of accumulation of bilirubin in skin
6. Elevation of conjugated bilirubin that causes urine to be dark (tea- or cola-colored); may be present before jaundice appears
7. Complete obstruction of flow of bile into duodenum causes light or clay-colored stools
8. Jaundice caused by an infectious process may be accompanied by fever and chills
9. Any client with liver dysfunction or injury may experience nausea, anorexia, and/or fatigue
10. Laboratory findings (see also Chapter 42)
    a. Increased indirect bilirubin: hepatocellular failure, hemolytic jaundice
    b. Increased direct bilirubin: obstructive causes of jaundice

c. An elevated urine bilirubin level is always caused by an increased level of direct bilirubin (it is water-soluble, and indirect bilirubin is not)
d. Alanine aminotransferase (ALT): elevation indicates damage to liver cells and helps rule out hemolysis as cause of jaundice
e. Aspartate aminotransferase (AST): elevated, but levels vary depending on type of jaundice; with hepatitis, levels can be elevated 20 times above normal, gallstones can cause levels ten times above normal
f. ALT and AST ratios; used to help diagnose causes of liver dysfunction
g. Alkaline phosphatase (ALP): increased with both extrahepatic and intrahepatic biliary obstruction
h. Radiologic procedures can help confirm infiltrative or cholestatic processes; abdominal ultrasound and CT scans can detect tumors, stones, and other focal liver lesions that may be causing jaundice

C. Therapeutic management

1. Aimed at symptom management and includes keeping client comfortable
2. *NCLEX®* Often clients are kept NPO pending diagnostic testing and because food increases pain secondary to stimulation of GI tract
3. *NCLEX®* IV hydration and pain management are important aspects of care
4. Management is aimed at treating cause of jaundice
5. *NCLEX®* Cool or tepid baths containing colloidal substances (oatmeal, cornstarch, soybean powder) can reduce or ease pruritus
6. Cool room (68–70°F) with 30–40% humidity
7. *NCLEX®* Use an emollient lotion rather than one containing alcohol, which is too drying
8. *NCLEX®* Medication therapy: there is no specific medication therapy for jaundice
   a. Topical corticosteroids may provide some relief
   b. Bile-sequestering agents remove excess bile from fat deposits under skin, decreasing pruritus

D. Reinforce client teaching

1. Required diagnostic tests
2. Disease process causing jaundice and future management
3. Causes of jaundice are usually correctable
4. Avoid alcohol and acetaminophen, since both can cause further liver damage

XIII. HEPATITIS

A. Overview

1. An inflammation of liver; ranges greatly in severity and can be caused by several different viruses, toxins, or disease states
2. Hepatitis viruses cause local necrosis of parenchymal cells of liver; inflammatory response leads to swelling and blockage of liver's drainage system
3. Hepatitis occurs in varying levels of severity from asymptomatic or mild cases, in which liver cells regenerate completely in 2–3 months, to more severe forms, in which hepatic necrosis and death may occur in 1–2 weeks
4. Forms of hepatitis (see Table 55–2)
5. Hepatitis A
   a. Sources include contaminated food, water, and shellfish; may also be contracted from contact with infected persons
   b. Highly contagious and easily spread throughout households and daycare centers
   c. Client is most contagious 10–14 days prior to onset of symptoms when fecal shedding of virus is greatest
   d. Is usually self-limiting
6. Hepatitis B
   a. Risk increases with multiple sex partners, in men who have sex with other men, and IV drug users; health care workers comprise a small percentage of cases
   b. Transmitted also through contaminated blood or blood products; clients who require hemodialysis are also at risk
   c. Can progress to a chronic form of disease; is a common cause of cirrhosis and hepatocellular carcinoma
7. Hepatitis C
   a. Is also called post-transfusion hepatitis; most common cause of chronic hepatitis
   b. Blood transfusions, sexual contact, sharing contaminated needles, and unintentional needlesticks account for a significant number of cases
   c. Up to 80% of clients develop chronic hepatitis, which is a risk factor for liver failure and hepatocellular carcinoma

Table 55-2 Forms of Hepatitis

Virus	Route of Transmission	Incubation Period	Lab Results	Vaccine Preventable	Carrier State
Hepatitis A (HAV)	Fecal–oral	2–6 weeks	Anti-HAV antibodies	Yes	No
Hepatitis B (HBV)	Blood and body fluids; perinatal	6–24 weeks	Positive HBsAG (surface antigen); anti-HBV antibodies	Yes	Yes
Hepatitis C (HCV)	Blood and body fluids	5–12 weeks	Anti-HCV antibodies	No	Yes
Hepatitis D (HDV)	Blood and body fluids; perinatal	3–24 weeks	Positive HDVAg (antigen); anti-HDV antibodies	No	Yes
Hepatitis E (HEV)	Fecal–oral	3–6 weeks	Anti-HEV antibodies	No	Yes

8. Hepatitis D is also known as Delta-agent hepatitis, and occurs only in people infected with hepatitis B (depends on HBV virus to replicate)
9. Hepatitis E is often transmitted by infected water supply; is uncommon in United States
10. Acute fulminating hepatitis: a rare but rapidly progressive form that leads to bleeding problems, hepatic encephalopathy, ascites and acute liver failure within 2–3 weeks of onset of symptoms

B. Nursing data collection

NCLEX® 1. A range of symptoms occurs, including anorexia, nausea, vomiting, malaise, fever, jaundice, and abdominal pain secondary to liver swelling; client may show signs of dehydration if vomiting is severe

NCLEX® 2. Course of acute viral hepatitis is divided into three phases
   a. Prodromal (preicteric) phase (most contagious) occurs before jaundice appears, about 2 weeks after exposure to virus, and includes flulike symptoms (general malaise, GI complaints such as nausea, vomiting, diarrhea, and anorexia), headache, fatigue, myalgia, joint pain, and low-grade fever; food odors, smoking, or alcohol may trigger nausea
   b. **Icteric** phase is marked by onset of jaundice; occurs about 2 weeks after prodromal phase and lasts 2–6 weeks; includes dark-colored urine and clay-colored stools before appearance of jaundice and pruritis; liver remains enlarged and possibly tender to touch
   c. Recovery (posticteric) phase begins with resolution of jaundice and lasts several weeks, during which symptoms improve, energy levels increase, and serum enzymes normalize

3. Acute infection with hepatitis C is generally asymptomatic, although some clients develop malaise, weakness, and anorexia
4. Diagnostic and laboratory test findings
   a. Antibodies to specific virus (see again Table 55–2)
   b. Alkaline phosphatase (ALP); nonspecific test to evaluate liver or bone dysfunction; can be elevated with hepatitis
   c. Gamma-glutamyl transferase (GGT); acutely elevated with alcohol consumption and hepatotoxic drugs
   d. Transaminases: ALT and AST; elevated to varying degrees with hepatitis caused by hepatocyte injury
   e. Bilirubin; both direct and indirect levels can be elevated secondary to liver cell injury
   f. Prothrombin time (PT); prolonged if liver is injured to point that it can no longer produce proteins necessary for blood coagulation

C. Therapeutic management

NCLEX® 1. Includes both pre- and postexposure prophylaxis for forms A and B as well as symptom management
   a. With cases of hepatitis A, controlling spread of infection is a major nursing focus; includes reporting to local public health department; exposed individuals should receive immune globulin as soon as possible; those at risk should receive vaccine
   b. With cases of hepatitis B, prevention is major health focus; hepatitis B vaccines are begun during neonatal period and are recommended for all infants as part of well-child care

NCLEX® 2. Use standard precautions and meticulous hand hygiene for all forms, but especially for hepatitis A (client, family, and staff)

NCLEX® 3. Hepatitis A precautions include private bathroom and proper bagging, cleansing, and disposal of contaminated items

NCLEX® 4. Provide antiemetic medications as ordered and encourage a diet high in CHO and low in fat

NCLEX® 5. Abstinence from alcohol is essential

6. If liver function is compromised, protein and salt should be restricted

NCLEX® 7. Encourage a good breakfast; clients tend to become more nauseous later in day
8. Initiate intravenous (IV) fluids as ordered
9. Monitor for signs of dehydration and monitor electrolyte status
NCLEX® 10. Encourage bedrest initially and very gradual increase of activity as tolerated
11. Plan nursing activities to allow for adequate rest
12. Inform clients they may never donate blood
13. Observe for blood in stool or urine, multiple ecchymosis, petechiae, or oozing of blood from gums or minor cuts, which may indicate a complication
14. Medication therapy
    a. Aimed at symptom relief; consists of antiemetics and analgesics; because most analgesics are metabolized in liver, their use must be limited
    b. IV fluids may be necessary if client is unable to tolerate oral fluids
    NCLEX® c. Prophylaxis may be considered if client has known HAV exposure and is early in incubation period
    NCLEX® d. Vaccination for hepatitis B is available; given as a series of three intramuscular injections to adults, children, and infants; second and third injections are given at 1 and 6 months after initial injection; efficacy of vaccination approaches 95%
    NCLEX® e. Postexposure vaccination for hepatitis B is recommended for clients in contact with infected blood or body fluids, those who have sexual contact with infected individuals, and infants exposed to a caregiver with known HBV infection or born to a mother with known HBsAg
    f. Hepatitis C: combination therapy is used for 12 to 18 weeks or as long as 48 weeks with interferon alfa-2b and ribavirin therapy
    g. Hepatitis D: there are no medications specific to treatment of HDV
    h. Vitamin K is indicated if PT is prolonged
    i. Antihistamines can be given for pruritis

D. Reinforce client teaching

1. Hepatitis A and E: detailed information about disease and prevention of transmission, need for meticulous hand hygiene, and need to avoid sharing eating utensils, bath towels, and other personal care items that are in contact with body fluids
2. Safe sex practices are a general health measure (hepatitis B, C, D) as well as vaccination and prevention of disease transmission according to type
NCLEX® 3. Avoid alcohol and any drugs that may be hepatotoxic (such as acetaminophen)
4. Importance of follow-up and possibility of developing chronic active hepatitis

XIV. CIRRHOSIS

A. Overview

1. Irreversible and chronic liver disease characterized by diffuse inflammation and fibrosis of liver tissue, which cause scarring and obstruction of hepatic blood flow
2. Three classifications: alcoholic, biliary, and postnecrotic
    a. Alcoholic cirrhosis (most prevalent type) is caused by prolonged, excessive alcohol intake with or without malnutrition; is directly related to toxic effects of alcohol on liver
    b. Biliary cirrhosis is caused by obstruction of bile canaliculi and ducts and results in necrosis and fibrosis; cause can be autoimmune or result from tumors, gallstones, or chronic pancreatitis
    c. Postnecrotic cirrhosis results from a chronic, severe liver disease such as hepatitis; is also caused by inherited metabolic liver disorders such as Wilson's disease
3. Regardless of cause, cirrhosis develops slowly; severity and rate of progression depend on cause and repeated injury to hepatocytes
4. Disruption of portal blood flow secondary to structural changes in liver results in edema, ascites, splenomegaly (from splanchnic venous congestion), portal hypertension (see next section), hemorrhoids, varicose veins, and esophageal varices (see section that follows)

B. Nursing data collection

NCLEX® 1. See Box 55–3
2. Vital signs: orthostatic measurement of BP and pulse, temperature and weight
3. Nutritional status: muscle atrophy and wasting
4. Decreased ability to metabolize CHOs leads to hypoglycemia, decreased energy, and alterations in glycogenolysis, glyconeogenesis, and glycogenesis
5. Altered fat metabolism causes increased synthesis of fatty acids and triglycerides leading to fatty liver and hepatomegaly

NCLEX®
6. Altered protein metabolism leads to low albumin levels and, with decrease in osmotic pressure and development of edema and ascites; decreased protein also decreases production of clotting factors, which increases risk of bleeding
7. Decreased metabolism of sex steroids (estrogen, progesterone, and testosterone) leads to gynecomastia, loss of body hair, development of palmar erythema and spider angiomata, erectile dysfunction, and menstrual disorders
8. Decreased metabolism of aldosterone results in sodium and water retention and worsening edema and **ascites** (fluid in peritoneal cavity)

NCLEX®
9. Decreased metabolism of ammonia leads to increased serum ammonia levels and hepatic encephalopathy (manifests as lack of coordination, decreased memory, lack of orientation, and coma)
10. Decreased stores of vitamins and minerals leads to malnutrition, fatigue, and anemia
11. Obstruction of bile flow leads to hyperbilirubinemia and jaundice, clay-colored stools, dark-colored urine
12. Splenomegaly leads to pancytopenia
13. Fibrosis and scarring continue, resulting in increased portal pressure that causes ascites, hemorrhoids, esophageal varices, caput medusa (superficial abdominal veins)

NCLEX®
14. Involuntary tremor or flapping of the hands is called liver flap or **asterixis**

NCLEX®
15. Liver biopsy is only definitive way to diagnose type of cirrhosis; may not be necessary if client has clinical manifestations with supportive risk factors; may not be advisable because prolonged PT would place client at increased risk for bleeding; see also Chapter 43
16. No laboratory tests will diagnose cirrhosis, but ordered tests are similar to those discussed for hepatitis
17. Findings include varying degrees of increased transaminases, decreased albumin, prolonged PT, hyperbilirubinemia, hyponatremia from excess free water, hypokalemia from diuretic therapy, and hypomagnesemia
18. Complete blood count (CBC) reflects pancytopenia (anemia, thrombocytopenia, leukopenia)

Box 55-3

Signs and Symptoms of Cirrhosis

- General malaise
- Skin
  - Pruritis
  - Jaundice and scleral icterus
  - Spider angiomata and telangiectasia
  - Ecchymoses, petechiae, hematomas, and propensity for bleeding
  - Edema
- Gastrointestinal
  - Nausea and vomiting
  - Anorexia, weight loss/malnutrition
  - Pyrosis
  - Clay-colored stools
  - Constipation
  - Flatulence, hemorrhoids
- Abdomen
  - Change in bowel sounds
  - Pain or tenderness in RUQ
  - Hepatomegaly, splenomegaly
  - Ascites (increasing abdominal girth)
  - Abdominal pain (RUQ)
  - Positive fluid wave
  - Shifting dullness
  - Caput medusa
- Neurological
  - Fatigue
  - Disorientation
  - Decreased level of consciousness
  - Encephalopathy
  - Asterixis (flapping tremor of hand from increased ammonia levels)
  - Decreased deep-tendon reflexes (DTRs)
- Pulmonary
  - Decreased breath sounds in bases (may indicate pleural effusion)
  - Crackles (might indicate development of heart failure)
- Reproductive
  - Gynecomastia
  - Testicular atrophy
  - Erectile dysfunction
  - Menstrual irregularities
- Palmar erythema
- Anemia
- Loss of body hair
- Dark urine

19. Elevated serum ammonia level
20. Liver ultrasound may reveal an enlarged fibrofatty liver or a small fibrotic and nodular liver; highly dense areas may reflect possible hepatocellular carcinoma

C. Therapeutic management

1. Abdominal **paracentesis** for only severe ascites; is an invasive procedure that drains fluid from abdomen via a needle; fluid is often sent for culture; ensure client is sitting in straight-back chair with bowel and bladder emptied before procedure
2. NCLEX® Surgical intervention to relieve portal hypertension and prevent reaccumulation of ascitic fluid: insertion of a LeVeen shunt or transjugular intrahepatic portosystemic shunt (TIPS)
3. NCLEX® Fluid-restriction to prevent further accumulation of ascitic fluid
4. NCLEX® Diet restrictions include decreased protein intake (to prevent encephalopathy) and low sodium intake to prevent worsening of ascites
5. NCLEX® Provide small, frequent meals
6. Weigh daily, and monitor I&O
7. NCLEX® Measure abdominal girth each day or shift as ordered to monitor ascites
8. NCLEX® For respiratory support, use high Fowler's position and use supplemental O_2 as ordered; encourage deep breathing; allow activity as tolerated; measure O_2 saturation and ABGs as ordered
9. Maintain skin integrity; remove moist linens promptly; keep skin clean and moistened with emollient; administer antihistamines as ordered for itching; encourage activity as tolerated, or reposition every 2 hours
10. NCLEX® Institute bleeding precautions as needed: prevent constipation, avoid injections, observe for signs of bleeding, encourage use of soft toothbrush, monitor labs (CBC, PT)
11. Determine understanding of illness; identify support system; determine coping skills; offer clergy support; encourage Alcoholics Anonymous for those with cirrhosis secondary to alcohol dependence; provide substance abuse referrals as indicated
12. Medication therapy
    a. NCLEX® Diuretics are given cautiously to promote excretion of excess fluid to decrease ascites; most commonly used drugs are spironolactone (Aldactone), a potassium-sparing diuretic, and furosemide (Lasix), a loop diuretic
    b. NCLEX® Lactulose (Cephulac) is a disaccharide laxative that is not absorbed by GI tract; it pulls water into bowel and helps to decrease absorption of ammonia
    c. Other medications include vitamin K to treat prolonged PT, antihistamines, and antiemetics

D. Reinforce client teaching

1. Lifestyle changes include dietary restrictions, abstinence from alcohol, fluid restrictions; suggest nutrition consultation
2. Reduce intake of foods high in sodium; avoid canned and frozen foods, highly processed cheeses, potato chips, and other salty foods
3. NCLEX® Limit intake of foods high in protein: eggs, cheese, milk, and meats
4. Avoid taking any OTC medications without checking with health care provider first because many are hepatotoxic (such as acetaminophen)
5. Signs and symptoms that require medical attention after discharge: weight gain, increased abdominal girth, respiratory distress, bleeding gums, blood in the stool or urine, fever, abdominal pain
6. How to adjust dose of lactulose according to number of loose stools per day (usually three)
7. Involve family and other support persons in client's care

E. Complications of cirrhosis

1. **Portal hypertension**
    a. An abnormally high BP within portal venous system; most commonly caused by cirrhosis but also caused by hepatitis or infection, hepatic vein thrombus, tumor, or right heart failure (any condition that impedes blood flow through portal venous system or vena cava)
    b. Clinical manifestations include all findings described with cirrhosis
    c. Other potentially fatal conditions that can develop as a result of portal hypertension are varices, ascites, hepatic encephalopathy leading to coma, and hepatorenal syndrome (see discussion of these conditions later in chapter)
    d. NCLEX® Most common clinical manifestation is vomiting of blood (**hematemesis**) secondary to rupture of esophageal varices; clients with oozing varices may present with anemia and melanotic stools
    e. Splenomegaly can result from increased pressure within splenic vein, which branches off portal vein
    f. Clients may report irritation from hemorrhoids or may present with bright red rectal bleeding secondary to hemorrhoids

g. Therapeutic management is same as treatment of cirrhosis and is based on symptomatic treatment of varices, ascites, encephalopathy, and hepatorenal syndrome

NCLEX® h. Medication therapy: aimed at decreasing portal venous pressure without causing hypotension; diuretics and fluid restriction are treatments of choice; propranolol (Inderal), a beta-blocker, has also been used to decrease portal venous pressures

2. **Esophageal varices**

a. Develop from increased portal pressure; are distended and tortuous vessels that can rupture secondary to coughing, sneezing, vomiting, or ingestion of foods high in roughage; bleeding can be abrupt and painless; ruptured esophageal varices are considered a medical emergency

NCLEX® b. Clinical manifestations: if bleeding is slow, melena and decreasing hemoglobin and hematocrit are present, but if bleeding is abrupt, severe hematemesis and signs of hypovolemic shock (tachycardia, hypotension) can occur

NCLEX® c. Therapeutic management: includes stopping bleeding either by **sclerotherapy** (injection of sclerosing drugs) or **esophageal tamponade** (direct pressure using Sengstaken-Blakemore or Minnesota tube with esophageal and gastric balloons); keep scissors at bedside to cut tube if tube position changes and airway is comprosmised; see also Chapter 27

NCLEX® d. Sclerotherapy and banding are accomplished via endoscopy; physician locates bleeding vessel via endoscope and injects a sclerosing agent (causes thrombosis and hemostasis); may be done emergently or as an elective procedure

e. Maintain airway, breathing, and circulation and measure VS

f. Start two large-bore IVs with infusion of normal saline (NS) as ordered

g. Draw serum laboratory tests (CBC, type and cross-match, chemistries)

h. Begin gastric **lavage** (irrigation) if ordered

i. Keep clients NPO for both sclerotherapy and esophageal tamponade (if elective); explain procedure and give a mild pre-procedure sedative as ordered

j. Prepare client for transfer to a setting with cardiac monitoring capability

NCLEX® k. Administer vasopressin via IV intermittent or continuous infusion, usually given once a cardiac monitor is in place; lowers portal pressure and controls bleeding by causing splanchnic vasoconstriction; use with caution in clients with cardiac disease

l. Administer propranolol (Inderal), a beta-blocker that reduces portal pressure, or sandostatin (Octreotide), which decreases splanchnic blood flow and subsequent bleeding from esophageal varices

3. **Ascites**

a. Accumulation of plasma-rich fluid within peritoneal cavity secondary to portal hypertension, increased aldosterone, and decreased oncotic pressure (from decreased circulating albumin levels, called **hypoalbuminemia**); cirrhosis is common cause; kidneys retain sodium and thus water, further increasing third-spaced fluid and anasarca (generalized body edema)

NCLEX® b. Clinical manifestations: abdominal distention, weight gain, increased abdominal girth, dilated abdominal veins (caput medusa), generalized edema, and respiratory distress if accumulation of ascitic fluid is large

NCLEX® c. Therapeutic management includes paracentesis to remove fluid; diuretics; shunting devices (to treat portal hypertension)

d. Monitor fluid and electrolyte status; give fluids as ordered

e. Monitor daily weights and measure abdominal girth every 8 to 24 hrs

f. Restrict intake of dietary protein and sodium

g. Provide education about disease process and diagnostic tests

h. Monitor for respiratory distress from upward pressure on diaphragm; monitor VS for hypotension and/or tachycardia

4. **Hepatic encephalopathy**

a. A neurological complication caused by accumulation of toxic substances (primarily ammonia) in blood

NCLEX® b. Clinical manifestations: loss of memory, irritability, confusion, lethargy, sleep disturbances, stupor, coma, and asterixis

NCLEX® c. Therapeutic management: aimed at reducing production of nitrogenous wastes (urea) and ammonia, correcting fluid and electrolyte imbalances, and eliminating use of sedating drugs and drugs metabolized by liver

d. Perform frequent neurologic observation to note progression of lethargy

e. Restrict dietary protein as ordered

f. Avoid sedating medications

g. Monitor for fluid and electrolyte imbalances and implement prescribed corrective measures
h. Treat cause of liver disease by implementing ordered therapies
NCLEX® i. Administer lactulose (Cephulac) as ordered, a hyperosmolar laxative that prevents absorption of ammonia and produces diarrhea
j. Neomycin is sometimes used to reduce bacteria in bowel, thus limiting further ammonia production; use with caution because of nephrotoxicity

5. **Hepatorenal syndrome**
a. Renal failure associated with advanced liver failure and caused by circulatory alterations without primary renal disease; most commonly found in alcoholic cirrhosis and fulminant hepatitis; results in sudden renal failure possibly from diuretics, characterized by intrarenal vasoconstriction, oliguria, azotemia, anorexia, and fatigue; is associated with a poor prognosis
NCLEX® b. Clinical manifestations include decreased urine output (UO), hyponatremia, decreased urine osmolality, hypotension, jaundice, ascites, possible GI bleeding, increased BUN and creatinine
c. Treat fluid and electrolyte imbalances and encephalopathy with aim of restoring renal and liver function
NCLEX® d. Eliminate nephrotoxic or hepatotoxic drugs (such as neomycin sulfate)
e. Liver transplantation is definitive treatment
NCLEX® f. Hemodialysis is used to treat hyperkalemia and fluid overload
g. Carefully note I&O and daily weights
h. Provide anticipatory teaching about treatments and procedures

XV. CANCER OF LIVER

A. Overview

1. Most commonly occurs as metastasis from lung, breast, kidney, and GI cancers
2. Primary liver cancer (hepatoma) is uncommon in United States and more prominent in areas with increased chronic liver disease (Africa, Asia); it carries a poor prognosis
3. Tumors arise in liver cell (hepatocellular) or bile duct (cholangiocellular)
4. Tumor can be diffuse, nodular, or single nodule; compresses surrounding cells and can invade blood supply, causing necrosis or hemorrhage
5. Most primary hepatic cancers in United States result from cirrhosis, hepatitis B or C, aflatoxin (toxin from *Aspergillus* mold exposure), chronic alcohol consumption, and nonalcoholic fatty liver

B. Nursing data collection

NCLEX® 1. RUQ pain or mass; feeling of fullness in epigastric region
NCLEX® 2. Fatigue and general malaise
NCLEX® 3. Anorexia and weight loss
NCLEX® 4. Later signs can include ascites, fever, jaundice, variceal bleeding, liver failure, and splenomegaly
5. Laboratory findings vary according to degree of liver damage
a. CBC: anemia
b. Hyperbilirubinemia
c. Prolonged PT
d. Elevated ESR due to liver inflammation
e. Hypoalbuminemia when there is malnutrition, liver failure
f. Elevated alkaline phosphatase, AST, ALT when there is liver failure or damage
g. Altered blood glucose due to liver damage
h. AFP (alpha-fetoprotein): high elevations in 70% of those with hepatocellular cancer
6. Ultrasound, CT scan, or MRI may reveal focal liver lesions
7. Definitive diagnosis is made through biopsy or aspiration of lesion

C. Therapeutic management

1. Partial hepatectomy for individuals with solitary lesions and without extrahepatic manifestations; serial AFPs are done postoperatively to determine effect on eradicating cancer
2. Liver transplant may be done for clients meeting established surgical criteria
NCLEX® 3. Radiation therapy (palliative measure) may shrink tumor or reduce pain or pressure on surrounding structures
4. Chemotherapy as a primary therapy has limited response; sometimes chemotherapy is infused via hepatic arterial pump
NCLEX® 5. Provide pain control measures and evaluate effectiveness
6. Provide care as outlined for other complications of liver failure or other disorders
NCLEX® 7. Medication therapy: chemotherapy and other medications commonly used to treat liver disease

D. Reinforce client teaching

1. Disease process, expected outcomes, and chemotherapy
2. Etiologic agents that cause or contribute to development of hepatic cancer
3. Refer to prior sections for other teaching points related to liver disease and its complications

XVI. CHOLELITHIASIS

A. Overview

1. Cholelithiasis (gallstones) can occur anywhere in biliary tree, although most are located within gallbladder; 80% are composed of cholesterol, 20% have a mixture of bile components (pigmented); may be asymptomatic
2. Cholesterol stones (usually several) develop slowly; are hard, white, or yellow-brown, radiolucent; can be up to 4 cm in size; are enhanced by production of mucin glycoprotein, which traps cholesterol and leads to stasis of bile
3. Pigmented stones form because of an increase in unconjugated bilirubin and calcium with a concurrent decrease in bile salts; usually develop within the intra- and extrahepatic ducts and are preceded by bacterial invasion
4. Increased bile concentration, bile stasis, and hypercholesterolemia contribute to stone formation
5. Risk factors associated with the formation of gallstones are listed in Box 55–4

B. Nursing data collection

1. *NCLEX®* Classic manifestations include severe and steady epigastric or RUQ pain that radiates to right scapula or shoulder; sudden onset, lasting 1–3 hours
2. *NCLEX®* May occur after a high-fat meal
3. *NCLEX®* Other symptoms include nausea, vomiting, heartburn, and flatulence
4. Fever and chills occur with acute cholecystitis
5. Biliary colic or cramping pain occurs when stone is lodged in cystic or common bile duct; if stone blocks duct, edema and inflammation of gallbladder (cholecystitis) occur and may be associated with jaundice
6. Physical exam findings include positive Murphy's sign (palpation of RUQ causes severe pain with inspiration); bowel sounds may be absent
7. Jaundice is not usually seen unless common bile duct is blocked
8. Laboratory findings include elevated WBC count (infection), increased serum bilirubin levels (stone in biliary ductal system causing obstruction), possible electrolyte depletion secondary to vomiting or anorexia; elevated liver function tests (LFTs) with hepatic involvement or damage caused by bile duct obstruction
9. Abdominal x-rays (flat plate) may reveal stones; however, most stones are not radiopaque
10. Ultrasonography is used to identify stones, gallbladder, and ductal dilatation in nonobese clients
11. Oral cholecystogram is not used as frequently as ultrasound for diagnosis of stones; involves ingestion of oral dye to determine ability of gallbladder to concentrate and excrete bile; outlines stones for visualization
12. Gallbladder scans: cholescintigraphy-nuclear medicine scan to evaluate for acute cholecystitis; also called HIDA, DIDA, or DISIDA scans

Box 55–4

Risk Factors for Gallstones

- Increasing age
- Female gender
- Family history (may relate to familial high dietary fat intake and sedentary lifestyle)
- Obesity and hyperlipidemia
- Rapid weight loss (very low calorie diet, bariatric surgery)
- Biliary stasis from pregnancy, prolonged TPN or fasting state
- Use of estrogen-containing medications (oral contraceptives, hormone replacement therapy)
- Comorbid medical diagnoses: Crohn's disease or ileal resection, diabetes mellitus, cirrhosis, sickle cell anemia
- Native American and Northern European ethnicity

C. Therapeutic management

1. Oral ursodiol (Actigall) or chenodiol (Chenix) reduce cholesterol in stones to help dissolve them; is useful for clients who are poor surgical risks or refuse surgery; effective for small cholesterol stones and not as effective for stones with high calcium content; full treatment can take 2 years or more and recurrence rate is high once drug therapy is stopped

NCLEX® 2. Extracorporeal shock wave **lithotripsy** uses shock waves to disintegrate stones; oral dissolution therapy is used postprocedure to dissolve stone fragments; clients may experience biliary colic postprocedure when gallbladder is contracting to pass stone fragments

NCLEX® 3. Endoscopic retrograde cholangiopancreatography (ERCP) uses a fiberoptic endoscope to visualize biliary tree, remove stones, drain bile sludge, and collect biopsies

NCLEX® 4. Laparoscopic cholecystectomy is less invasive than ERCP and involves shorter hospital stay; abdomen is insufflated with CO_2; laparoscope is introduced through a small incision, and gallbladder is deflated and removed through small abdominal incision

5. Cholecystectomy: surgical removal of gallbladder; occasionally a T-tube is placed in common bile duct to assist passage of bile until edema has decreased; bile collects in a bag by gravity drainage
6. Implement comfort measures, including prescribed analgesics and antiemetics
7. Provide education regarding diagnostic tests and disease process
8. Maintain NPO status preprocedure as ordered; institute IV fluids as ordered
9. Provide diet instruction regarding low-fat diet, frequent small meals
10. Encourage obese individuals to lose weight
11. Monitor fluid and electrolyte balance
12. Medication therapy
    a. Treatment of pain and nausea with prescribed analgesics (morphine as opioid during acute attack) and antiemetics
    b. Cholestyramine (Questran) is used for severe cases of pruritus; binds bile salts to hasten excretion through feces
    c. Ursodiol (Actigall) or chenodiol (Chenix) to dissolve cholesterol stones; ursodiol is often well tolerated but chenodiol frequently causes diarrhea and is hepatotoxic (requiring monitoring of liver enzymes)

D. Reinforce client teaching: disease process and gallstone formation; diagnostic procedures and expected outcomes; diet instruction to limit high-fat foods

XVII. CHOLECYSTITIS

A. Overview

1. An acute or chronic disorder, cholecystitis most often caused by gallstones obstructing cystic duct, resulting in a distended and inflamed gallbladder; pain is similar to that of gallstones
2. Approximately 5% of clients develop acalculous cholecystitis precipitated by trauma, prolonged TPN, fasting, or surgery

NCLEX® **B. Nursing data collection**

1. Clinical manifestations include all of those previously identified for cholelithiasis
2. Fever, leukocytosis, elevated serum bilirubin (possible jaundice) and alkaline phosphatase, elevated amylase with pancreatic duct involvement
3. Abdominal guarding, rigidity, and rebound tenderness suggest peritoneal involvement
4. Diagnostic and laboratory testing as outlined for cholelithiasis

NCLEX® **C. Therapeutic management**

1. NPO with IV fluids for hydration until the pain subsides
2. Opioid analgesics (usually morphine) are used for pain control
3. IV antibiotics are administered
4. Surgery is postponed until acute infectious process has subsided

D. Reinforce client teaching

1. Preoperative teaching
2. Some clients will be discharged to home and return after a period of convalescence for elective cholecystectomy

E. Surgical intervention for disorders of gallbladder

1. Laparoscopic cholecystectomy: removal of gallbladder through a small abdominal incision guided by a fiberoptic endoscope
2. Cholecystectomy: removal of gallbladder through a RUQ abdominal incision
3. Cholecystectomy with T-tube placement (less common): gallbladder is removed and a T-tube is placed within common bile duct to facilitate bile flow through edematous ducts postprocedure

NCLEX® 4. Postoperative nursing care
   a. Prevent infection: administer IV antibiotics as ordered, keep incision clean and dry; perform abdominal testing for peritonitis every 4 hours; monitor VS, report any temperature over 100°F
   b. Prevent pain: administer pain medication as ordered; instruct client to request pain medication before pain becomes too intense; medicate for pain prior to postoperative exercise/ambulation; keep client comfortable to promote pulmonary hygiene because incision is near diaphragm
   c. Prevent pulmonary infection: keep client comfortable to promote turning every 2 hours, coughing, deep breathing; reinforce importance of incentive spirometry every hour postoperatively
   NCLEX® d. Maintain clients with T-tube in Fowler's position to promote gravity drainage of bile; report bile drainage in excess of 500 mL in first 24 hours; should be less than 200 mL daily in 2 to 3 days
   e. Reinforce that T-tube is removed when bile drainage has subsided and stools have returned to a normal brown color
   f. Inspect surrounding skin for inflammation secondary to bile leakage
   g. Reinforce proper handling of tube for turning and ambulating
   h. Maintain NPO status as ordered; advance diet as tolerated
   i. Monitor bowel sounds and encourage ambulation to promote peristalsis
   j. Prevent deep-vein thrombosis with leg exercises, frequent ambulation, sequential compression devices, and elastic hosiery
   k. Provide general postoperative instruction before discharge about wound care, analgesia, diet, and signs of infection

XVIII. ACUTE PANCREATITIS

A. Overview

1. Obstruction to flow of pancreatic enzymes results in inflammation of pancreas
2. Can be mild, severe, or fulminant
3. Alcohol abuse and gallbladder disease (obstructive cholelithiasis causing reflux of bile into pancreas) are major causes; other causes are PUD, medications (thiazide diuretics, NSAIDs, estrogens, steroids, salicylates) and hyperlipidemia
4. Injury to pancreas or obstruction of pancreatic duct results in leakage of pancreatic enzymes into pancreatic tissue, leading to autodigestion of pancreas
5. Pain is caused by edema and stretching of pancreatic capsule and chemical irritation; pain may be referred to back because of retroperitoneal location of pancreas
6. Enzymes break down pancreatic tissue, causing inflammation, edema, damage to blood vessels, hemorrhage, and necrosis of pancreatic tissue (which can then form walled-off abscesses); leakage of enzymes into bloodstream can cause further systemic complications and possibly death
7. Excess hydrochloric acid secretion from chronic alcohol ingestion causes spasms of sphincter of Oddi and ampulla of Vater, which also obstruct flow of pancreatic enzymes
8. Fatty necrosis is normally present with fulminant disease and involves pancreas as well as thoracic and abdominal cavities
9. Types include acute interstitial edematous pancreatitis, necrotizing pancreatitis, biliary pancreatitis, and alcoholic pancreatitis

B. Nursing data collection

1. Clinical manifestations vary with severity of attack
2. NCLEX® Acute epigastric pain, steady and severe, can occur in umbilical area and radiate to back; it may be temporally associated with ingestion of alcohol or a fatty meal
3. NCLEX® Pain is greater when lying supine and improves with sitting up and leaning forward, flexion of knee, or fetal positioning
4. NCLEX® Nausea and vomiting is common and is worse with any oral intake; vomiting does not relieve abdominal pain
5. VS: fever (rarely above 102°F), hypotension, and tachycardia
6. NCLEX® Leukocytosis, hyperglycemia (as high as 500–900 mg/dL), and elevated amylase (for 48 hours) and lipase (for 5–7 days); increased urinary amylase
7. Abdominal tenderness, rigidity, progressive distention, and decreased bowel sounds
8. Fulminant disease can progress to hypovolemic shock, ascites, jaundice, and renal failure
9. NCLEX® Grey Turner sign is a bluish discoloration over flank area and represents accumulation of blood in that area
10. NCLEX® Cullen sign is a bluish discoloration around umbilicus
11. Hypocalcemia if calcium is sequestered by fat necrosis in abdomen, sign of severe pancreatitis
12. Elevated C-reactive protein indicates severity of disease

13. Alcohol abusers may have hypomagnesemia and hypoalbuminemia
14. Pancreatitis with liver involvement shows elevated bilirubin and LFTs
15. Abdominal x-ray identifies ascites, gallstones
16. Abdominal ultrasound identifies gallstones, pancreatic mass, or pseudocyst
17. NCLEX® CT scan is gold standard to visualize size of pancreas and to identify fluid collections, abscesses, masses, and areas of hemorrhage or necrosis
18. Chest x-ray identifies pleural effusion caused by enzymatic irritation from leaking pancreatic fluid

C. Therapeutic management

1. Treatment is aimed at supportive care, preventing further pancreatic autodigestion and preventing systemic complications
2. NCLEX® NPO status with NG tube if there is ileus or protracted vomiting or to decrease gastric secretions that stimulate pancreatic secretions
3. IV hydration to prevent hypotension and shock
4. NCLEX® TPN if needed for prolonged episodes; reverses catabolic state
5. Possible peritoneal lavage to remove toxic exudates from abdominal cavity
6. ERCP to remove retained or obstructing gallstones or to perform a sphincterotomy
7. Surgical removal of gallbladder for gallstones after acute pancreatitis is resolved
8. Surgical removal and drainage of pseudocyst or abscess may be needed
9. Administer pain medications as ordered and on regular schedule
10. NCLEX® Monitor VS, daily weights, hourly UO, bowel sounds, and stool chart (frequency, color, odor, and consistency)
11. NCLEX® Monitor respiratory function; provide pulmonary hygiene measures to prevent pneumonia
12. NCLEX® Provide diet instruction (several small meals; no alcohol allowed) when oral feeding is resumed (usually when amylase level returns to normal and abdominal pain subsides)
13. NCLEX® Maintain bedrest during acute phase and increase as tolerated
14. Medication therapy
    a. Opioids and antiemetics
    b. Gastric protection with IV H_2 blocker: ranitidine (Zantac) or proton pump inhibitiors such as pantoprazole (Protonix)
    c. Antispasmodics such as dicyclomine (Bentyl)
    d. Electrolyte replenishment as indicated by laboratory tests
    e. Insulin as required to regulate serum glucose levels
    f. Antibiotics as ordered for infection

D. Reinforce client teaching

1. Disease process and expected outcomes
2. Nutrition; explain necessity for NPO status during acute phase and rationale for several small meals with no alcohol allowed once diet resumes
3. NCLEX® Importance of taking enzyme replacement to prevent malnutrition and weight loss
4. Some clients (especially those with alcoholism) may develop chronic pancreatitis with recurrent epigastric and LUQ pain, anorexia, nausea, vomiting, weight loss, constipation, flatulence and steatorrhea (fatty stools); these clients may require long-term pancreatic enzyme replacement

XIX. CANCER OF PANCREAS

A. Overview

1. Most involve cancer of ductal epithelium and are adenocarcinomas; occurs most often after age 50
2. NCLEX® Is associated with cigarette smoking, environmental toxins, and a diet high in fat and/or meat
3. Other risk factors include diabetes mellitus, chronic pancreatitis, and hereditary pancreatitis
4. Usually located in head of pancreas, deep within tissue, often causing obstruction of common duct
5. Metastasis almost always occurs prior to symptoms with invasion of tumor into posterior wall of stomach, duodenal wall, colon, and common bile duct

B. Nursing data collection

1. NCLEX® Slow onset with anorexia, nausea, weight loss, flatulence, and dull epigastric pain
2. Later pain is severe, is worse when lying down, and is unrelated to meals
3. Jaundice, pruritis, clay-colored stools, and dark urine when bile duct is involved
4. NCLEX® Classic signs and symptoms with advanced disease include pain, jaundice, and weight loss
5. Some clients may have a palpable abdominal mass or ascites
6. Diarrhea and steatorrhea occur late in disease
7. Development of diabetes mellitus from impaired insulin production

8. Diagnostic tests same as for pancreatitis, jaundice, and cholelithiasis
9. MRI and CT scan reveal a mass, and CT-guided needle biopsy provides histological diagnosis

NCLEX® **C. Therapeutic management**

1. Most clients do not present for treatment until cancer is too advanced, and thus treatment is in many cases aimed at supportive or palliative care
2. ERCP may be performed to place stents within ductal system to facilitate bile drainage
3. Surgical management
   a. Gastrojejunostomy: bypasses duodenum
   b. Choledochojejunostomy: relieves biliary obstruction
   c. Pancreatoduodenectomy (Whipple's procedure): surgical removal of head of pancreas, entire duodenum, distal third of stomach, a portion of jejunum, and lower half of common bile duct
4. Chemotherapy and radiation therapy are usually adjuncts to surgery
5. *NCLEX®* Provide supportive care, reinforce information regarding treatment options and assist with educated decision making
6. Pain management is integral to quality of life; administer analgesics as ordered and determine effectiveness for appropriate discharge regimen
7. Provide preoperative teaching if client elects to have surgery
8. Provide information about support groups
9. Medication therapy
   a. No specific medications for treatment of pancreatic cancers
   b. All medications are aimed at controlling symptoms: pain, nausea, vomiting
   c. Chemotherapy is rarely effective and is used most often for palliative treatment

D. Reinforce client teaching: disease process and poor prognosis; importance of pain control and symptom relief; importance of abstinence from smoking and alcohol

XX. CLEFT LIP AND CLEFT PALATE

A. Overview

1. Cleft lip is a congenital anomaly involving one or more clefts in upper lip; degree of cleft varies from a small notch to a complete separation (see Figure 55–2)
2. Cleft palate is a congenital anomaly consisting of a cleft ranging from soft palate involvement alone to a defect including hard palate and portions of maxilla in severe cases
3. Causes include hereditary, environmental, and teratogenic factors
4. Both anomalies occur during embryonic development; cleft lip results from failure of fusion of lateral and medial tissues forming upper lip around 7 weeks gestation; cleft palate is a failure of fusion of tissues forming palate around 9 weeks' gestation

B. Nursing data collection (defects are readily apparent at birth)

1. *NCLEX®* Cleft lip involves a notched upper lip border, nasal distortion, and may include unilateral or bilateral involvement
2. *NCLEX®* Cleft palate is a visible or palpable gap in uvula, soft palate, hard palate, and/or incisive foramen with exposed nasal cavities and associated nasal distortion
3. Perform careful physical observation to rule out other midline birth defects

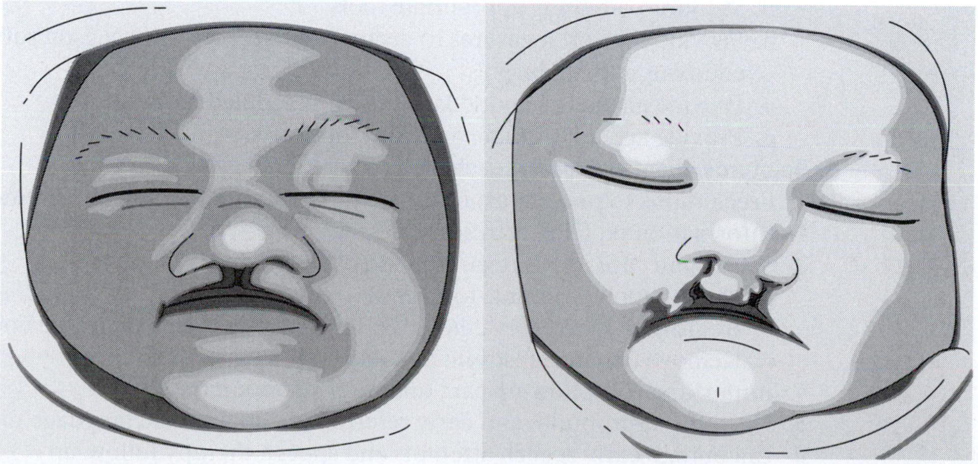

Figure 55–2

Cleft lip. *A.* Unilateral. *B.* Bilateral.

A B

C. Therapeutic management

NCLEX® 1. Depending on severity of defect and infant's general health, cleft lip is often surgically corrected around 3 months of age; cleft palate is generally repaired before age 18 months; cleft palate may be corrected through several operations performed in stages

2. Early correction of cleft palate enables development of more normal speech patterns and proper dentition; delayed closure of large defects may require use of orthodontic devices

3. Preoperative nursing care
   - a. Monitor respiratory status continuously during feedings (risk of aspiration)
   - NCLEX® b. Feed infant in upright position
   - c. Feed slowly and burp infant frequently

Memory Aid

Use ESSR: *E*nlarged nipple, *S*timulate suck by rubbing nipple on lower lip, *S*wallow, *R*est after each swallow to allow for complete swallowing.

   - NCLEX® d. Use alternate feeding devices such as elongated nipple (lamb's nipple) or breast shield
   - e. Note degree of cleft and ability to suck
   - f. Provide postoperative feeding instructions
   - g. Encourage parents to verbalize fears, concerns, negative emotions
   - h. Facilitate grief responses of shock, denial, anger, and mourning
   - i. Encourage touching, holding, cuddling, and bonding
   - j. Provide parents with pictures of other children before and after surgical repair
   - k. Discuss infant's positive characteristics
   - l. Describe community resources and parent support groups

4. Postoperative care
   - a. Monitor for respiratory distress; monitor lung sounds and encourage deep breathing without placing stress on suture line
   - b. No oral temperatures
   - c. Advance feedings as tolerated
   - NCLEX® d. No straws, pacifiers, spoons, or fingers in or around mouth for 7 to 10 days
   - NCLEX® e. For cleft lip, resume preoperative feeding techniques; a metal appliance or adhesive strips may be used to prevent tension on surgical site
   - NCLEX® f. For cleft palate, liquids can be taken from a cup; no straws are allowed; soft foods can be taken from side of spoon; to reduce risk of injury, child is not allowed to feed self
   - g. Clean lip from suture line out after feedings and prn
   - h. Apply antibacterial ointment as ordered
   - i. Use elbow restraints to keep infant from putting fingers in mouth or touching surgical site
   - NCLEX® j. No tooth brushing for 1–2 weeks
   - k. Place infant in side-lying position on unaffected side to avoid excessive contact with bed linens
   - NCLEX® l. Monitor site for redness, swelling, excess bleeding, purulent drainage, or fever
   - m. Monitor pain using appropriate tools
   - n. Provide comfort measures to decrease stress, such as crying, on suture line; encourage rocking, cuddling, and holding
   - o. Provide analgesics and sedatives on a scheduled basis
   - p. Provide age-appropriate activities for diversion

D. Reinforce client and family teaching

1. Precautions to prevent aspiration and phone numbers in case of emergency
2. Information on CPR certification
3. NCLEX® Safety and care issues regarding use of restraints
   - a. Do not apply restraints too tightly
   - b. Remove at least every 2 hours and play games to encourage flexion
   - c. Remove only one restraint at a time
4. Importance of follow-up care and referral appointments
5. Need for appropriate and early referrals for speech and language disabilities
6. Encourage early speech attempts and speech therapy follow-up
7. Encourage good dental hygiene and orthodontic follow-up

XXI. PYLORIC STENOSIS

A. Overview

1. Occurs when circular muscle of pyloric canal hypertrophies and impedes gastric emptying into the duodenum; inflammation and edema develop, which then lead to complete obstruction
2. Exact cause remains unknown; often there is a positive family history of disorder
3. Other risk factors are hypergastrinemia (too much gastrin in blood), infusion of prostaglandin E to treat patent ductus arteriosus, and treatment with oral erythromycin at less than one month of age
4. Pyloromyotomy (creation of an incision along anterior pylorus to split the muscle) is commonly performed to relieve obstruction

B. Nursing data collection

NCLEX® 1. Previously healthy infant with progressive, projectile, nonbilious vomiting
NCLEX® 2. Movable, palpable, firm, olive-shaped mass in RUQ
3. Visible, deep, peristaltic waves from LUQ to RUQ immediately before vomiting
4. Irritability, hunger, and crying
5. Sunken fontanels, poor skin turgor, dry mucous membranes, decreased urine output, constipation, jaundice, metabolic alkalosis
6. Ultrasonography and upper GI series may reveal delayed gastric emptying and an elongated pyloric canal
7. Laboratory findings: possible increased pH and bicarbonate level (metabolic alkalosis), decreased serum chloride, sodium, and potassium levels, and increased hematocrit and hemoglobin (hemoconcentration)

C. Therapeutic management

1. Monitor skin turgor, mucous membranes, and fontanels at least every shift, monitor urine specific gravity, weigh daily
NCLEX® 2. Maintain NPO status prior to surgery, monitor I&O hourly, administer IV fluids and electrolytes as ordered
3. Maintain NG tube patency and monitor NG output
4. Keep infant warm and quiet
NCLEX® 5. Initiate small, frequent feedings of clear liquids within 4–6 hours after surgery; follow strict diet regimen of gradual advancement of feedings until normal formula feedings have been resumed
6. Continue IV hydration until age- or weight-appropriate amounts of formula are tolerated
NCLEX® 7. Monitor incision for redness, swelling, and drainage; immediately report signs of infection to physician
8. Monitor VS at least every 4 hours
9. Encourage parental involvement and rooming-in

D. Reinforce client and family teaching

1. Explanation of what pyloric stenosis is and its treatment, including equipment such as NG tube and IV
2. Discharge instructions: report any vomiting, abdominal tenderness, fever, incisional redness, or drainage to physician
3. Verbal and written feeding instructions if child has not returned to full-strength formula feedings prior to discharge
4. Importance of follow-up care with physician

XXII. OMPHALOCELE AND GASTROSCHISIS

A. Overview

1. Omphaloceles are congenital malformations in which intra-abdominal contents herniate through umbilical cord
    a. Results from failure of abdominal contents to return to abdomen when abdominal wall begins to close by tenth week of gestation
    b. Viscera is outside of abdominal cavity but inside translucent sac covered with peritoneum and amniotic membrane
    c. May be associated with other congenital anomalies such as cardiac defects or an associated chromosomal anomaly
2. Gastroschisis occurs when bowel (usually small intestine and ascending colon) herniates through abdominal wall defect, usually to right of umbilical cord, and through rectus muscle; there is no membrane covering exposed bowel
    a. Uncertain etiology; tends to occur more often in young mothers who smoke
    b. Viscera is outside of abdominal cavity and not covered with peritoneal sac
    c. Rarely associated with other major congenital anomalies, but jejunoileal atresia, ischemic enteritis, and malrotation may occur as a result of defect itself

B. Nursing data collection

NCLEX® 1. With gastroschisis, there is obvious protrusion of abdominal contents present at time of delivery

NCLEX® 2. With omphocele, size of sac varies depending on extent of protrusion; rupture of sac results in evisceration of abdominal contents and needs to be prevented

3. Defect may be noted on prenatal ultrasound

C. Therapeutic management

1. Monitor body temperature continuously using skin probe; place infant in warmer immediately after birth

NCLEX® 2. Use sterile technique when handling or working with defect

NCLEX® 3. Immediately cover with sterile gauze soaked with warm sterile normal saline for irrigation, and place infant feet first into a "bowel bag" that extends to nipple line and is securely tied to preserve heat and allow visualization of defect

4. Minimize movement of infant and handling of intestines

5. Observe respiratory status continuously during immediate newborn period by placing on cardiac and apnea monitor with pulse oximetry

6. Monitor for circulatory compromise by monitoring temperature, pulses, capillary refill, skin color, and heart rate and respiratory rate

NCLEX® 7. Inspect mucous membranes for moisture and skin for elastic turgor; monitor I&O, weigh daily, inspect fontanels, monitor electrolytes, maintain IV, and administer fluids and TPN as ordered

8. Maintain NG tube for decompression and NPO status

NCLEX® 9. Monitor for signs of ileus by auscultating bowel sounds, measuring abdominal girth, assessing bowel movements

10. Anticipate surgical correction as single procedure or in stages depending on severity

11. Monitor parents' coping mechanisms and encourage them to verbalize feelings of loss of "perfect" child and guilt that may accompany congenital anomaly; encourage parental participation in infant's care

D. Reinforce family teaching

1. Written and verbal information on growth and developmental needs
2. Appropriate techniques for developmental stimulation
3. Information regarding support groups and other community resources
4. Signs of bowel obstruction and when to notify health care provider

XXIII. BILIARY ATRESIA

A. Overview

1. A progressive inflammation that causes both intrahepatic and extrahepatic bile duct fibrosis
2. Etiology is unknown; because problem originates during prenatal period, viruses, toxins, and chemicals are a few suspected causes
3. Obstruction of extrahepatic bile ducts causes obstruction of normal flow of bile from liver into gallbladder and small intestine
4. Bile plugs form and cause bile accumulation in liver
5. Inflammation, edema, and irreversible hepatic injury occur
6. Liver becomes fibrotic; cirrhosis and portal hypertension develop, leading to liver failure

NCLEX® 7. Because of lack of bile in intestines, fat and fat-soluble vitamins cannot be absorbed, resulting in malnutrition, fat-soluble vitamin deficiency, and growth failure

8. Without treatment, this disease is fatal
9. Treatment involves surgery (Kasai procedure) to temporarily correct obstruction and supportive care
10. Liver transplantation is eventually necessary

B. Nursing data collection

1. Healthy-appearing infant at birth

NCLEX® 2. Jaundice occurs within 2 weeks to 2 months

NCLEX® 3. **Acholic** stools: puttylike, clay-colored stools

4. Abdominal distention and hepatomegaly

NCLEX® 5. Increased bruising of the skin, prolonged bleeding time

NCLEX® 6. Intense itching

NCLEX® 7. Tea-colored urine

8. Increased bilirubin levels; ultrasound and liver biopsy confirm disorder

C. Therapeutic management

NCLEX® 1. Weigh daily

NCLEX® 2. Administer TPN with or without lipids as ordered

3. Administer fat-soluble vitamins A, D, E, and K as ordered

NCLEX® 4. Monitor stool pattern

5. Establish an open, caring relationship with family

6. Refer parents to support groups

D. Reinforce client and family teaching

1. Need for meticulous skin care
2. Verbal and written information regarding nutritional needs
3. Instructions on home medication regimen; allow time for return demonstration
4. Signs and symptoms for which to call the physician
5. If a transplant is performed, include detailed information on post-transplant medications

XXIV. HIRSCHSPRUNG'S DISEASE

A. Overview

1. A congenital anomaly resulting from an absence of ganglion cells in colon; also known as congenital aganglionic megacolon
2. Believed to be a familial, congenital defect; incidence is higher in children with congenital heart defects and chromosomal abnormalities such as Down syndrome
3. Rectosigmoid region is most commonly affected
4. Absence of autonomic parasympathetic ganglion cells in one portion of colon results in lack of innervation in that portion and absence of peristalsis
5. Lack of peristalsis causes accumulation of intestinal contents and distention of bowel proximal to defect

B. Nursing data collection

NCLEX® 1. Clinical manifestations in newborns include failure to pass meconium stool within 48 hours after birth, abdominal distention, and bile-stained emesis

NCLEX® 2. Clinical manifestations in infants include failure to thrive, constipation, abdominal distention, vomiting, and episodic diarrhea

NCLEX® 3. Clinical manifestations in toddlers and older children include chronic constipation, foul-smelling or pencil thin stools, abdominal distention, failure to gain weight, and malnutrition (including anemia and hypoproteinemia)

4. Rectal examination typically reveals an absence of stool
5. Diagnostic tests commonly reveal an enlarged portion of colon and a rectal biopsy confirms absence of ganglion cells

C. Therapeutic management

1. Involves removing aganglionic bowel through an endorectal pull-through procedure or if severe, by creation of a temporary colostomy that is later closed at 2–6 months of age if diagnosed at birth

NCLEX® 2. Preoperatively, monitor bowel function and stool characteristics; measure abdominal girth; monitor for vomiting and respiratory distress

3. Monitor electrolytes and urine specific gravity; note hydration status
4. Prepare child for surgery
5. Administer antibiotics as ordered

NCLEX® 6. Monitor VS; measure abdominal girth; inspect surgical site for redness, swelling, drainage after surgery

7. Observe stoma (if present) for color, bleeding, breakdown of surrounding skin; provide meticulous skin care, use appropriately sized stoma supplies
8. Inspect anal area after pull-through surgery for presence of stool, redness, drainage; do not place anything in rectum (thermometer or suppository) and place sign over bed alerting staff of this
9. Notify physician of any fever, unusual drainage, redness, or odor

NCLEX® 10. Keep child NPO until bowel sounds return or flatus is passed; maintain NG tube, administer IV fluids as ordered; monitor daily weights; begin diet with clear liquids and progress as tolerated

NCLEX® 11. Monitor pain using age-appropriate scales; provide comfort measures and involve parents; provide pain medications on regular basis as ordered; notify physician if pain is not managed

12. Involve child in quiet, age-appropriate activities for diversion
13. Encourage parents to share feelings, anxieties, and concerns about disorder and post-surgical care
14. Reinforce information about support groups and other appropriate referrals

D. Reinforce client and family teaching

1. Surgical repair procedure and recovery process
2. How to check for distention and obstruction and importance of reporting these findings to physician

3. Encourage preschool and early school-aged children to draw pictures, use dolls, and play to express concerns about bodily appearance, irrigations, and colostomy
4. NCLEX® Reinforce ostomy care in immediate postoperative period and encourage parents to participate and give return demonstration while in hospital; encourage child to learn and assume care as soon as appropriate

XXV. APPENDICITIS

A. Overview

1. Inflammation and infection of vermiform appendix, a small lymphoid, tubular blind sac at end of cecum
2. Exact cause is poorly understood but results from obstruction of lumen by hardened fecal material (**fecalith**), foreign bodies, microorganisms, or parasites
3. Obstruction of lumen causes accumulation of normal mucous secretions and distension of appendix, which causes capillary and venous engorgement and increased intraluminal pressure
4. Ischemia occurs and can lead to necrosis and perforation of intestinal wall; if perforation occurs, bacteria from bowel contaminate peritoneum and may lead to peritonitis and sepsis
5. Appendicitis is most common reason for abdominal surgery during childhood and adolescence

B. Nursing data collection

1. NCLEX® Generalized abdominal or periumbilical pain progressively worsening and then localizing in RLQ at **McBurney's point** (Figure 55–3), anorexia, possible nausea and vomiting, diarrhea or acute constipation
2. Signs of ruptured appendix include fever, chills, elevated WBC count (15,000 to 20,000 cells/mm^3), guarding, abdominal distention, rapid shallow breathing, irritability, and restlessness
3. Ultrasound indicates an enlarged incompressible appendix

C. Therapeutic management

1. Surgical removal (appendectomy) is done as soon as diagnosis made
2. Preoperative nursing care
   a. Reinforce information about procedure and postoperative care to client and family
   b. Keep client NPO and prevent dehydration with IV fluids as ordered
   c. NCLEX® Place client in semi-Fowler's or right-side lying position to help localize and prevent spread of any infection (used both preoperatively and postoperatively)
   d. Monitor for abdominal distention, auscultate bowel sounds, and observe elimination patterns
   e. NCLEX® Do nothing to stimulate peristalsis, which would hasten perforation; avoid laxatives, enemas, and heat applications
   f. Apply cold packs to client's abdomen to help relieve discomfort
   g. NCLEX® Sudden relief of pain usually indicates a ruptured appendix
3. Postoperative nursing care
   a. NCLEX® Monitor VS, observe for abdominal distention, and inspect surgical wound for signs of infection
   b. Encourage ambulation within 6 to 8 hours after surgery if not contraindicated
   c. Encourage client to turn, cough, and breathe deeply
   d. Monitor I&O and ensure that spontaneous voiding occurs
   e. Monitor for pain and administer analgesics as ordered
   f. NCLEX® If appendix ruptures, postoperative recovery is slowed; child will probably have an NG tube to decompress stomach and a Jackson-Pratt or Penrose drain; antibiotics may be administered

D. Reinforce client and family teaching

1. Diagnostic procedures, cause of appendicitis, surgical treatment, and anticipated postoperative care
2. How to inspect surgical incision for signs and symptoms of infection
3. Other problems to report to physician, such as fever, increased discomfort, and incision dehiscence (separation)
4. NCLEX® Child should avoid lifting, stretching, and strenuous activities until all follow-up care is completed
5. Information about fluids and nutrition during recovery process and advancement of diet; include symptoms to report to physician, such as vomiting, abdominal distention, and increased pain

XXVI. CELIAC DISEASE

A. Overview

1. An immunological disorder that is also known as gluten-sensitive enteropathy
2. Is characterized by a chronic inability to tolerate foods containing gluten, a protein present in wheat, rye, oats, and barley

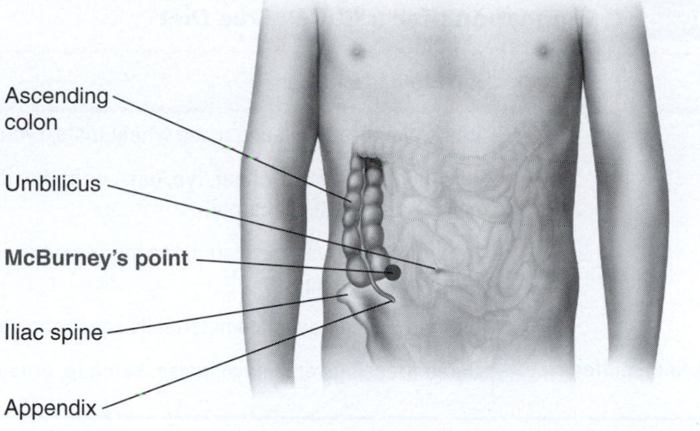

Figure 55–3
McBurney's point in right lower quadrant of abdomen with appendicitis.

NCLEX® 3. Results from inability to fully digest gliadin and glutenin (protein fractions); this leads to accumulation of amino acid glutamine, which is toxic to intestinal mucosa (leading to fatty stools initially and then malabsorption of protein, carbohydrates, calcium, iron, folate, and fat soluble vitamins as disease progresses)

NCLEX® 4. This deficiency in digestion requires lifelong dietary modifications

5. Exact cause is unknown; there may be a genetic predisposition possibly influenced by environmental factors and an immunologic abnormality

NCLEX® 6. Acute episodes (called celiac crises) are characterized by a general flare-up of symptoms and are precipitated by infections, prolonged fasting, ingestion of gluten, or anticholinergic drugs; can lead to electrolyte imbalance, rapid dehydration, and severe acidosis

B. Nursing data collection

1. Symptoms typically appear within 3 to 6 months after introduction of gluten (usually in form of grains) into child's diet

NCLEX® 2. Frequent bulky, greasy, malodorous stools with frothy appearance due to fat in stool (**steatorrhea**)

3. Abdominal distention, vomiting, and anorexia
4. Growth retardation with lack of fat deposits and muscle wasting
5. Anemia, irritability, edema

NCLEX® 6. In a celiac crisis, severe diarrhea and dehydration ensue; electrolyte imbalances and metabolic acidosis can create life-threatening disease

7. For unknown reasons, some children do not exhibit symptoms until after age 5 with growth retardation and delayed sexual maturation as predominant manifestations
8. Laboratory studies and diagnostic tests
   a. Flat mucosal surface, absence or atrophy of villi, and deep crypts visible on biopsy of small intestine

NCLEX® b. Steatorrhea on analysis of 72-hour quantitative fecal fat study

   c. Presence of serum IgA antiendomysial antibodies and IgA antitissue transglutaminase antibodies

C. Therapeutic management

NCLEX® 1. Nursing care focuses on supporting child and parents in maintaining a gluten-free diet; corn and rice become substitute grains (see Table 55–3)

2. Measure child's growth at each routine visit using a standard growth chart
3. Administer fluids for hydration; serum electrolytes and osmolality may be used as lab indicators of hydration status

NCLEX® 4. Monitor I&O, note skin turgor, mucous membranes, and urine specific gravity

5. Encourage participation in age-appropriate activities
6. Inform parents of organizations such as the American Celiac Society, the Celiac Sprue Association/United States of America, and the Gluten Intolerance Group

D. Reinforce client and family teaching

1. Written and verbal instructions on gluten-free diet

NCLEX® 2. Read labels of processed foods, because most contain gluten as a filler

3. Urgency of seeking medical care in the event of celiac crisis

NCLEX® 4. Importance of lifelong compliance with dietary modifications and follow-up medical care

Table 55-3 Suggestions for a Gluten-Free Diet

Unrestricted Food Items	Restricted Food Items
Beef, pork, poultry, fish	Items with bread coating using wheat, oats, rye or barley
Eggs	Any food made from wheat, rye, oats, or barley (bread, rolls, cookies, cakes, crackers, cereal, spaghetti, macaroni)
Milk, cream, cheese	Beer and ale, Ovaltine, instant tea mix, commercially prepared ice cream, malted milk, prepared puddings
Vegetables	Canned baked beans, commercially seasoned vegetable mixes or vegetables with sauce
Fruit	Salad dressings and mayonnaise, ketchup, gravy
Rice, corn, gluten-free wheat flour, puffed rice, corn flakes, corn meal	

XXVII. NECROTIZING ENTEROCOLITIS (NEC)

A. Overview

1. An intestinal inflammatory disease that occurs primarily in premature infants
2. Characterized by varying degrees of mucosal or transmural necrosis of intestine
3. Usual onset is in first 2 weeks of life but can be later in very low-birthweight infants
4. Caused by several factors, such as intestinal ischemia, bacterial or viral infection, and immaturity of GI tract; occurs most often in terminal ileum and colon
5. Pathology appears to begin when reduced blood flow to bowel leads to bowel wall ischemia; this ischemia allows bacteria to enter bowel wall and colonize
6. Damage to bowel can lead to perforation, which leads to need for bowel resection

B. Nursing data collection

NCLEX® 1. History may include prematurity, small for gestational age, maternal hemorrhage, preeclampsia, cocaine exposure in utero, exchange transfusions, umbilical catheters, low Apgar scores, or asphyxia

2. Typically, suspected NEC (stage I) consists of nonspecific clinical findings that represent physiologic instability or may resemble other common conditions in premature infants; these findings include the following:
   a. Temperature instability
   b. Lethargy
   c. Recurrent apnea and bradycardia
   d. Hypoglycemia
   e. Poor peripheral perfusion
   f. Increased pregavage gastric residuals
   g. Feeding intolerance, vomiting, abdominal distention
   h. Guaiac positive stools

NCLEX® 3. NEC (stage II) consists of nonspecific signs and symptoms plus the following:
   a. Severe abdominal distention
   b. Abdominal tenderness
   c. Grossly bloody stools
   d. Palpable bowel loops
   e. Edema of the abdominal wall
   f. Bowel sounds may be absent

NCLEX® 4. NEC (stage III) occurs when the infant becomes acutely ill; signs and symptoms include the following:
   a. Deterioration of VS
   b. Evidence of septic shock
   c. Edema and erythema of abdominal wall
   d. Right lower quadrant mass
   e. Acidosis (metabolic and/or respiratory)
   f. Disseminated intravascular coagulopathy (DIC)

5. Diagnostic testing includes an abdominal x-ray revealing free peritoneal gas, dilated bowel loops, bowel distention, and bowel thickening

C. Therapeutic management

NCLEX® 1. Nursing care focuses on early detection to minimize bowel necrosis

2. Measure abdominal girth frequently

3. Prepare feedings using aseptic technique
NCLEX® 4. Observe tolerance of feedings; monitor and maintain optimal hydration status
5. Monitor cardiac and respiratory status
6. Promote and maintain adequate body temperature
7. Administer antibiotics as ordered
8. Encourage family interaction and promote attachment process
9. Provide developmentally appropriate activities

D. Reinforce client and family teaching

1. Encourage parents to express concerns about outcomes of surgery
NCLEX® 2. Signs of intestinal obstruction, strictures, poor tolerance of feedings, and impaired healing processes
NCLEX® 3. Care of ostomy and IV central line

XXVIII. FAILURE TO THRIVE (FTT)

A. Overview

1. Is a syndrome in which infant or young child does not eat enough to be adequately nourished
2. Organic FTT results from a physical cause, such as congenital acquired immunodeficiency syndrome (AIDS), cystic fibrosis, celiac disease, congenital heart defects, chronic renal failure, gastroesophageal reflux, malabsorption syndrome, or endocrine dysfunction
3. Nonorganic FTT is called feeding disorder of infancy or early childhood; it is suspected in absence of evidence of organic disease; parental or caregiver risk factors include poverty, depression, substance abuse, psychosis, mental retardation, social or emotional isolation, and lack of knowledge of infant nurturing and nutrition; infant may not provide clear cues about hunger and is not easily soothed; preterm and small for gestational age infants are more frequently affected

B. Nursing data collection

NCLEX® 1. Physical findings
   a. Weight often below 5th percentile and weight-for-length is often less than 80%
   b. Delay in developmental milestones
   c. Decreased muscle mass and muscle hypotonia
   d. Abdominal distension
   e. Generalized weakness and **cachexia** (malnutrition accompanied by wasting)
2. Behavioral indicators
   a. Refuses food
   b. Erratic sleep patterns
   NCLEX® c. Disturbed manner, such as as being irritable or difficult to soothe
3. Diagnostic tests
   a. Developmental screening
   b. Tuberculin skin test
   c. Bone scan, chest x-ray, ECG, IV pyelogram, upper and lower GI series
   d. Urinalysis, complete blood count, sweat chloride test, stool tests, T_4 test
   e. Bowel and muscle biopsies

C. Therapeutic management

1. Document child's eating patterns and cues given about hunger or satiety
2. Document parent–child interaction patterns such as eye contact, touch, and cuddling
3. Encourage parents to discuss positive and negative feelings of care, procedures, and interaction with child
NCLEX® 4. Feed on demand or increase intake as tolerated; try to make mealtimes as stress-free as possible
NCLEX® 5. Offer high-protein, high-calorie snacks, and frequent, small portions of a wide variety of foods
6. Document I&O, daily weights and nutritional assessments
7. Provide consistency in nursing care
8. Upon discharge provide referral to agency that can continue to monitor child's home situation, family stress and behavior patterns, and feeding during meals

D. Reinforce client and family teaching

1. Normal growth and development
NCLEX® 2. How to recognize and respond to hunger and satiety cues, to hold and touch infant during feedings, and establish eye contact with infant or child

XXIX. VOMITING AND DIARRHEA

A. Overview

1. Vomiting is a forceful ejection of gastric contents through mouth
   a. Is common and usually self-limiting
   NCLEX® b. Requires no specific treatment unless complications occur (dehydration, electrolyte imbalances, malnutrition, and aspiration)
   c. Can be an associated symptom of an acute infectious disease, increased intracranial pressure, toxic ingestion, food intolerance and allergy, mechanical obstruction of GI tract, metabolic disorder, or a psychogenic problem
   NCLEX® d. Color and consistency of emesis suggests etiology: green bilious with bowel obstruction; coffee ground texture from blood mixing with stomach contents suggests GI bleeding; curdled stomach contents, mucus, or fatty foods several hours after eating suggest poor gastric emptying
   NCLEX® e. Associated symptoms also help to identify etiology: fever and diarrhea with infection; constipation with obstruction; localized abdominal pain with appendicitis, pancreatitis, or PUD; change in level of consciousness or headache with a central nervous system or metabolic disorder; forceful or projectile vomiting with pyloric stenosis
2. **Diarrhea** is defined as frequent, watery, loose stools and is actually a symptom rather than a disease
   a. Accompanies many disorders, including respiratory infections and GI disorders, and can also be caused by stress, food intolerance or sensitivity, medications, and surgical procedures that reduce absorptive surface of intestine
   b. Can be acute or chronic, inflammatory or noninflammatory, or viral or bacterial in nature
   c. Can lead to dehydration, electrolyte imbalance, hypovolemic shock, and even death in pediatric clients
   d. Increased intestinal motility and rapid emptying leads to impaired nutrient absorption and excessive excretion of water and electrolytes, especially sodium and potassium

B. Nursing data collection

NCLEX® 1. Monitor hydration status as highest priority (see Table 55–4 for signs of dehydration)
2. Note amount, color, consistency, and time of stools and vomitus
NCLEX® 3. Measure daily weights (best indicator of fluid balance) and I&O
4. Monitor client's activity level
5. Monitor for abdominal cramping, fever, and other related symptoms
6. Stool culture for bacteria, ova, parasites, or rotaviruses; stool examination for pH, leukocytes, glucose, and presence of blood; serum electrolytes, BUN, creatinine, and glucose; x-rays, ultrasound, or endoscopy

C. Therapeutic management

1. Priority nursing interventions focus on preventing and managing dehydration
NCLEX® 2. Weigh client on admission and daily using same scale at same time of day in same amount of clothing
NCLEX® 3. Monitor and document I&O hourly; weigh infant diapers after voiding and episode of diarrhea; monitor urine specific gravity
4. Monitor VS and avoid rectal temperatures
5. Client is usually NPO to allow bowel rest; administer IV fluids for severe dehydration
NCLEX® 6. Begin oral rehydration for mild to moderate dehydration and as supplement to IV fluid in severe dehydration
   a. Oral rehydration fluids (ORFs) include commercial preparations such as Infalyte, Rehydralyte, and Pedialyte for children
   b. Start with frequent, small amounts of liquids—1 to 3 teaspoons every 10 to 15 minutes (target goal for first 2–4 hours of treatment is 50 mL per kg weight); for older children and adults, offer sips to total up to 8 oz in an hour; offer 1 teaspoon every 2–3 minutes if vomiting since some fluid may still absorb
   c. Infants progress from clear liquids to their typical diet, although soy protein formula rather than milk-based formula may be recommended for formula-fed infants
   d. When diet resumes, advise intake of cereals, starches, soups, fruits and vegetables; avoid simple sugars and carbonated beverages, which could worsen diarrhea
7. Administer antidiarrheals, antibiotics, antiprotozoals as ordered based on cause
8. Monitor lab tests (electrolytes, hematocrit, pH, serum albumin)
9. Implement measures to reduce fever if needed
10. Cleanse diaper area (infants) or perianal skin with mild soap and water after each stool; avoid harsh astringent wipes that could further irritate reddened skin
NCLEX® 11. Practice standard precautions

D. Reinforce client and family teaching: causes of vomiting and diarrhea, oral rehydration therapy, skin care, and signs and symptoms requiring medical attention

Table 55-4 Severity of Clinical Dehydration

	Mild	Moderate	Severe
Percent of body weight lost	Up to 5%	6%–9% (60–90 mL/kg)	10% or more (100+ mg/kg)
Level of consciousness	Alert, restless, thirsty	Restless or lethargic (infants and very young children); alert, thirsty, restless (older children, adolescents, and adults)	Lethargic to comatose (infants and young children); often conscious and apprehensive (older children and adults)
Blood pressure	Normal	Normal or low; postural hypotension (older children and adults)	Low to undetectable
Pulse	Normal	Rapid	Rapid, weak to nonpalpable
Skin turgor	Normal	Poor	Very poor
Mucous membranes	Moist	Dry	Parched
Urine	May appear normal	Decreased output (<1 mL/kg/hr); dark color, increased specific gravity	Very decreased or absent output
Thirst	Slightly increased	Moderately increased	Greatly increased unless lethargic
Fontanel	Normal (children)	Sunken (children)	Sunken (children)
Extremities	Warm; normal capillary refill	Delayed capillary refill (>2 sec)	Cool, discolored; delayed capillary refill (>3–4 sec)
Respirations	Normal	Normal or rapid	Changing rate and pattern

Modified slightly from: Ball, J., & Bindler, R. *Child health nursing: Partnering with children & families.* © 2006, p. 730, Table 23–2. Reprinted by permission of Pearson Education, Inc., Upper Saddle River, NJ 07458.

Check Your NCLEX-PN® Exam I.Q.

You are ready for testing on this content if you can

- Identify basic structures and functions of the gastrointestinal system.
- Describe the pathophysiology and etiology of common gastrointestinal disorders.
- Discuss expected data and diagnostic test findings for selected gastrointestinal disorders.
- Discuss therapeutic management of a client experiencing a gastrointestinal disorder.
- Discuss nursing management of a client experiencing a gastrointestinal disorder.
- Identify expected outcomes for the client experiencing a gastrointestinal disorder.

PRACTICE TEST

1 A client has a total gastrectomy. The nurse explains to the client the need for long-term injections of which vitamin?

1. Thiamine
2. Folic acid
3. Cyanocobalamin
4. Niacin

2 A client with diverticular disease undergoes a colonoscopy. During abdominal data collection, the nurse looks for which sign to indicate a possible complication of the procedure?

1. Diarrhea
2. Nausea and vomiting
3. Guarding and rebound tenderness
4. Redness and warmth of the abdominal skin

3 The client who has ulcerative colitis is scheduled for an ileostomy. When the client asks the nurse what to expect related to bowel function and care after surgery, what response should the nurse make?

1. "You will be able to have some control over your bowel movements."
2. "The stoma will require that you wear a collection device all the time."
3. "After the stoma heals, you can irrigate your bowel so you will not have to wear a pouch."
4. "The drainage will gradually become semisolid and formed."

4 The nurse is conducting dietary education with a client who has dumping syndrome. The nurse encourages the client to avoid which foods that the client usually enjoys? Select all that apply.

1. Eggs
2. Cheese
3. Fruit
4. Pork
5. Cookies

5 A client is being evaluated for possible duodenal ulcer. The nurse monitors the client for which manifestation that would support this diagnosis?

1. Epigastric pain relieved by food
2. History of chronic aspirin use
3. Distended abdomen
4. Positive fluid wave

6 The client returning from a colonoscopy has been given a diagnosis of Crohn's disease. The nurse expects to note which manifestations in the client? Select all that apply.

1. Steatorrhea
2. Firm, rigid abdomen
3. Constipation
4. Enlarged hemorrhoids
5. Diarrhea

7 The nurse is reinforcing education to a client with gastroesophageal reflux disease (GERD) about ways to minimize symptoms. Which information in the client's history should the nurse address as an indicator that needs to be changed? Select all that apply.

1. Lifting weights for exercise
2. Being a vegetarian
3. Having a body mass index of 26
4. Taking calcium carbonate tablets
5. Drinking 2–4 cups of coffee daily

8 The client with a duodenal ulcer asks the nurse why an antibiotic is part of the treatment regimen. Which information should the nurse include in the response?

1. Antibiotics decrease the likelihood of a secondary infection.
2. Many duodenal ulcers are caused by the *Helicobacter pylori* organism.
3. Antibiotics are used in an attempt to sterilize the stomach.
4. Many people have *Clostridium difficile*, which can lead to ulcer formation.

9 The nurse should evaluate results of which laboratory tests while caring for a client who has postnecrotic cirrhosis of the liver? Select all that apply.

1. Prothrombin time
2. Urinalysis
3. Serum lipase
4. Serum troponin
5. Serum albumin

10 The nurse is caring for a client with a history of alcoholism. Which findings would indicate that the client has possibly developed chronic pancreatitis? Select all that apply.

1. Steady weight gain
2. Flank pain on left side only
3. Fatty stools
4. Excessive hunger
5. Constipation and flatulence

11 The nurse caring for a client with hemolytic jaundice anticipates which findings on laboratory test results?

1. Elevated serum indirect bilirubin
2. Decreased serum protein
3. Elevated urine bilirubin
4. Decreased urine pH

12 A client was admitted to the hospital with cholelithiasis. Which new finding indicates to the nurse that the stone has probably obstructed the common bile duct?

1. Nausea
2. Elevated cholesterol level
3. Right upper quadrant (RUQ) pain
4. Jaundice

13 The post-cholecystectomy client asks the nurse when the T-tube will be removed. Which response by the nurse would be appropriate?

1. "When your stool returns to a normal brown color, the tube can be removed."
2. "The tube will be removed at the same time as your staples."
3. "When the tube stops draining, it will be removed."
4. "The tube is usually removed the day after surgery."

14 Which findings made by the nurse could indicate the development of portal hypertension in a client with cirrhosis? Select all that apply.

1. Hemorrhoids
2. Bleeding gums
3. Muscle wasting
4. Splenomegaly
5. Ascites

15 The nurse is caring for a client who has ascites, and the health care provider prescribes spironolactone (Aldactone). The client asks why this drug is being used. What is the best response by the nurse?

1. "This drug will help increase the level of protein in your blood."
2. "The drug will cause an increase in the amount of the hormone aldosterone your body produces."
3. "This medication is a diuretic but does not make the kidneys excrete potassium."
4. "This will help you excrete larger amounts of ammonia."

16 When caring for a client who has cirrhosis, the nurse notices flapping tremors of the wrist and fingers. How should the nurse document this finding?

1. "Trousseau's sign noted."
2. "Caput medusa noted."
3. "Fetor hepaticus noted."
4. "Asterixis noted."

17 A mother arrives at the pediatric clinic with her 6-month-old infant. While the nurse monitors the child, the mother points to the umbilicus and says, "What am I going to do about this? When he cries, it looks like it's going to burst." What is the best response by the nurse?

1. "It's best if you don't let him cry."
2. "It probably won't rupture unless he gets excessively upset. I wouldn't worry about it at this time."
3. "I know it looks frightening, but it really won't burst."
4. "Put a binder around it, and that will keep it from bursting when he gets upset."

18 A 9-year-old male client with severe esophagitis is 12 hours status/post-Nissen fundoplication for gastroesophageal reflux. What action by the nurse would be appropriate while providing nursing care?

1. Encourage him to take small amounts of clear liquids every 4 hours.
2. Administer nasogstric or gastrostomy feedings every 4 hours.
3. Ask him to choose a face on the Wong FACES pain rating scale.
4. Insert a pH probe to monitor esophageal acidity.

19 Which laboratory test would the nurse expect to be ordered for a child with dehydration caused by vomiting and diarrhea? Select all that apply.

1. Serum sodium
2. Urine specific gravity
3. Serum ammonia
4. Serum amylase
5. Blood urea nitrogen (BUN)

20 The nurse is caring for a child with a history of severe diarrhea. Which notation about acid–base imbalance would the nurse expect to find in the medical record?

1. Respiratory acidosis
2. Respiratory alkalosis
3. Metabolic acidosis
4. Metabolic alkalosis

PRACTICE TEST

21 A child with Hirschsprung's disease is being discharged after Soave endorectal pull-through procedure for colostomy closure. Which item should the nurse include when reinforcing teaching at discharge?

1. Stools may be infrequent and uncomfortable for the first few weeks.
2. It will be necessary to perform weekly rectal irrigations for approximately 6 weeks.
3. Report fever, increasing pain or discomfort, or redness of the incision to the surgeon.
4. Stools will be fatty for a week or so and then gradually return to normal.

22 The mother of a child undergoing an emergency appendectomy tells the nurse, "If I had brought him in yesterday when he complained of an upset stomach, this wouldn't have happened." What is the best response by the nurse?

1. "It's okay; you got him here just in time before it ruptured."
2. "It is often difficult to predict when a simple complaint will become more serious."
3. "Next time he seems sick, you should bring him in immediately."
4. "Sometimes parents can make a mistake without meaning to do so."

23 The nurse is reinforcing teaching home feeding guidelines to the mother of a child with nonorganic failure to thrive. Essential information for the nurse to reinforce would be the importance of which item?

1. Restricting eating except at mealtimes
2. Allowing the child to eat alone to minimize distraction
3. Allowing the child to snack on finger foods, such as circular oat cereal and bananas
4. A relaxed mealtime with few limits on behavior

24 The nurse is admitting a child with a diagnosis of "rule out appendicitis." The nurse monitors this client for which manifestations? Select all that apply.

1. Generalized abdominal pain
2. Pain localizing in right lower quadrant
3. Fatty stools
4. Elevated white blood cell (WBC) count
5. Indigestion

25 A child who underwent cleft palate repair has just returned from surgery with elbow restraints in place. The parents question why their child must have the restraints. The nurse would give which explanation to the parents?

1. "This device is frequently used postoperatively to protect the intravenous (IV) site in small children."
2. "The restraints will help us maintain proper body alignment."
3. "Elbow restraints are used postoperatively to keep children's hands away from the surgical site."
4. "The restraints help maintain the child's NPO status."

26 The nurse is caring for an infant vomiting secondary to pyloric stenosis. The mother asks why the child's vomitus appears different from that of her other children when they have the flu. The nurse would explain that the emesis of an infant with pyloric stenosis does not contain bile for which reason?

1. The GI system is still immature in newborns and infants.
2. The obstruction is above the bile duct.
3. The emesis is from passive regurgitation.
4. The bile duct is obstructed.

27 The nurse is advising the parents of a child with celiac disease about the dietary restrictions. The nurse would explain that the most appropriate diet for their child is a diet that is free of which of the following? Select all that apply.

1. Rice
2. Wheat
3. Oats
4. Barley
5. Corn

28 A 4-month-old infant is admitted to the nursing unit with moderate dehydration. Which symptom does the nurse suspect led to the diagnosis of moderate dehydration in this child? Select all that apply.

1. Elevated heart rate
2. Urine specific gravity of 1.038
3. Weight gain
4. Polyuria
5. Slow capillary refill

29 While gathering admission data on a 16-month-old child, the nurse notes all the following abnormal findings. Which finding is related to a diagnosis of Hirschsprung's disease? Select all that apply.

1. Bile-stained vomitus
2. Decreased urine output
3. Poor weight gain since birth
4. Intermittent sharp pain
5. Alternating constipation and diarrhea

30 An older adult client presents with fever, leukocytosis, left lower quadrant pain, and diarrhea alternating with constipation. The nurse concludes that these symptoms are frequently seen in clients with which gastrointestinal disorder?

1. Appendicitis
2. Diverticulitis
3. Peptic ulcer disease
4. Irritable bowel syndrome

31 Which of the following findings would strongly indicate the possibility of cirrhosis?

1. Dry skin
2. Hepatomegaly
3. Peripheral edema
4. Pruritus

ANSWERS & RATIONALES

1 **Answer: 3** **Rationale:** The loss of parietal cells that secrete intrinsic factor results in vitamin B_{12} (cyanocobalamin) deficiency postgastrectomy, because intrinsic factor is needed for absorption of vitamin B_{12}. For this reason, clients require vitamin B_{12} injections for life. The other options identify other B-complex vitamins. **Cognitive Level:** Analyzing **Client Need:** Physiological Adaptation **Integrated Process:** Teaching and Learning **Content Area:** Adult Health **Strategy:** The core issue of the question is knowledge that gastric surgery results in loss of ability to produce intrinsic factor and subsequent vitamin B_{12} deficiency. Use nursing knowledge and the process of elimination to make a selection.

2 **Answer: 3** **Rationale:** Bowel perforation is a possible result of a colonoscopy if the colonoscope accidentally pierces the bowel wall. Perforation could lead to symptoms of peritonitis, such as guarding and rebound tenderness. The other options are incorrect, because diarrhea, nausea and vomiting as signs of obstruction, and redness and warmth of abdominal skin are of no concern. **Cognitive Level:** Analyzing **Client Need:** Physiological Adaptation **Integrated Process:** Nursing Process: Data Collection **Content Area:** Adult Health **Strategy:** The core issue of the question is data collection that correlates with complications of colonoscopy, such as peritonitis. Use nursing knowledge and the process of elimination to make a selection.

3 **Answer: 2** **Rationale:** A client with an ileostomy has no control over bowel movements and must always wear a collection device. The drainage tends to be liquid but becomes paste-like with intake of specific foods. **Cognitive Level:** Applying **Client Need:** Physiological Adaptation **Integrated Process:** Communication and Documentation **Content Area:** Adult Health **Strategy:** The core issue of the question is knowledge of stool characteristics and associated stoma appliance needs following ileostomy. Use nursing knowledge and the process of elimination to make a selection.

4 **Answer: 3, 5** **Rationale:** Dumping syndrome, in which gastric contents rapidly enter the bowel, can occur following gastrectomy. Dietary fats and proteins are increased, and carbohydrates, especially simple carbohydrates such as fruits and desserts, are reduced. This helps slow the GI transit time and reduce the GI cramping, diarrhea, and vasomotor symptoms associated with dumping syndrome. **Cognitive Level:** Applying **Client Need:** Physiological Adaptation **Integrated Process:** Nursing Process: Implementation **Content Area:** Adult Health **Strategy:** The core issue of the question is knowledge of foods to avoid when the client has dumping syndrome. Use nursing knowledge and the process of elimination to make a selection.

5 **Answer: 1** **Rationale:** The pain of a gastric ulcer is dull and aching, occurs after eating, and is not relieved by food as is the pain from duodenal ulcer. The pancreatic juices that are high in bicarbonate are released with food intake and relieve duodenal ulcer pain when the client eats. Chronic aspirin use is irritating to the stomach. Distended abdomen is a vague sign and is unrelated. A positive fluid wave is consistent with ascites and is unrelated. **Cognitive Level:** Applying **Client Need:** Physiological Adaptation **Integrated Process:** Nursing Process: Data Collection **Content Area:** Adult Health **Strategy:** The core issue of the question is expected findings in duodenal ulcer. Recall the effect of pancreatic juices on the duodenal ulcer surface and use the process of elimination to make a selection.

6 **Answer: 1, 5** **Rationale:** Steatorrhea is often present in the client with Crohn's disease. Diarrhea is a key feature, but unlike ulcerative colitis, the loose stool usually does not contain blood and is usually less frequent in number of episodes. A firm rigid abdomen is not a manifestation of Crohn's disease. Constipation is not a manifestation of Crohn's disease. Hemorrhoids are not a manifestation of Crohn's disease. **Cognitive Level:** Applying **Client Need:** Physiological Adaptation **Integrated Process:** Nursing Process: Data Collection **Content Area:** Adult Health **Strategy:** The core issue of the question is identification of common symptoms of Crohn's disease. Use nursing knowledge and the process of elimination to make a selection.

7 **Answer: 1, 3, 5** **Rationale:** Lifestyle modifications can minimize symptoms of GERD. Anything that increases intra-abdominal pressure should be avoided, such as lifting weights. Obesity or being overweight also aggravates symptoms, as indicated by a body mass index of 26. Coffee, cola, other sources of caffeine, and chocolate decrease lower esophageal sphincter tone and can increase symptoms of GERD. Being a vegetarian does not increase risk of GERD. Calcium carbonate tablets (Tums) often aid in symptom relief. **Cognitive Level:** Applying **Client Need:** Physiological Adaptation **Integrated Process:** Nursing Process: Planning **Content Area:** Adult Health **Strategy:** The core issue of the question is ability to identify risk factors that aggravate symptoms of GERD. Use nursing knowledge and the process of elimination to make a selection.

8 **Answer: 2 Rationale:** *Helicobacter pylori* infection is a major cause of peptic ulcers so treatment includes antibiotic therapy to eradicate the microorganisms. Antibiotics do not reduce the likelihood of a secondary infection; they treat the primary infection. Antibiotics are not used to sterilize the bowel, which would upset the normal flora of the GI tract. *Clostridium difficile* is a contagious microorganism that can lead to severe diarrhea. **Cognitive Level:** Applying **Client Need:** Physiological Adaptation **Integrated Process:** Nursing Process: Implementation **Content Area:** Adult Health **Strategy:** The core issue of the question is knowledge of etiology of peptic ulcers, including duodenal ulcers. Use nursing knowledge and the process of elimination to make a selection.

9 **Answer: 1, 5 Rationale:** Many clotting factors are produced in the liver, including fibrinogen (factor I), prothrombin (factor II), factor V, serum prothrombin conversion accelerator (factor VII), factor IX, and factor X. The client's ability to form these factors may be impaired with cirrhosis, putting the client at risk for bleeding. The prothrombin time will evaluate blood clotting ability. One function of the liver is to synthesize protein, which may be impaired with cirrhosis. Urinalysis is a general screening measure or can be used to diagnose problems with the urinary tract. Serum lipase is a useful indicator of disorders of the pancreas. Serum troponin is a common laboratory test used to diagnose myocardial infarction. **Cognitive Level:** Applying **Client Need:** Physiological Adaptation **Integrated Process:** Nursing Process: Data Collection **Content Area:** Adult Health **Strategy:** The critical word in the question is *cirrhosis*. With this in mind, the correct answers are those that could detect a complication of cirrhosis or disturbed liver function. Use nursing knowledge and the process of elimination to make a selection.

10 **Answer: 3, 5 Rationale:** Steatorrhea (fatty stools) results from a decrease in pancreatic enzyme secretion with pancreatitis. The client with chronic pancreatitis is likely to experience bouts of constipation and flatulence. The client with chronic pancreatitis is likely to experience weight loss rather than weight gain. The pain of pancreatitis is felt in the abdomen and is not limited to the left flank. Manifestations of chronic pancreatitis include nausea and vomiting rather than excessive hunger. **Cognitive Level:** Applying **Client Need:** Physiological Adaptation **Integrated Process:** Nursing Process: Data Collection **Content Area:** Adult Health **Strategy:** The core issue of the question is the ability to identify findings that are consistent with the development of chronic pancreatitis. Use nursing knowledge and the process of elimination to make a selection.

11 **Answer: 1 Rationale:** Hemolytic jaundice is caused by excessive breakdown of red blood cells, and the amount of bilirubin produced exceeds the ability of the liver to conjugate it, so there is an increase in indirect bilirubin. Serum protein is not measured to detect hemolytic jaundice. Unconjugated bilirubin is insoluble in water and is not found in the urine. Urine pH is not decreased by hemolytic jaundice. **Cognitive Level:** Applying **Client Need:** Physiological Adaptation **Integrated Process:** Nursing Process: Data Collection **Content Area:** Adult Health **Strategy:** The core issue of the question is knowledge of clinical indicators of hemolytic jaundice. Use nursing knowledge and the process of elimination to make a selection.

12 **Answer: 4 Rationale:** Nausea and RUQ pain occur in cholelithiasis, but obstruction of the common bile duct results in reflux of bile into the liver, which produces jaundice. Alkaline phosphatase increases with biliary obstruction but cholesterol level does not increase. **Cognitive Level:** Analyzing **Client Need:** Physiological Adaptation **Integrated Process:** Nursing Process: Data Collection **Content Area:** Adult Health **Strategy:** The core issue of the question is knowledge of clinical indicators of common bile duct obstruction. Think about the pathophysiology of blocked bile drainage and use the process of elimination to make a selection.

13 **Answer: 1 Rationale:** When T-tube drainage subsides and stools return to a normal brown color, the tube can be clamped 1 to 2 hours before and after meals in preparation for tube removal. If the client tolerates clamping, the tube will then be removed. The tube is not removed at the same time as the incisional staples. It is not necessary for drainage to completely stop before tube removal. The client may not be ready for tube removal the day after surgery. **Cognitive Level:** Applying **Client Need:** Physiological Adaptation **Integrated Process:** Communication and Documentation **Content Area:** Adult Health **Strategy:** The core issue of the question is the appropriate timeframe for use of a T-tube following gallbladder surgery. Use nursing knowledge and the process of elimination to make a selection.

14 **Answer: 1, 4, 5 Rationale:** Obstruction to portal blood flow causes a rise in portal venous pressure resulting in splenomegaly, ascites, and dilation of collateral venous channels predominantly in the paraumbilical and hemorrhoidal veins, the cardia of the stomach, and extending into the esophagus. Bleeding gums would indicate insufficient Vitamin K production in the liver. Muscle wasting commonly accompanies the poor nutritional intake commonly seen in clients with cirrhosis. **Cognitive Level:** Analyzing **Client Need:** Physiological Adaptation **Integrated Process:** Nursing Process: Data Collection **Content Area:** Adult Health **Strategy:** The wording of the question indicates that more than one option is likely to be correct. The core issue of the question is knowledge of associated findings in a client with portal hypertension. Use knowledge of the pathophysiology of the condition and the process of elimination to make appropriate selections.

15 **Answer: 3 Rationale:** Spironolactone is used in clients with ascites who show no improvement with bedrest and fluid restriction. It inhibits sodium reabsorption in the distal tubule and promotes potassium retention by inhibiting aldosterone. Spironolactone does not increase protein levels in the blood. Spironolactone does not increase production of aldosterone. Spironolactone does not aid in excreting ammonia, although lactulose (Cephulac) will do this. **Cognitive Level:** Applying **Client Need:** Pharmacological and Parenteral Therapies **Integrated Process:** Communication and Documentation **Content Area:** Adult Health **Strategy:** The core issue of the question is knowledge of medication effects in a client with ascites. Use nursing knowledge related to pharmacology and the process of elimination to make a selection.

16 **Answer: 4 Rationale:** Asterixis, also called liver flap, is the flapping tremor of the hands when the arms are extended. Trousseau's sign reflects hypocalcemia. Caput medusa refers to spiderlike abdominal veins that are also commonly found in clients with cirrhosis who have portal hypertension as a complication. Fetor hepaticus is a specific odor noted in liver failure. **Cognitive Level:** Applying **Client Need:** Physiological Adaptation **Integrated Process:** Communication and

Documentation **Content Area:** Adult Health **Strategy:** The core issue of the question is knowledge of typical findings in a client with cirrhosis. Use nursing knowledge and the process of elimination to make a selection.

17 **Answer: 3** **Rationale:** It is a common finding that when the infant with an umbilical hernia cries, the hernia protrudes but will not rupture. It is unnecessary to try to prevent the infant from crying. An umbilical hernia will not rupture because the infant gets upset and this response does not reassure the parent. The family is instructed not to apply tape, straps, or coins to the umbilicus to reduce the hernia. **Cognitive Level:** Applying **Client Need:** Physiological Adaptation **Integrated Process:** Communication and Documentation **Content Area:** Child Health **Strategy:** The core issue of the question is knowledge of the consequences of umbilical hernia and knowledge of therapeutic communication techniques. Use this knowledge and the process of elimination to make a selection.

18 **Answer: 3** **Rationale:** Pain management is a high priority following gastric surgery, and the nurse should use age-appropriate tools to monitor for pain, such as the Wong FACES rating scale. A gastrostomy tube or nasogastric tube placed during surgery is kept in place to maintain gastric decompression so drinking is not allowed. The child is kept NPO until bowel function returns. The use of a pH probe to measure gastric acidity is not necessary. **Cognitive Level:** Applying **Client Need:** Physiological Adaptation **Integrated Process:** Nursing Process: Implementation **Content Area:** Child Health **Strategy:** The core issue of the question is knowledge of appropriate interventions in the first 24 hours following gastric surgery. Use knowledge that the gastric tube should not be manipulated or used for feeding to eliminate some options. Use nursing knowledge of routine postoperative care and the process of elimination to make a final selection.

19 **Answer: 1, 2, 5** **Rationale:** Serum sodium would be expected to increase in a client with dehydration because of hemoconcentration. Measuring urine specific gravity provides data about the concentration of urine and provides information regarding hydration. The BUN rises with dehydration and is therefore a general indicator of hydration status, although it also reflects kidney function. Serum ammonia could be elevated in liver disease. Serum amylase could be elevated in pancreatic disorders. **Cognitive Level:** Applying **Client Need:** Physiological Adaptation **Integrated Process:** Nursing Process: Implementation **Content Area:** Child Health **Strategy:** The core issue of the question is dehydration and thus, the correct option is one that addresses fluid balance in the body in some way. Use nursing knowledge and the process of elimination to make a selection.

20 **Answer: 3** **Rationale:** In severe diarrhea, excess bicarbonate (base) is lost, which predisposes to metabolic acidosis. There is also carbohydrate malabsorption and depletion of glycogen stores, resulting in fat metabolism. Ketoacids are the by-products of fat metabolism, which adds to the metabolic acidosis. Diarrhea is not a respiratory problem. **Cognitive Level:** Analyzing **Client Need:** Physiological Adaptation **Integrated Process:** Nursing Process: Planning **Content Area:** Child Health **Strategy:** The core issue of the question is the ability to correlate acid–base imbalance with a diagnosis of diarrhea. Recall that bicarbonate is a base and that the respiratory system is not directly involved to make a selection.

21 **Answer: 3** **Rationale:** It is important that any signs of infection be reported at once. After the Soave procedure, normal bowel function is expected. No rectal irrigations are necessary. Stools are not fatty for a week or so following the Soave procedure. **Cognitive Level:** Applying **Client Need:** Physiological Adaptation **Integrated Process:** Nursing Process: Planning **Content Area:** Child Health **Strategy:** The core issue of the question is knowledge of routine discharge education following an abdominal surgical procedure. Use nursing knowledge and the process of elimination to make a selection.

22 **Answer: 2** **Rationale:** Parents often react to a child's illness with feelings of guilt for not recognizing the severity of the condition sooner. A response that provides emotional support and reduces parental anxiety encourages parents to feel confident in their abilities as caregiver. Telling the parent "it's OK" ignores the parent's feelings. Directing the parent to seek care immediately next time adds to the parent's stress. Using the word "mistake" adds to the parent's perceived guilt. **Cognitive Level:** Applying **Client Need:** Psychosocial Integrity **Integrated Process:** Communication and Documentation **Content Area:** Child Health **Strategy:** The core issue of the question is the ability to formulate a therapeutic response to a parent who indicates distress about not seeking help earlier for an ill child. Use nursing knowledge of therapeutic communication skills and the process of elimination to make a selection.

23 **Answer: 3** **Rationale:** Finger foods are helpful in encouraging children with failure to thrive to increase food intake. The parent should be taught to encourage increased food intake, including between meal snacks. The child does not need to eat alone; instead mealtimes should be structured family events. Although a relaxed atmosphere is good, there can be limits on behavior during mealtimes to provide structure. **Cognitive Level:** Applying **Client Need:** Physiological Adaptation **Integrated Process:** Teaching and Learning **Content Area:** Child Health **Strategy:** The core issue of the question is the intervention that will help to increase food intake in a child with nonorganic failure to thrive. Use nursing knowledge and the process of elimination to make a selection.

24 **Answer: 1, 2, 4** **Rationale:** Manifestations of appendicitis often begin with generalized abdominal pain. As abdominal pain progressively worsens, it tends to localize in the right lower quadrant at McBurney's point. WBC count can elevate to 15,000 to 20,000 cells/mm3 because of the inflammatory response. Fatty stools are not part of the clinical picture. Indigestion is not typical, although the client may have nausea and vomiting, fever, chills, anorexia, diarrhea, or acute constipation. **Cognitive Level:** Applying **Client Need:** Physiological Adaptation **Integrated Process:** Nursing Process: Data Collection **Content Area:** Child Health **Strategy:** The core issue of the question is knowledge of manifestations that are consistent with appendicitis. Use knowledge that the affected area is the large intestine to eliminate indigestion (stomach area, too vague) and fatty stools (small intestine absorption problem).

25 **Answer: 3** **Rationale:** Elbow restraints are used to keep hands away from the mouth after cleft palate surgery. This precaution will be maintained at home until the palate is healed, usually 4 to 6 weeks. They are not used to protect the IV site, maintain NPO status, or maintain body alignment. **Cognitive Level:** Applying **Client Need:** Physiological Adaptation **Integrated Process:** Nursing Process: Implementation **Content Area:** Child Health **Strategy:** Consider what movements elbow restraints will allow the child to determine the correct answer.

26 **Answer: 2** **Rationale:** In pyloric stenosis, bile is unable to enter the stomach from the duodenum because the pylorus muscle is hypertrophied, which causes the obstruction. **Cognitive Level:** Analyzing **Client Need:** Physiological Adaptation **Integrated Process:** Nursing Process: Implementation **Content Area:** Child Health **Strategy:** Consider the site of the pylorus to determine the correct answer.

27 **Answer: 2, 3, 4** **Rationale:** Most children who remain on a gluten-free diet remain healthy and free of symptoms and complications. Gluten is a protein found in wheat, barley, rye, and oats. For this reason, appropriate foods need to be free of these grains. **Cognitive Level:** Applying **Client Need:** Physiological Adaptation **Integrated Process:** Teaching and Learning **Content Area:** Child Health **Strategy:** Children with celiac disease can eat corn and rice. All other grains need to be eliminated from the diet.

28 **Answer: 1, 2, 5** **Rationale:** The nurse would expect an increased desire to drink fluids and a higher specific gravity caused by the concentration of urine. The heart rate would be elevated, and the fontanels sunken. The degree of dehydration is based on the percent of weight loss, so a weight gain would not be likely. Diminished urine output with elevated specific gravity is an expected normal finding in dehydration. Capillary refill is slowed, especially in children less than 2 years of age. **Cognitive Level:** Applying **Client Need:** Physiological Adaptation **Integrated Process:** Nursing Process: Data Collection **Content Area:** Child Health **Strategy:** Two of the options are age related and appropriate for the infant. Polyuria and weight gain would not be symptoms of dehydration.

29 **Answer: 1, 3, 5** **Rationale:** Infants with Hirschsprung's disease usually display failure to thrive, poor weight gain, and delayed growth. Vomiting is usually bile stained. The child will demonstrate alternating constipation and diarrhea, but the stools are not bloody. Decreased urine output and intermittent sharp pain are nonspecific symptoms that can be associated with many different diseases and disorders. **Cognitive Level:** Applying **Client Need:** Physiological Adaptation **Integrated Process:** Nursing Process: Data Collection **Content Area:** Child Health **Strategy:** Consider symptoms of Hirschsprung's disease without looking at the options. Then review the options to determine which options match those symptoms.

30 **Answer: 2** **Rationale:** Fever indicates an infection, ruling out two of the options. Appendicitis typically causes pain in the umbilical area or right lower quadrant and is not usually accompanied by diarrhea. Fever and diarrhea accompany diverticulitis. **Cognitive Level:** Applying **Client Need:** Physiological Adaptation **Integrated Process:** Nursing Process: Data Collection **Content Area:** Adult Health **Strategy:** Select an *-itis* as this indicates infection. Appendix pain is right sided.

31 **Answer: 2** **Rationale:** Hepatomegaly is an enlarged liver, which is correct. The spleen may also be enlarged. Dry skin can have many causes. Fluid accumulation is usually in the form of ascites in the abdomen. Peripheral edema can also occur, but there are other clinical conditions in which edema is present. Although pruritis is correct, it is not a strong indicator of cirrhosis. Pruritus can occur for many reasons. **Cognitive Level:** Applying **Client Need:** Physiological Adaptation **Integrated Process:** Nursing Process: Data Collection **Content Area:** Adult Health **Strategy:** Recall that hepatomegaly means enlarged liver, which is common in early cirrhosis.

Key Terms to Review

acholic p. 1010
ascites p. 999
asterixis p. 999
cachexia p. 1015
cholecystitis p. 1003
cholelithiasis p. 1003
cirrhosis p. 998
colostomy p. 985
diarrhea p. 1016
dumping syndrome p. 986
esophageal tamponade p. 1001
esophageal varices p. 1001
esophagogastroduodenoscopy (EGD) p. 984
fecalith p. 1012
hematemesis p. 1000
hepatic encephalopathy p. 1001
hepatorenal syndrome p. 1002
hernia p. 989
hyperbilirubinemia p. 1001
hypoalbuminemia p. 1001
icteric p. 997
ileostomy p. 986
jaundice p. 995
lavage p. 1001
lithotripsy p. 1004
McBurney's point p. 1012
paracentesis p. 1000
portal hypertension p. 1000
sclerotherapy p. 1001
steatorrhea p. 1013
Zollinger-Ellison syndrome p. 984

References

Ball, J., Bindler, R., & Cowen, K. (2010). *Child health nursing: Partnering with children and families* (2nd ed.). Upper Saddle River, NJ: Pearson Education.

Berman, A., & Snyder, S. (2012). *Kozier & Erb's fundamentals of nursing: Concepts, process, and practice* (9th ed.). Upper Saddle River, NJ: Pearson Education, Inc.

Ignatavicius, D., & Workman, L. (2010). *Medical-surgical nursing: Critical thinking for collaborative care* (6th ed.). Philadelphia: Saunders.

Kee, J. (2010). *Laboratory and diagnostic tests with nursing implications* (8th ed.). Upper Saddle River, NJ: Pearson Education.

LeMone, P., Burke, K., & Bauldoff, G. (2011). *Medical-surgical nursing: Critical thinking in patient care* (5th ed.). Upper Saddle River, NJ: Pearson Education.

Smith, S., Duell, D., & Martin, B. (2012). *Clinical nursing skills: Basic to advanced skills* (8th ed.). Upper Saddle River, NJ: Pearson Education.

Test Yourself

Are you ready for the NCLEX-PN® or course exams? Use the practice tests on the companion website to check.

Endocrine and Metabolic Disorders

56

In this chapter

Cross Reference

Other chapters relevant to this content area are

Meeting Nutritional Needs	Chapter 25
Endocrine Medications	Chapter 38
Common Laboratory Tests	Chapter 42
Common Diagnostic Tests and Procedures	Chapter 43
Fluid and Electrolyte Imbalances	Chapter 49

I. OVERVIEW OF ANATOMY AND PHYSIOLOGY OF ENDOCRINE SYSTEM

A. Basic structures of endocrine system

1. Exocrine glands secrete substances that reach their target tissue directly or via a duct; include sebaceous, salivary, mammary, and sweat glands
2. Endocrine glands secrete hormones directly into bloodstream to affect a variety of biological functions; neuronal stimulation, chemical substances, or hormones can control secretion of endocrine glands
3. Various conditions can cause endocrine glands to hypersecrete or hyposecrete, leading to altered body functions

4. **Hyposecretion** is a condition in which an insufficient amount of substance is secreted
5. **Hypersecretion** is a condition in which an excessive amount of substance is secreted

B. **Basic functions of endocrine system**

1. Endocrine glands: coordinate and regulate long-term changes in function of all body organs and tissues to maintain homeostasis
2. Hormones: chemical messengers that travel in circulatory system and alter cellular activities by changing enzymes and proteins in target cells
   a. **Receptor**: specially designed link on a target cell membrane or in cytoplasm for a specific hormone to contact and initiate an action response
   b. Regulation of secretion: effects on target tissue act as a negative-feedback mechanism to signal initiating gland to slow or stop secretion

C. **Major endocrine system glands**

1. Posterior pituitary gland: regulates fluid balance and facilitates childbirth and prostate gland function
   a. Releases antidiuretic hormone (ADH) and oxytocin, which are produced and stored in hypothalamus
   b. ADH stimulates kidneys to reabsorb water, decreasing urine output (UO) and supporting blood pressure (BP) and blood volume; also stimulates peripheral blood vessels (BVs) to constrict
   c. Oxytocin stimulates uterus to contract for childbirth, mammary glands for milk ejection, and smooth muscles of prostate gland to contract and eject secretions
2. Anterior pituitary gland: major role is to produce and release seven different hormones (most regulate secretion of other hormones): thyroid-stimulating hormone (TSH), adrenocorticotropic hormone (ACTH), follicle-stimulating hormone (FSH), luteinizing hormone (LH), prolactin (PRL), interstitial cell–stimulating hormone (ICSH), and growth hormone (GH), also called somatotropin
3. Thyroid gland: determines rate of cellular metabolism; in children, hormones are responsible for normal development of skeletal, muscular, and nervous systems
   a. Calcitonin targets bone and kidney cells to regulate calcium ion concentrations in body fluids
   b. Thyroxine (TX or tetraiodothyronine or T_4), and triiodothyronine (T_3) bind to mitochondria and nucleus of cells to increase rate of ATP production
4. Parathyroid glands: monitor and maintain circulating concentration of calcium (Ca^{++}) ions, by secreting parathyroid hormone (PTH), which increases serum Ca^{++} level; PTH stimulates osteoclasts, inhibits osteoblasts, promotes Ca^{++} absorption by intestines, and decreases renal excretion of Ca^{++}
5. Pancreas (islets of Langerhans): regulates blood glucose level
   a. Alpha cells produce glucagon to break down stored fat and carbohydrate (CHO) into glucose in response to low glucose level
   b. Beta cells produce insulin to transport glucose across cell membranes
   c. Delta cells produce somatostatin that inhibits production of glucagons and insulin
6. Adrenal medulla: increases cellular energy use and muscular strength endurance, and mobilizes energy reserves
   a. Secretes epinephrine (adrenaline) and norepinephrine (noradrenaline); receptors are on skeletal muscle fibers, adipose tissues, and liver
   b. Mobilizes glycogen reserves, metabolizes glucose for ATP, and increases cardiac rate and force of contraction
7. Adrenal cortex: hormones play a vital role for survival and affect metabolism of many different tissues
   a. Glucocorticoids: cortisol (hydrocortisone), corticosterone, and cortisone stimulate most cells to increase rate of glucose synthesis, glycogen formation, release of fatty acids, and break down fatty acids; exert an anti-inflammatory effect to suppress immune system
   b. Mineralocorticoids: aldosterone stimulates kidneys to increase reabsorption of sodium (Na^+) and water, and reduces Na^+ and water loss by sweat glands, salivary glands, and digestive tract
   c. Small amount of androgens
8. Female gonads (ovaries): regulate secondary sexual characteristics and reproduction
   a. Estrogens stimulate most cells to develop secondary sex characteristics and behaviors, follicle maturation, and growth of uterine lining
   b. Provide negative feedback to anterior pituitary gland to stop FSH secretion
   c. Progestins stimulate uterus to prepare for implantation and mammary glands for lactation
9. Male gonads (testes): regulate secondary sexual characteristics and reproduction
   a. Androgens, primarily testosterone, stimulate most cells for protein synthesis, maturation of sperm, secondary sexual characteristics and behaviors
   b. Inhibin secreted for negative feedback to anterior pituitary gland to stop secretion of FSH

II. DIAGNOSTIC TESTS AND DATA COLLECTION

A. Computed tomography (CT) scan: with or without contrast; see also Chapter 43

B. Studies of pituitary gland

1. Serum studies include GH or somatotropin, somatomedin C, GH release post-exercise, insulin-induced hypoglycemia, prolactin level, gonadotropin levels (FSH, LH), and water-deprivation test
2. Radiologic studies include skull x-ray to detect integrity of bone and bone tumors, CT scan and magnetic resonance imaging (MRI) to outline organ structure, tumors, edema, infarcts, blood flow patterns, and BV integrity

C. Studies of thyroid gland

NCLEX® 1. Serum studies
   a. L-thyroxine (total T_4): measures both free and protein-bound thyroxine; normal is 4.5–10.9 mcg/dL in adults
   b. Free T_4 is amount of thyroxine not bound to globulins; normal values are 0.8–2.7 ng/mL by actual assay or 4.6–11.2 by calculated method
   c. Triiodothyronine (T_3) (normal value 60–181 ng/dL), also called T_3 RIA, T_3 resin uptake (T_3RU)
   d. Additional tests are TSH or thyrotropin (normal value 0.5–5.0 units/mL) and serum calcitonin
2. Radiologic studies include thyroid scan or radioactive isotope uptake study to determine uptake of radionuclide by thyroid gland, and whole body scan to detect metastasis from a known malignant thyroid tumor

D. Studies of parathyroid glands

1. Serum studies
   a. PTH, which regulates serum Ca^{++} and phosphorus
   b. Total Ca^{++} (including free Ca^{++} and Ca^{++} bound to plasma proteins)
   c. Phosphorus: reported as phosphorus (P) or phosphate (PO_4) and 1,25 Dihydroxyvitamin D
2. Radiologic studies include skeletal x-ray and CT scan

E. Studies of adrenal glands

1. Serum cortisol: secreted by adrenal cortex, a larger amount in morning, then decreasing during day
2. Serum and/or urinary aldosterone: a mineralocorticoid secreted by adrenal cortex
3. Serum ACTH stimulation to confirm suspected disease of adrenal cortex
4. Dexamethasone suppression and metyrapone suppression
5. Urinary 17-Ketosteroids (17 KS): 24-hour urine is collected to measure amount of 17 KS or metabolites of steroids produced by adrenal cortex and testes

NCLEX® 6. Vanillylmandelic acid (VMA): a metabolite of catecholamines
   a. A 24-hour urine is collected in bottle containing HCL (a strong acid) obtained from lab
   b. Warn client about acid in bottle, to keep face away from opening when removing cap to add urine, and to avoid inhaling odor from bottle
   c. Instruct client to avoid exercise or exposure to stress
   d. Check with lab about specific foods to be avoided during testing period
   e. If possible client should not take any medication for 7 days before and during testing period
   f. Record BP, height, and weight on lab slip

F. Studies of pancreas

NCLEX® 1. Fasting blood glucose (FBG) levels or fasting plasma glucose; withhold food and insulin for at least 8 hours, (water is permitted); adult reference value: 70–110 mg/dL (whole blood: 60–100 mg/dL), older adults 70–120 mg/dL
2. Oral glucose tolerance test (GTT): tests for gestational glucose intolerance; medications, infection, trauma, bedrest, and stress can alter results; see Chapter 42

NCLEX® 3. Capillary glucose monitoring
   a. Warm extremity to encourage vasodilation; select digit to be used
   b. Cleanse site with soap and water or 70% alcohol; dry with a gauze sponge
   c. Avoid squeezing site to enhance blood flow since squeezing causes dilution with tissue fluid
   d. Avoid touching skin with reagent strip; skin oils may affect results
   e. Elevate digit and apply gentle pressure with dry sterile gauze to site until bleeding stops

NCLEX® 4. **Glycosylated hemoglobin**: prolonged **hyperglycemia** (elevated blood glucose) causes glucose to bind irreversibly to hemoglobin (Hgb) of red blood cell (RBC) for remaining life of RBC; HgbA1c determines control of blood glucose over past 3–5 weeks, generally; see Chapter 42, Table 42–3 for expected values

5. Urine studies
    a. Ketones: metabolic end-product of fatty acid metabolism; body uses fatty acids for energy when there is insufficient supply of glucose; ketones should be absent in urine (negative)
    b. Acetone: metabolite of fatty acid metabolism; should also be absent in urine

III. GROWTH HORMONE DEFICIENCY (GHD)

A. **Overview:** a disorder caused by deficiency of growth hormone (GH) production or release from anterior pituitary gland; may be inherited or caused by infection, pituitary gland infarction (such as in sickle cell disease), tumor in brain, cranial irradiation, chemotherapy, brain trauma, and psychosocial deprivation

B. **Nursing data collection**
1. Normal weight and length at birth
2. Below third percentile on growth chart by 1 year of age; child usually grows at rate less than 5 centimeters (cm) or 2 inches (in) per year
3. Infants: hypoglycemic seizures, hyponatremia, neonatal jaundice, pale optic discs, and in males, micropenis and undescended testes
4. *NCLEX®* Children: youthful facial features, high-pitched voice, delayed dentition, "ripply" abdominal fat, decreased muscle mass and skeletal maturation, delayed sexual maturation, and possible associated slipped capital femoral epiphysis
5. Diagnosed by low levels of IGF-1 (insulin like growth factor) on screening test; radiologic studies to determine bone age (skeletal maturation) or to rule out other disorders

C. **Therapeutic management**
1. Treatment of underlying disorder if present
2. *NCLEX®* GH therapy by subcutaneous injection daily or every other day until acceptable height is reached or growth velocity drops to less than 2 cm (1 in) per year
3. Monitor growth and document on growth chart at periodic health checkups (every 3 to 4 months)

D. **Reinforce client and family teaching**
1. Importance of optimal nutrition and adequate caloric and iron intake before and during therapy
2. Medication therapy: how to administer injections and information about course of therapy
3. Close monitoring and follow-up is important
4. Medication therapy is expensive, but drug companies may provide assistance if insurance is insufficient
5. Child can experience disturbed body image; use age-appropriate communication and style of dress (rather than according to body size)

IV. HYPERPITUITARISM

A. **Overview:** excessive secretion of GH from anterior pituitary gland that leads to gigantism (in children before long bone epiphyseal closure) or acromegaly (in adults after epiphyseal closure)

B. *NCLEX®* **Nursing data collection**
1. Tall stature if onset in childhood
2. Large hands and feet with prominent jawbone
3. Joint changes consistent with arthritis
4. Deep voice and possible dysphagia
5. Hypertension
6. Organomegaly
7. Skin changes leading to rough, oily texture

C. **Therapeutic management**
1. Monitor for Disturbed Body Image and provide emotional support to client and family
2. Provide measures to relieve joint pain
3. Possible radiation therapy to pituitary gland
4. Possible hypophysectomy (see next section)

D. **Hypophysectomy**
1. Transphenoidal hypophysectomy may be used to resect pituitary gland
2. Provide standard preoperative care
3. *NCLEX®* Reinforce client teaching about measures used to prevent rises in intracranial pressure (ICP) following surgery (see also Chapter 53)
4. *NCLEX®* Postoperative care
    a. Monitor vital signs (VS), level of consciousness (LOC), and neurological status
    b. Keep head of bed elevated to approximately 30 degrees
    c. Monitor "mustache" dressing taped under nose for drainage and test drainage for glucose to rule out cerebrospinal fluid (CSF) leakage

d. Monitor for postnasal drip, which could also indicate CSF leakage
e. Monitor intake and output (I&O) and observe for signs of diabetes insipidus (DI; water intoxication) as temporary postoperative complication; see next section
f. Keep oral mucous membranes moist; drying can occur because nasal packing after transphenoidal surgery can lead to mouth-breathing

5. Reinforce client teaching

NCLEX® **a.** Avoid activities that raise ICP, such as bending, lifting, sneezing, coughing, blowing nose, and any activity that closes glottis (Valsalva maneuver)
b. Medication teaching, including analgesics and possible antibiotic postoperatively, and possible hormone replacement therapy if entire gland is surgically removed

V. SYNDROME OF INAPPROPRIATE ANTIDIURETIC HORMONE (SIADH)

A. Overview

1. An excessive amount of serum ADH from posterior pituitary gland resulting in water intoxication and hyponatremia (serum Na^+ less than 135 mEq/L)
   a. Usual feedback mechanism does not work to decrease posterior pituitary secretion of ADH when there is decreased serum osmolality (indicating increased fluid)
   b. Elevated ADH leads to renal reabsorption of water and suppression of renin-angiotensin mechanism, causing renal excretion of Na^+
   c. Renal excretion of Na^+ leads to water intoxication, cellular edema, and dilutional hyponatremia
2. Causes include certain hormone-secreting malignant tumors; injury, infection, and medications; increased intrathoracic pressure that stimulates aortic baroreceptors; and activation of limbic system from trauma, pain, stress, and acute psychosis

NCLEX®
B. Nursing data collection

1. General manifestations of fluid volume excess, possibly including increased BP, crackles auscultated in lung fields, distended jugular neck veins, taut skin, and intake greater than output
2. Clinical manifestations: headache, fatigue, anorexia, nausea, muscle aches, abdominal cramps, weight gain without edema, progressive altered LOC, seizures, coma, and small amounts of concentrated amber-colored urine
3. Diagnostic and laboratory test findings: high urine osmolality (>1200 mOsm/kg H_2O) and specific gravity higher than 1.032, low serum osmolality (<275 mOsm/kg), and decreased hematocrit, BUN and serum Na^+ (dilutional effects)

C. Therapeutic management

NCLEX® 1. Restrict oral fluids, including ice chips, to 800 mL/day or less to prevent further hemodilution
2. Supplement Na^+ intake orally or by hypertonic saline IV infusion
NCLEX® 3. Flush all enteral and gastric tubes with normal saline instead of water to replace Na^+ and prevent further hemodilution
NCLEX® 4. Monitor I&O accurately
NCLEX® 5. Monitor for low serum Na^+ and BUN, and concentrated urine
NCLEX® 6. Weigh daily; a weight loss of 2.2 pounds (1 kilogram) indicates a loss of approximately 1 L of fluid
NCLEX® 7. Monitor for changes in LOC, mentation, cognition, nutrition, muscle twitching, and comfort
8. Medication therapy: IV hypertonic saline (3%) and demeclocycline (Declomycin) to replace electrolytes; diuretics to eliminate excessive fluid

D. Reinforce client teaching

1. SIADH and symptoms to report
2. Medication may be lifelong depending on cause
3. Identify hidden sources of water and fluids, such as ice and ice cream, to prevent accidental excessive intake
   a. Plan meal pattern and maintain fluid limitation and Na^+ prescription
   b. Weigh daily on same scale and report gain of 2 pounds in 1 day

VI. DIABETES INSIPIDUS (DI)

A. Overview

1. Results from excessive loss of water caused by hyposecretion of ADH from posterior pituitary gland or kidneys' inability to respond to ADH
2. Subsequent **polyuria** (excessive UO ranging from 4 to 30 L in 24 hours) can lead to severe dehydration if client does not replace lost water

3. Causes can be neurogenic (insufficient ADH secretion by posterior pituitary gland), nephrogenic (kidneys unable to respond to ADH), and medications (lithium carbonate and demeclocycline can cause kidneys to alter response to ADH)
4. Primary DI results from an inherited or idiopathic malfunction of posterior pituitary gland
5. Secondary DI is caused by brain tumors, head trauma, infection, surgery on or near pituitary gland, metastatic tumors from lung or breast, cerebrovascular hemorrhage, granulomatous disease, or cerebral aneurysm

B. Nursing data collection

1. History of head injury, brain surgery, infection, or tumor
2. Obtain a list of current and past medications
3. NCLEX® Monitor LOC, VS including orthostatic BP, skin turgor, I&O, weight, skin integrity, **polydipsia** (excessive thirst), tenting or sagging skin, bowel sounds, constipation
4. NCLEX® Clinical manifestations result largely from fluid volume deficit: polyuria; excessive thirst; dry, tented skin; dry mucous membranes; and severe hypotension leading to cardiovascular collapse (which can occur if the excessive water loss is not replaced)
5. NCLEX® Diagnostic and laboratory test findings: urine specific gravity less than 1.005, urine osmolality less than 300 mOsm/kg, positive water deprivation test, reduced serum ADH level in primary DI, serum sodium greater than 145 mEq/L

C. Therapeutic management

1. Water replacement orally is preferred or intravenous (IV) D_5W as needed to normalize lab values
2. For neurogenic DI, hormone replacement with desmopressin (DDAVP), a synthetic vasopressin; adjunctive medications, such as chlorpropamide (Diabinese), or carbamazepine (Tegretol), may increase ADH release or enhance effect of ADH on renal collecting duct
3. For nephrogenic DI, correct underlying disease or stop causative medication; begin a low-salt, low-protein diet to decrease net excretion of solute
4. NCLEX® Monitor I&O hourly; report UO over 200 mL/hour for 2 consecutive hours or 500 mL over 2 hours; monitor for continence and provide easy access to bathroom as appropriate
5. NCLEX® Weigh daily; report weight loss
6. NCLEX® Monitor urine specific gravity and report if it decreases; monitor serum osmolality and Na^+ for increases
7. NCLEX® Encourage fluid intake greater than UO; provide fluids within reach at all times; provide IV fluid replacement as ordered
8. Use skin protective barriers with incontinence

D. Reinforce client teaching

1. Information about DI, self-administration of medication, and possible need for lifelong medication
2. Wear a Medic-Alert bracelet listing DI and treatments
3. Drink fluid equal to amount of UO, keeping a log of I&O
4. Weigh self daily, on same scale at same time of day, and report weight loss
5. Consult practitioner before taking over-the-counter (OTC) medications

VII. HYPERTHYROIDISM (THYROTOXICOSIS)

A. Overview

1. Excessive secretion of thyroid hormone (TH) from thyroid gland leads to increased basal metabolic rate, cardiovascular function, GI function, neuromuscular function, weight loss, and heat intolerance; thyroid hormone affects metabolism of fats, carbohydrates (CHOs), and proteins
2. Hyperthyroidism can be caused by excess secretion of TSH from pituitary gland, autoimmune reaction (Graves' disease), thyroiditis (inflammation or viral infection of thyroid), tumor, side effects of certain drugs, and excessive dose of thyroid medication

B. Nursing data collection

1. NCLEX® Clinical manifestations: range from very minimal to severe depending on amount and time period of hypersecretion
   a. See Table 56–1
   b. Neck goiter and exophthalmos (bulging eyes) are characteristic in Graves' disease form of hyperthyroidism
2. NCLEX® **Thyroid crisis** or **thyroid storm**: life-threatening emergency occurring in extreme hyperthyroidism
   a. Usually occurs in clients with long-term, untreated hyperthyroidism or in clients with hyperthyroidism experiencing a stressor such as infection, trauma, or manipulation of thyroid gland

Table 56–1 Comparison of Signs of Hyperthyroidism and Hypothyroidism

Area of Function	Hyperthyroidism	Hypothyroidism
Cardiovascular	Tachycardia, dysrhythmias, palpitations, hypertension	Bradycardia, dysrhythmias, cardiomegaly, anemia, hypotension
Gastrointestinal	Diarrhea, possible abdominal pain	Constipation
Neurological	Nervousness, insomnia, hand and eye tremors, hyperactive reflexes, emotional lability	Lethargy, somnolence, confusion, memory impairment, hypoactive reflexes, hand and foot paresthesias
Sensory	Possible blurred vision, lacrimation, photophobia, exophthalmos (in Graves' disease)	Periorbital edema
Integumentary	Flushed moist skin and fine thin hair	Coarse dry skin, brittle nails, non-pitting edema, hair loss
Reproductive	Amenorrhea and decreased fertility (females), decreased libido and impotence (males)	Menorrhagia and decreased fertility (females), decreased libido (males)
General metabolic	Hyperthermia, hunger, weight loss, possible fluid volume deficit; high basal metabolic rate	Hypothermia, anorexia, weight gain, systemic edema, and low basal metabolic rate

NCLEX® **b.** Common manifestations of thyroid storm are temperature over 102°F (39°C), tachycardia, systolic hypertension, abdominal pain, nausea, vomiting, diarrhea, agitation, tremors, confusion, and possible seizures

3. Diagnostic and laboratory test findings: elevated serum T_3, T_4, free T_4; decreased TSH; positive RAI uptake scan and thyroid scan (depending on cause)

C. Therapeutic management

1. Consists of medical treatment or surgical removal of part of thyroid gland (partial or total thyroidectomy)

NCLEX® **2.** Ethionamide drugs for life to reduce secretion of thyroid hormone

NCLEX® **3.** Ablative therapy with radioactive Iodine 131: thyroid gland absorbs I-131, which destroys some thyroid cells over a period of 6 to 8 weeks

- **a.** Not recommended for pregnant women
- **b.** Radiation precautions are not required for small doses (<30 mCi) of I-131
- **c.** Instruct client to drink solution with straw to minimize exposure to buccal cavity
- **d.** Monitor lab values; report weight gain, fatigue, decreased pulse, and lowered BP (signs of excessive effects)
- **e.** Total or subtotal (partial) thyroidectomy may be indicated based on situation

NCLEX® **4.** Nursing care for non-surgical clients

- **a.** Keep environment cool and free of distractions and stress as able
- **b.** Encourage balance of rest with activity periods
- **c.** Monitor visual acuity, photophobia and corneal integrity, and ability to close eyes with exophthalmos; encourage eye protection measures such as tinted glasses, eye shields, cool moist compresses for irritation, and artificial tears to reduce dryness as needed
- **d.** Assist nutritional state by weighing client daily; provide diet high in carbohydrates, protein and between meal snacks (variation: six smaller meals may be better than three larger ones); monitor nutritional state with labs such as serum prealbumin, albumin, transferrin, and total lymphocyte count
- **e.** Assist client to cope with body image changes with goiter and exophthalmos

NCLEX® **5.** Preoperative preparation for thyroidectomy

- **a.** Review deep-breathing exercises and appropriate cough
- **b.** Instruct client to hold hands behind neck when coughing, sitting, turning, or getting up/back to bed to reduce postoperative pain and neck muscle strain
- **c.** Instruct client how to self-administer prescribed antithyroid drugs to decrease vascularity and size of thyroid and minimize risk of surgical hemorrhage

6. Postoperative care following thyroidectomy

- NCLEX® **a.** Provide comfort: analgesics, semi-Fowler's position with neck and head supported by pillows to prevent muscle strain, ice collar to wound area for comfort and to prevent edema
- NCLEX® **b.** Monitor for hemorrhage: tightness of dressing; sanguineous exudate on anterior or posterior neck dressing or on skin of neck, upper chest and upper back, shoulders, and back of neck; auscultate trachea for stridor (indicating edema and narrowed airway); first 24 hours postoperative is time of greatest risk

NCLEX® c. Promote patent airway: elevate head of bed 30 degrees; monitor for respiratory distress; keep oral and sterile suction supplies and emergency tracheostomy tray (with tracheostomy kit and IV calcium gluconate or calcium chloride) within immediate access; maintain humidification of inspired air if ordered; encourage deep-breathing exercises and incentive spirometer hourly; cough only if needed to clear secretions

NCLEX® d. Prevent tetany by early identification of hypocalcemia (serum calcium less than 8 mg/dL) evidenced by numbness or tingling of toes, extremities, and lips; muscle twitches; positive Chvostek's and Trousseau signs; see also Chapter 49

e. Maintain patent IV site

f. Monitor for laryngeal nerve damage, noting ability to speak loudly, quality and tone of voice (hoarseness may be temporary after surgery)

g. Analgesics to control surgical pain

D. Reinforce client teaching

1. Correct self-administration of lifelong medications with medical treatment
2. Hyperthyroidism, hypothyroidism, and symptoms to report; clients with underlying heart disease could experience chest pain and decreased cardiac output from increased workload
3. Postoperative conditions to report, including signs of hemorrhage, hypocalcemia, incisional infection, respiratory difficulty and discomfort
4. NCLEX® For exophthalmos, use methods to protect eyes and adapt to altered visual field
   a. Have regular eye exams
   b. Call practitioner immediately for any change in vision, appearance of eye, eyelid closure, eye pain or exudate, or **photophobia** (sensitivity to light)
   c. Protect eyes with tinted glasses or eye shields because lids do not cover eyes completely and corneal/blink reflex may be delayed
   d. Moisten eyes frequently with artificial tears to prevent dry irritation and corneal infection; use caution not to contaminate eyedropper
   e. Soothe dry-eye irritation with cool, moist compresses
   f. Sleep with head of bed elevated to minimize pressure on optic nerve, and wear eye patches to protect eyes during sleep if lids do not close
5. Surgical client
   a. Surgical procedure and expected outcomes
   b. NCLEX® Support neck with hands; position neck and head with pillows and maintain semi-Fowler's position; avoid hyperextension and sudden quick movements of head and neck
   c. Wound care
   d. NCLEX® Avoid/minimize talking and coughing until wound is healed to prevent strain on laryngeal nerve and vocal cords
6. Assist client to cope with lifestyle and self-image changes

VIII. HYPOTHYROIDISM

A. Overview

1. Insufficient secretion of TH by thyroid gland, causing decreased metabolic rate and heat production, and various effects on body systems
2. Primary hypothyroidism accounts for 99% of all cases, and 50% of cases are caused by cell-mediated and antibody-mediated destruction of thyroid gland
3. Other causes are thyroiditis, subacute postpartum, external irradiation of gland, iatrogenic (30 to 40%), infections, iodine deficiency, congenital or idiopathic
4. Secondary hypothyroidism, also called central hypothyroidism, is caused by insufficient secretion of TSH from pituitary gland or related to disease of hypothalamus
5. Thyroid gland gradually enlarges, forming a goiter (thickening of gland) in an attempt to secrete more thyroid hormone

NCLEX® **B. Nursing data collection**

1. See Table 56–1 again for common manifestations
2. Myxedema (a life-threatening crisis state of hypothyroidism): non-pitting edema in connective tissues throughout body, puffy face and tongue, severe metabolic disorders, hypothermia, cardiovascular collapse, and coma
3. Diagnostic and laboratory test findings: varies according to whether cause is thyroid gland or pituitary; may include decreased T_4 and free T_4, normal T_3, and increased TSH levels; elevated serum lipids

NCLEX® **C. Therapeutic management**

1. Medication therapy: thyroid hormone replacement, such as dessicated thyroid, thyroxine (Synthroid), or triiodothyronine (Cytomel)
2. Give medication in morning 1 hour before food intake or 2 hours after food intake to facilitate absorption
3. Adjust environmental temperature and use blankets as needed for warmth; chilling increases metabolic rate, cardiac workload, and O_2 demand
4. Pace activities with rest periods; instruct client to report shortness of breath, fatigue, dizziness, or any discomfort
5. Encourage intake of 2000 mL water daily and a high-fiber diet to promote regular bowel movements

D. Reinforce client teaching

1. Disorder and its management
2. Importance of wearing a Medic-Alert bracelet
3. NCLEX® Medication is needed for life and should be taken at same time every morning, 1 hr before a meal or 2 hrs after a meal
4. Take same brand of medication because brands vary in bioavailability
5. NCLEX® Report weight gain or loss of 5 pounds, activity intolerance, chest pain, heat or cold intolerance, and sleep pattern disturbance
6. Report symptoms of hypothyroidism and hyperthyroidism

IX. HYPERPARATHYROIDISM

A. Overview

1. Results from increased PTH secretion from parathyroid gland
   a. Primary type: hyperplasia or tumor of parathyroid gland, increasing absorption of Ca^{++} in GI tract
   b. Secondary type: gland enlargement caused by chronic hypocalcemia in presence of elevated PTH
2. Increased Ca^{++} reabsorption and increased phosphate excretion lead to hypercalcemia and hypophosphatemia
3. Kidneys increase bicarbonate excretion and decrease acid excretion, leading to metabolic acidosis and hypokalemia
4. Bones increase rate of Ca^{++} and phosphorus release, leading to bone decalcification
5. Hypercalcemia results in Ca^{++} deposits in soft tissues, renal calculi, altered neurological function with muscle weakness and atrophy, altered GI function with constipation, abdominal pain and anorexia

B. Nursing data collection

1. Polyuria (early sign) and renal calculi
2. Anorexia, constipation, abdominal pain, peptic ulcer disease (from hypercalcemia)
3. Generalized bone pain, pathologic fractures, and muscle weakness and atrophy
4. NCLEX® CNS signs (depressed deep tendon reflexes, **paresthesias** [altered sensations], depression, psychosis)
5. Elevated serum Ca^{++} and PTH; decreased phosphate
6. Possible bone changes on skeletal x-rays and CT scan

C. Therapeutic management

1. NCLEX® Decrease serum Ca^{++} level with IV normal saline (NS) infusions, diuretics, and phosphate replacement
2. Possible surgery to remove involved parathyroid glands
3. Promote comfort and safety; client may need to use walker to prevent falls
4. Strain all urine to detect calcium-based urinary stones
5. NCLEX® Provide 2000 to 3000 mL of fluids daily as tolerated and a high-fiber diet
6. Encourage progressive activity as tolerated, pacing activity with rest periods
7. Promote nutrition and fluid and electrolyte balance; weigh daily
8. NCLEX® Monitor for hypocalcemia to prevent tetany caused by surgery (removal of parathyroid gland) or aggressive excretion of Ca^{++}
   a. Numbness and tingling around mouth and fingertips
   b. Muscle twitching of extremities
   c. Change in voice
   d. Positive Chvostek sign (spasm of facial muscles when cheek touched) and Trousseau sign (spasm of hand when BP cuff inflated)
9. Medication therapy: analgesics to control pain; diuretics and NS by IV infusion to excrete excess calcium; phosphate and calcitonin (Miacalcin) may be used to inhibit bone reabsorption

D. Reinforce client teaching

1. Hyperparathyroidism and appropriate self-administration of medications
2. Symptoms to report, including those indicating hypocalcemia, activity intolerance, and infection

X. HYPOPARATHYROIDISM

A. Overview

1. Low PTH levels causing hypocalcemia, usually caused by surgical removal of all or part of gland
2. Hypocalcemia raises threshold for excitability in nerve and muscle fibers, causing fibers to be easily stimulated; could lead to life-threatening tetany

B. Nursing data collection

1. GI symptoms: abdominal pain, nausea, vomiting, diarrhea, anorexia
2. *NCLEX®* Signs of hypocalcemia (anxiety, headaches, paresthesias [hands, feet, lips], neuromuscular irritability with tremors, muscle spasms and hyperactive reflexes); positive Chvostek's or Trousseau's sign
3. *NCLEX®* Possible difficulty swallowing or hoarse voice, sensation of tightness in throat
4. Dry thin hair, patchy hair loss, ridged finger nails
5. Psychosis, mood disorders (anxiety, irritability, depression)
6. Decreased serum PTH, total calcium, free calcium; increased serum phosphate

C. Therapeutic management

1. *NCLEX®* Supplemental Ca^{++} and vitamin D
2. *NCLEX®* Promote comfort and safety; client may need to use walker to prevent falls
3. Encourage progressive activity as tolerated, pacing activity with rest periods
4. Promote nutrition and fluid and electrolyte balance
5. Medication therapy: Ca^{++} supplement orally or by IV infusion; vitamin D orally to promote intestinal absorption of Ca^{++}

D. Reinforce client teaching

1. Disorder and its management, to wear Medic-Alert bracelet listing disease and medications, and self-administration of medication
2. Symptoms to report (see again nursing data collection)
3. *NCLEX®* Diet high in Ca^{++} and vitamin D, identifying minimum daily intake; foods high in calcium are cheese, milk, turnip greens, almonds, collard greens, beans, peanuts, frankfurters, and bologna

XI. CUSHING'S DISEASE

A. Overview

1. Hyperfunction of adrenal cortex (AC) causing elevated serum cortisol or ACTH levels
2. Elevated serum cortisol causes life-threatening changes in physiological, psychological, and metabolic functioning
3. Incidence is greater in women; usual age of onset is 30 to 40 years
4. Primary Cushing's disease is caused by a tumor of adrenal cortex
5. Secondary Cushing's disease is caused by disorder of pituitary or hypothalamus (causing increased ACTH and hyperplasia of adrenal cortex) or by an ectopic tissue (such as an ACTH-producing cancer of lung, bronchus, or pancreas)
6. Iatrogenic: long-term use of glucocorticoid medication such as steroids

B. Nursing data collection

1. *NCLEX®* See Table 56–2
2. Elevated serum cortisol, Na^+, and glucose, and lowered Ca^{++} and potassium (K^+)
3. Serum ACTH can be elevated or decreased; positive ACTH suppression test
4. Elevated urine 17 KS; normal BUN

C. Therapeutic management

1. Possible radiation therapy to pituitary gland
2. *NCLEX®* Single or bilateral adrenalectomy or hypophysectomy (removal of pituitary gland)
3. Assist client to achieve fluid, electrolyte, glucose, and calcium balance
4. Analyze daily weights and I&O
5. *NCLEX®* Promote safety: uncluttered walking area, adequate lighting, assistive walking devices to prevent falls as needed, and use of stable, nonskid shoes or slippers
6. Assist client to pace activities and rest to prevent fatigue
7. *NCLEX®* Prevent infection before and after surgery: use standard precautions, provide aseptic wound care, and promote optimal nutrition
8. Assist client to use effective coping strategies and encourage client to discuss feelings about change in physical appearance
9. Preoperative care: ensure that client understands planned surgical procedure, postoperative routines, and expected outcomes

Table 56–2 Comparison of Signs of Adrenal Cortex Hyperfunction and Hypofunction

Area of Function	Cushing's Disease (Hyperfunction)	Addison's Disease (Hypofunction)
Fluid balance	Overhydration, hypervolemia, and weight gain	Dehydration, hypovolemia, and weight loss
Electrolytes	Hypernatremia, hypokalemia	Hyponatremia, hyperkalemia
Cardiovascular	Hypertension and possible signs of CHF (from overhydration)	Postural hypotension (from dehydration), tachycardia, dysrhythmias
Integumentary	Thin skin that bruises easily, striae, hirsutism, poor wound healing	Excess melatonin stimulating hormone, with skin pigmentation (eternal tan), delayed wound healing
Miscellaneous	Hyperglycemia, osteoporosis, emotional lability, abnormal fat deposits (truncal obesity, moon facies, fat pad on back of neck) generalized weakness with muscle wasting, possible amenorrhea, impotence, or decreased libido, susceptibility to infection	Hypoglycemia, anorexia, nausea, vomiting, diarrhea, depression, lethargy, emotional lability, confusion, muscle weakness, muscle and joint pain

10. Postoperative care
    a. NCLEX® Promote effective respirations with hourly coughing and deep-breathing exercises (clients with pituitary removal should avoid coughing)
    b. Assist with repositioning every 2 hours, and encourage ankle dorsiflexion exercises hourly
    c. Promote wound healing by minimizing stress on incision line
    d. NCLEX® After adrenalectomy, client should log roll to side to sit up at bedside and should do the reverse to recline
    e. NCLEX® Follow principles of postoperative care discussed previously if client underwent removal of pituitary gland
    f. Elevate head of bed 30 degrees, and use aseptic technique for wound care
11. NCLEX® Prevent Addisonian crisis: give NS by IV infusion bolus and cortisol per practitioner's order for these symptoms: dry, tenting skin; decreased BP; increased pulse; decreased LOC; anorexia; and weakness
12. Medication therapy: may include metapyrone (directly inhibits cortisol production and secretion by adrenal cortex); octreotide (Sandostatin), a somatostatin analog that suppresses ACTH secretion; and mitotane (Lysodren), which suppresses function of AC and decreases corticosteroid metabolism, thus decreasing serum cortisol

D. Reinforce client teaching

1. The disorder of Cushing's disease and its management
2. To wear Medic-Alert bracelet listing disease and medications
3. Self-administration of medication
4. NCLEX® Eat a diet high in protein and vitamins B and C to support immune system, and also take supplemental K^+ and Ca^{++}
5. NCLEX® Wound care and postoperative cortisol replacement for surgical clients (temporary replacement for 1 year or less for unilateral adrenalectomy; lifelong if surgery is bilateral)

XII. ADRENAL INSUFFICIENCY (ADDISON'S DISEASE)

A. Overview

1. Insufficient level of cortisol resulting from autoimmune disorder, tuberculosis, septicemia, acquired immunodeficiency syndrome (AIDS), bilateral adrenalectomy, infiltrative diseases, and sudden cessation of long-term high-dose steroid medication
2. Decreased aldosterone and cortisol levels lead to hyponatremia, hyperkalemia (high serum K^+), decreased extracellular fluid, decreased intravascular volume, decreased gluconeogenesis, hypoglycemia, and stress intolerance
3. High ACTH level leads to hyperpigmentation

NCLEX® **B. Nursing data collection**

1. See again Table 56–2
2. NCLEX® Addisonian crisis: a life-threatening response to sudden withdrawal of steroids or exposure to any form of stress, manifested by severe hypotension, circulatory collapse, shock, and coma
3. Decreased serum cortisol, glucose, Na^+, and urine 17 KS
4. Increased serum K^+, BUN, and ACTH levels
5. No increase in cortisol with ACTH stimulation test
6. CT scan can be positive

C. Therapeutic management

NCLEX®
1. Maintain fluid and electrolyte balance: analyze lab values, I&O, and daily weight; encourage 3000 mL of daily oral fluid intake and added Na^+ in diet

NCLEX®
2. Promote safety: appropriate walking assistive devices, adequate lighting, clear area for walking, and appropriate slippers or shoes
3. Medication therapy: hydrocortisone (Cortef) to replace cortisol; fludrocortisone (Florinef) to replace mineralocorticoids as needed

D. Reinforce client teaching

1. Addison's disease and symptoms to report (weight gain, easy bruising or bleeding, weakness, dizziness, lethargy, epigastric discomfort, and change in BP or pulse)

NCLEX®
2. Need for lifelong medication and disease management
3. Need to consult practitioner before taking any OTC medications
4. Self-administration of medication, and plan for medication adjustment upward during times of stress
5. Wear Medic-Alert bracelet listing Addison's disease, medications, and contact numbers
6. Diet to promote immune system function and foods to high in Na^+ and low in K^+ (see also Chapter 49)

XIII. DIABETES MELLITUS (DM)

A. Overview

1. Disorder of pancreas characterized by insufficient or absolute lack of insulin production, causing hyperglycemia (elevated blood glucose) and resulting in multisystem changes in health status
2. Type 1: results from autoimmune destruction of beta cells; has a genetic predisposition; is more common in males; can occur at any age but usually occurs in children and adolescents; is also characterized by hyperglycemia and **ketosis** (ketones in blood resulting from gluconeogenesis from fats)
3. Type 2: several proposed causes include compromised ability of beta cells to respond to hyperglycemia, abnormal insulin receptors on cells, and peripheral insulin resistance; it has a genetic predisposition, can occur at any age, and is more common in obesity, older adults, African Americans, Hispanic Americans, and Native Americans
4. Acute complications include hypoglycemia, diabetic ketoacidosis, and hyperglycemic hyperosmolar nonketotic (HHNK) coma, also called hyperosmolar coma (HOC) in type 2
5. Long-term or chronic complications (see Table 56–3)

NCLEX®

B. Nursing data collection

1. Type 1: polyuria, polydipsia (excess fluid intake), **polyphagia** (increased food intake), weight loss, malaise, and fatigue
2. Type 2: polyuria, polydipsia, blurred vision, fatigue, paresthesia (numbness, tingling, sensitivity), and skin infections
3. Elevated random and/or fasting blood glucose (BG)
4. Abnormal oral glucose tolerance test; elevated glycosylated hemoglobin (HgbA1c)
5. Positive serum ketones and possible urine ketones or acetone with ketoacidosis

Table 56–3 Chronic Effects or Complications of Diabetes Mellitus

Body System	Chronic Effect
Neurological	Somatic neuropathies (paresthesias, pain, and loss of sensation and motor control) and visceral neuropathies (pupil constriction, fixed heart rate, constipation or diarrhea, dysfunction of sweat glands, incomplete voiding, and sexual dysfunction)
Sensory	Cataracts, glaucoma, and diabetic retinopathy
Cardiovascular	Orthostatic hypotension, accelerated atherosclerosis leading to stroke, myocardial infarction (MI), and peripheral vascular disease (PVD), increased blood viscosity, and platelet disorders
Renal	Hypertension, edema, albuminuria, and chronic renal failure
Integumentary	Atrophic changes, foot ulcers or gangrene
Immune	Poor healing, periodontal disease, lung infections, chronic skin infections, urinary tract infections, vaginitis

C. Therapeutic management

NCLEX®

1. Diet
   a. Follow diet recommended in MyPyramid or exchange system diet from American Diabetes Association
   b. Caloric intake is based on individual needs, including possible weight loss needs for type 2 DM
   c. CHO in amounts tailored to individual need, avoiding simple sugars
   d. Protein at 10–20% of caloric intake
   e. Saturated fat less than 10% of calories with cholesterol intake equal to or less than 300 mg/day
   f. Sodium intake 2400 to 3000 mg/day (same as for general population)
   g. Dietary fiber 20 to 35 gm/day
   h. Tailor diet to individual and cultural preferences as possible to improve adherence

NCLEX®

2. Oral antidiabetic medications
   a. Used in type 2 DM only and indicated when diet and exercise alone fail to control BG levels
   b. Consist of oral sulfonylureas, alpha-glucosidase inhibitors, meglitinides, thiazolidinediones, a biguanide, and combination agents; see also Chapter 38
   c. Reinforce to clients taking oral sulfonylureas that concurrent use of alcohol can cause a disulfiram-type reaction (hypoglycemia, flushing, headache, nausea, and abdominal cramps)
   d. Reinforce to client about risk of metabolic acidosis and to discuss with primary care provider about need to discontinue medicine if severe diarrhea, infection, or dehydration occur
   e. Reinforce to all clients manifestations of both hyperglycemia and hypoglycemia, and appropriate corrective actions

NCLEX®

3. Insulin therapy
   a. Is used in type 1 DM or when diet, exercise, and oral agents are insufficient to control type 2 DM
   b. Different insulin preparations are available to maintain near-normal blood glucose levels; insulin is classified according to source, onset, peak, and duration of action
   c. Source: human insulin has a faster onset of action, a shorter peak, and a shorter duration than animal derived insulin; it is preferred to pork or beef insulin (higher incidence of allergic reaction)
   d. Preparations: include rapid-acting (e.g., Insulin lispro [Humalog], aspart [Novolog], and glulisine [Apidra]), short-acting (e.g., regular [Humulin R or Novolin R]) intermediate-acting, (e.g., isophane susp. NPH, Humulin N]), long-acting (e.g., zinc extended [Ultra lente], detemir [Levemir], glargine [Lantus]), mixtures of NPH and regular, and buffered insulin (e.g., Humulin BR); buffered preparations are used for external insulin pumps
   e. Insulin preparations can be combined to mimic pancreatic response to variations in BG levels; for example, rapid- and short-acting insulins are usually given to cover mealtimes, while intermediate- and long-acting insulins maintain basal insulin requirements between meals
   f. Insulin regimens combine short-acting, intermediate-acting, and long-acting preparations to maintain target BG levels
   g. Only regular insulin may be given IV; insulin preparations are usually given via subcutaneous (Subq) route; a continuous Subq insulin infusion (insulin pump) is also available to deliver a basal rate of insulin and allow for additional bolus doses based on requirements (e.g., before a meal)
4. Encourage an exercise plan that meets needs of growing child or enhances fitness and euglycemia in adult

NCLEX®

5. Promote safety: use appropriate lighting; have client wear protective slippers, socks, and shoes that do not rub or impinge on skin; analyze symptoms, activity tolerance, and coping effectiveness; monitor BG levels; give medication and appropriate food and fluids

NCLEX®

6. Prevent infection through appropriate foot care, aseptic injection technique, and fingerstick glucose monitoring technique
7. Identify appropriate glucose-monitoring protocol and medication administration process depending on client's vision, finances, finger dexterity, living environment, resources, literacy, lifestyle, personal values, work/school environment, and coping status
8. Coordinate continuing care as appropriate for client's school, work, and other schedules, such as health club
9. Promote acceptance and effective coping while living with DM

NCLEX®

10. Promote safety: explain early identification of hypoglycemia; check BG as scheduled; treat hypoglycemia with 15 gram CHO snack, such as 8 oz skim milk, 5 Lifesaver candies, 3 large marshmallows, 6 oz juice; and need to recheck BG after treatment of hypoglycemia

NCLEX®

11. Maintain hydration and avoid hyperglycemia; develop sick-day protocol and exercise protocol with client
12. See Table 56–4 for suggestions on promoting age-appropriate self-care for children with type 1 DM

Table 56–4 Developmental Care for Child with Type 1 Diabetes Mellitus

Infants and Toddlers	Preschoolers	School-Age	Teen
Allow toddler to make choices in food selection while monitoring CHO levels Toddler may wish to help with fingerstick by cleaning his or her finger Monitor temper tantrums as a possible sign of hypoglycemia	Allow preschooler to make food choices while monitoring CHO levels Be prepared to substitute snacks at birthday parties and at daycare Encourage guided independence during blood glucose/fingerstick procedure Have appropriate snacks available if needed during sports that require a high energy expenditure	Encourage independence of school-age child in food selection, glucose monitoring, and insulin injections; determine level of knowledge Assure that school personnel are available and knowledgeable if hypoglycemia should occur during school hours Encourage exercise but have snacks available for child Discourage fast food or snack machine selections	Observe teen's body image and sense of identity; monitor adherence to other tasks Encourage independence with food selection, blood glucose monitoring, and insulin injections Supervise diabetic tasks if teen is nonadherent to plan Discuss future plans with teen Include diabetic issues, but promote a normal lifestyle

D. Reinforce client teaching

1. Type of DM, symptoms to report, self-administration of medication, fingerstick glucose monitoring, plan for regular exam by practitioner, need to wear Medic-Alert bracelet indicating DM and medication prescription, need for lifelong medication management and lifestyle adjustments

NCLEX®

2. Foot care: keep feet clean and dry; inspect feet daily using mirror to see soles; protect feet by wearing shoes (allow ½- to ¾-inch toe room) or slippers at all times; avoid snug fitting socks or stockings; use cotton socks because they wick perspiration away from skin

NCLEX®

3. Sick-day management: maintain food and fluid intake, continue to take insulin; BG monitoring (up to q4h; report > 250 mg/dL); monitor urine for ketones
4. Diet plan, including considerations for traveling, sports, attendance at parties, and other alterations in daily routine

NCLEX®

5. Reinforce these instructions to clients receiving insulin
   a. Storage: store insulin in use at room temperature, away from direct sunlight, and replace after 4 weeks; administration of cold insulin causes subQ atrophy (lipoatrophy) or hypertrophy (lipodystrophy), which alters insulin absorption; store extra vials of insulin not being used in refrigerator
   b. Preparation: note date of expiration; discard vial and use new one if regular insulin appears cloudy; do not shake—may inactivate insulin and/or form bubbles that lead to dosage errors; roll nonregular insulin gently between hands to evenly disperse suspended particles; draw regular (clear) insulin first when mixing it with other types of insulin; only mix insulins of same concentration (e.g., U100 regular and U100 NPH) and from same source
   c. Injection: rotate injection sites to prevent lipoatrophy and lipodystrophy; do not inject insulin in an area that will be involved in exercise, as it will increase rate of absorption, onset, and peak action
   d. Monitor for signs of hypoglycemia; have candy or foods with simple carbohydrates available
   e. Avoid alcohol while taking insulin because it lowers BG levels and can cause hypoglycemia

NCLEX®

6. Reinforce signs of hypoglycemia (restlessness, irritability, weakness, hunger, nausea, pale diaphoretic skin, shakiness or trembling, headache, confusion, inability to concentrate, deteriorating LOC to coma, seizures), actions to take, causes of hypoglycemia, and methods to prevent
7. Reinforce how to prevent and manage acute complications of DM (hyperglycemia, hypoglycemia, diabetic ketoacidosis, and HHNK; and chronic complications of DM (diabetic retinopathy, nephropathy, and neuropathy); see Table 56–5 for comparison of hypoglycemia and hyperglycemia with ketoacidosis

NCLEX®

8. Develop with client a plan for wellness, including exercise
   a. Daily cardiovascular exercise decreases risk for insulin resistance, reduces risk for complications, and improves glucose management
   b. Check BG before exercise; check for urine ketones if fasting BG is 250 mg/dL; call practitioner if ketones are present and avoid exercise
   c. Monitor for signs of hypoglycemia for up to 24 hours after extensive exercise

Table 56-5 A Comparison of Hypoglycemia and Hyperglycemia with Ketoacidosis

	Hypoglycemia	Hyperglycemia with Ketoacidosis
Causes	Too much insulin; inadequate intake or missed meals; strenuous exercise without increased intake	Insufficient insulin; infection or other illness may contribute to its development
Symptoms	1. Blood glucose (BG) level drops below normal 2. Diaphoresis, tremors, hunger, weakness, pallor, dizziness, somnolence, coma, seizures, death	1. BG >250 mg/dL 2. Blood pH < 7.2; HCO_3^- < 15 mEq/L 3. Glycosuria, ketonuria, ↑ serum K^+ and chloride; ↓ serum Na^+, Ca^{++}, Mg^{++}, and phosphate (PO_4^-) 4. Kussmaul respirations, acetone breath, dehydration, weight loss, tachycardia, flushed facial skin, hypotension, decreased LOC, death 5. Reports of stomach ache or chest pain are common; vomiting may occur
Treatment	Depends on severity of symptoms but involves replacement of glucose Mild or moderate: juice or milk, graham crackers, glucose tablets or gel Severe: glucose paste; family may be taught to administer glucagon subQ	Normal saline is given IV until BG ↓ to 250–300 mg/dL; then is changed to 5% dextrose in 0.45% NaCl to avoid rebound hypoglycemia Potassium levels are monitored; initial hyperkalemia may become hypokalemia following fluid and insulin therapy

XIV. DIABETIC KETOACIDOSIS (DKA)

A. Overview

1. Life-threatening metabolic acidosis resulting from persistent hyperglycemia and breakdown of fats into glucose, leading to presence of ketones in blood
2. Can be triggered by emotional stress, uncompensated exercise, infection, trauma, or insufficient or delayed insulin administration
3. Hyperglycemia causes uncompensated polyuria, hemoconcentration, dehydration, hyperosmolarity, and electrolyte imbalance; a significant accumulation of serum ketones leads to acidosis

NCLEX® **B. Nursing data collection**

1. Thirst
2. Nausea and vomiting
3. Malaise and lethargy
4. Polyuria
5. Warm dry skin, flushed face
6. Acetone (fruity) odor to breath, Kussmaul respirations (deep, labored, rapid respirations)
7. Serum glucose above 250 mg/dL; plasma pH under 7.35; plasma bicarbonate (HCO_3^-) under 15 mEq/L; serum ketones present; urine positive for glucose and ketones; may have abnormal serum sodium and chloride levels and hyperkalemia

NCLEX® **C. Therapeutic management**

1. Consists of IV fluids, electrolytes, and regular insulin to correct hyperglycemia and dehydration; supportive care as indicated such as NPO status, vasopressors, and respiratory support
2. Insulin
   a. A bolus of IV regular insulin is given followed by a continuous IV drip (0.1 unit/kg body weight) until BG level drops to 250 mg/dL or pH is 7.30
   b. Once this blood level is reached, regular insulin is given on a sliding scale per BG results
   c. Bedside BG monitoring is done every 1–2 hours to evaluate effectiveness of therapy
3. Fluid therapy is needed for excessive dehydration that accompanies DKA
   a. As much as 1 to 2 L normal saline solution may be given during first hour, then IV rate is decreased to 500 mL/hr as tolerated by cardiac and respiratory systems
   b. When BG reaches 250–300 mg/dL, a 5% glucose solution (such as D_5½NS) is added to prevent hypoglycemia and cerebral edema
   c. Central venous pressure or hemodynamic monitoring may be needed to evaluate effectiveness of therapy

4. Potassium replacement is generally necessary in DKA
   a. The initial serum (K^+) level is usually elevated
   b. With reversal of acidosis and administration of insulin, K^+ shifts into cells and serum level can drop rapidly
   c. Institute replacement therapy based on serum K^+ level and urine output
   d. Institute cardiac monitoring to detect cardiac changes due to hyper- and hypokalemia and to monitor effects of therapy on serum K^+ level
   e. Replace other electrolytes such as phosphate based on laboratory results; bicarbonate is not given routinely in DKA because rapid correction of acidosis can cause severe hypokalemia
5. Analyze I&O, BG, urine ketones, VS, oxygenation, and breathing pattern
6. Maintain skin integrity; promote healing of impaired skin; prevent infection by repositioning client every 2 hours; provide pressure relief as indicated; manage incontinence and perspiration with skin protective barriers and cleansing; provide appropriate nutrition and oxygen support
7. Promote safety by analyzing VS, client communication, LOC and emotional response, and activity tolerance; implement measures to prevent falls
8. Assist client to verbalize concerns and cope effectively with illness and fears
9. Assist client to update Medic-Alert bracelet information as appropriate

D. **Reinforce client teaching:** nature and causes of DKA (excess glucose intake, insufficient medications, physiological and/or psychological stressors) and any new medications

XV. HYPERGLYCEMIC HYPEROSMOLAR NONKETOTIC SYNDROME (HHNK)

A. Overview

1. Life-threatening metabolic disorder of hyperglycemia; usually occurs with type 2 DM and triggered by stressors such as medications, infection, acute illness, invasive procedure, or chronic illness
2. Increased insulin resistance (caused by one or more triggers) along with increased CHO intake leads to hyperglycemia
3. Polyuria and decreased plasma volume occur
4. Subsequent decreased glomerular filtration rate (GFR) leads to glucose retention and Na^+ and water excretion
5. Hyperosmolarity causes dehydration and reduced intracellular water (cell shrinkage)

NCLEX®

B. Nursing data collection

1. Symptoms gradually occur over 24 hours to 2 weeks
2. Decreased LOC, dry mucous membranes, polydipsia, hyperthermia, impaired sensory and motor function, positive Babinski sign, and seizures
3. Elevated serum Na^+, serum osmolality greater than 340 mOsm/L, serum glucose greater than 600 mg/dL, abnormal serum K^+ and chloride, no serum ketones, and normal serum pH

NCLEX®

C. Therapeutic management

1. Determine and treat triggering situation; treat coexisting health deviations
2. Provide IV infusion of NS to replace fluids and Na^+, regular insulin IV to manage hyperglycemia, and K^+ to replace losses and shifts
3. Monitor I&O, weight, VS, lab values, sensory function, and cognitive function
4. Maintain intact skin by repositioning every 2 hours, using pressure relief aids, nutritional support, using skin moisturizers and barriers, and managing incontinence
5. Prevent aspiration by using appropriate feeding precautions, elevate head of bed (HOB) 15–30 degrees during and after feeding for 1 hour; if BP is too unstable to elevate HOB with feeding, then withhold oral feedings

D. **Reinforce client teaching:** HHNK symptoms to report, and administration of new medications

XVI. DELAYED PUBERTY

A. Overview

1. A condition noted in girls if there is no breast development by age 13, no pubic hair by age 14, or no menarche within 4 years after onset of breast development, usually by age 16
2. In boys, delayed puberty is a concern if there is no testicular enlargement or scrotal changes by age 13½ or 14, no pubic hair by age 15, or if genital growth is not complete by 4 to 5 years after testicular enlargement

3. Delayed puberty can be hereditary: other family members may have constitutional delay (delay of overall growth and puberty)
4. May be caused by hypogonadism (ovaries or testicles are not secreting hormones—estrogen or testosterone), which may result from abnormality of hypothalamus or pituitary gland (brain tumors, hypothyroidism, anorexia, and other chronic illnesses)
5. May also result from problem with testicle (Klinefelter's syndrome) or ovary (Turner's syndrome); these syndromes are secondary to chromosomal abnormalities that can be evaluated by studying child's karyotype (number and types of chromosomes)
   a. Klinefelter's syndrome is manifested by IQ scores below normal range, tall stature, and overly long arms and legs; usually there is one or more extra X chromosome, commonly 47 chromosomes with an XXY karyotype; clients are usually sterile
   b. Girls who have Turner's syndrome exhibit delayed puberty, short stature, webbed neck, and cubitus valgus (where forearm deviates laterally); karyotype shows a missing X chromosome (45XO); clients are usually infertile
6. Many clients with delayed puberty have short stature and may be treated as a child by teachers, coaches, and community members; during adolescent years, they may have difficulty in social situations

B. Nursing data collection

1. Obtain family growth history (especially growth patterns of parents)
2. Complete exam including measurements of arm span and (in males) testicular size and penile length
3. X-ray of left hand and wrist for bone age for skeletal growth and status of epiphyseal growth plate closure; beginning of puberty better correlates with bone age than chronological age
4. MRI or CT scan may determine a CNS lesion if a brain tumor is suspected
5. Possible blood levels of FSH, LH, and sex hormones; a complete blood count, thyroid function tests, and chemistry panel
6. A karyotype should be done for suspected Turner's or Klinefelter's syndromes; the gonadotropin-releasing hormone (GnRH) stimulation test may be used for diagnosis also

C. Therapeutic management

NCLEX® 1. Assure children with constitutional delay and delayed bone age that they usually do not require any treatment; medical intervention of low-dose injections of testosterone may be initiated if adolescent is over age 14

NCLEX® 2. If hypogonadism is present and other conditions are ruled out, child may receive hormone therapy to stimulate development of secondary sexual characteristics; boys receive testosterone enanthate injections, and girls take oral ethinyl estradiol with a combination of medroxyprogesterone

NCLEX® 3. Provide psychological support to child, especially if he or she has social concerns

D. Reinforce client and family teaching

1. Information regarding different stages of puberty and causes of delayed puberty; use language appropriate to child's chronological age
2. Administration of hormones if ordered; arrange for home nursing care to provide injections if needed

XVII. PRECOCIOUS PUBERTY

A. Overview

1. A condition characterized by early onset of puberty, usually before age 8 in girls and before age 9 in boys
2. Accompanied by appearance of secondary sexual characteristics and advanced growth rate and bone maturation, causing early fusion of epiphyseal plates and eventual short adult stature
3. Most cases of precocious puberty in both boys and girls are idiopathic; some are caused by benign hypothalamic tumors, other brain tumors, infection, cranial radiation, and head trauma
4. In normal puberty, hypothalamus secretes GnRH, which stimulates anterior pituitary gland to secrete hormones that result in development of secondary sexual characteristics
5. In precocious puberty, premature hormone secretion causes early onset of sexual characteristics; linear and skeletal growth is apparent because affected children appear very tall early on, but epiphyseal closure occurs because of hormone secretion, causing short stature as an adult

B. Nursing data collection

1. Signs of precocious puberty in females include breast development, pubic hair, axillary hair, and onset of menarche
2. Signs of precocious puberty in males include testicular enlargement, pubic hair, penile enlargement, axillary and chest hair, facial hair, and deepening voice

3. GnRH stimulation test stimulates secretion of FSH and LH; blood samples are obtained every 2 hours; if LH level is higher than FSH level, puberty has occurred
4. Bone age x-rays aid in determining epiphyseal maturation and closure; if bone age is more advanced than chronological age, skeletal growth acceleration is apparent

C. Therapeutic management

NCLEX®
1. Support children with precocious puberty by discussing their concerns about body image and sexuality
2. Offer support as family deals with sensitive issues such as premature appearance of secondary sexual characteristics and sexuality

NCLEX®
3. Encourage clients to express feelings about body changes; role-playing may help children cope with issues of peer teasing
4. Assure children that friends will go through same body changes
5. If synthetic form of LH-releasing factor is used to slow down or arrest progression of puberty, plan for monthly or daily injections with family

NCLEX®
6. Medication therapy: a synthetic form of LH-releasing factor (Lupron Depot) or nafarelin (Synarel) slows or stops progression of puberty and skeletal growth until a more typical age for puberty is reached, which will preserve adult height

D. Reinforce child and family teaching
1. Information about condition and possible referral to pediatric endocrinologist
2. If client is receiving synthetic LH, teach family subQ or intramuscular injection technique, and provide child and family with information about drug side effects as per product literature

XVIII. PHENYLKETONURIA (PKU)

A. Overview
1. An inherited autosomal recessive disorder affecting protein utilization that is caused by abnormal metabolism of essential amino acid phenylalanine, found in many natural protein foods; affects mostly white children; PKU is rare in African-American, Japanese, and Jewish populations
2. A deficiency in liver enzyme phenylalanine hydroxylase (which breaks down phenylalanine into tyrosine) causes serum phenylalanine metabolite levels to rise, leading to musty body and urine odor (excretion of phenol acids), seizures, hyperactivity, irritability, vomiting, and an eczema-type rash
3. Decreased levels of tyrosine cause a deficiency of pigment melanin, causing most children with PKU to have blond hair, blue eyes, and fair skin that is prone to eczema
4. Continued accumulation of phenylalanine affects protein synthesis and myelinization and results in seizure disorder and untreatable mental retardation if phenylalanine level is not decreased

B. Nursing data collection
1. Many infants with PKU appear healthy at birth; if treatment is not started to lower phenylalanine level immediately, infant's IQ can drop as many as 10 points within first month and will continue to decline
2. All 50 states require newborn screening
   a. The infant should ingest adequate protein (usually 24 hours of normal feedings of breast milk or formula) prior to test being performed

NCLEX®
   b. Heel blood should be used for specimen; sample should be collected after first 48 hours but no later than 7 days after birth
   c. A normal level is under 2 mg/dL; if level is elevated, a repeat test is performed to validate original results; a level higher than 15 mg/dL is considered dangerous
   d. If infant is discharged before 48 hours, test should be performed within 1 week after discharge from hospital or birthing center by a public health nurse, pediatrician, or pediatric nurse practitioner

NCLEX®
3. Symptoms arise over time and include failure to thrive, vomiting, irritability, and unpredictable behavior in infant; the urine will have a musty odor; the child may experience myoclonic or grand mal seizures

C. Therapeutic management
1. Ensure that test has been done correctly and results have been received; repeat blood test if phenylalanine levels are elevated on first test
2. Allow phenylalanines in diet based on weight of child and usually at a level of 20–30 mg/kg body weight or amount prescribed by physician; consult with registered nutritionist to aid in food calculations

NCLEX®
3. Place child on protein-restricted diet
   a. Encourage use of mature breast milk or modified-protein, phenylalanine-free, hydrolysate formula as a source of infant nutrition to keep phenylalanine level at 2 to 6 mg/dL
   b. Use special protein foods that are free of phenylalanine
4. Monitor serum phenylalanine levels periodically throughout child's life

5. Maintain restricted phenylalanine diet for life; is especially important before age 6 years (because of impact on IQ) and for adolescents and women before conception and during pregnancy (children of women with PKU may be born with congenital defects, including low birth weight, microcephaly, congenital heart defects, and mental retardation)
6. In young children inadequately screened after birth and who develop PKU, dietary modification at time of diagnosis usually improves behavioral and other symptoms; it prevents further mental retardation but does not raise IQ to previous level
7. Parents may be overwhelmed initially by diagnosis and dietary restrictions; emotional support is essential; suggest genetic counseling because each child born to this couple may have a 1 in 4 chance of having PKU
8. Medication therapy: antiepileptic medications if client is having seizures

D. Reinforce client and family teaching

1. Support parents and teach them disease and its management
2. Testing may need to be repeated if initial test was done before 48 hours of age or was positive initially
3. *NCLEX®* Review low-phenylalanine diet, including preparation of low-phenylalanine formula; avoid giving child meats, dairy products, and products containing aspartame because they contain large amounts of phenylalanine; it is important to read product labels, which may identify phenylalanine content
4. Offer emotional support and refer older child and parents to a support group for issues and problems related to chronic illness

Check Your NCLEX–PN® Exam I.Q.

You are ready for testing on this content if you can

- Identify basic structures and functions of the endocrine system.
- Describe the pathophysiology and etiology of common endocrine disorders.
- Discuss expected data and diagnostic test findings for selected endocrine disorders.
- Discuss therapeutic management of a client experiencing an endocrine disorder.
- Discuss nursing management of a client experiencing an endocrine disorder.
- Identify expected outcomes for the client experiencing an endocrine disorder.

PRACTICE TEST

1 A client recently diagnosed with hypothyroidism demonstrates understanding of prescribed levothyroxine (Synthroid) medication after making which statement?

1. "I should be able to become pregnant in a couple of months."
2. "This medication will help me lose all this excess weight."
3. "I should call the physician for nervousness, diarrhea, or increased pulse."
4. "This medication should be taken with food, preferably dairy products."

2 The client is post-transsphenoidal hypophysectomy and demonstrates understanding of methods for preventing increases in intracranial pressure by identifying which activity?

1. Sitting in a soft chair and leaning over slowly to tie shoes
2. Holding breath when reaching down to pick up something from the floor
3. Bending at the knees first before squatting down to reach something on the floor
4. Holding breath while using mouthwash, then leaning head down toward the sink to spit it out

3 The client with diabetes mellitus requests medication for headache soon after returning from an early morning x-ray procedure. The nurse observes the client is upset about the headache, angry at missing breakfast, and has moist hands. What priority action should the nurse take at this time?

1. Administer the medication for headache and arrange for a breakfast tray.
2. Check the blood glucose level and be prepared to give 4 ounces of juice immediately.
3. Acknowledge dissatisfaction, offer to obtain a snack, and give the medication.
4. Notify the charge nurse and instruct client to eat crackers.

PRACTICE TEST

4 A 70-year-old client with a blood glucose (BG) of 750 mg/dL is being treated for hyperosmolar hyperglycemic nonketotic coma (HHNK) with intravenous regular insulin at 10 units/hour, normal saline with 20 mEq of potassium per liter infusing at 250 mL/hr, and oxygen at 2 L/min. The client has been oriented when stimulated, and BG has dropped to 400 mg/dL. The client now demands to get out of bed and the skin feels cool and moist. What should the nurse do at this time?

1. Interpret this as a sign of hypoglycemia and check the blood glucose.
2. Recognize the client is feeling better and seeks control of the situation.
3. Auscultate breath sounds and monitor oxygen saturation.
4. Monitor the client for bladder distention and signs of imbalanced body temperature.

5 The client is recovering from a bilateral adrenalectomy as treatment for an adrenal cortex tumor. What is the nurse's highest priority action for this client in the immediate postoperative period?

1. Monitor fluid and electrolyte balance, signs of hypoglycemia, and hypotension.
2. Monitor for signs of hypoxia, cardiac arrhythmias, and peripheral edema.
3. Monitor the incision integrity, peripheral pulses, and magnesium level.
4. Monitor for hyperthermia, bed mobility, pupil reaction, and eye movement.

6 The client is 6 hours post-thyroid surgery. The unlicensed assistive person (UAP) reports that the client is upset because there is blood on the client's gown. What is the priority action of the nurse?

1. Monitor the client's breath sounds and respiratory effort.
2. State that it is normal to have some bleeding and ask the UAP to change the gown.
3. Reassure the client that some bleeding is normal, and then monitor the client's level of pain.
4. Reinforce the dressing, change the gown, and notify the registered nurse.

7 A client who was admitted with hyperglycemic hyperosmolar nonketotic coma (HHNK) asks how he can prevent recurrence of this illness. The nurse needs to reinforce with the client about which prevention measures? Select all that apply.

1. Use sliding-scale insulin to cover periodic snacks that are not part of the dietary plan.
2. Maintain fluid balance by drinking four glasses of water daily.
3. Monitor for signs of infection and treat infection early.
4. Consult primary care provider when fasting blood glucose is elevated.
5. Use stress management techniques to decrease blood glucose.

8 A female client newly diagnosed with hypothyroidism indicates that she no longer participates in evening social activities stating, "There is too much walking, and I prefer to go to bed early. I see enough of my friends at work every day." The nurse determines which priority nursing diagnosis for this client?

1. Social Isolation related to sleep rest needs as evidenced by desire to go to bed early
2. Disturbed Sleep Pattern related to excessive work as evidenced by desire to go to bed early and avoid evening activities
3. Fatigue related to reduced metabolic rate as evidenced by desire to avoid evening activities after work
4. Decreased Cardiac Output related to weak myocardium as evidenced by desire to avoid walking

9 A client with hyperparathyroidism is admitted with cardiac dysrhythmias, including bursts of supraventricular tachycardia (SVT) and occasional premature ventricular contractions (PVCs). The client asks why the cardiologist prescribed so much intravenous (IV) fluid and then furosemide (Lasix). What is the nurse's best explanation?

1. Improve cardiac output.
2. Eliminate metabolic wastes.
3. Replace missing electrolytes.
4. Promote excretion of calcium.

10 A client recently diagnosed with syndrome of inappropriate antidiuretic hormone (SIADH) is receiving continuous enteral nutrition. Considering the impact of the disorder on fluid balance, what action should the nurse take when working with the enteral feeding tube?

1. Discard the residual and replace it with water.
2. Flush the tube with 50 mL normal saline.
3. Count the flush but not the feeding in planning the fluid restriction.
4. Flush the tube with 30 mL water to maintain patency.

11 A client with a history of Cushing's syndrome is admitted with multiple contusions, lacerations and blood loss following a motor vehicle accident. Current laboratory values are BUN 30 mg/dL, creatinine 1.0 mg/dL, sodium 148 mEq/L, potassium 4.8 mEq/L, chloride 108 mEq/L, and cortisol 29 mcg/dL. Which nursing diagnoses would the nurse include when caring for this client? Select all that apply.

1. Impaired Urinary Elimination
2. Risk for Disuse Syndrome
3. Ineffective Airway Clearance
4. Risk for Infection
5. Deficient Fluid Volume

12 The client is being treated for Addison's disease with glucocorticoid replacement medication. The nurse determines that the client understands medication therapy when the client makes which statement? Select all that apply.

1. "I should take this medication every evening at bedtime."
2. "My irregular pulse should convert to a regular rate and rhythm."
3. "This medication will help me control my increased blood pressure."
4. "I should call my doctor if I gain 2 pounds."
5. "I should call my doctor if I feel weak or have a cold."

13 An 8-month-old infant is brought to the endocrine clinic with a musty body odor, seizures, and an eczema-like rash. The infant is diagnosed with phenylketonuria (PKU). What action should the nurse consider when caring for this infant?

1. Need for dietary information about a low-phenylalanine diet
2. Need for admission to a long-term care setting for handicapped infants
3. Preparing the family for the child's early demise
4. Providing instruction on medication management of PKU

14 A mother is quite concerned about her 7-year-old daughter after noticing breast development and the appearance of pubic hair. The mother asks the nurse if this is a cause for concern. What would be the nurse's best response?

1. "No. Some girls just develop earlier than boys."
2. "Yes, she may have precocious puberty. Let's talk to the pediatrician because she may need referral to an endocrinologist."
3. "Yes. She probably doesn't want the other children at school making fun of her."
4. "No. This early development may slow down when she reaches 9 years old."

15 The mother of an adolescent with diabetes mellitus tells the nurse that her son likes to eat cheeseburgers and french fries when he goes out with his friends. The son is aware he is exceeding the allowable carbohydrate exchanges on the diabetic diet. How could the nurse best explain why adolescents sometimes make choices that place their health at risk?

1. They want to be like their peers.
2. They have a self-destructive wish.
3. They eat foods with friends that they can't eat at home.
4. They want to show risk-taking behavior.

16 The nurse is caring for a pediatric client with a tentative diagnosis of hyperpituitarism. What findings should the nurse observe for in this client? Select all that apply.

1. Short stature
2. Large hands and feet with a prominent jawbone
3. Joint changes consistent with arthritis
4. Soft, high-pitched voice
5. Hypertension

17 A 14-year-old who was just diagnosed with type 1 diabetes mellitus has been taught to draw up and administer insulin. The client draws up in one syringe the following insulin before breakfast: 15 units of isophane (NPH) and 8 units of lispro (Humalog). Why does the nurse instruct the client to wait in administering the insulin?

1. Adolescents should not self-administer insulin until they have practiced drawing up the medication at least 10 times.
2. Lispro insulin is very fast-acting insulin. The breakfast tray should be at the bedside before insulin administration.
3. The child's mother should be present to witness the injection.
4. These two forms of medication should never be mixed.

PRACTICE TEST

18 The nurse is meeting with a child recently diagnosed with type 1 diabetes mellitus and his family to provide diet counseling. What information should be included in the discussion? Select all that apply.

1. As long as the child consumes 1200 calories a day, the food selection does not matter.
2. Stop eating snacks immediately; eat only three balanced meals a day.
3. Foods from all basic food groups are important, but do not overdo simple sugars and carbohydrates.
4. Sodas in any form must be avoided; the child should drink water and juices only
5. A high-fiber diet is recommended.

19 The nurse in the endocrine clinic is performing data collection on an adolescent. The nurse would suspect hyperthyroidism based on the presence of which data? Select all that apply.

1. Acne
2. Dilated pupils
3. Sleeping difficulties
4. Bulging eyes
5. Enlarged thyroid

20 After completing family education for the parents of a recently diagnosed infant with hypothyroidism, the nurse determines whether the teaching was effective. The nurse will need to reinforce instructions if the parents make which statement?

1. "If my child seems excessively tired, I know he will probably need a decrease in his medication."
2. "My child will need to take this medication for the rest of his life."
3. "I'm so glad that he was diagnosed soon after birth so that he will not develop mental delays."
4. "His tablets can be crushed and mixed with a small amount of his baby cereal."

21 A 2-month-old infant arrives at the pediatric clinic. Which characteristic does the nurse relate to a diagnosis of congenital hypothyroidism? Select all that apply.

1. Open fontanels
2. Protruding tongue
3. Tachycardia
4. Weight loss
5. Hypotonia

22 After being diagnosed with Graves' disease, a teenager begins taking propylthiouracil (PTU) for treatment of the disease. What symptom would indicate to the nurse that the dose may be too high?

1. Weight loss
2. Polyphagia
3. Lethargy
4. Difficulty with schoolwork

23 A client with Addison's disease is being discharged to home and will be taking hydrocortisone (Cortisol). The nurse concludes the client requires reinforcement of instructions about this medication after the client makes which statement?

1. "I will monitor closely for any signs of infection."
2. "I will wear a Medic-Alert bracelet indicating disease and treatment."
3. "I will report any rapid weight gain or fluid in my legs if it persists for over one week."
4. "I will take safety measures at home to prevent injuries."

24 The nurse concludes that a client newly diagnosed with type 1 diabetes mellitus requires reinforcement of teaching when the client makes which statement?

1. "I will notify my health care provider if my glucose levels run higher or lower than the target range."
2. "I will take my insulin as prescribed, and I will not miss a dose."
3. "I will check my glucose level 30 minutes before I eat, and at bedtime."
4. "I will not take my insulin if I am sick and cannot eat."

25 While administering an iodine preparation preoperatively to a client who is scheduled for a thyroidectomy to treat hyperthyroidism, the client asks the nurse to explain the purpose of the iodine. What explanation best describes the purpose of the iodine?

1. Iodine decreases the vascularity and size of the thryoid gland, thereby reducing the risk of intraoperative and post-operative hemorrhage.
2. Iodine reduces circulating hormone levels, thereby reducing the effects of elevated hormones.
3. Iodine is recommended in the treatment of cancer of the thyroid.
4. Iodine enlarges the thyroid gland and facilitates the surgeon's ability to locate the thyroid.

26 When providing discharge instructions to a client with Addison's disease, which of the following should the nurse include when reinforcing teaching?

1. Take prescribed prednisone (Deltasone) with food or milk.
2. Weigh self weekly and report changes.
3. Stop taking prednisone if stomach upset occurs.
4. Limit fluid intake to 1000 mL in 24 hours.

ANSWERS & RATIONALES

1 **Answer: 3 Rationale:** Nervousness, diarrhea, and increased pulse are indications of excessive effect of the medication, and the dosage may need to be adjusted downward. The client should report these to the health care provider. Levothyroxine is not ordered to affect pregnancy. After the client has reached normal serum T_4 levels, the normal metabolic rate may help the client lose the weight gained during the hypothyroid state, but this is not the purpose of the replacement medication. Usually, the medication should be taken on an empty stomach, 1 hour prior to a meal or 2 hours after a meal. **Cognitive Level:** Analyzing **Client Need:** Pharmacological and Parenteral Therapies **Integrated Process:** Teaching and Learning **Content Area:** Adult Health **Strategy:** The core issue of the question is knowledge of medications used to manage hypothyroidism. Use nursing knowledge and the process of elimination to make a selection.

2 **Answer: 3 Rationale:** Bending the knees and squatting is preferred to bending at the waist to reach the floor as a means of preventing rises in intracranial pressure (ICP) following pituitary surgery. Holding the breath as well as leaning over will increase ICP. To tie shoes, the client should sit on the couch or bed, bend the knee and place his or her foot on the couch or bed to reach the shoelaces. Alternatively, the client can sit on the floor to tie shoes or can avoid shoes that tie until there is no risk for increased ICP. Clients should be taught to avoid holding their breath for any reason and to avoid leaning forward or bending at the waist to prevent an increase in intracranial pressure. Holding the breath as well as leaning over will increase ICP. **Cognitive Level:** Applying **Client Need:** Physiological Adaptation **Integrated Process:** Nursing Process: Implementation **Content Area:** Adult Health **Strategy:** The core issue of the question is knowledge of measures to prevent rises in intracranial pressure following pituitary surgery. Use nursing knowledge and the process of elimination to make a selection.

3 **Answer: 2 Rationale:** Headache, restlessness, anxiety, sweating, and increased pulse are signs of hypoglycemia. Resolution of symptoms should occur after the client drinks the juice. Treating the headache and obtaining a breakfast tray fail to recognize the client's actual problem. Acknowledging dissatisfaction, obtaining a snack, and giving medication address the client's concerns but do not verify the client's blood glucose as a possible etiology for the symptoms. The nurse needs to check the blood glucose level first to determine if the client is hypoglycemic. Restlessness, anxiety and sweating are all signs of hypoglycemia. **Cognitive Level:** Analyzing **Client Need:** Physiological Adaptation **Integrated Process:** Nursing Process: Implementation **Content Area:** Adult Health **Strategy:** The core issue of the question is recognition that the client is at risk for hypoglycemia and the corrective actions that need to be taken. Use nursing knowledge and the process of elimination to make a selection.

4 **Answer: 3 Rationale:** Increased preload caused by the intravenous infusion at 250 mL/hr may exceed the myocardium's workload capacity, leading to signs of decreased cardiac output and congestive heart failure. There is no risk for hypoglycemia while the BG is still elevated to 400 mg/dL. The nurse should seek a physiological basis for the change in client's status rather than seeking control, especially since the skin is cool and moist. Checking for bladder distention or fever represents a failure to directly monitor for signs of possible fluid overload. **Cognitive Level:** Analyzing **Client Need:** Physiological Adaptation **Integrated Process:** Nursing Process: Implementation **Content Area:** Adult Health **Strategy:** The core issue of the question is recognition that rapid infusion of fluid in a 70-year-old client could lead to circulatory decompensation. Use nursing knowledge and the process of elimination to make a selection.

5 **Answer: 1 Rationale:** During the first 48 hours after adrenalectomy, clients are at risk for adrenal insufficiency and hypovolemic shock. The lack of cortisol production can cause fluid and electrolyte loss and hypoglycemia. Peripheral edema is more likely associated with excess fluid volume but the risk after adrenalectomy is deficient fluid volume caused by sudden decrease in circulating corticosteroids and mineralocorticoids. Incision integrity and peripheral pulses is routine data collection, and magnesium level is not of particular concern at this time. Monitoring for hyperthermia and bed mobility as part of routine postoperative data collection; neurological data collection of pupils and eye movements is not of particular concern after adrenalectomy. **Cognitive Level:** Analyzing **Client Need:** Physiological Adaptation

Integrated Process: Nursing Process: Implementation **Content Area:** Adult Health **Strategy:** The core issue of the question is knowledge that clients are at risk for adrenal insufficiency following adrenalectomy and how to monitor for its occurrence. Use nursing knowledge and the process of elimination to make a selection.

6 **Answer: 1 Rationale:** Blood on the gown indicates excessive incisional bleeding. Breath sounds, including auscultating over the tracheal area, and respiratory effort should be monitored first to determine if edema is present in the tissues, thus compromising the airway. After thoroughly monitoring the client and reinforcing or changing the dressing per protocol, the nurse should inform the registered nurse of the amount of bleeding and all other data. Usually, with thyroid surgery, there is minimal bleeding postoperatively and having the UAP change the gown fails to provide proper data collection. Focusing on the client's pain level does not address the bleeding, which is excessive rather than normal. Reinforcing the dressing and notifying the registered nurse fails to address the need for monitoring the client's airway, which is a critical oversight. **Cognitive Level:** Analyzing **Client Need:** Physiological Adaptation **Integrated Process:** Nursing Process: Implementation **Content Area:** Adult Health **Strategy:** The core issue of the question is possible threat to the airway and breathing with excessive bleeding following thyroid surgery. Use nursing knowledge, the ABCs, and the process of elimination to make a selection.

7 **Answer: 3, 5 Rationale:** HHNK is associated with hyperglycemic response to infection or other disease or illness, some medications, dehydration, stress-induced hyperglycemia, or a combination of these factors. The response to stress can increase blood glucose levels so stress management may be helpful as part of overall measures to prevent increased blood glucose. HHNK occurs in clients with type 2 diabetes mellitus, primarily older adults, and thus insulin is not part of the usual treatment plan. Drinking four glasses of water daily is insufficient; 6 to 8 glasses of water are recommended for general health. Consulting a health care provider for elevated blood glucose does not demonstrate an understanding of how to prevent HHNK. **Cognitive Level:** Applying **Client Need:** Physiological Adaptation **Integrated Process:** Nursing Process: Implementation **Content Area:** Adult Health **Strategy:** The critical word in the stem of the question is *prevent*. With this in mind, look for options that will reduce the likelihood of the client experiencing a recurrence. Use nursing knowledge and the process of elimination to make a selection.

8 **Answer: 3 Rationale:** Hypothyroidism is associated with fatigue, weight gain, and decreased activity tolerance. There is not enough data to conclude decreased cardiac output or sleep alterations. The client states she is able to socialize during the day at work. **Cognitive Level:** Analyzing **Client Need:** Physiological Adaptation **Integrated Process:** Nursing Process: Implementation **Content Area:** Adult Health **Strategy:** The core issue of the question is the etiology of the client's symptoms and applying a nursing diagnostic label to the problem. Use nursing knowledge and the process of elimination to make a selection.

9 **Answer: 4 Rationale:** Hyperparathyroidism causes hypercalcemia. Large volume saline infusion given concurrently with furosemide will stimulate the kidneys to excrete calcium. In acute situations requiring rapid reduction, clients could also be given IV calcitonin and phosphates. IV fluids and furosemide are not given to improve cardiac output, eliminate metabolic wastes, or replace missing electrolytes. **Cognitive Level:** Applying **Client Need:** Physiological Adaptation **Integrated Process:** Nursing Process: Implementation **Content Area:** Adult Health **Strategy:** The core issue of the question is knowledge of methods used to manage hypercalcemia in hyperparathyroidism. Use nursing knowledge and the process of elimination to make a selection.

10 **Answer: 2 Rationale:** Clients with SIADH are encouraged to drink fluids high in sodium, so they should have feeding tubes flushed with normal saline. To prevent electrolyte loss, all of the residual that is aspirated from a feeding tube should be returned to the client. Clients with SIADH are usually on a strict fluid restriction to correct water overload; therefore, all fluids (including enteral feeding and flush solution) should be considered when planning the fluid restriction. Because of the need for increased sodium, this client should not have the feeding tube flushed with water. **Cognitive Level:** Applying **Client Need:** Physiological Adaptation **Integrated Process:** Nursing Process: Implementation **Content Area:** Adult Health **Strategy:** The core issue of the question is proper fluid use and management in a client with SIADH. Use nursing knowledge about fluid imbalance in this disorder and the process of elimination to make a selection.

11 **Answer: 4, 5 Rationale:** Clients with Cushing's syndrome are at risk for infection because of impaired immune function related to an elevated cortisol level. The BUN and sodium are elevated because of deficient fluid volume caused by blood loss, and a potassium and chloride at the higher end of the normal range add further support to this conclusion. Because the creatinine is normal, the BUN and creatinine are not elevated because of kidney dysfunction. The client has no risk factors for impaired urinary elimination. The client's injuries do not predispose the client to risk for disuse syndrome. The client is not experiencing any difficulty with the airway. **Cognitive Level:** Analyzing **Client Need:** Physiological Adaptation **Integrated Process:** Nursing Process: Implementation **Content Area:** Adult Health **Strategy:** The core issue of the question is the ability to determine priorities of care for a client with Cushing's syndrome who experiences trauma. Use knowledge of pathophysiology and the process of elimination to make a selection.

12 **Answer: 4, 5 Rationale:** Glucocorticoid replacement medication can cause fluid and sodium retention, leading to weight gain and fluid volume excess. Doses need to be increased during times of stress and can impair the body's ability to recover from an infection. Therefore, the physician must be consulted for signs of a cold or infection. Glucocorticoids should be taken in the morning with food. The medication will not affect cardiac rhythm. Glucocorticoids will increase BP and thus are not safe for clients with hypertension. **Cognitive Level:** Applying **Client Need:** Pharmacological and Parenteral Therapies **Integrated Process:** Teaching and Learning **Content Area:** Adult Health **Strategy:** The core issue of the question is knowledge of adverse effects of drug therapy. Use nursing knowledge and the process of elimination to make a selection.

13 **Answer: 1 Rationale:** A low-phenylalanine diet reduces the amount of toxic metabolites in the body, thus reducing or preventing additional damage. There is no indication of a need to admit the child to a long-term care facility. Infants with PKU have normal life expectancy. No medications are currently being used to treat PKU. **Cognitive Level:** Applying **Client Need:** Physiological Adaptation **Integrated Process:** Nursing Process:

ANSWERS & RATIONALES

Implementation **Content Area:** Child Health **Strategy:** The core issue of the question is management of PKU in a newly diagnosed infant. Use nursing knowledge and the process of elimination to make a selection.

14 **Answer: 2** **Rationale:** The child should be seen by the physician because there might be secretion of sex hormones, and precocious puberty may affect linear growth. Stating that some girls develop earlier than boys ignores the clinical issue. Although she may be teased in school by the other children, the main reason for seeking treatment is health promotion. There is no reason to believe this process will slow down in a couple of years. **Cognitive Level:** Applying **Client Need:** Physiological Adaptation **Integrated Process:** Nursing Process: Implementation **Content Area:** Child Health **Strategy:** The core issue of the question is the priority need of a client with suspected precocious puberty. Use nursing knowledge and the process of elimination to make a selection.

15 **Answer: 1** **Rationale:** As part of normal psychosocial development, adolescents need to feel like part of their group, even if it means impairing their health. There is no information to support a self-destructive wish. Although some foods may not be allowed at home, it is not likely to be the motivating factor. Displaying risk-taking behaviors is not likely the primary motivation, but rather a secondary event. **Cognitive Level:** Analyzing **Client Need:** Physiological Adaptation **Integrated Process:** Nursing Process: Implementation **Content Area:** Child Health **Strategy:** The core issue of the question is knowledge of age-specific concerns of adolescents with diabetes mellitus. Use nursing knowledge and the process of elimination to make a selection.

16 **Answer: 2, 3, 5** **Rationale:** The client with hyperpituitarism will exhibit the following: tall stature if onset in childhood, large hands and feet with prominent jawbone, joint changes consistent with arthritis, deep voice and possible dysphagia, hypertension, organomegaly, and skin changes leading to rough, oily texture. The client would not have a soft voice or be short in stature. **Cognitive Level:** Analyzing **Client Need:** Physiological Adaptation **Integrated Process:** Nursing Process: Data Collection **Content Area:** Child Health **Strategy:** The core issue of the question is knowledge of findings with hyperpituitarism. Recall the functions of the pituitary gland and then correlate the functions with the logical signs of excess to make the appropriate selections.

17 **Answer: 2** **Rationale:** Lispro insulin has an onset of less than 15 minutes and peaks at one hour after administration. A food source should be available at the bedside to prevent the possibility of hypoglycemia shortly after administration. The client can perform medication self-administration as soon as the skill is learned. The child's mother does not need to be present. These insulins may be mixed and administered in one syringe. **Cognitive Level:** Applying **Client Need:** Pharmacological and Parenteral Therapies **Integrated Process:** Nursing Process: Implementation **Content Area:** Child Health **Strategy:** Consider the onset, peak, and duration of each time of insulin to determine the correct answer.

18 **Answer: 3, 5** **Rationale:** All basic food groups should be included; simple sugars and carbohydrates should be reduced to prevent spikes in blood glucose. A high-fiber diet is recommended for improved control of blood glucose. The dietary focus needs to include foods from the various food groups as well as overall caloric intake. Snacks may be an important part of the overall meal plan, especially in a growing child. Diet sodas are allowed. **Cognitive Level:** Applying **Client Need:** Health Promotion and Maintenance **Integrated Process:** Teaching and Learning **Content Area:** Child Health **Strategy:** Two options are opposites, so consider these options first as possible correct choices.

19 **Answer: 3, 4, 5** **Rationale:** Exophthalmos (bulging eyes) and an enlarged thyroid are evidence of hyperthyroidism. Other symptoms would include weight loss, tremors, tachycardia, and elevated basal body temperature. Some children may display behavior problems and have sleeping difficulties. The other symptoms are not associated with hyperthyroidism. **Cognitive Level:** Analyzing **Client Need:** Physiological Adaptation **Integrated Process:** Nursing Process: Data Collection **Content Area:** Child Health **Strategy:** Knowledge of the signs and symptoms of hyperthyroidism will help to determine the correct answer. Eliminate those options that are known to be wrong. The remaining options should be considered individually as to whether the physiology of hyperthyroidism would cause the problem.

20 **Answer: 1** **Rationale:** Symptoms of excessive fatigue may indicate inadequate medication, and the medication needs to be increased per health care provider direction. This statement indicates correct understanding of the management of hypothyroidism. This statement indicates correct understanding of hypothyroidism. This statement indicates correct understanding of the management of hypothyroidism. **Cognitive Level:** Applying **Client Need:** Physiological Adaptation **Integrated Process:** Teaching and Learning **Content Area:** Child Health **Strategy:** Since hypothyroidism results from insufficient thyroid hormones, the medication will supply the hormones. Insufficient dosage will result in hypothyroid symptoms, excessive dosage will cause hyperthyroid symptoms. Key words are *will need to provide additional instructions*, which indicate that the parent's response is incorrect. Therefore, choose the answer that indicates a misunderstanding on the part of the parents.

21 **Answer: 2, 5** **Rationale:** Most babies with congenital hypothyroidism exhibit a protruding tongue. Most babies with congenital hypothyroidism exhibit hypotonia. Open fontanels are normal for a 2-month-old infant. Most babies with congenital hypothyroidism exhibit bradycardia not tachycardia. Weight loss is a sign of hyperthyroidism not congenital hypothyroidism. **Cognitive Level:** Analyzing **Client Need:** Physiological Adaptation **Integrated Process:** Nursing Process: Data Collection **Content Area:** Child Health **Strategy:** Open fontanels are expected in a 2-month-old infant, so that is not a symptom of hypothyroidism. Weight loss and tachycardia would both be symptoms of hyperthyroidism.

22 **Answer: 3** **Rationale:** Lethargy may indicate an overdose of the drug, causing the child to exhibit signs of hypothyroidism. Weight loss is a sign of hyperthyroidism. Polyphagia is a sign of hyperthyroidism. Difficulty concentrating because of high energy level is a sign of hyperthyroidism. **Cognitive Level:** Analyzing **Client Need:** Pharmacological and Parenteral Therapies **Integrated Process:** Nursing Process: Data Collection **Content Area:** Child Health **Strategy:** Graves' disease is hyperthyroidism. Recall that the drug is used to suppress the thyroid. Oversuppression would be a symptom of too much drug.

23 **Answer: 3** **Rationale:** Weight must be monitored daily; any increase indicates fluid retention and should be reported immediately. Corticosteroids are immunosuppressants; therefore, careful monitoring for infection is necessary. Additionally, an increase in the medication may be required for stressors such as infection. A Medic-Alert bracelet is recommended to inform health care providers of Addison's disease and cortisol treatment. Safety measures are encouraged to prevent injuries. **Cognitive Level:** Analyzing **Client Need:** Pharmacological and Parenteral Therapies **Integrated Process:** Teaching and Learning **Content Area:** Adult Health **Strategy:** Recognize that questions asking for further instruction are looking for an incorrect answer. In other words, something which is wrong requiring continued teaching.

24 **Answer: 4 Rationale:** The client should inform the health care provider of illness and follow "sick-day rules," which may include taking insulin, or increasing insulin as prescribed, consuming extra fluids, resting, and monitoring glucose every 2 to 4 hours. This is a correct statement by the client. This is a correct statement by the client. This is a correct statement by the client. **Cognitive Level:** Analyzing **Client Need:** Physiological Adaptation **Integrated Process:** Teaching and Learning **Content Area:** Adult Health **Strategy:** The process of elimination is helpful with the three options that are correct. Choose the incorrect answer.

25 **Answer: 1 Rationale:** Iodine reduces the size and vascularity of the thyroid, reducing the risk of hemorrhage, which is a potential complication of thyroidectomy. Antithyroid medications, not iodine, are given to reduce hormone levels. The treatment for cancer of the thyroid is a total thyroidectomy. Iodine reduces the size and vascularity of the thyroid, reducing the risk of hemorrhage, which is a potential complication of thyroidectomy. **Cognitive Level:** Applying **Client Need:** Pharmacological and Parenteral Therapies **Integrated Process:** Nursing Process: Implementation **Content Area:** Adult Health **Strategy:** This question calls for knowledge of the relationship of iodine with thyroid function which may be transferred to the need for iodine treatment.

26 **Answer: 1 Rationale:** To decrease incidence of gastric ulcers, cortisol replacements (prednisone) should be taken with food or milk. Clients should weigh themselves daily and report changes. Abruptly discontinuing cortisol replacements can result in Addisonian crisis. Clients should increase fluid intake up to 3000 mL a day unless contraindicated. **Cognitive Level:** Applying **Client Need:** Physiological Adaptation **Integrated Process:** Nursing Process: Implementation **Content Area:** Pharmacology **Strategy:** Recall knowledge that prednisone increases the risk for gastrointestinal irritation and strategies to alleviate this.

Key Terms to Review

glycosylated hemoglobin p. 1027
hyperglycemia p. 1027
hypersecretion p. 1026
hyperthyroidism (Graves' disease) p. 1033
hyposecretion p. 1026
ketosis p. 1036
paresthesia p. 1033
photophobia p. 1032
polydipsia p. 1030
polyphagia p. 1036
polyuria p. 1029
receptor p. 1026
thyroid crisis (thyroid storm) p. 1030

References

Ball, J., Bindler, R., & Cowen, K. (2010). *Child health nursing: Partnering with children and families.* (2nd ed.). Upper Saddle River, NJ: Pearson Education.

Berman, A., & Snyder, S. (2012). *Kozier & Erb's fundamentals of nursing: Concepts, process, and practice* (9th ed.). Upper Saddle River, NJ: Pearson Education.

Ignatavicius, D., & Workman, L. (2010). *Medical-surgical nursing: Critical thinking for collaborative care* (6th ed.). Philadelphia: Saunders.

Kee, J. (2010). *Laboratory and diagnostic tests with nursing implications* (8th ed.). Upper Saddle River, NJ: Pearson Education.

LeMone, P., Burke, K., & Bauldoff, G. (2011). *Medical-surgical nursing: Critical thinking in patient care* (5th ed.). Upper Saddle River, NJ: Pearson Education.

Smith, S., Duell, D., & Martin, B. (2012). *Clinical nursing skills: Basic to advanced skills* (8th ed.). Upper Saddle River, NJ: Pearson Education.

Test Yourself

Are you ready for the NCLEX-PN® or course exams? Use the practice tests on the companion website to check.

ANSWERS & RATIONALES

Musculoskeletal Disorders

57

In this chapter

Cross Reference

Other chapters relevant to this content area are

Neurological and Musculoskeletal Medications	Chapter 35
Common Laboratory Tests	Chapter 42
Common Diagnostic Tests and Procedures	Chapter 43

I. OVERVIEW OF ANATOMY AND PHYSIOLOGY OF MUSCULOSKELETAL SYSTEM

A. Skeleton: consists of bones, joints, and cartilage; provides framework for body and protects soft tissue and vital organs; composed primarily of calcium (as Ca^{++} phosphate and Ca^{++} carbonate); provides points of attachment for muscles

B. Classification of bones

1. Two major classifications are based on structure: compact bone (dense) or cancellous bone (spongy)
2. A central shaft (**diaphysis**) and two end portions (**epiphyseals**) characterize long bones (e.g., humerus and radius)
3. Short bones are characterized by cancellous bone covered by a thin layer of compact bone (examples: carpals and tarsals)

4. Flat bones are characterized by two layers of compact bone separated by a layer of cancellous bone (e.g., skull, ribs, scapula, and sternum)

C. **Bone marrow**
1. Soft, spongy, highly cellular blood-forming tissue that fills cavities of bones and is site for hematopoiesis (red blood cell or RBC production) and storage of RBCs
2. Responsible also for production of white blood cells (WBCs), and platelets
3. Becomes predominantly fatty with age, particularly in long bones of limb

D. **Axial section**
1. Each vertebra is constructed like a ring, one on top of another, with a padding of cartilage between; vertebral rings are studded with bony projections called processes, which function as attachments for muscles and points of articulation with bones
2. Twelve pairs of ribs attach to thoracic vertebrae; upper 7 opposing pairs attach at front to sternum; 3 of remaining 5 pairs attach to rib immediately above by cartilage, and lowest 2 pairs are unattached

E. **Appendicular section**
1. Connected to axial skeleton by bones of upper and lower extremities
   a. Shoulder girdle supports arms; humerus is located in upper arm and ulna and radius in forearm
   b. Each innominate bone (hip bone) consists of 3 parts—ileum, ischium, and pubis; innominate bones unite with sacrum and coccyx of vertebral column to form pelvic girdle, which supports legs

F. **Joint articulations**
1. Result when two bones are joined together; categorized according to type of motion
2. Composed of fibrous connective tissue and cartilage (dense avascular connective tissue) that covers ends of bones making movement smooth
3. Joint cavity secretes synovial fluid, which lubricates joint and reduces friction

G. **Ligaments**: bands of rigid connective tissue that hold joints together, allowing for movement and stability; have a relatively poor blood supply, which significantly prolongs healing process after injury

H. **Muscles**
1. Primarily function as a source of power and pull against bones to move body
2. Three primary types of muscle: skeletal muscle (striated, voluntary) moves extremities and external areas of body; cardiac muscle (striated, involuntary) is found in heart; smooth muscle (nonstriated, involuntary) is found in walls of arteries and bowel

II. DIAGNOSTIC TESTS AND DATA COLLECTION

A. **Radiologic tests**: x-rays are widely used to identify musculoskeletal problems and effectiveness of treatment; radiological studies other than simple x-rays may be done with or without contrast

B. **EMG (electromyogram or myogram)**: records and evaluates electrical activity of muscles during contraction
1. There are two different types of EMG: intramuscular (IM) EMG (more commonly used) and surface EMG (SEMG)
2. *NCLEX®* Long, small-gauge needles are inserted through skin into muscle; client may feel mild to moderate discomfort during procedure
3. Needles detect electrical activity of muscle and transmit data to electromyogram machine, which displays electrical activity on an oscilloscope or transmits through an audiotransmitter (microphone)
4. SEMG: electrodes are placed above muscle to detect electrical activity

C. ***Arthroscopy***: surgical procedure done under local or general anesthesia to examine internal structure of a joint using an arthroscope (a pencil-sized device with optical fibers and lenses), which is inserted into very small skin incisions; device is connected to a video camera to allow visualization of interior of joint
1. Procedure may diagnose or treat musculoskeletal disorders such as osteoarthritis, rheumatoid arthritis, infectious types of arthritis, and internal joint injuries like meniscus tears, ligament strains or tears, and cartilage deterioration
2. Arthroscopic surgery can be done during procedure to repair joint tissue; arthroscopic surgery creates less tissue trauma, less pain, and allows for more rapid recovery than traditional joint surgery
3. *NCLEX®* Client education: postprocedure
   a. Take analgesics for comfort and limit activity as directed
   b. Observe site for hematoma or bleeding
   c. Perform neurovascular self-assessment (temperature, color, capillary refill, movement, and sensation) on affected extremity
   d. Report signs and symptoms of infection: elevated temperature, warmth at surgical site, purulent discharge, and redness

D. Arthrogram: contrast media or air is injected into joint cavity to visualize joint structures; client moves joint through a series of movements while a series of x-rays are taken; inquire about allergy to contrast media

NCLEX® 1. Client education preprocedure: if injected contrast dye is used, inform client that once dye is injected there may be a feeling of warmth, nausea, headache, salty taste in the mouth, itching, hives, and rash throughout body (symptoms are usually temporary and will be treated if necessary)

NCLEX® 2. Client education postprocedure
   - a. Temporary discoloration of skin and urine is normal after use of dye
   - b. Perform neurovascular self-assessment on affected extremity
   - c. Increase fluid intake to aid in dye excretion and protect kidneys from dye

E. CT scan (computerized axial tomography): combines x-rays with computer technology to produce a highly detailed, cross-sectional image of bones, joints, and other structures

F. MRI (magnetic resonance imaging): similar uses as CT Scan

G. Bone scan: creates images of bones on a computer screen or on a film using a small amount of radioactive material that travels through bloodstream; increased radioisotope uptake is seen with osteomyelitis, osteoporosis, fractures, Paget's disease, and cancer of bone

H. Bone densitometry (bone density): measurement of bone mineral density (BMD) that aids in diagnosis of osteoporosis, predicts fracture risk, and helps evaluate effectiveness of treatment

1. Non-invasive radiologic test that digitally images hip, spine, wrist, finger, tibia, or heel using photon energy beams
2. Takes 30 seconds to 4 minutes per site, and no preprocedure or postprocedure care is required
3. Client's scores include a T-score (compares client score with the score of a normal 30-year-old) and a Z-score (compares client normal to normal in a healthy, age-matched client)
4. Results are reported in standard deviations (SD) below normal and are expressed as negative numbers; scores within 1 standard deviation are considered normal; a score of –1 SD represents a 12% reduction in bone mass); treatment is initiated at –2.5 SD or lower
5. Results should be reassessed every 2 years

I. *Arthrocentesis* (joint aspiration) and analysis: fluid is removed from joint to reduce swelling and pain and/or obtain fluid for examination using a sterile needle and syringe

1. Postprocedure complications are uncommon but may include localized bruising, minor bleeding into joint cavity, and loss of pigment at injection site (septic arthritis is a rare but serious complication)

NCLEX® 2. Client education
   - a. If cortisone was injected into joint, monitor for inflammation of injected area, atrophy or loss of pigment at injection site, and increased blood glucose
   - b. Follow postprocedure activity restrictions as directed by health care provider and monitor for post-procedure complications; check dressing for excessive bleeding

III. LABORATORY STUDIES

A. Antinuclear antibodies (ANA): sensitive screening blood test used to detect autoimmune disease

1. ANAs destroy nucleus of cells
2. Test not definitive but suggests presence of autoantibodies (antibodies directed against body's own tissue)
3. Present in clients with a number of autoimmune diseases such as rheumatoid arthritis, systemic lupus erythematosus, scleroderma, and others

B. Calcium (Ca^{++}): an abundant electrolyte that causes neuromuscular irritability and contractions; adult normal reference value is 9 to 11 mg/dL; range varies slightly by laboratory; see also Chapter 49

1. Decreased calcium levels may be found in osteomalacia, inadequate dietary intake of calcium, renal disease, and hypoparathyroidism
2. Increased calcium levels may be seen in bone neoplasm, multiple fractures, immobilization, renal calculi, and hyperparathyroidism

C. Phosphorus (2.5 to 4.5 mg/dL is normal reference range); may be measured and compared to calcium level

1. Decreased levels can be seen with hypercalcemia, starvation, malabsorption syndrome, osteomalacia, and vitamin D deficiency
2. Increased levels can be seen with healing fractures, metastatic bone tumors, and hypocalcemia

D. Rheumatoid factor (RF) (Normal is negative or <1:20): screening blood test used to detect antibodies (IgM, IgG, or IgA) in rheumatoid arthritis; elevated RF level may indicate diseases other than rheumatoid arthritis

E. Erythrocyte sedimentation rate (ESR): normal is under 20 mm/hr; gender variations exist; nonspecific serologic test that measures rate at which RBCs settle out of unclotted blood in mm/hr; elevated levels indicate inflammatory process in diseases such as rheumatoid arthritis and osteomyelitis

F. Uric acid (normal male 4.5–6.5 mg/dL, female 2.5–5.5 mg/dL)

1. Elevated uric acid level is seen in gout

NCLEX® 2. Hyperuricemia (elevated urine or serum uric acid levels) occurs because of poor renal function, excessive purine metabolism, and/or excessive dietary intake of purine foods

IV. COMMON NURSING TECHNIQUES AND PROCEDURES

A. Crutch-walking

1. Crutch gaits: safe method of walking using crutches, alternating body weight on one or both legs and crutches

NCLEX® 2. See Box 57–1 for crutch-walking techniques

3. See Box 57–2 for transfer techniques (getting in and out of a chair) using crutches

NCLEX® 4. See Box 57–3 for negotiating stairs while using crutches

Memory Aid

Use the phrase "good leg up; bad leg down" to help remember which leg to place first when going up and down stairs with crutches.

Box 57–1

Instructions for Client on Use of Crutches

Four-Point Gait

- Slow gait
- Requires good coordination
- Weight-bearing is on both legs
- Move each foot and crutch forward separately (right crutch, left foot; left crutch, right foot)

Two-Point Gait

- Faster than four-point gait
- Requires more balance
- There is partial weight-bearing on each foot
- Arm movements simulate arm movement when walking
- Move left crutch and right foot forward together; move right crutch and left foot forward together

Three-Point Gait

- Fast gait
- Two crutches and unaffected leg bear weight alternately
- Weaker leg and both crutches move together followed by stronger leg

Swing-To Gait

- Fast gait
- Used by clients with paralysis of legs and hips
- Prolonged use may lead to atrophy of unused muscles
- Advance crutches forward together, lift body using arms, then swing to meet crutches

Swing-Through Gait

- Fast gait
- Good balance, skill, coordination, and strength required
- Move both crutches forward together
- Lift body using arms, then swing through and beyond crutches

Box 57-2

Transfer Techniques for Clients with Crutches

Getting Into a Chair

1. Use chair with armrests and support back of chair against a wall for stability.
2. Center back of unaffected leg against chair.
3. Transfer crutches to hand on affected side.
4. Hold crutches by horizontal hand bars.
5. Grasp arm of chair with hand on unaffected side.
6. Lean forward, flex knees and hips, and lower into chair.

Getting Out of a Chair

1. Move forward to edge of chair.
2. Place unaffected leg slightly under or at edge of chair (this position helps client to stand up from chair and achieve balance, since unaffected leg is supported against edge of chair).
3. Grasp crutches by horizontal hand bars using hand on affected side.
4. Grasp arm of chair using hand on unaffected side (body weight is placed on crutches and hand on armrest to support unaffected leg when client rises to stand).
5. Push down on crutches and chair armrest while raising body out of chair.
6. Assume a *tripod position* (crutches out laterally in front of feet, approximately 6 inches, with feet slightly apart creating a wide base of support) for balance before moving.

B. ***Traction***: direct pulling force applied to a fractured extremity that results in realignment of bone; see Figure 57–1, p. 1056

1. Reduces fracture, lessens muscle spasms, relieves pain, corrects deformities, promotes rest, and allows for exercise
2. Skin and skeletal traction are most commonly used; manual traction is used only briefly under physician direction

NCLEX®

3. Skin traction (using tape, boots, splints)
   - **a.** Generally used for short-term treatment (48–72 hours) and is applied directly to skin; used until skeletal traction or surgery are available to treat fracture

Box 57-3

Instructions for Clients with Crutches: Negotiating Stairs

Going Up Stairs (stand behind client slightly on affected side for support if needed)

1. Assume tripod position.
2. Transfer weight to crutches and move unaffected leg onto step.
3. Transfer weight to unaffected leg on step and move crutches and affected leg up to step.
4. Repeat steps 2 and 3 until client reaches top of stairs.

Going Down Stairs (stand one step below client on affected side for support if needed)

1. Assume tripod position at top of stairs.
2. Shift weight to unaffected leg.
3. Move crutches and affected leg down onto next step.
4. Transfer weight to crutches and move unaffected leg to that step.
5. Repeat steps 2 and 3 until client reaches bottom step.

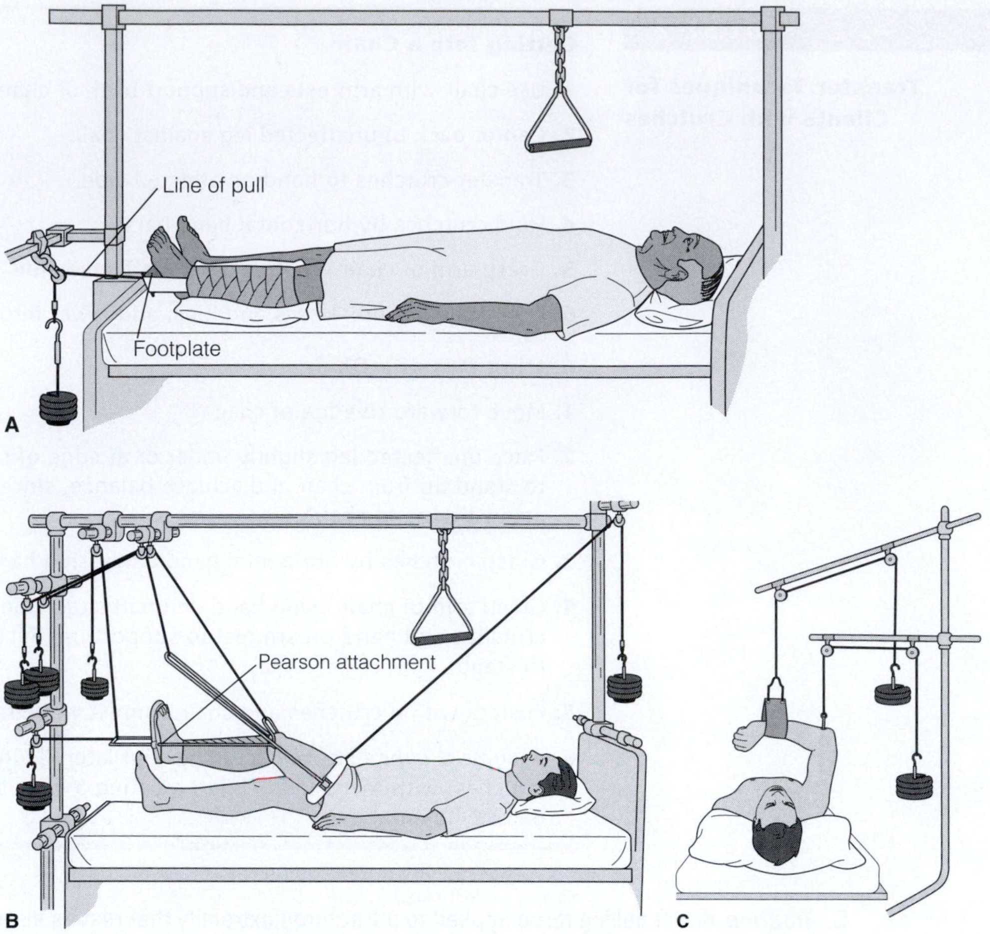

Figure 57–1

Types of traction. *A.* Skin traction (also called straight traction), such as Buck's traction for hip fracture. *B.* Balanced suspension traction, often used for fractures of the femur. *C.* Skeletal traction, in which pulling force is applied directly to bone, such as for a fracture of the humerus.

b. Assists in reduction of a fracture (does not primarily achieve reduction) and helps decrease muscle spasms

c. Weights range from 5 to 10 pounds

NCLEX®

4. Skeletal traction (using pins or wires inserted into bones)

a. Indicated for long-term use

b. Used to align injured bones and joints or to treat joint contractures and congenital hip dysplasia

c. Weights are usually 15–30 pounds and amounts of weight may be adjusted initially until full fracture reduction is achieved as noted on x-ray

5. Balanced suspension (traction that is a hanging support to immobilize body part in a desired position)

a. Used with skeletal traction to improve mobility while maintaining alignment of fracture

b. Body part is suspended using splints, ropes, and weights

c. Client can perform activities such as toileting and personal hygiene; bed linen can be changed without disturbing traction alignment

d. Risk for skin breakdown exists over bony prominences that are in contact with sheets (including back of head)

6. **Countertraction**: pulling force exerted in opposite direction to prevent client from sliding to end of bed; examples include client's weight, elevating foot of bed (Trendelenburg), and elevating head of bed with cervical traction

NCLEX®

7. See Box 57–4 for nursing care of client in traction

NCLEX®

C. **Cast care**: a cast is applied for immobilization to ensure stability of a fracture; see Box 57–5, p. 1058, for associated nursing care

D. **Splinting and immobilization**: like casts, splints are used to immobilize a fractured extremity to ensure stability after closed reduction and external fixation; teach client how to perform neurovascular examination (color, temperature, capillary refill less than 3 seconds, and pulses)

Box 57-4

Nursing Care of Client in Traction

- Ensure that all ropes, weights, and pulleys are hanging freely, not shredded or torn, in a straight line.
- Bed linen should be kept off traction ropes.
- Reinforce client teaching that weights should not be lifted for any reason (lifting weights alters line of pull and could potentially interfere with bone healing).
- Ensure that ordered amount of weight is maintained at all times.
- Avoid jarring bed or equipment.
- Ensure that knots are not lying on or near pulley.
- Perform neurovascular examination to monitor for superficial nerve damage (radial, median, ulnar, femoral, sciatic, peroneal nerves).
- Reinforce how to perform circulatory inspection on unaffected and affected limb, comparing observations (color, temperature, capillary refill, pulses).
- Perform skin inspection to monitor and prevent skin breakdown on bony prominence and pressure areas.
- Monitor client in skin traction for skin breakdown under traction boot or splint caused by friction and shear.
- Ensure that body is always kept in proper alignment to prevent complications such as external rotation of joint, increased pain, and poor healing of fracture.
- Provide pin care using normal saline solution or other agency approved solution if client is in skeletal traction, and teach client how to monitor for infection at pin sites (fever, localized warmth, redness, swelling, abnormal drainage, and odor).
- Inform client to avoid massaging calves or reddened areas to prevent clot dislodgment caused by venous stasis.
- Encourage client to increase fluid intake (2500 mL/day unless contraindicated) and roughage (fresh fruits and vegetables) in diet to prevent constipation, urinary tract infection, and renal calculi.
- Reinforce how to perform deep-breathing and coughing exercises to prevent respiratory complications.
- Encourage client to use overhead trapeze (and unaffected leg if possible) to reposition for comfort, shift weight to prevent skin breakdown, perform exercises, and assist with personal care, toileting, and bed linen changes.
- Encourage client to adhere to exercise regimen to maintain muscle tone, endurance, and prevent bone demineralization.
- Provide diversional activities and encourage social interaction with family and friends to prevent potential isolation.

V. NURSING MANAGEMENT OF CLIENT UNDERGOING MUSCULOSKELETAL SURGERY

A. *Laminectomy:* surgical incision of lamina done primarily to relieve symptoms related to herniated intervertebral disc

1. Monitor effectiveness of pain management
2. NCLEX® Perform neurological and neurovascular data collection monitor bowel and bladder function
3. Inquire with client about reports of severe headache or leakage of cerebrospinal fluid (CSF), nausea, abdominal discomfort, incontinence, amount and character of drainage on dressing
4. Use *logroll* technique (turning a client as a unit) to turn and reposition client; maintain proper alignment of spine at all times
5. NCLEX® Inform client that bedrest may be maintained for first 24–48 hours after procedure; pillows may be used for comfort under thighs in supine position and between thighs when in side-lying position
6. Help client to "rise as a unit" when getting out of bed (especially for first time)

Box 57-5

Nursing Care of Client in a Cast

- Reinforce client teaching that plaster cast should not get wet and that cast padding should not be removed; if cast becomes soiled with feces, clean with a damp cloth or rub baking soda on soiled area to limit odor.
- Reinforce client teaching that no foreign objects should be inserted into cast (sticks, food crumbs, etc.) to prevent skin breakdown; teach client how to smooth rough edges.
- Reinforce to client to avoid covering a new cast with blanket or plastic for extended periods (air cannot circulate, and heat builds up in the cast).
- Turn client from side to side (using palms, not fingertips) every 2 hours to facilitate drying for first 24–72 hours (use of fingertips causes indentation and pressure areas when cast is dry).
- Explain that casts made with newer synthetic materials dry more quickly and allow faster mobility (often can bear weight within 30 minutes).
- Reinforce to client to apply ice for first 24 hours over fracture site to control edema, ensuring that ice is securely contained so cast does not become wet.
- Reinforce to client to elevate extremity above level of heart to promote venous return for first 24 hours after application.
- Reinforce to client to perform active range of motion (AROM) to joints above and below immobilized extremity.
- Reinforce client teaching about signs and symptoms to report to health care provider: increasing pain in immobilized extremity, excessive swelling and discoloration of exposed limb, burning or tingling, sores, or foul odor under cast.

7. Reinforce to client that paresthesia (numbness and tingling of extremities) may not be relieved immediately after procedure

B. *Internal fixation*: fracture immobilization with a metal device (made of screws, pins, and/or plates) that is surgically inserted to realign and maintain a fracture

1. Perform neurovascular data collection regularly; report adverse changes in color, temperature, sensation or motion promptly
2. Monitor and treat postoperative pain promptly; report pain that becomes more severe or is unrelieved by analgesics
3. Perform standard postoperative data collection and care
4. Collaborate with physical therapy to aid client mobility
5. Reinforce signs and symptoms of infection to report: elevated temperature, localized pain and warmth, tenderness, chills, malaise, and changes in neurovascular status of affected extremity

C. External fixation: fracture immobilization using a frame connected to pins inserted perpendicular to long axis of bone

1. Monitor neurovascular status at least every 4 hours
2. Monitor for signs of infection and report promptly
3. Perform standard postoperative care measures
4. Explain that device allows greater mobility during healing

D. Joint replacement, total hip replacement (THR)

1. THR is frequently performed to treat conditions such as rheumatoid arthritis, malignant bone tumors, arthritis associated with Paget's disease, juvenile rheumatoid arthritis, and hip fractures
2. Advantages of THR: substantial relief of pain, improved function and quality of life
3. Reinforce client teaching about plan for effective pain management and side effects/adverse effects of pain medications

NCLEX®

4. Provide and teach client about dislocation precautions
   a. Avoid extremes of internal rotation, adduction, and 90-degree flexion of affected hip for at least 4–6 weeks after procedure
   b. Prevent adduction: use an abduction pillow, avoid crossing legs, avoid twisting to reach for objects behind, and avoid driving a car and taking tub baths for at least 4 to 6 weeks
   c. Modify equipment to avoid 90-degree hip flexion (raised toilet seats, platform under chair, use of reacher device, long-handled shoe horn, and sock puller)
5. Explain that passive range of motion (ROM) and physical therapy exercises will begin on first postoperative day to restore and maintain ROM, muscle strength, and mobility and to prevent complications such as deep vein thrombosis (DVT)

NCLEX® 6. Reinforce client teaching about signs and symptoms to report to health care provider
   a. Infection: redness, swelling, abnormal drainage, foul odor, and elevated temperature
   b. DVT: pain, sudden swelling in affected extremity, enlargement of superficial veins, skin discoloration, and localized warmth
7. Reinforce to client that home care management program will include the following:
   a. Ongoing nursing observation of pain management
   b. Periodic dressing changes and monitoring for infection
   NCLEX® c. Monitoring and adjustment of coagulation status weekly if taking warfarin (Coumadin) and less often if taking enoxaparin (Lovenox), a low-molecular-weight heparin
   d. An exercise program assisted by a physical therapist to monitor and restore muscle strength and ROM

NCLEX® 8. Reinforce to client to inform all health care providers (dentists, etc.) of history of joint replacement surgery so that prophylactic antibiotics can be prescribed as necessary
9. Inform client that periodic x-rays will be required as follow-up throughout lifetime

NCLEX® 10. Note for clients undergoing knee replacement: continuous passive motion (CPM) machine may be put in place immediately after surgery and accompanies client to surgical unit after postanesthesia recovery period; ensure that client's limb is positioned correctly and that pain medication is adequate; device should be used at least 8 of every 24 hours and increased as client can tolerate it

E. Amputation

1. Common levels of amputation of lower extremity includes toe, foot (part or all), Syme (ankle disarticulation), below knee and above knee
2. Two types of amputation are open (guillotine) and closed (flap)
   a. Open type is used when infection is present and wound is left open; a second surgery is done later to close wound
   b. Closed type involves covering end of wound with flap of skin
3. Provide standard postoperative care
4. Treat postoperative pain with opioid analgesics and provide client teaching about effective pain management techniques
5. Monitor for and teach client to report signs of infection or complications: redness, elevated temperature, and/or unusual, foul-smelling drainage; abrasions; and any other signs of skin breakdown
6. Monitor and maintain placement of residual limb shrinking devices, such as rigid plaster cast, elastic bandage, shrinker sock or elastic stockinette, to reduce postoperative edema
7. Use proper technique for wrapping residual limb with elastic bandage, if used (see Figure 57–2)
8. Reinforce client teaching to perform upper extremity active ROM exercises daily
9. Turn and reposition client every 2 hours
10. Assist client to lay prone for 30 minutes 3 to 4 times/day (if client is able and if part of standard of care) and avoid elevating or sitting with residual limb on pillows for prolonged amount of time to prevent flexion contractures; limb may be elevated above heart level for first 24 hours after surgery to reduce edema

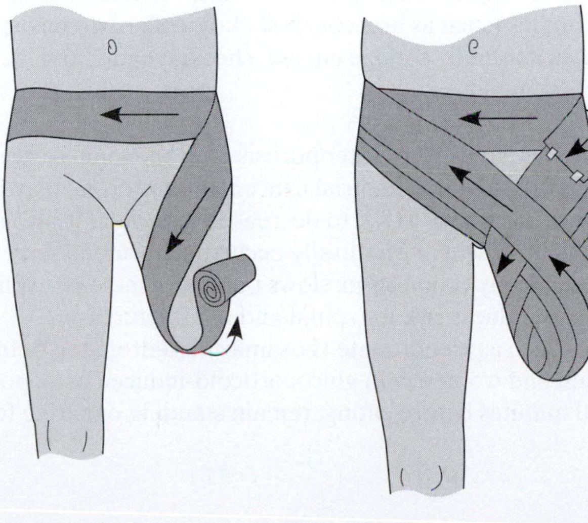

Figure 57–2

Residual limb wrapping in a distal to proximal direction reduces edema and allows conical shape to form in preparation for prosthesis.

NCLEX® 11. Tell client that phantom pain may persist in amputated extremity because of irritation of residual nerve endings; this is normal and real; discomfort will be treated with analgesics or other interventions

NCLEX® 12. Reinforce client teaching about how to care for residual limb
- a. Wash daily using warm water and bacteriostatic soap
- b. Rinse and gently pat dry thoroughly
- c. Expose to air for at least 20 minutes after washing
- d. Avoid use of lotions, alcohol, powder, or oils unless prescribed by health care provider
- e. Change cotton or wool limb sock daily, wash sock using mild soap and dry flat, and discard sock that is in poor condition

13. Assist client to cope with disturbed body image and actively participate in physical therapy to aid in rehabilitation

VI. OSTEOPOROSIS

A. Overview

1. Disease characterized by low bone mass and structural deterioration of bone tissue, causing bones (especially weight-bearing bones such as hip, spine, and wrist) to become fragile and more susceptible to fractures
2. Affects both women and men; however, women are at greater risk
3. As people age, bone resorption happens faster than bone formation, which causes bone to lose Ca^{++} and bone density; since most of body's Ca^{++} is stored in bones and teeth, this rapid bone resorption leads to porous bone or osteoporosis
4. When serum Ca^{++} decreases, body takes stored Ca^{++} from bone

NCLEX® B. Nursing data collection

1. Risk factors include caucasian or Asian ethnicity; family history; inadequate dietary intake of Ca^{++}; sedentary lifestyle; smoking; excessive alcohol intake; steroid medications; chronic liver disease; anorexia; and malabsorption
2. Females are at a higher risk for osteoporosis than men
   - a. Smaller body frames contribute to less bone density
   - b. Bone resorption begins at an earlier age and is accelerated in menopause
   - c. Breastfeeding and pregnancy deplete skeletal reserves unless Ca^{++} intake is increased to match demands
   - d. Longevity increases likelihood of osteoporosis (compared to men)

NCLEX® C. Therapeutic management

1. Provide client teaching about prevention
   - a. Take adequate amounts of Ca^{++} throughout lifetime to decrease incidence of osteoporosis
   - b. Proper nutrition for adequate Ca^{++} intake
   - c. Weight-bearing exercises to force Ca^{++} back into the bone
   - d. Safety measures to prevent falls that can result in fractures
   - e. BMD tests to measure bone mass in clients at risk for developing osteoporosis
   - f. Provide clients with information about recommended daily dietary intake of Ca^{++}: 1000–1200 mg/day for premenopausal and postmenopausal women taking estrogen replacement therapy (ERT), and 1500 mg/day for postmenopausal women who are not taking ERT
   - g. Provide information about foods high in Ca^{++} and importance of Ca^{++} intake with vitamin D: dark, green leafy vegetables (such as broccoli, bok choy, collard greens, spinach), sardines, salmon with bone, dairy products (such as milk, cottage cheese, cheese, yogurt, and ice cream); Ca^{++} supplements can also be added to dietary intake
2. Medication therapy
   - a. ERT is generally used to prevent osteoporosis after menopause; usually given in form of a pill or skin patch; can increase risk for endometrial cancer (progesterone may be given with estrogen, called hormone replacement therapy or HRT, to decrease risk); client is also at risk for developing DVT
   - b. Calcitonin (Micalcin, Calcimar): naturally occurring hormone secreted by thyroid gland; currently available as a nasal spray or injection; slows bone loss, increases spinal bone density, relieves pain from bone fractures, and reduces risk for spinal and hip fractures
   - NCLEX® c. Bisphosphonates such as alendronate (Fosamax), risedronate (Actonel) and others: prevent bone resorption in men and women with glucocorticoid-induced osteoporosis; take dose with a glass of water at least 30 minutes before eating; remain standing or sitting for 30 minutes after dose

d. Raloxifene (Evista): used to prevent or treat osteoporosis; selective receptor modulator (SERM) that prevents bone loss; side effects are rare but may include hot flashes or DVT; may be taken without regard to food

D. Reinforce client teaching

1. Importance of weight-bearing exercises (jogging, walking, hiking, stair climbing, tennis, dancing, and weight training)
2. Encourage client to stop smoking and avoid excessive intake of alcohol

VII. OSTEOMYELITIS

A. Overview

1. Acute or chronic infection of bone usually caused by *staphylococcus aureus* organism
2. Infection can occur from direct or indirect invasion of infectious organisms; see Figure 57–3
3. Direct invasion generally occurs from invasive procedures such as surgery (joint prosthesis, arthroplasty) and injuries such as fractures
4. Infection can also be caused by indirect invasion (also called hematogenous dissemination), where infection of bone or joint is caused by spread of organism through bloodstream from a pre-existing site of infection; course and virulence of infection is influenced by blood circulation to affected bone
5. Long bones are common sites of infection in children, and spine, hip, and foot are common sites of infection in adults
6. At-risk populations include children, older adults, and those with weakened immune systems
7. Osteomyelitis warrants aggressive immediate treatment with antibiotics or surgery (wound debridement) if infection of bone is extensive

NCLEX®

B. Nursing data collection

1. Observe for symptoms of local and/or systemic infection: elevated temperature, chills, restlessness, severe bone pain unrelieved by analgesics or rest and aggravated by movement, swelling, redness, and warmth at the infection site
2. Wound culture, bone scan, CT scan, and MRI diagnose problem and determine extent of infection

NCLEX®

C. Therapeutic management

1. Explain all therapies and interventions to client and family to decrease anxiety and enhance cooperation with plan of care
2. Use a rating scale to monitor pain and evaluate effectiveness of pain management measures
3. Provide ongoing education and emotional support since seriousness of infection, duration and uncertainty about recuperation time, potential complications, and associated risk can be a very fearful experience for client and family
4. NCLEX® Use sterile technique for all dressing changes and manipulation of affected limb; handle extremity very gently
5. NCLEX® Avoid activities that increase circulation to affected area or cause edema, pain, and pathologic fractures, such as exercise, application of heat, or keeping extremity in dependent position
6. Immobilize affected extremity as prescribed and keep body in proper alignment

Figure 57–3

Osteomyelitis. *A.* Site of initial infection. Bacteria enter bone and multiply, initiating inflammatory response. *B.* Acute phase, with spread of infection to other parts of bone. Pus forms, edema occurs, and vascular supply is compromised. If infection reaches outer margin of bone, periosteum lifts, and ischemia and necrosis occur eventually. *C.* Chronic phase. Necrotic bone separates, a new layer of bone forms around necrotic bone, and sinus develops to allow wound to drain.

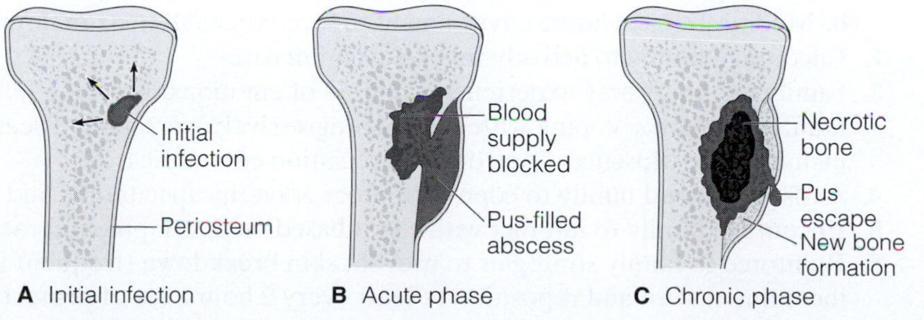

7. Monitor temperature at least every 2 hours
8. Provide cool environment, light clothing, antipyretic medication, antibiotics, and other therapies as prescribed and/or appropriate to keep temperature within client's baseline
9. Keep client well hydrated to prevent dehydration from insensible water loss
10. Instruct and assist client with interventions to prevent complications associated with immobility (turn and reposition every 2 hours, coughing and deep breathing exercises, etc.)
11. Medication therapy is indicated with or without surgical intervention; generally includes antibiotics and analgesics

D. Reinforce client teaching

1. Importance of taking antibiotic medications as prescribed (for full duration) and to report adverse medication effects to prescriber
2. Review medication regimen and check client understanding
3. Reinforce importance of rest and proper diet to facilitate healing and prevent constipation and dehydration
4. *NCLEX®* Reinforce importance of limb immobilization during treatment
5. If long-term management is required, provide instructions about wound care using sterile technique, medication regimen (including instruction on venous access devices if needed), antibiotic administration, proper diet, rest, follow-up visits, and laboratory tests
6. Provide information about adverse effects of antibiotic therapy such as ototoxicity and nephrotoxicity (aminoglycosides) and hepatotoxicity (cephalosporins)

VIII. MUSCULAR DYSTROPHY (MD)

A. Overview

1. Group of genetic sex-linked childhood disorders characterized by progressive muscle weakness, muscle wasting of symmetrical groups of muscles, and increasing disability and deformity
2. Types of MD include Duchenne (most common), myotonic, Becker's, facioscapulohumeral, and limb girdle
3. Significant risk factor is family history
4. Each type differs in regard to muscle groups affected, age at onset, rate of progression, and pattern of inheritance
5. Each type of MD affects specific muscle groups

B. Nursing data collection

1. Muscle biopsy confirms diagnosis (shows degeneration of muscle fibers)
2. EMG identifies origin of muscle weakness (muscle destruction, nerve damage)
3. *NCLEX®* Progressive muscle weakness, hypotonia (loss of muscle mass), and delayed development of motor skills such as walking may be noted
4. *NCLEX®* Ptosis (drooping of the eyelid), impaired chewing and swallowing, abnormal gait, fatigue with minimal activity, frequent falls may all be noted
5. Delayed intellectual development is seen with some forms of MD
6. Muscle contractures and deformities common
7. Abnormal curvature of spine (scoliosis or lordosis)
8. Enlargement of calf muscle (pseudohypertrophy) caused by fatty infiltration causing muscular enlargement
9. Cardiomyopathy or arrhythmia may be present with some forms of MD

C. Therapeutic management

1. Provide support and assist family with decision-making process surrounding:
   a. Development of a home care plan to support as much independence as possible
   b. Modifications in home environment to support client's maximal functional ability
2. Encourage family to actively involve client in care
3. *NCLEX®* Family members may experience a myriad of emotions, including fear, guilt, anger, and blame; support family to enhance coping with client's progressively worsening disease; refer to local support groups including the Muscular Dystrophy Association of America
4. Assist client and family to cope with progressive, incapacitating, and fatal nature of disease
5. *NCLEX®* Encourage family to interact with client based on developmental rather than chronological age
6. *NCLEX®* Reinforce to family strategies to prevent skin breakdown (frequent skin care and linen changes if incontinent, turn and reposition at least every 2 hours, use of protective skin barrier ointments, and adequate fluid intake)

7. Perform passive ROM exercises to maintain function in unaffected extremities and prevent or delay contractures in affected extremities
8. Medication therapy: there is no effective drug therapy; corticosteroids are often used to increase muscle strength

D. Reinforce client teaching

1. Information about health care team member roles, including those involved in home care program for client
2. NCLEX® Offer client soft foods and to cut into small pieces to prevent aspiration and choking
3. NCLEX® Seek genetic counseling (parents, female siblings, maternal aunts, and female offspring)
4. Appropriate clothing and footwear because of contractures and wheelchair-bound status
5. Information on community support groups and agencies with respite services to prevent role strain

IX. PAGET'S DISEASE (OSTEITIS DEFORMANS)

A. Overview

1. Chronic skeletal bone disease with insidious onset often diagnosed around fourth decade of life
2. Results in enlarged, deformed bones but does not affect normal bones
3. Generally affects skull, long bones, spine, and ribs
4. Cause is unknown, but viral infection is suspected as probable etiology
5. Hereditary factor: may be seen in more than one family member
6. Early diagnosis and treatment is important to prevent disease progression and deformity
7. Excessive bone resorption followed by bone formation leads to weakened bone, bone pain, arthritis, deformity, and potential pathologic fractures
8. Normal bone marrow is replaced by vascular, fibrous, connective tissue that leads to formation of larger, disorganized, and weaker bone tissue

B. Nursing data collection

1. X-ray is most definitive diagnostic test; serum alkaline phosphatase may be elevated
2. NCLEX® Bone scan may be done after positive serum alkaline phosphatase test (positive scan shows characteristic abnormally curved contours and thickened cortex); positive bone scan prompts x-ray for definitive diagnosis
3. Mild form of disease may be undetected because there may be no symptoms
4. NCLEX® Symptoms include bone pain (most common) and other symptoms depending on bones affected
   a. If skull is affected, headache and hearing loss may be reported as well as increasing head size
   b. Hip pain may be present if pelvis or femur is involved
   c. Bowing of lower extremities producing a waddling gait and curvature of spine may be seen in advanced stages
5. Arthritis may result because of damage to joint cartilage
6. Complications are pathologic fractures (may be first indicator of disease) and osteogenic sarcoma (form of bone cancer)

C. Therapeutic management

1. Prognosis is good especially if treatment is started before major deformity occurs
2. Provide analgesics and muscle relaxants for comfort
3. Administer medications as directed to control progression of disease (see Medication section) and teach to take as directed because deformity and loss of bone strength will continue without prescribed medications
4. If skull is affected, assist with diet modification, dentures, and eating utensils because teeth may become weak from disease
5. Hearing aid may be recommended if hearing loss results from disease
6. Refer client and family to support group
7. Medication therapy: goal is to control disease progression; FDA–approved drugs include calcitonin (Miacalcin) and bisphosphonates such as etidronate (Didronel), pamidronate (Aredia), alandronate (Fosamax), tiludronate (Skelid), and risedronate (Actonel)

D. Reinforce client teaching

1. Ensure that client understands plan for pain management and encourage client to take analgesics as prescribed
2. NCLEX® Reinforce importance of a balanced diet, high in Ca^{++} (1000–1500 mg/day) and vitamin D (at least 400 units/day); vitamin D can be obtained from exposure to sunlight
3. Inform health care provider of any history of kidney stones or disease before taking Ca^{++}

4. Participate in an exercise program to maintain skeletal muscle health, ideal body weight, and joint mobility
5. Sleep on a firm mattress if back discomfort is present; if back brace is needed, instruct client on prevention of skin breakdown under brace (undershirt) and safety measures (no driving with brace)
6. Modify environment at home to prevent falls that may lead to subsequent fractures
7. Participate in community support group according to need and preference

X. FRACTURES

A. Overview

1. A fracture is a break in continuity of a bone
2. May be classified as closed/simple fracture (bone breaks but skin remains intact) or open/compound (broken ends of bone penetrate skin)
3. Other classification of fractures (see Figure 57–4 and Table 57–1) *NCLEX®*
4. Fractures occur in all age groups, although older adults are more prone to fractures resulting from falls
5. When a bone breaks, healing process occurs in three phases
   a. A fracture initiates an inflammatory response (inflammatory phase)
   b. Ca^{++} eventually is deposited in area and osteoblasts promote new bone formation (reparative phase)
   c. Eventually ends of fracture reunite (remodeling phase)

NCLEX® **B. Nursing data collection**

1. Deformity: may be caused by break in continuity of bone itself and pull of muscles on fragmented bones
2. Edema and swelling (caused by bleeding into surrounding tissue)
3. Pain may be caused by muscle spasms and pressure on nerves
4. Crepitus may also be present on palpation; **crepitation** is a popping or grating sound created by movement of broken bone fragments
5. Muscle spasms may be noted near fractured bone
6. Ecchymosis or a bluish discoloration of area caused by blood extravasation into surrounding subcutaneous tissues
7. Pain that may be intense and possibly shock if blood loss is severe

NCLEX® **C. Therapeutic management**

1. Perform frequent neurovascular data collection; note and report abnormal findings
2. Immobilize joints above and below fracture; movement of affected area may cause a closed fracture to become open; splints may be used to immobilize fracture
3. Cover open wounds with sterile dressings
4. Manage fracture pain with prescribed analgesics
5. Elevate fractured extremity to reduce swelling and pain
6. Apply ice to affected extremity

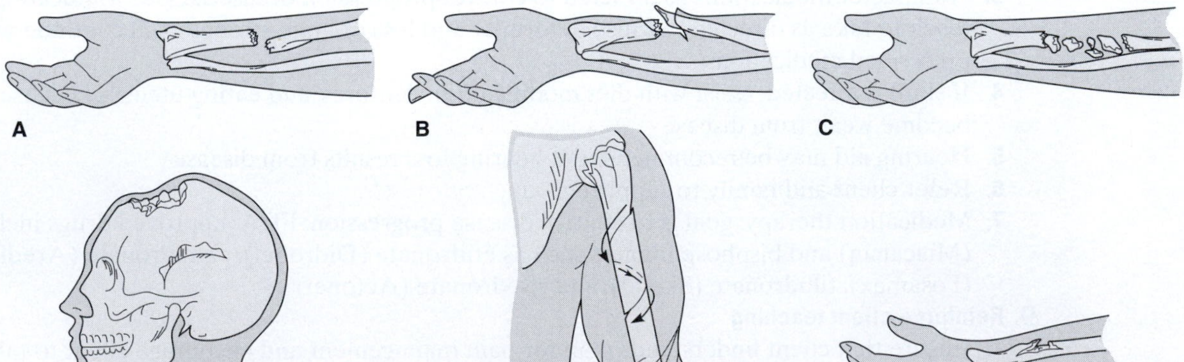

Figure 57–4

Types of fractures. *A.* Closed. *B.* Open. *C.* Comminuted. *D.* Depressed. *E.* Spiral. *F.* Greenstick.

Table 57–1 Types of Fractures

Type of Fracture	Description
Avulsion	Results from tearing of supporting tendons and ligaments
Comminuted	Broken bone fragments into more than two pieces
Compression	Bone is crushed
Impacted	Ends of broken bone are driven into each other
Depressed	A fracture in which bone structure is broken and pressed inward, such as in skull fracture
Spiral	Break spreads in a spiral fashion along bone shaft; is usually caused by sports injuries and child abuse
Greenstick	An incomplete break in bone where one side splinters leaving other side bent or intact; more common in children

7. Assist in fracture reduction: closed reduction involves external manipulation to realign bones; open reduction involves a surgical procedure to realign bones
8. Maintain traction as prescribed; see section on nursing care of client in traction
9. See also section on nursing care of a client in a cast

D. Complications

NCLEX® 1. **Compartment syndrome**
   a. Impairment of circulation within inelastic fascia caused by external pressure (>30 mmHg) that results in tissue death and nerve injury
   b. External pressure can be created by casts, splints, or dressings
   c. Manifestations include unrelieved pain, diminished or absent pulses distal to injury, cyanosis of extremity, tingling or diminished sensation (paresthesia), loss of sensation, pallor, coolness of extremity, and weakness
   d. Bivalving (splitting cast lengthwise and resecuring with elastic wrap) may be necessary if cast is too tight
2. Infection: wound drainage, fever, pain, and odor; treated with antibiotics

NCLEX® 3. Fat embolism: an emergency situation in which client experiences chest pain, dyspnea, tachycardia, decreased O_2 saturation, apprehension, changes in LOC, petechiae on upper trunk and axilla; aggressive diagnosis and treatment is necessary to save client's life
4. DVT: calf pain and tenderness, swelling or edema

E. Reinforce client teaching

1. Exercise extremities not immobilized to prevent muscle atrophy
2. Cast care, splint, and/or traction (see previous discussions)
3. Neurovascular self-assessments that need to be done
4. Pin care procedure and methods of preventing wound infection

XI. HIP FRACTURE

A. Overview

1. Hip can fracture at different sites: head, neck, and trochanteric areas; see Figure 57–5, p. 1066
2. Incidence of hip fracture increases with age; 90% of hip fractures are caused by falls
3. A hip fracture is a medical emergency

NCLEX® **B. Nursing data collection**

1. Monitor LOC and check for other injuries if fracture caused by a fall
2. Perform neurovascular examination on affected extremity (monitor for adverse changes such as cool, pale skin and delayed capillary refill more than 3 seconds)

Memory Aid

Use the 6 Ps to remember abnormal neurovascular findings: pain, pallor, paresthesia, pulselessness (or decreased pulses), paralysis (or weakness), and poikilothermia (reduced temperature).

3. Extremity of affected hip will be shorter than unaffected extremity and is often externally rotated

NCLEX® **C. Therapeutic management**

1. Prepare client for surgery (verify allergies, informed consent, etc.)
2. Instruct client that an abductor pillow or splint may be necessary to prevent disarticulation of femur

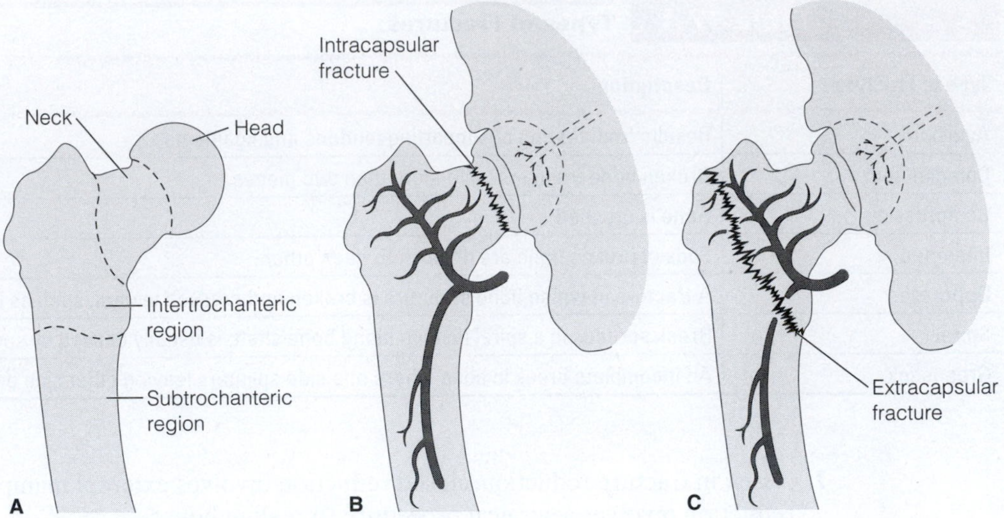

Figure 57-5

A. Hip fractures can occur in the head, neck, or trochanteric regions of the femur. *B.* An intracapsular fracture affects the femur head or neck. *C.* An extracapsular fracture occurs across the trochanteric region. All fractures disrupt the blood supply to the bone.

3. Place sandbags along external border of affected limb to prevent external rotation as ordered
4. Provide pain medication will be available for comfort postoperatively (generally, patient-controlled analgesia [PCA] is used)
5. Reinforce client teaching about pain rating scale and encourage client to report discomfort
6. Reinforce deep-breathing and coughing exercises preoperatively
7. Use aseptic technique for dressing changes and wound drainage
8. Provide information on therapies and equipment to expect postoperatively (indwelling urinary catheter, PCA, IV therapy, possible traction, incentive spirometer, etc.)
9. Monitor preoperative use of skin traction (Buck's traction) to immobilize limb until surgery is performed; inspect skin under traction boot/splint for breakdown each shift
10. Medication therapy: analgesics to manage pain

D. Reinforce client teaching

NCLEX®
1. Preoperatively teach client about postoperative precautions to prevent hip dislocation (no hip flexion greater that 90 degrees, internal rotation of affected hip, or adduction of affected hip); these include such activities as avoiding low chairs, using raised toilet seat, no excessive bending
2. Deep breathing and coughing exercises postoperatively
3. Reinforce teaching about postoperative course

XII. SPRAINS AND STRAINS

A. Overview

1. A **sprain** is a stretch and/or tear of a ligament
2. A **strain** is a twist, pull, and/or tear that may involve both muscles and tendons
3. Caused by direct or indirect trauma (fall, blow to body, muscle exhaustion), overuse or prolonged repetitive motion of muscles and tendons, inadequate rest periods during intensive training
4. Ankles, knees, and wrist are most vulnerable
5. Frequently seen in athletes and those with poor physical conditioning or who are overweight

B. Nursing data collection

1. Sprains are classified based on degree of ligament injury
2. Pain is aggravated by continuous use and influenced by degree of injury
3. *NCLEX®* Monitor for bruising, edema, joint swelling, muscle spasms, and inflammation
4. *NCLEX®* Monitor for changes in neurovascular status (pulse, temperature, capillary refill, and movement) of affected extremity
5. Decreased mobility in affected extremity

C. Therapeutic management

NCLEX®
1. Teach client about RICE approach to recovery
   a. *R*est affected extremity
   b. *I*ce for 15 to 30 minutes at a time for 2 to 3 days
   c. *C*ompression elastic support bandages or adhesive tape
   d. *E*levation

Memory Aid

Use RICE for musculoskeletal injuries (rest, ice, compression, and elevation).

2. Perform neurovascular data collection on affected extremity

NCLEX®
3. Encourage client to wrap affected extremity with elastic support bandages before strenuous activities
4. Inform client that x-rays of injured extremity may be necessary
5. Administer analgesics as needed

NCLEX®
6. Reinforce importance of stretching and warm-up exercises before athletic activities
7. Encourage client to adhere to exercise program to regain muscle tone and strength in collaboration with physical therapist
8. Medications: analgesics, muscle relaxants, anti-inflammatory agents as needed

D. Reinforce client teaching: information previously discussed

XIII. GOUT

A. Overview

1. Primary form of disease is hereditary; secondary form is acquired
2. Laboratory findings show elevated serum uric acid (hyperuricemia); see norms at beginning of chapter
3. Characterized by recurring attacks of acute joint inflammation; frequent sites affected are great toe or knee
4. Is an inherited abnormality in uric acid metabolism
5. Hyperuricemia is caused by increased purine synthesis and/or decreased renal excretion of uric acid; may also be caused by prolonged fasting and excessive alcohol intake

B. Nursing data collection

NCLEX®
1. Risk factors: obesity, excessive weight gain, excessive alcohol intake, impaired renal function, hypertension, chemotherapy for leukemia and certain lymphomas, certain thiazide diuretics, aspirin, and tuberculosis medications
2. Diagnosis includes analysis of synovial fluid, serum uric acid, and 24-hour urine

NCLEX®
3. Joint inflammation is extremely painful and is caused by deposits of uric acid crystals in synovial lining and fluid
4. Monitor for elevated temperature (may not always be present), tenderness and cyanosis of affected extremity, inflammation of small joints (commonly seen in great toe), and multiple joint involvement

NCLEX®
5. Precipitating factors generally include dehydration, fever, injury to joint, and excessive alcohol ingestion

NCLEX®

C. Therapeutic management

1. Prevent any bed linen from touching affected extremity because of extreme tenderness (bed cradle and/or footboard can be used)
2. Remind client to adhere to activity restriction such as bedrest and immobilization of affected extremity during periods of exacerbation
3. Monitor uric acid levels to prevent exacerbation and evaluate effectiveness of treatment
4. Reinforce client teaching about precipitating factors
5. Avoid foods high in purines (such as herring, sardines, sweetbreads, yeast)
6. Medication therapy: usually includes anti-inflammatory agents (such as colchicine, NSAIDs, or corticosteroids), an antihyperuricemic (such as allopurinol [Zyloprim]), and uricosurics (such as probenecid [Probalan])

D. Reinforce client teaching

1. Therapeutic management items outined above
2. Action, side/adverse effects of medication; take doses with meals to avoid gastric irritation
3. Avoid use of alcohol when taking medication and limit use if not on medications to avoid flares

NCLEX®
4. Drink at least 2.5 to 3 liters of fluid per day when taking medication

XIV. DEGENERATIVE JOINT DISEASE (DJD) OR OSTEOARTHRITIS (OA)

A. Overview

1. Slowly progressive disorder of articulating joints, especially weight-bearing joints
2. Commonly affects hands and weight-bearing joints (knees, hips, feet, and back)

3. Breakdown of articular cartilage occurs
4. Injury is usually limited to joint and surrounding tissue
5. Disease ranges from very mild to very severe
6. Cartilage degeneration causes bones to rub against each other, causing pain and decreasing joint function
7. Risk factors (NCLEX®)
   a. Age (most significant): primarily affects middle-aged to older adults
   b. Obesity (generally causes arthritis of knees)
   c. Repetitive joint injuries caused by sports, accidents, or work-related injuries
   d. Genetics (especially seen with OA of hands): client may be born with defective cartilage or slight defect in how joint fits together, and as client ages, joint cartilage continues to progressively degenerate and enzymes (hyaluronidase) are released, which cause further breakdown

B. Nursing data collection

1. Disease is diagnosed with physical exam and a history of symptoms
2. X-ray confirms disease
3. Joint pain is present with movement and weight-bearing and is relieved by rest (NCLEX®)
4. There is limited ROM with progressive loss of function
5. There is joint stiffness after rest (NCLEX®)
6. Crepitation (grating sensation when rough joint surfaces rub together) occurs
7. **Heberden's nodes** (raised bony growths over distal interphalangeal joints) are present (NCLEX®)
8. **Bouchard's nodes** (raised bony growths over proximal interphalangeal joint of hand) are noted (NCLEX®)

C. Therapeutic management

1. Encourage client to participate in an exercise program (approved by health care provider) to maintain joint flexibility and improve muscle strength
2. Encourage client to maintain ideal body weight to prevent excessive stress on joints
3. Have client apply heat/cold therapy to affected joint for temporary pain relief (NCLEX®)
4. Assist client in planning scheduled rest periods to relieve stress on joints (NCLEX®)
5. Assist client with activities of daily living (ADL) as needed
6. Provide information about complementary therapies such as visual imagery and relaxation techniques for pain control
7. Medication therapy (NCLEX®)
   a. Acetaminophen is generally used to control mild pain without inflammation
   b. Anti-inflammatory agents such as NSAIDs may also be used
   c. If NSAIDs are ineffective in controlling inflammation and pain, glucocorticosteroids may be injected directly into joint

D. Reinforce client teaching

1. Nature of and treatment for disease; principles of good body mechanics
2. Correct use of assistive devices; encourage use as needed
3. How to plan daily activities and tasks allowing for scheduled rest periods
4. Avoid activities that put excessive stress on joints and cause pain

XV. LOW BACK PAIN

A. Overview

1. Pain may result from acute or repeated stress on lower back over years
2. Pain occurs because of degeneration and/or acute or repeated injury to tissue of lower back
   a. Caused by sprain or strain of ligaments and muscles
   b. Pain may be felt at site of injury or referred
3. Overall health of lower back muscles determines degree of risk for injury as well as speed of recovery
4. Two most common causes of low back pain are mechanical strain (irritation or injury to disc causing degeneration) and herniation of nucleus pulposus (putting pressure on nerve roots)

B. Nursing data collection (NCLEX®)

1. Risk factors include but are not limited to: degenerative disc disease, poor muscle tone of lower back, sedentary lifestyle, obesity, poor body mechanics, smoking, and stress
2. Client will report pain caused by a shift of one vertebra on another or pinching and irritation of nerve root
3. Muscle spasms are a common symptom
4. Pain does not appear at time of injury but is related to gradual increase of muscle spasms of paravertebral tissue

5. Straight leg raise test may not be positive with acute injury but pain is present with radiation to buttock and leg along path of sciatic nerve with chronic injury

NCLEX®

C. Therapeutic management

1. Goal of treatment is to improve symptoms and slow progression of degenerative process
2. Include client and family in plan of care and provide emotional support
3. Medication therapy: includes but is not limited to analgesics, NSAIDs, and muscle relaxants; epidural corticosteroid injections may be used if conservative treatment is ineffective

D. Reinforce client teaching

1. Medication use, expected therapeutic effects, side/adverse effects, and contraindications
2. Use of pain rating scale; use of heat/cold therapy for comfort
3. Importance of adhering to activity restrictions such as bedrest initially
4. Importance of adhering to exercise plan and gradual increase in activity
5. Importance of maintaining ideal body weight
6. Physical therapy will help muscle strength and flexibility and improve muscle tone
7. Importance of using proper body mechanics to avoid excessive strain on lower back
8. Sleep on a firm mattress
9. Have client demonstrate correct sleeping position using principles of body mechanics (side lying or supine with knees and hips flexed)
10. Avoid or stop smoking
11. Use of prescribed brace or corset (if needed) to prevent flexion and extension motions of lower back

XVI. CONGENITAL MUSCULOSKELETAL HEALTH PROBLEMS

A. *Clubfoot*

1. Overview
   a. Foot is twisted and fixed in an abnormal position; may be one or a combination of four deformities: plantar flexion (foot is lower than heel), dorsiflexion (heel is lower than foot), varus deviation (foot turns in), or valgus deviation (foot turns out)
   b. Involves bone deformity and malposition with soft tissue contracture
   c. May be unilateral or bilateral
   d. Exact cause is unknown but may include abnormal intrauterine position or neuromuscular or vascular problems
   e. Strong familial tendency, with 1 in 10 chance that a parent with clubfoot will have an affected offspring
2. Nursing data collection
   a. Foot is twisted in a fixed abnormal position, which is easily recognized at birth; may be recognized on prenatal ultrasound
   b. (NCLEX®) Affected foot is usually smaller and shorter, with an empty heel pad and transverse plantar crease
   c. When defect is unilateral, affected limb is usually shorter with possible calf atrophy
3. Therapeutic management
   a. Correction is best achieved if begun in newborn period because small bones in foot begin to ossify shortly after birth
   b. (NCLEX®) Manipulation and serial casting are begun immediately and continued for 8 to 12 weeks, with foot placed in a cast in an overcorrected position; casts are changed every 1 to 2 weeks because of rapid growth
   c. Parents need to perform passive ROM exercises to foot and ankle several times a day for several months once cast is off
   d. Infant may need to sleep in Denis Browne splints (shoes attached to a metal bar to maintain position) or wear corrective shoes for up to 1 year
   e. Surgery is performed when manipulative therapy does not achieve full correction with casting; is often performed between 4 to 12 months of age; involves realigning foot bones and holding them in place with steel pins; foot is casted for 6 to 12 weeks
   f. (NCLEX®) Nursing care of child after casting and surgical repair of clubfoot includes neurovascular checks at least every 2 hours; observe for swelling around cast edges; elevate ankle and foot on pillows; monitor for cast drainage; pain management; and appropriate distraction
4. Reinforce client and family teaching
   a. (NCLEX®) Change diapers often to prevent soiled diapers from soiling cast
   b. (NCLEX®) Sponge-bathe infant to keep cast dry
   c. (NCLEX®) Evaluate crying episodes carefully because they may be caused by tingling sensation of circulatory compression
   d. Need for passive ROM exercises several times a day for several months

e. Use of Denis Browne splints or corrective shoes to maintain correction
f. Discuss options for clothing that accommodates casts
g. Reinforce care of a child in a brace or cast (see Box 57–6)

B. Developmental dysplasia of hip (DDH)

1. Overview
   a. Refers to a variety of conditions in which femoral head and acetabulum are improperly aligned
   b. Unilateral in 80% of affected children
   c. Cause is unknown, though certain factors are known to increase risk
   d. Family history increases risk ten-fold

Box 57–6

Child and Family Education for a Child in a Brace or a Cast

Perform Neurovascular Checks

- Observe fingers or toes for swelling, discoloration, and temperature.
- Check movement and sensation.
- Notify health care professional with any changes in neurovascular status.
- Show parents how to blanch nail bed and watch for capillary refill.

Observe for Infection

- Monitor for temperature increase.
- Monitor for drainage through cast or brace.
- Monitor for odors coming from beneath cast or brace.
- Notify health care professional of any of above.

Monitor and Maintain Skin around Cast or Brace Edges

- Perform frequent inspection of skin around cast or brace edges for irritation, rubbing, or blistering.
- Keep edges clean and dry; avoid use of lotions, powders, or oils near cast or brace.
- Petal cast edges as needed with tape to cover rough edges.
- Do not allow child to put anything down cast.
- If child is incontinent, protect cast edges with waterproof tape and plastic.
- Keep cast or brace clean and dry.

Activity

- Follow health professional's orders for activity level or restriction of activity.
- Avoid allowing affected extremity to hang in a dependent position for more than 30 minutes.
- Encourage frequent rest for first few days following brace or cast application, keeping injured extremity elevated while resting.
- Keep a clear path for ambulation, removing toys, hazardous floor rugs, pets, or other items over which child might stumble.
- If in a body cast or brace, assist child to be mobile using a wagon, cart, or large skateboard; do not move or reposition client using bar between lower extremities if present.

Comfort

- Monitor for discomfort and medicate according to health care provider's orders.
- Contact health care provider if pain is not relieved by any comfort measures.

Follow-up

- Encourage compliance with follow-up.
- Take child to health care provider if cast becomes too loose or becomes soft or cracked.

e. Prenatal conditions may affect development of DDH, such as frank breech position, maternal hormones (relaxin and estrogen may cause laxity of hip joint and capsule, leading to joint instability), twinning, and large infant size
f. Sociocultural methods of childrearing, such as way infants are carried, may promote or decrease extent of involvement; infants held with hips abducted have decreased involvement

2. Nursing data collection in infancy
a. Diagnosis should be made in newborn period; treatment is most successful if begun before 2 months of age
NCLEX® b. Shortening of affected limb
c. Allis' sign: child in supine position, thighs flexed to a 90-degree angle toward abdomen, unequal knee height
NCLEX® d. Uneven number and placement of skin folds on posterior thighs
e. Restricted abduction of hips after 6 to 10 weeks of age
f. Wide perineum in bilateral dislocation
NCLEX® g. Positive Ortolani up to 2 to 3 months of age; to examine for this, lie infant supine and flex knees and hips to 90 degrees; place middle fingers over greater trochanter and thumb in internal side of thigh over lesser trochanter; abduct hips while applying pressure over greater trochanter and listen for a clicking sound, which would indicate a positive Ortolani's sign; no sound will be heard with a normal hip
h. Positive Barlow's sign: with fingers in same position, hold knees and hips at 90 degrees, apply backward pressure, and adduct hips; positive Barlow's sign is present if able to feel hips dislocate

NCLEX® 3. Nursing data collection in an older child
a. Affected leg shorter than other
b. Telescoping or piston mobility of affected leg
c. History of delay in walking
d. Limp and toe walking
e. Trendelenburg's sign: when child bears weight on affected side, pelvis tilts downward on normal side instead of upward
f. Waddling gait and lordosis with bilateral dislocation

4. Therapeutic management
a. Correction involves positioning hip into a flexed, abducted (externally rotated) position to press femur head against acetabulum and deepen its contour
NCLEX® b. For infants under 3 months, most common treatment is use of a Pavlik harness, an adjustable chest halter that abducts legs; soft plastic stirrups hold hips flexed, abducted, and externally rotated; may or may not be removed for bathing; usually worn for 3 to 6 months (see Figure 57–6)

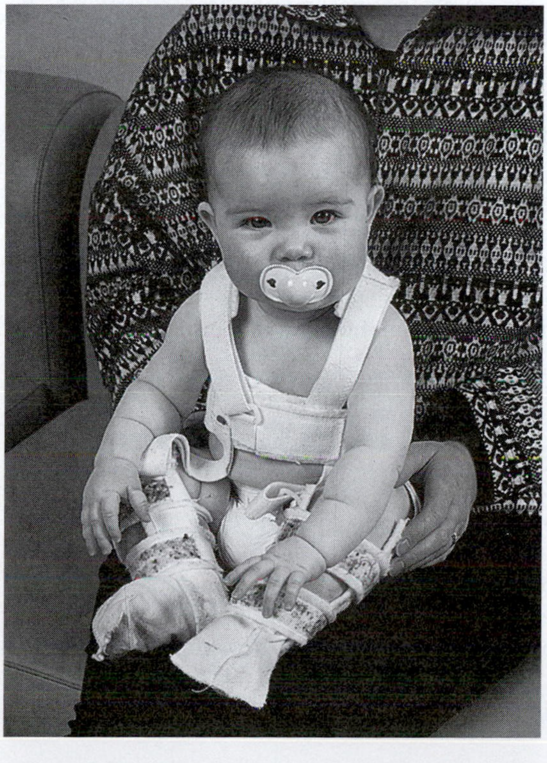

Figure 57–6

Pavlik harness.

Source: Ball, J., Bindler, R., & Cowen, K. (2010). *Child health nursing: Partnering with children and families* (2nd ed.). Upper Saddle River, NJ: Pearson Education, p. 1449.

c. For infants older than 3 months, skin traction followed by spica cast application may be required
d. Correction in child older than 18 months requires traction, operative reduction, and rehabilitation

NCLEX® 5. Reinforce client and family teaching
a. Pavlik harness: proper application, sponge bath, inspect skin under straps daily for irritation or redness; T-shirt and knee socks should be worn under brace to prevent skin irritation; diaper should be placed under straps and changed without taking harness off
b. For all abduction devices: modification of car seat, modification of positioning for nursing and eating
c. Parents need to ensure child has adequate stimulation with toys and activities at appropriate eye level; encourage activities that stimulate upper extremities
d. Children will catch up with developmental milestones once abduction splint is off

C. Osteogenesis imperfecta (OI)

1. Overview
a. Characterized by pathologic fractures resulting from connective tissue and bone defects
b. Occurs in several forms with variable degree of severity
c. Bones are so fragile that fractures result from trauma but also from simple walking or pressure of birth
NCLEX® d. A child with this diagnosis should not be confused with child with fractures because of abuse
e. Children with OI have normal Ca^{++} and phosphorus levels and abnormal precollagen type I, which prevents formation of collagen, a major component of connective tissue
f. Bone of children with OI consists of large areas of osseous tissue and increased numbers of osteoblasts
g. Genetically transmitted, generally in an autosomal dominant inheritance pattern, although some types are transmitted in a recessive pattern

2. Nursing data collection
NCLEX® a. Major clinical manifestations include multiple and frequent fractures, some of which may be present at birth
b. As child grows older, multiple breaks tend to cause limb and spinal column deformities, interfering with alignment or growth
c. Other clinical manifestations include blue sclera; thin, soft skin with easy bruising; increased joint flexibility; weak muscles; short stature; conductive hearing loss often by adolescence or young adulthood
d. May have dentinogenesis imperfecta: hypoplastic teeth with opalescent blue or brown discoloration

3. Therapeutic management
a. Keep floors dry; remove objects that could cause falls
NCLEX® b. Handle children gently: avoid lifting by a single arm or leg; use a blanket for extra support when lifting and moving
NCLEX® c. Never hold by ankles when being diapered, but gently lift by slipping a hand under buttocks
NCLEX® d. Lightweight leg braces, splints, casting, and physical therapy may be helpful
e. Intermedullary rods may be effective in strengthening bones
NCLEX® f. Medication therapy: calcitonin possibly (aids bone healing), bisphosphonates (to increase bone mass), possible growth hormone (stimulate growth)

4. Reinforce client and family teaching
a. Encourage a lifestyle that promotes growth and development yet minimizes risk of trauma
b. Show how to support when bathing, dressing, and moving
c. Encourage exercise, such as swimming, to improve muscle tone and prevent obesity
d. Encourage realistic occupational planning
e. Suggest genetic counseling
f. Educational materials and information can be obtained from the Osteogenesis Imperfecta Foundation (www.oif.org)

XVII. ACQUIRED CHILDHOOD MUSCULOSKELETAL HEALTH PROBLEMS

A. Legg-Calve-Perthes disease

1. Overview
a. A self-limiting disorder in which there is aseptic necrosis of femoral head
b. Affects children between ages of 2 and 12 years but is most common at 5 to 7 years
c. Caucasian children are affected 10 times more often than African-American children, and males more than females
d. Disease is bilateral in 10–15% of cases

e. Cause is unknown; familial predisposition present and possibly associated with preceding mild traumatic injury
f. Circulation to femoral capitol epiphysis is disturbed and produces an ischemic aseptic necrosis of femoral head
g. Stage I: avascular stage; aseptic necrosis of femoral capitol epiphysis with degenerative changes producing flattening of femoral head
h. Stage II: fragmentation or revascularization stage; old bone absorption and revascularization
i. Stage III: reparative stage; new bone formation
j. Stage IV: regeneration stage; gradual reformation of femoral head
k. Middle childhood is time when blood supply to femoral head is most tenuous, being supplied almost entirely by lateral retinacular vessels; these vessels can become obstructed by trauma, inflammation, coagulation defects, among other causes
l. Affected children may have delayed skeletal maturation and abnormal thyroid levels

NCLEX®
2. Nursing data collection
a. Mild pain in hip or anterior thigh and limp that are aggravated by increased activity and relieved by rest
b. Stiffness in morning or after rest
c. As disease progresses, there is limited ROM, weakness, muscle wasting, possible shortening of affected limb, and positive Trendelenburg sign

3. Therapeutic management
a. Prepare child for x-ray (usual diagnostic test); there may be no radiological findings early in disease, but bone scans and MRIs help diagnose early disease
b. Initial treatment includes rest to reduce inflammation and restore motion
NCLEX® c. Goal is to keep head of femur in contact with acetabulum, which serves as a mold of spherical shape of head of femur
NCLEX® d. Treatment may be conservative: rest; avoid weight bearing on lower extremities; traction and containment with abduction braces, leg casts, or leather harness slings
e. Conservative therapy may be needed for 2 to 4 years
f. Surgical correction may be done, which returns child to normal activities in 3 to 4 months
NCLEX® g. Assist in selecting suitable activities for a child unable to maintain usual level of physical activity
h. Ensure compliance with conservative devices
NCLEX® i. If surgery is done, postoperative care includes frequent neurovascular checks, pain management, and activity based on surgeon's orders
j. Assist family with appropriate activities for child during treatment

4. Reinforce client and family teaching
a. Purpose, function, application, and care of corrective device, and importance of compliance to achieve desired outcome
b. Importance of continuing school activities
c. Promote normal growth and development with appropriate diversional activities

B. Slipped capitol femoral epiphysis

1. Overview
a. A condition in which upper femoral epiphysis gradually slips from its functional position
b. Incidence is greatest during rapid growth spurt during adolescence; 13 to 16 years of age for males and 11 to 14 years of age for females
c. Occurs twice as often in African Americans as other races, and twice as often in males
d. Etiology is unknown and thought to be multifactorial; genetic predisposition possible
e. Is more common in obese or rapidly growing children, suggesting that growth hormone or trauma from excessive weight may have an influence on etiology
f. Slippage of femoral head occurs at proximal **epiphyseal plate**, and femur displaces from **epiphysis** (rounded end portion of long bones); this is usually a gradual process, but may result from trauma

2. Nursing data collection
NCLEX® a. Onset of symptoms may be gradual, with persistent hip pain that is aching or mild, and can be referred to thigh and/or knee, along with limp and decreased ROM and internal rotation of hip; child may hold leg in an externally rotated position to relieve stress and pain in hip joint
NCLEX® b. Child with an acute slip presents with sudden, severe pain and cannot bear weight
c. Prepare client for an x-ray, which will confirm diagnosis

3. Therapeutic management
NCLEX® a. As soon as diagnosis is made, place client on strict bedrest until surgery; adolescent may use crutches as long as affected leg is non-weight-bearing, but should not sit in a wheelchair, as this may increase slippage

b. Reinforce initial bedrest, as adolescents often do not see value of this measure
c. Provide appropriate diversional activities
d. Prepare for surgery with pinning or external fixation to stabilize femur head
e. Provide postoperative care, including frequent neurovascular checks and pain management
f. Provide adequate nutrition for healing

4. Reinforce client and family teaching
a. Reinforce ambulation and weight-bearing as ordered by surgeon
b. Contact sports are usually restricted until growth is complete
c. Reinforce compliance with followup visits until epiphyseal plates are closed

C. *Scoliosis*

1. Overview
a. Lateral curvature of spine; may be functional (occurs as a compensatory mechanism in children with unequal leg lengths) or poor posture; structural scoliosis is a permanent curvature of spine accompanied by damage to vertebrae
b. Structural scoliosis occurs most often during rapid growth spurt in adolescence, 11 to 14 years for females, 13 to 16 years for males
c. Female-to-male ratio is 5:1 for curves greater than 21 degrees
d. There is a familial predisposition; 70% of structural scoliosis is idiopathic
e. Scoliosis is common in diseases in which there is unequal muscle balance, such as CP, MD, and myelomeningocele

2. Nursing data collection
a. A painless and insidious onset is typical
NCLEX® b. Parent may first notice that skirts hang unevenly, or that bra straps are adjusted unevenly
NCLEX® c. On examination, there are unequal shoulder heights, waist angles, scapula prominences, rib prominences, and chest asymmetry
d. Screening by school nurse begins in fifth grade as mandated by law in many states
e. Scoliometer is used to document clinical deformity found on screening

3. Therapeutic management
a. Prepare adolescent for x-ray, which will identify extent of curvature and give baseline information for followup
NCLEX® b. If spinal curve is less than 15 to 20 degrees, teen is monitored every 3 to 6 months for change; exercises to improve posture and muscle tone and increase flexibility of spine are encouraged
c. If curve is greater than 24 degrees, treatment is provided by an orthopedic surgeon; if less than 40 degrees, conservative, nonsurgical treatment is indicated, with bracing, such as a Milwaukee brace; braces are made of leather and plastic and worn until spinal growth stops; see client teaching section
d. Electrical stimulation may be used for mild to moderate curvatures to cause regular and frequent muscle contractions, possibly helping to straighten spine
e. If curvature progresses or is greater than 40 degrees, surgery is warranted; instruments such as rods, screws, and wires are placed next to curvature; spine is then fused in correct position; bone from iliac crests may be used to strengthen fusion
f. Preoperative teaching includes deep breathing, coughing, turning every 2 hours, use of spirometry, pain medication, use of nasogastric (NG) tube and NPO status, ROM exercises, activity, possible ICU tour
NCLEX® g. Postoperative care includes ROM exercises, logrolling every 2 hours, encouraging coughing and deep breathing and use of incentive spirometer, NPO, NG tube, strict I&O, frequent VS and neurological checks, monitoring hematocrit, blood transfusions, pain management, antibiotic administration, antiembolism stockings, and gradual resumption of activity as ordered
h. Halo traction may be used for nonsurgical treatment of moderate curves or postoperatively in severe curves to provide stability for spine

4. Reinforce client and family teaching
a. Use of a Milwaukee or other brace: worn for 23 hours a day; off to shower, bathe, and swim; wear T-shirt under brace next to skin for protection; do exercises (such as pelvic tilt and lateral strengthening) several times daily while in brace to correct thoracic lordosis
b. Consistent use of brace will provide maximum benefit
c. Slight muscle aches may be noticed when first wearing brace
d. Encourage teens to be as active as possible while in brace
NCLEX® e. Discharge teaching: must not slump in chairs, bend or twist torso, or lift over 10 pounds; maintain activity restrictions for 6 to 8 months as ordered; address self-esteem issues; comply with follow-up visits

Check Your NCLEX-PN® Exam I.Q.

You are ready for testing on this content if you can

- Identify basic structures and functions of the musculoskeletal system.
- Describe the pathophysiology and etiology of common musculoskeletal disorders.
- Discuss expected data and diagnostic test findings for selected musculoskeletal disorders.
- Discuss therapeutic management of a client experiencing a musculoskeletal disorder.
- Discuss nursing management of a client experiencing a musculoskeletal disorder.
- Identify expected outcomes for the client experiencing a musculoskeletal disorder.

PRACTICE TEST

1 The nurse reinforces teaching to an adolescent after removal of a short leg cast. The nurse should include which instruction in discussions with this client? Select all that apply.

1. Wash the skin with undiluted hydrogen peroxide.
2. Vigorously scrub the legs to remove dead skin.
3. Gently wash the leg to remove dead skin over time.
4. Avoid touching the leg for 2 days after cast removal.
5. Use a lubricant to moisten the skin for easier removal of dead skin.

2 Which nursing diagnosis would the nurse anticipate as the priority for a client with Paget's disease?

1. Risk for Noncompliance
2. Disturbed Sleep Pattern
3. Impaired Physical Mobility
4. Disturbed Body Image

3 A client with a right arm cast for a fractured humerus states, "I haven't been able to straighten the fingers on my right hand since this morning." What action should the nurse take first?

1. Monitor neurovascular status to the hand.
2. Ask the client to massage the fingers.
3. Encourage the client to take the prescribed analgesic.
4. Elevate the right arm on a pillow to reduce edema.

4 A client with an open fracture is at risk for developing osteomyelitis. Which classic symptoms would the nurse monitor for to detect development of this complication? Select all that apply.

1. Increased pain at the fracture site
2. Elevated temperature
3. Acute respiratory distress
4. Shortening of the affected extremity
5. Increased swelling at the fracture site

5 A client who is obese has degenerative joint disease and is being treated with aspirin. The nurse concludes that teaching needs to be reinforced when the client makes which statement?

1. "I take aspirin only when I have extreme pain and stiffness."
2. "I use heat sometimes to help decrease my pain and joint stiffness."
3. "I frequently examine my stools for bleeding."
4. "I started an exercise program to lose weight."

6 A client underwent a lumbar laminectomy today. Which nursing diagnosis has highest priority for this client?

1. Disturbed Body Image
2. Social Isolation
3. Ineffective Role Performance
4. Impaired Physical Mobility

7 A client with a femoral fracture is in Buck's traction. While making rounds, the nurse notices that the client's foot is touching the footboard of the bed. What is the appropriate action by the nurse?

1. Wedge a pillow between the footboard and the client's foot.
2. Praise the client for maintaining countertraction.
3. Center the client on the bed.
4. Ask the client to pull up in bed while holding the weights.

8 A truck driver sees the primary care provider because of persistent back pain. The nurse explains that which client activity documented during the nursing history may contribute to further back injury?

1. Lifting objects close to the body
2. Shifting positions often when sitting for prolonged periods
3. Providing back support with a pillow when sitting
4. Prolonged standing or sitting

9 The nurse is assigned to the care of a client who underwent a lumbar laminectomy. Which activity would be appropriate 4 hours postoperatively?

1. Sitting up in a chair to watch television
2. Sitting at the side of the bed
3. Lying in bed in good alignment with the head of bed flat
4. Using the side-rails for support to get out of bed

10 A 50-year-old male with chronic low back pain visits the outpatient clinic. The client weighs 200 pounds, works as a truck driver, sits for prolonged periods, and exercises only occasionally. The client smokes one pack of cigarettes and drinks six cans of beer per day. What risk factors should the nurse focus on when reinforcing client teaching? Select all that apply.

1. Cigarette smoking
2. Age
3. Alcohol use
4. Insufficient exercise
5. Sitting for prolonged periods

11 The nurse is reinforcing teaching to a postmenopausal client about the use of calcium to reduce the risk of osteoporosis. The client asks: "Why do I have to take vitamin D with my calcium?" What is the nurse's best response?

1. "Vitamin D prevents osteoporosis."
2. "Vitamin D increases intestinal absorption of calcium."
3. "You are most likely to be deficient in vitamin D."
4. "Using calcium and vitamin D supplements is the only prevention for osteoporosis."

12 The nurse is caring for a client with a week-old cast. The client asks why the nurse touches the cast during the examination. What is the most appropriate response by the nurse?

1. "I am making sure that the cast has dried."
2. "I am determining the strength of the cast."
3. "I am feeling for hot spots that might indicate infection."
4. "I am making sure that the cast is not too tight."

13 A client is placed on a continuous passive motion (CPM) machine postoperatively after a total knee replacement. The nurse observes the client's knee is externally rotating during flexion. What should the nurse do next?

1. Move the client up in bed or move the CPM machine toward the foot of bed.
2. Support the knee with sandbags to prevent external rotation.
3. Assist the client to sit up in bed in a 45-degree position.
4. Do nothing because the client's knee is properly aligned.

14 A client in skeletal traction for a right femur fracture reports pain in the affected limb. After determining that the right foot is pale without a pulse, what should the nurse do next? Select all that apply.

1. Ensure that the leg is not raised above heart level.
2. Administer analgesics as ordered.
3. Release the traction.
4. Recheck the pulse in an hour.
5. Document findings and notify the registered nurse.

15 A nurse receives a client from the emergency department (ED) in Buck's traction following fracture of the right femur. The nurse documents which data as a priority in the client medical record?

1. Status of skin underneath the traction and over bony prominences
2. Type of pin, wire, or tongs used
3. The effectiveness of pain medication given in the field
4. Medications given in the emergency department

16 A client has been placed in balanced suspension traction after sustaining a fracture. The nurse explains to the family that which of the following is an advantage of this type of traction?

1. It eliminates the risk for skin breakdown.
2. It allows the client to raise the buttocks off the bed for bedpan use and skin care.
3. It is more effective in reducing hip contracture.
4. It requires only one weight to maintain traction.

17 A client taking colchicine (Novocolchine) for gout reports weakness, abdominal pain, and nausea and vomiting for the past 2 days. How should the nurse interpret these symptoms?

1. Therapeutic effects of the medication
2. Signs of toxicity
3. Expected side effects
4. An allergic response

18 An 87-year-old client who sustained a right hip fracture asks the nurse how long it will take for the fracture to heal. The nurse's response includes consideration of which client factor that influences the rate of bone healing?

1. Frequency of physical therapy
2. Age of the client
3. Weight of the client
4. Early ambulation

19 A client is scheduled to have a closed reduction of a right ankle fracture. The nurse determines the client understands the procedure when the client states that it involves which of the following?

1. Using an arthroscope to realign the bones
2. Realigning the bone using surgery
3. Correcting the bone alignment using manual manipulation
4. Inserting pins, rods, or other implantable devices

20 A child is admitted to the hospital with a diagnosis of osteomyelitis. Which data would the nurse likely obtain during a nursing history?

1. History of an upper respiratory infection
2. History of gastroenteritis
3. History of Legg-Calve-Perthes disease
4. History of congenital hip dysplasia

21 Two hours after a child had a cast applied for a fractured radius, the nurse monitors swelling in the hand, which is elevated higher than the heart. Ice has been applied continuously. The child denies an increase in pain but does report numbness and tingling. Which should the nurse do first?

1. Medicate the client for pain.
2. Elevate the injured extremity higher.
3. Notify the registered nurse.
4. Provide the child with diversional activities.

22 The pediatric nurse interprets that which infant is least likely to be diagnosed with developmental dysplasia of the hip (DDH)?

1. An infant with a family history of DDH
2. An infant with a birth weight of 10 pounds
3. The infant carried on the mother's hips
4. The infant who had frank breech position in utero

23 Which intervention would be essential for the nurse to implement to promote a stable respiratory status in an adolescent who recently had a spinal fusion for scoliosis?

1. Logrolling and repositioning every 4 hours
2. Coughing and deep breathing every 2 hours while awake
3. Monitoring pain status and ensuring adequate pain relief
4. Encouraging use of incentive spirometry every 4 hours while awake

24 An 8-year-old child presents to the emergency department with ankle pain and difficulty walking, although no injury is recalled. The triage nurse notes ankle redness, swelling, decreased mobility and range of motion, and pain with ankle movement. Temperature is 100.8°F and heart rate is 140 beats per minute. Which health problem would the triage nurse suspect?

1. Legg-Calve-Perthes disease
2. Slipped capital femoral epiphysis
3. Fracture of the ankle
4. Osteomyelitis

25 The nurse is preparing to help a pediatric client get up from a chair using crutches. Place in order the steps that the nurse outlines to the client to do this procedure correctly.

1. Place unaffected leg slightly under or at the edge of the chair.
2. Grasp the arm of the chair using the hand on the unaffected side.
3. Grasp the crutches by the horizontal hand bars using the hand on the affected side.
4. Move forward to the edge of the chair.
5. Push down on the crutches and the chair armrest while raising the body out of the chair.

26 The mother of a newborn is upset that her baby has congenital clubfoot. She asks the nurse what she did to cause her baby's deformity. Which answer is appropriate? Select all that apply.

1. Abnormal uterine positioning could have caused this deformity
2. A lack of good nutrition during pregnancy could have caused this defect
3. Having the baby before the due date could have caused this problem
4. There are no known etiologies of this defect
5. Neuromuscular and vascular problems may have caused the problem

ANSWERS & RATIONALES

1 **Answer: 3, 5 Rationale:** Dead skin and exudates often collect under the cast, and efforts to remove it should be done gradually. The client can use a lubricant which will soften dead skin cells for easier removal during cleansing. The use of undiluted peroxide is too harsh for the skin. The client should avoid any vigorous scrubbing of the skin to avoid interfering with skin integrity, which increases the risk for infection. There is no reason why the leg cannot be touched after removal of the cast. **Cognitive Level:** Applying **Client Need:** Physiological Adaptation **Integrated Process:** Nursing Process: Implementation **Content Area:** Adult Health **Strategy:** The core issue of the question is the knowledge of skin care following cast removal. Use nursing knowledge and the process of elimination to make a selection.

2 **Answer: 3 Rationale:** Impaired Physical Mobility is the appropriate priority nursing diagnosis for a client with Paget's disease. The client needs to remain active to decrease the complications associated with immobility and to maintain the ability to perform self-care activities. The other diagnoses, although they could be appropriate, are not the priority in clients with Paget's disease. **Cognitive Level:** Applying **Client Need:** Physiological Adaptation **Integrated Process:** Nursing Process: Planning **Content Area:** Adult Health **Strategy:** The core issue of the question is the knowledge of priorities for the client with Paget's disease. Use nursing knowledge and the process of elimination to make a selection.

3 **Answer: 1 Rationale:** This symptom suggests neurological injury caused by pressure on nerves and soft tissue because of swelling (compartment syndrome). Other symptoms of neurovascular compromise should be monitored and reported to the registered nurse. Massaging the fingers will not help alleviate the problem. An analgesic will not help with mobility caused by neurological injury and there is no evidence that the client is experiencing pain. Elevating the limb could worsen the symptoms at a time when circulation is already impaired from swelling, which led to the neurological injury. **Cognitive Level:** Analyzing **Client Need:** Physiological Adaptation **Integrated Process:** Nursing Process: Implementation **Content Area:** Adult Health **Strategy:** The core issue of the question is the knowledge of priority data collection in a client with possible compartment syndrome. Use nursing knowledge and the process of elimination to make a selection.

4 **Answer: 1, 2, 5 Rationale:** Increased pain could indicate development of osteomyelitis. Elevated temperature is a classic symptom seen with osteomyelitis as a systemic response to the invading organism. Increased swelling at the site of the fracture could indicate development of osteomyelitis. Acute respiratory distress is suggestive of fat embolism but not bone infection. The extremity does not shorten with osteomyelitis, although this is a classic finding with hip fracture. **Cognitive Level:** Applying **Client Need:** Physiological Adaptation **Integrated Process:** Nursing Process: Data Collection **Content Area:** Adult Health **Strategy:** The core issue of the question is the knowledge of manifestations of osteomyelitis. Use nursing knowledge and the process of elimination to make a selection.

5 **Answer: 1 Rationale:** Aspirin therapy for this condition is continuous and is effective only after a therapeutic level is reached. It should not be taken intermittently. Heat is a beneficial measure to increase client comfort. Aspirin is an antiplatelet agent and the client should monitor for blood in stools as an adverse effect of therapy. Losing weight is beneficial for the client because is decreases the stress on the joints, particularly in the lower limbs. **Cognitive Level:** Applying **Client Need:** Physiological Adaptation **Integrated Process:** Teaching and Learning **Content Area:** Adult Health **Strategy:** The core issue of the question is the knowledge of appropriate self-management techniques for degenerative joint disease. Use nursing knowledge and the process of elimination to make a selection. Note the wording of the question indicates the correct option is an incorrect statement by the client.

6 **Answer: 4 Rationale:** Immediately after surgery, the client may be hesitant to move because of pain and fear of disturbing the operative site. Minimal scarring results from this surgery, so body image disturbance is not likely to be appropriate. Social isolation would be a lesser problem in the immediate postoperative period, since the priority is physiological status rather than psychosocial status. Because the client has just had surgery, ineffective role performance is a low priority concern at this time. **Cognitive Level:** Analyzing **Client Need:** Physiological Adaptation **Integrated Process:** Nursing Process: Implementation **Content Area:** Adult Health **Strategy:** The core issue of the question is the knowledge of priority nursing diagnoses following musculoskeletal surgery. Use nursing knowledge and the process of elimination to make a selection.

7 **Answer: 3 Rationale:** The aim in traction is to maintain a constant force to align the distal and proximal ends of a fractured bone. To be effective, traction must have an opposing force (countertraction). Centering the client in bed maintains the line of pull and ensures that countertraction is maintained. Placing a pillow between the foot and the footboard attempts to relieve pressure on the foot but

ignores that this position interrupts the proper pull of the traction. The client's current position interrupts traction rather than maintaining proper countertraction. Holding the weight interrupts the line of pull of the traction and is contraindicated. **Cognitive Level:** Applying **Client Need:** Physiological Adaptation **Integrated Process:** Nursing Process: Implementation **Content Area:** Adult Health **Strategy:** The core issue of the question is the knowledge of proper use of traction. Use nursing knowledge and the process of elimination to make a selection.

8 **Answer: 4 Rationale:** Prolonged sitting or standing aggravates back injury because of the additional stress placed on structures supporting the back. Lifting objects close to the body, shifting positions frequently, and providing back support are appropriate actions to maintain good body mechanics. **Cognitive Level:** Analyzing **Client Need:** Physiological Adaptation **Integrated Process:** Nursing Process: Data Collection **Content Area:** Adult Health **Strategy:** The core issue of the question is the knowledge of risk factors and aggravating factors of back pain. Use nursing knowledge and the process of elimination to make a selection.

9 **Answer: 3 Rationale:** Physician orders after lumbar laminectomy include being kept flat or with head of bed slightly elevated to minimize stress on the suture line. The client is repositioned side to side using logrolling technique to maintain alignment of the vertebral column at all times. Using the side-rails to get out of bed causes shifting of the vertebral column. Sitting up in a chair or on the side of the bed is usually done the evening of the surgery or the first day following surgery, and it is for brief periods only. **Cognitive Level:** Applying **Client Need:** Safety and Infection Control **Integrated Process:** Nursing Process: Implementation **Content Area:** Adult Health **Strategy:** The core issue of the question is knowledge of postoperative activity that will not cause harm to the surgical area following laminectomy. Recall principles of proper body mechanics and use the process of elimination to make a selection.

10 **Answer: 1, 4, 5 Rationale:** Smoking has been found to contribute to intervertebral disc deterioration. Insufficient exercise predisposes the muscles of the back to strain and increases the risk of obesity, which places additional strain on back muscles. Occupations that require prolonged standing or sitting predispose to exacerbation of back pain. Although the risk of degenerative disk disease increases with age, this is not a priority when reinforcing client teaching because this is a nonmodifiable risk factor. Alcohol use is not a healthy pattern but does not increase the risk of degenerative disc disease that can lead to chronic low back pain. **Cognitive Level:** Analyzing **Client Need:** Physiological Adaptation **Integrated Process:** Nursing Process: Planning **Content Area:** Adult Health **Strategy:** The core issue of the question is the knowledge of factors that aggravate low back pain. Use nursing knowledge and the process of elimination to make a selection.

11 **Answer: 2 Rationale:** A combination of calcium and vitamin D is recommended for the prevention of osteoporosis. Vitamin D increases the intestinal absorption of calcium and mobilizes calcium and phosphorus into the bone. Vitamin D alone does not prevent osteoporosis. While some older adults may be deficient in Vitamin D, a postmenopausal state does not necessarily cause the deficiency. Lifestyle modifications, such as smoking cessation and exercise, may also help reduce the risk of osteoporosis. **Cognitive Level:** Applying **Client Need:** Health Promotion and Maintenance **Integrated Process:** Teaching and Learning **Content Area:** Adult Health **Strategy:** The core issue of the question is the knowledge of risk factors for and prevention of osteoporosis. Use nursing knowledge and the process of elimination to make a selection.

12 **Answer: 3 Rationale:** A complication of cast application is skin breakdown underneath the cast, which can lead to infection and subsequent heat in the infected area. A bad odor in the area may also be noted. A plaster cast dries in 24–48 hours and a fiberglass cast dries in 30 minutes to 1 hour. Determining cast strength is not part of a nursing examination and palpating the cast would not accomplish this anyway. If a cast is too tight, symptoms associated with neurovascular compromise will be noted, which include pain, paresthesia, pallor, diminished pulse distal to the cast, and paralysis. **Cognitive Level:** Applying **Client Need:** Physiological Adaptation **Integrated Process:** Communication and Documentation **Content Area:** Adult Health **Strategy:** The core issue of the question is the knowledge of various complications of casts. Use nursing knowledge and the process of elimination to make a selection.

13 **Answer: 1 Rationale:** The client's knee will externally rotate if there is insufficient space between the client's hip and the machine. The knee should be upright, facing the ceiling, as the machine moves the leg back and forth. Sandbags will not prevent external rotation because the issue is the position of the client relative to the CPM machine. Raising the head of bed will not correct external rotation of the leg. Taking no action places the client at risk for injury. **Cognitive Level:** Applying **Client Need:** Physiological Adaptation **Integrated Process:** Nursing Process: Implementation **Content Area:** Adult Health **Strategy:** The core issue of the question is the knowledge of appropriate care of the client using CPM. Use nursing knowledge and the process of elimination to make a selection.

14 **Answer: 1, 5 Rationale:** Pain and absent pulse indicate impaired circulation to the affected limb, which requires treatment to prevent damage to nerves and tissues, and necrosis requiring loss of limb (worst case). The nurse needs to ensure that the leg is not above heart level so no further damage occurs. Findings should always be documented and the registered nurse needs to be notified of the complication, so further medical treatment can be done. Pain caused by tissue ischemia will not be relieved by analgesics. Releasing the traction would be contraindicated. Rechecking the pulse in an hour delays treatment and also fails to assist the client, whose symptoms will not reverse without treatment. **Cognitive Level:** Applying **Client Need:** Physiological Adaptation **Integrated Process:** Nursing Process: Implementation **Content Area:** Adult Health **Strategy:** The core issue of the question is the knowledge of adverse neurovascular changes to a client in a cast. Recall principles of gravity and blood flow to aid in answering the question. Use nursing knowledge and the process of elimination to make a selection.

15 **Answer: 1 Rationale:** It is essential to monitor the condition of the skin under traction, as well as bony prominences, because these areas are at risk for breakdown due to continuous friction and pressure from the skin traction device. Skeletal tractions use pins, wires, or tongs to aid in realignment. Buck's traction is a type of skin traction. Effectiveness of medication given in the field is not pertinent to the client's status after admission from the ED. Evaluating effectiveness of analgesia is appropriate, but the most essential documentation for a client with skin traction is the condition

of the skin underneath the straps. **Cognitive Level:** Analyzing **Client Need:** Physiological Adaptation **Integrated Process:** Communication and Documentation **Content Area:** Adult Health **Strategy:** Use nursing knowledge about skin traction and the process of elimination to make selections.

16 **Answer: 2** **Rationale:** Balanced suspension allows for ease with bedpan use and skin care without disturbing the line of traction. In this type of traction, the client's injured extremity is lifted off the bed and a straight pull is accomplished by the application of several forces and several weights. Skin breakdown is not eliminated with this type of traction because any immobile client can be at risk. Because the extremity is lifted with the traction, the hip is flexed, making hip contracture possible. The number of weights is determined by the total pounds necessary to reduce the fracture. **Cognitive Level:** Applying **Client Need:** Physiological Adaptation **Integrated Process:** Nursing Process: Implementation **Content Area:** Adult Health **Strategy:** The core issue of the question is knowledge of balanced suspension traction as a type of skeletal traction. Use nursing knowledge and the process of elimination to make a selection.

17 **Answer: 2** **Rationale:** The symptoms described are signs of toxicity. The client should be instructed to stop the medication and be seen for follow-up treatment. The expected therapeutic effect of colchicine is to diminish the joint pain associated with the acute attack. The combination of symptoms is too severe to be expected side effects of the medication. The symptoms are not consistent with an allergic response. **Cognitive Level:** Applying **Client Need:** Pharmacological and Parenteral Therapies **Integrated Process:** Nursing Process: Evaluation **Content Area:** Adult Health **Strategy:** The core issue of the question is the knowledge of actions and adverse effects of colchicine. Use nursing knowledge and the process of elimination to make a selection.

18 **Answer: 2** **Rationale:** Age, site of the fracture, and blood supply to the affected area all affect the rate of bone healing. Younger and healthy clients will have faster bone healing than older adults and those with chronic illnesses. Although physical therapy will assist in mobility, it does not directly enhance bone healing. The weight of the client, unless accompanied by malnutrition, does not have a direct bearing on bone healing. The physician determines when ambulation is allowed and thus it is not a client factor. **Cognitive Level:** Applying **Client Need:** Physiological Adaptation **Integrated Process:** Nursing Process: Implementation **Content Area:** Adult Health **Strategy:** The core issue of the question is knowledge of possible threats to bone healing in an identified client. Use nursing knowledge and the process of elimination to make a selection.

19 **Answer: 3** **Rationale:** In a closed reduction procedure, the physician applies traction and manipulates the bone until the broken ends are realigned. Arthroscopy is a surgical procedure for treating some types of joint problems. Open reduction is a realignment of bone with surgery. Internal fixation devices are surgically inserted during an open reduction to immobilize the fracture during the healing process. **Cognitive Level:** Applying **Client Need:** Physiological Adaptation **Integrated Process:** Teaching and Learning **Content Area:** Adult Health **Strategy:** The core issue of the question is the knowledge of various approaches to correct bone fracture. Use nursing knowledge and the process of elimination to make a selection.

20 **Answer: 1** **Rationale:** The history of a child with osteomyelitis may include a recent upper respiratory infection (which may include an ear infection or sinus infection), skin infection, or blunt trauma to a bone. A recent history of gastroenteritis would not lead to osteomyelitis. Legg-Calve-Perthes disease is an aseptic necrosis of the femoral head that leads to pain and limping but osteomyelitis is a bone infection. Congenital hip dysplasia affects mobility but does not lead to osteomyelitis. **Cognitive Level:** Analyzing **Client Need:** Physiological Adaptation **Integrated Process:** Nursing Process: Data Collection **Content Area:** Child Health **Strategy:** The core issue of the question is the knowledge of risk factors for osteomyelitis. Use nursing knowledge and the process of elimination to make a selection.

21 **Answer: 3** **Rationale:** The client's symptoms are compatible with compartment syndrome, which can lead to neurological damage. This is a medical emergency and the registered nurse and physician should be notified immediately. Pain medication is not indicated based on the client's data and would not correct the current underlying problem. Elevating the arm further would worsen circulation to the area, which is already impaired. The nurse can provide diversional activities while waiting for definitive orders from the physician or registered nurse. **Cognitive Level:** Analyzing **Client Need:** Physiological Adaptation **Integrated Process:** Nursing Process: Implementation **Content Area:** Child Health **Strategy:** The core issue of the question is recognition of a complication, compartment syndrome, that can lead to neurological damage. The correct answer is the one that provides for definitive treatment of the problem, which in this case is to notify the registered nurse.

22 **Answer: 3** **Rationale:** The infant who is carried with the hips abducted is at decreased risk for developing DDH. A family history of DDH would possibly increase the incidence of this defect. A large infant size at birth has been associated with DDH. Breech position is associated with increased incidence of DDH. **Cognitive Level:** Analyzing **Client Need:** Physiological Adaptation **Integrated Process:** Nursing Process: Evaluation **Content Area:** Child Health **Strategy:** The core issue of the question is recognition of which situation allows the infant to keep the hips abducted. Evaluate each option according to this criteria to make a selection.

23 **Answer: 3** **Rationale:** Pain must be managed properly in the child after spinal fusion in order for the client to participate in respiratory exercises. Logrolling and repositioning, as well as coughing, deep breathing, and use of incentive spirometry should be done every 2 hours around the clock with this postoperative client. **Cognitive Level:** Analyzing **Client Need:** Physiological Adaptation **Integrated Process:** Nursing Process: Implementation **Content Area:** Child Health **Strategy:** The core issue of the question is the ability to prioritize nursing activities. While the ABCs are quite important, they must be timely. Also, the client cannot meet goals for the respiratory portion of ABCs unless pain relief is achieved. With this in mind, choose pain relief as the correct answer.

24 **Answer: 4** **Rationale:** The symptoms described are symptoms of osteomyelitis. This disease can result from a penetrating wound, but it also may result from an infection elsewhere in the body that traveled to the bone. Osteomyelitis may follow an upper respiratory infection, which is common in school-age children. Legg-Calve-Perthes disease affects the femoral head, not the ankle. Slipped capitol femoral epiphysis affects the hip. An ankle fracture is generally associated with injury. **Cognitive Level:** Analyzing **Client Need:** Physiological Adaptation **Integrated Process:** Nursing Process: Data Collection **Content Area:** Child Health **Strategy:** The issue of the question is the ability of the nurse to analyze data and compare it to typical data of childhood musculoskeletal problems. Note that the temperature is elevated to help choose the option related to infection.

25 **Answer: 4, 1, 3, 2, 5, Rationale:** The client moves first to the edge of the chair to move the center of gravity forward before trying to stand. Placing the unaffected leg slightly under or at the edge of the chair is done second to provide support to help the client to stand up from the chair and achieve balance. Grasping the crutches by the horizontal hand bars using the hand on the affected side is done third to provide support for the affected side before arising. Grasping the arm of the chair using the hand on the unaffected side is done fourth so that the body weight is supported on the armrest of the unaffected leg when the client rises to stand. Pushing down on the crutches and the chair armrest while raising the body out of the chair is done fifth once the body is fully positioned and supported. **Cognitive Level:** Analyzing **Client Need:** Physiological Adaptation **Integrated Process:** Nursing Process: Implementation **Content Area:** Child Health **Strategy:** Visualize the procedure and think about principles of joint support and balance to complete the ordered steps.

26 **Answer: 1, 5 Rationale:** The exact cause of clubfoot is unknown, though several possible etiologies exist. Abnormal intrauterine position may cause the deformity. The exact cause of clubfoot is unknown, though several possible etiologies exist. Abnormal intrauterine position may cause the deformity, along with neuromuscular or vascular problems. The exact cause of clubfoot is unknown, though several possible etiologies exist. However, nutrition during pregnancy is not considered a factor for this deformity. The exact cause of clubfoot is unknown, though several possible etiologies exist. However, having the baby early is not considered a factor for this deformity. The exact cause of clubfoot is unknown, though several possible etiologies exist. A positive family history increases the chance of this deformity. **Cognitive Level:** Analyzing **Client Need:** Physiological Adaptation **Integrated Process:** Nursing Process: Implementation **Content Area:** Child Health **Strategy:** Knowledge of the etiology of clubfoot will help to determine the correct response. Consider which response, in addition to being accurate, would be most comforting for the mother.

Key Terms to Review

References

Ball, J., & Bindler, R. (2010). *Child health nursing: Partnering with children and families* (2nd ed.). Upper Saddle River, NJ: Pearson Education.

Berman, A., & Snyder, S. (2012). *Kozier & Erb's fundamentals of nursing: Concepts, process, and practice* (9th ed.). Upper Saddle River, NJ: Pearson Education.

Ignatavicius, D., & Workman, L. (2010). *Medical-surgical nursing: Critical thinking for collaborative care* (6th ed.). Philadelphia: Saunders.

Kee, J. (2010). *Laboratory and diagnostic tests with nursing implications* (8th ed.). Upper Saddle River, NJ: Pearson Education.

LeMone, P., & Burke, K., & Bauldoff, G. (2011). *Medical-surgical nursing: Critical thinking in patient care* (5th ed.). Upper Saddle River, NJ: Pearson Education.

Smith, S., Duell, D., & Martin, B. (2012). *Clinical nursing skills: Basic to advanced skills* (8th ed.). Upper Saddle River, NJ: Pearson Education.

Test Yourself

Are you ready for the NCLEX-PN® or course exams? Use the practice tests on the companion website to check.

58 Integumentary Disorders

In this chapter

Cross Reference

Other chapters relevant to this content area are

Integumentary Medications	Chapter 39
Common Laboratory Tests	Chapter 42
Common Diagnostic Tests and Procedures	Chapter 43

I. OVERVIEW OF ANATOMY AND PHYSIOLOGY OF INTEGUMENTARY SYSTEM

A. *Epidermis* (see Figure 58–1): outer layer of skin made up of epithelial cells; protects body and internal structures from harm by providing a barrier to external environment

B. *Dermis*: second layer of skin made up of lymph vessels, blood vessels, and nerve fibers; papillary layer contains capillaries and receptor sites for touch and pain; reticular layer contains receptors for deep touch as well as sweat and sebaceous glandst

C. Subcutaneous (subQ) tissue: lies beneath dermis; is made up of adipose (fat) tissue and helps connect skin to structures below subQ tissue

D. Appendages: include hair, nails, and glands

1. Hair: composed of primarily dead cells; hair root begins in bulb of hair follicle and grows from dermis outward; pads scalp and protects from external objects; helps maintain body temperature
2. Nails: primarily made up of dead cells that cover nail bed; nail structure begins in epidermis and extends across and protects nail bed

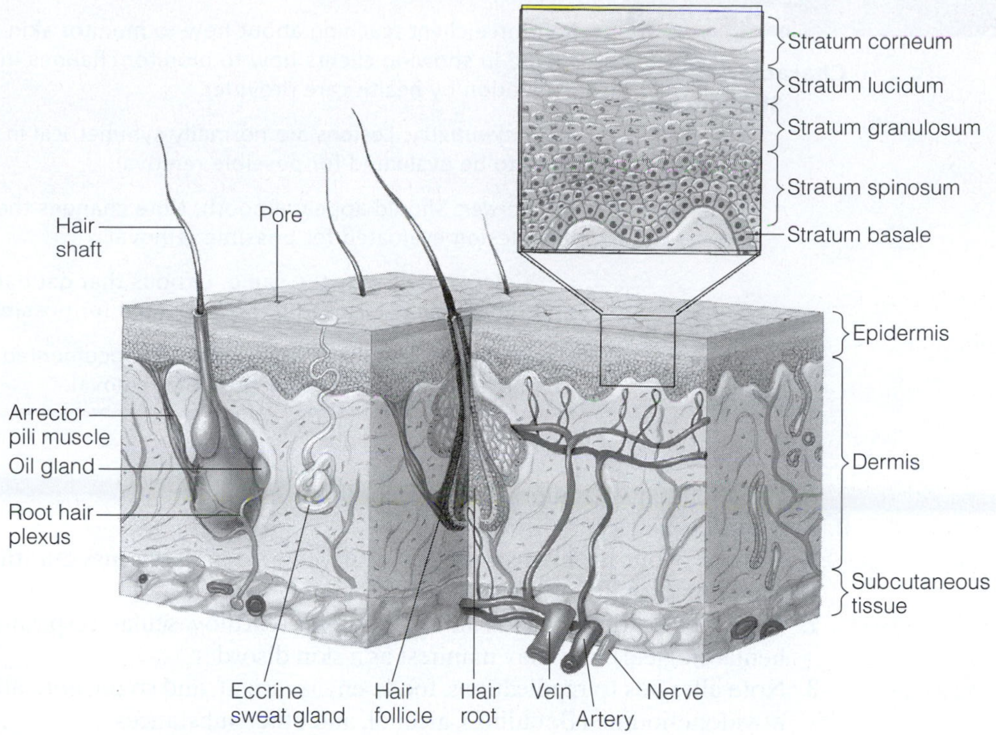

Figure 58–1

Layers and structures of the skin.

3. Glands
   a. Apocrine: sweat glands located in axilla, anus, and genital area; function unknown
   b. Eccrine: sweat glands located on forehead, hands, and soles of feet; maintain a stable body temperature through perspiration when body is overheated
   c. Sebaceous: oil glands located throughout body that secrete sebum to lubricate skin, decrease water loss, and aid in killing bacteria on skin surface (see Figure 58–1)

E. Skin functions
1. Sensitivity to pressure, pain, touch, and temperature
2. First line of defense against infectious organisms
3. Thermoregulation through sweating, shivering, and subQ insulation
4. Protects underlying tissues and organs from injury
5. Synthesizes vitamin D
6. Excretes water, salt, and electrolytes
7. Regenerates itself by shedding old cells and replacing with new cells

F. Pediatric variations in skin
1. Newborns are covered by lanugo—fine, soft hair that is shed in first month of life
2. Newborns have thin skin with little subQ fat that allows rapid heat loss and problems with thermoregulation
   a. Leads to increased absorption of harmful chemical substances
   b. Sweat glands not fully developed until middle childhood
3. Newborn skin contains more water than skin of older children
4. Dark-colored areas called Mongolian spots may be present on sacrum or buttocks of Native American, Asian, African-American, or Latino infants

II. DIAGNOSTIC TESTS AND DATA COLLECION

A. Skin cultures: non-invasive procedure in which a skin sample is obtained with a sterile applicator; used to identify viral, bacterial, or fungal causes of skin lesions

B. Skin scrapings: non-invasive procedure in which epithelial cells are scraped off and examined microscopically to identify viral, bacterial, fungal, or parasitic causes of skin lesion

C. Skin biopsy: invasive procedure in which a skin sample is removed for histological analysis
1. Requires informed consent
2. Apply pressure to site until bleeding stops; suture may be required

Box 58–1

Characteristics of Skin Lesions

Reinforce client teaching about how to monitor skin lesions. The ABCD rule is a useful aid in showing clients how to monitor changes in skin lesions and when to seek evaluation by health care provider.

A = Asymmetry: Lesions are normally symmetrical in shape. Any changes in symmetry need to be evaluated for possible removal.

B = Border: Should appear smooth. Note changes that appear rough and jagged, and have lesion evaluated for possible removal.

C = Color: Should stay the same. Lesions that get darker (brown or black) or have more than one color need to be evaluated for possible removal.

D = Diameter: Should be measured and documented. Lesions that enlarge need to be monitored and evaluated for possible removal.

3. Used to identify tumors or persistent dermatitis

D. Past medical history

1. Note previous problems with skin, hair, scalp, or nails; discuss duration of symptoms, associated symptoms, treatments used and results
2. Medical disorders: discuss all body systems (cardiovascular, respiratory, hepatic, endocrine/metabolic, hematological) that may manifest as a skin disorder
3. NCLEX® Note allergies to medications, foods, environment, and so on; note allergies to tape, latex, povidone-iodine (Betadine), alcohol, and other substances
4. Nutrition: note dietary changes, new foods introduced, and fluid intake
5. External exposure: note new products exposed to skin, such as soaps, lotions, sun, and chemicals
6. Activity: note daily physical activity and exercise routine
7. Sleep and rest: note number of hours of sleep each night and any rest periods
8. Coping: discuss skin disorders and how skin is affected when stress is experienced; note coping behaviors used and results
9. Current medications: list current medications, onset and dose of medications
10. NCLEX® Recent surgeries or treatments: note phototherapy, radiation therapy, or other therapy that may affect skin
11. NCLEX® Current problem: elicit data about current problem; for skin rash, obtain detailed data such as when rash began, how it has changed, medications or ointments used and results of treatment

E. Physical examination

1. Note color (pink, yellow, white, purple, bruising, etc.)
2. NCLEX® For lesions, document color, size, shape, symmetry, and border (see Box 58–1); note location and palpate texture, consistency, and mobility
3. Inspect hair for color, amount, distribution, lesions, and hygiene
4. Inspect nails for color, growth pattern, and thickness; inspect nail bed for inflammation or trauma
5. Note texture, temperature, and moisture of skin
6. Palpate skin turgor for hydration status
7. Palpate lower extremities (tibia and ankle) for edema
8. Palpate hair for texture (coarse, fine) and nails for texture and capillary refill

III. SKIN PROBLEMS CAUSED BY VASCULARITY

A. Spider angioma

1. A flat, bright red spot with radiating blood vessels (BVs) at edges
2. Commonly found on upper body; varies in size from a tiny dot up to 1.5 to 2 cm
3. Caused by vascular dilation of BVs commonly seen with high estrogen levels, pregnancy, liver disease, and/or vitamin B deficiency

B. Petechiae

1. NCLEX® Flat red spots, approximately 1–2 mm in diameter that do not change in color when blanched
2. NCLEX® Caused by tiny capillaries that have broken, possibly caused by thinning of blood (anticoagulant effect), liver disease, vitamin K deficiency, or septicemia

NCLEX® **C. Purpura**: purple or blue-appearing patch, varies in size and shape, caused by a bleeding disorder or broken BVs and may appear throughout body

IV. SKIN LESIONS

A. Primary skin lesions (see Figure 58–2)

1. **Macule**: nonpalpable, flat lesion that has color and measures less than 1 cm; examples: freckles, chloasma
2. **Papule**: elevated, palpable mass less than 0.5 cm; examples are warts and moles
   a. Management depends on diagnosis, such as cryotherapy for wart removal
   NCLEX® b. Mole removal may be recommended if premalignant; different methods of mole removal are available
   c. Excision of mole is one treatment that may be done in office setting; nursing care before treatment would be to explain procedure to client and obtain history of allergies (povidone–iodine, alcohol)
3. **Plaque**: elevated group of papules that have convalesced into one lesion larger than 0.5 cm; examples are actinic keratosis and psoriasis
4. **Nodule**: elevated, firm lesion with a circumscribed border that measures approximately 1–2 cm
5. **Vesicle**: fluid-filled, elevated mass less than 0.5 cm; a fluid mass more than 0.5 cm is called a bulla; examples of vesicles are chickenpox, small burns, and herpes virus lesion
6. **Wheal**: variable-sized, elevated **erythemic** (reddish) lesion with an irregular border that contains fluid in tissue of skin; examples include insect bites and hives
7. **Pustule**: elevated, pus-filled vesicle or bulla of any size; examples are acne and boils
8. **Cyst**: elevated, encapsulated fluid-filled or semisolid mass, often 1 cm or larger, in dermis or subQ tissue

B. Secondary skin lesions

1. Atrophy: dry, thin, taut skin that appears wasted from loss of collagen; an example is aged skin; hydration with fluids and keeping skin well-moisturized with emollients help this condition
2. Crusts: dried pus or blood on skin surface resulting from a ruptured vesicle; examples are impetigo or final stages of chickenpox lesions
3. Erosion: moist shallow skin depression that results from a previous lesion; an example is a ruptured vesicle; management includes warm, moist compresses to site for comfort; keep site clean and dry; clean with antibacterial soaps at least 3 to 4 times a day; may need topical antibiotic if site develops secondary bacterial infection
4. Fissure: linear break in skin with sharp edges, extending into dermis; examples are athlete's foot or cracks in corner of mouth from chapped lips; management of athlete's foot includes antifungal medications and keeping feet cool and dry (don't let sweat accumulate); encourage use of white, cotton socks; fissures of lips may be treated with topical ointments such as petroleum jelly or Blistex™ ointment
5. Scales: dry or greasy dead skin flakes that slough off skin surface; examples are dandruff or psoriasis
6. Scar: flat, irregular connective tissue remaining after a wound has healed; may vary in size, color, and shape; examples are healed surgical incisions or acne scars
7. Ulcer: deep excavations in skin that vary in size and shape and extend into dermis or subQ tissue; examples are chancres and pressure ulcers
8. Keloid: irregular elevated darker area of scar tissue from excess collagen formation during healing; extends beyond original area of injury

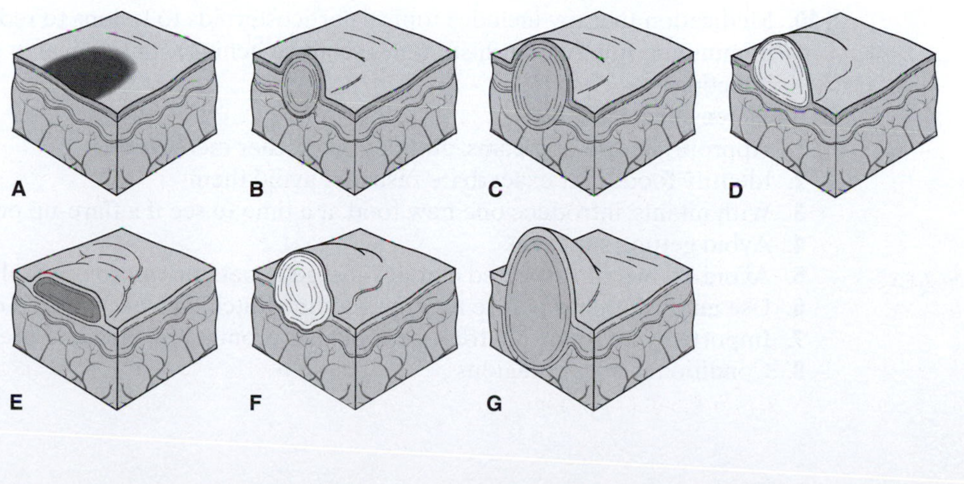

Figure 58–2

Primary skin lesions. *A.* Macule, patch. *B.* Papule, plaque. *C.* Nodule, tumor. *D.* Vesicle, bulla. *E.* Wheal. *F.* Pustule. *G.* Cyst.

V. ATOPIC DERMATITIS (ECZEMA)

A. Overview

1. **Atopic dermatitis (eczema)** is a chronic relapsing superficial inflammatory skin disorder that often begins in infancy, but can occur in early childhood and continue into adolescence and adulthood; is a risk factor for development of asthma and allergic rhinitis
2. Etiology is uncertain but involves a complex interaction of genetics, environmental exposure, infectious response, and defect in lipid barrier function of skin
3. Allergic form of disorder affects 70–85% of children with T-cell activation, increased IgE levels, and post-inflammatory skin lesions from cytokines and chemokines
4. Nonallergic form affects 15–30% of children and may have a later age at onset
5. Triggers include stress, changes in temperature and humidity, allergens (foods before age 3 and inhalants in older children), irritants (soaps, detergents, rough or wooly clothing) and autoantigens to human proteins

B. Data collection

NCLEX®

1. In infantile form (2 months–2 years), red papules (raised lesions) usually appear first on cheeks and then spread to forehead, scalp, and down extensor surfaces of arms and legs; is characterized by intense **pruritus** (itchiness), which causes skin excoriation that leads to exudate and crust formation

NCLEX®

2. Childhood form (2 years to puberty) may follow continuously from infancy, or may make first appearance later; is characterized by xerosis (dry skin that is more likely to crack and fissure) and dry, thickened, scaly, papular patches of skin on flexor and extensor surfaces of extremities, hands, feet, and folds of neck, perioral, periorbital and periauricular areas
3. In adolescent form (puberty onward), exudation is often caused by external irritation or secondary infection; is characterized by **lichenification** (large, dry, thickened lesions or plaques) on flexor folds, face, neck, back, upper arms, and dorsal aspects of hands, feet, fingers, and toes
4. Diagnosed by inspection of skin and history of asthma or hay fever (allergic rhinitis) in a child, or in a first-degree relative if child is under age 4
5. No diagnostic test exists for atopic eczema; skin prick tests or radioallergosorbent tests (RAST) may identify food allergies in allergic type; skin cultures diagnose secondary skin infection

C. Therapeutic management

NCLEX®

1. Goals are to identify and control triggers, keep skin dry and lubricated, and treat flares promptly to reduce risk of secondary infection
2. Bathe or shower daily with tepid to warm water using mild soap only on dirty areas; do not use bath additives such as baking soda, bubble bath, or bath oils

NCLEX®

3. Pat, rather than rub, skin dry
4. Immediately after bath (within 3 minutes), apply emollient such as Eucerin or Lubriderm to entire body to trap moisture in skin; reapply 3–4 times daily or whenever skin feels dry; avoid use of perfumed or scented lotions
5. Apply topical medications only to affected areas immediately after bath and put emollient on top
6. Use antibacterial soaps for handwashing
7. Keep fingernails clean and short; place cotton gloves or socks over hands of infants or young children to prevent scratching

NCLEX®

8. Avoid wool or constricting clothing, which can promote itching or trap perspiration
9. Provide support to child and family during flare-ups and reassurance that lesions do not produce scars unless excessively scratched and secondarily infected
10. Medication therapy includes topical corticosteroids to lesions to reduce inflammation during flare-ups, immunomodulators, antihistamines (control itching), and topical or oral antibiotics (used only for skin infection)

D. Reinforce client teaching

1. Appropriate use of creams, ointments, or other medications
2. Identify foods that exacerbate rash and avoid them
3. With infants, introduce one new food at a time to see if a flare-up occurs
4. Avoid getting sunburns

NCLEX®

5. Avoid known or suspected contact allergens, pets, or environmental factors
6. Use antihistamines before naps or bedtime if itching leads to sleep deprivation
7. Importance of following treatment plan to promote healing and prevent infections
8. Condition is not contagious

VI. PSORIASIS

A. Overview

1. A chronic, inflammatory skin disorder with raised, reddened, round plaques covered by silvery white scales, usually on scalp, knees, or elbows
2. Exact cause is unknown; is thought to include a T-lymphocyte–mediated dermal immune response, leading to increased growth of keratinocytes, dermal blood vessels, and inflammation; most clients with psoriasis have a positive family history

B. Data collection

NCLEX®

1. Dry, scaly rash that may appear as silvery scales or plaques usually found on scalp, knees, or elbows; may involve hands and feet
2. Diagnosed by clinical presentation, skin biopsy (if atypical manifestations or for differential diagnosis), or possibly ultrasound (to detect changes in dermis)

NCLEX®

C. Therapeutic management

1. Medications include topical corticosteroids used under an occlusive dressing, coal tar preparations (messy, cause staining, and have an unpleasant odor but remove scales and increase remission time), coal tar shampoos if scalp is affected, calcipotriene (Dovonex, a vitamin D derivative), and tazarotene (Tazorac, a synthetic retinoid)
2. Phototherapy for generalized psoriasis (more than 30% of body surface) with ultraviolet-B (UVB) 3 times weekly; is given for an increasing number of seconds of exposure time until an erythema response occurs about 8 hours later; eye shielding is needed during treatment
3. Photochemotherapy involves use of a light-activated form of drug methoxsalen; oral dose is followed 2 hours later by exposure to ultraviolet A (UVA) light; treatments are given 2–3 times weekly for total of 10–20 treatments; exposure to direct light for 8–12 hours after is avoided because treatment causes tanning; exposure to light is encouraged if UVA treatment not given
4. Skin care is similar to that described previously for atopic dermatitis
5. Assist client to cope with disturbed body image if lesions are large or visible to others; these clients may isolate themselves, withdraw from roles and responsibilities, and feel powerless

D. Reinforce client teaching: skin care, use of topical or systemic medications, and signs of complications of treatment to report (skin excoriation, increased erythema, increased skin peeling, or blister formation)

VII. SEBORRHEIC DERMATITIS

A. Overview

1. A chronic inflammatory skin condition in areas of active sebaceous glands, such as face, scalp, body folds, sternal area, and axilla
2. Appears as an erythematous scaling lesion that may appear dry or greasy
3. Etiology is unknown, but possible causes are believed to be hormonal influence, nutritional deficiency, neurogenic influence, dysfunction of sebaceous glands, and/or fungal infection

B. Data collection

1. Lesions with yellow or white plaques with scales (often yellow or orange) and crusts; skin may be oily or flaky and dry, pruritic, and may be at risk for secondary bacterial infections
2. Common sites include scalp, eyebrows, nose, ears, sternal area, and axillae
3. Is seen more frequently in cold weather, and may be triggered by decreased humidification and decreased exposure to sunlight

C. Therapeutic management: scalp treatment: selenium sulfide 2.5% suspension or coal tar shampoos and topical steroid creams; skin care and client teaching as discussed previously for atopic dermatitis

VIII. MALIGNANT NEOPLASMS

A. Actinic keratosis

1. Overview
   a. Premalignant macules on skin of fair-skinned clients age 50 years or older, but may occur in high-risk client at any age

   NCLEX®

   b. Occurs because of chronic sun exposure to skin; clients with light complexion are at highest risk
   c. Approximately 1% of these lesions will progress to squamous cell carcinoma
2. Data collection

   NCLEX®

   a. Erythematous, rough, and shiny-textured macules that appear singly or in groups
   b. Commonly seen on face, ears, scalp, lips, neck, and hands

3. Therapeutic management
   NCLEX® a. Protection from ultraviolet (UV) rays of sun with use of clothing and sunscreens are recommended when exposed to sunlight; these measures are both prophylactic against development and may slow or stop progression to carcinoma
   b. Biopsy and removal of lesion is recommended if changes in lesion occur; these changes include color, border, size, and shape of lesions; refer back to Box 58–1

B. Basal cell carcinoma

1. Overview
   a. Abnormal cell growth of basal layer of epidermal skin cells that do not mature properly into keratinocytes; neoplastic growth occurs and surrounding skin is also destroyed
   b. Most common contributor is UV rays from sunlight exposure
   c. Basal cell carcinoma is least aggressive type of skin cancer and rarely metastasizes to other organs
2. Data collection: types and characteristics of five types of basal cell carcinoma
   NCLEX® a. Nodular basal cell carcinoma: small, firm papule, which appears as pearly, white, pink, or flesh-colored and is commonly seen on face, neck, and/or head
   b. Superficial basal cell carcinoma: papule or plaque commonly seen on trunk and extremities (second most common lesion)
   c. Pigmented basal cell carcinoma: is less common and usually found on head, neck, or face; has ability to concentrate melanin, which causes deeper pigmentation of center of tumor
   d. Morpheaform basal cell carcinoma: least common form; found on head and neck, appearing like a tumor with fingerlike projections (usually ivory or flesh-colored) and typically resembles a scar; has ability to invade and destroy adjacent tissue and structures
   e. Keratotic basal cell carcinoma: found on preauricular or postauricular area; contains both basal cells and squamous cells that keratinize; if removed, this tumor is likely to recur; also has a high risk of metastasizing to other structures
3. Therapeutic management
   a. Monitor progress of growth of all lesions; lesions that measure more than 2 cm have a high reoccurrence rate; suspicious lesions are excised and sent for pathological examination
   NCLEX® b. Reinforce client teaching about importance of monitoring lesions and early identification of new lesions; suggest monthly self-assessment of skin and periodic screening by health care provider based on symptoms
   NCLEX® c. Encourage skin protection from UV light exposure by using sunscreens with SPF 15 or higher and wearing hats and and other protective clothing
   d. Medication therapy: none

C. Cutaneous T-cell lymphoma

1. Overview: a type of lymphoma involving skin that rarely invades lymph nodes; it is a thymus-derived helper cell cancer
2. Data collection: three stages exist; however, stages may occur in sequence or concurrently
   a. Stage 1—erythematous stage: erythemic, well-defined border patch that is pruritic and may resemble psoriasis or eczema; patch may become diffuse with severe itching
   b. Stage 2—plaque stage: erythemic, scaly patches that become indurated and/or elevated; center of plaque may appear healed with rough, ring-shaped borders; this stage may resemble tertiary syphilis or erythema multiforme perstans
   c. Stage 3—tumor stage: terminal stage in which tumor growth of plaques occur, often seen with secondary bacterial infection
3. Therapeutic management
   a. Initial stages may only require a tar cream and UVB light therapy
   NCLEX® b. Psoralen and UVA light (PUVA) has also been effective
   c. Nitrogen mustard treatment has been beneficial when used in earlier stages
   NCLEX® d. Medication therapy: systemic corticosteroids are used for first two stages; radiation therapy may be used at any point in disease; systemic chemotherapy has been used during plaque and tumor stage but may not always be successful

D. Kaposi's sarcoma

1. Overview
   a. A rare skin cancer of endothelial lining of small BVs, seen most often on face, nose, and ears
   b. May be related to infective agent such as a retrovirus (e.g., human immunodeficiency virus [HIV])

2. Data collection
   NCLEX®
   a. Vascular lesions (macules, papules, nodules) that can affect skin and viscera
   b. Over time, lesions enlarge and become confluent, forming large masses; as masses enlarge, tissue below mass becomes involved and tumor then invades lymphatic tissue, which may lead to lymphedema, primarily affecting genitalia and lower extremities
   c. As disease progresses, tumor may interfere with internal organ function and may even cause bleeding to point of hemorrhage (a late sign)
   d. Initially Kaposi's sarcoma may be symptom-free; however, pain maybe experienced in later stages

NCLEX®

3. Therapeutic management
   a. Isolated lesions may be removed by excision, cryotherapy, and/or local radiation for comfort and/or cosmetic treatment
   b. Medication therapy: single agent or combination chemotherapy

E. Nonmelanoma: Squamous cell carcinoma

1. Overview
   a. A cutaneous malignancy arising from keratinocytes; most common type of skin cancer; fair-skinned males tend to have a higher incidence of nonmelanoma skin cancer, with majority occurring from 30–60 years of age
   b. Occurs on skin frequently exposed to UV light, such as face, ears, nose, lips, and hands; of two nonmelanoma types of carcinoma, squamous cell carcinoma grows quicker, is more aggressive, and is more likely to metastasize than basal cell carcinoma
   c. Etiology of squamous cell carcinoma is multifactorial
   NCLEX®
   d. Environmental causes include UV radiation, chemicals, physical trauma, and pollution
   e. With exposure of UV light to skin, rays penetrate tissue and alter normal DNA and suppress body's T-cell and B-cell immunity, producing tumors of squamous epithelial or mucous membranes
   f. Tumors may proliferate with an irregular shape and invade dermal layer of skin
   g. Squamous cell carcinoma may also develop from pre-existing skin lesions, such as old scars; may proliferate into dermal structure and metastasize via lymphatic system

NCLEX®

2. Data collection: may present as a small, flesh-colored papule that is firm to touch; as tumor grows, color may change and appear erythemic and sore, and may even bleed if touched
3. Therapeutic management
   a. Recommended management is tumor removal by cryotherapy, surgical excision, electrodesiccation, or radiotherapy
   b. Cure rate with these methods is approximately 90%
   c. Tumor removal is recommended immediately to prevent metastasis
   NCLEX®
   d. Nursing management includes reinforcing methods to prevent further tumors from arising: minimize sun exposure, wear protective clothing, wear sunscreen with a SPF of 15 or higher, and avoid tanning booths
   e. Medication therapy: none

F. Malignant melanoma

1. Overview
   a. A less common skin cancer arising from melanocytes; is responsible for large majority of skin cancer deaths
   b. Risk factors include moles; fair skin with freckling, blond hair or blue eyes; having a close relative with melanoma or past history of melanoma; use of medications that suppress immune system; excess exposure to UV radiation via sunlight, tanning lamps or booths; age over 50 years; xeroderma pigmentosus (rare inherited disease with reduced ability to repair skin damage from sun)
   c. Major types: superficial spreading melanoma, lentigo maligna melanoma, nodular melanoma, and acral lentiginous melanoma; each is characterized by a radial and/or vertical growth phase; metastasis occurs during vertical growth phase
2. Data collection
   a. Lesions often found on trunk of men and legs of women
   b. Suspicious lesions often evaluated using the ABCDE rule

Memory Aid

Remember the alphabet—ABCDE—to remember the adverse changes in skin lesions that need to be reported: Asymmetry (one half doesn't match other half), Border (irregular), Color (variations or dark black), Diameter (greater than 6 mm-size of a pencil eraser), and Evolving or changing!

c. Diagnosis is with skin biopsy; other tests such as blood work, CT scan, x-rays, or MRI may be done to diagnose metastasis

3. Therapeutic management
   a. Surgery (with wide excision) is preferred treatment, but others include chemotherapy, immunotherapy and radiation therapy
   b. Maintain medical and surgical asepsis when changing surgical dressing or caring for incision
   c. Encourage adequate nutrition with sufficient calories, protein, and vitamins
   d. Assist client to cope with diagnosis of cancer and possibility or reality of metastasis

IX. BACTERIAL INFECTIONS

A. Impetigo

1. Overview
   a. A superficial skin infection that initially appears as an erythemic vesicle and later changes to a honey-colored crusted lesion
   b. Is most commonly seen in children but occasionally affects adults
   c. When skin integrity is interrupted, bacteria invade epidermis and cause an infection; most common organisms are *Staphylococcus aureas* and *group-A beta-hemolytic streptococcus*
2. Data collection
   a. Commonly found on face, arms, legs, and buttocks
   b. Appear as thin erythemic vesicles that become honey-colored crusts or erosions
   c. May occur as a single lesion or several lesions that have coalesced
3. Therapeutic management

NCLEX® a. Encourage frequent and thorough hand hygiene with warm soapy water to prevent spreading bacteria to others

b. For recurrent lesions, a culture of site is obtained to isolate pathogens

NCLEX® c. Medication therapy: topical or systemic antibiotics

d. Remind clients not to share toiletries, utensils, dishes, or towels with others; wash client's laundry and linens separately from others in hot water and detergent

e. Keep fingernails short to prevent scratching and spread of bacteria

B. Folliculitis

1. Overview
   a. A superficial bacterial infection of hair follicle; most common pathogens are *Staphylococcus aureus* and *Pseudomonas aeruginosa*
   b. Can occur at any age and is seen more often in males
   c. Can be aggravated by shaving, particularly skin on face (beard), legs, and axilla
2. Data collection
   a. Lesion appears as an erythemic, pruritic, mildly tender pustule located at hair follicle; various stages of folliculitis may occur, including a simple pustule, progressing to a furuncle or carbuncle
   b. In severe cases, fever and chills may be present
3. Therapeutic management
   a. Topical treatment includes cleaning site with warm soapy water 2–3 times a day
   b. Warm compresses may be used for comfort as needed
   c. If razors are being used, encourage client to use clean, sharp razors and to throw away old razors
   d. Do not use irritating lotions or creams at site
   e. Medication therapy: topical mupirocin (Bactroban) applied 3 times a day for simple folliculitis; for more severe cases, oral antibiotics may be needed

C. Furuncle

1. Overview
   a. An erythemic, warm, tender nodule of skin often caused by *Staphylococcus* organism; may be chronic problem in some cases
   b. Common sites are nares, neck, axilla, and genital area; are often seen in children, teens, and young adults
2. Data collection: warm, erythemic tender nodule of hair follicle
3. Therapeutic management
   a. Warm moist heat may be applied to site for comfort
   b. Occasionally, incision and drainage of site may be needed, in which case, Gram stain, culture, and sensitivity is obtained
   c. Medication therapy: oral antibiotics are not recommended except for immunocompromised clients

D. Furunculosis

1. Overview: an infection of an inflammatory nodule most commonly seen in children, adolescents, and young adults
2. Data collection: an erythemic, warm, hard, tender-to-touch nodule frequently found at site of a hair follicle
3. Therapeutic management: warm moist soaks to site; incision and drainage of site may be needed; keep lesions clean by washing site with warm soapy water several times a day
4. Medication therapy: simple furunculosis may be treated with topical antibiotics; complicated furunculosis with cellulitis requires systemic antibiotics; recurrent furunculosis may be controlled with prophylactic antibiotic therapy

E. Carbuncle

1. Overview
   a. An inflammatory lesion formed when several furuncles coalesce to form one larger infected lesion of skin
   b. Carbuncles are frequently seen in children, teens, and young adults; males are affected more frequently; common sites are hair follicles in nose, neck, face, buttocks, and axilla; *Staphylococcus* is a common causative organism
2. Data collection: erythemic, tender nodule that develops at a hair follicle area with possible malaise and low-grade fever
3. Therapeutic management
   a. Warm moist heat may be applied; incision and drainage of site is recommended
   b. Frequent use of antibacterial soaps and frequent showers are recommended for prevention
   c. Medication therapy: antibiotics

F. Cellulitis

1. Overview
   a. A bacterial infection of dermal and subQ tissues with lesions appearing in various stages, ranging from vesicles, bullae, abscesses, and plaques
   b. Most commonly seen in adults, with group-A beta-hemolytic *Streptococcus pyogenes* and *Staphylococcus aureus* being most frequent organisms
   c. Cellulitis occurs because of a break in skin integrity (abrasion, laceration, etc.); may also occur secondary to a skin lesion

NCLEX®

2. Data collection
   a. An erythemic, swollen, tender-to-touch area of skin at site of entry of bacteria
   b. Associated symptoms include fever, chills, malaise, and anorexia
   c. Regional lymphadenopathy

NCLEX®

3. Therapeutic management
   a. Rest and elevation of affected part; moist heat to site for comfort
   b. Culture and sensitivity of tissue site for severe cases
   c. For necrotic tissue, surgical excision and debridement are recommended along with antibiotic therapy
   d. Hospitalization is needed if cellulitis is on face or covers a large area; otherwise, management is done at home
   e. Medication therapy: antibiotic therapy

X. VIRAL INFECTIONS

A. Herpes simplex virus (Type 1, Type 2)

1. Overview
   a. A viral infection manifested by vesicles on oral mucosa (mouth or lips), which is HSV Type I, or in genital mucosa (HSV Type II)
   b. Herpes simplex virus (HSV) can occur at any age
   c. Is spread by direct contact of contaminated body fluids and has an incubation period range of 2 to 14 days
   d. Primary infection: initial outbreak in which blisters occur on mucosa or lips; malaise and fever are also common symptoms
   e. Recurrent infections: outbreaks may occur at any time and are commonly precipitated by stress and illness; symptoms are usually milder than primary outbreak; recurrent infection is commonly present with a prodrome of tingling, itching, or a burning sensation at site prior to outbreak of lesions
   f. Latency period: virus remains dormant in body during this time

NCLEX® 2. Data collection
- a. Primary symptoms include malaise, fever, and vesicles appearing on mucosa
- b. Secondary symptoms include prodrome of tingling, burning sensation prior to outbreak of vesicles on mucosa; latency period is asymptomatic

3. Therapeutic management
- a. Advise rest
- NCLEX® b. Encourage good hand hygiene technique to prevent spreading virus
- c. Comfort measures such as petroleum jelly or lip balm may be used for oral lesions
- NCLEX® d. To prevent spreading virus, reinforce that client avoid close contact with others while lesions are present; to prevent HSV Type 2, advise use of latex condoms to prevent spreading genital lesions
- e. Medication therapy: over-the-counter medications, such as acetaminophen (Tylenol) or camphophenique for comfort as needed; antiviral medications such as acyclovir (Zovirax), famciclovir (Famvir), or valacyclovir (Valtrex) may reduce further viral replication and diminish symptoms if started within 24 to 48 hours after initial onset of lesions

B. Herpes zoster

1. Overview
- a. A viral infection manifested by vesicles on skin and commonly seen in older adults and elderly
- b. Herpes zoster is a reactivation of varicella virus, which has been dormant for many years, in the dorsal root ganglia

NCLEX® 2. Data collection
- a. A vesicular rash on skin that usually follows one dermatome
- b. Clusters of vesicles are common along with symptoms of tingling, itching, burning, and even pain at site of lesions
- c. May also experience fatigue, malaise, fever, and headache in addition to local discomfort of rash

3. Therapeutic management
- NCLEX® a. Comfort measures include wet dressings or soaks (Burow's solution) on lesions 2 to 3 times a day
- NCLEX® b. Oatmeal baths (Aveeno™) are soothing and help to dry lesions
- c. Rest is recommended
- d. To prevent viral spread to others, take care to avoid persons at risk
- e. Monitor lesions for secondary bacterial infections
- NCLEX® f. Medication therapy: antiviral medications if therapy started within 24 to 48 hours after outbreak of vesicles; current medications include acyclovir (Zovirax), famciclovir (Famvir), and valacyclovir (Valtrex); acetaminophen (Tylenol) and ibuprofen (Motrin) may be used for discomfort

C. Warts

1. Overview
- a. An elevation in epidermal skin layer, commonly seen in children and young adults; seen more common in women than in men
- b. Caused by papillomavirus
- c. A tumor develops on skin within epidermal layer
- d. Virus may be transmitted from person to person by touch and is commonly seen on hands and feet

2. Data collection: a painless nodule on skin surface, which is flesh-colored and appears to have a rough surface with an irregular border; there are several types of warts
- a. Common wart—flesh-colored nodule commonly seen on hands or extremities, but can occur anywhere on body; commonly appears to have a "black seed" in the center of lesion; these warts may come and go, usually lasting approximately 6 to 12 months without treatment
- b. Flat wart—a tiny flesh-colored node, 1 to 3 mm in diameter, that may appear in clusters on dorsum of hand or forehead
- c. Filiform wart—a tiny, thin, projected nodule commonly seen on face, nose, or eyelids
- d. Plantar wart—a hard nodule found on bottom of foot; commonly projects into foot from constant pressure applied while walking on nodule; it measures approximately 2 to 3 cm and is frequently associated with discomfort or pain at site

3. Therapeutic management
- a. Sometimes no treatment is necessary for warts because viral lesions will resolve on their own
- NCLEX® b. Medication therapy: over-the-counter (OTC) therapy for wart removal includes salicylic acid (17%) and retinoic acid
- c. Laser therapy may be used for selected warts, such as those that are large or located in certain body areas (e.g., genital)
- d. Warts that are treated may reappear in same site or on other areas of skin

XI. FUNGAL INFECTIONS

A. *Candidiasis*

1. Overview
   - **a.** Infection caused by *candida albicans,* a yeast-like fungus that most often causes symptomatic superficial cutaneous or mucosal infections if local immunity is disturbed
   - **b.** Candida infections can affect all ages but often cause diaper rash in infants, summertime inframammary rash in women, vaginitis in premenopausal women, oral candidiasis in immunocompromised clients, and buttock and perineal rash in incontinent clients
   - *NCLEX®* **c.** Risk factors include moist, warm, or interrupted skin integrity; systemic antibiotics; pregnancy; birth control use; poor nutrition; diabetes mellitus or chronic illnesses; and immunosuppression
2. Data collection: lesions are bright red, smooth macules with a macerated appearance and a scaling, elevated border; characteristic "satellite" lesions are small, similar-appearing macules outside main lesion
   - *NCLEX®* **a.** Oral candidiasis (also called thrush) is characterized by white, milky plaques on oral mucosa; associated symptoms may include a burning sensation or decreased taste
   - *NCLEX®* **b.** Vulovaginitis is found on vaginal mucosa and can spread to perineum and groin; satellite lesions are usually present; other findings include excessive itching and a thick, white, curdlike vaginal discharge
   - **c.** Perineal/diaper and skin-fold rash occurs on perigenital and perianal areas and can extend to inner thighs and buttocks; other areas affected include axilla, umbilical area, and under breasts; erythema, papules, pustules, and a scaling border are characteristic
   - **d.** Balanitis is an inflammation of glans and prepuce of penis that typically present as flattened pustules with edema, scaling, erosion, burning, and tenderness
   - **e.** Paronychial infection presents as erythema, edema, and tenderness of nail folds; a creamy, purulent discharge may be expressed with pressure on nail; nails usually become discolored and have ridging
   - **f.** Candida organisms may also be a causative agent in otitis externa and scalp disorders
   - **g.** Diagnosis is made by culture of scrapings or by microscopic examination of scaling with potassium hydrochloride (KOH) preparation
3. Therapeutic management
   - *NCLEX®* **a.** Avoid sharing linens or personal items
   - *NCLEX®* **b.** Use clean towel and washcloth daily
   - **c.** Dry all skin folds, avoid frequent immersion of hands in water
   - **d.** Wear clean cotton underwear daily
   - **e.** For vaginal candida, avoid tight clothing and pantyhose, bathe more frequently, and dry genital area thoroughly; may need to treat sexual partner at same time to avoid reinfection or have partner use condoms until resolved; avoid douching, and change perineal pads frequently
   - **f.** For balanitis, carefully retract foreskin and perform careful cleaning and drying of glans penis
   - **g.** Encourage weight loss for obese clients and euglycemia in diabetic clients to decrease risk of infection
   - *NCLEX®* **h.** Medication therapy: antifungals (topical, shampoo, or vaginal suppository depending on site) or nystatin powder or ointment; systemic medications require monitoring of liver function tests (risk of hepatotoxicity)

B. Tinea corporis

1. Overview
   - **a.** A fungal infection of face, trunk, and extremities with exclusion of palms of hands, soles of feet, and groin; also known as ringworm of body
   - **b.** All species of dermatophytes can be causative agent; generally more prevalent in hot and humid climates
   - **c.** Can affect all age groups, but children are more often affected
   - **d.** Can be spread human-to-human, animal-to-human, and soil-to-human by direct contact; other risk factors include prolonged use of topical steroids or immunosuppression
2. Data collection
   - *NCLEX®* **a.** Classic lesions are annular (ringlike) plaques with an elevated border, sharp margins, and a clearing center
   - **b.** May occur singly or in groups of three to four
   - **c.** KOH preparation from these lesions is usually positive; woods lamp fluoresces yellow; dermatophyte test media changes medium from yellow to red
   - **d.** For most clinical purposes, classification by anatomic site is preferred
3. Therapeutic management
   - **a.** Avoid contact with suspected lesions
   - **b.** Topical creams are treatment of choice
   - **c.** Thoroughly clean environment to remove fungal scales that are shed from skin

d. Avoid sharing towels or other items that can transmit fungal scales

NCLEX® e. Search out infected animals/pets and treat appropriately

f. Apply creams after bathing and reapply after swimming and exercising

g. Keep skin dry

h. Monitor for superimposed bacterial infections

NCLEX® i. Medication therapy: topical drugs for superficial infections; eradication is slow and treatment may take 2 to 8 weeks; for added benefit, client should wash with an antifungal shampoo prior to using a cream

C. Tinea pedis

1. Overview

a. Also known as athlete's foot, is most common of all fungal infections; affects plantar surface of feet with mild to moderate erythema and scaly skin between toes

b. Caused by an infection by a dermatophyte (fungus that grows in nonliving, keratinized portions of skin)

c. Dermatophytes are commonly termed tinea and are named by affected location

d. Pustules may be present in severe cases with a foul odor, possibly indicating a secondary bacterial or yeast infection

e. Risk factors include communal showers and pools, occlusive footwear, excessive sweating, sharing of footwear, and hot, humid weather, immunocompromised status, and prolonged use of topical steroids; both feet often involved

NCLEX® 2. Data collection

a. Interdigital scaling, crusting, and maceration; pruritis may or may not be present

b. Plantar and lateral surfaces of feet may also be affected

c. Vesicles, pustules, and interdigital blisters may provide entry for secondary bacteria such as *Streptococcus* organisms

3. Therapeutic management

NCLEX® a. Keep involved areas clean, dry, and exposed to air when possible

b. Wear light cotton socks and change frequently throughout day

c. Wear sandals or open-toed shoes when possible; avoid plastic or occlusive shoes

d. Carefully dry between toes after showering or bathing

e. Apply drying or dusting powers, topical antiperspirants

f. Put socks on before underwear to avoid spreading to groin

g. Reinforce teaching about signs of bacterial infection such as pain, increased inflammation, pustules, or purulent exudates

NCLEX® h. Medication therapy: antifungal creams; powders may be used as an adjunct treatment and aid in keeping areas dry; for severe cases, Burow's solution soak for lesions that are oozing, and oral antifungals such as griseofulvin, fluconazole, itraconazole, and tervinafine

XII. INFESTATIONS AND INSECT BITES

A. Bees and wasps

1. Stings that contain poison cause local tissue inflammation and destruction

2. Allergic reaction can occur from previous sensitization or toxic reaction from large inoculation of poison; IgE-mediated hypersensitivity to insect venom may be confirmed by skin testing done by an allergist

3. Data collection

a. Local reactions include erythema, pain, heat, swelling, itching, blisters, secondary infection, necrosis, ulceration, and drainage

b. Toxic reactions include nausea, vomiting, headache, fever, diarrhea, lightheadedness, syncope, drowsiness, muscle spasms, edema, and/or seizures

NCLEX® c. Systemic reactions include allergic/itching eyes, facial flushing, generalized urticaria, dry cough, chest/throat constriction, wheezing, dyspnea, cyanosis, abdominal cramps, diarrhea, nausea, vomiting, vertigo, chills/fever, stridor, shock, loss of consciousness, involuntary bowel/bladder action, frothy sputum, respiratory failure, cardiovascular collapse, and death

d. Delayed reactions include serum sickness–like reactions, fever, malaise, headache, urticaria, lymphadenopathy, polyarthritis

e. Unusual reactions include encephalopathy, neuritis, vasculitis, nephrosis, extreme fear/anxiety

4. Therapeutic management

a. Includes first-aid measures, local treatment, or activation of emergency services for severe reactions

NCLEX® b. Remove stinger by scraping—do not squeeze with a tweezer—then cleanse wound

NCLEX® **c.** Ice packs to bite or sting—alternate 10 minutes on and 10 minutes off
d. Elevate and rest affected part
e. Maintain adequate airway
NCLEX® **f.** Persons with known sensitivity should wear medical ID tag; prevent reexposure and teach use of Epi-pen or anaphylactic kit
g. Explain risks of increasing severity of responses in future
h. Instruct to use insect repellants when outdoors or in infested areas
i. Medication therapy: local analgesics, diphenhydramine (Benadryl) or other antihistamines; topical or oral steroids; if severe systemic reaction, Epinephrine 1:1000 subQ to combat urticaria, wheezing, angioedema; medications to treat shock if indicated; antivenom for black widow spider or scorpion
j. Consider desensitization with immunotherapy in severe cases

B. Pediculosis

1. Overview
a. An infestation of skin or hair by species of blood-sucking lice capable of living as external parasites on human host
b. ***Pediculosis capitis*** is head louse, size of a sesame seed, clear in color when hatched but becomes grayish-white to red/brown after maturing
c. Head lice infestation is very common among school-age children of all socioeconomic backgrounds and is spread by sharing combs, hats, and scarves
d. *Pediculosis pubis,* also known as "crabs," infests genital area and is a common sexually transmitted infection because it spreads by sexual contact
e. Nits/eggs attach to hair shaft by a cementlike or cocoonlike structure and are difficult to remove
f. Lice live up to 30 days, and a female can lay up to 100 eggs

NCLEX® **2.** Data collection
a. Intensive pruritis is most common symptom that may result in excoriations
b. Head lice may resemble dandruff flakes, but are not easily brushed off
c. Papular urticaria may be found at neck or pubic area

3. Therapeutic management
a. Nits must be mechanically removed; a 50/50 white vinegar/water solution may loosen nits; olive oil may also be used; a nit comb removes nits from hair shafts (best effect by back-combing hair); lice may also be removed by fingers or tweezers
b. To treat eyelashes, apply petrolatum to lashes twice daily for 10 days; lice either suffocate or slide off
NCLEX® **c.** Inform children and parents about mode of transmission (person to person) and preventive measures, such as not sharing combs, brushes, hats, scarves, helmets, headphones, bedding, or sleeping bags
d. Coats and hats should be hung separately and not touching each other
e. Sleeping material should be labeled and kept separately in plastic bags, not stacked
NCLEX® **f.** All family members need to be examined and treated at same time
g. Soak personal hair items or any item in contact with hair in 2% Lysol or pediculocide for 1 hour
h. Shaving hair is not found to be helpful
NCLEX® **i.** Machine-wash all washable clothing used in last 48 hours and dry in hot dryer for at least 20 minutes
j. Place unwashable items in airtight plastic bags for 1 week to kill lice
k. Upholstered furniture or pillows may be ironed with a hot iron
l. Vacuum mattresses, rugs, upholstered furniture, and stuffed animals regularly
NCLEX® **m.** For *pediculosis capitis*: permethrin (Nix), pyrethrin shampoo (Rid), or lindane (Kwell) shampoo left on 5 to 10 minutes and then washed off; lindane can be repeated in 1 week, but due to neurotoxicity lindane should not be used by children, nursing or pregnant women, clients with known seizure disorders, or on open skin
n. For pediculosis pubis: treatment includes lindane, pyrethrin (Rid) or permethrin (Nix) as a shampoo left on for 10 minutes or as a lotion left on for several hours
o. Trimethoprim/sulfamethoxazole (Bactrim DS) has been shown to be effective for cases of resistance to pediculicides (non-FDA approved)

C. *Scabies*

1. Overview
a. A contagious disease caused by infestation of skin by mite *Sarcoptes scabiei var hominis*; impregnated mite burrows into skin and remains there for life (approximately 30 days), laying 2 to 3 eggs per day; eggs hatch in 3 to 4 days and reach maturity in 4 days, migrate to skin surface, mate, and repeat cycle

b. Is spread by skin-to-skin or sexual contact; is easily transmitted within a household; casual contact is not likely to cause infection because mite takes 45 minutes to burrow into skin; mites can live in clothing fibers and can be transmitted by contact with infected clothing or bed linens
c. Diagnosis is usually made by clinical presentation of burrows, vesicles, and nodules; although rarely performed, skin biopsy of a nodule will reveal portions of mite

2. Data collection

NCLEX® a. Presents as a generalized pruritic rash particularly of webs of fingers, intergluteal folds, axillae, palms, wrists, elbows, inner thighs and waist; head, neck, face, palms, soles and insteps of feet may also be affected in children under age 2
b. Itching may become intense; increased warmth of skin and nocturnal itching is a classic symptom, since mites tend to have increased movment at night; exposure to hot water or steam also can increase pruritis
c. Lesions may be erythematous, crusted papules, vesicles, pustules or nodules, and may be accompanied by flesh-colored, raised burrows (threadlike linear ridges with a pinpoint vesicle at one end); clients develop itch approximately 10 to 14 days after exposure

3. Therapeutic management

a. Close family members and personal contacts must be treated as well, even if there are no apparent signs or symptoms
NCLEX® b. All bed clothing, linens, unwashed worn clothing, and stuffed animals should be washed and dried in a hot dryer to kill mites
NCLEX® c. Mites and eggs may be killed by placing items in airtight plastic bags for 7 days since mite cannot live away from host more than 3 days; mites can live 24–36 hours in room conditions and longer in humid environments
d. Relief from itching may not occur for 3 to 6 weeks after treatment because of hypersensitivity of skin to debris left in burrow
NCLEX® e. Scabicide lotions/creams should be applied to entire body but avoiding eyes and mucous membranes, using a toothbrush to get under fingernails and toenails; lotion is showered off 8 to 12 hours later
f. Permethrin 5% lotion (Elimite) or malathion (ovide) is treatment of choice; a second application one week later is recommended
g. Crotamiton 10% (Eurax) is less toxic but is also slightly less effective; therefore, application for 2 nights is advised
NCLEX® h. Lindane 1% cream or lotion (Kwell) is least expensive but has potential for neurotoxicity and should not be used by children, nursing or pregnant women, people with a known seizure disorder, or any widespread excoriations/open skin; treatment may be repeated after 1 week
i. An oral antihistamine may be needed to relieve itching
j. May require emollients and midpotency corticosteroids after using scabicide to suppress hyperreactivity caused by mites; antibiotics may be needed if secondary infection occurs

XIII. ALLERGIC REACTIONS

A. *Contact dermatitis*

1. Overview

a. A skin inflammation caused by an external irritant or an allergic reaction mediated by IgE; epidermal reaction is caused by T-lymphocytes; location of rash helps provide clues to offending substance or antigen
b. Common irritants include chemicals, dyes, metals, poisonous plants (ivy, sumac, oak) and latex; allergic contact dermatitis affects only those previously sensitized and is a delayed hypersensitivity reaction

2. Data collection

NCLEX® a. Acute: papules, vesicles, bullae with surrounding erythema; crusting, oozing, and pruritis may be present
b. Chronic: erythematous base, thickening with lichenification, scaling, and fissuring

3. Therapeutic management

a. Identify and remove causative agents
b. Topical emollients in combination with mid- to high-potency corticosteroids
c. Drainage of large vesicles may be necessary without removing tops
d. Apply wet dressings to oozing, pruritic lesions to aid in drying and debridement; cool tap water, Burow's solution 1 to 40, saline 1 tsp/pint water, and silver nitrate solution can be used
e. Suppress inflammation with antibacterial solution
NCLEX® f. May use topical corticosteroid creams but do not use on face

g. Aveeno (oatmeal) baths are helpful to decrease itching
h. Antihistamines of choice may be used to decrease itching and edema
i. Use calamine lotion to aid drying
j. Mid-potency or high potency topical corticosteroids

B. *Urticaria*

1. Overview

NCLEX® a. An itchy rash; single or multiple superficial raised pale macules with red halo; subsides rapidly, with no scars or change in pigmentation, but may reoccur
b. Acute urticaria is a response to many stimuli; IgE-mediated histamine release from mast cells is sometimes seen in response to drug exposure and subsides over several hours
c. Chronic urticaria persists over 6 weeks; it is not mediated by IgE; it is also associated with fever, chills, arthralgia, myalgia, and headache

NCLEX® d. Urticaria is a response to massive histamine release from mast cells in superficial dermis; can be caused by multiple agents such as drug reaction, food or food-additive allergy, inhalant, contact or ingestion allergy, transfusion reaction, insect bite or sting, bacterial, viral, fungal or helminthic infection, collagen vascular disease, lupus, heat, cold, sunlight, or emotional stress
e. True urticarial lesions do not remain in same area of skin longer than 24 hours; lesions that are present 72 hours or longer suggest cutaneous vasculitis as a possible cause

2. Data collection

NCLEX® a. Single or multiple raised, blanched, central wheals surrounded by red flare that is intensely pruritic; may occur anywhere on body
b. Variable size of 1–2 mm to 15–20 cm or larger
c. Resolves spontaneously in less than 48 hours

3. Therapeutic management

a. Cool moist compresses help to control itching
b. Avoidance if etiology is known
c. Antihistamine if accidentally reexposed

NCLEX® d. Reinforce to client that there is risk of life-threatening reaction on reexposure
e. SubQ administration of epinephrine 1:1000 for intense itching
f. Antihistamines; histamine (H_2) receptor antagonists may enhance effectiveness of conventional antihistamines
g. Cyprohepadine (Periactin) 4 mg every 6 hours for cold urticaria
h. Corticosteroids for pressure urticaria
i. Topical sunscreens and hydroxyzine (Vistaril) for solar urticaria

XIV. BENIGN CONDITIONS

A. *Acne*

1. Overview

a. Androgenically stimulated, inflammatory disorder of sebaceous glands resulting in comedones, papules, inflammatory pustules, cysts, and occasional scarring; acne cannot occur without a hair follicle
b. Has many causes including increased sebum production, abnormal keratinization of follicular epithelium, proliferation of *propionibacterium acnes*, and inflammation
c. Rate of sebum production is determined genetically and is increased by presence of androgens; earliest changes in acne may be seen in prepubescent years

2. Data collection

a. Lesions may occur on forehead, cheeks, nose, and may extend over central back and chest
b. Presence of closed comedones (whiteheads) and open comedones (blackheads)
c. Nodules or papules, pustules, with or without redness and edema, scars
d. Grades of acne (see Box 58–2)

3. Therapeutic management

a. Is intended to control disease and is not curative
b. Use a gentle antibacterial soap and wash affected areas with fingertips
c. Avoid cosmetics containing oil and use moisturizing lotions only on dry patches of skin
d. Instruct not to pick lesions, which would increase scarring
e. Six to eight weeks of treatment is usual before obvious improvement occurs
f. Explain that diet does not cause acne
g. Stress-management if acne flares with stress

Box 58-2

Stages and Grades of Acne

Stages of Acne

Mild: few to several papules, no nodules, on face and neck only

Moderate: several papules to many papules and pustules; few to several nodules on face, back, chest, or upper arms

Severe: numerous and extensive papules and pustules; many nodules with acne-induced scarring

Grades of Acne

Grade 1: comedonal—closed and open

Grade 2: papular—over 25 lesions on face and trunk

Grade 3: pustular—over 25 lesions with mild scarring

Grade 4: nodulocystic—inflammatory nodules and cysts with extensive scarring

NCLEX® h. Topical retinoids are usually prescribed for all types of acne

i. For mild acne, combination therapy of a topical retinoid plus one or more of the following: benzoyl peroxide, topical antibiotics, or azelaic acid

j. For moderate acne, topical agents and oral antibiotics such as tetracycline for a specified period of time and then antibiotic is discontinued

k. For severe acne, isotretinoin (Accutane) may be prescribed for up to 20 weeks

l. Antiandrogens such as birth control pills and spironolactone inhibit sebum production

B. Lentigo

1. Overview

a. A brown macule resembling a freckle except that border is usually irregular

b. Benign lentigo resembles a freckle; lentigo maligna (premelanoma) is a brown or black mottled, irregularly outlined, slowly enlarging lesion with an increased number of scattered atypical melanocytes; it usually occurs on face; one third progress to melanoma but transition may take 10–15 years

c. Senile lentigo (liver spot) occurs on exposed skin of older white individuals

2. Data collection

a. Benign lentigo: freckle, pigmented, flat, or slightly elevated macule

b. Lentigo maligna: brown/black uneven macule with irregular border which slowly extends

c. Senile lentigo: pigmented flat areas usually on sun-exposed areas

3. Therapeutic management

NCLEX® a. Ask client to report changes in existing skin lesions; these need evaluation by a health care provider

b. Explain to inspect skin routinely and seek professional advice for changes

NCLEX® c. Remind clients to use sunscreens, hats, and protective clothing when out in sun to avoid overexposure

d. No medication needed for lentigo

e. Lentigo maligna: follow-up by a dermatologist is recommended

C. Seborrheic keratosis

1. Overview

a. Benign plaques, beige to brown or even black in color, ranging in diameter from 3–20 mm with a velvety or warty surface

b. Involves proliferation of immature keratinocytes and melanocytes totally within dermis; it affects mainly males 30 years and older

2. Data collection

a. "Stuck-on" brown spots that may bleed when irritated by clothing or picked; usually present on face, neck, scalp, back, and trunk

b. Size varies from 1–3 cm; may be skin-colored, tan, brown, or black and are usually oval-shaped with a warty, greasy feel

3. Therapeutic management

a. Use sunscreens, decrease sun exposure, and avoid tanning; wear hats when outdoors

NCLEX® b. Reinforce ABCD of skin lesions that indicate need for evaluation by a health care provider

c. No medications indicated for seborrheic keratosis

d. May be removed by electrocautery or frozen with liquid nitrogen; the area may be hypopigmented after removal

D. *Vitiligo*

1. Overview
   a. Totally white macules with an absence of melanocytes
   b. An acquired, slowly progressive depigmentation in small or large areas of skin caused by a decrease in active melanocytes
   c. Type A: nondermatomal and widespread involvement in 75% of cases
   d. Type B: dermatomal and segmental; 50% of cases begin between ages 10 to 30
2. Data collection
   a. Loss of pigment with increased sunburning of areas; more often occurs around eyes, mouth, and anus
   b. May be pruritic and associated with premature graying
3. Therapeutic management
   a. Avoid sun exposure, which may increase differentiation between normal and abnormal skin
   b. Skin dyes/cosmetics for blending purposes
   c. Localized areas treated with midpotency corticosteroids
   d. Oral systemic corticosteroids are effective in arresting disease progression
   e. Depigmenting of normal skin with hydroquinone cream (Melanex)

XV. PRESSURE ULCERS

A. Overview

1. Ischemic lesions of skin and underlying tissue caused by external pressure that impairs flow of blood and lymph
2. A common and serious complication affecting frail, disabled, acutely ill, or immobile clients
3. Most common sites are over bony prominences, such as elbows, hips, heels, outer ankles, and base of spine; over 95% of ulcers develop on lower part of body
4. Causes include an uneven application of pressure over a bony site: high pressure applied for 2 hours (produces irreversible tissue ischemia and necrosis), shearing forces that develop when a client slides toward floor or foot of bed, frictional forces that develop when pulling a client across a bed sheet, and moisture from incontinence or perspiration

B. Data collection

1. *NCLEX®* Stage pressure ulcers according to their characteristics; see Box 58–3
2. *NCLEX®* Monitor for risk factors (see Box 58–4)
3. Monitor ulcer routinely for location, dimensions, stage, exudate, visible necrotic tissue, or abnormal pathways in wound (sinus tract, tunneling, undermining)
4. Diagnostic and laboratory test findings: culture of wound, WBC with differential and sedimentation rate to diagnose primary or secondary infection; if no progression of ulcer, albumin levels may be obtained to determine dietary needs

C. Therapeutic management

1. *NCLEX®* Reposition client every 2 hours
2. *NCLEX®* Provide relief of pressure on wound; use support devices such as padding (gel pads), flotation pads, mattress overlays, and specialized (such as air-fluidized, oscillating, or kinetic) beds as indicated
3. Perform passive range of motion (ROM) and encourage active ROM exercises
4. *NCLEX®* Improve overall nutritional status—adequate protein intake; encourage oral high-calorie and high-protein supplements and oral zinc, vitamins A and C, and iron to aid in tissue healing
5. Clean wound with each dressing change to remove dead tissue, excess fluid, and debris; monitor healing and document
6. Maintain body temperature and acidic pH

Box 58–3

Pressure Ulcer Stages

Stage 1: Nonblanching erythema, warmth, and tenderness

Stage 2: Skin breakdown limited to dermis, excoriation, blistering, drainage, more sharply defined erythema, variable skin temperature, local swelling, and edema

Stage 3: Ulcer formation into subcutaneous tissues, crater formation, slough, eschar, and/or drainage

Stage 4: Ulcers extend beyond deep fascia into muscle or bone, decayed area may be larger than visible wound, osteomyelitis or sepsis may be present, granulation tissue and epithelialization may be present at wound margins

Box 58-4

Risk Factors for Pressure Ulcers

Immobility
Malnutrition, hypoalbuminemia, or vitamin C deficiency
Low body weight
Fecal and/or urinary incontinence
Bone fracture
Low diastolic blood pressure
Age-related skin changes such as diminished pain perception, thinning of epidermis, loss of dermal vessels, and altered barrier properties
Reduced immunity and slowed wound healing
Disorders such as anemia, infections, peripheral vascular insufficiency, dementia, malignancies, diabetes mellitus, or cerebrovascular accident (CVA)
Dry skin
Edema

7. Never use antiseptics and harsh skin cleansers that may harm tissue; provide gentle but thorough skin care and avoid drying
8. Avoid agents that delay wound healing such as topical corticosteroids, hydrogen peroxide, povidone iodine, and hypochlorite
9. Control fecal and urine incontinence; use a moisture barrier on skin
10. Avoid massage over bony prominences
11. *NCLEX®* Inspect site every 8–12 hours; carefully document healing (e.g., "healing stage III ulcer" rather than "stage II ulcer" if ulcer was stage III and exhibits healing)
12. *NCLEX®* Use appropriate type of dressing, which may include hydrocolloid, alginate, hydrofibers, hydrogel, transparent adhesive, wet-to-moist, or vacuum assisted closure

D. Medication therapy

1. Clindamycin (Cleocin) or gentamycin (Garamycin) may be ordered for complications such as cellulitis, osteomyelitis, or sepsis
2. Vitamin C 500 mg twice daily and zinc sulfate supplements aid healing
3. Antibiotic prophylaxis will eradicate bacterial component
4. A 2-week trial of topical antimicrobials should be used only for a clean, superficial ulcer that is either not healing or is producing a moderate amount of exudates—cultures are necessary to determine whether antifungal or specific antibacterial agents are indicated
5. *NCLEX®* Enzymatic debriding agents such as collagenase (Santyl, Granulex), fibinolysin-desoxyribonuclease (Elase), or sutilains (Travase) are used with a moisture barrier to protect surrounding tissue

E. Reinforce client teaching

1. Need for frequent evaluation of clients with a history of pressure ulcers, especially if they have limited mobility
2. Nutritional requirements (adequate protein, vitamins, minerals, and calories) and meal planning
3. Early identification of skin redness to prevent breakdown
4. Skin cleansing routine
5. Underpads to absorb moisture
6. Repositioning techniques and frequency
7. Need to evaluate and ensure continence and access to bathroom facilities
8. Use of pressure relief devices such as mattress overlays, seat cushions or special mattresses
9. Ways to avoid injuries

XVI. BURN INJURY

A. Overview

1. A break in skin integrity leading to tissue loss or injury caused by heat, chemicals, electricity, or radiation
2. *NCLEX®* Types of burn injury: thermal, chemical, electrical, and radiation
   a. Thermal burn (most common): results from dry heat (flames) or moist heat (steam or hot liquids); causes cell destruction that results in vascular, bony, muscle, or nerve complications; can also lead to inhalation injury if head and neck area is affected

b. Chemical burn: caused by direct contact with either acidic or alkaline agents; alters tissue perfusion and leads to necrosis

c. Electrical burn: severity depends on type and duration of current and amount of voltage; electricity follows path of least resistance (muscles, bone, blood vessels, and nerves); sources of electrical injury include direct current, alternating current, and lightning

d. Radiation burn: usually associated with sunburn or radiation treatment for cancer; usually superficial; extensive exposure to radiation may lead to tissue damage and multisystem injury

B. Emergent/resuscitative phase: lasts from onset of injury through successful fluid resuscitation; during this phase, it is determined whether client requires care in a burn center based on onset of injury, burn source, and complicating factors

NCLEX® 1. Classification of burn depth: made according to depth of damaged tissue (Table 58–1)

NCLEX® 2. An estimate of burn size is calculated using Rule of Nines (see Figure 58–3) or Lund and Browder method; each chart accounts for 100% of total body surface area (TBSA), although Lund and Browder method takes into account client's age when estimating body surface area

Table 58–1 Classification of Burn Injury by Depth of Burn

Superficial thickness (formerly first-degree)	Involves epidermis only and is recognized by characteristics of erythema, absence of blisters for 24 hours, local pain; healing occurs spontaneously in 3 to 5 days with no scar formation
Superficial partial thickness (formerly second-degree)	Involves epidermis and dermis, characterized by moist areas that are red to ivory white in color, blisters form immediately; area is painful because touch and pain receptors are intact; area heals with greater or lesser amounts of scarring within 21 to 28 days
Deep partial thickness (formerly second-degree)	Involves possibly entire layer of dermis and is more severe than a superficial partial-thickness burn; skin appendages are left intact; area has a dry, waxy, whitish appearance and may be difficult to differentiate initially from full-thickness burns; may heal spontaneously in about 1 month, although skin grafting is often done to close wound, accelerate healing, and reduce scarring and risk of infection
Full thickness (formerly third- or fourth-degree)	Involves destruction of all skin elements with coagulation of subdermal plexus; muscle and tendons may be involved

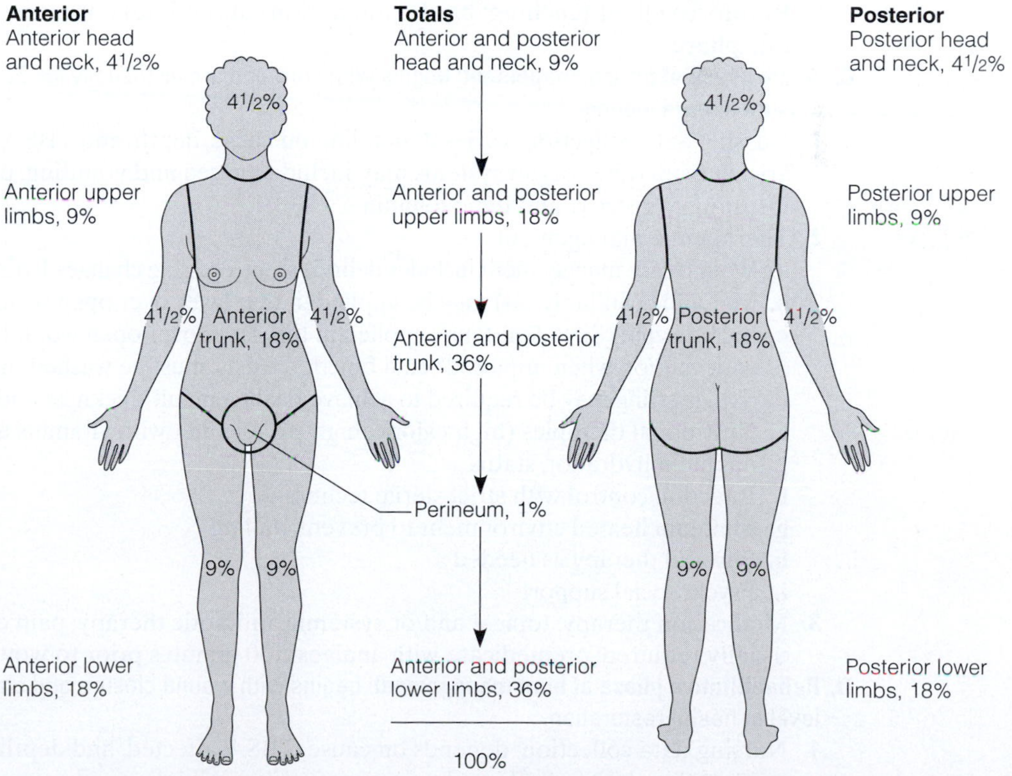

Figure 58–3

Calculating burn injury using the Rule of Nines.

3. Severity of burn is classified using American Burn Association criteria as minor burn, moderate uncomplicated burn, and major burn; these categories help determine treatment
   a. Burns of hands, feet, face, and perineum are at higher risk for functional impairment
   NCLEX® b. Circumferential burns (surrounding an extremity or trunk) are considered major burns
NCLEX® 4. Nursing data collection: history of injury, estimate burn extent and depth, past medical history and medication history including date of last tetanus prophylaxis; note other concurrent injuries
NCLEX® 5. Systemic effects of severe burns include asphyxia from smoke inhalation that causes edema of respiratory passages; shock from fluid shifts; renal failure from shock; protein loss from open wound; potassium excess from tissue destruction and renal failure
NCLEX® 6. Diagnostic and laboratory test findings: may have elevated hematocrit (Hct) and decreased hemoglobin (Hgb) caused by fluid shift, decreased sodium (Na^+) and increased potassium (K^+) caused by damage to capillary and cell membranes, elevated BUN and creatinine caused by dehydration, myoglobin in urine, and possible deterioration of arterial blood gases (ABGs) and oxygen (O_2) saturation readings depending on respiratory status
7. Therapeutic management
   NCLEX® a. First aid: douse flames with water or smother with a blanket, coat, or other similar object; cool a scald burn with cool water; flush chemical burns copiously with water or other appropriate irrigant after dusting away any dry powder if present; remove client from contact with an electrical source only after current has been shut off
   NCLEX® b. Priority care is on ABCs: airway, breathing, and circulation; observe for smoke inhalation injury (singed nares, eyebrows or lashes; burns on face or neck; stridor, increasing dyspnea) and give O_2 (up to 100% as prescribed), being prepared for possible intubation and mechanical ventilation if severe inhalation injury or carbon monoxide inhalation has occurred; monitor for signs of shock caused by fluid shifts (decreased urine output, increased pulse, falling BP, pallor, cool clammy skin, deteriorating level of consciousness [LOC])
   NCLEX® c. Fluid resuscitation: Brooke formula uses 2 mL/kg/% TBSA burned (3/4 crystalloid plus 1/4 colloid) plus maintenance fluid of 2000 mL D_5W per 24 hours; Parkland (Baxter) formula uses 4 mL/kg/% TBSA burned per 24 hours (crystalloid only—lactated Ringer's); both formulas give half of 24-hour total in first 8 hours and second half over next 16 hours
   d. Other considerations: remove all rings and jewelry to avoid tourniquet effect from swelling of burn site; provide cardiac monitoring for first 24 hours after an electrical burn
NCLEX® 8. Medication therapy: analgesics—usually morphine sulfate IV, tetanus booster (> 5–10 years since last dose), topical antimicrobials, systemic antibiotics
9. Reinforce client teaching: brief explanations about injury, treatments, and ongoing nursing care in this phase

C. Acute phase of burn management: begins with start of diuresis (usually 48–72 hours postburn) and ends with closure of burn wound

1. Nursing data collection: varies depending on cause, depth, and TBSA of burn; associated symptoms arising from other organ systems may include nausea and vomiting, pain, skin redness, chills, respiratory distress, and hypovolemia
NCLEX® 2. Therapeutic management
   a. Wound care management includes debridement, dressing changes, hydrotherapy, and possible escharotomy
   b. Mafenide (Sulfamylon) may be applied in thin layer over open wound and covered with dressing
   c. Sulfadiazine (Silvadene) may applied in thin layer over open wound and covered with dressing; use with caution when impaired renal function exists; must be washed off and reapplied every 8 to 12 hours
   d. Skin grafting may be required to achieve healing in full-thickness and large, deep partial-thickness burns
   e. Nutritional therapies (high-calorie, high-protein diet with vitamins and minerals) and continue to maintain hydration status
   f. Infection control with strict sterile technique
   g. Maintain heated environment to prevent chilling
   h. Physical therapy as needed
   i. Psychosocial support
3. Medication therapy: topical and/or systemic antibiotic therapy; pain control with opioid analgesics is usually required; premedicate with analgesic 30 minutes prior to wound care

D. Rehabilitative phase of burn management: begins with wound closure and ends when client returns to highest level of health restoration

1. Nursing data collection: depends on cause, TBSA affected, and depth; may have immobility or restricted mobility of affected area; scarring is possible

2. Therapeutic management
   a. Obtain psychosocial evaluation; provide support and management; arrange counseling if necessary
   NCLEX® b. Prevent immobility contractures with exercises or ongoing physical therapy
   c. Assist in returning to work, family, and social life
   d. Use preventative measures for scar formation (such as burn garments)
   e. Review home environment for needs and accessibility
3. Medication therapy: ongoing pain management and antibiotic therapy as necessary
4. Reinforce client teaching
   NCLEX® a. Environmental safety: use low temperature setting for hot water heater, ensure access to and adequate number of electrical cords/outlets, isolate household chemicals, avoid smoking in bed
   b. Use of household smoke detectors with emphasis on maintenance, especially battery replacement
   c. Proper storage and use of flammable substances
   d. Evacuation plan for family
   e. Care of burn at home
   f. Signs and symptoms of infection
   g. How to identify risk of skin changes
   NCLEX® h. Use of sunscreen to protect healing tissue and other protective skin care measures

Check Your NCLEX-PN® Exam I.Q.

You are ready for testing on this content if you can

- Identify basic structures and functions of the integumentary system.
- Describe the pathophysiology and etiology of common integumentary disorders.
- Discuss expected data and diagnostic test findings for selected integumentary disorders.
- Discuss therapeutic management of a client experiencing an integumentary disorder.
- Discuss nursing management of a client experiencing an integumentary disorder.
- Identify expected outcomes for the client experiencing an integumentarydisorder.

PRACTICE TEST

1 A nurse is assisting with teaching a group of young adults about skin lesions. Which item would be appropriate to include in discussions with these clients? Select all that apply.

1. Benefits of sun tanning
2. Importance of monthly skin self-inspection
3. Examination of skin lesions using the ABCD method
4. Need to seek professional advice regarding lesions
5. Use of sunscreen with an SPF of 8 or higher

2 A client with psoriasis has a follow-up visit with the health care provider. The nurse concludes that the client is receiving first-line therapy after seeing a medical record notation for which treatments? Select all that apply.

1. An emollient
2. Phototherapy
3. Topical corticosteroid
4. Methotrexate
5. Dermabrasion

3 The health care provider documents in a client record that the adolescent has closed comedones. The nurse explains to the client that this means the lesions are what type of skin eruption?

1. Whiteheads
2. Blackheads
3. Pustules
4. Cysts

4 The nurse determines that the clinical management of seborrheic keratosis is understood when the client explains the use of which therapy? Select all that apply.

1. Antibiotics
2. Antifungal creams
3. Liquid nitrogen
4. Corticosteroids
5. Electrocautery

5 A client with contact dermatitis asks the nurse how the condition could have developed. Which etiology should the nurse include in a response to the client?

1. Allergic reaction mediated by IgE
2. Poor hygiene
3. Reactivation of IgA antibodies
4. Side effect of oral medication

6 When explaining the disorder to a client with tinea corporis, the nurse should include which information about this skin disorder?

1. It requires no treatment.
2. It can be passed human to human.
3. It should be exposed to sunlight.
4. It is a malignant skin condition.

7 A client with burn injury asks the nurse what the term "full thickness" means. The nurse should respond that burns classified as full thickness involve tissue destruction down to which level?

1. Epidermis
2. Subcutaneous tissue
3. Internal organs
4. Dermis

8 The client comes to the office for a skin rash. Which question would the nurse include when obtaining a client history?

1. "Have you ever had a skin rash like this before?"
2. "Do you smoke?"
3. "How long have you had that mole on your left arm?"
4. "Do you have a family history of skin cancer?"

9 The nurse is examining the client's skin. What technique can the nurse perform to evaluate a site for petechiae?

1. Rub the site and watch for bleeding
2. Apply pressure to the site to monitor for blanching of the skin
3. Look for other lesions that are similar to that lesion
4. Apply a tourniquet in a limb and watch for the development of petechiae

10 A client has been diagnosed with eczema. Which statement made by the client indicates an understanding of its management?

1. "I will avoid excessive use of soap and water and keep my skin well-hydrated with emollients."
2. "I will take daily baths and use strong antibacterial soaps to prevent skin infections."
3. "I will make sure to expose my skin to the sun at least 1 hour a day."
4. "I will wait 3 hours after bathing to apply lotion to my skin."

11 The nurse should reinforce which instruction when teaching a client measures to reduce the risk of developing basal cell carcinoma?

1. Limit use of tanning beds.
2. Use sunscreen with SPF protection of 15 or higher when in the sun.
3. Limit exposure of skin to the sun to between the hours of 10 a.m. and 2 p.m.
4. Eat a balanced diet as the most important means of preventing skin cancer.

12 The client with cellulitis is being discharged from the hospital. What statement should the nurse include in discharge instructions to the client?

1. "If pustules develop, squeeze the lesions gently each day to remove the pus."
2. "If the lesion looks healed, stop taking the antibiotic so you will not develop resistance."
3. "Monitor for signs of infection such as fever, chills, malaise, and redness or tenderness at the site."
4. "Drainage from the site is an expected finding and is no cause for concern."

13 Which nursing diagnosis is a priority for a client experiencing cellulitis of the arm?

1. Disturbed Sleep Pattern related to skin infection
2. Social Isolation related to skin infection
3. Powerlessness related to inability to control the infection
4. Pain related to skin infection

---

14 The client receives a prescription to treat a skin condition affecting the scalp and neck. The medications prescribed are coal tar shampoo and topical steroids. The nurse concludes that this client has which probable diagnosis?

1. Folliculitis
2. Cellulitis
3. Psoriasis
4. Furuncles

---

15 A client has just been diagnosed with herpes simplex virus Type 2. The nurse should share with the client which item of information?

1. "The initial outbreak of herpes is often the most uncomfortable. Recurrent infections usually present with a tingling and burning sensation prior to outbreak of the vesicle."
2. "Each outbreak of herpes is uncomfortable, with the amount of pain at the genital area worsening each time."
3. "You can only have one outbreak of herpes, so you will never experience another."
4. "You should never experience discomfort with herpes; thus, if you have pain in the genital area, you probably have a sexually transmitted infection."

---

16 A client presents for removal of a skin lesion after it is determined that it meets all four criteria for removal according to the ABCD rule. The nurse interprets this to mean which of the following?

1. The lesion is symmetrical, with a smooth border, a single color, and the diameter has stayed the same.
2. The lesion is symmetrical with an irregular border, a single color, and the diameter has increased.
3. The lesion is asymmetrical with a regular border, two colors, and the diameter is smaller.
4. The lesion is asymmetrical with an irregular border, two colors, and has increased in diameter.

---

17 The nurse examining the skin of a client notes vascular skin lesions that are flat, bright red in color, with tiny vessels that radiate out from its center. The nurse concludes that the lesions are probably which of the following?

1. Petechiae
2. Spider angiomas
3. Venous stars
4. Port wine stains

---

18 A client presents on admission with pressure ulcers extending into the bone. The nurse documents this ulcer at stage ____. Provide a numerical answer.

Fill in your answer below:

Stage _______

---

19 A child was admitted to the emergency department with a thermal burn to the right arm and leg. Which data collected by the nurse requires immediate action?

1. Coughing and wheezing
2. Bright red skin with small blisters on the burn sites
3. Thirst
4. Singed hair

---

20 A school-age child develops atopic dermatitis secondary to food allergies. An appropriate nursing diagnosis for this child would be which of the following?

1. Imbalanced Nutrition: Less Than Body Requirements
2. Disturbed Body Image
3. Risk for Ineffective Thermoregulation
4. Impaired Tissue Perfusion

21. An infant has a positive family history of allergies. To reduce the risk of the infant developing eczema, the nurse reinforces teaching to the family to do which of the following?

1. Avoid synthetic clothing—use natural fibers like cotton and wool.
2. Keep up with the schedule of childhood immunizations.
3. Avoid contact with infected personnel.
4. Introduce only one new food a week so food allergies can be recognized and eliminated.

22. The parents of an 18-month-old with eczema are concerned that a secondary infection that has developed will permanently disfigure their child. How can the nurse best support the parent's feelings?

1. Divert the conversation to another topic.
2. Let them know that they are not being blamed for their feelings.
3. Encourage them to discuss their fears and concerns.
4. Tell them not to worry because scarring is unlikely with eczema.

23. A parent of a child with a full thickness burn asks why the nurse keeps spreading "that white cream" on the child's burns. The nurse explains that the cream is mafenide (Sulfamylon), which is being applied to the burned area for which reason?

1. Lubricant that will keep the area well hydrated.
2. Topical antibiotic that inhibits infection.
3. Tissue hormone that stimulates new tissue growth.
4. Steroid that reduces edema at the site.

24. A child has been diagnosed with scabies. The nurse reinforces to the parents that, in addition to 5% permethrin lotion, appropriate medical therapy for this child would include which of the following? Select all that apply.

1. Antihistamines
2. Narcotic analgesics
3. Non-steroidal anti-inflammatory drugs (NSAIDs)
4. Antibiotics
5. Scabicides

25. The nurse is providing home care instructions for a family with a toddler diagnosed with lice. The nurse reinforces which instructions when teaching? Select all that apply.

1. Immerse combs and brushes in boiling water for 30 minutes to kill lice.
2. Vacuum floor and furniture to remove hair that might have live nits.
3. Use a bright light and magnifying glass to check the hair for lice.
4. Launder bedding and clothing in hot water with detergent and dry in a hot dryer for 20 minutes.
5. Instruct children to not share combs, brushes, and hats.

ANSWERS & RATIONALES

1 **Answer: 2, 3, 4** **Rationale:** Monthly skin inspection will aid in detecting skin lesions. Examining skin lesions for asymmetry, border, color, and diameter is important to help detect early changes consistent with skin cancer. Health professionals can accurately diagnose skin conditions as well as determine which ones are benign versus cancerous. Tanning and sun exposure can increase susceptibility to skin cancers. For best protection against ultraviolet light rays, sunscreens should have an SPF factor of 15 or higher. **Cognitive Level:** Applying **Client Need:** Health Promotion and Maintenance **Integrated Process:** Teaching and Learning **Content Area:** Adult Health **Strategy:** The wording of the question tells you that more than one option is likely to be correct. Use the process of elimination and knowledge about prevention and monitoring of skin lesions to evaluate each option.

2 **Answer: 1, 2, 3** **Rationale:** Emollients, phototherapy, and topical corticosteroids are first-line treatments for psoriasis. Methotrexate is used for severe and nonresponsive cases of psoriasis; it is not a first-line form of therapy. Dermabrasion is not a treatment used for psoriasis. **Cognitive Level:** Applying **Client Need:** Physiological Adaptation **Integrated Process:** Communication and Documentation **Content Area:** Adult Health **Strategy:** The core issue of the question is knowledge of the sequence of treatments for psoriasis. The wording of the question tells you that more than one option is likely to be correct. Use the process of elimination and nursing knowledge to make a selection.

3 **Answer: 1** **Rationale:** Whiteheads are classified as closed comedones. Blackheads are open comedones. Pustules are a type of primary skin lesion. Cysts are fluid-filled lesions. **Cognitive Level:** Applying **Client Need:** Physiological Adaptation **Integrated Process:** Nursing Process: Data Collection **Content Area:** Child Health **Strategy:** The core issue of the question is knowledge of various skin eruptions. The wording of the question tells you that the correct response is also a true statement of fact. Use the process of elimination and nursing knowledge to make a selection.

4 **Answer: 3, 5** **Rationale:** No medications are indicated for treatment of seborrheic keratosis. The lesions of seborrheic keratosis may be removed with liquid nitrogen or electrocautery. **Cognitive Level:** Applying **Client Need:** Physiological Adaptation **Integrated Process:** Teaching and Learning **Content Area:** Adult Health **Strategy:** The core issue of the question is knowledge of treatments for seborrheic keratosis. The wording of the question tells you that more than one option is likely to be correct. Use the process of elimination and nursing knowledge to make a selection.

5 **Answer: 1** **Rationale:** Contact dermatitis is an inflammatory response of the skin following prior sensitization to an antigen with production of a specific IgE antibody. Skin manifestations occur with subsequent exposures. Contact dermatitis is not caused by poor hygiene, reactivation of IgA antibodies, or as a side effect of an oral medication. **Cognitive Level:** Applying **Client Need:** Physiological Adaptation **Integrated Process:** Nursing Process: Data Collection **Content Area:** Adult Health **Strategy:** The core issue of the question is the ability to correctly describe contact dermatitis. The wording of the question tells you the correct answer is also a true statement. Use the process of elimination and nursing knowledge to make a selection.

6 **Answer: 2** **Rationale:** Fungal infections such as tinea corporis may be transmitted by direct contact with animals and other persons. Tinea corporis does require treatment. Tinea corporis is not treatable by sunlight. Tinea corporis is not malignant. **Cognitive Level:** Applying **Client Need:** Physiological Adaptation **Integrated Process:** Nursing Process: Implementation **Content Area:** Adult Health **Strategy:** The core issue of the question is knowledge of the characteristics of infection with tinea corporis. The wording of the question tells you the correct statement is the correct answer. Use the process of elimination and nursing knowledge to make a selection.

7 **Answer: 2** **Rationale:** A full-thickness burn involves all skin layers, including the epidermis and dermis, and may extend into the subcutaneous tissue and fat; it does not involve internal organs. **Cognitive Level:** Applying **Client Need:** Physiological Adaptation **Integrated Process:** Nursing Process: Implementation **Content Area:** Adult Health **Strategy:** The core issue of the question is knowledge of the various depths of burn injury. The critical words *down to* indicate that the correct option is the deepest level of involvement possible. Use the process of elimination and nursing knowledge to make a selection.

8 **Answer: 1** **Rationale:** The most important questions would be aimed at obtaining information about the chief complaint, which in this case is the skin rash. Questions about smoking involve general health and could be asked at a later time. Questions about a skin mole involve a different skin condition and could be asked at a later time. Although important for general health screening, family history of skin cancer is unrelated to the current skin problem. **Cognitive Level:** Applying **Client Need:** Physiological Adaptation **Integrated Process:** Nursing Process: Data Collection **Content Area:** Adult Health **Strategy:** The issue of the question is appropriate questions to ask when obtaining a nursing history about a skin disorder. The wording of the question tells you the correct statement is the correct answer. Use the process of elimination and knowledge of data collection to make a selection.

9 **Answer: 2** **Rationale:** When monitoring for petechiae, pressure is applied to the site but will not produce blanching of the skin. For other types of lesions, blanching may occur. The site should not be rubbed to try to elicit bleeding. Identifying similar lesions will not aid in monitoring current petechiae. Tourniquets interrupt arterial and venous circulation and are not used to monitor for petechiae. **Cognitive Level:** Applying **Client Need:** Physiological Adaptation **Integrated Process:** Nursing Process: Data Collection **Content Area:** Adult Health **Strategy:** The issue of the question is knowledge of data collection techniques for the skin. The wording of the question tells you the correct statement is the correct answer. Use the process of elimination and nursing knowledge to make a selection.

10 **Answer: 1** **Rationale:** Skin care for eczema should include keeping the skin well hydrated, which is aided by the use of emollients. The client should avoid using harsh soaps. Sun exposure will not aid in keeping skin hydrated and could exert a drying effect. Emollients should be applied immediately after bathing. **Cognitive Level:** Applying **Client Need:** Physiological Adaptation **Integrated Process:** Teaching and Learning **Content Area:** Adult Health **Strategy:** The core issue of the question is knowledge of appropriate care to the skin when the client has eczema. The wording of the question tells you the answer is a true statement. Use the process of elimination and nursing knowledge to make a selection.

11 **Answer: 2** **Rationale:** Protecting the skin with sunscreen SPF 15 or higher, along with avoiding the sun during the peak hours of 10:00 a.m. to 2:00 p.m. is recommended to help prevent basal cell carcinoma. Avoiding the use of tanning beds is recommended to help prevent basal cell carcinoma. While a balanced diet is important for general health, other factors such as ionizing radiation play a key role in development of basal cell carcinoma. **Cognitive Level:** Applying **Client Need:** Health Promotion and Maintenance **Integrated Process:** Nursing Process: Implementation **Content Area:** Adult Health **Strategy:** The core issue of the question is knowledge of behaviors that can reduce the risk of developing basal cell carcinoma. The wording of the question tells you the correct option is a true statement. Use the process of elimination and nursing knowledge to make a selection.

12 **Answer: 3** **Rationale:** Infection may be manifested by fever, chills, malaise, erythema, and tenderness at the site. Squeezing pustules is not recommended. Antibiotics should be taken for the full prescribed course of therapy. Infection may be manifested by drainage at the site, especially if it is cloudy. The physician must be notified if signs of infection occur. **Cognitive Level:** Applying **Client Need:** Physiological Adaptation **Integrated Process:** Nursing Process: Implementation **Content Area:** Adult Health **Strategy:** The core issue of the question is recognition of signs of infection that are important to note after being treated for cellulitis. The wording of the question tells you the correct option is a true statement. Use the process of elimination and nursing knowledge to make a selection.

13 **Answer: 4** **Rationale:** Clients with cellulitis experience pain at the local site. Controlling the pain is the priority nursing diagnosis for this client. The client's sleep may be disturbed by pain but this would not be the priority nursing diagnosis. There is insufficient information to determine whether the client is experiencing social isolation. Cellulitis can be treated with appropriate antibiotic therapy. **Cognitive Level:** Analyzing **Client Need:** Physiological Adaptation **Integrated Process:** Nursing Process: Data Collection **Content Area:** Adult Health **Strategy:** Recall that pain relief is high priority for many clients and is included in the physiological needs on Maslow's hierarchy. Use the

process of elimination and nursing knowledge to make a selection, considering that physiological needs take priority over psychosocial needs in most cases.

14 **Answer: 3** **Rationale:** Current treatments for psoriasis include coal tar shampoo and topical steroids. Folliculitis, cellulitis, and furuncles are bacterial infections of the skin and would be treated with antimicrobial therapy. **Cognitive Level:** Analyzing **Client Need:** Physiological Adaptation **Integrated Process:** Nursing Process: Implementation **Content Area:** Adult Health **Strategy:** The core issue of the question is knowledge of the uses of medication therapy for psoriasis. The wording of the question tells you the correct option is a true statement. Use the process of elimination and nursing knowledge to make a selection.

15 **Answer: 1** **Rationale:** The initial outbreak of herpes is the most uncomfortable or painful. Recurrent episodes present with a prodrome of symptoms, such as tingling and burning. The pain of herpes does not increase over time. Repeated episodes may occur during periods of stress. Herpes is characterized by discomfort with each outbreak. **Cognitive Level:** Applying **Client Need:** Physiological Adaptation **Integrated Process:** Nursing Process: Implementation **Content Area:** Adult Health **Strategy:** The core issue of the question is knowledge of the characteristics and presentation of this type of viral infection. The wording of the question tells you the correct option is a true statement. Recall that the first outbreak is the most severe to make a selection.

16 **Answer: 4** **Rationale:** To meet all four criteria for removal of a lesion, the lesion will be asymmetrical (A) with an irregular border (B), have color change or more than one color (C), along with an increased diameter (D). **Cognitive Level:** Applying **Client Need:** Physiological Adaptation **Integrated Process:** Nursing Process: Data Collection **Content Area:** Adult Health **Strategy:** The core issue of the question is knowledge of criteria that determine the need to remove a skin lesion. The wording of the question tells you the correct option is a true statement. Use the process of elimination and nursing knowledge to make a selection.

17 **Answer: 2** **Rationale:** Spider angiomas are red lesions with vessels radiating from the center. Petechiae appear as red "freckles" or dots. A venous star is a flat blue lesion with radiating linear veins. A port wine stain is a flat, irregular-shaped lesion that does not have radiating vessels. **Cognitive Level:** Applying **Client Need:** Physiological Adaptation **Integrated Process:** Nursing Process: Data Collection **Content Area:** Adult Health **Strategy:** The core issue of the question is knowledge of various types of skin lesions. The wording of the question tells you the correct option is a true statement. Use the process of elimination and nursing knowledge to make a selection.

18 **Answer: 4** **Rationale:** Stage 4 ulcers result in full-thickness skin loss with extensive damage to the muscle and bone. **Cognitive Level:** Applying **Client Need:** Physiological Adaptation **Integrated Process:** Communication and Documentation **Content Area:** Adult Health **Strategy:** The core issue of the question is knowledge of various stages of ulcer development. The wording of the question guides you to a decision. Use nursing knowledge to supply an answer.

19 **Answer: 1** **Rationale:** Coughing and wheezing may indicate that the child has inhaled smoke or toxic fumes. Maintaining airway patency is the highest nursing priority in this situation. Skin color changes are expected. Thirst may be present but does not require immediate nursing action. Singed hair warrants attention because of the risk of inhalation injury, but is not as high priority as actual respiratory symptoms. **Cognitive Level:** Analyzing **Client Need:** Physiological Adaptation **Integrated Process:** Nursing Process: Data Collection **Content Area:** Child Health **Strategy:** The core issue of the question is the ability to determine that the client's airway could be in jeopardy. Use the ABCs whenever a question deals with burn injury as a first method to determine priority setting.

20 **Answer: 2** **Rationale:** Atopic dermatitis is a chronic inflammatory skin disorder. School-age children are very aware of their own and others' skin appearance. Children with atopic dermatitis will feel different from other children and this may affect their body image. Food allergies do not relate to decreased nutrition. Atopic dermatitis does not affect the skin's ability to maintain temperature. Atopic dermatitis does not affect blood flow to the area. **Cognitive Level:** Analyzing **Client Need:** Psychosocial Integrity **Integrated Process:** Nursing Process: Implementation **Content Area:** Child Health **Strategy:** The core issue of the question is recognition of key concerns of a child with atopic dermatitis. The wording of the question tells you the correct option is a true statement. Use the process of elimination and nursing knowledge to make a selection.

21 **Answer: 4** **Rationale:** Infants with eczema frequently have food sensitivities. Slow introduction of new foods allows the parents to recognize food sensitivities and eliminate the offending item from the diet. The mother is taught to avoid scratchy clothing such as wool. Childhood immunizations would be given as scheduled but do not reduce risk. Eczema is not an infectious disease. Avoiding infectious personnel is appropriate for all children but does not prevent development of eczema. **Cognitive Level:** Applying **Client Need:** Physiological Adaptation **Integrated Process:** Nursing Process: Implementation **Content Area:** Child Health **Strategy:** The core issue of the question is the appropriate client teaching to reinforce to reduce risk of developing eczema. Recall the risk factors and use the process of elimination to make a selection.

22 **Answer: 3** **Rationale:** The nurse should encourage parents to identify and discuss their feelings and concerns. Changing the topic is not therapeutic. Merely not blaming parents does not give them the opportunity to discuss what is important to them. Giving false reassurance by telling them not to worry is inappropriate. **Cognitive Level:** Applying **Client Need:** Psychosocial Integrity **Integrated Process:** Communication and Documentation **Content Area:** Child Health **Strategy:** The core issue of the question is the ability to use basic communication techniques in responding to the concerns of a parent. Choose the option that directly addresses the client's or family's issues and concerns.

23 **Answer: 2** **Rationale:** Sulfamylon is a topical antibiotic that is used on burns to prevent bacteria from infecting the burn site. Sulfamylon is not a lubricant. Sulfamylon is not a tissue hormone. Sulfamylon is not a steroid. **Cognitive Level:** Applying **Client Need:** Pharmacological and Parenteral Therapies **Integrated Process:** Nursing Process: Implementation **Content Area:** Child Health **Strategy:** Knowledge of the actions for the medications used to treat burns will aid in choosing the correct answer.

24 **Answer: 1, 5** **Rationale:** The saliva, ova, and feces of the scabies mite trigger an antigenic response that causes intense pruritus. Scabicides are used to kill the mites causing scabies. Pain is not present so the need of narcotic analgesics is not needed. Pain and inflammation is not present so the need of NSAIDs is not needed. Antibiotics would only be added to the regimen if the itching leads to scratching and breaks in the skin with development of a bacterial infection. **Cognitive Level:** Analyzing **Client Need:** Physiological

Adaptation **Integrated Process:** Nursing Process: Implementation **Content Area:** Child Health **Strategy:** Consider the symptoms of scabies to determine the correct response.

25 **Answer: 2, 3, 4, 5 Rationale:** Live nits can hatch up to 8 to 10 days later, so it is important to remove them from the environment. Each member of the family should be examined so those infested can be treated. Washing and drying on hot settings will be sufficient to kill lice and nits. Sharing of hair care material spreads lice and should be avoided. Soaking combs in a Lysol or anti-lice shampoo mixture will kill lice or nits. **Cognitive Level:** Applying **Client Need:** Safety and Infection Control **Integrated Process:** Teaching and Learning **Content Area:** Child Health **Strategy:** Knowledge of the spread of lice and the home care necessary to prevent reinfestation is necessary to choose the correct answer. Identify those options that are absolutely incorrect first. Then consider the remaining options.

Key Terms to Review

acne p. 1097
actinic keratosis p. 1087
atopic dermatitis (eczema) p. 1086
candidiasis p. 1093
cellulitis p. 1091
contact dermatitis p. 1096
cyst p. 1085
dermis p. 1082
epidermis p. 1082
erythemic p. 1085
lichenification p. 1086
macule p. 1085
nodule p. 1085
papule p. 1085
pediculosis capitis p. 1095
plaque p. 1085
pressure ulcers p. 1099
pruritus p. 1086
pustule p. 1085
scabies p. 1095
urticaria p. 1097
vesicle p. 1085
vitiligo p. 1099
wheal p. 1085

References

Ball, J., Bindler, R., & Cowen, K. (2010). *Child health nursing: Partnering with children and families* (2nd ed.). Upper Saddle River, NJ: Pearson Education.

Berman, A., & Snyder, S. (2012). *Kozier & Erb's fundamentals of nursing: Concepts, process, and practice* (9th ed.). Upper Saddle River, NJ: Pearson Education.

Ignatavicius, D., & Workman, L. (2010). *Medical-surgical nursing: Critical thinking for collaborative care* (6th ed.). Philadelphia: W. B. Saunders.

Kee, J. (2010). *Laboratory and diagnostic tests with nursing implications* (8th ed.). Upper Saddle River, NJ: Pearson Education.

LeMone, P., Burke, K., & Bauldoff, G. (2011). *Medical-surgical nursing: Critical thinking in patient care* (5th ed.). Upper Saddle River, NJ: Pearson Education.

Smith, S., Duell, D.,& Martin, B. (2012). *Clinical nursing skills: Basic to advanced skills* (8th ed.). Upper Saddle River, NJ: Pearson Education.

Test Yourself

Are you ready for the NCLEX-PN® or course exams? Use the practice tests on the companion website to check.

59 Eye, Ear, Nose and Throat Disorders

In this chapter

Cross Reference

Other chapters relevant to this content area are

Eye and Ear Medications	Chapter 40
Common Laboratory Tests	Chapter 42
Common Diagnostic Tests and Procedures	Chapter 43

I. OVERVIEW OF ANATOMY AND PHYSIOLOGY OF EYE AND EAR

A. Eye structures

1. Outer protective layer, also called fibrous coat; consists of sclera and cornea
2. Middle vascular layer, also called uveal tract; contains pigmented iris surrounding pupil, which regulates amount of light entering eye, and ciliary body that surrounds lens and produces aqueous humor to maintain intraocular pressure (IOP) (flows from posterior to anterior chamber and drains into Schlemm's canal); also contains choroid that has blood vessels to supply eye tissues

3. Inner layer, the retina: thin, semitransparent layer containing rods and cones, responsible for vision in dim light and for perception of fine details, respectively

B. Eye functions

1. Eye receives light waves through cornea; waves are refracted by aqueous humor, lens, and vitreous humor as they are transmitted to retina; retinal images formed by light rays are inverted and reversed by biconvex lens
2. Rods and cones of retina translate light waves into neural impulses for relay to optic nerve and then to brain's occipital lobes for interpretation as vision
3. Fusion of images from each eye into a single image is called binocular vision

NCLEX®

C. Age-related changes of eye that affect vision

1. Decreased ability of pupil to dilate, which reduces night vision and increases light needed for reading and small motor tasks, such as sewing
2. Development of **presbyopia**, a decreased elasticity of lens that makes focusing for near vision more difficult and results in farsightedness
3. Lens becomes discolored and opacified, which reduces color perception (especially green, blue, and violet)
4. Decreased eye motility and senile enophthalmos (sinking in) of eyes limits peripheral vision upward, downward, and to sides
5. Degenerative changes to choroid, retina, and optic nerve reduce depth perception and ability to see lines of demarcation (stair edges, doorframes)

D. Ear structures

1. External ear: outer visible ear or auricle and external auditory canal
2. Middle ear: tympanic membrane; malleus, incus, and stapes bones; and window membranes
3. Inner ear: semicircular canals, cochlea, distal portion of cranial nerve VIII (vestibulocochlear nerve)

E. Ear functions

1. Hearing: sound is transferred from tympanic membrane to malleus, incus, and stapes and through cochlea; vibrations are changed by transduction into action potentials that are sent to brain as neural impulses
2. **Proprioception** (balance): sensation about body's position in space is transferred to brain after changes in body position trigger fluid movement and bending of hair cells in vestibular structures

F. Age-related changes of ear that affect hearing

1. External auditory canal narrows; cerumen glands atrophy and produce thicker, drier cerumen
2. Tympanic membrane is less flexible, and ossicle joints calcify
3. Cochlear hair cell degeneration and loss of auditory neurons in organ of Corti lead to **presbycusis**, an age-related sensorineural hearing loss characterized by decreased ability to hear high-frequency sounds; results in difficulty hearing and localizing normal speech

II. DIAGNOSTIC TESTS AND DATA COLLECTION

A. Fluorescein angiography: injection of sodium fluorescein into arm blood vessel (BV), followed by serial imaging to detect disorders in retinal vessels, such as with diabetic retinopathy and eye tumors

1. Preprocedure care
   a. Question for allergies and/or history of reactions to dye
   b. Ensure client has signed consent form
   c. Give prescribed mydriatic medication 1 hour prior to test to dilate pupil

NCLEX®

2. Postprocedure care
   a. Encourage rest and increased fluid intake (aids in dye excretion)
   b. Explain that dye causes temporary skin discoloration in injected area and temporary green discoloration of urine that resolves when dye is fully excreted
   c. Remind client to avoid sunlight or other bright light sources for several hours until pupil dilation returns to normal

B. Corneal staining: instillation of dye into conjunctival sac to highlight irregularities caused by trauma, abrasions, or ulcers; damaged corneal epithelium appears green when viewed through a blue filter

1. Ensure that contact lenses are removed prior to procedure, if worn
2. Tell client to blink to distribute dye evenly over cornea
3. Wipe excess dye from cheeks and instruct client not to rub eyes

C. Tonometry: measurement of IOP to detect glaucoma by determining resistance of eyeball to an applied force

NCLEX®

1. Normal IOP ranges from 12 to 21 mm Hg
2. Eye may be anesthetized, and client stares forward
3. Applanation: most accurate, measures force needed to flatten a small area of cornea; eye is anesthetized

4. Indentation: measures change in form of globe after standard weight (Schiøtz tonometer) is applied to cornea; eye is anesthetized
5. Noncontact: calculates IOP by measuring deflection of a puff of air applied to cornea; no anesthetic needed
6. NCLEX® Tell client not to rub eyes after test if anesthetic was used to avoid possible corneal scratches or injury

D. Physical examination of eye and vision

1. Acuity of distance vision: measures vision using Snellen chart hung 20 feet away
   a. Client reads chart lines with one eye covered, moving downward from row that is most clear to last line that is completely read
   b. Findings are recorded as a fraction: numerator is client's distance from chart (20 feet), and denominator is number identified at end of smallest line read, which corresponds to distance at which normal eye can read that line; normal vision is 20/20; a larger denominator indicates myopia (nearsightedness)
   c. Red and green lines on Snellen chart can provide a quick test of color blindness
2. NCLEX® Acuity of near vision: measures vision using a Rosenbaum chart or a card with newsprint 12 to 14 inches from client's eyes; impairment indicates hyperopia (farsightedness) in a young client or presbyopia in an adult after approximately 45 years of age
3. Refraction test: uses Snellen chart to test visual acuity while client reads through various strengths of corrective lenses; used to prescribe correction for errors with *myopia* (nearsightedness), *hyperopia* (farsightedness), and *astigmatism* (irregularity of corneal surface that inhibits light rays from focusing clearly on retina)
4. NCLEX® Visual fields: measures peripheral vision, often called confrontation test
   a. Client and examiner face each other with client looking into examiner's eyes; both cover own eye on same side
   b. Examiner raises a finger or other small object at arm's length midway between client and examiner, and brings it in from periphery into line of vision; procedure is repeated from above and below on same side
   c. Client states "now" when able to see object; examiner should see object at about same time (test assumes examiner has normal peripheral vision); test is repeated on other eye
5. Color vision
   a. Tested for driver's license, employment requiring color discrimination, or with history of difficulty distinguishing colors; sensitive for red/green blindness, but not for blue
   b. NCLEX® Involves picking colored numbers or letters out of plates with multiple colors in background (such as an Ishihara chart) or noting green and red lines on Snellen chart; results recorded as a fraction of correct identifications divided by total number shown
6. Extraocular muscle movements
   a. Client's eyes follow a small object through six cardinal positions of gaze: to right, upward and right, down and right, left, upward and left, and down and left
   b. NCLEX® Client should have parallel eye movement and absence of **nystagmus**, involuntary rhythmic oscillating eye movements (vertical, horizontal, rotary, or mixed)
   c. As last step, client follows finger as it moves in to bridge of nose; eyes should sustain convergence to within 5–8 centimeters
7. Outer eye structures
   a. Sclera is white in color, although dark-skinned clients may have slight yellow cast or pigmented dots; yellow discoloration (or heightened yellow) can indicate jaundice
   b. Cornea is normally transparent, smooth, and shiny; opacities (cloudy areas) or specks may indicate prior injury
   c. Pupils should be round, equal in size, and constrict in response to direct light or to light shone in opposite pupil (consensual response); should constrict and converge when looking at object over examiner's shoulder and then shifting gaze to an object 4 to 6 inches from own nose (accommodation)
8. Ophthalmoscopy
   a. Used to examine retina, optic disk, optic blood vessels, fundus, and macula
   b. NCLEX® As light shines on pupil, reflection of light on retina causes a red glare (red reflex); absence of red reflex may indicate lens opacity

E. Otoscopic examination

1. NCLEX® Tilt client's head slightly away, pull pinna up and back in an adult (down and back in a child) to straighten external auditory canal, and insert speculum while visualizing canal
2. Normal findings
   a. Pink, intact external canal with no lesions and variable amount of cerumen and fine hairs; absence of inflammation, deviations, or foreign bodies

b. Tympanic membrane should be transparent, opaque, pearly gray, slightly concave, intact, and free of lesions or perforations

F. Whisper test

1. Have client occlude one ear at a time with a finger; stand 1–2 feet away from client on side of unoccluded ear
2. Whisper numbers or a statement and ask client to repeat; perform again with other ear; alternatively, a ticking watch can be held 5 inches from each ear
3. Note whether it is necessary to stand closer or raise voice to be heard

NCLEX®

G. Rinne test

1. Place stem of an activated tuning fork on mastoid bone and ask client to signal when sound is no longer heard
2. Quickly place vibrating end of tuning fork in front of ear close to ear canal and have client indicate when sound is no longer heard
3. With no conductive hearing loss, sound is heard twice as long by air conduction as by bone conduction
4. With conductive hearing loss, bone conduction is greater than air conduction in affected ear

NCLEX®

H. Weber test

1. Especially valuable when hearing in one ear is reported as better than other
2. Place stem of vibrating tuning fork on midline of forehead or vertex of head (skull) and ask whether sound is heard equally in both ears or if one side is better than other
3. Sound that lateralizes to one ear indicates conductive hearing loss in that ear or sensorineural hearing loss in opposite ear

I. Audiometry: quantifies hearing deficits by presenting various sound frequencies to each ear by either sound or bone conduction

J. Speech audiometry: identifies intensity at which speech is identifiable

K. Tympanometry: indirectly monitors compliance and impedance of middle ear to sound transmission after neutral, positive, and negative air pressure is applied to external auditory meatus

L. Tests of vestibular function

1. Romberg test: stand close to client to ensure safety; ask client to close eyes while feet are together and arms are resting at sides; observe for a normal slight sway; significant sway is a positive test
2. Past pointing test
   a. Client sits facing examiner, closes eyes, and points both index fingers at examiner; examiner places own index fingers under client's as a reference point; then client raises both arms and then lowers them to original spot with eyes closed
   b. With normal response, client can return to reference point easily; with vestibular dysfunction, fingers deviate to left or right
3. Gaze nystagmus test: observe client's eyes as they look straight ahead, 30 degrees to each side, upward, and downward; with vestibular problems, eyeballs exhibit nystagmus
4. Hallpike maneuver: client lies supine and rotates head to side for 1 minute; is positive for positional vertigo or induced dizziness if nystagmus occurs

III. COMMON NURSING TECHNIQUES AND PROCEDURES

A. Ocular medications

NCLEX®

1. Eye drops
   a. Ensure that medication is sterile and treat each eye separately, if both are being medicated, to prevent cross-contamination
   b. Follow procedure as outlined in Chapter 28
   c. Wait 2–5 minutes between drops as per manufacturer's directions
2. Eye ointments: as per procedure outlined in Chapter 28
3. Medicated eye disk
   a. Position client with head tilted back and expose lower conjunctival sac
   b. Press tip of index finger of gloved hand against convex part of disk, place disk horizontally in sac between iris and lower eyelid
   c. Pull lower eyelid out and up over disk and ask client to blink until disk is not visible and have client press fingers against closed lids without moving eyes or disk to secure disk in position
   d. To remove disk, expose lower conjunctival sac and use thumb and index finger to pinch and lift disk from sac

B. Ocular irrigation

1. Position client with head tilted toward side to be irrigated and place waterproof pad and curved basin under affected side
2. Cleanse eyelids and lashes with gloved hand and moistened cotton ball, discarding each cotton ball after one wipe
3. Draw up ordered irrigant into sterile irrigation set or bulb syringe
4. Using non-dominant hand to hold eyelids open, hold syringe 1 inch above eye and push fluid gently into conjunctival sac (fluid flows across eye from inner to outer canthus)

NCLEX®
5. Avoid flushing directly onto eyeball to avoid damage to cornea

C. Eye patches and shields

1. Have client close both eyes during application of patch or shield

NCLEX®
2. Position patch and secure with two strips of tape extending from midforehead to lateral cheekbone (medial top to lateral bottom) on same side
3. Do not use pressure unless specifically ordered, and then use 2–3 pads and extra tape
4. Change only with physician order
5. Apply shield alone or over eye patch to protect eye from pressure or other type of irritation

NCLEX®
6. Place shield on bony prominences of cheek, nose, and brow; secure with transparent tape in same manner as for eye patch

D. Eye prosthesis (artificial eye) care

1. Allow client to perform own artificial eye care if preferred; some prostheses are permanently implanted; others are removable
2. Remove prosthesis by retracting lower eyelid and exerting pressure just below eye to break suction and lift it from socket; can also use rubber bulb syringe or medicine dropper bulb to create suction effect
3. Cleanse with normal saline (NS) or tap water according to client's routine
4. Irrigate eye socket with NS using aseptic technique if ordered (such as for infection)
5. Cleanse edges of eye socket and surrounding area with moistened gauze
6. Reinsert by retracting upper and lower eyelids and slipping prosthesis into eye socket comfortably under upper eyelid
7. Store prosthesis in labeled container with NS or tap water

E. Otic medications

1. Use clean technique unless tympanic membrane is damaged, then use sterile technique
2. Follow procedure as outlined in Chapter 28

F. Otic irrigation

1. Assist client to a sitting or lying position with head tilted toward affected ear; place a waterproof pad and drainage receptacle under affected ear
2. Check that temperature of irrigant is 37°C or 98°F
3. Determine that tympanic membrane is intact before beginning an otic irrigation

NCLEX®
4. Straighten ear canal and gently insert syringe tip into auditory meatus; direct solution slowly and steadily along wall of canal (not center, which could damage tympanic membrane); use no more than 50 to 70 mL at one time
5. After solution drains, dry outside of ear with cotton balls and place a dry one in auditory meatus lightly to absorb remaining excess fluid
6. Assist client to a side-lying position on affected side for further drainage, and monitor client for discomfort

G. Hearing aid prosthesis care

1. There are several types of hearing aids available; they improve quality of hearing with conductive hearing loss but only intensify distortions heard with sensorineural hearing loss (they may be useful in signaling client of danger, enabling client to hear alarms, for example)
2. Wash hands before handling an external hearing aid
3. Make sure battery is working properly and is inserted correctly; have client keep an extra battery on hand
4. Do not drop hearing aid or twist cord

NCLEX®
5. To insert a hearing aid: inspect to ensure it is intact, turn down volume, insert ear mold first into ear canal, then secure rest of device; once in place, turn up volume slowly until comfortable, and check for structural problems or placement problems if feedback occurs
6. Remove a hearing aid after turning it off and lowering volume; remove earmold by rotating it forward slightly and pulling outward

7. After removal, clean a detachable earmold with mild soap and water, rinse and dry well; avoid excessive wetting or use of alcohol, which can cause damage; wipe nondetachable earmolds with a damp cloth

NCLEX® 8. Avoid using aerosol sprays, oils, or cosmetic products near hearing aid, because earmold opening could become clogged

9. Remove battery to prevent corrosion and leakage if aid will not be used for more than 24 hours; store in a safe place away from moisture and heat

IV. NURSING MANAGEMENT OF CLIENT HAVING EYE SURGERY

A. Preoperative care

1. Reduce anxiety by teaching about procedure and postoperative course and care
2. Evaluate client's support systems, ability to care for self after surgery, and environmental safety (such as hand rails, absence of throw rugs)
3. Shampoo or scrub around eyes if ordered; remove eye makeup; store contact lens or eyeglasses (needed to aid vision in other eye) so they are available after surgery

NCLEX® 4. Administer preanesthetic medications and eyedrops as ordered, which commonly include **mydriatic** eye drops (to dilate pupils) and **cycloplegic** eye drops (to paralyze ciliary muscles); see Chapter 40 for overview of commonly ordered eye medications

B. Postoperative care

1. Perform baseline examination as for all postoperative clients (vital signs [VS], level of consciousness [LOC], status of dressing); changes may be minimal if surgery done under local anesthesia
2. Maintain eye patch or shield in place to prevent eye injury, and instruct client not to rub or touch area

NCLEX® 3. Elevate head to 30–45 degrees and have client lie on back or unaffected side (to reduce IOP) after surgery to treat cataracts or glaucoma; use small pillows at sides of head to immobilize head when lying on back

NCLEX® 4. Position client with repair of detached retina as prescribed so that area of detachment is dependent/inferior (to maintain pressure on repaired retinal area and improve its contact with choroid)

5. Remind and assist client to avoid activities that increase IOP, such as coughing, sneezing, vomiting, or straining at stool; if it is necessary to cough or sneeze, client should do so with mouth open and use tissues

NCLEX® 6. Maintain client safety: orient to environment, keep articles and call bell on unaffected side, use side-rails with bed in low position, and assist with ambulation

7. Give antibiotic, anti-inflammatory, and other prescribed topical (eye) or systemic medications
8. Give analgesics as ordered, avoiding or using caution with opioids to prevent postoperative nausea, vomiting, and constipation; discomfort may be described as achy or scratching; avoid morphine, which can cause miosis

NCLEX® 9. Monitor for and report immediately possible surgical complications to preserve sight:
   a. Sudden sharp eye pain, possibly indicating hemorrhage, sudden rise in IOP, or other ocular emergency
   b. Hemorrhage, with blood noted in anterior chamber of eye
   c. Retinal detachment, noted by client sensations of flashes of light, floaters, or a curtain being drawn over eye
   d. Corneal edema, noted by a cloudy appearance to cornea

10. Reinforce client and family teaching about postdischarge care (see Box 59–1)
11. Refer to community health agency for assistance with home care if needed

V. NURSING MANAGEMENT OF CLIENT HAVING EAR SURGERY

A. Preoperative care: principles same as before eye surgery

1. Complete a baseline evaluation of hearing for comparison postoperatively

NCLEX® 2. Shampoo or scrub around ear if ordered; complete usual preoperative activities and checklist; administer preanesthetic medications as ordered

B. Postoperative care

1. Perform baseline evaluation as for all postoperative clients (VS, LOC, bleeding or drainage from dressing, pain, recovery from anesthesia)

NCLEX® 2. Implement standard postoperative interventions (pain control, mobility, prevention of postoperative complications)

NCLEX® 3. Keep client on bedrest for 24 hours with head either elevated or flat (depending on surgeon's order) and lying on nonoperative side (operative ear upward) for 12–24 hours

4. Change internal or external dressings if ordered; wipe away discharge from ear with dry sterile dressing material

Box 59-1

Client Education Following Eye Surgery

Include the following points in discharge instructions for client and family after eye surgery:

- Leave eye shield in place until surgeon's office visit on day after surgery; then use eye shield at night during sleep for eye protection as prescribed
- Avoid rubbing, scratching, touching, squeezing, or putting pressure on surgical eye
- Avoid activities that increase intraocular pressure, such as sneezing, coughing, vomiting, straining, moving rapidly, bending, or lifting more than 5 pounds
- Maintain sedentary lifestyle for approximately 2 weeks or as prescribed by surgeon; avoid heavy work, such as gardening, mowing lawn, or moving furniture
- Avoid reading until allowed by surgeon, and then read in moderation during healing
- Use measures to prevent constipation, such as adequate fiber and fluid intake, maintaining mobility as able, and possible use of stool softener
- Wear sunglasses with side shields when out of doors (photophobia commonly occurs)
- New corrective lenses (if needed) will not be prescribed until vision stabilizes, which may take several weeks; make and keep all recommended follow-up appointments with physician
- Use proper techniques for applying and removing eye patch or shield and for instillling eye drops
- Understand medication names, dose, schedule, side effects, purpose, and anticipated duration of use
- Symptoms to report to physician include new, increased, or severe eye pain or pressure; decreased vision; redness; cloudiness; drainage; floaters or light flashes; and halos around brightly lit objects

NCLEX® 5. Monitor for nausea and vomiting; medicate with antiemetics prn to prevent vomiting, which can disrupt surgical site by increasing pressure in middle ear

NCLEX® 6. Monitor for dizziness and vertigo; avoid unnecessary movements or turning in bed; provide antivertigo medications; provide assistance when client is allowed to ambulate to reduce falls

7. Monitor client's hearing postoperatively and compare to baseline; use alternate communication means as needed

8. Remind client that decreased hearing immediately after surgery may be caused by edema and drainage at operative site; permanent hearing loss may be expected if cochlea is involved or no middle ear reconstruction is done

NCLEX® 9. Reinforce client and family teaching about post-discharge care (see Box 59–2)

VI. STRABISMUS

A. Overview

1. Misalignment of eyes; two types are esotropia (inward deviation or "crossed eyes," most common type) or exotropia (outward deviation or "wall eyes")
2. Caused by lack of coordination of eye muscles
3. Can be congenital or acquired; leads to amblyopia in 30–50% of cases

B. Data collection:

1. Symptoms may occur only when tired; include squinting when reading, closing one eye to see, and difficulty in picking up objects
2. **Cover-uncover test**: client fixes gaze straight ahead, focusing on a distant object; cover one eye with an opaque card while observing uncovered eye for movement; remove card while observing eye just uncovered for movement; this test screens for deviation in eye alignment and eye muscle weakness (weakness is seen as movement of "lazy eye" when it attempts to refocus during cover test)
3. **Corneal light reflex (Hirschberg test)**: checks for parallel symmetry of eyes; examiner shines a penlight directly onto corneas of both eyes, holding penlight about 12 inches away from client's nasal bridge while client focuses on a distant object; light should be reflected at same spot in both eyes; an asymmetric light reflex indicates a deviation in alignment of client's eyes

Box 59-2

Client Education Following Ear Surgery

Include the following points in discharge instructions given to client and family after ear surgery:

- Keep outer ear dressing clean and dry; change it as ordered if needed; do not remove inner ear dressing until allowed by surgeon; do not insert small objects to clean external ear canal
- Whenever possible, avoid activities that increase middle ear pressure, such as blowing nose, sneezing, coughing, straining
- If necessary, cough or sneeze with mouth open; wipe nostril with tissue or blow nose one nostril at a time with mouth open; avoid drinking through a straw for 2–3 weeks; avoid air travel until allowed by surgeon
- Use measures to prevent constipation, such as adequate fiber and fluid intake, maintaining mobility as able, and possible use of stool softener
- Do not shower or shampoo hair until allowed by surgeon (usually 1 or more weeks)
- Keep ear dry for 6 weeks with use of petrolatum-coated cotton ball placed in external auditory canal as ordered; if used, change it daily; do not swim or dive until allowed by surgeon (when full healing occurs)
- Reduce risk of infection by avoiding those with respiratory infections
- Understand medication names, dose, schedule, side effects, purpose, and anticipated duration of use (antibiotics, antiemetics, antivertigo agents)
- Symptoms to report to physician include persistent postoperative headache, increased drainage or bleeding from site, fever, new or increased ear pain or dizziness, and decreasing hearing

C. Therapeutic management

NCLEX®

1. Includes occlusion therapy ("good eye" is patched 1–2 hours daily, forcing client to focus with weaker eye, thus strengthening eye muscles), corrective lenses in eyeglasses, eye drops to cause blurred vision in "good eye," eye muscle exercises
2. Surgical treatment
   - **a.** Strabismus can be corrected surgically if conservative treatment fails; surgery on rectus muscles of eyes can achieve normal eye alignment
   - **b.** Congenital strabismus should be corrected before 24 months of age to prevent amblyopia

D. Reinforce client and family teaching

1. Provide explanation of eye patching to parents
2. Preoperative teaching about maintaining NPO status prior to surgery and general preoperative and postoperative care

VII. AMBLYOPIA

A. Overview

1. Reduction in vision in one or both eyes, usually with one eye having poorer vision than the other, causing loss of binocular vision; also known as "lazy eye"
2. Results from anything causing visual deprivation to eye, including untreated strabismus (most common), congenital cataract, or uncorrected refractive errors

B. Data collection

1. Is diagnosed with vision testing by optometrist or ophthalmologist
2. Nursing data collection depends upon age of child

NCLEX®

   - **a.** Manifestations of visual impairment for infants include lack of tracking objects or lights with eyes and poor or no eye contact
   - **b.** Signs of visual impairment in toddlers and older children are excessive tearing, rubbing, and squinting of eyes; frequent blinking; and holding objects close to eyes to see them or to read
3. Vision changes may be accompanied by dizziness and headache
4. Diagnosis is confirmed by corneal light reflex and cover-uncover tests

C. Therapeutic management

NCLEX®
1. Medical treatment options include corrective lenses in eyeglasses, occluding unaffected eye with a patch 2–6 hours daily (occlusion therapy), eye muscle exercises
2. Treatment is discontinued when vision has improved; however, 20/20 visual acuity is rarely attained
3. Treatment is most successful when done by age 7 to 8 years
4. Untreated amblyopia can lead to permanent visual impairment
5. Nursing care involves instruction about need to complete treatment

D. Reinforce client and family teaching: how to patch unaffected eye while maintaining skin integrity; therapy and long-term benefits

VIII. GLAUCOMA

A. Overview

1. Damage to optic nerve caused by increased IOP, usually because of an imbalance between aqueous humor production and drainage, can be of two types: open-angle or angle-closure (narrow-angle, closed-angle)
2. Risk factors are family history, older age, African-American race, eye trauma, prolonged corticosteroid use, thin cornea, myopia, and disorders such as diabetes mellitus, cardiovascular disease, and migraine syndromes
3. Open-angle glaucoma: most frequent form with unknown cause, although heredity is suspected; angle of anterior chamber between iris and cornea is normal; flow of aqueous humor through trabecular network to canal of Schlemm is obstructed; usually is a bilateral process
4. Angle-closure (narrow-angle, closed-angle) glaucoma: less common form, is often unilateral, although other eye can be affected at a later time
   a. Anterior chamber narrows because of corneal flattening or bulging of iris
   b. When iris thickens (pupil dilation) or lens thickens (during visual accommodation), angle can close completely, blocking outflow and causing sudden elevation of IOP

NCLEX®
   c. Damage to neurons in retina and optic nerve can occur, rapidly lead to loss of vision if not treated quickly

B. Data collection

NCLEX®
1. Open-angle
   a. Loss of peripheral vision, mild headaches, difficulty adapting to dark, seeing halos around lights, and difficulty focusing on near objects
   b. Symptoms may be vague with client unaware of them for a time; visual acuity deteriorates over time with rising IOP

NCLEX®
2. Angle-closure
   a. Triggered by pupil dilation, such as with high emotions and darkness, among others
   b. Symptoms include severe eye and face pain, nausea and vomiting, malaise, colored halos around lights, and episodes of sudden decline in vision; possible reddened eye, cloudy cornea from edema, and pupil fixed at midpoint
3. Diagnosed by history; presenting symptoms; tonometry (IOP > 21 mmHg); ophthalmoscopy; **gonioscopy** (measurement of anterior chamber angle, differentiates open-angle from angle-closure glaucoma)

C. Therapeutic management

NCLEX®
1. Acute glaucoma: medical emergency; vision loss can occur within 1–2 days if untreated; provide information to client and administer ordered therapies such as osmotic diuretics or carbonic anhydrase inhibitors such as acetazolamide (Diamox) to lower IOP (see Chapter 40); surgery may be needed

NCLEX®
2. Chronic glaucoma: provide medication therapy and client education
3. Provide pre- and postoperative care as previously outlined if eye surgery is needed; surgical procedures to facilitate drainage of aqueous humor can include trabeculectomy, laser trabeculoplasty, iridectomy, or laser iridotomy
4. Medication therapy
   a. **Miotic** drugs that constrict pupils
   b. Carbonic anhydrase inhibitors to decrease production of aqueous humor
   c. Beta-adrenergic blockers to constrict pupils and reduce production of aqueous humor

D. Reinforce client teaching

NCLEX®
1. Drug therapy is needed for life; nonadherence can lead to permanent vision loss
2. Avoid mydriatic medications such as atropine that dilate pupils
3. Obtain Medic-Alert card or bracelet specifying type of glaucoma

NCLEX®
4. Use safety precautions at night (lighting, hand rails) to compensate for reduced pupil dilation because of miotics, and remove obstacles in environment for safety
5. Follow general instructions following eye surgery; see previous discussion
6. Review specific drug information and procedures for self-administration

IX. CATARACTS

A. Overview

1. Progressive cloudiness or opacity in lens or lens capsule that results in vision loss

NCLEX® 2. Risk factors include age (most common), long-term exposure to ultraviolet light (UV-B rays), cigarette smoking, heavy alcohol use, eye injury or inflammation, congenital defect, diabetes mellitus, and medications such as systemic corticosteroids
3. Fibers and proteins of lens degenerate with age or following insult; opacity often begins at periphery of lens and moves to center
4. Partial opacity is termed *immature cataract*; opacity of entire lens is termed *mature cataract*
5. Opacity tends to occur bilaterally but is asymmetric in development, with one maturing faster than other

B. Data collection

NCLEX® 1. Decline in close and distance vision, blurred vision, changes in color vision (loss), glare, halos around lights, object distortion, white or cloudy gray pupil
2. Diagnosed by history and physical exam, results of visual acuity tests and slit-lamp exam; absence of red reflex with ophthalmoscopy

C. Therapeutic management

1. Provide emotional support because impaired vision is anxiety-producing
2. Identify and correct safety concerns in environment related to impaired vision
3. Surgical removal of lens is sole treatment option and is accompanied by lens implant or is treated with contact lenses or aphakic corrective lenses (rare)
4. Assist client in decision making about surgery, which is indicated when vision or activities of daily living (ADLs) are affected or if cataract is causing secondary problems such as uveitis or glaucoma
5. Reinforce explanations about surgical extraction of lens
   a. Cryoextraction: forceps or supercooled probe used to extract lens after making small incision in cornea
   b. Phacoemulsification: ultrasound vibrations break lens into fragments that are aspirated (suctioned) from eye
   c. Intracapsular extraction: removal of entire lens and surrounding capsule (see Figure 59–1A)
   d. Extracapsular extraction: removal of lens nucleus and cortex, leaving posterior capsule intact to support lens implant; currently most popular method (see Figure 59–1B)

NCLEX® 6. Surgery is done on one eye at a time, on an outpatient basis using local anesthesia
7. Lens implant rapidly restores binocular vision and depth perception
8. Provide preoperative and postoperative care as outlined in previous section
9. Medication therapy: includes postoperative eyes drops (combined antibiotic, antiinflammatory and/or corticosteroid eye drops or ointment) and mild analgesic such as acetaminophen (Tylenol)

D. Reinforce client teaching

1. Adaptive strategies to compensate for changes in vision and depth perception if surgery is not currently indicated or desired
2. Postoperative instructions as outlined in previous section on eye surgery
3. Leave eye patch or shield in place until changed or removed by surgeon at postoperative visit, usually within 24–48 hours
4. Protect eye using sunglasses with side shields during day and eye shield at night

NCLEX® 5. Information and procedures for medication use after surgery, such as acetaminophen for general discomfort, combination steroid (anti-inflammatory) and antibiotic eye drops, and others as needed by individual client
6. Insertion and care of postoperative contact lenses if prescribed

NCLEX® 7. Permanent eyeglasses will be prescribed several weeks after surgery when healing is complete and vision has stabilized

X. DETACHED RETINA

A. Overview

1. Separation of sensory layer of retina from choroid (pigmented vascular layer)
2. Retina may tear and fold back onto itself or remain intact and be pulled away from choroid by shrinking of vitreous humor
3. Most frequently an age-related condition with shrinkage of vitreous humor, which pulls on retina at points of attachment, such as the optic disk, macula, and periphery of eye; other causes are trauma, inflammation, tumor, or complication of eye surgery (lens removal)
4. With a retinal break or tear, fluid enters defect, possibly leading to further rapid tearing and separation due to pressure

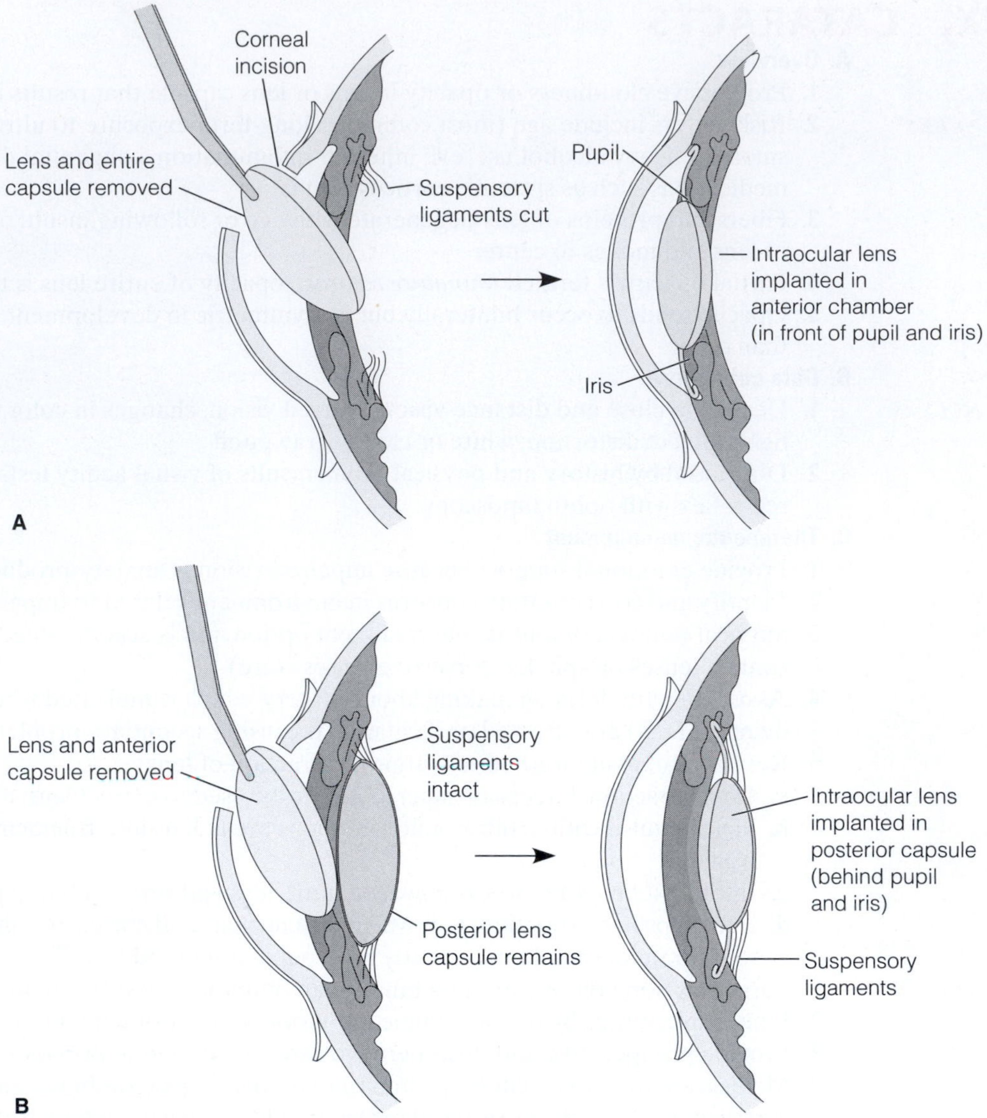

Figure 59–1

A. Intracapsular cataract extraction removes entire lens and capsule, with lens implantation in anterior chamber. *B.* Extracapsular cataract extraction removes lens and anterior capsule, with lens implantation within the intact posterior capsule.

5. Incomplete area of detachment can progress slowly or can enlarge quickly and become complete

NCLEX®
6. Will lead to permanent blindness if untreated so is considered a medical emergency

NCLEX®
B. Data collection
1. Initial: presence of floating spots (floaters) and/or flashing lights
2. Progressive blurring of vision, visual field deficits corresponding to area of damage, sense of curtain or veil coming down, up or across field of vision, painless
3. Ophthalmic exam shows area of gray opaque retina, with possible accompanying tears, holes, or folds

C. Therapeutic management
1. Surgical repair (see Box 59–3)
2. Preoperative care

NCLEX®
a. Protect eye from further damage: bedrest, cover both eyes with eye patches to limit movement and prevent eye stress, instruct client not to bend forward or make sudden or jerking head movements

NCLEX®
b. Position client with detached area dependent/inferior so gravity pushes detachment closer to choroid (e.g., with left eye superior temporal detachment, keep client supine with head turned toward left)

NCLEX®
c. Protect client from injury by keeping bed low, side-rails up, call bell within reach; talk to client before approaching bed, assist with self-care

d. Provide support to alleviate anxiety associated with sudden loss of vision; reassure client most detachments are successfully treated (often on outpatient basis); reinforce explanations about surgical repair

e. Provide preoperative care as described in previous section

3. Postoperative care

a. Provide standard postoperative care as described in previous section

Box 59-3

Surgical Procedures for Detached Retina

- Laser photocoagulation or cryotherapy (cold probe): creates a local inflammation that will locally adhere retina onto the choroid
- Scleral buckling: holds retina and choroid together with an implant or encircling strap or "buckle"
- Pneumatic retinopexy: injects air/gas into vitreous with adjustment of client's head position to push detached portion of retina back into contact with choroid
- Surgical instrument manipulation to move detached segment of torn retina into place, followed by laser therapy or injection of gas or silicone oil to create a bond

NCLEX®
b. Stress importance of maintaining prescribed position (affected eye inferior or dependent to maintain contact between retina and choroid)
c. Usually includes antibiotic, anti-inflammatory, and analgesic medications

D. **Reinforce client teaching**: as previously described

XI. MACULAR DEGENERATION

A. Overview

1. Degeneration of macular area (center area) of retina, which normally receives light from center of visual field and has greatest visual acuity
2. Most common type is age-related macular degeneration (ARMD), a leading cause of vision loss in clients over age 60 in developed countries
3. Causes of ARMD are unknown, although heredity, smoking, injury, inflammation, and nutritional factors may play a role; males and females are affected equally
4. In ARMD, there is gradual failure of outer layer of retina (pigmented epithelium that attaches retina to choroid layer and removes cellular wastes); in this process, photoreceptor cells are lost, metabolic wastes accumulate in subretinal space, leading to cell death
5. There are two types of macular degeneration
   a. Atrophic ("dry") form: bilateral and gradual but progressive loss of vision occurs because of atrophy and degeneration of macula (85–90% of cases)
   b. Exudative ("wet") form: serous fluid or blood leaks from abnormally proliferative blood vessels (neovascularization) and accumulates in subretinal space; leads to more rapid, severe loss of vision; scar tissue forms and leads to cell death and vision loss (10–15% of cases but more likely to result in legal blindness)

B. Data collection

NCLEX®
1. Clinical manifestations include loss of central vision with intact peripheral vision, pale yellow spots called *drusen* on macula, visual distortion of images (i.e., straight lines may appear crooked or wavy), and difficulty with activities requiring focused and close central vision (i.e., sewing, needlepoint, reading)
2. Diagnostic tests: vision testing, fundoscopy (examination of fundus of eye); fluorescein angiography (for wet form only); and electroretinography (ERG) to measure retinal responses to light

C. Therapeutic management

1. Currently there is no treatment for dry macular degeneration and no curative therapy for either wet or dry macular degeneration
2. Wet macular degeneration may be treated by:
   a. Laser photocoagulation
   b. Photodynamic therapy in which a light-activated drug is injected into vein and circulates to retinal blood vessels; a low-intensity laser light is shone on retina; light activates drug to eventually occlude blood vessel and stop leakage; it is possible for disorder to recur in another area

NCLEX®
3. Nursing care
   a. Standard nursing measures to prevent falls and other injuries caused by impaired vision
   b. Standard measures to assist those with impaired vision
   c. Obtain home safety evaluation before discharge to minimize risk of injuries and falls in home setting
4. No medications are available to treat this condition

NCLEX®
D. Reinforce client teaching

1. Need for regular eye examinations to determine disease progression
2. Use of Amsler grid for self-monitoring of central vision (available from eye care professionals or on Internet)

3. Measures to maintain safety at home and adapt to visual changes
   a. Obtain aids to enhance vision and promote safety (i.e., magnification devices, enhanced lighting)
   b. Determine availability of large-print books and newspapers and audio books
4. Postprocedure self-care for photodynamic therapy includes use of dark glasses and protective clothing as well as avoiding bright indoor light for a few days

XII. EYE INFECTIONS OR INFLAMMATIONS

A. Overview and data collection (see Table 59–1)

NCLEX®

B. Therapeutic management

1. Medications: topical or systemic antibiotics or antivirals, antihistamines, and corticosteroids
2. Promote infection control through diligent hand hygiene; teach client and family that conjunctivitis can be highly contagious
3. Cleanse eye with warm water and remove any crusting or exudate before instilling eye drops or eye ointment
4. Reduce pain or discomfort with warm compresses, dark sunglasses, and analgesics (acetaminophen and/or codeine)
5. If corneal perforation is suspected, have client lie supine, close eye, and cover with dry, sterile dressing to avoid loss of eye contents until surgery is done

C. Reinforce client and family teaching

1. How to instill antibiotic drops or ointment into conjunctival sac
2. (NCLEX®) Prevention measures to limit spread of infection to other eye or other people, including not to share face cloths or towels, not to rub eyes or wear contact lenses during infection, not to cross-contaminate infection to other eye, and discard eye makeup and purchase new after infection clears

XIII. EYE INJURY

A. Overview and data collection

1. Corneal abrasion (disruption of superficial cornea from drying, contact lenses, eyelashes, or foreign bodies such as dust, dirt, or fingernails): pain, photophobia, tearing
2. Burns (from chemicals, heat, radiation, explosion): eye pain, decreased vision, swollen eyelids, burns, reddened and edematous conjunctiva, possible corneal haziness or cloudiness, ulcerations
3. Blunt trauma (caused by sports injuries, motor vehicle accidents, falls, physical assault): includes lid ecchymosis (black eye), conjunctival hemorrhage (painless erythema), hyphema (bleeding into anterior chamber with eye pain, decreased vision, and seeing a reddish hue), and orbital fractures (diplopia/double vision, pain with upward eye movement, limited eye movements, sunken appearance to eye, and decreased sensation on affected cheek)

Table 59–1 Overview and Data Collection for Eye Inflammation or Infection

Condition	Description	Manifestations
Blepharitis	Inflammation of eyelid margin glands and lash follicles	Red-rimmed eyes; irritation, burning, itching of eyelid margins; mucous discharge with crusting and scaling of lid margins
Hordeolum or sty	Infection of sebaceous glands of eyelid	Raised area of lid, pain, redness, tenderness, possible photophobia, tearing, and sensation of foreign body in eye
Chalazion	Granulomatous eyelid cyst or nodule	Hard swelling, painless, reddened local conjunctival tissue, may be due to inadequately treated hordoleum
Conjunctivitis (also called pink eye)	Infection or inflammation of conjunctiva caused by allergen, toxin, viruses, bacteria, or other irritant	Eye redness and itching; possible scratchy, burning, or gritty sensation; photophobia, tearing, discharge (watery, purulent, or mucoid; yellow, white or green color); usually not painful; if severe, possible conjunctival edema, bleeding, or perforation
Corneal ulcer	Local necrosis of cornea caused by infection, trauma, or misuse of contact lenses	Photophobia, discomfort ranging from gritty sensations to severe pain, excessive tearing; possible discharge; decreased vision; unable to open eye or spasm of eyelid; visible area of ulceration
Keratitis	Inflammation of cornea	Similar to conjunctivitis; can lead to ulceration and blindness
Uveitis	Inflammation of uveal tract, e.g., vascular layer	Pupillary constriction, erythema around limbus, severe eye pain, photophobia, blurred vision

NCLEX®

B. Therapeutic management

1. If chemical burn present, irrigate eye with copious amounts of normal saline (preferred) or water (if necessary) until pH of eye is in range of 7.2 to 7.4; use topical anesthetic to make irrigation easier; then evaluate vision with and without any corrective eyeglasses
2. Remove loose foreign bodies quickly using a sterile, moistened cotton-tipped applicator or by irrigation to prevent corneal abrasion
3. If no foreign substances are present, first evaluate vision with and without eyeglasses to provide data about extent of injury and for use as a baseline
4. Apply eye patches or sterile gauze dressings over both eyes if severe or penetrating eye injury occurs to reduce eye movements; stabilize any penetrating objects until surgery is done to help preserve vision; institute bedrest

C. Reinforce client teaching

1. Purpose, effects, and use of medications
2. Use of eye patch or shield
3. Avoid activities that increase IOP during healing (lifting, bending, straining); teach how to avoid future injury

XIV. LEGAL BLINDNESS

A. Overview

1. Visual acuity that is no better than 20/200 even with correction in better eye, or a visual field of less than 20 degrees (instead of 180 degrees)
2. Common causes in United States are glaucoma and cataracts, macular degeneration, diabetic retinopathy, and congenital disorders

B. Therapeutic management

1. Assist client with grieving process that accompanies vision loss, because of loss of sight and interference with mobility, self-sufficiency, and possibly finances
2. Support client who is experiencing changes in roles and relationships, communication patterns (through loss of ability to perceive nonverbal cues), and possibly sexual expression

NCLEX®

3. Foster independence in hospital environment
   a. Verbally and physically orient client to room using bed as a reference point
   b. Keep room and hallway free of clutter
   c. Introduce self when entering client's room and state when leaving
   d. Use increased verbal communication: describe activities in environment and provide stimuli such as radio or television; ask client what assistance is needed
   e. Ensure that call bell and other needed articles are within client's easy reach and that client knows their location
   f. Describe location of food on plate using a clock face description (for a client who was previously sighted and knows what a clock face is)
   g. Assist with ambulation, walking slightly ahead and allowing client to hold your arm (not the reverse); describe environment that lies ahead, such as turns or stairs

NCLEX®

C. Reinforce client teaching: measures to minimize risk of injury in home setting and adapt to performing ADLs with impaired vision

XV. HEARING IMPAIRMENT

A. Overview

1. Condition that interferes with ability to receive auditory signals from environment
2. Three types of hearing loss: conductive, sensorineural, and mixed
3. Conductive: occurs when tympanic membrane cannot vibrate freely or when sounds cannot reach middle ear; common causes are otitis media, impacted cerumen, and foreign body in ear canal
4. Sensorineural: occurs with damage to cochlea or auditory nerve; may be congenital (as in congenital rubella syndrome) or acquired (ototoxic drugs); may also be genetic, such as with Tay-Sachs disease
5. Mixed: involves a combination of conductive and sensorineural hearing losses

NCLEX®

B. Data collection for hearing impairment

1. In infants and young children with hearing loss, language development is affected; it should be diagnosed as early as possible to promote optimal development
2. Infant: does not startle to loud noises, arouses to touch and not noise, does not turn head to sounds or localize sounds, little or no babbling or vocalizations

3. Toddler and preschooler: communicates through gestures; little or no speech, unintelligible speech; developmental delay; no response to doorbell, telephone
4. School-age child and adolescent: sits close to speaker or turns up TV volume loudly, poor school performance, speech problems, cannot correctly respond except when able to view speaker's face
5. Adult or older adult: watches speaker's face during conversation; does not respond to noises if not in line of vision; uses loud volume with TV, radio, and other entertainment equipment
6. Diagnosed by otoscopic examination, tympanography, and audiography

C. Therapeutic management

1. Prevent acquired hearing loss by client education to avoid exposure to loud noises
2. Advocate prompt treatment of otitis media
3. Assist with developmental assessment for early identification of infants and children with hearing loss to prevent significant delays in development and school performance
4. If hearing loss is correctable in child, therapeutic goal is treatment of cause, such as removal of a foreign body in conductive loss
5. If hearing loss cannot be corrected, a multidisciplinary team consisting of otolaryngologist, audiologist, pediatrician, nurse, and speech-language pathologist works with child and family to obtain appropriate therapies and enhance communication
6. Hearing aids may be prescribed; see previous section on hearing aid care (NCLEX®)
7. Advocate for clients with hearing impairment and their families; provide support and appropriate referrals to child and family

D. Reinforce client teaching

1. Means of communicating with children or adults who have hearing loss
2. Encourage parents to enroll child in early intervention program to promote speech development

XVI. OTOSCLEROSIS

A. Overview

1. Hereditary disorder of labyrinthine capsule in which abnormal bone growth occurs around ossicles
2. Causes fixation of stapes, leading to conductive hearing loss
3. Is an autosomal dominant hereditary disorder most common in whites and females; onset is in adolescence or early adulthood; pregnancy exacerbates condition
4. Stapes do not vibrate as they should because of stiffening, which reduces sound transmission to inner ear

NCLEX® **B. Data collection**

1. Bilateral conductive hearing loss that is progressive and asymmetrical, tinnitus, possible retention of bone conduction (so client has difficulty in ordinary conversation but can use telephone adequately)
2. Reddish or pinkish orange tympanic membrane from increased vascularity (Schwartz's sign)
3. Rinne test results: bone sound conduction equal to or longer than air conduction (abnormal finding) if hearing loss is greater than 25 decibels (dB)
4. Weber test results: lateralization to ear with greater conductive hearing loss

NCLEX® **C. Therapeutic management**

1. Encourage use of a hearing aid(s) to augment sound
2. Administer sodium fluoride as ordered to slow bone resorption and overgrowth
3. Implement strategies to enhance communication with a hearing-impaired client (see Box 59–4)
4. Surgical intervention
   a. Stapedectomy with fenestration: microsurgical removal of diseased stapes, with drill or laser creation of a hole in footplate, followed by insertion of a steel or synthetic prosthesis to restore hearing
   b. Stapedotomy: insertion of a wire or platinum ribbon prosthesis into a small hole created in stapes footplate

D. Reinforce client teaching: referral to appropriate community agencies; postoperative care as previously outlined

XVII. EAR INFECTIONS

A. Overview

1. Otitis externa: infectious, inflammatory, or allergic response in external auditory canal or auricle; also called "swimmer's ear"; more frequent in warm, humid areas
2. **Otitis media**
   a. Acute or chronic infection or inflammation of middle ear; greatest incidence is between 6 and 36 months of age during winter months
   b. Related to dysfunction of eustachian tube, which provides drainage and ventilation of middle ear; when blocked from edema in upper respiratory infection, fluid can accumulate in middle ear, providing a medium for bacterial growth and infection

Box 59-4

Communication with a Hearing Impaired Client

- Approach client from within client's line of vision or tap client lightly on shoulder to get attention before speaking
- Reduce background noise, such as radio or TV, before beginning to speak
- Avoid covering mouth with hands or other objects while speaking
- Face client and speak slowly and clearly—pronounce words clearly without overarticulating them; speak using low pitch and normal loudness
- Use nonverbal cues and written messages to enhance communication
- Repeat sentences using different words if client has difficulty understanding
- Ask client to repeat directions or teaching that was done to ensure understanding

c. Children with facial malformations such as cleft palate and Down syndrome have anatomic variations of their eustachian tubes, making them more vulnerable to otitis media

d. Causative organisms: most common are *Streptococcus pneumoniae, Haemophilus influenzae,* and *Neisseria catarrhalis*

3. Mastoiditis: infection of mastoid process (temporal bone adjacent to middle ear), usually results from untreated or inadequately treated otitis media

NCLEX® **B. Data collection**

1. Otitis externa: redness, swelling, and exudate in external auditory canal, earache, itching, sensation that ear is "plugged" or "blocked," hearing loss in affected ear

2. Otitis media

a. Children (acute): ear pain, irritability, diarrhea, fever, and vomiting are common; possible pulling at the affected ear; some children are asymptomatic; diagnosis is based on otoscopic examination of tympanic membrane; a red, bulging, nonmobile tympanic membrane indicates otitis media

b. Adults (acute): severe earache or ear pain (classic), ear pressure, fever, malaise, diminished hearing, dizziness or vertigo, nausea and possible vomiting, possible tinnitus (ringing in ears), presence of fluid behind a bulging tympanic membrane

c. Chronic: slight fever, diminished hearing, chronic ear discharge

3. Mastoiditis: fever, malaise, possible tinnitus and headache, persistent throbbing ear pain worsened by head movement, tenderness behind ear over mastoid process, local cellulitis of skin, drainage from ear, diminished hearing in affected ear

C. Therapeutic management in adults

NCLEX® 1. Apply local heat 3 times per day for 20 minutes at a time as prescribed

2. Encourage bedrest as applicable to reduce head movements and pain

NCLEX® 3. Administer prescribed antibiotics (otic or systemic), decongestants, antihistamines, analgesics (acetaminophen or aspirin), and antivertigo agents

4. Encourage client to use caution while hearing is diminished

5. Provide care to clients undergoing ear surgery as previously outlined

6. Surgical procedures

a. Myringotomy: surgical perforation of tympanic membrane to allow drainage of middle ear secretions and relieve pain and pressure (otitis media)

b. Tympanocentesis: insertion of a 20-gauge spinal needle through inferior portion of tympanic membrane to drain secretions, possibly to obtain culture, and relieve pain and pressure (otitis media)

c. Mastoidectomy: surgical removal of infected mastoid air cells, bone, and pus; radical mastoidectomy involves removal of middle ear structures such as incus and malleus as well as diseased tissue (conductive hearing loss then occurs unless reconstructive surgery is done as well)

d. Tympanoplasty: surgical reconstruction of ossicles and tympanic membrane of middle ear to help restore hearing

D. Therapeutic management in children

NCLEX® 1. Nursing management of child with tympanostomy tubes: usually surgery is accomplished in a day-surgery center, not an inpatient hospital setting

a. Reinforce to parents to give acetaminophen (Tylenol) for discomfort following myringotomy and insertion of tympanostomy tubes

b. Parents should follow physician's directions for postoperative ear care; eardrops are often prescribed

c. Some physicians require parents to insert earplugs for bathing and swimming and avoid water in ear canal; others do not
d. Explain that ear tubes will spontaneously extrude and fall out; they may note presence of spool-shaped tube in child's ear canal; ear tubes usually fall out in about 1 year

2. Medication therapy
   a. Oral antibiotic therapy for 10–14 days; first-line drugs are amoxicillin (Amoxil), and trimethoprim-sulfamethoxazole (Bactrim, Septra)
   b. Recurrent or chronic otitis media infections may require prophylactic antibiotics as a 6-month trial
3. Surgical procedures: as described in previous section for adults
4. Reinforce client and family teaching: signs and symptoms of otitis media; need to monitor and treat temperature; how to administer medication safely and effectively (complete full course of antibiotic therapy even if feeling better; give doses on time)

XVIII. MÉNIÈRE'S DISEASE

A. Overview

1. A disorder of inner ear in which excessive endolymphatic fluid accumulates in membranous labyrinth because of malabsorption or blocked endolymphatic duct; also called idiopathic endolymphatic hydrops
2. Impaired reabsorption of endolymph leads to dilation of lymph channels, which causes symptoms
3. Has an unknown etiology; possibly heredity, viral influence, and immune dysfunction play a role; affects men and women equally; average age at onset is in 40s

NCLEX®

B. Data collection

1. Recurrent severe attacks of vertigo accompanied by sense of fullness in ears, roaring or ringing tinnitus, nausea, headache, and gradual but progressive sensorineural hearing loss (often unilateral)
2. Attacks may last minutes to hours with possible associated symptoms of hypotension, diaphoresis, and nystagmus
3. Attacks may be triggered by increased sodium (Na^+) intake, vasoconstriction, premenstrual fluid retention, stress, or allergies (sometimes no trigger is identified)
4. Diagnosed by electronystagnography (including caloric testing), Rinne and Weber tests, x-ray, CT scan, evaluation of response to a test dose of an osmotic or loop diuretic

NCLEX®

C. Therapeutic management

1. Low-Na^+ diet, avoidance of sugars, and, if symptoms are severe, fluid restriction
2. Avoid use of alcohol, caffeine, nicotine
3. Bedrest to control vertigo; assist with ambulation for safety
4. Medication therapy: diuretics, antihistamines to suppress vestibular system, antivertigo and antiemetic drugs
5. Endolymphatic sac decompression: relieves pressure in labyrinth and creates shunt between membranous labyrinth and subarachnoid space for fluid drainage (preserves hearing in most cases, relieves vertigo in approximately 70% of cases, relieves tinnitus and sensations of ear fullness in 50% of cases)
6. Vestibular nerve sectioning: severing of portion of CN VIII that controls balance and sensation of vertigo (relieves vertigo in about 98% of cases)
7. Labyrinthectomy: complete removal of labyrinth, destroying cochlear function, relieving vertigo but causing loss of any minimal remaining hearing as well ("last resort")
8. Cochlear implant: for sensorineural hearing loss
   a. An electrode is implanted in cochlea to receive stimuli from a processor worn on body; used for a client with intact neurons capable of stimulation (see Figure 59–2)
   b. A second type of device, used for clients with no excitable auditory fibers, amplifies and transmits a signal to a receiver implanted in brainstem
   c. Devices do not restore normal hearing but allow perception of sound to alert a client to conversation or dangers in the environment
9. Complications of all inner ear surgical procedures include infection and cerebrospinal fluid (CSF) leakage

D. Reinforce client teaching

NCLEX®
1. Follow restrictions in Na^+, sugar, fluid, nicotine, alcohol, and caffeine
2. Take medications as prescribed

NCLEX®
3. Learn signs of an impending attack: fullness in affected ear, increasing tinnitus, headache; lie down in bed in a dark quiet room if at home when an attack begins, or pull off the road for safety if driving

NCLEX®
4. Avoid sudden movements or position changes; move head slowly, and do not get up unassisted during an attack

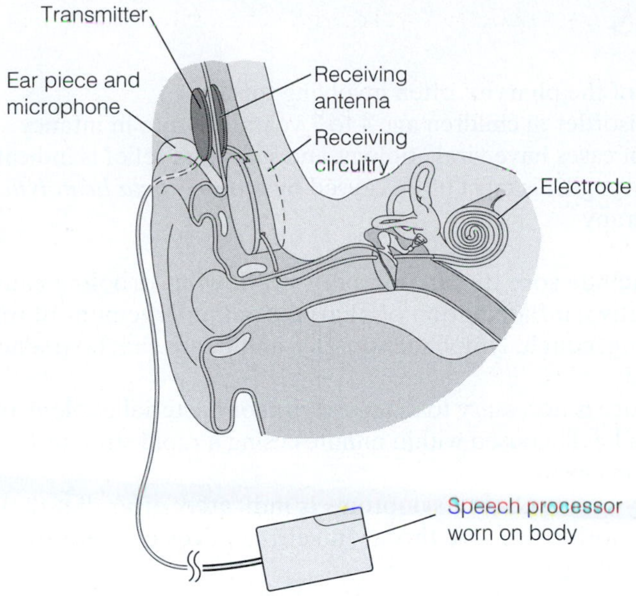

Figure 59-2

Cochlear implant used in sensorineural hearing loss in which excitable auditory neurons remain.

5. Wear a Medic-Alert identification
6. Learn stress reduction techniques of choice to help reduce severity of attacks
7. If tinnitus persists between attacks, use white noise or ambient sound machine to mask tinnitus and promote sleep; consider use of medication most commonly effective—oral antidepressant nortriptyline (Pamelor) taken at bedtime
8. Practice balance training exercises to help brain learn to compensate for damage to vestibular system; exercises consist of moving head up and down, side to side, and tilting head to left and right; repeated 10 times each twice a day

XIX. EPISTAXIS

A. Overview

1. Also known as nosebleed; very common in children, especially boys
2. Superficial veins in nares are a common source of bleeding
3. Bleeding can occur from irritation, drying of mucosa from low humidity, increased blood pressure, or picking nose

B. Data collection

1. Monitor vital signs of client in emergency department or clinic with uncontrolled epistaxis while simultaneous efforts to control bleeding are being performed
2. If client has had significant blood loss, hemoglobin and hematocrit may be measured

C. Therapeutic managment

NCLEX® 1. Remind client or parents to humidify air (especially during winter months and nighttime hours) and have child sleep with head elevated to prevent recurrence

NCLEX® 2. Following an episode of nosebleed, client is prone to rebleeding; client should not bend forward, drink hot liquids, exercise excessively, or take hot baths or showers for 3–4 days following a significant nosebleed

3. If bleeding cannot be controlled using pressure, topical vasoconstrictive agents may be used, such as Neo-Synephrine, epinephrine, or thrombin
4. Cautery may be required with silver nitrate or electrocautery
5. If bleeding cannot be stopped, nose may be packed with absorbent packing material by health care provider to stop bleeding

D. Reinforce child and family teaching

NCLEX® 1. Stop a nosebleed by applying steady pressure to both nostrils just below nasal bone for 10 to 15 minutes

2. Have client sit upright and slightly forward for best results when applying pressure to nostrils and to prevent excessive swallowing of blood
3. Seek health care if bleeding cannot be stopped
4. Client should avoid picking at nose or forcefully blowing nose; client should also release sneezes through open mouth covered with tissues

XX. PHARYNGITIS

A. Overview

1. An infection of the pharynx, often involving tonsils
2. A common disorder in children age 4 to 7 years, but rare in infancy
3. About 80% of cases have viral etiology, and symptom relief is indicated
4. Bacterial pharyngitis is most often caused by *group A beta-hemolytic streptococcus* and requires antibiotic therapy

NCLEX®

B. Data collection

1. Symptoms include sore throat, difficulty swallowing, drooling caused by sore throat, and inability to swallow saliva; inflammation of pharynx and enlargement of tonsils (with or without exudate), fever, vomiting, cough, lymphadenopathy, and headache; hoarseness or a change in voice quality may be noted
2. A throat culture is necessary to diagnose viral or bacterial etiology of pharyngitis; streptococcal infections can be diagnosed within minutes using a rapid strep test

NCLEX®

C. Therapeutic management

1. In viral pharyngitis, relief of symptoms is indicated; offer diet that is easy to swallow (soft or liquids) and soothing to sore throat (no citrus juices or other foods that could cause burning or increased irritation)
2. Saltwater gargles, throat lozenges, or anesthetic sprays promote pain relief
3. Medications: analgesics (acetaminophen); antibiotics for bacterial infections

D. Reinforce client and family teaching

1. Importance of completing antibiotic therapy to eradicate microorganisms
2. Untreated or inadequately treated streptococcal infections can result in acute rheumatic fever, glomerulonephritis, or other serious sequelae

XXI. TONSILLITIS

A. Overview

1. Inflammation of tonsils in posterior pharynx from viral or bacterial infection
2. Causative organism in bacterial infection can be *group A beta-hemolytic streptococcus,* which is particularly virulent

NCLEX®

B. Data collection

1. Diagnosis of etiology is made by throat culture
2. Streptococcal infection can be diagnosed within minutes using a rapid strep test
3. Symptoms
   a. Enlarged, reddened tonsils, with or without exudate
   b. Sore throat, difficulty swallowing because of severe sore throat
   c. Drooling, caused by the inability to swallow saliva secretions
   d. Lymphadenopathy
   e. Mouth breathing

NCLEX®

C. Therapeutic management

1. Management for viral tonsillitis is symptom relief: promoting comfort, pain relief with acetaminophen (Tylenol); is similar to management of viral pharyngitis
2. Management for bacterial tonsillitis is antibiotic therapy as well as symptom relief
3. Nursing management: offer diet that is easy to swallow (soft or liquids, including ice pops) and soothing to sore throat (no citrus juices or other foods that could cause burning or increased irritation)
4. Use of saltwater gargles, throat lozenges, or anesthetic sprays for pain relief
5. Medication therapy: analgesics (acetaminophen) for comfort and fever; antibiotics as ordered for bacterial infections

D. Reinforce child and family teaching: complete full course of antibiotic therapy; how to manage symptoms

E. Tonsillectomy

1. Surgical removal of tonsils; may be indicated for recurrent tonsillitis, peritonsillar abcess, or respiratory compromise from airway obstruction
2. Commonly performed in a day-surgery setting, ambulatory surgical setting, or may require an overnight hospital stay
3. Client should not have symptoms of tonsillitis for at least 1 week before surgery
4. Preoperative nursing management: includes client and family preoperative teaching, baseline lab data, including bleeding and clotting times

NCLEX®

5. Postoperative nursing management
   a. Provide pain control with analgesics and ice collar
   b. Most common complication is excessive bleeding or hemorrhaging from operative site; observe child for frequent or continual swallowing, vomiting bright red blood, and changes in vital signs
   c. Offer clear, chilled fluids or ice pops to relieve pain and reduce inflammation when awake and alert; avoid red-colored fluids because emesis of these fluids could be mistaken for blood
   d. Teach child and parents that a sore throat is to be expected for approximately 1 week postoperatively

F. Reinforce client and family teaching

1. Analgesic medications to be given at home
2. Observe child for signs of complications such as hemorrhage from operative site
3. Ensure adequate fluid intake to prevent dehydration; advance child's diet as tolerated to include soft, nonirritating foods; avoid citrus (acidic) foods and foods that are rough in texture for 10–14 days
4. Avoid strenuous activity for about 1 week; child may return to school in 10 days, when operative site is adequately healed

Check Your NCLEX-PN® Exam I.Q.

You are ready for testing on this content if you can

- Identify basic structures and functions of the eye and ear.
- Describe the pathophysiology and etiology of common eye and ear disorders.
- Discuss expected data and diagnostic test findings for selected eye and ear disorders.
- Discuss therapeutic management of a client experiencing an eye and ear disorder.
- Discuss nursing management of a client experiencing an eye and ear disorder.
- Identify expected outcomes for the client experiencing an eye and ear disorder.

PRACTICE TEST

1 To communicate effectively with a client who has hearing loss caused by presbycusis, the nurse should use which strategy to improve communication with the client? Select all that apply.

1. Approach the client from the front.
2. Use the mouth to exaggerate word pronunciation.
3. Shout initially to get the client's attention.
4. Turn down background noise from radio or TV before speaking.
5. Speak very loudly but in an even tone of voice.

2 A client has completed a full course of antibiotics for acute otitis media. The nurse conducting a follow-up examination to determine whether medication therapy was effective by questioning the client about relief from which most common presenting symptom?

1. Dizziness
2. Impaired hearing
3. Nausea and vomiting
4. Ear pain

3 A client has undergone myringotomy. The nurse working in an ambulatory surgery center would reinforce to the client to avoid which activity while healing is occurring?

1. Gardening
2. Swimming
3. Softball
4. Bowling

4 A 68-year-old female client tells the ambulatory care nurse during a routine visit that she has recently noticed a decline in her ability to hear. The nurse documents this information on the client's health record, suspecting that this client most likely is exhibiting which disorder?

1. Presbycusis
2. Otitis externa
3. Otalgia
4. Ménière's disease

5 After a client has undergone outpatient surgery for a right eye cataract removal, the nurse reinforces client teaching to avoid which activity when the client gets home? Select all that apply.

1. Walking about the house unassisted
2. Lying on the right side
3. Picking up objects that are at waist level
4. Washing dishes in the sink
5. Mowing the lawn

6 A client has hearing loss characterized by distortion of sounds that are heard. The client asks the nurse about the benefits of obtaining a hearing aid. The nurse would include in a response that a hearing aid will have which effect for this client?

1. It will intensify the already distorted sounds.
2. It will improve the client's ability to distinguish words from background noises.
3. It will make sounds louder and clearer.
4. It will have no effect on hearing.

7 A client reports ongoing problems with vertigo. The nurse should question the client about which accompanying manifestations to determine whether the client has developed Ménière's disease? Select all that apply.

1. Tinnitus
2. Hearing loss
3. Headache
4. Sense of fullness in the ear
5. Purulent discharge

8 The nurse prepares to reinforce client teaching for which medication commonly used to treat Ménière's disease?

1. Meclizine (Antivert)
2. Dexamethasone (Decadron)
3. Acetaminophen (Tylenol)
4. Propranolol (Inderal)

9 What should be the initial intervention by the nurse for a client in the emergency department who suffered a chemical burn to the eyes?

1. Administer an analgesic as prescribed.
2. Determine vision with and without prescription eyeglasses.
3. Administer an antibiotic as prescribed.
4. Irrigate the eyes with normal saline solution or water.

10 The nurse is caring for a client who is in the recovery area following cataract surgery. The nurse would ask the client about which manifestations that would indicate onset of retinal detachment as a postoperative complication? Select all that apply.

1. Increased lacrimation
2. Flashing lights
3. Sudden, severe eye pain
4. Inability to move the eye
5. Part loss of visual field in the eye

11 A client who was diagnosed with chronic open-angle glaucoma has been started on medication therapy with timolol maleate (Timoptic). The nurse monitors for which possible adverse systemic response to the drug?

1. Tachycardia
2. Anxiety
3. Bradycardia
4. Hypertension

12 The daughter of an older adult client diagnosed with dry macular degeneration asks the nurse to explain the disorder. In formulating a response, the nurse would include which characteristics of this condition?

1. Atrophy and degeneration of outer pigmented layer of the retina
2. Scar formation between the retina and the choroid
3. Rapid and severe loss of vision
4. Separation of the retina from the choroids

13 The nurse is determining the effectiveness of preoperative teaching for a client who will undergo repair of a detached retina using scleral buckling. The nurse identifies that the client understands the procedure after the client gives which description of the surgery?

1. Using a piece of silicone to indent the sclera to increase contact between retinal layers
2. Injecting a gas into the vitreous humor to push the detached retina against the choroid
3. Removing the torn segment of retina
4. Replacing the torn segment of the retina with donor retinal tissue

14 The nurse would take which action when the client first comes into the emergency department with blunt trauma to the eye?

1. Irrigate the eye to remove foreign substances.
2. Administer miotics.
3. Place the client in semi-Fowler's position.
4. Prevent loss of intraocular contents.

15 The nurse receives an order to do an otic irrigation to the left ear of an assigned client. The nurse uses which technique to perform this procedure correctly?

1. Direct the stream into the center of the ear canal.
2. Draw up 250 mL of solution.
3. Pack the external ear tightly with cotton balls after instilling the irrigant.
4. Help the client to lie on the left side after the irrigation is finished.

16 Which actions would be beneficial for the nurse to use as part of collaborative management of a client who has conjunctivitis? Select all that apply.

1. Cold eye compresses
2. Careful handwashing
3. Antibiotic therapy
4. Dark sunglasses
5. Opioid analgesics

17 The nurse needs to administer an ophthalmic medication to a client. What action by the nurse is the correct way to administer this medication?

1. Drop the medication onto the eyeball.
2. Apply pressure to the inner canthus while administering the medication.
3. Rub the eye with a cotton ball after instillation.
4. Wait 10 seconds between drops.

18 The nurse has administered a dose of antibiotic intramuscularly to a 5-year-old client with tonsillitis. The child cries for an adhesive bandage over the injection site. What is the best action by the nurse?

1. Apply an adhesive bandage.
2. Ask the child why he wants the bandage.
3. Explain to the child that an adhesive bandage is not necessary.
4. Show the child that the site is not bleeding.

19 What is the most appropriate intervention by the nurse who is caring for an infant with acute otitis media and a fever of 102.7°F?

1. Provide sponging with cool water to reduce fever.
2. Encourage the baby's intake of solids to maintain adequate caloric intake.
3. Swaddle the baby in layers of blankets to promote comfort and prevent chills.
4. Offer fluids frequently to prevent dehydration.

20 Which nursing diagnosis would be most appropriate for the nurse to use when caring for a child with pharyngitis?

1. Anxiety
2. Risk for Ineffective Airway Clearance
3. Risk for Deficient Fluid Volume
4. Impaired Growth and Development

21 The nurse recommends a humidified atmosphere for a child with recurrent epistaxis. When questioned by the parent, the nurse explains that which of the following is a benefit of humidity for the child?

1. Liquefies secretions
2. Improves oxygenation
3. Increases ventilation
4. Prevents drying of mucous membranes

22 The nurse would reinforce which instruction to a client after fluorescein angiography to diagnose an eye condition? Select all that apply.

1. Encourage reduced fluid intake to limit intraocular pressure.
2. The dye causes temporary green discoloration to urine.
3. Avoid sunlight until pupil size returns to normal.
4. Lie down with eyes closed for 12 hours postprocedure after returning home.
5. Expect headache and blurred vision for approximately 24 hours after the procedure.

23 The nurse reinforces teaching to the parents of an infant with chronic otitis media. What should the nurse recommend to prevent future infections? Select all that apply.

1. The parents should routinely administer nasal decongestant drops to their infant.
2. The parents should position the child supine for all feedings.
3. The parents should avoid exposing their infant to tobacco smoke.
4. The parents should apply warm compresses to the ear daily.
5. The parent should not allow the baby to fall asleep with a pacifier.

24 A 4-year-old has been diagnosed with amblyopia. The nurse who is providing the parents with information about this diagnosis should reinforce which items of information? Select all that apply.

1. The eye itself has lost the cells that send the visual data to the brain.
2. The child will need to wear a patch over his unaffected eye.
3. If not treated, the child may become permanently blind in the affected eye.
4. The brain shuts off the signal from both eyes because of misalignment of the eyes.
5. Amblyopia is diagnosed with the Snellen E chart.

25 The nurse working in a pediatric clinic concludes that which finding in a child indicates a risk for visual impairment?

1. Delayed language development
2. Excessive rubbing of the eyes
3. Disinterest in watching television
4. Bilateral symmetric corneal light reflex

ANSWERS & RATIONALES

1 **Answer: 1, 4** **Rationale:** The client should be approached from the front so as not to startle the client. An effective method to improve communication with the client is to eliminate background noises that could interfere with hearing. The nurse should use normal pronunciation of words to assist the client's understanding. The nurse should refrain from shouting, which is demeaning and not helpful. The nurse should speak in normal tones to aid hearing; speaking very loudly is not necessarily helpful and can be perceived as demeaning. **Cognitive Level:** Analyzing **Client Need:** Physiological Adaptation **Integrated Process:** Communication and Documentation **Content Area:** Adult Health **Strategy:** The core issue of the question is the appropriate strategy for communicating with a client who is hearing impaired. Recall that clients rely on visual cues and can benefit from reduced background noise to aid in answering the question.

2 **Answer: 4** **Rationale:** Ear pain is the most common symptom of otitis media that motivates clients to seek health care. Secondary or associated symptoms include fever, nausea and vomiting, dizziness, and hearing impairment. **Cognitive Level:** Analyzing **Client Need:** Physiological Adaptation **Integrated Process:** Nursing Process: Data Collection **Content Area:** Adult Health **Strategy:** The critical words in the question are *most common*, which tell you it is necessary to prioritize the options by the frequency of their occurrence. Use nursing knowledge and the process of elimination to make this selection.

3 **Answer: 2** **Rationale:** Myringotomy is a surgical procedure that perforates the tympanic membrane to allow drainage from the middle ear. Postoperatively, the client should avoid getting water into the ear canal, which could potentially enter the middle ear. Activities such as gardening, softball, and bowling do not risk water getting into the surgical ear pose no risk to the client. **Cognitive Level:** Applying **Client Need:** Physiological Adaptation **Integrated Process:** Nursing Process: Implementation **Content Area:** Adult Health **Strategy:** The core issue of the question is identification of activities that could be harmful to the client while healing is occurring after surgery. Recall that it is necessary to avoid getting the surgical area wet to make the appropriate selection.

4 **Answer: 1** **Rationale:** Presbycusis is the most common form of sensorineural hearing loss in older adults. Otitis externa is infection in the external auditory canal and can occur in clients of any age. Otalgia is an earache. Ménière's disease is an inner ear disorder characterized by tinnitus and vertigo that primarily affects middle-aged adults. **Cognitive Level:** Applying **Client Need:** Physiological Adaptation **Integrated Process:** Nursing Process: Data Collection **Content Area:** Adult Health **Strategy:** The core issue of the question is the ability to identify age-related changes in hearing in an older adult. Use nursing knowledge and the process of elimination to make a selection.

5 **Answer: 2, 5** **Rationale:** The client should avoid lying on the operative side following eye surgery to minimize edema and intraocular pressure. Activities that involved pushing or straining, such as mowing the lawn, can increase intraocular pressure and should be avoided in the postoperative period. Walking unassisted is not a problem given the information in the question. Some clients with severe visual impairment or other health problems may need assistance to move about in the environment. Picking up objects at waist level

is acceptable because it does not raise intraocular pressure. Washing dishes in the sink poses no risk to the client as it does not increase intraocular pressure. **Cognitive Level:** Analyzing **Client Need:** Physiological Adaptation **Integrated Process:** Nursing Process: Implementation **Content Area:** Adult Health **Strategy:** The core issue of the question is reinforcing client teaching about safe and unsafe activities following cataract surgery. Recall that it is important to avoid positions in which gravity can lead to increased edema or pressure to make the correct selection.

6 **Answer: 1 Rationale:** When hearing loss is characterized by distortion of sounds, amplification of sound is of little help because it only increases the intensity of distorted sounds, and a hearing aid will not help the client distinguish words from background noises or make words louder and clearer. A hearing aid will have some effect for this client but it will not be helpful. **Cognitive Level:** Applying **Client Need:** Physiological Adaptation **Integrated Process:** Nursing Process: Implementation **Content Area:** Adult Health **Strategy:** The core issue of the question is the ability to correlate the types of hearing loss that can be improved with the use of a hearing aid. To do this, reflect on the types of hearing loss and the likely effect of a hearing aid for that condition. Use nursing knowledge and the process of elimination to make a selection.

7 **Answer: 1, 2, 4 Rationale:** Vertigo, tinnitus, hearing loss, and a sense of fullness in the ear are classic symptoms of Ménière's disease. Nystagmus also occurs with acute attacks. Headache is not part of this clinical picture. Purulent drainage suggests infection. **Cognitive Level:** Applying **Client Need:** Physiological Adaptation **Integrated Process:** Nursing Process: Data Collection **Content Area:** Adult Health **Strategy:** The core issue of the question is identification of signs and symptoms of Ménière's disease. Recall that this is a disorder of the inner ear, thus making symptoms related to balance as well as hearing important to identify. Use nursing knowledge and the process of elimination to make a selection.

8 **Answer: 1 Rationale:** Antivertigo and antiemetic medications, such as meclizine, are used to control symptoms associated with Ménière's disease. Diuretics are used between acute attacks to reduce the volume of endolymph and prevent attacks. Glucocorticoids such as dexamethasone are not used to treat Ménière's disease. Analgesics such as acetaminophen, which work at the level of the peripheral nervous system, are not part of the treatment plan. Beta-blockers such as propranolol have no role in the treatment of Ménière's disease. **Cognitive Level:** Analyzing **Client Need:** Physiological Adaptation **Integrated Process:** Teaching and Learning **Content Area:** Adult Health **Strategy:** The core issue of the question is the ability to anticipate medications that will be effective in relieving the symptoms associated with Ménière's disease. To answer correctly, it is necessary to have a core body of knowledge related to pharmacology. Use nursing knowledge and the process of elimination to make a selection.

9 **Answer: 4 Rationale:** The immediate priority for clients with chemical burns is flushing the affected eye with copious amounts of normal saline or water. Analgesics, with the exception of topical anesthesia, are not indicated. Determination of visual acuity is an appropriate intervention after flushing. Antibiotics may be administered after the initial actions have been taken. **Cognitive Level:** Applying **Client Need:** Safety and Infection Control **Integrated Process:** Nursing Process: Implementation **Content Area:** Adult Health **Strategy:** The critical word in the question is *initial*, which indicates more than one or all options could be correct and it is necessary to prioritize the most important or immediate action needed. Whenever there is an injury involving chemicals, the priority action is to remove the offending substance.

10 **Answer: 2, 5 Rationale:** Clients with retinal detachment frequently report flashing lights and loss of vision, commonly described as a veil or curtain being drawn across the eye. Retinal detachment is not associated with increased lacrimation or tearing, eye pain, or change in ocular movements. **Cognitive Level:** Applying **Client Need:** Physiological Adaptation **Integrated Process:** Nursing Process: Data Collection **Content Area:** Adult Health **Strategy:** The core issue of the question is knowledge of complications of cataract surgery. Use nursing knowledge and the process of elimination to make a selection.

11 **Answer: 3 Rationale:** Medications that end in *-olol* are beta-adrenergic blocking agents. When taken as ophthalmic preparations, they can produce systemic effects such as bradycardia, hypotension, and bronchospasm. Beta-adrenergic blockers may also be used to treat adrenergic symptoms associated with anxiety, but this does not relate to glaucoma. **Cognitive Level:** Applying **Client Need:** Physiological Adaptation **Integrated Process:** Nursing Process: Data Collection **Content Area:** Adult Health **Strategy:** The core issue of the question is the ability to identify adverse effects of medication used to treat glaucoma. To answer correctly, it is necessary to have a core body of knowledge related to pharmacology. Use nursing knowledge and the process of elimination to make a selection.

12 **Answer: 1 Rationale:** Atrophic or dry macular degeneration results from atrophy and degeneration of the outer layer of the retina. In exudative, or wet macular degeneration, blood leaks into the subretinal space and scar tissue gradually forms. The resulting loss of vision occurs rapidly and is more profound. Exudative macular degeneration accounts for 90% of all cases of legal blindness. Separation of the retina from the choroid describes retinal detachment. **Cognitive Level:** Applying **Client Need:** Physiological Adaptation **Integrated Process:** Nursing Process: Implementation **Content Area:** Adult Health **Strategy:** The core issue of the question is the ability to discriminate correct information to be reinforced in teaching clients and/or families about disease processes. Thus, to answer this question, it is necessary to understand the two types of macular degeneration and how they present in terms of symptoms.

13 **Answer: 1 Rationale:** Scleral buckling involves using a piece of silicone, which is used to indent the sclera to increase contact between the retinal layers. It is used in conjunction with laser photocoagulation or cryothermy to achieve the best results. A gas is injected into the vitreous humor during pneumatic retinopexy as treatment for detached retina. Scleral buckling does not involve removing the torn segment of retina, which would result in permanent vision loss in that area of the eye. Scleral buckling does not include use of donor retinal tissue. **Cognitive Level:** Applying **Client Need:** Physiological Adaptation **Integrated Process:** Teaching and Learning **Content Area:** Adult Health **Strategy:** The core issue of the question is determination of a client's understanding of a surgical procedure. To select correctly, it is necessary to be able to identify how the surgery will be performed. Use nursing knowledge and the process of elimination to make a selection.

14 **Answer: 3 Rationale:** Prevention or reduction of intraocular pressure (that may accompany blunt trauma to the eye) can

be accomplished by the use of semi-Fowler's position and administration of a carbonic anhydrase inhibitor, such as acetazolamide (Diamox). Semi-Fowler's position also reduces edema formation at the site of injury when compared to lying flat. It is unnecessary to irrigate the eye because no foreign body is present. Constriction of the pupil with miotics is not indicated. Blunt trauma does not cause loss of intraocular contents. **Cognitive Level:** Applying **Client Need:** Physiological Adaptation **Integrated Process:** Nursing Process: Implementation **Content Area:** Adult Health **Strategy:** The core issue of the question is identification of a correct action in the treatment of eye trauma. Recall that injuries typically cause formation of edema at the site, and thus early actions for an injury may involve proper client positioning to reduce edema formation.

15 **Answer: 4 Rationale:** The client should lie on the affected side following the irrigation to allow gravity to further assist in draining the ear canal. The irrigant should be directed along the wall of the external canal, not the center (which could damage the tympanic membrane). Usually 50 to 70 mL of solution is used, according to the size of the syringe used for the procedure. A single cotton ball is placed loosely into the external meatus to absorb any remaining irrigant after the procedure. **Cognitive Level:** Applying **Client Need:** Physiological Adaptation **Integrated Process:** Nursing Process: Implementation **Content Area:** Adult Health **Strategy:** The core issue of the question is the ability to correctly perform the nursing procedure of ear irrigation. Use nursing knowledge and the process of elimination to make a selection.

16 **Answer: 2, 3, 4 Rationale:** Careful hand hygiene is effective in reducing the risk of transmitting the infection to others. Antibiotic therapy kills the bacteria that are responsible for the eye infection. Dark sunglasses are helpful in reducing photophobia. Warm compresses, not cold, should be used as part of the management of conjunctivitis. Warm compresses help relieve discomfort and reduce inflammation by increasing circulation to the area. Although there is eye discomfort, there is no need for strong analgesics such as opioids. **Cognitive Level:** Applying **Client Need:** Physiological Adaptation **Integrated Process:** Nursing Process: Implementation **Content Area:** Adult Health **Strategy:** A critical word in the stem of the question is *useful*, indicating that the correct answer is an option that is either correct or high priority. Use nursing knowledge about care of the client with conjunctivitis and the process of elimination to make selections.

17 **Answer: 2 Rationale:** The nurse should apply pressure to the inner canthus (nasolacrimal duct) during and for at least 30 seconds after instillation, according to agency procedure, to prevent systemic absorption of the medication. The medication should be dropped into the lower conjunctival sac. The eye should not be rubbed after instillation of the medication. The nurse should wait from 1 to 5 minutes between drops, depending on the medication and manufacturer's recommendations. **Cognitive Level:** Applying **Client Need:** Physiological Adaptation **Integrated Process:** Nursing Process: Implementation **Content Area:** Adult Health **Strategy:** The core issue of the question is the ability to administer eye medication correctly. Use nursing knowledge and the process of elimination to make a selection.

18 **Answer: 1 Rationale:** It is appropriate to comfort the child following a painful procedure and applying the bandage provides support and comfort. There is no reason to question the child. By fulfilling the child's request, the nurse allows the child to regain some control over the situation. The child may be looking for comfort rather than concerned about bleeding. **Cognitive Level:** Analyzing **Client Need:** Psychosocial Integrity **Integrated Process:** Nursing Process: Implementation **Content Area:** Child Health **Strategy:** The core issue of the question is the best response to a 5-year-old client who is responding to a painful procedure such as an injection. Eliminate options that do not meet the client's immediate need for comfort following the injection.

19 **Answer: 4 Rationale:** A febrile infant is at risk for deficient fluid volume deficit from larger-than-normal insensible fluid losses and decreased fluid intake. It is contraindicated to sponge with cool water, which could lead to shivering and higher temperature. Intake of solid food is less important than preventing dehydration. A febrile infant will experience a higher fever if blankets are added. **Cognitive Level:** Analyzing **Client Need:** Physiological Adaptation **Integrated Process:** Nursing Process: Implementation **Content Area:** Child Health **Strategy:** The core issue of the question is an appropriate nursing intervention when a client has fever caused by ear infection. Use nursing knowledge and the process of elimination to make a selection.

20 **Answer: 3 Rationale:** A symptom of pharyngitis is sore throat and difficulty swallowing, which could lead to the refusal to drink. Thus, risk for deficient fluid volume is an appropriate diagnosis. The client may have anxiety because of pain associated with pharyngitis, but this will resolve with treatment of the infection. Risk for ineffective airway clearance would apply if the client cannot clear secretions from the respiratory tract, which is not evident in this question. Impaired growth and development is not a concern with this brief health problem. **Cognitive Level:** Analyzing **Client Need:** Physiological Adaptation **Integrated Process:** Nursing Process: Planning **Content Area:** Child Health **Strategy:** The core issue of the question is the ability to determine priority concerns for a client with pharyngitis by selecting a nursing diagnosis. Whenever the airway is involved, first think about the ABCs and then think about hydration/food intake as the next priority of physiological needs using Maslow's hierarchy.

21 **Answer: 4 Rationale:** Humidifying the air can prevent dry mucous membranes and recurrence of epistaxis. Liquefying secretions is not a concern for a client with recurrent nosebleed. Humidification does not increase the oxygen percentage of ambient air, which is 21%. Humidifying the air does not increase the client's ventilation. **Cognitive Level:** Applying **Client Need:** Physiological Adaptation **Integrated Process:** Nursing Process: Implementation **Content Area:** Child Health **Strategy:** The core issue of the question is an understanding of the rationale for nursing actions for a client with recurrent epistaxis. Use nursing knowledge and the process of elimination to make a selection.

22 **Answer: 2, 3 Rationale:** The client should know that the dye causes temporary skin discoloration in the injected area and temporary green discoloration of urine that resolves when dye is fully excreted. The client should avoid sunlight or other bright light sources until pupil dilation returns to normal. Typical instructions after fluorescein angiography include increased fluid intake to aid in dye excretion. Although the client should rest after the procedure, it is not necessary to lie down with eyes closed for 12 hours. Headache and blurred vision are not expected. **Cognitive Level:** Analyzing **Client Need:** Physiological Adaptation **Integrated Process:** Teaching and Learning **Content Area:** Adult Health **Strategy:** The core issue of

ANSWERS & RATIONALES

the question is knowledge of postprocedure instructions to a client following fluorescein dye eye examination. Use nursing knowledge and general concepts of procedures that utilize contrast dye to make your selections.

23 **Answer: 3, 5 Rationale:** Exposure to secondhand smoke increases incidence of otitis media so this should be avoided to reduce the risk of future episodes of otitis media. Preventing the infant from falling asleep with a pacifier will also help because saliva from sucking cannot accumulate and enter the Eustachian tube. Medications such as a nasal decongestant would have side effects and should be avoided unless specifically needed. Infants who feed in the supine position have an increased risk of otitis media. Warm compresses will not prevent future infection. **Cognitive Level:** Analyzing **Client Need:** Physiological Adaptation **Integrated Process:** Teaching and Learning **Content Area:** Child Health **Strategy:** Consider which options will have an effect on the middle ear. Warm compresses cannot be applied to the middle ear, so that option is incorrect. From this point, recall risk factors for otitis media to aid in choosing the correct options.

24 **Answer: 2, 3 Rationale:** Without treatment, including patching, corrective lenses, and muscular exercises, the damage will become permanent. Without treatment, including patching, corrective lenses, and muscular exercises, the damage will become permanent. The pathophysiology is misalignment of the eyes causing the brain to stop receiving the signal of the affected eye. The pathophysiology is misalignment of the eyes causing the brain to stop receiving the signal of the affected eye. Vision testing is done with the Snellen chart not the Snellen E chart. **Cognitive Level:** Applying **Client Need:** Physiological Adaptation **Integrated Process:** Teaching and Learning **Content Area:** Child Health **Strategy:** Knowledge of amblyopia, its causes and treatment, will assist in correctly answering this straight forward question.

25 **Answer: 2 Rationale:** Symptoms of decreased visual acuity are squinting to focus, excessive tearing of the eyes, and rubbing of the eye. **Cognitive Level:** Applying **Client Need:** Physiological Adaptation **Integrated Process:** Nursing Process: Data Collection **Content Area:** Child Health **Strategy:** Language would not be affected by diminished vision. To distinguish among the other options, recall signs of visual impairment at various ages.

Key Terms to Review

amblyopia p. 1117
cataract p. 1119
corneal light reflex (Hirschberg test) p. 1116
cover-uncover test p. 1116
cycloplegic p. 1115
epistaxis p. 1127
glaucoma p. 1118
gonioscopy p. 1118
Ménière's disease p. 1126
miotic p. 1119
mydriatic p. 1115
nystagmus p. 1112
otitis media p. 1124
otosclerosis p. 1124
pharyngitis p. 1128
presbycusis p. 1111
presbyopia p. 1111
proprioception p. 1111
strabismus p. 1116
tonometry p. 1111
tonsillitis p. 1128

References

Ball, J., Bindler, R., & Cowen, K. (2010). *Child health nursing: Partnering with children and families* (2nd ed.). Upper Saddle River, NJ: Pearson Education.

Berman, A., & Snyder, S. (2012). *Kozier & Erb's fundamentals of nursing: Concepts, process, and practice* (9th ed.). Upper Saddle River, NJ: Pearson Education.

Ignatavicius, D., & Workman, L. (2010). *Medical-surgical nursing: Critical thinking for collaborative care* (6th ed.). Philadelphia: Saunders.

Kee, J. (2010). *Laboratory and diagnostic tests with nursing implications* (8th ed.). Upper Saddle River, NJ: Pearson Education.

LeMone, P., Burke, K., & Bauldoff, G. (2011). *Medical-surgical nursing: Critical thinking in patient care* (5th ed.). Upper Saddle River, NJ: Pearson Education.

Smith, S., Duell, D., & Martin, B. (2012). *Clinical nursing skills: Basic to advanced skills* (8th ed.). Upper Saddle River, NJ: Pearson Education.

Test Yourself

Are you ready for the NCLEX-PN® or course exams? Use the practice tests on the companion website to check.

60 Hematological Disorders

In this chapter

Cross Reference

Other chapters relevant to this content area are

I. OVERVIEW OF ANATOMY AND PHYSIOLOGY OF HEMATOLOGICAL SYSTEM

A. Blood components

1. Plasma: straw-colored liquid portion of blood; comprises 50–55% of a blood sample; consists of water (approximately 92%), amino acids, proteins, carbohydrates, lipids, vitamins, hormones, electrolytes, and cellular wastes
2. Serum is essentially same as plasma but without fibrinogen and clotting factors
3. Blood cells (red blood cells [RBCs], white blood cells [WBCs]) and platelets comprise remaining blood sample; see Chapter 42 for detailed discussion of blood cells
4. Volume of blood is approximately 8% of total body weight

B. Normal clotting mechanisms

1. **Hemostasis** and coagulation are a series of reactions leading to clot formation in an injured or damaged area

2. Involves three mechanisms: vascular constriction and spasm, formation of platelet plug, and activation of clotting factors; fibrin clot is produced through either intrinsic or extrinsic pathway; both pathways end in common coagulation cascade
   a. Intrinsic pathway: stimulated by contact with foreign surfaces without tissue damage; initiated by activation of Hageman factor which, in presence of calcium (Ca^+) ions, triggers a series of changes leading to formation of prothrombin activator
   b. Extrinsic pathway: triggered by release of tissue thromboplastin from damaged tissues
3. After a clot forms, **fibrinolysis** (clot breakdown) occurs; plasminogen from blood clot is transformed into plasmin, which dissolves fibrin strands of clot; peak action is 7 to 10 days after clot formation

II. DIAGNOSTIC TESTS AND DATA COLLECTION

A. RBC count (see Table 60–1)

B. Hemoglobin and hematocrit

1. Hemoglobin (Hgb) measures oxygen-carrying capacity of an erythrocyte
2. Hematocrit (Hct) is ratio of RBC volume to volume of whole blood

C. RBC indexes

1. MCV (mean corpuscular volume): estimates size of RBC
2. MCH (mean corpuscular hemoglobin): measures content of Hgb in RBCs from a single cell
3. MCHC (mean corpuscular hemoglobin concentration): more accurate measurement of Hgb content of RBC because it measures entire volume of RBCs

D. Serum ferritin, transferrin, and total iron-binding capacity (TIBC): evaluate iron levels; ferritin measures iron in plasma, which is also a direct reflection of total iron stores; transferrin is major iron-transport protein

E. WBC count (see Table 60–2)

1. Abnormal elevation of WBC count is referred to as **leukocytosis**
2. **Leukopenia** is a decrease in number of WBCs
3. Differential count refers to breakdown of different types of cells

F. Coagulation studies (Table 60–3)

1. *Bleeding time:* used to evaluate platelet function; extended bleeding times are seen with **thrombocytopenia** (decrease or cessation of platelet production) and aspirin therapy, as well anticoagulants and several other drugs
2. *Prothrombin Time (PT)*: measures speed of blood clotting; PT evaluates extrinsic coagulation pathway, which includes factors I, II, V, VII, X; International normalized ratio (INR) is often used instead of PT because it is a standardized value (therapeutic range is often 2 to 3 depending on condition) *NCLEX®*
3. *Partial thromboplastin time (PTT)*: evaluates intrinsic coagulation pathway or fibrin clot formation

Table 60–1 Normal Laboratory Values for Red Blood Cells and Platelets

Laboratory Test		Normal Value
Red blood cell count	Men	4.2–5.4 million/mm^3
	Women	3.6–5.0 million/mm^3
Reticulocytes		1.0–1.5% of total RBC
Hemoglobin (Hgb)	Men	14–16.5 grams/dL
	Women	12–15 grams/dL
Hematocrit (Hct)	Men	40–50%
	Women	37–47%
Mean corpuscular volume (MCV)		85–100 fL/cell
Mean corpuscular hemoglobin concentration (MCHC)		31–35 grams/dL
Mean corpuscular hemoglobin (MCH)		27–34 pg/cell
Platelet count		150,000–400,000/mm^3

Source: Adapted from Lemone, P., & Burke, K. *Medical-surgical nursing: Critical thinking in client care* (3rd ed.), © 2004, p. 934. Reprinted by permission of Pearson Education, Inc., Upper Saddle River, NJ 07458.

Table 60–2 Normal Laboratory Values: White Blood Cells

Laboratory Test	Value
WBC count	5000–10000/mm^3
Differential	
Neutrophils	60–70% or 3000–7000/mm^3
Eosinophils	1–3% or 50–400/mm^3
Basophils	0.3–0.5% or 25–200/mm^3
Lymphocytes	20–30% or 1000–4000/mm^3
Monocytes	3–8% or 100–600/mm^3

Source: LeMone, P., Burke, K., & Bauldoff, G. *Medical-surgical nursing: Critical thinking in client care* (5th ed.), © 2011, p. 1084. Reprinted by permission of Pearson Education, Inc., Upper Saddle River, NJ 07458.

Table 60–3 Coagulation Studies

Laboratory Test	Normal Value
Bleeding time	1 to 4 minutes
Prothrombin time (PT)	11 to 16 seconds
International normalized ratio (INR)	2 to 3 (usual therapeutic value)
Partial thromboplastin time (PTT)	60 to 70 seconds
Activated partial thromboplastin time (aPTT)	30 to 45 seconds
Fibrinogen	150 to 400 mg/dL
Fibrin degradation products (FDP	Less than 10 mcg/mL
Fibrin D-dimer	0 to 0.5 mcg/mL

NCLEX®
4. *Activated partial thromboplastin time (aPTT)*: is a modified PTT, preferred because it is quicker to perform; aPTT is used in heparin therapy and when evaluating hemophilia; aPTT is increased in anticoagulation therapy, liver disease, vitamin K deficiency, and disseminated intravascular coagulopathy (DIC)
5. *Fibrinogen:* is a soluble plasma protein necessary for clotting that is decreased in DIC and fibrinogen disorders and increased in acute infections, hepatitis, and oral contraceptive use
6. *Fibrin degradation products (FDP)*: FDP is increased in fibrinolysis, thrombolytic therapy, and DIC
7. *Fibrin D-dimer:* D-dimer is the most sensitive indicator to differentiate DIC from primary fibrinolysis; it is elevated in DIC

G. Bone marrow examination

1. Specimens may be obtained by aspiration (most common) or biopsy
2. NCLEX® Sites for bone marrow aspiration may include sternum, iliac crest (most common), and tibia; most common site for bone marrow biopsy is posterosuperior iliac spine (sternum also is used)
3. Position client based on site selected; skin and periosteum are anesthetized to decrease pain with anesthetic such as procaine; marrow aspiration needle is then inserted; after marrow cavity is entered, marrow stylet is removed from needle and a sterile syringe is attached; syringe plunger is drawn back until marrow appears in syringe
4. NCLEX® During withdrawal of aspirate, client will experience sharp pain often described as burning
5. NCLEX® After needle is removed, apply pressure dressing over puncture site, where only minimal bleeding should occur; if client has thrombocytopenia, apply pressure for 3 to 5 minutes
6. Check agency procedure for handling specimens
7. Most clients experience little, if any, pain or discomfort after procedure; some report tenderness and ache at aspiration site for a few days
8. NCLEX® Procedure for a bone marrow biopsy is essentially same as for aspiration; after procedure, monitor clients for bleeding from puncture site

H. Lymphangiography: visualization of lymph system radiographically after injection of a dye; used primarily to stage Hodgkin's and non-Hodgkin's lymphoma

I. Lymph node biopsy: obtains lymph tissue for histologic analysis; a closed-needle biopsy can be done at bedside, or open biopsy can be performed in operating room

III. IRON-DEFICIENCY ANEMIA (IDA)

A. Overview: anemia that results when iron supply is inadequate for optimal RBC formation because of excessive iron loss from bleeding, decreased dietary intake, or malabsorption

1. Accounts for 60% of anemias in clients over age 65; most common cause is blood loss from GI or GU system
2. Normal iron excretion is less than 1 mg/day through urine, sweat, bile, feces, and from desquamated cells of the skin; an average woman loses 0.5 mg of iron daily or 15 mg monthly during menstruation (most common cause of iron deficiency in women); GI bleeding is most common cause in men
3. Anemia reduces O_2-carrying capacity of blood, producing tissue hypoxia
4. Iron is stored in body tissues (primarily in reticuloendothelial cells of liver, spleen, and bone marrow) as ferritin after being formed in intestinal mucosa
5. Anemia develops slowly through 3 phases: depletion of body stores of iron; insufficient iron transport to bone marrow, and onset of iron-deficient erythopoiesis
6. Average diet supplies body with 12 to 15 mg/day of iron, of which only 5–10% is absorbed; minimum daily needs are approximately 6 mg/day (infants under 6 months), 10 mg/day (6 months to adolescence, and over age 50), 12 mg/day (adolescent males), and 15 mg/day (females from adolescence to age 50)

NCLEX® **B. Nursing data collection**

1. Fatigue and weakness, dizziness
2. Shortness of breath
3. Pallor (ear lobes, palms, and conjunctiva)
4. Brittle spoonlike nails
5. **Cheilosis** (cracks in the corners of the mouth)
6. Smooth, sore tongue
7. Pica (craving to eat unusual substances such as clay or starch)
8. Blood sample shows **microcytic** and **hypochromic** anemia (small RBC diameter with decreased pigmentation) and an increase in red cell size distribution width (RDW)
   a. Decreased MCV, MCH, and MCHC; analyzed only when Hgb is low
   b. Low serum iron level and elevated serum iron-binding capacity or low serum ferritin levels

C. Therapeutic management

1. Review history for cause
2. *NCLEX®* Examine stools for occult blood; endoscopic examination and other diagnostic procedures may be done to detect possible sources of bleeding
3. *NCLEX®* Increase intake of iron-rich foods, such as organ meats, meat, beans, green leafy vegetables, molasses, and raisins
4. *NCLEX®* Administer iron supplements
   a. Give oral iron preparation with orange juice or vitamin C to increase absorption; antacids interfere with absorption of iron
   b. Oral liquid form of iron can stain teeth; clients should use a straw or place spoon at back of mouth to take supplement and rinse mouth thoroughly afterward
   c. Usual therapy is oral ferrous sulfate ($FeSO_4$) 300 to 325 mg t.i.d., given 1 hour before meals for 6 months; other oral forms may include ferrous gluconate (Fergon) and ferrous fumarate (Ircon, Femiron)
5. *NCLEX®* Administer parenteral iron dextran (InFed) by deep IM route via Z-track method
   a. Use separate needles for withdrawing and injecting medication
   b. There is risk of anaphylaxis with parenteral administration, so give small test dose before giving full dose
   c. Monitor for systemic (allergic) reactions (flushing, nausea/vomiting, myalgias) and report promptly if they occur
6. Identify and implement energy conservation techniques (e.g., shower chair, sitting to perform tasks)
7. Promote quiet environment to facilitate sleep and rest
8. Monitor for dizziness; suggest position changes be made slowly
9. Provide assistance with activities and ambulation as needed, allowing client independence as much as safely possible

10. Monitor laboratory studies (e.g., Hgb/Hct, RBC count)
11. Administer medications, blood, or blood products as indicated; monitor closely for transfusion reactions
12. Encourage and assist with good oral hygiene before and after meals, using soft-bristled toothbrush for gentle brushing of fragile gums
13. NCLEX® Determine stool color, consistency, frequency, and amount; may appear greenish black and tarry; caution client that iron supplements usually cause constipation and client should take preventive measures (fluids, fiber)
14. Encourage fluid intake of 2500 to 3000 mL day unless contraindicated by another medical condition, such as heart or renal failure
15. Discuss use of stool softeners, bulk-forming laxatives, mild stimulants, or enemas if indicated; monitor effectiveness
16. Refer to appropriate community resources when indicated (e.g., social services for food stamps, Meals on Wheels)
17. Transfusion of packed RBCs may be necessary if anemia is severe

D. Reinforce client teaching

1. Maintain good nutrition; older adults and those with limited economic means may have dietary deficiencies requiring referrals to appropriate agencies (e.g., Meals on Wheels)
2. NCLEX® Take iron on an empty stomach; absorption of iron is decreased with food; absorption may be enhanced when taken with an acidic beverage (such as one with vitamin C), but avoid grapefruit juice
3. Stools will appear black with oral iron intake
4. Report persistent GI symptoms secondary to iron intake
5. Iron preparations cause constipation; use stool softeners and increase oral intake of fluids and fiber as preventive measures
6. NCLEX® Foods high in iron include organ meats (beef or calf liver, chicken liver), other meats, beans (black, pinto, and garbanzo), leafy green vegetables, raisins, and molasses

IV. MEGALOBLASTIC ANEMIA

A. Vitamin B_{12} deficiency anemia (pernicious anemia)

1. Overview
   a. A type of anemia characterized by macrocytic RBCs
   b. Inevitably develops after total gastrectomy, 15% of clients develop pernicious anemia after partial gastrectomy or gastrojejunostomy
   c. Lack of vitamin B_{12} alters structure and disrupts function of peripheral nerves, spinal cord, and brain; its lack also impairs cellular division and maturation, especially in rapidly proliferating RBCs
   d. Pernicious anemia inhibits ability to absorb vitamin B_{12} because of lack of intrinsic factor, a substance secreted by parietal cells of gastric mucosa
2. NCLEX® Nursing data collection
   a. Pallor or slight jaundice with a complaint of weakness
   b. Smooth, sore, beefy red tongue (**glossitis**), and cheilosis (cracking of lips)
   c. Diarrhea
   d. Paresthesias (numbness or tingling in extremities)
   e. Impaired proprioception (difficulty identifying one's position in space, which may progress to difficulty with balance)
   f. Clients with this anemia tend to be fair-haired or prematurely gray
   g. Macrocytic (megaloblastic) anemia (RBC diameter > 8) with increase in MCV and MCHC
   h. Gastric secretion analysis reveals achlorhydria: absence of free hydrochloric acid in a pH maintained at 3.5
   i. Twenty-four-hour urine for Schilling test (a vitamin B_{12} absorption test that indicates lack of intrinsic factor by measuring excretion of orally administered radionuclide-labeled B_{12}) confirms diagnosis of pernicious anemia
3. Therapeutic management
   a. Review required diet alterations to meet specific dietary needs; if deficiency is caused by vegetarian diet, fortified soy milk may be added, or oral supplements of B_{12} may be added
   b. Monitor client carefully for neurologic deficits and assist client to prevent injury
   c. If deficiency is caused by gastric malabsorption such as deficiency of intrinsic factor, lifelong replacement therapy is required
   d. NCLEX® Medication therapy: parenteral vitamin B_{12}, 100 to 1000 mcg subcutaneously daily for 7 days, then once a week for 1 month, then monthly for lifetime is usually prescribed; a nasal form is now available also

4. Reinforce client teaching
   a. A burning sensation felt after a parenteral dose of vitamin B_{12} is temporary

NCLEX®
   b. Dietary sources of vitamin B_{12} include dairy products, animal proteins, and eggs
   c. A regular schedule of replacement vitamin B_{12} and importance and necessity for continued treatment are important for clients who have pernicious anemia

B. Folic acid–deficiency anemia

1. Overview
   a. Anemia caused by a deficiency of folic acid, which interrupts DNA synthesis and normal maturation of RBCs; frequently accompanies iron-deficiency anemia
   b. Causative etiologies: poor nutrition, malabsorption syndrome, medications that impede absorption (oral contraceptives, antiepileptics, methotrexate), alcohol abuse, and anorexia
   c. Clients at risk include those with alcoholism, receiving total parenteral nutrition (TPN), pregnant women, infants, teenagers, and clients on hemodialysis
   d. Lack of folic acid causes formation of megaloblastic cells, which are fragile

NCLEX®

2. Nursing data collection
   a. Pallor, progressive weakness, fatigue
   b. Shortness of breath
   c. Cardiac palpitations
   d. GI symptoms are similar to B_{12} deficiency but usually more severe (glossitis, cheilosis, and diarrhea)
   e. Neurological symptoms seen in B_{12} deficiency are not seen in folic acid deficiency and therefore assist in differentiating these two types of anemia
   f. RBC analysis shows macrocytic (megaloblastic) anemia (RBC diameter > 8), high MCV with low hemoglobin, low serum folate level
3. Therapeutic management

NCLEX®
   a. Includes dietary counseling and administration of folic acid
   b. Identify and implement energy conservation techniques (e.g., shower chair, sitting to perform tasks)
   c. Monitor for dizziness; suggest position changes be made slowly
   d. Provide assistance with activities and ambulation as needed, allowing client independence as much as safely possible
   e. Monitor laboratory studies (e.g., Hgb/Hct, RBC count)
   f. Encourage and assist with good oral hygiene before and after meals, using soft-bristled toothbrush for gentle brushing of fragile gums
   g. Refer to appropriate community resources when indicated (e.g., social services for food stamps, Meals on Wheels, Alcoholics Anonymous)
   h. Medication therapy: oral folate, 1 to 5 mg/day for 3 to 4 months; folate should be given along with vitamin B_{12} when both are deficient
4. Reinforce client teaching

NCLEX®
   a. Dietary sources of folic acid such as green leafy vegetables, fish, citrus fruits, yeast, dried beans, grains, nuts, and liver
   b. Increase intake through diet selection and supplements for those at risk
   c. Strategies to reduce pain associated with glossitis such as eating bland and soft foods

V. APLASTIC ANEMIA

A. Overview

1. A form of anemia with decreased production of RBCs, WBCs, and platelets; may be congenital or acquired
2. Congenital aplastic anemia is caused by a chromosomal alteration
3. Acquired form may be caused by radiation, chemical agents and toxins, drugs, viral and bacterial infections, pregnancy, and idiopathic; in about 50% of cases, cause is unknown
4. There is a decrease or cessation of production of RBCs (**anemia**), WBCs (leukopenia), and platelets (thrombocytopenia); may result from damage to bone marrow stem cells, bone marrow itself, and replacement of bone marrow with fat; depending on causative factor, condition may be acute or chronic

NCLEX®

B. Nursing data collection

1. Pallor and fatigue
2. Palpitations and exertional dyspnea
3. Infections of the skin and mucous membranes
4. Bleeding from gums, nose, vagina, or rectum

5. Purpura (bruising)
6. Retinal hemorrhage
7. Blood counts reveal pancytopenia (decreased RBC, WBC, and platelets)
8. Decreased reticulocyte count
9. Bone marrow examination reveals decreased or absent bone marrow cell activity

C. Therapeutic management

1. Identification of cause of bone marrow suppression
2. Bone marrow transplantation
3. Immunosuppression
4. Transfusion of leukocyte-poor RBCs
5. Splenectomy
6. NCLEX® Institute reverse isolation to protect client from infection
7. Limit visitors and potential sources of infection
8. NCLEX® Monitor for evidence of bleeding; avoid invasive procedures including rectal temperatures
9. Provide frequent rest periods; monitor tolerance to activities
10. Medication therapy: antilymphocyte globulin (ALG), antithymocyte globulin (ATG), and cyclosporine (Sandimmune), immunosuppresive agents such as prednisone and cyclophosphamide (Cytoxan)

D. Reinforce client teaching

1. NCLEX® Methods to prevent infection such as avoiding crowds, maintaining good hygiene, hand hygiene, and elimination of uncooked foods from diet
2. NCLEX® Methods to prevent hemorrhage such as using a soft toothbrush, avoiding contact sports, and use of an electric razor
3. NCLEX® Avoid drugs that increase bleeding tendency, such as aspirin
4. Balance activity with adequate rest periods to avoid fatigue
5. Symptoms to report to health care provider, including signs of infection, bleeding, and decreasing tolerance to activity

VI. SICKLE CELL DISEASE

A. Overview

1. A hereditary, chronic form of hemolytic anemia that predominantly affects clients of African descent
2. Sickle cell trait (heterozygous state) is a generally mild condition that produces few, if any, manifestations
3. Sickle cell anemia is caused by an autosomal genetic defect (one gene affected) that results in synthesis of hemoglobin S
4. Produced by a mutation in beta chain of Hgb molecule through a substitution of amino acid valine for glutamine in both beta chains
5. When there is decreased O_2 tension in plasma, hemoglobin S causes RBCs to elongate, become rigid, and assume a crescent, sickled shape; curved shape causes cells to clump together, obstructing capillary blood flow and leading to ischemia and possible tissue infarction
6. Conditions likely to trigger a sickle cell crisis include hypoxia, low environmental and/or body temperature, excessive exercise, high altitudes, and inadequate oxygen during anesthesia
7. Other causes of sickle cell crisis include elevated blood viscosity and decreased plasma volume, infection, dehydration, and increased hydrogen ion concentration (acidosis)
8. With normal oxygenation, sickled RBCs resume normal shape; repeated episodes of sickling and unsickling weaken cell membranes, causing them to hemolyze
9. Crisis is extremely painful and can last from 4 to 6 days

NCLEX® **B. Nursing data collection**

1. Pallor and jaundice
2. Fatigue and possible irritability
3. Large joints and surrounding tissue may become swollen during crisis
4. Priapism (abnormal, painful, continuous erection of penis) may occur if penile veins are obstructed
5. Severe pain
6. Anemia with sickled cells noted on a peripheral smear
7. Hemoglobin electrophoresis to detect presence and amount of hemoglobin S is used for a definitive diagnosis
8. Elevated serum bilrubin levels
9. Elevated reticulocyte count

C. Therapeutic management

1. Bone marrow transplantation
2. Blood transfusions
3. Management of pain
4. Use of chemotherapy drug hydroxyurea (Droxia) to increase hemoglobin F and decrease sickling
5. Refer to appropriate agency for genetic counseling and family planning
6. NCLEX® Care of client in sickle cell crisis
   a. Recognize that client may have severe pain and medicate accordingly, usually with opioid analgesics
   b. Administer O_2 to increase oxygenation to cells
   c. Promote hydration to decrease blood viscosity; provide oral intake of at least 6 to 8 quarts daily or IV fluids of 3 liters daily
   d. Monitor for complications such as vaso-occlusive disease (thrombosis), hypoxia, CVA, renal dysfunction, priapism leading to impotence, acute chest syndrome (fever, chest pain, cough, pulmonary infiltrates, and dyspnea), and substance abuse
   e. Manage infection if appropriate
7. Medication therapy
   a. Nifedipine (Procardia) for priapism
   b. Hydroxyurea (Droxia) to increase hemoglobin F and decrease sickling
   c. NCLEX® Narcotic (opioid) analgesics during the acute phase of sickle cell crisis, often at large doses
   d. Broad-spectrum antibiotics to manage acute chest syndrome
   e. Folic acid supplements

D. Reinforce client teaching

1. NCLEX® Ways to prevent sickle cell crisis
   a. Maintain an oral intake of at least 4 to 6 quarts a day; avoid conditions that might predispose to dehydration
   b. Avoid high altitudes
   c. Prevent and promptly treat infections
   d. Use stress-reduction strategies
   e. Avoid exposure to cold or overexertion
2. Importance of adhering to vaccination schedules for pneumococcal pneumonia, haemophilus influenza type B
3. Importance of regular medical follow-up

VII. POLYCYTHEMIA

A. Overview

1. An increased number of circulating RBCs and Hgb concentration in blood; also known as polycythemia vera (PV), or myeloproliferative red cell disorder; can be a primary or secondary disorder
2. Primary
   a. Neoplastic stem cell disorder characterized by increased production of RBCs, granulocytes, and platelets; more common in men of European Jewish descent over age 50
   b. With overproduction of RBCs, increased blood viscocity leads to congestion of blood in tissues, liver, and spleen
   c. Thrombi form, acidosis develops, and tissue infarction occurs because of diminished blood flow caused by increased viscosity
3. Secondary
   a. Most common form; disturbance is not in RBC development but in excessive erythropoiesis as a physiologic response to hypoxia
   b. Chronic hypoxic states may be produced by prolonged exposure to high altitudes, pulmonary diseases, hypoventilation, and smoking
   c. Result of an increased RBC production is increased viscosity of blood, which alters circulatory flow

B. Nursing data collection

1. NCLEX® **Plethora**: a ruddy (dark, flushed) color of face, hands, feet, ears, and mucous membranes resulting from engorgement or distention of blood vessels
2. NCLEX® Symptoms associated with increased blood volume, including headaches, vertigo, blurred vision, and tinnitus
3. Distended superficial veins
4. Itching unrelieved by antihistamines
5. Symptoms associated with impaired tissue oxygenation, including angina, claudication, or dyspnea

6. Erythromyalgia, or burning sensation of the fingers and toes
7. Splenomegaly in majority of those with primary polycythemia vera
8. Epistaxis, GI bleeding
9. Elevated Hgb, Hct, RBC and WBC counts, basophils, and platelets
10. Decreased MCHC
11. Elevated leukocyte alkaline phosphatase, uric acid, cobalamin levels, and histamine levels
12. Bone marrow examination shows hypercellularity

C. Therapeutic management

NCLEX®
1. Manage underlying condition (such as COPD) causing chronic hypoxia
2. Repeated phlebotomy to decrease blood volume; goal is to keep hematocrit at 45–48% or lower

NCLEX®
3. Hydration to decrease blood viscosity
4. Measures to relieve pruritus, including cool and tepid baths
5. Accurate monitoring of fluid intake and output (I&O)

NCLEX®
6. Nursing measures to prevent thrombotic events, including early ambulation, passive leg exercises when on bedrest, encouraging client to keep legs uncrossed and maintain adequate hydration
7. Medication therapy
   a. Myelosuppressive agents to inhibit bone marrow activity including hydroxyurea (Hydrea), melphalan (Alkeran), and radioactive phosphorus
   b. Allopurinol to manage gout caused by increased uric acid levels (see also Chapter 57)
   c. Antiplatelet agents to prevent thrombotic complications

D. Reinforce client teaching

NCLEX®
1. Maintain good hydration; drink at least 3 liters of fluid per day
2. Disease and methods of control, such as smoking cessation
3. Signs and symptoms of complications, including signs of vaso-occlusive states (MI, CVA) and bleeding, which require immediate medical attention

NCLEX®
4. Prevent bleeding states such as by using electric razor and soft-bristled toothbrush, not flossing, and avoiding use of aspirin and aspirin-containing products
5. Importance of a regular medical check-up
6. Avoid products that contain iron
7. Ways to prevent thrombosis

VIII. THROMBOCYTOPENIA

A. Overview

1. Platelet count of less than 100,000/mL blood
2. Decreased circulating platelets may result from three mechanisms: decreased production, increased destruction, or increased consumption
3. Cause of decreased platelet production may be inherited or acquired; inherited form is known as autoimmune or idiopathic thrombocytopenic purpura (ITP), and usually follows viral infection such as measles, rubella, or chicken pox
4. Causes of increased destruction of platelets include non–immune-related factors such as infection or drug-induced effects

NCLEX®
5. A decrease in number of functional platelets leads to bleeding disorders; high risk for bleeding if platelet count is below 20,000/mm^3; cerebral and pulmonary hemorrhage can occur when platelet counts drop below 10,000/mm^3

NCLEX®
B. Nursing data collection

1. Petechiae (pinpoint hemorrhages on skin and mucous membranes) and purpura (purplish discolored areas) most commonly found in mucous membranes, anterior thorax, arms, and neck
2. Epistaxis, gingival bleeding, menorrhagia, hematuria, and gastrointestinal bleeding (bloody or tarry stools)
3. Signs of internal hemorrhage
4. Decreased hemoglobin and hematocrit if bleeding is present
5. Decreased platelet count; platelet antibodies present if ITP
6. Prolonged bleeding time
7. Bone marrow examination may reveal decreased platelet activity or increased megakaryocytes

C. Therapeutic management

1. Treat underlying cause or remove causative agent in acquired thrombocytopenia

NCLEX®
2. Platelet transfusions if there is active bleeding; little benefit in ITP

3. If medications are not effective, a splenectomy may be done in older child with 1 year of thrombocytopenia

NCLEX® 4. Institute bleeding (thrombocytopenic) precautions
   a. Avoid intramuscular or subcutaneous injections
   b. Avoid indwelling catheters
   c. If absolutely necessary, use smallest gauge needles for injections or venipunctures; apply pressure on injection sites for 5 minutes or until bleeding stops
   d. Discourage straining at stool, vigorous coughing, and nose blowing
   e. Avoid rectal manipulation such as rectal temperatures, suppositories, or enemas
   f. Discourage the use of razors; use only electric shavers
   g. Use soft-bristled toothbrush or toothettes and avoid flossing
   h. Pad siderails if necessary and avoid tissue trauma
   i. Avoid use of aspirin and drugs that interfere with blood coagulation

NCLEX® 5. Monitor for signs of bleeding; test stools for occult blood
6. Monitor CBC and platelet counts
7. Monitor neurological status every shift and PRN
8. Medication therapy
   a. Steroids and immunoglobulins to suppress immune response in ITP
   b. Immunosuppressive agents such as vincristine (Oncovin) and cyclophosphamide (Cytoxan)
   NCLEX® c. Platelet growth factor such as oprelvekin (Neumega)

D. Reinforce client and family teaching

1. Monitor for signs of bleeding and when to contact primary care provider

NCLEX® 2. Bleeding precautions such as using soft-bristled toothbrush, avoiding flossing, preventing tissue trauma and injury (including vigorous sexual intercourse), and using an electric razor for shaving
3. Methods of controlling bleeding and to seek medical assistance if severe

NCLEX® 4. Avoid drugs that contain aspirin and others that interfere with coagulation
5. Medication dosing, schedule, and side effects
6. Importance of regular medical follow-up and platelet monitoring

IX. HEMOPHILIA

A. Overview

1. A group of hereditary clotting factor disorders characterized by prolonged coagulation time that results in prolonged and sometimes excessive bleeding
2. Hemophilia A and B are **X-linked recessive traits** transmitted by female carriers and displayed almost exclusively in males
   a. *Hemophilia A* (classic hemophilia) is a deficiency in factor VIII (an alpha-globulin that stabilizes fibrin clots; is the most common form of hemophilia
   b. *Hemophilia B* (Christmas disease) is a deficiency in factor IX (a vitamin-dependent beta-globulin essential in stage 1 of intrinsic coagulation system; is an influence on amount of thromboplastin available)
3. In clients with hemophilia A and B, platelet plugs are formed at site of bleeding, but clotting factor impairs coagulation response and capacity to form a stable clot
4. *Von Willebrand's disease* is a related disorder caused by deficiency of von Willebrand's factor (vWF) necessary for factor VIII activity and platelet adhesion

NCLEX® **B. Nursing data collection**

1. Persistent and prolonged bleeding from small cuts and injuries
2. Subcutaneous **ecchymosis** (purplish color) and subcutaneous hematomas
3. Gingival bleeding
4. GI bleeding, manifested by hematemesis (vomiting blood), occult blood in stools, gastric pain, or abdominal pain
5. Urinary tract bleeding (hematuria)
6. Pain, paresthesia, or paralysis resulting from nerve compression by hematomas
7. **Hemarthrosis** (joint bleeding, swelling and damage)
8. APTT is increased in all types of hemophilia
9. Bleeding time is prolonged in von Willebrand's disease
10. Decreased factor VIII in hemophilia A, vWF in von Willebrand's disease, and factor IX in hemophilia B

C. Therapeutic management

1. Replacement of deficient coagulation factor(s)
2. NCLEX® Hemophilia A: cryoprecipitate containing 8 to 100 units of factor VIII per bag at 12-hour intervals until bleeding ceases; freeze-dried concentrate of factor VIII may also be given
3. NCLEX® Hemophilia B: plasma or factor IX concentrate given every 24 hours or until bleeding ceases
4. NCLEX® Von Willebrand's disease: cryoprecipitate containing 8 to 100 units of factor VIII per bag at 12-hour intervals until bleeding ceases; desmopressin (DDAVP) may also be used
5. Supportive treatment for hemarthrosis, including arthrocentesis and physiotherapy
6. Control of topical bleeding with hemostatic agents, pressure, and application of ice
7. Management of complications associated with hemorrhage
8. Refer for genetic counseling and family planning and to National Hemophilia Foundation for support and counseling
9. Monitor for signs of complications, including hemarthrosis and intracranial bleeding
10. NCLEX® Assist in managing pain associated with hemarthrosis; measures include immobilizing joint, applying ice, and administering analgesics; avoid aspirin and drugs affecting coagulation
11. Control bleeding and maintain hemostasis through direct pressure, applying topical hemostatic agents, and applying ice

D. Reinforce client teaching

1. Disease and therapeutic regimen
2. NCLEX® Signs and symptoms requiring immediate medical attention, such as severe joint pain, trauma or injury, and signs of uncontrolled internal bleeding
3. NCLEX® Precautions to prevent bleeding, as previously described
4. Wear a Medic-Alert bracelet indicating hemophilia; notify all health care providers of condition
5. Maintain good dental hygiene to decrease need for invasive dental procedures
6. Importance of continued follow-up care with health care provider
7. Encourage genetic counseling if appropriate

X. DISSEMINATED INTRAVASCULAR COAGULOPATHY (DIC)

A. Overview

1. A syndrome characterized by abnormal initiation and acceleration of clotting and simultaneous hemorrhage; also called consumption coagulopathy
2. Precipitated by conditions such as widespread tissue damage, hemolysis, hypotension, hypoxia, and metabolic acidosis (see Box 60–1)
3. Clotting process initiated either through activation of factor XII, factors II and X, or release of tissue thromboplastin
4. Clotting factors II, V, VIII, fibrinogen, and platelets needed for clotting are consumed more rapidly than they can be replaced
5. Body begins to break down clots with release of fibrin degradation products (FDPs), which are potent anticoagulants used to lyse clots further; anticoagulants worsen bleeding state
6. With depletion of clotting factors and increase in FDPs, stable blood clots no longer form and hemorrhage occurs

B. Nursing data collection

1. NCLEX® Clinical manifestations (see Box 60–2)
2. NCLEX® Prolonged aPTT, PT, and thrombin time
3. NCLEX® Decreased fibrinogen and platelets

Box 60–1

Risk Factors for DIC

Venomous snakebite	Acute hemolysis
Tissue necrosis	Neoplasms
Sepsis	Extensive burns
Drug reactions	Vascular disorders
Trauma	Prosthetic devices
Liver disease	Hypoxia
Obstetric complications	

Box 60–2

Clinical Manifestations of DIC

Integumentary
- Decreased skin temperature
- Pallor
- Purpura
- Ecchymosis
- Hematomas
- Acral cyanosis
- Altered sensation
- Superficial gangrene
- Gingival bleeding
- Bleeding from puncture sites

Gastrointestinal
- Hemoptysis
- Melena
- Occult blood in stool or vomitus
- Abdominal distention
- Abdominal pain

Respiratory
- Dyspnea
- Tachypnea
- Orthopnea
- Decreased breath sounds
- Chest pain

Cardiovascular
- Decreased pulses
- Decreased capillary filling time
- Tachycardia
- Venous distention

Genitourinary
- Hematuria
- Oliguria

Nervous System
- Vision changes
- Dizziness
- Headache
- Irritability
- Anxiety
- Confusion
- Seizures

Musculoskeletal
- Joint pain
- Bone pain
- Weakness

NCLEX® 4. Elevated fibrin degradation products
5. Factor assays (factors V, VII, VIII, X, XIII): reduced
6. D-dimer elevated

C. Therapeutic management
1. Initiate treatment of underlying precipitating medical condition is a priority
2. Supportive treatment includes control of bleeding
NCLEX® 3. Life-threatening hemorrhage may be treated with platelets for thrombocytopenia; cryoprecipitate to replace fibrinogen, and factors V and VII; and fresh frozen plasma (FFP) to replace all clotting factors except platelets
4. Observe client carefully for evidence of bleeding and reduced tissue oxygenation
NCLEX® 5. Institute thrombocytopenic/bleeding precautions (refer to previous discussion on thrombocytopenia)
NCLEX® 6. Monitor I&O hourly
7. Monitor for signs of complications such as renal failure, pulmonary embolism, cerebrovascular accident, and acute respiratory distress syndrome
8. Provide emotional support to client and family
9. Medication therapy
   a. Heparin and antithrombin III, although their use is controversial; are usually indicated to manage thrombosis
   b. Epsilon aminocaproic acid (Amicar) to inhibit fibrinolysis

D. Reinforce client teaching
1. Disorder, its treatments and interventions
2. Report symptoms of complications, including abdominal pain, headache, visual disturbances, and pain
3. Thrombocytopenic/bleeding precautions (see previous client teaching section in thrombocytopenia)

XI. NEUTROPENIA

A. Overview
1. Neutrophils constitute about 70% of total circulating WBCs
2. Neutropenia is a neutrophil count of less than 2000/mm^3 (normal > 2000/mm^3)
3. Absolute neutrophil count (ANC) is determined using this formula:

$$\frac{\%\text{neutrophils} + \%\text{bands}}{100} \times \text{total WBC count} = \text{ANC}$$

4. Caused by either decreased production or increased destruction of neutrophils

5. Because neutrophils play a major role in phagocytosis of microorganisms, neutropenia increases risk for infection
6. Neutropenia may occur as a primary hematologic disorder but may also be caused by drugs (such as cancer chemotherapy), autoimmune disorders, infections, and other medical conditions such as severe sepsis and nutritional deficiencies

NCLEX® **B. Nursing data collection**

1. Clinical manifestations: there are no real symptoms associated with neutropenia; it may not be discovered until client presents with signs of infection
2. Diagnostic and laboratory tests
   a. Absolute neutrophil count less than 1000 to 1500
   b. Examination of bone marrow cell morphology helps determine etiology

NCLEX® **C. Therapeutic management**

1. If etiology is drug-induced, medication should be discontinued whenever possible
2. Corticosteroids are used if etiology is immunologic
3. If etiology is decreased production, growth factors (granulocyte/macrophage colony–stimulating factor or GM-CSF) may be used
4. NCLEX® Monitor for signs of infection; monitor temperature elevations
5. Obtain cultures suspected as sites of infection
6. Infections are treated with antimicrobial therapy
7. NCLEX® Enforce strict hand hygiene by all individuals in contact with client
8. NCLEX® Institute reverse isolation (also called protective isolation); use private room with HEPA filtration if possible; do not allow those with infections to visit; use gloves and masks when entering client's room; prohibit known sources of microorganisms (plants, flowers, fresh unpeeled fruits and vegetables, standing water—such as water pitcher or vase)
9. Avoid invasive procedures whenever possible

D. Reinforce client teaching

1. What neutropenia is and rationale for therapeutic interventions
2. Report signs of fever
3. NCLEX® Strict hand hygiene and reverse-isolation procedure (for client and those who come in contact with client)
4. Maintain good personal hygiene to decrease microbes on skin

XII. LEUKEMIA

A. Overview

1. Malignancy of blood-forming tissues of bone marrow, spleen, and lymph system characterized by unregulated proliferation of WBCs and their precursors
2. Classified by type of WBC affected (granulocyte, lymphocyte, monocyte) and by cell differentiation (acute if majority of cells are primitive or poorly differentiated and chronic if mature or well differentiated)
3. Acute lymphocytic/lymphoblastic leukemia (ALL)
   a. Peak incidence at 2 to 4 years of age
   b. Immature granulocytes proliferate and accumulate in bone marrow
4. Chronic lymphocytic leukemia (CLL)
   a. More common in men and mainly between ages of 50 and 70
   b. Abnormal and incompetent lymphocytes proliferate and accumulate in lymph nodes and spread to other lymphatic tissues and spleen; most circulating cells are mature lymphocytes
5. Acute myelogenous/myelocytic leukemia (AML)
   a. All age groups are affected with a peak incidence at age 60
   b. There is uncontrolled proliferation of myeloblasts, which are precursors of granulocytes; they accumulate in bone marrow
6. Chronic myelogenous leukemia (CML)
   a. Uncommon in people under 20 years of age; incidence rises with age
   b. Uncontrolled proliferation of granulocytes results in increased circulating blast (immature) cells; marrow expands into long bones and also extends into liver and spleen
   c. NCLEX® In most cases, Philadelphia chromosome, a characteristic chromosomal abnormality, is present
7. Abnormal or immature WBCs do not function properly; abnormal cells continue to multiply, infiltrate, and damage bone marrow, spleen, lymph nodes, liver, kidneys, lungs, gonads, skin, and CNS

8. Normal bone marrow becomes diffusely replaced with abnormal or immature WBCs, interfering with production of cells such as RBCs and platelets; bone marrow becomes functionally incompetent with resulting bone marrow suppression
9. Acute leukemia has rapid onset and progression with a short clinical course; left untreated, death results in days or months; symptoms relate to depressed bone marrow, infiltration of leukemic cells into other organ systems, and hypermetabolism of leukemic cells
10. Chronic leukemia has more insidious onset and prolonged clinical course; usually asymptomatic early in disease; life expectancy may be more than 5 years; symptoms relate to hypermetabolism of leukemic cells infiltrating other organ systems; cells are more mature and function more effectively

NCLEX® **B. Nursing data collection**

1. Fever and night sweats
2. Bleeding such as ecchymoses, gingival bleeding, and epistaxis
3. Lymphadenopathy, splenomegaly, and hepatomegaly
4. Weakness and fatigue
5. Pruritic vesicular lesions
6. Anorexia and weight loss
7. Shortness of breath and decreased activity tolerance
8. Bone or joint pain
9. Visual disturbances
10. Pallor
11. Diagnostic and laboratory tests
    a. Increased WBC (in CLL and CML)
    b. A normal, decreased or increased WBC (in ALL and AML)
    c. Decreased reaction to skin sensitivity tests (**anergy**)
    d. Bone marrow tests reveal excessive blast cells in AML
    e. NCLEX® Philadelphia chromosome found in 90–95% of clients with CML; BCR/ABL gene is present in virtually all clients with CML
    f. Bone marrow biopsy and aspirate is the definitive diagnostic test

C. Therapeutic management

1. NCLEX® Induction of remission with chemotherapy and radiation therapy
2. Bone marrow and stem cell transplantation
3. NCLEX® Assist in bone marrow biopsy; apply pressure to site for 5 minutes or until bleeding stops; frequently inspect site for signs of bleeding up to 4 hours after procedure
4. NCLEX® Maintain neutropenic and bleeding precautions (see previous discussions)
5. NCLEX® Schedule activities to prevent fatigue; provide measures for uninterrupted rest and sleep
6. Provide for diversionary activities
7. Maintain good nutrition; consult dietitian as needed to meet nutritional needs
8. Assist client in maintaining good personal hygiene and promote good oral hygiene
9. Refer to appropriate agencies such as Meals on Wheels, American Cancer Society (ACS), and the Leukemia Society
10. Provide emotional support to client and family; refer to appropriate agency, organization, or professional for counseling and support
11. Administer prescribed drugs and monitor for side effects
12. Monitor laboratory results to evaluate effectiveness of interventions and therapy
13. Prepare client for bone marrow transplantation if part of treatment plan
14. NCLEX® Medication therapy: chemotherapeutic drugs include alkylating agents (Busulfan, Myleran), anthracyclines (Doxorubicin, Adriamycin), antimetabolites (Fludarabine, Fludara), corticosteroid (Prednisone), plant alkaloids (Vincristine, Oncovin), and others

D. Reinforce client teaching

1. Thrombocytopenic/bleeding precautions; see previous discussion
2. Neutropenic precautions; see previous discussion
3. Maintain good oral hygiene; keep oral cavity moist: rinse mouth with saline, lubricate lips and oral mucosa with water-soluble lubricants every 2 hours; avoid alcohol-based mouthwash; use sponge-tipped applicators for oral hygiene if neutrophil and/or platelet counts are low
4. Measures to prevent perirectal complications: wash and clean perineal area thoroughly after each bowel movement
5. Therapeutic plans and interventions

XIII. MALIGNANT LYMPHOMAS

A. Overview

1. A group of malignant neoplasms that affect lymphatic system, resulting in proliferation of lymphocytes; can be classified as Hodgkin's lymphoma (Hodgkin's disease) and non-Hodgkin's lymphoma
2. Hodgkin's disease
   - **a.** More common in men than in women; has two peaks, at 15 to 35 and at 55 to 75 years of age; incidence is higher in whites than in African Americans
   - **b.** Etiology unknown but several identified factors contribute to development, including infection with Epstein-Barr virus (EBV), familial pattern, and exposure to toxins
   - **c.** Characterized by presence of Reed-Sternberg cell, a multinucleated and gigantic tumor cell thought to be of lymphoid origin
   - **d.** Originates in a lymph node (majority of cases in cervical nodes) and infiltrates spleen, lungs, and liver
3. Non-Hodgkin's lymphoma
   - **a.** Most common form of lymphoma; usually affects adults from 50 to 70 years old; is more common in men than in women and in whites than in other races
   - **b.** No known cause but incidence is linked to viral infections, immune disorders, genetic abnormalities, exposure to chemicals, and infection with *Helicobacter pylori*
   - **c.** Has a similar pathophysiology to Hodgkin's disease, although Reed-Sternberg cells are absent and method of lymph node infiltration is different
   - **d.** Often involves malignant B cells; usually originates outside lymph nodes; normal cells are crowded out by malignant cells in affected lymphoid tissues

B. Nursing data collection

NCLEX®

1. Hodgkin's disease
   - **a.** Often firm, painless enlargement of one or more lymph nodes on one side of neck
   - **b.** Fatigue and weakness
   - **c.** Anorexia and dysphagia
   - **d.** Dyspnea and cough
   - **e.** Pruritus and jaundice
   - **f.** Severe but brief pain at site after ingestion of alcohol
   - **g.** Abdominal pain and bone pain
   - **h.** Enlarged lymph nodes, liver, and spleen
   - **i.** B symptoms: fever without chills; night sweats, and unintentional 10% weight loss
   - **j.** Normocytic, normochromic anemia
   - **k.** Neutrophilia, monocytophilia, and lymphopenia
   - **l.** Presence of Reed-Sternberg cells in excisional bone biopsy
   - **m.** Mediastinal lymphadenopathy seen on chest x-ray, CT scan, and radioisotope studies
   - **n.** Mediastinal mass and pulmonary infiltrates may be seen on chest x-ray
   - **o.** Absent or decreased response to skin sensitivity testing known as anergy

NCLEX®

2. Non-Hodgkin's lymphoma
   - **a.** Painless lymph node enlargement
   - **b.** B symptoms (see above)
   - **c.** Abdominal pain, nausea, vomiting
   - **d.** Hematuria
   - **e.** Peripheral neuropathy, cranial nerve palsies, headaches, visual disturbances, changes in mental status, and seizures
   - **f.** Lymphocytopenia
   - **g.** X-ray may reveal pulmonary infiltrates
   - **h.** Lymph node biopsy helps to identify the cell type and pattern

C. Therapeutic management

1. Hodgkin's disease
   - **a.** Lymphangiography to evaluate abdominal nodes
   - **b.** Staging laparotomy to obtain specimen of retroperitoneal lymph nodes and remove spleen
   - **c.** Staging of disease to determine extent and appropriate therapy; stage I involves single lymph node region; stage IV (for Hodgkin's disease only) indicates diffuse or disseminated involvement of one or more extralymphatic organs, with or without lymph node involvement (liver, lung, marrow, skin)

NCLEX®

   - **d.** Treatment may include radiation therapy and/or chemotherapy

2. Non-Hodgkin's lymphoma
   a. Staging of disease is based on results of CT scans and bone marrow biopsies
   b. Combination chemotherapy
   c. Radiation alone or in combination with chemotherapy for stage I and II
   d. Biologic therapy with alpha-interferon, interleukin-2, and tumor necrosis factor
   e. Administration of rituximab (Rituxan), a monoclonal antibody against the CD20 of malignant B lymphocytes, which causes cell lysis and death

NCLEX® 3. Carry out nursing interventions for clients on chemotherapy or radiation therapy
NCLEX® 4. Assist in balancing activity with periods of rest
NCLEX® 5. Provide and assist in maintaining good nutritional state
6. Provide measures to diminish the discomfort associated with pruritus
7. Help client to cope with bodily changes such as alopecia, weight loss, and sterility
8. Refer client and family to appropriate agencies for support, such as ACS
NCLEX® 9. Implement care to prevent infection
NCLEX® 10. Medication therapy: chemotherapy drugs and biologic therapy agents

D. Reinforce client teaching
1. Nature of disease, course of therapy, and associated interventions
2. Medications prescribed, precautions, and side effects
NCLEX® 3. Symptoms necessitating immediate medical intervention, such as bleeding, infection, or fever

XIV. THALASSEMIA

A. Overview
1. Another of group of hereditary blood disorders of hemoglobin synthesis, characterized by mild to severe anemia
2. Most common type is beta-thalassemia, also known as Cooley anemia; there are three types of beta-thalassemia:
   a. Thalassemia minor is also known as thalassemia trait and produces mild anemia
   b. Thalassemia intermedia produces severe anemia
   c. Thalassemia major produces anemia that requires transfusions
3. Commonly seen in those of Mediterranean descent; however, may also be seen among African, Asian, and Middle Eastern populations
4. Condition is autosomal recessive; when both parents carry gene, there is a 25% chance of passing disorder to child; if child acquires one gene, child will be a carrier
5. Thalassemia causes synthesis of defective hemoglobin; RBCs are fragile with shortened life span, which leads to anemia and chronic hypoxia
6. Body conserves iron from aged and broken down RBCs; when blood is administered, iron is retained also from transfused cells; this leads to high iron levels or **hemosiderosis**, which causes cellular damage and long-term complications, such as the following:
   a. Splenomegaly
   b. Cardiac complications
   c. Gallbladder disease
   d. Liver enlargement and cirrhosis
   e. Growth retardation and endocrine complications
   f. Jaundice and brown skin pigmentation
   g. Skeletal changes including enlarged head, thickened cranial bones, enlarged maxilla, and malocclusion of the teeth
7. If untreated, child may die

NCLEX® **B. Nursing data collection**
1. Thalassemia can be diagnosed early in infancy when child presents with pallor, failure to thrive (FTT), hepatosplenomegaly, and severe anemia; see Box 60–3 for clinical manifestations of beta-thalassemia
2. Signs and symptoms of chronic hypoxia such as lethargy, headache, bone pain, exercise intolerance, and anorexia
3. Hemoglobin electrophoresis shows decreased production of one hemoglobin chain; RBC changes may be detected as early as 6 weeks of age
4. Decreased Hgb, Hct, and reticulocyte count
5. Folic acid deficiency may be present

NCLEX® **C. Therapeutic management**
1. Administer blood products as ordered, observing for complications of multiple transfusions

Box 60-3

Clinical Manifestations of Beta-Thalassemia

Anemia

Hypochromic and microcytic changes

Folic acid deficiency

Frequent epistaxis

Skeletal Changes

Osteoporosis

Delayed growth

Susceptibility to pathologic fractures

Facial deformities: enlarged head, prominent forehead and cheek bones, broadened and depressed bridge of nose, enlarged maxilla with protruding front teeth, eyes with mongolian slant and epicanthal fold

Heart

Chronic congestive heart failure

Myocardial fibrosis

Murmurs

Liver/Gallbladder

Hepatomegaly

Hepatic insufficiency

Spleen

Splenomegaly

Endocrine System

Delayed sexual maturation

Fibrotic pancreas, resulting in diabetes mellitus

Skin

Darkening of skin

Source: Ball, J., Bindler, R., & Cowen, K. *Child health nursing: Partnering with children and families* (2nd ed.), ©2010, p. 1049. Reprinted by permission of Pearson Education, Inc., Upper Saddle River, NJ 07458.

2. Monitor for signs of iron overload (hemosiderosis) and hepatitis
3. Observe for signs of infection and prevent infection through good hand hygiene, avoiding those with infection, proper rest and nutrition
4. Administer folic acid as ordered
5. Work toward fracture prevention by encouraging and providing opportunities for physical activities that do not increase risk of fractures, such as swimming and walking
6. Implement iron chelation therapy (desferoxamine) as ordered to help eliminate excessive iron
7. Provide support and opportunity for child and family to discuss feelings regarding chronic life-threatening illness
8. Encourage child and family to allow child to live as normal a life as possible
9. Bone marrow transplantation may be offered to cure disease

D. Reinforce child and family teaching

1. Nature of disease and its medical management
2. Possible complications, including iron overload, as well as signs of infection
3. Activity restrictions to reduce risk of fractures secondary to excessive iron stores
4. Encourage genetic counseling if appropriate

Check Your NCLEX–PN® Exam I.Q.

You are ready for testing on this content if you can

- Identify basic structures and functions of the hematological system.
- Describe the pathophysiology and etiology of common hematological disorders.
- Discuss expected data and diagnostic test findings for selected hematological disorders.
- Discuss therapeutic management of a client experiencing a hematological disorder.
- Discuss nursing management of a client experiencing a hematological disorder.
- Identify expected outcomes for the client experiencing a hematological disorder.

PRACTICE TEST

1 The nurse is reinforcing teaching to a client with polycythemia vera on ways to maintain nutrition. The nurse should include which measure when teaching?

1. Increase intake of foods high in iron.
2. Encourage small, frequent meals rather than three big meals.
3. Increase the amount of red meats and organ meats in the diet.
4. Encourage the use of hot spices in foods to stimulate appetite.

2 The nurse is administering oral care to a client with disseminated intravascular coagulopathy (DIC). Which action is most appropriate for this client?

1. Limit flossing to once a day.
2. Use an alcohol-based mouthwash to prevent infection.
3. Use swabs to administer oral care.
4. Encourage tooth brushing at least once a shift.

3 A client with stomatitis and on neutropenic precautions is ordered to have mouthwashes every 2 hours. The nurse would provide mouthwashes containing which ingredients as most helpful to this client? Select all that apply.

1. Viscous lidocaine (Xylocaine)
2. Normal saline solution
3. Hydrogen peroxide
4. Diluted baking soda
5. A liquid antacid

4 A client with acute myelogenous leukemia (AML) is scheduled for a bone marrow transplant (BMT). When reinforcing teaching to the client's family about BMT, which statement by the nurse is best?

1. "The client will be in the operating room with the donor so that immediate transplantation can occur."
2. "The specially prepared marrow is infused intravenously to the client."
3. "The client will be brought to the radiology department to transplant the marrow."
4. "A large bore needle will be inserted into the client's bone marrow where the donor marrow will be infused."

5 A client has undergone a lymph node biopsy. The nurse anticipates that the report will reveal which result if the client has Hodgkin's lymphoma?

1. Reed-Sternberg cells
2. Philadelphia chromosome
3. Epstein-Barr virus
4. Herpes simplex virus

6 During a physical examination, the nurse finds a non-tender, moveable cervical node on a client. The nurse makes which interpretation of this finding?

1. Normal, since the node is moveable
2. Abnormal and may suggest the presence of a malignancy
3. Normal, since the node is non-tender
4. Abnormal and a positive indicator of a malignancy

7 A client with anemia has a nursing diagnosis of Activity Intolerance. Which intervention should the nurse incorporate into the client's care? Select all that apply.

1. Space interventions during the day.
2. Educate the client about the basics of good nutrition.
3. Promote active or passive range of motion activities.
4. Reinforce teaching to a client to change position slowly to prevent dizziness.
5. Encourage defined rest periods during the day.

8 The nurse is reinforcing teaching to a client with hemophilia A about home management. Which strategy should the nurse include when teaching?

1. Increase iron-rich foods in the diet.
2. Avoid contact sports.
3. Use aspirin when severe pain occurs.
4. Minimize joint pain by walking and weight-bearing.

9 The nurse is obtaining a health history on a client admitted with a diagnosis of "rule out aplastic anemia." Considering the diagnosis, which data is most important for the nurse to elicit during the interview?

1. Recent travel outside the country
2. Exposure to chemicals and drugs
3. History of blood transfusion
4. Medication allergies

10 The nurse is reinforcing teaching to family members about precautions to take in visiting a client who has neutropenia. Which instructions should the nurse include in the discussion? Select all that apply.

1. People who have colds or infectious diseases should not visit.
2. Visitors must wash their hands before and after a visit.
3. Fresh fruits and vegetables will help fortify the client's immune system.
4. Fresh flowers will help to provide a cheerful environment.
5. It is helpful to keep the client's water pitcher full to prevent dehydration.

11 A client has a platelet count of 18,000/mm^3. What intervention must the nurse include when caring for this client?

1. Institute bleeding precautions.
2. Institute reverse isolation.
3. Schedule medications by intramuscular route when able.
4. Obtain temperatures rectally.

12 A nurse is assisting a physician with a bone marrow aspiration on a client with anemia. After the procedure, the nurse should take which action?

1. Apply pressure on the site to stop bleeding.
2. Massage the area to decrease pain.
3. Apply heat to the area to diminish the discomfort.
4. Cover the area with a light dressing.

13 The white blood cell (WBC) differential on a client indicates a shift to the left. The nurse makes which accurate interpretation of this report?

1. There is an increase in the number of segmented neutrophils.
2. There is an increase in the number of bands released into the circulation.
3. The number of lymphocytes increased in number.
4. The number of lymphocytes exceeds the total WBC count.

14 A client with iron-deficiency anemia is scheduled for a complete blood count. The nurse anticipates that the report will show which characteristics of the red blood cells (RBCs)?

1. Normocytic, normochromic
2. Macrocytic, normochromic
3. Microcytic, hypochromic
4. Normocytic, hyperchromic

15 The nurse in the hematology clinic is reviewing laboratory findings for a 2-year-old being treated for anemia. Which finding is the best indication that the treatment is successful?

1. The child is no longer cyanotic.
2. The reticulocyte count is rising.
3. The child is more active.
4. Stools are black, indicating iron intake.

16 A pregnant woman tells the nurse that she has a family history of sickle cell anemia and is afraid her baby will be born with the disease. The nurse would provide which information during a discussion with this client?

1. Sickle cell anemia is a male disease and would be passed on through the man's family.
2. Genetic testing will be needed to determine if her fetus is affected.
3. Both mother and father must carry the defective gene for the child to have sickle cell anemia.
4. The child only needs one parent to be a carrier in order for the child to be affected.

17 A young child admitted to the hospital with a bleeding disorder is diagnosed with idiopathic thrombocytopenic purpura (ITP). The child's mother says to the nurse, "I have a friend who has a son with hemophilia. When he bleeds, they give him a 'factor,' which they keep in their home refrigerator. Can we just give my child this factor?" Which response by the nurse would be best?

1. "Your friend's child has a natural deficiency in clotting factors; your child does not."
2. "Factor therapy has a lot of negative side effects, and the doctors would rather not use it on your child."
3. "The amount of factor that would be required to treat your child would be excessive."
4. "That treatment may be tried later if your child does not respond to steroids."

18 The nurse has admitted a child newly diagnosed with anemia of unknown origin. Which nursing diagnosis is most appropriate?

1. Decreased Cardiac Output related to abnormal platelet count
2. Activity Intolerance related to generalized weakness and fatigue
3. Imbalanced Nutrition: Less Than Body Requirements related to poor food intake
4. Risk for Pain related to vaso-occlusion

19 The nurse is caring for a child with beta-thalassemia who has received many blood transfusions. The nurse monitors for which data as a priority at this time?

1. Neutropenia
2. Petechiae
3. Hemosiderosis
4. Hemoglobin S formation

20 A client with vitamin B_{12} deficiency needs to increase dietary intake of foods that are good sources of this vitamin. The nurse recommends that the client increase intake of which foods? Select all that apply.

1. Apples
2. Spinach
3. Carrots
4. Oranges
5. Liver

21 An 8-year-old is being admitted in vaso-occlusive crisis. To which actions should the nurse give priority when caring for this client?

1. Administer high concentration of oxygen to provide adequate oxygenation
2. Determine the acid-base status and administer sodium bicarbonate as necessary
3. Monitor for pain and administer pain medication as necessary
4. Replace Factor 8

22 The pediatric clinic nurse receives a call from the mother of a child who was started on iron supplements 2 weeks ago. The mother is panicked because this morning her daughter's stools were a black, tarry color. How should the nurse respond?

1. "This is an expected symptom of the iron deficiency anemia."
2. "This is a normal sign that the iron preparation is working properly."
3. "This is a sign that the dose of iron is more than required."
4. "This is a sign that the child is experiencing bleeding and needs to come to the office immediately."

23 A child with sickle cell anemia is admitted to the hospital. The nurse anticipates that laboratory evaluation of the client's red blood cells would reveal which of the following?

1. Polycythemia
2. Hematopoiesis
3. Crescent-shaped red blood cells
4. Hypochromatic red blood cells

24 A 2-year-old has just been diagnosed with sickle cell anemia. The nurse has explained the diagnosis to the family as well as provided information about the treatment plan. The nurse will anticipate the need to reinforce teaching to promote child safety when the mother makes which statement?

1. "My husband loves to fly his small plane. I guess we'll have to take a commercial plane for our trips from now on."
2. "If my child gets the flu bug, she might develop a sickling crisis."
3. "My child will need extra iron tablets because of her anemia."
4. "During a sickling crisis, my child will probably be hospitalized for pain control and hydration therapy."

25 The nurse is working with the family of an 8-month-old infant who has severe nutritional anemia. In reinforcing dietary recommendations, the nurse should instruct the family to take which action?

1. Switch the baby to cow's milk.
2. Delay the introduction of solid food in the diet.
3. Restrict the amount of milk or formula in the baby's diet to 1 quart per day.
4. Provide dietary iron sources such as peanuts and unsweetened chocolates.

26 The nurse is administering a liquid iron preparation to a 3-year-old with iron deficiency anemia. What appropriate method should the nurse use?

1. Mix the medication in the child's milk and give it at lunch.
2. Give the medication after lunch with a sweet dessert to disguise the taste.
3. Give the medication in a small cup and allow the child to sip it through a straw.
4. Allow the child to decide whether to take the medicine with breakfast or dinner.

ANSWERS & RATIONALES

1 **Answer: 2 Rationale:** Clients with polycythemia experience satiety and fullness resulting from hepatomegaly and splenomegaly. Frequent, small meals will help maintain adequate nutrition. Foods rich in iron are not appropriate because there is an increase in erythrocytes in this condition. Red meats and organ meats may be higher in animal blood content which is not helpful for this condition. Spicy foods will increase the gastrointestinal symptoms, which also include dyspepsia and increased gastric secretions. **Cognitive Level:** Applying **Client Need:** Physiological Adaptation **Integrated Process:** Teaching and Learning **Content Area:** Adult Health **Strategy:** The core issue of the question is knowledge of an appropriate diet for a client with polycythemia. Use nursing knowledge and the process of elimination to make a selection.

2 **Answer: 3 Rationale:** Clients with DIC should be protected from injury that will result in bleeding. An oral swab is least likely to cause tissue injury to the oral cavity during mouth care. Flossing, even once daily, can increase the risk of bleeding from the gums. Mouthwashes containing alcohol should be avoided because they may cause discomfort and tend to dry the mucous membranes. Toothbrushes may be used only if they are soft-bristled, but a swab or toothette is the best option. **Cognitive Level:** Applying **Client Need:** Physiological Adaptation **Integrated Process:** Nursing Process: Implementation **Content Area:** Adult Health **Strategy:** The core issue of the question is appropriate methods of providing mouth care to a client with stomatitis. Use nursing knowledge and the process of elimination to make a selection.

3 **Answer: 1, 2, 4, 5 Rationale:** Viscous lidocaine helps to ease the pain of stomatitis. Normal saline is isotonic and is therefore less irritating to the oral tissues. Diluted solution with baking soda is soothing and acceptable in a mouthwash solution. A solution containing an antacid tends to be soothing for a client with mouth pain due to stomatitis. Hydrogen peroxide is not a good choice because it tends to dry the oral mucosa and further aggravate the discomfort. **Cognitive Level:** Applying **Client Need:** Physiological Adaptation **Integrated Process:** Nursing Process: Implementation **Content Area:** Adult Health **Strategy:** The core issue of the question is a mouth care product that would be irritating to a client with stomatitis. Use nursing knowledge and the process of elimination to make a selection.

4 **Answer: 2 Rationale:** Harvested bone marrow is infused into the recipient intravenously. The transplantation is usually preceded by chemotherapy and radiation therapy. During this period and up to when the client's response to the transplantation has been successful, nursing interventions should focus on prevention of infection. **Cognitive Level:** Applying **Client Need:** Physiological Adaptation **Integrated Process:** Teaching and Learning **Content Area:** Adult Health **Strategy:** The core issue of the question is knowledge of bone marrow transplantation as a treatment method. Use nursing knowledge and the process of elimination to make a selection.

5 **Answer: 1 Rationale:** Histological isolation of Reed-Sternberg cells in lymph node biopsy examination is a diagnostic feature of Hodgkin's lymphoma. Philadelphia chromosome is attributed to chronic myelogenous leukemia. Viruses are much smaller than can be visualized with cytology. **Cognitive Level:** Applying **Client Need:** Physiological Adaptation **Integrated Process:** Nursing Process: Data Collection **Content Area:** Adult Health **Strategy:** The core issue of the question is knowledge of characteristic findings in the diagnosis of lymphoma. Use nursing knowledge and the process of elimination to make a selection.

6 **Answer: 2 Rationale:** A non-tender and moveable cervical node may suggest the presence of malignancy and even lymphoma. Palpable nodes do not confirm the diagnosis of a malignancy. Biopsy and histological examination will aid in interpreting the significance of enlarged nodes. **Cognitive Level:** Analyzing **Client Need:** Physiological Adaptation **Integrated Process:** Nursing Process: Data Collection **Content Area:** Adult Health **Strategy:** The core issue of the question is the ability to interpret data related to lymph nodes. Use nursing knowledge and the process of elimination to make a selection.

7 **Answer: 1, 4, 5 Rationale:** Activity intolerance in clients with anemia results from the imbalance between oxygen demand and supply. Activities should be planned to intersperse activity with periods of rest to decrease hypoxemic episodes and to decrease tissue demand for oxygen. A client with anemia

may experience dizziness if there is insufficient oxygenation of red blood cells supplying the brain, which could then interfere with tolerance of activity. Providing for rest periods aids in energy conservation. Education on nutrition to a client with anemia is appropriate but does not directly relate to the nursing diagnosis of activity intolerance. Promoting range of motion would be helpful for the nursing diagnosis of impaired mobility. **Cognitive Level:** Applying **Client Need:** Physiological Adaptation **Integrated Process:** Nursing Process: Implementation **Content Area:** Adult Health **Strategy:** The core issue of the question is knowledge that anemia causes fatigue and that measures to prevent fatigue need to be incorporated in planning care. Use this knowledge and the process of elimination to make a selection.

8 **Answer: 2 Rationale:** Clients with hemophilia should be taught to participate in noncontact sports and to avoid any activities that increase the risk of tissue injury and bleeding. Iron-rich foods are not appropriate in clients with this condition unless there is an accompanying anemia. Clients with hemophilia should never use aspirin because of the risk of bleeding. Joint pain may be caused by hemarthrosis (bleeding in the joints), a situation in which the client should be taught to seek medical care immediately. **Cognitive Level:** Applying **Client Need:** Physiological Adaptation **Integrated Process:** Teaching and Learning **Content Area:** Adult Health **Strategy:** The core issue of the question is an appropriate element of client education with hemophilia. Use concepts related to prevention of bleeding and the process of elimination to make a selection.

9 **Answer: 2 Rationale:** Aplastic anemia may be congenital or acquired, but most cases do not have an identifiable etiology. It is known that aplastic anemia may follow exposure to chemicals (e.g., Benzene, DDT) or drugs (chloramphenicol, sulfonamides). Recent travel outside the country is not pertinent. Aplastic anemia is not a sequela of blood transfusion. Aplastic anemia is not caused by allergies to medications. **Cognitive Level:** Analyzing **Client Need:** Physiological Adaptation **Integrated Process:** Nursing Process: Data Collection **Content Area:** Adult Health **Strategy:** The core issue of the question is knowledge of the possible etiologies of aplastic anemia. Use knowledge about the possible causes of this disorder and the process of elimination to make a selection.

10 **Answer: 1, 2 Rationale:** A client with neutropenia has a compromised immune system and is predisposed to infections. Hand hygiene will reduce the risk of infection to the client. Fresh fruits and vegetables carry microorganisms that could lead to infection in a neutropenic client. Fresh flowers are not allowed in the client's room because they tend to harbor bacteria. The client should not have standing water in the room because it can attract and harbor bacteria that could lead to infection in a neutropenic client. **Cognitive Level:** Applying **Client Need:** Reduction of Risk Potential **Integrated Process:** Teaching and Learning **Content Area:** Adult Health **Strategy:** The core issue of the question is knowledge of the components of neutropenic precautions. The wording of the question tells you the correct options are correct statements. Use nursing knowledge and the process of elimination to make a selection.

11 **Answer: 1 Rationale:** A platelet count below 20,000 indicates that the client is at risk for bleeding and necessitates the avoidance of activities and interventions that increase this risk. Nursing interventions such as the use of intramuscular injections, rectal temperatures, and shaving with a razor are activities that predispose the client to further injury. Reverse isolation is not appropriate for this client unless there is accompanying evidence of neutropenia. **Cognitive Level:** Applying **Client Need:** Reduction of Risk Potential **Integrated Process:** Nursing Process: Implementation **Content Area:** Adult Health **Strategy:** The core issue of the question is appropriate interpretation of a low platelet count and interpreting the appropriate intervention to protect the client from bleeding. Use nursing knowledge and the process of elimination to make a selection.

12 **Answer: 1 Rationale:** Application of direct pressure and pressure dressing should follow the withdrawal of the aspiration needle after a bone marrow aspiration. If the client has thrombocytopenia, pressure should be applied on the site for at least 3 to 5 minutes or until hemostasis has been achieved. The area should not be massaged. Heat increases local blood flow and could increase the risk of bleeding. Covering the area with a light dressing fails to provide the necessary pressure after the procedure. **Cognitive Level:** Applying **Client Need:** Physiological Adaptation **Integrated Process:** Nursing Process: Implementation **Content Area:** Adult Health **Strategy:** The core issue of the question is knowledge of specific care following bone marrow aspiration that will prevent complications of the procedure. Use nursing knowledge and the process of elimination to make a selection.

13 **Answer: 2 Rationale:** A shift to the left indicates an increase in immature neutrophils or bands. An increase in the number of bands indicates an increase in the production of granulocytes, which could be a compensatory mechanism in response to infection. **Cognitive Level:** Analyzing **Client Need:** Physiological Adaptation **Integrated Process:** Nursing Process: Data Collection **Content Area:** Adult Health **Strategy:** The core issue of the question is the ability to make an accurate interpretation of findings on a laboratory report of WBC count and morphology. Use nursing knowledge and the process of elimination to make a selection.

14 **Answer: 3 Rationale:** The morphologic characteristics of RBCs in iron-deficiency anemia is microcytic and hypochromic. Aplastic anemia, hemolysis, and acute blood loss will reveal RBCs with normocytic and normochromic characteristics. Vitamin B_{12} anemia produces a macrocytic and normochromic morphology. Anemias would be hypochromic rather than hyperchromic. **Cognitive Level:** Applying **Client Need:** Physiological Adaptation **Integrated Process:** Nursing Process: Data Collection **Content Area:** Adult Health **Strategy:** The core issue of the question is the pathophysiological changes of RBCs in specific anemias. Use nursing knowledge and the process of elimination to make a selection.

15 **Answer: 2 Rationale:** Reticulocytes are immature RBCs. An increase in the number of reticulocytes indicates the body is producing new RBCs. A child with anemia is not cyanotic but pale. An increase in activity is hard to measure subjectively and would be a late finding. Evidence of iron intake does not assure an improvement in anemia status. **Cognitive Level:** Analyzing **Client Need:** Physiological Adaptation **Integrated Process:** Nursing Process: Data Collection **Content Area:** Child Health **Strategy:** The core issue of the question is the ability to evaluate outcomes of care for a client with anemia. Use nursing knowledge and the process of elimination to make a selection.

16 **Answer: 3 Rationale:** Sickle cell is inherited as an autosomal recessive disorder. Both parents must carry the defective gene. The other statements are factually incorrect.

Cognitive Level: Applying **Client Need:** Physiological Adaptation **Integrated Process:** Teaching and Learning **Content Area:** Child Health **Strategy:** The core issue of the question is the ability to educate a client about genetics as they relate to sickle cell disease. Use nursing knowledge and the process of elimination to make a selection.

17 **Answer: 1 Rationale:** Hemophilia is characterized by a deficiency in one or more clotting factors, while ITP is a platelet disorder. Because the child with ITP is not deficient in clotting factors, this treatment would not be beneficial. **Cognitive Level:** Applying **Client Need:** Physiological Adaptation **Integrated Process:** Communication and Documentation **Content Area:** Child Health **Strategy:** The core issue of the question is an understanding of the differences between hemophilia and bleeding disorders caused by platelet problems. Use nursing knowledge and the process of elimination to make a selection.

18 **Answer: 2 Rationale:** Clients with anemia will experience activity intolerance with even the simplest activities of daily living. There may be insufficient cardiac output, but it will not be related to platelet count. There is no information in the question to indicate that the anemia is secondary to poor diet. There is no vaso-occlusion with anemia. **Cognitive Level:** Analyzing **Client Need:** Physiological Adaptation **Integrated Process:** Nursing Process: Implementation **Content Area:** Child Health **Strategy:** The core issue of the question is knowledge of typical pathophysiology and client data in anemia and using this information to identify the most important nursing diagnosis. Use nursing knowledge about anemia and the process of elimination to make a selection.

19 **Answer: 3 Rationale:** Frequent blood transfusion will lead to an overload of iron in the body. This iron is stored in tissues and organs and is called hemosiderosis. Blood transfusions do not lower the white blood count, cause petechiae, or hemoglobin S formation. **Cognitive Level:** Analyzing **Client Need:** Physiological Adaptation **Integrated Process:** Nursing Process: Data Collection **Content Area:** Child Health **Strategy:** The core issue of the question is identification of a complication of chronic blood transfusion therapy. Use nursing knowledge of thalassemia and the process of elimination to make a selection.

20 **Answer: 2, 4, 5 Rationale:** Clients with nutritional anemias require dietary sources of folic acid, such as green, leafy vegetables; fish; citrus fruits; yeast; dried beans; grains; nuts; and liver. Apples and carrots are not as rich in folic acid as the other food sources listed. **Cognitive Level:** Analyzing **Client Need:** Physiological Adaptation **Integrated Process:** Nursing Process: Implementation **Content Area:** Adult Health **Strategy:** The core issue of the question is knowledge of foods that are rich in Vitamin B_{12}. Use nursing knowledge and the process of elimination to make your selections.

21 **Answer: 3 Rationale:** A vaso-occlusive crisis is a very painful experience and proactive examination and pain control are imperative. Although oxygen will help in pain control by preventing more sickling, high concentrations are not needed. Acid-base balance is not routinely disrupted in a vaso-occlusive crisis. Factor 8 replacement therapy is utilized with hemophilia. **Cognitive Level:** Analyzing **Client Need:** Physiological Adaptation **Integrated Process:** Nursing Process: Implementation **Content Area:** Child Health **Strategy:** First, eliminate activities not related to sickle cell then determine priority of those remaining options.

22 **Answer: 2 Rationale:** A change in the stools to a black, tarry color is an expected side effect of the medication and a sign that the medication is working properly. A change in the stools to a black, tarry color is not a symptom of the anemia. A change in the stools to a black, tarry color is not a sign that the dose is high. A change in the stools to a black, tarry color is not a sign that the child is experiencing bleeding. **Cognitive Level:** Analyzing **Client Need:** Pharmacological and Parenteral Therapies **Integrated Process:** Communication and Documentation **Content Area:** Child Health **Strategy:** The core concept in this stem is the addition of an oral iron preparation. Consider common side effects of this drug in making a selection.

23 **Answer: 3 Rationale:** Children with sickle cell anemia develop sickling of the red cells when exposed to low oxygen tension; this means that the cells become crescent-shaped. Polycythemia is not a finding with sickle cell anemia. Hematopoiesis is the formation of new cells, which occurs at a rapid rate in children with sickle cell anemia due to the rapid destruction of RBCs; however, this process is not visible under the laboratory microscope. Children with sickle cell anemia have adequate iron stores so the cells are not pale in color. **Cognitive Level:** Analyzing **Client Need:** Reduction of Risk Potential **Integrated Process:** Nursing Process: Data Collection **Content Area:** Child Health **Strategy:** Compare each of the responses with what is known about sickle cell anemia. The fact that it is an anemia eliminates polycythemia.

24 **Answer: 3 Rationale:** The child with sickle cell anemia does not need more iron supplements than the regular child. The cause of the child's anemia is fragile red blood cells, which are broken down more rapidly than the normal cell. Children with sickle cell anemia must guard against low oxygen tension in the air. For that reason, they should not fly in unpressurized planes. Because infections increase the basal metabolic rate (BMR) and oxygen requirements, infections often precipitate a crisis. During a sickling crisis, the child will need hydration therapy and pain management to break the sickling cycle. **Cognitive Level:** Analyzing **Client Need:** Coordinated Care **Integrated Process:** Teaching and Learning **Content Area:** Child Health **Strategy:** Knowledge of the management of sickle cell disease will help to choose the correct answers. The wording of the question indicates the need for an option that would be inappropriate for a child with sickle cell anemia.

25 **Answer: 3 Rationale:** Many infants with nutritional anemia rely primarily on the milk/formula for dietary intake and refuse solid foods. When the milk/formula is limited, the child will be more willing to take solid foods. Cow's milk is a poor source of iron. Delaying introduction of solid foods will not help. Peanuts and unsweetened chocolates are sources of iron but are not appropriate for this child's diet. **Cognitive Level:** Applying **Client Need:** Health Promotion and Maintenance **Integrated Process:** Nursing Process: Implementation **Content Area:** Child Health **Strategy:** Nutritional anemia means a diet with inadequate iron. Milk is a poor source of iron.

26 **Answer: 3 Rationale:** Iron preparations should be taken through a straw in order to prevent staining the teeth. Iron is best absorbed on an empty stomach. Iron is best absorbed on an empty stomach. While it is best to give toddlers choices in the hospital setting, iron is best absorbed on an empty stomach. **Cognitive Level:** Applying **Client Need:** Pharmacological and Parenteral Therapies **Integrated Process:** Nursing Process: Implementation **Content Area:** Child Health **Strategy:** Consider attributes of the medication to choose the best answer.

Key Terms to Review

anemia p. 1141
anergy p. 1149
cheilosis p. 1139
ecchymosis p. 1145
fibrinolysis p. 1137
glossitis p. 1140
hemarthrosis p. 1145
hemosiderosis p. 1151
hemostasis p. 1136
hypochromic p. 1139
leukocytosis p. 1137
leukopenia p. 1137
microcytic p. 1139
plethora p. 1143
thrombocytopenia p. 1137
X-linked recessive trait p. 1145

References

Ball, J., Bindler, R., & Cowan, K. (2010). *Child health nursing: Partnering with children and families* (2nd ed.). Upper Saddle River, NJ: Pearson Education.

Berman, A., & Snyder, S. (2012). *Kozier & Erb's fundamentals of nursing: Concepts, process, and practice* (9th ed.). Upper Saddle River, NJ: Pearson Education, Inc.

Ignatavicius, D., & Workman, L. (2010). *Medical-surgical nursing: Critical thinking for collaborative care* (6th ed.). Philadelphia: Saunders.

Kee, J. (2010). *Laboratory and diagnostic tests with nursing implications* (8th ed.). Upper Saddle River, NJ: Pearson Education.

LeMone, P., Burke, K., & Bauldoff, G. (2011). *Medical-surgical nursing: Critical thinking in patient care* (5th ed.). Upper Saddle River, NJ: Pearson Education.

Smith, S., Duell, D., & Martin, B. (2012). *Clinical nursing skills: Basic to advanced skills* (8th ed.). Upper Saddle River, NJ: Pearson Education.

Test Yourself

Are you ready for the NCLEX-PN® or course exams? Use the practice tests on the companion website to check.

61 Oncological Disorders

In this chapter

Cross Reference

Other chapters relevant to this content area are

Promoting Healthy Lifestyle Choices	Chapter 16
Meeting Nutritional Needs	Chapter 25
Common Laboratory Tests	Chapter 42
Common Diagnostic Tests and Procedures	Chapter 43
Respiratory Disorders	Chapter 51
Gastrointestinal Disorders	Chapter 55
Hematological Disorders	Chapter 60

I. OVERVIEW OF CANCER

A. ***Cancer***: mutation of normal cells into abnormally proliferating cells; a neoplasm is an abnormal growth or **tumor** (solid mass functioning independently and serving no useful purpose)

1. **Benign neoplasms**: slow-growing, localized, and encapsulated nonmalignant growths with well-defined borders; are generally easily removed and only cause tissue damage by compressing tissues and interfering with circulation

2. **Malignant neoplasms**: aggressive growths that invade and destroy surrounding tissues; can lead to death unless aggressively treated
3. Invasion occurs when cancer cells infiltrate adjacent tissues surrounding neoplasm
4. **Metastasis** occurs when malignant cells travel through blood or lymph system and invade other tissues and organs to form a secondary tumor

B. Characteristics of malignant cells

1. Rapid cell division and growth: regulation of rate of mitosis is lost
2. No contact inhibition: cells do not respect boundaries of other cells and invade their tissue areas
3. Loss of differentiation: cells lose specialized characteristics of function for that cell type and revert back to an earlier, more primitive cell type
4. Ability to migrate (metastasize): cells move to distant areas of body and establish new site malignant lesions (tumors)
5. Alteration in cell structure: cell membrane, cytoplasm, and overall cell shape
6. Self-survival
   a. May develop ectopic sites to produce hormones needed for own growth
   b. Can develop a connective tissue stroma to support growth
   c. May develop own blood supply by secreting angiotensin growth factor to stimulate local blood vessels to grow into tumor

II. RISK FACTORS FOR DEVELOPMENT OF CANCER

A. Age

1. Increased risk for people over age 65 years
2. Factors attributed to cancer in older adults include hormonal changes, decreased immune responses, and accumulation of free radicals
3. Age has been identified as single most important factor related to development of cancer

B. Gender: certain cancers are more commonly seen in specific genders; for example, breast cancer occurs more often in females

C. Geographic location

1. Risks for cancer vary according to environment and location
2. Rates for specific cancer sites, morbidity, and mortality vary from state to state, nation to nation, and in urban versus rural living

D. Genetics

1. Accounts for approximately 15% of cancers
2. Cancers demonstrating a familial relationship include breast, colon, lung, ovarian, and prostate
3. Clients with a genetic predisposition to cancer should be counseled and screened according to American Cancer Society (ACS) guidelines

E. Immune disturbance: some viruses tend to increase risk, such as Epstein-Barr, genital herpes, papillomavirus, hepatitis B, and human cytomegalovirus (CMV)

F. Chemical agents: over 1000 chemicals are known to be carcinogenic; exposure in some occupations heightens risk over decades

G. Race

1. Cancer can affect any population
2. African Americans experience a higher rate of cancer and higher mortality rates than other racial or ethnic groups, possibly because of more advanced state when seeking treatment

H. Tobacco

1. A strong correlation exists between smoking and lung cancer
2. Other cancers associated with tobacco use include bladder, esophageal, gastric, laryngeal, oropharyngeal, and pancreatic
3. Smokeless tobacco (snuff and chewing tobacco) increases risk of oral and esophageal cancers
4. Long-term exposure to secondhand smoke increases risk for lung and bladder cancers

I. Alcohol: serves as a promoter in cancers of liver and esophagus; when combined with tobacco, risks for other cancers are even higher

J. Diet: has been shown to correlate with some cancers; diets high in fat, low in fiber, and those containing nitrosamines and nitrosindoles (in preserved meats and pickled foods) promote certain cancers such as colon, breast, esophageal, and gastric

K. Miscellaneous factors studied that might correlate with increased incidence of cancer: stress, occupation involving exposure to carcinogens (such as miners and asbestos workers), viruses

Box 61–1

American Cancer Society's Seven Warning Signs of Cancer

*C*hange in bowel or bladder habits

A sore that does not heal

*U*nusual bleeding or discharge

*T*hickening or lump in breast or elsewhere

*I*ndigestion or difficulty in swallowing

*O*bvious change in wart or mole

*N*agging cough or hoarseness

III. AMERICAN CANCER SOCIETY RECOMMENDATIONS FOR EARLY CANCER DETECTION

NCLEX® **A. American Cancer Society's seven warning signs of cancer (see Box 61–1 and Memory Aid)**

Memory Aid

Remember to use CAUTION to recall risk factors for cancer.

NCLEX® **B. Detection of breast cancer**

1. Beginning at age 20, routinely perform monthly breast self-examination (BSE)
2. Women ages 20 to 39 should have breast examination by a health care provider every 3 years
3. Women age 40 and older should have a yearly mammogram and breast examination by a health care provider

NCLEX® **C. Detection of colon and rectal cancer**

1. All persons age 50 and older should have a yearly fecal occult blood test
2. Digital rectal examination and flexible sigmoidoscopy should be done every 5 years
3. Colonoscopy with barium enema should be done every 10 years

NCLEX® **D. Detection of uterine cancer**

1. Yearly Papanicolaou (Pap) smear for sexually active females and those over age 18
2. At menopause, high-risk women should have an endometrial tissue sample

NCLEX® **E. Detection of prostate cancer**

1. Beginning at age 50, have a yearly digital rectal examination
2. Beginning at age 50, have a yearly prostate-specific antigen (PSA) test

F. Self detection of cancer: see Chapter 16 for breast and testicular self examinations

IV. DIAGNOSTIC METHODS, TESTS, AND DATA COLLECTION

A. Grading

1. Classifies cancer based on degree of abnormality of cells when examined under microscope
2. Grading utilizes a Roman numeral rating of I through IV, with I being least abnormal and IV being most abnormal (see Box 61–2)

B. *Staging*: TNM system is used to classify solid tumors (see Box 61–2)

C. *Tumor markers*

1. Are protein substances found in blood or body fluids
2. Are released either by tumor itself or by body as a defense in response to tumor (called host response)
3. Tumor markers are derived from tumor itself and include the following:
   a. *Oncofetal antigens*, present normally in fetal tissue, may indicate an anaplastic process in tumor cells; carcinoembryonic antigen (CEA) and alpha-fetoprotein (AFP) are examples
   b. *Hormones* at high levels may indicate a hormone-secreting malignancy; hormones that may be used as tumor markers include antidiuretic hormone (ADH), calcitonin, catecholamines, human chorionic gonadotropin (HCG), and parathyroid hormone (PTH)
   c. *Isoenzymes* normally present in a tissue may be released into bloodstream if tissue is experiencing rapid, excessive growth because of tumor; examples include neuron-specific enolase (NSE) and prostatic acid phosphatase (PAP)
   d. *Tissue-specific proteins* identify type of tissue affected by malignancy; an example is prostatic-specific antigen (PSA) used to identify prostate cancer
4. Host-response tumor markers include C-reactive protein, interleukin-2, lactic dehydrogenase, serum ferritin, and tumor necrosis factor

Box 61–2

Grading and Staging of Solid Tumors

Grading

Grade I: cells slightly different than normal, well differentiated (mild dysplasia)

Grade II: cells more abnormal, moderately well differentiated (moderate dysplasia)

Grade III: cells clearly abnormal, poorly differentiated (severe dysplasia)

Grade IV: cells anaplastic (immature) and undifferentiated (cell origin difficult to determine)

Staging

T indicates tumor size

T0: no evidence of tumor

Tis: tumor in situ

T1, T2, T3, T4: progressive degrees of tumor size and involvement

N indicates lymph node involvement

N0: no abnormal lymph nodes detected

N1a, N2a: regional nodes involved with increasing degree from N1a to N2a; no metastasis detected

N1b, N2b, N3b: progressive regional lymph nodes involvement; metastasis suspected

Nx: inability to assess regional nodes

M indicates distant metastasis

M0: no evidence of distant metastasis

M1, M2, M3: increasing degrees of distant metastasis and includes distant lymph nodes

D. *Biopsy* and cytology

1. Histologic and cytologic examination of cells collected by needle aspiration of solid tumors, exfoliation from epithelial surface, or aspiration of fluid from blood or body cavities; examples include specimens from Pap smear, bone marrow, or tissue biopsy
2. Tissues for biopsy may be obtained by excisional, incisional, and needle biopsy methods
3. By examining these tissues, tumor name, grade, and stage can be identified

E. Laboratory tests: see Table 61–1

F. Diagnostic studies: include such tests as x-rays, radionuclide and nuclear imaging scans, CT scans, MRI

V. COMMON TREATMENT TECHNIQUES AND PROCEDURES

A. *Radiation therapy*

1. Use of ionizing rays for therapeutic purposes in cancer therapy
2. Used to kill a tumor, reduce tumor size, relieve obstruction, or decrease pain
3. Causes lethal injury to DNA so it can destroy rapidly multiplying cancer cells; radiation therapy kills normal cells as well
4. Classified as internal radiation therapy (brachytherapy) or external radiation therapy (teletherapy)

B. Brachytherapy (internal radiation)

1. Sources of internal radiation
   a. Implanted into affected tissue or body cavity
   b. Ingested as a solution
   c. Injected as a solution into bloodstream or body cavity
   d. Introduced through a catheter into tumor
2. Side effects of internal radiation
   a. Fatigue
   b. Anorexia

Table 61–1 Laboratory Tests Used in Diagnosing Cancer

Lab Test	Cancer-Related Abnormality
Acid phosphatase (ACP)	Elevated in bone, breast, and prostate cancers and in multiple myeloma
Adrenocorticotropic hormone (ACTH)	Decreased in adrenal cancer; elevated in pituitary cancer or tumor that secretes ACTH (bronchogenic cancer)
Alanine aminotransferase (ALT)	Elevated in liver cancer
Albumin	Decreased in metastatic liver cancer and malnutrition
Alkaline phosphatase (ALP)	Elevated in bone, breast, liver, and prostate cancers and in leukemia and multiple myeloma
Alpha-fetoprotein (AFP)	Elevated in testicular cancer and in germ cell tumors
Aspartate aminotransferase (AST)	Elevated in liver cancer
Bilirubin	Elevated in liver and gallbladder cancers
Bleeding time	Prolonged in leukemia and metastatic liver cancer
Blood urea nitrogen (BUN)	Increased in renal cancer; decreased in malnutrition
Calcitonin	Elevated in breast, lung, and thyroid medullary cancers
Calcium (Ca)	Elevated in bone cancer
Carcinoembryonic antigen (CEA)	Elevated in GI, lung, breast, bladder, kidney and cervical cancers, and leukemia
C-reactive protein	Elevated in metastatic cancer and Burkitts's lymphoma
Creatinine	Decreased in malnutrition; elevated in most cancers
Dexamethasone suppression test	Nonsuppression in adrenal cancer and ACTH-producing tumors, severe stress
Estradiol-serum	Elevated in estrogen-producing tumors and testicular tumor
Fibrinogen	Decreased in leukemia and as side effect of chemotherapy
Gamma glutamyltransferase (GGT)	Elevated in liver, pancreas, prostate, breast, kidney, lung, and brain cancers
Haptoglobin	Elevated in Hodgkin's disease and lung, large intestine, stomach, breast, and liver cancers
Hematocrit (Hct)	Decreased in anemia, leukemia, Hodgkin's disease, lymphosarcoma, multiple myeloma, and malnutrition and as a side effect of chemotherapy
Hemoglobin (Hgb)	Decreased in anemia, many cancers, Hodgkin's disease, leukemia, and malnutrition and as side effect of chemotherapy
Human chorionic gonadotropin (HCG)	Elevated in choriocarcinoma
Lactic dehydrogenase (LDH)	Elevated in liver, brain, kidney, and muscle cancers, acute leukemia, anemia
Occult blood	Positive in gastric and colon cancers
Parathyroid hormone (PTH)	Increased in PTH-secreting tumors
Platelet count (thrombocytes)	Decreased in bone, gastric, and brain cancers, in leukemia, and as a side effect of chemotherapy
Prostate-specific antigen (PSA)	Elevated from 10 to 120+ in prostate cancer
Red blood cells (RBCs)	Decreased in anemia, leukemia, infection, multiple myeloma
Uric acid	Increased in leukemia, metastatic cancer, multiple myeloma, Burkitt's lymphoma, after vigorous chemotherapy
White blood cells (WBCs); Total leukocytes	Elevated in acute infection, leukemias, tissue necrosis; decreased as a side effect of chemotherapy
Neutrophils	Elevated in bacterial infection, Hodgkin's disease; decreased in leukemia and malnutrition and as a side effect of chemotherapy
Eosinophils	Elevated in bone, ovary, testes, and brain cancers
Basophils	Elevated in leukemia and healing stage of infection
Monocytes	Elevated in infection, monocytic leukemia, and cancer; decreased in lymphocytic leukemia and as a side effect of chemotherapy
Lymphocytes	Elevated in lymphocytic leukmemia, Hodgkin's disease, multiple myeloma; decreased in cancer and other leukemias, and as a side effect of chemotherapy

Adapted from LeMone, P., Burke, K., & Bauldoff, G. (2012). *Medical-surgical nursing: Critical thinking in patient care* (5th ed.). Upper Saddle River, NJ: Pearson.

c. Immunosuppression
d. Other side effects similar to external radiation (see section C2)

NCLEX®

3. Reinforce client teaching
   a. Avoid close contact with others until treatment is completed because of radioactivity
   b. Maintain daily activities unless contraindicated, allowing for extra rest periods as needed
   c. Maintain balanced diet; may tolerate food better if consumed in small, frequent meals
   d. Maintain fluid intake to ensure adequate hydration (2–3 liters/day)
   e. If implant is temporary, maintain bedrest to avoid dislodging it
   f. Excreted body fluids may be radioactive; double-flush toilets after use
   g. Radiation therapy may lead to bone marrow suppression (refer to precautions for anemia, thrombocytopenia, and immunosuppression later in chapter)

NCLEX®

4. Nursing management of client receiving internal radiation
   a. Exposure to small amounts of radiation is possible during close contact with persons receiving internal radiation; understand principles of protection from exposure to radiation: time, distance, and shielding
   b. Time: minimize time spent in close proximity to radiation source; a common standard is to limit contact time to 30 minutes total per 8-hour shift; minimum distance of 6 feet used when possible
   c. Distance: maintain maximum distance possible from radiation source
   d. Shielding: use lead shields/aprons and other precautions to reduce exposure to radiation
   e. Place client in private room
   f. Instruct visitors to maintain at least a distance of 6 feet from client and limit visits to 10 to 30 minutes
   g. Ensure proper handling and disposal of body fluids, assuring containers are marked appropriately
   h. Ensure proper handling of bed linens and clothing
   i. In event of a dislodged implant, use long-handled forceps and place implant into a lead container; never directly touch implant
   j. Do not allow pregnant women to come into any contact with radiation sources; screen visitors and staff for pregnancy
   k. If working routinely near radiation sources, wear a monitoring device to measure exposure
   l. Educate client in all safety measures
   m. Provide emotional support to client who may feel isolated because of necessary precautions and to family who are concerned for client and unable to assist client at this time

C. External radiation therapy (teletherapy)

1. Radiation oncologist marks specific treatment area using a semipermanent type of ink or tattoo
   a. Treatment is usually given 15–30 minutes per day, 5 days/week, for 2–7 weeks
   b. Client does not pose a risk for radiation exposure to other people
2. Side effects of external radiation therapy
   a. Tissue damage to target area (erythema, sloughing, hemorrhage)
   b. Ulcerations of oral mucous membranes
   c. Gastrointestinal effects such as nausea, vomiting, and diarrhea
   d. Radiation pneumonia
   e. Fatigue
   f. Alopecia
   g. Immunosuppression

NCLEX®

3. Client teaching for external radiation
   a. Wash marked area of skin with plain water only and pat skin dry; do not use soaps, deodorants, lotions, perfumes, powders or medications on site during duration of treatment; do not wash off treatment site marks
   b. Avoid rubbing, scratching, or scrubbing treatment site; do not apply extreme temperatures (heat or cold) to treatment site; if shaving, use only an electric razor
   c. Wear soft, loose-fitting clothing over treatment area
   d. Protect skin from sun exposure during treatment and for at least 1 year after treatment is completed; when going outdoors, use sun-blocking agents with sun protection factor (SPF) of at least 15
   e. Maintain proper rest, diet, and fluid intake as essential to promoting health and repair of normal tissues
   f. Hair loss may occur; choose a wig, hat, or scarf to cover and protect head (refer to care of client with alopecia later in chapter)

NCLEX®

4. Nursing management of client receiving external radiation
   a. Monitor for adverse side effects of radiation (see preceding section)
   b. Monitor for significant decreases in white blood cell (WBC) and platelet counts
   c. Reinforce client teaching (refer to later sections for management of immunosuppression, thrombocytopenia, and anemia)

D. ***Chemotherapy***

1. Chemotherapy: administration of cytotoxic medications and chemicals to promote tumor cell death; IV route is preferred, but drugs may also be administered by oral, intrathecal, topical, intra-arterial, intracavity, and intravesical routes
   a. Chemotherapy disrupts cell cycle in various phases, interfering with cellular metabolism and reproduction
   b. According to **cell-kill hypothesis**, during each cell cycle a fixed percentage of cells are killed by chemotherapy, leaving some tumor cells remaining; this necessitates repeated doses to reduce number of cells, allowing body's immune system to destroy any remaining tumor cells
2. Classified according to mechanism of action
   a. *Alkylating agents* are non-phase-specific and act by interfering with DNA replication
   b. *Antimetabolites* interfere with metabolites or nucleic acids necessary for RNA and DNA synthesis
   c. *Cytotoxic antibiotics* disrupt or inhibit DNA or RNA synthesis
   d. *Hormones and hormone antagonists* are phase-specific (G1 or first growth stage) and act by interfering with RNA synthesis
   e. *Plant alkaloids* interfere with cell division
   f. *Miscellaneous agents* may be cell-cycle phase-specific or non-phase-specific and interfere with DNA replication

NCLEX®

3. Side effects of chemotherapeutic agents
   a. **Bone marrow suppression**: decreased WBC count (immunosuppression), platelet count (thrombocytopenia), and Hgb and Hct (anemia)
   b. Gastrointestinal (GI) effects: anorexia, nausea, vomiting, and diarrhea
   c. **Stomatitis** (inflammation of mouth) and mucositosis
   d. **Alopecia** (hair loss)
   e. Fatigue
   f. **Xerostomia** (dry mouth)
   g. Other side effects specific to chemotherapeutic agent

NCLEX®

4. Management and client teaching for immunosuppression
   a. Risk for infection is high when WBC count is low
   b. Avoid crowds, people with infections, and small children when WBC is low
   c. Use meticulous personal hygiene to avoid infection
   d. Wash hands before and after eating, after toileting, and after contact with other people and pets
   e. Consume a low-bacteria diet; avoid undercooked meat and raw fruits and vegetables
   f. Be aware of signs and symptoms of infection and report them immediately to primary care provider
   g. Monitor laboratory values: CBC with differential, platelets, BUN, liver enzymes
   h. Monitor for infection; monitor vital signs for early indication of infection: fever, tachycardia, and tachypnea
   i. Utilize neutropenic precautions: low-bacteria diet, no fresh plants or flowers in room, no pets, no visitors with infections when WBC level falls below predetermined level (such as 2000 mm^3)

NCLEX®

5. Management and client teaching for thrombocytopenia
   a. Monitor stools and urine for bleeding; stools may be dark or tarry and urine will have pinkish to red tinge
   b. Avoid use of straight razors; use electric shaver only
   c. Avoid contact sports and other activities that may cause trauma
   d. If trauma does occur, apply ice to area and seek medical assistance
   e. Avoid dental work or other invasive procedures unless absolutely necessary
   f. Inform all health care providers of chemotherapy and/or radiation treatments
   g. Avoid aspirin and aspirin-containing products
   h. Safety precautions for oral hygiene: use soft toothbrushes and do not floss; avoid alcohol-based mouthwashes
   i. There is a high risk for spontaneous hemorrhage when platelet count is below 20,000; bleeding precautions are necessary for platelet count below 50,000
   j. Monitor for bleeding, monitor stools and urine for occult blood

k. Inspect skin for ecchymosis, petechiae, and trauma
l. Reinforce client teaching about ways to reduce risk of bleeding and measures that are part of bleeding precautions during times of high risk
m. Avoid intramuscular (IM) injections and limit venipunctures

NCLEX®
6. Management and client teaching for stomatitis and mucositosis
   a. Use a soft toothbrush; mouth swabs may be needed during acute episode
   b. Avoid mouthwashes containing alcohol; do not use lemon glycerin swabs or dental floss
   c. Consider using chlorhexidine mouthwash (Peridex) to decrease risk of hemorrhage and protect gums from trauma
   d. Observe daily for lesions, infection, bleeding, or irritation
   e. For xerostomia, apply lubricating and moisturizing agents to protect mucous membranes from trauma and infection
   f. May consider using "artificial saliva" and hard candy or mints to help with dryness
   g. Avoid smoking and alcohol, which can further irritate oral mucosa
   h. Reinforce signs and symptoms of oral infection and to report to health care provider
   i. Drink cool liquids, and avoid hot (very warm) and spicy or otherwise irritating foods
   j. Inspect oral mucous membranes every 4 hours
   k. Teach and implement proper oral care (see client teaching above)

NCLEX®
7. Management and client teaching for inadequate nutrition and fluid and electrolyte imbalance
   a. Eat frequent, small, low-fat meals
   b. Avoid spicy and fatty foods
   c. Avoid extremely hot, spicy, or extremely cold foods
   d. Perform oral hygiene before and after meals
   e. Maintain fluid intake as prescribed
   f. Take nutritional supplements as prescribed (vitamins, liquid nutrition)
   g. Maintain a daily journal of food and fluid intake
   h. Monitor for adequate hydration; for duration of treatment, encourage daily fluid intake of 2 to 3 liters unless contraindicated
   i. Administer antiemetics *prior* to chemotherapy
   j. Weigh client routinely such as weekly, monitor for weight loss; daily weights are not necessary and could increase client anxiety or depression about weight loss
   k. Monitor lab values indicative of nutritional status (Hgb, Hct, albumin, prealbumin)
   l. Monitor for diarrhea or constipation and nausea or vomiting
   m. Encourage adequate nutritional intake with meals that are served attractively and in an environment free of noxious stimuli (bedpan, urinal, perfumes, air fresheners, and other odors)

NCLEX®
8. Management and client teaching for fatigue
   a. Fatigue is a normal response to chemotherapy and does not necessarily indicate disease progression
   b. Continue daily activities as much as possible, allowing for rest periods in between
   c. Assist client in self-care needs when indicated
   d. Allow for periods of rest; cluster activities

NCLEX®
9. Nursing management and client teaching for alopecia (hair loss)
   a. Chemotherapy and radiation therapy may cause hair loss; chemotherapy–induced hair loss is temporary and hair will grow back, usually beginning about a month after completion of chemotherapy, although texture and color of new hair growth may be different; hair loss during radiation therapy to head may be permanent
   b. Encourage client to choose a wig *before* hair loss occurs in order to match texture and hair color; an alternative is to wear colorful scarf or turban if client wishes
   c. Care of hair and scalp includes washing hair two to three times a week with a mild shampoo; pat hair dry, and do not use a blow dryer
   d. Allow client to express feelings concerning altered body image

E. Bone marrow transplant (BMT)

1. BMT is used in treatment of leukemias, usually in conjunction with radiation or chemotherapy
   a. *Autologous BMT*: client is infused with own bone marrow harvested during remission of disease
   b. *Allogenic BMT*: client is infused with donor bone marrow harvested from a healthy individual
2. Bone marrow is usually harvested from iliac crests, then frozen and stored until transfusion

3. Before receiving BMT, client must first undergo a phase of dose-intensive chemotherapy or radiation therapy to destroy cancer cells, such as leukemic cells; this process also severely suppresses immune system; infection, bleeding, and death are major complications during this conditioning phase
4. After immunosuppression, bone marrow is transfused IV through a central line
5. Side effects of BMT
   a. Malnutrition
   b. Infection related to immunosuppression
   c. Bleeding related to thrombocytopenia
6. Reinforce client teaching: refer to previous sections on client teaching for altered nutrition, immunosuppression, and thrombocytopenia
7. Nursing management of client undergoing a BMT
   a. Monitor for graft-versus-host disease (in which T lymphocytes in donated marrow identify client tissue as foreign, leading to attack on liver, skin, and GI tract, and resulting in skin rashes and desquamation, diarrhea, GI bleeding, and liver damage)
   b. Provide private room for client (will be hospitalized 6 to 8 weeks)
   c. Encourage contact with significant others using telephone, computer, and other means to reduce feelings of isolation
   d. Refer to nursing management for imbalanced nutrition, immunosuppression, and thrombocytopenia

F. Other therapeutic interventions

1. Immunotherapy/biologic response modifiers (BMR); see also Chapter 41
   a. Enhances client's immune responses to modify biologic processes responsible for malignant cells
   b. Currently considered experimental in use
   c. *Monoclonal antibodies*: antibodies are recovered from an inoculated animal with a specific tumor antigen, then given to person with that type of cancer; goal is destruction of tumor
   d. *Cytokines*: normal growth-regulating molecules that have antitumor abilities, such as interleukin-2, interferons, hematopoietic growth factors such as erythropoietin, and granulocyte colony–stimulating factors (GCSF)
   e. *Natural killer cells* (NK cells): exert a spontaneous cytotoxic effect on specific cancer cells; they also secrete cytokines and provide resistance to metastasis
2. Gene therapy: investigational; increases susceptibility of cancer cells to destruction by other treatments; insertion of specific genes enhances ability of client's immune system to recognize and destroy cancer cells
3. Photodynamic therapy
   a. Used to treat specific superficial tumors such as those of surface of bladder, bronchus, chest wall, head, neck, and peritoneal cavity
   b. Photofrin, a photosensitizing compound, is administered IV, where it is retained by malignant tissue
   c. Three days after injection, drug is activated by a laser treatment, which continues for 3 more days
   d. Drug produces a cytotoxic O_2 molecule (singlet oxygen)
   e. During IV administration, monitor for chills, nausea, rash, local skin reactions, and temporary photosensitivity
   f. Drug remains in tissues 4 to 6 weeks after injection; direct or indirect exposure to sun activates drug, resulting in chemical sunburn; educate client to protect skin from sun exposure

VI. ONCOLOGIC EMERGENCIES: DIAGNOSIS AND MANAGEMENT

A. Spinal cord compression

1. Occurs because of pressure in epidural space of spinal cord from expanding tumor (lung, breast, GI) or lymphoma
2. NCLEX® Early symptoms include back and leg pain, coldness, numbness, tingling, paresthesia; progression leads to bowel and bladder dysfunction, weakness, and paralysis
3. Early detection is essential: investigate all reports of back pain or neurological changes
4. Treatment is aimed at reducing tumor size by radiation and/or surgery to relieve compression and prevent irreversible paraplegia; client may receive cortico steroids to reduce cord edema
5. NCLEX® Nursing interventions include early recognition of symptoms, monitoring vital signs, neurological checks, and medication administration

B. Superior vena cava (SVC) syndrome

1. Compression or obstruction of SVC by a tumor
2. Usually associated with cancer of lung, non-Hodgkin's lymphomas, and Hodgkin's disease
3. Signs and symptoms result from blockage of venous circulation of head, neck, and upper trunk

NCLEX® 4. Early signs and symptoms are periorbital edema, facial edema, and jugular vein distention (JVD)

NCLEX® 5. Symptoms progress to edema of neck, arms, and hands; difficulty swallowing; shortness of breath

NCLEX® 6. Late signs and symptoms are cyanosis, altered mental status, headache, hypotension, and possible seizures

7. Death may occur if compression is not relieved
8. Treatment includes high-dose radiation to shrink tumor and relieve symptoms and possible adjuvant chemotherapy

NCLEX® 9. Nursing interventions include monitoring vital signs (VS), providing O_2 support, preparing for tracheostomy if necessary, initiating seizure precautions, and administering corticosteroids to reduce edema

C. Disseminated intravascular coagulopathy (DIC)

1. Severe disorder of coagulation, often triggered by sepsis, whereby abnormal clot formation occurs in microvasculature; clotting factors and platelets become depleted, allowing extensive bleeding to occur; tissue hypoxia occurs from occlusion of blood vessels from clots
2. Signs and symptoms are related to decreased blood flow to major organs (tachycardia, oliguria, dyspnea) and depleted clotting factors (abnormal bleeding and hemorrhage)

NCLEX® 3. Treatment includes anticoagulants to decrease stimulation of coagulation and transfusion of one or more of the following: fresh frozen plasma (FFP), cryoprecipitate, platelets, and packed red blood cells (RBCs)

NCLEX® 4. Nursing interventions include observing client, monitoring for bleeding, applying pressure dressings to venipuncture sites, and preventing risk of sepsis

D. Cardiac tamponade

1. Pericardial effusion secondary to metastases or esophageal cancer can lead to compression of heart, restricting heart movement and resulting in cardiac tamponade

NCLEX® 2. Signs and symptoms are related to cardiogenic shock or circulatory collapse: anxiety, cyanosis, dyspnea, hypotension, tachycardia, tachypnea, impaired LOC, and increased central venous pressure

3. Pericardiocentesis is performed to remove fluid from pericardial sac

NCLEX® 4. Nursing interventions include administering O_2, maintaining IV line, monitoring VS, hemodynamic monitoring, and administration of vasopressor agents

VII. NEUROBLASTOMA

A. Overview

1. Solid tumor outside cranium originating in primitive neurocrest cells, which give rise to adrenal medulla, paraganglia, and sympathetic nervous system cervical chain and thoracic chain
2. In children, most common tumor located outside cranium; usual age at onset is 22 months
3. Prognosis based on client age and staging of tumor; children under 1 year of age have a better prognosis
4. Cause unknown, although environmental factors, such as prenatal drug exposure, may be implicated
5. Oncogenes have been found in neuroblastoma cells; DNA sequence responsible for this is called *N-myc*; high *N-myc* level is associated with rapid disease progression and poorer prognosis
6. Tumor is often silent, leading to late diagnosis and poor prognosis

B. Nursing data collection

NCLEX® 1. Symptoms represent location and stage of disease
   a. A peritoneal tumor may present as an abdominal mass or may be evidenced by bowel and bladder dysfunction; typical signs include weight loss, abdominal fullness, irritability, fatigue, and fever
   b. Mediastinal tumors cause dyspnea and lead to neck and facial edema if tumor is large
   c. Bone metastasis may lead to limp, fever, and malaise; ptosis and ecchymosis of eyes can also occur

2. CT of skull, neck, chest, abdomen, and bone locate tumor
3. Bone marrow aspiration helps to locate mass and determine metastasis
4. Urine testing detects breakdown products of adrenal catecholamines (epinephrine and norepinephrine), which some tumors secrete; these breakdown products are vanillylmandelic acid (VMA) and homovanillic acid (HVA)

C. Therapeutic management

1. Surgery to remove tumor following biopsy
2. Radiation therapy
3. Chemotherapy

NCLEX® 4. If surgery is performed, monitor surgical site for hemorrhage and infection; use temperature as most accurate indicator of infection

5. Monitor skin integrity at radiation site

NCLEX® 6. Monitor mucous membrane integrity; use appropriate nursing interventions to prevent and treat mouth ulcers

7. Minimize exposure to infection as previously discussed
8. Monitor bleeding as previously discussed

D. Reinforce client and family teaching

1. Disease process as well as treatment modalities
2. Blood dyscrasias and actions they can take to improve child's condition
3. Need for good nutrition and management of nausea

VIII. BRAIN TUMORS

A. Overview

1. Over half of brain tumors in children are **infratentorial** (below tentorium cerebelli in the posterior third of the brain), primarily in cerebellum and brainstem
2. Most adult tumors and some tumors in children are **supratentorial** (above tentorial notch in anterior part of brain) and are mainly in cerebrum
3. The terms benign and malignant are of little value; benign brain tumors can also be fatal because of solid skull that allows no room for expansion of tumor and thus causes increased intracranial pressure (ICP)
4. Cause is unknown, although radiation and environmental factors may play a role
5. Supporting cells of brain, such as glias and astrocytes, frequently account for pediatric brain tumors

B. Nursing data collection

1. Symptoms depend upon location of tumor and age of client
2. Since an infant's sutures are open, symptoms may be found late

NCLEX® 3. Increased ICP occurs with brain tumors because of presence of the tumor and obstructions in flow of CSF; symptoms related to increased ICP include headache, especially on awakening, and vomiting unrelated to eating

NCLEX® 4. Visual symptoms include diplopia and papilledema

NCLEX® 5. Supratentorial tumors lead to symptoms such as personality changes and seizures

NCLEX® 6. Infratentorial tumor symptoms include ataxia, visual disturbances, delayed or precocious puberty, and growth failures

7. Diagnosis is based on results of MRI, CT scans, and radiographic studies with IV contrast; angiography is done when CT scans are positive
8. Surgery is used for biopsy (diagnosis), to completely remove a tumor, or to **debulk** an unremovable tumor (palliative procedure to surgically remove part of a neoplasm when complete excision is impossible); surgery may also be performed to restore patency of ventricles
9. Laser surgery can be used for more sensitive areas, where greater precision is needed
10. Radiation therapy may be used at the site postoperatively
11. Chemotherapy is commonly used, sometimes intrathecally
12. Complications such as hydrocephalus, seizures, sensorimotor deficits, and endocrine disorders may also need management

NCLEX® 13. Maintain nutritional support; if client vomits from increased ICP, provide hygiene and refeed

NCLEX® 14. Monitor LOC and observe for signs of increased ICP (increasing systolic BP, widening pulse pressure, bradycardia, irregular respirations); regulate fluid status to prevent rises in ICP; observe for seizures and provide nursing care should they occur; protect client from injury and have suction and O_2 available at bedside

NCLEX® 15. Monitor I&O and measure urine specific gravity (to detect diabetes insipidus [DI] or syndrome of inappropriate ADH [SIADH] from pituitary involvement)

NCLEX® 16. Postoperatively, position of head is critical; with an infratentorial incision, head position is flat with neck slightly extended; with supratentorial incision, head is elevated; surgeon orders degree of head elevation, often 30 degrees; keep head and neck midline to promote arterial and venous blood flow

NCLEX® 17. If a ventriculoperitoneal (VP) shunt has been placed to restore ventricle drainage, nursing care includes maintaining suture line and skin integrity over shunt

18. Provide eye care to prevent dryness if client cannot blink or close eyes because of postoperative orbital edema
19. Monitor pain and provide relief; avoid medications that sedate client, which could interfere with evaluation of LOC
20. Monitor sensory-perceptual status and assist with loss of function
21. Monitor surgical site for hemorrhage and infection

C. Reinforce client and family teaching

1. Information provided by physician about diagnosis and treatment; prepare client and family for craniotomy if indicated, including need to shave head and to expect ecchymosis of eyes (common postoperatively)
2. Activities that can reduce pain preoperatively and postoperatively
3. Encourage client and family to talk honestly about diagnosis and their feelings
4. Medication (desmopressin [DDAVP]) to control symptoms if DI occurs secondary to brain tumor

IX. WILMS TUMOR (NEPHROBLASTOMA)

A. Overview

1. Intrarenal tumor that most commonly occurs between 2 and 5 years of age
2. A small proportion of Wilms tumors show a genetic basis with family members being at increased risk of development
3. Tumor may be unilateral or bilateral; bilateral tumors have poorer prognosis
4. Tumor is often encapsulated until relatively late; it metastasizes to lungs and liver

B. Nursing data collection

1. Usually asymptomatic
2. *NCLEX®* Most frequent admitting symptom is abdominal mass, which parent often finds on one side of midline of abdomen
3. *NCLEX®* Pain and hematuria may be present in some children
4. *NCLEX®* Hypertension is present in approximately 25% of children because of increased renin production
5. Diagnosis is made by abdominal ultrasound and intravenous pyelogram (IVP)
6. CT scan and MRI of the lungs are done to detect metastasis
7. *NCLEX®* Avoid palpating abdomen preoperatively to reduce risk of rupturing capsule and causing tumor spillage; place a sign over child's bed with instruction "No abdominal palpations"

C. Therapeutic management

1. If unilateral tumor is present, surgery is performed to remove affected kidney and check for metastasis
2. Radiation to abdomen and chemotherapy can be used before and/or after surgery
3. *NCLEX®* Postoperatively, monitor functioning of remaining kidney
   a. Measure I&O
   b. Monitor daily weight and urine specific gravity
   c. Monitor fluid levels, IV infusions, and BP
4. *NCLEX®* Monitor pain when measuring VS; provide pain relief with medications and nursing interventions; in addition to incisional pain, pain may result from postoperative shift of internal organs to compensate for loss of kidney
5. *NCLEX®* Monitor bowel sounds, abdominal distention, and bowel movements
6. *NCLEX®* Monitor for infection, observing surgical wound and body temperature

D. Reinforce client and family teaching

1. Need to avoid unnecessary palpation of abdomen prior to surgical removal
2. Nature of disease, treatment options, and therapeutic and side effects of chemotherapy in use (to parents)
3. Need to protect remaining kidney; signs and symptoms of urinary tract infections; and avoid contact sports, during which injury to kidney might occur

X. BONE TUMORS

A. Osteogenic sarcoma

1. Tumor that arises from a bone cell, probably osteoblast
   a. Most common bone cancer in children
   b. Most frequently affects metaphysis of long bones
   c. Osteogenic sarcoma usually occurs in adolescent boys; tumor growth is detected at time of rapid bone growth
   d. Most frequently affects distal portion of femur; also affects humerus, tibia, pelvis, jaw, and phalanges
   e. Malignant tumor that frequently metastasizes to lungs; metastasis may be present at time of diagnosis
   f. Etiology is unknown, but increased incidence is noted in children who have had retinoblastoma; an abnormal gene may also be implicated, as familial tendency for osteogenic sarcoma has been noted
2. Nursing data collection
   a. *NCLEX®* Pain and swelling are initial symptoms
   b. X-rays following traumatic injury may be first indication of disease
   c. Follow-up tests include CT or MRI imaging to detect areas of metastasis

3. Therapeutic management
   a. Treatment may include radical resection or amputation
   b. Selected clients may have limb-salvaging procedures with prosthetic replacement
   c. Thoracotomy may be performed for metastasis to lung
   d. Chemotherapy may be administered pre- and postoperatively
   e. Emotional support of child is important before and after surgery, because child and family deal with life-threatening disease, and treatment affects body image and mobility
   f. Employ a straightforward approach when amputation is indicated; allow for verbal expression of feelings
   NCLEX® g. Postoperative care includes sterile residual limb care and special bandaging as ordered
   NCLEX® h. Elevate residual limb for 24 hours, if prescribed, but avoid prolonged elevation
   i. Maintain body alignment
   j. Perform ROM to joints proximal to amputation
   k. Provide opioid analgesics to relieve postoperative pain as ordered; be aware that phantom pain can occur in amputated limb because of irritation of residual nerve endings; use opioid analgesics for this type of pain also
   l. Assist with early ambulation; assist with temporary prosthesis use
   m. Reinforce appropriate use of assistive devices
   n. Encourage early interaction with peers
4. Reinforce client and family teaching
   a. Disease process and treatment options
   NCLEX® b. Residual limb care (wash daily; use clean cotton or woolen sock; examine daily for intact skin)
   c. Demonstrate safe use of prosthesis; teach child to monitor condition of residual limb
   d. Phantom limb pain and its management; possibility of phantom limb sensation

B. Ewing's sarcoma

1. Overview
   a. A malignant, small, round cell tumor that usually involves diaphysial (shaft) portion of long bones; commonly found in femur, pelvis, tibia, fibula, ribs, scapula, humerus, and clavicle
   b. Tumor arises in marrow spaces of bone
   c. Tends to occur between ages of 4 and 25
   d. Is a highly malignant tumor that metastasizes to lung
2. NCLEX® Nursing data collection
   a. Pain
   b. Soft tissue mass
   c. Secondary symptoms of anorexia, malaise, fever, fatigue, and weight loss
   d. Diagnosed with x-rays of affected area
   e. Radionuclide bone scans and CT scans of chest test for metastasis
3. NCLEX® Therapeutic management
   a. Amputation usually not recommended
   b. Treatment includes extensive radiation along with chemotherapy
   c. Emotional support of child is important, as radiation therapy can affect appearance and mobility of extremity
   d. Encourage mobility of extremity as tolerated
   e. Allow open communication with child and family about disease and prognosis
4. Reinforce client and family teaching: disease process and treatment options; skin care related to radiation therapy

XI. COLON CANCER

A. Overview

1. Develops in bowel wall or begins as polyps in colon or rectum that deteriorate
2. Metastasizes via circulatory or lymphatic system or by direct extension to other areas of bowel or adjacent organs
3. Can cause abscesses or fistulas, bowel obstruction, hemorrhage or perforation of bowel, leading to peritonitis

NCLEX® **B. Nursing data collection**

1. Client may have no signs early in course of disease, making screening tests such as fecal occult blood and colonoscopy so important
2. Anorexia, vomiting, and weight loss; cachexia are late signs
3. Malaise

4. Anemia
5. Abdominal distention and possible guarding
6. Hematest positive or bloody stools with altered bowel pattern
    a. Tumor in ascending colon: diarrhea
    b. Tumor in descending colon: constipation or diarrhea; possible flat, ribbonlike stools from partial obstruction
    c. Tumor in rectum: alternating diarrhea and constipation
7. Abdominal mass (late sign)

NCLEX®

C. Therapeutic management

1. Monitor for development of complications
    a. Bowel perforation: distended abdomen; fever; weak, rapid pulse; and hypotension
    b. Intestinal obstruction: abdominal pain and distention, constipation, vomiting (may be fecal), hyperactive bowel sounds early (attempt to push past obstruction) followed by hypoactive then absent bowel sounds
2. Preoperative or postoperative radiation therapy to shrink tumor and reduce associated symptoms or to prevent recurrence
3. Surgery: bowel resection, ileostomy or colostomy; see Chapter 55 for highlights of colostomy and ileostomy care
4. Note characteristics of stool following ostomy creation
    a. Ileostomy: liquid dark green stool progressing to yellow
    b. Ascending colostomy: liquid stool that is greenish then brown
    c. Transverse colostomy: liquid to semiformed brown
    d. Descending colostomy: semiformed to almost normal brown
5. Provide routine postoperative care including pain management and assessment of stoma and return of bowel function

D. Reinforce client teaching

1. Ostomy care
2. Dietary needs with ostomy (foods that loosen or thicken stool; foods that reduce or cause odor of stool)
3. Activity, medications, and follow-up care
4. Signs and symptoms of complications to report (such as infection, delayed wound healing)

XII. TESTICULAR CANCER

A. Overview

1. Unregulated growth of abnormal cells within testicles
2. Exact cause is unknown, but risk factors include cryptorchidism (undescended testicles at birth), maternal treatment with DES during pregnancy, mumps orchitis, trauma, environmental factors, and age
3. (NCLEX®) Most common cancer among males age 15 to 35, making sperm banking important to preserve ability to produce offspring
4. Testicular cancer is usually slow-growing and localized, with a good prognosis

NCLEX®

B. Nursing data collection

1. Painless, hardened area or lump found during testicular self-examination (TSE) is common
2. Dull ache in pelvis or scrotum
3. Testicular pain may occur with associated infection, necrosis, or hemorrhage
4. Weight loss and fatigue
5. Metastatic signs such as respiratory symptoms, GI disturbances, lumbar back pain, lymphadenopathy, and gynecomastia
6. Scrotal ultrasound; CT or MRI scan of chest, abdomen, and pelvis may rule out metastasis
7. IVP to determine kidney involvement
8. (NCLEX®) AFP and beta unit of HCG are tumor markers; elevated levels strongly suggest testicular cancer; markers are measured after surgery to determine residual disease, possibly in lymph nodes
9. Serum lactic dehydrogenase (LDH) is elevated with testicular cancer

C. Therapeutic management

1. Prepare client for screening tests to determine type of cancer and stage
2. Provide emotional support for client and family; respond to questions and encourage client to express feelings
3. Prepare client for surgery if indicated (orchiectomy and exploration of adjacent area to identify cancer cell type and stage disease; lymphadenectomy if indicated)

4. Prepare client for chemotherapy after surgery and possible radiation therapy if cancer has spread to lymph nodes

NCLEX® 5. After surgery: provide analgesics, ice packs, and scrotal support to control pain and swelling; monitor for complications, such as bleeding or infection

D. Reinforce client teaching

1. Reinforce explanation of type and extent of cancer, and plans for treatment
2. Importance of monthly TSE, because malignancy may develop in remaining testis; see Chapter 16 for procedure

NCLEX® 3. Possibility of preserving sperm in a bank before surgery to help relieve client's fears about infertility

4. Orchiectomy should have no lasting effects on sexual or reproductive function
5. Signs of complications: bleeding, gaping incision, or purulent drainage from incision
6. Methods to control pain, such as ice bags and scrotal support
7. Remain at home for about 5 days and avoid driving for 1 week
8. Avoid strenuous physical activity for 3 weeks
9. Follow health care provider's instructions for resuming sexual activity
10. Importance of follow-up, especially if retroperitoneal lymph nodes were not surgically explored; client will need periodic physical examinations, tumor markers, and CT scans of retroperitoneal nodes for 5 to 10 years after surgery

XIII. PROSTATE CANCER

A. Overview

1. Unregulated growth of abnormal cells in prostate gland
2. Adenocarcinoma is most common type; high levels of testosterone may play a role; is most common after 40 years of age
3. Usually begins in peripheral tissue on back and sides of gland
4. Metastasis via lymph and venous channels is common; bony tissue is major site of distant metastasis—especially pelvic bones and spine

B. Nursing data collection

1. Often no symptoms in early stages; tumor may be found during digital prostate exam

NCLEX® 2. Genitourinary: dysuria, frequency, reduced force of stream, hematuria, nocturia, abnormal prostate found on digital rectal exam

3. Musculoskeletal: back pain, migratory bone pain, bone or joint pain
4. Neurological: nerve pain, muscle spasms, bowel or bladder dysfunction, bilateral weakness of lower extremities

NCLEX® 5. Systemic: fatigue and weight loss

NCLEX® 6. Diagnostic and laboratory tests: elevated PSA levels, transrectal ultrasound (obtained if PSA results are abnormal), tissue biopsy, bone scan; MRI, or CT scans to detect metastasis

C. Therapeutic management

1. Treatment options include hormone therapy, radiation therapy, brachytherapy (radioactive seeds implanted in prostate), prostatic cryosurgery, and conventional surgery
2. Surgical procedures
   a. Orchiectomy decreases androgen production
   b. Radical prostatectomy procedures include removal of gland, capsule, ampulla, vas deferens, seminal vesicles, adjacent lymph nodes, and cuff of bladder neck
   c. Suprapubic prostatectomy: abdominal and bladder incisions to remove prostate tissue; abdominal dressing may leak copious urine; change dressing as needed and maintain continuous bladder irrigation (see next section); risk of hemorrhage and bladder spasms
   d. Retropubic prostatectomy: low abdominal incision without opening bladder; less bleeding and fewer bladder spasms than suprapubic route
   e. Perineal prostatectomy: incision between scrotum and anus (perineal area); minimal bleeding but increased risk of infection; urinary incontinence common; surgery causes sterility; avoid rectal tubes, enemas, and temperatures
   f. Homium laser: laser treatment; less bleeding, fewer complications, and shorter hospital stay
3. Encourage annual prostate examination for men 40 years old and above
4. Medication therapy: estrogen therapy or luteinizing hormone antagonist (Lupron) given to slow rate of tumor growth and extension

D. Care of client having prostate surgery

NCLEX® **1.** Monitor VS closely for 24 hours, observing for signs of hemorrhage (frank blood in urine, large blood clots, decreased Hgb and Hct, tachycardia, and hypotension)

2. Collect usual postoperative data, including lung and bowel sounds, IV fluid infusions, pain, urine output

NCLEX® **3.** If dressings are present, monitor for drainage and change as needed

NCLEX® **4.** Clients have a urinary catheter following surgery; surgeon may apply traction against prostatic fossa to prevent bleeding; balloon at tip of catheter exerts pressure to prevent hemorrhage (surgeon positions external end of catheter by anchoring it tightly to client's inner thigh to maintain traction; do not reposition catheter)

5. A client who has a large indwelling catheter may feel urge to void, which results from stimulation of micturition center; explain to client this is a normal sensation; efforts by client to void or strain will increase risk of bleeding and aggravate pain

NCLEX® **6.** Continuous bladder irrigation (CBI) postoperatively

- **a.** Purpose is to prevent formation of blood clots
- **b.** If blood clots do form, urinary catheter will become plugged and prevent outflow of urine; obstruction will also cause bladder spasms and pain
- **c.** Titrate flow rate of irrigating solution to maintain outflow light pink (early) or pale yellow (later) in color with no visible clots; it is essential to calculate both intake and output from catheter to determine true urine output; subtract CBI inflow from output for shift or 24-hour period to determine actual urine output
- **d.** Indications that irrigation rate is inadequate (slow) include decreased outflow from catheter; bladder spasms; and dark-colored, "punch-colored," or frankly bloody drainage
- **e.** Maintain sterile technique while changing irrigation bags

7. Monitor client for signs of hemorrhage; bladder spasms and frank bloody output may indicate bleeding

NCLEX® **8.** The irrigating solution used during and after surgery may be absorbed, causing fluid shifts and dilutional hyponatremia, referred to as TURP syndrome

- **a.** Monitor client for signs of hyponatremia and bradycardia, nausea, and vomiting
- **b.** Monitor serum sodium and Hgb and Hct (lowered with dilutional effect)
- **c.** Other signs of volume excess will also be evident, including hypertension and confusion

9. If manual irrigations are ordered, maintain sterile technique

NCLEX® **10.** Medicate as needed for surgical pain with opioids and use suppositories such as belladonna and opium (B&O) to relieve sudden severe pain caused by bladder spasm

E. Reinforce client teaching

1. Information about illness and treatment plan
2. Methods to deal with urinary incontinence, which occurs temporarily after surgery, but could be permanent if bladder sphincters have been permanently damaged
3. Care of urinary catheter
4. Methods of pain control
5. Impact of surgery on sexual function (temporary or permanent impotence, permanent infertility after radical prostatectomy)
6. Importance of follow-up tests for recurrence of disease
7. Signs of spinal cord compression (back pain and lower extremity weakness) because of high incidence of metastasis to spinal cord
8. Activity levels as prescribed
9. Refer client to support groups, such as American Cancer Society

XIV. CERVICAL CANCER

A. Overview

1. Unregulated growth of abnormal cells in female cervix
2. Most common reproductive system cancer; often seen between ages of 30 and 50
3. May become invasive and spread to tissue outside cervix, uterine fundus, and lymph glands
4. Treatment depends on extent of disease
5. Squamous cell carcinoma accounts for 90% of cervical cancers; have gradual onset; spread by direct invasion of accessory structures

NCLEX® **B. Nursing data collection**

1. Thin, watery, blood-tinged vaginal discharge, which may go unnoticed by client
2. Painless bleeding between periods, often seen after intercourse, douching, or other contact
3. Late symptoms occur as cancer progresses to other organs, including referred pain in back and thighs, hematuria, bloody stools, anemia, and weight loss
4. Early diagnosis is critical, because cervical cancer can be cured in early stages
5. Cervical Pap test; abnormal results call for repeat test, colposcopic exam of cervix, and tissue biopsy; diagnosis is based on biopsy results

C. Therapeutic management

1. NCLEX® Treatment methods consist of chemotherapy, radiation therapy, and surgery
2. Assist client in dealing with psychological effects of illness; provide information and emotional support
3. Explore treatment options with client and family
4. Develop strategies for pain control
5. Maintain skin and tissue integrity during radiation treatment and following surgery
6. NCLEX® Observe for fistula formation between vagina and bladder or rectum, a possible complication of radiation therapy; signs include voiding or having bowel movement through vagina
7. NCLEX® Recommend a high-carbohydrate, high-protein diet
8. Medication therapy: chemotherapy for tumors unresponsive to other therapy or that cannot be removed, or as adjunct therapy for metastasis; and analgesics for pain control

D. Reinforce client teaching

1. Explanations of diagnostic tests and treatments, allowing client time to express feelings and ask questions
2. Wound and skin care if surgery and/or radiation therapy are performed
3. Importance of regular screening exams and follow-up after treatment is completed

XV. OVARIAN CANCER

A. Overview

1. Unregulated growth of abnormal cells in the ovaries
2. Most lethal of gynecologic cancers; etiology not understood; risk increases after age 40
3. Often asymptomatic, leading to late diagnosis; usually detected by chance, not through screening
4. May involve one or both ovaries; staged according to tissue involvement
5. Four stages of ovarian cancers: I—limited to ovaries; II—pelvic extension; III—metastasis outside pelvis or positive lymph nodes; IV—distant metastasis

B. Nursing data collection

1. Symptoms are rare until extensive tumor growth is present
2. NCLEX® Feeling of pelvic pressure or heaviness, vague abdominal discomfort, dyspepsia, bloating, constipation, urinary frequency, and increased abdominal size
3. NCLEX® Palpable, hard, fixed, firm mass in the area of ovaries during pelvic exam
4. No definitive diagnostic tool is available; diagnosis is made during surgery (exploratory laparotomy)
5. NCLEX® CA125 antigen level (tumor marker) sometimes aids in detecting ovarian cancer

C. Therapeutic management

1. NCLEX® Treatment options include surgery, radiation therapy, and chemotherapy
2. Explore treatment options with client and family; surgery is treatment of choice, radiation is used for palliative purposes to shrink tumor
3. Assist client in dealing with psychological effects of illness; provide information and emotional support
4. Develop strategies for pain control
5. Maintain skin and tissue integrity during radiation treatment and following surgery
6. Medication therapy: chemotherapy may be used to achieve remission, but is not a cure

D. Reinforce client teaching

1. Information about diagnostic tests and treatments, giving client time to express feelings and ask questions
2. Wound and skin care if surgery or radiation therapy is performed
3. Importance of regular screening exams and follow-up after treatment is completed
4. Not to ignore vague symptoms, such as indigestion, nausea, or urinary frequency

XVI. BREAST CANCER

A. Overview

1. Unregulated growth of abnormal cells in breast tissue
2. Cause unknown, but many risk factors influence development
   - a. Female gender and Caucasian race
   - b. Family history of mother or sister with breast cancer
   - c. Medical history of cancer of other breast, endometrial cancer, or atypical hyperplasia
   - d. Menarche before age 12 (early) or menopause after age 50 (late)
   - e. First birth after 30 years of age, oral contraceptive use (early or prolonged), prolonged use of estrogen replacement therapy
   - f. Lifestyle factors: high-fat diet, obesity, high socioeconomic status, breast trauma, smoking, ingesting more than two alcoholic drinks daily
   - g. Exposure to radiation through chest x-ray, fluoroscopy
3. Begins as a single, transformed cell and is hormone-dependent; does not develop in women without functioning ovaries who never received hormone replacement therapy
4. Most often occurs in ductal areas of breasts
5. non-invasive: does not penetrate surrounding tissues; may be ductal or lobular; usually diagnosed through mammogram or nipple discharge
6. Invasive: penetration of tumor into surrounding tissue; there are five subtypes of invasive cancers, but they have only slight differences in prognosis
7. Staging depends on size of tumor, lymph node involvement, and metastasis to distant sites

NCLEX® **B. Nursing data collection**

1. Lump may be palpable in breast tissue, usually non-tender, but may be tender
2. Dimpling of breast tissue surrounding nipple or bleeding from the nipple may be present
3. Possible asymmetry, with affected breast being higher
4. Possible swollen and tender regional lymph nodes
5. Diagnostic and laboratory tests: mammography, ultrasonography, MRI, PET, tissue biopsy, sentinel node biopsy (uses radionuclides to locate sentinel node for removal and analysis rather than a chain of nodes)

C. Therapeutic management

1. Treatment options include surgery, radiation therapy, chemotherapy, and hormonal therapy
2. Explore treatment options with client and family; prepare client for treatment, which is based on stage of disease
3. Radiation therapy is used to destroy remaining cancer cells after surgery or to shrink tumor prior to surgery
4. Various types of mastectomy may be performed
   - a. Segmental mastectomy or lumpectomy: removes tumor and a margin of breast tissue surrounding tumor
   - b. Simple mastectomy: removal of complete breast but no other structures
   - c. Modified radical mastectomy: removal of breast and axillary lymph nodes, but not chest wall muscles
   - d. Radical mastectomy: removal of breast, axillary lymph nodes, and underlying chest wall muscles; seldom done anymore
   - *NCLEX®* e. Breast reconstruction: may be performed at time of mastectomy or at a later time; can be accomplished through submuscular breast implant, placing an implant after using a tissue expander, using muscles with intact blood supply from back or abdomen, or creating a free muscle flap with gluteus maximus muscle
5. *NCLEX®* Assist client in dealing with psychological effects of illness; provide information and emotional support, including information about breast reconstruction surgery
6. Maintain skin and tissue integrity during radiation treatment and following surgery
7. Medication therapy: tamoxifen (Novadex) interferes with estrogen activity for treating advanced breast cancer, and chemotherapy when axillary nodes are involved

D. Nursing management of client undergoing a mastectomy

1. Maintain usual postoperative examinations
2. Begin emotional support before surgery and continue in postoperative period
3. Turn, cough, and deep-breathe to prevent respiratory complications; restrictive surgical dressing may decrease chest expansion
4. Position client on back or unaffected side

NCLEX® 5. Maintain Jackson-Pratt drain or Hemovac to drain fluid that accumulates when lymph nodes are removed

6. Note signs of bleeding on dressing and reinforce pressure dressing as needed

NCLEX® 7. Encourage early gentle ROM exercise to prevent contractures and lymphedema

NCLEX® 8. Use only unaffected arm for IV therapy and venipuncture and to measure BP

NCLEX® 9. Position affected arm with each distal joint higher than proximal one before it (shoulder, elbow, wrist, and fingers)

E. Reinforce client teaching

1. Information about diagnostic tests and treatments, giving client time to express feelings and ask questions
2. Information about mastectomy surgery and what to expect afterward
3. Wound care if surgery is performed, including care of short-term wound drains
4. NCLEX® Discharge instructions postmastectomy
   a. Use caution when lifting heavy objects with arm on affected side
   b. Avoid injury and infection on affected side; wear rubber gloves when washing dishes and garden gloves when working outside; use potholders and oven mitts when using warm or hot cooking items
   c. Do not allow procedures, such as BP or venipuncture, on affected side
   d. Availability of support groups for psychosocial support
   e. Avoid heavy lifting for at least 6 weeks or until approved by surgeon
5. Techniques for proper skin care if radiation therapy is performed
6. Encourage client to meet others who have had treatment, if appropriate
7. Postoperative exercises and monthly SBE
8. Self-care during radiation and chemotherapy treatments
9. Importance of regular screening exams and follow-up after treatment is completed

Check Your NCLEX–PN® Exam I.Q.

You are ready for testing on this content if you can

- Describe the pathophysiology and etiology of common oncological disorders.
- Discuss expected data and diagnostic test findings for selected oncological disorders.
- Discuss therapeutic management of a client experiencing an oncological disorder.
- Discuss nursing management of a client experiencing an oncological disorder.
- Identify expected outcomes for the client experiencing an oncological disorder.

PRACTICE TEST

1 A 4-year-old child is receiving postoperative care for surgical resection of a Wilms tumor. In addition to urinary functioning, the nurse makes which priority postoperative examination?

1. Bowel function
2. Neurological status
3. Presence of bone pain
4. Activity level

2 A child with a brain tumor has shown symptoms of diabetes insipidus. What would the nurse monitor to provide ongoing data of this condition?

1. Blood glucose level
2. Urine specific gravity
3. Adrenocorticotropic hormone (ACTH) levels
4. Serum amylase

3 The nurse determines that the client with Ewing's sarcoma understands instruction related to radiation therapy when the client states that side effects include which of the following?

1. An increased risk of infection
2. Constipation
3. An increased appetite
4. Hemorrhagic cystitis

4 A 6-month-old infant is being treated for neuroblastoma. Because of chemotherapy, the infant feeds poorly and vomits frequently. The nurse would use which finding to best determine the child's fluid status?

1. Daily weight
2. Urinary output
3. Specific gravity of urine
4. Hemoglobin and hematocrit

5 A child has been diagnosed with a brain tumor, but surgery cannot be scheduled for several days. The mother asks what she can do to ease her child's headaches. What suggestion should the nurse give the mother?

1. Help the child to drink plenty of liquids
2. Discourage the child from having a bowel movement
3. Encourage the child to sleep in a semi-Fowler's position
4. Encourage the child to blow the nose when headaches become severe

6 A client with squamous cell carcinoma of the lung comes to the emergency department with shortness of breath and respiratory difficulty. The nurse notes cyanosis and edema of the face and arms. Based on these findings, the nurse suspects the client is probably experiencing which complication?

1. Spinal cord compression
2. Syndrome of inappropriate antidiuretic hormone (SIADH)
3. Superior vena cava syndrome
4. Sepsis

7 A client with lung cancer is admitted to the oncology clinic for radiation therapy to treat spinal cord compression. The client's spouse asks why radiation is being done. The nurse's response would include that radiation therapy should have which effect?

1. To eradicate the tumor
2. To reduce size of the tumor
3. To effectively treat all oncological emergencies
4. Provide an alternative to chemotherapy for the lung tumor

8 A client with esophageal cancer arrives in the emergency department with shortness of breath, tachycardia, hypotension, and cyanosis. Cardiac tamponade is diagnosed. Which intervention would the nurse expect to include in this client's care? Select all that apply.

1. Administer a vasodilator agent orally
2. Assist registered nurse in inserting an intravenous catheter for IV access
3. Prepare to assist physician with a thoracentesis
4. Prepare the client for radiation therapy
5. Initiate oxygen therapy

9 The clinic nurse is discussing risk factors for cancer with a male client, who asks which cancers have the highest incidence in men. In order of occurrence, the nurse should reply that the client has greatest risk for which cancers based on gender?

1. Lung, prostate, and colorectal cancers
2. Prostate, lung, and colorectal cancers
3. Colorectal, lung, and prostate cancers
4. Prostate, colorectal, and lung cancers

10 After completing a health risk examination on an adult client, the nurse determines health education is necessary because of an increased risk for laryngeal cancer caused by which risk factors? Select all that apply.

1. Past infection with Epstein-Barr virus
2. Past exposure to asbestos
3. Cigarette smoking
4. Heavy daily alcohol consumption
5. Recreational use of marijuana

11 A client newly diagnosed with breast cancer is scheduled for lymph node biopsy and asks the nurse why it is necessary when cancer has already been diagnosed. The nurse's response is based on which purpose?

1. It will determine what types of cancer cells are present
2. It is performed on all females with cancer
3. It is performed to determine if cancer has metastasized
4. It is performed to determine what type of chemotherapy is indicated

12 A 65-year-old postmenopausal client tells the nurse that she has recently experienced painless vaginal bleeding. What is the appropriate interpretation by the nurse?

1. Do not be concerned because postmenopausal bleeding is normal
2. Be concerned because painless uterine bleeding is a sign of uterine cancer
3. Be concerned because the client may develop anemia
4. Do not be concerned because the client does not complain of pain

PRACTICE TEST

13 A client is brought to the surgical unit after a suprapubic prostatectomy for prostate cancer. The client has a three-way Foley catheter. The nurse notices a very dark red output via the catheter. What is the priority nursing intervention?

1. Report the finding immediately to the registered nurse
2. Increase the irrigation flow rate
3. Check the latest hemoglobin and hematocrit count
4. Chart the observation in the medical record

14 The nurse who is screening female clients for cancer anticipates what finding as an early sign of ovarian cancer?

1. Painful urination is a common complaint
2. Pelvic pain radiating to thighs may occur
3. Usually no symptoms are seen
4. Low back pain is a common complaint

15 A client has stage 2 ovarian cancer documented as a diagnosis on the medical record. The nurse determines care based on which characteristic of this tumor at this stage?

1. Tumor growth is limited to the ovaries
2. Tumor growth involves one or both ovaries, with pelvic extension
3. Tumor growth involves the ovaries and peritoneum, with positive lymph nodes
4. Tumor growth involves distant metastasis

16 A client is scheduled for a radical mastectomy. When reinforcing the surgeon's explanation of the procedure, the nurse would include that the surgery involves removal of which tissue?

1. Breast tissue and lymph nodes under the arm
2. Entire breast, underlying chest muscles, and lymph nodes
3. Complete breast only
4. Tumor and surrounding tissues

17 A client returns to the medical unit after a transurethral resection of the prostate (TURP) for prostate cancer. The client wants the three-way Foley catheter to be removed because it is causing bladder spasms. What is the best response by the nurse?

1. "Spasms are painful but expected because of the wide diameter catheter and retention balloon in the bladder."
2. "This must be a complication because the catheter is supposed to evacuate clots that cause the spasms."
3. "The spasm is an unexpected finding because the procedure does not invade the urethra."
4. "Foley catheters tend to cause bladder spasms because of the silicone used in the catheter."

18 The client who underwent prostate cancer surgery is approaching the time of discharge from the hospital. What instruction should the nurse reinforce to this client as part of discharge teaching? Select all that apply.

1. "Maintain a high fluid intake after you go home."
2. "Call the doctor immediately if you notice blood in your urine."
3. "You may drive yourself home."
4. "Avoid strenuous activity for 4 to 8 weeks."
5. "Avoid heavy lifting for 2 to 4 weeks."

19 The nurse should include which interventions in caring for a client following a left mastectomy for breast cancer? Select all that apply.

1. Use warm, moist compresses on left arm for comfort
2. Allow lab draws from the left arm only in the antecubital area
3. Wait for the third postoperative day to begin any arm exercises
4. Keep left arm elevated above heart level
5. Take blood pressures on the right arm only

20 A client has a continuous bladder irrigation running after prostatectomy. During the shift, 600 mL of one bag of irrigant infused and 1500 mL of the next also infused. Upon draining the urine bag three times during the shift, the nurse measures volumes of 800 mL, 1050 mL, and 950 mL. The nurse records the client's true urine output as _____ mL. Provide a numerical answer.

Fill in your answer below:

_____ mL

21 A 6-year-old child is being admitted for surgical removal of a brain tumor. The nurse anticipates that what finding will be present during the preoperative period?

1. Bulging fontanels
2. Vomiting
3. Drainage from the ear or nose
4. Elevated blood glucose levels

22 An 18-month-old client is brought in for a well-child visit. The parent reports feeling a lump to the right of the "bellybutton" during bathing. What intervention should the nurse include during the initial examination? Select all that apply.

1. Measuring weight and height
2. Palpation of the area
3. Routine urine testing
4. Vital signs
5. Question the parents about abuse

23 A child diagnosed with Ewing's sarcoma is being treated with chemotherapy. The results of a complete blood count (CBC) indicate severe thrombocytopenia. What is the priority nursing intervention related to this finding? Select all that apply.

1. Encouraging foods high in iron
2. Limiting physical contact with the child
3. Removing fresh flowers from the child's room
4. Clearing the floor of the child's room to prevent falls and bruises
5. Minimizing needle sticks and intrusive procedures

24 When reinforcing teaching about safety precautions to the client with an internal radiation implant, the nurse would include which statement?

1. "No precautions are necessary for internal radiation implants."
2. "You pose a risk of radiation exposure to others."
3. "You must remain in solitary isolation for the entire hospitalization."
4. "Visitors should maintain a distance of 3 feet from you at all times."

25 A nurse is educating a client who will likely experience alopecia (hair loss) as a result of the current chemotherapy treatment. Which client statement indicates the need for the nurse to reinforce the instructions?

1. "I will wash my hair every day."
2. "I will pat my hair dry and avoid the use of hairdryers."
3. "My hair will begin to grow back after the chemotherapy is completed."
4. "I will choose a wig or hairpiece before the loss of hair occurs."

ANSWERS & RATIONALES

1 **Answer: 1** **Rationale:** There is great risk for altered bowel function (adynamic ileus) because of surgery and possible radiation to the abdominal area and use of chemotherapeutic agents. Wilms tumor is an intrarenal tumor, so neurological status is not a related manifestation. Bone pain is not associated with Wilms tumor. Activity level would not be a specific finding to make with this diagnosis. **Cognitive Level:** Analyzing **Client Need:** Physiological Adaptation **Integrated Process:** Nursing Process: Data Collection **Content Area:** Child Health **Strategy:** The core issue of the question is knowledge that Wilms tumor affects the kidney, and therefore principles related to care after abdominal surgery applies to this client. Use nursing knowledge and the process of elimination to make a selection.

2 **Answer: 2** **Rationale:** Diabetes insipidus presents with symptoms of increased urinary output and very dilute urine. Urinary specific gravity will measure the concentration of the urine. Blood glucose is unrelated to a pituitary gland problem. ACTH levels are not routinely monitored in any client. Serum amylase would be monitored with a pancreatic disorder such as pancreatitis. **Cognitive Level:** Analyzing **Client Need:** Physiological Adaptation **Integrated Process:** Nursing Process: Data Collection **Content Area:** Child Health **Strategy:** The core issue of the question is knowledge of diabetes insipidus as a complication of brain tumor and methods to monitor the status of this complication. Use nursing knowledge and the process of elimination to make a selection.

3 **Answer: 1** **Rationale:** Bone marrow suppression occurs with radiation therapy, which can lead to risk of infection when white blood cells are affected, bleeding when platelets are affected, and anemia when red blood cells are affected. Diarrhea would be more likely to occur than constipation as a side effect of cancer therapy. If appetite is affected, it decreases rather than increases. Hemorrhagic cystitis occurs after chemotherapy. **Cognitive Level:** Applying **Client Need:** Physiological Adaptation **Integrated Process:** Nursing

Process: Data Collection **Content Area:** Child Health **Strategy:** The core issue of the question is knowledge of bone marrow suppression in a client receiving radiation therapy. Use basic nursing knowledge and the process of elimination to make a selection.

4 **Answer: 1 Rationale:** Because infant kidneys do not concentrate urine as well as the kidneys of adults, urine volume and specific gravity may not indicate fluid volume as accurately as will daily weight. Weight loss can be directly tied to fluid loss. Hemoglobin and hematocrit could rise and fall because of hemodilution or hemoconcentration, depending on fluid status, but these levels would be indirect indicators with large changes in fluid status and therefore not specific fluid balance measurements. **Cognitive Level:** Analyzing **Client Need:** Physiological Adaptation **Integrated Process:** Nursing Process: Implementation **Content Area:** Child Health **Strategy:** The core issue of the question is the most reliable method of determining fluid balance in an infant who is not feeding well because of neuroblastoma. Use nursing knowledge of fluid balance measurement and the process of elimination to make a selection.

5 **Answer: 3 Rationale:** When a client is lying flat, the blood flow to the brain is greater, increasing the intracranial pressure. If the client sleeps in a semi-Fowler's position, less pressure will develop, which in turn should ease headaches. Excess liquids could aggravate headache. Discouraging bowel movements will reduce straining but is not a helpful measure from a gastrointestinal perspective. Blowing the nose could aggravate headache by further increasing intracranial pressure. **Cognitive Level:** Analyzing **Client Need:** Physiological Adaptation **Integrated Process:** Nursing Process: Implementation **Content Area:** Child Health **Strategy:** Recall principles of gravity to answer this question. When a client lies flat, blood can accumulate to a greater extent in the cranium, resulting in vasodilation, increased pressure, and worsening headache. Placing the client's head in an elevated position allows gravity to drain blood to the heart and thereby keeps intracranial pressure rises to a minimum.

6 **Answer: 3 Rationale:** While all identified problems are potential risks to clients with cancer depending on site, edema of the face and arms results from obstruction of blood flow, which is indicative of superior vena cava syndrome. Spinal cord compression would give rise to neurological symptoms. SIADH would result in general fluid overload. Sepsis would be noted by signs of infection. **Cognitive Level:** Analyzing **Client Need:** Physiological Adaptation **Integrated Process:** Nursing Process: Data Collection **Content Area:** Adult Health **Strategy:** The core issue of the question is knowledge of various oncological emergencies. Use nursing knowledge about which body systems are affected by each and then use the process of elimination to make a selection.

7 **Answer: 2 Rationale:** Radiation is palliative treatment for spinal cord compression to reduce the tumor size and relieve compression. Radiation therapy will not eradicate the tumor. Radiation therapy is not effective for all oncological emergencies. Radiation is not a new modality to treat the lung cancer. **Cognitive Level:** Applying **Client Need:** Physiological Adaptation **Integrated Process:** Teaching and Learning **Content Area:** Adult Health **Strategy:** The core issue of the question is the rationale for using radiation therapy in a client with spinal cord compression secondary to cancer. Recall that radiation therapy is often used as a supplement to shrink tumors to aid in making a selection.

8 **Answer: 2, 5 Rationale:** Inserting an IV catheter for IV access is an immediate intervention for the client with cardiac tamponade. The client requires immediate oxygen therapy to treat the respiratory symptoms and relieve the cyanosis. Vasopressor agents will be administered to manage hypotension. A pericardiocentesis is performed, not a thoracentesis. Radiation therapy is not indicated for cardiac tamponade. **Cognitive Level:** Analyzing **Client Need:** Physiological Adaptation **Integrated Process:** Nursing Process: Implementation **Content Area:** Adult Health **Strategy:** The stem of the question indicates that the client has an ineffective airway (shortness of breath and cyanosis). Look for the option that first addresses airway (oxygen) and circulation (IV access) as correct answers.

9 **Answer: 2 Rationale:** Prostate cancer has surpassed lung cancer in order of occurrence; colorectal cancer is the third-most common cancer. The other options are partially incorrect. **Cognitive Level:** Applying **Client Need:** Physiological Adaptation **Integrated Process:** Teaching and Learning **Content Area:** Adult Health **Strategy:** Specific knowledge of the risks associated with various cancers in men is needed to answer the question. Use nursing knowledge related to epidemiology of cancer and the process of elimination to make a selection.

10 **Answer: 3, 4 Rationale:** Cigarette smoking increases the risk of upper airway, esophageal and lung cancers. Drinking large quantities of alcohol daily increase the risk of several cancers. Epstein-Barr virus does not increase the risk of laryngeal cancer. Past exposure to asbestos increases risk of mesothelioma. Recreational use of marijuana is not associated with increased risk of laryngeal cancer. **Cognitive Level:** Analyzing **Client Need:** Physiological Adaptation **Integrated Process:** Nursing Process: Data Collection **Content Area:** Adult Health **Strategy:** The core issue of the question is risk factors for laryngeal cancer. Consider that alcohol and cigarette smoking are irritants to the upper airway to help choose correctly.

11 **Answer: 3 Rationale:** The lymph node biopsy is performed to determine any metastasis from the primary site of cancer, and a common metastatic site for breast cancer is regional lymph nodes. The biopsy of the tumor itself will determine the type(s) of cancer cells that are present. The lymph node biopsy is performed when indicated regardless of gender. The types of cancer cells determine what cancer chemotherapy drugs will be used. **Cognitive Level:** Analyzing **Client Need:** Physiological Adaptation **Integrated Process:** Teaching and Learning **Content Area:** Adult Health **Strategy:** The core issue of the question is knowledge that a biopsy procedure is used to diagnose a primary tumor or to evaluate lymph node involvement or metastasis. Use nursing knowledge and the process of elimination to make a selection.

12 **Answer: 2 Rationale:** The nurse should be concerned because painless bleeding not related to the menstrual cycle is often the only symptom of uterine cancer. Postmenopausal bleeding is not normal. Anemia is not an immediate concern. Pain is often considered to be a late sign related to the diagnosis of cancer. **Cognitive Level:** Analyzing **Client Need:** Physiological Adaptation **Integrated Process:** Nursing Process: Data Collection **Content Area:** Adult Health **Strategy:** The core issue of the question is the significance of painless vaginal bleeding in a client who is postmenopausal. Use nursing knowledge and the process of elimination to make a selection.

13 **Answer: 2 Rationale:** A very dark red output character following prostatectomy may indicate venous bleeding or inadequate dilution of the urine. The Foley catheter is at risk for

occlusion. Increasing the irrigation flow will prevent the formation of blood clots and occlusion of the catheter. If the urine does not clear after increasing the rate of bladder irrigation, then it would be appropriate to notify the registered nurse. Although reviewing the latest hemoglobin and hematocrit may be appropriate, it is not the most pressing intervention the nurse must do for this client. Charting is a routine care activity but further action to clear the urine is indicated immediately. **Cognitive Level:** Analyzing **Client Need:** Physiological Adaptation **Integrated Process:** Nursing Process: Implementation **Content Area:** Adult Health **Strategy:** The core issues of the question are interpreting the significance of dark red urine flow following prostatectomy and the ability to choose a corrective action. Interpret that the dark color is due to bleeding and then select an intervention that will reduce clot formation.

14 **Answer: 3 Rationale:** Ovarian cancer generally causes no warning signs or symptoms in the early stages, which is why screening is important. Painful urination, pelvic pain radiating to the thighs, and low back pain are not associated with this health problem. **Cognitive Level:** Applying **Client Need:** Physiological Adaptation **Integrated Process:** Nursing Process: Data Collection **Content Area:** Adult Health **Strategy:** The core issue of the question is knowledge of early signs of ovarian cancer. Use nursing knowledge and the process of elimination to make a selection.

15 **Answer: 2 Rationale:** In stage 2 ovarian cancer, tumor growth involves one or both ovaries with pelvic extension. In stage 1, tumor growth is limited to the ovaries. In stage 3, lymph nodes become positive along with tumor growth that involves ovaries and the peritoneum. In stage 4, there is distant metastasis. **Cognitive Level:** Applying **Client Need:** Physiological Adaptation **Integrated Process:** Nursing Process: Implementation **Content Area:** Adult Health **Strategy:** The core issue of the question is knowledge of the staging system for ovarian cancer. Use nursing knowledge and the process of elimination to make a selection.

16 **Answer: 2 Rationale:** Radical mastectomy includes removal of the entire breast, underlying chest muscles, and lymph nodes. Modified radical mastectomy involves removal of breast tissue and lymph nodes under the arm. A simple mastectomy involves removal of the complete breast only. A lumpectomy involves removal of the tumor and surrounding tissues. **Cognitive Level:** Applying **Client Need:** Physiological Adaptation **Integrated Process:** Teaching and Learning **Content Area:** Adult Health **Strategy:** The core issue of the question is the ability to discriminate among various types of mastectomy procedures. Use nursing knowledge and the process of elimination to make a selection.

17 **Answer: 1 Rationale:** Clients with three-way Foley catheters may report bladder spasms, which are caused by the presence of the wide diameter catheter and the pressure of the retention balloon on the catheter. Blood is irritating to the bladder wall but the catheter is often responsible for bladder spasm. The surgical procedure does involve the urethra. The silicone in the catheter is not responsible for bladder spasms. **Cognitive Level:** Analyzing **Client Need:** Physiological Adaptation **Integrated Process:** Communication and Documentation **Content Area:** Adult Health **Strategy:** The core issue of the question is knowledge of the significance of bladder spasms following prostate surgery. Recall that spasms are not expected findings to help narrow the plausible options. Then use nursing knowledge and the process of elimination to make a selection.

18 **Answer: 1, 4 Rationale:** Continued increased fluid intake will help the urine to remain dilute and reduce the risk of clot formation. The healing period after prostate surgery is 4 to 8 weeks, and the client should avoid strenuous activity during this period. Blood in the urine is fairly common after surgery but only needs to be reported if it increases in amount instead of decreasing. The client should not drive for 2 weeks, except for short rides. The client should avoid heavy lifting for 4 to 8 weeks after surgery while healing continues. **Cognitive Level:** Applying **Client Need:** Physiological Adaptation **Integrated Process:** Teaching and Learning **Content Area:** Adult Health **Strategy:** The core issue of the question is knowledge of postdischarge care to a client following prostate surgery. Use nursing knowledge and the process of elimination to make a selection.

19 **Answer: 4, 5 Rationale:** The arm should be elevated above heart level following mastectomy to reduce the risk of edema after lymph node removal on the affected side. Blood pressures and lab draws should be performed on the unaffected side. Warm, moist compresses could enhance edema formation. Lab draws should not be done on the affected side at any location. Gentle, simple range of motion exercises can be started immediately after surgery. **Cognitive Level:** Applying **Client Need:** Physiological Adaptation **Integrated Process:** Nursing Process: Implementation **Content Area:** Adult Health **Strategy:** The core issue of the question is knowledge that edema is a risk following mastectomy and of nursing measures that can reduce this risk. Use nursing knowledge and the process of elimination to make a selection.

20 **Answer: 700 Rationale:** The total infused is 600 + 1500 = 2100 mL. The total drained was 800 + 1050 + 950 = 2800 mL. Subtract 2100 from 2800 to obtain 700 mL, the true urine output for the shift. **Cognitive Level:** Applying **Client Need:** Physiological Adaptation **Integrated Process:** Nursing Process: Implementation **Content Area:** Adult Health **Strategy:** The principles for intake and output calculation are the same as for any other client. Tally first the intake, then the output, and subtract the difference to determine how much of the output is actually because of urinary drainage. Use knowledge of basic nursing procedures to calculate the answer.

21 **Answer: 2 Rationale:** Vomiting is a symptom of increased intracranial pressure. Bulging fontanels would not be present in a school-age child. Drainage from the ear or nose might indicate a basilar skull fracture, not a brain tumor. Some brain tumors display the symptom of diabetes insipidus, not diabetes mellitus, thus the symptom would be dilute urine rather than elevated blood glucose. **Cognitive Level:** Applying **Client Need:** Physiological Adaptation **Integrated Process:** Nursing Process: Data Collection **Content Area:** Child Health **Strategy:** Consider two items in answering the question: normal growth and development of the school-age child, and typical symptoms of a brain tumor.

22 **Answer: 1, 3, 4 Rationale:** Since Wilms' tumor is a cancer of the kidney, it is important to monitor growth and development. Since Wilms' tumor is a cancer of the kidney, it is important to monitor kidney function. Since Wilms' tumor is a cancer of the kidney, it is important to monitor blood pressure, which may be elevated due to increased renin production. This is the usual presentation of Wilms' tumor (nephroblastoma), and palpating the area may cause the tumor to spread. There is no evidence of abuse. **Cognitive Level:** Applying **Client Need:** Physiological Adaptation **Integrated Process:** Nursing Process: Implementation **Content Area:** Child

Health **Strategy:** Consider what conditions are common in the abdomen of toddlers. All normal examinations would be performed as well as examinations related to the possible condition. Knowledge of Wilms' tumor and the contraindication for palpating the abdomen will also help to identify the correct answer.

23 **Answer: 4, 5 Rationale:** Preventing falls and bruises would be appropriate for an individual with platelet deficiencies. Thrombocytopenia refers to a decrease in platelets. Minimizing needle sticks and other intrusive procedures would be appropriate for an individual with platelet deficiencies. Providing foods high in iron would be appropriate to restore red blood cells. Limiting contact with the child could affect his or her body image and self-esteem. Contact is acceptable as long as the individual is not infectious. Fresh flowers may contain molds and fungus that can lead to infection and would be a concern for a child with neutropenia. **Cognitive Level:** Analyzing **Client Need:** Physiological Adaptation **Integrated Process:** Nursing Process: Implementation **Content Area:** Child Health **Strategy:** The learner will need to understand which blood cell is deficient in thrombocytopenia.

24 **Answer: 2 Rationale:** The client is a risk to others as long as the radiation implant is present. While the client has the internal implant, certain radiation precautions must be taken to protect others. The client may not need isolation for the entire period of hospitalization; rather just while the implant is in place. The client should have a private room, and visitors should maintain a distance of 6 feet and limit visits to 10 to 30 minutes. **Cognitive Level:** Applying **Client Need:** Reduction of Risk Potential **Integrated Process:** Nursing Process: Implementation **Content Area:** Adult Health **Strategy:** This question requires knowledge of the means to protect the client and others.

25 **Answer: 1 Rationale:** Washing the hair daily will promote further hair loss. Hair washing should be limited to 2 to 3 times per week. Patting the hair dry and avoiding the use of hairdryers is a helpful measure for the client experiencing alopecia. Hair generally grows back after chemotherapy is completed, although the hair may have a slightly different texture or color. Choosing a wig or a hairpiece before starting chemotherapy is a useful strategy to help a client cope with hair loss during chemotherapy. **Cognitive Level:** Analyzing **Client Need:** Physiological Adaptation **Integrated Process:** Teaching and Learning **Content Area:** Adult Health **Strategy:** Use the process of elimination to determine the correct answer, in this case the incorrect option requiring further instruction.

Key Terms to Review

References

Ball, J., & Bindler, R. (2010). *Child health nursing: Partnering with children and families* (2nd ed.). Upper Saddle River, NJ: Pearson Education.

Berman, A., & Snyder, S. (2012). *Kozier & Erb's fundamentals of nursing: Concepts, process, and practice* (9th ed.). Upper Saddle River, NJ: Pearson Education, Inc.

Ignatavicius, D., & Workman, L. (2010). *Medical-surgical nursing: Critical thinking for collaborative care* (6th ed.). Philadelphia: Saunders.

Kee, J. (2010). *Laboratory and diagnostic tests with nursing implications* (8th ed.). Upper Saddle River, NJ: Pearson Education.

LeMone, P., Burke, K., & Bauldoff, G. (2011). *Medical surgical nursing: Critical thinking in patient care* (5th ed.). Upper Saddle River, NJ: Pearson Education.

Lewis, S., Dirksen, S. Heitkemper, M. & Bucher, L. (2011). *Medical surgical nursing: Assessment and management of clinical problems* (8th ed.). St. Louis, MO: Elsevier.

Smeltzer, S., Bare, B., Hinkle, J., & Cheever, K. (2010). *Textbook of medical-surgical nursing* (12th ed.). Philadelphia: Lippincott Williams & Wilkins.

Test Yourself

Are you ready for the NCLEX-PN® or course exams? Use the practice tests on the companion website to check.

Immunological Disorders

62

In this chapter

Cross Reference

Other chapters relevant to this content area are

Immunological and Anti-Infective Medications	Chapter 41
Common Laboratory Tests	Chapter 42
Common Diagnostic Tests and Procedures	Chapter 43
Respiratory Disorders	Chapter 51

I. OVERVIEW OF ANATOMY AND PHYSIOLOGY OF IMMUNE SYSTEM

A. Basic structures of immunologic system

1. Lymphoid system
   - **a.** Lymphoid system consists of lymphoid organs (lymph nodes, spleen, thymus, and tonsils), lymphoid tissues (lymphocytes and plasma cells in mucosa and connective tissues) and *bone marrow* (myeloid tissue involved in blood cell formation)
   - **b.** Lymphatic system consists of a communication network of vessels, lymph nodes, lymph node clusters, and circulating and resident lymphocytes that function as a primary component in immune system response
2. Central lymphoid organs
   - **a.** *Thymus gland*, which assists in T lymphocyte formation, is located in superior mediastinum behind sternum
   - **b.** Bone marrow sources can be found in iliac crest, sternum, and in bone cavities throughout body
3. Peripheral organs
   - **a.** Tonsils are a group of lymphoid tissue found in palatine area of oropharynx
   - **b.** A lymph node is a small, rounded mass of tissue from which lymph fluid drains; lymph nodes are found throughout body

c. Mucosa-associated lymph tissue (MALT) consists of a group of lymph tissue found in many organs of body that work together to promote an immune response; specific locators identify source of tissue; for example: bronchial-associated lymph tissue (BALT), gut-associated lymph tissue (GALT), skin-associated lymph tissue (SALT)
d. Spleen, located in left upper quadrant of abdomen, is composed of white and red pulp; white pulp is composed of B and T lymphocytes; red pulp is composed of erythrocytes

4. Mononuclear phagocyte system (MPS)
   a. Monocytes are largest component of the white blood cells (WBCs) and have one nucleus and very little cytoplasm; they are considered to be agranulocytes
   b. Macrophages are mature cells of MPS that migrate to different areas of body, becoming specialized cells to perform function of defense
   c. MPS protects body by participating in immune response; it secretes chemical components and factors (enzymes, complement proteins, and interleukins)

B. Basic functions of immunologic system

1. Thymus gland produces T lymphocytes, which are involved in **cell-mediated immunity**; secretes thymic hormones such as thymosin (stable from birth to age 25 and then gradually decreases as gland atrophies with age)
2. Bone marrow
   a. Is a diagnostic predictor for immunologic, hematologic, and oncologic disorders
   b. Provides for analysis of chemical markers that identify specific disease processes
   c. Is a primary lymphoid action that helps to initiate and maintain immune response; marrow gives rise to cellular components of blood and stores stem cells
   d. Gives rise to B lymphocytes and humorally mediated responses (**humoral immunity**) that involve production of **antibodies** (specific substances produced in response to specific antigens)
3. Spleen
   a. Site of RBC destruction, a storage site for blood, and a reservoir for B lymphocytes to develop into mature plasma cells
   b. Filters and removes foreign material, worn-out cells and forms of cellular debris

II. NORMAL IMMUNE RESPONSE

A. Defense

1. Communication network of protection that involves both nonspecific and specific forms of defense
2. Nonspecific defense relates to external reactions that include anatomic and chemical barriers such as skin and mucous membranes; nonspecific defenses are activated against any foreign substance that body encounters
3. Specific defense relates to internal physiological reactions that include both cell-mediated and humorally mediated antibodies; antibodies are unique substances that require activation
4. Immune response is activated in presence of an **antigen**, a protein substance that triggers antibody production

B. Homeostasis: body seeks to maintain a balanced response of circulating and resident lymphocytes to maintain adequate protection

C. Surveillance

1. Body's ability to use memory and recognition to maintain an immune response
2. Body remembers activation response even if person does not remember a specific insult

III. TYPES OF IMMUNITY

A. Acquired immunity

1. Long-term response that leads to development of antibodies that offer protection
   a. Individual develops antibodies in response to having a disease process or by a response to artificial antigens such as a vaccine or toxoid
   b. Response can be boosted and maintained via repeated injections
   c. Titer serum levels can be monitored to indicate status of immunity
2. *NCLEX®* Passive acquired immunity requires an antibody be introduced to individual, either by maternal transfer (placenta and/or colostrum) or immune serum antibody injection, to promote a specific antigen response

B. Natural immunity: is related to a species, race, or genetic trait; an individual is born with natural immunity

Table 62–1 Types of Immunoglobulins

Class	Location	Characteristic
IgA	Body secretions, tears, saliva Colostrum and breast milk	Lines mucous membranes; protects body surfaces
IgD	Plasma	Present on lymphocytes
IgE	Plasma, interstitial fluid Exocrine secretions	Allergic response, anaphylaxis; bound to mast cells
IgG	Plasma, interstitial fluid	Crosses placenta; complement fixation; secondary immune response
IgM	Plasma	Complement fixation; primary immune response; involved in ABO antigens

C. Humoral immunity

1. Involves recognition of antigens by B lymphocytes
2. B lymphocytes differentiate into plasma cells and memory cells
3. Memory cells lead to a more rapid response by remembering an original insult
4. Plasma cells secrete **immunoglobulins**, a group of glycoproteins, each of which has four polypeptide chains (two heavy and two light chains); the FAB fragment, which is different in each immunoglobulin, denotes specific antigen-binding sites
5. Immunoglobulins are identified as IgA, IgD, IgE, IgG, and IgM; see Table 62–1 for listing and characteristics of immunoglobulins

D. Cell-mediated immunity

1. T lymphocytes recognize a specific **major histocompatibility complex (MHC)**, a group of proteins that participate in autoimmune recognition and tissue rejection, and bind to them to elicit an immune response
2. Protein markers on surface of T-cell help define specific function receptor sites; these are called CD antigens or clusters of differentiation; CD markers serve as an important prognostic indicator of immune function and are used to diagnose and manage human immunodeficiency virus (HIV) and acquired immunodeficiency syndrome (AIDS)
3. *NCLEX®* Humoral immunity is considered a long-term process whereby T lymphocytes help protect body against bacterial, viral, and fungal infections
4. *NCLEX®* Cell-mediated immunity is also responsible for mediation of transplant rejection

E. Other immune system participants

1. Natural killer cell (null cell, NK cell) activity is present at birth, increases as individual reaches adulthood and decreases gradually in old age; null cells do not require prior sensitization and are not considered T or B lymphocytes
2. Cytokines (also referred to as lymphokines and monokines) are soluble protein mediators of immune response; interleukins, tumor necrosis factor, and interferon are examples of these chemical messengers, which are treatment options in boosting immune response

F. Complement system

1. Group of glycoproteins activated in sequential order; provide a link to humoral response
2. IgG and IgM are responsible for activating complement cascade; once activated, complement has been fixed or **complement fixation** has taken place
3. Complement assays diagnose immunodeficiencies and autoimmune diseases
4. There is a classic pathway and an alternate pathway whereby complement system can be activated

G. Biological response modifiers (BRMs)

1. Group of substances that can elicit, modify, and restore biological response between an individual and a tumor cell
2. Examples
   a. *NCLEX®* **Monoclonal antibodies** (produced by a specific group of identical cells), may be used to treat tumors because of their specific targeting effect
   b. *NCLEX®* **Colony-stimulating factors** (a group of proteins that stimulate growth of either RBCs or WBCs), prevent or help reduce a client's adverse response to disease; these types of BRMs are used in a variety of hematologic and immunologic diseases

IV. COMMON TESTS AND PROCEDURES OF IMMUNE SYSTEM

A. Skin testing

1. A small quantity of allergen is introduced into skin by scratching or intradermal (ID) injection
2. A scratch test is used to test many antigens at a single time; has lower sensitivity than injection, but many allergens can be tested at once and results can be obtained in 30 minutes
3. ID injection is more accurate but leads to higher incidence of systemic reactions
4. Patch test evaluates contact allergens by applying allergen directly to skin and covering with a dressing
5. NCLEX® Antihistamines that could impair immune response should be discontinued 72 hours prior to skin testing
6. NCLEX® Immediate positive reaction usually occurs within 10 to 30 minutes and consists of wheal formation and erythema formation greater than 3 millimeters of a positive control (histamine)
7. NCLEX® Minor itching at site can be relieved by cool compresses, topical steroids, and topical or oral antihistamines

B. Radioallergosorbent test (RAST)

1. Reveals elevated levels of IgE associated with **atopy** (allergic reactions stemming from hereditary disposition)
2. Allergen is usually planted on a surface such as a paper disk
3. Client blood is then applied to surface and incubated
4. Antibodies specific to an allergen bind to allergen, but others wash away, and level of IgE can be measured
5. More sensitive than skin testing but also more time consuming and expensive

C. Pulmonary function tests to diagnose asthma; see Chapter 51

D. Blood assays reveal increased circulating IgE in presence of allergic disease

E. Eosinophilia may be present with allergic disease

V. HYPERSENSITIVITY REACTIONS

A. ***Hypersensitivity*** is an abnormal exaggerated immune response to a specific substance

B. The Gell and Coombs Classification of Hypersensitivity Reactions categorizes a reaction according to type, class, and immunity (see Table 62–2)

C. Type I: anaphylactoid reactions

1. Involves an immediate response; however, potential responses can be cumulative; for example, initial or sensitizing dose may not elicit a strong response, but subsequent contacts, even if not long term in nature, may cause a stronger response
2. Involves activation of IgE bound to mast cells, with release of histamine
3. NCLEX® Clinical manifestations range from bronchospasm, wheezing, rhinorrhea, and urticaria to angioedema and finally anaphylaxis; there may be progression from local to systemic reactions; characteristic allergic "gape" and allergic "shiner" can be seen in individuals with atopy
4. Diagnostic and laboratory test findings: immunoglobulin titers are predictive of potential allergen response; skin and patch testing determine potential allergens
5. NCLEX® Therapeutic management
   a. **Antihistamine** medications such as diphenhydramine (Benadryl) block chemical release of mediators (histamines)
   b. Mast cell degradation inhibitors such as cromolyn sodium (Intal) also block chemical response
   c. Decongestants and corticosteroids help minimize immune response; however, in potential anaphylactic reactions, use of epinephrine is warranted; an Epipen may be prescribed for those at profound risk for hypersensitivity reactions and are available in adult and pediatric dosages
   d. Immediately withdraw offending allergen in presence of documented or suspected reaction
   e. Manage client according to ABC (airway, breathing, and circulation) protocol

Table 62–2 Gell and Coombs Classification

Type	Class	Immunity
I	Immediate hypersensitivity	Humoral
II	Cytotoxic reactions	Humoral
III	Immune complex related	Humoral
IV	Delayed hypersensitivity	Cell-mediated

D. Type II: cytotoxic and cytolytic reactions

1. Involves activation of complement and is considered a form of humoral immunity
    a. Involves production of autoantibodies that destroy own cells or tissues
    b. IgA and IgM are involved with this type of response

NCLEX®
2. Clinical manifestations: range from hemolytic reactions (such as transfusion, erythroblastosis fetalis, hemolytic anemia, and drug-induced hemolysis) to target cell destruction as in Goodpasture's syndrome (autoimmune disease affecting pulmonary and renal systems) and other autoimmune disease processes such as myasthenia gravis and Graves' disease
3. Diagnostic and laboratory test findings: Coombs blood test can define presence of hemolytic anemia and identify potential ABO incompatibility

NCLEX®
4. Therapeutic management
    a. Use proper identification during blood product administration to prevent exposure and sensitization
    b. Detect reactions early by awareness that certain blood types and potential drug interactions can cause antigen complex activation
    c. Remain with client during first 15 minutes of any blood product administration because clients are more likely to experience a reaction during this time
    d. Make sure to follow agency policy and procedure when monitoring all blood products

E. Type III: immune complex reactions

1. Involves formation of **antigen–antibody complexes** (a binding together of an antibody and an antigen)
    a. Leads to activation of serum factors, causing inflammation and leading to activation of complement cascade
    b. Rheumatoid arthritis (RA) and systemic lupus erythematosus (SLE) are examples of Type III reactions
    c. Deposits of antigen–antibody complexes in body tissues are not localized and can result in extensive tissue or organ destruction
2. Complement activation impacts vulnerable organs and leads to intravascular changes

NCLEX®
3. Clinical manifestations
    a. Arthrus reaction involves a localized inflammatory response with excess IgG causing edema and necrotic lesions
    b. Serum sickness involves a systemic response leading to deposit and activation of complement throughout body manifested as joint pain, pyrexia, and/or lymphadenopathy
    c. Reactions can be acute or chronic in nature
4. Diagnostic and laboratory test findings: complement assays indicate acute and/or chronic process; erythrocyte sedimentation rate (ESR) is elevated; proteinuria may be found on urinalysis

NCLEX®
5. Therapeutic management
    a. Analgesics, antihistamines and topical steroids may provide symptom relief; disease process is usually self-limiting because of use of human antitetanus serum and availability of antibiotics
    b. Monitor for localized inflammatory reactions that may develop at site of serum injections after 1 week; this can be followed by a more systemic response involving both regional as well as generalized lymphadenopathies
    c. If symptoms arise, monitor client for potential complications, because organ damage can occur and kidneys can be compromised

F. Type IV: delayed hypersensitivity reactions

1. A form of cell-mediated immunity involving T lymphocytes; considered a delayed response
2. Involve recognition and response of T lymphocytes to foreign substances

NCLEX®
3. Clinical manifestations
    a. Wide range of presentations from tuberculin response, poison ivy, and contact dermatitis to transplant or graft rejection; edema, ischemia, and eventual tissue destruction may ensue
    b. Pyrexia, pain, edema, and failure of transplanted organ characterize transplant rejection
4. Diagnostic and laboratory test findings: purified protein derivative (PPD) test result of induration more than 5 mm identifies type IV hypersensitivity to tubercle bacillus; abnormal test results indicating declining function of transplanted organ are used to diagnose transplant rejection

NCLEX®
5. Therapeutic management
    a. Monitor client for evidence of potential transplant rejection
    b. Medicate client with immunosuppressive drugs to prevent tissue rejection
    c. Identify potential irritants that can cause contact dermatitis and avoid exposure
    d. Remind client to avoid offending irritant if a past exposure has been documented
    e. Use topical and oral medications as indicated to alleviate many symptoms and increase client comfort

VI. ANAPHYLAXIS

A. Overview

1. Sudden, severe allergic reaction mediated by massive histamine release from cells
2. Common causes are drugs, foods (especially nuts and shellfish), latex exposure, insect bites, and stings
3. Can lead to shock state and death if not treated immediately
4. Onset of symptoms can be within minutes to an hour, with more rapid onset associated with severe episode

NCLEX®

B. Nursing data collection

1. Hives and urticaria (itching), angioedema (swelling of face, lips, neck, and/or tongue)
2. Dyspnea and wheezing, respiratory obstruction
3. Difficulty swallowing
4. Skin flushing
5. Syncope, hypotension, shock
6. Circulatory collapse and possible death

NCLEX®

C. Therapeutic management

1. Maintain patent airway
2. Subcutaneous epinephrine injection
3. Remove or discontinue causative agent
4. Administer oxygen
5. Place in modified Trendelenburg position for shock
6. Give IV fluids such as normal saline or lactated Ringer's to support circulation
7. Provide antihistamines or corticosteroids as ordered
8. Provide supportive care to stabilize client and emotional support

D. Reinforce client teaching

1. Avoid future contact with allergen
2. Wear Medic-Alert identification listing allergy
3. Tell all future caregivers about allergy and symptoms
4. Learn how to use epinephrine auto-injector pen

VII. AUTOIMMUNE DISORDERS

A. Overview

1. Concept of autoimmunity
   - **a.** An abnormal immune system response whereby body perceives "self" as a threat
   - **b.** Several mechanisms of action can affect autoimmune process, such as cell-mediated, antibody-mediated, and immune complex reactions
2. Genetic component of autoimmune response: **Human leukocyte antigens (HLAs)**, genetic markers found on chromosome 6, are involved with diagnosis of many autoimmune diseases and are also used for tissue typing
3. Cell-mediated autoimmunity
   - **a.** Associated with an abnormal T-cell response
   - **b.** Overabundance of T-cytotoxic (killer) cells or deficiency of T-suppressor (helper) cells may occur
4. Antibody-mediated autoimmunity
   - **a.** Autoantibodies develop that affect specific receptor sites, causing tissue and organ damage
   - **b.** Complement activation causes inflammatory reactions and leads to cell damage
   - **c.** Graves' disease and myasthenia gravis are examples of antibody-mediated autoimmunity
5. Immune complex disease
   - **a.** Associated with deposition of immune complexes at serum level
   - **b.** Complement activation causes inflammatory reactions and leads to further damage
6. Diagnostic testing for autoimmunity
   - **a.** Autoantibody assays, complement fixation, and complement assays diagnose disorder
   - **b.** Identification of HLA antigens provides indication of genetic inheritance
7. Treatment for autoimmunity
   - **a.** Immunosuppressive agents and corticosteroids suppress abnormal immune response
   - **b.** Symptom management can be achieved with anti-inflammatory agents to minimize pain from tissue damage caused by immune complex deposits
   - **c.** **Plasmapheresis** removes circulating immune complexes; in this treatment, plasma is removed from body, sent through a machine membrane that traps immune complexes, and returned to body

8. Progression of disease

a. Autoimmune diseases are characterized by acute exacerbation of a chronic condition

b. They affect a large percent of population and, depending on specific disease, can be seen across lifespan, affecting both children and adults

c. Splenectomy has been performed as part of therapeutic management of many autoimmune diseases; a client can live without a spleen but its removal is not guaranteed as a form of therapeutic management; current therapeutic regimens being explored are chemotherapy and use of biological response modifiers, instead of splenectomy

B. Systemic lupus erythematosus (SLE)

1. Overview

a. Multisystem autoimmune disease with a fluctuating, chronic course

b. Multiple organ involvement results in eventual major organ system failure

c. Two forms: systemic and discoid; systemic involves entire system response, and discoid involves characteristic skin rash without systemic disease

d. Specific HLA antigens indicate this type of disease (HLA-B8, HLA-DR2, HLA-DR3); C_2 and C_4 complement deficiencies are also seen

e. Estrogen inhibits suppressor T-cell function leading to abnormal immune response; primarily affects women of childbearing age (30–50 years most common)

NCLEX® **2.** Nursing data collection

a. Environmental triggers such as ultraviolet (UV) light, infection or other stressor, and/or drugs

b. Arthritis (joint pain) is most common symptom presentation

c. Butterfly rash (malar rash) across bridge of nose and cheeks or erythema of face is most common dermatologic expression; palmar erythema also possible

d. Weakness, fatigue, and general malaise; anorexia and weight loss

e. Pleural manifestations such as pleuritis and pleural effusions

f. Renal involvement may lead to renal failure

g. Central nervous system (CNS) involvement: photosensitivity, subtle behavioral changes, possible stroke or seizure activity

h. Hematologic involvement: altered immune responses with anemia (decreased RBC count), leukopenia (noted by infection and fever), thrombocytopenia (low platelet count), and even hemolytic anemia (positive Coombs test)

i. Pregnancy and use of oral contraceptives can affect estrogen level and may pose an increased risk for disease flare-ups

j. A positive ANA titer

k. During flare-ups, complement (C_3 and C_4) may be decreased and ESR and C reactive protein (CRP) may be elevated

l. A positive rheumatoid factor (+RF) may be seen with a titer of higher than 1:40

m. Urinalysis may reveal presence of casts and sediment; creatinine levels may rise as renal involvement progresses

NCLEX® **3.** Therapeutic management

a. Aimed at recognizing flare-ups and preventing further complications

b. Adjusted to disease activity; client receives individualized care

c. Conservative measures include rest and general supportive pharmacotherapy; aggressive measures include splenectomy and chemotherapy

d. Collaborate with dietitian to support metabolic needs and immune functions

e. Plan for rest periods to avoid fatigue and lessen client's stress levels

f. Avoid environmental triggers such as prolonged UV light exposure that may cause client to develop skin eruptions; consider possibility of photosensitivity when planning care

g. Monitor for symptoms and medicate as ordered to promote symptom relief

h. Institute with other health care providers a long-term treatment plan that offers anticipatory guidance and emotional support

i. Monitor for potential complications of treatment measures (glucocorticoids) or disease progression

j. Clients with SLE should try to have a planned pregnancy; alternative birth control methods such as diaphragm and condoms should be used because oral contraceptives can affect estrogen level

k. Nonsteroidal anti-inflammatory drugs (NSAIDs) and acetylsalicylic acid (aspirin, ASA) are used to control joint pain experienced by most clients

l. Hydroxychloroquine (Plaquenil) is used to treat dermatologic symptoms

m. Glucocorticoids suppress disease activity and provide symptom management; dosing can be adjusted in response to flare-ups; oral or IV route is preferred; tapered dose therapy (pulse dose) is usually initiated to achieve best results to arrive at lowest possible dosage and to prevent side effects
n. Immunosuppressive agents such as cyclophosphamide (Cytoxan) and azathiopine (Imuran) may modulate immune response; however, client will be at increased risk for **myelosuppression** (inhibition or destruction of bone marrow) with this regimen and must be monitored accordingly
o. Gamma globulin can be given IV to promote specific immune function
p. Plasmapheresis removes immune complexes to help relieve symptoms

4. Reinforce client teaching
a. Likelihood of flare-ups and chronic nature of disease
b. Self-monitoring of condition to identify potential health problems more quickly
c. Potential dynamic life changes such as pregnancy and childbearing may influence disease activity
d. Medication therapy

C. Rheumatoid arthritis (RA)

1. Overview
a. Systemic disorder involving symmetrical inflammation of synovial membranes and joints that leads to deformities and loss of joint function
b. Clinical course has periods of remission and exacerbation, but underlying disease process is chronic
c. Thought to be associated with deposits of antigen–antibody complexes and development of rheumatoid nodules
d. RA has a bimodal appearance: there is a juvenile form (JRA) as well as more common adult form

NCLEX®

2. Nursing data collection
a. Fatigue, general malaise, and anorexia and weight loss
b. Persistent joint pain lasting more than 3 months that is more evident on motion, but pain at rest can occur
c. Characteristic morning stiffness lasting more than 1 hour; note onset, duration, and joints involved
d. Tenderness, swelling, and restricted range of motion in affected joints
e. With disease progression and less stable joints, characteristic deformities such as swan neck deformity, Boutonniere deformity, subcutaneous nodules, and ulnar deviation or drift (see Figure 62–1) develop
f. Systemic signs range from fever to splenomegaly and reflect extra-articular findings
g. Possible joint effusions
h. +RF is a nonspecific finding because it may be found in healthy population as well
i. Elevated ESR, CRP, and serum complement
j. CBC with differential may reveal anemia as well as leukocytosis
k. X-rays reveal a narrowing of joint spaces and erosive changes at bone margins as disease progresses
l. Aspiration of synovial fluid reveals turbidity, elevated cell counts, and formation of a poor mucin clot

NCLEX®

3. Therapeutic management
a. Major treatment goal: help client maintain ability to function
b. Treatment measures are aimed at decreasing joint pain and swelling
c. Support client as diagnosis of disease is made and as disease progresses
d. Identify assistive devices needed in client's environment to aid function
e. Modify client's schedule as needed to incorporate rest periods
f. Include nonpharmacologic pain relief measures such as imagery and biofeedback
g. Use heat and cold applications to affected joints to provide relief; individualize these measures to provide maximum comfort
h. Include foods high in omega-3 fatty acids, since current research shows that these are beneficial to clients who have RA and other diseases such as heart disease; suggested food items include fish oils and salmon
i. ASA and NSAIDS decrease joint inflammation and control symptoms
j. Disease-modifying antirheumatic drugs (DMARDS) slow rate of disease progression; examples include antimalarial agent hydroxychloroquine (Plaquenil), sulfasalazine (Azulfidine), leflunomide (Arava), and minocycline (Minocin)

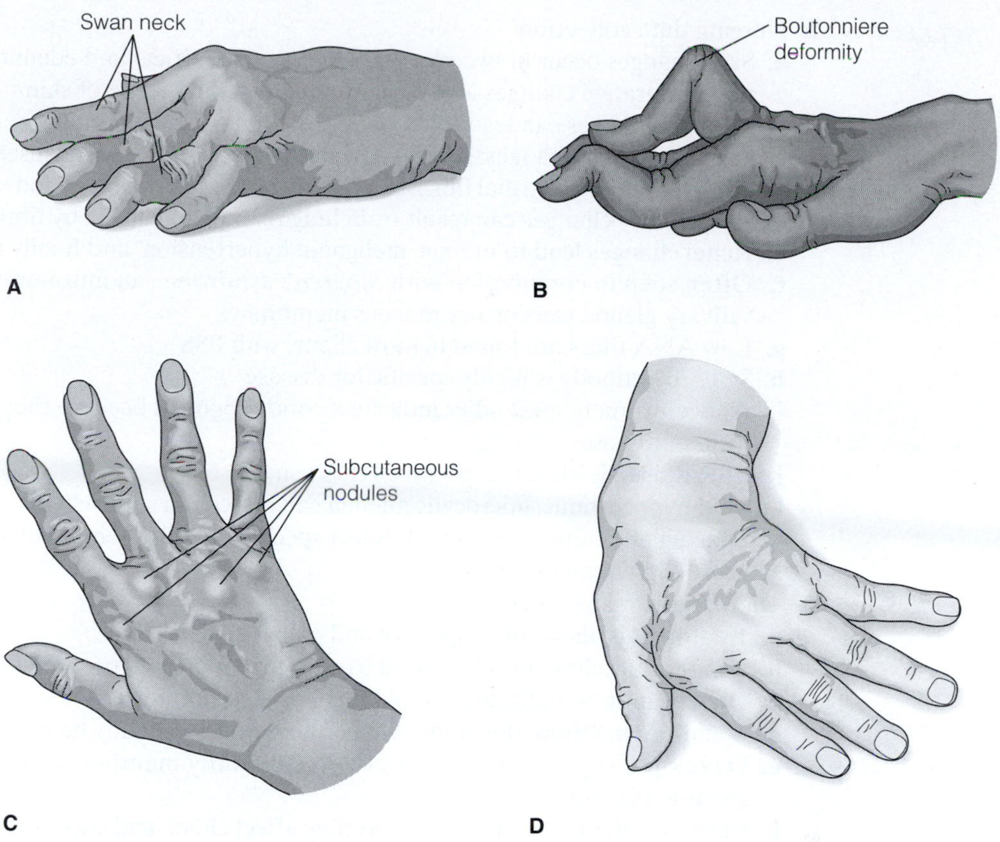

Figure 62–1

Characteristic hand deformities in rheumatoid arthritis. *A.* Swan neck deformity. *B.* Boutonniere deformity. *C.* Subcutaneous nodules. *D.* Ulnar deviation.

- **k.** Methotrexate (Rheumatrex), an immunosuppressive agent, is widely used in treatment of RA; onset of action is similar to other DMARDs; dosage is adjusted to get maximum response at lowest dose; relief effect continues during course of treatment; may be used in combination with etanercept (Enbrel), a tumor necrosis factor to optimize response
- **l.** Other immunosuppressive agents such as azathioprine (Imuran) and cyclophosphamide (Cytoxan) are also used in severe, disabling RA or RA refractory to other treatments

4. Reinforce client teaching
- **a.** Rheumatologist will coordinate care
- **b.** Occurrence of flare-ups and chronic nature of disease process
- **c.** Importance of adequate symptom management for optimal level of function
- **d.** Importance of client self-monitoring and adherence to treatment plan
- **e.** Potential dynamic life changes that might occur as a result of progression of deformity and loss of function

D. Scleroderma: progressive systemic sclerosis (PSS)

1. Overview
- **a.** A multisystem disease with fibrosis (hardening) of visceral organs and skin; leads to inability of involved organs to function with normal motility
- **b.** CREST syndrome is a specific, more limited form of disease

Memory Aid

C = Calcium deposits
R = Raynaud's syndrome
E = Esophageal dysmotility
S = Sclerodactyly (scleroderma digits)
T = Teleangiectasia (spider nevi)

- **c.** Systemic sclerosis morphea is a specific disease form that affects only skin
- **d.** Mild disease may go unrecognized unless it progresses or other medical issues bring it to forefront
- **e.** Has unknown etiology with underlying common factors: inflammation, vasoconstriction, and abnormal immune function and connective tissue
- **f.** Usually presents during third to fifth decade and affects females more than males

NCLEX®

2. Nursing data collection
   a. Skin changes occur in two phases; painless, symmetrical and edematous changes occur first, then indurative changes lead to hardening and thickening of skin
   b. GI tract changes can lead to dysphagia, esophageal reflux, malabsorption, and bowel obstruction
   c. Cardiovascular changes: Raynaud's phenomenon (vasospastic disease), secondary bacterial endocarditis, myocardial fibrosis, left ventricular (LV) dysfunction, and heart failure
   d. Respiratory changes can result from lung restriction caused by fibrosis
   e. Renal changes lead to uremia, malignant hypertension, and finally renal failure
   f. Often seen in conjunction with *Sjögren's syndrome*, an autoimmune disease affecting lacrimal and salivary glands, causing dry mucous membranes
   g. Low ANA titers are found in most clients with PSS
   h. SCL-70 antibody is highly specific for disease
   i. Anticentromere antibodies indicate a good prognosis because they are associated with a more limited form of disease
   j. ESR is usually elevated; positive RF is usually seen
   k. Mild hypochromic, microcytic anemia can be seen in some clients
   l. Imaging and other studies may detect specific organ system involvement, such as GI, pulmonary, heart, kidney, and skin

NCLEX®

3. Therapeutic management
   a. Treatment is aimed at supportive and palliative measures
   b. Long-term follow-up is indicated to monitor for disease progression
   c. Dialysis may be indicated if renal function deteriorates
   d. If end-organ failure develops, renal or lung transplant may be indicated
   e. Develop a support system for client and family members to help them cope with stressors of chronic disease
   f. Identify potential complications as they affect client, and coordinate health care team approach to manage developing risk situations
   g. Protect client's extremities from temperature changes that can exacerbate Raynaud's syndrome; encourage client to use gloves during activities that can affect temperature changes (such as washing dishes)
   h. Calcium channel blockers and peripheral alpha$_1$-adrenergic blocking agents treat symptoms of Raynaud's
   i. Anti-inflammatory agents treat joint pain
   j. H_2 receptor antagonists and proton pump inhibitors treat esophageal reflux
   k. Angiotensin converting enzyme (ACE) inhibitors treat hypertension and prevent development of resultant renal crisis
   l. Antibiotics treat potential secondary bowel infections caused by decreased motility
   m. O_2 therapy is used to support pulmonary function
4. Reinforce client teaching
   a. Importance of adequate symptom management
   b. Chronic nature of disease process
   c. Support client and family members with diagnosis and impact that no known cause exists; provide anticipatory guidance
   d. Client may be referred to a rheumatologist to coordinate care management

E. Polyarteritis nodosa

1. Overview
   a. Collagen disease that leads to inflammation of arteries and subsequent thickening with impaired circulation
   b. Etiology is unknown and often affects middle-aged men
   c. Cardiac and renal sequelae are most serious complications
2. Nursing data collection
   a. Low-grade fever
   b. Weakness and fatigue
   c. Weight loss, abdominal pain, and bloody diarrhea
   d. Elevated ESR
3. Therapeutic management
   a. Provide supportive care, emotional support, and anticipatory guidance
   b. Initiate support services depending on need
   c. Corticosteroids and analgesics manage inflammation and pain

4. Reinforce client teaching
   a. Importance of well-balanced diet
   b. Need for follow-up care
   c. Medication therapy
   d. Energy conservation measures

F. Pemphigus

1. Overview
   a. Skin disorder beginning with lesions on oral mucosa that spread to generalized body areas
   b. Rare with unknown etiology
   c. Occurs mostly in middle-aged and older adults
2. Nursing data collection
   a. Bullae that are fragile and appear flaccid; rupturing of bullae leads to partial thickness lesions that weep, form crusts, and may bleed
   b. Malaise
   c. Pain
   d. Impaired chewing and swallowing
   e. Nikolsky's sign: when skin is rubbed, epidermis separates from underlying skin
   f. Foul-smelling skin discharge
   g. Leukocytosis and eosinophilia
3. Therapeutic management
   a. Oral hygiene and measures to soothe oral lesions
   b. Baths with oatmeal or potassium permanganate for relief of skin symptoms
   NCLEX®
   c. Medication therapy including topical or systemic antibiotics (secondary infections), and corticosteroids or cytotoxic agents (as immunosuppressants)
   d. Provide general supportive care
4. Reinforce client teaching: need for follow-up care and medication therapy

VIII. PRIMARY IMMUNODEFICIENCY DISORDERS

A. Overview

1. Caused by a primary defect or deficiency involving B lymphocytes, T lymphocytes, complement or phagocytic cells that results in severe recurrent or chronic infection (see Table 62–3 for a listing of selected primary immunodeficiency diseases)
2. Involve specific genetic alterations in immune response seen in infants and young children

B. Nursing data collection

1. Overall immune response is abnormal, leading to opportunistic infections that cause tissue and organ damage to heart and lungs over time because immune response cannot be supported

NCLEX®

2. Signs and symptoms of infection and inflammation: fever, chills, cough (nonproductive or productive), difficulty swallowing or breathing, erythema, edema, or drainage
3. Diarrhea either due to overwhelming infection by offending agents or in response to antimicrobial therapy
4. CBC with differential, ESR, antibody titers, ANA, ANC (absolute neutrophil count), and culture and sensitivity of pertinent areas may all provide a baseline and identify potential source(s) of infection
5. Immunoglobulin and complement assay levels provide an overview of immune system function

C. Therapeutic management

NCLEX®

1. Therapy is most effective when aimed at infection prophylaxis, early treatment of infections, and replacement of immunologic factors
2. Bone marrow transplant (BMT) and/or thymus transplant may be indicated depending on the severity of presentation
3. Identify clients who present with repeated infections

Table 62–3 Selected Primary Immunodeficiency Disorders

Disorder	Immune Cell Problem
Bruton's X-linked disorder	B lymphocytes
DiGeorge's syndrome	T lymphocytes
Graft-versus-host disease	B, T lymphocytes
Wiskott-Aldrich syndrome	B, T lymphocytes

4. Support family members with impending diagnosis of chronic medical condition
5. Collaborate with health care team members to establish treatment goals
6. Refer clients of childbearing families for genetic counseling
7. Assist client and family in decisions regarding lifestyle changes to reduce infection
8. Collaborate with health care team members to support the client's ADLs and lifestyle changes during this hospitalization and after discharge
9. Antimicrobial therapy may be started to prevent infection or treat current infection

NCLEX® 10. Depending on nature of organism, antifungals may be warranted

NCLEX® 11. Gamma globulins may be needed to support and maintain deficient immunoglobulin levels

NCLEX® 12. Colony-stimulating factors may be used to boost immune response

D. Reinforce client teaching

1. Benefits of genetic counseling
2. Antimicrobial therapy, including treatment, response, and need for long-term compliance

NCLEX® 3. Importance of prevention and protection from high-risk environments that could lead to further infection

IX. HUMAN IMMUNODEFICIENCY VIRUS (HIV)

A. Overview

1. An RNA retrovirus attacks immune system at CD4 antigen, causing cell mutation that leads to eventual disease progression
2. HIV infection involves a process whereby course of disease progresses
3. Primary infection is followed by a clinical latency period when client may appear asymptomatic
4. Infecting virus is transmitted through contact with blood and/or body fluids

NCLEX® **B. Data collection**

1. Primary HIV can manifest with flu-like symptoms
2. Symptomatic HIV presentation leads to decreased CD4 cell counts and progressive weight loss
3. Systemic constitutional symptoms such as fatigue, fever, night sweats, and skin lesions may become apparent with further viral progression; once latency period ends, HIV infection progresses to acquired immunodeficiency syndrome (AIDS)
4. History of "high-risk" exposures (IV drug use, sexual contact, contaminated blood products, and perinatal transmission—in utero, during delivery and/or breastfeeding)
5. Enzyme-linked immunosorbent assay (ELISA) is screening test used to detect development of antibodies to HIV; results are described as positive or negative
6. Western blot is used to confirm HIV infection because it detects both HIV antibodies and individual viral components that cause reactive bands; results are described as positive or negative
7. Polymerase chain reaction (PCR) detects proviral DNA by identifying specific gene sequences of HIV proviral DNA molecule
8. Nonspecific markers of disease progression include blood counts, albumin levels, and ESR
9. Specific markers include CD4 and viral load (VL) levels to indicate client's current status and response to treatment
10. Other lab and diagnostic tests, such as skin biopsy, serum chemistries, and imaging studies, may be indicated depending on organ or system involvement and disease progression

NCLEX® **C. Therapeutic management**

1. Periodic clinical reevaluation of client: physical examination and laboratory testing
2. Vaccination against preventable illnesses
3. Assist client to manage life issues that will be affected by disease process
4. Maintain awareness of current CDC recommendations, which affect client during course of treatment
5. Establish an early working relationship with a dietitian to deal with client's altered taste perception, and prevent or delay **wasting syndrome** (unexplained weight loss of more than 10% ideal body weight [IBW] associated with a cycle of malnutrition and subsequent wasting) later in disease process
6. Monitor for potential fluid and electrolyte imbalances during course of disease or in response to therapy
7. Antiretroviral therapy is used to attack virus at a basic level
8. Nucleoside analogue reverse transcriptase inhibitors (NRTIs) are aimed at specific processes to prevent the replication process; see also Chapter 41
9. Protease inhibitors are aimed at specific processes to prevent viral replication
10. Nonnucleoside analogue reverse transcriptase inhibitors (NNRTIs) are used to treat emerging viral mutations

11. Fusion inhibitor (enfuvirtide [Fuzeon]) inhibits ability of HIV to bind to CD4 cells
12. Prophylactic medications are recommended based on CDC guidelines to provide primary and secondary prophylaxis of opportunistic infections
13. Oral progesterones (Megace, Winstrol) stimulate appetite, thereby assisting with treatment of weight loss and loss of taste perception

D. Reinforce client teaching

1. Course of disease and disease progression
2. *NCLEX®* Importance of compliance with long-term treatment regimen and adherence to complex drug regimen; noncompliance could lead to drug resistance over time
3. Need for follow-up physical examination and diagnostic tests to monitor response to treatment and disease progression
4. Risk of increased infection caused by disease-related immunodeficiency
5. Confidentiality and issues with releasing health information in business and personal relationships
6. Importance of nutritional support and maintaining IBW in early phase of treatment
7. *NCLEX®* Importance of balanced nutrition to support immune system function
8. *NCLEX®* Measures to prevent transmission, such as use of latex condoms and any measures that prohibit blood and body fluid contact with others

X. ACQUIRED IMMUNODEFICIENCY SYNDROME (AIDS)

A. Overview

1. AIDS is a progression of HIV
2. *NCLEX®* CD_4 count is under 200/mm^3 in presence of an AIDS-defining disease, such as opportunistic infections, malignancies, and/or neurologic diseases; pulmonary TB, recurrent pneumonia, and invasive cervical cancer are also considered AIDS-defining diseases (see Table 62–4 for a listing of AIDS infections and malignancies)
3. Since AIDS affects total individual, all body organs and tissues are affected
4. *NCLEX®* **Opportunistic infections** are nonpathogenic infections that become pathogenic because of a baseline immunosuppressive state; refer to Table 62–4 again for testing for opportunistic infections

B. Nursing data collection

1. Depending on organ system affected, there can be a wide range of presentations
2. Non-Hodgkin's lymphoma, Kaposi's sarcoma, and invasive cervical cancer are secondary malignancies often associated with AIDS
3. *NCLEX®* Wasting syndrome is seen in all clients who have AIDS; aggressive nutritional support at time of HIV-positive diagnosis may prevent or deter possible effects of wasting and malnutrition
4. *NCLEX®* Continued observation of client's skin and mucous membranes reveals early signs of infection
   a. Clients with HIV are at risk for oropharyngeal candida infections, leading to stomatitis
   b. Clients can experience pain when eating and benefit from soft, nonspicy and nonacidic foods, and beverages that are neither too warm nor too cold
5. *NCLEX®* Monitor nutritional status and hydration level, carefully noting baseline weight changes and alterations in taste perceptions
6. Monitor for potential fluid and electrolyte imbalances, especially hyponatremia
7. Obtain CD4, VL, and PCR levels as ordered
8. Obtain pertinent imaging studies as determined by client's presentation
9. Biopsies and other invasive procedures help diagnose secondary malignancies

Table 62–4 AIDS Infections and Malignancies

Classification	Type
Bacterial infection	Mycobacterium avium complex (MAC)
Fungal infection	Candidiasis, cryptococcus neoformans, histoplasmosis
Protozoan infection	Pneumocystic carinii, toxoplasmosis, cryptosporidium
Viral infection	Cytomegalovirus (CMV)
Dementia	HIV encephalopathy
Nutritional/malnutrition	Wasting syndrome
Cancer	Kaposi's sarcoma, associated lymphomas

C. Therapeutic management

1. Provide ongoing care coordinated with health care team to provide optimal assistance to client during this time of stress and crisis
2. Have dietitian analyze client's nutritional requirements and make recommendations to maintain IBW
3. NCLEX® Provide specific nutrition-related measures, such as small, frequent meals, fluids between meals, and dry crackers to help with mealtime nausea
4. NCLEX® Premedicate with antiemetics to reduce risk of nausea
5. Use sorbets as palate cleansers, zinc supplementation, and plastic instead of metal utensils to reduce altered taste perception
6. NCLEX® Dairy products, fish, and poultry are tolerated better than red meat when client experiences altered taste
7. Encourage counseling and guidance for both client and immediate support systems
8. Monitor total impact of disease on client and family support group
9. Allow for expression of feelings relative to life situation
10. Maintain client advocacy
11. Provide prescribed antibiotic therapy if client develops an infection
12. Chemotherapy and/or surgery may be needed if secondary malignancies occur
13. Pain management may be required as disease progresses
14. NCLEX® Antiemetics and appetite stimulants may relieve nausea and vomiting and loss of appetite
15. NCLEX® Antifungal medications may treat active or chronic opportunistic infections; topical medications may be used for palliative care

D. Reinforce client teaching

1. Measures to maintain nutrition
2. NCLEX® Energy conservation measures
3. Continue to emphasize how new symptoms will be managed and how client is active member of health care team
4. NCLEX® Discuss life issues with client and support system members as disease progresses and prognosis worsens

Check Your NCLEX–PN® Exam I.Q.

You are ready for testing on this content if you can

- Identify basic structures and functions of the immunological system.
- Describe the pathophysiology and etiology of common immunological disorders.
- Discuss expected data and diagnostic test findings for selected immunological disorders.
- Discuss therapeutic management of a client experiencing an immunological disorder.
- Discuss nursing management of a client experiencing an immunological disorder.
- Identify expected outcomes for the client experiencing an immunological disorder.

PRACTICE TEST

1 Which suggestion by the nurse would be most helpful to a human immunodeficiency virus (HIV) positive client who has altered taste perception?

1. "Drink plenty of salty broths and other fluids to stimulate taste buds."
2. "Try zinc supplementation to improve taste perception."
3. "Increase intake of meat to at least one serving per day."
4. "Avoid using plastic eating utensils."

2 Which suggestion would the nurse give to a client with human immunodeficiency virus (HIV) infection to best alleviate nausea?

1. "Drink liquids with meals."
2. "Eat high-fat foods."
3. "Eat small, frequent meals."
4. "Lie down after eating."

3 A client diagnosed with scleroderma reports painful fingers that change colors (pale to red) when washing dishes. Which suggestion by the nurse might help the client with this symptom?

1. Increase the water temperature.
2. Use gloves during dishwashing.
3. Start physical therapy to increase blood flow to the hands.
4. Take over-the-counter H_2 receptor antagonist medications.

4 A client is to start taking prednisone for treatment of rheumatoid arthritis (RA). Which client statement indicates that medication teaching was successful?

1. "I will take the medication on an empty stomach to maximize absorption."
2. "I will take the specific dose ordered at the same time every day."
3. "I will not have to limit my sodium intake."
4. "I will not have to adjust my insulin regimen."

5 In determining care to manage pain for a client with rheumatoid arthritis (RA), what intervention would the nurse use to increase the client's mobility?

1. Have the client work through pain by continuing exercise in order to establish endurance.
2. Have the client use pain medication only when pain is present.
3. Inform the client that both heat and cold applications may help to relieve pain.
4. Educate the client to flex muscle groups when pain is felt in an extremity.

6 The nurse looks for results of what laboratory measurement that provides a reliable indicator of lymphocyte status in a client with HIV infection?

1. B lymphocytes
2. T-helper cells (CD_4)
3. Natural killer cells (NK)
4. T-cytotoxic cells

7 The nurse who is providing care to a group of clients concludes that the client with which health problem exhibits a type 3 immune-complex–mediated hypersensitivity reaction?

1. Transfusion reaction
2. Goodpasture's syndrome
3. Transplant rejection
4. Systemic lupus erythematosus

8 A male client who has acquired immunodeficiency syndrome (AIDS) asks why oral progesterone (Megace) is being prescribed for treatment. What is the nurse's best response?

1. "Megace is used to treat the nausea associated with this infection."
2. "Megace is used as an appetite stimulant to boost nutritional support."
3. "Megace provides symptomatic relief of constipation."
4. "Megace is used as an antineoplastic agent for palliative treatment."

9 The nurse would monitor for which electrolyte imbalance as a common finding in a client with acquired immunodeficiency syndrome (AIDS)?

1. Hyponatremia
2. Hypernatremia
3. Hyperkalemia
4. Hypocalcemia

10 Which finding by the nurse warrants further investigation to determine if the client has rheumatoid arthritis (RA)?

1. Negative family history
2. Reports of prolonged morning stiffness lasting for 1 hour
3. Occasional use of NSAIDs for aches and pains
4. Reports of pain with movement

11 The nurse reinforces to a client that which factor might increase risk of developing an exacerbation of systemic lupus erythematosus (SLE)?

1. Pregnancy
2. Hypotension
3. Fever
4. Gastrointestinal (GI) upset

PRACTICE TEST

12. A client will undergo scratch tests for allergies. In explaining to the client about the planned tests, the nurse should include which statement?

1. "This test allows us to rule out one or two specific antigens."
2. "The scratch test is the most sensitive allergy test."
3. "Results can be obtained in 30 minutes."
4. "It involves drawing a small amount of blood for testing."

13. A client presents with dyspnea, pruritis, and localized swelling of the forearm after being stung by a bee. What is the priority nursing intervention?

1. Remove the stinger from the client's arm.
2. Keep the client warm with soft blankets.
3. Check the tongue for swelling and listen for stridor.
4. Place client in the Trendelenburg position.

14. The nurse determines that which nursing diagnosis is a priority early in the care of a client with scleroderma?

1. Impaired Skin Integrity
2. Disturbed Body Image
3. Activity Intolerance
4. Hopelessness

15. The nurse is caring for a pediatric client with acquired immunodeficiency syndrome (AIDS). Which activity by the nurse should be reported to the employee health department as an exposure for the nurse?

1. While flushing out the used bedpan, fluid splashes in the nurse's eyes.
2. The nurse does not wear a mask while in the client's room.
3. During the bath, the nurse removes gloves when giving a backrub on intact skin.
4. The nurse is stabbed with a sterile syringe to be used to draw up the client's medications.

16. A 5-year-old child is brought into the clinic after being stung by an insect. The child appears to be going into anaphylactic shock. Which nursing action is of highest priority?

1. Monitor urinary output to determine renal perfusion.
2. Apply cold, wet compresses to the site.
3. Position the child's head to maintain an open airway.
4. Assist registered nurse to determine intravenous access.

17. A 12-year-old boy is diagnosed with early human immunodeficiency virus (HIV) infection secondary to factor transfusions for hemophilia. The family is very concerned about its ability to manage his care, risk of infection to family members, and whether the child should remain in the home. Which action by the nurse will best promote family coping at this time?

1. Explain to the family that the infection cannot be spread by casual contact.
2. Demonstrate positive acceptance of the child with each contact.
3. Explain that prophylactic drugs will prevent the virus from spreading.
4. Show the family members how to wash their hands properly.

18. A client who must undergo skin testing for allergies takes an antihistamine to control symptoms. The nurse explains that the client must discontinue use of the antihistamine for _____ days before the skin testing to avoid false negative results. Provide a numerical answer.

Fill in your answer below:

_____ days

19. The nurse has explained allergy-proofing the home to the mother of a child with dust allergies. Which statement by the mother indicates a clear understanding of appropriate allergy-proofing? Select all that apply.

1. "I'm going to replace the cotton curtains on the window with blinds."
2. "The only toys allowed in his bedroom are his stuffed toys."
3. "I should store out-of-season clothes in the bedroom."
4. "The mattress and box springs both need to be enclosed in a thick plastic cover."
5. "I will try to clean and vacuum the bedroom frequently to limit dust collection."

PRACTICE TEST

20 A child is in the clinic for a scratch test. Because of the risk of anaphylaxis, the nurse has which medication available for emergency treatment?

1. Epinephrine (Adrenalin)
2. Prednisone (Deltasone)
3. Naloxone (Narcan)
4. Cromolyn sodium (Intal)

21 A child is admitted to the hospital with an allergic reaction. The physician orders a complete blood count (CBC) with differential. The nurse would expect to see an elevation in which value?

1. Red blood cells (RBCs)
2. Hemoglobin
3. Leukocytes
4. Eosinophils

22 A sexually active teenager with flu-like symptoms is given an ELISA test that returns negative. After the physician informs her that the ELISA test will be repeated in several weeks, the client asks the nurse why. What is the best explanation by the nurse?

1. The first test may be inaccurate.
2. The antibodies do not always show up initially.
3. The test is sensitive and can give false positives.
4. It is standard practice.

23 In addition to a viral load of 25,000, which would indicate that the medications being taken by a client with acquired immunodeficiency virus (AIDS) are working?

1. Rare occurrence of symptoms
2. Negative ELISA test
3. CD_4 cell count of 490
4. WBC of 1700 mm

24 In examining a client with a suspected latex allergy, which question should the nurse ask?

1. "Are your hands usually moist or dry?"
2. "What drug allergies do you have?"
3. "Are you allergic to bananas or kiwi fruit?"
4. "What types of surgeries have you had?"

25 The white blood cell (WBC) count of a client with systemic lupus erythematosus (SLE) shows a shift to the left. Which nursing diagnosis reflects the highest priority for this client?

1. Ineffective Health Maintenance
2. Impaired Skin Integrity
3. Ineffective Individual Coping
4. Ineffective Protection

ANSWERS & RATIONALES

1 **Answer: 2 Rationale:** Zinc deficiency is associated with taste changes; therefore, supplementation may benefit a client experiencing altered taste perception. Drinking salty broth and fluids will not help with taste changes but may help restore electrolyte balance in clients experiencing diarrhea. Dairy products, fish, and poultry are better food choices than meat when taste is altered. Substituting plastic utensils for metal ones is suggested to decrease possibility of taste perception of "metal." **Cognitive Level:** Applying **Client Need:** Physiological Adaptation **Integrated Process:** Nursing Process: Implementation **Content Area:** Adult Health **Strategy:** The core issue of the question is knowledge of measures to minimize taste alterations in a client with HIV infection. Use nursing knowledge and the process of elimination to make a selection.

2 **Answer: 3 Rationale:** Small, frequent meals help lessen nausea because they require less work of digestion and do not overwhelm the client with food odors from a lengthy meal. Drinking liquids can give a sensation of fullness. High-fat foods are more difficult to digest and may distend the stomach. Lying down after eating can encourage reflux. **Cognitive Level:** Applying **Client Need:** Physiological Adaptation **Integrated Process:** Nursing Process: Implementation **Content Area:** Adult Health **Strategy:** The core issue of the question is the ability to reinforce teaching to minimize nausea in a client with HIV. Use nursing knowledge and the process of elimination to make a selection.

3 **Answer: 2 Rationale:** Clients who have scleroderma usually have Raynaud's phenomenon, which can be triggered by temperature changes, such as with prolonged contact with water. Use of gloves when washing dishes may prevent temperature changes yet still allow the client to participate in ADLs. Hotter water may increase the risk of scalding and so is not suggested. Physical therapy is indicated for treatment of esophageal problems associated with scleroderma. H_2 receptor blockers help to treat esophageal problems associated with scleroderma. **Cognitive Level:** Analyzing **Client Need:** Physiological Adaptation **Integrated Process:** Nursing Process: Implementation **Content Area:** Adult Health **Strategy:** The core issue of the question is recognition of Raynaud's syndrome as part of scleroderma and the ability to select an appropriate intervention for that problem. Use nursing knowledge and the process of elimination to make a selection.

4 **Answer: 2 Rationale:** Steroid therapy is usually done as part of a tapered-dose treatment plan. It is important to take this

ANSWERS & RATIONALES

medication at the same time each day and to become aware of tapered-dose effect. Steroids are usually taken with foods to minimize GI upset. Steroids cause fluid retention, and therefore sodium intake may be restricted. Steroids increase blood glucose, so insulin therapy dosages may have to be adjusted. **Cognitive Level:** Applying **Client Need:** Pharmacological and Parenteral Therapies **Integrated Process:** Teaching and Learning **Content Area:** Adult Health **Strategy:** The core issue of the question is knowledge of client teaching related to steroid therapy. Use nursing knowledge and the process of elimination to make a selection.

5 **Answer: 3 Rationale:** Heat and cold applications can provide analgesia and relieve muscle spasms. The individual client will have to determine whether heat, cold, or alternation of both is most effective. Exercising in the presence of pain may only further exacerbate pain. Pain medication should be taken on a regular schedule if the client has chronic pain so that the pain threshold can be raised and pain relief maintained at a constant level. Flexing of muscle groups is not related to effective pain control. **Cognitive Level:** Applying **Client Need:** Physiological Adaptation **Integrated Process:** Nursing Process: Implementation **Content Area:** Adult Health **Strategy:** The core issue of the question is knowledge of measures that relieve the symptoms of RA. Use nursing knowledge and the process of elimination to make a selection.

6 **Answer: 2 Rationale:** CD4 cells are indicative of a client's HIV status. As the disease progresses, the T-helper cells decrease in number and lose their ability to function effectively. B lymphocytes indicate the status of humoral immunity and are not directly associated with HIV infection. NK cells are not directly related to HIV infection. T-cytotoxic cells are not directly related to HIV infection. **Cognitive Level:** Applying **Client Need:** Physiological Adaptation **Integrated Process:** Nursing Process: Data Collection **Content Area:** Adult Health **Strategy:** The core issue of the question is knowledge of which laboratory measure will provide information about the status of the immune system of a client with HIV. Use nursing knowledge and the process of elimination to make a selection.

7 **Answer: 4 Rationale:** Transfusion and Goodpasture's are examples of type 2 cytotoxic hypersensitivity reactions and are involved with the activation of complement. Lupus is an example of a type 3 hypersensitivity reaction, which involves IgG and IgM with the activation of complement. Transplant rejection is a type 4 hypersensitivity reaction. **Cognitive Level:** Applying **Client Need:** Physiological Adaptation **Integrated Process:** Nursing Process: Evaluation **Content Area:** Adult Health **Strategy:** The core issue of the question is the ability to associate various types of hypersensitivity reactions with their etiologies. Use nursing knowledge and the process of elimination to make a selection.

8 **Answer: 2 Rationale:** While Megace is used as a palliative treatment for clients with advanced cancers, this is not the rationale for its use with AIDS. In clients with AIDS, it provides appetite enhancement. Side effects of Megace can include nausea and constipation. **Cognitive Level:** Applying **Client Need:** Pharmacological and Parenteral Therapies **Integrated Process:** Communication and Documentation **Content Area:** Adult Health **Strategy:** The core issue of the question is the purpose of oral progesterone in a client with AIDS. Use nursing knowledge about anorexia as a symptom of AIDS and the process of elimination to make a selection.

9 **Answer: 1 Rationale:** Hyponatremia is a common finding in clients with AIDS. The incidence of opportunistic infections may contribute to this decrease in sodium. Hypernatremia, hyperkalemia, and hypocalcemia are not usually seen in clients who have AIDS. **Cognitive Level:** Analyzing **Client Need:** Physiological Adaptation **Integrated Process:** Nursing Process: Data Collection **Content Area:** Adult Health **Strategy:** The core issue of the question is identification of an electrolyte disturbance that is more common to clients with AIDS. Use nursing knowledge and the process of elimination to make a selection.

10 **Answer: 2 Rationale:** Prolonged morning stiffness is associated with RA. A negative family history does not increase the risk of RA. Occasional use of NSAIDs is not by itself a direct link to the development of RA. Reports of pain with movement are more likely to be associated with degenerative joint disease (osteoarthritis). **Cognitive Level:** Analyzing **Client Need:** Physiological Adaptation **Integrated Process:** Nursing Process: Data Collection **Content Area:** Adult Health **Strategy:** The core issue of the question is the ability to identify symptoms that are possibly associated with RA. Use nursing knowledge and the process of elimination to make a selection.

11 **Answer: 1 Rationale:** Pregnancy can be associated with an exacerbation because of increased estrogen levels. Hypotension, fever, and GI upset do not exacerbate SLE. **Cognitive Level:** Applying **Client Need:** Physiological Adaptation **Integrated Process:** Teaching and Learning **Content Area:** Adult Health **Strategy:** The core issue of the question is risk factors and triggers for SLE. Use nursing knowledge and the process of elimination to make a selection.

12 **Answer: 3 Rationale:** A scratch test tests many allergens at once. It is of low sensitivity, but many allergens can be tested at once, and the results can be obtained in 30 minutes. Because it is a skin scratch test, no blood needs to be drawn. **Cognitive Level:** Applying **Client Need:** Physiological Adaptation **Integrated Process:** Nursing Process: Implementation **Content Area:** Adult Health **Strategy:** The core issue of the question is identification of appropriate concepts to reinforce to a client about scratch tests for allergies. Use nursing knowledge and the process of elimination to make a selection.

13 **Answer: 3 Rationale:** The priority intervention is to maintain a patent airway in a potential anaphylactic reaction. Therefore, the nurse should monitor for swelling of the tongue and stridor, which could indicate impending respiratory obstruction. The other interventions are supportive measures that can be used during an allergic response. **Cognitive Level:** Analyzing **Client Need:** Physiological Adaptation **Integrated Process:** Nursing Process: Implementation **Content Area:** Adult Health **Strategy:** Remember in emergency or near-emergency situations to use the ABCs (airway, breathing, and circulation) to plan priorities of care. Use the process of elimination to make a selection.

14 **Answer: 1 Rationale:** Skin manifestations are a common finding in clients with scleroderma and therefore require preventative and supportive nursing care as the priority. As the disease progresses, dermatologic effects may lead to disturbances in body image. With disease progression, there may be an impact on respiratory and musculoskeletal function, leading to activity intolerance. Hopelessness can develop with worsening symptoms later in the disease process.

Cognitive Level: Applying **Client Need:** Physiological Adaptation **Integrated Process:** Nursing Process: Planning **Content Area:** Adult Health **Strategy:** The core issue of the question is knowledge that scleroderma is primarily a skin disorder in many cases and thus the primary nursing diagnosis needs to address loss of skin as a protective barrier. Use nursing knowledge and the process of elimination to make a selection.

15 **Answer: 1 Rationale:** Body fluid-contaminated liquids may contain the human immunodeficiency virus (HIV) and can be absorbed through the eye mucosa. The other activities do not expose the nurse to blood and/or body fluids of the client and therefore poses no risk of contracting HIV. **Cognitive Level:** Applying **Client Need:** Safety and Infection Control **Integrated Process:** Nursing Process: Implementation **Content Area:** Child Health **Strategy:** The core issue of the question is the ability to identify a breach in standard precautions. Use nursing knowledge about transmission of HIV via body fluids and the process of elimination to make a selection.

16 **Answer: 3 Rationale:** Maintaining an open airway is always the highest priority. With anaphylactic shock, the airway may constrict, mucous membranes swell, and air trapping occurs. The second priority would be IV access, followed by urine output, and finally site care. **Cognitive Level:** Analyzing **Client Need:** Physiological Adaptation **Integrated Process:** Nursing Process: Implementation **Content Area:** Child Health **Strategy:** Use the ABCs (airway, breathing, and circulation) to answer questions related to anaphylaxis. Airway is always the first priority in life-threatening situations.

17 **Answer: 2 Rationale:** The family has stated multiple concerns, and demonstrating acceptance of the child is the best way to foster acceptance of the child and development of further coping skills. Prevention of transmission, handwashing, and drug therapy are all important, but none of these individually targets the global concerns of the family. **Cognitive Level:** Analyzing **Client Need:** Psychosocial Integrity **Integrated Process:** Nursing Process: Implementation **Content Area:** Child Health **Strategy:** The core issue of the question is the best nursing action to model acceptance of the child and enhances coping skills of the family. Select the option that is the most global in nature because the family has multiple concerns, and use the process of elimination to make a selection.

18 **Answer: 3 Rationale:** The client needs to discontinue use of antihistamines for 72 hours (3 days) prior to allergy testing to avoid false negative readings. **Cognitive Level:** Applying **Client Need:** Reduction of Risk Potential **Integrated Process:** Nursing Process: Implementation **Content Area:** Adult Health **Strategy:** The core issue of the question is knowledge of the time frame that antihistamine drugs need to be withheld so as not to interfere with the results of allergy testing. Use specific nursing knowledge to determine the correct answer.

19 **Answer: 4, 5 Rationale:** Both the mattress and the box spring should be enclosed in special plastic covers to eliminate a source of dust. Frequent vacuuming helps to keep dust levels reduced. Cotton curtains would be preferred over blinds because cotton curtains can be washed frequently. Stuffed animals retain dust and should be removed from the bedroom. Cloth items hold dust. Only essential items should be stored in the child's bedroom, and those should be in drawers or closets. **Cognitive Level:** Analyzing **Client Need:** Health Promotion and Maintenance **Integrated Process:** Teaching and Learning **Content Area:** Child Health **Strategy:** Consider what objects would hold dust and eliminate them from the environment.

20 **Answer: 1 Rationale:** Prick tests determine allergens. Should the child have an allergy, epinephrine might be needed to counteract anaphylaxis. Corticosteroids such as prednisone are helpful in minimizing allergic response, but would not be effective in the management of anaphylaxis. In addition, pretreatment with prednisone would make test results invalid. Naloxone reverses the effects of opioid analgesics. Cromolyn sodium is useful in managing asthma. **Cognitive Level:** Applying **Client Need:** Pharmacological and Parenteral Therapies **Integrated Process:** Nursing Process: Planning **Content Area:** Child Health **Strategy:** Eliminate naloxone immediately after associating it with narcotic overdose. The other three drugs are related to allergies, but the correct answer is one that will work quickly and have a systemic response rather than a local one.

21 **Answer: 4 Rationale:** Eosinophils are the type of white blood cell that is associated with allergic reactions. RBCs carry oxygen to tissues. Hemoglobin is present in red blood cells. Leukocytes fight infection. **Cognitive Level:** Applying **Client Need:** Reduction of Risk Potential **Integrated Process:** Nursing Process: Data Collection **Content Area:** Child Health **Strategy:** The RBCs and the hemoglobin level are not related to the immune system, so these can be eliminated immediately. Choose between the remaining two to select the type of WBC that is associated with allergies.

22 **Answer: 2 Rationale:** The ELISA test may be negative upon initial testing and positive at the time of seroconversion, which takes 6 to 12 weeks after infection. The ELISA test may be negative upon initial testing. This time period when the antibodies are negative is called the seroconversion window and virally infected individuals may have negative antibody tests. A test that is negative would not be repeated because of the risk of false positive results. The ELISA test is repeated based on need. **Cognitive Level:** Analyzing **Client Need:** Reduction of Risk Potential **Integrated Process:** Nursing Process: Implementation **Content Area:** Adult Health **Strategy:** This question requires knowledge about the ELISA tests. Note the wording of the question indicates the correct answer is also a true statement.

23 **Answer: 3 Rationale:** A CD4 cell count between 200 and 500 is in the "suppressed immune state" but certainly above the 200 mark that is indicative of severe depression of the immune system. A client with AIDS will have exacerbations and remissions with opportunistic infections, therefore symptoms may vary. With a diagnosis of AIDS, an ELISA test would remain positive for antibodies. A WBC of 1700 shows neutropenia which does not indicate improvement. **Cognitive Level:** Analyzing **Client Need:** Physiological Adaptation **Integrated Process:** Nursing Process: Data Collection **Content Area:** Adult Health **Strategy:** Use the process of elimination to answer this question.

24 **Answer: 3 Rationale:** Clients with a history of allergies to fruit such as bananas or kiwi tend to have latex allergies. The degree of moistness of the skin will not determine a latex allergy. Although drug allergies should be asked, this information does not help in determining a latex allergy. Surgical history is part of general data collection, but the focus for a latex allergy would be any problems after the surgery similar to the one being exhibited now. **Cognitive Level:** Applying **Client Need:** Reduction of Risk Potential **Integrated Process:** Nursing Process: Data Collection **Content Area:** Adult Health **Strategy:** Use the process of elimination to determine the correct answer.

25 **Answer: 4 Rationale:** All identified nursing diagnoses are of concern for a client with SLE. However, the results of the laboratory test demonstrate an increased risk for infection that is due to the disease process and/or possible treatment measures such as steroids and immunosuppressive agents. A shift to the left in a WBC differential indicates an increased number of immature cells, suggesting infection. **Cognitive Level:** Analyzing **Client Need:** Physiological Adaptation **Integrated Process:** Nursing Process: Planning **Content Area:** Adult Health **Strategy:** The core issue of the question is the ability to analyze WBC differential count data to determine risk of infection. Use nursing knowledge and the process of elimination to make a selection.

Key Terms to Review

antibody p. 1186
antigen p. 1186
antigen–antibody complexes p. 1189
antihistamine p. 1188
atopy p. 1188
cell-mediated immunity p. 1186
colony-stimulating factors p. 1187
complement fixation p. 1187
human leukocyte antigens (HLA) p. 1190
humoral immunity p. 1186
hypersensitivity p. 1188
immunoglobulins p. 1187
major histocompatibility complex (MHC) p. 1187
monoclonal antibodies p. 1187
myelosuppression p. 1192
opportunistic infection p. 1197
plasmapheresis p. 1190
wasting syndrome p. 1196

ANSWERS & RATIONALES

References

Ball, J., Bindler, R., & Cowen, K. (2010). *Child health nursing: Partnering with children and families* (2nd ed.). Upper Saddle River, NJ: Pearson Education.

Berman, A., & Snyder, S. (2012). *Kozier & Erb's fundamentals of nursing: Concepts, process, and practice* (9th ed.). Upper Saddle River, NJ: Pearson Education, Inc.

Ignatavicius, D., & Workman, L. (2010). *Medical-surgical nursing: Critical thinking for collaborative care* (6th ed.). Philadelphia: Saunders.

Kee, J. (2010). *Laboratory and diagnostic tests with nursing implications* (8th ed.). Upper Saddle River, NJ: Pearson Education.

LeMone, P., Burke, K., & Bauldoff, G. (2011). *Medical surgical nursing: Critical thinking in patient care* (5th ed.). Upper Saddle River, NJ: Pearson Education.

Lewis, S., Dirksen, S. Heitkemper, M. & Bucher, L. (2011). *Medical surgical nursing: Assessment and management of clinical problems* (8th ed.). St. Louis, MO: Elsevier.

Smeltzer, S., Bare, B., Hinkle, J., & Cheever, K. (2010). *Textbook of medical-surgical nursing* (12th ed.). Philadelphia: Lippincott Williams & Wilkins.

Test Yourself

Are you ready for the NCLEX-PN® or course exams? Use the practice tests on the companion website to check.

Communicable or Infectious Diseases

63

In this chapter

Cross Reference

Other chapters relevant to this content area are

I. CHICKENPOX (VARICELLA)

A. Overview

1. Organism: varicella zoster virus
2. *NCLEX®* Mode of transmission: airborne and direct contact with contaminated objects (fomites)
3. Source: respiratory secretions and vesicular skin lesions (scabs not infectious)
4. Incubation period: often 13 to 17 days
5. Communicability: from 1 day before lesions erupt to crusting of all lesions

NCLEX® **B. Nursing data collection**

1. Fever
2. Malaise and anorexia for first 24 hours
3. Rash beginning on scalp and trunk and spreading to extremities; may involve oral mucous membranes or genital and rectal areas
4. Rash rapidly progresses to papules and vesicles that break and form crusts

NCLEX® **C. Therapeutic management**

1. Prevention: **immunization** with varicella vaccine (see Chapter 14)
2. Maintain airborne and contact precautions in hospital
3. Isolate child in home until vesicles have crusted over and dried

4. Skin care: bathe and change clothes and bed linens daily; use oatmeal soaps, soaks, or lotions, and calamine lotion or topical antihistamines to prevent scratching of pruritic lesions; encourage child not to scratch; use mittens on young child
5. Administer acetaminophen for fever; avoid aspirin to prevent Reye's syndrome

D. **Complications**: encephalitis, varicella pneumonia, secondary bacterial infections (abscesses, cellulitis, sepsis)

II. DIPHTHERIA

A. Overview

1. Organism: *Corynebacterium diphtheriae*
2. NCLEX® Mode of transmission: direct contact with infected client, carrier, or contaminated objects
3. Source: nasal and respiratory secretions, skin, other lesions
4. Incubation period: 2 to 5 days, possibly slightly longer
5. Communicability: variable until virulent bacilli absent in three negative cultures; usually 2 to 4 weeks

NCLEX® **B. Nursing data collection**

1. Low-grade fever, sore throat, malaise, anorexia
2. Foul mucopurulent nasal discharge (as in common cold); may have epistaxis
3. Smooth, adherent, white or gray membrane on tonsils and pharynx
4. Hoarseness, cough, apprehension, dyspnea with retractions, possible airway obstruction and cyanosis

NCLEX® **C. Therapeutic management**

1. Prevention: diphtheria **vaccine** (see Chapter 14)
2. Maintain strict isolation and bedrest in hospital
3. Administer antibiotic therapy and antitoxin as prescribed (do skin or conjunctival test first to rule out sensitivity to horse serum)
4. Provide suction and oxygen as needed to maintain airway
5. Be prepared for emergency tracheostomy if airway obstruction occurs

D. **Complications**: myocarditis, neuritis, toxemia and septic shock; death possible

III. ERYTHEMA INFECTIOSUM (FIFTH DISEASE)

A. Overview

1. Organism: human parvovirus B19 (HPV)
2. NCLEX® Mode of transmission: unknown; possibly respiratory secretions and blood
3. Source: infected individuals; direct contact with contaminated secretions
4. Incubation period: 4 to 14 days, but possibly up to 20 days
5. Communicability: uncertain, but usually before onset of symptoms

B. Nursing data collection

1. NCLEX® Rash that occurs in three stages
   a. Erythema of face (mainly cheeks, giving a "slapped cheeks" appearance); disappears in 1 to 4 days
   b. Symmetrical, maculopapular "lacy" red rash on trunks and limbs (proximal to distal); lasts 1 week or longer; rash may itch
   c. Rash subsides but can reappear with skin irritation or trauma, as with sunlight, heat, cold, or friction
2. Possible joint swelling of hands, wrists, and knees bilaterally that resolves within 1 or 2 weeks
3. With aplastic crisis, rash is often absent but child has prodromal signs of fever, lethargy, myalgia, and GI symptoms including nausea, vomiting, and abdominal pain

NCLEX® **C. Therapeutic management**

1. Treat respiratory secretions that can transmit infection with care; place hospitalized child on respiratory precautions
2. Provide antipyretics, analgesics, anti-inflammatory drugs as ordered
3. Provide supportive care; transfuse blood to clients with aplastic anemia as ordered

D. Complications

1. Self-limited or chronic arthritis
2. Aplastic crisis in clients with hemolytic disease or immune deficiency
3. Rarely myocarditis or encephalitis
4. Possible low risk of fetal death if mother is infected during pregnancy

IV. INFECTIOUS MONONUCLEOSIS

A. Overview

1. Organism: Epstein-Barr virus (EBV)
2. NCLEX® Mode of transmission: direct contact with infected blood or secretions
3. Source: oral secretions

4. Incubation period: 4 to 6 weeks
5. Communicability: unknown; viral shedding occurs before onset of symptoms until 6 months or longer after recovery

NCLEX® **B. Nursing data collection**

1. Fever, sore throat, headache
2. Malaise and fatigue
3. Nausea and abdominal pain
4. Lymphadenopathy and hepatosplenomegaly

NCLEX® **C. Therapeutic management**

1. Supportive care including rest
2. Assess for abdominal pain, left upper quadrant or left shoulder pain (signs of ruptured spleen)

D. Complication: ruptured spleen

V. MUMPS (PAROTITIS)

A. Overview

1. Organism: paramyxovirus
2. Mode of transmission: direct contact or via droplets from infected client (NCLEX®)
3. Source: saliva
4. Incubation period: 2 to 3 weeks
5. Communicability: greatest immediately before and after swelling begins

NCLEX® **B. Nursing data collection**

1. First 24 hours: fever, headache, malaise, and anorexia
2. Jaw pain and/or ear pain aggravated by chewing
3. Unilateral or bilateral swelling of parotid glands with pain and tenderness

NCLEX® **C. Therapeutic management**

1. Prevention: mumps vaccine (see Chapter 14)
2. Maintain respiratory precautions during hospitalization
3. Maintain bedrest
4. Encourage fluids and soft, bland foods that require little chewing
5. Comfort measures: analgesics, antipyretics, warm or cool compresses to neck, warmth and local support (snug-fitting underwear) for orchitis

D. Complications

1. Sensorineural deafness, meningitis, or encephalitis
2. Myocarditis or arthritis
3. Hepatitis
4. Epididymo-orchitis and possible sterility

VI. PERTUSSIS (WHOOPING COUGH)

A. Overview

1. Organism: *Bordetella pertussis*
2. Mode of transmission: direct contact or droplet; contact with freshly contaminated articles (NCLEX®)
3. Source: respiratory tract secretions
4. Incubation period: range of 5 to 21 days, usually 10 days
5. Communicability: greatest during catarrhal stage before paroxysms of coughing begin and may extend to fourth week after paroxysms begin

NCLEX® **B. Nursing data collection**

1. Catarrhal stage: sneezing, runny nose, lacrimation, low-grade fever, and cough that gradually worsens over 1 to 2 weeks
2. Paroxysmal stage: coughing occurs frequently at night, with a series of short rapid coughs followed by inspiration with a high-pitched "whooping" sound; cheeks become flushed or cyanotic; attack often followed by vomiting; lasts 4 to 6 weeks, then convalescent stage begins

NCLEX® **C. Therapeutic management**

1. Prevention: pertussis vaccine (see Chapter 14)
2. Maintain bedrest during fever
3. Encourage small amounts of fluids frequently, especially after vomiting
4. Provide humidity via humidifier or tent; also humidify any oxygen given
5. Place on respiratory precautions
6. Administer antimicrobial such as erythromycin and also give pertussis immune globulin

D. Complications

1. Atelectasis and pneumonia
2. Otitis media
3. Dehydration
4. Hemorrhage (subarachnoid, epistaxis, subconjunctival)
5. Hernia and/or prolapsed rectum
6. Seizures

VII. POLIOMYELITIS

A. Overview

1. Organism: three types of enterovirus—abortive or unapparent, nonparalytic, and paralytic—each associated with varying severity of paralysis
2. *NCLEX®* Mode of transmission: direct contact or transmission by fecal–oral or oropharyngeal routes
3. Source: feces and oropharyngeal secretions
4. Incubation period: usually 1 to 2 weeks, with range of 5 to 35 days
5. Communicability: uncertain; virus present in throat and feces shortly after infection and lasts about 1 week in throat and 4 to 6 weeks in feces

NCLEX® **B. Nursing data collection**

1. Abortive or unapparent type: fever, uneasiness, sore throat, headache, anorexia, vomiting, abdominal pain (lasts a few hours to a few days)
2. Nonparalytic type: similar to abortive poliomyelitis, but more severe, with pain and stiffness in back, neck, and legs
3. Paralytic type: initially similar to nonparalytic type, followed by recovery and then CNS paralysis

NCLEX® **C. Therapeutic management**

1. Prevention: inactivated polio vaccine (IPV); see Chapter 14
2. Maintain complete bedrest
3. Monitor for impending respiratory paralysis: shallow rapid respirations, dyspnea, difficulty talking, ineffective cough
4. Mechanical ventilation for respiratory paralysis, manual resuscitation bag at bedside, tracheostomy insertion tray at bedside
5. Care of immobilized client: range of motion exercises, proper positioning for body alignment, use footboard; prevent skin breakdown
6. Physical therapy for muscles after acute stage; moist heat to muscles

D. Complications

1. Kidney stones from bone demineralization during immobility
2. Hypertension
3. Respiratory arrest
4. Permanent paralysis

VIII. ROCKY MOUNTAIN SPOTTED FEVER

A. Overview

1. Organism: *Rickettsia rickettsii*
2. *NCLEX®* Mode of transmission: bite of infected tick
3. Source: tick; mammal source such as dog or rodent
4. Incubation period: 2 days to 2 weeks
5. Communicability: contact with tick or infected animal

NCLEX® **B. Nursing data collection**

1. Chills, fever, malaise, myalgia
2. Anorexia, nausea
3. Headache, mental confusion
4. Maculopapular or petechial rash often on extremities (ankles or wrists) that may spread over trunk, and face; characteristic locations are palms and soles

NCLEX® **C. Therapeutic management**

1. Prevention: avoid contact with ticks or infected animals; use insect repellents and protective clothing; immunize children at risk; inspect skin for ticks (do not crush on skin if found; remove with tweezers)
2. Provide supportive care
3. Administer antimicrobials (doxycycline or tetracycline) as prescribed

D. Complication: can be fatal

IX. ROSEOLA (EXANTHEM SUBITUM)

A. Overview

1. Organism: human herpesvirus type 6

NCLEX®

2. Mode of transmission: unknown
3. Source: unknown
4. Incubation period: 5 to 15 days
5. Communicability: unknown, but usually occurs between 6 months and 3 years of age

NCLEX® **B. Nursing data collection**

1. Fever above 102°F for 3 to 4 days in child who appears well
2. Sudden drop in fever accompanied by appearance of rose pink macules or maculopapules
3. Nonpruritic rash begins on trunk, then spreads to neck, face, and extremities; lasts 1 to 2 days
4. May be associated with lymphadenopathy in cervical area and behind ears, cough, runny nose, and injected pharynx

NCLEX® **C. Therapeutic management**

1. Supportive care
2. Antipyretics to control fever
3. Seizure precautions for child at risk of recurrent febrile seizures

D. Complications: recurrent febrile seizures; meningitis and rarely encephalitis; hepatitis

X. RUBEOLA (MEASLES)

A. Overview

1. Organism: rubeola virus

NCLEX®

2. Mode of transmission: direct contact with droplets
3. Source: respiratory secretions, blood, and urine
4. Incubation period: 10 to 20 days
5. Communicability: 4 days before to 5 days after appearance of rash but mainly communicable during prodromal (catarrhal) stage

NCLEX® **B. Nursing data collection**

1. Prodromal stage
   - **a.** Fever, malaise, coryza (upper respiratory or cold symptoms), cough, and conjunctivitis
   - **b.** Appearance of Koplik spots (small, irregular red spots with tiny, bluish white center) on oral mucosa that last from 2 days before rash appears until about 2 days after
2. Rash
   - **a.** Onset is 3 to 4 days after prodromal stage; erythematous maculopapular rash appears on face and spreads downward
   - **b.** Original or earlier sites have more extreme and confluent rash (blending together), while later (lower) sites have less severe, discrete rash (rash that affects separate or unconnected skin areas)
   - **c.** Rash becomes brownish 3 to 4 days later, and moist desquamation occurs over areas extensively involved

NCLEX® **C. Therapeutic management**

1. Prevention: measles vaccine (see Chapter 14)
2. Isolate child at home until fifth day of rash; institute respiratory precautions for hospitalized child
3. Maintain bedrest with quiet activity during prodromal stage
4. Provide supportive care: antipyretics for fever (no aspirin, to prevent Reye's syndrome), seizure precautions if prone to febrile seizures, cool-mist vaporizer, and adequate fluid intake; tepid baths for skin care and warm saline to remove eye crusts; dim lights if photophobia present

D. Complications: otitis media, pneumonia, bronchiolitis, obstructive laryngitis or laryngotracheitis encephalitis

XI. RUBELLA (GERMAN MEASLES)

A. Overview

1. Organism: rubella virus

NCLEX®

2. Mode of transmission: direct contact or contact with objects freshly contaminated with nasopharyngeal secretions, urine, or feces
3. Source: respiratory secretions, virus also present in urine, stool, and blood
4. Incubation period: 2 to 3 weeks
5. Communicability: 7 days before to about 5 days after appearance of rash

NCLEX® **B. Nursing data collection**

1. Low-grade fever, headache, malaise, anorexia, mild conjunctivitis, coryza, sore throat, and lymphadenopathy lasting 1 to 5 days in adolescents and adults until 1 day after appearance of rash; often children do not have this prodromal stage
2. Discrete pinkish red maculopapular rash on face and spreading downward to neck, arms, trunk, and legs within 1 day
3. Rash disappears in the order it began and is usually gone by third day

NCLEX® **C. Therapeutic management**

1. Prevention: rubella vaccine (see Chapter 14)
2. Antipyretics for fever and analgesics for comfort
3. Comfort measures since illness is benign in children
4. Isolate child from pregnant women

D. Complications: rare, but include arthritis, encephalitis, or purpura; greatest risk is teratogenic effect on fetus (fetal deformity)

XII. SCARLET FEVER

A. Overview

1. Organism: group A beta-hemolytic streptococci
2. NCLEX® Mode of transmission: direct contact, droplets, indirect contact with contaminated objects, ingestion of contaminated milk or food
3. Source: respiratory secretions
4. Incubation period: 2 to 4 days with range of 1 to 7 days
5. Communicability: approximately 10 days during incubation period and clinical illness; also during first 2 weeks to perhaps months in carrier phase

NCLEX® **B. Nursing data collection**

1. Sudden-onset high fever, headache, chills, malaise, vomiting, abdominal pain
2. Pharyngeal or tonsillar redness, swelling and enlargement, tonsils are covered with gray white exudate
3. Tongue is coated, and papillae become red and swollen (white strawberry tongue) followed by sloughing of white after 4 to 5 days
4. Red, pinhead-sized rash appears 12 hours after prodromal stage, which rapidly progresses to generalized rashes in axillae, groin, and neck; desquamation begins at end of first week and may last for 3 weeks or longer
5. Rash is characteristically absent on face, which has flushed appearance with circumoral pallor

NCLEX® **C. Therapeutic management**

1. Respiratory precautions for 24 hours after beginning antibiotic therapy (penicillin or erythromycin if allergic to penicillin)
2. Provide supportive care, including bedrest with quiet environment, and comfort measures for sore throat (gargles, lozenges, cool mist, throat sprays)
3. Increase fluid intake while avoiding irritating citrus juices; provide soft diet (no rough foods) during acute phase

D. Complications: otitis media, sinusitis, or peritonsillar abscess, glomerulonephritis, carditis, polyarthritis (uncommon)

XIII. SMALLPOX

A. Overview

1. Organism: variola major or variola minor virus
2. NCLEX® Mode of transmission: droplets and contact with contaminated objects
3. Source: frozen stores in U.S. Centers for Disease Control and Prevention (CDC); other sources unknown but is a potential agent for biological warfare

B. Nursing data collection

1. Fever and malaise, headache
2. Vomiting
3. Vesicular, pustular rash initially on face and extremities that develops 2 days after onset of symptoms

C. Therapeutic management

1. Prevention: immunization with vaccinia (a related poxvirus) for laboratory workers or those at risk for exposure (such as military)
2. Supportive care

D. Complication: death

PRACTICE TEST

XIV. ANTHRAX

A. Overview

1. Organism: *Bacillus anthracis* (spore-forming bacteria usually seen in cattle, sheep, and goats)
2. *NCLEX®* Mode of transmission: direct skin contact, inhalation, digestive system
3. Source: infected animal hides that come in contact with broken skin, airborne spores, or spores impregnated in carrier agent such as a powder (biological warfare); ingestion of contaminated undercooked meat
4. Incubation period: 2 to 60 days
5. Highly contagious

B. Nursing data collection *NCLEX®*

1. Cutaneous form: reddish brown lesion ulcerates and forms scab surrounded by brawny edema; toxin destroys surrounding tissue
2. GI: internal hemorrhage, abdominal pain, headache, fever, nausea and vomiting, severe diarrhea
3. Pulmonary form: fever, muscle aches and fatigue, rapidly developing respiratory distress and shock

C. Therapeutic management

1. *NCLEX®* Ciprofloxacin or erythromycin for all types
2. Clean contaminated surfaces with 5% hypochlorite solution
3. Provide vaccine to those at occupational high risk (animal workers)
4. Mechanical ventilation as needed and supportive treatment for shock
5. Institute contact and respiratory precautions because of resistant spores

D. Complications: respiratory form more likely to be fatal

Check Your NCLEX-PN® Exam I.Q.

You are ready for testing on this content if you can

- Identify basic structures and functions of the immunological system.
- Describe the pathophysiology and etiology of common infectious diseases.
- Discuss data and diagnostic test findings for selected infectious diseases.
- Discuss therapeutic and nursing management of a client experiencing an infectious disease.
- Identify expected outcomes for the client experiencing an infectious disease.

PRACTICE TEST

1 After reinforcing client teaching with the mother of a 4-year-old child exposed to chickenpox, the nurse determines the mother needs additional information when the mother makes which statement?

1. "I should monitor my child for Reye's syndrome, which is a complication of chickenpox."
2. "My child should not visit my pregnant sister at this time."
3. "During the prodomal period, my child will have pox all over his body."
4. "Chickenpox is a viral infection that can be spread to other children."

2 A mother overhears two nurses discussing the incubation period for a measles outbreak. The mother asks the nurses why it is important to know this. The nurse's reply would include which statement about the incubation period?

1. It describes a period when the child might be contagious
2. It determines the severity of the infection
3. It varies depending on the age of the child
4. It is a time when medications can prevent the development of symptoms

3 A 2-year-old child is in the hospital for a fractured femur breaks out with chickenpox. Which nursing intervention will best prevent secondary skin infections?

1. Caladryl lotion to lesions
2. Acetylsalicylic acid
3. Immune globulin for the first 3 days
4. Nubaine every 4 hours as needed for pain

PRACTICE TEST

4 A child is being treated at home for chickenpox. The home-health nurse is visiting and notes an elevated temperature. To prevent a common complication of fever the nurse recommends which of the following?

1. Tepid sponge baths
2. Aspirin as needed for fever control
3. Keep child well covered to prevent chilling
4. Antibiotics as ordered

5 A child has been diagnosed with mumps and the mother has been given instructions on caring for the child during the acute period. Which statement by the mother indicates a need for additional education?

1. "I can give my child acetaminophen for fever."
2. "My child will be more comfortable if I give him fluids and soft foods."
3. "I should watch my child for headache and vomiting."
4. "I will give my child antibiotics every 4 hours around the clock."

6 A child is exposed to a playmate who contracted chickenpox. Two days later, the child is admitted to the hospital for another problem, and the parents inform the nurse of the exposure on admission. How long after the exposure should the child be watched for signs of upper respiratory illness?

1. 5 to 10 days
2. 10 to 21 days
3. 21 to 25 days
4. One month

7 The nurse sees a child with mumps. The mother says that the child is not eating well and asks for suggestions. The nurse most appropriately makes which suggestion?

1. Provide warm, chopped foods
2. Provide cool table foods with spices
3. Provide cool fluids with minimum of acids
4. Provide a regular diet tray at frequent intervals

8 The mother of a 3-year-old child with measles calls the nurse at the clinic and asks what she can do to help decrease the redness and itching. The nurse responds that which action is likely to be helpful?

1. Overdress the child and cause him to perspire
2. Keep the child out of drafts
3. Bathe the child in an oatmeal (Aveeno) bath
4. Provide adequate oral fluids

9 The clinic nurse is working with a toddler diagnosed with roseola (exanthem subitum) after being seen for fever and a skin rash. The nurse makes which response to the mother who asks how to reduce the risk of infecting other children at home?

1. "There is no way to reduce risk because the route of transmission is unknown."
2. "Do not allow the child to cough or sneeze in the presence of others whenever possible."
3. "Use disposable dishes and eating utensils, and dispose of them in a separate trash bag."
4. "Select one bathroom to be used exclusively by the toddler until the rash clears."

10 A college student was hospitalized following onset of a severe case of pertussis. In preparing for discharge, the nurse would correct which client statement that indicates a misconception about postdischarge care?

1. "Irritants that I breathe, such as smoke or dust, could make me have coughing spells again."
2. "I will try to avoid being around people for a full week after going home so I don't spread this to others."
3. "I will be very careful to wash my hands often."
4. "It will still be important to try to drink a lot of fluids when I go home."

11 A child who may have scarlet fever is being evaluated in the urgent care clinic. The nurse recognizes that the client's presentation is not consistent with scarlet fever after noting which of the following during data collection?

1. Rash in the axillae and groin
2. Pharyngeal redness and swelling
3. Koplik's spots in the oral mucosa
4. Red strawberry tongue

12 The nurse is examining a child in the outpatient clinic who has fever, lethargy, nausea, and vomiting. The nurse notes that the child's cheeks have the appearance of being windburned or slapped. The nurse suspects which of the following childhood communicable diseases?

1. Chickenpox
2. Measles
3. Diphtheria
4. Fifth disease

13 The spouse of a postal worker who contracted cutaneous anthrax asks the nurse whether this communicable disease can be treated. Which response by the nurse is most appropriate?

1. "No, there is only supportive care available for the itching associated with skin lesions."
2. "No, although we will be ready to provide aggressive respiratory support measures if needed."
3. "Yes, the infection can be treated with antiviral agents and immune globulin."
4. "Yes, the infection can be treated with antibiotics such as ciprofloxacin or erythromycin."

14 The nurse is providing health teaching to a group of high school students about infectious mononucleosis. When discussing timing of disease transmission, the nurse explains that the incubation period for this infection is up to ____ weeks. Provide a numeric answer.

Fill in your answer below:

_____ weeks

15 A child with chickenpox has an elevated temperature. To prevent a common complication of an elevated temperature, the nurse recommends which of the following? Select all that apply.

1. Antipyretics such as acetaminophen and ibuprofen
2. Aspirin as needed for fever control
3. Keeping child well covered to prevent chilling
4. Giving antibiotics as ordered
5. Providing tepid baths

16 The child has been diagnosed with mumps. The nurse has reinforced with the mother instructions on caring for the child during the acute period. Which statement by the mother indicates a need for additional information?

1. "I can give my child acetaminophen for fever."
2. "My child will be more comfortable if I give him fluids and soft foods."
3. "I should watch my child for headache and vomiting."
4. "I will give my child antibiotics every four hours around the clock."

ANSWERS & RATIONALES

1 **Answer: 3** **Rationale:** The prodromal period is the time between the initial symptoms and the presence of the full-blown disease. The rash would not be apparent during this time. All the other statements are correct. **Cognitive Level:** Analyzing **Client Need:** Physiological Adaptation **Integrated Process:** Nursing Process: Evaluation **Content Area:** Child Health **Strategy:** The core issue of the question is knowledge of client teaching points related to chickenpox, particularly related to the timing of symptoms. Use nursing knowledge and the process of elimination to make a selection.

2 **Answer: 1** **Rationale:** The incubation period is the time between exposure and outbreak of the disease. It is often a period when the child can be contagious without others being aware of the possible exposure. The incubation period has nothing to do with the severity of the infection. The incubation period is constant and does not vary from child to child. Measles can be prevented by vaccination early in life. **Cognitive Level:** Applying **Client Need:** Physiological Adaptation **Integrated Process:** Nursing Process: Implementation **Content Area:** Fundamentals **Strategy:** The core issue of the question is knowledge of the significance of the prodromal period in a communicable disease. Use nursing knowledge and the process of elimination to make a selection.

3 **Answer: 1** **Rationale:** Caladryl will reduce itching and discomfort and therefore diminish scratching and skin breakdown. Acetylsalicylic acid should not be given to young children with a viral disease because of the relationship to Reye's syndrome. Immunoglobin will not decrease skin eruptions. Nubaine is a narcotic analgesic. **Cognitive Level:** Applying **Client Need:** Physiological Adaptation **Integrated Process:** Nursing Process: Implementation **Content Area:** Child Health **Strategy:** The core issue of the question is knowledge of various products used in the care of children and which one will reduce the likelihood of itching or pruritus with skin lesions. Use nursing knowledge and the process of elimination to make a selection.

4 **Answer: 1** **Rationale:** Tepid baths allow heat to be removed from the body. Aspirin use is avoided because of the risk of Reye's syndrome. The child should wear only light clothing to allow heat to escape. Antibiotics are not usually ordered for this viral infection. **Cognitive Level:** Applying **Client Need:** Physiological Adaptation **Integrated Process:** Nursing Process: Implementation **Content Area:** Child Health **Strategy:** The core issue of the question is an effective measure to prevent febrile seizures as a complication of fever in a child. Use nursing knowledge and the process of elimination to make a selection.

5 **Answer: 4** **Rationale:** Mumps is a viral infection and thus antibiotics will not be effective. The other statements are true. Acetaminophen, fluids, and soft foods are helpful, and the mother should watch for vomiting and headache. **Cognitive Level:** Analyzing **Client Need:** Physiological Adaptation **Integrated Process:** Nursing Process: Evaluation **Content Area:** Child Health **Strategy:** The core issue of the question is knowledge of supportive measures for a child with mumps. Use nursing knowledge and the process of elimination to make a selection.

6 **Answer: 2** **Rationale:** The upper respiratory symptoms may be early prodromal symptoms of chickenpox. The incubation period of chickenpox is 10 to 21 days. The other responses are either too short or too long. **Cognitive Level:** Applying **Client Need:** Physiological Adaptation **Integrated Process:** Nursing Process: Data Collection **Content Area:** Child Health **Strategy:** The core issue of the question is knowledge of the incubation period for chickenpox. Use nursing knowledge and the process of elimination to make a selection.

7 **Answer: 3** **Rationale:** Cool fluids will help decrease the swelling of the glands around the mouth and neck. Acidic foods are too irritating and difficult to swallow, which is why they should be avoided. Warm, chopped foods may be difficult to swallow. Although cool foods may be soothing, spices are likely to be irritating. The child should be given small, frequent meals with soft foods rather than a regular diet. **Cognitive Level:** Applying **Client Need:** Physiological Adaptation **Integrated Process:** Nursing Process: Implementation **Content Area:** Child Health **Strategy:** The core issue of the question is knowledge of foods and beverages that will be helpful to the child with mumps. Use principles of diet therapy that utilize cool, soft, and nonirritating food items to make a selection.

8 **Answer: 3** **Rationale:** Soothing the skin with an oatmeal-based substance will decrease the itching and redness. Overdressing the child will increase perspiration and thereby increase the itching. Keeping the child out of drafts has nothing to do with itching. Although drinking adequate fluids is helpful, it does not directly affect the itching. **Cognitive Level:** Applying **Client Need:** Physiological Adaptation **Integrated Process:** Nursing Process: Implementation **Content Area:** Child Health **Strategy:** The core issue of the question is an effective measure to treat itching caused by a communicable disease such as measles. Use nursing knowledge and the process of elimination to make a selection.

9 **Answer: 1** **Rationale:** The route of transmission of roseola is unknown. It is not known to be transmitted by the respiratory tract, contact with contaminated articles, or body secretions such as urine or stool. **Cognitive Level:** Analyzing **Client Need:** Physiological Adaptation **Integrated Process:** Teaching and Learning **Content Area:** Child Health **Strategy:** The core issue of the question is knowledge of transmission of roseola. The wording of the question tells you the correct answer is also a true statement. Use nursing knowledge and the process of elimination to make a selection.

10 **Answer: 2** **Rationale:** Pertussis is most infectious early in the course of the disease, so it is not necessary for the client to self-isolate following discharge from the hospital. Coughing bouts may still be triggered by irritants, so these should be avoided. Frequent handwashing is a generally helpful measure that should also be continued after discharge. Increased fluid intake is a generally helpful measure that should also be continued in the home setting. **Cognitive Level:** Analyzing **Client Need:** Physiological Adaptation **Integrated Process:** Teaching and Learning **Content Area:** Adult Health **Strategy:** The core issue of the question is knowledge of care for a client recovering from pertussis. The wording of the question tells you the correct answer is an incorrect client statement. Use nursing knowledge and the process of elimination to make a selection.

11 **Answer: 3** **Rationale:** Koplik's spots are seen with roseola, not scarlet fever. Reddened edematous pharynx, red strawberry tongue, and rash in the axillae and groin are findings consistent with scarlet fever. **Cognitive Level:** Analyzing **Client Need:** Physiological Adaptation **Integrated Process:** Nursing Process: Data Collection **Content Area:** Adult Health **Strategy:** The core issue of the question is the ability to discriminate between clinical findings associated with scarlet fever and roseola. The wording of the question tells you the correct answer is an incorrect client statement. Use nursing knowledge and the process of elimination to make a selection.

12 **Answer: 4** **Rationale:** Fifth disease is characterized by flu-like symptoms such as fever, malaise, nausea, and vomiting, and by the characteristic *slapped cheeks* appearance. This finding is not characteristic of chickenpox, measles, or diphtheria. **Cognitive Level:** Analyzing **Client Need:** Physiological Adaptation **Integrated Process:** Nursing Process: Data Collection **Content Area:** Child Health **Strategy:** The core issue of the question is the ability to discriminate the classic sign of Fifth disease from other childhood communicable diseases. Use nursing knowledge and the process of elimination to make a selection.

13 **Answer: 4** **Rationale:** Anthrax is caused by a bacterium and is therefore amenable to treatment with antibiotics. Antivirals and immune globulin play no role in treating this disease. Inhaled anthrax leads to respiratory symptoms, not cutaneous anthrax. **Cognitive Level:** Analyzing **Client Need:** Physiological Adaptation **Integrated Process:** Communication and Documentation **Content Area:** Adult Health **Strategy:** The core issue of the question is knowledge of available treatment methods for anthrax. Use nursing knowledge and the process of elimination to make a selection.

14 **Answer: 6** **Rationale:** The incubation period for infectious mononucleosis is up to 6 weeks (with a minimum of 4 weeks). This has important implications for the nurse and the client, since the source of the exposure may be difficult to determine after several weeks. **Cognitive Level:** Analyzing **Client Need:** Safety and Infection Control **Integrated Process:** Teaching and Learning **Content Area:** Adult Health **Strategy:** The core issue of the question is knowledge of the incubation period for infectious mononucleosis. Specific knowledge is needed to answer this type of question. Note that the question asks for the number of weeks, which suggests that the number to be provided is not excessively large.

15 **Answer: 1, 5** **Rationale:** These are allowed but aspirin products are avoided because of the risk of Reye's syndrome. Tepid baths allow heat to be removed from the body. Aspirin products are avoided because of the risk of Reye's syndrome. The child should have only light clothing to allow heat to escape. Antibiotics are not usually ordered for this viral infection. **Cognitive Level:** Applying **Client Need:** Physiological Adaptation **Integrated Process:** Nursing Process: Implementation **Content Area:** Child Health **Strategy:** Knowledge of the nursing management of a child with fever will help to choose the correct answer.

16 **Answer: 4** **Rationale:** Antibiotics are not prescribed. Non-aspirin analgesics and antipyretics can be given to control fever and pain. Swallowing and chewing may be painful so giving fluids and soft foods is helpful. Signs of complications such as headache, stiff neck, vomiting, and photophobia may indicate meningeal irritation. **Cognitive Level:** Analyzing **Client Need:** Physiological Adaptation **Integrated Process:** Nursing Process: Evaluation **Content Area:** Child Health **Strategy:** Critical words are *indicates a need for additional teaching*. Look for an answer that is incorrect. Knowledge of the nursing management of a child with mumps will aid in choosing the correct answer.

Key Terms to Review

immunization p. 1205

vaccine p. 1206

References

Ball, J., Bindler, R., & Cowen, K. (2010). *Child health nursing: Partnering with children and families* (2nd ed.). Upper Saddle River, NJ: Pearson Education.

Berman, A., & Snyder, S. (2012). *Kozier & Erb's fundamentals of nursing: Concepts, process, and practice* (9th ed.). Upper Saddle River, NJ: Pearson Education, Inc.

Ignatavicius, D., & Workman, L. (2010). *Medical-surgical nursing: Critical thinking for collaborative care* (6th ed.). Philadelphia: Saunders.

LeMone, P., Burke, K., & Bauldoff, G. (2011). *Medical surgical nursing: Critical thinking in patient care* (5th ed.). Upper Saddle River, NJ: Pearson Education.

Lewis, S., Dirksen, S.,Heitkemper, M. & Bucher, L. (2011). *Medical surgical nursing: Assessment and management of clinical problems* (8th ed.). St. Louis, MO: Elsevier.

Smeltzer, S., Bare, B., Hinkle, J., & Cheever, K. (2010). *Textbook of medical-surgical nursing* (12th ed.). Philadelphia: Lippincott Williams & Wilkins.

Test Yourself

Are you ready for the NCLEX-PN® or course exams? Use the practice tests on the companion website to check.

64 Basic Life Support

In this chapter

Cross Reference

Other chapters relevant to this content area are

Respiratory Disorders	**Chapter 51**
Cardiovascular Disorders	**Chapter 52**

I. OVERVIEW OF BASIC LIFE SUPPORT (BLS)

A. *Basic Life Support (BLS)* consists of a set of guidelines for use with respiratory or cardiac arrest

B. Commonly called *cardiopulmonary resuscitation (CPR)*

1. Is a mechanical attempt to perfuse vital organs, especially brain

NCLEX® 2. Follows a series of steps newly referred to as CAB (circulation, airway, and breathing), which is the American Heart Association 2010 revision to the old ABC (airway, breathing, circulation)

> ***Memory Aid***
>
> Remember the new CAB of basic life support!
> **C**—Chest compressions
> **A**—Airway
> **B**—Breathing
> The usual mnemonic ABC (airway, breathing, circulation) still applies for a client who has not experienced respiratory or cardiac arrest, but whose status is beginning to deteriorate or become unstable.

II. BARRIER MASKS AND DEVICES

A. Purpose: provide a barrier against contracting communicable disease such as HIV or hepatitis during resuscitation efforts

B. Face shield

1. A clear plastic or silicon sheet that can be placed over victim's mouth
2. Has an opening or tube in center sheet to permit air flow into airway during ventilations
3. Advantage: small and portable; fits on a key ring

C. Face mask

1. Rigid plastic device that fits over mouth and nose; more effective than face shield
2. Is bulky, costs more than face shield, and may not always be available

D. Bag-valve-mask ventilation

1. Utilizes a combination of a rigid plastic mask with manual resuscitation bag (Ambu bag)
2. Can be attached to oxygen (O_2) source for more effective oxygenation

3. Eliminates risk of communicable disease transmission
4. Is preferred method for providing respiratory support during respiratory insufficiency or arrest

NCLEX® 5. Ensure that mouth and nose are covered completely and firmly with mask to make an effective seal

III. ADULT BLS FOR HEALTH CARE PROVIDERS

A. Used for resuscitating individuals at age of puberty and older when following American Heart Association healthcare provider guidelines; BLS for laypersons includes using adult CPR guidelines for adults and children age 8 and older

B. Recognition of need for CPR and emergency cardiac care

1. Check client to determine unresponsiveness by tapping or gently shaking shoulder and asking loudly, "Are you okay?"
2. Briefly check for absence of breathing or abnormal breathing while checking unresponsiveness
3. Call for help or activate emergency medical system (EMS); dial 911 if outside a health care facility; use institutional policy for calling a code or inhouse response team if inside a health care agency
4. Retrieve an automatic external defibrillator (AED) if readily available or send someone else to do so
5. Place client on flat firm surface in supine position

C. Circulation

1. Place two or three fingers on Adam's apple and slide fingers into groove between Adam's apple and neck muscle
2. Palpate for carotid pulse for minimum of 5 seconds but not longer than 10 seconds
3. If pulse is present, observe airway and breathing; provide rescue breathing at rate of 10 to 12 breaths per minute if needed
4. If no pulse is present, begin external cardiac compressions
   a. Using hand closest to client's feet, place heel of hand at nipple line and place second hand on top of first
   b. Place middle finger on notch and index finger next to middle finger
   c. Place heel of opposite hand next to index finger (hand position is now on lower half of sternum); proper positioning is critical for success of CPR and to avoid injuring client
   d. Position own body directly over hands, with shoulders above hands, and elbows straight

   NCLEX® e. Provide compressions at rate of at least 100/minute and at depth of at least 2 inches; 2010 AHA guidelines state to "push hard, push fast," and allow chest to recoil after each compression (AHA, 2010, p. 5).

   f. Use a 30:2 compression to ventilation ratio for either 1- or 2-rescuer CPR; change positions for "switch" as needed after 5 cycles of 30:2
5. Do not interrupt chest compressions for more than 10 seconds at a time except for defibrillation or intubation; interruptions for rescue breaths should take less than 10 seconds; "switches" during two-person CPR should take less than 5 seconds
6. When automated external defibrillator (AED) is available, continue CPR while AED pads are being initially placed on chest and stop CPR only when AED is analyzing cardiac rhythm

D. Airway

1. Use gloves and barrier device if available

NCLEX® 2. Open airway using **head tilt-chin lift** method by lifting chin with two fingers while pushing down on forehead with other hand; kneel parallel to client's sternum

NCLEX® 3. If head or neck (cervical spine) injury is suspected or has occurred, use **jaw thrust maneuver** to open airway by lifting mandible on both sides with fingertips while positioning hands on sides of client's face; kneel at client's head

E. Breathing

1. Inadequate or absent breathing
   a. If client is not breathing adequately, maintain head tilt-chin lift and give two rescue breaths at rate of 1 second/breath; use breath sufficient to produce a rise in chest
   b. If chest does not rise with breath, reposition airway and try again (incorrect airway position is most common cause of obstructed rescuer ventilations)
   c. If chest still does not rise and fall, perform finger sweep of mouth to check for foreign body; clear airway and try again; remove dentures only if obstructing airway

   NCLEX® d. Provide one breath every 5 to 6 seconds or 10 to 12 breaths per minute; allow time for client to exhale between ventilations; this is called rescue breathing
2. Breathing client
   a. If client is breathing adequately and has suspected or actual head or neck trauma, do not move client
   b. If client is breathing adequately and does not have suspected head or neck trauma, logroll client onto side as a unit (maintaining alignment of spine) and continue to monitor; this position is also called recovery position

3. Improper ventilation technique could lead to ineffective ventilations or gastric distention
4. Use mouth-to-nose ventilation if mouth cannot be sealed, has serious injuries, or cannot be opened for any reason
5. Use mouth-to-stoma ventilation after temporary tracheostomy or laryngectomy; seal client's mouth and nose to ensure adequate ventilation

IV. PEDIATRIC BLS FOR HEALTH CARE PROVIDERS

A. Overview

1. Principles are same as for adult CPR; differences relate to smaller body size and needs of client

NCLEX® 2. Use child CPR if client is age 1 to 8

NCLEX® 3. Use infant CPR for clients less than 1 year old

B. Circulation

NCLEX® 1. Check carotid or femoral pulse for child and brachial or femoral pulse for infant (health care providers only, not lay rescuers)

2. Provide compressions at ratio of 30 compressions to two breaths for both child and infant CPR; when there are two health care provider rescuers, may use a 15:2 ratio

NCLEX® 3. Maintain rate of at least 100 compressions per minute for both child and infant CPR; same as for adult

4. Use heel of one hand or two hands for compressions to child with compression depth of at least ⅓ of anterior-posterior (AP) diameter of chest (about 2 inches or 5 cm); use same hand placement as adult
5. Use middle and ring fingers for compressions to infant at a depth of at least ⅓ AP diameter of chest (about 1.5 inches or 4 cm)
6. Determine correct hand placement for infant by placing index finger of hand farthest from infant's head on sternum just below an imaginary line between nipples; lower middle and ring fingers onto sternum and then lift index finger; provide compressions with middle and ring fingers

C. Airway: open airway using head tilt-chin lift method for both infant and child

D. Breathing

1. After checking breathing, if needed, provide two rescue breaths initially for both infant and child CPR with visible chest rise (same as for adult client); cover mouth and nose with infant breaths

NCLEX® 2. After initial two breaths, provide two breaths after each 30 compressions for both child and infant with single rescuer

NCLEX® 3. Deliver a breath every 3 to 5 seconds for a total ventilation rate of 12 to 20 breaths per minute

V. AUTOMATED EXTERNAL DEFIBRILLATOR (AED) USE

A. Overview

1. **Automated External Defibrillator (AED)** is a computerized defibrillator that analyzes cardiac rhythm of client, recognizes rhythm amenable to shock, and uses synthesized voice and flashing lights to indicate if shock is warranted

NCLEX® 2. Apply AED when client has signs of cardiac arrest: unresponsive, absence of respirations, absence of pulse (or signs of circulation for laypeople)

3. Place AED machine near client's left ear to allow room for reaching AED controls easily, applying pads without excessive reaching, and performing CPR without interference

B. Steps of AED operation

1. Turn power on
2. Apply AED electrode pads to client's chest
   a. Attach connecting cables to electrode pads (if not preconnected) before applying to client's chest
   b. Attach electrodes to chest as indicated on pad backing or packaging; placement does not have to be exact but should be within an inch or two of placement shown on package diagram
   c. Apply first pad to upper right side of chest (to right of sternum between nipple and clavicle)
   d. Apply second pad to outside of left nipple, with top margin of pad several inches below left axilla
3. Analyze rhythm

NCLEX® a. Do not touch client in any way, and do not allow others to do so; announce loudly to stand clear of client

   b. Do not push button to analyze rhythm until all contact with client has stopped; some machines analyze automatically without activation by button

4. Charge AED and, if indicated, deliver shock

NCLEX® a. Stay clear of client while charging; most models charge automatically

   b. Look to see that no one is touching client; announce to stand clear
   c. AED will analyze rhythm and provide direction to either deliver a shock or continue CPR
   d. Push button to deliver shock when instructed to do

e. If shock is ineffective, leave AED paddles attached and perform CPR for 2 minutes or 5 cycles of CPR; then reanalyze

f. If shock is effective, follow CPR guidelines according to client need

C. Special circumstances

1. If available, use child pads and a pediatric dose attenuator system for children ages 1 to 8; if not available, use standard AED and pads
2. Use a manual defibrillator for infants less than one year of age, if available; if not available, then use an AED with pediatric dose attenuation; if neither is available, an AED without a pediatric dose attenuator may be used
3. NCLEX® Do not use AED on client lying in standing water until client is removed and chest is dried
4. Avoid placing AED electrodes directly over an implantable defibrillator
5. Remove transdermal medication before placing an AED electrode on that site; wipe skin dry and then position electrode
6. Use a prep razor if needed for hairy chest to ensure good contact between client's skin and AED electrodes

VI. FOREIGN BODY AIRWAY OBSTRUCTION

A. Adult or child who is choking

1. Conscious
   a. Ask client, "Are you choking?" (will not be able to cough or speak if choking with severe or complete airway obstruction; will also have increasing respiratory distress and developing cyanosis)
   b. Encourage client to cough if crowing noise is heard (partial obstruction)
   c. NCLEX® Use **Heimlich maneuver** (see Box 64–1) until client becomes unconscious or blockage is relieved
2. Unconscious (health care provider directions)
   a. Place client on back
   b. Proceed to sequence for chest compressions
   c. Observe for breathing; if chest does not rise, return to compressions
   d. Repeat sequence until obstruction is cleared

B. Infant who is choking

1. Conscious
   a. Observe respiratory difficulty in infant
   b. Use series of five back blows and five chest thrusts on infant (positioned with head lower than trunk) until relieved
   c. Check mouth of infant for foreign object after each series, but avoid blind finger sweeps that could push obstruction further into airway
2. Unconscious
   a. Evaluate unconsciousness of infant
   b. Institute sequence of chest compressions
   c. Check breathing and observe for foreign object; remove if seen
   d. Attempt ventilation
   e. Repeat CAB sequence until successful or EMS personnel arrive

C. Pregnant or obese client who is choking

1. Conscious
   a. Stand behind client and put own arms around client's chest
   b. NCLEX® Place fist on middle of sternum between nipples (be sure to avoid xiphoid process)
   c. Grasp fist with other hand and deliver firm backward thrusts until object is removed or victim becomes unconscious

Box 64–1

Heimlich Maneuver

1. Stand behind client and encircle client's waist with own arms.
2. Make a fist with one hand.
3. Place thumb side of fist on abdomen above umbilicus but below xiphoid process of sternum.
4. Grasp fist with other hand and give quick inward and upward thrusts until victim becomes unconscious or obstruction is expelled.

PRACTICE TEST

2. Unconscious

NCLEX®

a. Position victim lying on back; use a small pillow or wedge under right hip of pregnant client to shift uterus to left side of abdomen
b. Institute chest compressions using ratio of 30 compressions to 2 ventilations
c. Check breathing and observe for obstruction; remove if seen
d. Attempt to ventilate
e. Repeat CAB sequence until successful or EMS personnel arrive

Check Your NCLEX–PN® Exam I.Q. *You are ready for testing on this content if you can*

- Recognize and intervene when client requires cardiopulmonary resuscitation or Heimlich maneuver/abdominal thrusts.
- Monitor and document response to resuscitation efforts.
- Explain emergency interventions to client and family when necessary.

PRACTICE TEST

1 A client is brought to the emergency department awake and alert following a fall from a ladder from a height of 15 feet. During an initial examination, the client becomes unresponsive and stops breathing. Which method should the nurse use to open the airway?

1. Head-tilt chin-lift
2. Jaw thrust
3. Tongue-jaw lift
4. None; client needs emergency intubation

2 The nurse has begun cardiopulmonary resuscitation (CPR) on a 5-year-old child. The nurse times the rate of ventilation to achieve up to how many breaths per _______ minute? Provide a numeric answer.

Fill in your answer below:

_______ minute

3 A nurse has begun to resuscitate a 10-month-old infant. In what location would the nurse check the infant's pulse?

1. Brachial
2. Radial
3. Carotid
4. Temporal

4 The nurse on a surgical nursing unit has just called a code blue using the telephone in the room of an unresponsive client who had abdominal surgery. Which of the following actions would be appropriate during initiation of CPR?

1. Open the airway using the jaw thrust method
2. Deliver one deep breath before checking for a pulse
3. Depress the sternum at least 2 inches during cardiac compressions
4. Reevaluate status every 2 to 3 minutes until the code team arrives

5 The nurse who is doing the documentation during a code blue on an adult client observes an unlicensed assistive person (UAP) doing CPR. The nurse interprets that the UAP is performing CPR correctly after noting that the UAP is depressing the sternum at least _______ inches? Provide a numeric answer.

Fill in your answer below:

_______ inches

6 The nurse is performing cardiopulmonary resuscitation (CPR) on a 10-month-old infant. The nurse times the rate of compressions to achieve a total number of approximately _______ compressions per minute? Provide a numeric response.

Fill in your answer below:

_______ compressions per minute

7 A nurse witnesses an adult male collapse at the airport, and an automated external defibrillator (AED) is brought to the scene. The nurse should perform which action in utilizing the device?

1. Press the electrodes down firmly because the client has a hairy chest
2. Instruct another person at the scene to keep the airway open during delivery of the electric shock
3. Initiate CPR after 5 minutes if the AED has not restored a perfusing cardiac rhythm
4. Quickly wipe up the spilled coffee under the victim's chest before using the AED

8 A nurse is eating in a restaurant when a woman who is 8 months pregnant at the next table begins to choke. Which hand placement should the nurse use to perform the Heimlich maneuver?

1. Midsternum
2. Lower sternum
3. Midway between umbilicus and xiphoid process
4. Midway between umbilicus and symphysis pubis

9 The long-term-care nurse has been called to the aid of a resident who has become unconscious after choking in the dining room. After positioning the client on the back, which action should the nurse take next?

1. Attempt to ventilate the client
2. Observe the oral cavity; carry out a finger sweep of the mouth if object seen
3. Perform five abdominal thrusts
4. Perform five chest thrusts

10 A nurse enters an adult client's room and says, "Good morning!" while doing initial shift rounds after receiving report. The client does not respond. Put the nurse's actions in order of priority.

1. Call for someone to announce a code blue
2. Check for a carotid pulse
3. Gently shake the client's shoulder and ask, "Are you okay?"
4. Begin chest compressions

ANSWERS & RATIONALES

1 **Answer: 2 Rationale:** The jaw thrust maneuver is used whenever head or cervical spine injury is suspected to avoid causing further physiological damage. The head-tilt-chin-lift method is the standard method for opening the airway when there is no suspected cervical spine injury. The tongue-jaw lift aids in visualizing foreign bodies in the airway. The client does not need emergency intubation. **Cognitive Level:** Applying **Client Need:** Physiological Adaptation **Integrated Process:** Nursing Process: Implementation **Content Area:** Adult Health **Strategy:** Note critical information in the stem, which indicates that the client had a traumatic injury and is therefore at risk of cervical spine injury. Next use knowledge of basic CPR procedures to select the option for opening the airway in a client with suspected head or neck injury.

2 **Answer: 20 Rationale:** The proper ventilation rate for a child or infant is 12 to 20 breaths per minute, which is the same as delivering one breath every 3 to 5 seconds. The correct answer is 20 based on the words *up to*. **Cognitive Level:** Applying **Client Need:** Physiological Adaptation **Integrated Process:** Nursing Process: Implementation **Content Area:** Child Health **Strategy:** Recall basic CPR procedures to identify the correct rate. Remember that compressions and ventilation rates need to be higher in children than in adults.

3 **Answer: 1 Rationale:** The brachial artery is the correct location for determining whether an infant under one year of age has a pulse. The radial artery would not generate enough pulsation in an infant to be reliable and is also more difficult to palpate. The carotid pulse is not as easily located in an infant with a small neck and neck folds. The temporal pulse is not used in CPR for an individual of any age. **Cognitive Level:** Applying **Client Need:** Physiological Adaptation **Integrated Process:** Nursing Process: Implementation

Content Area: Child Health **Strategy:** First eliminate radial and temporal because they are not used in CPR. Choose brachial over carotid using knowledge of infant anatomy and accessibility of the site.

4 **Answer: 3 Rationale:** In an adult, the sternum should be depressed during CPR to a depth of at least 2 inches. The head-tilt-chin-lift method of opening the airway is used for the client who has no head or neck injury. After determining unresponsiveness while simultaneously checking quickly for breathing, the nurse begins chest compressions. The nurse should reevaluate the client's status after approximately 1 minute. **Cognitive Level:** Applying **Client Need:** Physiological Adaptation **Integrated Process:** Nursing Process: Implementation **Content Area:** Adult Health **Strategy:** Use knowledge of basic CPR procedures to answer the question. Recall 2010 changes to aid in making the correct selection.

5 **Answer: 2 Rationale:** On an adult client, chest compressions should be done to a depth of at least 2 inches to be effective. **Cognitive Level:** Applying **Client Need:** Physiological Adaptation **Integrated Process:** Nursing Process: Implementation **Content Area:** Adult Health **Strategy:** Use the process of elimination and knowledge of basic CPR procedures to answer the question. Recall that compressions are at least 2 inches to answer correctly.

6 **Answer: 100 Rationale:** The rate of compressions for an infant during CPR is at least 100 per minute. **Cognitive Level:** Applying **Client Need:** Physiological Adaptation **Integrated Process:** Nursing Process: Implementation **Content Area:** Child Health **Strategy:** Use knowledge of basic CPR procedures to answer the question. Memorize the number 100 to answer correctly.

7 **Answer: 4 Rationale:** The client should not be lying in water or other liquid, which could lead to burns or to defibrillating another individual who comes in contact with the liquid during AED shock delivery. The electrodes should not be placed on hairy areas, or the site should be shaved. All people should stand clear of the individual during an AED shock to avoid being defibrillated themselves. CPR is initiated after 1 minute or whenever the series of shocks is terminated, as indicated by client condition. However, 5 minutes is too excessive and could lead to permanent brain damage if the client survives. **Cognitive Level:** Applying **Client Need:** Physiological Adaptation **Integrated Process:** Nursing Process: Implementation **Content Area:** Adult Health **Strategy:** First recall that hair interferes with good skin contact of any type of electrode to eliminate that option. Next recall that brain death can occur within 4 to 6 minutes if CPR is not initiated. Use general principles of electrical safety to choose between the remaining two options.

8 **Answer: 1 Rationale:** In a pregnant client, the Heimlich maneuver is performed in a manner that avoids causing injury to the fetus. For this reason, the hand placement is at the midsternum. The lower sternum should be avoided to prevent accidental fracture of the xiphoid process, which could lead to internal injury. Midway between the umbilicus and the xiphoid process is the abdomen, which is contraindicated in the pregnant client. Midway between the umbilicus and the symphysis pubis is the lower abdomen, which is contraindicated in the pregnant client. **Cognitive Level:** Applying **Client Need:** Physiological Adaptation **Integrated Process:** Nursing Process: Implementation **Content Area:** Adult Health **Strategy:** Note the key information in the question that the client is pregnant. Then use knowledge of basic CPR procedures to answer the question.

9 **Answer: 2 Rationale:** After positioning the client on the back, the nurse would observe the oral cavity to detect any foreign body that may be removed immediately. The nurse would attempt to ventilate after inspecting the mouth. The nurse would perform abdominal thrusts third. Chest thrusts are performed on the adult only for pregnant or obese clients. **Cognitive Level:** Analyzing **Client Need:** Physiological Adaptation **Integrated Process:** Nursing Process: Implementation **Content Area:** Adult Health **Strategy:** Remember the ABCs of life support to answer this question. Choose the option that attempts to clear the airway before taking any other actions.

10 **Answer: 3, 1, 2, 4 Rationale:** The first action of the nurse is to establish unresponsiveness. This can be done by shaking the shoulder and asking if the client is okay. The second action of the nurse is to call for help. The third action of the nurse is to address circulation by checking the client's pulse. If no pulse is present, the nurse should begin chest compressions. The 2010 CPR guidelines use the mnemonic CAB (chest compressions, airway, and breathing). **Cognitive Level:** Analyzing **Client Need:** Physiological Adaptation **Integrated Process:** Nursing Process: Implementation **Content Area:** Adult Health **Strategy:** Specific knowledge of the sequence of events is needed to answer the question. Using the mnemonic CAB (chest compressions, airway, and breathing) will be of assistance once unresponsiveness has been determined.

Key Terms To Review

automated external defibrillator (AED) p. 1218
basic life support (BLS) p. 1216
cardiopulmonary resuscitation (CPR) p. 1216
head tilt-chin lift p. 1217
Heimlich maneuver p. 1219
jaw thrust maneuver p. 1217

C

D

E

H

I

J

K

L

M

O

Q

R

S

T

V

W